The Complete Directory
for
People with Disabilities

2017
Twenty-Fifth Edition

The Complete Directory
for
People with Disabilities

A Comprehensive Source Book for
Individuals and Professionals

A SEDGWICK PRESS Book

Grey House
Publishing

PUBLISHER: Leslie Mackenzie
EDITORIAL DIRECTOR: Laura Mars

PRODUCTION MANAGER & COMPOSITION: Kristen Thatcher
MARKETING DIRECTOR: Jessica Moody

A Sedgewick Press Book
Grey House Publishing, Inc.
4919 Route 22
Amenia, NY 12501
518.789.8700
FAX 845.373.6390
www.greyhouse.com
e-mail: books@greyhouse.com

First edition published 1991
Twenty-fifth edition published 2016

The complete directory for people with disabilities : products, resources, books, services.-1992-2015

1. People with disabilities-Services for-United States-Directories. 2. People with disabilities-Services for-United States-Periodicals. 3. Disabled Persons-United States-Bibliography. 4. Disabled Persons-United States-Directory. 5. Information Services-United States-Bibliography. 6. Information Services-United States-Directory. 7. Mental Retardation-Rehabilitation-United States-Bibliography. 8. Mental Retardation-Rehabilitation-United States-Directory. 9. Rehabilitation-United States-Bibliography. 10. Rehabilitation-United States-Directory. I. Title: Directory for people with disabilities.

HV1553.C58
362.4/048/02573   92-658843

Printed in Canada
ISBN 13: 978-1-61925-927-0 Softcover

Table of Contents

Introduction xi
Glossary of Disability-Related Terms xxiii
User Guide xxix
User Key xxxi

General Resources for People with Disabilities

Arts & Entertainment
Resources for the Disabled 1

Assistive Devices
Automobile 9
Bath 15
Bed 17
Communication 19
Chairs 23
Cushions & Wedges 25
Dressing Aids 28
Health Aids 29
Hearing Aids 31
Kitchen & Eating Aids 32
Lifts, Ramps & Elevators 35
Major Catalogs 40
Miscellaneous 46
Office Devices & Workstations 50
Scooters 52
Stationery 55
Visual Aids 57
Walking Aids: Canes, Crutches & Walkers 58
Wheelchairs: Accessories 61
Wheelchairs: General 62
Wheelchairs: Pediatric 65
Wheelchairs: Powered 66
Wheelchairs: Racing 67

Associations
General Disabilities 68

Camps
Alabama 88
Alaska 89
Arizona 89
Arkansas 90
California 91

Table of Contents

Colorado 95
Connecticut 97
Delaware 98
District of Columbia 98
Florida 98
Georgia 100
Hawaii 101
Idaho 101
Illinois 101
Indiana 103
Iowa 105
Kansas 107
Kentucky 107
Louisiana 108
Maine 108
Maryland 110
Massachusetts 111
Michigan 114
Minnesota 115
Mississippi 116
Missouri 116
Montana 117
Nebraska 118
Nevada 119
New Hampshire 119
New Jersey 119
New Mexico 121
New York 121
North Carolina 124
North Dakota 125
Ohio 125
Oklahoma 128
Oregon 128
Pennsylvania 129
Rhode Island 132
South Carolina 132
South Dakota 132
Tennessee 133
Texas 134
Utah 135
Vermont 136
Virginia 137
Washington 138
West Virginia 139
Wisconsin 139
Wyoming 140

Clothing
Dresses & Skirts 141
Footwear 141

Miscellaneous & Catalogs 142
Robes & Sleepwear. 143
Shirts & Tops 144
Slacks & Pants 144
Undergarments 145

Computers
Assistive Devices 146
Braille Products 149
Information Centers & Databases. 150
Keyboards, Mouses & Joysticks. 156
Scanners 157
Screen Enhancement. 158
Speech Synthesizers 158
Software: Math 159
Software: Miscellaneous. 162
Software: Professional 172
Software: Reading & Language Arts 174
Software: Vocational 178
Word Processors. 179

Conferences & Shows
General 181

Construction & Architecture
Associations 187
Publications & Videos 188

Education
Aids for the Classroom 190
Associations 201
Directories 204
Educational Publishers 206

State Agencies
Alabama 209
Alaska 209
Arkansas 209
California 209
Colorado 209
Connecticut. 209
Delaware. 210
DC 210
Florida. 210
Hawaii. 210
Illinois. 210
Indiana 211
Iowa 211
Kansas. 211
Kentucky. 211
Louisiana. 211

Table of Contents

Massachusetts 211
Maryland 211
Michigan 212
Minnesota 212
Missouri 213
Mississippi 213
Montana 213
North Carolina 213
North Dakota 213
Nebraska 213
New Hampshire 214
New Jersey 214
New Mexico 214
Nevada 214
New York 214
Ohio 214
Oklahoma 214
Oregon 214
Pennsylvania 215
Rhode Island 215
South Carolina 215
South Dakota 215
Tennessee 215
Texas 215
Utah 216
Virginia 216
Washington 216
West Virginia 216
Wyoming 216
Magazines & Journals 216
Newsletters 222
Professional Texts 226
Testing Resources 263
Treatment & Training 270

Exchange Programs
General 274

Foundations & Funding Resources
Alabama 278
Alaska 278
Arizona 278
Arkansas 279
California 279
Colorado 285
Connecticut 286
Delaware 287
District of Columbia 287
Florida 289
Georgia 290

Hawaii. 291
Illinois. 292
Indiana 296
Iowa 296
Kansas. 297
Kentucky. 297
Louisiana. 297
Maine 297
Maryland. 298
Massachusetts 300
Michigan. 301
Minnesota 303
Mississippi 304
Missouri 304
Nebraska 305
Nevada 305
New Hampshire 306
New Jersey 306
New Mexico 307
New York 308
North Carolina 314
North Dakota 315
Ohio 315
Oklahoma 317
Oregon 318
Pennsylvania. 318
Rhode Island 320
South Carolina 321
Tennessee 322
Texas. 323
Utah. 326
Vermont 326
Virginia. 326
Washington. 327
West Virginia 328
Wisconsin 328
Wyoming 329
Funding Directories 329

Government Agencies

Federal 333
Alabama 335
Alaska 336
Arizona 337
Arkansas 338
California 339
Colorado 341
Connecticut. 341
Delaware. 342
District of Columbia 343

Florida. 344
Georgia 345
Hawaii. 347
Idaho. 348
Illinois. 349
Indiana 350
Iowa 351
Kansas. 352
Kentucky. 353
Louisiana. 354
Maine 355
Maryland. 355
Massachusetts 356
Michigan. 357
Minnesota 359
Mississippi 361
Missouri 362
Montana 362
Nebraska 363
Nevada 365
New Hampshire 366
New Jersey 367
New Mexico 368
New York 369
North Carolina 372
North Dakota 373
Ohio 374
Oklahoma 375
Oregon 376
Pennsylvania. 377
Rhode Island 378
South Carolina 379
South Dakota 380
Tennessee 381
Texas. 382
Utah. 385
Vermont 386
Virginia. 388
Washington. 389
West Virginia 390
Wisconsin 391
Wyoming 392

Independent Living Centers
Alabama 394
Alaska. 394
Arizona 395
Arkansas 396
California 397
Colorado 404

Connecticut 406
Delaware 406
District of Columbia 407
Florida 407
Georgia 410
Hawaii 411
Idaho 412
Illinois 413
Indiana 417
Iowa 418
Kansas 419
Kentucky 424
Louisiana 424
Maine 425
Maryland 426
Massachusetts 427
Michigan 429
Minnesota 431
Mississippi 433
Missouri 434
Montana 436
Nebraska 437
Nevada 438
New Hampshire 438
New Jersey 439
New Mexico 440
New York 441
North Carolina 445
North Dakota 446
Ohio 447
Oklahoma 448
Oregon 448
Pennsylvania 449
Rhode Island 452
South Carolina 452
South Dakota 453
Tennessee 454
Texas 454
Utah 457
Vermont 458
Virginia 459
Washington 461
West Virginia 462
Wisconsin 462
Wyoming 464

Law

Associations & Referral Agencies 465
Resources for the Disabled 467

Libraries & Research Centers

Alabama 476
Alaska 476
Arizona 476
Arkansas 477
California 477
Colorado 479
Connecticut 479
Delaware 480
District of Columbia 480
Florida 481
Georgia 483
Hawaii 484
Idaho 484
Illinois 485
Indiana 486
Iowa 487
Kansas 487
Kentucky 489
Louisiana 489
Maine 489
Maryland 490
Massachusetts 491
Michigan 492
Minnesota 494
Mississippi 495
Missouri 495
Montana 496
Nebraska 496
Nevada 497
New Hampshire 497
New Jersey 497
New Mexico 498
New York 498
North Carolina 500
North Dakota 500
Ohio 500
Oklahoma 501
Oregon 502
Pennsylvania 502
Rhode Island 502
South Carolina 503
South Dakota 503
Tennessee 503
Texas 503
Utah 504
Vermont 504
Virginia 505
Washington 506

West Virginia 507
Wisconsin 507
Wyoming 508

Media, Print
Children & Young Adults. 509
Community 511
Employment 512
General Disabilities 512
Parenting: General 533
Parenting: Specific Disabilities 539
Parenting: School 540
Parenting: Spiritual 541
Professional. 542
Specific Disabilities 545
Vocations 545

Media, Electronic
Audio/Visual. 546
Web Sites 554

Support Groups & Hotlines
General 562

Toys & Games
General. 563

Travel & Transportation
Newsletters & Books 566
Associations & Programs 567
Tours. 569
Vehicle Rentals. 571

Veteran Services
National Administrations 573
Alabama 574
Alaska 574
Arizona 574
Arkansas 575
California 575
Colorado 577
Connecticut. 577
Delaware 578
District of Columbia 578
Florida. 578
Georgia 579
Hawaii. 580
Idaho 580
Illinois. 581
Indiana 581
Iowa 582
Kansas. 582

Table of Contents

Kentucky. 583
Louisiana. 583
Maine 583
Maryland. 584
Massachusetts 584
Michigan. 585
Minnesota 586
Mississippi 586
Missouri 586
Montana 587
Nebraska 587
Nevada 588
New Hampshire 588
New Jersey 588
New Mexico 589
New York 589
North Carolina 590
North Dakota 591
Ohio 591
Oklahoma 592
Oregon 592
Pennsylvania. 592
Rhode Island 593
South Carolina 594
South Dakota 594
Tennessee 594
Texas. 595
Utah. 596
Vermont 596
Virginia. 596
Washington. 597
West Virginia 597
Wisconsin 597
Wyoming 598

Vocational & Employment Programs

Alabama 599
Alaska 601
Arizona 601
Arkansas 602
California 602
Colorado 606
Connecticut. 607
Delaware. 608
District of Columbia 609
Florida. 609
Georgia 613
Hawaii. 613
Idaho 614
Illinois. 614

Indiana 616
Iowa 619
Kansas 620
Kentucky 620
Louisiana 621
Maine 621
Maryland 622
Massachusetts 623
Michigan 624
Minnesota 624
Mississippi 625
Missouri 625
Montana 626
Nebraska 626
Nevada 626
New Hampshire 626
New Jersey 627
New Mexico 630
New York 630
North Carolina 631
North Dakota 632
Ohio 632
Oklahoma 633
Oregon 633
Pennsylvania 634
Rhode Island 634
South Carolina 635
South Dakota 635
Tennessee 636
Texas 636
Utah 637
Vermont 637
Virginia 637
Washington 638
West Virginia 639
Wisconsin 639
Wyoming 639

Rehabilitation Facilities, Acute

Alabama 641
Arkansas 641
Arizona 641
California 642
Colorado 645
Connecticut 646
District of Columbia 646
Florida 646
Georgia 648
Hawaii 648
Idaho 648

Table of Contents

Illinois. 648
Indiana 649
Iowa 651
Kansas. 651
Kentucky. 652
Louisiana. 652
Maine 653
Maryland. 653
Massachusetts 653
Michigan 654
Minnesota 654
Missouri 654
Montana 655
Nebraska 655
Nevada 655
New Hampshire 655
New Jersey 655
New Mexico 656
New York 656
North Carolina 657
Ohio 657
Oklahoma 658
Oregon 659
Pennsylvania. 659
South Carolina 661
Tennessee 661
Texas. 662
Utah. 665
Vermont 666
Virginia. 666
Washington. 666
West Virginia 667
Wisconsin 667
Wyoming 667

Rehabilitation Facilities, Post-Acute
Alabama 668
Alaska. 669
Arizona 670
Arkansas. 672
California 672
Colorado 685
Connecticut. 687
Delaware. 688
District of Columbia 689
Florida. 690
Georgia 695
Hawaii. 697
Idaho 697
Illinois. 697

Indiana 704
Iowa 705
Kansas 706
Kentucky 707
Louisiana 708
Maine 710
Maryland 710
Massachusetts 712
Michigan 715
Minnesota 716
Mississippi 717
Missouri 717
Montana 718
Nebraska 718
New Hampshire 718
New Jersey 719
New Mexico 720
New York 720
North Carolina 722
Ohio 723
Oklahoma 726
Oregon 727
Pennsylvania 727
Rhode Island 729
South Carolina 729
Tennessee 729
Texas 730
Utah 732
Vermont 732
Virginia 732
Washington 733
Wisconsin 735

Rehabilitation Facilities, Sub-Acute

Alabama 736
Alaska 736
Arizona 736
California 736
Colorado 737
Connecticut 738
Delaware 738
Florida 738
Georgia 739
Hawaii 740
Idaho 740
Illinois 741
Indiana 741
Iowa 743
Kentucky 743
Louisiana 743

Table of Contents

Maine 743
Maryland 744
Massachusetts 744
Michigan 745
Minnesota 745
Missouri 745
Montana 746
Nebraska 746
Nevada 746
New Hampshire 746
New Jersey 746
New York 747
North Carolina 748
Ohio 749
Oregon 750
Pennsylvania 750
Rhode Island 751
South Carolina 751
Tennessee 751
Texas 752
Utah 753
Virginia 753
Washington 754
West Virginia 755
Wisconsin 755
Wyoming 756

Aging
Associations 758
Print: Books 763
Print: Journals 767
Print: Magazines 768
Print: Newsletters 768
Non Print: Newsletters 768
Support Groups 770

Blind & Deaf
Associations 772
Camps 774
Print: Books 774
Print: Magazines 775
Print: Newsletters 775
Non Print: Newsletters 775
Non Print: Software 776
Non Print: Video 776
Sports 777
Support Groups 777

Cognitive
Associations 778
Camps 783

Print: Books 788
Print: Journals 801
Print: Magazines 801
Print: Newsletters 802
Non Print: Newsletters 802
Non Print: Software 803
Non Print: Video 804
Support Groups 806

Dexterity
Associations 807
Print: Books 808
Print: Magazines 809
Print: Newsletters 809
Non Print: Newsletters 809

Hearing
Associations 810
Camps 815
Print: Books 818
Print: Journals 829
Print: Magazines 830
Print: Newsletters 831
Non Print: Newsletters 832
Non Print: Video 833
Sports 835
Support Groups 835

Mobility
Associations 836
Camps 840
Print: Books 841
Print: Magazines 843
Print: Newsletters 844
Non Print: Newsletters 845
Non Print: Video 846
Sports 847
Support Groups 849

General Disorders
Associations 851
Camps 857
Print: Books 870
Print: Journals 890
Print: Magazines 890
Print: Newsletters 891
Non Print: Newsletters 894
Non Print: Video 895
Sports 895
Support Groups 895

Table of Contents

Speech & Language

Associations 899
Camps 903
Print: Books 904
Print: Journals 909
Print: Magazines 910
Print: Newsletters 910
Non Print: Newsletters 911
Non Print: Video 911
Support Groups 912

Visual

Associations 913
Camps 923
Print: Books 925
Print: Journals 942
Print: Magazines 942
Print: Newsletters 943
Non Print: Newsletters 948
Non Print: Video 948
Sports 950
Support Groups 951

Indexes

Entry & Publisher Index 953
Geographic Index 1007
Subject Index 1023

Introduction

This 25th edition of the award-winning *Complete Directory for People with Disabilities* is an invaluable resource for all those living with a disability and all those committed to empowering these individuals. It offers thousands of ways for people with disabilities to succeed at work, in school, and in their community. Coverage includes Associations, Products, Camps, Living Facilities, Print and Electronic Resources and much more. The comprehensive Table of Contents guides you through the 31 chapters and more than 100 subchapters contained in this rich resource.

Careful research and compilation of the best data available maintains the reputation of *The Complete Directory for People with Disabilities* among educators, librarians and the disability community. This resource is a repeat recipient of the **National Mature Media Award** and the **National Health Information Award**.

Sure to save hours of Internet research time, *The Complete Directory for People with Disabilities* provides comprehensive, critical and immediate information in one source that can be accessed quickly and easily. This edition provides **9,145 descriptive listings**, **24,629 key contacts**, **8,069 fax numbers**, **7,101 email addresses**, and **8,705 web sites**. Following this Introduction is a Glossary of Disability-Related terms.

Three indexes provide quick, easy access to the data:
- **Entry & Publisher Index** lists all directory listings alphabetically.
- **Geographic Index** organizes listings alphabetically by state.
- **Subject Index** alphabetically organizes directory listings by relevant topics, i.e. autism, language disorders.

In addition to the print directory, *The Complete Directory for People with Disabilities* is available for subscription on G.O.L.D., Grey House OnLine Databases. This gives you immediate access to the most valuable disability industry contacts in the United States, plus offers easy-to-use keyword searches, organization type and subject searches, hotlinks to web sites and emails, and so much more. Call 800-562-2139 for a free trial or visit http://gold.greyhouse.com for more information.

We welcome your comments, and look forward to another year of serving the disability community.

Praise for previous editions:

> *"The strength of this source is in the information referral portion for each entry: the wide range of resources and organizations presented that can assist with additional information and support."*
>
> —ARBA

> *"...thousands of resources...covering a diverse range of services...separate section for specific disabilities...from aging to mobility and from the blind and deaf to speech and language disorders. Libraries...will want to consider..."*
>
> —Against the Grain

Glossary of Disability-Related Terms

Accessible: In the case of a facility, readily usable by a particular individual; in the case of a program or activity, presented or provided in such a way that a particular individual can participate, with or without auxiliary aids(s); in the case of electronic resources, accessible with or without the use of adaptive computer technology.

Access barrier: Any obstruction that prevents people with disabilities from using standard facilities, equipment and resources.

Accessible Web design: Creating World Wide Web pages according to universal design principles to eliminate or reduce barriers, including those that affect people with disabilities.

Accommodation: An adjustment to make a workstation, job, program, facility, or resource accessible to a person with a disability.

Adaptive technology: Hardware or software products that provide access to a computer that is otherwise inaccessible to an individual with a disability.

ALT attribute: HTML code that works in combination with graphical tags to provide alternative text for graphical elements.

Americans with Disabilities Act of 1990 (ADA): A comprehensive Federal law that prohibits discrimination on the basis of disability in employment, telecommunications, public services, public accommodations and services.

American Standard Code for Information Interchange (ASCII): Standard for unformatted text which enables transfer of data between platforms and computer systems.

Assistive technology: Technology used to assist a person with a disability (e.g., a handsplint or computer-related equipment).

Auxiliary aids and services: May include qualified interpreters or other effective methods of making aurally delivered materials available to individuals with hearing impairments; qualified readers, taped texts, or other effective methods of making visually delivered materials available to individuals with visual impairments; acquisition or modification of equipment or devices; and other similar services and actions.

Braille: A system of embossed characters formed by using a Braille cell, a combination of six dots consisting of two vertical columns of three dots each. Each simple Braille character is formed by one or more of these dots and occupies a full cell or space.

Browser: A program that runs on an Internet-connected computer and provides access to the World Wide Web. Web browsers may be text-only, such as Lynx, or graphical, such as Internet Explorer and Netscape Navigator.

Captioned film or videos: Transcription of the verbal portion of films or videos is displayed to make them accessible to people who have hearing impairments.

Closed Circuit TV Magnifier (CCTV): A camera used to magnify books or other materials on a monitor.

Cooperative education: Programs that work with students, faculty, staff, and employers to help students clarify career and academic goals, and expand classroom study by allowing students to participate in paid, practical work experiences.

Compensatory tools: Adaptive computing systems that allow people with disabilities to use computers to complete tasks that would be difficult without a computer (e.g., reading, writing, communicating, accessing information).

Disability: A physical or mental impairment that substantially limits one or more major life activities; a record of such an impairment; or being regarded as having such an impairment (Americans with Disabilities Act of 1990).

Discrimination: The act of treating a person differently in a negative manner based on factors other than individual merit.

Dymo Labeller: A device used to create raised print or Braille labels.

Electronic information: Any digital data for use with computers or computer networks, including disks, CD-ROMs, and World Wide Web resources.

Essential job functions: Those functions of a job or task which must be completed with or without an accommodation.

Facility: All or any portion of a physical complex, including buildings, structures, equipment, grounds, roads, and parking lots.

FM sound amplification system: An electronic amplification system consisting of three components: a microphone/transmitter, monaural FM receiver and a combination charger/carrying case. It provides wireless FM broadcasts from a speaker to a listener who has a hearing impairment.

Frame tags: A means of displaying Web pages. The browser reads the frame tags and produces an output that subdivides output within a browser into discrete windows.

Graphical user interface (GUI): Program interface that presents digital information and software programs in an image-based format as compared to a character-based format.

Hardware: Physical equipment related to computers.

Hearing impairment: Complete or partial loss of the ability to hear, caused by a variety of injuries or diseases, including congenital causes. Limitations, including difficulties in understanding language or other auditory messages and/or in production of understandable speech, are possible.

Independent study: A student works one-on-one with individual faculty members to develop projects for credit.

Informational interview: An activity where students meet with people working in careers to ask questions about their jobs and companies, allowing students to gain personal perspectives on career interests.

Input: Any method by which information is entered into a computer.

Internet: Computer network connecting governmental, educational, commercial, other organizations, and individual computer systems.

Internship: A time-limited, intensive learning experience outside of the typical classroom.

Interpreter: Professional person who assists a person who is deaf in communicating with hearing people.

Job shadowing: A short work-based learning experience where students visit businesses to observe one or more specific jobs to provide them with a realistic view of occupations in a variety of settings.

Keyboard emulation: Uses hardware and/or software in place of a standard keyboard.

Kinesthetic: Refers to touch-based feedback.

Large-print: Most ordinary print is six to ten points in height (about 1/16 to 1/8 of an inch). Large-print type is fourteen to eighteen points (about 1/8 to 1/4 of an inch) and sometimes larger.

Link: a connection between two electronic files or data items.

Lynx: A text-based World Wide Web browser.

Macro: A mini-program that, when run within an application, executes a series of predetermined keystrokes and commands to accomplish a specific task. Macros can automate tedious and often-repeated tasks or create special menus to speed data entry.

Mainstreaming: The inclusion of people with disabilities, with or without special accommodations, in programs, activities, and facilities with non-disabled people.

Major life activities: Functions such as caring for oneself, performing manual tasks, walking, seeing, hearing, speaking, breathing, learning, working, and participating in community activities (Americans with Disabilities Act of 1990).

Multimedia: A computer-based method of presenting information by using more than one medium of communication, such as text, graphics, and sound.

Optical Character Recognition (OCR): Machine recognition of printed or typed text. Using OCR software with a scanner, a printed page can be scanned and the characters converted into text in an electronic format.

Output: Any method of displaying or presenting electronic information to the user through a computer monitor or other device (e.g., speech synthesizer).

Portable Document Format (PDF): The file format for representing documents in a manner that is independent of the original application software, hardware and operating system used to create the documents.

Physical or mental impairment: Any physiological disorder or condition, cosmetic disfigurement, or anatomical loss affecting one or more, but not necessarily limited to, the following body systems: neurological; musculoskeletal; special sense organs; respiratory, including speech organs; cardiovascular; reproductive; digestive; genitourinary; hemic and lymphatic; skin and endocrine; or any mental or psychological disorder, such as mental retardation, organic brain syndrome, emotional or mental illness, and specific learning disabilities (Americans with Disabilities Act of 1990).

Plug-ins: Programs that work within a browser to alter, enhance, or extend the browser,s operation. They are often used for viewing video, animation or listening to audio files.

Proprietary software: Privately owned software based on trade secrets, privately developed technology, or specifications that the owner refuses to divulge, thus preventing others from duplicating a product or program unless an explicit license is purchased. The opposite of proprietary is open (publicly published and available for emulation by others).

Qualified individual with a disability: An individual with a disability who, with or without reasonable modification to rules, policies or practices, the removal of architectural, communication, or transportation barriers, or the provision of auxiliary aids and services, meets the essential eligibility requirements for the receipt of services or participation in programs or activities provided by a public entity (Americans with Disabilities Act of 1990).

Reader: Volunteer or employee of a blind or partially sighted individual who reads printed material in person or records to audiotape.

Relay service: A third-party service (usually free) that allows a hearing person without a TTY/TDD device to communicate over the telephone with a person who has a hearing impairment. The system also allows a person with a hearing impairment who has a TTY/TDD to communicate in voice through a third party, with a hearing person or business.

Screen reader: A text-to-speech system intended for use by computer users who are blind or have low vision that speaks the text content of a computer display using a speech synthesizer.

Service learning: A structured, volunteer work experience where students provide community service in non-paid, volunteer positions to give them opportunities to apply knowledge and skills learned in school while making a contribution to local communities.

Sign language: Manual communication commonly used by people who are deaf. Sign language is not universal; deaf people from different countries speak different sign languages. The gestures or symbols in sign language are organized in a linguistic way. Each individual gesture is called a sign. Each sign has three distinct parts: the hand shape, the position of the hands, and the movement of the hands. American Sign Language (ASL) is the most commonly used sign language in the United States.

Specific learning disability (SLD): A disorder of one or more of the basic psychological processes involved in understanding or in using language, spoken or written, which may manifest itself in difficulties listening, thinking, speaking, reading, writing, spelling, or doing mathematical calculations. Limitations may include hyperactivity, distractibility, emotional instability, visual and/or auditory perception difficulties and/or motor limitations, depending on the type(s) of learning disability.

Speech output system: A system that provides the user with a voice alternative to the text presented on the computer screen.

Speech impairment: A problem in communication and related areas, such as oral motor function, ranging from simple sound substitutions to the inability to understand or use language or use the oral-motor mechanism for functional speech and feeding. Some causes of speech and language disorders include hearing loss; neurological disorders; brain injury; mental retardation; drug abuse; physical impairments, such as cleft lip or palate; and vocal abuse or misuse.

Speech input system: A computer-based system that allows the operator to control the system using his/her voice.

Sticky keys: Enables a computer user to do multiple key combinations on a keyboard using only one finger at a time. The sticky keys function is usually used with the Ctrl, Alt, and Shift keys. Simultaneous keystrokes can be entered sequentially.

Telecommunications Device for the Deaf (TDD) or Teletypewriter (TTY): A device which enables someone who has a speech or hearing impairment to use a telephone when communicating with someone else who has a TDD/TTY. TDD/TTYs can be used with any telephone, and one needs only a basic typing ability to use them.

Trackball: A pointing device consisting of a ball housed in a socket containing sensors to detect the rotation of the ball " like an upside down mouse. The user rolls the ball with his thumb or the palm of his hand to move the pointer.

Traumatic Brain Injury (TBI): An open or closed head injury resulting in impairments in one or more areas, such as cognition; language; memory; attention; reasoning; abstract thinking; judgment; problem-solving; sensory, perceptual, and motor abilities; psychosocial behavior; physical functions; information processing; and speech. The term does not apply to brain injuries that are congenital or degenerative, or brain injuries induced by birth trauma.

Undue hardship: An action that requires significant difficulty or expense in relation to the size of the employer, the resources available, and the nature of the operation (Americans with Disabilities Act of 1990).

Universal design: Designing programs, services, tools, and facilities so that they are usable, without additional modification, by the widest range of users possible, taking into account a variety of abilities and disabilities.

Vocational Rehabilitation Act of 1973: An act prohibiting discrimination on the basis of disability which applies to any program that receives federal financial assistance. Section 504 of the act is aimed at making educational programs and facilities accessible to all people with disabilities. Section 508 of the act requires that electronic office equipment purchased through federal procurement meets disability access guidelines.

Voice input system: A computer-based system that allows the operator to control the system using his/her voice.

Vision impairments: A complete or partial loss of the ability to see, caused by a variety of injuries or diseases including congenital causes. Legal blindness is defined as visual acuity of 20/200 or less in the better eye with correcting lenses, on the widest diameter of the visual field subtending an angular distance no greater than 20 degrees.

World Wide Web (WWW, W3, or Web): Hypertext and multimedia gateway to the Internet.

DO-IT
University of Washington
Box 354842
Seattle, WA 98195-4842
doit@uw.edu
http://www.washington.edu/doit/
206-685-DOIT (3648) (voice/TTY)
888-972-DOIT (3648) (toll free voice/TTY)
206-221-4171 (FAX)
509-328-9331 (voice/TTY) Spokane

Director: Sheryl Burgstahler, Ph.D.

User Guide

Descriptive listings in *The Complete Directory for People with Disabilities* are organized into 31 chapters, by either resource type or disability category type. You will find the following types of listings throughout the book:

- National Agencies & Associations
- State Agencies & Associations
- Camps & Exchanges Programs
- Manufacturers of Assistive Devices, Clothing, Computer Equipment & Supplies
- Print & Electronic Media
- Living Centers & Facilities
- Libraries & Research Centers
- Conferences & Trade Shows

Below is a sample listing illustrating the kind of information that is or might be included in an Association entry. Each numbered item of information is described in the paragraphs on the following page.

---

1 ➡ 1234
2 ➡ **Advocacy Center for Seniors with Disabilities**
3 ➡ 1762 South Major Drive
New Orleans, LA 98087

4 ➡ **800-000-0000**

5 ➡ **058-884-0709**

6 ➡ **Fax: 058-884-0568**

7 ➡ **TDD: 800-000-0001**

8 ➡ **email: info@sadvoc.com**

9 ➡ **www.sadvoc.com**

10 ➡ Barbara Pierce, Executive Director
Diane Watkins, Marketing Director
Robert Goldfarb, Administrative Assistant

11 ➡ The mission of the Center is to advance the dignity, equality, self-determination and choices of senior citizens with disabilities. It provides referrals, publishes information, including a monthly newsletter, offers workshops and consultation on legal, social, travel, and medical issues. The Center works with various local organizations to help seniors with disabilities stay active in their community.

12 ➡ Founded 1964

13 ➡ 18 pages

14 ➡ Monthly

User Key

1 ➤ **Record Number**: Entries are listed alphabetically within each category and numbered sequentially. The entry numbers, rather than page numbers, are used in the indexes to refer to listings.

2 ➤ **Organization Name**: Formal name of company or organization. Where organization names are completely capitalized, the listing will appear at the beginning of the alphabetized section. In the case of publications, the title of the publication will appear first, followed by the publisher.

3 ➤ **Address**: Location or permanent address of the organization.

4 ➤ **Toll Free Number**: This is listed when provided by the organization.

5 ➤ **Phone Number**: The listed phone number is usually for the main office of the organization, but may also be for the sales, marketing, or public relations office as provided by the organization.

6 ➤ **Fax Number**: This is listed when provided by the organization.

7 ➤ **TDD Number**: This is listed when provided. It refers to Telephone Device for the Deaf.

8 ➤ **E-Mail**: This is listed when provided by the organization and is generally the main office e-mail.

9 ➤ **Web Site**: This is also referred to as an URL address. These web sites are accessed through the Internet by typing *http://* before the URL address.

10 ➤ **Key Personnel**: Name and titles of department heads of the organization.

11 ➤ **Organization Description**: This paragraph contains a brief description of the organization and their services.

12 ➤ **Year Founded:** The year in which the organization was established or founded. If the organization has changed its name, the founding date is usually for the earliest name under which it was known.

13 ➤ **Number of Pages**: Number of pages if the listing is a publication.

14 ➤ **Frequency:** The frequency of the listing if it is a publication.

Arts & Entertainment

Resources for the Disabled

1   AbleArts
P.O. Box 831
Bear, DE 19701
302-368-7477
AbleArts@AbleArts.org
ablearts.org

2   American Art Therapy Association (AATA)
4875 Eisenhower Avenue
Suite 240
Alexandria, VA 22304
703-548-5860
888-290-0878
FAX: 703-783-8468
info@arttherapy.org
www.americanarttherapyassociation.org
Sarah P. Deaver, PhD, ATR-BC, President
Michele Basham, Director, Membership Information & Programs
Barbara Florence, Director, Communication, Education & Conference
Dean Sagar, Director of Public Policy
Organization of professionals who believe the art process is a beneficial and healing process.

3   American Council of the Blind
2200 Wilson Boulevard
Ste 650
Arlington, VA 22201-3354
202-467-5081
800-424-8666
FAX: 703-465-5085
info@acb.org
www.acb.org
Kim Charlson, President
Jeff Thom, First Vice President
Marlaina Lieberg, Second Vice President
Ray Campbell, Secretary
Aims to enlarge the art experience of blind people, encourages blind people to visit museums, galleries, concerts, the theater and other enjoyable public places, offers consultation to program planners in establishing accessible art and museum exhibits and presents Performing Arts Showcases at the American Council of the Blind's national convention.

4   American Dance Therapy Association (ADTA)
10632 Little Patuxent Pkwy
Ste 108
Columbia, MD 21044- 6258
410-997-4040
FAX: 410-997-4048
info@adta.org
www.adta.org/
Sharon Goodill, President
Jody Wager, MS, BC-DMT, Vice President
Gail Wood, Secretary
Meghan Dempsey, Treasurer
Dance-movement therapy is a psychotherapeutic use of movement as a process which furthers the emotional, cognitive and physical integration of the individual.

5   American Music Therapy Association (AMTA)
8455 Colesville Road
Suite 1000
Silver Spring, MD 20910-3392
301-589-3300
FAX: 301-589-5175
info@musictherapy.org
www.musictherapy.org
Andrea H. Farbman, Executive Director
Miss Angie K Elkins, Director of Membership Services & Information Systems
Al Bumanis, Director of Communications & Conferences
Jane P. Creagan, Director of Professional Programs
AMTA's purpose is the progressive development of the therapeutic use of music in rehabilitation, special education and community settings. Predecessors to the American Music Therapy Association included the National Association for Music Therapy founded in 1950 and the American Association for Music Therapy founded in 1971. AMTA is committed to the advancement of education, training, professional standards, credentials and research in support of the music therapy profession.

6   Arena Stage
The Mead Center for American Theater
1101 Sixth St. SW
Washington, DC 20024
202-554-9066
arenastage.org
Edgard Dobie, Executive Director
Molly Smith, Artistic Director
Anita Maynard Losh, Director, Community Engagement
Holly K. Oliver, Chief Development Officer
Arena Stage has played a pioneering role in providing access to all productions for people with disabilities. Access services and programs include wheelchair accessible seating; infrared assistive listening devices; Braille, large print, audio description and sign interpretation at designated performances.

7   Art Therapy SourceBook
McGraw-Hill Company
2 Penn Plaza
New York, NY 10121-101
212-904-2000
www.mhhe.com/hper/physed
Cathy Malchiodi, Author
An overview of the uses of art as a mentally therapeutic tool.
$18.00
272 pages
ISBN 1-565658-84-1

8   Art and Disabilities
Brookline Books
8 Trumbull Rd
Suite B-001
Northampton, MA 01060
413-584-0184
800-666-2665
FAX: 413-584-6184
brbooks@yahoo.com
www.brooklinebooks.com
Florence Ludins-Katz, Author
A step-by-step guide to establishing creative arts centers for people with disabilities. Includes philosophy and making creative arts centers happen.

9   Art and Healing: Using Expressive Art to Heal Your Body, Mind, and Soul
Three Rivers Press/Crown Publishing-Random House
1745 Broadway
New York, NY 10019
212-782-9000
crownpublicity@randomhouse.com
www.randomhouse.com/crown/trp.html
Barbara Ganim, Author
Markus Dohle, Chairman & CEO
Melanie Fallon-Houska, Dir., Corporate Contributions
The author believes creating a visual image through any medium can produce physical and emotional benefits for both the creator as well as those who view it. *$17.00*
256 pages
ISBN 0-609803-16-6

10 Art for All the Children: Approaches to Art Therapy for Children with Disabilities
Charles C. Thomas
2600 S First St
Springfield, IL 62704-4730
217-789-8980
800-258-8980
FAX: 217-789-9130
books@ccthomas.com
www.ccthomas.com
Frances E Anderson, Author
Sharon Moorman, Editorial Assistant
This second edition is for art therapists in training and for in-service professionals in art therapy, art education and special educa-

tion who have children with disabilities as a part of their case/class load. *$56.95*
398 pages Paperback
ISBN 0-398060-07-7

11 **Arts Unbound**
542/544 Freeman Street
Orange, NJ 07050
973-675-2787
FAX: 973-678-4408
info@artsunbound.org
www.artsunbound.org
Margaret Mikkelsen, Executive Director
Catherine Lazen, Founder and Board Chair
Alan Hirsh, Executive Vice President
Tashea Patterson Carless, Director of Agency Operations
Arts Unbound is a nonprofit organization dedicated to the artistic achievement of youth, adults, and senior citizens with disabilities.

12 **Association of Mouth and Foot Painting Artists (AMPFA)**
2070 Peachtree Court
Suite 101
Atlanta, GA 30341
770-986-7764
877-637- 872
FAX: 770-986-8563
mfpausa@bellsouth.net
www.mfpausa.com
Erich Stegmann, Founder
The AMPF is an international, for-profit association wholly owned and run by disabled artists to help them meet their financial needs. Members paint with brushes held in their mouths or feet as a result of a disability sustained at birth or through an accident or illness that prohibits them from using their hands.

13 **Awakenings Project, The**
PO Box 177
Wheaton, IL 60187
www.awakeningsproject.org
Robert Lundin, Co-Director
Irene O'Neill, President and Co-Director
Mary Lou Lowry, Secretary
John Rakow, Vice President
The Awakenings Project is an organization whose mission is to assist those artists with psychiatric illnesses in developing their talent and finding an outlet for their creative abilities through art in all forms.

14 **Brookline Books**
8 Trumbull Rd
Suite B-001
Northampton, MA 01060
413-584-0184
800-666-2665
FAX: 413-584-6184
brbooks@yahoo.com
www.brooklinebooks.com

15 **Clinical Applications of Music Therapy in Developmental Disability, Pediatrics and Neurolog**
Taylor & Francis
400 Market Street
Suite 400
Philadelphia, PA 19106-4738
215-922-1161
866-416-1078
FAX: 215-922-1474
hello.usa@jkp.com
www.jkp.com
Tony Wigram, Editor
Jessica Kingsley, Chairman, Managing Director
Jemima Kingsley, Director
Octavia Kingsley, Production Director
More and more, music therapy is being practiced as an intervention in medical and special educational settings. This book describes and explains the planning and evaluation of music therapy intervention and how it can be used for assessing complex organic and emotional disabilities. *$34.95*
312 pages
ISBN 1-853027-34-0

16 **Contemporary Art Therapy with Adolescents**
Taylor & Francis
400 Market Street
Suite 400
Philadelphia, PA 19106-4738
215-922-1161
866-416-1078
FAX: 215-922-1474
hello.usa@jkp.com
www.jkp.com
Shirley Riley, Author
Jessica Kingsley, Chairman, Managing Director
Jemima Kingsley, Director
Octavia Kingsley, Production Director
Reviews contemporary theories on adolescent development and therapy and offers solutions to the treatment of young people. *$ 26.95*
285 pages
ISBN 1-853026-37-9

17 **Creative Arts Resources Catalog**
MMB Music
9051 Watson Road
Ste 161
St. Louis, MO 63126
314-531-9635
80 -54 -377
FAX: 314-531-8384
info@mmbmusic.com
www.mmbmusic.com
Norm Goldberg, Founder & Chair
Publisher and distributor of creative arts therapy materials in the areas of music, dance, art, drama, and poetry. Free catalog contains hundreds of books, recordings, and videos.

18 **Creative Growth Art Center**
355 - 24th St
Oakland, CA 94612
510-836-2340
FAX: 510-836-0769
info@creativegrowth.org
www.creativegrowth.org
Becki Couch-Alvarado, Executive Director
Tom Di Maria, Director
Jennifer Strate O'Neal, Partnerships & Communications Manager
Creative Growth Art Center serves adult artists with developmental, mental and physical disabilities, providing a professional studio environment for artistic development, gallery exhibition and representation and a social atmosphere among peers.

19 **Creativity Explored**
3245 16th Street
San Francisco, CA 94103
415-863-2108
FAX: 415-863-1655
info@creativityexplored.org
www.creativityexplored.org
Jeff Spicer, President
Nina Sazevich, Vice President
Amy Taub, Executive Director
Ann Kappes, Marketing & Business Development Director
Creativity Explored is a nonprofit visual arts center for artists with developmental disabilities.

20 **Dancing from the Inside Out**
Fanlight Productions
c/o Icarus Films
32 Court Street, 21st Floor
Brooklyn, NY 11201
718-488-8900
800-876-1710
FAX: 718-488-8642
info@fanlight.com
www.fanlight.com
Ben Achtenberg, Founder
This eloquent video looks at the lives and work of three talented dancers who dance professionally with the acclaimed AXIS Dance Troupe, which includes both disabled and non-disabled dancers. They discuss the process they went through in adapting to their disability and how they came to re-discover physical expression through dance.

21 Deaf West Theatre
5114 Lankershim Blvd.
Los Angeles, CA 91601

818-762-2998
FAX: 818-762-2981
info@deafwest.org
deafwest.org

Ed Waterstreet, Founding Artistic Director
David Kurs, Artistic Director
Mark Freund, President
Deaf West Theatre, Inc., was founded in 1991 to directly improve and enrich the cultural lives of the 1.2 million deaf and hard-of-hearing individuals who live in the Los Angeles area. DWT provides exposure and access to professional theatre, filling a void for deaf artists and audiences.

22 Dionysus Theatre
4930 W. Bellfort
Houston, TX 77035

713-728-0041
FAX: 713-779-7483
Deb@Dionysustheatre.org
www.dionysustheatre.net

Deborah E. Nowinski, Founder & Executive Director
Dionysus Theatre is a non profit organization bringing the theatre experience to actors with disabilities and those that are non-disabled together using the theatre as our creative venue.

23 Disability and Social Performance: Using Drama to Achieve Successful Acts
Brookline Books
8 Trumbull Rd
Suite B-001
Northampton, MA 01060

413-584-0184
800-666-2665
FAX: 413-584-6184
brbooks@yahoo.com
www.brooklinebooks.com

Bernie Warren, Author
This book makes a major contribution to the understanding of disability, people with disabilities and the creative power they possess which can be unleashed through performance. The books name is Disability and Social Performance: Using Drama to Achieve Successful Acts of Being. *$17.95*

24 Expressive Arts for the Very Disabled and Handicapped of All Ages
Charles C. Thomas
2600 S First St
Springfield, IL 62704-4730

217-789-8980
800-258-8980
FAX: 217-789-9130
books@ccthomas.com
www.ccthomas.com

Marilyn Wannamaker, Co-Author
Jane G. Cohen, Co-Author
The ideas presented are not only designed to hold the interest of the children and adults, but to meet the needs of professionals and volunteers working with the disabled artists. All crafts are rated on a sliding scale, are of a low difficulty rating, use inexpensive and safe materials, and include explicit instructions. *$ 49.95*
236 pages Spiral-Paper 1996
ISBN 0-398067-04-5

25 Fanlight Productions
c/o Icarus Films
32 Court Street, 21st Floor
Brooklyn, NY 11201

718-488-8900
800-876-1710
FAX: 718-488-8642
info@fanlight.com
www.fanlight.com

Ben Achtenberg, Founder
Fanlight Productions is a leading distributor of innovative film and video works on the social issues of our time, with a special focus on healthcare, mental health, professional ethics, aging and gerontology, disabilities, the workplace, and gender and family issues. Select titles include Acting Blind, Autism: A World Apart, Dancing from the Inside Out, and Able to Laugh.

26 Fountain House Gallery
702 Ninth Ave at 48th St
New York, NY 10019

212-262-2756
fountaingallerynyc.com

Ariel Wilmott, Director
Camille Tibaldeo, Communications Director
Fountain House Gallery provides an environment for artists living and working with mental illness to pursue their personal visions and to challenge the stigma that surrounds mental illness.

27 Friends In Art (FIA)
4317 Vermont Court
Columbia, MO 65203

573-445-5564
paltschul@centurytel.net
www.friendsinart.com

Peter Altschul, President
Lynn Hedl, Vice President
Don Horn, Corresponding Secretary
Arlo Monthei, Treasurer
Friends in Art is a national organization for blind, visually impaired, and deaf-blind artists, musicians and writers, and art enthusiasts. The organization is dedicated to enhancing the skills and broadening the opportunities of the individuals involved with the organization.

28 Future Horizons
721 West Abram Street
Arlington, TX 76013-6995

817-277-0727
800-489-0727
FAX: 817-277-2270
www.fhautism.com

R. Wayne Gilpin, President
Jennifer Gilpin, VP, Foreign Translations
Kelly Gilpin, Editorial Dir.
Teresa Corey, Conference Administration
Founded in 1996, Future Horizons is devoted to supporting and fostering works and programs for those who live and work with autism and asperger's syndrome.

29 Guide to the Selection of Musical Instruments
MMB Music
9051 Watson Road
Ste 161
St. Louis, MO 63126

314-531-9635
800-543-3771
FAX: 314-531-8384
info@mmbmusic.com
www.mmbmusic.com

Norm Goldberg, Founder & Chair
A marvelous resource book to aid therapists teaching those who are disabled to play musical instruments. *$7.75*

30 In-Definite Arts Society
8038 Fairmount Drive SE
Calgary, AB T2H0Y

403-253-3174
FAX: 403-255-2234
ida@indefinitearts.com
www.indefinitearts.com

Darlene Murphy, Executive Director
Dijana Andric, Client Services Manager
Peter Kelsch, Accountant
Bernice Webb, Facility Coordinator
Promotes opportunities for people with developmental disabilities to express themselves and to grow and develop through their involvement in art.

31 Infinity Dance Theater
220 W 93rd St
New York, NY 10025

212-877-3490
info@infinitydance.com
infinitydance.com

Kitty Lunn, RDE, Founder/Artistic Director
Michael A. Fitch, Executive Director
Infinity Dance Theater is a non-traditional dance company committed to expanding the boundaries of dance by featuring dancers with and without disabilities. The company aims to inspire people with and without disabilities, encourage their artistic and other

professional aspirations, and empower them through the organization's educational and performance programs.

32   Instrumental Music for Dyslexics: A Teaching Handbook
Wiley & Sons
111 River Street
Hoboken, NJ 07030-5774   201-748-6000
                                     FAX: 201-748-6088
                                          info@wiley.com
                                          www.wiley.com
Sheila Oglethorpe, Author
Stephen M. Smith, President and CEO
Ellis E. Cousens, Executive Vice President, Chief Operations Officer
MJ O'Leary, Senior Vice President, Human Resources
Describes dyslexia in layman's terms and explains how the various problems that a dyslexic may have can affect all aspects of learning to play a musical instrument. It alerts the music teacher with a problem pupil to the possibilities of that pupil having some form of dyslexia. It offers suggestions as to how to teach dyslexics, with particular reference to piano teaching, and it suggests ways in which the music teacher may contribute to the welfare of a dyslexic pupil. *$ 34.95*
200 pages
ISBN 1-861562-91-8

33   Interact Center for the Visual and Performing Arts
Interact Center
1860 Minnehaha Ave W
St. Paul, MN 55401   651-209-3575
                                     FAX: 651-209-3579
                                   info@interactcenter.com
                                     interactcenter.com
Jeanne Calvit, Artistic & Executive Director
Shannon Forney, Managing Director
Beth Bowman, Director, Advancement
Creates art in a spirit of radical inclusion; Inspires artists and audiences to explore the full spectrum of human potential; Transforms lives by expanding ideas of what is possible.

34   Kaleidoscope: Exploring the Experience of Disability through Literature & the Fine Arts
United Disability Services
701 South Main Street
Akron, OH 44311-1019   330-762-9755
                                     FAX: 330-379-3342
                               kaleidoscope@udsakron.org
                         www.udsakron.org/services/kaleidoscope
Gail Willmott, Editor in Chief
Gary Knuth, President/CEO
Howard Taylor, Vice President
Kay Shellenberger, Director of Adult Services
This magazine explores the experiences of disability through the lens of creative arts. Unlike rehabilitation, advocacy or independent living journals, this journal challenges and transcends stereotypical, patronizing and sentimental attitudes about disability. It offers a variety of articles, fiction, art and poetry relating to issues of disability, literature and the fine arts. *$10.00*
64 pages BiAnnually

35   Keshet Dance Company
4121 Cutler Ave NE
Albuquerque, NM 87110   505-224-9808
                                      info@keshetarts.org
                                        keshetarts.org
Shira Greenberg, Artistic Director
Randy Trask, President
Julia Maccini, Vice President
Keshet's professional dancers conduct youth and adult classes and workshops for individuals with varying levels of physical disabilities and dance experience. Keshet pairs dancers with physical disabilities with able-bodied dancers, which often include siblings, parents, and peers, to create professional-quality dance works.

36   Learning Disabilities Sourcebook, 3rd Ed.
Omnigraphics
Order Department
PO Box 8002
Aston, PA 19014-8002   610-461-3548
                                          800-234-1340
                                     FAX: 800-875-1340
                                   contact@omnigraphics.com
                                     www.omnigraphics.com
Joyce Brennfleck Shannon, Editor
Fred Ruffner, Founder
Peter Ruffner, Co-Founder
Learning Disabilities Sourcebook, Third Edition provides updated information about specific learning disabilities and other conditions that make learning difficult. These include dyscalculia, dysgraphia, dyslexia, auditory and visual processing, communication disorders, autism spectrum disorders, attention deficit/hyperactivity disorder, hearing and visual impairments, and brain injury. *$84.00*
600 pages Hard cover
ISBN 0-780810-39-6

37   Manual of Sequential Art Activities for Classified Children and Adolescents
Charles C. Thomas
2600 S First St
Springfield, IL 62704-4730   217-789-8980
                                          800-258-8980
                                     FAX: 217-789-9130
                                    books@ccthomas.com
                                      www.ccthomas.com
Rocco A L Fugaro, Author
Offers information to the special education professional on art therapy and management. *$41.95*
246 pages Softcover
ISBN 0-39805 -85-6

38   Mozart Effect: Tapping the Power of Music to Heal the Body, Strengthen the Mind
Harper Collins Publishers
10 E 53rd St
New York, NY 10022-5244   212-207-7000
                                      www.harpercollins.com
Don Campbell, Author
Brian Murray, President and CEO
Michael Morrison, President and Publisher, U.S. General Books and Canada
Susan Katz, President and Publisher, HarperCollins Children's Books
Offers dramatic accounts of how doctors, shamans, musicians, and others use music to deal with everything from anxiety, cancer, and chronic pain, to dyslexia and mental illness. *$14.95*
352 pages
ISBN 0-060937-20-3

39   Music Therapy
Future Horizons, Inc.
721 West Abram St
Arlington, TX 76013-6995   817-277-0727
                                          800-489-0727
                                     FAX: 817-277-2270
                                        www.fhautism.com
Betsey King Brunk, Author
R. Wayne Gilpin, President
Jennifer Gilpin, VP, Foreign Translations
Kelly Gilpin, Editorial Dir.
Music therapy is the use of music to address non-musical goals. Parents and professionals are finding that music can break down barriers for children with autism in areas such as cognition, socialization, and communication. *$19.95*
123 pages
ISBN 1-885477-53-8

40 Music Therapy and Leisure for Persons with Disabilities
Sagamore Publishing
1807 N Federal Drive
Urbana, IL 61801

217-359-5940
800-327-5557
FAX: 217-359-5975
books@sagamorepub.com
www.sagamorepub.com

Alicia L. Barksdale, Author
Joseph J. Bannon, Sr., Ph.D., Publisher & CEO
Peter L. Bannon, MBA, President
William Anderson, M.S., Director of Sales and Marketing
Explores the use of musical therapy in order to enhance the development of independent leisure skills with a variety of special populations. Suggestions are provided for alternative avenues through musical experiences enabling individuals to achieve their greatest potential for independence and a high quality of life. *$19.95*

ISBN 1-571675-11-6

41 Music Therapy for the Developmentally Disabled
Sage Publications
2455 Teller Road
Thousand Oaks, CA 91320

805-499-9774
800-818-7243
FAX: 800-583-2665
info@sagepub.com
www.sagepub.com

S. Venkatesan, Author
Included are practical guidelines, case samples and step-by-step instructions that enable a music therapist to bring about dramatic improvements in developmentally disabled adults and children. *$40.00*
269 pages Hardcover
ISBN 0-890791-90-2

42 Music Therapy in Dementia Care
Jessica Kingsley Publishers
400 Market Street
Suite 400
Philadelphia, PA 19106-4738

215-922-1161
866-416-1078
FAX: 215-922-1474
hello.usa@jkp.com
www.jkp.com

David Aldridge, Editor
Jessica Kingsley, Chairman, Managing Director
Jemima Kingsley, Director
Octavia Kingsley, Production Director
A comprehensive look at music therapy as a means of improving memory, health, and identity in those suffering from dementia, particularly Alzheimer's. For music therapists and those involved in psychogeriatry. *$29.95*
256 pages
ISBN 1-853027-76-6

43 Music Therapy, Sensory Integration and the Autistic Child
Jessica Kingsley Publishers
400 Market Street
Suite 400
Philadelphia, PA 19106-4738

215-922-1161
866-416-1078
FAX: 215-922-1474
hello.usa@jkp.com
www.jkp.com

Dorita S. Berger, Author
Jessica Kingsley, Chairman, Managing Director
Jemima Kingsley, Director
Octavia Kingsley, Production Director
Examines the human physiologic function, the brain, information processing, functional adaption, and how that might be affected by music interventions in persons with sensory integration difficulties. *$23.95*
256 pages
ISBN 1-843107-00-7

44 Music and Dyslexia: A Positive Approach
Wiley & Sons
111 River Street
Hoboken, NJ 07030-5774

201-748-6000
FAX: 201-748-6088
info@wiley.com
www.wiley.com

John Westcombe, Editor
Stephen M. Smith, President and CEO
Ellis E. Cousens, Executive Vice President, Chief Operations Officer
MJ O'Leary, Senior VP, Human Resources
This book shows how some people who have Dyslexia can be gifted musicians. The main point this books makes is that Dyslexic musicians can succeed provided only that they are given sufficient encouragement and understanding. *$34.95*
200 pages
ISBN 1-861562-05-5

45 Music for the Hearing Impaired
MMB Music
9051 Watson Road
Ste 161
St. Louis, MO 63126

314-531-9635
800-543-3771
FAX: 314-531-8384
info@mmbmusic.com
www.mmbmusic.com

Norm Goldberg, Founder & Chair
A resource manual and curriculum guide. It is the product of a four-year developmental music program, placing emphasis on the needs of those with severe and profound losses. *$29.95*

46 Music: Physician for Times to Come
Quest Books
P.O.Box 270
Wheaton, IL 60187-270

630-665-0130
800-669-9425
FAX: 630-665-8791
submissions@questbooks.net
www.questbooks.net

Don Campbell, Author
A resource guide for various types of music and their therapeutic outcome.
365 pages
ISBN 0-835607-88-7

47 National Arts and Disability Center (NADC)
Tarjan Center at UCLA
760 Westwood Plaza
Los Angeles, CA 90095-8346

310-825-2631
800-825-2631
FAX: 310-794-1143
oraynor@mednet.ucla.edu
www.semel.ucla.edu/nadc

Peter Whybrow, Director
Fawzy Fawzy, Associate Director
Alan Han, Director of Development
Monica Rodriguez, Director of Human Resources
NADC has a database and website which deals with access to and participation in the arts by people with disabilities.

48 National Association for Drama Therapy
1450 Western Avenue
Suite 101
Albany, NY 12203

571-223-6440
888-416-7167
FAX: 518-463-8656
office@nadta.org
www.nadt.org

Nadya Trytan, MA, RDT/BCT, President
Jeremy Segall, MA, RDT, LCAT, Vice President
Jason Butler, RDT/BCT, LCAT, President-Elect
Whitney Sullivan, RDT, LCSW, Secretary
The National Association for Drama Therapy (NADT) was incorporated in 1979 to establish and uphold rigorous standards of pro-

fessional competence for drama therapists. The NADT promotes drama therapy through information and advocacy.

49   National Endowment for the Arts: Office for AccessAbility
1100 Pennsylvania Ave NW
Washington, DC 20506-0001
                                        202-682-5034
                                        FAX: 202-682-5666
                                        TTY:202-682-5496
                                        webmgr@arts.gov
                                        www.arts.gov/
Jane Chu, Chairman
Beth Bienvenu, Accessibility Director
Wendy Clark, Director of Museums, Visual Arts, and Indemnity
Ayanna N. Hudson, Arts Education Director
The National Endowment for the Arts Office for AccessAbility is the advocacy-technical assistance arm of the Arts Endowment to make the arts accessible for people with disabilities, older adults, veterans, and people living in institutions.

50   National Institute of Art and Disabilities
551 23rd St
Richmond, CA 94804-1626
                                        510-620-0290
                                        FAX: 510-620-0326
                                        admin@niadart.org
                                        www.niadart.org
Deborah Dyer, Exec. Dir.
Tim Buckwalter, Director of Exhibitions and Marketing
Belinda Sifford, Director of Client Services
Judith Zoon, Administrative Coordinator
The National Institute of Art & Disabilities (NIAD) provides an art program that promotes creativity, independence, dignity, and community integration for people with developmental and other disabilities.

51   National Library Service for the Blind And Physically Handicapped
1291 Taylor St NW
Washington, DC 20011
                                        202-707-5100
                                        FAX: 202-707-0712
                                        TTY:202-707-0744
                                        nls@loc.gov
                                        www.loc.gov/nls
Karen Keninger, Dir.
Erica Vaughns, Exec. Assistant to the Dir.
Michael Martys, Automation Officer
Neil Bernstein, R & D Officer
Administers a national library service that provides Braille and recorded books and magazines on free loan to anyone who cannot read standard print because of visual or physical disabilities.
Annual

52   National Theatre Workshop of the Handicapped (NTWH)
535 Greenwich Street
New York, NY 10013-1004
                                        212-206-7789
                                        FAX: 212-206-0200
                                        admissions@ntwh.org
                                        www.ntwh.org
Jason Matthews, Director of Admissions
Rick Curry, President & CEO
John Spalla, General Manager
A non-profit organization that provides individuals within the disabled community with the communication skills and the artistic discipline necessary to pursue a life in professional theatre.

53   National Theatre of the Deaf
139 N Main St
West Hartford, CT 06107-1264
                                        860-236-4193
                                        FAX: 860-574-9107
                                        Info@NTD.org
                                        www.ntd.org
Betty Beekman, Executive Director
William C. Martin, Marketing/PR Director
George Ghista, Accountant
Kathy Strauss, Company Interpreter
The mission of the National Theatre of the Deaf is to produce theatrically challenging work of the highest quality, drawing from as wide a range of the world's literature as possible and to perform these original works in a style that links American Sign Language with the spoken word.

54   New Music Therapist's Handbook, 2nd Ed. Berklee School of Music
Berklee Press Publications
1140 Boylston Street
Boston, MA 02215
                                        617-747-2146
                                        866-237-5533
                                        www.berkleepress.com
Suzanne B. Hanser, Author
Dr. Hanser's well-respected Music Therapist's Handbook has been revised and thoroughly updated to reflect the latest developments in the field of music therapy. *$29.95*
256 pages
ISBN 0-634006-45-2

55   No Limits
9801 Washington Blvd
2nd Fl
Culver City, CA 90232
                                        310-280-0878
                                        FAX: 310-280-0872
                                        michelle@nolimitsfordeafchildren.org
                                        nolimitsfordeafchildren.org
Michelle Christie, Founder & Executive Director
Juliana Scott, Director, Operations & Development
The mission of No Limits is to meet the auditory, speech and language needs of deaf children and enhance their confidence through the theatrical arts and individual therapy as well as provide family support and community awareness on the needs and talents of deaf children who are learning to speak.

56   Non-Traditional Casting Project
Ste 1600
1560 Broadway
New York, NY 10036-1518
                                        212-730-4750
                                        FAX: 212-730-4820
                                        TTY:212-730-4913
                                        info@ntcp.org
                                        www.ntcp.org/
Nancy Kim, Manager
The Non-Traditional Casting Project (NTCP) is a not-for-profit advocacy organization whose purpose is to address and seek solutions to the problems of racism and exclusion in theatre, film and television. NTCP's principal concerns are those of artists of color, female artists, Deaf and hard of hearing artists, and artists with disabilities.

57   Nuvisions For Disabled Artists, Inc.
C/O Rose Marcus
1319 Magee Street
Philadelphia, PA 19111
                                        hbedelstein@att.net
                                        www.hbedelstein.home.att.net
Kaye E Schonbach, Executive Director
Nuvisions was established to enable physically challenged artists to pursue professional and semi-professional artistic opportunities. Nuvisions supports these artists by sponsoring accessible exhibitions, special projects and educational opportunities in Southeastern Pennsylvania and Southern New Jersey.

58   Open Circle Theatre
102-500 King Farm Blvd
Rockville, MD 20850
                                        240-683-8934
                                        info@opencircletheatre.org
                                        opencircletheatre.org
Suzanne Richard, Artistic Director
Ian Armstrong, Executive Producer
Open Circle Theatre is a professional theatre dedicated to producing productions that integrate the considerable talents of artists with disabilities. OCT was formed by a group of people with and without disabilities, who possess professional theater experience, love of the theater, and a commitment to full access for all persons in every opportunity our community has to offer.

59 Pied Piper: Musical Activities to Develop Basic Skills
Jessica Kingsley Publishers
400 Market Street
Suite 400
Philadelphia, PA 19106-4738

215-922-1161
866-416-1078
FAX: 215-922-1474
hello.usa@jkp.com
www.jkp.com

John Bean, Author
Jessica Kingsley, Chairman, Managing Director
Jemima Kingsley, Director
Octavia Kingsley, Production Director
Describes 78 enjoyable music activities for groups of children or adults who may have learning difficulties. The emphasis is on using music, rather than learning songs or rhythms, so group members do not need any special skills to be able to participate. Full details are given about any equipment required for the games, as well as suggestions for variations or modifications. *$21.95*
96 pages
ISBN 1-853029-94-

60 Project Onward Gallery
Bridgeport Art Center
1200 W. 35th St
4th Fl
Chicago, IL 60609

773-940-2992
info@projectonward.org
projectonward.org

61 Pure Vision Arts
The Shield Institute
114 W 17th St
3rd Fl
New York, NY 10011

212-366-4263
FAX: 718-269-2059
progers@shield.org
purevisionarts.org

Pamala Rogers, Director
Pure Vision Arts mission is to provide people with autism and developmental disabilities opportunities for artistic expression and to build public awareness of their important creative contributions.

62 Reaching the Child with Autism Through Art
Future Horizons, Inc.
721 W Abram St
Arlington, TX 76013-6995

817-277-0727
800-489-0727
FAX: 817-277-2270
www.fhautism.com

Toni Flowers, Author
R. Wayne Gilpin, President
Jennifer Gilpin Yacio, Vice President and Editorial Director
David Reasor, CPA and Administrative Director
This book uncovers how art encourages communication, positive self-image, concept development, spatial relationships, fine-motor skills, and many more facets of health child development. *$19.95*
130 pages

63 Survivors Art Foundation
PO Box 383
Westhampton, NY 11977

safe@survivorsartfoundation.com
www.survivorsartfoundation.org

Michael Herships, Ph.D, Project Leader & Board President
Candyce Brokaw, Art Director
Candyce M. Brokaw, Executive Director
Margaret Ashe Magistro, Secretary/Treasurer
Dedicated to encourage healing through the arts, committed to empowering Trauma-Survivors with Effective Expressive Outlets via Internet Art Gallery, Outreach Programs, National Exhibitions, Publications and Development of Employment Skills.

64 Teaching Asperger's Students Social Skills Through Acting
Future Horizons, Inc.
721 W Abram St
Arlington, TX 76013-6995

817-277-0727
800-489-0727
FAX: 817-277-2270
www.fhautism.com

Amelia Davies, Author
R. Wayne Gilpin, President
Jennifer Gilpin Yacio, Vice President and Editorial Director
David Reasor, CPA and Administrative Director
This book provides the theories and activities needed for setting up acting classes that double as social skills groups for individuals with Asperger's or high-functioning autism. Using these skills, students will be able to develop social understanding through repetition and generalization. *$19.95*
211 pages

65 Teaching Basic Guitar Skills to Special Learners
MMB Music
9051 Watson Road
Ste 161
St. Louis, MO 63126

314-531-9635
800-543-3771
FAX: 314-531-8384
info@mmbmusic.com
www.mmbmusic.com

Norm Goldberg, Founder & Chair
The first-of-its-kind guitar book for use with persons who have difficulty learning to play via traditional methods. *$16.00*

66 The Arts of Life
2010 W. Carroll Ave
Chicago, IL 60612

312-829-2787
info@artsoflife.org
artsoflife.org

Denise Fisher, Co-Founder & Executive Director
Sara Bemer, Development Coordinator
An organization comprised of people with and without disabilities seeking to promote artistic expression, community building, self-respect, and independence.

67 Theatre Without Limits
P.O.Box 4002
Portland, ME 04101

207-607-4016
FAX: 207-761-4740
www.vsartsmaine.org

Kippy Rudy, Executive Director
VSA Maine is a 501(c)(3) non-profit organization providing educational, arts, and cultural opportunities to children and adults with disabilities in Maine.

68 VSA - The International Organization on Arts and Disability
2700 F Street, NW
Washington, DC 20566

202-467-4600
800-444-1324
FAX: 202-429-0868
TTY: 202-737-0645
info@vsarts.org
www.kennedy-center.org/education/vsa/

Ambassador J Kennedy Smith, Founder
David M. Rubenstein, Chair
Michael M. Kaiser, President
Christoph Eschenbach, Music Director, NSO and Kennedy Center
VSA offers a large selection of guides, publications, and other resources dealing with a wide variety of subject matter in education, arts, and disabilities.

69   **VSA arts**
2700 F Street, NW
Washington, DC 20566
                              202-467-4600
                              800-444-1324
                         FAX: 202-429-0868
                         TTY: 202-737-0645
                           info@vsarts.org
          www.kennedy-center.org/education/vsa/

Ambassador J Kennedy Smith, Founder
David M. Rubenstein, Chair
Michael M. Kaiser, President
Christoph Eschenbach, Music Director, NSO and Kennedy Center

VSA arts is an international, nonprofit organization founded in 1974 by Ambassador Jean Kennedy Smith whose mission is to create a society where all people with disabilities learn through, participate in, and enjoy the arts. Most states offer local programs, such as Arts in Action, that showcases the accomplishments of artists with disabilities and promotes increased access to the arts for people with disabilities.

70   **We Are PHAMALY**
Fanlight Productions
c/o Icarus Films
32 Court Street, 21st Floor
Brooklyn, NY 11201
                              718-488-8900
                              800-876-1710
                         FAX: 718-488-8642
                           info@fanlight.com
                           www.fanlight.com

Ben Achtenberg, Owner
Stands for Physically Handicapped Musical Actors League. This dynamic troupe doesn't cut any corners or make any compromises. The musicals they perform are chosen for their appeal to the audience, not because they are easy for the performers, who have a variety of sensory and mobility handicaps. *$199.00*

ISBN 1-572954-08-6

Assistive Devices

Automobile

71   Ability Center
Contact Technologies
11600 Western Ave
Stanton, CA 90680-3436

866-405-6806
FAX: 714-901-1492
info@abilitycenter.com
www.abilitycenter.com

Darrell Heath, CEO
Dan Monahan, Manager
Offers rear or side entry designed with painstaking craftsmanship using steel.

72   Acc-u-trol
Ahnafield Corporation
9850 E. 30th Street
Indianapolis, IN 46229

877-223-5301
info@acemobility.us
www.acemobility.us

73   All View Mirror
4335 S Santa Fe Dr
Englewood, CO 80110-5417

303-781-2062
800-782-4335
FAX: 303-761-6811
info@handicapsinc.com
www.handicapsinc.com

74   Arcola Mobility
51 Kero Rd
Carlstadt, NJ 07072-2601

201-507-8500
800-272-6521
FAX: 201-507-5372
info@arcolasales.com
www.arcolasales.com

Andrew Rolfe, Exec VP
Jeff Krane, Sales Mgr/Nat'l Accounts
John Akerlind, General Mgr
Teresa Smeriglio, Comml Bus Sales Coord
Arcola sells new and used accessible vehicles and adaptive driving equipment including hand controls, wheelchair lifts and securement systems. Daily, weekly and monthly vehicle rentals available. Stairway lift, porch elevators and ramps for the home sold and rented.

75   Automobile Lifts for Scooters, Wheelchairs and Powerchairs
Bruno Independent Living Aids
P.O.Box 84
Oconomowoc, WI 53066

262-567-4990
800-882-8183
FAX: 262-953-5501
www.bruno.com

Michael R. Bruno, II, President and CEO
Mike Krawczyk, Marketing Manager
Andrew Bayer, Product Manager
Over 18 different styles of automobile lifts for scooters, wheelchairs and power chairs for nearly any car, van, truck or sport utility vehicle that can raise most scooters or wheelchairs under 200 pounds and power chairs up to 300 pounds. All Bruno lifts are eligible for reimbursement of up to $1000.00 from GM, Saturn, Ford, and Chrysler under the terms of their Mobility Programs.

76   Blinker Buddy II Electronic Turn Signal
HARC Mercantile
5413 S. Westnedge Ave.
Suite A
Portage, MI 49002-5317

269-324-1615
800-445-9968
FAX: 269-324-2387
TTY: 800-445-9968
info@harc.com
www.harc.com

77   Braun Corporation
631 West 11th Street
Winamac, IN 46996

574-946-6153
800-THE-LIFT
FAX: 574-946-4670
mediaquestions@braunlift.com
www.braunability.com

Ralph Braun, Founder
Manufactures wheelchair lifts and lowered floor minivans as well as many other mobility products.

78   Chevy Lowered Floor
Ahnafield Corporation
9850 E. 30th Street
Indianapolis, IN 46229

877-223-5301
info@acemobility.us
www.acemobility.us

79   Classic
Ricon
1135 Aviation Place
San Fernando, CA 91340

818-267-3000
800-322-2884
FAX: 818-962-1201
sales@riconcorp.com
www.riconcorp.com

80   DW Auto & Home Mobility
1208 N Garth Ave
Columbia, MO 65203-4056

573-449-3859
800-568-2271
FAX: 573-449-4187
contactus@dwauto.com
www.dwauto.com

Shawn Bright, Owner
Don Rothwell, General Manager
Brian Lutz, Service Manager
Paratransit conversions and personalized conversions for the physically challenged. Home elevators and lifts. Scooter, wheelchairs and DME.

81   Dodge Lowered Floor
Ahnafield Corporation
9850 E. 30th Street
Indianapolis, IN 46229

877-223-5301
info@acemobility.us
www.acemobility.us

82   Drive Master Company
37 Daniel Rd West
Fairfield, NJ 07004-2521

973-808-9709
FAX: 973-808-9713
sales@drivemaster.net
www.drive-master.com

Peter B. Ruprecht, President
Adrienne Ruprecht, Bookkeeping
Christina M. Knapik, General Office Manager
Vinnie Dalli-Cardillo, Dealer Relations
Full service mobility center, raised tops/doors, drop floors, custom driving equipment, distributor of name brand devices and systems for full sized and mini vans. Sister company Van Master rents mobility equipped vans.

83   Driving Systems Inc.
16139 Runnymede St
Van Nuys, CA 91406-2913   818-782-6793
                                   FAX: 818-782-6485
                          info@drivingsystems.com
                          www.drivingsystems.com

Rudolf Schinz, President
William C Butt, VP
DSI is the manufacturer of the Scott Driving Controls for the severely disabled driver. Also manufacture the 'Wave Grip' grab rails and bathroom accessories for the disabled and elderly. DSI is also the importers of the Carospeed Menox Hand Controls, Left Foot Pedals and other handicapped driving aids.

84   Dual Brake Control
Kroepke Kontrols
104 Hawkins Street
Bronx, NY 10464   718-885-2100
                                   FAX: 337-235-4181
                             kroepke@mail.idt.net

85   Entervan
Braun Corporation
631 West 11th Street
Winamac, IN 46996   574-946-6153
                                     800-THE-LIFT
                                   FAX: 574-946-4670
                    mediaquestions@braunlift.com
                          www.braunability.com

Ralph Braun, Founder
The Entervan accessible features are designed to blend seamlessly into the original design of the Chrysler minivan. In fact, you'll find the Entervan to be virtually indistinguishable from other minivans on the road, with the only differences being the easily accessible qualities of the van.

86   Escort II XL
Worldwide Mobility Products
Mesa, AZ   480-497-4692
                                     800-848-3433
                                   FAX: 480-497-3834
                   service@worldwide-mobility.com
                        www.worldwide-mobility.com

87   Foot Pedal Extensions
4335 S Santa Fe Dr
Englewood, CO 80110-5417   303-781-2062
                                     800-782-4335
                                   FAX: 303-761-6811
                          info@handicapsinc.com
                          www.handicapsinc.com

88   Foot Steering
Drive Master Company
37 Daniel Rd West
Fairfield, NJ 07004-2521   973-808-9709
                                   FAX: 973-808-9713
                             sales@drivemaster.net
                           www.drive-master.com

Peter B. Ruprecht, President
Adrienne Ruprecht, Bookkeeping
Christina M. Knapik, General Office Manager
Vinnie Dalli-Cardillo, Dealer Relations
Custom installed system to steer a vehicle with your foot.

89   Foot Steering System
Ahnafield Corporation
9850 E. 30th Street
Indianapolis, IN 46229
                                       877-223-5301
                            info@acemobility.us
                             www.acemobility.us

90   Ford Lowered Floor
Ahnafield Corporation
9850 E. 30th Street
Indianapolis, IN 46229
                                       877-223-5301
                            info@acemobility.us
                             www.acemobility.us

91   Gear Shift Adaptor By Handicaps, Inc.
4335 S Santa Fe Dr
Englewood, CO 80110-5417   303-781-2062
                                     800-782-4335
                                   FAX: 303-761-6811
                          info@handicapsinc.com
                          www.handicapsinc.com

Jeanenne Phillips, Executive Director
Allows column mounted gear shift to be used with the left hand.
$90.00

92   Gresham Driving Aids
30800 S Wixom Rd
Wixom, MI 48393-2418   248-624-1533
                                     800-521-8930
                                   FAX: 248-624-6358
                     dave@greshamdrivingaids.com
                        www.greshamdrivingaids.com

David Ohrt, General Manager
Craig Wigginton, Sales Consultant
Dexter Jackson, Service Manager
Joyce Martell, Customer Service
Offers a full-service package to physically challenged individuals including lowered floors, raised roofs and doors and high-quad driver control systems. Dealer for Braun, Ricon, Crow River and Bruno wheelchair lifts.

93   HANDYBAR, The
Maxi Aids
42 Executive Blvd
Farmingdale, NY 11735-4710   631-752-0521
                                     800-522-6294
                                   FAX: 631-752-0689
                                   TTY: 800-281-3555
                             sales@maxiaids.com
                             www.maxiaids.com

Elliot Zaretsky, Founder & President
For those who have trouble getting in and out of a car. Sturdy bar slides into door striker and allows you better support to lift yourself out of the car. Stores easily under car seat. *$39.95*

94   Hand Brake Control Only
Kroepke Kontrols
104 Hawkins Street
Bronx, NY 10464   718-885-2100
                                   FAX: 337-235-4181
                             kroepke@mail.idt.net

95   Hand Dimmer Switch
Gresham Driving Aids
30800 S Wixom Rd
Wixom, MI 48393-2418   248-624-1533
                                     800-521-8930
                                   FAX: 248-624-6358
                     dave@greshamdrivingaids.com
                        www.greshamdrivingaids.com

David Ohrt, General Manager
Craig Wigginton, Sales Consultant
Dexter Jackson, Service Manager
Joyce Martell, Customer Service
This switch is recommended for left leg handicaps or when a right leg handicap uses a left foot throttle. *$36.25*

96   Hand Dimmer Switch with Horn Button
Gresham Driving Aids
30800 S Wixom Rd
Wixom, MI 48393-2418   248-624-1533
                                      800-521-8930
                                 FAX: 248-624-6358
                          dave@greshamdrivingaids.com
                             www.greshamdrivingaids.com

David Ohrt, General Manager
Craig Wigginton, Sales Consultant
Dexter Jackson, Service Manager
Joyce Martell, Customer Service
Attaches to the handle of control with a chrome plated steel insulated switch box, giving an instant warning without removing your hand from the steering wheel. *$28.75*

97   Hand Gas & Brake Control
Kroepke Kontrols
104 Hawkins Street
Bronx, NY 10464-288   718-885-2100
                                 FAX: 337-235-4181
                              kroepke@mail.idt.net
                             www.kroepkekontrols.com

98   Hand Operated Parking Brake
Gresham Driving Aids
30800 S Wixom Rd
Wixom, MI 48393-2418   248-624-1533
                                      800-521-8930
                                 FAX: 248-624-6358
                          dave@greshamdrivingaids.com
                             www.greshamdrivingaids.com

David Ohrt, General Manager
Craig Wigginton, Sales Consultant
Dexter Jackson, Service Manager
Joyce Martell, Customer Service
Converts foot parking brake to a hand operation for easy access and maneuverability. *$30.20*

99   Hand Parking Brake
Kroepke Kontrols
104 Hawkins Street
Bronx, NY 10464-288   718-885-2100
                                 FAX: 337-235-4181
                              kroepke@mail.itd.net
                             www.kroepkekontrols.com

100   Handicapped Driving Aids
Handicapped Driving Aids of Michigan
3990 2nd Street
Wayne, MI 48184-1715   734-728-8808
                                 FAX: 734-595-4520

Jim Bishop, President
Automobiles and vans customized, modified and equipped with industry approved handicapped equipment for ease of operation.

101   Handicaps, Inc.
4335 S Santa Fe Dr
Englewood, CO 80110-5417   303-781-2062
                                      800-782-4335
                                 FAX: 303-761-6811
                              info@handicapsinc.com
                             www.handicapsinc.com

Jeanenne Phillips, Executive Director
Manufacturer of 'Superarm' wheelchair lifts, hand driving controls, and left foot gas pedals for vans & motor homes. *$120.00*

102   Headlight Dimmer Switch
Kroepke Kontrols
P.O.Box 288
Bronx, NY 10464-288   718-885-2100
                                 FAX: 337-235-4181
                              kroepke@mail.idt.net
                             www.kroepkekontrols.com

103   Horizontal Steering
Drive Master Company
37 Daniel Rd West
Fairfield, NJ 07004-2521   973-808-9709
                                 FAX: 973-808-9713
                              sales@drivemaster.net
                              www.drive-master.com

Peter B. Ruprecht, President
Adrienne Ruprecht, Bookkeeping
Christina M. Knapik, General Office Manager
Vinnie Dalli-Cardillo, Dealer Relations
Horizontal steering system is customized to meet the needs of the high-level, spinally injured and all others who experience limited arm strength and range of motion.

104   Horn Control Switch
Kroepke Kontrols
P.O.Box 288
Bronx, NY 10464-288   718-885-2100
                                 FAX: 337-235-4181
                              kroepke@mail.idt.net
                             www.kroepkekontrols.com

105   Joystick Driving Control
Ahnafield Corporation
9850 E. 30th Street
Indianapolis, IN 46229   877-223-5301
                              info@acemobility.us
                              www.acemobility.us

106   Kessler Institute for Rehabilitation
1199 Pleasant Vallely Way
West Orange, NJ 07052   973-731-3600
                                      888-KES-SLER
                                 FAX: 973-243-6819
                              www.kessler-rehab.com

Robert H. Brehm, President
Bruce M. Gans, MD, Executive Vice President and Chief Medical Officer
Karen Liszner, Chief Nurse Executive
Kim Ratner, AVP, Rehabilation Services
Driver evaluation training for the physically/mentally challenged offering state certified driving instructors. Door-to-door pickup at home, work or rehab centers.

107   Key Holders, Ignition & Door Keys
Gresham Driving Aids
30800 S Wixom Rd
Wixom, MI 48393-2418   248-624-1533
                                      800-521-8930
                                 FAX: 248-624-6358
                          dave@greshamdrivingaids.com
                             www.greshamdrivingaids.com

David Ohrt, General Manager
Craig Wigginton, Sales Consultant
Dexter Jackson, Service Manager
Joyce Martell, Customer Service
Easy for arthritic hands to handle. Easily installed. *$18.70*

108   Kneelkar
Mednet
923 E. Michigan Avenue
Battle Creek, MI 49014   269-660-1002
                                      888-625-6335
                                 FAX: 269-660-1296
                              kneelvan@fminow.com
                              http://www.freedommotors.com

Mike Thompson, Vice President
Chet Baranski, Mobility Specialist-Midwest Vans
Danielle Baughman, Product Manager
Offers the ultimate van conversions with equipment that is easily installed and accessible for the physically challenged.

109 Latchloc Automatic Wheelchair Tiedown
Ahnafield Corporation
9850 E. 30th Street
Indianapolis, IN 46229

877-223-5301
info@acemobility.us
www.acemobility.us

110 Left Foot Accelerator
Gresham Driving Aids
30800 S Wixom Rd
Wixom, MI 48393-2418

248-624-1533
800-521-8930
FAX: 248-624-6358
dave@greshamdrivingaids.com
www.greshamdrivingaids.com

David Ohrt, General Manager
Craig Wigginton, Sales Consultant
Dexter Jackson, Service Manager
Joyce Martell, Customer Service
A custom pedal designed for left-foot usage. Stainless steel cross bar attaches above the throttle pedal and leaves right pedal free for right foot use. *$80.50*

111 Left Foot Gas Pedal
Kroepke Kontrols
P.O. Box 288
Bronx, NY 10464-288

718-885-2100
FAX: 337-235-4181
kroepke@mail.itd.net
www.kroepkekontrols.com

112 Left Foot Gas Pedal by Handicaps, Inc.
4335 S Santa Fe Dr
Englewood, CO 80110-5417

303-781-2062
800-782-4335
FAX: 303-761-6811
info@handicapsinc.com
www.handicapsinc.com

113 Left Hand Shift Lever
Gresham Driving Aids
30800 S Wixom Rd
Wixom, MI 48393-2418

248-624-1533
800-521-8930
FAX: 248-624-6358
dave@greshamdrivingaids.com
www.greshamdrivingaids.com

David Ohrt, General Manager
Craig Wigginton, Sales Consultant
Dexter Jackson, Service Manager
Joyce Martell, Customer Service
Converts steering wheel lever or automatic transmission selector lever to left hand usage for right arm handicaps. *$34.50*

114 Low Effort and No Effort Steering
Drive Master Company
37 Daniel Rd West
Fairfield, NJ 07004-2521

973-808-9709
FAX: 973-808-9713
sales@drivemaster.net
www.drive-master.com

Peter B. Ruprecht, President
Adrienne Ruprecht, Bookkeeping
Christina M. Knapik, General Office Manager
Vinnie Dalli-Cardillo, Dealer Relations
Reduced effort steering modifications available for nearly all vehicles. Additional products are pedal extensions which are 1 inch to 4 inch clamp-on aluminum blocks and 6 inch to 12 inch adjustable fold-down pedals.

115 Mini-Bus and Mini-Vans
Arcola Bus Sales
51 Kero Rd
Carlstadt, NJ 07072-2604

201-507-8500
800-272-6521
FAX: 201-507-5372
JudyLongo@alliancebusgroup.com
www.arcolamobility.com

Andrew Rolfe, Exec VP
John Akerlind, General Mgr
Sam Garcia, Parts Manager
Cory Mahady, Vehicle Service & Repair
Offers a virtually unlimited choice of chassis size, body style, floor plan and optional features. We provide transporters for almost every use, including school buses, vans, mini-coaches, medium-duty buses and personalized vans for the disabled.

116 Mini-Rider
Ricon
1135 Aviation Place
San Fernando, CA 91340-6090

818-267-3000
800-322-2884
FAX: 818-962-1201
sales@riconcorp.com
www.riconcorp.com

117 Mobility Vehicle Stairlifts and Ramps
Arcola Bus Sales
51 Kero Rd
Carlstadt, NJ 07072-2604

201-507-8500
800-272-6521
FAX: 201-507-5372
JudyLongo@alliancebusgroup.com
www.arcolamobility.com

Andrew Rolfe, Exec VP
John Akerlind, General Mgr
Sam Garcia, Parts Manager
Cory Mahady, Vehicle Service & Repair
Arcola Mobility is a leading dealer of personal, accessible mini and full-size vans with custom conversions and modifications available. We offer a complete line of adaptive driving equipment, including wheelchair lifts, ramps, hand controls, steering devices, scooter lifters, car top wheelchair carriers and power transfer seats. In addition to new custom vehicles, we also have an extensive selection of used vehicles for the physically challenged.

118 Monarch Mark 1-A
Access Mobility Systems
7202 Evergreen Way
Everett, WA 98203

425-353-6563
800-854-4176
FAX: 425-355-6159
info@accessams.com
www.accessams.com

119 Monmouth Vans, Access and Mobility
5105 New Jersey RT-33
Farmingdale, NJ 07727-4003

877-275-4907
ask@mobilityworks
www.mobilityworks.com/

Gene Morton, President
Ray Morton, General Manager
Don Dufty, Certified Mobility Consultant
Nathan Ahrens, Care Center Director
Full vehicle modifications for driving and for transport of people with disabilities. Access equipment for buildings, e.g. ramps, stair lifts, pool lifts, automatic door openers and patient transfer lifts, pride jazzy portable and modular wheelchairs and scooters. Large selection of modified vans in stock.

120 New Quad Grip
Gresham Driving Aids
30800 S Wixom Rd
Wixom, MI 48393-2418
248-624-1533
800-521-8930
FAX: 248-624-6358
dave@greshamdrivingaids.com
www.greshamdrivingaids.com

David Ohrt, General Manager
Craig Wigginton, Sales Consultant
Dexter Jackson, Service Manager
Joyce Martell, Customer Service
Automobile aids for the disabled. *$40.25*

121 PAC Unit
Ahnafield Corporation
9850 E. 30th Street
Indianapolis, IN 46229
877-223-5301
info@acemobility.us
www.acemobility.us

122 Park Brake Extension By Handicaps, Inc.
4335 S Santa Fe Dr
Englewood, CO 80110-5417
303-781-2062
800-782-4335
FAX: 303-761-6811
info@handicapsinc.com
www.handicapsinc.com

123 Pedal Ease
Ahnafield Corporation
9850 E. 30th Street
Indianapolis, IN 46229
877-223-5301
info@acemobility.us
www.acemobility.us

124 Portable Hand Controls
Ahnafield Corporation
9850 E. 30th Street
Indianapolis, IN 46229
877-223-5301
info@acemobility.us
www.acemobility.us

125 Portable Hand Controls By Handicaps, Inc.
4335 S Santa Fe Dr
Englewood, CO 80110-5417
303-781-2062
800-782-4335
FAX: 303-761-6811
info@handicapsinc.com
www.handicapsinc.com

126 Portable Vehicle Controls
Contact Technologies
1033 Business Center Cir
Newbury Park, CA 91320-1128
805-498-8157
FAX: 805-498-2747

127 Power Seat Base (6-Way)
Ricon
1135 Aviation Place
San Fernando, CA 91340-6090
818-267-3000
800-322-2884
FAX: 818-962-1201
sales@riconcorp.com
www.riconcorp.com

128 Quad Grip with Pin
Gresham Driving Aids
30800 S Wixom Rd
Wixom, MI 48393-2418
248-624-1533
800-521-8930
FAX: 248-624-6358
dave@greshamdrivingaids.com
www.greshamdrivingaids.com

David Ohrt, General Manager
Craig Wigginton, Sales Consultant
Dexter Jackson, Service Manager
Joyce Martell, Customer Service
Automobile aids for the disabled. *$40.25*

129 Rampvan
Independent Mobility Systems
631 West 11th Street
Winamac, IN 46996
574-946-6153
800-THE-LIFT
FAX: 574-946-4670
mediaquestions@braunlift.com
www.braunability.com

Ralph Braun, Founder
Fully accessible minivan conversions with automatic doors and ramps, manufactured by Toyota, Chrysler, Dodge and Ford minivans.

130 Reduced Effort Steering
Ahnafield Corporation
9850 E. 30th Street
Indianapolis, IN 46229
877-223-5301
info@acemobility.us
www.acemobility.us

131 Right Hand Turn Signal Switch Lever
Gresham Driving Aids
30800 S Wixom Rd
Wixom, MI 48393-2418
248-624-1533
800-521-8930
FAX: 248-624-6358
dave@greshamdrivingaids.com
www.greshamdrivingaids.com

David Ohrt, General Manager
Craig Wigginton, Sales Consultant
Dexter Jackson, Service Manager
Joyce Martell, Customer Service
Converts signal switch to right hand usage for left arm handicaps. *$34.50*

132 Slim Line Brake Only
Gresham Driving Aids
30800 S Wixom Rd
Wixom, MI 48393-2418
248-624-1533
800-521-8930
FAX: 248-624-6358
dave@greshamdrivingaids.com
www.greshamdrivingaids.com

David Ohrt, General Manager
Craig Wigginton, Sales Consultant
Dexter Jackson, Service Manager
Joyce Martell, Customer Service
A chrome plated steel handle, contour shaped, with a left hand or right hand unit available. *$155.25*

133 Slim Line Control
Gresham Driving Aids
30800 S Wixom Rd
Wixom, MI 48393-2418
248-624-1533
800-521-8930
FAX: 248-624-6358
dave@greshamdrivingaids.com
www.greshamdrivingaids.com

David Ohrt, General Manager
Craig Wigginton, Sales Consultant
Dexter Jackson, Service Manager
Joyce Martell, Customer Service

A plated, strong, compact unit designed to be easily transferred from car to car. Built of heavy steel tubing, welded and chrome plated and contour-shaped for maximum driving room. *$201.25*

134   Slim Line Control: Brake and Throttle
Gresham Driving Aids
30800 S Wixom Rd
Wixom, MI 48393-2418
                                              248-624-1533
                                              800-521-8930
                                         FAX: 248-624-6358
                             dave@greshamdrivingaids.com
                                   www.greshamdrivingaids.com

David Ohrt, General Manager
Craig Wigginton, Sales Consultant
Dexter Jackson, Service Manager
Joyce Martell, Customer Service
Brake is actuated by pushing the control lever directly towards the brake. Throttle is actuated by moving the lever at right angles to the brake movement, toward the seat. The weight of the operator's hand is sufficient to hold the throttle at any designed speed. *$300.00*

135   Steering Backup System
Ahnafield Corporation
9850 E. 30th Street
Indianapolis, IN 46229

                                              877-223-5301
                                         info@acemobility.us
                                         www.acemobility.us

136   Steering Device By Handicaps, Inc.
4335 S Santa Fe Dr
Englewood, CO 80110-5417
                                              303-781-2062
                                              800-782-4335
                                         FAX: 303-761-6811
                                   info@handicapsinc.com
                                   www.handicapsinc.com

137   Super Grade 4 Hand Controls By Handicaps, Inc.
4335 S Santa Fe Dr
Englewood, CO 80110-5417
                                              303-781-2062
                                              800-782-4335
                                         FAX: 303-761-6811
                                   info@handicapsinc.com
                                   www.handicapsinc.com

138   Super Grade IV Hand Controls
4335 S Santa Fe Dr
Englewood, CO 80110-5417
                                              303-781-2062
                                              800-782-4335
                                         FAX: 303-761-6811
                                   info@handicapsinc.com
                                   www.handicapsinc.com

139   Tim's Trim
25 Bermar Park
Rochester, NY 14624-1542
                                              585-429-6270
                                              888-468-6784
                                         FAX: 585-429-6355
                                         Info@TimsTrim.com
                                         www.timstrim.com/

Tim Miller, Owner
Offers vehicle modifications, drop floors, raised tops/doors, driving equipment, touch pads and lifts. Also is a member of NEMDA and QAP certified

140   Transportation Equipment for People with Disabilities
Drive Master Company
30800 S Wixom Rd
Wixom, MI 48393-2418
                                              248-624-1533
                                              800-521-8930
                                         FAX: 248-624-6358
                             dave@greshamdrivingaids.com
                                   www.greshamdrivingaids.com

David Ohrt, General Manager
Craig Wigginton, Sales Consultant
Dexter Jackson, Service Manager
Joyce Martell, Customer Service

Wheelchair lifts and ramps, hand and foot controls, steering and braking modifications, complete van conversions, home modifications, wheelchairs and scooters and wheelchair accessible van rentals.

141   Tri-Post Steering Wheel Spinner
Gresham Driving Aids
37 Daniel Rd West
Fairfield, NJ 07004-2521
                                              973-808-9709
                                         FAX: 973-808-9713
                                         sales@drivemaster.net
                                         www.drive-master.com

Peter B. Ruprecht, President
Adrienne Ruprecht, Bookkeeping
Christina M. Knapik, General Office Manager
Vinnie Dalli-Cardillo, Dealer Relations
Three nylon posts, adjustable for proper fit to drivers hand, to control the wheel, for use by persons with weak or limp wrists. *$40.25*

142   Turn Signal Adapter By Handicaps, Inc.
Handicaps
4335 S Santa Fe Dr
Englewood, CO 80110-5417
                                              303-781-2062
                                              800-782-4335
                                         FAX: 303-761-6811
                                   info@handicapsinc.com
                                   www.handicapsinc.com

143   Ultra-Lite XL Hand Control
Drive Master Company
30800 S Wixom Rd
Wixom, MI 48393-2418
                                              248-624-1533
                                              800-521-8930
                                         FAX: 248-624-6358
                             dave@greshamdrivingaids.com
                                   www.greshamdrivingaids.com

David Ohrt, General Manager
Craig Wigginton, Sales Consultant
Dexter Jackson, Service Manager
Joyce Martell, Customer Service
Allows the driver to operate gas and brake by hand— push for brake— pull for gas. Can be installed in nearly every vehicle.

144   United Access
Wright-Way
175 E Interstate 30
Garland, TX 75043-4021
                                              972-240-8839
                                              877-503-9399
                                              888-939-1010
                                         FAX: 972-240-0412
                                         info@unitedaccess.com
                                         www.unitedaccess.com

145   Vantage Mini-Vans
Vantage Mini-Vans
5202 S 28th Pl
Phoenix, AZ 85040-3799
                                              602-243-2700
                                              800-348-VANS
                                         FAX: 602-304-3290
                                         www.vantagemobility.com

146   Velcro Peel-Off Shoes
4335 S Santa Fe Dr
Englewood, CO 80110-5417
                                              303-781-2062
                                              800-782-4335
                                         FAX: 303-761-6811
                                   info@handicapsinc.com
                                   www.handicapsinc.com

147   Voice Choice
Ahnafield Corporation
9850 E. 30th Street
Indianapolis, IN 46229

                                              877-223-5301
                                         info@acemobility.us
                                         www.acemobility.us

148 **Voice Scan**
Ahnafield Corporation
9850 E. 30th Street
Indianapolis, IN 46229

877-223-5301
info@acemobility.us
www.acemobility.us

149 **Warp Drive**
Ahnafield Corporation
9850 E. 30th Street
Indianapolis, IN 46229

877-223-5301
info@acemobility.us
www.acemobility.us

150 **Wheelers Accessible Van Rentals**
Wheelers Accessible Van Rental
6614 West Sweetwater
Glendale, AZ 85304

623-776-8830
800-456-1371
FAX: 623-412-9920
info@WheelersVanRentals.com
www.WheelersVanRentals.com

151 **XL Steering**
Ahnafield Corporation
9850 E. 30th Street
Indianapolis, IN 46229

877-223-5301
info@acemobility.us
www.acemobility.us

Bath

152 **ARJO Inc.**
2349 West Lake Street
Suite 250
Addison, IL 60101

630-785-4490
800-323-1245
FAX: 888-389-2756
usa.info@ArjoHuntleigh.com
www.arjohuntleigh.com

153 **Adjustable Bath Seat**
Arista Surgical Supply Company/AliMed
297 High St
Dedham, MA 02026-2852

781-329-2900
800-225-2610
FAX: 781-329-8392
info@alimed.com
www.alimed.com

Julian Cherubini, President
Bath seat that fits easily in any size tub. Easily adjustable to any height for easier maneuverability. *$44.00*

154 **Adjustable Raised Toilet Seat & Guard**
Frohock-Stewart
1 Invacare Way
Elyria, OH 44035-4190

440-329-6000
800-333-6900
FAX: 877-619-7996
www.invacare.com

A Malachi Mixon III, Chairman
Gerald B. Blouch, President & CEO
Joseph B. Richey III, President - Invacare Technologies Division and SVP
Robert K. Gudbranson, Senior Vice President and Chief Financial Officer
The seat features an exclusive pivot locking system so it won't slip or tip and the adjustable guard rail fits all toilets.

155 **Bath Fixtures**
Crane Plumbing/Fiat Products
1000 Industrial Dr
Unit 2A
Bensenville, IL 60106-1260

630-350-7575
FAX: 630-350-7775
www.deery-pardue.com

Dave Pardue, Chairman Emeritus
Greg Pardue, Sales
Mark Nasuta, Sales
Matt Pardue, Sales
Manufacturers plumbing fixtures for the disabled. Products include toilets, lavatories, showers and tub/shower units.

156 **Bath Products**
Snug Seat
12801 E. Independence Blvd.
P.O. Box 1739
Matthews, NC 28106-1739

800-336-7684
FAX: 704-882-0751
information@snugseat.com
www.snugseat.com

Kirk MacKenzie, President
Scott Crosswhite, Vice President
Greg Tilley, Controller
Angela Stegall, Purchasing
Offers a wide range of products to meet the transportation, mobility, seating and bath aid needs for people of all ages. From car seats and standers for children with special needs to versatile wheelchairs that offer adults customized options and the freedom to go anywhere with confidence.

157 **Bath Shower & Commode Chair**
7830 Steubenville Pike
Oakdale, PA 15071-9226

724-695-2122
888-347-4537
FAX: 724-695-2922
info@clarkehealthcare.com
www.clarkehealthcare.com

158 **Bath and Shower Bench 3301B**
Mada Medical Products
625 Washington Ave
Carlstadt, NJ 07072-2901

201-460-0454
800-526-6370
FAX: 201-460-3509
dianelind@mail.madamedical.com
www.madainternational.com

Jeffrey Adam, President
The bath and shower bench is corrosion resistant, has a cross brace design and angled legs to prevent tipping, and seat height adjustments.

159 **BathEase**
3815 Darston St
Palm Harbor, FL 34685-3119

727-786-2604
888-747-7845
FAX: 727-786-2604
bathease@aol.com
www.bathease.com

Terry , Director of Design & Development
Gerry , Supervisor of Manufacturing
Bill , Supervisor of Operations
BathEase is the original, standard size, residential style, acrylic bathtub with a door. Ideal for use in private homes by all who are ambulatory, the award winning design was specially created as an aid to daily living for the elderly and physically challenged. *$1897.00*

160 **Bathroom Transfer Systems**
Columbia Medical Manufacturing
11724 Willake Street
Santa Fe Springs, CA 90670-5032

562-282-0244
800-454-6612
FAX: 310-305-1718
info@columbiamedical.com
www.columbiamedical.com

Gary Werschmidt, CEO
Keith Wright, Dir. of Sales & Mktg
Sue Johnson, Dir. of Finance
Reese Regan, Dir. of Engineering
Offers a complete line of bathroom transfer systems, bath lifts, reclining bath chairs, bath/shower/commode chairs, wrap-around bath supports, toilet supports, positioning commodes, premium air, foam and gel seat cushions, giant trainers and positioning restraint car seats that accommodate individuals from 20-130 pounds.

161 **Bathtub Safety Rail**
Arista Surgical Supply Company/AliMed
297 High St
Dedham, MA 02026-2852

781-329-2900
800-225-2610
FAX: 781-329-8392
info@alimed.com
www.alimed.com

Julian Cherubini, President
Made of stainless steel, this safety rail fits in any size bathtub and offers safety and independence at bathing time. *$55.00*

162 **Braun Corporation**
Braun Corporation
631 West 11th Street
Winamac, IN 46996

574-946-6153
800-843-5438
FAX: 574-946-4670
mediaquestions@braunlift.com
www.braunability.com

Ralph Braun, Founder
Offers a variety of assistive devices for the bath and surrounding environment.

163 **Can-Do Products Catalog**
Independent Living Aids
137 Rano Rd
Buffalo, NY 14207

516-937-1848
800-537-2118
FAX: 516-937-3906
can-do@independentliving.com
www.independentliving.com

Irwin Schneidmill, President
Fran Hennelly, Sales Director
Russell Pennington, Marketing Director
Provide essential aids and products for the blind and visually impaired.
84 pages Quarterly

164 **Clarke Healthcare Products, Inc.**
Clarke Health Care Products
7830 Steubenville Pike
Oakdale, PA 15071-9226

724-695-2122
888-347-4537
FAX: 724-695-2922
info@clarkehealthcare.com
www.clarkehealthcare.com

165 **Commode**
Maxi Aids
42 Executive Blvd
Farmingdale, NY 11735-4710

631-752-0521
800-522-6294
FAX: 631-752-0689
TTY: 800-281-3555
sales@maxiaids.com
www.maxiaids.com

Elliot Zaretsky, Founder & President

Adjustable seat height for patient comfort. *$65.95*

166 **Deluxe Bath Bench with Adjustable Legs**
Maxi Aids
42 Executive Blvd
Farmingdale, NY 11735-4710

631-752-0521
800-522-6294
FAX: 631-752-0689
TTY: 800-281-3555
sales@maxiaids.com
www.maxiaids.com

Elliot Zaretsky, Founder & President
Bath bench with back support and adjustable legs. *$ 49.95*

167 **Electric Leg Bag Emptier and Tub Slide Shower Chair**
RD Equipment
230 Percival Dr
West Barnstable, MA 02668-1244

508-362-7498
FAX: 508-362-7498
info@rdequipment.com
www.rdequipment.com

Richard Dagostino, Owner and Founder
Designed for independence, this small, lightweight, battery-operated valve attaches to the bottom of the leg bag. A simple flip of the switch empties the leg bag, allowing the user to take in unlimited amounts of fluids. Tub Slide Shower Chair is a complete bathroom care system, with no need of costly renovations. Eliminates all transfers in the bathroom. *$200.00*

168 **Freedom Bath**
Arjo Inc
2349 West Lake Street
Suite 250
Addison, IL 60101

630-785-4490
800-323-1245
FAX: 888-389-2756
usa.info@ArjoHuntleigh.com
www.arjohuntleigh.com

169 **Great Big Safety Tub Mat**
Maxi Aids
42 Executive Blvd
Farmingdale, NY 11735-4710

631-752-0521
800-522-6294
FAX: 631-752-0689
TTY: 800-281-3555
sales@maxiaids.com
www.maxiaids.com

Elliot Zaretsky, Founder & President
Tub mat provides security against falls in the bath and shower. *$16.95*

170 **Long Handled Bath Sponges**
Therapro, Inc.
225 Arlington St
Framingham, MA 01702-8723

508-872-9494
800-257-5376
FAX: 508-875-2062
info@therapro.com
www.therapro.com

Karen Conrad, Owner
Plastic-handled, 18-inch bath sponge. Handle may be heated and bent for easy reach. *$2.50*

171 **Mariner Shower and Commode Chair**
Maxi Aids
42 Executive Blvd
Farmingdale, NY 11735-4710

631-752-0521
800-522-6294
FAX: 631-752-0689
TTY: 800-281-3555
sales@maxiaids.com
www.maxiaids.com

Elliot Zaretsky, Founder & President
The all aluminum frame and stainless steel hardware provides optimum rust resistance making it ideal for use in the shower. Lightweight; folds easily for transport or storage. Padded 4-position

seat with easy access, swing-away front riggings with tool-less adjustable height footrests. *$699.95*

172 **Modular Wall Grab Bars**
Frohock-Stewart
1 Invacare Way
Elyria, OH 44035-4190   440-329-6000
                                      800-333-6900
                                FAX: 877-619-7996
                                  www.invacare.com

A Malachi Mixon III, Chairman
Gerald B. Blouch, President & CEO
Joseph B. Richey II, President, Invacare Technologies Division
Robert K. Gudbranson, Senior Vice President and Chief Financial Officer
Engineered for strength and beauty, these bars can be assembled in various combinations to fit any bath or shower.

173 **Portable Shampoo Bowl**
Ambulatory Cosmetology Technicians
JK Designs
4004 NE 4th Street suite #107-456
Renton, WA 98059   206-999-8226
                        info@portableshampoobowl.com
                        www.portableshampoobowl.com

174 **Prelude**
Arjo Inc
2349 West Lake Street
Suite 250
Addison, IL 60101   630-785-4490
                                     800-323-1245
                                FAX: 888-389-2756
                         usa.info@ArjoHuntleigh.com
                               www.arjohuntleigh.com

175 **SLIDER Bathing System**
Assistive Technology
21279 Protecta Dr
Elkhart, IN 46516-9539   574-522-7201
                                     800-478-2363
                                FAX: 574-293-0202
                                   info@pvcdme.com
                                    www.pvcdme.com

176 **Suregrip Bathtub Rail**
Frohock-Stewart
1 Invacare Way
Elyria, OH 44035-4190   440-329-6000
                                     800-333-6900
                                FAX: 877-619-7996
                                  www.invacare.com

A Malachi Mixon III, Chairman
Gerald B. Blouch, President & CEO
Joseph B. Richey II, President, Invacare Technologies Division
Robert K. Gudbranson, Senior Vice President and Chief Financial Officer
Compact and versatile, the bars have a soft-touch, contoured, white vinyl gripping area for added safety.

177 **Talking Bathroom Scale**
Independent Living Aids
137 Rano Rd
Buffalo, NY 14207   516-937-1848
                                     800-537-2118
                                     855-746-7452
                                FAX: 516-937-3906
                     can-do@independentliving.com
                        www.independentliving.com

Irwin Schneidmill, President
Michael Gutierrez, Director of Operations
Pamela Strauss, Director of Marketing
Ursula Izurieta, Director of Merchandising
Talking scale. *$59.95*

178 **Terry-Wash Mitt: Medium Size**
Therapro, Inc.
225 Arlington St
Framingham, MA 01702-8723   508-872-9494
                                     800-257-5376
                                FAX: 508-875-2062
                                   info@therapro.com
                                    www.therapro.com

Karen Conrad, Owner
Includes a thumb socket and a palm pocket to hold a bar of soap. *$8.00*

179 **Toilet Guard Rail**
Maxi Aids
42 Executive Blvd
Farmingdale, NY 11735-4710   631-752-0521
                                     800-522-6294
                                FAX: 631-752-0689
                                TTY: 800-281-3555
                                sales@maxiaids.com
                                   www.maxiaids.com

Elliot Zaretsky, Founder & President
Made of chrome-plated, heavy gauge steel. Fits securely to the toilet for maximum sturdiness. *$43.95*

180 **Transfer Tub Bench**
Arista Surgical Supply Company/AliMed
297 High St
Dedham, MA 02026-2852   781-329-2900
                                     800-225-2610
                                FAX: 781-329-8392
                                    info@alimed.com
                                     www.alimed.com

Julian Cherubini, President
Curved padded backrest for comfortable support. Backrest also assists patient during lateral transfer. *$64.00*

181 **Tri-Grip Bathtub Rail**
Maxi Aids
42 Executive Blvd
Farmingdale, NY 11735-4710   631-752-0521
                                     800-522-6294
                                FAX: 631-752-0689
                                TTY: 800-281-3555
                                sales@maxiaids.com
                                   www.maxiaids.com

Elliot Zaretsky, Founder & President
Two gripping heights for easy bathtub entrance or exit. *$36.95*

182 **Tub Slide Shower Chair**
RD Equipment
230 Percival Dr
West Barnstable, MA 02668-1244   508-362-7498
                                FAX: 508-362-7498
                                info@rdequipment.com
                                 www.rdequipment.com

Richard Dagostino, Owner and Founder
The tub slide shower chair was designed for the elderly and disabled to make any bathroom (at home or when travelling) accessible with little or no renovations. Go from the bed, to the commode and over to the bathtub for a shower using one product. No transfers in the bathroom whatsoever. *$2000.00*

Bed

183 **ASSISTECH Special Needs**
4801 W Calle Don Miguel
Tucson, AZ 85757-1400   520-883-8600
                                     866-674-3549
                                FAX: 520-883-5926
                                TTY: 520-883-5926
                                   www.assistech.com

Oliver Simoes, Owner
Sells hearing, visual and mobility aid devices. *$39.00*

184 Adjustable Bed
Golden Technologies
401 Bridge St
Old Forge, PA 18518-2323

570-451-7477
800-624-6374
FAX: 800-628-5165
www.goldentech.com

Richard Golden, CEO
Robert Golden, Co-Founder and Chairman
Fred Kiwak, Co-Founder and VP
Trouble-free gear motor, safety features, dual massage, variable speed timer and more, for the ultimate sleep experience.

185 Bye-Bye Decubiti Air Mattress Overlay
Ken McRight Supplies
401 Linden Center Drive
Fort Collins, CO 80524

970-484-7967
800-467-7967
FAX: 970-484-3800
info@randscot.com
www.randscot.com

Joel Lerich, Co-Founder
Barbara , Co-Founder
Originally designed for hospital beds, converts any bed into an exceptionally therapeutic, flotation unit when used between the conventional mattress and pad. The complete overlay is comprised of five individually inflatable, 100 percent natural rubber, ventilated sections enclosed within separate pockets of a soft fleece cover. Conforms to any configuration of electric or manual beds. *$731.50*

186 Cervical Support Pillow
Wise Enterprises
5017 El Don Dr
Rocklin, CA 95677-4417

916-624-3848
888-947-3368
sales@winsent.com
www.wisent.com

Tom Wise, Owner
These hypoallergenic, antimicrobial fiber pillows support the neck in a natural position. Standard, midsize and petite pillows support the neck while sleeping on the back or side. The compact travel pillow offers support while sitting or lying down. The cervical roll has a gentle center and firm ends to ensure maximum comfort and proper support. Position the roll under the neck, back or knees. Standard and midsize fits adults, petite fits children and small adults.

187 Dual Security Bed Rail
Maxi Aids
42 Executive Blvd
Farmingdale, NY 11735-4710

631-752-0521
800-522-6294
FAX: 631-752-0689
TTY: 800-281-3555
sales@maxiaids.com
www.maxiaids.com

Elliot Zaretsky, Founder & President
Sleep without worry! Dual rails for double the safety. Steel with Powder Coat. Rails adjust up and down.

188 Foam Decubitus Bed Pads
Profex Medical Products
P.O. Box 140188
Memphis, TN 38114

800-325-0196
FAX: 901-454-9850
customercare@ProfexMed.com
www.profexmed.com

Robert Gates Watel, Founder
Convoluted foam provides extra back support and comfort for wheelchair users.

189 Global Assistive Devices, Inc.
1121 East Commercial Blvd. #39
Oakland Park, FL 33334-3920

954-776-1373
888-778-4237
FAX: 954-776-8136
TTY:954-776-1373
sales@GlobalAssistive.com
www.GlobalAssistive.com

Manufacturer of assistive devices designed to make life easier. Products include: vibrating watches/countdown timers, extra loud alarm clocks with adjustable tone and bed shaker option, door signalers, telephone ring signaler and caller identification for the television.

190 Hard Manufacturing Company
230 Grider St
Buffalo, NY 14215-3797

800-873-4273
www.hardmfg.com

191 Jackson Cervipillo
Wise Enterprises
5017 El Don Dr
Rocklin, CA 95677-4417

916-624-3848
888-947-3368
sales@winsent.com
www.wisent.com

Tom Wise, Owner
The Jackson Cervipillo comfortably supports the neck vertebrae when sleeping on the side or on the back. Pillow measures 7 in diameter and is 17 long. A machine-washable cover is available separately.

192 NeckEase
Wise Enterprises
5017 El Don Dr
Rocklin, CA 95677-4417

916-624-3848
888-947-3368
sales@winsent.com
www.wisent.com

Tom Wise, Owner
Microwave NeckEase for penetrating heat that sooths stiff necks and shoulders, easing tension. NeckEase features a unique filling of organic, long grain rice and aromatic herbs and spices. When heated, this filling provides soothing, moist aromatherapy. Heat lasts about 30-45 minutes. Available in two sizes: small fits snugly around the neck, applying gentle pressure at the base of the skull; Large may be worn for a snug fit, or loosely for application on the shoulder and upper back.

193 Permaflex Home Care Mattress
BG Industries
8550 Balboa Blvd
Ste 214
Northridge, CA 91325-3564

818-894-0744
FAX: 818-894-7972
maxifloat@bgind.com
www.bgind.com

Larry Lankard, Director
Arnie Balonick, CEO/Director
Mattress with flame retardant upholstery material, water-repellant, anti-microbial and tear-resistant cover, for extra comfort.

194 SleepSafe Beds
3629 Reed Creek Drive
Bassett, VA 24055

276-627-0088
866-852-2337
FAX: 276-627-0234
SleepSafeBed@SleepSafeBed.com
www.sleepsafebed.com

Gregg Weinschreider, President
Edward Hettig, Marketing
Casey Collins, Office Manager
Al Flora, Sales
Perfect for adult home or home care use. Offering twin or full size bed frames in classic style, these beds offer an attractive alterna-

tive to a hospital bed. Keeps the user safe during rest and electrically adjusts smoothly for user comfort and caregiver ease of use.

195 **Sonic Alert Bed Shaker**
ASSISTECH
4801 W Calle Don Miguel
Tucson, AZ 85757-1400
520-883-8600
866-674-3549
FAX: 520-883-5926
TTY: 520-883-5926
www.assistech.com

Oliver Simoes, Owner
Sells hearing, visual and mobility aid devices. *$49.00*

196 **Vibes Bed Shaker**
ASSISTECH
4801 W Calle Don Miguel
Tucson, AZ 85757-1400
520-883-8600
866-674-3549
FAX: 520-883-5926
TTY: 520-883-5926
www.assistech.com

Oliver Simoes, Owner
Sells hearing, visual and mobility aid devices.

197 **Waterproof Sheet-Topper Mattress and Chair Pad**
Pillow Talk
260 Madison Avenue
New York, NY 10016
732-780-9483
FAX: 732-780-0279
info@PTIproductmarketing.com
www.pillowtalkusa.com

Dorothy Fajerman, President
Jack Fajerman, Marketing Director
This soft pad lies on the top sheet, absorbing accidents from incontinence, pregnancy or medical problems. Waterproof barrier locks out moisture, soiling and stains and eliminates midnight linen changes and the resulting laundry. Available in bed sizes W/4 Anchor, twin, full, queen, king, and crib.

Communication

198 **ADA Hotel Built-In Alerting System**
HARC Mercantile
5413 S. Westnedge Ave.
Suite A
Portage, MI 49002
269-324-1615
800-445-9968
FAX: 269-324-2387
TTY: 269-324-1615
info@harc.com
www.harc.com

199 **Access Control Systems: NHX Nurse Call System**
Aiphone Corporation
1700 130th Ave NE
Bellevue, WA 98005-2203
425-455-0510
800-692-0200
FAX: 425-455-0071
tech@aiphone.com.
www.aiphone.com

Futoshi Tanaka, President/CEO
AIPHONE manufactures audio and video intercom systems for home or business to help the physically disabled answer doors and communicate through physical barriers; also ADA-compliant emergency call intercom stations for use in public facilities and an Environmental Control System for persons with limited mobility.

200 **Adaptek Systems**
14224 Plank Street
Fort Wayne, IN 46818
260-637-8660
FAX: 260-637-8597
info@adapteksystems.com
www.adapteksystems.com

201 **Akron Resources**
20 La Porte St
Arcadia, CA 91006-2827
626-254-9005
800-841-0884
FAX: 626-254-9266
www.arkon.com

Paul Brassard, Owner
Aaron Roth, VP, Marketing & Sales
Benjamin Arana, Sr. Account Manager
Cleber Gandra, Account Manager
Manufacturers of infrared amplification systems for televisions or stereos. $29-$69.00. The company name is Arkon Resources.

202 **Amplified Handsets**
HARC Mercantile
5413 S. Westnedge Ave.
Suite A
Portage, MI 49002
269-324-1615
800-445-9968
FAX: 269-324-2387
TTY: 269-324-1615
info@harc.com
www.harc.com

203 **Amplified Phones**
HARC Mercantile
5413 S. Westnedge Ave.
Suite A
Portage, MI 49002
269-324-1615
800-445-9968
FAX: 269-324-2387
TTY: 269-324-1615
info@harc.com
www.harc.com

204 **Amplified Portable Phone**
HARC Mercantile
5413 S. Westnedge Ave.
Suite A
Portage, MI 49002
269-324-1615
800-445-9968
FAX: 269-324-2387
TTY: 269-324-1615
info@harc.com
www.harc.com

205 **Artificial Larynx**
HARC Mercantile
5413 S. Westnedge Ave.
Suite A
Portage, MI 49002
269-324-1615
800-445-9968
FAX: 269-324-2387
TTY: 269-324-1615
info@harc.com
www.harc.com

206 **Assistive Technology**
333 Elm St
Dedham, MA 02026-4530
781-461-8200
800-793-9227
FAX: 781-461-8213
sales@tobiiATI.com
www.tobii.com/

Henrik Eskilsson, CEO
John Elvesjo, CTO and deputy CEO
Mårten Skogo, Chief Science Officer
Torbjorn Moller, Chief Operating Officer
A premiere developer of innovative technology solutions for people with physical and learning disabilities. Breakthrough products enable people of all ages and abilities to live and learn independently. Supportive material for teachers, clinicians and those with disabilities.

207   **Big Red Switch**
AbleNet
2625 Patton Road
Roseville, MN 55113-1308   651-294-2200
800-322-0956
FAX: 651-294-2222
customerservice@ablenetinc.com
www.ablenetinc.com

Bill Sproull, Chairman
Jennifer Thalhuber, CEO/President
William Mills, Board of Director
Five inches across the top and activates no matter where on its surface it is touched. It is made of shatterproof plastic and contains a cord storage compartment. Also available in green, yellow and blue. *$42.00*

208   **Cornell Communications**
7915 N 81st St
Milwaukee, WI 53223-3830   414-351-4660
800-558-8957
FAX: 414-351-4657
sales@cornell.com
www.cornell.com

George , Management Staff
Gary , Management Staff
Jim , Management Staff
Cornell's Rescue Assistance Systems allow personnel to request emergency assistance. Applications include handicapped evacuations, parking garages and elevators. Voice, intercom and visual only signaling systems are available.

209   **Davis Center**
19 State Rte 10 E
Ste 25
Succasunna, NJ 07876   862-251-4637
FAX: 862-251-4642
npdunn@thedaviscenter.com
www.thedaviscenter.com

Dorinne S. Davis, MA, CCC-A, FAAA, President
Elizabeth Meade, Head Sound Therapist
Nancy Puckett-Dunn, Office Manger
Offers sound-based therapies supporting positive change in learning, development and wellness. All ages/all disabilities. The Davis Model of Sound Intervention-an alternative approach. The company name is The Davis Center.

210   **Flashing Lamp Telephone Ring Alerter**
Independent Living Aids
137 Rano Rd
Buffalo, NY 14207   516-937-1848
800-537-2118
855-746-7452
FAX: 516-937-3906
can-do@independentliving.com
www.independentliving.com

Irwin Schneidmill, President
Michael Gutierrez, Director of Operations
Pamela Strauss, Director of Marketing
Ursula Izurieta, Director of Merchandising
Once your phone is plugged into the Telephone Ring Alerter, the lamp light will flash with each ring, alerting you that there is a phone call. *$62.00*

211   **Harc Mercantile Ltd**
HARC Mercantile
5413 S. Westnedge Ave.
Suite A
Portage, MI 49002   269-324-1615
800-445-9968
FAX: 269-324-2387
TTY: 269-324-1615
info@harc.com
www.harc.com

212   **Ideal-Phone**
IDEAMATICS
1364 Beverly Road
Suite 101
McLean, VA 22101-3617   703-903-4972
800-247-IDEA
FAX: 703-903-8949
ideamatics@ideamatics.net
www.ideamatics.com

David L Danner, President
Michael A. Schwartz, Vice President
Mark A. Moore, Vice President of Operations
John R. Kaplar, Director of Applications Development
Integrates the personal computer and the telephone into a single, efficient workstation. It is ideal for mobility-impaired persons and others who need a hands-free operation of the phone. The Ideal-Phone includes one PC Board, a Plantronics headset, software for access and logging and complete documentation. It can be integrated into programs or pops-up over any application. MS-DOS based, version 3.0 or higher are available. *$195.00*

213   **IntelliKeys**
IntelliTools
24 Prime Parkway
Natick, MA 01760   303-651-2829
800-547-6747
FAX: 720-382-7438
customerservice@cambiumlearning.com
www.intellitools.com

Arjan Khalsa, CEO
Card and cable to create keyboard port on Apple IIe computer to allow use of IntelliKeys alternative keyboard.

214   **LPB Communications**
960 Brook Rd
Norristown, PA 19401   856-365-8080
FAX: 856-365-8999
info@LPBInc.om
www.lpbinc.com

John Devecka, VP Sales
Limited area AM and FM broadcast systems for hearing assistance and language translation manufacturing since 1960. Systems for small conference halls, churches and Olympic stadiums. Components or complete system. *$400.00*

215   **Language, Learning & Living**
Prentke Romich Company
1022 Heyl Rd
Wooster, OH 44691-9786   330-262-1984
800-262-1984
FAX: 330-263-4829
info@prentrom.com
www.prentrom.com

David L Moffatt, President
Barry Romich, Co-Founder
Dave Moffatt, President & COO
A Minspeak application program designed for adolescent and adult individuals with developmental disabilities and associated learning difficulties. The software is used with Prentke Romich Company augmentative communication devices. *$355.00*

216   **Large Button Speaker Phone**
HARC Mercantile
5413 S. Westnedge Ave.
Suite A
Portage, MI 49002   269-324-1615
800-445-9968
FAX: 269-324-2387
TTY: 269-324-1615
info@harc.com
www.harc.com

217 Large Print Telephone Dial
Maxi Aids
42 Executive Blvd
Farmingdale, NY 11735-4710

631-752-0521
800-522-6294
FAX: 631-752-0689
TTY: 800-281-3555
sales@maxiaids.com
www.maxiaids.com

Elliot Zaretsky, Founder & President
Pressure sensitive dial with numbers that are easy to see for the disabled. *$69.00*

218 Large Print Touch-Telephone Overlays
Maxi Aids
42 Executive Blvd
Farmingdale, NY 11735-4710

631-752-0521
800-522-6294
FAX: 631-752-0689
TTY: 800-281-3555
sales@maxiaids.com
www.maxiaids.com

Elliot Zaretsky, Founder & President
Pressure-sensitive and easy to apply overlays that make everyday phones accessible. *$49.00*

219 Liberator
Prentke Romich Company
1022 Heyl Rd
Wooster, OH 44691-9786

330-262-1984
800-262-1984
FAX: 330-263-4829
info@prentrom.com
www.prentrom.com

David L Moffatt, President
Barry Romich, Co-Founder
Dave Moffatt, President & COO
A portable electronic communication device that uses Minspeak so that symbols are used to represent words, sentences or phrases. Liberator can be accessed by pressing keys, optical headpointing and a wide variety of switch activated scans. It can be configured with 8, 32 or 128 locations. It offers a variety of unique features to permit the most effective communication possible. $7,345-$8,575.

220 Metropolitan Washington Ear
12061 Tech Road
Silver Spring, MD 20904-7826

301-681-6636
FAX: 301-625-1986
information@washear.org
www.washear.org

Brother Hilary Mettes, Chairman
Freddie L Peaco, President Pro Tem
Dr. George Long, Vice President
Neely Oplinger, Executive Director
Multi-media reading service for blind and visually impaired. Offering 24 hour audio radio reading, dial-in newspapers and web casting, as well as audio description at theaters, museums and films.

221 Mini Teleloop
HARC Mercantile
5413 S. Westnedge Ave.
Suite A
Portage, MI 49002

269-324-1615
800-445-9968
FAX: 269-324-2387
TTY: 269-324-1615
info@harc.com
www.harc.com

222 Multiple Phone/Device Switch
HARC Mercantile
5413 S. Westnedge Ave.
Suite A
Portage, MI 49002

269-324-1615
800-445-9968
FAX: 269-324-2387
TTY: 269-324-1615
info@harc.com
www.harc.com

223 Personal FM Systems
HARC Mercantile
5413 S. Westnedge Ave.
Suite A
Portage, MI 49002

269-324-1615
800-445-9968
FAX: 269-324-2387
TTY: 269-324-1615
info@harc.com
www.harc.com

224 Personal Infrared Listening System
HARC Mercantile
5413 S. Westnedge Ave.
Suite A
Portage, MI 49002

269-324-0301
800-445-9968
FAX: 269-324-2387
TTY: 269-324-1615
info@harc.com
www.harc.com

225 Prentke Romich Company
1022 Heyl Rd
Wooster, OH 44691-9786

330-262-1984
800-262-1984
FAX: 330-263-4829
info@prentrom.com
www.prentrom.com

David L Moffatt, President
Barry Romich, Co-Founder
Dave Moffatt, President / COO
The Prentke Romich Company is a full service company offering easy, yet powerful communication aids. The company believes in supporting customers before and after the sale by offering funding assistance, distance learning training, extended warranty, service assistance and much more. Visit our website to view our full line catalog, read about our success stories and to sign up for our online newsletter.

226 Push to Talk Amplified Handset
HARC Mercantile
5413 S. Westnedge Ave.
Suite A
Portage, MI 49002

269-324-0301
800-445-9968
FAX: 269-324-2387
TTY: 269-324-1615
info@harc.com
www.harc.com

227 Room Valet Visual-Tactile Alerting System
HARC Mercantile
5413 S. Westnedge Ave.
Suite A
Portage, MI 49002

269-324-0301
800-445-9968
FAX: 269-324-2387
TTY: 269-324-1615
info@harc.com
www.harc.com

228 **Silent Call Communications**
5095 Williams Lake Rd
Waterford, MI 48329-3553
248-673-7353
800-572-5227
FAX: 248-673-7360
TTY: 800-572-5227
customerservice@silentcall.com
www.silentcall.com

George Elwell, President
Diana Elwell, President
Lisa DeLeuil, Director of Sales & Marketing
Alerting devices such as paging systems and smoke detectors for deaf and deaf-blind people.

229 **Sonic Alert**
Harris Communications
15155 Technology Dr
Eden Prairie, MN 55344-2273
952-906-1180
800-825-6758
FAX: 952-906-1099
TTY: 800-825-9187
info@harriscomm.com
www.harriscomm.com

Dr.Robert Harris, Owner
Lori Foss, Marketing Director
Offers visual alerting devices that provide safety and convenience by turning vital sound into flashing light: telephone ring signalers, doorbell signalers, baby cry signalers and wake up alarms. Free catalog available.

230 **Sound Induction Receiver**
HARC Mercantile
5413 S. Westnedge Ave.
Suite A
Portage, MI 49002
269-324-0301
800-445-9968
FAX: 269-324-2387
TTY: 269-324-1615
info@harc.com
www.harc.com

231 **SpeakEasy Communication Aid**
AbleNet
2625 Patton Road
Roseville, MN 55113-1308
651-294-2200
800-322-0956
FAX: 651-294-2259
customerservice@ablenetinc.com
www.ablenetinc.com

Bill Sproull, Chairman of the Board
Jennifer Thalhuber, President/CEO
William Mills, Board of Director
SpeakEasy is a digitalized voice output communication Aid that is ideal for anyone who is beginning to develop communication skills such as making choices and identifying symbols. It holds 12 messages totaling four minutes and 20 seconds of recording time. It measures 7 1/2 inch by 1 3/4 inch and weighs only one pound. Activate messages using the built-in keyboard or via external switch. *$399.00*

232 **Speech Discrimination Unit**
HARC Mercantile
5413 S. Westnedge Ave.
Suite A
Portage, MI 49002
269-324-0301
800-445-9968
FAX: 269-324-2387
TTY: 269-324-1615
info@harc.com
www.harc.com

233 **Speechmaker-Personal Speech Amplifier**
HARC Mercantile
5413 S. Westnedge Ave.
Suite A
Portage, MI 49002
269-324-0301
800-445-9968
FAX: 269-324-2387
TTY: 269-324-1615
info@harc.com
www.harc.com

234 **Standard Touch Turner Sip & Puff Switch**
Access to Recreation
8 Sandra Ct
Newbury Park, CA 91320-4302
805-498-7535
800-634-4351
FAX: 805-498-8186
customerservice@accesstr.com
www.accesstr.com

Don Krebs, President /Founder
A page turning device.

235 **Step-by-Step Communicator**
AbleNet
2625 Patton Road
Roseville, MN 55113-1308
651-294-2200
800-322-0956
FAX: 651-294-2259
customerservice@ablenetinc.com
www.ablenetinc.com

Bill Sproull, Chairman of the Board
Jennifer Thalhuber, President/CEO
William Mills, Board of Director
Allows you to record a series of messages (as many as you want up to the 75 second limit). It has a 2 1/2 inches diameter switch surface and is 3 inches at its tallest point. Angled switch surface makes it easy to see and access. *$129.00*

236 **Strobe Light Signalers**
5413 S. Westnedge Ave.
Suite A
Portage, MI 49002
269-324-0301
800-445-9968
FAX: 269-324-2387
TTY: 269-324-1615
info@harc.com
www.harc.com

237 **TTY's: Telephone Device for the Deaf**
HARC Mercantile
5413 S. Westnedge Ave.
Suite A
Portage, MI 49002
269-324-0301
800-445-9968
FAX: 269-324-2387
TTY: 269-324-1615
info@harc.com
www.harc.com

238 **TalkTrac Wearable Communicator**
Ablenet
2625 Patton Road
Roseville, MN 55113-1308
651-294-2200
800-322-0956
FAX: 651-294-2259
customerservice@ablenetinc.com
www.ablenetinc.com

Bill Sproull, Chairman of the Board
Jennifer Thalhuber, President/CEO
William Mills, Board of Director
The TalkTrac Wearable Communicator is a personal, portable communication aid that is wearable on the wrist. TalkTrac features: simple to use, 75 seconds of recording time, four 3/4 x 1/2 message locations, rechargeable, water resistant, adjustable 9 inch band, Boardmaker compatible.

239 Talking Calculators
ASSISTECH
4801 W Calle Don Miguel
Tucson, AZ 85757-1400

520-883-8600
866-674-3549
FAX: 520-883-5926
TTY: 520-883-5926
www.assistech.com

Oliver Simoes, Owner
Marsha Neilson, Sales Representative
Carries a complete line of assistive products for the deaf and hard
of hearing, blind and visually impaired, speech impaired, and
physically challenged . They also feature products for everyone
such as medicine reminder watches and electronic language
translators.

240 Talking Clocks
HARC Mercantile
5413 S. Westnedge Ave.
Suite A
Portage, MI 49002

269-324-0301
800-445-9968
FAX: 269-324-2387
TTY: 269-324-1615
info@harc.com
www.harc.com

241 Talking Watches
HARC Mercantile
5413 S. Westnedge Ave.
Suite A
Portage, MI 49002

269-324-0301
800-445-9968
FAX: 269-324-2387
TTY: 269-324-1615
info@harc.com
www.harc.com

242 Telecaption Adapter
HARC Mercantile
5413 S. Westnedge Ave.
Suite A
Portage, MI 49002

269-324-0301
800-445-9968
FAX: 269-324-2387
TTY: 269-324-1615
info@harc.com
www.harc.com

243 Touch Turner-Page Turning Devices
Touch Turner Company
13621 103rd Ave NE
Arlington, WA 98223-8827

360-651-1962
888-811-1962
FAX: 360-658-9380
touchturner@worldnet.att.net
www.touchturner.com

244 Unity
Prentke Romich Company
1022 Heyl Rd
Wooster, OH 44691-9786

330-262-1984
800-262-1984
FAX: 330-263-4829
info@prentrom.com
www.prentrom.com

David L Moffatt, President
Barry Romich, Co-Founder
Dave Moffatt, President / COO
A Minspeak application program available for the Liberator and
Delta Talker communication devices. Provides single word vo-
cabulary to people of all ages at varying stages of language devel-
opment, who may be either cognitively intact or challenged.
$355.00

245 Vantage
Prentke Romich Company
1022 Heyl Rd
Wooster, OH 44691-9786

330-262-1984
800-262-1984
FAX: 330-263-4829
info@prentrom.com
www.prentrom.com

David L Moffatt, President
Barry Romich, Co-Founder
Dave Moffatt, President / COO
Vantage is a portable communication aid that features the Unity
Enhanced vocabulary software and a large high quality dynamic
display. Vantage also employs the recently upgraded 4.0 operating system that makes system settings quick and easy. Vantage
has synthesized speech powered by DECtalk Software, Spelling
and Word Protection software, built-in visor (flip-up protective
cover), digitized speech capability and built-in computer access
and ECU controls. 15 and 45 location keyguards available.
$6295.00

246 Vibrotactile Personal Alerting System
HARC Mercantile
5413 S. Westnedge Ave.
Suite A
Portage, MI 49002

269-324-0301
800-445-9968
FAX: 269-324-2387
TTY: 269-324-1615
info@harc.com
www.harc.com

247 Voice Amplified Handsets
HARC Mercantile
5413 S. Westnedge Ave.
Suite A
Portage, MI 49002

269-324-0301
800-445-9968
FAX: 269-324-2387
TTY: 269-324-1615
info@harc.com
www.harc.com

248 WalkerTalker
Prentke Romich Company
1022 Heyl Rd
Wooster, OH 44691-9786

330-262-1984
800-262-1984
FAX: 330-263-4829
info@prentrom.com
www.prentrom.com

David L Moffatt, President
Barry Romich, Co-Founder
Dave Moffatt, President / COO
A portable direct selection communication device for active persons. The 16 location keyboard and speakers are carried in a belt
that straps comfortably around the waist. The keyboard can be re-
moved from its pouch to use by activating keys. Two versions are
available, standard memory and expanded memory. *$1195.00*

Chairs

249 Adjustable Chair
Bailey Manufacturing Company
P.O.Box 130
Lodi, OH 44254-130

330-948-2655
800-321-8372
FAX: 800-224-5390
baileymfg@baileymfg.com
www.baileymfg.com

Larry Strimple, President
Sandy Mooney, Customer Service
Judie Butler, Dealer Contact
The seat and footboard of this versatile chair can be adjusted to
accommodate children of various sizes. A classroom-suitable
variation of this model is also available.

250 Adjustable Clear Acrylic Tray
Bailey Manufacturing Company
P.O.Box 130
Lodi, OH 44254-130
330-948-2655
800-321-8372
FAX: 800-224-5390
baileymfg@baileymfg.com
www.baileymfg.com

Larry Strimple, President
Sandy Mooney, Customer Service
Judie Butler, Dealer Contact
Adjusts for height and depth and is equipped with a spill rim for easy to clean edges.

251 Adjustable Rigid Chair
Kuschall North America
1811 Lefthand Cir
Ste B
Longmont, CO 80501-6785
303-682-2571
888-682-2571
FAX: 866-651-6973
www.kuschallna.com

Terry Mulkey, Owner
The Champion 3000 is a fully adjustable rigid frame chair weighing only 21 pounds with a new clamping system that adjusts seat height and angle without tools.

252 Adjustable Tee Stool
Bailey Manufacturing Company
P.O.Box 130
Lodi, OH 44254-130
330-948-2655
800-321-8372
FAX: 800-224-5390
baileymfg@baileymfg.com
www.baileymfg.com

Larry Strimple, President
Sandy Mooney, Customer Service
Judie Butler, Dealer Contact
May be used to encourage balance as well as develop integrative and perceptual motor skills.

253 BackSaver
BackSaver Products Company
53 Jeffrey Ave
Holliston, MA 01746-2084
508-893-6990
800-251-2225
FAX: 508-429-8698
stevek@backsaver.com
www.backsavercorp.com

Ed Foye, Owner
Eliminates slouching and extra pressure on your back and thighs which impairs circulation.

254 Better Back
Orthopedic Products Corporation
4100 1/2 Glencoe Ave
Marina Del Rey, CA 90292
323-584-6977
FAX: 310-306-0177

255 Carendo
Arjo Inc
2349 West Lake Street
Addison, IL 60101
630-785-4490
800-323-1245
FAX: 888-389-2756
usa.info@ArjoHuntleigh.com
www.arjo.com

Philip M. Croxford, President/ CEO
The Carendo hygiene chair has been designed for caregivers.

256 Century 50/60XR Sit
Arjo Inc
2349 West Lake Street
Addison, IL 60101
630-785-4490
800-323-1245
FAX: 888-389-2756
usa.info@ArjoHuntleigh.com
www.arjo.com

Philip M. Croxford, President/ CEO
This bathing system has a built-in cleaning/disinfectant injection system with adjustable flowmeter. The incorporation of an automatic hot water alarm/shut-off system, and digital temperature monitors, helps to assure resident safety and comfort.

257 Convert-Able Table
REAL Design
187 S Main St
Dolgeville, NY 13329-1455
315-429-3071
800-696-7041
FAX: 315-429-3071
rdesign@twcny.rr.com
www.realdesigninc.com

Sam Camardello, Owner
This table has push button height adjustment and interchangeable tops so it can become a desk, art easel or a sensory stimulation bowl.

258 Evac + Chair Emergency Evacuation Chair
Evac + Chair North America LLC
3000 Marcus Ave
Ste 3E6
Lake Success, NY 11042-1012
516-502-4240
FAX: 516-327-8220
sales@evac-chair.com
www.evac-chair.com

Richard Perl, VP Business Dev.
David Egen, Founder
Gravity driven evaluation chair allows one nondisabled person to smoothly glide a seated passenger down fire stairs and across landings to exit on a combination of wheels and track belts. Pivots in own width for tight landing turns. Aluminum; weight 19 pounds. Compactly stores on wall mount, 38 by 20 by 9 inches. Maximum capacity 330 pounds. Self braking features. No installation, works on all fire exit stairs. *$950.00*

259 Golden Technologies
401 Bridge St
Old Forge, PA 18518-2323
570-451-7477
800-624-6374
FAX: 800-628-5165
johngcei@excite.com
www.goldentech.com

Richard Golden, CEO
Robert Golden, Chairman of the Board
Fred Kiwak, VP of R & D
The largest facility in the world dedicated solely to the manufacture of lift chairs.

260 High-Low Chair
Rehab and Educational Aids for Living
NY
800-696-7041
rdesign@twcny.rr.com
www.realdesigninc.com/

Sam Camardello, President
Kris Wohnsen, Vice President
A high chair and mobile floor sitter in one. The high-low chair comes with colorful upholstered wipe clean seat and height adjustable tray. The chair has a single lever adjustment to change the seat height. Lateral and head supports are available as options. *$1199.00*

261 Ladybug Corner Chair
Rehab and Educational Aids for Living
NY

800-696-7041
rdesign@twcny.rr.com
www.realdesigninc.com/

Sam Camardello, President
Kris Wohnsen, Vice President
For children 0-3 years. This chair is adjustable for long legs for conventional sitting.

262 Lumex Recliner
Graham-Field Health Products
2935 Northeast Pkwy
Atlanta, GA 30360-2808

678-291-3207
800-347-5678
FAX: 770-368-4702
cs@grahamfield.com
www.grahamfield.com

Kenneth Spett, President & Chief Executive Officer
Cherie Antoniazzi, SVP Quality, Regulatory and Risk Management
Ivan Bielik, Senior Vice President, Business Analyst
Marc Bernstein, Senior Vice President, Consumer Sales
Combines therapeutic benefits of position change with attractive appearance.

263 Modular QuadDesk
Gpk
535 Floyd Smith Dr
El Cajon, CA 92020-1228

619-593-7381
800-468-8679
FAX: 888-755-5603
sales@gpk.com
www.gpk.com

264 Mulholland Positioning Systems
P.O. Box 70
839 Albion Avenue
Burley, ID 83318

208-878-3840
800-543-4769
FAX: 208-878-3841
info@mulhollandinc.com
www.mulhollandinc.com

Larry Mulholland, Owner
Dick Stepan, Sales Manager
Provides a full line of standing aids, seating systems, adaptive components and bath aids.

265 Prime Engineering
Prime Engineering
4202 W Sierra Madre Ave
Fresno, CA 93722-3932

559-276-0991
800-827-8263
FAX: 800-800-3355
info@primeengineering.com
www.primeengineering.com

Bruce Boegel, CFO
Mary Wilson Boegel, President
Mark Allen, Vice President
Dawn Smith Cobb, Customer Service
Prime Engineering is a leading manufacturer of adult and pediatric standing devices and patient transfer equipment. Products include the all-new Support Standing System, Granstand III MSS Standing System Kidstand III MSS Standing System Superstand Multi-Position Pediatric Stander, the Lift, the CindyLift and the Original Lift Walker.

266 Roll Chair
Bailey Manufacturing Company
P.O. Box 130
Lodi, OH 44254-130

330-948-2655
800-321-8372
FAX: 800-224-5390
baileymfg@baileymfg.com
www.baileymfg.com

Larry Strimple, President
Sandy Mooney, Customer Service
Judie Butler, Dealer Contact

The padded roll helps maintain proper hip abduction and prevents scissoring of the legs.

267 Safari Tilt
Convaid Products
2830 California Street
Torrance, CA 90503

310-618-0111
888-266-8243
FAX: 310-618-2166
www.convaid.com

Chris Braun, President
A semi-contour seat provides positioning with 5-45 degree tilt adjustment. One step design folds compactly into a lightweight chair.

268 Spatial Tilt Custom Chair
Redman Powerchair
Suite 107
1601 S Pantano Road
Tucson, AZ 85710-6791

520-546-6002
800-727-6684
FAX: 520-546-5530
info@redmanpowerchair.com
www.redmanpowerchair.com

Don Redman, CEO
Paula Redman, CFO
Scott Evans, Regulatory affairs
Samuel Redman, General manager
Custom chair designed for comfort with a solid seat and back with modifications available for seat depth, height or width.

269 Transfer Bench with Back
Frohock-Stewart
1 Invacare Way
Elyria, OH 44035-4190

440-329-6000
800-333-6900
FAX: 877-619-7996
www.invacare.com

A. Malachi Mixon III, Chairman of the Board
Gerald B. Blouch, President and Chief Executive Officer
Joseph B. Richey, II, President - Invacare Technologies Division
Robert K. Gudbranson, Senior Vice President and Chief Financial Officer
This bench with air-cushioned seat sections has a full, reversible backrest for safety and comfort.

Cushions & Wedges

270 Action Products
954 Sweeney Drive
Hagerstown, MD 21740-4910

301-797-1414
800-228-7763
FAX: 301-733-2073
service@actionproducts.com
www.actionproducts.com

Mistie Witt, President
Janet Kaplan, Marketing Director
Wheelchair pads, mattress pads, positioning cushions and insoles that aid in the prevention and cure of pressure sores by reducing pressure. All products are made of Akton viscoelastic polymer that does not leak, flow or bottom out. Manufacturer of the Xact line of positioning cushions for patients with high risk of skin breakdown.

271 Adjustable Wedge
Bailey Manufacturing Company
P.O. Box 130
Lodi, OH 44254-130

800-321-8372
FAX: 800-224-5390
baileymfg@baileymfg.com
www.baileymfg.com

272   **Back-Huggar Pillow**
Bodyline Comfort Systems
3730 Kori Rd
Jacksonville, FL 32257-6036

904-262-4068
800-874-7715
FAX: 904-262-2225
info@bodyline.com
www.bodyline.com

Dr. John W. Fiore, Owner
Exclusive design makes almost any seat more comfortable by exerting soothing pressure against back muscles and discs.

273   **Bye-Bye Decubiti (BBD)**
Ken McRight Supplies
7456 S Oswego Ave
Tulsa, OK 74136-5903

918-492-9657
FAX: 918-492-9694

Ken McRight, President
The BBD therapeutic wheelchair cushions have been market-proven since 1951 — in the prevention and cure of pressure sores (decubiti). These natural rubber inflatable products have recently been expanded to include pediatric, sports and double-valve models. Moderately priced, they offer a viable and cost-effective alternative in the market. $84.00-$112.00.

274   **Dynamic Systems**
104 Morrow Branch Rd
Leicester, NC 28748-9635

828-683-3523
855-786-6283
FAX: 844-270-6478
dsi@sunmatecushions.com
www.sunmatecushions.com

Charles A Yost, CEO
Lewis McCrain, General Manager
SunMate orthopedic foam sheets and cushions, pudgee pads for pressure relief and skin breakdown prevention, laminar wheelchair cushions and Foam-in-Place Seating for custom molding seat inserts. Sample packs and literature available upon request.

275   **Econo-Float Water Flotation Cushion**
Jefferson Industries
1985 Rutgers Blvd
Lakewood, NJ 08701-4569

732-905-9001
800-257-5145
FAX: 732-905-9899

Charles Landa, General Manager
An inexpensive, yet effective approach to the problem of pressure ulcers for patients confined to wheelchairs, geriatric chairs, etc. *$15.00*

276   **Econo-Float Water Flotation Mattress**
Jefferson Industries
1985 Rutgers Blvd
Lakewood, NJ 08701-4569

732-905-9001
800-257-5145
FAX: 732-905-9899

Charles Landa, General Manager
Helps prevent and treat pressure ulcers by reducing and distributing pressure over the patient's bony prominences while supporting the body evenly over a greater surface area. *$39.00*

277   **Enhancer Cushion**
ROHO Group
100 North Florida Avenue
Belleville, IL 62221-5429

618-277-9173
800-851-3449
FAX: 618-277-9561
tomb@therohogroup.com
www.therohogroup.com

Tom Borcherding, President
Bobby Graebe, CEO
Tim Richter, Vice President of Finance
Dave McCausland, Sr. VP of Planning & Gov Affairs
Uses AIR IN PLACE progressive positioning for enhanced midline channeling of the femurs, lateral stability and tissue protection.

278   **Functional Forms**
Consumer Care Products
1446 Pilgrim Rd
Plymouth, WI 53073-4969

920-893-4614
FAX: 800-977-2256
ccpi@consumercareinc.com
www.consumercareinc.com

Terry Grall, Owner
These blocks, wedges, rolls, cervical pillows, head and leg supports and barrel rolls in resilient high density foam covered with durable antibacterial, antistatic, flame resistant, nonabsorbent vinyl are used to attain individualized support for the most difficult positioning needs for children and adults. Unique sizes allow fitting for almost any person. Use during exercise, feeding, therapy, recreation and rest at home, school and health care facilities. Packages available.

279   **Gaymar Industries**
Gaymar Industries
10 Centre Dr
Orchard Park, NY 14127-2295

716-662-2551
800-828-7341
FAX: 716-662-0748
webmaster@gaymar.com
www.gaymar.com

Dan Kormowicz, International Sales & Mktg
Cindy Sylvia, Educational Svcs Administrator
Heather Lindstrom, Medical Res
Brian McLaughlin, International Order Coordinator
Gaymar offers a complete line of support surfaces, including low-air-loss mattresses, specialty foam mattresses, turning mattresses, air overlays and fluid therapy beds. These products economically prevent and treat bedsores. Clinical and reimbursement professionals are available to answer any question related to bedsores (decubitus ulcers). Also offers a complete line of temperature control devices. The T-Pump delivers warm therapy to effectively dilate vessels and increase blood flow.

280   **Geo-Matt for High Risk Patients**
Span-America Medical Systems
70 Commerce Ctr
Greenville, SC 29615-5814

864-288-8877
800-888-6752
FAX: 864-288-8692
www.spanamerica.com

James D Ferguson, CEO
Helps prevent pressure sores in high risk patients.

281   **High Profile Single Compartment Cushion**
ROHO Group
100 North Florida Avenue
Belleville, IL 62221-5429

618-277-9173
800-851-3449
FAX: 618-277-9561
tomb@therohogroup.com
www.therohogroup.com

Tom Borcherding, President
Bobby Graebe, CEO
Tim Richter, Vice President of Finance
Dave McCausland, Sr. VP of Planning & Gov Affairs
With 4 inch cells, the HIGH PROFILE is the cushion of choice for individuals who suffer from ischemic ulcers (pressure sores) or who have a history of tissue breakdown.

282   **Inflatable Back Pillow**
Corflex
669 East Industrial Park Dr
Manchester, NH 03109-5625

603-623-3344
800-426-7353
FAX: 603-623-4111
sales@corflex.com
www.corflex.com

Paul Lorenzetti, CEO
Folds flat to fit into its own carrying case, this inflatable back pillow ensures comfort while at home or traveling.

283   **Jobri**
520 N Division St
Konawa, OK 74849-2223
580-925-3500
800-432-2225
FAX: 580-925-3501
support@jobri.com
www.jobri.com

Brian Gourley, CEO
Jobri manufactures ergonomic back supports, ergonomic chairs, orthopedic soft goods and sleep products.

284   **Lumex Cushions and Mattresses**
Graham-Field Health Products
2935 Northeast Pkwy
Atlanta, GA 30360-2808
678-291-3207
800-347-5678
FAX: 770-368-4702
cs@grahamfield.com
www.grahamfield.com

Kenneth Spett, President & Chief Executive Officer
Cherie Antoniazzi, SVP Quality, Regulatory and Risk Management
Ivan Bielik, Senior Vice President, Business Analyst
Marc Bernstein, Senior Vice President, Consumer Sales
Line of cushions and pillows give comfort and independence to the physically challenged.

285   **Medpro Static Air Chair Cushion**
Medpro
1950 Rutgers Blvd
Lakewood, NJ 08701-4537
800-257-5145
FAX: 732-905-9899

Jody Gorran, President
Provides a protective layer of air beneath the patient helping prevent and treat pressure ulcers. *$94.95*

286   **Medpro Static Air Mattress Overlay**
Medpro
1950 Rutgers Blvd
Lakewood, NJ 08701-4537
800-257-5145
FAX: 732-905-9899

Jody Gorran, President
Supports the patient on a cushioned network of air designed to redistribute the patient's weight reducing tissue interface pressure. Medpro's design incorporates a series of 65 air-breather vents that maintain air circulation. Medpro effectively reduces pressure and helps prevent and treat pressure ulcers. *$164.95*

287   **Mini-Max Cushion**
ROHO
100 North Florida Avenue
Belleville, IL 62221-5429
618-277-9173
800-851-3449
FAX: 618-277-9561
tomb@therohogroup.com
www.therohogroup.com

Tom Borcherding, President
Bobby Graebe, CEO
Tim Richter, Vice President of Finance
Dave McCausland, Sr. VP of Planning & Gov Affairs
Designed for the active individual with low risk of skin breakdown. The unique air cells of the MINI-MAX provide significant shock and impact absorption, skin protection and stability.

288   **NEXUS Wheelchair Cushioning System**
ROHO
100 North Florida Avenue
Belleville, IL 62221-5429
618-277-9173
800-850-7646
FAX: 618-277-9561
tomb@therohogroup.com
www.therohogroup.com

Tom Borcherding, President
Bobby Graebe, CEO
Tim Richter, Vice President of Finance
Dave McCausland, Sr. VP of Planning & Gov Affairs

A unique modular cushion that mates a contoured polyurethane foam base with a dry flotation support pad. It is designed to give the user positioning and stability, while offering maximum protection to the ischia, sacrum and coccyx.

289   **Pediatric Seating System**
ROHO
100 N Florida Ave
Belleville, IL 62221-5429
618-277-9173
800-851-3449
FAX: 618-277-9561
tomb@therohogroup.com
www.therohogroup.com

Tom Borcherding, President
Bobby Graebe, CEO
Tim Richter, Vice President of Finance
Dave McCausland, Sr. VP of Planning & Gov Affairs
ROHO Cushions for kids use individual air cells, creating the most versatile and dynamic cushioning products available. These cushions are designed to specifically fit pediatric wheelchairs.

290   **Quadtro Cushion**
ROHO
100 North Florida Avenue
Belleville, IL 62221-5429
618-277-9173
800-851-3499
FAX: 618-277-9561
tomb@therohogroup.com
www.therohogroup.com

Tom Borcherding, President
Bobby Graebe, CEO
Tim Richter, Vice President of Finance
Dave McCausland, Sr. VP of Planning & Gov Affairs
For individuals who require special positioning of the pelvis or thighs and are at risk of skin breakdown, the Quadtro, with 4 inch cell height and air in place, progressive positioning is the cushion of choice.

291   **Silicone Padding**
Spenco Medical Group
P.O.Box 2501
Waco, TX 76702-2501
254-772-6000
800-877-3626
spenco@spenco.com
www.spenco.com

Jeff Antonioli, VP Sales
Ryan Cruthirds, Vice President
For the management of pressure sores, this padding provides a special support system which allows even distribution of pressure and cool, comfortable, well-ventilated support.

292   **Soft-Touch Convertible Flotation Mattress**
Medpro
1950 Rutgers Blvd
Lakewood, NJ 08701-4537
800-257-5145
FAX: 732-905-9899

Jody Gorran, President
Gives the patient the option to choose between water and gel flotation depending on the needs of the patient. The mattress helps prevent and treat pressure ulcers by spreading the patient's weight over a greater surface area. $164.95-$239.95.

293   **Soft-Touch Gel Flotation Cushion**
Medpro
1940 Rutgers Blvd
Lakewood, NJ 08701-4537
732-905-9001
800-257-5145
FAX: 732-905-9899

Jody Gorran, President
Acts like an additional layer of fatty tissue beneath the patient to help prevent and treat pressure sores. *$99.95*

294   Spenco Medical Group
P.O. Box 2501
Waco, TX 76702-2501
254-772-6000
800-877-3626
spenco@spenco.com
www.spenco.com

Jeff Antonioli, VP Sales
Ryan Cruthirds, Vice President
Wheel chair cushions, silicone mattress pads, wound dressings, second skin blister and burn pads, polysorb insoles, elbow, knee and wrist supports and walking shoes.

295   Stop-Leak Gel Flotation Mattress
Jefferson Industries
1989 Rutgers Blvd
Lakewood, NJ 08701-4538
732-905-9001
800-257-5145
FAX: 732-905-9899

Charles Landa, General Manager
Protects persons from messy leaks while it protects from pressure ulcers. *$54.00*

296   Sun-Mate Seat Cushions
Dynamic Systems
104 Morrow Branch Rd
Leicester, NC 28748-5710
828-683-3523
855-786-6283
FAX: 844-270-6478
dsi@sunmatecushions.com
www.sunmatecushions.com

Charles A Yost, CEO
Lewis McCrain, General Manager
Line of cushions, pads and accessory items for personal comfort of the disabled. SunMate Orthopedic foam cushions and sheets that contours slowly to give uniform pressure distribution and soft spring back. Liquid SunMate for Foam-in-Place Seating (FIPS) to make custom molded seat inserts.

297   Twin-Rest Seat Cushion & Glamour Pillow
Better Sleep
57 Industrial Rd
Berkeley Heights, NJ 07922-1501
908-464-6568
FAX: 908-464-0058

William Emery Jr, President
Makes any seat more comfortable because it is ingeniously designed to soothe sensitive areas while at work, in the car or at home.

Dressing Aids

298   Button Aid
Maxi Aids
42 Executive Blvd
Farmingdale, NY 11735-4710
631-752-0521
800-522-6294
FAX: 631-752-0689
TTY: 800-281-3555
sales@maxiaids.com
www.maxiaids.com

Elliot Zaretsky, Founder / President
Makes buttoning possible with the use of only one hand. *$9.95*

299   Deluxe Sock and Stocking Aid
Therapro, Inc.
225 Arlington St
Framingham, MA 01702-8723
508-872-9494
800-257-5376
FAX: 508-875-2062
info@therapro.com
www.therapro.com

Karen Conrad, ScD, OTR/L, Owner
Flexible plastic, lined with blue nylon to reduce friction and outside with beige terry cloth to hold sock firmly until it is on the foot. *$12.95*

300   Dressing Stick
Maxi Aids
42 Executive Blvd
Farmingdale, NY 11735-4710
631-752-0521
800-522-6294
FAX: 631-752-0689
TTY: 800-281-3555
www.maxiaids.com

Elliot Zaretsky, Founder / President
Helps put on coats, sweaters and garments even when arm and shoulder movement is limited. *$7.95*

301   Elastic Shoelaces
Therapro, Inc.
225 Arlington St
Framingham, MA 01702-8723
508-872-9494
800-257-5376
FAX: 508-875-2062
info@therapro.com
www.therapro.com

Karen Conrad, ScD, OTR/L, Owner
The elastic laces allow the wearer to slip tied shoes on and off. *$4.25*

302   Featherweight Reachers
Therapro, Inc.
225 Arlington St
Framingham, MA 01702-8723
508-872-9494
800-257-5376
FAX: 508-875-2062
info@therapro.com
www.therapro.com

Karen Conrad, ScD, OTR/L, Owner
Useful in dressing or retrieving objects. *$17.95*

303   Mirror Go Lightly
AbleNet
2625 Patton Road
Roseville, MN 55113-1308
612-379-0956
800-322-0956
FAX: 612-379-9143
customerservice@ablenetinc.com
www.ablenetinc.com

Bill Sproull, Chairman of the Board
Jennifer Thalhuber, President/CEO
William Mills, Board of Director
Framed in plastic, the mirror can be tilted to provide either a normal or magnified image or to direct its lights at, or away from, the user. *$22.00*

304   Molded Sock and Stocking Aid
Therapro, Inc.
225 Arlington St
Framingham, MA 01702-8723
508-872-9494
800-257-5376
FAX: 508-875-2062
info@therapro.com
www.therapro.com

Karen Conrad, ScD, OTR/L, Owner
Sock or stocking is pulled over the molded plastic and then can be put on more easily. *$13.25*

305   Say What
Maxi Aids
42 Executive Blvd
Farmingdale, NY 11735-4710
631-752-0521
800-522-6294
FAX: 631-752-0689
TTY: 800-281-3555
www.maxiaids.com

Elliot Zaretsky, Founder / President
Braille the tag with information that the wearer wants on the tag and place the tag on a hanger. The custom-identification program makes it easier for the user to remember and identify just the right clothes. *$4.95*

306   Shoe and Boot Valet: Decreased Mobility Aid
Maxi Aids
42 Executive Blvd
Farmingdale, NY 11735-4710   631-752-0521
                                         800-522-6294
                                    FAX: 631-752-0689
                                    TTY: 800-281-3555
                                         www.maxiaids.com

Elliot Zaretsky, Founder / President
This is the perfect device to alleviate and in many cases eliminate
the pain and embarrassment for millions of people who have a
problem doing the simple everyday task of putting on and taking
off their footwear. It works perfectly with shoes, boots, galoshes
and slippers. *$49.95*

Health Aids

307   AMI
P.O.Box 808
Groton, CT 06340-808   860-536-3735
                                         800-248-4031
                                    FAX: 860-536-3735
                                    sales@aquamassage.com
                                         www.aquamassage.com

David M. Cote, President
Dow Cote, Vice President Sales
Hilaire Cote, Senior Vice President
Scott Gilbert, Customer Service Manager
The Aqua PT provides the major benefits of Hydrotherapy, Massage Therapy and Dry Heat Therapy. 36 water jets provide continuous full body or localized massage while the client remains
CLOTHED AND DRY! Adjustable water pressure, temperature
and pulsation frequency can massage in either a two direction
travel mode for musculoskeletal pain management or a one direction mode, flowing water from head to foot for a contrast mas-
sage-relax therapy. $25,000 to $30,000.

308   American Medical Industries
Ste 2
330 E 3rd St
Dell Rapids, SD 57022-1918   605-428-5501
                                         801-618-0444
                                    FAX: 605-428-5502
                                    info@ezhcare.com
                                         www.ezhealthcare.com

Koby Jackson, Founder
Rick Martin, CEO
Kerina Blauer, VP Client Services
Jim Cannon, SVP Sales and Marketing
EZ-Swallow, EZ-Health, EZ-Home Care, Kleen-Handz,
Kleen-Scent, EZ-Irrigator, EZ-VU, Pureshark, Gobot and AMI
are all trademarks of American Medical Industries. Healthcare
products made easy.

309   BIPAP S/T Ventilatory Support System
Respironics
1010 Murry Ridge Ln
Murrysville, PA 15668-8517   724-387-5200
                                    FAX: 724-387-5010
                                    customerservice@respironics.com
                                         www.respironics.com

John L Miclot, CEO
Gerald McGinnis, Chairman
Daniel Bevevino, VP/CFO
Craig Reynolds, Executive VP/COO
Respironics, a recognized resource in the medical device market,
provides innovative products and unique designs to the health
care provider while helping them to grow and manage their busi-
ness efficiently.

310   Bed Rails
Mada Medical Products
625 Washington Ave
Carlstadt, NJ 07072-2901   201-460-0454
                                         800-526-6370
                                    FAX: 201-460-3509
                                    dianelind@mail.madamedical.com
                                         www.madainternational.com

Jeffrey Adam, President
Chrome plated steel rails and crossbars, all welded construction,
telescopic side rail length adjustable, and a standard rail height of
16 inches.

311   Coast to Coast Home Medical
Ste 4d
3381 Fairlane Farms Rd
Wellington, FL 33414-8711   561-792-4009
                                         800-330-6316

Keri Suess, Owner
Home-delivered medical supplies for diabetes, respiratory, arthritis and impotence supplies.

312   Drew Karol Industries
P.O.Box 1066
Greenville, MS 38702-1066   662-378-2188
                                    FAX: 601-378-3188
                                    dki@techinfo.com

Andrew K Hoszowski, Owner
Orally operated toothbrush and dental care system for persons
with limited or complete loss of hand or arm use - wheelchair accessible. *$600.00*

313   Duraline Medical Products Inc.
P.O.Box 67
324 Werner Street
Leipsic, OH 45856-1039   419-943-2044
                                         800-654-3376
                                    FAX: 419-943-3637
                                    duraline@fairpoint.net
                                         www.dmponline.com

Kathy Peck, General Manager
An assortment of quality incontinence products for adults and
children.

314   Duro-Med Industries
1931 Norman Drive
Waukegan, IL 60085
                                         800-526-4753
                                         800-622-4714
                                    FAX: 800-479-7968
                                         www.mabisdmi.com

Mike Mazza, President
Tony D'Antonio, Senior VP of Sales
Alan Yefsky, Exec VP, Sales & Mktg
Manufacturers of a complete line of home health care products.
Featured products are patient gowns, back and seat cushions, pil-
lows and a complete line of aids for daily living.

315   Easy Ply
BioMedical Life Systems
P.O.Box 1360
Vista, CA 92085-1360
                                         800-726-8367
                                    FAX: 760-727-4220
                                    information@bmls.com
                                         www.bmls.com

316   Electronic Stethoscopes
HARC Mercantile
5413 S. Westnedge Ave.
Suite A
Portage, MI 49002   269-324-0301
                                         800-445-9968
                                    FAX: 269-324-2387
                                    TTY: 269-324-1615
                                    info@harc.com
                                         www.harc.com

317 Fold-Down 3-in-1 Commode
Mada Medical Products
625 Washington Ave
Carlstadt, NJ 07072-2901   201-460-0454
      800-526-6370
      FAX: 201-460-3509
      dianelind@mail.madamedical.com
      www.madainternational.com
Jeffrey Adam, President
The Fold-Down commode is constructed of heavy duty, 1 inch diameter, steel tubing with X frame, has folding features convenient for storage and transport, easily removable back rest, and full length armrests.

318 Healing Dressing for Pressure Sores
Baxter Healthcare Corporation
1 Baxter Pkwy
Deerfield, IL 60015-4625   800-422-9837
      FAX: 800-568-5020
      www.baxter.com
Robert L Parkinson Jr, Chairman of the Board/CEO
Jean-Luc Butel, Corporate Vice President - President, International
Ludwig N. Hantson, Corporate Vice President - President, BioScience
Robert J. Hombach, Corporate VP/CFO
A dressing specifically designed to promote healing of pressure sores and other dermal ulcers.

319 Invacare Corporation
1 Invacare Way
Elyria, OH 44035-4190   440-329-6000
      800-333-6900
      FAX: 877-619-7996
      info@invacare.com
      www.invacare.com
A Malachi Mixon Iii, Chairman of the Board
Robert Gudbranson, Interim President & CEO; SVP & CFO
Joseph B. Richey, II, President - Invacare Technologies Division
Anthony C. LaPlaca, Senior Vice President /General Counsel
The world's leading manufacturer and distributor of innovative home and long-term care medical products which promote recovery and active lifestyles.

320 MADAMIST 50/50 PSI Air Compressor
Mada Medical Products
625 Washington Ave
Carlstadt, NJ 07072-2901   201-460-0454
      800-526-6370
      FAX: 201-460-3509
      dianelind@mail.madamedical.com
      www.madainternational.com
Jeffrey Adam, President
The new compressor rated at 50 PSI is designed to drive humidifiers, nebulizers, mist tents and is ideal to administer pentamidine aerosol therapy.

321 MedDev Corporation
730 N Pastoria Ave
Sunnyvale, CA 94085-3522   408-730-9702
      800-543-2789
      FAX: 408-730-9732
      info@meddev-corp.com
      www.meddev-corp.com

322 Medi-Grip
Therapro, Inc.
225 Arlington St
Framingham, MA 01702-8723   508-872-9494
      800-257-5376
      FAX: 508-875-2062
      info@therapro.com
      www.therapro.com
Karen Conrad, ScD, OTR/L, Owner
Reasonably priced, nonskid material. This nonslip material is available in marine blue, desert sand and burgundy rolls 12 inches x 144 inches. *$11.95*

323 Pocket Otoscope
HARC Mercantile
5413 S. Westnedge Ave.
Suite A
Portage, MI 49002   269-324-0301
      800-445-9968
      FAX: 269-324-2387
      TTY: 269-324-1615
      info@harc.com
      www.harc.com

324 Standard 3-in-1 Commode
Mada Medical Products
625 Washington Ave
Carlstadt, NJ 07072-2901   201-460-0454
      800-526-6370
      FAX: 201-460-3509
      dianelind@mail.madamedical.com
      www.madainternational.com
Jeffrey Adam, President
The standard commode is constructed of a heavy duty anodized aluminum frame, seat adjustment and an easily removable back rest.

325 Strider
Osborn Medical Corporation
7022 S. Revere Pkwy
Suite 240
Centennial, CO 80112   507-932-5028
      800-535-5865
      FAX: 507-932-5044
      info@osbornmedical.com
      www.osbornmedical.com
Bill Davis, President and CEO
Keith Walli-Ware, Vice President of Sales and Marketing
Ian MacDonald, COO
Strider allows you to exercise in most chairs found in your home. No more small, uncomfortable bicycle seats to sit on while exercising. With Strider, your hands are free to read the paper or your favorite book while you exercise.

326 Talking Clinical Thermometer
Maxi Aids
42 Executive Blvd
Farmingdale, NY 11735-4710   631-752-0521
      800-522-6294
      FAX: 631-752-0689
      TTY: 800-281-3555
      www.maxiaids.com
Elliot Zaretsky, Founder / President
Audible clinical thermometer. *$199.95*

327 Talking Thermometers
Maxi Aids
42 Executive Blvd
Farmingdale, NY 11735-4710   631-752-0521
      800-522-6294
      FAX: 631-752-0689
      TTY: 800-281-3555
      www.maxiaids.com
Elliot Zaretsky, Founder / President
Clearly announces temperature in Fahrenheit or Celcius. *$17.95*

328 Transfer Bench
Mada Medical Products
625 Washington Ave
Carlstadt, NJ 07072-2901   201-460-0454
      800-526-6370
      FAX: 201-460-3509
      dianelind@mail.madamedical.com
      www.madainternational.com
Jeffrey Adam, President
The transfer bench is a one piece bench with a wide base for stability, 1 inch diameter aluminum framework, corrosion resistant, and an adjustable seat.

Hearing Aids

329 Auditech: Personal PA Value Pack System
P.O.Box 821105
Vicksburg, MS 39182-1105

800-229-8293
FAX: 800-221-8639
info@auditechusa.com
www.auditechusa.com

330 Auditech: Pocketalker Pro
P.O.Box 821105
Vicksburg, MS 39182-1105

800-229-8293
FAX: 800-221-8639
info@auditechusa.com
www.auditechusa.com

331 Battery Device Adapter
AbleNet
2625 Patton Road
Roseville, MN 55113-1308

612-379-0956
800-322-0956
FAX: 651-294-2259
customerservice@ablenetinc.com
www.ablenetinc.com

Bill Sproull, Chairman of the Board
Jennifer Thalhuber, President/CEO
William Mills, Board of Director
A cable which connects to and adapts battery-operated devices for external switch control. Two sizes are available to adapt devices with either AA or C and D size batteries. *$8.00*

332 Custom Earmolds
Lloyd Hearing Aid Corporation
P.O.Box 1645
4435 Manchester Dr
Rockford, IL 61109-1645

815-964-4191
800-323-4212
FAX: 815-964-8378
info@lloydshearingaid.com
www.lloydhearingaid.com

Andy PalmQuist, President
Hearing aid molds, custom built to the exact fit of the customer. *$29.95*

333 Digital Hearing Aids
Lloyd Hearing Aid Corporation
P.O.Box 1645
4435 Manchester Dr
Rockford, IL 61109-1645

815-964-4191
800-323-4212
FAX: 815-964-8378
info@lloydshearingaid.com
www.lloydhearingaid.com

Andy PalmQuist, President
Latest hearing technology. *$7.50*

334 Doorbell Signalers
HARC Mercantile
5413 S. Westnedge Ave.
Suite A
Portage, MI 49002

269-324-0301
800-445-9968
FAX: 269-324-2387
TTY: 269-324-1615
info@harc.com
www.harc.com

335 Double Gong Indoor/Outdoor Ringer
HARC Mercantile
5413 S. Westnedge Ave.
Suite A
Portage, MI 49002

269-324-0301
800-445-9968
FAX: 269-324-2387
TTY: 269-324-1615
info@harc.com
www.harc.com

336 Duracell & Rayovac Hearing Aid Batteries
Lloyd Hearing Aid Corporation
P.O.Box 1645
4435 Manchester Dr
Rockford, IL 61109-1645

815-964-4191
800-323-4212
FAX: 815-964-8378
info@lloydhearingaid.com
www.lloydhearingaid.com

Andy PalmQuist, President
Batteries for hearing aids at discounted prices. As low as 45 cents each.

337 Harris Communications
Harris Communications
15155 Technology Dr
Eden Prairie, MN 55344-2273

800-825-6758
FAX: 952-906-1099
TTY:800-825-9187
info@harriscomm.com
www.harriscomm.com

Dr.Robert Harris, Owner and President
A national distributor of assistive devices for the deaf and hard-of-hearing with many manufacturers represented. Catalog includes a wide range of assistive devices as well as a variety of books and video tapes related to deaf and hard-of-hearing issues. Products available for children, teachers, hearing professionals, interpreters and anyone interested in deaf culture, hearing loss and sign language.
180 pages Yearly

338 Hearing Aid Batteries
HARC Mercantile
5413 S. Westnedge Ave.
Suite A
Portage, MI 49002

269-324-0301
800-445-9968
FAX: 269-324-2387
TTY: 269-324-1615
info@harc.com
www.harc.com

339 Hearing Aid Battery Testers
HARC Mercantile
5413 S. Westnedge Ave.
Suite A
Portage, MI 49002

269-324-0301
800-445-9968
FAX: 269-324-2387
TTY: 269-324-1615
info@harc.com
www.harc.com

340 Hearing Aid Dehumidifier
HARC Mercantile
5413 S. Westnedge Ave.
Suite A
Portage, MI 49002

269-324-0301
800-445-9968
FAX: 269-324-2387
TTY: 269-324-1615
info@harc.com
www.harc.com

341   In the Ear Hearing Aid Battery Extractor
HARC Mercantile
5413 S. Westnedge Ave.
Suite A
Portage, MI 49002   269-324-0301
                                                     800-445-9968
                                               FAX: 269-324-2387
                                               TTY: 269-324-1615
                                                     info@harc.com
                                                     www.harc.com

342   Micro Audiometrics Corporation
655 Keller Rd
Murphy, NC 28906-5890   828-644-0771
                                                     800-729-9509
                                                     866-327-7226
                                               FAX: 866-683-4447
                                               sales@microaud.com
                                                     www.microaud.com

Jason Keller, President
Manufacturer and distributor of hearing testing instruments, including the complete line of Earscan.

343   Mushroom Inserts
Lloyd Hearing Aid Corporation
P.O.Box 1645
4435 Manchester Drive
Rockford, IL 61109- 1645   815-964-4191
                                                     800-323-4212
                                               FAX: 815-964-8378
                                          info@lloydhearingaid.com
                                               www.lloydhearingaid.com

Andy PalmQuist, President
A universal earplug useful in wearing behind the ear type hearing instruments. *$2.50*

344   Oval Window Audio
33 Wildflower Ct
Nederland, CO 80466-9638   303-447-3607
                                               FAX: 303-447-3607
                                               TTY:303-447-3607
                                          info@ovalwindowaudio.com
                                               www.ovalwindowaudio.com

Norman Lederman, Dir. of R & D
Paula Hendricks, Educational Dir.
Manufacturer of induction loop hearing assistance technologies compatible with hearing aids already used by many hard of hearing people. Also multisensory sound systems for use in speech and music therapy and science classes.

Kitchen & Eating Aids

345   Bagel Holder
Maxi Aids
42 Executive Blvd
Farmingdale, NY 11735-4710   631-752-0521
                                                     800-522-6294
                                               FAX: 631-752-0689
                                               TTY: 800-281-3555
                                                     www.maxiaids.com

Elliot Zaretsky, Founder / President
Holds bagels in place for easy slicing. *$3.95*

346   Big Bold Timer Low Vision
Maxi Aids
42 Executive Blvd
Farmingdale, NY 11735-4710   631-752-0521
                                                     800-522-6294
                                               FAX: 631-752-0689
                                               TTY: 800-281-3555
                                                     www.maxiaids.com

Elliot Zaretsky, Founder / President
Sixty-minute mechanical timer with large, easy-to-read numbers for the vision impaired. *$9.95*

347   Box Top Opener
Sammons Preston Rolyan
W68 N158 Evergreen Blvd.
Cedarburg, WI 53012   630-378-6000
                                                     800-228-3693
                                               FAX: 262-387-8748
                                          sp@pattersonmedical.com
                                               www.pattersonmedical.com

David P Sproat, President
Bruce Curtis, Sales Representative
This handy device exerts the pressure on those hard-to-open boxes of laundry/dishwasher soap, rice and prepared dinners. *$2.95*

348   Capscrew
Access with Ease
P.O.Box 1150
Chino Valley, AZ 86323-1150   928-636-9469
                                                     800-531-9479
                                               FAX: 928-636-0292
                                               KMJC@northlink.com

349   Cool Handle
Maxi Aids
42 Executive Blvd
Farmingdale, NY 11735-4710   631-752-0521
                                                     800-522-6294
                                               FAX: 631-752-0689
                                               TTY: 800-281-3555
                                                     www.maxiaids.com

Elliot Zaretsky, Founder / President
A specially designed, heat-resistant handle, available in three sizes which can be affixed to the handles of most fry, sauce and saute pans. *$7.95*

350   Cordless Receiver
AbleNet
2625 Patton Road
Roseville, MN 55113-1308   612-379-0956
                                                     800-322-0956
                                               FAX: 651-294-2259
                                          customerservice@ablenetinc.com
                                               www.ablenetinc.com

Bill Sproull, Chairman of the Board
Jennifer Thalhuber, President/CEO
William Mills, Board of Director
The Cordless Receiver in conjunction with the Cordless Big Red Switch, can be used anywhere a switch is currently used to control battery or electrically-operated toys, games or appliances; augmentative communication systems; and computers (through a computer switch interface). *$79.00*

351   Deluxe Long Ring Low Vision Timer
Maxi Aids
42 Executive Blvd
Farmingdale, NY 11735-4710   631-752-0521
                                                     800-522-6294
                                               FAX: 631-752-0689
                                               TTY: 800-281-3555
                                                     www.maxiaids.com

Elliot Zaretsky, Founder / President
Bold black numerals on white background allows for easy reading at any distance. *$17.95*

352   Deluxe Roller Knife
Sammons Preston Rolyan
28100 Torch Parkway
Suite 700
Warrenville, IL 60555-3938   630-378-6000
                                                     800-323-5547
                                               FAX: 630-393-7600
                                          sp@pattersonmedical.com
                                               www.pattersonmedical.com

David P Sproat, President
Bruce Curtis, Sales Representative
Stainless steel blade rolls smoothly, cutting food cleanly. *$10.95*

353 Dual Brush with Suction Base
Sammons Preston Rolyan
28100 Torch Parkway
Suite 700
Warrenville, IL 60555-3938   630-378-6000
                                     800-323-5547
                          FAX: 630-393-7600
                          sp@pattersonmedical.com
                          www.pattersonmedical.com

David P Sproat, President
Bruce Curtis, Sales Representative
Two brushes clean the inside and outside of bottles and glasses at
the same time using just one hand. *$14.50*

354 Easy Pour Locking Lid Pot
Maxi Aids
42 Executive Blvd
Farmingdale, NY 11735-4710   631-752-0521
                                     800-522-6294
                          FAX: 631-752-0689
                          TTY: 800-281-3555
                          www.maxiaids.com

Elliot Zaretsky, Founder / President
Baked enamel and dishwasher safe, the pot comes with an easy lid
that locks in place for extra safety. *$24.95*

355 Electric Can Opener & Knife Sharpener
Maxi Aids
42 Executive Blvd
Farmingdale, NY 11735-4710   631-752-0521
                                     800-522-6294
                          FAX: 631-752-0689
                          TTY: 800-281-3555
                          www.maxiaids.com

Elliot Zaretsky, Founder / President
Features include a powerful magnetic lid holder, the ability to
open odd-shaped cans, and easy operation for the physically challenged. *$19.95*

356 Evio Plastics
P.O.Box 2295
Sandusky, OH 44871-2295   419-621-1105
                          FAX: 419-626-2183

Doug Didion, Adminintrator Director
Danny Thomas, Owner
Handi Holder is a plastic holder for 1/2 gallon paper cartons of
milk or juice. It is used to pour milk or juice without spills by using the handle.

357 Food Markers/Rubberbands
Maxi Aids
42 Executive Blvd
Farmingdale, NY 11735-4710   631-752-0521
                                     800-522-6294
                          FAX: 631-752-0689
                          TTY: 800-281-3555
                          www.maxiaids.com

Elliot Zaretsky, Founder / President
These are durable plastic markers, easily identified by touch, tex-
ture, shape and form which help the visually impaired orient
themselves to food location on the plate. *$11.95*

358 Good Grips Cutlery
Therapro, Inc.
225 Arlington St
Framingham, MA 01702-8723   508-872-9494
                                     800-257-5376
                          FAX: 508-875-2062
                          info@therapro.com
                          www.therapro.com

Karen Conrad, ScD, OTR/L, Owner
Stainless steel utensils have a special twist built into the metal to
facilitate bending of a spoon or fork at any angle for right or left
handed people. *$7.50*

359 H.E.L.P. Knife
Maxi Aids
42 Executive Blvd
Farmingdale, NY 11735-4710   631-752-0521
                                     800-522-6294
                          FAX: 631-752-0689
                          TTY: 800-281-3555
                          www.maxiaids.com

Elliot Zaretsky, Founder / President
Adjustable food slicing system guides the knife for even, uniform
slices while protecting the user. *$11.95*

360 Handy-Helper Cutting Board
Maxi Aids
42 Executive Blvd
Farmingdale, NY 11735-4710   631-752-0521
                                     800-522-6294
                          FAX: 631-752-0689
                          TTY: 800-281-3555
                          www.maxiaids.com

Elliot Zaretsky, Founder / President
Laminated cutting board with unique features to hold food in
place with corner ledge for cutting and spreading. *$19.95*

361 Innerlip Plates
Therapro, Inc.
225 Arlington St
Framingham, MA 01702-8723   508-872-9494
                                     800-257-5376
                          FAX: 508-875-2062
                          info@therapro.com
                          www.therapro.com

Karen Conrad, ScD, OTR/L, Owner
Food may be pushed to the side of the plate, then scooped up with
a fork and spoon. Available in beige or blue. *$5.00*

362 Long Oven Mitts
Sammons Preston Rolyan
28100 Torch Parkway
Suite 700
Warrenville, IL 60555-3938   630-378-6000
                                     800-323-5547
                          FAX: 630-393-7600
                          sp@pattersonmedical.com
                          www.pattersonmedical.com

David P Sproat, President
Bruce Curtis, Sales Representative
Protect hands and forearms from heat, flames and oven grates
with these practical mitts that allow a longer reach and less bending. *$8.95*

363 Magnetic Card Reader
Maxi Aids
42 Executive Blvd
Farmingdale, NY 11735-4710   631-752-0521
                                     800-522-6294
                          FAX: 631-752-0689
                          TTY: 800-281-3555
                          www.maxiaids.com

Elliot Zaretsky, Founder / President
Produces audible labels so a recorded card can be taped on cans of
food or a box of cake mix; even adding instructions for baking.
$159.95

364 Maxi-Aids Braille Timer
Maxi Aids
42 Executive Blvd
Farmingdale, NY 11735-4710   631-752-0521
                                     800-522-6294
                          FAX: 631-752-0689
                          TTY: 800-281-3555
                          www.maxiaids.com

Elliot Zaretsky, Founder / President
Three raised dots at 15, 30 and 45, two raised dots at remaining
five minute intervals and one raised dot at remaining two and a
half minute intervals, offers ease of operation to make this a helpful aid for the visually impaired. *$12.95*

365   Nosey Cup
Therapro, Inc.
225 Arlington St
Framingham, MA 01702-8723

508-872-9494
800-257-5376
FAX: 508-875-2062
info@therapro.com
www.therapro.com

Karen Conrad, ScD, OTR/L, Owner
For those with a stiff neck or persons who can't tip their head back while drinking. *$6.00*

366   Paring Boards
Therapro, Inc.
225 Arlington St
Framingham, MA 01702-8723

508-872-9494
800-257-5376
FAX: 508-875-2062
info@therapro.com
www.therapro.com

Karen Conrad, ScD, OTR/L, Owner
Suction feet stabilize board and stainless steel prongs hold food in place for easy, one-handed cutting. *$32.50*

367   PowerLink 2 Control Unit
AbleNet
2625 Patton Road
Roseville, MN 55113-1308

612-379-0956
800-322-0956
FAX: 651-294-2259
customerservice@ablenetinc.com
www.ablenetinc.com

Bill Sproull, Chairman of the Board
Jennifer Thalhuber, President/CEO
William Mills, Board of Director
The PowerLink 2 Control Unit allows switch operation of electrical appliances. It can be used to activate 1 or 2 appliances (up to 1700 watts combined). If 2 appliances are used, they will activate simultaneously. There are four modes of control on the PowerLink 2; direct mode, timed (seconds) mode, timed (minutes) mode and latch mode. Meets safety standards from Underwriters Laboratory (UL) and Canadian Standards Association (CSA) for electrical appliances. *$159.00*

368   Sammons Preston Rolyan
28100 Torch Parkway
Suite 700
Warrenville, IL 60555-3938

630-378-6000
800-323-5547
FAX: 630-393-7600
sp@pattersonmedical.com
www.pattersonmedical.com

David P Sproat, President
Bruce Curtis, Sales Representative
Sammons Preston Rolyan is a leading provider of rehabilitation and assistive devices to help those with disabilities meet daily physical challenges and achieve their greatest level of independence. With one of the industry's largest catalogs, Sammons Preston Rolyan offers a wide range of products available.
Annually

369   Slicing Aid
Snug Seat
12801 E. Independence Blvd.
P.O. Box 1739
Matthews, NC 28106-1739

704-882-0666
800-336-7684
FAX: 704-882-0751
information@snugseat.com
www.snugseat.com

Scott Crosswhite, Vice President
Kirk Mackenzie, President
Greg Tilley, Controller
Angela Stegall, Purchasing
The design of these knives allows a better working posture and makes optimal use of strength in the arms and hands.

370   Small Appliance Receiver
AbleNet
2625 Patton Road
Roseville, MN 55113-1308

612-379-0956
800-322-0956
FAX: 651-294-2259
customerservice@ablenetinc.com
www.ablenetinc.com

Bill Sproull, Chairman of the Board
Jennifer Thalhuber, President/CEO
William Mills, Board of Director
The Small Appliance Receiver, in conjunction with the Cordless Big Red Switch, allows you to control small electrical appliances in the environment without a cord. It should only be used with low-wattage appliances (under 500 watts) which have two prong plugs (i.e., radios, fans, lamps, blenders, etc.). It should not be used with heat generating appliances. *$32.00*

371   Steel Food Guard
Maxi Aids
42 Executive Blvd
Farmingdale, NY 11735-4710

631-752-0521
800-522-6294
FAX: 631-752-0689
TTY: 800-281-3555
www.maxiaids.com

Elliot Zaretsky, Founder / President
Provides stable area to push against while eating. *$ 10.95*

372   Thick-n-Easy
Therapro, Inc.
225 Arlington St
Framingham, MA 01702-8723

508-872-9494
800-257-5376
FAX: 508-875-2062
info@therapro.com
www.therapro.com

Karen Conrad, ScD, OTR/L, Owner
Instant food thickener that sets in 30 seconds and will not become thicker even after refrigeration. *$6.50*

373   Thumbs Up Cup
Therapro, Inc.
225 Arlington St
Framingham, MA 01702-8723

508-872-9494
800-257-5376
FAX: 508-875-2062
info@therapro.com
www.therapro.com

Karen Conrad, ScD, OTR/L, Owner
This cup is designed for those with limited strength or coordination or arthritis. The two backward-tilt handles and thumb rests allow finger joints to be used to their greatest mechanical advantage. *$9.50*

374   Undercounter Lid Opener
Sammons Preston Rolyan
28100 Torch Parkway
Suite 700
Warrenville, IL 60555-3938

630-378-6000
800-323-5547
FAX: 630-393-7600
sp@pattersonmedical.com
www.pattersonmedical.com

David P Sproat, President
Bruce Curtis, Sales Representative
The gripper of this unit which installs under the counter can help unscrew any cap. *$5.75*

375 Uni-Turner
Sammons Preston Rolyan
28100 Torch Parkway
Suite 700
Warrenville, IL 60555-3938
630-378-6000
800-323-5547
FAX: 630-393-7600
sp@pattersonmedical.com
www.pattersonmedical.com

David P Sproat, President
Bruce Curtis, Sales Representative
Odd shaped handles can be turned easily with one-handed, L-shaped Uni-Turner. *$16.50*

376 Universal Hand Cuff
Therapro, Inc.
225 Arlington St
Framingham, MA 01702-8723
508-872-9494
800-257-5376
FAX: 508-875-2062
info@therapro.com
www.therapro.com

Karen Conrad, ScD, OTR/L, Owner
Comfortable cuff with Velcro strap holds utensils, toothbrushes, etc. *$9.95*

Lifts, Ramps & Elevators

377 Accessibility Lift
Inclinator Company of America
601 Gibson Blvd
Harrisburg, PA 17104-3215
717-939-8420
800-343-9007
FAX: 717-939-8075
isales@inclinator.com
www.inclinator.com

Stephen Nock, President
An economical lift for restricted usage that provides barrier-free access that can be used by churches, schools, lodging halls and meeting halls to meet compliance requirements, with the dignified convenience and freedom they deserve.

378 Adjustable Incline Board
Bailey Manufacturing Company
P.O. Box 130
Lodi, OH 44254-130
800-321-8372
FAX: 800-224-5390
baileymfg@baileymfg.com
www.baileymfg.com

379 AlumiRamp
855 E Chicago Rd
Quincy, MI 49082-9450
800-800-3864
FAX: 517-639-4314
sales@alumiramp.com
www.alumiramp.com

Doug Cannon, General Manager
Complete line of modular, aluminum and portable ramps for both home and vehicle use. Welded construction and non-skid extruded surfaces are featured on all our ramps.

380 Area Access
7131 Gateway Court
Manassas, VA 20109-1015
703-396-4949
800-333-2732
FAX: 703-207-0446
www.areaaccess.com

381 Basement Motorhome Lift By Handicaps, Inc.
4335 S Santa Fe Dr
Englewood, CO 80110
303-781-2062
800-782-4335
FAX: 303-761-6811
info@handicapsinc.com
www.handicapsinc.com

382 Braun Corporation, The
631 West 11th Street
Winamac, IN 46996-310
574-946-6153
800-843-5438
FAX: 574-946-4670
mediaquestions@braunlift.com
www.braunability.com

Nick Gutwein, President
Greg Cook, Vice President Sales & Marketing
Joe Garnett, Director Of Marketing
Ralph Braun, Founder/ CEO
The Braun Corporation is the world's largest manufacturer of wheelchair-accessible vans, ramps and wheelchair lifts. Our products enable people with physical disabilities to regain their mobility and to lead active and independent lives. Our companies broad product line includes the Chrysler/Dodge Entervan, the Honda Odyssey Entervan, and the Toyota Sienna Rampvan.

383 Bruno Independent Living Aids
P.O.Box 84
1780 Executive Drive
Oconomowoc, WI 53066
262-567-4990
800-882-8183
FAX: 262-953-5510
www.bruno.com

Michael R. Bruno, II, President/CEO
Andrew Bayer, Product Mgr, Automotive Div.
Mike Krawczyk, Mktg Svcs Mgr
An ISO 9001 Certified Manufacturer of automotive lifts for scooter, wheelchairs, and power chairs, three and four wheel scooters, and straight and custom curve stairlifts.

384 Butlers Wheelchair Lifts
Flinchbaugh Company
629 Lowther Road #C
Lewisberry, PA 17339
717-938-4253
888-847-0804
FAX: 717-938-4238
hal@butlermobility.com
www.butlermobility.com

Hal Feinstein, VP Sales / Marketing
This wheelchair lift can be equipped with an end ramp and guard. Automatically retractable, it locks firmly into place when the lift is in operation.

385 Classique
Handi-Lift
730 Garden St
Carlstadt, NJ 07072-1625
201-933-0111
800-432-5438
FAX: 201-933-0050
sales@handi-lift.com
www.handi-lift.com

Douglas Boydston, President
The Classique elevator answers access problems in churches, schools and small offices.

386 Columbus McKinnon Corporation
140 John James Audubon Pkwy
Amherst, NY 14228-1197
716-689-5400
800-888-0985
FAX: 716-689-5644
www.cmworks.com

Timothy T. Tevens, President/CEO
Gregory P. Rustowicz, VP/CFO
Charles R. Giesige, VP, Corporate Dev.
Richard A. Steinberg, VP, Human Resources
Supplies various lift and transfer systems for independent or attended applications including ceiling mounted or freestanding overhead track lifts and mobile floorbase units for homes,

schools and healthcare facilities. Lift Systems for transferring between bed, chair, commode or bath are available with a variety of slings, scales and accessories.

387   Curb-Sider
Bruno Independent Living Aids
PO Box 84
1780 Executive Drive
Oconomowoc, WI 53066

262-567-4990
800-882-8183
FAX: 262-953-5501
www.bruno.com

Michael R. Bruno, II, President/CEO
Andrew Bayer, Product Mgr, Automotive Div.
Mike Krawczyk, Mktg Svcs Mgr
The lift of choice for storing your fully or partially assembled scooter or power chair weighing up to 400 pounds in the rear of your van or minivan, SUV, pickup truck or some station wagon applications.

388   Curb-Sider Super XL
P.O.Box 84
1780 Executive Drive
Oconomowoc, WI 53066

262-567-4990
800-882-8183
FAX: 262-953-5510
www.bruno.com

Michael R. Bruno, II, President/CEO
Andrew Bayer, Product Mgr, Automotive Div.
Mike Krawczyk, Mktg Svcs Mgr

389   Custom Lift Residential Elevators
Waupaca Elevator Company
1726 N Ballard Rd
Appleton, WI 54911-2444

920-991-9082
800-238-8739
FAX: 920-991-9087
info@waupacaelevator.com
waupacaelevator.com

Bill Mc Michael, Owner
Waupaca Elevator residential elevators and dumbwaiters add value, convenience and reliability to today's homes.

390   Deluxe Convertible Exercise Staircase
Sammons Preston Rolyan
28100 Torch Parkway
Suite 700
Warrenville, IL 60555-3938

630-378-6000
800-323-5547
FAX: 630-393-7600
sp@pattersonmedical.com
www.pattersonmedical.com

David P Sproat, President
Bruce Curtis, Sales Representative
Here's an exercise staircase to fit any department configuration. Just reposition a few nuts and bolts to change from a straight to a corner type staircase.

391   E-Z Access Van Ramp
Maxi Aids
42 Executive Blvd
Farmingdale, NY 11735-4710

631-752-0521
800-522-6294
FAX: 631-752-0689
TTY: 800-281-3555
www.maxiaids.com

Elliot Zaretsky, Founder / President
Telescopic ramps for manual and electric wheel chairs. Bridges gaps over steps and curbs and makes vans more accessible. Extends 7'ft. in length, locking securely in place with snap-button catches. Easy to store. Holds up to 600lbs. *$299.95*

392   Easy Pivot Transfer Machine
Rand-Scot
401 Linden Center Dr
Fort Collins, CO 80524-2429

970-484-7967
800-467-7967
FAX: 970-484-3800
info@randscot.com
www.randscot.com

Joel Lerich, President
The Easy Pivot Patient Lifting System allows for strain-free, one-caregiver transfers of the disabled individual.

393   Easy Stand
Altimate Medical
262 W. 1st St.
Morton, MN 56270-180

507-697-6393
800-342-8968
FAX: 507-697-6900
info@easystand.com
www.easystand.com

Andrew Gardeen, International Sales Manager
Designed to make standing fast and simple. The easy to operate, hydraulic lift system provides a controlled lifting and lowering. With the convenience of simply transferring to the chair and reaching a standing position in seconds with no straps to struggle with.

394   Economical Liberty
Handi-Lift
730 Garden St
Carlstadt, NJ 07072-1625

201-933-0111
800-432-5438
FAX: 201-933-0050
sales@handi-lift.com
www.handi-lift.com

Douglas Boydston, President
Installs quickly and easily on most straight stairways. It uses regular household current and mounts over the carpet or directly to the stairs without marring.

395   Electra-Ride
Bruno Independent Living Aids
PO Box 84
1780 Executive Drive
Oconomowoc, WI 53066

262-567-4990
800-882-8183
FAX: 262-953-5501
www.bruno.com

Michael R. Bruno, II, President/CEO
Andrew Bayer, Product Mgr, Automotive Div.
Mike Krawczyk, Mktg Svcs Mgr
Bruno stairlifts can fit almost any custom curve or straight rail application and require no structural modification to the stairway. Plus, battery power allows for uninterrupted operation even during a power outage.

396   Electra-Ride Elite
Bruno Independent Living Aids
P.O.Box 84
1780 Executive Drive
Oconomowoc, WI 53066

262-567-4990
800-882-8183
FAX: 262-953-5510
www.bruno.com

Michael R. Bruno, II, President/CEO
Andrew Bayer, Product Mgr, Automotive Div.
Mike Krawczyk, Mktg Svcs Mgr
The new Electra-Ride Elite installs to within 5 inches of the wall and has a 350 pound weight capacity. Bruno stairlifts can fit almost any custom curve or straight rail application and require no structural modification to the stairway. Plus, battery power allows for uninterrupted operation even during a power outage.

397 Electra-Ride III
P.O.Box 84
1780 Executive Drive
Oconomowoc, WI 53066   262-567-4990
                             800-882-8183
                        FAX: 262-953-5510
                           www.bruno.com

Michael R. Bruno, II, President/CEO
Andrew Bayer, Product Mgr, Automotive Div.
Mike Krawczyk, Mktg Svcs Mgr

398 Freedom Wheels
580 Tc Jester Blvd
Houston, TX 77007   713-864-1460
                             888-422-5337
                        FAX: 713-864-1469
                     info@freedomwheels.com
                      www.freedomwheels.com

Carlos Saez, Owner
An assistive technology and mobility equipment provider and is committed to people with disabilities and personal transportation options for an independent lifestyle.

399 Handi Home Lift
Handi-Lift
730 Garden St
Carlstadt, NJ 07072-1625   201-933-0111
                             800-432-5438
                        FAX: 201-933-0050
                        sales@handi-lift.com
                         www.handi-lift.com

Douglas Boydston, President
An outdoor lift designed to provide access over porch stairs or other steps that impede movement.

400 Handi Lift
730 Garden St
Carlstadt, NJ 07072-1625   201-933-0111
                             800-432-5438
                        FAX: 201-933-0050
                        sales@handi-lift.com
                         www.handi-lift.com

Douglas Boydston, President
Accessibility with Dignity. We create solutions that enable people with mobility impairments to live freely with products like wheelchair lifts and home elevators.

401 Handi Prolift
Handi-Lift
730 Garden St
Carlstadt, NJ 07072-1625   201-933-0111
                             800-432-5438
                        FAX: 201-933-0050
                        sales@handi-lift.com
                         www.handi-lift.com

Douglas Boydston, President
Provides dependable vertical transportation for multi-level buildings.

402 Handi-Ramp
Handi-Ramp
510 North Ave
Libertyville, IL 60048-2025 847-680-7700
                             800-876-7267
                        FAX: 847-816-7689
                         info@handiramp.com
                          www.handiramp.com

Thomas Disch, President/ CEO
Alicia C. Johns, Program Manager
Provides a complete line of economical, ADA Compliant access ramping products. Line includes van attachable and wheelchair tie downs; aluminum or expanded metal folding portables; aluminum channels; portable, sectional ramp systems; semi-permanent ramps, platforms and systems. All ramp series are available in varied lengths and widths in combination with platforms and op-

tional hand railing, single or double bar construction with return ends. Special Order ramps and ramp systems.

403 Homewaiter
Inclinator Company of America
601 Gibson Blvd
Harrisburg, PA 17104-3215   717-939-8420
                             800-343-9007
                        FAX: 717-939-8075
                       isales@inclinator.com
                         www.inclinator.com

Stephen Nock, President
With its roller truck riding in a specially formed monorail, it is easy to install and highly adaptable to existing conditions. It can travel up to 35 feet, opening on any or all three sides at different stations, whether at counter level or floor level.

404 Horcher Lifting Systems
324 Cypress Rd
Ocala, FL 34472-3102   352-687-8020
                             800-582-8732
                        FAX: 866-378-3318
                      us-office@horcher.com
                          www.horcher.com

David Schultz, General Manager
Sharon Harbert, Administrative Assistant
Barrier Free Lifts by Horcher leads the industry for excellence in patient transfers and technology for over 18 years. They offer state of the art ceiling track systems, floor base lifts and bathing systems such as the Unilift, PC-2, Diana, Lexa, and Raisa to achieve greater mobility.

405 Inclinette
Inclinator Company of America
601 Gibson Blvd
Harrisburg, PA 17104-3215   717-939-8420
                             800-343-9007
                        FAX: 717-939-8075
                       isales@inclinator.com
                         www.inclinator.com

Stephen Nock, President
Inclinette provides comfort and convenience in providing multi-floor access to persons who have difficulty climbing stairs.

406 Independent Driving Systems
580 T.C. Jester
Houston, TX 77007   713-864-1460
                             888-422-5337
                        FAX: 713-864-1469
              info@independentdrivingssystems.com
               www.independentdrivingsystems.com

Chad Donnelly, Owner
Provides adaptive driving systems for individuals with disabilities with more severe higher levels of injury that require more sophisticated types of assistive technology to enable them to drive safely.

407 Joey Interior Platform Lift
Bruno Independent Living Aids
PO Box 84
1780 Executive Drive
Oconomowoc, WI 53066   262-567-4990
                             800-882-8183
                        FAX: 262-953-5501
                           www.bruno.com

Michael R. Bruno, II, President/CEO
Andrew Bayer, Product Mgr, Automotive Div.
Mike Krawczyk, Mktg Svcs Mgr
Lifts and stores your unoccupied scooter or powerchair in the back of your minivan at the touch of a button.

408 Lectra-Lift
La-Z-Boy
1284 N Telegraph Rd
Monroe, MI 48162-5138

734-242-1444
800-375-6890
FAX: 734-457-2005
www.lazboy.com

Kurt L Darrow, CEO
David M Risley, SVP/CFO
Patrick H Norton, Chairman
Kurt Darrow, CEO
This power recliner has a single motor drive that operates three distinct cycles: lifting, leg elevation and full power recline.

409 Liberty LT
Handi-Lift
730 Garden St
Carlstadt, NJ 07072-1625

201-933-0111
800-432-5438
FAX: 201-933-0050
sales@handi-lift.com
www.handi-lift.com

Douglas Boydston, President
Stair lift with dual armrests that lock into position. The comfortable, contoured seat is designed to swivel and move forward at the bottom or top landings to facilitate transfer.

410 Lift-All
Amigo Mobility International
6693 Dixie Highway
Bridgeport, MI 48722-9725

989-777-0910
800-692-6446
800-248-9131
FAX: 800-334-7274
info@myamigo.com
www.myamigo.com

Al Thieme, Chairman and Founder
Beth Thieme, CEO
Tim Drumhiller, President
Sandy Humpert, Sales Rep
Leading manufacturer of electric mobility; Amigo's Lift-All transports your wheelchair easily into the trunk of an automobile and neatly stores it for easy access. Also available is the Lift-It. $965.00

411 Lifts for Swimming Pools and Spas
Aquatic Access
1921 Production Dr
Louisville, KY 40299-2110

502-425-5817
800-325-5438
FAX: 502-425-9607
info@AquaticAccess.com
www.aquaticaccess.com

Linda Nolan, President
David Nolan, Vice President
Aquatic Access manufacturers and sells water-powered lifts providing access to in-ground and above-ground swimming pools, spas, boats and docks. $2310.00

412 Mac's Lift Gate
2801 South Street
Long Beach, CA 90805-3751

562-634-5962
800-795-6227
FAX: 562-529-3466
sales@macsliftgate.com
www.macsliftgate.com

Randy Maner, Training Mgr
Sales and service of van and truck lifts. Sales and service of wheel chair lifts for vans and automobiles. Sales, installation and service of vertical home lifts, scooter lifts and pool lifts. Sales of scooters.

413 Mecalift Sling Lifter
Arjo Inc
2349 West Lake Street
Addison, IL 60101

630-785-4490
800-323-1245
FAX: 888-389-2756
usa.info@ArjoHuntleigh.com
www.arjo.com

Philip M. Croxford, President/ CEO

414 Motorhome Lift By Handicaps, Inc.
4335 S Santa Fe Dr
Englewood, CO 80110

303-781-2062
800-782-4335
FAX: 303-761-6811
info@handicapsinc.com
www.handicapsinc.com

415 One for All Lift All
6693 Dixie Highway
Bridgeport, MI 48722-9725

989-777-0910
800-692-6446
800-248-9131
FAX: 800-334-7274
info@myamigo.com
www.myamigo.com

Al Thieme, Chairman and Founder
Beth Thieme, CEO
Tim Drumhiller, President
Amigo Mobility designs and manufactures a complete line of power operated vehicles/mobility scooters and accessories in Bridgeport, Mich.

416 Out-Sider III
P.O.Box 84
1780 Executive Drive
Oconomowoc, WI 53066

262-567-4990
800-882-8183
FAX: 262-953-5510
www.bruno.com

Michael R. Bruno, II, President/CEO
Andrew Bayer, Product Mgr, Automotive Div.
Mike Krawczyk, Mktg Svcs Mgr

417 Out-Sider Meridian
Bruno Independent Living Aids
P.O. Box 84
1780 Executive Drive
Oconomowoc, WI 53066

262-567-4990
800-882-8183
FAX: 262-953-5501
www.bruno.com

Michael R. Bruno, II, President/CEO
Andrew Bayer, Product Mgr, Automotive Div.
Mike Krawczyk, Mktg Svcs Mgr
Lets you carry your scooter fully assembled and keeps your trunk space available for other things.

418 Parker Bath
Arjo Inc
2349 West Lake Street
Addison, IL 60101

630-785-4490
800-323-1245
FAX: 888-389-2756
usa.info@ArjoHuntleigh.com
www.arjo.com

Philip M. Croxford, President/ CEO
Ross Scavuzzo, President
This involves no manual lifting, strain or stress for the caregiver.

419   Patient Lifting & Injury Prevention
Arjo Inc
2349 West Lake Street
Addison, IL 60101   630-785-4490
                                            800-323-1245
                                       FAX: 888-389-2756
                              usa.info@ArjoHuntleigh.com
                                            www.arjo.com

Philip M. Croxford, President/ CEO
Aids in patient lifting while protecting the caregiver from the risk
of backstrain.

420   Ramplette Telescoping Ramp
Graham-Field Health Products
2935 Northeast Pkwy
Atlanta, GA 30360-2808   678-291-3207
                                            800-347-5678
                                       FAX: 770-368-4702
                                      cs@grahamfield.com
                                      www.grahamfield.com

Kenneth Spett, President & Chief Executive Officer
Cherie Antoniazzi, SVP Quality, Regulatory and Risk Management
Ivan Bielik, Senior Vice President, Business Analyst
Marc Bernstein, Senior Vice President, Consumer Sales
A multi-functional, easily moved, economical ramp weighing 25
pounds.

421   Rickshaw Exerciser
Access to Recreation
8 Sandra Ct
Newbury Park, CA 91320-4302   805-498-7535
                                            800-634-4351
                                       FAX: 805-498-8186
                              customerservice@accesstr.com
                                            www.accesstr.com

Don Krebs, President/ Founder
This Exerciser develops the muscle used most by those in wheelchairs. It develops the strength you need to lift yourself for pressure relief, doing transfers and pushing your wheelchair.

422   Ricon Corporation
1135 Aviation Place
San Fernando, CA 91340-6090   818-267-3000
                                            800-322-2884
                                       FAX: 818-962-1201
                                      sales@riconcorp.com
                                            www.riconcorp.com

John Condon, National Sales Manager
Mike O'Neill, Eastern Saler Manager
Peter Buckley, Central Area Sales Manager
Ricon corporation is a world leader in the manufacture of lifts and
other mobility products for people with disabilities. The Ricon
product line features the Activan (R) a lowered floor minivan
conversion, wheelchair lifts power seat base and automatic door
openers.

423   Smart Leg
Invacare Corporation
1 Invacare Way
Elyria, OH 44035-4190   440-329-6000
                                            800-333-6900
                                       FAX: 877-619-7996
                                      info@invacare.com
                                            www.invacare.com

A Malachi Mixon Iii, Chairman of the Board
Gerald B. Blouch, President and Chief Executive Officer
Joseph B. Richey, II, President - Invacare Technologies Division
*Robert K. Gudbranson, Senior Vice President and Chief Financial
Officer*
An ingenious elevating leg rest that automatically extends to cor-
rectly fit every outstretched leg.

424   Smooth Mover
Dixie EMS
10101 Foster Ave
Brooklyn, NY 11236-3425   718-257-6400
                                            800-347-3494
                                       FAX: 718-257-6401
                              customerservice@dixieems.com
                                            www.dixieems.com

Eva Silverstein, President
Patient mover is a board designed to transfer patients from bed to
stretcher or table with one or two people. *$199.95*

425   SpectraLift
Inclinator Company of America
601 Gibson Blvd
Harrisburg, PA 17104-3215   717-939-8420
                                            800-343-9007
                                       FAX: 717-939-8075
                                      isales@inclinator.com
                                            www.inclinator.com

Stephen Nock, President
A newly designed hydraulic wheelchair lift made of fiberglass
construction suitable for commercial and residential use.

426   Spectrum Aquatics
7100 Spectrum Ln
Missoula, MT 59808-8416   406-543-6823
                                            800-791-8056
                                       FAX: 800-791-8057
                              nkhaled@spectrumproducts.com
                                            www.spectrumproducts.com

Nabil Khaled, Director of Sales
Rob Nelson, Manager of Logistics and Customer Service
Philip Frandsen, Customer Service Representative
Josh Hartley, Business Development Specialist (Southeast Region)

427   Spectrum Products Catalog
Spectrum Products
982 County Route 1
Pine Island, NY 10969-1205   406-542-9781
                                            800-724-5305
                                       FAX: 800-791-8057
                              info@spectrumproducts.com
                                            www.spectrumproducts.com

Nabil Khaled, Dir. of Sales
Chris Rhyne, Business Dev. Specialist
Rob Nelson, Mgr of Logistics
Manufacturers of swimming pool disabled access products such
as lifts, ramps, railings, ladders, and stainless steel hydrotherapy
tanks for the swimming pool and medical therapy markets.

428   StairLIFT SC & SL
Inclinator Company of America
601 Gibson Blvd
Harrisburg, PA 17104-3215   717-939-8420
                                            800-343-9007
                                       FAX: 717-939-8075
                                      isales@inclinator.com
                                            www.inclinator.com

Stephen Nock, President
Simple, self-contained and efficient stair units.

429   Stairway Elevators
Bruno Independent Living Aids
P.O. Box 84
1780 Executive Drive
Oconomowoc, WI 53066   262-567-4990
                                            800-882-8183
                                       FAX: 262-953-5510
                                            www.bruno.com

Michael R. Bruno, II, President/CEO
Andrew Bayer, Product Mgr, Automotive Div.
Mike Krawczyk, Mktg Svcs Mgr
Bruno offers a full line of stairway elevators, including the
Electra-Ride II featuring access during power interruptions, con-
venient installation, comfort and a powerful drive system. The

Electra-Ride which features battery-powered technology, a rail width of 25 inches and seat rotation for easy transfers. The Comfort-Ride AC stair lift which is battery operated, has a rail width of 7.25 inches and folded width of less than 14.5 inches.

430 Straight and Custom Curved Stairlifts
Bruno Independent Living Aids
P.O.Box 84
1780 Executive Drive
Oconomowoc, WI 53066

262-567-4990
800-882-8183
FAX: 262-953-5501
www.bruno.com

Michael R. Bruno, II, President/CEO
Andrew Bayer, Product Mgr, Automotive Div.
Mike Krawczyk, Mktg Svcs Mgr
Bruno stairlifts can fit almost any curve or straight rail application and requires little or no structural modification to the stairway. Normal rail position for a Bruno inside turn is 7 to 8 inches from the wall or obstruction which is the tightest radius of any stairlift manufacturing company in the world. The Bruno inside turn is ideal for bi-level homes or staircases with mid-level doors. Bruno's unique battery power allows for uninterrupted operation even during a power outage.

431 Superarm Lift for Vans By Handicaps, Inc.
4335 S Santa Fe Dr
Englewood, CO 80110

303-781-2062
800-782-4335
FAX: 303-761-6811
info@handicapsinc.com
www.handicapsinc.com

432 SureHands Lift & Care Systems
982 County Route 1
Pine Island, NY 10969-1205

845-258-6500
800-724-5305
FAX: 845-258-6634
info@surehands.com
www.surehands.com

Thomas F Herceg, President
Joyce Moraczewski, Marketing Coordinator
SureHands specializes in lift & care systems for both homecare and professional settings where the user's safety is most important. Offering a variety of lift and transfer options, SureHands provides the necessary tools to overcome physical and architectural barriers to deliver a system designed to meet the specific needs of the user.

433 Thyssen Krupp Access
4001 E 138th St
Grandview, MO 64030-2837

816-200-1954
800-829-9760
FAX: 816-763-4467
dealerinfo@tkaccess.com
www.tkaccess.com

Jurrien van Akker, CEO
Scott Zoetewey, Vice President of Operations
Thomas Hance, President
Whether you want to open your facility or stay in the home you love, Thyssen Krupp Access has the perfect wheelchair lift, stair lift or elevator to suit your budget and needs. Our lifts have the best warranties. Our nationwide network of dealers are close by and ready to help.

434 Turning Automotive Seating (TAS)
Bruno Independent Living Aids
P.O.Box 84
Oconomowoc, WI 53066-84

262-567-4990
800-882-8183
FAX: 262- 95- 550
info@bruno.com
www.bruno.com

Michael R. Bruno, II, President/CEO
Cindy Schmidt, Customer Relations
Steve Nelson, Service Manager
Thomas Jacobson, Senior Vice President

Transfer in and out of a car, minivan, pickup truck and full size van without any lifting!

435 Vangater, Vangater II, Mini-Vangater
631 West 11th Street
Winamac, IN 46996-310

800-THE-LIFT
FAX: 574-946-4670
mediaquestions@braunlift.com
www.braunability.com

Ralph Braun, Founder
Tri-fold and fold-in-half lifts represent a major innovation in the field of adapted van transportation.

436 Versatrainer
Pro- Max/ Division Of Bow- Flex Of America
2200 NE 65th Ave
Vancouver, WA 98661-6978

800-618-8853
800-952-7205
FAX: 360-993-3610
customerservice@bowflex.com
www.bowflex.com

437 Vestibular Board
Bailey Manufacturing Company
P.O. Box 130
Lodi, OH 44254-130

800-321-8372
FAX: 800-224-5390
baileymfg@baileymfg.com
www.baileymfg.com

438 Wheelchair Carrier
7325 Douglas Road
Lambertville, MI 48144-2624

734-568-6084
800-541-3213
FAX: 734-568-6705
admin@WheelChairCarrier.com
wheelchaircarrier.com

David Makulinsky, President
Mike Siler, Engineer
Christina Makulinski, Office Manager
Wheelchair, scooter and powerchair carriers for hitch mount on vehicles, priced from $199 to $999.

Major Catalogs

439 Access Store Products for Barrier Free Environments
Access Store.Com
820 W 7th St
Chico, CA 95928-5011

530-893-1596
800-497-2003
FAX: 530-893-1560
sales@accessstore.com
www.accessstore.com

Tim Vander Heiden, Owner
Lisa Bantum, Sales Administrator
One of the largest online ADA Compliance Catalogs available. Offers everything from innovative barrier removal products to survey equipment, to unique specialty products.

440 Access to Recreation
8 Sandra Ct
Newbury Park, CA 91320-4302

805-498-7535
800-634-4351
FAX: 805-498-8186
customerservice@accesstr.com
www.accesstr.com

Don Krebs, President
The Access to Recreation catalog is full of recreation and exercise equipment. One can find items such as electric fishing reels and other fishing and hunting equipment for the disabled sportsman. There are also adapted golf clubs, swimming pool lifts, wheelchair gloves and cuffs and bowling equipment. There are devices to help with embroidery, knitting and card playing, vid-

eos, books and practical aides such as wheelchair ramps and book.

64 pages Bi-Annually

441 Achievement Products
P.O. Box 6013
Carol Stream, IL 60197-6013

800-373-4699
FAX: 800-766-4303
Bids@achievement-products.com
www.specialkidszone.com

Teresa Cardon, VP
Offer a wide range of pediatric rehabilitation equipment and special education products including handwriting aids, weighted vests, positioning equipment, sensory integration products and adaptive furniture. Call for your free catalog.

442 Adaptive Clothing: Adults
Special Clothes
P.O. Box 333
E Harwich, MA 02645-333

508-430-2410
FAX: 508-430-2410
TTY:508-430-2410
SPECIALCLO@aol.com
www.special-clothes.com

Judith Sweeney, President
Special Clothes produces a catalogue of garments for adults with disabilities and/or incontinence. Offerings include: undergarments, snap-crotch tee shirts, sleepwear, jumpsuits, bibs and some footwear. The catalogue is available without charge. Comparable to department store prices. Special Clothes produces a catalog of adaptive clothing for children in sizes from toddler through young adults. A full line of clothing is included from undergarments through wheelchair jackets and ponchos.

443 Adaptive Technology Catalog
Synapse Adaptive
14 Lynn Ct
San Rafael, CA 94901-5114

415-455-9700
800-317-9611
FAX: 415-455-9801
info@synapse-ada.com
www.synapseadaptive.com

Martin Tibor, President
Adaptive technology for individuals with disabilities, ADA compliant workstations, and ergonomic furniture. Products accommodate blindness, low vision, mobility impairments or learning differences.

444 Adult Long Jumpsuit with Feet
Special Clothes
P.O. Box 333
E Harwich, MA 02645-333

508-896-7939
FAX: 508-896-7939
specialclo@aol.com
www.special-clothes.com

Judith Sweeney, President
Line of clothing for people with disabilities. Child and adult catalog available.

445 Adult Short Jumpsuit
Special Clothes
P.O. Box 333
E Harwich, MA 02645-333

508-896-7939
FAX: 508-896-7939
specialclo@aol.com
www.special-clothes.com

Judith Sweeney, President
This pull-on jumpsuit provides comfort and full coverage without bulk. Wide leg ribbing ends at mid-thigh, with snaps at the crotch. We use fine quality, comfortable cotton knit. 100% cotton knit. Made in USA. Option: long sleeves - add $3.00. Colors: white, navy, teal, light blue, light pink, red, burgundy, royal blue and black. Sm & Med: $36.50/3 for $104.00; L & XL: $39.00/3 for $111.25; and XXL: $42.00/3 for $119.25.

446 AliMed
297 High St
Dedham, MA 02026

781-329-2900
800-225-2610
FAX: 781-329-8392
customerservice@alimed.com
alimed.com

447 American Discount Medical
459 Main St
Ste 101-417
Trussville, AL 35173

205-467-6995
800-877-9100
FAX: 888-809-3029
Sales@AmericanDiscountMed.com
www.americandiscountmed.com

Tom Ruf, General Manager
Offers deep discounts for all major brands of medical products.

448 Apria Healthcare
26220 Enterprise Ct
Lake Forest, CA 92630-8405

949-639-2000
800-277-4288
contact_us@apria.com
www.apria.com

Dan Starck, Chief Executive Officer
Nichola Denney, Executive Vice President, Revenue Management
Lisa M. Getson, EVP, Government Relations, Investor Relations and Compliance
Bill Guidetti, Executive Vice President, East Zone
Lifts, chairs, bathroom aids, bedroom aids, eating utensils and independent living aids for the physically challenged.

449 Armstrong Medical
575 Knightsbridge Parkway
P.O. Box 700
Lincolnshire, IL 60069-700

847-913-0101
800-323-4220
FAX: 847-913-0138
csr@armstrongmedical.com
www.armstrongmedical.com

Armstrong, CEO
Diane Joseph, customer representative
Training aids, anatomical models, medical equipment, pediatrics equipment and rehabilitation equipment.

450 Assistive Technology Journal
1700 N Moore St
Suite 1905
Rosslyn, VA 22209-1905

703-243-1975
FAX: 703-524-6630
info@technologistsinc.com
www.technologistsinc.com

Bi-Annually

451 Assistive Technology Sourcebook
Special Needs Project
Ste H
324 State St
Santa Barbara, CA 93101-2364

805-962-8087
818-718-9900
FAX: 818-349-2027
editor@specialneeds.com
www.specialneeds.com

Hod Gray, Owner
Marian Hall, Editor
Provides you with 18 chapters of practical information on all aspects of assistive technology for individuals with functional limitations. *$60.00*
576 pages

452   Bailey
Bailey Manufacturing
P.O.Box 130
Lodi, OH 44254-130

800-321-8372
FAX: 800-224-5390
baileymfg@baileymfg.com
www.baileymfg.com

70 pages

453   Best 25 Catalog Resources for Making Life Easier
Meeting Life's Challenges
9042 Aspen Grove Ln
Madison, WI 53717-2700

608-824-0402
FAX: 608-824-0403
help@meetinglifeschallenges.com
www.meetinglifeschallenges.com

Shelley Peterman Schwarz, President
Deborah , Dir. of Mktg & Dev.
Unique reference guide to locate thousands of useful and hard-to-find adaptive devices to make dressing, eating, cooking, grooming, communicating, playing, exercising, etc. easier, safer and less frustrating for people of all ages and disabilities. A comprehensive, up-do-date reference for people with disabilities, caregivers and healthcare professionals. *$8.95*
36 pages
ISBN 1-891854-03-8

454   Body Suits
Special Clothes
P.O.Box 333
E Harwich, MA 02645-333

508-430-2410
FAX: 508-430-2410
specialclo@aol.com
www.special-clothes.com

Judith Bari, President
Bodysuits, Jumpsuits, back opening garments, incontinence wear, bibs. Features include snap crotches and g-tube pockets.

455   Cambridge Career Products Catalog
Cambridge Educational
132 West 31st Street
17th Floor
New York, NY 10001

800-322-8755
800-468-4227
FAX: 609-679-0266
custserv@films.com
www.cambridge.films.com/

Lisa Schmuclei, Marketing Director
A full color catalog featuring hundreds of products designed to aid people in career exploration, selecting specific occupations and obtaining these jobs through resume and interview preparation.
64 pages BiAnnual

456   Carex Health Brands
P.O. Box 2526
Sioux Falls, SD 57101-2526

800-328-2935
FAX: 888-616-4297
customerservice@carex.com
carex.com

457   Carolyn's Low Vision Products
3938 S Tamiami Trl
Sarasota, FL 34231-3622

941-373-9100
800-648-2266
FAX: 941-739-5503
info@carolynscatalog.com
www.carolynscatalog.com

John Colton, Owner
Free mail-order catalog of items for visually impaired people. We also have a retail store.

458   Communication Aids for Children and Adults
Crestwood Communication Aids
6589 N
Crestwood Drive
Milwaukee, WI 53209

414-351-0311
FAX: 414-351-0311
crestcomm@aol.com
www.communicationaids.com

Ruth B Leff, President
A free catalog of communication aids for children and adults with disabilities. Over 300 light and high tech switches and aids, and a large selection of adapted and voice-activated toys. Talking Pictures and Passports communication boards, easy to use and moderately priced talking aids.
32 pages Yearly

459   Danmar Products
221 Jackson Industrial Drive
Ann Arbor, MI 48103-9104

734-761-1990
800-783-1998
FAX: 734-761-8977
sales@danmarproducts.com
www.danmarproducts.com

Dan Russo, President
Karen Green, Sales
Hidie Bowman, Sales
Manufactures adaptive equipment for persons with physical and mental disabilities, from seating and positioning equipment, flotation devices, toileting aids to hard and soft shell helmets.

460   Dayspring Associates
2111 Foley Rd
Havre De Grace, MD 21078-1703

410-939-5900
FAX: 410-939-6252

Benedict Schwartz, Manager
This publisher provides a directory of 1,000 rehabilitation aids.

461   Disabilities Sourcebook
Omnigraphics
155 West Congress
Suite 200
Detroit, MI 48226

313-961-1340
800-234-1340
FAX: 313-961-1383
contact@omnigraphics.com
www.omnigraphics.com

Paul Rogers, Publicity Associate
Georgiann Fratoni, Customer Service Manager
Peter Ruffner
$78.00
616 pages
ISBN 0-780803-89-2

462   Disability Bookshop Catalog
P.O.Box 129
Vancouver, WA 98666-129

360-694-2462
800-637-2256
FAX: 360-696-3210
twinpeak@pacifier.com
www.disabilitybookshop.virtualave.net/

40 pages

463   Dressing Tips and Clothing Resources for Making Life Easier
Attainment Company
504 Commerce Parkway
P.O.Box 930160
Verona, WI 53593-160

608-845-7880
800-327-4269
FAX: 608-845-8040
info@attainmentcompany.com
www.attainmentcompany.com

Don Bastian, Founder and CEO
Scott Meister, Director of Software Development
Sue Lockard, Director of Operations/Dealer Sales
Karen Riley, Shipping/Receiving Manager

Learn hundreds of simple tips and techniques to make dressing easier. Learn how to adapt/modify ready-to-wear garments to accommodate your special dressing needs. Find out how to locate more than 100 resources offering specially designed or easy-on/easy-off clothing for men, women, children and/or wheelchair users. You'll find everything you need to look your best. An invaluable resource for people with special dressing needs, people with disabilities, caregivers and healthcare professionals. *$19.00*
144 pages 2000
ISBN 1-578611-19-9

464   Enrichments Catalog
Sammons Preston Rolyan
28100 Torch Parkway
Suite 700
Warrenville, IL 60555-3938
630-378-6000
800-323-5547
FAX: 630-393-7600
sp@pattersonmedical.com
www.pattersonmedical.com

David P Sproat, President
Bruce Curtis, Sales Representative
Provides people with physical challenges with the products they need to help live their lives to the fullest. Includes items for everyday tasks and personal care; assistive products for home use; toileting and bathing aids; grooming and dressing devices; kitchen and dining aids. Also items for range of motion, mobility and exercise such as weights, therapy putty and exercise equipment; ergonomic gloves and supports; canes, crutches, walkers and wheelchair accessories. 36-page catalog.

465   Equipment Shop
34 Hartford Street
Bedford, MA 01730-33
781-275-7681
800-525-7681
FAX: 781-275-4094
info@equipmentshop.com
www.equipmentshop.com

Ken Larson, Owner
Barbara Johnston, General Manager
Specializing in oral motor therapy equipment including flexi cut cups, maroon spoons, chewy tubes, ARK grabbers and z-vibes. Also tricycle foot peal attachments and trike back supports as well as fat wheels.

466   Essential Medical Supply, Inc.
6420 Hazeltine National Dr
Orlando, FL 32822
407-770-0710
800-826-8423
FAX: 407-770-0624
essentialmedicalsupply.com

467   Everest & Jennings
Division of Graham-Field
2935 Northeast Parkway
Atlanta, GA 30360
678-291-3207
800-347-5678
FAX: 770-368-2386
cs@grahamfield.com
www.grahamfield.com

Kenneth Spett, President & Chief Executive Officer
Cherie Antoniazzi, SVP Quality, Regulatory and Risk Management
Ivan Bielik, Senior Vice President, Business Analyst
Marc Bernstein, Senior Vice President, Consumer Sales
Manufactures more than 200 items for persons with physical disabilities, including wheelchairs, seat cushions, shower chairs, grab bars and more.

468   Express Medical Supply
218 Seebold Spur
Fenton, MO 63026
636-349-8448
800-633-2139
FAX: 800-633-9188
sales@exmed.net
www.exmed.net

Bill Nahm, President

Offers a full line of medical and ostomy supplies at discounted prices. Order by phone or online.

469   FlagHouse Rehab Resources
601 FLAGHOUSE DRIVE
Hasbrouck Heights, NJ 07604-3116
201-288-7600
800-793-7900
FAX: 800-793-7922
www.flaghouse.com

George Carmel, President

470   FlagHouse Special Populations
601 FLAGHOUSE DRIVE
Hasbrouck Heights, NJ 07604-3116
201-288-7600
800-793-7900
FAX: 800-793-7922
sales@flaghouse.com
www.flaghouse.com

Brigid de Lime, Sr Brand Manager
Diana Hohman, Brand Manager
Contains over 2,000 products of interest to therapy professionals.
Bi-Annually

471   Freedom Rider
Freedom Rider
5225 Tudor Ct
Naples, FL 34112
603-540-0933
888-253-8811
FAX: 866-522-4708
info@freedomrider.com
www.freedomrider.com

Victoria Surr, President
A catalog of equipment for people with disabilities who ride and drive horses which includes instructional aids, vaulting equipment, and lots of hard to find items.

472   HAC Hearing Aid Centers of America: HARC Mercantile
Hearing Center
1111 W Centre Ave
Portage, MI 49024
269-324-0301
800-445-9968
888-426-6632
FAX: 269-324-2387
info@harc.com
www.hacofamerica.com

473   Health and Rehabilitation Products
Luminaud
8688 Tyler Blvd
Mentor, OH 44060
440-255-9082
800-255-3408
FAX: 440-255-2250
info@luminaud.com
www.luminaud.com

Thomas M Lennox, President
Dorothy Lennox, VP
Switches for limited capability, stoma and trach covers, shower protectors and thermo-stim oral motor stimulator. Personal voice amplifiers for people with weak voices. Artificial larynges for people with no voices. Small electronic communication boards. Books for laryngectomies and speech pathologists.

474   HealthCare Solutions
Blue Chip II
3478 Hauck Rd
Cincinnati, OH 45241
513-271-5115
800-417-5115
FAX: 513-527-3686

Michael Leabhart, Manager
Quality rehabilitation equipment sales and rental. Available equipment includes manual and powered mobility, positioning/seating equipment, vehicle modification, environmental controls, augmentative and alternative communication devices, adaptive computer access, ambulance aids and aids for daily living. Equipment provision is carried out through a total team approach. .

475 Hear You Are
98 Us Highway 46
Budd Lake, NJ 07828-1818
973-347-7662
FAX: 973-691-0611

Dorinne S Davis, President
A large catalog of various assistive and communication devices for people who are hearing impaired. *$3.00*
42 pages

476 Hig's Manufacturing
8375 Sunset Rd Ne
Minneapolis, MN 55418-3238
763-795-9478
FAX: 612-788-1926

Jim Murphy, Owner
Factory direct, lightweight aluminum, portable, 2 & 4-way folding, telescoping tracks, threshold, van, scooter and approach ramps.

477 Huntleigh Healthcare
2349, W Lake Street
Suite 250
Addison, IL 60101
630-785-4490
800-323-1245
FAX: 888-389-2756
us.info@ArjoHuntleigh.com
www.huntleigh-healthcare.com

478 Invacare Corporation
1 Invacare Way
Elyria, OH 44035-4190
800-333-6900
FAX: 877-619-7996
info@invacare.com
invacare.com

Matthew E. Monaghan, Chair, President & CEO
Dean Childers, Senior Vice President & General Manager, North America
The global leader in the manufacture and distribution of innovative home and long-term care medical products that promote recovery and active lifestyles.

479 Kleinert's
433 Newton St
Elba, AL 36323
800-498-7051
FAX: 305-937-0825
customercare@kleinerts.com
www.kleinerts.com

Michael Brier, President
Offers a complete line of sweat and odor protection products, incontinence products, and skin care products consisting of disposable and reusable panties for women and pants for men. Also disposable liners, diapers and underpads.

480 LS&S
145 River Rock Drive
Buffalo, NY 14207
716-348-3500
800-468-4789
FAX: 877-498-1482
TTY: 800-317-8533
www.LSSproducts.com

Melissa Balbach, President
John K Bace, Executive Vice President.
Specializes in products for the blind, visually impaired, hearing impaired, and deaf. Free catalog upon request.

481 Lighthouse Low Vision Products
Lighthouse International
111 E 59th St
New York, NY 10022-1202
212-821-9200
800-829-0500
FAX: 212-821-9707
info@lighthouse.org
www.lighthouse.org

Mark Ackermann, Chief Executive Officer
Joseph A Ripp, Chairman
Sarah Smith, Treasurer

This organization provides health care services related to vision loss; Career and academic services for people with vision loss; Music instruction and pre K curriculum for visually impaired students.

482 Luminaud
8688 Tyler Blvd
Mentor, OH 44060-4348
440-255-9082
800-255-3408
FAX: 440-255-2250
info@luminaud.com
www.luminaud.com

Thomas M Lennox, President
Dorothy Lennox, VP
Offers a line of artificial larynx, personal voice amplifiers, special switches, stoma covers and other communication, health and safety items.

483 MOMS Catalog
9385 Dielman Ind Dr
Saint Louis, MO 63132-2214
800-269-4663
FAX: 314-997-0047
custcare@hdis.com
www.hdis.com

Bruce Grench, President
MOMS catalog features high quality, incontinence supplies, mobility products, bath safety products urological products, aids for daily living products, ostomy supplies and many other adaptive items. MOMS offers low prices, excellent customer service and convenient home delivery to your doorstep.
52 pages

484 Maddak Inc.
661 Route 23 S
Wayne, NJ 07470
973-628-7600
800-443-4926
FAX: 973-305-0841
custservice@maddak.com
maddak.com

485 Maxi Aids
42 Executive Blvd
Farmingdale, NY 11735-4710
631-752-0521
800-522-6294
FAX: 631-752-0689
TTY: 800-281-3555
sales@maxiaids.com
www.maxiaids.com

Elliot Zaretsky, Founder/ President
Products specially designed for the blind, low vision, visually impaired, deaf, deaf-blind, hard of hearing, arthritic, diabetic and individuals with special needs.

486 New Vision Store
919 Walnut Street
Philadelphia, PA 19107
215-627-0600
FAX: 215-922-0692
asbinfo@asb.org
www.asb.org

Patricia C. Johnson, President & Chief Executive Officer
Derby Ewing, Director, Human Services
Brian Rusk, Public Relations Officer
Richard Forsythe, Director, Braille Division and Custom Audio
Catalog for individuals with visual impairments, listing visual aids, magnifiers, large print books and more.
30 pages

487 Patterson Medical
28100 Torch Parkway
Ste 700
Warrenville, IL 60555-3938
630-393-6000
800-323-5547
FAX: 630-393-7600
sp@pattersonmedical.com
pattersonmedical.com

488   Pearson Performance Solutions
1 North Dearborn
Suite 1150
Chicago, IL 60602

800-922-7343
FAX: 312-242-4403
HCM.info@vangent.com
hcrm.gdit.com

David Fabianski, Senior VP and General Mgr
Cindy Hotsky, finance Dir.
Julia McClung, VP, Talent Management Solutions
Publishes human resource assessment instruments for employment settings. The instruments include job analysis procedures to identify important characteristics for job success and objective assessment procedures to evaluate applicants and employees on these characteristics.

489   Pearson Reid London House
1 North Dearborn Street
Chicago, IL 60602-4335

FAX: 312-242-4403
HCM.info@vangent.com
www.pearsonreidlondonhouse.com/index.htm
David Fabianski, Senior VP and General Mgr
Cindy Hotsky, finance Dir.
Julia McClung, VP, Talent Management Solutions

490   Potomac Technology
1500 Olympic Boulevard
Santa Monica, CA 90404

310-656-4924
800-233-9130
FAX: 310-450-9918
TTY: 800-233-9130
www.weitbrecht.com/

24 pages

491   Prentke Romich Company Product Catalog
1022 Heyl Rd
Wooster, OH 44691-9786

330-262-1984
800-262-1984
FAX: 330-263-4829
info@prentrom.com
www.prentrom.com

David L Moffatt, President
Dave Moffatt, President/ COO
Barry Romich, Co-Founder
A full line, product catalog containing information on speech-output communication devices, environmental controls and computer access products.

492   Products for People with Disabilities
LS&S
145 River Rock Drive
Buffalo, NY 14207

716-348-3500
800-468-4789
FAX: 877-498-1482
TTY: 866-317-8533
info@LSSproducts.com
www.LSSproducts.com

John K Bace, Executive Vice President
LS&S, LLC has a free catalog of products for the blind, deaf, visually and hearing impaired including: TTYs, computer adaptive devices, CCTVs, talking blood pressure, blood glucose and talking scales.

493   Rehabilitation Engineering and Assistive Technology Society of North America (RESNA)
1700 North Moore Street
Suite 1540
Arlington, VA 22209- 1903

703-524-6686
FAX: 703-524-6630
TTY:703-524-6639
membership@resna.org
www.resna.org

Alex Mihailidis, PhD, P.Eng, President
Ray Grott, ATP, RET, President-Elect
Paul J. Schwartz, Treasurer
Jamie Arasz Prioli, ATP, Secretary
RESNA improves the potential of people with disabilities to achieve their goals through the use of technology. RESNA promotes research, development, education, advocacy and provision of technology; and by supporting the people engaged in these activities.

494   Sammons Preston Enrichments Catalog
Sammons Preston Rolyan
28100 Torch Parkway
Suite 700
Warrenville, IL 60555-3938

630-378-6000
800-323-5547
FAX: 630-393-7600
sp@pattersonmedical.com
www.pattersonmedical.com

David P Sproat, President
Bruce Curtis, Sales Representative
Our Enrichments Catalog offers products that make the tasks and challenges of living at home— bathing, getting dressed, getting around— a little easier. Choose from personal care items to kitchen and dining aids, household helpers to mobility devices, plus a complete selection of pain-reducing products, exercise items, health monitoring equipment and more.
40 pages Yearly

495   Sportaid
78 Bay Creek Rd
Loganville, GA 30052

770-554-5033
800-743-7203
FAX: 770-554-5944
stuff@sportaid.com
www.sportaid.com

Stacy Green, Owner
jimmy green, Owner
Offers an assortment of wheelchairs (everyday and racing), wheelchair sports equipment, replacement tires, hubs, spokes, pushrims, cushions and more. Call for free catalog.
68 pages Yearly

496   Store @ HDSC Product Catalog
Hearing, Speech & Deafness Center (HDSC)
1625 19th Ave
Seattle, WA 98122-2848

206-323-5770
888-222-5036
800-761-2821
FAX: 206-328-6871
TTY:206-452-7953
seattle@hsdc.org
www.hsdc.org

Pamela Anderson, President
Ken Block, Vice President
Dan Bridge, Interim Executive Director
Deanna Aberle, Director of Speech

32 pages Yearly

497   Ultratec
450 Science Dr
Madison, WI 53711-1166
608-238-5400
800-482-2424
FAX: 608-238-3008
TTY: 800-482-2424
service@ultratec.com
www.ultratec.com

Jackie Morgan, Marketing Director
Robert M Engelke, CEO
Works to make telephone access more convenient and reliable for people with hearing loss.
Yearly

498   WCI/Weitbrecht Communications
1500 Olympic Boulevard
Santa Monica, CA 90405
310-656-4924
800-233-9130
FAX: 310-450-9918
TTY: 800-233-9130
www.weitbrecht.com

24 pages

499   Walgreens Home Medical Center
7173 Cermak Rd
Berwyn, IL 60402-2103
708-795-1295
800-323-2828
FAX: 708-795-1308

Stan Kozlowski, Manager
Hospital supplies and home medical equipment with nationwide direct mail delivery. .

500   Walton Way Medical
1225 Walton Way
Augusta, GA 30901-2141
706-722-0276
FAX: 706-722-0279

Michael Bower, President
Offers medical, therapeutic, urological, hygiene and skin care products for disabled persons.

Miscellaneous

501   Access-USA
242 James St
PO Box 160
Clayton, NY 13624-160
800-263-2750
FAX: 800-563-1687
info@access-usa.com
www.access-usa.com

Deborah Haight, PICOE
Access-USA provides one-stop alternate format transcription services for almost any type of document-reports, schedules, menus, monthly statements, brochures, reports, etc. Items may be submitted on computer disk, hard copy or email. Alternate formats include Braille, large print, Braille and print, audio recordings, adapted disks as well as video services-open/closed captioning and video descriptions. Accessible products also include Braille Business Cards and ADA signage.

502   Access-USA: Transcription Services
242 James St
PO Box 160
Clayton, NY 13624-160
800-263-2750
FAX: 800-563-1687
info@access-usa.com
www.access-usa.com

Deborah Haight, PICOE
Access-USA produces Braille business cards as well as offering alternate format services and products to enhance accessibility. Braille, large print, captioning, audio-descriptive forms are available. We help business, government, education, corporations by providing brochures, menus, manuals, books, collateral materials, videos, specialties and promotion items that can be more accessible to more people.

503   BeOK Key Lever
Sammons Preston Rolyan
28100 Torch Parkway
Suite 700
Warrenville, IL 60555-3938
630-378-6000
800-323-5547
FAX: 630-393-7600
sp@pattersonmedical.com
www.pattersonmedical.com

David P Sproat, President
Bruce Curtis, Sales Representative
Handy accessory helps position key to provide maximum leverage enabling the user to work the most stubborn lock. *$11.50*

504   Big Lamp Switch
Maxi Aids
42 Executive Blvd
Farmingdale, NY 11735-4710
631-752-0521
800-522-6294
FAX: 631-752-0689
TTY: 800-281-3555
sales@maxiaids.com
www.maxiaids.com

Elliot Zaretsky, President
This big, three-spoke knob replaces small rotating knobs which are a problem for those with arthritis or other limitations of the fingers. *$6.75*

505   Bookholder: Roberts
Therapro, Inc.
225 Arlington St
Framingham, MA 01702-8723
508-872-9494
800-257-5376
FAX: 508-875-2062
info@therapro.com
www.therapro.com

Karen Conrad , ScD, OTR/L, Owner
Gray plastic, ideal for hand free reading, adjusts to all sizes of books and prevents pages from flipping for the physically challenged. *$27.50*

506   Brandt Industries
4461 Bronx Blvd
Bronx, NY 10470-1496
718-994-0800
800-221-8031
FAX: 718-325-7995
brandtequip@yahoo.com
www.brandtind.com

507   Bus and Taxi Sign
Maxi Aids
42 Executive Blvd
Farmingdale, NY 11735-4710
631-752-0521
800-522-6294
FAX: 631-752-0689
TTY: 800-281-3555
sales@maxiaids.com
www.maxiaids.com

508   Care Electronics
3301 W 151 Court
Broomfield, CO 8002
303-444-2273
888-444-8284
FAX: 303-447-3502
tmoody@careelectronics.com
www.medicalshoponline.com

Tom Moody, President
Care Electronics manufactures safety monitoring systems for caregivers, home-health care, and nursing homes. WanderCARE monitors loved ones who tend to wander away from home. Care Deluxe Occupancy systems monitor patients in bed and in wheelchairs to help prevent falls. WetSENSE provides incontinence monitors.

509   Child Convertible Balance Beam Set
Bailey Manufacturing Company
P.O. Box 130
Lodi, OH 44254-130

800-321-8372
FAX: 800-224-5390
baileymfg@baileymfg.com
www.baileymfg.com

510   Child Variable Balance Beam
Bailey Manufacturing Company
P.O. Box 130
Lodi, OH 44254-130

330-948-1080
800-321-8372
FAX: 330-948-4439
baileymfg@baileymfg.com
www.baileymfg.com

511   Child's Mobility Crawler
Bailey Manufacturing Company
P.O. Box 130
Lodi, OH 44254-130

800-321-8372
FAX: 800-224-5390
baileymfg@baileymfg.com
www.baileymfg.com

512   Choice Switch Latch and Timer
AbleNet
2625 Patton Road
Roseville, MN 55113-1308

651-294-2200
800-322-0956
FAX: 651-294-2259
customerservice@ablenetinc.com
www.ablenetinc.com

Bill Sproull, Chairman of the Board
Jennifer Thalhuber, President/CEO
William Mills, Board of Director
A Choice Switch Latch and Timer allows one user to learn to make choices. It has two switch inputs and can control two devices. Once one device has been activated, the other will not function until the first one is turned off or completes its timed cycle. *$83.00*

513   Cordless Big Red Switch
AbleNet
2625 Patton Road
Roseville, MN 55113-1308

651-294-2200
800-322-0956
FAX: 651-294-2259
customerservice@ablenetinc.com
www.ablenetinc.com

Bill Sproull, Chairman of the Board
Jennifer Thalhuber, President/CEO
William Mills, Board of Director
The Cordless Big Red Switch, when used in conjunction with either the Cordless Receiver or the Small Appliance Receiver, gives you cordless control of toys, games, and appliances in your environment. *$89.00*

514   DEUCE Environmental Control Unit
APT Technology
236a N Main St
Shreve, OH 44676

330-567-2001
888-549-2001
FAX: 330-567-3073
sales@apt-technology.com
www.apt-technology.com

Grace Miller, Office Manager
Allows a severely disabled person to control a variety of useful devices via a dual switch. DEUCE controls phone, 4 AC powered devices such as a radio, 4 switch controlled devices such as a page turner and up to 16 lights and or appliances distributed around the environment. Starts at $1,500. .

515   Dazor Manufacturing Corporation
2079 Congressiona
Saint Louis, MO 63146

314-652-2400
800-345-9103
FAX: 314-652-2069
info@dazor.com
www.dazor.com

Kirk Cressey, Marketing Director
Bob Smith, National Sales Manager
Mark Hogrebe, President
Dazor is a US manufacturer of quality task lighting. Products include fluorescent, incandescent and halogen lighting fixtures. Illuminated magnifiers combine light and magnification to greatly enhance activities such as reading and make hobbies more enjoyable. All lamps come in a variety of mounting options to include desk bases, clamp on, floor stands and wall tracks. $95 - $450.

516   Digi-Flex
Therapro, Inc.
225 Arlington St
Framingham, MA 01702-8723

508-872-9494
800-257-5376
FAX: 508-875-2062
info@therapro.com
www.therapro.com

Karen Conrad , ScD, OTR/L, Owner
This is a unique hand and finger exercise unit. Recommended for use of individuation of fingers, web space and general strengthening of work hands. Available in a variety of resistances. *$ 17.50*

517   Dorma Architectural Hardware
DORMA Drive, Drawer AC
Reamstown, PA 17567-411

717-336-3881
866-401-6063
FAX: 717-336-2106
archdw@dorma-usa.com
www.dorma-usa.com

Larry O'Toole, CEO
Gary Phillips AHC, VP Regional Sales, East
Ken Theaker, VP Regional Sales West
DORMA provides a complete line of door controls, including barrier-free units that comply with the Americans with Disabilities Act. A wide variety of surface applied and concealed closers, low energy operators, exit devices and electronic access control systems are available to address these equipments.

518   Dual Switch Latch and Timer
AbleNet
2625 Patton Road
Roseville, MN 55113-1308

651-294-2200
800-322-0956
FAX: 651-294-2259
customerservice@ablenetinc.com
www.ablenetinc.com

Bill Sproull, Chairman of the Board
Jennifer Thalhuber, President/CEO
William Mills, Board of Director
A Dual Switch Latch and Timer allows two users to activate two devices at a time in the latch. Timed seconds or timed minutes mode of control. *$88.00*

519   Enabling Devices
50 Broadway
Hawthorne, CA 10532

914-747-3070
800-832-8697
FAX: 914-747-3480
customer_support@enablingdevices.com
www.cnablingdevices.com

Elizabeth Bell, Marketing Manager
Karen O'Connor, VP Operations
Steven Kanor, Owner
For more than 25 years, Enabling Devices has been dedicated to providing affordable learning and assistive devices for the physically challenged. Products include augmentative communicators, adapted toys, capability switches, training and sensory devices and activity centers. Call for a free catalog.

520 Foot Inversion Tread
Bailey Manufacturing Company
P.O. Box 130
Lodi, OH 44254-130

800-321-8372
FAX: 800-224-5390
baileymfg@baileymfg.com
www.baileymfg.com

521 Foot Placement Ladder
Bailey Manufacturing Company
P.O. Box 130
Lodi, OH 44254-130

800-321-8372
FAX: 800-224-5390
baileymfg@baileymfg.com
www.baileymfg.com

522 HealthCraft SuperPole Traveller
Maxi Aids
42 Executive Blvd
Farmingdale, NY 11735-4710

631-752-0521
800-522-6294
FAX: 631-752-0689
TTY: 800-281-3555
sales@maxiaids.com
www.maxiaids.com

Elliot Zaretsky, President
Central to the system is a stylish floor-to-ceiling grab bar, which provides a secure structure that can be installed in minutes between a floor and ceiling. Use it beside a bed, bath, toilet or chair. *$193.00*

523 Home Bed Side Helper
Maxi Aids
42 Executive Blvd
Farmingdale, NY 11735-4710

631-752-0521
800-522-6294
FAX: 631-752-0689
TTY: 800-281-3555
sales@maxiaids.com
www.maxiaids.com

Elliot Zaretsky, President
The extra support you need getting in and out of bed is within your grasp with this easy to install Home Bed Side Helper. The rail itself features four easily accessible grasping points for the secure support you need when getting in or out of bed. *$126.75*

524 Hospital Environmental Control System
Prentke Romich Company
1022 Heyl Rd
Wooster, OH 44691-9786

330-262-1984
800-848-8008
800-262-1933
FAX: 330-263-4829
sales@prentrom.com
www.prentrom.com

David L Moffatt, President
Permits the non-ambulatory patient to operate a variety of electrical items in a single room. A large liquid crystal display is mounted in front of the user and they scan through the menu of operations and make a selection using a sip-puff switch. Options include nurse call, standard telephone functions, electric bed control, hospital television operation and electrical appliance on and off. *$3860.00*

525 Knock Light
HARC Mercantile
5413 S. Westnedge Ave.
Suite A
Portage, MI 49002

269-324-0301
800-445-9968
FAX: 269-324-2387
TTY: 269-324-1615
info@harc.com
www.harc.com

526 Leg Elevation Board
Bailey Manufacturing Company
P.O. Box 130
Lodi, OH 44254-130

800-321-8372
FAX: 800-224-5390
baileymfg@baileymfg.com
www.baileymfg.com

527 Leveron
Lindustries
21 Shady Hill Rd
Weston, MA 02193-1407

781-237-8177
877-794-9511
FAX: 651-989-2131
www.trademarkia.com/leveron-73486756.html

Willard H Lind, Owner
Louise T Lind, VP
Leveron is a doorknob lever handle for ease of operation. Leveron converts standard doorknobs to lever action without removing existing hardware. No gripping, twisting or pinching when hands are wet, arthritic or arms are full. Leveron provides convenience. Available in five colors: almond, satin brass, silver metallic, dark bronze and Hi-Glow (glows in the dark) at low cost to comply with ADA access requirements in public and private places. *$16.95*

528 Longreach Reacher
Therapro, Inc.
225 Arlington St
Framingham, MA 01702-8723

508-872-9494
800-257-5376
FAX: 508-875-2062
info@therapro.com
www.therapro.com

Karen Conrad , ScD, OTR/L, Owner
Reacher is useful when reaching, sitting or when standing. *$18.95*

529 Loop Scissors
Therapro, Inc.
225 Arlington St
Framingham, MA 01702-8723

508-872-9494
800-257-5376
FAX: 508-875-2062
info@therapro.com
www.therapro.com

Karen Conrad , ScD, OTR/L, Owner
Pliable, plastic handles that allow for easy and controlled cutting. *$14.25*

530 Pedal-in-Place Exerciser
Thoele Manufacturing
475 County Road 100 N
Montrose, IL 62445-3019

217-924-4553
FAX: 217-924-4553
www.axistive.com/thoele-manufacturing.html

531 Pet Partners
Delta Society National Service Dog Center
875 124th Ave NE
Ste 101
Bellevue, WA 98005-2531

425-679-5550
FAX: 425-379-5539
info@deltasociety.org
www.petpartners.org

Annie Peters Magnant, President & CEO
Mary Margaret Callahan, Senior National Director, Program Development
Evan Wight, National Director, Marketing
Linda Dicus, Executive Assistant
Pet Partners, formerly Delta Society, is a 501(c)(3) non-profit organization that helps people live healthier and happier lives by incorporating therapy, service and companion animals into their lives.

532   Plastic Card Holder
Therapro, Inc.
225 Arlington St
Framingham, MA 01702-8723
508-872-9494
800-257-5376
FAX: 508-875-2062
info@therapro.com
www.therapro.com

Karen Conrad , ScD, OTR/L, Owner
For those with reduced finger control. *$4.00*

533   Power Door
11240 Gemini Ln
Dallas, TX 75229-4710
800-688-1758
FAX: 972-620-9875
info@powerdoor.com
www.powerdoor.com

Jim Goldthwaite, National Sales Manager
Power door, low energy door operators.

534   ProtectaCap, ProtectaCap+PLUS, ProtectaChin Guard and ProtectaHip
Plum Enterprises
P.O. Box 85
Valley Forge, PA 19481-85
610-783-7377
800-321-PLUM
FAX: 610-783-7577
info@PlumEnt.com
www.plument.com

Janice Carrington, CEO
Plum Enterprises award winning, exquisite, ergonomic protective wear keeps you safe from the dangers of falls. ProtectCap+Plus and ProtectHips are engineered for superior shock-absorption and designed for exquisite simplicity and amazing lightweight comfort. The perfect blend of style and function.

535   Quad Commander
Gpk
535 Floyd Smith Dr
El Cajon, CA 92020-1228
619-593-7381
800-468-8679
FAX: 888-755-5603
info@gpk.com
www.gpk.com

536   Rocker Balance Square
Bailey Manufacturing Company
P.O. Box 130
Lodi, OH 44254-130
800-321-8372
FAX: 800-224-5390
baileymfg@baileymfg.com
www.baileymfg.com

537   Scott Sign Systems
7525 Pennsylvania Ave
Suite 101
Sarasota, FL 34243
941-355-5171
800-237-9447
FAX: 941-351-1787
info@scottsigns.com
www.scottsigns.com

Kathy Hannon, VP
Evelyn Brown, Sales
Call for a brochure.

538   Series Adapter
AbleNet
2625 Patton Road
Roseville, MN 55113-1308
651-294-2200
800-322-0956
FAX: 651-294-2259
customerservice@ablenetinc.com
www.ablenetinc.com

Bill Sproull, Chairman of the Board
Jennifer Thalhuber, President/CEO
William Mills, Board of Director
Allows two-switch operation of any battery-operated device or electrical devices. *$13.00*

539   Signaling Wake-Up Devices
HARC Mercantile
5413 S. Westnedge Ave.
Suite A
Portage, MI 49002
269-324-1615
800-445-9968
FAX: 269-324-2387
TTY: 269-324-1615
info@harc.com
www.harc.com

Ron Slager, Owner
Wake up devices. Vibrating alarm clocks, available with flashing lights, louder alarm noises and more. *$29.50*

540   Smoke Detector with Strobe
HARC Mercantile
5413 S. Westnedge Ave.
Suite A
Portage, MI 49002
269-324-1615
800-445-9968
FAX: 269-324-2387
TTY: 269-324-1615
info@harc.com
www.harc.com

Ron Slager, Owner
Most of the smoke alarms are twice as loud, and have a 120+ candela strobe that will wake a person from a sound sleep. Mounting hardware for ceiling or wall. *$165.95*

541   Spinal Network: The Total Wheelchair Resource Book
No Limits Communications & New Mobility
75-20 Astoria Blvd.
East Elmhurst, NY 11370
800-404-2898
888-850-0344
www.newmobility.com

Josie Byzek, Managing Editor
Jean Dobbs, Editorial Director
Tim Gilmer, Editor
Ian Ruder, Senior Editor
Nearly 600 pages of profiles, articles and resources on every topic of interest to wheelchair users. Subjects include health, coping, relationships, sexuality, parenthood, computers, sports, recreation, travel, personal assistance services, legal rights, financial strategies, employment, and media images. *$34.95*
400 pages

542   SteeleVest
Steele
P.O. Box 7304
Kingston, WA 98346-7304
360-297-4555
888-783-3538
FAX: 360-297-2816
www.steelevest.com

Sandra Steele, President
Vest developed by NASA provides an external cooling system.

543   TV & VCR Remote
AbleNet
2625 Patton Road
Roseville, MN 55113-1308

651-294-2200
800-322-0956
FAX: 651-294-2259
customerservice@ablenetinc.com
www.ablenetinc.com

Bill Sproull, Chairman of the Board
Jennifer Thalhuber, President/CEO
William Mills, Board of Director
Controls a TV, a VCR or a TV that is connected through a VCR tuner. It may be programmed to control functions such as on and off, channel up, preprogrammed TV channels and, if desired, other TV functions such as mute and pause. *$82.00*

544   Tactile Thermostat
Sense-Sations
919 Walnut Street
Philadelphia, PA 19107-5237

215-627-0600
FAX: 215-922-0692
asbinfo@asb.org
www.asb.org

Patricia C. Johnson, President & Chief Executive Officer
Derby Ewing, Director, Human Services
Brian Rusk, Public Relations Officer
Richard Forsythe, Director, Braille Division and Custom Audio
Large embossed numbers on cover ring and raised temperature setting knob. *$31.50*

545   Therapy Putty
Therapro, Inc.
225 Arlington St
Framingham, MA 01702-8723

508-872-9494
800-257-5376
FAX: 508-875-2062
info@therapro.com
www.therapro.com

Karen Conrad , ScD, OTR/L, Owner
Designed to exercise and strengthen hands, ranging from soft to firm for developing a stronger grasp. Available in two, four and six ounce sizes. Three ounce putty in unique clear fist shaped container.

546   Uppertone
535 Floyd Smith Dr
El Cajon, CA 92020-1228

619-593-7381
800-468-8679
FAX: 888-755-5603
info@gpk.com
www.gpk.com

547   Visual Alerting Guest Room Kit
HARC Mercantile
5413 S. Westnedge Ave.
Suite A
Portage, MI 49002

269-324-1615
800-445-9968
FAX: 269-324-2387
TTY: 269-324-1615
info@harc.com
www.harc.com

Ron Slager, Owner
ADA compliant visual alerting guest room kit for the hard of hearing and deaf. Includes visual smoke detector, phone alert, door knock sensor, tactile alarm clock and telephone amplifier. Variations include TTY.

548   Window-Ease
A-Solution
5505 Barranca Oso Ct NE
Albuquerque, NM 87111

505-856-6632
FAX: 505-856-6652
info@windowease.com
www.windowease.com

Robert Gorrell, President
Jeff Dodd, Sales

Device adapts horizontally and vertically sliding windows to ANSI A117.1 standards. 10:1 mechanical advantage at the crank arm opens a 50lb window with 5lbs force. Price ranges from $350.00-$450.00.

Office Devices & Workstations

549   Combination File/Reference Carousel
Center for Rehabilitation Technology
Ste 118
490 10th St NW
Atlanta, GA 30318-5754

404-712-5667
800-457-9555
FAX: 404-875-9409
rerc-br@scsn.net

TW Gannaway, Executive VP
Anthony Stringer PhD
Offers two reading platforms and file holders joined on one easily rotated carousel. The carousel is easily rotated by head, mouth or handstick. Page retainer adjusts to hold open a variety of books and magazines. *$299.00*

550   Don Johnston
26799 W Commerce Dr
Volo, IL 60073-9675

847-740-0749
800-999-4660
800-889-5242
FAX: 847-740-7326
info@donjohnston.com
www.donjohnston.com

Don Johnston, President
A provider of quality products and services that enable people with special needs to discover their potential and experience success. Products are developed for the areas of Physical Access, Augmentative Communication and for those who struggle with reading and writing.

551   Extensions for Independence
6100 Center Drive
Suite 1190
Los Angeles, CA 90045

757-416-6575
888-321-4678
FAX: 866-632-7149
support@inmotionhosting.com
www.mouthstick.net

Ted Sakis, Director of Operations
Develops, manufactures and markets special vocational equipment for the physically handicapped. Products: mouthsticks, computer mechanical aids: key locks and diskette loaders. Also, turntable desks, wheelchair portable desks, filing trays with slanted sides, telephone adapters, and motorized artist easel. All these products have been designed to solve the functional limitations of people with little or no use of hands and/or arms.

552   Fairway Spirit Adaptive Golf Car: Model4852
Fairway Golf Cars
Ste 300
3225 Gateway Rd
Brookfield, WI 53045-5139

262-790-9363
888-320-4850
888-320-4850
FAX: 262-790-9396
bob_hansen@fairwaygolfcars.com
www.fairwaygolfcars.com

553   Freedom Ryder Handcycles
Brike International
20589 SW Elk Horn Ct
Tualatin, OR 97062-9518

503-692-1029
800-800-5828
FAX: 970-221-4308
Mike@Freedomryder.com
www.freedomryder.com

Mike Lofgren, Owner
Brian Stewart, VP

The finest handcycle in the world. The cycles incorporate body, lean steering and the finest bicycle components to make this a three-wheeled vehicle without equal. Suitable for both recreation and competition. *$1995.00*

554   Golf Xpress
Emotorsports
4400 West M-61
Standish, MI 48658

989-846-6255
FAX: 989-846-6255
mitch@golfxpress.com
www.golfxpress.com

555   Infogrip: AdjustaCart
1899 E. Main Street
Ventura, CA 93001-3411

805-652-0770
800-397-0921
FAX: 805-652-0880
tech@infogrip.com
www.infogrip.com

556   Infogrip: BAT Personal Keyboard
1899 E. Main Street
Ventura, CA 93001-3411

805-652-0770
800-397-0921
FAX: 805-652-0880
tech@infogrip.com
www.infogrip.com

557   Maxi Marks
Maxi Aids
42 Executive Blvd
Farmingdale, NY 11735-4710

631-752-0521
800-522-6294
FAX: 631-752-0689
TTY: 800-281-3555
sales@maxiaids.com
www.maxiaids.com

Elliot Zaretsky, President
Braille writing and identification products. *$2.50*

558   Pencil/Pen Weighted Holders
Therapro, Inc.
225 Arlington St
Framingham, MA 01702-8723

508-872-9494
800-257-5376
FAX: 508-875-2062
info@therapro.com
www.therapro.com

Karen Conrad , ScD, OTR/L, Owner
Securely hold any pencil or pen. These weighted holders allow for more control along with proprioceptive feedback to encourage better writing skills.

559   Perkins Brailler
Maxi Aids
42 Executive Blvd
Farmingdale, NY 11735-4710

631-752-0521
800-522-6294
FAX: 631-752-0689
TTY: 800-281-3555
sales@maxiaids.com
www.maxiaids.com

Elliot Zaretsky, President
Can emboss 25 lines with 42 cells on an 11 x 11 1/2 sheet. *$495.00*

560   PhoneMax Amplified Telephone
Assistech
2738 N Campbell Ave
Tucson, AZ 85719-3141

520-883-8600
866-674-3549
FAX: 520-883-3172
www.assistivedevices.net

Oliver Simoes, Owner

561   Raised Line Drawing Kit
Maxi Aids
42 Executive Blvd
Farmingdale, NY 11735-4710

631-752-0521
800-522-6294
FAX: 631-752-0689
TTY: 800-281-3555
sales@maxiaids.com
www.maxiaids.com

Elliot Zaretsky, President
For writing script or drawing graphs by the use of special plastic paper. *$24.45*

562   Reizen Braille Labeler
Maxi Aids
42 Executive Blvd
Farmingdale, NY 11735-4710

631-752-0521
800-522-6294
FAX: 631-752-0689
TTY: 800-281-3555
sales@maxiaids.com
www.maxiaids.com

Elliot Zaretsky, President
Label everything in Braille with 3/8 or 1/2 wide labeling tape. *$47.95*

563   Sharp Calculator with Illuminated Numbers
Independent Living Aids
137 Rano Rd
Buffalo, NY 14207

516-937-1848
800-537-2118
855-746-7452
FAX: 516-937-3906
can-do@independentliving.com
www.independentliving.com

Irwin Schneidmill, President
Michael Gutierrez, Director of Operations
Pamela Strauss, Director of Marketing
Ursula Izurieta, Director of Merchandising
A trim desktop calculator with large illuminated numbers that can be carried anywhere. *$34.95*

564   Signature and Address Self-Inking Stamps
Independent Living Aids
137 Rano Rd
Buffalo, NY 14207

516-937-1848
800-537-2118
855-746-7452
FAX: 516-937-3906
can-do@independentliving.com
www.independentliving.com

Irwin Schneidmill, President
Michael Gutierrez, Director of Operations
Pamela Strauss, Director of Marketing
Ursula Izurieta, Director of Merchandising
Gives thousands of impressions before requiring re-inking. *$11.95*

565   Steady Write
Maxi Aids
42 Executive Blvd
Farmingdale, NY 11735-4710

631-752-0521
800-522-6294
FAX: 631-752-0689
TTY: 800-281-3555
sales@maxiaids.com
www.maxiaids.com

Elliot Zaretsky, President
Furnishes the writer with increased holding capacity and stabilizes the hand. *$6.95*

566 **Talking Desktop Calculators**
Maxi Aids
42 Executive Blvd
Farmingdale, NY 11735-4710

631-752-0521
800-522-6294
FAX: 631-752-0689
TTY: 800-281-3555
sales@maxiaids.com
www.maxiaids.com

Elliot Zaretsky, President
Unique voice synthesizers call out numerals and functions as they are keyed in or read out data stored in memory. *$467.95*

567 **Talking Electronic Organizers**
Independent Living Aids
137 Rano Rd
Buffalo, NY 14207

516-937-1848
800-537-2118
855-746-7452
FAX: 516-937-3906
can-do@independentliving.com
www.independentliving.com

Irwin Schneidmill, President
Michael Gutierrez, Director of Operations
Pamela Strauss, Director of Marketing
Ursula Izurieta, Director of Merchandising
Electronic, portable, personal organizers that talk the user through all the functions and are totally voice interactive. $199.95 and up.

568 **Television Remote Controls with Large Numbers**
Independent Living Aids
137 Rano Rd
Buffalo, NY 14207

516-937-1848
800-537-2118
855-746-7452
FAX: 516-937-3906
can-do@independentliving.com
www.independentliving.com

Irwin Schneidmill, President
Michael Gutierrez, Director of Operations
Pamela Strauss, Director of Marketing
Ursula Izurieta, Director of Merchandising
Large 5 1/2 inch x 8 1/2 inch unit that has easy to see and use buttons. Can be used on nearly every TV, VCR and cable boxes. *$39.95*

569 **Wheelchair Activity/Computer Table**
Maxi Aids
42 Executive Blvd
Farmingdale, NY 11735-4710

631-752-0521
800-522-6294
FAX: 631-752-0689
TTY: 800-281-3555
sales@maxiaids.com
www.maxiaids.com

Elliot Zaretsky, President
This powered height-adjustable table is a wheelchair accessible activity table or computer workstation that's as stylish as it is functional. Adjusts with the push of a button from 27-39 inches, powered by an extremely quiet motor. ADA compliant computer workstation for assistive technology and school computer labs.

Scooters

570 **Aerospace Compadre**
Aerospace America
900 Harry Truman Pkwy.
Bay City, MI 48706-4171

989-684-2121
800-237-6414
FAX: 989-684-4486
www.aerospaceamerica.com

Mike Alley, President
Fully customized golf cart type vehicle for the physically impaired person. Fully equipped with hand controls, wheelchair rack, storage racks, head and tail lights and full safety belts. *$2500.00*

571 **Alante**
Golden Technologies
401 Bridge St
Old Forge, PA 18518-2323

800-624-6374
FAX: 800-628-5165
www.goldentech.com

Robert Golden, Chairman
Richard Golden, CEO
Fred Kiwak, President
Rear-wheel-drive vehicle that represents the best in powered mobility.

572 **Amigo Mobility International**
Amigo Mobility International
6693 Dixie Highway
Bridgeport, MI 48722

989-777-0910
800-248-9131
800-692-6446
FAX: 800-334-7274
info@myamigo.com
www.myamigo.com

Al Thieme, Chairman and Founder
Beth Thieme, CEO
Tim Drumhiller, President
An industry leader in power operated vehicles/scooters, Amigo provides innovative, durable, and customized mobility solutions for the disabled, injured, and seniors worldwide. Other services include healthcare, travel and transportation services. *$1295.00*

573 **Amigo Mobility International Inc.**
6693 Dixie Hwy
Bridgeport, MI 48722-9725

989-777-0910
800-692-6446
888-892-2580
FAX: 800-334-7274
info@myamigo.com
myamigo.com

Al Thieme, Chairman & Founder
Beth Thieme, Chief Executive Officer
Amigo Mobility designs and manufactures a complete line of power operated vehicles/mobility scooters and accessories in Bridgeport, Michigan.

574 **Bravo! + Three-Wheel Scooter**
EZ-International
W194 N11301 McCormick Drive
Germantown, WI 53022

262-250-7740
800-824-1068
FAX: 262-250-7741
sales@ek-tech.com
www.ek-tech.com

575 **Cruiser Bus Buggy 4MB**
Convaid Products
2830 California Street
Torrance, CA 90503

310-618-0111
888-266-8243
FAX: 310-618-2166
www.convaid.com

rocio , Inside Sales Manager
In sizes from infant through young adult, this positioning buggy is crash-tested.

576 **Cub, SuperCub and Special Edition Scooters**
1780 Executive Dr
Oconomowoc, WI 53066

262-567-4990
FAX: 262-953-5502
www.bruno.com

Michael R. Bruno, II, President/CEO
Michael R Bruno II, President/CEO
Steve Nelson, Service Manager

577   Electric Mobility Corporation
P.O.Box 156
Sewell, NJ 08080-156   856-468-0083
                                       800-257-7955
                                  FAX: 856-468-3426
                                  www.rascalscooters.com

Linda Autore, CEO
Manufactures Rascal Scooters.

578   Explorer+ 4-Wheel Scooter
EZ-International
W194 N11301 McCormick Drive
Germantown, WI 53022   262-250-7740
                                       800-824-1068
                                  FAX: 262-250-7741
                                  sales@ek-tech.com
                                  www.ek-tech.com/

579   Featherlite
No Boundaries
1 Monster Way
Corona, CA 92879   714-891-5899
                                       800-426-7367
                                  FAX: 714-891-0658
                                  info@hansens.com
                                  www.hansens.com

Hubert Hansen, Founder
Lightweight scooter folds in seconds without tools or bending
down for hassle free travel on airplanes, cruise ships, trains, RVs,
buses and more! Heaviest component weighs 27 pounds. Fits easily in almost any vehicle trunk.

580   Invacare Fulfillment Center
Invacare Corporation
1 Invacare Way
Elyria, OH 44035-4190   440-329-6000
                                       800-333-6900
                                  FAX: 877-619-7996
                                  www.invacare.com

A Malachi Mixon Iii, Chairman of the Board
Gerald B. Blouch, President and Chief Executive Officer
Joseph B. Richey, II, President - Invacare Technologies Division
*Robert K. Gudbranson, Senior Vice President and Chief Financial
Officer*
Invacare Corporation is the world's leading manufacturer and
distributor of non-acute medical products which promote recov-
ery and active lifestyles for people requiring home and other
non-acute health care.

581   Invacare Lynx L-3 Scooter
Maxi Aids
42 Executive Blvd
Farmingdale, NY 11735-4710   631-752-0521
                                       800-522-6294
                                  FAX: 631-752-0689
                                  TTY: 800-281-3555
                                  sales@maxiaids.com
                                  www.maxiaids.com

Elliot Zaretsky, President
The L-3 model conveniently disassembles into four compact
pieces for easy transport. With an estimated seven miles of range,
a plug-in battery charger and flat-free tires, consumers can plan
their schedule around what they want to do, not around the limitations of their scooter. *$795.00*

582   Leisure Lift
Leisure Lift
1800 Merriam Ln
Kansas City, KS 66106-4714   913-722-5658
                                       800-255-0285
                                  FAX: 913-722-2614
                                  Leisure-Lift@Leisure-Lift.com
                                  www.pacesaver.com

Bill Burke, Founder
Leisure Lift offers light three wheel scooter models and seven
power wheelchair models. *$2695.00*

583   MVP+ 3-Wheel Scooter
EZ-International
W194 N11301 McCormick Drive
Germantown, WI 53022   262-250-7740
                                       800-824-1068
                                  FAX: 262-250-7741
                                  sales@ek-tech.com
                                  www.ek-tech.com/contact.php

584   Moxie
No Boundaries
1 Monster Way
Corona, CA 92879   714-891-5899
                                       800-426-7367
                                  FAX: 714-891-0658
                                  info@hansens.com
                                  www.hansens.com

Hubert Hansen, Founder
Disassembles into three parts in less than a minute. Heaviest component weighs 41 pounds. Portable, affordable and downright
snazzy!

585   Outdoor Independence
Palmer Industries
P.O.Box 5707
Endicott, NY 13763-5707   607-754-2957
                                       800-847-1304
                                  FAX: 607-754-1954
                                  palmer@palmerind.com
                                  www.palmerind.com

Jack Palmer, President
The futuristic, one, two and three seater, electric three-wheeler
designed to take you almost anywhere.

586   Pace Saver Plus II
Leisure-Lift
1800 Merriam Ln
Kansas City, KS 66106-4714   913-722-5658
                                       800-255-0285
                                  FAX: 913-722-2614
                                  Leisure-Lift@Leisure-Lift.com
                                  www.pacesaver.com

Bill Burke, Founder
The scooter combines outdoor ruggedness with indoor maneuverability at a low price.

587   Palmer Independence
Palmer Industries
P.O.Box 5707
Endicott, NY 13763-5707   607-754-2957
                                       800-847-1304
                                  FAX: 607-754-1954
                                  palmer@palmerind.com
                                  www.palmerind.com

Jack Palmer, President
Futuristic electric outdoor three wheeler designed to take the
rider almost anywhere.

588   Palmer Twosome
Palmer Industries
P.O.Box 5707
Endicott, NY 13763-5707   607-754-2957
                                       800-847-1304
                                  FAX: 607-754-1954
                                  palmer@palmerind.com
                                  www.palmerind.com

Jack Palmer, President
All electric two seat vehicle for those who can't pedal.

589 Phantom Compact Size Scooter
Maxi Aids
42 Executive Blvd
Farmingdale, NY 11735-4710 631-752-0521
800-522-6294
FAX: 631-752-0689
TTY: 800-281-3555
sales@maxiaids.com
www.maxiaids.com

Elliot Zaretsky, President
Travel in style-ideal/affordable compact scooter. Great for both indoor and outdoor use. Three wheel design allows for small 32.3 turning radius. Top speed 4 miles per hour and a cruising range of 15 miles. Large carry basket.

590 Polaris Trail Blazer
Polaris Industries
2100 Highway 55
Medina, MN 55340-9770 763-542-0500
888-704-5290
FAX: 763-542-0599
www.polarisindustries.com

Scott Wine, Chairman and Chief Executive Officer
Bennett J. Morgan, President and Chief Operating Officer
Michael W. Malone, Vice President - Finance and Chief Financial Officer
Todd-Michael Balan, Vice President - Corporate Development
A four-wheeler that has many engineered innovations, features such as: full floorboards for full comfort, single lever breaking with auxiliary foot brake, electronic throttle control, parking brake and adjustable handlebars.

591 Quickie 2
Sunrise Medical/Quickie Designs
2842 Business Park Avenue
Fresno, CA 93727 800-333-4000
800-300-7502
www.sunrisemedical.com

Pete Coburn, President
Randi Binstock, VP- Business Dev.
Peter Riley, Senior VP - Corporate CFO
Kevin Marshman, North American Controller
This custom, ultralight, folding, everyday scooter offers portability and performance plus modular flexibility.

592 Rascal 3-Wheeler
Electric Mobility Corporation
P.O.Box 156
Sewell, NJ 08080-156 856-468-1000
800-257-7955
FAX: 856-468-3426
www.emobility.com

Scott Patrick, Manager
For primarily outdoor use, this three wheeler provides extra strength, durability and reliability.

593 Rascal ConvertAble
Electric Mobility Corporation
P.O.Box 156
Sewell, NJ 08080-156 856-468-1000
800-257-7955
FAX: 856-468-3426
www.emobility.com

Scott Patrick, Manager
An electric vehicle that's a compact mobile chair one minute and a rugged outdoor scooter the next. Use both indoors and outdoors. Also available with joystick controls.

594 Regal Scooters
Bruno Independent Living Aids
Ste 84
1780 Executive Dr
Oconomowoc, WI 53066-4830 262-567-4990
800-882-8183
FAX: 262-953-5510
webmaster@bruno.com
www.bruno.com

Michael R. Bruno, II, President/CEO
This line includes the Regal Standard, the Regal Large Adult, the Regal Small Adult, the Regal Pediatric, The Regal Ten models 65 and 75, and The Regal Four. These scooters offer adjustable flip-up armrests, pneumatic tires front and rear, and more.

595 Regent
Golden Technologies
401 Bridge St
Old Forge, PA 18518-2323 570-451-7477
800-624-6374
FAX: 800-628-5165
info@goldentech.com
www.goldentech.com

Richard Golden, CEO
Lisa Miller, Senior Customer Service
Top-rated performance scooter, with extra features and economically priced.

596 Roadster 20
ATV Solutions
Unit 4
4700 W 60th Ave
Arvada, CO 80003-6928 303-450-2881
866-777-9727
888-867-1159
FAX: 303-450-2880
sales@atvsolutions.com
www.atvsolutions.com

Andrew Miro, Owner
Great for indoor or outdoor use. The powerful, quiet drive system, independent front suspension and fully reclining high-back seat make for a smooth, quiet ride. The Roadster is loaded with great features at a bargain price.

597 Safari Scooter
Ranger All Seasons Corporation
P.O.Box 132
George, IA 51237-132 712-475-2811
800-225-3811
FAX: 712-475-2810
www.rangerallseason.com

598 Scoota Bug
Golden Technologies
401 Bridge St
Old Forge, PA 18518-2323 570-451-7477
800-624-6324
FAX: 800-628-5165
info@goldentech.com
www.goldentech.com

Richard Golden, CEO
A lightweight, completely modular scooter, that disassembles and fits into most auto trunks.

599 Sierra 3000/4000
EZ-International
W194 N11301 McCormick Drive
Germantown, WI 53022 262-250-7740
800-824-1068
FAX: 262-250-7741
Sales@EK-Tech.com
www.ek-tech.com/

Assistive Devices / Stationery

600 Solo Scooter

Ranger All Seasons Corporation
P.O.Box 132
George, IA 51237-132

712-475-2811
800-225-3811
FAX: 712-475-2810
sales@rangerallseason.com
www.rangerallseason.com

601 SoloRider Industries

Regal Research & Manufacturing Company
1200 East Plano Parkway
Plano, TX 75074

972-422-5324
800-898-3353
FAX: 972-422-8010
info@solorider.com
www.solorider.com

Roger Pretekin, Founder
Manufacturer and distributor of the Solorider Golf Cart. This revolutionary single rider adaptive cart is specifically designed to meet the needs of individuals with mobility impairments.

602 Sportster 10

ATV Solutions
Unit 4
4700 W 60th Ave
Arvada, CO 80003-6928

303-450-2881
866-777-9727
888-867-1159
FAX: 303-450-2880
sales@atvsolutions.com
www.atvsolutions.com

Andrew Miro, Owner
Sportster 10 is our most maneuverable scooter, ideal for riders who must operate in tight spaces. Equipped with all of the great features of the Roadster 20, this three-wheeler is an exceptional buy.

603 Systems 2000

BioMedical Life Systems
P.O.Box 1360
Vista, CA 92085-1360

760-727-5600
800-726-8367
FAX: 760-727-4220
information@bmls.com
www.bmls.com

604 Terra-Jet: Utility Vehicle

TERRA-JET USA
P.O.Box 918
Junction Hwy. 417 & 419
Innis, LA 70747-918

225-492-2249
800-864-5000
FAX: 225-492-2226
Terra-Jet@Terra-Jet.Com
www.terra-jet.com

Larry Rabalais, President, General Manager and CEO
Shawn Oubre, Sales
TERRA-JET utility vehicles are unique in their ability to traverse many different types of terrain in remote areas otherwise inaccessible. It has a multitude of uses for industry, sportsmen or the whole family. Uniquely designed, industrial duty construction of low maintenance and low fuel consumption. $8,675-$21,995.

605 Terrier Tricycle

TRIAID
P.O.Box 1364
Cumberland, MD 21501-1364

301-759-3525
800-306-6777
FAX: 301-759-3525
sales@triaid.com
www.triaid.com

606 Trekker 40

ATV Solutions
Unit 4
4700 W 60th Ave
Arvada, CO 80003-6928

303-450-2881
866-777-9727
888-867-1159
FAX: 303-450-2880
sales@atvsolutions.com
www.atvsolutions.com

Andrew Miro, Owner
Our biggest, toughest scooter. With a huge 450 pound capacity and five inches of ground clearance, this machine is ideal for the daily outdoor user. The high top speed means you get there fast and the four-wheel suspension makes the ride smooth and comfortable.

607 Tri-Lo's

TRIAID
P.O.Box 1364
Cumberland, MD 21501-1364

301-759-3525
800-306-6777
FAX: 301-759-3525
sales@triaid.com
www.triaid.com

608 Triumph 3000/4000

EZ-International
W194 N11301 McCormick Drive
Germantown, WI 53022

262-250-7740
800-824-1068
FAX: 262-250-7741
Sales@EK-Tech.com
www.ek-tech.com/

609 Triumph Scooter

EZ-International
W194 N11301 McCormick Drive
Germantown, WI 53022

262-250-7740
800-824-1068
FAX: 262-250-7741
Sales@EK-Tech.com
www.ek-tech.com/

Stationery

610 Access-USA

242 James St
PO Box 160
Clayton, NY 13624-160

800-263-2750
FAX: 800-563-1687
info@access-usa.com
www.access-usa.com

Deborah Webster, PICOE
Access-USA provides one-stop alternate format transcription services for almost any type of document-reports, schedules, menus, monthly statements, brochures, reports, etc. Items may be submitted on computer disk, hard copy or email. Alternate formats include Braille, large print, Braille and print, audio recordings, adapted disks as well as video services-open/closed captioning and video descriptions. Accessible products also include Braille Business Cards and ADA signage.

611 Address Book

Sense-Sations
919 Walnut Street
Philadelphia, PA 19107-5237

215-627-0600
FAX: 215-922-0692
asbinfo@asb.org
www.asb.org

Patricia C. Johnson, President & Chief Executive Officer
Derby Ewing, Director, Human Services
Brian Rusk, Public Relations Officer
Richard Forsythe, Director, Braille Division and Custom Audio

The big print address book is the first personal book to provide enlarged writing spaces, making it easier to write down and retrieve information. *$12.50*

612   Big Print Address Book
Access with Ease
42 Executive Blvd
Farmingdale, NY 11735-4710   631-752-0521
                                               800-522-6294
                                          FAX: 631-752-0689
                                          TTY: 800-281-3555
                                          sales@maxiaids.com
                                          www.maxiaids.com

Elliott Zaretsky, Founder and President
Rods supported by two rubber blocks facilitate writing. *$16.95*

613   Bold Line Paper
Sense-Sations
919 Walnut Street
Philadelphia, PA 19107-5237   215-627-0600
                                          FAX: 215-922-0692
                                          asbinfo@asb.org
                                          www.asb.org

Patricia C. Johnson, President & Chief Executive Officer
Derby Ewing, Director, Human Services
Brian Rusk, Public Relations Officer
Richard Forsythe, Director, Braille Division and Custom Audio
This pad consists of 100 sheets of paper with bold lines to help guide the writing of an individual with limited vision. *$2.50*

614   Braille Notebook
Maxi Aids
42 Executive Blvd
Farmingdale, NY 11735-4710   631-752-0521
                                               800-522-6294
                                          FAX: 631-752-0689
                                          TTY: 800-281-3555
                                          sales@maxiaids.com
                                          www.maxiaids.com

Elliott Zaretsky, Founder and President
Made of heavy-duty board, covered with waterproof imitation leather and three rings for binding, including Braille paper and titles. *$12.95*

615   Braille: Desk Calendar
Maxi Aids
42 Executive Blvd
Farmingdale, NY 11735-4710   631-752-0521
                                               800-522-6294
                                          FAX: 631-752-0689
                                          TTY: 800-281-3555
                                          sales@maxiaids.com
                                          www.maxiaids.com

Elliott Zaretsky, Founder and President
Schedule appointments, remember birthdays or write messages for a particular day. *$39.95*

616   Braille: Greeting Cards
Sense-Sations
919 Walnut Street
Philadelphia, PA 19107-5237   215-829-9997
                                          FAX: 215-922-0692
                                          asbinfo@asb.org
                                          www.asb.org

Patricia C. Johnson, President & Chief Executive Officer
Derby Ewing, Director, Human Services
Brian Rusk, Public Relations Officer
Richard Forsythe, Director, Braille Division and Custom Audio
Birthday, anniversary, get well, sympathy and Christmas cards offering Braille print for the blind. *$.95*

617   Clip Board Notebook
Sense-Sations
919 Walnut Street
Philadelphia, PA 19107-5237   215-627-0600
                                          FAX: 215-922-0692
                                          asbinfo@asb.org
                                          www.asb.org

Patricia C. Johnson, President & Chief Executive Officer
Derby Ewing, Director, Human Services
Brian Rusk, Public Relations Officer
Richard Forsythe, Director, Braille Division and Custom Audio
Kit includes a pack of Bold Line paper and black ink pen. *$5.95*

618   Deluxe Signature Guide
Maxi Aids
42 Executive Blvd
Farmingdale, NY 11735-4710   631-752-0521
                                               800-522-6294
                                          FAX: 631-752-0689
                                          TTY: 800-281-3555
                                          sales@maxiaids.com
                                          www.maxiaids.com

Elliott Zaretsky, Founder and President
Rods supported by two rubber blocks facilitate writing. *$1.25*

619   Highlighter and Note Tape
Therapro, Inc.
225 Arlington St
Framingham, MA 01702-8723   508-872-9494
                                               800-257-5376
                                          FAX: 508-875-2062
                                          info@therapro.com
                                          www.therapro.com

Karen Conrad, Owner
A great way to highlight and draw attention to words without damaging original. Price ranges from $4.00-$7.00.

620   Letter Writing Guide
Independent Living Aids
137 Rano Rd
Buffalo, NY 14207
                                               800-537-2118
                                               855-746-7452
                                          FAX: 516-937-3906
                                          www.independentliving.com

Irwin Schneidmill, President
Michael Gutierrez, Director of Operations
Pamela Strauss, Director of Marketing
Ursula Izurieta, Director of Merchandising
Sturdy plastic sheet with 13 apertures corresponding to standard line spacing. *$3.49*

621   Lettering Guide Value Pack
Independent Living Aids
137 Rano Rd
Buffalo, NY 14207
                                               800-537-2118
                                               855-746-7452
                                          FAX: 516-937-3906
                                          www.independentliving.com

Irwin Schneidmill, President
Michael Gutierrez, Director of Operations
Pamela Strauss, Director of Marketing
Ursula Izurieta, Director of Merchandising
Included in this useful pack are four durable plastic lettering and number guides for tracing letters when the individual is unable to write letters unassisted. *$6.29*

Visual Aids

622 Aluminum Adjustable Support Canes for the Blind
Maxi Aids
42 Executive Blvd
Farmingdale, NY 11735-4710

631-752-0521
800-522-6294
FAX: 631-752-0689
TTY: 800-281-3555
sales@maxiaids.com
www.maxiaids.com

Elliott Zaretsky, Founder and President
Adjustable canes for the visually impaired. *$17.95*

623 Audio Book Contractors
P.O. Box 96
Riverdale, MD 20738-96

301-439-5830
FAX: 301-439-5830
info@audiobookcontractors.com
www.audiobookcontractors.com

Flo Gibson, President
Over 950 titles of unabridged classic books on audio cassettes in
sturdy vinyl covers with picture and spine windows. Discounted
prices for disabled patrons.

624 Beyond Sight
5650 S Windermere St
Littleton, CO 80120-1240

303-795-6455
FAX: 303-795-6425
jim@beyondsight.com
www.beyondsight.com

Scott Chaplick, Owner & President
Gina Whetzel, Sales & Merchandise Specialist
Products for the blind and visually impaired including talking
clocks, watches and calculators, also carry a large selection of
Braille products, magnifiers, reading machines and computer
equipment.

625 Big Number Pocket Sized Calculator
Independent Living Aids
137 Rano Rd
Buffalo, NY 14207

516-937-1848
800-537-2118
855-746-7452
FAX: 516-937-3906
can-do@independentliving.com
www.independentliving.com

Marvin Sandler, President
A handy pocket size calculator with big numbers that fits easily
into purse or pocket. *$14.95*

626 Braille Compass
Maxi Aids
42 Executive Blvd
Farmingdale, NY 11735-4710

631-752-0521
800-522-6294
FAX: 631-752-0689
TTY: 631-752-0738
sales@maxiaids.com
www.maxiaids.com

Elliott Zaretsky, Founder and President
The visually impaired can tell the direction by using this compass. *$42.95*

627 Braille Plates for Elevator
Maxi Aids
42 Executive Blvd
Farmingdale, NY 11735-4710

631-752-0521
800-522-6294
FAX: 631-752-0689
TTY: 800-281-3555
sales@maxiaids.com
www.maxiaids.com

Elliott Zaretsky, Founder and President
The plates have curing type pressure sensitive material applied
for metal to metal bonding. *$79.95*

628 Braille Touch-Time Watches
Independent Living Aids
137 Rano Rd
Buffalo, NY 14207

516-937-1848
800-537-2118
855-746-7452
FAX: 516-937-3906
can-do@independentliving.com
www.independentliving.com

Marvin Sandler, President
White dial with black numerals and hands makes telling time possible quickly and easily for the visually impaired. *$44.95*

629 Circline Illuminated Magnifier
Dazor Manufacturing Corporation
2079 Congressional Dr.
St. Louis, MO 63146

314-652-2400
800-345-9103
FAX: 314-652-2069
info@dazor.com
www.dazor.com

Mark Hogrebe,Ph.D, Past President
Provides even, shadow free light under the magnifying lens with
a 22-watt circline fluorescent. The magnifier is mounted on a
floating arm that allows you to position the light source and lens
with the touch of a finger.

630 Extra Loud Alarm with Lighter Plug
HARC Mercantile
5413 S. Westnedge Ave.
Suite A
Portage, MI 49002

269-324-1615
800-445-9968
FAX: 269-324-2387
TTY: 269-324-1615
info@harc.com
www.harc.com

Ron Slager, Owner
Battery operated, easy to read, digital clock with extra loud
alarm. *$45.00*

631 Low Vision Telephones
2738 N Campbell Ave
Tucson, AZ 85719-3141

520-883-8600
866-674-3549
FAX: 520-883-3172
info@assistivedevices.net
www.assistivedevices.net

Oliver Simoes, Owner

632 Magni-Cam & Primer
Innoventions
9593 Corsair Dr
Conifer, CO 80433-9317

303-797-6554
800-854-6554
FAX: 303-727-4940
magnicam@magnicam.com
www.magnicam.com

Mark Freeman, President
Magni-Cam and Primer are hand-held, light weight, inexpensive
auto-focus electronic magnification systems designed to meet the
reading and writing needs of those with low vision. The systems
present the image in black and white or in color with three different view modes. Connects to any TV monitor in minutes. Systems
read any surface with no distortion. A battery powered system is
available, providing total portability and flexibility.

633 Magnifier Bookweight
Levenger
420 S Congress Ave
Delray Beach, FL 33445-4693

901-566-5771
800-544-0880
FAX: 561-274-0263
cservice@levenger.com
www.levenger.com

Steve Leveen, CEO

The Magnifier Bookweight features an optical quality magnifier and is long enough to enlarge the full width of most book pages while holing the pages open. This magnifier is encased in embossed leather and enlarges approximately four lines of text at a time to twice the original size.

634   Man's Low-Vision Quartz Watches
Independent Living Aids
137 Rano Rd
Buffalo, NY 14207

516-937-1848
800-537-2118
855-746-7452
FAX: 516-937-3906
can-do@independentliving.com
www.independentliving.com

Marvin Sandler, President
An inexpensive, easy-to-read watch with chrome case. *$27.95*

635   Men's/Women's Low Vision Watches & Clocks
Maxi Aids
42 Executive Blvd
Farmingdale, NY 11735-4710

631-752-0521
800-522-6294
FAX: 631-752-0689
TTY: 800-281-3555
sales@maxiaids.com
www.maxiaids.com

Elliott Zaretsky, Founder and President
Choose from a wide range of watches from Braille automatic to quartz pocket watches.

636   MonoMouse Electronic Magnifiers
Maxi Aids
42 Executive Blvd
Farmingdale, NY 11735-4710

631-752-0521
800-522-6294
FAX: 631-752-0689
TTY: 800-281-3555
sales@maxiaids.com
www.maxiaids.com

Elliott Zaretsky, Founder and President
Simple and affordable magnifier for people with Low Vision. Just about the size of a standard computer mouse. Allows you to read books, newspapers, product labels, etc. on either a computer or TV screen.

637   Rigid Aluminum Cane with Golf Grip
Maxi Aids
42 Executive Blvd
Farmingdale, NY 11735-4710

631-752-0521
800-522-6294
FAX: 631-752-0689
TTY: 800-281-3555
sales@maxiaids.com
www.maxiaids.com

Elliott Zaretsky, Founder and President
A straight, tubular, heavy gauge aluminum rigid cane for blind and visually impaired persons. *$12.95*

638   Stretch-View Wide-View Rectangular Illuminated Magnifier
Dazor Manufacturing Corporation
2079 Congressional Dr.
St. Louis, MO 63146

314-652-2400
800-345-9103
FAX: 314-652-2069
info@dazor.com
www.dazor.com

Mark Hogrebe,Ph.D, Past President
Provides even, shadow free light under the magnifying lens with a 22-watt circline fluorescent. The magnifier is mounted on a floating arm that allows you to position the light source and lens with the touch of a finger.

639   Timex Easy Reader
Independent Living Aids
137 Rano Rd
Buffalo, NY 14207

516-937-1848
800-537-2118
855-746-7452
FAX: 516-937-3906
can-do@independentliving.com
www.independentliving.com

Marvin Sandler, President
An easy-to-read large face watch that's water resistant. *$29.95*

640   Unisex Low Vision Watch
Independent Living Aids
137 Rano Rd
Buffalo, NY 14207

516-937-1848
800-537-2118
855-746-7452
FAX: 516-937-3906
can-do@independentliving.com
www.independentliving.com

Marvin Sandler, President
Unisex watch with large numbers and wide hands. Gold-toned case with either expansion or leather band. *$31.95*

Walking Aids: Canes, Crutches & Walkers

641   Air Lift Oxygen Carriers
Air Lift Unlimited
1212 Kerr Gulch Rd
Evergreen, CO 80439-6397

800-776-6771
888-343-3352
FAX: 303-526-4700
info@airlift.com
www.meridianmedicalusa.com

642   Aluminum Crutches
Arista Surgical Supply Company
297 High Street
Dedham, MA 02026-2852

781-329-2900
800-225-2610
FAX: 781-329-8392
info@alimed.com
www.alimed.com

Julian Cherubini, President
Lightweight aluminum crutches with wood underarms and handgrips. *$25.00*

643   Aluminum Walking Canes
Maxi Aids
42 Executive Blvd
Farmingdale, NY 11735-4710

631-752-0521
800-522-6294
FAX: 631-752-0689
TTY: 800-281-3555
sales@maxiaids.com
www.maxiaids.com

Elliott Zaretsky, Founder and President
Lightweight but strong, these walking canes are made of a heavy gauge aluminum tube with safety locknuts and heavy-duty rubber tips. *$10.75*

644   Compact Folding Travel Rollator
Maxi Aids
42 Executive Blvd
Farmingdale, NY 11735-4710

631-752-0521
800-522-6294
FAX: 631-752-0689
TTY: 631-752-0738
sales@maxiaids.com
www.maxiaids.com

Elliott Zaretsky, Founder and President
Is perfect for someone on the go. Pull strap for quick folding and disassembly. Folds down to half its assembled size in seconds, to

a manageable 26 inch L x 22 inch W x 8 inch D for easy storage. *$149.95*

645   Crutches
Mada Medical Products
625 Washington Ave
Carlstadt, NJ 07072-2901   201-460-0454
                                             800-526-6370
                                        FAX: 201-460-3509
                    dianelind@mail.madamedical.com
                           www.madainternational.com

Jeffrey Adam, President
All aluminum construction, underarm crutch with double pushbutton height adjustment.

646   Dapper Folding Adustable Cane
Maxi Aids
42 Executive Blvd
Farmingdale, NY 11735-4710   631-752-0521
                                             800-522-6294
                                        FAX: 631-752-0689
                                        TTY: 631-752-0738
                                    sales@maxiaids.com
                                        www.maxiaids.com

Elliott Zaretsky, Founder and President
The Dapper walking stick can be folded and unfolded with only one hand and with minimum effort. The durable lanyard attached prevents loss and allows trailing of staff. Features a non-slip handle, non-skid rubber tip and is made of high quality sturdy aluminum. *$ 34.95*

647   Dapper Walking Stick
Maxi Aids
42 Executive Blvd
Farmingdale, NY 11735-4710   631-752-0521
                                             800-522-6294
                                        FAX: 631-752-0689
                                        TTY: 631-752-0738
                                    sales@maxiaids.com
                                        www.maxiaids.com

Elliott Zaretsky, Founder and President
The Dapper walking stick is safe durable and sturdy allowing the user to conveniently store it when not in use. It can be folded and unfolded with only one hand and with minimum effort. The durable lanyard attached prevents loss and allows trailing of staff. Features a non-slip handle, non-skid rubber tip and is made of high quality sturdy aluminum construction. *$34.95*

648   Deluxe Nova Wheeled Walker & Avant Wheeled Walker
Sammons Preston Rolyan
W68n158 Evergreen Blvd
Cedarburg, WI 53012-2637   262-387-8720
                                             800-323-5547
                                        FAX: 800-547-4333
                    CustomerSupport@PattersonMedical.com
                           www.pattersonmedical.com/

Bruce Curtis, Sales Representative
David.P Sproat, President
Lightweight and simple to handle with an easy-to-operate braking system. *$425.40*

649   Deluxe Standard Wood Cane
Arista Surgical Supply Company/AliMed
297 High Street
Dedham, MA 02026-2852   781-329-2900
                                             800-225-2610
                                        FAX: 781-329-8392
                                        info@alimed.com
                                          www.alimed.com

Julian Cherubini, President
A standard old-fashioned wooden cane for the physically challenged. *$10.00*

650   EasyStand 6000 Glider
Access To Recreation
8 Sandra Ct
Newbury Park, CA 91320-4302   800-634-4351
                                        FAX: 805-498-8186
                    customerservice@accesstr.com
                                      www.accesstr.com

Don Krebs, President
Provides dynamic leg motion for individuals who are unable to stand upright or walk on their own.

651   Freedom Three Wheel Walker
Mada Medical Products
625 Washington Ave
Carlstadt, NJ 07072-2901   201-460-0454
                                             800-526-6370
                                        FAX: 201-460-3509
                    dianelind@mail.madamedical.com
                           www.madainternational.com

Jeffrey Adam, President
The freedom walker has ultra light touch, locking loop brakes and sure grip hand grips.

652   Liberty Lightweight Aluminum Stroll Walker
Mada Medical Products
625 Washington Ave
Carlstadt, NJ 07072-2901   201-460-0454
                                             800-526-6370
                                        FAX: 201-460-3509
                    dianelind@mail.madamedical.com
                           www.madainternational.com

Jeffrey Adam, President
The Liberty walker has a spring loaded push down braking system, adjustable handle height with locking system, a 12in wide fully padded seat, and a removable shopping basket.

653   Maxi Superior Cane
Maxi Aids
42 Executive Blvd
Farmingdale, NY 11735-4710   631-752-0521
                                             800-522-6294
                                        FAX: 631-752-0689
                                        TTY: 800-281-3555
                                    sales@maxiaids.com
                                        www.maxiaids.com

Elliott Zaretsky, Founder and President
Convenient folding cane designed for optimum balance. Tapered joints provide rigidity when open, and are made of heavy gauge aluminum. *$17.50*

654   Out-N-About American Walker
742 Market St
Oregon, WI 53575-1059   608-835-9255
                                        FAX: 608-835-5234

Luann Smith, President
The lightweight Out-N-About is easy to handle. The four wheel design provides greater support and stability than any other walking aids. Its large rubber tires move effortlessly over most surfaces, indoors and out. The small turning radius makes it ideal for getting through confined spaces and narrow doorways. The attractive, burgundy colored, tubular steel frame is extremely durable. The Out-N-About folds flat and stands alone for easy storage. Made in USA.

655   Patriot Extra Wide Folding Walkers
Mada Medical Products
625 Washington Ave
Carlstadt, NJ 07072-2901   201-460-0454
                                             800-526-6370
                                        FAX: 201-460-3509
                    dianelind@mail.madamedical.com
                           www.madainternational.com

Jeffrey Adam, President
The extra wide walkers have padded foam hand grips, two-stage push button folding mechanism, dual width adjustment, height adjustment, and nonskid tips.

656   Patriot Folding Walker Series
Mada Medical Products
625 Washington Ave
Carlstadt, NJ 07072-2901
    201-460-0454
    800-526-6370
    FAX: 201-460-3509
    dianelind@mail.madamedical.com
    www.madainternational.com

Jeffrey Adam, President
The patriot walker has high density, padded foam hand grips, high strength 1in lightweight, anodized, dull silver aluminum tube construction, adjustable height with push-button lock security, nonskid tips, and a single button folding mechanism.

657   Patriot Reciprocal Folding Walkers
Mada Medical Products
625 Washington Ave
Carlstadt, NJ 07072-2901
    201-460-0454
    800-526-6370
    FAX: 201-460-3509
    dianelind@mail.madamedical.com
    www.madainternational.com

Jeffrey Adam, President
The reciprocal folding walkers have padded foam hand grips, adjustable height with snap-in security, double front cross brace, and nonskid tips.

658   Prone Support Walker
Consumer Care Products
W282 N7109 Main Street
Merton, WI 53056
    262-820-2300
    info@consumercarellc.com
    www.consumercarellc.com

659   Push-Button Quad Cane
Arista Surgical Supply Company/AliMed
297 High Street
Dedham, MA 02026-2852
    781-329-2900
    800-225-2610
    FAX: 781-329-8392
    info@alimed.com
    www.alimed.com

Julian Cherubini, President
A reliable walking cane offering independence to the physically challenged user. *$25.00*

660   Quad Canes
Mada Medical Products
625 Washington Ave
Carlstadt, NJ 07072-2901
    201-460-0454
    800-526-6370
    FAX: 201-460-3509
    dianelind@mail.madamedical.com
    www.madainternational.com

Jeffrey Adam, President
There are large and small base quad canes with high density foam grips.

661   Rand-Scot
401 Linden Center Dr
Fort Collins, CO 80524-2429
    970-484-7967
    800-467-7967
    FAX: 970-484-3800
    TTY: 800-467-7967
    info@randscot.com
    www.randscot.com

Joel Lerich, President
Barbara Hoehn, President
Manufactures the Easy Pivot patient lift, the BBD wheelchair cushion line and Saratoga Exercise products for the disabled. Offers a line of patient lifts and standers for the disabled. Rand-scot products are designed to help the disabled achieve independence, comfort, and stamina. A video or dvd is available at no charge for potential users. $800-$3,000.

662   Secret Agent Walking Stick
Gold Violin
PO BOX 147
Jessup, PA 18434
    877-648-8466
    FAX: 800-821-1282
    goldviolin.blair.com

Connie Hallquist, CEO
The Secret Agent Walking Stick features a built-in flashlight, a red reflector and a built-in secret pill compartment. this folding aluminum cane is height adjustable and has a derby-style handle and a non-skid rubber tip. A nylon carrying case is included. The walking stick comes in a choice of gold, bronze, or black shaft with a faux burled walnut handle. . It has been taken over by Orchard Brands.

663   StairClimber
Martin Technology
29 N Main St
Gloversville, NY 12078-3006
    518-725-1837
    800-800-1410
    FAX: 518-725-9522

Michael Lewy, Owner
A walker-capable person can climb and descend stairs with this walker-designed StairClimber.

664   Standing Aid Frame with Rear Entry
Consumer Care Products
W282 N7109 Main Street
Merton, WI 53056
    262-820-2300
    FAX: 920-459-9070
    www.consumercarellc.com

665   Stick Canes
Mada Medical Products
625 Washington Ave
Carlstadt, NJ 07072-2901
    201-460-0454
    800-526-6370
    FAX: 201-460-3509
    dianelind@mail.madamedical.com
    www.madainternational.com

Jeffrey Adam, President
Mada's stick canes are adjustable with a locking security system.

666   Torso Support
Grandmar
5635 Peck Rd.
Arcadia, CA 91006-20
    626-443-3143
    800-447-6739
    FAX: 800-767-3933
    info@posey.com
    www.posey.com

Ernest Posey, CEO
Bob Kelleher, Senior Vice President of Supply Chain and Administration
Tracey Bertolina, CFO
Dale Clendon, President
An aid for people who are unable to maintain an upright position in an automobile or a wheelchair.

667   U-Step Walking Stabilizer: Walker
Maxi Aids
42 Executive Blvd
Farmingdale, NY 11735-4710
    631-752-0521
    800-522-6294
    FAX: 631-752-0689
    TTY: 631-752-0738
    sales@maxiaids.com
    www.maxiaids.com

Elliott Zaretsky, Founder and President
If you want to feel as stable as you would while holding onto another person's arm, the U-Step Walking Stabilizer is for you. The innovative braking system is easy to use and puts you in complete control; roll only when you want to. Plus, it easily folds for transport. *$ 539.95*

668 Ventura Enterprises
4431 S. Eastern Avenue
Las Vegas, NV 89119
702-457-7676
FAX: 317-745-3179
info@venturaenterprises.com
www.venturaenterprises.com

Sam Ventura, President, CEO
Ron Ventura, Vice President of Development
Galit Rozen, Vice President of Acquisitions
Ofir Ventura, ESQ., In House General Council
Manufacturer of everyday living mobility aids. Products include carrying aids for walkers and wheelchairs and also wheelchair cushions.

669 WCIB Heavy-Duty Folding Cane
Maxi Aids
42 Executive Blvd
Farmingdale, NY 11735-4710
631-752-0521
800-522-6294
FAX: 631-752-0689
TTY: 800-281-3555
sales@maxiaids.com
www.maxiaids.com

Elliott Zaretsky, Founder and President
A four section aluminum folding cane with a golf-type grip handle and flexible wrist loop. Available in 34-60 lengths. *$17.95*

670 Walker Leg Support
Sammons Preston Rolyan
W68 N158 Evergreen Blvd
Cedarburg, WI 53012-2637
262-387-8720
800-228-3693
FAX: 262-387-8748
CustomerSupport@PattersonMedical.com
www.pattersonmedical.com/

Bruce Curtis, Sales Representative
David.P Sproat, President
For lower extremity trauma. An alternative to crutches that allows safe, stable ambulation and frees hands and arms for daily tasks. *$11.50*

Wheelchairs: Accessories

671 Advantage Wheelchair & Walker Bags
Laurel Designs
TORRANCE, CA 90505
800-556-6307
FAX: 310-316-2561
advantagebag@verizon.net
www.advantagebag.com/

672 Automatic Wheelchair Anti-Rollback Device
Alzheimer's Store
3197 Trout Place Rd
Cumming, GA 30041-8260
678-947-4001
800-752-3238
FAX: 678-947-8411
cs@alzstore.com
www.alzstore.com

Ellen Warner, President
As a wheelchair user transfers to and from the chair, a pair of brake arms grabs the tires to prevent the chair from rolling backwards. Once the individual is seated, the device switches to stand-by mode and the wheelchair returns to standard function.

673 Battery Operated Cushion
DA Schulman
3827 Creekside Lane
Holmen, WI 54636
608-782-0031
866-782-9658
FAX: 608-782-0488
aquila@aquilacorp.com
www.aquilacorp.com

674 Dual-Mode Charger
Lester Electrical
625 West A Street
Lincoln, NE 68522-1794
402-477-8988
FAX: 402-474-1769
sales@lesterelectrical.com
www.lesterelectrical.com

675 Equalizer 1000 Series
Helm Distributing
P.O Box 25105 Deer Park P.O, Rd Dee
Alberta, T4R 2
403-309-5551
FAX: 403-342-5509
james@equalizerexercise.com
www.equalizerexercise.com

676 Equalizer 5000 Home Gym
Helm Distributing
P.O Box 25105
Deer Park P.O.
Red Deer, AB, Canada T4R- 2M2
403-309-5551
FAX: 403-342-5509
info@equalizerexercise.com
www.equalizerexercise.com

677 Featherspring
105 W Lincoln Hwy
DeKalb, IL 60115
800-628-4693
FAX: 800-261-1164
customerservice@luxis.com
www.luxis.com

678 Gem Wheelchair & Scooter Service: Mobility & Homecare
176-39 Union Turnpike
Flushing, NY 11366-1515
718-969-8600
800-943-3578
help@gemwheelchairservice.com
www.gemwheelchairservice.com/

679 Lifestand
Frank Mobility Systems
300 Duke Drive
Lebanon, TN 37090
800-736-0925
FAX: 800-231-3256
techsupport@permobil.com
www.lifestandusa.com

Larry Jackson, President and CEO
Tom Rolick, VP Sales North America
Darin Lowery, VP of Operations
Rick Haynes, Senior HR Manager
Lifestand offers a full line of standing wheelchairs for manual operation. Power assisted are fully motorized. *$7000.00*

680 Mat Factory
6726 North Figueroa Street
Los Angeles, CA 90042
800-628-7626
FAX: 323-254-4545
www.matfactoryinc.com

681 One Thousand FS
Fortress
P.O.Box 489
Clovis, CA 93613-489
559-322-5437
FAX: 559-323-0299

682 Pac-All Wheelchair Carrier
Pac-All Carriers
2321 Carolton Rd
Maitland, FL 32751-3624
407-830-6604
800-628-6672
FAX: 407-339-2847

LE Angel

No more lifting and no more pain wheelchair carrier. VA approved. Made in USA.
$158 - $226.40

683   **Safety Deck II**
Mat Factory
6726 North Figueroa Street
Los Angeles, CA 90042

800-628-7626
FAX: 323-254-4545
www.matfactoryinc.com

684   **Scooter & Wheelchair Battery Fuel Gauges and Motor Speed Controllers**
Curtis Instruments, Inc.
200 Kisco Ave
Mount Kisco, NY 10549-1407

914-666-2971
FAX: 914-666-2188
gomezj@curtisinst.com
www.curtisinst.com

Stuart E Marwell, President and CEO
David Matthews, VP Sales Americas
Cheryl Leonaggeo, Customer Service Manager
Richard McFarlane, Customer Support Engineer
Provides a readable, accurate indication of battery in easy to read type of display. Innovative, efficient motor speed controllers for single or dual PM motor vehicles.

685   **Softfoot Ergomatta**
Mat Factory
6726 North Figueroa Street
Los Angelesa, CA 90042

949-645-3122
800-628-7626
FAX: 323-254-4545
www.matfactoryinc.com

686   **Tilt-N-Table**
Osterguard Enterprises c/o Jim's Shop
3228 W Olive Ave
Fresno, CA 93722-5733

559-275-4695

Jim Ostergaard Ii, Owner
These are lightweight tables for wheelchairs that are angle and height adjustable to your changing needs.

687   **Wheel Life News**
University of Virginia, Rehab Engineering Centers
3363 University Sta
Charlottesville, VA 22903

434-924-5118
www.medicine.virginia.edu

Kristine M. Garza, Ph.D., Executive Director of SACNAS
Steven T. DeKosky, Dean
Features tie downs and other adaptive technology for persons with disabilities.

688   **Wheelchair Accessories**
Diestco Manufacturing Company
P.O.Box 6504
Chico, CA 95927-6504

800-795-2392
info@diestco.com
www.diestco.com

689   **Wheelchair Aide**
Graham-Field
400 Rabro Dr
Hauppauge, NY 11788-4258

631-348-1364

690   **Wheelchair Back Pack and Tote Bag**
Med Covers
320 Roebling Street
Suite 515
Brooklyn, NY 11211

718-302-1923
800-320-7140
FAX: 866-522-6967
info@1800wheelchair.com
www.1800wheelchair.com

691   **Wheelchair Roller**
Access To Recreation
8 Sandra Ct
Newbury Park, CA 91320-4302

800-634-4351
FAX: 805-498-8186
customerservice@accesstr.com
www.accesstr.com

Don Krebs, President
The McClain Wheelchair Roller allows you to build strength and stamina in the comfort of your own home.

692   **Wheelchair Work Table**
Bailey Manufacturing Company
P.O. Box 130
Lodi, OH 44254-130

800-321-8372
FAX: 800-224-5390
baileymfg@baileymfg.com
www.baileymfg.com

Wheelchairs: General

693   **21st Century Scientific, Inc.Bounder Power Wheelchair**
4931 N Manufacturing Way
Coeur D Alene, ID 83815-8931

208-667-8800
800-448-3680
FAX: 208-667-6600
21st@wheelchairs.com
wheelchairs.com

Ronald E. Prior, Ph.D., President and Founder
RD Davidson, Sales/Marketing Director
Susan Harris, CFO and Webmaster

High performance power chairs for active individuals. Very fast (11+ MPH), OFF-ROAD and Bariatric options available. Power seating options include tilt, recline, 13-inch seat elevator, reverse tilt, leg rests, standing and front load (latitude). 6-drive programmable electronics standard; lights, horn, electric leg bag emptier and many other options available. Customization is our specialty.

694   **Arcoa Travel Chair**
Maxi Aids
42 Executive Blvd
Farmingdale, NY 11735-4710

631-752-0521
800-522-6294
FAX: 631-752-0689
TTY: 631-752-0738
sales@maxiaids.com
www.maxiaids.com

Elliott Zaretsky, Founder and President
The unique Comfort Travel Chair collapses into an easy to manage 25in x 26in x 11in and includes a strap for easy carrying. It weighs just 16 lbs. but can hold up to 200 lbs., making it the perfect travel companion. You can rest assured that it will 'stay put' with a dual wheel lock, while you enjoy the comfort and support of the padded swing-back armrests and 16in seat. *$197.00*

695 Bariatric Wheelchairs Regency FL
Gendron
520 W. Mulberry St.
Suite 100
Bryan, OH 43506

800-537-2521
FAX: 419-636-9261
sales@gendroninc.com
www.gendroninc.com

Roberta Jacobs, National Sales Manager
Bariatric wheelchairs, for users weighing up to seven hundred pounds. Manual and power styles built to order for specific needs.

696 Breezy
Sunrise Medical/Quickie Designs
2842 Business Park Avenue
Fresno, CA 93727

800-333-4000
800-300-7502
webmaster@sunmed.com
www.sunrisemedical.com

Pete Coburn, President
Randi Binstock, VP, Business Dev.
Peter Riley, Senior VP/Corporate CFO
Roxane Cromwell, SVP, Operations North America
This lightweight chair is durable, comfortable and flexible enough to meet the needs of a wide range of wheelchair users.

697 Champion 1000
Kuschall of America
3601 Rider Trl S
Earth City, MO 63045-1116

314-512-7000
800-654-4768
FAX: 800-542-3567

698 Champion 2000
Kuschall of America
3601 Rider Trl S
Earth City, MO 63045-1116

314-512-7000
800-654-4768
FAX: 800-542-3567

699 Champion 3000
Kuschall of America
3601 Rider Trl S
Earth City, MO 63045-1116

314-512-7000
800-654-4768
FAX: 800-542-3567

700 Choosing a Wheelchair: A Guide for Optimal Independence
Patient-Centered Guides
1005 Gravenstein Hwy N
Sebastopol, CA 95472-3836

707-827-7019
800-889-8969
FAX: 707-824-8268
order@oreilly.com
www.patientcenters.com

Linda Lamb, Series Editor
Shawnde Paull, Marketing
Tim O'Reilly, Publisher
Gary Karp, Author
With the right wheelchair, quality of life increases dramatically and even people with severe disabilities can have a considerable degree of independence and activity. Choosing the wrong chair can indeed the tantamount to confinement. This book describes technology, options, and the selection process to help you identify the chair than can provide you with optimal independence.
$9.95
186 pages Paperback
ISBN 1-565924-11-8

701 Convaid
2830 California Street
Torrance, CA 90503

310-618-0111
888-266-8243
FAX: 310-618-2166
convaid@convaid.com
www.convaid.com

Rocio , Sales Manager
Monica , National Account Representative
Veronica , Export Department
Five different styles of wheelchairs.

702 Custom
Fortress
P.O.Box 489
Clovis, CA 93613-489

559-322-5437
FAX: 559-323-0299

703 Custom Durable
21279 Protecta Dr
Elkhart, IN 46516-9539

574-522-7201
800-478-2363
FAX: 574-293-0202
info@pvcdme.com
www.pvcdme.com

704 Edge
Fortress
P.O.Box 489
Clovis, CA 93613-489

559-322-5437
FAX: 559-323-0299

705 Etac USA: F3 Wheelchair
Ste J
2325 Parklawn Dr
Waukesha, WI 53186-2938

262-717-9910
800-678-3822
FAX: 262-796-4605
etac1usa@execpc.com
www.execpc.com/~etac1usa

Mark Samolyk, Manager
A Swedish wheelchair designed to provide function, comfort and flexibility. Seat frame and upholstery are adjustable to fit each individual. Swing away, detachable footrests are standard. Available in frame widths from 14, 18 and 20 inch. Numerous accessories are available in order to individualize each chair. Lifetime warranty on frame for original user.

706 Evacu-Trac
Garaventa Canada
7505 - 134 A Street, Surrey, BC V3W
Blaine, WA 98231-1769

866-824-8314
productinfo@evacutrac.com

707 Folding Chair with a Rigid Feel
Kuschall of America
3601 Rider Trl S
Earth City, MO 63045-1116

314-512-7000
800-654-4768
FAX: 800-542-3567

708 Formula Series Active Mobility Wheelchairs
Everest & Jennings
3233 Mission Oaks Blvd
Camarillo, CA 93012-5047

805-389-7450

709 Freestyle II
Fortress
P.O.Box 489
Clovis, CA 93613-489

559-322-5437
FAX: 559-323-0299

710 Gadabout Wheelchairs
Gadabout Wheelchairs
1165 Portland Ave
Rochester, NY 14621-3945   585-338-2110
                                         800-828-4242
                                    FAX: 585-338-2696

Michael Fonte, Owner
Enjoy independence with the wheelchair that is lightweight, portable, convenient, comfortable and sturdy.

711 Gem Wheelchair & Scooter Service: Mobility & Homecare
176-39 Union Tpke
Flushing, NY 11366-1515   718-969-8600
                                         800-943-3578
                                    FAX: 718-969-8300
                            help@gemwheelchairservice.com
                            www.gemwheelchairservice.com/

712 Gendron
520 W. Mulberry St. Suite 100
Bryan, OH 43506   419-445-6060
                                         800-537-2521
                                    FAX: 419-636-9261
                            rbell@gendroninc.com
                            www.gendroninc.com

Roberta Jacobs, National Sales Manager
Manufacturer of wheelchairs for a variety of other applications, specializing in bariatric mobility products.

713 HiRider
Gaymar Industries
10 Centre Dr
Orchard Park, NY 14127-2280   716-662-2551
                                        800-828-7341
                                   FAX: 800-993-7890
                            www.gaymar.com

Frank L Lumbar, CEO
John.K Whitney, Founder
Cindy Sylvia, Educational Svcs Administrator
Dan Kormowicz, International Sales Coordinator
A wheelchair that provides mobility in both sitting and standing positions.

714 Innovative Products
4351 W College Ave
Appleton, WI 54914-3928   920-738-9090
                                        800-424-3369
                                   FAX: 920-738-9050
                            www.att.com

Fritz H Heerdt, President
Wheelchairs; accessories.

715 Liberty
Fortress
P.O.Box 489
Clovis, CA 93613-489   559-322-5437
                                   FAX: 559-323-0299

716 Lightweight Breezy
Motion Design
2842 Business Park Avenue
Fresno, CA 93727

                                        800-333-4000
                                   FAX: 800-300-7502
                            webmaster@sunmed.com
                            www.sunrisemedical.com

Pete Coburn, President
Randi Binstock, VP, Business Dev.
Peter Riley, Senior VP/Corporate CFO
Roxane Cromwell, SVP, Operations North America
A lightweight wheelchair. $750.00

717 Majors Medical Equipment
415 W Wilshire Blvd., Suite A
Oklahoma City, OK 73116   405-840-5272
                                        1 8-8 4-4 01
                                   FAX: 405-840-5274
                            help@mmedsupply.com
                            www.majorsmedicalequipment.com

Pat Metz, Owner
America's largest selection of wheelchairs and homecare equipment.

718 Natural Access
PO Box 5729
Santa Monica, CA 90409   310-392-9864
                                        800-411-7789
                                   FAX: 310-392-3874
                            john_egan_2000@yahoo.com
                            www.landeez.com

John Egan, Owner
Provides the Landeez all-terrain wheelchair, that can roll easily on sand, gravel and snow for outdoor fun. The entire chair can fit inside a travel bag!

719 Patient Transport Chair
Mada Medical Products
625 Washington Ave
Carlstadt, NJ 07072-2901   201-460-0454
                                        800-526-6370
                                   FAX: 201-460-3509
                            dianelind@mail.madamedical.com
                            www.madainternational.com

Jeffrey Adam, President
Mada's lightweight design transport chair is constructed of heavy gauge chrome-plated, steel tubing with reinforced cross braces.

720 Posture-Glide Lounger
Graham-Field Health Products
2935 Northeast Pkwy
Atlanta, GA 30360-2808   678-291-3207
                                   FAX: 770-368-2386
                            cs@grahamfield.com
                            www.grahamfield.com

Kenneth Spett, President & CEO
Marc Bernstein, Senior Vice President, Consumer Sales
Cherie Antoniazzi, Senior Vice President, Quality, Regulatory & Risk Management
Ivan Bielik, Senior Vice President, Business Analyst
Provides all day comfort and safe, independent mobilization with feet or hands. The ergonomically engineered seat back provides correct support.

721 Prairie Cruiser
Wheelchairs of Kansas
204 West 2nd Street P.O.Box 32
Ellis, KS 67637-32   785-726-4885
                                        800-537-6454
                                   FAX: 800-337-2447
                            workinfo@go2wok.com
                            www.wheelchairsofkansas.com

722 Redman Apache
Redman Powerchair
1601 S Pantano Road Suite 107
Tucson, AZ 85710   520-546-6002
                                        800-727-6684
                                   FAX: 520-546-5530
                            info@redmanpowerchair.com
                            www.redmanpowerchair.com

Don Redman, CEO
Paula Redman, CFO
Scott Evans, Regulatory affairs
Samuel Redman, General Manager
These ultralight, active use wheelchairs offer quick release rear wheels, adjustable arm height and detachable arm swing-away.

723 Redman Crow Line
Redman Powerchair
1601 S Pantano Road Suite 107
Tucson, AZ 85710
520-546-6002
800-727-6684
FAX: 520-546-5530
info@redmanpowerchair.com
www.redmanpowerchair.com

Don Redman, CEO
Paula Redman, CFO
Scott Evans, Regulatory affairs
Samuel Redman, General Manager
Reclining wheelchair that reclines a full 90 degrees to flat and can be stopped anywhere on the axis.

724 Rolls 2000 Series
Invacare Corporation
1 Invacare Way
Elyria, OH 44035-4107
440-329-6000
800-333-6900
FAX: 877-619-7996
info@invacare.com
www.invacare.com

A. Malachi Mixon, III, Chairman of the Board
Gerald B. Blouch, President and Chief Executive Officer
Joseph B. Richey, II, President - Invacare Technologies Division & SVP
Robert K. Gudbranson, Senior Vice President and Chief Financial Officer
These wheelchairs are the first light-weight wheelchairs designed for rental use.

725 Skyway
Skyway Machine
4451 Caterpillar Rd
Redding, CA 96003-1496
530-243-5151
800-332-3357
FAX: 530-243-5104
sales@skywaywheels.com
www.skywaytuffwheels.com

Ken Coster, Sales Department
Parrey Cremeans, Sales Department
Rein Stolz, Engineering Department
Patrick McEachen, Customer Service
For over 20 years Skyway has been the world leader in composite wheels. Supplying over 650 different wheel combinations for wheelchairs, lawn and garden products, bicycles and a large assortment of wheeled devices. Wheel sizes range from 4 inch to 24 inch diameter.

726 Stand-Up Wheelchairs
Lifestand
P.O.Box 232171
Encinitas, CA 92023-2171
800-782-6324
FAX: 610-586-0847
dallery@msn.com

Jacques A Dallery, President
Offers a complete line of manual, electric and stand-up wheelchairs for the disabled.

727 Standard Wheelchair
Mada Medical Products
625 Washington Ave
Carlstadt, NJ 07072-2901
201-460-0454
800-526-6370
FAX: 201-460-3509
dianelind@mail.madamedical.com
www.madainternational.com

Jeffrey Adam, President
Mada's standard wheelchairs are designed and built for long-lasting, reliable operation. Each wheelchair is constructed of heavy gauge, chrome plated, steel framework and tube in tube construction at stress points. Mada's state-of-the art engineering uses the most modern components to provide the strength needed while keeping the chair's weight down.

728 Super Light Folding Transport Chair with Carry Bag
Maxi Aids
42 Executive Blvd
Farmingdale, NY 11735-4710
631-752-0521
800-522-6294
FAX: 631-752-0689
TTY: 631-752-0738
sales@maxiaids.com
www.maxiaids.com

Elliott Zaretsky, Founder and President
Folds like a conventional folding chair for added convenience and includes carry bag, fold-down footrests, padded flip back armrests, standard rear wheel locks and an attractive frame with durable lightweight nylon upholstery and limited lifetime warranty. Weighs only 18 pounds. Easy to push or transport. *$319.95*

729 Surf Chair
2052 S Peninsula Dr
Daytona Beach, FL 32118-5237
386-253-0986
800-841-6610
FAX: 386-253-7600

730 Vista Wheelchair
Arista Surgical Supply Company/AliMed
297 High Street
Dedham, MA 02026-2852
781-329-2900
800-225-2610
FAX: 781-329-8392
info@alimed.com
www.alimed.com

731 Wheelchair with Shock Absorbers
Iron Horse Productions
3114 Strawberry Ln
Port Huron, MI 48060-1727
810-987-6700
800-426-0354

Wheelchairs: Pediatric

732 Commuter & Kid's Commuter
Fortress
P.O.Box 489
Clovis, CA 93613-489
559-322-5437
FAX: 559-323-0299

733 Convaid
2830 California St
Torrance, CA 90503-3908
310-618-0111
888-266-8243
FAX: 310-618-2166
convaid@earthlink.net
www.convaid.com

Rocio , Sales Manager
Monica , National Account Representative
Veronica
Convaid manufactures Mobile Positioning Systems for children. The Expedition, Safari Tilt, Cruiser, EZ Rider and Metro offer a non-institutional styling and are lightweight and compact-folding. The steel/aluminum structure is engineered for maximum comfort and durability. The mobile positioning lines come with more than 20 positioning features and a full range of positioning adaptations. All chairs have been successfully crash-tested and offer a limited lifetime warranty (except the Metro).

734 Imp Tricycle
TRIAID
P.O.Box 1364
Cumberland, MD 21501-1364
301-759-3525
800-306-6777
FAX: 301-759-3525
sales@triaid.com
www.triaid.com

735 Kid's Custom
Fortress
P.O.Box 489
Clovis, CA 93613-489
559-322-5437
FAX: 559-323-0299

736 Kid's Edge
Fortress
P.O.Box 489
Clovis, CA 93613-489
559-322-5437
FAX: 559-323-0299

737 Kid's Liberty
Fortress
P.O.Box 489
Clovis, CA 93613-489
559-322-5437
FAX: 559-323-0299

738 Kid-Friendly Chairs
Vector Mobility
5030 E Jensen Ave
Fresno, CA 93725-4010
559-431-3334
800-441-0358
FAX: 559-431-5535

Dave Deatherage, Owner
Manual base offers the lowest available floor to seat height, growth capability, one-third the parts of a conventional chair and no welds to break. The power unit features standard shapes and personality designs from elephants to inch worms and autos to rainbows, lowest seat height, and smallest turning radius on the market.

739 Koala Miniflex
Permobil USA
300 Duke Dr
Lebanon, TN 37090
800-736-0925
FAX: 800-231-3256
info@permobilus.com
permobilus.com

740 Seven Fifty-Five FS
Fortress
P.O.Box 489
Clovis, CA 93613-489
559-322-5437
FAX: 559-323-0299

741 TMX Tricycle
TRIAID
P.O.Box 1364
Cumberland, MD 21501-1364
301-759-3525
800-306-6777
FAX: 301-759-3525
sales@triaid.com
www.triaid.com

Wheelchairs: Powered

742 Bounder Plus Power Wheelchair
21st Century Scientific
4931 N Manufacturing Way
Coeur D Alene, ID 83815-8931
208-667-8800
800-448-3680
FAX: 208-667-6600
21st@wheelchairs.com
wheelchairs.com

Ronald E. Prior, Ph.D., President and Founder
RD Davidson, Sales/Marketing Director
Susan Harris, CFO and Webmaster
Available in widths of 16 to 20 inches for users up to 500 pounds with a 2 year warranty on the entire chair. It offers all the standard features of a BOUNDER, plus reinforced rear wheel mounts, reinforced caster barrels, and super duty upholstery (with double liner and web straps under every screw). The BOUNDER Plus also features tandem cross struts, middle vertical support strut,

seat rails supported at five points and back upholstery attached with machine screws.

743 Bounder Power Wheelchair
21st Century Scientific
4931 N Manufacturing Way
Coeur D Alene, ID 83815-8931
208-667-8800
800-448-3680
FAX: 208-667-6600
21st@wheelchairs.com
wheelchairs.com

Ronald E. Prior, Ph.D., President and Founder
RD Davidson, Sales/Marketing Director
Susan Harris, CFO and Webmaster
Available in a variety of widths from 16 to 18 inches for users up to 250 pounds. The rugged frame is constructed with steel tubing. The standard 12 position Adjustable Front Forks, made of 1/4 inch thick steel, provides impact dampening and seat tilt adjustment. A Dual Group 27 Sliding Battery Box provides extended range and easy battery maintenance. *$8695.00*

744 Breez 1025
Electro Kinetic Technologies
W194 N11301 McCormick Dr
Germantown, WI 53022
262-250-7740
800-824-1068
FAX: 262-250-7741
info@ek-tech.com
ek-tech.com

745 Damaco D90
Damaco
28918 Hancock Parkway
Valencia, CA 91355
661-775-2020
877-528-2288
FAX: 661-775-2025
www.atbatt.com

746 Gem Wheelchair & Scooter Service: Mobility & Homecare
176-39 Union Turnpike
Flushing, NY 11366-1515
718-969-8600
800-943-3578
FAX: 718-969-8300
help@gemwheelchairservice.com
www.gemwheelchairservice.com/

747 Geronimo
Redman Powerchair
Ste 202
3840 S Palo Verde Rd
Tucson, AZ 85714-2076
520-294-1466
800-727-6684
FAX: 520-294-1460

Arnie Johnson, Owner
Wheelchair offering direct drive, two year electronic guarantee and micro controls.

748 Invacare IVC Tracer EX2 Wheelchair with Legrest
Maxi Aids
42 Executive Blvd
Farmingdale, NY 11735-4710
631-752-0521
800-522-6294
FAX: 631-752-0689
TTY: 631-752-0738
sales@maxiaids.com
www.maxiaids.com

Elliott Zaretsky, Founder and President
Bob Messenger, Clinical Respiratory Specialist
The Tracer EX2 combines the design and technology of the Invacare 9000 A true dual axle position allows for repositioning the 24 inch rear wheels and 8 inch casters for adult and hemi seat-to-floor heights. The new design also makes it possible to interchange components with the 9000 series chairs. *$189.95*

749 Jet 3 Ultra Power Wheelchair
Maxi Aids
42 Executive Blvd
Farmingdale, NY 11735-4710   631-752-0521
                                          800-522-6294
                                          FAX: 631-752-0689
                                          TTY: 800-281-3555
                                          sales@maxiaids.com
                                          www.maxiaids.com

Elliott Zaretsky, Founder and President
Delivers a broad range of standard performance features like Active-Trac Suspension and a powerful 50 amp PG VSI controller on a very compact and maneuverable frame.

750 One Thousand FS
Fortress
P.O.Box 489
Clovis, CA 93613-489   559-322-5437
                                          FAX: 559-323-0299

751 Permobil Max 90
Permobil
4020 Christopher Way
Plano, TX 75024   877-394-3941
                                          mumu.moorthi@sigmabatteries.com
                                          www.sigmabatteries.com

752 Permobil Super 90
Permobil
4020 Christopher Way
Plano, TX 75024   877-394-3941
                                          mumu.moorthi@sigmabatteries.com
                                          www.sigmabatteries.com

753 Power Wheelchairs
LaBac Systems
3845 Forest St
Denver, CO 80207-2516
                                          800-370-6808
                                          www.falconrehab.net

Power tilt and recline seating systems for wheelchairs, offering more comfort and dependability for the physically challenged.

754 Power for Off-Pavement
Redman Powerchair
1601 S Pantano Road
Suite 107
Tucson, AZ 85710-2076   520-546-6002
                                          800-727-6684
                                          FAX: 520-546-5530
                                          info@redmanpowerchair.com
                                          www.redmanpowerchair.com

Don Redman, CEO
Paula Redman, CFO
Scott Evans, Regulatory Affairs
Samuel Redman, General manager
Power-drive wheelchair has a solid seat and can handle safely and securely knolls and off-pavement terrain.

Wheelchairs: Racing

755 Eagle Sportschairs, LLC
2351 Parkwood Rd
Snellville, GA 30039-4003   770-972-0763
                                          800-932-9380
                                          FAX: 770-985-4885
                                          eaglesportschairs@gmail.com
                                          www.eaglesportschairs.com

Barry Ewing, Owner
The Eagle line of custom lightweight performance chairs includes a range of options to fit all racing and sport needs including; track, baseball, quad-rugby, tennis, field events and waterskiing. Also popular for daily use. We are able to customize any chair to accommodate size and disability and all frames have a full five year warranty.

756 East Penn Manufacturing Company
East Penn Manufacturing Company
Deka Road P.O.Box 147
Lyon Station, PA 19536-147   610-682-6361
                                          FAX: 610-682-4781
                                          contactus@eastpenn-deka.com
                                          www.eastpenn-deka.com

Harold DeLight, Breidegam
Chairman
Specially engineered for demanding deep-cycle applications Gelled electrolyte Deka Dominator Batteries provides maintenance-free operation, longer battery life and hours of reliable performance. Their excellent recharge characteristics provide quick turn around time.

757 Invacare Top End
1 Invacare Way
Elyria, OH 44035-4107   440-329-6000
                                          800-333-6900
                                          FAX: 877-619-7996
                                          info@invacare.com
                                          www.invacare.com

A. Malachi Mixon, III, Chairman of the Board
Gerald B. Blouch, President and Chief Executive Officer
Joseph B. Richey, II, President - Invacare Technologies Division & SVP
Robert K. Gudbranson, Senior Vice President and Chief Financial Officer
Manufacturers of light weight, rigid, sport-specific wheelchairs such as the Eliminator line of racing chairs, T-3 tennis and softball chairs, and the Terminator for quad rugby and basketball. The Excelerator, XLT three-wheel hand cycle for adults and juniors. Check out our full line of wheelchairs to fit every need. $1,895-$2,495

758 Invacare Top End Excelerator XLT Gold Handcyle
Maxi Aids
42 Executive Blvd
Farmingdale, NY 11735-4710   631-752-0521
                                          800-522-6294
                                          FAX: 631-752-0689
                                          TTY: 631-752-0738
                                          sales@maxiaids.com
                                          www.maxiaids.com

Elliott Zaretsky, Founder and President
It's been completely re-designed to be light and faster with more control than ever before. The 27 speeds operated by Shimano Rapid fire hands-on-shifter/brake delivers smooth, responsive shifting and braking right at your fingertips. No foot pedaling! *$3036.00*

Associations

General Disabilities

759 ACS Federal Healthcare
5270 Shawnee Rd
Alexandria, VA 22312-2310   703-941-4387
                                    FAX: 703-310-0126

Helene Fisher, VP
Project RSVP supports the SSA's initiative to expand operations vocational rehabilitation services through a national network of private providers. Rehabilitation companies interested in gaining access to a new client base, acquiring a new funding stream, and developing creative service delivery and entrepreneurial partnerships, may benefit from such a program.

760 AHEAD Association
107 Commerce Centre Drive
Suite 204
Huntersville, NC 28078   704-947-7779
                                    FAX: 704-948-7779
                                information@ahead.org
                                        www.ahead.org

Bea Awoniyi, President
Stephan Smith, Executive Director
Michael Johnson, Treasurer
Terra Beethe, Secretary
The premiere professional association committed to full participation of persons with disabilities in postsecondary education. AHEAD values diversity, personal growth and development and creativity. Promotes leadership and exemplary practices. Provides professional development and disseminates information. Orchestrates resources through partnership and collaboration. AHEAD dynamically addresses current and emerging issues with respect to disability, and education to achieve universal access.

761 APSE
416 Hungerford Drive
Suite 418
Rockville, MD 20850   301-279-0060
                                    FAX: 301-279-0075
                                membership@apse.org
                                            apse.org

Susie Rinne, President
Derek Nord, Vice President
Allison Wohl, Executive Director
Jeannine Pavlak, Secretary
Through advocacy and education, the Association of People Supporting EmploymentFirst advances employment and self-sufficiency for all people with disabilities.

762 Abilities!
201 I.U. Willets Road
Albertson, NY 11507   516-465-1400
                                    FAX: 516-465-3358
                                info@viscardicenter.org
                                www.abilitiesonline.org

Gerard O'Connor, Chairperson
John D. Kemp, Esq., President & CEO
Michael Caprara, Chief Technology Officer
Lauren M. Mazo, Chief Development Officer
Dedicated to creating a world in which people with disabilities will live simply as people.

763 Acupressure Institute
1533 Shattuck Ave
Berkeley, CA 94709-1516   510-845-1059
                                        800-442-2232
                                info@acupressure.com
                                    www.acupressure.com

Michael Gach, Ph. D., Exec. Dir.
Joseph Carter, B.S., L.Ac., Dir. of Acupressure Institute
Kathleen Davis, B.A., C.M.T. Di, Teacher
Katie Carrin, Instructor

Since 1976 the Acupressure institute has offered comprehensive acupressure trainings in the traditional Asian Bodywork Therapy (ABT)such as Thai massage and Shiatsu massage to students from around the world. In comparing other Acupressure schools, our trainings provide high quality education to support each student'sprofessional and personal goals, in a setting that encourages communication, respect, and confidentiality and safety for everyone.

764 Advocacy Center
1650 South Avenue
Suite 200
Rochester, NY 14620-1371   585-546-1700
                                        800-650-4967
                                    FAX: 585-546-7069
                                    TTY: 585-546-1700
                                info@starbridgeinc.org
                                www.starbridgeinc.org

Paul Shew, Executive Director
Joyce Steel, Director
Stepen G. Schwarz, President
Adam Anolik, Vice President
Is a non profit organization located in New York State that educates, supports, and advocates with people who have disabilities, their families and circles of support. A diverse consumer-driven organization leading New York State in shaping the future through the development of innovative, outcome-oriented, and quality initiatives for people with disabilities, their families, and circle of support.

765 Advocacy Center for Persons with Disabilitites
2671 Executive Center Circle, W.
Suite 100
Tallahassee, FL 32301-5092   850-488-9071
                                        800-342-0823
                                    FAX: 850-488-8640
                                    TTY: 800-346-4127
                                info@advocacycenter.org
                        www.flspedlaw.com/Advocacy_Cntr.html

Bob Whitney, Executive Director
Paige Morgan, Executive Assistant
A non-profit organization providing protection and advocacy services in the State of Florida. The Center's mission is to advance the dignity, equality, self-determination and expressed choices of individuals with disabilities.

766 Advocates for Children of New York
151 West 30th Street
5th Floor
New York, NY 10001   212-947-9779
                                    FAX: 212-947-9790
                                info@advocatesforchildren.org
                                www.advocatesforchildren.org

Eric F. Grossman, President
Jamie A. Levitt, Vice President
Kim Sweet, Executive Director
Harriet Chan King, Secretary
AFC works on behalf of children from infancy to age 21 who are at greatest risk for school-based discrimination and/or academic failure. These include children with disabilities, ethnic minorities, immigrants, homeless children, foster care children, limited English proficient children and those living in poverty.

767 Alliance for Technology Access
1119 Old Humboldt Rd
Jackson, TN 38305   731-554-5282
                                        800-914-3017
                                    FAX: 731-554-5283
                                    TTY: 731-554-5284
                                atainfo@ataccess.org
                                    www.ataccess.org

James Allison, President
Bob Van der Linde, Vice President
Margaret Doumitt, Executive Director
Mike Hewitt, Secretary/Treasurer
The ATA is a growing national network of technology resource centers, organizations, individuals and companies. ATA encourages and facilitates the empowerment of people with disabilities

to participate fully in their communities. Through public education, information and referral, capacity building in community organizations, and advocacy/policy efforts, the ATA enables millions of people to live, learn, work, define their futures, and achieve their dreams.

768   American Academy of Disability Evaluating Physicians
PO Box 1537
Elk Grove Village, IL 60009-1537   312-663-1171
                                        FAX: 312-663-1175
                                        aadep@aadep.org
                                        www.aadep.org

James L. Williams, MD, FAADEP, Secretary/Treasurer
Ellen Goldrick, MPA, Member Services Representative
Sandra L. Yost, MBA, Veritas Medicus Executive Dir
Debra Frigo, Interim Executive Director

AADEP is the premiere society serving physicians involved in disability management. There activities include ongoing teaching of the management of disabled patients as well as impairment and disability evaluation to physicians, other health care providers, attorneys, regulators, legislators and others involved in the care of the injured person.

769   American Academy of Environmental Medicine
6505 E Central Ave #296
Wichita, KS 67206-1924   316-684-5500
                              FAX: 316-684-5709
                              defox@aacmonline.org
                              www.aaemonline.org

De Rogers Fox, Executive Director
William A. Ingram, M.D., President
Martha Grout, M.D., MD(H), President-Elect
Alvis L. Barrier, M.D., FAAOA, Secretary

Environmental Medicine is the comprehensive, proactive and preventive strategic approach to medical care dedicated to the evaluation, management, and prevention of the adverse consequences resulting from Environmentally Triggered Illnesses.

770   American Academy of Pediatrics
141 NW Point Blvd
Elk Grove Village, IL 60007-1098   847-434-4000
                                        800-433-9016
                                        FAX: 847-434-8000
                                        kidsdocs@aap.org
                                        www.aap.org

Rober.W. Block,MD,FAAP, President
Thomas K. McInerny, MD, FAAP, President-Elect
Errol Alden, MD, Executive Director/CEO
O. Marion Burton, MD, FAAP, Immediate Past President

Organization of 60,000 pediatricians committed to the attainment of optimal physical, mental, and social health and well-being for all infants, children, adolescents and young adults.

771   American Association of Children's Residential Centers
11700 W Lake Park Dr
Milwaukee, WI 53224-3021   877-332-2272
                                FAX: 877-362-2272
                                ksisson@aacrc-dc.org
                                www.aacrc-dc.org

Okpara Rice, President
Kari Sisson, Executive Director
Keith Polan, Treasurer
Brenton Diers, Secretary

The American Association of Children's Residential Centers believes that children and adolescents, and their families, are entitled to treatment which offers the maximum opportunity for growth and change. AACRC believes that clinically crafted residential treatment options, ranging from community based homes through institutional environments, are essential components in a comprehensive system of behavioral health care.

772   American Association of Oriental Medicine
PO Box 96503
Suite 44114
Washington, DC 20090-6503   866-455-7999
                                 FAX: 866-455-7999
                                 mjabbour@aaaomonline.org
                                 www.aaaomonline.org

Don Lee, President
Jacob Godwin, Vice President
Anne Biris, Lac, Secretary
Carlos Chapa, Treasurer

Dedicated to the promotion and advancement of high ethical, educational, and professional standards in the practice of acupuncture and Oriental medicine (AOM) in the U.S.

773   American Association of People with Disabilities
2013 H Street, NW
5th Floor
Washington, DC 20006   202-457-0046
                            800-840-8844
                            FAX: 866-536-4461
                            TTY: 800-840-8844
                            referrals@aapd.com
                            www.aapd.com

Fred Maahs, Chair
Mary P. Davis, Vice Chair
Helena Berger, President/CEO
TaKeisha Bobbitt, Managing Director

The largest national nonprofit cross-disability member organization in the United States, dedicated to ensuring economic self-sufficiency and political empowerment for the more than 56 million Americans with disabilities. AAPD works in coalition with other disability organizations for the full implimentation and enforcement of disability nondiscrimination laws, particularly the Americans With Disabilities Act (ADA) of 1990 and the Rehabilitation Act of 1973.

774   American Association on Health and Disability
110 N. Washington Street
Suite 328-J
Rockville, MD 20850   301-545-6140
                           FAX: 301-545-6144
                           contact@aahd.us
                           www.aahd.us

Roberta Carlin, MS, JD, Executive Director
E. Clarke Ross, DPA, Public Policy Director
Karl Cooper, Esq., NDNRC Project Associate
Wanda C. Smith, MSA, Program Associate

The mission of AAHD is to advance health promotion and wellness initiatives for children and adults with disabilities.

775   American Board of Clinical Metal Toxicology
4889 Smith Rd
West Chester, OH 45069   419-358-0273
                              80-35 -222
                              FAX: 513-942-3934
                              treasurer@abcmt.org
                              www.abcmt.org

Rashid A Buttar, Chairman
James M. Holbert, MD, PhD, Vice Chairman
James Smith, DO, Treasurer
J Joseph Holliday, MD, Director

Dedicated to establishing and maintaining guidelines and standards for the practice of Clinical Metal Toxicology and to the assurance of a superior level of competence on the part of physicians treating patients with this psectrum of expanding global afflictions.

776   American Board of Professional Disability Consultants
Belle Meade Office Park
4525 Harding Road, 2nd Fl
Nashville, TN 37205   615-327-2984
                           FAX: 615-327-9235
                           americanbd@aol.com
                           www.americandisability.org

777 American Botanical Council
6200 Manor Rd
Austin, TX 78723
512-926-4900
800-373-7105
FAX: 512-926-2345
abc@herbalgram.org
www.herbalgram.org

Mark Blumenthal, Executive Director/Founder
Hannah Bauman, Assistant Editor
Janie Carter, Membership Coordinator
Gayle Engels, Special Projects Director
The American Botanical Council (ABC) is the leading independent, nonprofit, international member-based organization providing education using science-based ad traditional information to promote the responsible use of herbal medicine.

778 American Camping Association
5000 State Road 67 N
Martinsville, IN 46151-7902
765-342-8456
800-428-2267
FAX: 765-342-2065
jalbarran@ACAcamps.org
www.acacamps.org

Tisha Bolger, Chair
Rue Mapp, Vice Chair
Tom Holland, Chief Executive Officer
Craig Whiting, Treasurer
The American Camp Association is a community of camp professionals who, for nearly 100 years, have joined together to share our knowledge and experience and to ensure the quality of camp programs. Because of our diverse 7,000 plus emmbership and exceptional programs, children and adults have the opportunity to learn powerful lessons in cmmunity, character-building, skill development, and healthy-living—-lessons that can be learned nowhere else.

779 American Chiropractic Association
1701 Clarendon Blvd
Suite 200
Arlington, VA 22209
703-276-8800
FAX: 703-243-2593
memberinfo@acatoday.org
www.acatoday.org

Richard Bruns,DC, Chair
Anthony W. Hamm,DC, President
David Herd, DC, Vice President
Kelli K. Pearson, DC, Director, Gov. District 1
The ACA is a professional organization representing Doctors of Chiropratic. Its mission is to preserve, protect, improve, and promote the chiropractic profession and the services of Doctors of Chiropratic for the benefit of the patients they serve. The purpose of the ACA is to provide leadership in health care and a positive vision for the chiropractic profession and its natural approach to health and wellness.

780 American College of Advancement in Medicine
380 Ice Center Lane
Suite C
Bozeman, MT 59718
949-309-3520
800-LEA- OUT
FAX: 406-587-2451
info@acam.org
www.acam.org

Allen Green, MD, President
Michael Bauerschmidt, MD, Vice President/ Secretary
Veronica Haynes, Executive Director
W.A. Shrader, Jr., MD, Treasurer
The American College for Advancement in Medicine (ACAM)is a not-for-profit society dedicated to educating physicians and other health care professionals on the latest findings and emerging procedures in preventive/nutritional medicine. ACAM's goals are to improve skills, knowledge and diagnostic procedures as they relate to complimentary and alternative medicine; to support research; and to develop awareness of alternative methods of medical treatment.

781 American College of Nurse Midwives
8403 Colesville Rd
Ste 1550
Silver Spring, MD 20910
240-485-1800
FAX: 240-485-1818
info@acnm.org
www.midwife.org

Elaine M. Moore, President
Lorrie Kaplan, Chief Executive Officer
Nicholas Kroll, Office Associate
Carol Ann Ross, Executive Assistant
The American College of Nurse-Midwives (ACNM) is the oldest women's health care organization in the U.S. ACNM provides research, accredits midwifery education programs, administers and promotes continuing education programs, establishes clinical practice standards, creates liasons with state and federal agencies and members of Congress.

782 American Counseling Association
6101 Stevenson Ave
Alexandria, VA 22304
703-823-9800
800-347-6647
FAX: 703-823-0252
TTY: 703-823-6862
webmaster@counseling.org
www.counseling.org

Robert L. Smith, President
Richard Yep, Chief Executive Officer
Thelma Duffey, President-Elect
Brian Canfield, Treasurer
The American Counseling Association is a not-for-profit, professional and educational organization that is dedicated to the growth and enhancement of the counseling profession.

783 American Disability Association
815 First Avenue
Suite 280
Seattle, WA 98104
205-328-9090
freeman@adanet.org
www.adanet.org

784 American Disabled Golfers Association
1295 SE Port St. Lucie Blvd
Port St. Lucie, FL 34952
772-335-3820
FAX: 772-335-3822
Info@theADGA.com
www.americandisabledgolfersassociation.com

785 American Herbalists Guild
125 South Lexington Avenue
Suite 101
Asheville, NC 28801
617-520-4372
office@americanherbalistsguild.com
www.americanherbalistsguild.com

Bevin Clare, M.S., R.H., CN, President
Phyllis D. Light, Vice President
Richard Mandelbaum RH (AHG), Secretary
David N. Harder, RH (AHG), Treasurer
Founded in 1989 as a non-profit, educational organization to represent the goals and voices of herbalists specializing in the medicinal use of plants. Our primary goal is to promote a high level of professionalism and education in the study and practice of theraputic herbalism.

786 American Holistic Medical Association
5313 Colorado Street
Duluth, MN 55804
218-525-5651
FAX: 218-525-5651
info@aihm.org
aihm.org

Mimi Guarneri, President
Daniel Friedland, MD, Chair
Daniel M. Asimus, MD, MSEd, Vice President
Scott M. Shannon, MD, Secretary
The Academy of Integrative Health & Medicine unites the many voices in integrative health - from family doctors to psychologists, acupuncturists to nurses and every practitioner in between to build bridges between professions and offer credible educa-

tional and certification programs for licensed healthcare providers. There's a place for you, no matter your profession.

787   American Massage Therapy Association
500 Davis St
Ste 900
Evanston, IL 60201-4695

847-864-0123
877-905-0577
FAX: 847-864-5196
info@amtamassage.org
www.amtamassage.org

Jeff Smoot, President
Dolly Wallace, Vice President
Kathie Lea, Vice President
Joan Nichols, Vice President

AMTA works to establish massage therapy as integral to the maintenance of good health and complementary to other therapeudic processes; to advance the profession through ethics and standards, certification, school accreditation, continuing education, professional publications, legislative efforts, public education, and fostering the development of members.

788   American Occupational Therapy Association
4720 Montgomery Lane
Suite 200
Bethesda, MD 20814-3449

301-652-6611
800-789-2682
FAX: 240-762-5150
TTY: 800-377-8555
praota@aota.org
www.aota.org

Florence Clark, President
Ginny Stoffel, President-Elect
Amy Lamb, VP
Paul A Fontana, Secretary

Advances the quality, availability, use and support of occupational therapy through standard setting, advocacy, education, and research on behalf of its members.

789   American Organization for Bodywork Therapies of Asia
PO Box 343
West Berlin, NJ 08091

856-809-2953
FAX: 856-809-2958
office@aobta.org
www.aobta.org

Wayne Mylin, President
Deborah Overholt, Legislative Director
Deborah Valentine Smith, Treasurer/Secretary
Cindy Banker, Director of COSP

The American Organization for Bodywork Therapies of Asia (AOBTA) is a professional membership organizaton which promotes Asian Bodywork Therapy and its practitioners while honoring a diversity of disciplines. AOBTA serves its community of members by supporting appropriate credentialing; defining scope of practice and educational standards; and providing resources for training, professional development and networking. AOBTA advocates public policy to protect its members.

790   American Public Health Association
800 I St NW
Washington, DC 20001

202-777-2742
FAX: 202-777-2534
TTY: 202-777-2500
comments@apha.org
www.apha.org

Pamela Aaltonen, PhD, RN, Chair
Georges C. Benjamin, MD, Executive Director
James Carlo, Executive Office
Kemi Oluwafemi, MBA, CPA, Finance & Systems

Founded in 1872, APHA is the oldest, largest and most diverse organization of public health professionals in the world. The association works to protect all Americans and their communities from preventable, seruious health threats. APHA represents a broad array of health officials, educators, environmentalists, policy-makers and health providers at all levels working both within and outside governmental organizations and educational institutions.

791   American Red Cross
2025 E Street, NW
Washington, DC 20006

202-303-5214
800-733-2767
FAX: 518-459-8268
news@redcrossneny.org
www.redcross.org/contact-us

Gary Striar, CEO
Susan Rounds, COO
Gary Ferris, Executive Director
Lynn Gilbert, Executive Director

Today, in addition to domestic disaster relief, the American Red Cross offers compassionate services in five other areas: community services that help the needy; support and comfort for military members and their families; the collection, processing and distribution of lifesaving blood and blood products; educational programs that promote health and safety; and international relief and development programs.

792   American Self-Help Clearinghouse
50 Morris Avenue
St Clares Health Services
Denville, NJ 07834

973-625-7107
800-367-6274
FAX: 973-326-9467
info@selfhelpgroups.org
www.selfhelpgroups.org

Edward J Madara MS, Director

Provides information on national self-help groups and offers training and technical assistance to exisiting and new self-help groups and clearinghouses. It has compiled a national database of over 800 of these model groups. Provides information on resource groups such as Violence Anonymous, Batterers Anonymous, and Stalkers' Victims Support Groups.

793   American Society for the Alexander Technique
PO Box 2307
Dayton, OH 45401-2307

937-586-3732
800-473-0620
FAX: 937-586-3699
webteam@AmSATonline.org
www.amsat.ws

Rick Carbaugh, Chair
Alan Bowers, Treasurer
Susan Overton, Secretary
Michele Drivon, Member at Large

The Alexander Technique is a proven, effective self help method for improving balance and coordination and increasing movement awareness by eliminating habitual reactions of misuse in every day activities. AmSats mission is to define, maintain and promote the Alexander Technique at its highest standard of professional practice and conduct.

794   American Society of Bariatric Physicians
2821 S Parker Rd
Ste 625
Aurora, CO 80014-2735

303-770-2526
FAX: 303-779-4834
info@asbp.org
www.asbp.org

David Bryman, DO, FASBP, Chair
Eric C. Westman, MD, MHS, President
Wendy Scinta, Vice President
Laurie Traetow, CPA, CAE, Executive Director

The American Society of Bariatric Physicians is an international association and allied health care professionals with special interest and experience in the comprehensive treatment of overweight, obesity and related disorders.

795   American Society of Clinical Hypnosis
140 N Bloomingdale Rd
Bloomingdale, IL 60108

630-980-4740
FAX: 630-351-8490
info@asch.net
www.asch.net

Michael White, Communication/Marketing Director
Erickson, MD Founder

To provide and encourage education programs to further, in every ethical way, the knowledge, understanding, and application of hypnosis in health care; to encourage research and scientific publication in the field of hypnosis; to promote the further recognition and acceptance of hypnosis as an important tool in clinical health care and focus for scientific research; to cooperate with other professional societies that share mutual goals, ethics, and interests

796   Association for Applied Psychophysiology and Biofeedback
10200 W 44th Ave
Ste 304
Wheat Ridge, CO 80033   303-422-8436
                                     800-477-8892
                                     info@aapb.org
                                     www.aapb.org

Richard Harvey, PhD, President
David Stumph, CAE, Executive Director
Michelle Cunningham, Associate Director
Fred B. Shaffer, PhD, Treasurer
Provides names and phone numbers of local chapters. Mission is to advance the development, dissemination and utilization of knowledge about applied psychophysiology and biofeedback to improve health and the quality of life through research, education, and practice.

797   Association for Persons in Supported Employment
416 Hungerford Drive
Suite 418
Rockville, MD 20850   301-279-0060
                                     FAX: 301-279-0075
                                     membership@apse.org
                                     www.apse.org

Susie Rinne, President
Derek Nord, Vice President
Allison Wohl, Executive Director
Jeannine Pavlak, Secretary
Supported employment enables people with disabilities who have not been successfully employed to work and contribute to society. Focuses on a person's abiliities and provides the supports the individual needs to be successful on a long-term basis.

798   Association for Persons with Severe Handicaps (TASH)
2013 H Street, NW
Ste 715
Washington, DC 20036   202-540-9020
                                     FAX: 202-540-9019
                                     info@tash.org
                                     www.tash.org

Ralph Edwards, President
Jean Trainor, Vice President
Barb Trader, Executive Director
Trri Ward, Secretary
International association of people with disabilities, their family members, other advocates and professionals, fighting for a society in which inclusion of all people in all aspects of society is the norm.

799   Association of Assistive Technology Act Programs
1 W Old State Capitol Plaza
Suite 100
Springfield, IL 62701
                                     linda.jaco@okstate.edu
                                     www.ataporg.org

Linda Jaco, Chair
Sachin Pavithran, Vice Chair
Alan Knue, Treasurer
Wade Wingler, Secretary
The Association of Assistive Technology Act Programs (ATAP) is a national, member-based organization, comprised of state Assistive Technology Act Programs funded under the Assistive Technology Act (AT Act).

800   Association of Disability Advocates, The
Fayetteville, AR   479-442-8558
                                     888-350-1247
                                     associationofdisabilityadvocates.com

801   Association of Educational Therapists
7044 S. 13th St.
Oak Creek, WI 53154   414-908-4949
                                     FAX: 414-768-8001
                                     customercare@AETOnline.org
                                     www.aetonline.org

Alice Pulliam, MA, BCET, President
Susan Grama, MA, Treasurer
Vicki Bergoff, JD, ET/P, Secretary
Jose Chavez, MA, ET/P, Director
Educational Therapy offers children and adults with learning disabilities and other learning challenges a wide range of intensive, individualized interventions designed to remediate learning problems.

802   Association of University Centers on Disabilities
AUCD
1100 Wayne Ave
Ste 1000
Silver Spring, MD 20910   301-588-8252
                                     FAX: 301-588-2842
                                     aimparato@aucd.org
                                     www.aucd.org

Olivia Raynor, PhD., President
Andrew J. Imparato, JD, Executive Director
Harold Kleinert, EdD, Treasurer
Brent Askvig, PhD, Secretary
The central office for the 61 University Centers for Excellence programs and 21 Mental Retardation and Developmental Disabilities Research Centers and is their representative to the federal government. UCEDD's are located at major universities and teaching hospitals in all 50 states, the District of Columbia and many US territories. UCCED's target their activities to support the independence, productivity and integration into the community of individuals with developmental disabilities.

803   Association on Higher Education and Disability (AHEAD)
107 Commerce Centre Drive
Suite 204
Huntersville, NC 28078   704-947-7779
                                     FAX: 704-948-7779
                                     information@ahead.org
                                     www.ahead.org

Bea Awoniyi, President
Stephan Smith, Executive Director
Michael Johnson, Treasurer
Terra Beethe, Secretary
International, multicultural organization of proessionals committed to full participation in higher education for persons with disabilities. Plans and develops training programs, workshops, publications and conferences. Founded in 1977 to address the need and concern for upgrading the quality of services and support available to persons with disabilities in higher education.

804   Bastyr University Natural Health Clinic
3670 Stone Way N
Seattle, WA 98103   206-834-4100
                                     FAX: 206-834-4131
                                     www.bastyrcenter.org

805   Beach Center on Families and Disability
University of Kansas
1200 Sunnyside Ave
Rm 3136
Lawrence, KS 66045-7534   785-864-7600
                                     866-783-3378
                                     FAX: 785-864-7605
                                     TTY: 785-864-3434
                                     beachcenter@ku.edu
                                     www.beachcenter.org

Shonda Anderson, Project Coordinator
Barbara Miller, Accountant
Susan Palmer, Research Professor
Peter Griggs, Evaluation Coordinator
A federally funded center that conducts research and training in the factors that contribute to the successful functioning of families with members who have disabilities.

806   **Birth Defect Research for Children**
976 Lake Baldwin Lane, Suite 104
Orlando, FL 32814

407-895-0802
staff@birthdefects.org
www.birthdefects.org

Betty Mekdeci, Manager/Founder

A nonprofit organization that provides information about birth defects of all kinds to parents and professionals. Offers a library of medical books and files of information on less common categories of birth defects and is involved in research to discover possible links between environmental exposures and birth defects.

807   **Bonnie Prudden Myotherapy**
4330 E. Havasu Road
Tucson, AZ 85718

520-529-3979
800-221-4634
FAX: 520-529-6679
info@bonnieprudden.com
www.bonnieprudden.com

Enid Whittaker, Associate Director

Myotherapy is a method for relaxing muscle spasm, improving circulation and alleviating pain. Pressure is applied using elbows, knuckled or fingers, and held for several seconds to defuse trigger points. The success of this method depends upon the use of specific corrective exercises of the freed muscles.

808   **Brain Injury Association of America**
1608 Spring Hill Rd
Ste 110
Vienna, VA 22812

703-761-0750
800-444-6443
FAX: 703-761-0755
shconnors@biausa.org
www.biausa.org

Daniel S. Chamberlain, Esq., Chairman
Brant A. Elkind, MS, Vice Chairman
Susan H Connors, B.A., President/CEO
Ira Sherman, Esq., Treasurer

Founded in 1980, the Brain Injury Association of America (BIAA) is the leading national organization serving and representing individuals, families and professionals who are touched by a life-altering, often devistating, traumatic brain injury (TBI) Together with its network of more then 40 charted state affiliates, as well as hundreds of local chapters and support groups across the country, the BIAA provides information, education and support to assist the 5.3 million living with brain injuries

809   **CAPP National Parent Resource Center Federation for Children with Special Needs**
45 Bromfield St
10th Fl
Boston, MA 02108

866-815-8122
FAX: 617-542-7832
info@ppal.net
www.ppal.net

Earl N. Stuck, Chair
Lisa Lambert, Executive Director
Anne Silver, Operations Director
Anne Metzger, Treasurer

A parent-run resource system designed to further the needs and goals of family-centered, community-based coordinated care for children with special health needs and their families. Offers written materials, training packages, workshops and presentations for parents and professionals on special education, health care financing and other topics.

810   **CARF Rehabilitation Accreditation Commission**
6951 E Southpoint Rd
Tucson, AZ 85756-9407

888-281-6531
888-281-6531
FAX: 520-318-1129
info@carf.org
www.carf.org

Brian J Boon, Ph.D., President/CEO
Di Shen, PhD, Chief research officer
Cindy L. Johnson, CPA, Chief Resource Officer
Darren M. Lehrfeld, Chief Accreditation Officer

CARF serves as the standards-setting and accrediting body for rehabilitation and life enhancement programs and services. The independent, not-for-profit commission provides accrediation of human service providers in the areas of aging services, behavioral health, child and youth services, DMEPOS, employment and community services, medical rehabilitation, and opioid treatment programs.

811   **Canine Companions for Independence**
National Offices
P.O.Box 446
Santa Rosa, CA 95402-0446

866-224-3647
800-572-2275
TTY:707-577-1756
info@cci.org
www.cci.org

John Miller, Chair
John McKinney, Vice Chair
Paul Mundell, Chief Executive Officer
Alan Feinne, Chief Financial Officer

A nonprofit organization that enhances the lives of people with disabilities by providing highly trained assistance dogs and ongoing support to ensure quality partnerships.

812   **Canine Helpers for the Handicapped**
5699 Ridge Rd
Lockport, NY 14094

716-433-4035
FAX: 716-439-0822
chhdogs@aol.com
www.caninehelpers.org

Beverly D. Underwood, Executive Director

A nonprofit organization devoted to custom training Assistance Dogs to assist people with disabilities to lead more independent, secure lives.

813   **Cape Organization for Rights of the Disabled (CORD)**
106 Bassett Ln
Hyannis, MA 02601-3800

508-775-8300
800-541-0282
FAX: 508-775-7022
TTY: 800-541-0282
cordinfo@cilcapecod.org
www.cilcapecod.org

Cathy Taylor, ADA Specialist

The Cape Organization for the Rights of the Disabled (CORD) has been aggresively working since 1984 to advance the independence, productivity, and integration of people with disabilities into mainstream society. CORD is the Center for Independent Living (CIL) and is a member of the Aging and Disability Resources Consortium (ADRC) serving Cape Cod and the Islands.

814   **Case Management Society of America**
6301 Ranch Dr
Little Rock, AR 72223

501-225-2229
800-216-2672
FAX: 501-221-9068
cmsa@cmsa.org
www.cmsa.org

Nancy Skinner, RN-BC, CCM, President
Betty Overbey, RN-BC, CRRN,, Secretary
Jose Alejandro, RN-BC, MSN, Treasurer
Cheri A Lattimer, Executive Director

The Case Management Society of America is an international, non-profit organization founded in 1990 dedicated to the support and development of the profession of case management through

73

educational forums, networking opportunities and legislative involvement.

815 Center for Assistive Technology and Environmental Access
490 Tenth St NW
Atlanta, GA 30332-0156
404-894-4960
800-726-9119
FAX: 404-894-9320
TTY: 404-894-4960
catea@coa.gatech.edu
www.catea.org

Carrie Bruce, Research Scientist II
Karen Milchus, Research Engineer II
Charlie Drummond, Administrative Assistant
Sarah Endicott, Research Scientist I
CATEA supports individuals with disabilities of any age within the State of Georgia and beyond through expert services, research, design and technological development, information dissemination, and educational programs.

816 Center for Disability Resources
Pediatrics, School Of Medicine,Univ Of S. Carolina
8301 Farrow Rd
Columbia, SC 29208
803-935-5231
FAX: 803-935-5059
David.Rotholz@uscmed.sc.edu
uscm.med.sc.edu/cdrhome/directions.asp
Jerome D. Odom Ph.D., Exec. Dir.
Susan Greer, Fiscal/Foundation Coordinator
Mechelle English, Senior Dev. Dir.
Kim E. Creek, PhD., Dir.
A University Affiliated Program which develops model programs designed to serve persons with disabilities and to train students in fields related to disabilities.

817 Center for Mind/Body Studies
5225 Connecticut Ave NW
Suite 415
Washington, DC 20015
202-966-7338
FAX: 202-966-2589
center@cmbm.org
www.cmbm.org
James S. Gordon. MD, President
Mark Hyman, MD, Director
Ann Hopes, Director
Herman Bluestein, Secretary
The Center for Mind-Body Medicine is a non-profit educational organization dedicated to reviving the spirit and transforming the practice of medicine. The Center is working to create a more effective, comprehensive and compassionate model of healthcare and education. The Center's model combines the precision of modern science with the best of the world's healing traditions.

818 Center for Universal Design
NC State University
College of Design, NC State Uni
Campus Box 8613
Raleigh, NC 27695-8613
919-515-3082
800-647-6777
FAX: 919-515-8951
cud@ncsu.edu
www.ncsu.edu/ncsu/design/cud/
Sean Vance, AIA, Acting Director
Sharon Joines, Ergonomist
Leslie Young, M.S.,, Director of Design
Angela Brockelsby, Director of Communications
A federally funded resource center that works toward improving housing for people with disabilities. Provides technical assistance, training and publications on accessible housing and universal design.

819 Change
1413 Park Rd NW
Washington, DC 20010-2801
202-387-3725
FAX: 202-387-3729
changeinc@hotmail.com
Gracie Rolling, Executive Director
Therman Walker, President
Preston Hursey Jr., VP
Offers counseling/assessment, emergency food and clothing referrals, rental assistance and job assistance to disabled persons in the District of Columbia area.

820 Child and Parent Resource Institute
600 Sanatorium Road
London, ON, Canada N6H-3W7
519-858-2774
877-494-2774
FAX: 519-858-3913
TTY: 519-858-0257
Gillian.Kriter@ontario.ca
www.cpri.ca
Dr. Shannon Stewart, Program Manager
Kim Arbeau, Research Coordinator
Liz Willits, Research Project Assistant
Melissa Currie, Manager (A)
Provides highly specialized services to children and youth from 0-18 years of age with complex mental health and/or developmental challenges on a short term inpatient and community basis.

821 Children's Alliance
420 Capitol Ave
Frankfort, KY 40601
502-875-3399
FAX: 502-223-4200
dlocey@rameyestep.com
www.childrensallianceky.org
Denny Locey, Chair
Jeff Hardin, Vice-Chair
Michelle Sanborn, President
Chris Peck, Treasurer
An association of individuals and human services organizations committed to being a voice for at-risk children and families. Interacts with the legislative and executive branches of government and assists members in developing services that most effectively meet the needs of at-risk children and families.

822 Children's National Medical Center
111 Michigan Ave NW
Washington, DC 20010
202-476-5000
888-884-BEAR
FAX: 202-476-2270
tbear@childrensnational.org
www.cnmc.org
Kurt Newman, President/CEO
Gerard Martin, SVP
Douglas Myers, Exec VP, CFO
Mark Batshaw, MD, Chief Academic Officer
Our mission is to be preeminent in providing health care services that enhance the health and well-being of children regionally, nationally and internationally. Through leadership and innovation, Children's will create solutions to pediatric health care problems. To meet the unique health care needs of children, adolescents and their families, Children's will excel in Care, Advocacy, Research and Education.

823 Clay Tree Society
838 Old Victoria Road
Nanaimo, BC V9R-6A1
250-753-5322
FAX: 250-753-2749
claytree@shaw.ca
www.claytree.org
Veronica Harrison, President
Joan Gibson, Vice President
Glenys Patmor, Executive Director
Darryl Racine, General Manager
Non-profit society providing day programming for 75 adults with various developmental disabilities governed by an elected Board of Directors and funded by Community Living British Columbia and BC Gaming.

824   Community Enterprises
441 Pleasant Street
Northampton, MA 01060   413-584-1460
FAX: 413-586-1121
TTY:413-584-1460
info@communityenterprises.com
www.communityenterprises.com

W8illiaqm Donohue, Chair
Donald Miner, Vice-Chair
Stephanie Burbine, Treasurer
Joanne Carlisle, Clerk
Provide supported education services in a community college setting; supported employment including job training, placement and follow-up; transitional services from group homes and other settings to supported living within the community.

825   Council For Exceptional Children
2900 Crystal Drive, Suite 1000
Arlington, VA 22202-3557   888-232-7323
888-232-7733
agraham@cec.sped.org
www.cec.sped.org/

James P. Heiden, President
Antonis Katsiyannis, President-Elect
Sharon Raimondi, Treasurer
Alexander T. Graham, Secretary
The Council for Exceptional Children (CEC) is the largest international professional organization dedicated to improving the educational success of individuals with disabilities and/or gifts and talents.

826   DB-Link
National Consortium on Deaf-Blindness
345 N. Monmouth Ave.
Monmouth, OR 97361   503-838-8754
800-438-9376
FAX: 503-838-8150
TTY: 800-854-7013
info@nationaldb.org
www.nationaldb.org

Brenda Baroncelli, Administrative Assistant
Megan Cote, Project Specialist
Jeff Denton, Lead Web Developer
D. Jay Gense, Senior Advisor
Found at the National Consortium of Deaf-Blindness, DB-LINK is the largest collection of information related to deaf-blindness worldwide. A team of information specialists makes this extensive resource available in response to direct requests, via the NCDB website, through conferences, and via a variety of electronic medium.

827   Davis Center, The
110 Wesley St
PO Box 508
Manlius, NJ 13104   862-251-4637
FAX: 862-251-4642
info@thedaviscenter.com
www.thedaviscenter.com

Dorinne S Davis MA CCC-A FAAA, Director
Elizabeth Meade, Head Sound Therapist
Nancy Puckett-Dunn, Office Manager
Donna Warr, Office Assistant
Offers sound-based therapies supporting positive change in learning, development, and wellness. All ages/all disabilities. The Davis Model of Sound Intervention-an alternative approach.

828   Department of Physical Medicine & Rehabilitation at Sinai Hospital
2401 W Belvedere Ave
Baltimore, MD 21215-5271   410-601-9000
FAX: 410-601-9692
www.lifebridgehealth.org

Jason A. Blavatt, Esq., Chairman
Barry F. Levin, Esq., Vice Chairman
Leonard Stoler, Treasurer
Jeffery A. Wothers, Esq., Secretary
As one of largest, most comprehensive and most highly respected providers of health-related services to the people of the North-

west Baltimore region, LifeBridge heath advocates preventive services, wellness and fitness services and programs to educate and support the communities it serves. LifeBridge is dedicated to advancing the health of the community through a variety of health and wellness programs and services.

829   DisAbility LINK
1901 Montreal Road
Suite 102
Tuckr, GA 30084   404-687-8890
800-239-2507
FAX: 404-687-8298
info@disabilitylink.org
www.disabilitylink.org

Garrick Scott, Chairman
Barbaraann Bongiovani, Vice Chairman
Kim Gibson, Executive Director
Larry Brown, Finance Director
This center for rights and resources is committed to promoting the rights of all people with disabilities in allowing them to be independent, achieve goals, have access to their community and make decisions for themselves.

830   Disability Funders Network
14241 Midlothian Turnpike
#151
Midlothian, VA 23113   703-795-9646
info@disabilityfunders.org
www.cof.org

Sherry P. Magill, Ph.D., Chairman
Javier Soto, Vice Chairman
Vikki Spruill, President/CEO
Eugene W. Cochrane, Jr., Treasurer
Disability-inclusive grantmaking is the mission of DFN: inclusion of the disability in grantmaking programs and inclusion of people with disabilities in grantmaking organizations.

831   Disability Rights Bar Association
900 S. Crouse Avenue
Crouse-Hinds Hall, Suite 300
Syracuse, NY 13244-2130   FAX: 315-443-9725
DRBA-Law@law.syr.edu
disabilityrights-law.org

832   Disabled Athlete Sports Association
1236 Jungermann Rd.
Suite A
St. Peters, MO 63376   636-477-0716
meghang@dasasports.org
www.dasasports.org

Fred Schlichting, President
Bryan Krueger, Treasurer
Mike Schulte, Secretary
Kelly Behlmann, Executive Director, Founder
The Disabled Athlete Sports Association (DASA) is a 501 (c)(3) nonprofit organization specializing in adaptive sport and fitness opportunities. DASA relies heavily upon fundraising events, grants, and individual and corporate donations to sustain its mission.

833   Disabled Businesspersons Association
6367 Alvarado Court
Suite 350
San Diego, CA 92120   619-594-8805
info@disabledbusiness.com
disabledbusiness.org

834   Disabled Children's Relief Fund
PO Box 89
Freeport, NY 11520   516-377-1605
FAX: 516-377-3978
www.dcrf.com

835 Disabled Drummers Association
18901 NW 19 Avenue
Miami Gardens, FL 33056   305-621-9022
DDAFathertime@comcast.net
www.disableddrummers.org

836 Disabled and Alone/Life Services for the Handicapped
1440 Broadway
23rd Floor
New York, NY 10018-2326   212-532-6740
800-995-0066
FAX: 212-532-6740
info@disabledandalone.org
www.disabledandalone.org

Leslie D. Park, Chairman
Rex L. Davidson, Vice President
Lee Alan Ackerman, B.A., Executive Director
William G. Shannon, J.D., Treasurer

A national nonprofit humanitarian organization whose primary concern is the well-being of handicapped persons, particularly when their families can no longer care for them. Disabled and Alone 1) Helps families do sensible planning for and with their disabled children; 2) Provides advocacy and oversight when the parents cannot do so; 3) Advises families, attorneys and financial planners about life planning for a family member with a disability.

837 Easter Seals
233 South Wacker Drive
Suite 2400
Chicago, IL 60606
800-221-6827
easterseals.com

Rick Davidson, Chair
Eileen Howard Boone, First Vice Chairman
Joseph G. Kern, Second Vice Chairman
Edward L. Wenzel, Secretary

Easter Seals provides exceptional services, education, outreach and advocacy so that people living with autism spectrum disorders and other disabilities can live, learn, work, and play in our communities.

838 Educational Accessibility Services
Wayne State University
5155 Gullen Mall
1600 Undergraduate Library
Detroit, MI 48202   313-577-1851
FAX: 313-577-4898
TTY:313-577-3365
studentdisability@wayne.edu
studentdisability.wayne.edu/

Jane DePriester-Morandini,, Interim Dir.
Randie Kruman, M.A., University Counselor II
Kimberly Werth, M.A., LLPC, Professional Technician
Fran Marlowe, Program Specialist

To ensure a university experience in which individuals with disabilities have equitable access to programs and to empower students to self advocate i norder to fulfill their academic goals.

839 Elwyn
111 Elwyn Road
Elwyn, PA 19063   610-891-2000
info@elwyn.org
elwyn.org

Joseph E. Pappano Jr.,M.D., Chair
J. Richard Leaman, Jr., Vice Chairman
Linnette W. Black, Vice Chairman
Sandra S. Cornelius, Ph.D, President

our organization is recognized as a pioneer in developing groundbreaking programs for children and adults with disabilities and disadvantages.

840 Enable America Inc.
101 E. Kennedy Boulevard
Suite 3250
Tampa, FL 33602   877-362-2533
FAX: 813-222-3298
richard.salem@enableamerica.org
enableamerica.org

Richard J. Salem, Founder/CEO
Chris Jadick, Executive Director
Sandy Moonert, Program Director

Enable America's objective is to increase employment among people with disabilities in the United States.

841 Esalen Institute
55000 Highway 1
Big Sur, CA 93920   831-667-3000
888-837-2536
FAX: 831-667-2724
info@esalen.org
www.esalen.org

Gordon Wheeler, President
Tricia McEntee, Chief Executive Officer
Cheryl Franzel, Director of Programs
Patrick Sheridan, Operations Director

Founded in 1962 as an alternative education center devoted to the exploration of the world of unrealized human capacities that lies beyond the imagination. Blends East/West philosophies, experiential/didactic workshops, and a steady influx of philosophers, psychologists, artists, and religious thinkers.

842 Family Resource Center on Disabilities
11 E. Adams St.
Suite 1002
Chicago, IL 60603   312-939-3513
800-952-4199
FAX: 312-854-8980
TTY: 312-939-3519
info@frcd.org
www.frcd.org

843 Family Voices
3701 San Mateo Blvd. N.E.
Suite 103
Albuquerque, NM 87110   505-872-4774
888-835-5669
FAX: 505-872-4780
lkeene@familyvoices.org
www.familyvoices.org

Molly Cole, President
Marcia O'Malley, Vice-President
Leolinda Parlin, Treasurer
Grace P. Williams, Secretary

Not-for-profit voluntary organization dedicated to ensuring that children's health issues are addressed as public and private healthcare systems undergo change in communities, states and the nation. National grassroots clearinghouse for information and education in ways to assure and improve health care for children with disabilities and chronic conditions. Provides materials including pamphlets, a newsletter and one-page papers on important topics.

844 Favarh/Farmington Valley ARC
225 Commerce Dr
Canton, CT 06019-2478   860-693-6662
FAX: 860-693-8662
favarh@favarh.org
www.favarh.org

George Kral, President
Ernest E. Mack, Vice President
Fran Traceski, Treasurer
Augusto Russell, Secretary

Provides a variety of programs and services to adults with developmental, physical or mental disabilities and their families throughout the Farmington Valley communities of Avon, Burlington and more. Favarh's programs are designed to enhance the personal, social, emotional, vocational and living capabilities of persons with disabilities.

845   Fedcap Rehabilitation Services
633 Third Avenue
6th Floor
New York, NY 10017   212-727-4200
                                 FAX: 212-727-4374
                                 TTY:212-727-4384
                                     info@fedcap.org
                                     www.fedcap.org

Mark O'Donoghue, Chair
Laurence Ach, Vice Chair
Christine McMahon, President and CEO
Joseph Giannetto, Chief Operating Officer
Fedcap helps people with barriers achieve economic independence through employment. Through evaluation, vocational and soft-skills training, job placement, job creation and support programs, each year Fedcap helps thousands of Americans overcome obstacles, rebuild their lives, and find and keep meaningful employment.

846   Federation for Children with Special Needs
529 Main Street
Suite 1102
Boston, MA 02129   617-236-7210
                                      800-331-0688
                                 FAX: 617-241-0330
                                     fcsninfo@fcsn.org
                                        www.fcsn.org

James F. Whalen, President
Rich Robison, Executive Director
Maureen Jerz, Director of Development
Michael Weiner, Treasurer
The Federation for Children with Special Needs provides information, support, and assistance to parents of children with disabilities, their professional partners, and their communities. We are committed to listening to and learning from families, and encouraging full participation in community life by all people, especially those with disabilities.

847   Federation of Families for Children's Mental Health
15883-A Crabbs Branch Way
Suite D23A
Rockville, MD 20855   240-403-1901
                                 FAX: 240-403-1909
                                     ffcmh@ffcmh.org
                                        www.ffcmh.org

Teka Dempson, President
Sherri Luthe, Vice President
Diana Autin, Board Member
Kristin Melton, Secretary
The FFCMH, a nationally family-run organization serves to provide advocacy at the national level for the rights of children and youth with emotional, behavioral and mental health challenges and their families. Provide leadership and technical assistance to a nation-wide network of family run organizations. Collaborate with family run and other child serving organizations to transform mental health care in America. The correct name is National Federation of Families for Children's Mental Health.

848   Feingold Association of the US
11849 Suncatcher Drive
Fishers, IN 46037   631-369-9340
                                      800-321-3287
                                 FAX: 631-369-2988
                                     help@feingold.org
                                        www.feingold.org

Annette Miller, President
Kathleen Bratby MSN, RN, Secretary
Larisa Scarbrough, Vice President
Gail Wachsmuth, Treasurer
An organization of families and professionals, the Feingold Association of the United States is dedicated to helping children and adults apply proven dietary techniques for better behavior, learning and health.

849   Feldenkrais Guild of North America (FGNA)
401 Edgewater Place
Suite 600
Wakefield, MA 01880   781-876-8935
                                      800-775-2118
                                 FAX: 781-645-1322
                            executivedirector@feldenkrais.com
                                     www.feldenkrais.com

Susan Marshall, Executive Director
Robert Black, BA, MSc, President
Jaclyn Boone, Vice President
Tom Bode, Treasurer
This is the organization which sets the standards for and certifies all FELDENKRAIS practitioners in North America. In order to practice, a practitioner must be a graduate of an FGNA accredited program (a minimum of 800 instruction hours over a three to four year period), and agree to follow both the Code of Professional Conduct and the Standards of Practice. FGNA may be contacted for further information about the FELDENKRAIS METHOD or for a list of FELDENKRAIS practitioners sorted by region.

850   Focus Alternative Learning Center
126 Dowd Avenue
PO Box 452
Canton, CT 06019   860-693-8809
                                 FAX: 860-693-0141
                            info@focuscenterforautism.org
                               www.focuscenterforautism.org

Marcia Bok, President
Claudia Godburn, Secretary
Rita Barredo, Treasurer
Carol Doiron, LCSW, Dir. of Education Svcs
A private non profit, licensed clinical and learning center specialized in the treatment of creatively wired and socially challenged kids. We treat kids on the autism spectrum who suffer from high anxiety, experience processing difficulties and learning problems. The name has been changed to FOCUS Center for Autism.

851   George Washington University Health Resource Center
2134 G St NW
Washington, DC 20052-0001
                                     askheath@gwu.edu
                                     www.heath.gwu.edu

Stephen J Trachtenberg, CEO
Timothy W. Tong, Ph.D., Dean-School of Engineering
Rachelle Heller, Ph.D., Assoc. Dean, Academic Affairs
William Roper, Ph.D., Civil & Env Engineer
National clearinghouse for information about education after high school for people with disabilities. Also serves as an information exchange about educational support services, policies, procedures, adaptations and opportunities on American campuses, vocational-technical schools, adult education programs, independent living centers and other training entities after high school.

852   Goodwill Industries International
15810 Indianola Dr
Rockville, MD 20855   301-530-6500
                                      800-GOO-WILL
                                 FAX: 301-530-1516
                                 TTY: 301-530-9759
                                  contactus@goodwill.org
                                      www.goodwill.org

Jim Gibbons, President/CEO
Lauren Lawson, Public Relations Director
Pat Boelter, Vice President of Marketing
Paul Spears, SCSEP Program Manager
Strives to achieve the full participation in society of disabled persons and other individuals with special needs by expanding their opportunities and occupational capabilities through a network of autonomous, nonprofit, community-based organizations providing services throughout the world in response to local needs.

853 HRSA Information Center
5600 Fishers Lane
Rockeville, MD 20857

301-443-3376
877-464-4772
888-275-4772
FAX: 703-821-2098
TTY:877-489-4772
press@hrsa.gov
www.ask.hrsa.gov

Jim Macrae, MA, MPP, Acting Administrator
Diana Espinosa, Deputy Administrator
Martin Kramer, Communications Director
Leslie Atkinson, Legislation Director

Provides publications, information, resources, and referrals about health care services for medically underserved individuals and populations.

854 Haldimand-Norfolk Resource Education and Counseling
101 Nanticoke Creek Parkway
Townsend, ON, Canada N0A-1S0

519-587-2441
800-265-8087
FAX: 519-587-4798
info@hnreach.on.ca
www.hnreach.on.ca

Ronelda Smith, President
Clarence Wheaton, Vice President
Jeff Lefler, Secretary/Treasurer
Lisa Wallace, Member at Large

Promote and support community well-being by providing co-ordinated access, planning, programs and services for individuals and families.

855 Health Action
5276 Hollister Ave
Ste 257
Santa Barbara, CA 93111

805-617-3390
FAX: 805-685-4710
ha@healthaction.net
www.healthaction.net

Dr. Roger Jahnke, Co Founder and CEO
Rebecca Mclean, Co Founder

Our mission is to foster innovation in health care that will increase health status, increase customer satisfaction, increase profitability, increase clinical efficacy and eliminate error, support provider efficiency and enhance clinical outcomes, and empower consumer self-managed care.

856 Health Resource Center for Women with Disabilities
Rehabilitation Institute of Chicago
345 E Superior St
Chicago, IL 60611

312-238-1000
800-354-7342
FAX: 312-238-1616
webmaster@ric.org
www.ric.org

Jude Reyes, Chair
Thomas A. Reynolds III, Esq., Vice Chair
Mike P. Krasny, Vice Chair
Joanne C. Smith, MD, President/CEO

RIC has earned a worldwide reputation as being a leader in patient health care, advocacy, research and educating health professionals in physical medicine and rehabilitation. People from around the globe choose RIC because of our expertise in treating a range of conditions, from the most complex conditions including cerebral palsy, spinal cord injury, stroke and traumatic brain injury, to the more common, such as arthritis, chronic pain, and sports injuries.

857 Homeopathic Educational Services
2124B Kittredge St
Berkeley, CA 94704

510-649-0294
800-359-9051
FAX: 510-649-1955
email@homeopathic.com
www.homeopathic.com

Dana Ulman, MPH, Owner

Resource center for homeopathic products and services including books, tapes, research, medicines, medicine kits, software for the general public and the health professional and correspondence courses.

858 Human Ecology Action League (HEAL)
PO Box 509
Stockbridge, GA 30281

770-389-4519
FAX: 770-389-4520
HEALNatnl @aol.com / HEAL3@aol.com
www.healnatl.org

859 Institute for Scientific Research
1000 Technology Dr
Ste 1000
Fairmont, WV 26554

304-366-2577
877-363-5482
FAX: 304-366-2699
jestep@wvhtf.org
www.wvhtf.org

James R. Haney, Chair
James L. Estep, President/CEO
Dr. Brian Lemoff, VP, Advanced Technologies
Nancy E. Trudel, Esquire, General Counsel & Corporate Sec

Institute for Scientific Research, Inc. performs cutting-edge research across a variety of scientific and engineering disciplines. Our people participate in world-class projects from concept through development, in some of today's most fascinating scientific fields.

860 Institute of Transpersonal Psychology
1069 E Meadow Cir
Palo Alto, CA 94303

650-493-4430
FAX: 650-493-6835
Student_Services@sofia.edu
sofia.edu/

Qiaoyun Li, Ph.D., President
Sara Javid, VP of Strategic Planning
Barbara Hecker, J.D., Ph.D., Dean of Faculty
Olga Louchakova-Schwartz, Director of Research

The Institute of Transpersonal Psychology is a private, non-sectarian graduate school accredited by the Western Association of Schools and Colleges. For over twenty-five years the Institute has remained a leader at the forefront of psychological research and education, probing the mind, body, spirit connection. The Institute's challenging and transformative educational paradigm has attracted students from all over the world.

861 International Association of Machinists
9000 Machinists Place
Upper Marlboro, MD 20772-2687

301-967-4500
FAX: 301-967-4588
websteward@iamaw.org
www.goiam.org

R Thomas Buffenbarger, President
Robert Martinez, Jr., General Vice President
Diane Babineaux, Executive Council
Robert Roach, Jr., General Secretary-Treasurer

Placement programs for persons with disabilities.

862 International Association of Yoga Therapists
PO Box 251563
Little Rock, AZ 72225

928-541-0004
FAX: 928-541-0182
mail@iayt.org
www.iayt.org

Dilip Sarkar, MD, FACS, CAP, President
John Kepner, MA, MBA, CYTh, Executive Director
Kelly Birch, Editor-in-Chief
Matra Raj, OTR, E-RYT 500, Treasurer & Secretary

IAYT supports research and education in Yoga and serves Yoga practitioners, Yoga teachers, Yoga therapists, health care professionals, and researchers worldwide. Our mission is to establish Yoga as a recognised and respected therapy in the Western world. IAYT also serves members, the media, and the general public as a comprehensive source of information about contemporary Yoga education, research, and statistics.

863 International Chiropractors Association
6400 Arlington Blvd
Ste. 800
Falls Church, VA 22042   703-528-5000
                                           800-423-4690
                                      FAX: 703-528-5023
                                 chiro@chiropractic.org
                                    www.chiropractic.org

Huygo V. Gibson, DC, FICA, Chair
George B. Curry, DC, FICA, President
Stephen P. Welsh, DC, FIFA, Vice President
Sharon Gorman, DC, Director
Established in 1926 to empower humanity in the expression of
maximum health, wellness and human potential through the universal chiropractic expression and utilization. Strives to advance
chiropractics throughout the world as a distinct health care profession predicated upon its unique philosophy, science and art.

864 International Clinic of Biological Regeneration
PO Box 509
Florissant, MO 63032   314-921-3997
                                           800-826-5366
                                      FAX: 314-921-8485
                                         icbr@aol.com
                                          www.icbr.com

Dr. C. Tom Smith, Medical Director
Judith A. Smith, Co Founder & Director
Dr. William Johnson, Director of Medical Services
The International Clinic of Biological Regeneration (ICBR) is a
leading international cell therapy center that has been in continuous operation since 1981. During this time, Dr. Smith has constantly improved theraputic results of the treatment by selecting
newer, safer and more effective formulations as delveloped by
leading European research centers.

865 International Women's Health Coalition
333 7th Ave
6th Fl
New York, NY 10001   212-979-8500
                                      FAX: 212-979-9009
                                         info@iwhc.org
                                          www.iwhc.org

Marlene Hess, Chair
Debora Diniz, Vice Chair
Susan Nitze, Vice Chair
Francoise Girard, President
Information and pamphlets on sexually transmitted diseases and
other health concerns. IWHC works to generate health and popu-
lation policies, programs, and funding that promote and protect
the rights and health of girls and women worldwide.

866 Invisible Disabilities Association
P.O. Box 4067
Parker, CO 80134
                                          800-223-TALK
                                 invisibledisabilities.org

Wayne Connell, President/Founder
Steve Tonkin, Vice President
Ann Speer, Treasurer
Jim Calanni, JD, Secretary
The Invisible Disabilities Association (IDA) encourages, edu-
cates and connects people and organizations touched by illness,
pain and disability around the globe.

867 Job Accommodation Network
PO Box 6080
Morgantown, WV 26506-6080   304-293-7186
                                           800-526-7234
                                      FAX: 304-293-5407
                                      TTY: 877-781-9403
                                        jan@askjan.org
                                         www.jan.wvu.edu

Anne Hirsh, Co-Director
Louis Orslene, Co-Director
Linda Carter Batiste, Principal Consultants
Beth Loy, Principal Consultants
JAN's mission is to facilitate the employment and retention of
workers with disabilities by providing employers, employment

providers, people with disabilities, their family members and
other interested parties with information on job accomodations,
self-employment and small business opportunities and related
subjects. JAN's efforts are in support of the employment, including self-employment and small business ownership, of people
with disabilities.

868 Joni and Friends
PO Box 3333
Agoura Hills, CA 91376-3333   818-707-5664
                                           800-736-4177
                                      FAX: 818-707-2391
                                      TTY: 818-707-9707
                                 jafmin@joniandfriends.org
                                    www.joniandfriends.org

Joni Eareckson-Tada, Founder and CEO
Doug Mazza, President & COO
Billy Burnett, VP/CFO
Lorraine Mazza, VP of Development
A nonprofit organization seeking to accelerate Christian ministry
with people affected by disabilities. JAF educates churches and
the community worldwide concerning the needs of the disabled
and how those needs can be met. We sponsor family retreats for
families with disabled members. Wheels for the World collects,
restores and distributes used wheelchairs to disadvantaged
populations around the world.

869 Juvenile Diabetes Research Foundation International
26 Broadway
14th Fl
New York, NY 10004   212-785-9500
                                           800-533-2873
                                      FAX: 212-785-9595
                                         info@jdrf.org
                                          www.jdrf.org

Mary Tyler Moore, International Chairman
Stephen Newman, MD, Vice Chairman
Karen Case, Treasurer/ Chair, Finance
Max C. Chapman, Secretary
The world's leading nonprofit, nongovernmental funder of diabetes research. It was founded in 1970 by parents of children with
diabetes. JDF's mission is to find a cure for diabetes and its complications through the support of research. JDF also sponsors international workshops and conferences for biomedical
researchers, individual chapters offer support groups and other
activities for families affected by diabetes. JDF has more than
110 chapters and affiliates worldwide. Quarterly newsletter.

870 Lambton County Developmental Services
339 Centre Street
PO Box 1210
Petrolia, ON, Canada N0N- 1R0   519-882-0933
                                      FAX: 519-882-3386
                                 administration@lcds.on.ca
                                      www.lcds.on.ca

Adrian Vermeiren, President
Tony Hogervorst, 1st Vice-President
Kari Lupton, 2nd Vice-President
Frank Backx, Treasurer
A network of caring people, working together to provide services
for people with developmental disabilities to facilitate the
achievement of their life dreams.

871 Learning Disabilities Association of America
4156 Library Rd
Pittsburgh, PA 15234-1349   412-341-1515
                                      FAX: 412-344-0224
                                    info@ldaamerica.org
                                      www.ldaamerica.org

Mary-Clare Reynolds, Executive Director
Stephanie Fedro-Byrom, Operations Manager
Joyce Kraemer, Conference Coordinator
Ericka Pardun, Communications Coordinator
LDA's mission is to create opportunities for success for all indi-
viduals affected by learning disabilities and to reduce the inci-
dence of learning disabilities in future generations.

872   Learning Disabilities Association of New York State
Learning Disabilities Association of America
1190 Troy-Schenectady Rd
Latham, NY 12110   518-608-8992
                                                   FAX: 518-608-8993
                                                      www.ldanys.org

Michael Helman, President
Charles Giglio, Vice President
The Learning Disabilities Association (LDA) is a non-profit organization advocating for children and adults with learning disabilities. LDA is a three-tiered organization comprised of a national organization, state affiliates and local chapters. In New York, LDA's state affiliate, the Learning Disabilities Association of New York State and its network of 8 local chapters serve as the conduit of information, advocacy and services for individuals with learning disabilities and their families.

873   Learning Disabilities Worldwide
14 Nason St.
Maynard, MA 1754   978-897-5399
                                                   FAX: 978-897-5355
                                                   info@ldworldwide.org
                                                   www.ldworldwide.org
Teresa Allissa Citro, Chief Executive Officer
Michael Stressenger, Business Manager
Deanne Arcuri, Conferences & Events Coordinator
Joseph Citro, Environmental Health Director
Learning Disabilities Worldwide, Inc. (LDWr), established in 1965, is an international professional organization dedicated to improving the educational, professional, and personal outcomes for individuals with learning disabilities (LD) and other related disorders.

874   LoSeCa Foundation
215-1 Carnegie Drive
St Albert, AB T8N-5B1   780-460-1400
                                                   FAX: 780-459-1380
                                                   rbourret@telus.net
                                                   www.loseca.ca
Ron Bourret, Program Manager
Raymond Nkorimana, Program Manager
Francois Busque, Program Manager
Jules Lefebvre, Human Resources Manager
A non-profit organization that provides support services to adults with developmental disabilities

875   MCC Supportive Care Services
103-2776 Bourquin Cres. West
Abbotsford, BC V2S-6A4   604-850-6608
                                                        800-622-5455
                                                   FAX: 604-850-2634
                                                   office@communitascare.com
                                                   www.communitascare.com/
Marlyce Friesen, Board Chair
Jacquie Lepp, Treasurer
Karyn Santiago, Chief Executive Officer
Gillian Viljoen, Chief Program Officer
A service provider, advocate and resource for persons living and dealing with mental, physical and/or emotional disabilities. The correct name is Communitas Supportive Care Society.

876   Mainstream
300 S Rodney Parham Rd
Ste 5
Little Rock, AR 72205-4774   501-280-0012
                                                        800-371-9026
                                                   FAX: 501-280-9267
                                                   TTY: 501-280-9262
                                                   www.mainstreamilrc.com

877   March of Dimes Birth Defects Foundation
1275 Mamaroneck Ave
White Plains, NY 10605-5201   914-997-4488
                                                   FAX: 914-428-8203
                                                   nbrown@marchofdimes.com
                                                   www.marchofdimes.com/
Dr. Jennifer Howse, President
Richard Mulligan, Exec VP
Lisa Bellsey, Esq., SVP & General Counsel
The mission of the March of Dimes is to improve the health of babies by preventing birth defects and infant mortality.

878   Mental Health America
2000 N Beauregard Street
6th Floor
Alexandria, VA 22311   703-684-7722
                                                        800-969-6642
                                                   FAX: 703-684-5968
                                                   dshern@mentalhealthamerica.net
                                                   www.mentalhealthamerica.net
Paul Gionfriddo, President and CEO
Peter Carson, Senior VP of Operations
Julie Nicholson Burke, VP of Finance
Mike Turner, VP of Dev
Nonprofit organization addressing all issues related to mental health and mental illness. With more than 340 affiliates nationwide, NMHA works to improve the mental health of all Americans, especially the 54 million individuals with mental disorders, through advocacy, education, research and service.

879   Metametrix Clinical Laboratory
63 Zillicoa Street
Asheville, NC 28801-2552   828-253-0621
                                                        800-522-4762
                                                   FAX: 828-252-9303
                                                   inquiries@metametrix.com
                                                   www.gdx.net
Chris Smith, President and CEO
Andrew Church, Vice President
Darryl Landis, Chief Medical Officer
Ceco Ivanov, Chief Information Officer
Metametrix Clinical Laboratory has been a pioneer and leader in the development of nutritional, metabolic, and toxicant analyses since 1984. Metametrix is committed to helping health care professionals identify nutritional influences on health and disease, and is recognized internationally for its laboratory procedures in nutritional and biochemical testing.

880   Mind, Body, Health Sciences
PO Box 1300
Tesuque, NM 87574-9769   303-440-8460
                                                   FAX: 303-440-7580
                                                   luzie@joanborysenko.com
                                                   www.joanborysenko.com
Joan Borysenko, Founder
publish free annual newsletter/cataloge:Circle of Healing. Information about the works of Joan Borysenko.

881   Muscular Dystrophy Association - USA
222 S. Riverside Plaza
Suite 1500
Chicago, IL 85718-3299   520-529-2000
                                                        800-572-1717
                                                   FAX: 520-529-5454
                                                   mda@mdausa.org
                                                   www.mda.org
Steven M. Derks, President and CEO
Valerie A. Cwik, Executive Vice President
Julie Faber, Chief Financial Officer
Steven G. Ford, Marketing Officer
MDA provides comprehensive medical services to tens of thousands of people with neuromuscular diseases at some 230 hospital-affiliated clinics across the country. The Association's worldwide research program, which funds over 400 individual scientific investigations annually, represents the largest single effort to advance knowledge of neuromuscular diseases and to find cures and treatments for them. In addition, MDA conducts

far-reaching educational programs for the public and professionals.

882   National Association for Holistic Aromatherapy
PO Box 27871
Raleigh, NC 27611-7871   919-894-0298
                                   FAX: 919-894-0271
                                   info@naha.org
                                   www.naha.org

Annette Davis, President
Jennifer Pressimone, Vice President
Rose Chard, Secretary
Eric Davis, Treasurer

The NAHA is an educational, nonprofit organization dedicated to enhancing public awareness of the benefits of true aromatherapy. It offers aromatherapy Tele-classes & membership benefits, and acts as a referral service.

883   National Association of Blind Merchants
1837 S Nevada Ave
PMB #243
Colorado Springs, CO 80905   719-423-4384
                                   888-691-1819
                                   kevanwirkey@blindmerchants.org
                                   www.blindmerchants.org

Nicky Gacos, President

Membership organization of blind persons employed in either self-employment work or the Randolph-Sheppard vending program. Provides information regarding rehabilitation, social security, tax and other issues which directly affect blind merchants. Serves as advocacy and support group.

884   National Association of Councils on Developmental Disabilities
1825 K Street NW
Suite 600
Washington, DC 20006   202-506-5813
                                   info@nacdd.org
                                   www.nacdd.org

885   National Association of Developmental Disabilities Councils
1825 K Street, NW
Suite 600
Washington, DC 20006   202-506-5813
                                   FAX: 202-506-5846
                                   info@nacdd.org
                                   www.nacdd.org

Claire Mantonya, President, Exec. Dir.
Michael Brogioli, CEO
John Morris, Treasurer, Exec. Dir.
Sheryl Matney, Senior Mgr, Council Svcs

The National Association of Councils on Developmental Disabilities (NACDD) is a national, member-driven organization consisting of 55 State and Territorial Councils. NACDD places high value on meaningful participation and contribution by Council members.

886   National Association of Disability Representatives
PO Box 96503 #30550
Washington, DC 20090-6503   202-822-2155
                                   800-747-6131
                                   FAX: 972-245-6701
                                   www.nadr.org

Robert McDowell, President
Steven Skinner, Vice President
Philip Litteral, Secretary
Michael Wener, Treasurer

For many years, Professional Social Security Claimants Representatives have wanted to have an organization that would be interested in their issues, educational opportunities, and interests. In March of 2000, 35 Professional Social Security Claimants Representatives met in St. Louis, MO and formed NADR, Inc.

887   National Association of State Directors of Developmental Disabilities Services (NASDDDS)
301 N Fairfax Street
Suite 101
Alexandria, VA 22314-2633   703-683-4202
                                   FAX: 703-684-1395
                                   cmosely@nasddds.org
                                   www.nasddds.org

Laura L. Nuss, President
Bernard Simons, Vice President
John Martin, Secretary
Jane Gallivan, Past President

The association's goal is to promote and assist state agencies in developing effective, efficient service delivery systems that furnish high-quality supports to people with developmental disabilities.

888   National Business & Disability Council
201 I U Willets Rd
Albertson, NY 11507-1516   516-465-1400
                                   FAX: 516-465-3730
                                   info@viscardicenter.org
                                   www.viscardicenter.org/services/nbdc

John D. Kemp, President/CEO
Michael C. Pascucci, Exec. Leadership Team
Brandon M. Macsata, General Consultant
Gary Karp, Training Consultant

The NBDC is the leading resource for employers seeking to integrate people with disabilities into the workplace and companies seeking to reach them in the consumer marketplace.

889   National Center for Education in Maternal and Child Health
Georgetown University
PO Box 571272
Washington, DC 20057-1272   202-784-9770
                                   877-624-1935
                                   FAX: 202-784-9777
                                   mchlibrary@ncemch.org
                                   www.ncemch.org

Rochelle Mayer, Research Professor and Director
John Richards, Co-director
Jeanne Anastasi, Senior program specialist
Sarah Riehl, Researcher

Provides information on children with special health needs, child health and development, adolescent health, nutrition, violence and injury prevention and other issues of maternal and child health for health professionals and the public.

890   National College of Naturopathic Medicine
049 SW Porter St
Portland, OR 97201-4848   503-552-1555
                                   FAX: 503-226-8133
                                   jstanard@ncnm.edu
                                   www.ncnm.edu

Ellen Goldsmith, Board Chair
Willow Moore, Board Vice Chair
Brian Camastral, Board Secretary
Don Drake, Chair Strategic Pathways Comm

NCNM offers two graduate professional degrees in accredited and recognized programs that prepare you for licensed practice in many states and provinces: Doctor of Naturopathic Medicine, a four-year program of clinical sciences and holistic methods of heal

891   National Council on Disability
1331 F Street Northwest
Suite 850
Washington, DC 20004- 1138   202-272-2004
                                   FAX: 202-272-2022
                                   TTY:202-272-2074
                                   ncd@ncd.gov
                                   www.ncd.gov

Aaron Bishop, Exec. Dir.
Anne Sommers, Dir. of Legislative Affairs
Joan M. Durocher, General Counsel & Dir. of Policy
Sylvia Menifee, Dir. of Administration

NCD is a small, independent federal agency charged with advising the President, Congress, and other federal agencies regarding policies, programs, practices, and procedures that affect people with disabilities.

892 National Council on Independent Living
2013 H St. NW
6th Floor
Washington, DC 20006   202-207-0334
877-525-3400
FAX: 202-207-0341
TTY: 202-207-0340
ncil@ncil.org
www.ncil.org

Kelly Buckland, Executive Director
Lou Ann Kibbee, President
Mark Derry, Vice President
Ann McDaniel, Secretary
NCIL advances independent living and the rights of people with disabilities through consumer-driven advocacy.

893 National Deaf Education Network and Clearinghouse/Info To Go
Deaf Education Center/Gallaudet University
800 Florida Ave NE
Washington, DC 20002-3695   202-651-5051
FAX: 202-651-5704
TTY:202-651-5052
clerc.center@gallaudet.edu.
www.gallaudet.edu/clerc_center

Dr T Alan Hurwitz, President
Edward Bosso, VP, National Deaf Education
Dr. Lynne Murray, VP for Dev. and Alumni Relations
Dr. Cynthia King, Chief Information Officer
Info to Go, from the Laurent Clerc National Deaf Education Center, provides information on topics dealing with deafness and hearing loss in children and young people under 21 years of age.

894 National Disability Rights Network
820 1st Street NE
Suite 740
Washington, DC 20002-3560   202-408-9514
FAX: 202-408-9520
TTY:202-408-9521
info@ndrn.org
www.ndrn.org

Rocky Nichols, President
Kim Moody, Vice President
Teresa Larsen, Secretary
Elmer Cerano, Treasurer
Voluntary national membership association of protection and advocacy systems and client assistance programs. Promoting and strengthening the role and performance of its members in providing quality legally based advocacy services.

895 National Dissemination Center for Children and Youth with Disabilities (NICHCY)
35 Halsey St.
Fourth Floor
Newark, NJ 07102   202-884-8200
800-695-0285
FAX: 202-884-8441
TTY: 800-695-0285
nichcy@aed.org
www.parentcenterhub.org/nichcy-gone

Myriam Alizo, project assistant
Carol Valdivieso, Principal Investigator
Theresa Rebhorn, Writer / Designer
Lisa Kupper, Writer / Designer
NICHCY is the center that provides information to the nation on disabilities in children and youth; programs and services for infants, children, and youth with disabilities; IDEA, the nation's special education law; and research-based information on effective practices for children with disabilities.

896 National Early Childhood Technical Assistance Center
CB 8040
Chapel Hill, NC 27599-8040   919-962-2001
FAX: 919-966-7463
ectacenter@unc.edu
ectacenter.org

Lynne Kahn, Dir. & Principal Investigator
Joan Danaher, Associate Dir. Information
Christina Kasprzak, Associate Dir. Evaluation
Martha Diefendorfer, Associate Director
Assists states and other designated governing jurisdictions as they develop multidisciplinary, coordinated and comprehensive services for children with special needs.

897 National Easter Seal Society
233 S Wacker Drive
Ste 2400
Chicago, IL 60606-4851   312-726-6200
800-221-6827
FAX: 312-726-1494
TTY: 312-726-4258
www.easterseals.com

Rick Davidson, Chairman
Eileen Howard Boone, 1st Vice Chairman
Edward L. Wenzel, Treasurer
Nancy Goguen, Secretary
Easter Seals provides exceptional services, education, outreach, and advocacy so that people living with autism and other disabilities can live, learn, work and play in our communities.

898 National Guild of Hypnotists
PO Box 308
Merrimack, NH 03054-0308   603-429-9438
FAX: 603-424-8066
ngh@ngh.net
www.ngh.net

Dr. Dwight F Damon, DC, DNGH, OB, President
Don Mottin, NGH VP, CMI, D, Vice President
Melody Damon-Bachand, BCH, Executive Director
Dawn Huard, CH, Membership / Member Services
The National Guild of Hypnotists, Inc.is a not-for-profit, educational corporation in the State of New Hampshire. Officially founded in Boston, Massachusetts in 1950 the Guild is a professional organization comprised of dedicated individuals committed to advancing the field of hypnotism.

899 National Information Center for Children
35 Halsey St.
Fourth Floor
Newark, NJ 07102   202-884-8200
800-695-0285
FAX: 202-884-8441
TTY: 800-695-0285
nichcy@fhi360.org
www.parentcenterhub.org/nichcy-gone

Myriam Alizo, project assistant
Carol Valdivieso, Principal Investigator
Theresa Rebhorn, Writer / Designer
Lisa Kupper, Writer / Designer
Information on disabilities and disibility-related issues for family, educators and professionals related to children and youth.

900 National Institute on Disability and Rehabilitation Research
Potomac Center Building
550 12 St., SW
Washington, DC 20202-7100   202-245-7640
800-872-5327
FAX: 202-245-7643
TTY: 800-437-0833
nidrr-mailbox@ed.gov
www.ed.gov

Charlie Lakin, Dir.
Ruth Brannon, Acting Deputy Dir.
Tim Muzzio, Dir. Program Budget
Conducts comprehensive and coordinated programs of research and related activities to maximize the full inclusion, social integration, employment and independent living of individuals of all ages with disabilities. NIDRR's focus includes research in areas

such as employment, health and function, technology for access and function, independent living and community integration, and other associated disability research areas.

901   National Organization on Disability
77 Water Street
Ste 204
New York, NY 10005   646-505-1191
                                 FAX: 646-505-1184
                          kbitting@weareneiman
                                    www.nod.org

Carol Glazer, President
Kate Brady, Dir. of Res
Anne Fitzsimmons, Project & Business Associate
Howard Green, Deputy Director
The National Organization on Disability promotes the full and equal participation of men, women and children with disabilities in all aspects of American life. Founded in 1982, NOD is the leading national disability organization concerned with all disabil

902   National Rehabilitation Association (NRA)
P.O Box 150235
Alexandria, VA 22315-4109   703-836-0850
                                      888-258-4295
                                 FAX: 703-836-0848
                                 TTY: 703-836-0849
                              info@nationalrehab.org
                                www.nationalrehab.org

Beverlee Stafford, Executive Director
Sandra Mulliner, Administrative Assistant
Patricia Leahy, Governmental Affairs Director
Brian Coupe, Membership Director
NRA members work to eliminate barriers and increase employment opportunities for people with disabilities. We provide our members opportunities for advocacy and increased awareness of issues through professional development and access to current research topics.

903   National Rehabilitation Information Center(NARIC)
8400 Corporate Drive
Suite 500
Landover, MD 20785-2245   301-459-5900
                                      800-346-2742
                                 FAX: 301-459-4263
                          naricinfo@heitechservices.com
                                    www.naric.com

Mark Odum, Director
Mark X. Odum, Project Director
Jessica H. Chaiken, Information Services Manager
Catherine E. Graves, Media/Information Specialist
NARIC is a federally-funded library and information center that focuses on disability and rehabilitation information.

904   National Vaccine Information Center
21525 Ridgetop Circle
Suite 100
Sterling, VA 20166-4737   703-938-3783
                                 FAX: 571-313-1268
                             contactnvic@gmail.com
                                    www.nvic.org

Barbara Loe Fisher, Co-Founder/President
Kathi Williams, Co-Founder/VP
Theresa Wrangham, Executive Director
Paul Arthur, Director of Operations
A national nonprofit educational organization dedicated to preventing, through public education, vaccine injuries and deaths. NVIC represents vaccine consumers and health care providers, including parents whose children suffered illness or died following vaccination. NVIC supports the right of vaccine consumers to have access to the safest and most effective vaccine as well as the right to make informed, independent vaccination decisions.

905   National Women's Health Network
1413 K St NW
4th Floor
Washington, DC 20005-3459   202-682-2640
                                 FAX: 202-682-2648
                                 nwhn@nwhn.org
                                    www.nwhn.org

Cynthia Pearson, Executive Director
Heidi Gider, Director of Advancement
Christina Cherel, Program Coordinator
Coco Jervis, Program Director
The National Women's Health Network improves the health of all women by developing and promoting a critical analysis of health issues in order to affect policy and support consumer decision-making. The Network aspires to a health care system that is guided by social justice and reflects the needs of diverse women.

906   Native American Protection and Advocacy
PO Box 306
Window Rock, AZ 86515   928-871-4151
                                      800-789-7287
                                 FAX: 928-871-5036
                              www.nativelegalnet.org

Levon Henry, Executive Director
Sylvia Struss, Administrative Director
Kathy Gallagher, Development Director
Victoria Lee, Executive Assistant .
The Native American Protection & Advocacy which helps protect, promote, and expand the legal and human rights of Native Americans with disabilities. There are several goals for this organization, including quality legal representation for individuals with disabilities in various areas such as abuse and neglect, special education, civil rights and discrimination and employment.

907   New York Therapeutic Riding Center-Equestria
                                      212-535-3917
                                 FAX: 212-535-3917
                              info@equestria.org
                                    www.equestria.org

Richard Brodie, Board Of Director
Patricia Neal, Board Of Director
Karen Nielsen Esq., Board Of Director
Peter Rajsingh Esq., Board Of Director
The Therapeutic Riding Center has been conducting therapeutic horseback riding progams for children and adults with disabilities living in New York City for 11 years. Its riding facility is located at the well-equipped Chateau Stables, and staffed by volunteers with experience in physical therapy, osteopathy, art therapy and other areas designed to deal with various aspects of disabled individuals.

908   North America Riding for the Handicapped Association
7475 Dakin Street
Suite #600
Denver, CO 80233-150   303-452-1212
                                      800-369-7433
                                 FAX: 303-252-4610
                                 pathintl@pathintl.org
                                    www.pathintl.org

Kathy Alm, CEO
Kaye Marks, Dir. of Mktg & Comm.
Carolyn Malcheski, Finance/Human Resources Dir.
Jaime Covington, Conference & Events Manager
National nonprofit equestrian organization dedicated to serving individuals with disability by giving disabled individuals the opportunity to ride horses. Establishes safety standards, provides continuing education and offers networking opportunities for both its individuals and center members. Produces educational materials including fact sheets, brochures, booklets, audio-visual tapes, a directory and NARHA's magazine Strides.

909 North Hastings Community Integration Association
2 Alice Street
Box 1508
Bancroft, ON, Canada K0L-1C0 613-332-2090
FAX: 613-332-4762
communityliving@nhcia.ca
www.nhcia.ca

John Muro, President
Cathy Fulford, Vice President
Peter Stone, Treasurer
Aaron Hill, Executive Director
Supports people with an intellectual disability and their families.

910 Nurse Healers: Professional Associates International
TTIA Box 130
Delmar, NY 12054-419 518-325-1185
FAX: 509-693-3537
info@therapeutic-touch.org
www.therapeutic-touch.org

Sue Conlin, QTTT, President
Marjorie Anderson, Communications
Marilyn Johnston-Svoboda, Education & Practice
Denise Coppa, Membership
Cooperative among health professionals interested in healing. Sets the standards for the practice and teaching of Therapeutic Touch. Voluntary, not-for-profit organization.

911 PACER Center (Parent Advocacy Coalition for Educational Rights)
8161 Normandale Blvd
Bloomington, MN 55437-1044 952-838-9000
800-537-2237
FAX: 952-838-0199
TTY: 952-838-0190
pacer@pacer.org
www.pacer.org

Paula F. Goldberg, Executive Director
Mary Schrock, Chief Operating/Development Off
Paul Luehr, Board President
Jessica Broyles, Board Treasurer
Mission is to expand opportunities and enhance the quality of life of children and young adults with disabilities and their families based on the concept of parents helping parents. Offers workshops, individual assistance and written information. Provides programs and materials that assist multicultural families, programs for students, schools and professionals with disability awareness puppet and child abuse prevention programs. Computer Resource Center/Software Lending Library available.

912 PEAK Parent Center
611 N Weber St
Suite 200
Colorado Springs, CO 80903-1072 719-531-9400
800-284-0251
FAX: 719-531-9452
info@peakparent.org
www.peakparent.org

Barbara Buswell, Executive Director
Kent Willis, President Attorney
Janet Brugger, Vice President
Brandi Young, Secretary
PEAK Parent Center is Colorado's federally-designated Parent Training and Information Center (PTI). As a PTI, PEAK supports and empowers parents, providing them with information and strategies to use when advocating for their children with disabilities. PEAK works one-on-one with families and educators helping them realize new possibilities for children with disabilities by expanding knowledge of special education and offering new strategies for success.

913 Pacific Institute of Aromatherapy
PO Box 6723
San Rafael, CA 94903 415-479-9120
FAX: 415-479-0614
contact@osapia.com
www.pacificinstituteofaromatherapy.com

914 Parent Professional Advocacy League
15 Court Square
Suite 660
Boston, MA 02108 617-542-7860
866-815-8122
FAX: 617-542-7832
info@ppal.net
www.ppal.net

Lisa Lambert, Executive Director
Anne Metzger, Treasurer
Anne Silver, Director of Operations
Jessica Childs, Project Coordinator
An organization that promotes a strong voice for families of children and adolescents with mental health needs. PAL advocates for supports, treatment and policies that enable families to live in their communities in an environment of stability and respect.

915 Parents Helping Parents (PHP)
1400 Parkmoor Ave
Ste 100
San Jose, CA 95126-3797 408-727-5775
855-727-5775
FAX: 408-286-1116
info@php.com
www.php.com

Mary Ellen Peterson, M.A., CEO/Executive Director
Suzanne Cistulli, Board Chair
James Quaranta, Board Treasurer
Joyce Uggla, Board Secretary
Dedicated to assisting children with any type of special need: mental, physical, emotional, or learning disability. Mission is to help children with special needs receive love, hope, respect, and services needed to achieve their full potential by strengthening their families and the professionals who serve them. Developed and implemented numerous programs; produce a variety of educational and support materials, including information packets, brochures, database and a quarterly newletter.

916 People First of Canada
120 Maryland St
Suite 5
Winnipeg, MB R3G-1L1 204-784-7362
866-854-8915
FAX: 204-784-7364
info@peoplefirstofcanada.ca
www.peoplefirstofcanada.ca

Kory Earle, President
Shelley Fletcher, Executive Director
Catherine Rodgers, National Coordinator
Lora Beddall, Administrative Assistant
People First of Canada is the national voice for people who have been labeled with an intellectual disability. People First is a movement of people who want all citizens to live equally in the country.

917 People First of Oregon
PO Box 12642
Salem, OR 97309-642 503-362-0336
FAX: 503-585-0287
people1@people1.org
www.people1.org

Steven Kramer, President
Self-advocacy organization of developmentally disabled people who have joined together to learn how to speak for themselves. People first offers support, a united voice and advocacy to its members. Offers information and helps develop service projects in the communities they live in. Offers information and assistance to countries around the world in starting new chapters. Offers participation on DD boards, ARC boards, Transit Boards, and other boards in the community. .

918   People-to-People Committee on Disability
2405 Grand Blvd
Suite 500
Kansas City, MO 64108   816-531-4701
                                         800-676-7874
                                    FAX: 816-561-7502
                                         ptpi@ptpi.org
                                         www.ptpi.org

Mary Eisenhower, President and CEO
Dr. Micah Kubic, Chairman
Anita Manuel, Vice Chairman
Dr. Joyce Ann Miller, Secretary
Individuals concerned about the circumstances of handicapped people throughout the world. Disseminates information, acts as a consultant in promoting exchange activities, coordinates special assistance projects in developing countries and more.

919   People-to-People International: Committee for the Handicapped
2405 Grand Blvd
Suite 500
Kansas City, MO 64108   816-531-4701
                                         800-676-7874
                                    FAX: 816-561-7502
                                         ptpi@ptpi.org
                                         www.ptpi.org

Mary Eisenhower, President and CEO
Dr. Micah Kubic, Chairman
Anita Manuel, Vice Chairman
Dr. Joyce Ann Miller, Secretary
Goals of this committee include: betterment of the handicapped through international unity; educating those with and without handicaps through technical assistance; opening access doors through sensory aids, prosthetic devices and travel tips; and coordination of major international cultural exchanges.

920   Quan Yin Healing Arts Center
965 Mission St
Ste 405
San Francisco, CA 94103-3416   415-861-4964
                                    FAX: 415-644-0614
                                         quanyinone@aol.com
                                         www.quanyinhealingarts.com
Carla Wilson, Exec. Dir.
Colin Howard, President
Hulda Brown, VP
Misha Cohen, Chair, Res & Education
The mission of Quan Yin Healing Arts Center is to provide accessible high quality, affordable acupuncture and Chinese medicine regardless of income. Collaborating with other healthcare providers, we support a holistic philosophy, empowering the individual to take responsibility for their health and well being.

921   Rehabilitation International
1 Liberty Plaza
Office 2342
New York, NY 10006   212-420-1500
                                    FAX: 212-505-0871
                                         info@riglobal.org
                                         www.riglobal.org
Venus Ilagan, Secretary General
Iris Reiss, Rehabilitation Expert
Anne President
RI and its members develop and promote initiatives to protect the rights of people with disabilities and improve rehabilitation and other crucial services for disabled people and their families. RI also works toward increasing international collaboration and advocates for policies and legislation recognizing the rights of people with disabilities and their families, including the establishment of a UN Convention on the Rights and Dignity of Persons with Disabilities.

922   Rehabilitation Services
3075 Orchard Vista Drive SE
PO Box 890
Grand Rapids, MI 49546   616-301-8000
                                         800-695-7273
                                    FAX: 616-301-8010
                                    TTY: 800-649-3777
                                         mtanis@hopenetwork.org
                                         www.hopenetwork.org
Dana DeVos, Chair
Joanne Voorhees, Vice Chair
Patrick A. Miles, jr., Secretary/Treasurer
Wilbur Lettinga, Ex Offico
An office of Hope Netowrk, one of the largest, private, nonprofit organization of its kind in Michigan. The purpose is to assist people with brain injuries and/or physical disabilities in achieving an optimal level of self determinations, dignity, and independence as they develop and attain goals to overcome environmental barriers and mobilize adaptive skills.

923   Rolf Institute
5055 Chaparral Ct
Ste 103
Boulder, CO 80301-3326   303-449-5903
                                         800-530-8875
                                    FAX: 303-449-5978
                                         www.rolf.org
Ida P Rolf, Founder
Diana Yourell, Executive Director
Heidi Hauge, Membership Services Coordinator
Jim Jones, Director of Education
Established in 1971, The Rolf Institute is a nonprofit corporation, organized and existing under the laws of California and Colorado. It is recognized by the US Government as a tax-exempt educational and scientific research organization.

924   Ronald McDonald House
1500 17th St
Huntington, WV 25701-3956   304-529-1122
                                    FAX: 304-529-2970
                                         margaret@mchouse.org
                                         www.mchouse.org
Susan Barnes, Board President
Paul E. Smith, Board Vice President
Robert E. Yost, Board Secretary
Daniel Yon, Board Treasurer
A home-away-from-home, a temporary lodging facility for the families of seriously ill children being treated at nearby hospitals. Each house is run by a local nonprofit agency comprised of members of the medical community, McDonald's owners, businesses and civic organizations and parent volunteers.

925   St. Paul Abilities Network
4637-45 Avenue
St Paul, AB T0A-3A3   780-645-3441
                                         866-645-3900
                                    FAX: 780-645-1885
                                         mail@spanet.ab.ca
                                         www.stpaulabilitiesnetwork.ca
Tim Bear, Executive Director
Dave Lashuk, Finance Controller
Eugene McCafferty, Human Resources
Daina Foerster, Dir. of Residential Svcs
Provides support and opportunities to encourage the development of an individual's full potential through education, advocacy and community partnerships.

926   Student Disability Services
Wayne State University
5155 Gullen Mall
1600 UGL
Detroit, MI 48202-3919   313-577-1851
                                           877-978-4636
                                      FAX: 313-577-4898
                                      TTY: 313-577-3365
                             studentdisability@wayne.edu
                             www.studentdisability.wayne.edu

Randie Kruman, Director
Cherise Frost, Disability Specialist
Fran Marlowe, Program Specialist
Claressa Adams, M. A., Administrative Assistant II
Their mission is to ensure a university experience in which individuals with disabilities have equitable access to programs and to empower students to self-advocate in order to fulfill their academic goals.

927   Teacher Preparation and Special Education
2136 G St NW
Ste 416
Washington, DC 20052   202-994-9283
                                          800-449-7343
                                     FAX: 202-994-8613
                                       gsehdcom@gwu.edu
                                       www.gsehd.gwu.edu

Michael J. Feuer, Dean
Carol Kochhar-Bryant, Senior Associate Dean
Maxine Freund, Associate Dean for Research
Phoebe Stevenson, Administrative Dean
Administers the Education of the Handicapped Act and related programs for the education of handicapped children, including grants to institutions of higher learning and fellowships to train educational personnel. Grants to states for the education of handicapped children, research and demonstration.

928   Technology and Media Division
Council For Exceptional Children
2900 Crystal Drive
Suite 1000
Arlington, VA 22202-3557   866-509-0218
                                          888-232-7733
                                     FAX: 703-264-9454
                                     TTY: 866-915-5000
                                      service@cec.sped.org
                                      www.cec.sped.org

James P Heiden, President
Antonis Katsiyannis, President Elect
Sharon Raimondi, Treasurer
Alexander T Graham, Executive Director
To support educational participation and improved results for individuals with disabilities and diverse learning needs through the selection, acquisition, and use of technology. The secondary purpose is to provide services to members and other units of CEC, to federal, state and local education agencies, and to business and industry regarding the current and future uses if technology and media with individuals with exceptionalities

929   Thresholds Psychiatric Rehabilitation Centers
4101 N Ravenswood Ave
Chicago, IL 60613-2196   773-572-5500
                                          888-997-3422
                                     FAX: 773-880-6279
                                     TTY: 773-880-6263
                                   thresholds@thresholds.org
                                   www.thresholds.org

Jana Barbe, President
Marianne Doan, Vice President
Harold E. D'Orazio, Treasurer
Kathy Graham, Secretary
A nationally-recognized psychosocial rehabilitation agency serving persons with severe and persistent mental illness. The agency offers its programming at 22 service locations and more than 40 residential facilities throughout Chicago and Northern Illinois. Also offers specialized programming for older adults, young adults, parents, the homeless and the hearing impaired and mentally ill.
Sliding scale

930   United States Disabled Golf Association
598 Dixie Road
Clinton, NC 28328   910-214-5983
                                          info@USDGA.net
                                          www.usdga.net

Jason Faircloth, Founder
There mission is to provide people with physical,sensory, and mental disabilities an opportunity to play golf at the highest level in the USA.

931   United States Trager Association
13801 W Center St
Ste C, P.O. Box 1009
Burton, OH 44021-9005   440-834-0308
                                     FAX: 440-834-0365
                                       info@tragerus.org
                                       www.tragerus.org

Anna Marie Bowers, Executive Director
Carla Keene, President
Sharon King Green, Vice President
Deborah Haber, Treasurer
The Trager approach is a pleasurable, gentle and effective approach to movement education and mind/body integration. The Trager approach helps release deep-seated physical and mental patterns and facilitates deep relaxation, increased physical mobility, and mental clarity. The benefits of a Trager session are long-lasting and cumulative, with subsequent sessions allowing for deeper and longer lasting changes.

932   Universal Pediatric Services
6750 Westown Parkway
Suite 115A
West Des Moines, IA 50266   515-280-2160
                                          800-383-0303
                                          www.upsi.net

Tucker Anderson, President
Universal Pediatric Services, provides high tech care to medically fragile children and adults in the home setting. Emphasis is placed on the provision of services in the rural areas, the ability to service high tech needs and the promotion of primary nurse concept.

933   Upledger Institute
11211 Prosperity Farms Rd
Ste D-325
Palm Beach Gardens, FL 33410   561-622-4334
                                          800-233-5880
                                     FAX: 561-622-4771
                                      upledger@upledger.com
                                      www.upledger.com

John M Upledger, CEO
Roy Desjarlais, VP
Alex Jozefyk, Chief Financial Officer
Steve Keller, Director of Distributions
A healthcare resource center recognized worldwide for its comprehensive education programs, advanced treatment options and unique outreach initiatives. The Institute has trained more than 100,000 healthcare professionals throughout the globe in the therapeutic approach.

934   Women to Women
PO Box 306
Portland, ME 04112-306   800-540-5906
                                     FAX: 207-846-6167
                             personalprogram@womentowomen.com
                             www.womentowomen.com

Marcelle Pick OB/GYN, NP, Co Founder/Director
Combination of alternative and conventional medicine in women's health, bring science and disipline to natural and preventative methods. Publishes the Creating Health Guide, a quarterly collection of articles written by the health care professionals at Women to Women.

935   World Institute on Disability
3075 Adeline Street
Suite 155
Berkeley, CA 94703   510-225-6400
                                                FAX: 510-225-0477
                                                TTY:510-225-0478
                                                     wid@wid.org
                                                     www.wid.org

Anita Shafer Aaron, Executive Director
Thomas Foley, Deputy Dir/Access to Assets
Julia Day, Content Production Mgr
Loretta Herrington, Program Director
The mission of the World Institute on Disability (WID) in communities and nations worldwide is to eliminate barriers to full social integration and increase employment, economic security and health care for persons with disabilities. WID creates innovative programs and tools; conducts research, public education, training and advocacy campaigns; and provides technical assistance.

936   YAI: National Institute for People with Disabilities
460 W 34th St
New York, NY 10001-2382   212-273-6100
                                                FAX: 212-273-6200
                                                     www.yai.org

Matthew Sturiale, CEO
Stephen Freeman, President/COO
Sanjay Dutt, Chief Financial Officer
Thomas A. Dern, L.C.S.W., Chief Operating Officer
Mission is to build brighter futures for people with developmental and learning disabilities and thier families. Every person, at every age and level of disability, has the potential for growth. Each individual is entitled to the same dignity, respect, and opportunities as all other members of society. Firmly committed to helping the people we serve to achieve their potential for independence, individuality, productivity, and inclusion in their communities.

Camps

Alabama

937   ADA Teen Adventure Camp
American Diabetes Association
4000 Ridgeway Drive
Birmingham, AL 35209

800-900-8086
FAX: 205-313-7475
email@nchpad.org
www.nchpad.org

Sue Apsey, Program Director
Camping for teenagers with diabetes. Coed, ages 14 to 18. Camp dates are early in August. Located at the YMCA Camp Duncan in Ingleside, Illinois. Featured activities include archery and crafts, singing, outdoor movie night, and roller skating.

938   ADA Triangle D Camp
American Diabetes Association
4000 Ridgeway Drive
Birmingham, AL 35209

800-900-8086
FAX: 205-313-7475
email@nchpad.org
www.nchpad.org

Sue Apsey, Program Director
Triangle D Camp is a resident camp program located at the YMCA Camp Duncan in Ingleside, Illinois. Activities include swimming, row boating, canoeing, high ropes (11-13 yr. olds), climbing tower (9-10 yr. olds), Camp games, singing, archery, campfires, soccer, basketball, volleyball and diabetes education.

939   Camp Evoked Potential @ Camp ASCCA
Epilepsy Foundation of Alabama
310-273 Azalea Rd
Office Park 3
Mobile, AL 36609-1970

251-341-0170
800-626-1582
ddodson@efala.org
www.efala.org/camp-evoked-potential/

Donna Dodson, Executive Director
Paige Norris, Outreach/Program Director
Camp Evoked Potential is a 5-day overnight camp for children and teens aged 6 to 18 years old living with epilepsy. The camp provides a great opportunity for kids to experience the fun of camp activities—swimming, fishing, sports, hiking and more—in a safe, medically monitored setting. Camp activities are designed to be accessible and adapted to campers' individual needs and abilities.

940   Camp Merrimack
Merrimack Hall Performing Arts Center
3320 Triana Blvd.
Huntsville, AL 35805

256-534-6455
FAX: 212-397-4684
info@merrimackhall.com
www.merrimackhall.com

Debra Jenkins, Founder and President
Alan Jenkins, Vice President
Joe Ritch, Secretary / Treasurer
Kay Harrington, Financial Advisor
For children ages 3-12 with special needs including Down Syndrome, Cerebral Palsy, Autism and others. Camp includes theatre, visual arts and dance.

941   Camp Rap-A-Hope
2701 Airport Blvd
Mobile, AL 36606-2319

251-476-9880
FAX: 251-476-9495
info@camprapahope.org
www.camprapahope.org

Sandy Blount, President
Bob Stewart, President Elect
Melissa McNichol, Executive Director
Roz Dorsett, Assistant Director
Camp Rap-A-Hope is a one-week summer camp for children and teenagers who are battling cancer or have ever been diagnosed with cancer and are 7 to 17 years of age. It is free of charge. Camp Rap-A-Hope strives to make sure every camper gets the opportunity to develop new skills and self-confidence. Camp activities are appropriate for our campers' ages and abilities and include, but are not limited to: swimming, music, arts and crafts, archery, fishing, canoeing and horseback riding.

942   Camp Seale Harris
Southeastern Diabetes Education Services
500 Chase Park S
Ste 104
Birmingham, AL 35244

205-402-0415
FAX: 205-402-0416
info@campsealeharris.org
www.campsealeharris.org

Tip McAlpin, Chair
David Jamieson, Vice Chairman
Rhonda McDavid, Executive Director
John Latimer, Camp & Community Programs Director
Camp Seale Harris for a medically-supervised, fun camp experience and family connection to year-round support that helps them fight diabetes every day.

943   Camp Shocco for the Deaf
AL Baptist State Board of Missions
1314 Shocco Springs Road
Talladega, AL 35160

256-761-1111
TTY:256-474-0109
campshocco@albcdeaf.org
www.campshocco.org

Chad Fleming, Director
Linnea Elliott, Assistant Dir. - Youth Camp
Mathew Dixon, Co-Director
Adam Schrimsher, Secretary / Director of Recreati
Camp Shocco gives each child and teenager attending camp the opportunity to have an unforgettable one week of fun, games, and spiritual growth. Campers also learn the essence of teamwork, while developing their own unique abilities and talents that can often be overlooked.

944   Camp Smile-A-Mile
P.O.Box 550155
Birmingham, AL 35255-155

205-323-8427
888-500-7920
FAX: 205-323-6220
info@campsam.org
www.campsam.org

Bruce Hooper, Executive Director
Jennifer Amundsen, Program Director
Savannah Lanler, Development Director
Katie Langley, Administrative & Development Assistant
Camp Smile-A-Mile is a non-profit organization for children who have or had cancer in Alabama. Camp Smile-A-Mile's mission is to provide challenging, unforgettable recreational and educational experiences for young cancer patients from across Alabama at no cost to their families. Our purpose is to provide these children with avenues for fellowship, to help them cope with their disease, and to prepare them for life.

945 Camp WheezeAway
YMCA Camp Chandler
1240 Jordan Dam Rd
Wetumpka, AL 36092
334-229-0035
jreynolds@ymcamontgomery.org
ymcamontgomery.org/camp/wheezeaway
Jeff Reynolds, Executive Director
Art Mason, Operations Director
Suzy Stewart, Program Director
Kids age 8-12 suffering from moderate to severe asthma can apply for this FREE summer camp program offered at YMCA Camp Chandler. Kids experience all the fun of summer camp while learning confidence building skills in asthma management from medical professionals.

946 Easter Seals Camp ASCCA
Easter Seals
5278 Camp ASCCA Drive
Jackson's Gap, AL 36861
256-825-9226
FAX: 256-825-8332
info@campascca.org
campascca.org
Matt Rickman, Camp Director
John Stephenson, Administrator
Jocelyn Jones, Secretary
Enis Higgs, Food Service Director
Camp ASCCA is Alabama's Special Camp for Children and Adults. ASCCA is a nationally recognized leader in therapeutic recreation for children and adults with both physical and intellectual disabilities. Providing weekend and week long sessions, Camp ASCCA is open year round.

Alaska

947 ADA Camp Kushtaka
American Diabetes Association
201 West Fireweed Lane
Suite 103
Anchorage, AK 99503- 1893
907-272-1424
800-342-2383
FAX: 907-272-1428
askada@diabetes.org
www.childrenwithdiabetes.org
Michelle Cassano, Executive Director
Pam Bell, Organizer
ADA Camp Kushtaka is a five day camp for children & teens age 7-17 and their families (space permitting) and is held on the shores of Kenai Lake on the Kenai Peninsula in Cooper Landing. The camp combines ongoing and informal diabetes management and education along with the fun of outdoor activities such as hiking, canoeing, crafts and swimming.

948 Camp Alpine
Alpine Alternatives
2518 E. Tudor Road
Suite 105
Anchorage, AK 99507-1105
907-561-6655
800-361-4174
FAX: 907-563-9232
alpinealternatives@arctic.net
www.alpinealternatives.org
Margaret Webber, Executive Director
Nancy Burnette, Bookkeeper/Program Administrator
Vanessa Hartley, Downhill Ski Program Director
LaVerne Lee, Day Outings Director & Camp Alpi
Our programs are designed to help people expand their horizons, master new skills, make new friends, and increase motor coordination. Most importantly, participants experience growth in self-confidence and independence that affects all aspects of an individual's life. Our services are open to all, regardless of type of disability or age. Activities include canoeing, hiking, swimming, outdoor games, sports, nature identification and much more.

949 Camp Birchwood
Muscular Dystrophy Association
17161 David Blackburn Drive
Chugiak, AK 99567
907-688-2734
FAX: 907-688-2734
stay@birchwoodcamp.org
www.birchwoodcamp.org
Marie Sweezey, Camp Director
Stephen Sweezey, Program Director & Camp Manager
A summer camp at Birchwood Camp in Chugiak, Alaska for individuals ages 6-21 who are affected by any of the 40-plus neuromuscular diseases in MDA's program. Common activities include: swimming, hockey, baseball, soccer, football, boating, horseback riding, fishing, music, cooking, arts and crafts, movies, dancing, talent shows, Harley-Davidson motorcycle sidecar or three-wheeled cycle rides, a visit from fire fighters and time for socializing and laughing.

Arizona

950 Arizona Camp Sunrise
American Cancer Society
PO Box 27872
Tempe, AZ 85285
602-952-7550
FAX: 602-404-1118
barb.nicholas@cancer.org
www.azcampsunrise.org
Barbara Nicholas, Dir.
Leigh Ansley, Mgr of Childhood Cancer Support
Melissa Lee, Camp Dir.
Jason Poulter, Technical Media Dir.
Provides one-week summer camping sessions to children aged 8-16 who have had, or currently have, cancer. The classes range from sports and outdoor games to dance and drama, arts, crafts, and cooking. Other activities planned for the campers include horseback riding, a trip to a lake, a dance, and learning to make friendship bracelets.

951 Camp Abilities Tucson
1200 West Speedway Boulevard
P.O. Box 86838
Tucson, AZ 85754-6838
520-235-2582
campabilitiestucson@gmail.com
www.campabilitiestucson.org
Murry Everson, Camp Director
One week camp offering comprehensive developmental sports for children in middle and high school who are blind, deaf-blind or multiply disabled.

952 Camp Candlelight
Epilepsy Foundation Arizona
3033A N. 7th Ave
Ste 104
Phoenix, AZ 85013
602-406-3581
800-332-1000
info@epilepsyaz.org
epilepsyaz.org/programs/camp-candlelight/
Suzanne Matsumori, Executive Director
Min Skivington, Program Manager
Camp Candlelight provides children ages 8 to 15 a unique camp experience that mixes traditional summer camp with special sessions that teach campers about their seizures and gives them resources to manage the challenges that the seizures represent. Staff inclues a neurologist, several nurses, and a school psychologist, in addition to traditional camp staff who are given specialized training in responding appropriately to the needs of kids with epilepsy.

953   Camp Civitan
Civitan Foundation
12635 North 42nd Street
Phoenix, AZ 85032-3339   602-953-2944
                                                    FAX: 602-953-2946
                                            info@campcivitan.org
                                    www.civitanfoundationaz.com
John W Day, President
Frank S. Nightingale, Vice President
Bo Larsen, Director
Trapp Dawn, Chief Executive Officer
We are the premier camp for developmentally disabled individu-
als of all ages. People from around Arizona and neighboring
states come to Camp Civitan to enhance their quality of life, enjoy
the multitude of outdoor experiences we offer and make lifelong
friends.

954   Camp Honor
Hemophilia Association
826 North 5th Avenue
Phoenix, AZ 85003   602-955-3947
                                                    888-754-7017
                                            info@hemophiliaz.org
                                    www.arizonahemophilia.org
Steven Helm, President
Jim Durr, Vice President
Victor Alonzo, Treasurer
Cindy Komar, Executive Director
Camp is located in Payson, Arizona at the Whispering Hope
Ranch. One-week sessions for children with hemophilia or HIV
and their siblings, as well as children of hemophiliacs. Coed, ages
7-17. Activities include swimming, canoeing, sports, archery and
arts and crafts (to name a few fun things).

955   Camp Not-A-Wheeze
American Lung Association
Friendly Pines
933 East Friendly Pines Road
Prescott, AZ 86303-8202   928-445-2128
                                                    888-281-2267
                                                    FAX: 928-445-6065
                                            info@friendlypines.com
                                                    www.lung.org
Larry Blumenthal, Chair
George Walker, Regional Dir.
Cindy Liverance, VP of Programs
Liz Toohey, Dir. of Dev
Camp Not-A-Wheeze is designed especially for kids ages 7-14
with moderate to severe asthma and was created to provide a tra-
ditional residential camp experience and teach children how to
manage their asthma.

956   Camp Rainbow
Phoenix Childrens Hospital
1919 East Thomas Road
Phoenix, AZ 85016-7710   602-933-1000
                                                    888-908-5437
                                    msalloom@phoenixchildrens.com
                                    www.phoenixchildrens.com/
Robert Meyer, President and CEO
David Cavazos, Chairman of the Board
Larry Clemmensen, Chairman of the Board
Steven S. Schnall, Senior VP
Camp is located in Prescott, Arizona. Offers one-week sessions
for children who have had, or currently have, cancer. Boys and
girls ages 7-17. Camp activities include swimming, horseback
riding, arts and crafts, canoeing, performing arts, archery,
rollerskating, fishing, an overnight camping trip and much more!
It's a week filled with laughter, new experiences and new friends.

957   Lions Camp Tatiyee
Arizona Lions Clubs Multiple District 21
5283 W White Mountain Blvd
Lakeside, AZ 85216-6910   480-380-4254
                                                    800-246-9771
                                                    FAX: 602-244-8667
                                    director@arizonalionscamp.com
                                    www.arizonalionscamp.com
Pamela Swanson, Executive Director
Desirae Bender, RN BSN, Lead Nurse
Megan Anderson, Assistant Program Director
Camp is located in Lakeside, Arizona. Sessions are provided for
campers of all ages, with a wide variety of disabilities/special
needs and are divided by age and disability. Featured activities include arts and crafts, ceramics/pottery, climbing/rappelling,
counselor training (CIT), drama, fishing, football, hiking, na-
ture/environmental studies and team building.

958   Triangle Y Ranch YMCA
YMCA Of Southern Arizona
PO Box 1111
Oracle, AZ 85623   520-623-5511
                                                    FAX: 520-624-1518
                                            camp@tucsonymca.org
                                                    www.tucsonymca.org
Dane Woll, President and CEO
Kerry Dufour, V.P. Chief Dev. Officer
Cathy Scheirman, Chief Financial Officer
Amanda Thomas, Human Resources Director
For children and young adults ages 6-17. The camp offers nature
programs, swimming, horseback riding, sports, arts & crafts.

Arkansas

959   Camp Aldersgate
Camp Aldersgate, Inc.
2000 Aldersgate Road
Little Rock, AR 72205   501-225-1444
                                                    FAX: 501-225-2019
                                            info@campaldersgate.net
                                                    www.campaldersgate.net
Sarah C. Wacaster, CEO
Bill Faggard, Chief Operating Officer
Ali Miller, Program Manager
Regina Riehl, Director of Finance and Human Re
A non-profit camp for children and young adults with medical or
physical conditions such as cerebral palsy, diabetes, arthritis,
asthma, kidney disorders.

960   Camp Funshine
Camp Funshine Foundation, Inc.
P.O. Box 576
Pea Ridge, AR 72751
                                                    www.campfunshine.com
Jeff Brown, President
Aimee Albright, Vice President
Holly Floyd, Treasurer
Rain Sheppard, Secretary
A free camp for children ages 7 and up who have cystic fibrosis.
The mission of the camp is to provide a fun, safe environment in
which the kids can talk openly about themselves or their disease.

961   Camp Kota
Junior League Of Little Rock
401 South Scott Street
Little Rock, AR 72201   501-375-5557
                                                    FAX: 501-907-5296
                                                    www.jllr.org
Marisha DiCarlo, President
Amanda M. Richardson, President Elect
Sabrina Lewellen, Community Vice President
Mickey Willett, Membership Vice President
Camp Kota is for disabled and non-disabled children ages 6-16.
Some of the activities include fishing, canoeing, swimming, ar-
chery, music and arts & crafts.

962 Camp Quality Arkansas
PO Box 9095
Jonesboro, AR 72403
870-931-2844
FAX: 866-285-5208
chris.jennings@campqualityusa.org
www.campqualityusa.org/ar

Chris Jennings, Director
Camp Quality is for children with cancer and their siblings. The camp offers a stress-free environment that offers exciting activities and fosters new friendships, while helping to give the children courage, motivation and emotional strength.

California

963 ASCCA
Alabama Easter Seal Society
44 Montgomery St.
Suite 1605
San Francisco, CA 94104- 4602
415-296-6952
FAX: 415-296-6901
socca@iars.org
www.socca.org/

Aryeh Shander, President
Laureen L. Hill, Director
Daniel R. Brown, Treasurer
Miguel A. Cobas, Secretary
The Society of Critical Care Anesthesiologists (SOCCA) formerly ASCCA, was founded in 1986 to address the unique concerns of intensivists before the American Society of anesthesiologists (ASA). The founding members of SOCCA believed and continue to believe that multidisciplinary critical care medicine is a desirable goal.

964 Bearskin Meadow Camp
Diabetic Youth Foundation
5167 Clayton Road
Suite F
Concord, CA 94521-3163
925-680-4994
FAX: 925-680-4863
info@dyf.org
www.dyf.org

Janet Kramschuster, Executive Director
Mark McComb, President
Jim Simpson, Treasurer
Merilee Silverstein, Secretary
Bear Skin Meadow Camp is for children, teens and families who are affected by diabetes. The Camp also teaches the children and teens diabetes management and education, skills for blood glucose checking and techniques for adjusting insulin, as well as food choices and how to have a fun, active life while living with diabetes.

965 Camp Beyond The Scars
Burn Institute
8825 Aero Drive
Suite 200
San Diego, CA 92123-2269
858-541-2277
FAX: 858-541-7179
dkuhn@burninstitute.org
www.burninstitute.org

Chief David Ott, President
Chief Bob Pfohl, VP Chief Financial Officer
Susan Day, Executive Director
Brittany Bachmann, Director of Marketing
Summer camp for children who have suffered burns. The camp provides a relaxed social setting and helps to enhance the children's self esteem.

966 Camp Bloomfield
Junior Blind of America
5300 Angeles Vista Blvd.
Los Angeles, CA 90043
323-295-4555
800-352-2290
FAX: 323-296-0424
info@juniorblind.org
www.juniorblind.org

Mike Jordan, President & CEO
Jay Allen, EVP & COO
Laura M Hardy, SVP of Development & Marketing
Kami Mann, SVP, Finance & CFO
Offers children and youth's who are blind, visually impaired or multi-disabled with a safe and natural environment where they can develop self esteem and build independence. The camp offers swimming, horseback riding, fishing, hiking, track and field, arts and crafts and more.

967 Camp Christian Berets
Christian Berets, Inc.
1317 Oakdale Road
Suite 340
Modesto, CA 95355
209-524-7993
FAX: 209-524-7979
www.christianberets.org

James Woodhead, President
Carletta Evans Steele, Treasurer
Kelly Luth, Secretary
Brian Robison, Facilities Manager
Camp for children, students and adults with special needs.

968 Camp Coelho
Epilepsy Foundation Of Northern California
155 Montgomery Street
Suite 309
San Francisco, CA 94104
416-677-4011
800-632-3532
FAX: 416-677-4190
www.epilepsynorcal.org

Katherine Keeney, President and CEO
Olivia Salfiti, Office Manager
Prakash Arunachalam, Treasurer
Heather Berry, Secretary
Camp for children and young adults ages 5-15 with epilepsy and seizure disorders.

969 Camp Conrad-Chinnock
Diabetic Youth Services
12045 E. Waterfront Drive
Playa Vista, CA 90094
310-751-3057
FAX: 888-800-4010
rocky.wilson@dys.org
www.diabetescamping.org

Rocky Wilson, Ph.D., Executive And Camp Director
Dale Lissy, Camp Manager
Ryan Martz, Program Director
Tom Jenkins, Chief Operating Officer
Camp conrad-chinnock offers social, recreational and educational opportunities for youth and families with diabetes. Campers are taught diabetes self-management skills in an interactive, fun & safe environment.

970 Camp Costanoan
VIA Services West
2851 Park Avenue
Santa Clara, CA 95050
408-243-7861
info@viaservices.org
www.viaservices.org

John Heagerty, Chair
Laura Beth DeHority, Vice Chair
Brad Baron, Senior Vice President
Sandi Conniff, Community Volunteer
Camp Costanoan is a residential, outdoor education, and recreational camp for children and adults, ages 5 and older, with physical and/or developmental disabilities and special needs. Camp Costanoan enhances camper self-esteem, improves socialization skills and provides hands-on learning and therapeutic recreation opportunities.

971 Camp Del Corazon
11615 Hesby St
North Hollywood, CA 91601-3620   818-754-0312
888-621-4800
FAX: 818-754-0377
info@campdelcorazon.org
www.campdelcorazon.org
Lisa Knight, RN, Exec. Dir. and Co-Founder
Kevin Shannon, MD, Medical Dir. & Co-Founder
Tom Klitzner, MD, Exec. Board Member
Carl Schuster, Exec. Board Member
Active program for campers with heart disease, Camp del Corazon provides summer activities free of charge that include hiking and archery, arts and crafts, court and field games, waterfront activities and a beach barbecue.

972 Camp Firefly
The Firefly Foundation
5737 Kanan Road
Suite 180
Agoura Hills, CA 91301
CampFirefly89@gmail.com
www.campfirefly.com

973 Camp Forrest
Angel View Crippled Children's Foundation
12379 Miracle Hill Rd
Desert Hot Springs, CA 92240-4010   760-329-6471
FAX: 760-329-9024
angelview44@aol.com
www.angelview.org
David Thorton, Executive Director
Shelly Lee, Resale Shops
Catherine Rips, Director of Development
DeAnn Lubell Ames, Director of Public Relations
Camp is located in Joshua Tree, California. Offers to one-week sessions June-August to both able-bodied campers and those with a wide variety of disabilities. Coed, ages 10-25. Activities include archery, arts and crafts, cookouts, swimming, sports and games, hiking and star study.

974 Camp Grizzly
NorCal Services For Deaf & Hard Of Hearing, Inc.
4708 Roseville Road
Suite 111
North Highlands, CA 95660-5172   916-349-7500
FAX: 916-349-7580
TTY:916-349-7500
info@nocalcenter.org
www.norcalcenter.org/
Sheri Farinah, CEO
Cheryl Bella, Chair
Michael D. Wilson, Vice Chair
Yim Orsi, Secretary
This camp is designed the deaf and hard of hearing youth or hearing youth with deaf or hard of hearing parent. The camp helps with social interaction, building self esteem, leadership skills while enriching the lives of the deaf and hard of hearing.

975 Camp Kindle
28245 Avenue Crocker
Suite 104
Santa Clarita, CA 91355   877-800-2267
FAX: 702-995-9186
info@projectkindle.org
projectkindle.org
Eva Payne, Founder/Executive Director
Mandy Nickolite, Vice President/PsychoSocial Lead
Erin FitzGerald, Program Coordinator
The purpose of Camp Kindle is to enhance the overall well-being of children and young people living with a chronic or life threatening illness, disability, or other life challenge. Camp Kindle's primary mechanism for achieving its purpose is through camping events held in Nebraska and California.

976 Camp Krem
Camping Unlimited
102 Brook Lane
Boulder Creek, CA 95006   510-222-6662
campkrem@gmail.com
campingunlimited.org
Judy Simmons, President
Alex J. Krem, Treasurer
Christina Krem, Program Director
Katie Giampa, Program Director
Year-round camp offering recreational activities and camping for children and adults with developmental disabilities.

977 Camp Okizu
Okizu Foundation
16 Digital Drive
Suite 130
Novato, CA 94949-5755   415-382-9083
FAX: 415-382-8384
info@okizu.org
www.okizu.org
John H. Bell, Chairman
Michael D. Amylon, M.D., Vice-Chairman
Suzanne B. Randall, Secretary
James Halow, Treasurer
Camp Okizu is located in Berry Creek, California, and offers children who are struggling with life threatening illnesses and their families a place to go and explore and enjoy a normal life experience. The camp also offers peer support, respite, mentoring as well as other programs designed to meet the needs of all members of families whom are affected by childhood cancer. The camp is open from April through October.

978 Camp Pacifica, Inc.
California Lions Camp
45895 CA-49
Ahwahnee, CA 93601-209-   559-683-4660
ilybrookeb@yahoo.com
camppacifica.org
Russ Custer, President
Jill Loving, Secretary
Ted Allan, Treasurer
Dee Heller, Vice President
Camp Pacifica has been developed to provide a unique environment where special needs children have opportunities to grow and understand themselves. The camp is open to special needs children ages 7-17 years old, and strives to promote greater independence and self confidence and provides opportunities for social interaction, further development of social skills and the opportunity to develop friendships.

979 Camp Paivika
AbilityFirst
1300 E. Green Street
Pasadena, CA 91106   626-396-1010
877-768-4600
FAX: 626-396-1021
sramirez@abilityfirst.org
www.abilityfirst.org
Lori Gangemi, President and CEO
Keri Castaneda, Chief Program Officer
Kevin Schaffels, Chief Financial Officer
Oscar Franco, Director of Safety
AbilityFirst has 24 locations throughout So. California, including a camp, serving children and adults with disabilities.

980 Camp Quest
The Epilepsy Foundation Of Northern California
155 Montgomery Street
Suite 309
San Francisco, CA 94104   416-677-4011
800-632-3532
FAX: 416-677-4190
www.epilepsynorcal.org
Katherine Keeney, President and CEO
Olivia Salfiti, Office Manager
Prakash Arunachalam, Treasurer
Heather Berry, Secretary

Summer camp for children and young adults ages 5-15 with epilepsy and seizure disorders.

981 Camp Ramah In California
17525 Ventura Blvd. #201
Encino, CA 91316
310-476-8571
888-226-7726
FAX: 310-472-3810
info@ramah.org
www.ramah.org

Rabbi Joe Menashe, Executive Director
Randy Michaels, Director of Finance & Admin
Ariella Moss Peterseil, Associate Director
Ilana Ormond, Director of Development
Camp for young adults ages 11-18 with learning, emotional and developmental disabilities.

982 Camp ReCreation
2110 Broadway
Sacramento, CA 95818
916-733-0136
FAX: 916-733-0195
CampRec@scd.org
www.camprecreation.org

Marisa Bender, President
Alex Nelson, Vice President
Peter Mendenhall, Secretary
Ann Theobald, Treasurer
A residential summer camp program for adults and children with developmental disabilities.

983 Camp Reach for the Sky
American Cancer Society c/o CR4TS
Ste 100
2655 Camino Del Rio N
San Diego, CA 92108-1633
619-682-7427
800-227-2345
FAX: 404-417-5974
TTY: 866-228-4327
www.cancer.org

Kimberly Wright, Dir., Mission Solutions & Tools
Kristina Thomson, LCSW, Division Director
Sheila G. Williamson, Regional VP
Tawana Thomas Johnson, Dir., Health Disparities
One-week sessions for children who have had, or currently have, cancer, and are residents of San Diego and Imperial counties. Coed, ages 4-18. Siblings are also invited to participate in activities.

984 Camp Ronald McDonald for Good Times
Ronald McDonald House Charities - Southern Calif.
1250 Lyman Place
Los Angeles, CA 90029
626-744-9449
800-625-7295
FAX: 626-744-9969
bbaillie@campronaldmcdonald.org
rmhcsc.org/camp

Edward Lodgen, Esq., President
Jodie Lesh, Vice President
Sarah Orth, Executive Director
Chad Edwards, Program Director
Free year-round residential camping for children with cancer and their families.

985 Camp Ronald McDonald® at Eagle Lake
2555 49th Street
Sacramento, CA 95817
916-734-4230
FAX: 530-825-3158
vflaig@rmhcnc.org
www.campronald.org

Vicky Flaig, MEd, RD, Camp Director
Supported by Ronald McDonald House Charities® Northern California-a fully accessible residential camp for kids with special needs. The goal of the camp is to provide confidence building experiences to children who are at risk, disadvantaged and/or living with physical, developmental or emotional disabilities.

986 Camp Rubber Soul
325A East Redwood Avenue
Fort Bragg, CA 95437
707-962-0906
camp@camprubbersoul.org
www.camprubbersoul.org

Rachel Miller, Camp contact person
Sayre Statham, Camp contact person
The camp offers five one-week camping stays for children and young adults with special needs. Some of the activities include sports, wood working, painting, theatre, music and arts and crafts.

987 Camp Sunburst
Sunburst Projects
1025 19th Street
Suite 1A
Sacramento, CA 95811
916-440-0889
FAX: 916-440-1208
admin@sunburstprojects.org
www.sunburstprojects.org

Geri DeLaRosa , PhD, Founder/Executive Director
Mireya Herrara-Bayard, LCSW, Director of Client Services
Kathryn Nevard, Deputy Director
Jolene Ford, MSW, Clinical Case Manager
At Camp Sunburst, our acclaimed national model residential summer camp, HIV/AIDS children and their families enjoy the companionship of others without the social stigma and isolation associated with the AIDS epidemic.

988 Camp Sunshine Dreams
P.O. Box 28232
Fresno, CA 93729-8232
559-301-5419
contact@campsunshinedreams.com
www.campsunshinedreams.com

Bryan Wood, Camp contact person
Anthony Aiello, Camp contact person
Pam Aiello, Board Of Director
Jeff Clem, Board Of Director
Camp Sunshine Dreams is open for children and young adults ages 8-15 years and their siblings. The camp focuses on providing an enjoyable, stimulating and supportive camping experience while also providing for each child's special emotional and physical needs.

989 Camp Taylor, Inc.
5424 Pirrone Road
Salida, CA 95368-9094
209-545-4715
FAX: 209-543-1861
camp@kidsheartcamp.org
www.kidsheartcamp.org

Kimberlie Gamino, Executive Director and Founder
Rollin A. Podwys, Camp Director
Steven Barbieri, Camp Counselor
Kavin H. Desai, Camp Medical Director
Camp Taylor is open to children and young adults and their families who have heart disease and offers many recreational activities.

990 Camp Trinity
Star Route Box 150
Hayfork, CA 96041
530-628-5992
FAX: 530-628-9392
camptrinity@bar717.com
www.bar717.com/

Nora Bundy, Program Coordinator
Casey Zarnes, Barn Director
Lucy A. Newell, Counseling Staff
Mitch Carter, Counseling Staff
Offers two, three and four-week camping sessions May-September. Accepts campers with diabetes and mobility limitation. Coed, ages 8-16. Also families, single adults and seniors.

991 Camp-A-Lot And Leisure Express (PALS Program)
Arc of San Diego
3030 Market Street
San Diego, CA 92102
619-685-1175
FAX: 619-234-3759
info@arc-sd.com
www.arc-sd.com

Gerald W. Hansen, Chair
David W. Schneider, President and CEO
Anthony J. DeSalis, Esq, EVP & COO
Chad Lyle, VP of Finance/CFO
Recreational opportunities for children, teens and adults with developmental and intellectual disabilities. Programs include summer resident camp, San Diego local activities and trip/travel vacations.

992 Camping Unlimited
102 Brook Ln
Boulder Creek, CA 95006-9320
510-222-6662
FAX: 831-338-3210
campkrem@gmail.com
campingunlimited.org

Judy Simmons, President
Christina Krem, Program Director
Alex J. Krem, Treasurer
Katie Giampa, Program Director
Camping Unlimited is a non-profit organization providing special needs children and adults a full program of recreation, education, fun and adventure. Our program encourages independence, nurtures responsibility, develops competence and builds lifelong friendships in a warm supportive atmosphere of planned permissiveness.
2 pages Monthly

993 Camping Unlimited-Camp Krem
Camping Unlimited for Children & Adults
102 Brook Ln
Boulder Creek, CA 95006
510-222-6662
campkrem@gmail.com
campingunlimited.org

Judy Simmons, President
Christina Krem, Program Director
Alex J. Krem, Treasurer
Katie Giampa, Program Director
Camp is located in Boulder Creek, California in the Santa Cruz mountains. Offers one and two-week sessions June-August to campers with a variety of disabilities. Coed, ages 5-50. Camping unlimited also offers weekend programs and travel camps, year round programs and recreation. Boulder Creek is located 15 minutes from Santa Cruz, CA, and Pacific Ocean Beach.

994 Deaf Kid's Kamp
Sproul Ranch, Inc.
42263 50th Street West
Suite 610
Quartz Hill, CA 93536
661-675-3323
deafkidskamp@earthlink.net
www.deafkidskamp.com

Buffy Sproul, Executive Director
Our purpose is to meet the needs of deaf children outside of the classroom setting. These needs, as we have defined them, would include but are not limited to: social contact with peers; contact with the culture of the Deaf Community; educational and recreational programs not available in most school settings.

995 Dream Street Camp
Dream Street Foundation
324 S. Beverly Drive
Suite 500
Beverly Hills, CA 90212
424-333-1371
FAX: 310-388-0302
dreamstreetca@gmail.com
www.dreamstreetfoundation.org

Patty Grubman, Director
Louise Gonzales, Office Manager
Tiffany Alfaro, Director
For children and young adults with life threatening and chronic illnesses.

996 Easter Seals Camp Harmon
Easter Seals Central California
16403 Highway 9
Boulder Creek, CA 95006-9696
831-338-3383
800-400-0671
FAX: 831-338-0200
campharmon@es-cc.org
www.centralcal.easterseals.com

Ruth Hutchison, Board Chair
Robert Guerin, Board Vice Chair
Tom Conway, CEO
Judy Anderson, Secretary / Treasurer
Camp is located in Boulder Creek, California. 6-10 day sessions for children and adults with physical and developmental disabilities. Coed, ages 8-65.

997 Enchanted Hills Camp for the Blind
Lighthouse for the Blind
214 Van Ness Ave
San Francisco, CA 94102
415-431-1481
888-400-8933
FAX: 415-863-7568
info@lighthouse-sf.org
lighthouse-sf.org/

Joshua A. Miele, Ph.D., President
Chris Downey, 1st Vice President
Kathleen Knox, 2nd Vice President
Lisa Carvalho, 3rd Vice President
Camp is located in Napa, California. Half-week, one and two-week sessions for blind, deaf/blind children and adults, ages 5 and up. This program offers a basic camping experience. Activities include music, art, dance, hiking and riding. Camperships are available to California residents.

998 Firefighters Kids Camp
Firefighters Burn Institute
3101 Stockton Blvd.
Sacramento, CA 95820
916-739-8525
FAX: 916-455-4376
website@ffburn.org
ffburn.org/

Brian Rice, President
Jim Doucette, Executive Director
Pat Cook, Secretary-Treasurer
Ka Vue, Programs Manager
Provides children and young adults ages 6-17 who have had serious burn injuries the opportunity to continue their rehabilitation and recovery in an outdoor environment where they are safe and can have fun.

999 Lions Wilderness Camp for Deaf Children, Inc.
Lions Clubs of California and Nevada
P.O.Box 195
Knightsen, CA 94548
877-896-1598
888-613-1557
campdirector@lionswildcamp.org
www.lionswildcamp.org

Richard A. Wilmot, President
Rachel Mix, Camp Program Director
Robin L. Nichol, Camp Manager
Dana Johnson, Secretary
A camp experience where a deaf child age 7 to 15 can learn outdoor skills and enjoy the wonder and beauty of nature to the fullest extent.

1000 New Horizons Summer Day Camp
YMCA
13821 Newport Avenue
Suite 200
Tustin, CA 92780
714-549-9622
FAX: 714-838-5976
www.ymcaoc.org

Robert Traut, Board Chair
Jeff Black, Vice Chair
John Rochford, Vice Chair
Jeff McBride, President/CEO

One-week sessions for children with ADD and speech/communication impairment. Coed, ages 5-14.

1001   Painted Turtle, The
1300 4th Street
Suite 300
Santa Monica, CA 90401   310-451-1353
                                       866-451-5367
                                       FAX: 310-451-1357
                            info@thepaintedturtle.com
                            www.thepaintedturtle.org/

Page Adler, Founder/Chair
Lou Adler, Producer
Shelly Brown, Board Member
Tom Amster, Board Member
This camp is the sixth edition to the 'Hole in the Wall' camps and is for seriously ill children in the California area. The Painted Turtle offers swimming, boating, fishing, horseback riding, art and crafts, and nature activities.

1002   Pilgrim Pines Camp & Conference Center
United Church of Christ
39570 Glen Road
Yucaipa, CA 92399   909-797-1821
                                       800-616-6612
                                       800-678-5102
                                       FAX: 909-797-2691
                            info@pilgrimpinescamp.org
                            www.pilgrimpinescamp.org

June Boutwell, Executive Director
Christian camp offering one-week sessions for campers with developmental disabilities. Coed, ages 10-Adult. Also families.

1003   Quest Camp
907 San Ramon Valley Blvd.
Suite 202
Danville, CA 94583   925-743-2900
                                       800-313-9733
                                       FAX: 925-820-9761
                            questcamps@mac.com
                            www.questcamps.com

Dr. Robert B Field, PhD., Founder/Executive Director
Debra Forrester-Field, M.A., Administrative Director
Aprilyn Artz, Clinical Director
Jodie Knott, Ph.D., Director
Camp is located in Alamo, California. Day camp offering three to eight-week sessions including psychological treatment for children with ADD and other mild to moderate psychological disorders. Coed, ages 6-15.

1004   Special Camp For Special Kids
31641 La Novia Avenue
San Juan Capistrano, CA 92675   949-661-0108
                                       FAX: 949-661-8637
                            lindsay.eres@smes.org
                            www.specialcamp.org

Lindsay Eres, Executive Director
Stefani Baker, Camp Operations Director
Patty Canright, RN, Nursing Director
Sabine Scott, Development Coordinator
Day camp for youths with disabilities offering arts & crafts, games, reading, and entertainment.

1005   Tuolumne Trails
22988 Ferretti Road
Groveland, CA 95321   209-962-7534
                            info@tuolumnetrails.org
                            tuolumnetrails.org

Colorado

1006   Adam's Camp
6767 South Spruce Street
Suite 102
Centennial, CO 80112   303-563-8290
                                       FAX: 303-563-8291
                            laura@adamscamp.org
                            adamscamp.org/

Bill Harmon, President
Cindy Wells, Vice President
Jay L Clark, Executive Director
Laura Johnson, Finance Director
Adam's camp is designed for infants and children with special needs and their families, as well as young adults with mild to moderate developmental disabilities. The camp offers a variety of intensive, therapeutic programs and recreational programs.

1007   Aspen Camp of the Deaf & Hard of Hearing
4862 Snowmass Creek Rd.
Snowmass, CO 81654   970-315-0513
                                       FAX: 970-923-0643
                                       TTY:970-315-0513
                            office@aspencamp.org
                            www.aspencamp.org/

Kelly Krumrie, President
Ellen Roth, Board Member
Nick Stark, Board Member
Tim Whitsitt, Board Member
Provide enriching experiential educational and recreational experiences for Deaf and Hard of Hearing individuals.

1008   Breckenridge Outdoor Education Center
P.O.Box 697
Breckenridge, CO 80424   970-453-6422
                                       800-383-2632
                                       FAX: 970-453-4676
                            boec@boec.org
                            www.boec.org

Tim Casey, Chair
John Ebright, Vice Chair
Bruce Fitch, Executive Director
Bill Gillilan, Treasurer
Provides year-round adventure based wilderness and adaptive ski programs for people with disabilities. The Center excels in offering challenging, rewarding outdoor experiences individually designed to the abilities and needs of participants.

1009   CNI Cochlear Kids Camp
Colorado Neurological Institute
701 East Hampden Avenue
Suite 415
Englewood, CO 80113   303-783-4010
                                       855-463-6264
                                       FAX: 303-788-5469
                            info@thecni.org
                            www.thecni.org

Tami Lack, MA, CFRE, Executive Director
Greg Seal, President
Troy Talbert, Senior VP
Molly Hagan, Vice President
Designed to bring together children ages 1-18 with cochlear implants and their families. Campers enjoy both indoor and outdoor recreational and educational programs.

1010   Camp Paha Rise Above
City of Lakewood
480 S. Allison Pkwy
Lakewood, CO 80226   303-987-7000
                                       FAX: 303-987-7832
                                       TTY:303-987-7057
                            marsno@lakewood.org
                            www.lakewood.org

Bob Murphy, Mayor
Kathy Hodgson, City Manager
Nanette Neelan, Deputy City Manager

Camp Paha is a City of Lakewood day camp for children ages 6-17 and young adults ages 18-25 with disabilities. We provide programs for campers with all disability types: developmental, physical, emotional, behavioral, and learning. Camp Paha offers safe, quality, fun and challenging activities. Camp provides campers an opportunity to participate in aquatics, sports, games, nature, music, drama, hiking, arts and crafts, and field trips into the community.

1011 Camp Rocky Mountain Village

Easter Seals Colorado
5755 West Alameda Avenue
Lakewood, CO 80226-3500
303-233-1666
FAX: 303-569-3857
campinfo@eastersealscolorado.org
www.easterseals.com/co

Chris Whitley, Chair
Lynn Robinson, President/CEO
Nancy Hanson, VP, Human Resources
Bill Evert, Co-Treasurer

For children and adults with disabilities. Campers enjoy swimming, fishing, day trips, sports and recreation, arts and crafts.

1012 Camp Wapiyapi

191 University Boulevard
Box 294
Denver, CO 80206
303-534-0883
FAX: 303-534-0874
Wapiyapi@wapiyapi.org
www.wapiyapi.org

Jeff Druck, President
Caryl Wojcik, Vice President
Chris Watts, Treasurer
Jason Elbot, Engineering Manager

A no-cost respite for children with cancer and their families. The camp offers a wide variety of group and individual activities

1013 Challenge Aspen

P.O.Box 6639
Snowmass Village, CO 81615
970-923-0578
FAX: 970-923-7338
possibilities@challengeaspen.com
www.challengeaspen.org

Jimmy Yeager, President
Jack Kennedy, VP
Kevin Berg, Board Member
Grayson Stover, Secretary

Challenge Aspen provides recreational and cultural experiences for individuals who have cognitive or physical challenges. Challenge Aspen offers a variety of recreational programs to fit a diversity of needs and interests. We offer both summer, winter and special events for both adults and children.

1014 Champ Camp

American Lung Association
Glacier View Ranch
8748 Overland Rd
Ward, CO 80481
303-847-0279
champcamp@lungcolorado.org
www.lung.org/

Ashley Seder, Director

Champ Camp is an educational program and week-long summer camp for children ages 7-14 with asthma. At camp, children gain confidence in themselves and their ability to take control of their asthma.

1015 Cheley/Children's Hospital Burn Camps Program

The Children's Hospital
Anschultz Medical Campus
13123 East 16th Avenue
Aurora, CO 80045
720-777-1234
800-624-6553
boulter.trudy@tchden.org
www.thechildrenshospital.org

Jim Shmerling, DHA, FACHE, President and CEO

Camp is open for children ages 8 to 18 who have been hospitalized at The Children's Hospital or other burn units across the country. Campers gain life skills and confidence whether they are on a challenge course, catching a fish or climbing onto a horse.

1016 Colorado Lions Camp

28541 HWY 67N
P.O.Box 9043
Woodland Park, CO 80863
719-687-2087
FAX: 719-687-7435
dsmith@coloradolionscamp.org
www.coloradolionscamp.org

Sharla F Westerman, President
Barbara Guest, VP
Sharron Nickerson, Executive Director
Michelle Werner, Executive Administrative Assista

Outdoor recreational camping for the visually and hearing impaired and developmentally delayed. All normal camp activities are offered at the year-round facility. Summer and winter programs. 1 to 4 staff supervision with a nurse or doctor in attendance.

1017 First Descents

3001 Brighton Boulevard
Suite 623
Denver, CO 80216
303-945-2490
FAX: 303-474-3005
info@firstdescents.org
firstdescents.org

Brent Goldstein, Chairman
Ryan O'Donoghue, Executive Director
Brad Ludden, Founder
Sarah Hubbard, Marketing Director

First Descents offers young adult cancer fighters and survivors a free outdoor adventure experience designed to empower them to climb, paddle, and surf beyond their diagnosis, defy their cancer, reclaim their lives and connect with others doing the same.

1018 Rocky Mountain Village

Easter Seals Colorado
5755 West Alameda Avenue
Lakewood, CO 80226-3500
303-233-1666
FAX: 303-569-3857
campinfo@eastersealscolorado.org
www.easterseals.com/co

Chris Whitley, Chair
Lynn Robinson, President/CEO
Nancy Hanson, VP, Human Resources
Bill Evert, Co-Treasurer

An 11 week summer camp for people with disabilities. After the summer season there is respite weekends for people with disabilities - once a month.

1019 Roundup River Ranch

8333 Colorado River Road
PO Box 8589
Gypsum, CO 81620
970-748-9983
FAX: 877-619-0323
info@rounduptriverranch.org
www.rounduptriverranch.org

Lia Gore, Chair
Dick O'Loughlin, Vice Chair
Ruth B. Johnson, J.D., President/CEO
Tammy Argenbright, Chief Administrative Officer/Chi

Roundup River Ranch is a medically supported camp for kids with chronic and life-threatening illnesses- the place where they can truly feel incredible, no matter what illness they're battling. We put the focus on their fun, not their conditions. And most importantly, we give kids an experience that encourages their lives, allowing them to simply enjoy the fun, games, and joys of childhood- for free.

1020 **YMCA Camp Shady Brook**
YMCA of the Pikes Peak Region (PPYMCA)
316 N. Tejon Street
Colorado Springs, CO 80903   719-329-7266
                                     FAX: 719-272-7258
                                     campinfo@ppymca.org
                                     www.campshadybrook.org

Sonny Adkins, Executive Director
Lillian Cross, Business Manager Child
Chris Chambers, Facility Director
Mark Bowers, Conference & Retreat Director
Camp is located in Sedalia, Colorado. One-week sessions for campers with HIV. Boys and girls 7-16. Also families, seniors and single adults.

Connecticut

1021 **Arthur C. Luf Children's Burn Camp**
Connecticut Burns Care Foundation
601 Boston Post Road
Milford, CT 06460   203-878-6744
                                     FAX: 203-878-4044
                                     ctburnscare@optonline.net
                                     www.ctburnsfoundation.org

Frank Szivos, Executive Director
Susan M. Howard, Foundation Secretary
Frank Szivos, Executive Director
A safe outdoor environment for children ages 8-18 from around the world who have survived life altering burn injuries. Children learn to build self-confidence and self-esteem.

1022 **Camp Harkness**
Arc of New London County
P.O. Box 2545
Hartford, CT 06146-2545

                                     www.sbacct.tripod.com/

1023 **Camp Hemlocks**
Easter Seals: Connecticut
733 Summer Street
Suite 104
Stamford, CT 6901   203-388-2192
                                     800-832-4409
                                     FAX: 203-388-2196
                                     campinfo@eastersealsct.org
                                     www.easterseals.com/cfc

Chris Whitley, Chair
Bill Evert, Co-Treasurer
Nancy Hanson, Corporate Secretary
Lynn Robinson, President/CEO
Camp is located in Hebron, Connecticut. One and two-week sessions June-August for campers with a variety of disabilities. Coed, ages 6 and up. Families, seniors, single adults. Campers can enjoy nature walks, swimming, boating arts & crafts and sing-a-longs around the campfire.

1024 **Camp Horizons**
127 Babcock Hill Rd
South Windham, CT 06266   860-456-1032
                                     FAX: 860-456-4721
                                     scott.lambeck@camphorizons.org
                                     horizonsct.org

Adam Milne, Board Chairperson
Chris McNaboe, President
Kathleen McNaboe, Board Vice President
L. Sanford (Sandy) Rice, Board Treasurer
Bordering Lake Probus, the facilities at the camp are equipped to accommodate a wide range of activities and programs for campers with developmental disabilities, or other challenging emotional and social needs. There is a 5:1 camper-counselor ratio with a schedule of three programs in the morning and four in the afternoon.

1025 **Camp Isola Bella**
American School for the Deaf
139 N Main St
West Hartford, CT 06107   860-570-2300
                                     FAX: 860-824-4276
                                     TTY:860-570-2222
                                     IBDirector@asd-1817.org
                                     www.campisolabella.org

Alyssa Pecorino, Director
Jenilee Terry, Camp Registrar
Ed Peltier, Executive Director
Tom Wood, CFO
Hearing-impaired children, ages 6-19, blend educational instruction in communications with recreational activities. Qualified deaf and hearing staff members with experience in education, child care and counseling are employed at the camp.

1026 **Hole in the Wall Gang Camp**
565 Ashford Center Rd
Ashford, CT 06278   860-429-3444
                                     FAX: 860-429-7295
                                     ashford@holeinthewallgang.org
                                     www.holeinthewallgang.org

Raymond Lamontagne, Chairman
Ken Alberti, Chief Development Officer
James H. Canton, Chief Executive Officer
Kevin M. Magee, Chief Financial Officer
Low-cost eight-week sessions June-August for children with cancer and HIV. Coed, ages 7-15.

1027 **Marvelwood Summer**
Marvelwood School
476 Skiff Mountain Road
P.O. Box 3001
Kent, CT 06757- 3001   860-927-0047
                                     FAX: 860-927-0021
                                     summerschool@marvelwood.org
                                     www.marvelwood.org

Arthur F. Goodearl, Head of School
Bettyann Haskell, Business Office
Katherine Almquist, Director of Admission
Richard Becker, CFO
The emphasis in this summer program is on diagnosis and remediation of individual reading, spelling, writing, mathematics and study problems. Offered to ages 12-16.

1028 **YMCA Camp Jewell**
YMCA of Greater Hartford
6 Prock Hill Road
P.O. Box 8
Colebrook, CT 06021   860-379-2782
                                     888-412-2267
                                     FAX: 860-379-8715
                                     TTY: 888-412-2267
                                     camp.jewell@ghymca.org
                                     www.ghymca.org

Harold Sparrow, President and CEO
Jim Scherer, Chief Operating Officer
Liz Whitty, Vice President of development
Joseph Weist, Chief Financial Officer
Camp is located in Colebrook, Connecticut. Two-week sessions for children with cancer. Coed, ages 8-16. Also families.

Delaware

1029 Camp Fairlee Manor
Easter Seals DE/MD Eastern Shore
61 Corporate Circle
New Castle, DE 19720
302-324-4444
800-677-3800
FAX: 302-324-4441
contact@esdel.org
www.de.easterseals.com

Cynthia Morgan, Chair
Martha Rees, Vice Chair
Kenan Sklenar, President/CEO
Jeffery Gosnear, Treasurer
Residential camp at Fairlee Manor serves an average of 50 to 75 children and adults each week with physical disabilities and/or cognitive, behavioral impairments throughout the summer and on select weekends year-round.

1030 Camp Manito/Camp Lenape
United Cerebral Palsy Of Delaware
700 A River Road
Wilmington, DE 19809-2746
302-764-2400
FAX: 302-764-8713
ucpde@ucpde.org
www.ucpde.org

Donna M. Hopkins, President
D. Bruce McClenathan, Vice President
Michele M. Zonick, Recording Secretary
Daniel Edgar, Treasurer
For children & young adults aged 3-21 with orthopedic disabilities. Campers find a structured program of arts, crafts, sports, swimming, music and nature studies.

1031 Childrens Beach House
1800 Bay Ave
Lewes, DE 19958
302-645-9184
FAX: 302-655-4216
www.cbhinc.org

Martha P. Tschantz, President
Linda K. Berdine, Vice President
Linda M. Fischer, Secretary
Charles H. Sterner, Treasurer
Camp is located in Lewes, Delaware. Four-week sessions June-August for Delaware children with hearing impairment or speech/communication impairment, also fine or gross motor delays. Coed, ages 7-18. Also, serves children year round on weekends only.

1032 Sandcastle Day Camp
Children's Beach House
1800 Bay Ave
Lewes, DE 19958
302-645-9184
FAX: 302-655-4216
www.cbhinc.org

Martha P. Tschantz, President
Linda K. Berdine, Vice President
Linda M. Fischer, Secretary
Charles H. Sterner, Treasurer
Camp is located in Lewes, Delaware. Four-week sessions June-August for Delaware children with hearing impairment or speech/communication impairment. Coed, ages 6-12.

District of Columbia

1033 Columbia Lighthouse for the Blind Summer Camp
Columbia Lighthouse for the Blind
1825 K Street NorthWest
Suite 1103
Washington, DC 20006
202-454-6400
FAX: 877-595-6401
info@clb.org
www.clb.org

Tony Cancelosi, K.M.,, President and CEO
Anthony Cancelosi, CEO
Jocelyn Hunter, Director of Communications
Cathy Miller, Director of Development
Helps enable the blind or visually impaired to obtain and maintain independence at home, school, work and in the community. Programs and services include early intervention services, training and consultation in assistive technology, career placement services, comprehensive low vision care and a wide range of rehabilitation services. Highly acclaimed summer camp, picnics and holiday activities encourage blind and visually impaired children to make new friends and experience the joys of childhood

1034 Lab School of Washington
4759 Reservoir Rd NW
Washington, DC 20007-1921
202-965-6600
labschool@webmail.org
www.labschool.org

Mimi W. Dawson, Chair
Mac Bernstein, Vice Chair
Mike Tongour, Secretary
Bill Tennis, Treasurer
The Lab School six week summer session includes individualized reading, spelling, writing, study skills and math programs. A multisensory approach addresses the needs of bright learning disabled children. Related services such as speech/language therapy and occupational therapy are integrated into the curriculum. Elementary/Intermediate; Junior High/High School.

Florida

1035 Camp Amigo Burn Camp
Children's Burn Camp Of North Florida, Inc.
P.O. Box 368
Tallahassee, FL 32302
850-509-6200
www.campamigo.com

Rusty Roberts, President
Stephanie Powell, Treasurer
Camp Amigo is open to burn survivors ages 6-18 living in North or Central Florida. The camp is free of charge and provides children who have physical and emotional scarring a place to be themselves and build a network of support.

1036 Camp Boggy Creek
30500 Brantley Branch Rd
Eustis, FL 32736
352-483-4200
866-462-6449
FAX: 352-483-0589
info@campboggycreek.org
www.boggycreek.org

J. Patterson Cooper, Chair
Wendy Durden, Vice Chair
June Clark, President/CEO
David Mann, Camp Director
Year-round sessions for children with a variety of chronic or life-threatening illnesses including cancer, hemophilia, epilepsy, heart defects, HIV, spina bifida and asthma/respiratory ailments. Coed, ages 7-16.

1037 Camp Challenge
Easter Seals Of Florida
31600 Camp Challenge Road
Sorrento, FL 32776
352-383-4711
camp@fl.easterseals.com
www.easterseals.com/florida/

1038 Camp Thunderbird
Quest, Inc.
P.O. Box 531125
Orlando, FL 32853 407-218-4300
888-423-7700
FAX: 407-218-4301
webadmin@questinc.org
www.questinc.org/

David Canora, Chair
James Gallagher, Vice Chair
John Gill, President / CEO
Brooke Eakins, COO
Residential summer camping program for children and adults
with a developmental disability. Located on 19-acres of Wekiwa
Springs State Park. Campers enjoy swimming, sports, nature
hikes, an outdoor amphitheater, etc. One and two-week sessions
June-August. Coed, ages 8-80.

1039 Center Academy at Pinellas Park
6710 86th Ave
Pinellas Park, FL 33782 727-541-5716
FAX: 727-544-8186
infopp@centeracademy.com
www.centeracademy.com

Mack R Hicks PhD, Founder/Chairman of the Board
Eric V. Larson, Ph. D.,, President & COO
Andrew P Hicks PhD, CEO/Clinical Dir.
Lisa Hartmann, Dir. Education
Specifically designed for the learning disabled child and other
children with difficulties in concentration, strategy, social skills,
impulsivity, distractibility and study strategies. Programs offered
include: attention training, visual-motor remediation, socialization skills training, relaxation training, horseback riding and
more. The day camp meets weekdays from 9-3 for 3,4 or 5 week
sessions.

1040 Dream Oaks Camp
Foundation For Dreams, Inc.
16110 Dream Oaks Place
Bradenton, FL 34212 941-746-5659
FAX: 941-745-1409
jfranke@foundationfordreams.org
www.foundationfordreams.org

Jodi Franke, Executive Director
Elena Cassella, Director of Development
Gilda Poe, Administrative Assistant
Weekend camps and day residential programs open to children
with physical and developmental disabilities and serious illnesses. Activities include horseback riding, nature programs,
sports, game, swimming, talent shows, and arts and crafts.

1041 Florida Diabetes Camp
P.O. Box 14136
Gainesville, FL 32604 352-334-1321
FAX: 352-334-1326
fccyd@floridadiabetescamp.org
www.floridadiabetescamp.org

Gary Cornwell, Executive Director
Chris Stakely, Assistant Director
Amy Soileau, Outreach Director
Robena Cornwell, Finance
Camp is located in Florida. One and two-week sessions June-Au-
gust for children with diabetes. Coed, ages 6-18 and families.
Camps throughout the year.

1042 Florida Lions Camp
Lions of Multiple District 35
2819 Tiger Lake Rd
Lake Wales, FL 33898 863-696-1948
FAX: 863-696-2398
jrv113@gmail.com
www.lionscampfl.org

Barbara Cage, Executive Director
Liz Cage, Program Director/ Rentals
Carissa Moen, Bookkeeping/Registrar
One-week sessions June-August for youths and adults with vi-
sual impairments and other challenging disabilities. Coed, ages 5
and up. A variety of traditional summer camp activities which in-

clude: swimming, canoeing, fishing, hiking, camping out and
cooking over a fire, games, arts & crafts, singing & dancing,
hay-wagon rides, challenge course and much more. Activities are
adapted to the age and ability of each camper to ensure maximum
participation, safety and fun.

1043 Florida Sheriffs Caruth Camp
Florida Sheriffs Youth Ranches
2486 Cecil Webb Place
Live Oak, FL 32060 386-842-5501
800-765-3797
FAX: 386-842-2429
youthranches.org

Sheriff B. Stewart, Chair
Dan Hager, Vice Chairman
Roger Bouchard, President
Bill Frye, EVP
Camp is located in Inglis, Florida. One-week sessions for chil-
dren with ADD. Coed, ages 10-15.

1044 Hands To Love
165 Montgomery Road
P.O. Box 140572
Altamonte, FL 32714 352-273-7382
FAX: 352-273-7388
info@handstolove.org
www.handstolove.org

Jackie Hadala, President
Hands to Love (affectionately nicknamed H2L) is an organization for children with upper limb differences and their families.

1045 Kris' Camp
1132 Green Hill Trace
Tallahassee, FL 32317 850-445-4821
FAX: 877-267-9451
kberger62@gmail.com
www.kriscamp.org

Kathy Berger, PT, Executive Director
Michelle Hardy, MT-BC, NMT, Music Therapist
Sue Yudovin, Board of Director
Chris McHorney, Board of Director
For children with autism.

1046 Sertoma Camp Endeavor
Sertoma Camp Endeavor
P.O. Box 910
Dundee, FL 33838-0910 863-439-1300
db4storm@aol.com
www.sertomacampendeavor.net

David Ball, Chair
Ronald Bochenek, Director
Misti Carman, Secretary
Charles Lake, President
The integration of deaf, hard of hearing and hearing youngsters is
a unique characteristic of our camping program. Both hearing,
deaf and hard of hearing children have the opportunity to learn
about themselves and each other in an informal and empowering
setting.

1047 VACC Camp
Miami Childrens Hospital
3200 S.W. 60 Ct.
Suite 203
Miami, FL 33155-4076 305-662-8222
FAX: 786-268-1765
bela.florentin@mch.com
www.vacccamp.com

Bela Florentin, Camp Coordinator
Free week-long overnight camp for ventilation assisted children
and their families.

Georgia

1048 Aerie Experiences
Aerie Experiences
969 Golden Avenue
Dahlonega, GA 30533

404-285-0467
mdweneta@aerieexperiences.com
aerieexperiences.com

Matthew D. Weneta, M.Ed.
We offer experiential, adventure-based, wilderness and therapeutic activities for children, individuals and families navigating Neurobiological Disorders, Aspergers, High Functioning Autism, Learning Disabilities and other special needs.

1049 Camp Breathe Easy
American Lung Association
2452 Spring Rd
Smyrna, GA 30080-3828

404-231-9887
annie@camptwinlakes.org
www.campbreatheeasy.com/

Annie Garrett, Camp Director
Camp Breathe Easy is a seven-day, six-night overnight camp for children, ages 7-13, with asthma who need medication and are limited in summer camping opportunities. The children learn asthma self-management techniques and coping strategies to better handle their illness. Campers swim, repel off trees, fish, canoe, play soccer, basketball and miniature golf, and participate in ceramics and arts and crafts.

1050 Camp Caglewood
Caglewood, Inc.
P.O. Box 158
Flowery Branch, GA 30542

678-405-9000
FAX: 770-441-3406
info@caglewood.org
www.caglewood.org

1051 Camp Dream
Camp Dream Foundation
4355 Cobb Parkway
Suite J117
Atlanta, GA 30339

www.campdreamga.org

JR Clark, President
Gary Marshall, Vice President
Beverly Taylor, Programs Director
Valarie Dunn, Secretary
Camp Dream is a free camp where special needs children can camp and have fun regardless of their physical and/or mental condition. The camp offers many recreational activities and programs.

1052 Camp Esperanza
Southern California Chapter
1330 W. Peachtree St
Suite 100
Atlanta, GA 30309

404-872-7100
800-954-2873
FAX: 323-954-5790
jziegler@arthritis.org
www.arthritis.org

Manuel Loya, CEO
Victoria Fung, Chief Program Officer
Amy Daugherty, Chief Development Officer
Angele Price, VP, Development
A one-week camp in August that allows children with arthritis to participate in such activities as horseback riding, swimming, etc. in a fun-filled environment.

1053 Camp Hawkins
GA Baptist Childrens Homes & Family Ministries,Inc
P.O. Box 329
Palmetto, GA 30268

770-463-3800
ksewell@gbchfm.org
www.gbchfm.org

James Harper, D.Min, President/CEO
Kendra Sewell, Contact Person
Brian Hawkins, Administrator
Alan Mccumber, Vice President - Finance
Residential summer camp for youth's ages 8-12 coping with varying developmental disabilities such as down's syndrome, traumatic brain injuries, cerebral palsy, and learning disorders and/or developmental delays. Staff works one-on-one with each camper.

1054 Camp Juliena
Georgia Council for the Hearing Impaired
4151 Memorial Drive
Suite 103B
Decatur, GA 30032-1511

404-292-5312
866-873-2485
FAX: 404-299-3642
info@fullcirclegrp.com
http://www.fullcirclegrp1.com

Thomas Galey, Executive Director
Bonna Lenyszyn, Camp Director
Ron Vickery, President
Deborah Douglin, Treasurer
A weeklong residential summer camp for youths and teens who are deaf or hard of hearing. Through challenging, team-oriented activities, campers form lasting friendships and acquire valuable leadership, social and communication skills.

1055 Camp Kudzu
Camp Kudzu, Inc.
5885 Glenridge Drive
Suite 160
Atlanta, GA 30328

404-250-1811
FAX: 404-250-1812
info@campkudzu.org
www.campkudzu.org

Chris Kane, Chairman
Seth Tuttle, Development Director
Alexandra Allen, Executive Director
Ashley Conant, Camp Director
Camp for children, teens and families with type 1 diabetes. Besides teaching diabetes management, campers learn that they are not alone in their struggles and enjoy climbing, swimming and many other outdoor activities.

1056 Camp Sunshine
1850 Clairmont Road
Decatur, GA 30033-3405

404-325-7979
866-786-2267
FAX: 404-325-7929
www.mycampsunshine.com

Dorothy H. Jordan, Founder
Beth Abernathy, Chair
Randall Kirsch, Vice Chair
J. Preston Byers, Treasurer
Camp sunshine gives children with cancer the opportunity to enjoy normal activities such as horseback riding, swimming, and arts & crafts.

1057 Camp Twin Lakes
1391 Keencheefoonee Rd
Rutledge, GA 30663

706-557-9070
FAX: 706-557-9147
contact@camptwinlakes.org
www.camptwinlakes.org

Doug Hertz, Chairman and Founder
Elizabeth C. Richards, President
Adrian J. Powell, Treasurer
Jeffrey S. Sloan, Secretary
One-week sessions June-August for children with serious illnesses and life challenges. Works with over 40 different special needs organizations. Coed, ages 8-18. Two locations: Rutledge and Will-A-Way in Winder, GA.

1058 Squirrel Hollow Summer Camp
The Bedford School
5665 Milam Rd
Fairburn, GA 30213
770-774-8001
FAX: 770-774-8005
bbox@thebedfordschool.org
www.thebedfordschool.org

Michael Vigil, Chairman
Todd Weaver, Board Member
Aaron Turner, Board Member
Jimmy Collins, Board Member
A remedial summer program for children with academic needs held on the campus of The Bedford School in Fairburn, Georgia. It is a five week day camp held from June 19 to July 21 and serves ages 6-16. For more information contact Betsy Box at (770) 774-8001.

Hawaii

1059 Camp Anuenue
American Cancer Society
Waialua, HI 96791
818-788-9900
FAX: 808-595-7502
editor@specialneeds.com
www.specialneeds.com/directory/camp/cancer/hi
Debra Glowik, Director
Camp Anuenue is for children ages 7-17 who have or have had cancer.

1060 YMCA Camp Erdman
YMCA Of Honolulu
1441 Pali Highway
Honolulu, HI 96813
808-531-9622
FAX: 808-533-1286
info@ymcahonolulu.org
www.ymcahonolulu.org

Lance Wilhelm, Chair
Keith Sakamoto, Vice Chair
Bruce Coppa, Vice Chair
Tim John, Vice Chair
Traditional Resident Camp program is five nights and six days of fun-filled activities that will create positive lifetime memories. Camp activities include: arts & crafts, swimming, kayaking, hiking, challenge course, snorkeling, athletics, nature, dance & drama, beach writing and archery. Traditional Resident Camp Experience (Ages 6-17) serving the needs of the disabled.

Idaho

1061 Camp Hodia
1701 N 12th St
Boise, ID 83702
208-891-1023
FAX: 208-891-1023
lisa1@hodia.org
www.hodia.org

Natalie B. DelRio, Chair
Richard Christensen, Vice Chair
Lisa Gier, Executive Director
Vicki Cutshall, R.N., Director, Hodia Kids Camp
Camp is located in Alturas Lake, Idaho. One-week sessions for children with diabetes. Coed, ages 8-18. Ski Camp in Sun Valley in January, ages 12-18.

1062 Camp Rainbow Gold
216 West Jefferson Street
Boise, ID 83702
208-350-6435
info@camprainbowgold.org
camprainbowgold.org

Tim Tyree, President
Elizabeth Lizberg, Executive Director
Doris F. Tunney, M.D., Treasurer
Meg Omel-Tyree, Secretary
Camp Rainbow Gold provides year round programs such as medically supervised camps, college scholarships and other emotionally empowering experiences to children diagnosed with cancer, their families and support network.

1063 Camp Sawtooth
Oregon-Idaho Conference Center
HC 64 BOX 8290
Ketchum, ID 83340
208-726-1155
directorscampsawtooth@yahoo.com
www.campsawtooth.org/

Illinois

1064 Camp Callahan
Camp Callahan, Inc.
P.O. Box 5253
Quincy, IL 62305
217-833-2707
www.campcallahan.com

1065 Camp Christmas Seal
American Lung Association of Oregon
55 W. Wacker Drive
Suite 1150
Chicago, IL 60601-7790
503-924-4094
FAX: 202-452-1805
info@lungoregon.org
www.lung.org/associations/states/oregon/
Kathryn A Forbes, Chairman
John F. Emanuel, Vice Chair
Harold Wimmer, President and Chief Executive Of
Penny J. Siewert, Secretary/Treasurer
Camp is located in Sisterhood, Oregon. Sessions for children with asthma/respiratory ailments. Coed, ages 8-15.

1066 Camp Discovery
American Academy Of Dermatology
930 E. Woodfield Road
Schaumburg, IL 60173
847-240-1280
866-503-SKIN
866-503-7546
FAX: 847-240-1859
jmueller@aad.org
www.campdiscovery.org

Brett M. Coldiron, MD, President
Elise A. Olsen, VP
Suzanne M. Olbricht, Secretary-Treasurer
Neal D. Bhatia, Director
Free camp for ages 8-16 with chronic skin conditions such as psoriasis, eczema, scleroderma, epidermolysis bullosa, alopecia, Vitiligo, congenital nevus. Campers can enjoy boating, fishing, water skiing, swimming, arts and crafts.

1067 Camp Easter Seals
Easter Seals: Oregon
233 South Wacker Drive
Suite 2400
Chicago, IL 60606-3765
503-228-5108
800-221-6827
FAX: 503-228-1352
www.easterseals.com
Rick Davidson, Chairman
Eileen Howard Boone, 1st Vice Chairman
Edward L. Wenzel, Treasurer
Nancy Goguen, Secretary
Camp is located in Corbett, Oregon. Summer sessions for children and adults with a variety of disabilities. Coed, ages 6-90.

1068 Camp Hug The Bear
Northern Suburban Special Recreation Association
3105 MacArthur Blvd.
Northbrook, IL 60062
    847-509-9400
    FAX: 847-509-1177
    info@nssra.org
    www.nssra.org

Mary V. Arsdale, Chair
Steve Wilson, Vice Chair
Craig Culp, Executive Director
Caitlin Deptula, Registrar
For children who have sensory integration disorder or children who are on the autism spectrum. Children have the opportunity to take part in a unique camp experience which is vital in their growth and development. Recreation based programs include sports, arts and crafts, swimming, and games.

1069 Camp I Am Me
Illinois Fire Safety Alliance
P.O. Box 911
Mount Prospect, IL 60056
    847-390-0911
    800-634-0911
    FAX: 847-390-0920
    ifsa@ifsa.org
    www.ifsa.org

Jim Kreher, President
Chris Logston, VP
Michelle Nabor, Secretary/Treasurer
Philip Zaleski, Executive Director
Camp is held during the third week of June for children who are burn survivors. The children are able to share their common experiences, have fun and not feel self conscious about what others think. Some of the activities include swimming, boating, fishing, archery, basketball and volleyball.

1070 Camp Little Giant
SIU:Carbondale Therapeutic Recreation Prgm
Southern Illinois University
Mail Code 6888
Carbondale, IL 62901
    618-453-1121
    FAX: 618-453-1188
    tonec@siu.edu
    www.ton.siu.edu

Mary Anne Cunningham, Manager
Camp Little Giant is a summer program but the Therapeutic Program runs all year round. One and two week sessions for campers with a variety of disabilities. Coed, ages 8-80.

1071 Camp New Hope
P.O.Box 764
Mattoon, IL 61938-764
    217-895-2341
    FAX: 217-895-3658
    cnhinc@rr1.net
    www.cnhinc.org

Kim Carmack, Executive Director
Terri Taylor, Camp Director
Weekend Respite, advocacy services, social and recreational services and a summer camp for the disabled. The camp accommodates people of widely diverse needs and abilities including access for wheelchair users. Co-ed, for those 8 years and older, including adults. Facilities include a mini golf area; pontoon boat; fishing deck; playground; trails; swimming pool; and sleeping cabins with air conditioning.

1072 Camp Quality Illinois
PO Box 641
Lansing, MI 60438
    708-895-8311
    FAX: 866-285-5208
    illinois@campqualityusa.org
    www.campqualityusa.org/il

Mary Lockton, Executive Director
Dawn Winters, Treasurer
Linda Reece, Secretary/Staff Coordinator
Beverly Bonnema-Ream, Companion Coordinator
Camp Quality is for children with cancer and their siblings. The camp offers a stress-free environment that offers exciting activities and fosters new friendships, while helping to give the children courage, motivation and emotional strength.

1073 Easter Seals Camp Sunnyside
Easter Seals Iowa
233 South Wacker Drive
Suite 2400
Chicago, IL 60606
    515-309-2375
    800-221-6827
    FAX: 515-289-1281
    TTY: 515-289-4069
    krumpf@eastersealsia.org
    www.easterseals.com

Rick Davidson, Chairman
Nancy Goguen, Secretary
Eileen Howard Boone, 1st Vice Chairman
Joseph G. Kern, 2nd Vice Chairman
Each summer from June through August, campers with disabilities ages five and up, take part in one week camping sessions, gaining skills and independence by participating in activities like swimming, horseback riding, canoeing, fishing, camping and more. Coed, ages 4-95. Accepts seniors and single adults. Financial assistance available.

1074 JCYS Camp Red Leaf
Jewish Council for Youth Services
180 W Washington St.,
Suite 1100
Chicago, IL 60602
    312-726-8891
    FAX: 312-726-7920
    jthomason@jcys.org
    www.jcys.org

Jeffery Friedman, President
Adam Tarantur, President Elect
Stefanie Wolfson, VP of Operations
Aaron Turner, VP of Development
Our special needs camp, serves adults and children with developmental disabilities in 8- one week sessions during the summer, several travel adventures for adults and ten respite weekends during the year for children and young adults.

1075 Muscular Dystrophy Association Free Camp
222 S. Riverside Plaza
Suite 1500
Chicago, IL 85718-3208
    800-572-1717
    mda@mdausa.org
    www.mda.org

Steven M. Derks, President and CEO
Valerie A. Cwik, Executive Vice President
Julie Faber, Chief Financial Officer
Steven G. Ford, Marketing Officer
MDA Camp provides a wide range of activities for those with limited mobility or are in wheelchairs. The camp offers many outdoor sporting events, arts & crafts and talent shows.

1076 One Step At A Time Camp
213 West Institute Place
Suite 306
Chicago, IL 60610
    312-924-4220
    FAX: 312-878-7374
    jeff@onestepcamp.org
    onestepcamp.org

Jeff Infusino, President
Darryl Winston Perkins, Jr., Director Of Programs
Katie Weil, Development Officer
Hailey Danisewicz, Development Coordinator
Through our One Step programs, we offer camp experiences and other programs throughout the year that allow children with cancer to just be kids. Our programs offer fun, friendship and support in a safe and nurturing environment. Through the magic of childhood experiences, we help kids diagnosed with cancer reclaim their lives.

1077 Rimland Services for Autistic Citizens
1265 Hartrey Ave
Evanston, IL 60202

847-328-4090
FAX: 847-328-8364
TTY:847-328-4090
rimland.org/

Lorraine Ganz, President
Bernice Gryczan, VP
Barbara Cooper, Secretary
Wiliam Egan, Board Member

An accessible camp facility that can be utilized by groups for day use or overnight camping experiences. Six winterized cabins, a meeting facility, indoor pool, full food service, and an excellent staff are available. Educational programs can be arranged or you can utilize the facility to manage your own programs.

1078 Shady Oaks Camp
16300 Parker Rd
Homer Glen, IL 60491

708-301-0816
FAX: 708-301-5091
soc16300@sbcglobal.net
www.shadyoakscamp.org

Harry Burroughs, Chairman
Robert Szajkovics, President
Lori McAleavy, Vice President
Scott Steele, Executive Director

Shady Oaks Camp provides outdoor fun and recreation for children and adults with cerebral palsy and similar disabilities. Our camp is organized with the goal of providing stimulating life experiences that our campers may not have the opportunity to engage in elsewhere.

1079 Summer Camp for Children with Muscular Dystrophy
Muscular Dystrophy Association - USA
222 S. Riverside Plaza
Suite 1500
Chicago, IL 85718-3208

520-529-2000
800-572-1717
FAX: 520-529-5300
mda@mdausa.org
www.mda.org

Steven M. Derks, President and CEO
Valerie A. Cwik, Executive Vice President
Julie Faber, Chief Financial Officer
Steven G. Ford, Marketing Officer

The MDA Summer Camp offers a wide range of activities specifically designed for young people with limited mobility or who use a wheelchair. Some of the activities include boating and canoeing, swimming, adaptive sports, fishing, archery, karaoke, scavenger hunts, arts & crafts, dances, talent shows and campfires.

1080 Summer Wheelchair Sport Camps
University of Illinois
1207 S Oak St
Champaign, IL 61820-6901

217-333-4607
FAX: 212-333-0248
sportscamp@illinois.edu
www.illinoiswheelchairathletics.com

Maureen Gilbert, Camp Director

Rigorous camps designed for individuals with lower extremity physical disabilities. Camp attendees will spend an average of 8-9 hours a day, focusing on development and refinement of fitness, techniques and strategies. Strength training, nutrition and mental training sessions will also be included in all camps. The camp staff is comprised of athletic staff and local wheelchair athletes with coaching experience from the University of Illinois Wheelchair Athletics Program.

1081 Timber Pointe Outdoor Center
Easter Seals UCP
507 East Armstrong Avenue
Peoria, IL 61603-3197

309-686-1177
FAX: 309-687-2035
www.ci.easterseals.com

Brad Halverson, Chair
Don Young, 1st Vice Chair
Wes Blumenshine, 2nd Vice Chair
Jeff White, Treasurer

One and two-week sessions for campers with a wide variety of disabilities. Coed, ages 6-99. Campers experience different activities each day such as arts and crafts, music, horses, field sports, outdoor nature, swimming, canoeing and fishing. Every night there is a different activity: skit night, casino night, boat night (campers go out on the lake on pontoon boats), night swim, camp fires, and of course, everyone's favorite - a dance on the last night.

1082 YMCA Camp Duncan
32405 N Highway 12
Ingleside, IL 60041

847-546-8086
FAX: 847-546-3550
www.ymcacampduncan.org

Art Catrambone, Chair
Kim Kiser, Executive Director
Rona Roffey, Camp Director
Danielle Kiessel, Day Camp Director

The Tourette Syndrome/TS Camp USA, founded in 1994, is a residential camping program designed for girls and boys ages 8 - 16+ whose primary diagnosis is TS, and to a lesser degree, OCD and ADD/ADHD. The TS Camp is held at YMCA Camp Duncan which is located 30 miles north of Chicago. The goal of the camp is to allow children with TS an opportunity to meet other children, share similar experiences and coping mechanisms in a fun, safe and positive environment.

Indiana

1083 Anderson Woods
4630 Adyeville Rd
Bristow, IN 47515

812-639-1079
andersonwoodspsci.net
www.andersonwoods.org

Judy Colby, Administrative Office

Provides camping experience and residential services to persons with mental and/or physical disabilities. Campers learn self confidence, trust and responsibilities through working together, tending gardens, feeding animals all while enjoying natures beauty.

1084 Autism Day Camp
Hillcroft Services: Isanogel
114 East Streeter Avenue
Muncie, IN 47304

765-284-4166
bwilliamson@hillcroft.org
www.hillcroft.org

Ted Baker, Chair
Brenda Llyod, Vice Chair
Bruce Baldwin, Director
Julie Bering, Secretary/ Treasurer

The camp is designed to improve the academic, social skills, and behaviors of children with autism spectrum disorders. The day camp is an 8-week intensive experience for children classified with autism spectrum disorders.

1085 Bradford Woods: Camp Riley
Indiana University
5040 State Road 67 N
Martinsville, IN 46151

765-342-2915
FAX: 765-349-1086
bradwood@indiana.edu
www.bradwoods.org

Shay Dawson, CTRS, Director
Melanie Wills, Director of Outdoor Education
Tim Street, Associate Director
Sheryl McGlory, Retreats Coordinator

One and two-week sessions for children with a variety of disabilities. Coed, ages 8-18.

1086 Brave Heart's Camp
The People's Burn Foundation
6337 Hollister Drive
Suite 2H
Indianapolis, IN 46224
317-803-2876
FAX: 317-692-0876
www.peoplesburnfoundation.org

Daryl Mickens, President
Matt Godbout, VP
Cindy Allison, Camp Director
Lora Hays, Adult, Child & Family Counselor
Specialized residential summer camp for burn survivor children. The camp gives the children an opportunity to heal from the physical and emotional scars by giving them the opportunity to just be kids.

1087 CHAMP Camp
6271 Coffman Road
Indianapolis, IN 46268
317-679-1860
FAX: 317-245-2291
admin@champcamp.org
www.champcamp.org

Scott Beaty, President
Rick Adams, VP
Karen Mellen, Secretary
Scott Black, Treasurer

1088 Camp About Face
The Head's Up Foundation
P.O. Box 167
Medora, IN 47260
812-966-2761
FAX: 812-966-2927
headsupfoundation2012@gmail.com
http://www.headsupfoundation.org

1089 Camp Alexander Mack
Indiana Deaf Camps Foundation
1113 E. Camp Mack Rd.
Milford, IN 46542
574-658-4831
www.campmack.org

Galen Jay, Interim Executive Director
Lauren Carrick, Director of Development/Facility
Amber Barrett, Food Service
Norma Miller, Ordained Minister
Our program is intentionally designed to provide campers with life changing experiences that lead to a formation of personal faith within a safe faith community.

1090 Camp Brave Eagle
Indiana Hemophilia And Thrombosis Center
8402 Harcourt Road
Suite 500
Indianapolis, IN 46260
219-834-2331
800-241-2873
www.campbraveeagle.org/

Angel Couch, Program Director
Jennifer Maahs, Pediatric Nurse Practitioner
Summer camp for children with bleeding disorders and their siblings. Campers participate in a traditional summer camp experience with swimming, canoeing, fishing, and nature education. The goal is to encourage the children to have fun while learning to be self-sufficient, building their self confidence and self-esteem and promoting a positive outlook.

1091 Camp Challenge
8914 Us Highway 50 East
Bedford, IN 47421
812-834-5159
info@gocampchallenge.com
www.gocampchallenge.com

Brian Klein, Executive Director
Kevin Wilson, President
Brian Allison, Vice-President
Trent Freed, Secretary
One and two-week sessions for campers with developmental and or physical disabilities, hearing impairment and the blind/visually impaired. Ages 6-99 and families.

1092 Camp Crosley YMCA
165 Ems T2 Ln
North Webster, IN 46555-9378
574-834-2331
877-811-6189
FAX: 574-834-3313
info@campcrosley.org
campcrosley.org/

Richard Armstrong, Executive Director
Mark Battig, Associate Executive Director
Naomi Thompson, Program Director
Pam Endicott, Office Manager/Registrar
Camp is located in North Webster, Indiana. Half-week, one, two and three-week sessions for campers with asthma/respiratory ailments and diabetes. Coed, ages 7-17. Also families and seniors.

1093 Camp John Warvel
Camp Crosley YMCA
165 EMS T2 Lane
North Webster, IN 46555
317-352-9226
FAX: 317-913-1592
cdixon@diabetes.org
www.diabetes.org

Janel Wright, JD, Chair
Kevin L. Hagan, CEO
Debbie Johnson, CFO
Greg Elfers, Chief Field Development Officer
Camp is located in North Webster, Indiana. Provides an enjoyable, safe and educational out-of-doors experience for children with insulin-dependent diabetes. A unique learning atmosphere for children to acquire new skills in caring for their disease. The camp experience instills confidence for the child's self-management of diabetes. Offers one-week sessions and can accommodate 200 campers, boys and girls aged 7-16.

1094 Camp Little Red Door
Little Red Door Cancer Agency
1801 North Merideian Street
Indianapolis, IN 46202-1411
317-925-5595
FAX: 317-925-5597
www.littlereddoor.org

Jeff Henry, Chair
Erika Rager, Vice Chair
Jim Schulz, Treasurer
Nicole Morgan, Secretary
Camp for pediatric cancer patients ages 8-19. The program is open to children diagnosed with or receiving treatment for cancer in the state of Indiana. Activities include swimming, fishing, canoeing, nature hikes, astronomy, arts and crafts.

1095 Camp Millhouse
25600 Kelly Rd
South Bend, IN 46614
574-233-2202
FAX: 574-233-2511
campmillhouse@gmail.com
www.campmillhouse.org

Diana Breden, Executive Director
Scarlett Russell, Camp Director
Nestled in a rustic clearing surrounded by 45 acres of woods, Camp Millhouse is a retreat for children and young adults with mental and physical disabilities. Hiking trails, nature studies, crafts, swimming, and stories around the bonfire make up activities campers long remember. One-week session. Co-ed, ages 4 to 30.

1096 Camp Red Cedar
3900 Hursh Road
Fort Wayne, IN 46845
260-637-3608
FAX: 260-637-5483
redcedar@awsusa.com
http://www.awsredcedar.com

Carrie Perry, Director
Shelly Detcher, HR Recruiter/Program Manager
Theresa Prentice, Barn Manager
Mallory Leatherman, Riding Instructor
Camp Red Cedar is open for children and adults with or without disabilities. Activities include, fishing, hiking, swimming and arts and crafts.

1097 **Camp Riley**
Camp Riley/Riley's Children Foundation
Attn: Camp Coordinator
30 S. Meridian Street, Suite 200
Indianapolis, IN 46204-3509　　　　317-634-4474
　　　　　　　　　　　　　　　　877-867-4539
　　　　　　　　　　　　　　　FAX: 317-634-4478
　　　　　　　　　　　　　riley@rileykids.org
　　　　　　　　　　　　www.rileykids.org/camp

James T Morris, Chairman
Kristin G Fruehwald, Treasurer
Rebecca Kubacki, Secretary
Kevin O'Keefe, President and CEO
Camp Riley is for youth's ages 8-18 with physical disabilities. The camp helps them to realize their potential as they become increasingly independent. Some of the activities that the camp offers is horseback riding and swimming.

1098 **Englishton Park Academic Remediation**
Englishton Park Presbyterian
P.O. Box 228
Lexington, IN 47138　　　　　　　812-889-2046
　　　　　　　　　　　　　　　FAX: 812-934-4322
　　　　　　　　　　ThomasLisaBarnett@etczone.com
　　　　　　　　　　　　www.englishtonpark.org

Lisa Barnett, Co-Directors
Thomas Barnett, Co-Director
Camp is located in Lexington, Indiana. Two-week sessions for children with ADD. Boys and girls, ages 7-12.

1099 **Happiness Bag**
3833 Union Rd
Terre Haute, IN 47802　　　　　　812-234-8867
　　　　　　　　　　　　　　　FAX: 812-238-0728
　　　　　　　　　　　　　　jmexdir@aol.com
　　　　　　　　　　　　www.happinessbag.org/

Trudy Rupska, President
Cari Rohrmayer, VP
Jodi Moan, Executive Director
Caren Elrod, Program Director
Serves developmentally disabled age 5-adult; day and residential camp program; after school program; scouting; Special Olympic anticipation (basketball, athletics, bowling, softball and aquatics); and a bowling league.

1100 **Hoosier Burn Camp**
P.O. BOX 233
Battle Ground, IN 47920　　　　　765-567-0115
　　　　　　　　　　　　　　　800-254-2878
　　　　　　　　　　　　　　　FAX: 765-567-0195
　　　　　　　　markkoopman@hoosierburncamp.org
　　　　　　　　　　　www.hoosierburncamp.org

Mark Koopman, Director
Mark Koopman, Executive Director
Abby James, Program Manager
Kim Jones, Administrative Assistant
Held at Camp Tecumseh in Brookston, IN., the camp is for burn survivors ages 8-18. Campers learn how to have fun and just be kids, while building their self-esteem and self confidence, learning independence and the life skills they need to fully recover from burn injuries.

1101 **Indiana Children's Deaf Camp**
The Indiana Deaf Camps Foundation, Inc.
100 West 86th Street
Indianapolis, IN 46260　　　　　317-846-3404
　　　　　　　　　　　　　　　FAX: 317-844-1034
　　　　　　　　　　　　deafcamp@hotmail.com
　　　　　　　　　　　　www.deafcamps.org

1102 **Residential Camp**
Hillcroft Services: Isanogel
114 East Streeter Avenue
Muncie, IN 47303　　　　　　　765-284-4166
　　　　　　　　　　　　　TTY:765-288-1073
　　　　　　　　　　　bwilliamson@hillcroft.org
　　　　　　　　　　　　www.hillcroft.org

Ted Baker, Board Chair
Brenda Lloyd, Vice Chair
Julie Bering, Secretary/Treasurer
Debbie Bennett, Chief Executive Officer
Programming at Isanogel includes creative arts, nature, recreation and aquatics. Individuals age 8 and older participate in one and two week programs.

1103 **Twin Lakes Camp**
1451 E Twin Lakes Rd
Hillsboro, IN 47949-8004　　　　765-798-4000
　　　　　　　　　　　　　　　FAX: 765-798-4010
　　　　　　　　　　outdoors@twinlakescamp.com
　　　　　　　　　　　www.twinlakescamp.com

Jon Beight, Executive Director
Dan Daily, Program Director
Ashley Nierman, Outdoor Education Coordinator
Donna Beight, Secretary
Provides a summer camp program for special needs children and young adults. Campers suffer from a wide range of maladies including crippling accidents, Spina Bifida, epilepsy, Cerebral Palsy, Muscular Dystrophy, Quadriplegia, Paraplegia, and other disabling diseases. Campers range in age from 8 to 27.

Iowa

1104 **Camp Albrecht Acres**
14837 Sherrill Rd
PO Box 50
Sherrill, IA 52073　　　　　　　563-552-1771
　　　　　　　　　　　　　　　FAX: 563-552-2732
　　　　　　　　　　　info@albrechtacres.org
　　　　　　　　　　　www.albrechtacres.org

Terry Mozena, President
Randy Judge, Vice President
Paul Gorrell, Treasurer
Greg Malm, Secretary
For children and adults with special needs. Campers enjoy swimming, fishing, nature studies, cookouts and dances.

1105 **Camp Courageous of Iowa**
P.O.Box 418
12007 190 th Street
Monticello, IA 52310- 0418　　　319-465-5916
　　　　　　　　　　　　　　　FAX: 319-465-5919
　　　　　　　　　　　info@campcourageous.org
　　　　　　　　　　　www.campcourageous.org

Jeanne Muellerleile, Camp Director
Charlie Becker, Executive Director
Shannon Poe, Respite Care/Volunteers Director
A year round residential and respite care facility for individuals with special needs and their families. Campers range in age from 1-99 years old. Activities include traditional activities like canoeing, hiking, swimming, nature and crafts plus adventure activities like caving, rock climbing, etc. Campers with disabilities have opportunities to succeed at challenging activities. This feeling of self-worth can transfer to home, work or school environments.

1106 **Camp Hertko Hollow**
501 Grand Avenue
Des Moines, IA 50309-1720　　　515-471-8523
　　　　　　　　　　　　　　　855-502-8500
　　　　　　　　　　　　　　　FAX: 515-288-2531
　　　　　　　v.murray@camphertkohollow.com
　　　　　　　　　www.camphertkohollow.com

Ann Wolf, Executive Director
Vivian Murray, Camp Director Emeritus
Deb Holwegner, Camp Director

Camp Hertko Hollow is a resident camp held at the Des Moines YMCA Camp site, located along the Des Moines River north of Boone, Iowa. Activities include horseback riding, swimming, canoeing, rappelling, crafts, ropes course, archery and riflery to name a few, plus special activities for different ages. Half-week and one-week sessions for children with diabetes. Coed, ages 6-16.

1107 Camp L-Kee-Ta
1308 Broadway Street
P.O. Box 190
West Burlington, IA 52655-190   319-752-3639
                                         FAX: 319-753-1410
                                         girlscoutstoday.org

Teresa Colgan, Chair
Jill Dashner, First Vice-Chair
Lee Mowers, Treasurer
Theresa Dunkin, Secretary
Camp is located in Danville, Iowa. Half-week and one-week sessions June-August for children with asthma/respiratory ailments. Girls, ages 7-18 and families.

1108 Camp Quality Heartland
PO Box 402
Council Bluffs, IA 51502   330-671-0167
                                         FAX: 866-285-5208
                                 caleb.rogers@campqualityusa.org
                                    www.campqualityusa.org/htl
Caleb Rogers, Camp Director
Camp Quality is for children with cancer and their siblings. The camp offers a stress-free environment that offers exciting activities and fosters new friendships, while helping to give the children courage, motivation and emotional strength.

1109 Camp Sunnyside
Easter Seals Of Iowa
401 N.E. 66th Avenue
Des Moines, IA 50313   515-289-1933
                                     krumpf@easterseals.org
                                       www.easterseals.org
Duncan Hawthorne, Chair
Kelsey Rumpf, Program Assistant
John M. Herhalt, Treasurer
The camp is open year-round and is a place for children and adults with or without disabilities to gather and enjoy themselves while exploring their potentials. Activities include swimming, boating arts and crafts and games.

1110 Camp Tanager
Tanager Place
1614 W Mount Vernon Rd
Mount Vernon, IA 52314-9533   319-363-0681
                                         FAX: 319-365-6411
                                     dpirrie@tanagerplace.org
                                        www.camptanager.org
Donald Pirrie, Executive Director
Offers camp experiences for children 7 to 11 whose special social, economic or medical needs might not otherwise allow them to enjoy a summer camp experience. This private, non-profit camp serves over 600 children each summer with the staff-camper ratio being 1:6.

1111 Camp Wyoming
Presbyterian Church USA
9106 42nd Ave
Wyoming, IA 52362-7647   563-488-3893
                                         FAX: 563-488-3895
                                     office@campwyoming.net
                                        www.campwyoming.net
Kevin Cullum, Executive Director
Rev. Beth Hilkerbaumer, Board President
Eric Norton, Board Vice President
Amy Saskowski, Board Secretary
Youth and adults, ages 16 and up, with mild to moderate mental and physical disabilities can take part in a one week experience of fun and fellowship in early July.

1112 Diabetes Camp
Tanager Place
1614 W Mount Vernon Rd
Mount Vernon, IA 52314-9533   319-363-0681
                                         FAX: 319-365-6411
                                     dpirrie@tanagerplace.org
                                        www.camptanager.org
Donald Pirrie, Executive Director
Provides children and adolescents with Diabetes a safe and healthy environment and healthy environment to enjoy a variety of recreational activities designed for fun and fitness. The camp held each July has an on-site 24-hour physician and nursing staff. Ages 6-13.

1113 Wendell Johnson Speech And Hearing Clinic
University Of Iowa
250 Hawkins Dr
Iowa City, IA 52242-1025   319-335-8736
                                         FAX: 319-335-8851
                                     kathy-miller@uiowa.edu
                                     www.uiowa.edu/~comsci/
Linda Souke, Clinic Director
Kathy Miller, Clinic Assistant
The clinic offers assessment and remediation for communication disorders in adults and children. The clinic also offers services during the Summer for school age children needing intervention services because of speech, language, hearing and/or reading problems.

1114 Wesley Woods Camp and Retreat Center
Iowa Conference United Methodist
10896 Nixon St
Indianola, IA 50125-7301   515-961-4523
                                         866-684-7753
                                         FAX: 515-961-4162
                                   wesleywoods.camp@iaumc.org
                                      www.wesleywoodsiowa.org
Deke Rider, Executive Director
Suzanne Rider, Equestrian Coordinator
Camp is located in Indianola, Iowa. Half-week and one-week sessions June-August for campers with developmental disabilities. Coed, ages 18-99. Horses Helping People program is also available for developmentally and physically challenged persons age 4 and older.

1115 Y Camp
YMCA of Greater Des Moines
1192 166th Drive
Boone, IA 50036-1720   515-432-7558
                                         FAX: 515-432-5414
                                       ycamp@dmymca.org
                                          www.y-camp.org
Mike Havlik, Program Director- Environmental
David Sherry, Executive Director
Alex Kretzinger, Program Director- Summer Camp
Tom Monroe, Program Director- Retreats and C
Camp is located in Boone, Iowa. Year-round one and two-week sessions for boys and girls with cancer, diabetes, asthma, cystic fibrosis, hearing impaired and other disabilities. Coed, ages 6-16 and families.

Kansas

1116   **Camp Discovery - Kansas**
American Diabetes Association
Rock Springs 4-H Center
1168 K-157 Highway
Junction City, KS 66441

316-684-6091
800-362-1355
888-342-2838
FAX: 316-684-5675
lthomas@diabetes.org
www.diabetescamps.org

Mark Moyer, Chairperson
Janet Kramschauster, Vice-Chairperson
Andrea Schnelten, Secretary
John Latimer, Treasurer
Camp is located in Junction City, Kansas. Offers young people with diabetes a week of fun at rock springs 4-H Center. Special attention to diabetes makes Camp Discovery a safe environment for active youth while providing valuable diabetes management education. Call the American Diabetes Association Kansas area office for more information. Coed, ages 8-17.

1117   **Camp Quality Kansas**
2617 N 75th Street
Kansas City, KS 66109

913-424-8355
FAX: 913-334-2802
Susie.Mooney@CampQualityUSA.org
www.campqualityusa.org/ks

Patricia Harris, Executive Director
Vicki Irey, President
Anneliese Kulakofsky, Vice-President
Dennis Hart, Secretary
Camp Quality is for children with cancer and their siblings. The camp offers a stress-free environment that offers exciting activities and fosters new friendships, while helping to give the children courage, motivation and emotional strength.

1118   **Summer Camp for Physically & Mentally Challenged Children & Adults**
Kansas Jaycees' Cerebral Palsy Foundation
P.O.Box 267
Augusta, KS 67207-267

316-775-2421
execdirector@cpranch.org
http://cpranch.cfsites.org

Cheryl Schmeidler, Executive Director
Sarah Walker, Camp Director
Our mission is to provide a program which will allow individuals to enjoy their highest level of functioning and independence, consistent with their abilities, in a summer camp setting.

Kentucky

1119   **Bethel Mennonite Camp**
2773 Bethel Church Rd
Clayhole, KY 41317-9028

606-666-4911
FAX: 606-666-4216
grow@bethelcamp.org
www.bethelcamp.org

Mark Driskill, Summer Camp Pastor
Roger Voth, Camp Director
Mary Driskill, Summer Camp Pastor
A Christ-centered ministry with an emphasis on Bible study and personal commitment to Christ. We offer a week long Special Needs Camp in June, with lodging for caregivers.

1120   **Camp Quality Kentuckiana**
PO Box 35474
Louisville, KY 40232

502-507-3235
FAX: 866-285-5208
charlie.obranowicz@campqualityusa.org
www.campqualityusa.org/ki

Charlie Obranowicz, Executive Director
Paul Bobbitt, Development Director
Amanda McClung, Secretary
Stefanie Nguyen, Treasurer
Camp Quality is for children with cancer and their siblings. The camp offers a stress-free environment that offers exciting activities and fosters new friendships, while helping to give the children courage, motivation and emotional strength.

1121   **Cedar Ridge Camp**
4010 Old Routt Road
Louisville, KY 40299

502-267-5848
FAX: 502-297-0116
info@cedarridgecamp.com
www.cedarridgecamp.com

Peter Ruys de Perez, Owner & Executive Director
Grayson Burke, Director
Jodie Campbell, Assistant Director
Alexandra Campbell, Director of Operations
Half-week, one and two-week sessions for children with diabetes, developmental disabilities and muscular dystrophy. Coed, ages 6-17.

1122   **Center For Courageous Kids, The**
1501 Burnley Road
Scottsville, KY 42164

270-618-2900
FAX: 270-618-2902
info@courageouskids.org
courageouskids.org

Roger Murtie, President/Executive Director
Emily Cosby, Program Director
Joanie O'Bryan, Development Director
Stormi Murtie, Communications Director
The Center for Courageous Kids is a year round medical camp for children who have chronic or life threatening illnesses by creating experiences that are memorable, exciting, fun, build self-esteem, are physically safe and medically sound. Family retreats serve children 3-17 and summer camps serve children 7-15. No child or family will pay to attend camp.

1123   **Indian Summer Camp**
P.O. Box 24337
Louisville, KY 40224

502-365-1538
Shelby.Dehner@gmail.com
www.iscamp.org

Shelby Dehner, Executive Director
Jon Dubins, Board President
David Power, Vice President
Dewey Minton, Treasurer
Indian Summer Camp is open to boys and girls aged 6-18 years old who have had or are currently receiving treatment for cancer. Children can come to have fun, while having the opportunity to grow, learn and build self reliance.

1124   **Lions Camp Crescendo, Inc.**
1480 Pine Tavern Road
P.O. Box 607
Lebanon Junction, KY 40150-0607

502-833-3554
888-879-8884
FAX: 502-833-4249
wibblesb@aol.com
www.lccky.org

Billie Flannery, Administrator
Lion Mel Gilbert, Secretary
Lion Barbara Walker, Chairperson
Lion Scott Skinner, Vice-Chairperson
The enhancement of the quality of life for youth, especially those with disabilities, through the delivery of a traditional camp experience by caring individuals and to enable others to use our camping and retreat facilities to serve the larger communities humanitarian needs.

1125 Medical Camping
The Center For Courageouos Kids
1501 Burnley Road
Scottsville, KY 42164
270-618-2900
FAX: 270-618-2902
info@courageouskids.org
www.courageouskids.org

Ed Collins, Camp Director
Roger Murtie, President and Executive Director
Joanie O'Bryan, Development Director
Stormi Murtie, Communications Director
A year-round, fun, safe camping experience for seriously ill and disabled children and their families.

Louisiana

1126 Camp Bon Coeur
Bon Coeur, Inc.
405 W. Main St.
Lafayette, LA 70501
337-233-8437
FAX: 337-233-4160
info@heartcamp.com
www.heartcamp.com

Susannah Craig, Executive Director
Two-week sessions June-July for children with heart defects. Coed, ages 8-16.

1127 Camp Challenge
P.O.Box 10591
New Orleans, LA 70181
504-347-2267
campdirector@campchallenge.org
www.campchallenge.org

Cathy Allain, Camp Director
Alaina Wertz, Public Relations
Camp Challenge is a grass roots non-profit organization dedicated to giving ill children and their siblings ages 6 through 18 a summer camp experience. Camp is open to all children who reside in Louisiana and have a form of cancer and chronic hematological disorders. These children do not have to pay for camp, it is free for all campers.

1128 Camp Pelican
Louisiana Lions Camp
292 L. Beauford Dr.
Anacoco, LA 71403
504-466-7124
800-348-6567
FAX: 337-239-9975
tbone333@aol.com
www.lionscamp.org

Cathy Allain, Assistant Camp Director
Reverend R. Tony Ricard, Camp Director
Camp Pelican is an overnight residential camp for children with moderate to severe asthma or other pulmonary problems. Founded in 1977, Camp Pelican is jointly sponsored by the Louisiana Pulmonary Disease Camp Inc and the Louisiana Lions Camp. Over 100 children attend annually and participate in education, sports, arts and crafts, swimming and other camping activities. Medical staff including physicians, nurses, respiratory therapists and social workers participate in camp. Coed, ages 5-17.

1129 Camp Quality Louisiana
1800 Forsythe Avenue
Suite 2, Box 307
Monroe, LA 71201
800-734-2752
FAX: 866-285-5208
louisiana@campqualityusa.org
www.campqualityusa.org/la

Matthew Matusiak, Executive Director
Camp Quality is for children with cancer and their siblings. The camp offers a stress-free environment that offers exciting activities and fosters new friendships, while helping to give the children courage, motivation and emotional strength.

1130 Camp Victory
Lions Club And American Diabetes Association
292 L. Beauford Drive
Suite 122
Anacoco, LA 71403
800-348-6567
FAX: 337-239-9975
www.lionscamp.org

Lori Koonce, Manager
Treva Lincoln, Contact Person
Camp is for children with diabetes age 6-14 years old. The camp offers many outdoor activities as well as daily diabetes education classes.

1131 Louisiana Lions Camp
LA Lions League for Crippled Children
292 L. Beauford Drive
Anacoco, LA 71403
800-348-6567
FAX: 337-239-9975
lalions@lionscamp.org
www.lionscamp.org

Raymond E Cecil III, Camp Director
Susan Todd, President
Free camp for boys and girls with mental and physical challenges, diabetes and pulmonary disorders.

1132 Louisiana Lions Camp - Camp Pelican
Lions Club Of Louisiana
292 L. Beauford Drive
Anacoco, LA 71403
800-348-6567
FAX: 337-239-9975
www.lionscamp.org

Jerry Adams, President
Free, residential summer camp for children with special needs, diabetes and pulmonary disorders.

1133 Med-Camps of Louisiana
102 Thomas Road
Suite 615
West Monroe, LA 71291
318-329-8405
info@medcamps.com
www.medcamps.com

Caleb Seney, Executive Director
Erin Harper, Nursing Director
Bethany Gerfers, Administrative Assistant
Kacie Hobson, Events & Volunteer Coordinator
Serves children with severe asthma and allergies and many more.

Maine

1134 Camp Waban
Waban Projects, Inc.
5 Dunaway Drive
Sanford, ME 04073
207-324-7955
FAX: 207-324-6050
www.waban.org

Isabel Schmedemann, President
Denise Allaire, Vice President
Neal Meltzer, Executive Director
Blaine Boudreau, Treasurer
Recreational opportunities in fully handicapped accessible waterfront facilities for children and adults with developmental disabilities. Activities include swimming, kayaking, pontoon boat rides, fishing and nightly camp fires.

1135 Camp Bishopswood
Diocese of Maine Episcopal
98 Bishopswood Rd.
Hope, ME 4847-3701
207-772-1953
800-244-6062
mike@bishopswood.org
www.bishopswood.org

Laurie Kazilionis, President
Robert Johnston, Vice President
Jeff Mansir, Treasurer
Pam Waite, Secretary
Camp is located in Hope, Maine. One to seven-week sessions for hearing impaired children June-August. Coed, ages 7-16.

1136 Camp Capella
8 Pearl Point Road
Delham, ME 04429
207-843-5104
dana@campcapella.org
www.campcapella.org

Dana Mosher, Religious Leader
Provides an opportunity for children with disabilities to engage in various recreational and social experiences.

1137 Camp Lawroweld
Northern New England Conference
228 West Side Road
Weld, ME 04285
207-585-2984
FAX: 207-585-2985
www.lawroweld.org

Harry Sabnani, Executive Director
Camp is located in Weld, Maine. Week sessions July for campers who are blind or visually impaired, all ages. Other camps coed, ages 9-16 and families, single adults, June - September.

1138 Camp No Limits
No Limits Limb Loss Foundation
265 Centre Road
Wales, ME 04280
207-240-5762
campnolimits@gmail.com
www.nolimitsfoundation.org

Mary Leighton, Founder/ Occupational Therapist
Kim Furlong, Physical Therapist
Loi Ho, Adult Amputee Volunteer/Prosthet
Missy Moreau, Volunteer Coordinator/Office Adm
Camp No Limits is the leading camp for young people with limb loss and their families. The camp also has several other locations in California, Florida, Idaho, Maryland and Missouri.

1139 Camp Pinecone
Pine Tree Society
149 Front Street
P.O. Box 518
Bath, ME 04530-518
207-443-3341
FAX: 207-443-1070
TTY:207-443-3341
info@pinetreesociety.org
www.pinetreesociety.org

Paul Jacques, Chair
Dean Paterson, 1st Vice Chair
Penny Plourde, 2nd Vice Chair
Timothy J. Kittredge, Secretary
A day camp for children with physical and/or developmental disabilities, ages 5 to 12. May through September.

1140 Camp Sunshine
35 Acadia Road
Casco, ME 04015
207-655-3800
FAX: 207-655-3825
info@campsunshine.org
www.campsunshine.org

Anna Gould, Board Chair
Albert Ragucci, Board President
Joseph Pappalardo, Board Treasurer
Les Tager, Board Secretary
This year round program provides respite, support, hope & joy to children with life threatening illnesses and their immediate families. The camp is open to families of children diagnosed with kid-

ney disease, cancer, lupus, solid organ transplants and other life threatening illnesses. The camp is free of charge and includes onsite medical and psychosocial support, and bereavement groups.

1141 Camp Waziyatah
530 Mill Hill Rd
Waterford, ME 04088
207-583-2267
FAX: 509-357-2267
info@wazi.com
www.wazi.com

Gregg Parker, Owner/Director
Mitch Parker, Owner/Director
Joseph Pappalardo, Board Treasurer
Carl Acosta, New Family Liaison/Pines Divisio
Camp is located in Waterford, Massachusetts. Three, four and seven-week sessions June-August for campers with cancer and diabetes. Coed, ages 8-15 and families, single adults.

1142 Camp Winnebago
19708 Camp Winnebago Road
Caledonia, MN 55921
507-724-2351
FAX: 507-724-3786
andy@campwinnebago.org
www.campwinnebago.org

Tommy Means, Co-Director, Program Director
Heather Johnson, RN, Co-Director, Health Center Direc
Elise Hynek, Volunteer Coordinator
Michele Thompson, Office Assistant
A non profit organization specializing in the recreational needs of adults and children with developmental disabilities.

1143 Indian Acres Camp for Boys
1712 Main St
Fryeburg, ME 04037-4327
207-935-2300
geoff@indianacres.com
www.indianacres.com

Michael Burness, Assistant Director
Lisa Newman, Director
Geoff Newman, Director
Mary Beth Wiig, Head Counselor, Camp Forest Acre
Camp is located in Fryeburg, Florida. Four and seven-week sessions June-August for boys with ADD ages 7-16.

1144 Pine Tree Camp
Pine Tree Society
149 Front Street
P.O. Box 518
Bath, ME 04530
207-443-3341
FAX: 207-397-5324
ptcamp@pinetreesociety.org
www.pinetreesociety.org

Paul Jacques, Chair
Dean Paterson, 1st Vice Chair
Diane Gilbert, Treasurer
Timothy J. Kittredge, Secretary
Offers Maine children and adults with disabilities an extraordinary summer camp experience. The barrier-free setting and commitment of our staff allow campers to fully participate in activities that normally aren't available to them including swimming, fishing, boating, outdoor games, kayaking, arts and crafts and even camping in a tent under the stars. May through September.

1145 YMCA Camp of Maine
305 Winthrop Center Rd
P.O. Box 446
Winthrop, ME 04364
207-395-4200
FAX: 207-395-7230
info@maineycamp.org
www.maineycamp.org

Barry W Costa, Executive Director
Activities include arts and crafts, nature study, hiking, and overnight camping, dancing, and singing. Summer session dates run from June through August; for ages 8-16.

Maryland

1146 ASL Camp
417 Oak Court
Catonsville, MD 21227
443-739-0716
deafcampsinc@gmail.com
deafcampsinc.wordpress.com

Kathy MacMillan, President
Louise Rollins, Secretary
TJ Waters, Treasurer
Erin Krug, Director
For ages 7-18; August 2-7, 2015 at Manidokan Camp and Retreat Center.

1147 Camp Fairlee Manor
Easter Seals Of Delaware
61 Corporate Circle
New Castle, DE 19720
302-324-4444
FAX: 302-324-4441
contact@esdel.org
www.de.easterseals.com

Martha Rees, Chair
Jeffrey Gosnear, Vice Chair
Christine Sauers, Treasurer
David Dougherty, Secretary
For children and adults with physical disabilities and/or cognitive impairments. Activities include arts and crafts, sports and games, nature walks, swimming, and fishing

1148 Camp Glyndon
American Diabetes Association
PO Box 56
Nanjemoy, MD 20662
301-870-5858
FAX: 301-246-9108
info@LionsCampMerrick.org
www.lionscampmerrick.org

Wayne Magoon, President
Ray Shumaker, Vice President
Frank Culhane, Treasurer
Marcia Holpuch, Secretary
Camp is located in Nanjemoy, Maryland. One and two-week sessions July-August for children with diabetes and their families. Coed, ages 8-16.

1149 Camp JCC
Jewish Community Center of Greater Washington
6125 Montrose Rd
Rockville, MD 20852-4860
301-881-0100
FAX: 301-881-6549
fgold@jccgw.org
www.jccgw.org

Bradley C. Stillman, President
Brian Pearlstein, Vice President for Admin
Heidi Hookman Brodsky, Vice President for Development
Mindy Berger, Vice President for Member & Gues
Camp JCC serves children with disabilities alongside their neighbors and friends. The American Camping Association has presented a National award to Camp JCC for its extraordinary model inclusion program. We also offer a program designed especially for 13-21 year olds with severe to profound disabilities. In order for us to afford to do these things, we count on contributions to our Inclusion Fund. Four and eight-week sessions general day camp program offering June-August for children.

1150 Camp Joy
9812 Falls Road
Ste. 114-331
Potomac, MD 20854-1518
610-754-6878
888-694-6735
FAX: 610-754-7880
contact@DomainMarket.com
www.campjoy.com

1151 Camp Milldale
Jewish Community Center
3506 Gwynnbrook Avenue
Owings Mills, MD 21117
410-559-2390
FAX: 410-581-0561
info@campmilldale.org
www.campmilldale.org

Amy Bram, Camp Director
Stacy Deems, Camp Administrator
Jalen Thomas Chichester, Assistant Camp Director
Shawnise Crawford, Aquatics Director
Camp is located in Reisterstown, MD. Four and eight week sessions, June - August. Inclusion program for children entering grades 5-13 with learning, developmental, social, emotional and physical disabilities. Self-contained program for teenagers with disabilities ages 14-21 focusing on recreational and vocational activities, including weekly field trips.

1152 Camp Quality George Washington University
1600 Harpers Ferry Road
Knoxville, MD 21758
301-834-7244
FAX: 866-285-5208
manidokan@gmail.com
www.campqualityusa.org/gwu

Chris Willis, RN, Medical Director
Shivali Choxi, Executive Director
Chris Schlieckert, Camp Director
Camp Quality is for children with cancer and their siblings. The camp offers a stress-free environment that offers exciting activities and fosters new friendships, while helping to give the children courage, motivation and emotional strength.

1153 Camp Roehr
Epilepsy Foundation Greater Southern Illinois
8301 Professional Place East
Suite 200
Landover, MD 20785-2353
301-459-3700
800-332-1000
FAX: 301-459-1569
ContactUs@efa.org
www.epilepsyfoundation.org

Warren Lammert, Chair
Phil Gattone, President and CEO
May J. Liang, Secretary
Roger Heldman, Treasurer
A seven day residential camp for children diagnosed with epilepsy. The camp is held at the Pere Marquette State Park where children enjoy swimming, horseback riding, arts and crafts, nightly entertainment and the camaraderie of other children with epilepsy.

1154 Camp Sunrise
John Hopkins Hospital
750 East Pratt Street
Suite 1700
Baltimore, MD 21201
410-516-2385
mscalf19@yahoo.com
www.hopkinsmedicine.org/kimmel_cancer_center/

Marilyn Scalf, Staffing Director
Jaclyn Young, Activities
Stephanie Davis, Donations!
Jack Shipkoski, CEO
Camp Sunrise is open to children ages 6-18 who have or have had cancer. The camp also has a 'day camp' program for children ages 4-5 years old. Some of the camps activities include swimming, arts & crafts, nature walks, sports and games.

1155 Camp Superkids
John Hopkins Bayview Medical Center
P.O. Box 96
Maryland Line, MD 21105
410-550-0374
campsuperkids@gmail.com
www.hopkinsbayview.org/campsuperkids

Ceal Curry, Camp Director
Heather Dougherty, Camp Administrator
Camp Superkids is an overnight camp for children between the ages of 8-14 with asthma.

1156   Deaf Camp
417 Oak Court
Catonsville, MD 21227   443-739-0716
deafcampsinc@gmail.com
deafcampsinc.wordpress.com

Kathy MacMillan, President
Louise Rollins, Secretary
TJ Waters, Treasurer
Kelley Finck, Volunteer
For ages 7-19; August 2-7, 2015 at Manidokan Camp and Retreat
Center.

1157   Kamp A-Komp-Plish
9035 Ironsides Rd
Nanjemoy, MD 20662-3432   301-870-3226
301-934-3590
FAX: 301-870-2620
recreation@melwood.org
http://www.melwoodrecreation.org

Michael Glanz, VP, Community Services
Doria Fleisher, Program Director
Caitlin Holden, Equestrian Coordinator
Hannah Rutt, Travel Coordinator
Camp is located in Nanjemoy, Maryland. Half-week, one-week
and two-week sessions for blind/visually impaired children and
those with developmental disabilities and mobility limitation.
Coed, ages 8-16.

1158   League at Camp Greentop
The League for People with Disabilities
1111 E. Cold Spring Lane
Baltimore, MD 21239   410-323-0500
FAX: 410-323-3298
TTY:410-435-4298
vfoster@leagueforpeople.org
www.leagueforpeople.org

Bill Morgan, VP, Camping & Therapeutic Recrea
David A. Greenberg, President/ CEO
Margy Ryan, Vice President, Finance
Tom Schniedwind, Vice President, Marketing & Deve
Camp is located in Thurmont, Maryland. Summer residential
camp located in the Catoctin Mountain National Park. Since
1937, Greentop has been serving children and adults with physical and multiple disabilities in a completely accessible camp setting. Campers enjoy a traditional camping program. Medical
facilities staffed 24 hours a day. Half-week/one/two-week sessions June-August. ACA/MD Youth Camp.

1159   Lions Camp Merrick
Lions Clubs of District 22-C
3650 Rick Hamilton Place
P.O. Box 56
Nanjemoy, MD 20662-56   301-870-5858
FAX: 301-246-9108
info@LionsCampMerrick.org
www.lionscampmerrick.org

Wayne Magoon, President
Ray Shumaker, Vice President
Frank Culhan, Treasurer
Marcia Holpuch, Secretary
This recreational camp for special needs children offers a complete waterfront program including swimming, canoeing and
fishing for ages 6-16. Designed for children who are deaf and
hard of hearing, children of deaf parents, and children with diabetes. Also helps children to learn to deal with their special
conditions.

1160   Raven Rock Lutheran Camp
17912 Harbaugh Valley Road
P.O.Box 136
Sabillasville, MD 21780-136   800-321-5824
ravenrock@innernet.net
www.campinglist.us

1161   TLC's Summer Programs
2092 Gaither Road
Suite 100
Rockville, MD 20850   301-424-5200
FAX: 301-424-8063
enyang@ttlc.org
www.ttlc.org

Bill McDonald, President
Michael Cogan, Vice President
James LaGrone, Treasurer
Betty Anne Aschenbach, Secretary
For children ages 3-13 and high school students in grades 9-12,
who have special needs in the areas of speech, language, perceptual motor, sensory processing, academic development, and/or
skill maintenance. Some programs also fulfill the requirements
for Extended School Year Services (ESY). Extended Day is available for children 5 years or older in all programs (excluding the
high school program). Extended day hours are 8:00 am to 9:00 am
and 3:00 pm to 5:00 pm.

1162   Young Adult Deaf Camp
417 Oak Court
Catonsville, MD 21227   443-739-0716
deafcampsinc@gmail.com
deafcampsinc.wordpress.com

Kathy MacMillan, President
Louise Rollins, Secretary
TJ Waters, Treasurer
Kelley Finck, Volunteer
For ages 18 and up; June 14-19, 2014 at West River Camping Cen-
ter .

1163   Youth Leadership Camp
National Association of the Deaf
8630 Fenton Street
Suite 820
Silver Spring, MD 20910- 3819   301-587-1788
FAX: 301-587-1791
TTY:301-587-1789
infor@nad.org
www.nad.org

Howard Rosenblum, Chief Executive Officer
Christopher Wagner, President
Melissa S. Draganac-Hawk, Vice-President
Joshua Beckman, Secretary
Sponsored by the National Association of the Deaf, this camp em-
phasizes leadership training for deaf teenagers and young adults.
In addition to many recreational activities and sports, there are
academic offerings and camp projects.

Massachusetts

1164   Agassiz Village Camp
Easter Seals: Massachusetts
484 Main St
Worcester, MA 01608
800-244-2756
FAX: 508-831-9768
TTY:800-564-9700
info@eastersealsma.org
www.eastersealsma.org

Thomas Sanglier II, Chairman
Peter Mahoney, Vice Chair
Kelley Hippler, Treasurer
Pauline Hamel, Secretary
Operates a full inclusion residential summer camp that serves
campers with disabilities (ages 8-13). Camp activities are facili-
tated with consideration to the needs of youth with disabilities.

1165 Becket Chimney Corners YMCA Camps and Outdoor Center
748 Hamilton Rd
Becket, MA 1223-9686

413-623-8991
FAX: 413-623-5890
cburke@bccymca.org
www.bccymca.org

Phil Connor, CEO
Jim Brown, Chief Operations Officer
Christine Kalakay, Chief Financial Officer
Steve Turner, Director of Property & Maintenan
Half-week and one-week sessions for campers with asthma/respiratory ailments. Coed, ages 3 and up, families, seniors, single adults.

1166 Bright Horizons Summer Camp
Sickle Cell Disease Association of Illinois
200 Talcott Avenue South
Watertown, MA 02472

617-673-8000
parents@brighthorizons.com
www.brighthorizons.com

David Lissy, CEO
Linda Mason, Chairman and Founder
Mary Ann Tocio, President and COO
Elizabeth Boland, CFO
Camping for children with blood disorders, ages 7-13. The joys of learning include instruction in first aid, swimming and water safety, boating, horseback riding and bowling plus arts and crafts. In addition, there is a traditional menu of camp pleasures, like hayrides, cookouts, nature hikes and sing-a-longs.

1167 Camp Howe
P.O. Box 326
Goshen, MA 01032

413-549-3969
office@camphowe.com
www.camphowe.com

Heidi Gutekenst, Camp Director
Douglas Mollison, President
Edlin Black, Vice President
Stephanie Martin, Secretary
One and two-week sessions June-August for children with a variety of disabilities. Coed, ages 7-17.

1168 Camp Jabberwocky
200 Greenwood Avenue Ext.
P.O. Box 1357
Vineyard Haven, MA 02568

508-693-2339
info@campjabberwocky.org
www.campjabberwocky.org

Kristin LB Oseychik, Chair
Liana Mccabe, Vice Chair
Corby Reese, Treasurer
Linda Leahy, Secretary
Residential vacation camp for people with disabilities.

1169 Camp Joslin
Barton Center for Diabetes Education
30 Ennis Road
PO Box 356
North Oxford, MA 01537-0356

508-987-2056
FAX: 508-987-2002
info@bartoncenter.org
www.bartoncenter.org

David A. Harned, Chair
Mark W. Fuller, Treasurer
John Peri-Okonny, M.D., 1st Vice Chair
Kristyn Dyer, 2nd Vice Chair
Camp is located in Charlton, Massachusetts. For boys, ages 7-16, with diabetes. This program offers active summer sports and activities, supplemented by medical treatment and diabetes education. Coed Winter Camp and Coed Weekend Retreats are offered during the school year.

1170 Camp New Connections
McLean Hospital
115 Mill Street
Belmont, MA 02478

617-855-2000
kamadden@partners.org
www.mclean.harvard.edu/

Scott Rauch, MD, President and Psychiatrist in Ch
Joseph Coyle, Chief Scientific Officer
Joseph Gold, Chief Medical Officer
Michele L. Gougeon, Chief Operating Officer
A four-week, summer day camp for children ages 7-17 who have Asperger's Syndrome, autism spectrum disorders, pervasive developmental disorders and non-verbal learning disabilities. Recreational activities include arts & crafts, swimming, field trips and communication games.

1171 Camp Ramah in New England
39 Bennett St
Palmer, MA 01069-9514

413-283-9771
FAX: 413-283-6661
info@campramahne.org
www.campramahNE.org

Rabbi Ed Geld, Executive Director
Josh Edelglass, Assistant Director
Ed Pletman, Director of Finance & Operation
Talya Kalender, Director of Camper
8 week sleep-away camp for Jewish adolescents with developmental disabilities. Full camping program includes swimming, Hebrew singing and dancing, sports, arts and crafts, daily services, Kosher food and Jewish studies classes. Some mainstreaming and vocational opportunities.

1172 Camp Starfish
1121 Main Street
Lancaster, MA 01523

978-368-6580
FAX: 978-368-6578
info@campstarfish.org
www.campstarfish.org

Emily Golinsky, Executive Director
Michele Cyr, MSW, Associate Director
Jill Connell, Administrative & Development Ass
Fosters the growth and success of children with emotional, behavioral and learning problems.

1173 Camp Wee-Kan-Tu
127 Worcester Street
Watertown, MA 02472

info@campweekantu.org
www.campweekantu.org

Leslie G Brody, Ph.D, President and CEO
Charlene Sturgis, Director of Operations
Susan Welby, Director of Programs
Kristine Binette, Maine Field Service Coordinator
The camp offers children and teenagers aged 8-17 with epilepsy an overnight camping program full of fun and adventure. The camp strives to enhance the child's self esteem, confidence and independence.

1174 Carroll School Summer Programs
25 Baker Bridge Rd
Lincoln, MA 01773-3199

781-259-8342
FAX: 781-259-8842
info@carrollscholl.org
www.carrollschool.org

Sam Foster, Chair
Josh Levy, Co-Vice-Chair
Brad Watts, Treasurer
Richard Waters, Co-Vice-Chair
Academic and recreational programs designed to improve learning skills and build self-confidence. The school is a tutorial program for students not achieving their potential due to poor skills in reading, writing and math. The summer camp complements the summer school offering outdoor activities in a supportive, non-competitive environment.

1175 **Clara Barton Diabetes Camp**
Clara Barton for Girls with Diabetes
30 Ennis Road
PO Box 356
North Oxford, MA 01537-0356 508-987-2056
FAX: 508-987-2002
info@bartoncenter.org
www.bartoncenter.org

David A. Harned, Chair
John Peri-Okonny, 1st Vice Chair
Kristyn Dyer, 2nd Vice Chair
Mark W. Fuller, Treasurer
Girls, ages 3-17, with diabetes participate in a well-rounded camp program with special education in diabetes, health and safety. Activities include swimming, boating, sports, dance, music and arts and crafts. Two week adventure camp for high school girls offering camping, hiking, canoeing, etc. Also a minicamp (one week) for girls 6-12. Day camps are offered in Worcester, Boston, and New York City.

1176 **Eagle Hill School: Summer Program**
242 Old Petersham Road
P.O. Box 116
Hardwick, MA 01037- 0116 413-477-6000
FAX: 413-477-6837
admission@ehs1.org
www.ehs1.org

Jim Richardson, Chairman
Marilyn Waller, President
Alden Bianchi, Vice President
Arthur Langhaus, Treasurer
For children ages 9-19 with specific learning (dis)abilities and/or Attention Deficit Disorder, this summer program is designed to remediate academic and social deficits while maintaining progress achieved during the school year. Electives and sports activities are combined with the academic courses to address the needs of the whole person in a camp-like atmosphere.

1177 **Edward J Madden Open Hearts Camp**
250 Monument Valley Road
Great Barrington, MA 01230 413-528-2229
888-611-1113
hearts@openheartscamp.org
www.openheartscamp.org

David Zaleon, Executive Director
Jill Helme, Assistant Director
Jacqueline Reasor, Counselor
David Andrew, Counselor
Eight week program for children who have had and are fully recovered from open heart surgery or a heart transplant. Four two week sessions by age group. Small camp - 25 campers per session.

1178 **Handi Kids**
The Bridge Center
470 Pine St
Bridgewater, MA 02324-2112 508-697-7557
FAX: 508-697-1529
info@TheBridgeCtr.org
www.bridgectr.com

Anita Howards, Director of Administration
Karen Ellis, Office Manager
Spencer Nichols, Program Director
Sarah Norris, Riding Programs Coordinator
A therapeutic recreational facility in Bridgewater, Massachusetts offering after-school programs, special events, school vacation full-week and summer day camp programs. Every individual is welcome. Two-week sessions July-August.

1179 **Kamp for Kids: Camp Togowauk**
Abilities Unlimited of Western New England
55 Lake Avenue North
S3-301
Worcester, MA 01655 413-562-5678
TTY:800-764-0200
info@disabilityinfo.com
www.disabilityinfo.org

Anne Benoit, Director
Ben Amankwata, Business Analyst
Phil Chase, Instructional Designer
Derek Chaves, IT Director
Two-week sessions July-August for children and young adults with a variety of disabilities. Coed, ages 3-22.

1180 **PKU Camp**
YMCA Camp Burgess & Hayward
75 Stowe Road
Sandwich, MA 02563 508-428-2571
FAX: 508-420-3545
pgorman@ssymca.org
www.ssymca.org

Paul Gorman, President
John Ireland, Executive Vice President
Jim Jarosz, Vice President of Finance and Sy
Jeanette Paul, Vice President of Human Resource
Coed camp in August where children with PKU join other campers with or without PKU. This opportunity allows children to meet other children facing the same issues. Recreational activities include tennis, sailing, horseback riding and performing arts.

1181 **TSA CT Kid's Summer Event**
Tourette Syndrome Association of Connecticut (TSA)
39 Godfrey Street
Taunton, MA 02780 617-277-7589
info@tsa-ma.org
www.tsact.org

Peter Tavolacci, Vice Chairman
Paul Nazario, Treasurer
Jeanette Nazario, Board Member
Mike Tavolacci, Board Member
TSA of Connecticut sponsors summer events for children with TS/Tourette Syndrome activities of which include miniature golf in addition to an Annual Conference. The kids' program at this annual conference provides children who have TS a unique opportunity to meet other children like them who also struggle with TS. Entertainment includes puppeteers, magicians, learning karate from the experts, getting face paintings and more.
uniqu pages

1182 **Tower Program at Regis College**
Regis College
235 Wellesley St
Weston, MA 2493-1545 781-768-7000
FAX: 781-899-7209
admission@regiscollege.edu
www.regiscollege.edu

Joan Shea, Chair
Lee Hogan, Vice Chair
Maureen Doherty, Secretary
Michael Halloran, Treasurer
Helps average and above average college-bound students, ages 16-17, having a diagnosed dyslexic learning disability, to adjust to a college setting. Emphasis is on instruction and academic reinforcement, affective support, awareness of support services available on most college campuses and strategy training.

Michigan

1183 Camp Barakel
P.O. Box 159
Fairview, MI 48621-0159
989-848-2279
FAX: 989-848-2280
info@campbarakel.org
www.campbarakel.org

Paul Gardner, Resident Missionary Staff
Hannah Gardner, Resident Missionary Staff
Dan Haines, Resident Missionary Staff
Sarah Haines, Resident Missionary Staff
Five-day Christian camp experience in mid-August for campers ages 18-55 who are physically disabled, visually impaired, upper trainable mentally impaired or educable mentally impaired, bus transportation provided from locations in Lansing, Flint and Bay City, Michigan.

1184 Camp Barefoot
The Fowler Center For Outdoor Learning
2315 Harmon Lake Rd
Mayville, MI 48744-9737
989-673-2050
FAX: 989-673-6355
info@thefowlercenter.org
www.thefowlercenter.org

Kyle L Middleton, CTRS, Executive Director
Lynn M Seeloff, CTRS, Assistant Director
Pat Jordan, Office Manager
Farrah Wojcik, Events Supervisor
Offered to adults with traumatic brain injuries/closed head injuries. A wide variety of activities are offered. The participants in Camp Barefoot request their week's activities, allowing each participant to design their own activity schedule.

1185 Camp Catch-a-Rainbow
American Cancer Society
6941 Stony Lake Road
Jackson, MI 49201
517-536-8607
800-227-2345
FAX: 517-536-4922
kwilson@ymcastorercamps.org
www.ymcastorercamps.org

Katie Wilson, Camp-Catch-A-Rainbow (CCAR) Coor
Becky Spencer, Vice President of Camping
Abimbola Fajobi, Program Executive
Nancy Burger, Director of Outdoor Education
Camp Catch-a-Rainbow's programs are available completely free to any child in MI or IN who has or has had cancer, between the ages of 4 and 20, with their doctor's approval. Family Camp is reserved for those campers who have attended camp during that year's summer sessions and their families. Day, week, adult retreat, and family camp are available options.

1186 Camp Chris Williams
Lions 11 B-2 and MADHH
PO BOX 16234
Suite C
Lansing, MI 48901-6234
586-932-6090
800-968-7327
info@michdhh.org
www.michdhh.org

Nancy Asher, Executive Director
Office Manag
An exciting summer camp experience for deaf and hard of hearing youth and their siblings ages 8-14.

1187 Camp Grace Bentley
8250 Lakeshore Rd
Burtchville Township, MI 48059
313-962-8242
campgrace@hotmail.com
www.campgracebentley.org

Nancy Perri, Director
Camp Grace Bentley hosts campers with a range of physical and mental challenges. Campers ages seven through sixteen are invited to sign up for a nine day session beginning late June and running through mid-August.

1188 Camp Nissokone
YMCA Camping Services
1401 Broadway
Suite 3A
Detroit, MI 48226
313-267-5300
FAX: 248-887-5203
camp@ymcadetroit.org
www.miymcacamps.org

Scott Landry, President and CEO
Scott Walters, EVP, COO
Michelle Kotas, CFO
Latitia McCree, SVP
A six week summer resident camp program for boys and girls whose learning and behavior styles have made successful participation in the traditional camp program difficult. All camp activities have a special emphasis on building self-esteem and peer relationships. Strong in waterfront, nature, campcrafts and a special arts program.

1189 Camp Quality Michigan
PO Box 345
Boyne City, MI 49712
231-582-2471
FAX: 866-564-7637
mioffice@campqualityusa.org
www.campqualityusa.org/MI

Kristyn Balog, Michigan Executive Director
Jean McDonough, North Camp Director
Jeff Cram, South Camp Director
Camp Quality is for children with cancer and their siblings. The camp offers a stress-free environment that offers exciting activities and fosters new friendships, while helping to give the children courage, motivation and emotional strength.

1190 Camp Roger
8356 Belding Road
Rockford, MI 49341-9628
616-874-7286
FAX: 616-874-5734
doug@camproger.org
www.camproger.org

Doug Vanderwell, Executive Director
Jon Swets, Chairperson
Bonnie Mulder, Vice Chairperson
Shaun Bredeweg, Treasurer
Camp Roger provides a fun top-notch summer program for disabled campers. Campers learn to love the woods, the water and the trails, getting to enjoy a wide variety of activities all designed to be fun, to build friendships, and develop self confidence.

1191 Camp Tall Turf
816 Madison Ave SE
Grand Rapids, MI 49507
616-452-7906
FAX: 616-452-7907
info@turf.org
www.tallturf.org

Jack Kooyman, President
Camp is located in Walkerville, Michigan. Summer camping sessions for youth with asthma/respiratory ailments and ADD. Coed, ages 8-16.

1192 Echo Grove Camp
Salvation Army
1101 Camp Rd
Leonard, MI 48367-2812
248-628-3108
FAX: 248-628-7055
vicky_purkey@usc.salvationarmy.org
www.echogrove.org

Mark Mc Clenaghan, Camp Director
Sharon McClenaghan, Associate Camp Director
Jeanie Engle, Program Director
Martin Soffran, Site & Facility Manager
Since 1921, the Army's Echo Grove Camp has offered a structured camping program for children, adults and seniors referred through Corps Community Centers. During the course of Echo Grove's 12 week season, the camp includes programs geared for every need and interest. In addition to outdoor recreation, camps may include religious, musical and skill-building instruction.

1193 Indian Trails Camp
0-1859 Lake Michigan Drive
Grand Rapids, MI 49534
616-677-5251
FAX: 616-677-2955
info@indiantrailscamp.org
www.indiantrailscamp.org

Brett Hoover, President
Cameron Young, Vice President
Karol Belk, Treasurer
Nate Herrygers, Secretary
Year round residential camping program for children and adults
with physical disabilities. One and two-week sessions. Coed,
ages 6-70.

1194 Sherman Lake YMCA Outdoor Center
6225 N 39th St
Augusta, MI 49012-9722
269-731-3000
FAX: 269-731-3020
shermanlakeymca@ymcasl.org
www.shermanlakeymca.org

Luke Austenfeld, Executive Director
Lorrie Syverson, Director of Camping, Education &
Karen Stanley, Assist. Camp Director
Jean Henderson, Business Manager
Summer camping sessions for campers with ADD and spina
bifida. Coed, ages 6-15 and families, seniors.

1195 St. Francis Camp On The Lake
10120 Murrey Road
Jerome, MI 49249
517-688-9212
FAX: 517-688-9298
campadmin@saintfranciscamp.org
www.saintfranciscamp.org

Russell Kreinbring, President
Connie Quinn, Vice President
Don Collom, Secretary
Bob Steinberger, Treasurer
The camp runs one-week sessions from June through August for
cognitively impaired children and adults and is staffed with a
3-to-1 camper ratio. Campers are encouraged to plan their own
activities and can partake in swimming, hiking, volleyball, and
basketball. Camp staff also helps to emphasize the importance of
daily living and socialization skills, and other activities such as
helping in the kitchen, and making beds.

1196 Trail's Edge Camp
Mott Respiratory Care
500 S. State Street
Ann Arbor, MI 48109-0208
734-764-1817
mdekeon@umich.edu
www.umich.edu/~tecamp

Mary Dekeon
Summer camp for children and young adults between the ages of
3-18 with special medical needs. Campers have tracheotomies or
need ventilator assistance. Some of the camp activities include
fishing, hiking, horseback riding, boating, swimming, nature &
outdoor living skills.

1197 YMCA Camp Copneconic
10407 North Fenton Road
Fenton, MI 48430
810-629-9622
FAX: 810-629-2128
request@campcopneconic.org
www.campcopneconic.org

John Carlson, Branch Executive Director
Brandon Dreffs, Associate Executive Director
Tom Correll, Director of School Programs/Over
Katie O'Toole, Retreats and Partnership Manager
Camp is located in Fenton, Michigan. Summer sessions for camp-
ers with diabetes. Coed, ages 3-16 and seniors.

Minnesota

1198 Camp Benedict
12459 Upper Sylvan Road SW
Pillager, MN 56473
612-424-2267
FAX: 763-592-8098
campbenedict.org

Rob Andrews, President
Sheila DeChantal, Vice President
Camp Benedict is an educational/recreational family Camp. We
strive to improve the quality of life for households who are infected or affected by HIV/AIDS.

1199 Camp Buckskin
PO Box 389
Ely, MN 55731
218-365-2121
FAX: 218-365-2880
info@campbuckskin.com
www.campbuckskin.com

Thomas R Bauer CCD, Camp Director
Mary Bauer, Co-Director
Jared Griffin, Program Director
Camp is located in Ely, Minnesota. Buckskin assists LD, AD/HD,
Asperger's, and adopted individuals to realize and develop the
potentials and abilities which they possess. Teaches a combina-
tion of traditional camp, academic activities and social skills so
the campers experience success in many areas. Ages 6-18.

1200 Camp Confidence
1620 Mary Fawcett Drive W
East Gull Lake, MN 56401
218-828-2344
info@campconfidence.com
www.campconfidence.com

Jeff Olson, Executive Director
Bob Slaybaugh, Program Director
Mary Harder, Volunteer Director
Jenni Bailey, Programs & Camp Sertoma Director
Confidence Learning Center otherwise known as Camp Confidence is an outdoor center for persons with developmental disabilities. The program at Camp Confidence is aimed at promoting
self-confidence and self-esteem, and the necessary skills to become full, contributing members of society.

1201 Camp Courage North
Courage Center
800 E. 28th St.
Minneapolis, MN 55407-4249
612-863-4200
866-880-3550
TTY:763-520-0245
couragekenny@allina.com
www.couragecenter.org

Jan Malcolm, CEO
Camp is located in Lake George, Minnesota. Summer sessions for
campers who have blood disorders, hearing impairment, mobility
limitation or are blind/visually impaired. Coed, ages 7-70.

1202 Camp Friendship
Friendship Ventures
10509 108th St NW
Annandale, MN 55302
952-852-0101
800-450-8376
FAX: 320-852-0123
fv@friendshipventures.org
www.friendshipventures.org

Floyd Adelman, Chairman
Camp Friendship offers resident camp programs for children,
teenagers and adults with developmental, physical or multiple
disabilities, special medical conditions, Down Syndrome, Williams Syndrome, autism or other conditions. Summer camp offers
archery, sailing, horseback riding, biking, fishing, creative arts,
adventure challenge programs and other activities. Weekend
camps and longer available. Other services available throughout
the year. Coed, ages 5-90, families, seniors.

1203 Camp Heartland
One Heartland
2101 Hennepin Avenue
Suite 200
Minneapolis, MN 55405
　　　　　　　612-824-6464
　　　　　　　888-216-2028
　　　　　　　FAX: 612-824-6303
　　　　　　　helpkids@oneheartland.org
　　　　　　　www.oneheartland.org

Colleen Brennan, President
John Adams, Vice President
W. Morgan Burns, Treasurer
Katherine Kellett, Secretary
Non-profit organization committed to improving the lives of children, youth and their families who have been impacted by HIV/AIDS.

1204 Camp Knutson
Camp Knutson And Knutson Point Retreat Center
1169 Whitefish Avenue
Crosslake, MN 56442
　　　　　　　218-543-4232
　　　　　　　www.lssmn.org/camp/

Rob Larson, Camp Director
Mary (Kate) Williams, Assistant Director
Susann Zeug-Hoese, Chairperson
Camp for children with autism, down syndrome, heart disease and skin disease. Activities include boating, swimming and other water activities.

1205 Confidence Learning Center
Confidence Learning Center
1620 Mary Fawcett Memorial Drive We
East Gull Lake, MN 56401
　　　　　　　218-828-2344
　　　　　　　FAX: 218-828-2618
　　　　　　　info@campconfidence.com
　　　　　　　www.campconfidence.com/

Jeff Olson, Executive Director
Bob Slaybaugh, Program Director
Mary Harder, Volunteer Director
Jenni Bailey, Specialty Programs, Outdoor Educ
A year-round outdoor center for persons with developmental disabilities. Some of the summer activities include fishing, archery, beach activities, water volleyball and basketball. Also a specialty camps for deaf and hearing impaired campers.

1206 Courage Center Camps
Courage Center
3915 Golden Valley Road
Minneapolis, MN 55422
　　　　　　　763-588-0811
　　　　　　　866-734-3273
　　　　　　　FAX: 320-963-3698
　　　　　　　TTY: 763-520-0245
　　　　　　　couragekenny@allina.com
　　　　　　　www.couragecenter.org/camps

Jan Malcolm, CEO
Pamela J. Lindemoen, Exec VP of Operations
Stephen Bariteau, Chief Dev. Officer
Alice Johnson, Chief Financial Officer
Camp is located in Maple Lake, Minnesota. Summer sessions for campers with a variety of disabilities. Coed, ages 6-99, families, seniors.

1207 YMCA Camp Ihduhapi
Minneapolis YMCA Camping Services
3425 Ihduhapi Rd
Loretto, MN 55357-9512
　　　　　　　763-479-1146
　　　　　　　FAX: 612-823-2482
　　　　　　　Kerry.pioske@ymcatwincities.org
　　　　　　　www.ymcatwincities.org/camps/camp_ihduha pi/

Kerry Pioske, Camp Executive
Josh Cobb, Overnight Camp Director
Eric Wobschall, Building Superintendent
Camp is located in Loretto, Minnesota. Summer sessions for campers with asthma/respiratory ailments and epilepsy. Coed, ages 7-16.

Mississippi

1208 Camp Dream Street
Camp Dream Street, MS
3863 Morrison Road
Utica, MS 39175
　　　　　　　601-885-6042
　　　　　　　info@dreamstreetms.org
　　　　　　　www.dreamstreetms.org

Kimberly Evans, Program Director
Molly Fargotstein, Assistant Program Director
Scott Levy, Chairman
Cynthia Huff, Administrator
For children with physical disabilities. The camp is full of fun and excitement and offers activities such as swimming, art's and crafts, horseback riding and more.

Missouri

1209 Camp Barnabas
901 Teas Trail 2060
Purdy, MO 65734
　　　　　　　417-476-2565
　　　　　　　FAX: 417-486-2980
　　　　　　　info@campbarnabas.org
　　　　　　　www.campbarnabas.org

Robin Walker, Chairman
Janie Bennoch, Owner
David Ross, Director of Operations
Myron Mizell, Cardiology
Camp for people with developmental challenges, post traumatic burns, blood disorders, cancer, low vision/blindness, and physical challenges. The camp runs from June to August and provides activities such as canoeing, horseback riding and swimming.

1210 Camp Encourage
208 West Linwood Boulevard
Kansas City, MO 64111
　　　　　　　816-830-7171
　　　　　　　info@campencourage.org
　　　　　　　www.campencourage.org

Jenny Hines, President
Marita Burrow, Ph.D., Secretary
Kelly Lee, M.S.Ed., Executive Director
Alissa Jensen, MPA, Development Coordinator
Encourages social growth, independence and self esteem in children and young adults with autism spectrum disorders.

1211 Camp Hickory Hill
Central Missouri Diabetic Childrens Camp
P.O.Box 1942
Columbia, MO 65205-1942
　　　　　　　573-445-9146
　　　　　　　camphickoryhill@yahoo.com
　　　　　　　www.camphickoryhill.com

David Bernhardt, President
Pete Bakutes, Treasurer
Myia Custer, Vice President
Michael Gardner MD, Medical Director
Educates diabetic children concerning diabetes and its care. In addition to daily educational sessions on some aspects of diabetes, campers participate in swimming, sailing, arts and crafts and overnight camping. Coed, ages 7-17.

1212 Camp MITIOG
Share, Inc
7615 N. Platte Purchase Drive
Suite 116
Kansas City, MO 64118
　　　　　　　913-522-9516
　　　　　　　877-221-4450
　　　　　　　FAX: 816-221-1420
　　　　　　　midlands@midlandsmc.org
　　　　　　　www.campmitiog.org

1213 Camp Quality Central Missouri
PO Box 953
Jefferson City, MO 65012-0953   636-795-7229
                                    FAX: 866-285-5208
                            cmo@campqualityusa.org
                            www.campqualityusa.org/cmo

Casey Bucher, Co-Director
Erin Carl, Co-Director
Camp Quality is for children with cancer and their siblings. The camp offers a stress-free environment that offers exciting activities and fosters new friendships, while helping to give the children courage, motivation and emotional strength.

1214 Camp Quality Greater Kansas City
434 NE Station Dr.
Lee's Summit, MO 64086   816-809-8600
                            FAX: 888-456-1611
                    crystal.davison@campqualityusa.org
                    www.campqualityusa.org/gkc

Crystal Davison, Executive Director
Camp Quality is for children with cancer and their siblings. The camp offers a stress-free environment that offers exciting activities and fosters new friendships, while helping to give the children courage, motivation and emotional strength.

1215 Camp Quality Northwest Missouri
1325 Village Dr.
St. Joseph, MO 64506   816-232-2267
                            FAX: 816-232-2920
                    nwmo@campqualityusa.org
                    www.campqualityusa.org/nwmo

Adam Nelson, Director
Gabe Bailey, Director
Camp Quality is for children with cancer and their siblings. The camp offers a stress-free environment that offers exciting activities and fosters new friendships, while helping to give the children courage, motivation and emotional strength.

1216 Camp Quality Ozarks
PO Box 302
Joplin, MO 64802   330-671-0167
                        FAX: 866-285-5208
                Ozarks@campqualityusa.org
                www.campqualityusa.org/oz

Vicki Irey, President
Anneliese Kulakofsky, Vice-President
Dennis Hart, Secretary
Lois Hartje, Treasurer
Camp Quality is for children with cancer and their siblings. The camp offers a stress-free environment that offers exciting activities and fosters new friendships, while helping to give the children courage, motivation and emotional strength.

1217 Concerned Care, Inc.
320 Armour Rd
North Kansas City, MO 64116-3506   816-474-3026
                                        FAX: 816-474-3029
                                www.concernedcarekc.org

Janet White, President
Marilyn Barth, Vice President
Candyce Kuebler, Secretary
Sharlea Leatherwood, Treasurer
Summer sessions for campers with developmental disabilities. Coed, ages 7-16. Residential facilities & programs; therapeutic recreation programs.

1218 Kiwanis Camp Wyman
Wyman Center
600 Kiwanis Dr
St. Louis, MO 63025-2212   636-938-5245
                                FAX: 636-938-5289
                        info@wymancenter.org
                        www.wymancenter.org

Dave Hilliard, President/CEO
Allison Williams, Sr. VP, Programs
Claire Wyneken, Senior VP & Dir. of Partner Svcs
Mindy Sharp, VP, Finance & Administration

Summer sessions for youth with diabetes. Coed, ages 8-16, run in conjunction with the American Diabetes Association. Call for program description.

1219 Lions Den Outdoor Learning Center
600 Kiwanis Dr
St. Louis, MO 63025-2212   636-938-5245
                                FAX: 636-938-5289
                        info@wymancenter.org
                        wymancenter.org

Dave Hilliard, President/CEO
Allison Williams, Sr. VP, Programs
Claire Wyneken, Senior VP & Dir. of Partner Svcs
Mindy Sharp, VP, Finance & Administration
Varied programs for mentally retarded children, ages 6 and up, includes daily living, socialization and language skills. Sports, tent camping, crafts, and nature study are also offered. Sliding scale tuition for 2 weeks.

1220 Sunnyhill Adventure Center
Council for Extended Care
6555 Sunlit Way
Dittmer, MO 63023-3306   636-274-9044
                            FAX: 636-285-1305
                    dropin4fun@aol.com
                    www.sunnyhilladventures.org

Vicky James, President/CEO
Kathleen Branson, Director of Finance
Amy Reitz, Director of Human Resources
Rob Darroch, Director of Sunnyhill Adventures
Camp is located in Dittmer, Missouri. Summer sessions for campers with developmental disabilities and autism. Coed, ages 8-99. Sunnyhill Adventures is program that offers campers fun, exciting, educational experiences in a beautiful outdoor setting. Our residential summer camp combines traditional camping activities plus specially selected and adapted events to meet the needs of each camper group.

1221 Wonderland Camp Foundation
18591 Miller Circle
Rocky Mount, MO 65072-2400   573-392-1000
                            info@wonderlandcamp.org
                            www.wonderlandcamp.org

Lori Miller, President
Dan Volmert, Vice President
Jill Wilke, Vice President
Jason Hynson, Executive Director
A residential camp for children and adults with mental and physical disabilities. 12 one week sessions. Coed. All Ages starting at age 6 through adult.

Montana

1222 Big Sky Kids Cancer Camps
Eagle Mount-Bozeman
6901 Goldenstein Lane
Bozeman, MT 59715   406-586-1781
                        FAX: 406-586-5794
                eaglemount@eaglemount.org
                www.eaglemount.org

Mary Peterson, Executive Director
Maggee Harrison, Equestrian Program Director
Chad Biggerstaff, Big Sky Program Director
Tracey Wheeler, Finance Director
Provides recreational opportunities for people of all ages with disabilities and children with cancer. Big Sky offers skiing, swimming, fishing, ice-skating, golf, cycling, and so much more.

1223 Camp Mak-A-Dream
P.O. Box 1450
Missoula, MT 59806
406-549-5987
FAX: 406-549-5933
info@campdream.org
www.campdream.org

Dan Ortt, President
Margot O'Leary, Vice President
Laura Bianco Hanna, Executive Director
Bill Simmel, Treasurer

A unique experience for young children in various stages of cancer therapy. The camp gives the children a chance to make new friends, try new things and experience how fun camp can be. Some of the activities include art projects, swimming, archery and campouts.

1224 Charles Campbell Childrens Camp
The Billings Lions Club
PO Box 23342
Billings, MT 59104
406-670-2496
campbellcamp@msn.com
www.billingslions.org/ccc.htm

Doug Hanson, Director
Sue Hanson, Director

Camp is open to young adults with physical disabilities that include sight or hearing impairment, spina bifida, cerebral palsy, gross motor skill impairments and other disabilities. Campers enjoy hiking, swimming, fishing, dances, campfires and much more.

Nebraska

1225 Camp Comeca & Retreat Center
United Methodist Church
75670 Road 417
Cozad, NE 69130-4117
308-784-2808
comeca@greatplainsumc.org
www.campcomeca.com

John Butler, Site Director

Camp is located in Cozad, Nebraska. Summer sessions for campers with diabetes and hearing impairment. Coed, ages 6-19, families, seniors, single adults.

1226 Camp Floyd Rogers
Floyd Rogers Foundation
PO BOX 541058
Omaha, NE 68154-536
402-885-9022
director@campfloydrogers.com
www.campfloydrogers.com

1227 Camp Kindle
Project Kindle/Camp Kindle
PO BOX 81147
Lincoln, NE 68501
661-257-1901
877-800-2267
FAX: 702-995-9186
info@projectkindle.org
www.campkindle.org

Eva Payne, Founder and Executive Director
Mandy Nickolite, Vice President and PsychoSocial
Erin FitzGerald, Program Coordinator
Nikki Wiener, Medical Director

The camp offers children with HIV and AIDS a safe environment where they can go to strengthen their self esteem through interactive participation in educational and recreational programming.

1228 Easter Seals Nebraska
Easter Seals Nebraska
12565 West Center Road
Suite 100
Omaha, NE 68144-8144
402-345-2200
800-650-9880
FAX: 402-345-2500
www.ne.easterseals.com

James C. Summerfelt, President & CEO
Angela Howell, Vice President Easter Seals Nebr
Lily Sughroue, Director of Camp, Respite & Recr

Offers a variety of services to help people with disabilities address life's challenges and achieve personal goals. Terrific fun for campers and a much needed respite for families and caregivers from the daily challenges of caring for special needs individuals.

1229 Kamp Kaleo
46872 Willow Springs Rd
Burwell, NE 68823-8805
308-346-5083
FAX: 308-346-5083
kampkaleo@gmail.com
www.kampkaleo.com

Gaylene O'Brien, Facilities Administrator
Sandy Denton, Minister of Faith Dev.
Jim Becker, Chairperson

Camp is located in Burwell, Nebraska. Summer sessions for campers who are blind/visually impaired or have developmental disabilities. Coed, ages 9-18 and families, seniors, single adults.

1230 National Camps for Blind Children
Christian Record Services
4444 S 52nd Street
Lincoln, NE 68516-1302
402-488-0981
FAX: 402-488-7582
info@christianrecord.org
www.christianrecord.org

Larry Pitcher, President
Matthew Orian, VP for Finance
Dan Jackson, Chair
Tom Lemon, Vice Chair

Provides free Christian publications and programs, as well as new opportunities for people with visual impairments. Free services include subscription magazines available in Braille, large print and audio cassette, full-vision books combining Braille and print, lending library, gift bibles and study guides in Braille, large print and audio cassette, national camps for blind children and scholarship assistance for blind young people trying to obtain a college education.

1231 YMCA Camp Kitaki
Lincoln YMCA
570 Fallbrook Blvd.
Suite 210
Lincoln, NE 68521-3110
402-434-9200
FAX: 402-434-9226
info@ymcalincoln.org
www.ymcalincoln.org

Barb Bettin, President/CEO
J.P. Lauterbach, Chief Operations Officer
Misty Muff, Chief Administrative Officer
Renee Yost, Chief Financial Officer

Camp is located in Louisville, Nebraska. Summer sessions for children with cystic fibrosis. Coed, ages 7-17 and families.

Nevada

1232   Camp Buck
Nevada Diabetes Association
18 Stewart Street
Reno, NV 89501   775-856-3839
                                       800-379-3839
                                       FAX: 775-348-7591
                                       camp@diabetesnv.org
                                       www.diabetesnv.org

Sarah Gleich, Associate State Exec. Dir.
Mylan Hawkins, State Exec. Dir.
Diana Kern, State Dir. of Dev.
Lynn Wexler, Southern Nevada Dir. Of dev.
Co-ed summer camp for children with diabetes ages 8-17. While
at the camp, the children develop a better understanding of their
diabetes while enjoying a week filled with recreational and athletic activities such as swimming, kayaking, fishing and arts &
crafts.

1233   Camp Lotsafun
164 Hubbard Way
Suite D
Reno, NV 89502   775-827-3866
                                       FAX: 775-827-0334
                                       camp@camplotsafun.com
                                       www.camplotsafun.com

Gayla Ouellette, Director
Stephanie Rice, Chairwoman
Linda Barnes, Director
Alan Herak, Treasurer
Provides therapeutic, educational, and recreational opportunities
for individuals with developmental disabilities, while providing
respite care for their families. Children, teens and adults with autism, down syndrome, traumatic brain injury, cerebral palsy and
attention deficit hyperactive disorder are among some of the individuals who attend camp for fun and recreational activities such
as swimming, kayaking, pet therapy, arts & crafts, drama and
music.

1234   Camp SignShine
DHHARC
1150 Corporate Blvd.
Suite 1
Reno, NV 89502   775-434-0290
                                       FAX: 775-355-8996
                                       TTY:775-355-8994
                                       www.dhharc.org

J. Farrell Cafferata Jenkins, President
Sean Meredith, Treasurer
Sean Mulholland, Vice President
Jennifer Montoya, SVP of Camp
Week long camp for children ages 7-19 who are deaf or hard of
hearing and their siblings. Campers enjoy recreational and educa-
tional activities in a safe and comfortable environment.

1235   CampCare
P.O. Box 12155
Reno, NV 89510-2155   775-323-3737
                                       FAX: 775-323-1019
                                       cmoore@campcarenevada.org
                                       www.campcarenevada.org

New Hampshire

1236   Camp Allen
56 Camp Road
Bedford, NH 03110-6606   603-622-8471
                                       FAX: 603-626-4295
                                       mary@campallennh.org
                                       www.campallennh.org

Mary Constance, Executive Director
Michael Constance, Summer Camp Director
John Cronin, Director
Deb Schulte, Office Manager

A residential summer camp for individuals with disabilities. All
of the activities are conducted by individual coordinators under
the supervision of Program Director. Some of the activities include, aquatics, arts, crafts, games and nature programs. All camp
events, special events, evening programs, and field trips are
scheduled throughout the summer and are structured to meet the
individual abilities and needs of each camper.

1237   Camp Sno Mo
Easter Seals: New Hampshire
555 Auburn St
Manchester, NH 03103-4803   603-623-8863
                                       800-870-8728
                                       FAX: 603-625-1148
                                       rkelly@eastersealsnh.org
                                       www.easterseals.com/nh/

Jim Bee, Chairman
Christine Gordon, Vice Chairman
Andrew MacWilliam, Treasurer
Renee Walsh, Secretary
Mission is to create solutions that change the lives of children and
adults with disabilities or special needs or their families. From
campfire sing-a-longs and late night ghost stories, to boating, nature walks, swimming, and arts and crafts, Easter Seals camps
provide the same excitement and activity available at other summer camp programs. Easter Seals campers experience the joys
and challenges of camp in a fully-accessible setting.

**1238   Windsor Mountain American Sign Language Camp
Program**
Windsor Mountain International
One World Way
Windsor, NH 03244   603-478-3166
                                       800-862-7760
                                       FAX: 603-478-5260
                                       Jake@WindsorMountain.org
                                       www.windsormountain.org

Jake Labovitz, Director
Kerry Labovitz, Director
Pam Butler, Administrative Assistant
Richard Herman
Camp Windsor is for children from around the world who are deaf
or hard of hearing.

New Jersey

1239   Camp Chatterbox
200 Portland Rd A-20
P.O. Box 8310
Highlands, NJ 07732- 2015   908-301-5451
                                       CampChatterbox@gmail.com
                                       www.campchatterbox.org

Joan Bruno, Ph.D., Director
Camp Chatterbox is an overnight camp for children who use
augmentative communication devices. The camp offers recreational activities such as swimming, boating, sports and being
with nature, and the camp activities programs are designed to facilitate device use throughout the day.

1240   Camp Dream Street
Kaplen JCC On The Palisades
411 East Clinton Avenue
Tenafly, NJ 07670   201-569-7900
                                       FAX: 201-569-7448
                                       info@jccotp.org
                                       www.jccotp.org

Tina Guberman, President
Jordan B. Shenker, CEO
Michael Kollender, Vice President
Barry Zeller, Secretary
A one-week camp for children ages 4-14 who have cancer and
other blood disorders. Campers and their siblings can enjoy a
wide variety of activities such as arts and crafts, sports, nature,
swimming, entertainment and music.

1241 Camp Jotoni
ARC of Somerset County
141 S Main St
Manville, NJ 08835-1803
908-725-8544
lauraz@thearcofsomerset.org
www.thearcofsomerset.org

Ron Slahetka, President
Timothy McKeown, Vice President
Stefanie Irwin, Treasurer
Debra Albanese, Secretary
Sponsored by the Arc of Somerset County, Camp Jotoni is a day and residential camp for children and adults with developmental disabilities. Campers are ages five to adult. Set on 15 acres in Somerset County, the camp features a junior Olympic size pool, cabins, dining hall, playgrounds, open air pavilions, unspoiled woods, and wildlife. Coed, ages 5-99.

1242 Camp Lou Henry Hoover
Girl Scouts of Washington Rock Council
201 E Grove St
Westfield, NJ 07090-5614
908-518-4400
FAX: 908-725-4933
girlscouts@gshnj.org
www.gshnj.org

Nancy Faulks, Chairman
Lydia Whitefield, 1st Vice Chairman
Andrea Hawkins, Secretary
Michael Kzirian, Treasurer
Camp is located in Middleville, New Jersey. Sessions for girls who are blind/visually impaired, ages 7-18.

1243 Camp Merry Heart
Easter Seals: New Jersey
25 Kennedy Blvd
Suite 600
East Brunswick, NJ 08816
732-257-6662
FAX: 732-257-7373
camp@nj.easterseals.com
www.easterseals.com/nj/

Michael Bisesti, Chairman
Frank Lavadera, Vice Chairman/Operations
Ken Tsoi-A-Sue, Vice Chair/Treasurer
Eric Kunkel, Board Member
An organized program of swimming, arts and crafts, boating, nature study and travel offered to campers with a variety of disabilities. Coed, ages 5-80, families, seniors. Fall and spring travel programs for adults.

1244 Camp Nejeda
Camp Nejeda Foundation
910 Saddlebrook Road
P.O. Box 156
Stillwater, NJ 07875- 156
973-383-2611
FAX: 973-383-9891
information@campnejeda.org
www.nejeda.convio.net

Henry Anhalt, DO, President
Scott Ross, Vice President
Bill Vierbuchen, Executive Director
Jim Daschbach, Camp Director
For children with diabetes, ages 7-15. Provides an active and safe camping experience which enables the children to learn about and understand diabetes. Activities include boating, swimming, fishing, archery, as well as camping skills.

1245 Camp Oakhurst
New York Service for the Handicapped
111 Monmouth Rd
Oakhurst, NJ 07755-1514
732-531-0215
FAX: 732-531-0292
info@nysh.org
www.nysh.org/

Robert Pacenza, Executive Director
Charles Sutherland, Camp Director
Andy Arno, Board Member
Julian Bach, Board Member

Camp is located in Oakhurst, New Jersey. Summer sessions for campers with cerebral palsy, mobility limitation and spina bifida. Coed, age 8-18.

1246 Camp Quality New Jersey
PO Box 264
Adelphia, NJ 07710
330-671-0167
FAX: 866-285-5208
al.passy@campqualityusa.org
www.campqualityusa.org/nj

Al Passy, Director
Mindy Rosenthal, Personnel Coordinator
Camp Quality is for children with cancer and their siblings. The camp offers a stress-free environment that offers exciting activities and fosters new friendships, while helping to give the children courage, motivation and emotional strength.

1247 Camp Sun'N Fun
ARC of Gloucester
1555 Gateway Blvd.
West Deptford, NJ 08096-3486
856-848-8648
FAX: 856-875-1499
camp@thearcgloucester.org
www.thearcgloucester.org

Robert H. Weir, Charter President
Dottie Weir, Charter President
Charles Funk, Vice President
Terri Wilson, Camp Director
Camp is located in Williamstown, New Jersey. Summer sessions for campers with developmental disabilities. Coed, ages 8-88. Activities include swimming, arts & crafts, nature, sports, games, music, dance and drama.

1248 Camp Vacamas
256 Macopin Rd
West Milford, NJ 07480-3718
973-838-0942
877-428-8222
info@vacamas.org
www.vacamas.org

Felix A. Urrutia Jr, Executive Director
Kevin Ervin, Bronx Borough Supervisor
Seth Friedman, MPA., Director of Programs
Jennifer Thompson, MSW., Director of Strategic Developmen
Disadvantaged children with asthma or sickle cell anemia, ages 8-16, are offered special programs in canoeing, backpacking, camping, music and leadership training. Sliding scale tuition. Year round programs for youth at risk groups. Conference center facility open for group rentals.

1249 Happiness Is Camping
62 Sunset Lake Road
Hardwick, NJ 07825-2201
908-362-6733
FAX: 908-362-5197
hicoffice@happinessiscamping.org
www.happinessiscamping.org

Louis D'Agostino, President of the Board
James Kramer, Secretary/Treasurer
Kenneth Bertholf, Officer
Martin Elson, Esq., Counsel
Camp is located in Blairstown, New Jersey. Free camping sessions for children with cancer. Coed, ages 6-15. June 30 - July 31, 2008.

1250 New Jersey Camp Jaycee
The Arc of New Jersey
223 Ziegler Road
Effort, PA 18330-1843
570-629-3291
FAX: 570-620-9851
info@campjaycee.org
www.campjaycee.org

Frank Pirrello, President
John O'Brien, Vice President
Patricia Rhein, Secretary
James Sandham, Treasurer
Camp Jaycee is located on 185 acres of forests, fields and streams located in the lovely Pocono Mountains, a short distance from the New Jersey border. Sessions for children and adults with autism and developmental disabilities. Goals of Camp Jaycee are cen-

tered around developing social skills, improving self esteem, increasing confidence, learning in a fun environment, developing physical fitness, and establishing meaningful relationships with new friends. Coed, ages 7-85.

1251 New Jersey YMHA/YWHA Camps Milford
21 Plymouth St
Fairfield, NJ 07004-1686
973-575-3333
800-776-5657
FAX: 973-575-4188
info@njycamps.org
www.njycamps.org

Bruce L. Nussman, President
Silvio Berlfein, Assistant Director
Leonard Robinson, Executive Director
Hylton Wener, Director
Camp is located in Milford, Pennsylvania. Summer sessions for children with ADD. Coed, ages 6-17 and families.

1252 Rolling Hills Country Day Camp
P.O.Box 172
Marlboro, NJ 07746
732-308-0405
FAX: 732-780-4726
info@rollinghillsdaycamp.com
www.rollinghillsdaycamp.com
Billy Breitner
Summer sessions for children with ADD. Coed, ages 3-12.

1253 Round Lake Camp
21 Plymouth Street
Fairfield, NJ 07004
973-575-3333
FAX: 973-575-4188
rlc@njycamps.org
www.roundlakecamp.org

1254 Summit Camp
322 Route 46 West
Suite 210
Parisppany, NJ 07054
973-732-3230
800-323-9908
FAX: 973-732-3226
info@summitcamp.com
www.summitcamp.com

Eugene Bell, Senior Director
Leah Love, Assistant Director
Kim Daum, Travel Director
Maryann Santora, Clinical Social Worker/Admission
Camp is located in Honesdale, Pennsylvania. Summer sessions for children with ADD. Coed, ages 8-17.

New Mexico

1255 Camp for Kids With Diabetes
American Diabetes Association
Manzano Mountain Retreat
County Road AO03, Post 210
Torreon, NM 87061
505-266-5716
FAX: 877-684-7907
rguerrero@diabetes.org
www.diabetes.org

Ron Guerrero, Director
The main goal of the program at American Diabetes Association Camp for Kids is to allow the campers the ability to feel at ease and accepted in a community where having diabetes is the rule, not the exception. The campers learn to understand diabetes and the process of self-management, unde skilled and continuous medical supervision. It is the hope of the staff that these children go home feeling more self-confident, self-reliant and having gained the invaluable knowledge.

New York

1256 ADA Camp Sunshine
American Diabetes Association
160 Allens Creek Rd
Rochester, NY 14618-3309
FAX: 585-458-3810
dhumphreys@diabetes.org
www.diabetescamp.org

Terry Ackley, Exec. Dir.
Lorne Abramson, Consultant
Shelley Yeager, Dir. of Outreach & Dev.
Kathy Latimer, Administrative Assistant
The American Diabetes Association New York Area's Camp is a residential camp for children with diabetes. The program is held on the Rotary Sunshine Campus in Rush, only 15 miles from Rochester. The camp is located on 133 acres of land in a rural setting including modern year round cabins, an Olympic-sized swimming pool, nature trails, athletic fields and a fishing pond. Ages 8-16; held during July.

1257 Camp Abilities Brockport
The College At Brockport, State Univ Of New York
350 New Campus Drive
Brockport, NY 14420
585-395-5361
FAX: 585-395-2771
llieberm@brockport.edu
www.campabilitiesbrockport.org

Dr. Lauren Lieberman, PhD, Camp Director
Tiffany Mitrakos, MEd, Assistant Director
Gina Pucci, Aquatic and Boating Director
Timothy Busch, Graduate Assistant
A one-week sports camp for children who are visually impaired, blind or deaf blind. Children learn to be more physically active, which in turn improves their health and well being.

1258 Camp Glengarra
Girl Scouts - Foothills Council
93 Birmingham Drive
Camden, NY 13316-4715
nbrown@girlscoutsfoothills.org
www.cartervilleacres.com

Karen Lubecki, Director
Camp Glengarra is located on 500+ acres of fields and forests, about eight miles west of Camden. This Girl Scout Camp hosts a myriad of programs throughout the year as well as summer day and resident camp. Summer sessions for girls 5-17 with ADD or asthma/respiratory ailments.

1259 Camp Good Days and Special Times
1332 Pitsford-Mendon Rd
PO Box 665
Mendon, NY 14506
585-624-5555
800-785-2135
FAX: 585-624-5799
www.campgooddays.org

J. Robert Bleier, Board President
Donald DeBlase, Board Vice-President
Michael Mercier, Board Treasurer
Wendy Bleier-Mervis, Executive Director
The camp is dedicated to improving the quality of life for children, adults and their families whose lives have been touched by cancer and/or other life challenges.

1260 Camp Huntington
56 Bruceville Road
P.O. Box 37
High Falls, NY 12440
845-687-7840
855-707-2267
FAX: 845-213-4313
mbednarz@camphuntington.com
www.camphuntington.com

Michael Bednarz, Executive Director
Alex Mellor, Program Director
Margaret Short, Health Director
Cathy Crowley, Program Supervisor

A co-ed residential summer camp specifically designed to focus on Adaptive and Therapeutic Recreation. Campers include those with learning and developmental disabilities, ADD/HD, Autism Spectrum Disorders, Asperger's, PDD, and other special needs. Three programs are offered that focus on: recreation and social skills; independence; and participation. Campers may attend for a week at a time with a full summer lasting nine weeks.

1261   Camp Independence
National Kidney Foundation
30 East 33rd Street
New York, NY 10016
770-452-1539
855-653-2273
855-NKF-CARE
FAX: 212-689-9261
nkfcares@kidney.org
www.kidney.org

Gregory w. Scott, Chairman
Beth Piranio, President
Petros Gregoriou, VP, Finance
Ellie Schlam, VP, Communications
Camp Independence is Georgia's a overnight, week-long summer camp providing essential medical care, treatment & fun for kids with kidney disease and transplants. Camp Independence recognizes that campers are normal children but have special needs providing these children with opportunities for development & individual growth, peer support & normal life experiences. Activities include swimming, arts & crafts, fishing and horseback riding, in addition to archery, games and sports, and ceramics.

1262   Camp Jened
United Cerebral Palsy Association New York
P.O. Box 483
Rock Hill, NY 12775-483
845-434-2220
FAX: 845-434-2253
www.campjened.org

1263   Camp Mark Seven
Mark Seven Deaf Foundation
144 Mohawk Hotel Rd
Old Forge, NY 13420-4010
315-207-5706
registrar@campmark7.org
www.campmark7.org

Andrew Brinks, Ph.D., Executive Director
Dr. Kim Kurz, Board Chair
P.J. Mattiacci, Assistant Chair
Jane Moran-Breiter, Board Secretary
Adirondack Mountain camp for hard-of-hearing, deaf and hearing people. Coed, ages 1-99, families, seniors and single adults.

1264   Camp Northwood
132 State Route 365
Remsen, NY 13438-5700
315-831-3621
FAX: 315-831-5867
northwoodprograms@hotmail.com
www.nwood.com

Gordon W Felt, Director
Donna Felt, Director
Summer sessions for children with ADD. Coed, ages 8-18.

1265   Camp Ramapo
Route 52 Salisbury Turnpike
PO Box 266
Rt. 52 / Salisbury Turnpike
Rhinebeck, NY 12572
845-876-8403
FAX: 845-876-8414
office@ramapoforchildren.org
www.ramapoforchildren.org

Adam Weiss, CEO
Teri Goldberg Horowitz, President
David Ross, VP & Secretary
Bob Dean, Treasurer
Ramapo's specific focus is adventure-based, experiential learning programs that promote positive character values in children and teens with special needs.

1266   Camp Sisol
Jewish Community Center of Greater Rochester/JCC
1200 Edgewood Ave
Rochester, NY 14618-5408
585-461-2000
jshellman@jccrochester.org
www.jccrochester.org

Matthew Ryen, President
Daniel Goldstein, Vice President
Staci Henning, Secretary
Justin Goldman, Treasurer
Camp is located in Honeoye Falls, New York. Summer sessions for children with autism. Coed, ages 5-16.

1267   Camp Tova
92nd Street Y
1395 Lexington Ave
New York, NY 10128-1612
212-415-5500
www.92y.org

Stuart J. Ellman, President
Sol Adler, Executive Director
Laurence D. Belfer, Vice President
Cheryl Minikes, Vice President
Children with learning and developmental disabilities thrive in Camp Tova's small group setting. Making friends and developing a wide variety of creative, social, and physical skills are the goals for Tova campers.

1268   Camp Venture, Inc.
25 Smith Street
Suite 510
Nanuet, NY 10954-2970
845-624-3860
www.campventure.org

John Murphy, President
Daniel Lukens, Exec. Dir.
Dorothy Cox, Deputy Exec. Dir.
Lisa Nolte, Associate Exec. Dir.
In more than a dozen Rockland neighborhoods, residential, employment, rehabilitation or recreation programs have arisen to help people with disabilities contribute to the life of the community. There are, for instance, more than a dozen Community Residential Facilities, Venture Industries, Venture Day Treatment, Day Habilitation, Venture Chorus, after school programs and more.

1269   Camp Whitman on Seneca Lake
Presbyterian Church USA
150 Whitman Road
Penn Yan, NY 14527-278
703-201-4345
FAX: 315-536-2128
camp@campwhitman.org
www.campwhitman.org

Lindsey Jensen, Pine Camp Program Coordinator
Rhonda Everdyke, Communications and Interim Camp
Karen Jensen, Camp Registrar
Darwyn Jepsen, Property Manager
To give the developmentally disabled youth/adult, ages 10-60, the opportunity to enjoy him/herself in a camping program. Campers are encouraged to participate in a full range of activities including games, sports, swimming, singing, and dancing. Because the camps are fairly small, we have a low camper to counselor ratio, and all have a chance to know one another and form close friendships.

1270   Casowasco Camp, Conference and Retreat Center
158 Casowasco Dr
Moravia, NY 13118-3498
315-364-8756
855-414-6400
FAX: 315-364-7636
info@campsandretreats.org
www.campsandretreats.org/index.php/casowasco/

David Little, Chair
Carmen Vianese, Vice Chair
Mike Huber, Executive Director, CRM
Demetrio Beach, Program Director, Casowasco
Camp is located in Moravia, New York. Summer sessions for children with ADD. Coed, ages 6-18 and families.

1271 Clover Patch Camp
Center for Disability Services
55 Helping Hand Ln
Glenville, NY 12302-5801

518-384-3081
FAX: 518-384-3001
cloverpatchcamp@cfdsny.org
www.cloverpatchcamp.org

Laura Taylor, Camp Director
Christopher Schelin, Program Administrator
Camp is located in Scotia, NY. Summer sessions for campers with a variety of disabilities. Coed, ages 5-85.

1272 Double H Ranch
A Hole In The Wall Camp
97 Hidden Valley Road
Lake Luzerne, NY 12846

518-696-5676
FAX: 518-696-4528
myurenda@doublehranch.org
www.doublehranch.org

Victor Hershaft, Chairman
Ed Lewi, Vice Chairman
Max Yurenda, CEO/Executive Director
Jacqui Royael, Director Of Operations
Summer residential camp and winter sports programs for children and young adults ages 6-16 who have cancer and other life threatening illnesses. The programs are free of charge and some of the recreational activities include bead making, arts & crafts, kickball, tennis, soccer, and volleyball.

1273 Father Drumgoole Connelly Summer Camp
MIV Mount Loretto
6581 Hylan Blvd
Staten Island, NY 10309-3830

718-317-2803
srynn@mountloretto.org
www.mountloretto.org

Anne Tommaso, CEO
Stephen Rynn, Exec. Director
Maryann Virga, Executive Assistant
Loretta Polanish, Exec. Secretary
Summer sessions for children with epilepsy, hearing impairment and developmental disabilities. Coed, ages 5-13.

1274 Friends Academy Summer Camps
Duck Pond Rd
Locust Valley, NY 11560

516-393-4207
FAX: 516-465-1720
camp@fa.org
www.fasummercamp.org

Rich Mack, Camp Director
Summer sessions for children with diabetes. Coed, ages 3-14, families.

1275 Friendship Circle Summer Camp
121 West 19th Street
121 West 19th Street
New York, NY 10011

646-820-1066
www.friendshipnyc.com

1276 Gow School Summer Programs
2491 Emery Road
P.O. Box 85
South Wales, NY 14139-0085

716-652-3450
FAX: 716-652-3457
summer@gow.org
www.gow.org

Robert Garcia, Director of Admissions
Gayle Hutton, Director of Development
Eric Bray, Summer Program Director
Rosemary Shields, CPA, Director of Finance
Co-ed summer programs for students ages 8-16 with dyslexia or similar learning disabilities offer a balanced blend of morning academics, afternoon/evening traditional camp activities and weekend overnights. The primary purpose of these programs is to provide a positive experience while balancing these three elements. Committed to the creation of a positive and enjoyable experience for each participant by defining and merging the goals of the camp and the school with those of camper students.

1277 Hemophilia Camp
Tanager Place
116 West 32nd Street, 11th Floor
New York, NY 10001-9533

212-328-3700
FAX: 212-328-3777
dpirrie@tanagerplace.org
www.hemaware.org/story/hemophilia-summer-camp

Donald Pirrie, Executive Director
John Indence, Executive Editor
January Payne, Managing Editor
During the six-day camp children with Hemophilia and their siblings participate in individual and group activities designed for fun and fitness. The camp held each year in mid-June has a 24-hour physician and nursing staff. Ages 5-16.

1278 Kamp Kiwanis
New York District Kiwanis Foundation
9020 Kiwanis Rd
Taberg, NY 13471-2727

315-336-4568
FAX: 315-336-3845
kamp@kampkiwanis.org
www.kamp-kiwanis.org

Rebecca O. Lopez, Executive Director
Kamp Kiwanis is a mainstream camp for underprivileged youth with and without special needs. 20 campers with disabilities are integrated into weekly sessions. Coed, ages 8-14, seniors and single adults.

1279 Maplebrook School
5142 Route 22
Amenia, NY 12501-5357

845-373-9511
FAX: 845-373-7029
jscully@maplebrookschool.org
www.maplebrookschool.org

Mark J. Metzger, Chairman
Robert Audia, Vice Chairman
George T. Whalen, Jr, Treasurer
Charles F. Chiusano, Secreaty
A coeducational boarding school which offers a six week camp for children with learning differences and ADD.

1280 Marist Brothers Mid-Hudson Valley Camp
P.O.Box 197
Esopus, NY 12429-197

212-555-1234
info@maristbrotherscenter.org
www.maristretreathouse.net

Michelle Flemen-Tung, Camp Director, Special Children
Brother Owen Ormsby, Executive Director
Matt Fallon, Director of Operations
Mike Trainor, Facilities Director
Serves special people: children who have cancer or who are HIV positive, deaf or mentally retarded.

1281 Sunshine Campus
Rochester Rotary Club
180 Linden Oaks
Suite 200
Rochester, NY 14625

585-533-2080
tdreisbach@rochesterrotary.org
www.sunshinecampus.org

Tracey Dreisbach, Executive Director
Brandi Koch, Sunshine Campus Partner Director
Amy Nicolis
Camp is located in Rush, New York. Camping sessions for children and young adults with a variety of disabilities. Ages 7-21.

1282 VISIONS Vacation Camp for the Blind
VISIONS Center on Blindness
500 Greenwich Street
3rd Floor
New York, NY 10013-1354

212-625-1616
888-245-8333
FAX: 212-219-4078
info@visionsvcb.org
www.visionsvcb.org

Nancy T. Jones, President
Richard P. Simon, Vice President
Burton M. Strauss, Jr., Treasurer
Carol Spawn Desmond, Secretary
Is a non profit agency that promotes the independence of people of all ages who are blind or visually impaired. Camp offers Braille classes, computers with large print and voice output, support groups, discussions, mobility lesions, cooking classes, personal and home management training, large print and Braille books.

1283 Wagon Road Camp
Children's Aid Society
105 East 22nd Street
New York, NY 10010-2000

212-949-4800
FAX: 914-238-0714
webmaster@childrensaidsociety.org
www.childrensaidsociety.org

Mark M. Edmiston, Chair
Bart J. Eagle, Vice Chair
Kevin J. Watson, Treasurer
Martha Bicknell Kellner, Secretary
Wagon Road Day Camp is a co-ed program for children ages 6-13 with a variety of disabilities held within Chappaqua, New York. Uniquely qualified specialists in Project Adventure activities, athletics, horsemanship, theater arts, nature/ecology studies and arts/crafts complement the day camp staff. Special events including Carnival, Olympics, Crazy Hat Day, Western Day, and optional sleepovers add to the summer excitement providing children with an enriching multicultural experience.

1284 YMCA Camp Chingachgook on Lake George
Capital District YMCA
1872 Pilot Knob Rd
Kattskill Bay, NY 12844-1802

518-656-9462
FAX: 518-656-9362
chingachgook@cdymca.org
www.cdymca.org

George Painter, Executive Director
Billy Rankin, Senior Program Director
Lesley Munshower, Summer Camp Program Director
Heather Siegel-Sawma, Groups Director
Sailing programs for people with disabilities. Sessions for campers who are blind/visually impaired. Coed, ages 7-16, families, seniors and single adults.

1285 YMCA Camp Weona
YMCA of Greater Buffalo
301 Cayuga Rd
Suite 100
Buffalo, NY 14225-1912

716-565-6000
FAX: 716-565-6007
jczochara@ymcabuffaloniagara.org
www.ymcabuffaloniagara.org

Jeff Burghardt, Finance/Financial Dev. Chair
A.L. Ferreira, Camp Exec. Dir.
Tim Marble, Camp Ranger
Julie Czochara, Business and Sales Coordinator
Camp is located in Gainesville, New York. Camping sessions for children and adults with epilepsy. Coed, ages 7-16, families and single adults. Nestled in 1,000 acres of hardwood and pine forests, Weona has miles of picturesque hiking trails, brooks, a heated outdoor pool and a world class adventure ropes course. Our indoor facilities include arts and crafts studios, environmental classrooms and a challenging rock climbing wall. It is the ideal setting for hands-on fun, adventure and learning.

North Carolina

1286 Camp Carefree
275 Carefree Lane
Stokesdale, NC 27357

336-427-0966
carefreedirectors@gmail.com
www.campcarefree.org

Lynn Tuttle, Chair
Diane Samelak, Vice Chair
Carol Wright, Secretary
Rhonda Rodenbough, Treasurer
A free, one-week camp for youngsters with serious health problems. The camp gives the children a chance to have the freedom to play, learn and enjoy all the recreational and craft activities the camp has to offer.

1287 Camp Carolina Trails
American Diabetes Association
YMCA Camp Hanes
Camp Hanes Road
King, NC 27021

919-743-5400
888-342-2383
FAX: 919-783-7838
jthomas@diabetes.org
www.diabetes.org

Justin Thomas, Director
The American Diabetes Association is the nation's leading nonprofit health organization providing diabetes research, information, advocacy and year round programs for children with diabetes.

1288 Camp New Hope
FriendshipVentures
4805 N Carolina 86
Chapel Hill, NC 27514

919-942-4716
FAX: 919-942-3266
info@newhopeccc.org
www.newhopeccc.org

Richard Stevens, Executive Director
Gerald Sigleton, Facilities Manager
Suzanne Blankfard, Office Staff
Minnilue Braverman, Office Administrator
A place for children, teens and adults to have the time of their lives. The program focuses on building self esteem, independence and provides opportunities to practice social skills specifically designed for persons with developmental, physical and multiple disabilities, special medical needs, Down Syndrome, autism, or other conditions.

1289 Camp Royall
Autism Society of North Carolina
505 Oberlin Road
Suite 230
Raleigh, NC 27605

919-743-0204
800-442-2762
info@autismsociety-nc.org
www.autismsociety-nc.org

Sharon Jeffries-Jones, Chairman
Elizabeth Phillippi, Vice Chairman
Tracey Sheriff, Chief Executive Officer
Darryl R. Marsch, Secretary
The best source in North Carolina for connecting people who live with autism (and those who care about them) with resources, support, advocacy and information tailored to their unique needs.

1290 Camp Sertoma
1105 Camp Sertoma Dr
Westfield, NC 27053

336-593-8057
www.campsertoma.org

Keith Russell, Center Director
Mike Bowman, Property Director
Camp Sartoma is a place where deaf and hard of hearing children can come to meet people just like them, with out communication barriers. Activities include swimming, canoeing, fishing, hiking, hayrides, campfires, games, astronomy, and nature crafts.

1291   Camp Sky Ranch
634 Sky Ranch Rd
Blowing Rock, NC 28605-8231

828-264-8600
FAX: 828-265-2339
jsharp1@triad.rr.com
www.campskyranchevents.com

Jack Sharp, Owner
A private, residential camp for the developmentally delayed. This season is the camp's 56th year of providing a real camping experience for the handicapped. Camp Sky Ranch was the first private camp for the handicapped in the Southeast. Activities include: swimming, boating, horseback riding, and more. Campers must be able to walk, dress and feed themselves, and toilet trained.

1292   Camp Tekoa UMC
Western NC Conference/United Methodist Church
United Methodist Camp Tekoa
P.O. Box 160
Hendersonville, NC 28793-0160

828-692-6516
FAX: 828-697-3288
ecampbell@camptekoa.org
www.camptekoa.org

James Johnson, Exec. Dir.
John Isley, Assistant Director
Karen Rohrer, Business Mgr
Melisa Coates, Administrative Assistant
Camping for children with asthma/respiratory ailments, hearing impairment and developmental disabilities. Coed, ages 6-17.

1293   SOAR Summer Adventures
NC Base Camp
226 SOAR Lane
P.O.Box 388
Balsam, NC 28707-388

828-456-3435
FAX: 828-456-3449
admissions@soarnc.org
www.soarnc.org

Jonathan Jones, Dir. Emeritus
Wandajean Jones, Dir. Emeritus
John Willson, M.S., LRT/CTR, Exec. Dir.
Laura Pate, Dir. of North Carolina Programs
A nonprofit adventure program working with disadvantaged youth diagnosed with learning disabilities in an outdoor, challenge based environment. Focuses on esteem building and social skills development through rock climbing, backpacking, whitewater rafting, mountaineering, sailing, snorkeling, and much more. Offers two week, one month, and semester programs available. SOAR programs utilize North Carolina, Florida, Colorado, American Southwest, Alaska, and Jamaica as program areas.

1294   Talisman Summer Camp
64 Gap Creek Rd
Zirconia, NC 28790-8791

828-697-6313
855-588-8254
FAX: 828-697-6249
info@talismancamps.com
talismancamps.com

Doug Smathers, Camp Director & Owner
Linda Tatsapaugh, Operations Director & Owner
Robiyn Mims, Admissions Director
Lee Kisselburg, Facilities Manager
Camp is located in Black Mountain, North Carolina. Offers a program of hiking, rafting, climbing, and caving for learning disabled ADD/ADHD and autistic young people. Coed, ages 9-18.

1295   Victory Junction Gang Camp
4500 Adam's Way
Randleman, NC 27317

336-498-9055
877-854-2268
info@victoryjunction.org
www.victoryjunction.org

Pattie Petty, Founder, Chairman & CEO
Kyle Petty, Founder; Vice-Chairman
Brian Flynn, Treasurer/ COO
Carolyn Bechtel, Member
The camp serves children with Autism, cancer, Craniofacial Anomalies, Diabetes, Sickle Cell and Spina Bifida.

North Dakota

1296   Camp Sioux
American Diabetes Association
106 Solid Rock Circle
Park River, ND 58270

763-593-5333
800-342-2383
FAX: 952-582-9000
rbarnett@diabetes.org
www.diabetes.org

Kevin L. Hagan, CEO
Shereen Arent, Exec VP, Govt Affairs
Mary Vaneeda Bennett, Chief Revenue Officer
Becky Barnett, Camp Dir.
Camp Sioux, located in Park River, ND, is a week-long residential summer camp for children ages 8-14 who are living with diabetes. Programs encourage independence and self management with appropriate medical supervision to ensure the best possible experience for every camper. Nutrition activities, blood glucose monitoring, and injections/medications are integrated into the camp program.

Ohio

1297   CYO Day Camp: Wickliffe
Catholic Charities Health and Human Services
7911 Detroit Avenue
Cleveland, OH 44102-2815

216-334-2963
contactus@clevelandcatholiccharities.org
ccdocle.org

Gerald Elliot, Chairman
Kathleen Homyock, Vice Chairman
John P. Albert, Treasurer
Kathleen Petrulis, Secretary
Welcomes children and young adults ages 6-21 with cognitive (mr/dd) and other developmental disabilities, regardless of race, religion, culture or economic background.

1298   Camp Allyn
Stepping Stones Center
5650 Given Rd
Cincinnati, OH 45243-3426

513-831-4660
FAX: 513-831-5918
info@steppingstonescenter.org
www.steppingstonescenter.org

Jeremy Vaughan, President
John Mongelluzzo, Vice President
Whitney Eckert, Treasurer
Mark Robertson, Secretary
A residential camp in Batavia, Ohio for children and adults with disabilities. Coed, ages 7-60. Campers participate in crafts, swimming, hiking, nature, sports and motor activities. Camp sessions range from 3 to 10 days, are theme oriented, and geared to individual abilities and interests. Also offers day camps for children ages 5-22.

1299   Camp Cheerful
Achievement Centers For Children
15000 Cheerful Ln
Strongsville, OH 44136-5420

440-238-6200
FAX: 440-238-1858
connie.boros@achievementctrs.org
www.achievementcenters.org

Mozelle Jackson, Chairwoman
Julie Boland, Vice Chairwoman
Marvin A. Thomas, Jr, Treasurer
Jennifer Vergilli, Secretary
Sessions for campers with developmental disabilities, mobility limitation and speech/communication impairment. Coed, ages 7-99.

1300 Camp Courageous
12701 Waterville-Swanton Rd
Whitehouse, OH 43571-9551
419-875-6828
FAX: 419-875-5598
camping@campcourageous.com
www.campcourageous.com

Steve Kiessling, Executive Director
Chelsea Banas

Camp Courageous provides residential camping services for people with developmental disabilities from ages 7-75 years old. Our six day, 5 night programs give campers a chance to experience activities such as: aquatics, arts and crafts, animal programs, sports skills, hiking, recreational and leisure education programs, nature studies, drama, cookouts and campfires.

1301 Camp Emanuel
P.O. Box 752343
Dayton, OH 45475
937-477-5504
nan33@sbcglobal.net
www.campemanuel.weebly.com

Brian Demarke, President
Stephanie Ackner, Vice President
Mary Foreman, Secretary
Nan Crawford, Executive Director

Camp for hearing impaired and normal hearing youth.

1302 Camp Happiness
Catholic Charities Health & Human Services
7911 Detroit Road
Cleveland, OH 44102-2815
216-334-2963
contactus@clevelandcatholiccharities.org
ccdocle.org

Gerald Elliot, Chairman
Kathleen Homyock, Vice Chairman
John P. Albert, Treasurer
Kathleen Petrulis, Secretary

Offers a summer camp program for persons with developmental disabilities. Camp Happiness is a six-week day camp at several sites throughout the Diocese for individuals six years of age to 21 years of age.

1303 Camp Ho Mita Koda
Diabetes Association Of Greater Cleveland
3601 South Green Road
Suite 100
Cleveland, OH 44122-5719
216-591-0800
FAX: 216-591-0320
information@diabetespartnership.org
www.dagc.org

Roger Ruch, Chair
William Murman, Chair Elect
Alenka Winslett, Treasurer
Jeffrey Malbasa, Secretary

Camp is located in Newbury, Ohio. Summer sessions for children with type 1 diabetes. Coed, ages 6-15. Type 2 diabetes, coed, ages 12-17. Bicycle adventure, coed, ages 13-19. Mini-day camp, ages 4-7, coed.

1304 Camp Ko-Man-She
American Diabetes Association
2555 S Dixie Drive
Suite 112
Dayton, OH 45409
937-220-6611
FAX: 937-224-0240
dada@diabetesdayton.org
www.diabetesdayton.org

Tyler Starline, President
Michael Martens, Vice President
Becky Roberts, Secretary
Bill Shepard, Treasurer

Camp is located in Bellefontaine, Ohio. Summer sessions for children with diabetes. Coed, ages 8-17. Held in July.

1305 Camp Libbey
Maumee Valley Girl Scout Center
2244 Collingwood Blvd
Toledo, OH 43620-1147
419-243-8216
800-860-4516
FAX: 419-245-5357
roniluckenbill@girlscoutsofwesternohio.org
www.girlscoutsofwesternohio.o rg

Jody Wainscott, Chair
Ellen Lobst, 1st Vice Chair
Ann Hartmann, 2nd Vice Chair
Kimber Fender, Secretary

Camp for girls 7-18 with asthma/respiratory ailments, diabetes, epilepsy and muscular dystrophy is located in Defiance, Ohio.

1306 Camp Nuhop
404 Hillcrest Dr
Ashland, OH 44805-4152
419-289-2227
info@campnuhop.org
www.nuhop.org

Trevor Dunlap, CEO
Ann Bell, Summer Camp Director
Chris Clyde, Associate Director
Kristin Feldman, Director of Outdoor Education

A summer residential program for any youngster from 6 to 18 with a learning disability, behavior disorder or Attention Deficit Disorder. 84 campers and 41 staff members live on site in groups of to seven campers to every three counselors. Activities focus on positive self-concept and behaviors and teaches children to learn how to find their strengths, abilities and talents from a positive, yet realistic viewpoint.

1307 Camp Quality Ohio
PO Box 2462
Akron, OH 44309
330-819-3008
FAX: 888-300-8541
ohiooffice@campqualityusa.org
www.campqualityusa.org/oh

Kerri Franks, Executive Director
Brian Krebs, Public Relations
Sharon Quinn, Camper Registrar
Allison Whoroski, Companion Coordinator

Camp Quality is for children with cancer and their siblings. The camp offers a stress-free environment that offers exciting activities and fosters new friendships, while helping to give the children courage, motivation and emotional strength.

1308 Camp Stepping Stone
Stepping Stones Center
5650 Given Rd
Cincinnati, OH 45243-3499
513-831-4660
FAX: 513-831-5918
www.steppingstonescenter.org

Jeremy Vaughan, President
John Mongelluzzo, Vice President
Whitney Wckert, Treasurer
Mark Robertson, Secretary

Day camp for children ages 5-22, serving persons with autism, cognitive deficits, Down Syndrome, cerebral palsy, brain injury, and multiple disabilities.

1309 Echoing Hills
36272 County Road 79
Warsaw, OH 43844-9770
740-327-2311
800-419-6513
FAX: 740-327-6371
info@ehvi.org
www.echoinghillsvillage.org/

Buddy Busch, President
Larry Armentrout, Board of Director
Charles Bethel, Board of Director
Todd Imhoff, Board of Director

Summer camp for children and adults with cerebral palsy. Coed, ages 7-70.

1310 Highbrook Lodge
Cleveland Sight Center
1909 East 101st Street
P.O.Box 1988
Cleveland, OH 44106-188   216-791-8118
                                                             877-776-9563
                                         camp@clevelandsightcenter.org
                                            www.clevelandsightcenter.org

Thomas P. Furnas, Chairman
Robert L. Englander, Vice Chairman
Gary W. Latz Poth, Treasurer
Sheryl King Benford, Secretary
Camp is located in Chardon, Ohio. Summer sessions for children,
adults and families who are blind or have low vision. There are
seven sessions held annually through June, July and August with
an wide range of outdoor camp activities. Camp activities focus
on gaining independent skills, mobility, orientation and self confidence in an accessible and traditional camp setting.
220-660/session

1311 Leo Yassenoff JCC Specialty Day Camp
Jewish Community Center of Greater Columbus
1125 College Ave
Columbus, OH 43209-7802   614-231-2731
                                                      FAX: 614-231-8222
                                            cfolkerth@columbusjcc.org
                                                www.columbusjcc.org

Carol Folkerth, Executive Director
Mike Klapper, Assistant Executive Director
Louise Young, Finance Director
Melanie Butter, Program Director
Summer camping sessions for children and young adults with de-
velopmental, physical, emotional, mental and learning disabili-
ties. Coed, ages 3-25.

1312 Recreation Unlimited: Day Camp
Recreation Unlimited Foundation
7700 Piper Rd
Ashley, OH 43003-9741   740-548-7006
                                                      FAX: 740-747-2640
                                            info@recreationunlimited.org
                                               www.recreationunlimited.org

Paul L. Huttlin, Executive Director & CEO
Chris Link, Operations Manager
David D. Hudler, Business Development Manager
Michelle Higgins, Billing Coordinator
Camping sessions for children and adults with a variety of dis-
abilities. Coed, ages 5-99, families, seniors and single adults.

1313 Recreation Unlimited: Residential Camp
Recreation Unlimited Foundation
7700 Piper Rd
Ashley, OH 43003-9741   740-548-7006
                                                      FAX: 740-747-2640
                                            info@recreationunlimited.org
                                               www.recreationunlimited.org

Paul L. Huttlin, Executive Director & CEO
Chris Link, Operations Manager
David D. Hudler, Business Development Manager
Michelle Higgins, Billing Coordinator
Camping sessions for children and adults with a variety of dis-
abilities. Coed, ages 5-99, families, seniors and single adults.

1314 Recreation Unlimited: Respite Weekend Camp
Recreation Unlimited Foundation
7700 Piper Rd
Ashley, OH 43003-9741   740-548-7006
                                                      FAX: 740-747-2640
                                            info@recreationunlimited.org
                                               www.recreationunlimited.org

Paul L. Huttlin, Executive Director & CEO
Chris Link, Operations Manager
David D. Hudler, Business Development Manager
Michelle Higgins, Billing Coordinator
Camping sessions for children and adults with a variety of dis-
abilities. Coed, ages 5-99, families, seniors and single adults.

1315 Recreation Unlimited: Specialty Camp
Recreation Unlimited Foundation
7700 Piper Rd
Ashley, OH 43003-9741   740-548-7006
                                                      FAX: 740-747-2640
                                            info@recreationunlimited.org
                                               www.recreationunlimited.org

Paul L. Huttlin, Executive Director & CEO
Chris Link, Operations Manager
David D. Hudler, Business Development Manager
Michelle Higgins, Billing Coordinator
Camping sessions for children and adults with a variety of dis-
abilities. Coed, ages 5-99, families, seniors and single adults.

1316 Rotary Camp
Akron Area YMCA
50 S. Main Street
Ste. LL 100
Akron, OH 44308-3430   330-376-1355
                                                      FAX: 330-644-1013
                                               aso@akronymca.org
                                                 www.akronymca.com

Grady P. Appleton, President/CEO
Laura Bennett, VP & COO
Robert R. Beiswenger, President
Cindy Dormo, Vice President
Offers camping experiences for children and adults with disabilities. Rotary Camp is American Camping Association (ACA) accredited and provides a nurturing and enriching atmosphere
where campers develop friendships, skills and memories that will
last a lifetime. Coed, ages 6-17.

1317 St. Augustine Rainbow Camp
Disability Ministries at St. Augustine Parish
2486 W 14th St
Cleveland, OH 44113-4407   216-781-5530
                                                      FAX: 216-781-1124
                                               staugch@earthlink.net
                                            www.staugustine-west14.org

Sr. Corita Ambro, CSJ, Program Dir.
Terry Hogan, Dir. of Special Religious Ed
Mary Ellen Czelusniak, Education Specialist
Mary Smith, Disability Advocate
Day camp for all children, disabled and non-disabled working to-
gether.

1318 Triangle D Camp
American Diabetes Association
8216 Princeton-Glendale Rd.
PMB200
West Chester, OH 45069-1675   907-272-1424
                                                             800-342-2383
                                                      FAX: 907-272-1428
                                               JRoss@diabetes.org
                                            www.childrenwithdiabetes.com

1319 YMCA Outdoor Center Campbell Gard
105 North Second Street
P.O. Box 13029
Hamilton, OH 45011   513-887-0001
                                                             877-224-9622
                                                      FAX: 513-887-0960
                                               contact@gmvymca.org
                                                   www.gmvymca.org

Jim Sexstone, Exec. Dir.
Pete Fasano, Outdoor School Program Dir.
Darren Corns, Special Needs Coordinator
Tom Andrews, Properties & Facilities Mgr
Camp is located in Hamilton, Ohio. Camping sessions for chil-
dren with ADD, autism, developmental disabilities and blind-
ness/visual impairment. Coed, ages 6-17 and families.

Oklahoma

1320 Camp Classen YMCA
YMCA of Greater Oklahoma City
500 North Broadway
Suite 500
Okhlama City, OK 73102-9405
405-297-7777
FAX: 580-369-2284
bdoherty@ymcaokc.org
www.ymcaokc.org

Jack Talley, Chair
Tricia Everest, Chair Elect
David Houston, Vice Chair
Alfred C. Branch, President
Camp is located in Davis, Oklahoma. Sessions for children and adults with diabetes. Coed, ages 8-17, families, seniors and single adults.

1321 Camp Perfect Wings
3800 N. May Avenue
Oklahoma City, OK 73112
405-942-3800
info@bgco.org
www.bgco.org/campperfectwings

Amanda Davis, Camp Director
Becka Johnson, Camp Director
Keith Burkhart, BGCO Family Ministry
Jeremy Davis, BGCO Family Ministry
Specifically for children ages 8-17 with special needs. Campers enjoy canoeing, pool games, low ropes challenges, and crafts.

1322 Easter Seals Oklahoma
701 NE 13th St
Oklahoma City, OK 73104-5003
405-239-2525
FAX: 405-239-2278
vwasinger@easterealsoklahoma.org
www.ok.easterseals.com/

Rodney Burgamy, Chairman
Matt Vance, Chairman-Elect
Paula K. Porter, President & CEO
Jeb Reid, Treasurer
A nationally accredited, full-day program welcoming all children, including those with disabilities and those at risk of disability. The center offers developmentally appropriate learning activities and services to meet the unique needs of each child. Our Adult Day Health Center provides solutions to meet the physical, social and emotional needs of adults from the ages of 21 to 100+.

Oregon

1323 Adventures Without Limits
1341 Pacific Avenue
Forest Grove, OR 97116
503-359-2568
FAX: 503-359-4671
awloutdoors.com

Brad Bafaro, Volunteer Executive Director
Katie Jack, Program Director
Lartz Stewart, Ass. Exe. Dir.
Adventures Without Limits facilitates inclusive, outdoor adventure for people of all ages and ability levels.

1324 Camp Latgawa Special Needs, Inc.
Oregon-Idaho Conference Center
13250 S Fork Little Butte Cr Rd
Eagle Point, OR 97524-5593
541-826-9699
camplatgawa@hotmail.com
www.latgawa.gocamping.org/

Eva LaBonty, Camp Director
Greg Clensy, Camp Director
We are located in a beautiful, wooded area of the Rogue National Forest. Two gentle flowing creeks and towering evergreens provide a peaceful setting just 35 miles east of Medford, Oregon.

1325 Camp Magruder
Oregon-Idaho Conference Center
17450 Old Pacific Hwy
Rockaway Beach, OR 97136-9609
503-355-2310
FAX: 503-355-8701
steve@campmagruder.org
www.campmagruder.org

Steve Rumage, Camp Director
Rik Gutzke, Facilities Manager
Angie Nebeker, Guest Services Manager
Troy Taylor, Assistant Camp Director
Camp is located in Rockaway Beach, Oregon. Sessions for children and adults with cancer and developmental disabilities. Coed, ages 9-18, families, seniors and single adults.

1326 Camp Starlight
P.O. Box 80666
Portland, OR 97280
503-964-1516
info@camp-starlight.org
camp-starlight.org

Angie Raffaele, Camp Director
Kit Noble, Operations Director
Melanie Smith-Wilusz, Program Director
Mark Duell, Mental Health Director
Camp Starlight is a week-long sleep-away summer camp for children in Oregon and Washington whose lives are affected by HIV/AIDS. Some of our campers are HIV+ themselves while others have someone in their immediate family- a parent, a sibling, a care-taker- who is infected.

1327 Camp Taloali
Lions Club of Oregon and Washington
P.O. Box 32
Stayton, OR 97383-9619
971-239-8153
FAX: 503-769-6415
TTY:503-400-6547
camptaloali@comcast.net
www.taloali.org

Audrey Mortensen, Chair
Elaine Wyatt, Vice Chair
Doug Fiala, Secretary
Anna Meliza, Treasurer
Summer sessions for children with hearing impairment. Coed, ages 9-17.

1328 Gales Creek Diabetes Camp
Gales Creek Camp Foundation
7110 SW Fir Loop
Suite 170
Portland, OR 97223-8136
503-968-2267
FAX: 503-443-2313
info@galescreekcamp.org
www.galescreekcamp.org

Steve Tagmyer, President
Angie Evans, Vice President
Scott Sloan, Secretary
Michael Sause, Treasurer
Camp is located in Forest Grove, Oregon. Summer sessions for children with diabetes. Coed, ages 6-16, family and pre-school family camps also available.

1329 Hull Park
PO Box 157
Sandy, OR 97055
503-668-6195
oralhull@gmail.com
oralhull.org

Gilbert Rivero, President
The Oral Hull Foundation for the Blind is dedicated to providing a special place for persons with blindness or low vision and their friends to get away for a day, weekend, or week for an exceptional experience.

1330 Meadowood Springs Speech and Hearing Camp
Institute for Rehab., Research, & Recreation Inc
316-A SE Emigrant
P.O. Box 1025
Pendleton, OR 97801-30
541-276-2752
FAX: 541-276-7227
info@meadowoodsprings.org
www.meadowoodsprings.org

Michael Ashton, Executive Director
Kathy Hosek, Administrative Assistant
Cliff Story, Property Manager
Missy Newcomb, MS, CCC-SLP, Clinical Director
On 143 acres in the Blue Mountains of Eastern Oregon, this camp is designed to help young people who have diagnosed clinical disorders of speech, hearing or language. A full range of activities in recreational and clinical areas is available.

1331 Mt Hood Kiwanis Camp
Kiwanis Club of Montavilla
10725 Sw Barbur Blvd.
Suite 50
Portland, OR 97219
503-452-7416
FAX: 503-452-0062
Kenney@mhkc.org
www.mhkc.org

Erik Marter, President
Kaleen Deatherage, Exec. Dir.
Terri Hammond, Mktg/Communications Dir.
Skye Burns, Development Director
Camp is located in Government Camp, Oregon. Summer sessions for children and adults with a variety of disabilities. Coed, ages 9-35.

1332 Strength for the Journey
Oregon-Idaho Conference Center
1505 SW 18th Ave
Portland, OR 97201-2524
800-593-7539
FAX: 503-228-3196
camping@gocamping.org
www.getmorestrength.org/

Rev. Lisa Jean Hoefner, Executive Director
Geneva Cook, Registrar
Susan Delaney, Camping Office Assistant
Camp is located near Sisters, Oregon. For adults living with HIV/AIDS.

1333 Suttle Lake Camp
Oregon/Idaho Conference Center
29551 Suttle Lake Rd
Sisters, OR 97759-9508
541-595-6663
FAX: 503-228-3196
suttlelake@gocamping.org
www.gbgm-umc.org/suttlelake/

Jane Petke, Camp Director
Daniel Petke, Facilities Director
Wendy White, Food Service
Steven Willson, Camping Ministry Intern
Camp is located in Sisters, Oregon. Camping sessions for children and adults with HIV. Coed, ages 6-18, families, seniors and single adults.

1334 Upward Bound Camp for Persons With
P.O.Box C
Stayton, OR 97383-90
503-897-2447
FAX: 503-897-4116
upward.bound.camp@gmail.com
www.upwardboundcamp.org

1335 Wallowa Lake Camp
Oregon-Idaho Conference Center
84522 Church Ln
Joseph, OR 97846
541-432-1271
wallowa@gocamping.org
www.wallowalakecamp.org

David Cook, Manager
Ingrid Cook, Manager

Camp offers volleyball, baseball, badminton, horseshoes, crafts, nature viewing and more

1336 YWCA Camp Westwind
YWCA of Greater Portland
1111 SW 10th Ave
Portland, OR 97205-2496
503-294-7400
FAX: 503-794-7399
connect@ywcapdx.org
www.ywcapdx.org

Robert Mccarthy, President
Susan Stoltenberg, Executive Director
Patricia Martin, Program Manager
Sarah Keplinger, Camp Westwind Office Manager
Promotes the understanding of racism and all forms of discrimination and fosters value, respect, and enjoyment of each person's unique contribution.

Pennsylvania

1337 Achieva
711 Bingham St
Pittsburgh, PA 15203-1007
412-995-5000
888-272-7229
FAX: 412-995-5001
nmurray@achieva.info
www.achieva.info

Marsha S. Blanco, President and CEO
Gary K. Horner, Executive Vice President
Reid Wolfe, Senior Vice President
Nancy J. Murray, President
Life-long services for people with disabilities.

1338 Camp AIM
South Hills YMCA
51 McMurray Road
Pittsburgh, PA 15241
412-833-5600
FAX: 412-653-7115
campaiminfo@gmail.com
www.campaim.org

Paulette Colonna, Camp Administrator
Tom DiPietro, Camp Director
Julie Blanc, Administrative Assistant
Sarah Kettell, Activities Director
It is the goal of our program to create an environment that offers a variety of activities centered on positive recreational and social interactions that enrich the lives of our campers. Our staff and volunteers are dedicated to this endeavor.

1339 Camp Akeela
314 Bryn Mawr Avenue
Bala Cynwyd, PA 19004
866-680-4744
FAX: 866-462-2828
info@campakeela.com
www.campakeela.com

Eric Sasson, Camp Director
Debbie Sasson, Camp Director
Kevin Trimble, Assistant Director and Program D
Rob Glyn-Jones, Head Counselor
Co-ed, overnight camp for children and young adults ages 9-17 who have been diagnosed with Asperger's Syndrome or a non verbal learning disability.

1340 Camp Can Do
3 Unami Trail
Chalfont, PA 18914
info@campcandoforever.com
campcandoforever.org

Tom Prader, Board
Sharon Maerten, Board
Stephanie Cole, Board
Amy McGonigal, Board
Camp Can Do is for children, ages 8-17, who have been diagnosed with cancer in the last 5 years.

1341 Camp Dunmoreia
Easter Seals: Southeastern Pennsylvania
3975 Conshohocken Avenue
Philadelphia, PA 19131-5506
215-879-1000
FAX: 610-565-5256
recreation@easterseals-sepa.org
www.easterseals-sepa.org

Roy Yaffe, President
Linda A. McDevitt, Vice President
Cummins Catherwood, Secretary
Linda A. McDevitt, Treasurer
Summer sessions for children and young adults with a variety of disabilities. Coed, ages 5-21.

1342 Camp Kweebec
P.O.Box 511
Narberth, PA 19072-511
610-667-2123
FAX: 610-667-6376
info@kweebec.com
www.kweebec.com

Les Weiser, Director
Maddy Weiser, Director
Josh Weiser, Associate Director
Amy Weiser, Associate Director
Camp is located in Schwenksville, Pennsylvania. Sessions for children and adults with diabetes. Coed, ages 6-16, families, seniors and single adults.

1343 Camp Lee Mar
805 Redgate Rd
Dresher, PA 19025-1432
215-658-1708
FAX: 215-658-1710
gtour400@aol.com
www.leemar.com

Ari Segal, Exec. Dir.
Lee Morrone, Dir. and Founder
Laura Leibowitz, Assistant Director
Lynsey Trohoske, Program Director
Seven week summer camp for children and young adults with mild to moderate developmental disabilities. 5-21 years of age

1344 Camp Ramah in the Poconos Education, Inc.
2100 Arch Street
Philadelphia, PA 19103
215-885-8556
FAX: 215-885-8905
info@ramahpoconos.org
www.ramahpoconos.org

Rabbi Joel Seltzer, Director
Michelle Sugarman, Assistant Director
Bruce Lipton, Director of Finance & Operation
Susan Ansul, Director
The Camp Ramah Tikvah Family Camp is located in Lakewood, Pennsylvania. It has a week-long camp in mid-August for families who have children with special needs.

1345 Camp Setebaid
Setebaid Services
P.O.Box 196
Winfield, PA 17889-196
570-524-9090
info@setebaidservices.org
www.setebaidservices.org

Mark Moyer, Executive Director
Suzanne Lee, Director
David E. Keefer, Vice President
Peggy Coleman, Director
Camping sessions for children with diabetes. Coed, ages 3-13 years. Family retreat for children with diabetes and their families.

1346 Camp Surefoot Center
Easter Seals: Southeastern Pennsylvania
233 South Wacker Drive
Suite 2400
Chicago, IL 60606-5426
215-263-7000
800-221-6827
FAX: 215-945-4073
recreation@easterseals-sepa.org
www.easterseals.com

Rick Davidson, Chairman
Eileen Howard Boone, 1st Vice Chairman
Joseph G. Kern, 2nd Vice Chairman
Edward L. Wenzel, Treasurer
Camp is located in Levittown, Pennsylvania. Sessions for children and young adults with a variety of disabilities. Coed, ages 5-21.

1347 Camp Victory
58 Camp Victory Road
Millville, PA 17846
570-458-6530
www.campvictory.org

Dennis Wolff, President
Paul Kettlewell, Vice President
Art Girio, Vice President
Tara Holdren, Secretary
At Camp Victory, partner groups with specialized knowledge and training provide camping opportunities for children with chronic health problems or physical or mental challenges. We believe that by sharing their challenges with each other in the relaxed atmosphere of a summer camp, the children become mutually supportive, teaching each other confidence, courage, and self-esteem.

1348 Camp Wesley Woods: Northeastern Pennsylvan
Western PA United Methodist Church
1001 Fiddlersgreen Rd
Grand Valley, PA 16420-4429
814-436-7802
FAX: 814-436-7669
info@wesleywoods.com
www.wesleywoods.com

Rick Frederick, Exec. Dir.
Marie Goodwill, Mktg Asst.
Andy Blystone, Programs and Mktg Dir.
Exceptional children's camp for children with emotional and intellectual handicaps.

1349 Camp Woodlands
134 Shenot Road
Wexford, PA 15090
724-935-6533
FAX: 724-935-6511
www.woodlandsfoundation.org

Douglas A. Clark, Chairman
Andrew J. Morrison, Vice Chairman
William P. Rydell, Treasurer
Edward A. Vargo, Secretary
Camp Woodlands is a one-of-a-kind camp for youth and teens, ages 8-18 with varying disabilities and chronic illness where the emphasis is on the campers Abilities rather than their disabilities.

1350 Dragonfly Forest Summer Camp
1100 E. Hector Street
Suite 333
Conshohocken, PA 19428
610-298-1820
FAX: 267-434-0100
info@dragonflyforest.org
www.dragonflyforest.org

Dennis Wolff, President
Paul Kettlewell, Vice President
Art Girio, Vice President
Kathy Fries, Secretary
Dragonfly Forest Summer Camp program, provides children with Autism and medical needs the opportunity to enjoy an overnight camp experience in an environment that is safe, equipped to meet a variety of physical, medical, and psychological needs, nurturing, and filled with activities that allow each child to reach their full fun.

1351 Elling Camps
1635 State Route 2036
Thompson, PA 18465-9100
570-756-2660
FAX: 570-756-3083
info@camptioga.com
www.camptioga.com

Ron Kuznetz, President
Dale Kuznetz, Camp Director
Mike Wagenberg, Camp Director
Mike Kuznetz, Camp Director
For youth ages 6-21 with learning disabilities and accompanying difficulties. This camp allows them to learn to adjust socially in a community atmosphere. The structured camp program includes land and water sports, nature and forestry, industrial arts, construction and work programs, and arts and crafts.

1352 Handi Camp
Handi Vangelism Ministries International
P.O.Box 122
Akron, PA 17501-122
717-859-4777
FAX: 717-721-7662
info@hvmi.org
www.hvmi.org

Tim Sheetz, Exec. Dir.
Steve Gentino, Chief Financial Officer
Kathy Sheetz, Exec. Secretary
Brian Robinson, Assistant Director
Christian, overnight camping program for people with disabilities, ages 7-50, in Eastern PA and Southern NJ. Sponsored by Handi Vangelism Ministries International.

1353 Innabah Camps
United Methodist Church: Eastern Pennsylvania
712 Pughtown Rd
Spring City, PA 19475-3311
610-469-6111
FAX: 610-469-0330
camp@innabah.org
www.innabah.org

Dan Lebo, Director
Katie MacFarlan, Program Manager
Erin Slye, Registrar
Gina L. James, Business Manager
Sessions for children and young adults with developmental disabilities. Ages 4-18, families and seniors.

1354 Lions Camp Kirby
1735 Narrows Hill Rd
Upper Black Eddy, PA 18972-9712
610-982-5731
info@lionscampkirby.org
www.lionscampkirby.org

Alice Breon, Camp Director
Offers 4-week camps for deaf and hearing impaired children and their siblings in eastern Pennsylvania.

1355 Mainstay Life Services Summer Program
200 Roessler Road
Pittsburgh, PA 15220
412-344-3640
FAX: 412-344-5486
mainstaylifeservices.org

James R. Kirk, CEO
Henry Johnston III, Chair
Bryan Cox, Vice Chair
Steven Dobis, Treasurer
Mainstay Life Services' Summer program is a unique, urban camping experience. The program runs for four weeks in July with extended, overnight stay on a college campus in Pittsburgh, Pennsylvania. One and two week sessions are offered.

1356 Outside In School Of Experiential
P.O.Box 639
Greensburg, PA 15601-639
724-837-1518
FAX: 724-837-0801
administration@outsideinschool.com
www.myoutsidein.org

Michael C. Henkel, Executive Director

Camp is located in Bolivar, Pennsylvania. Sessions for children with ADD and substance abuse problems. Boys 11-18 and girls 13-18.

1357 Phelps School Summer School
583 Sugartown Rd
Malvern, PA 19355-2800
610-644-1754
FAX: 610-644-6679
admis@thephelpsschool.org
www.thephelpsschool.org

Michael J. Reardon, Head of School
Stephany Phelps Fahey, President
Gerald D. Fahey, Treasurer
Andrew Wilmerding, Secretary
Open for grades 7-11 to make up academic deficiencies or complete studies in English, math and reading. Sports include riding, tennis and swimming. A program is also available to a limited number of international students in English as a Second Language.

1358 Sequanota Lutheran Conference Center and Camp
P.O. Box 245
Jennerstown, PA 15547
814-629-6627
FAX: 814-629-0128
contact@sequanota.com
www.sequanota.com/

Rev. Carol Custead, President
David Shoemaker, Vice President
Bob Coleman, Treasurer
Megan Will, Secretary
Summer sessions for adults with developmental disabilities and speech/communication impairment.

1359 Variety Club Camp & Developmental
2950 Potshop Road
P.O.Box 609
Worcester, PA 19490-609
610-584-4366
FAX: 610-584-5586
www.varietyphila.org

Douglas I. Zeiders, Esq., President
John Bruke, Vice President
Donald F. Faul, Treasurer
Robert J. George Jr., Secretary
Year-round camping and recreation facility for children with special needs and their families. Includes summer camping, aquatics, weekend retreats and other specialty programs. Coed, ages 5-21.

1360 YMCA Camp Fitch
The YMCA's Camp Fitch On Lake Erie
2950 Potshop Road
Worcester, PA 19490-1014
610-584-4366
877-863-4824
FAX: 610-584-5586
info@campfitchymca.org
www.varietyphila.org

Douglas I. Zeiders, Esq., President
John Bruke, Vice President
Donald F. Faul, Treasurer
Robert J. George Jr., Secretary
Camp is located in North Springfield, Pennsylvania. Camping sessions for children and adults with diabetes, hearing impairment, developmental disabilities, mobility limitation and speech/communication impairment. Ages 8-16, families and seniors.

Rhode Island

1361 Camp Mauchatea
Rhode Island Lions Sight Foundation, Inc.
PO Box 19671
Johnston, RI 02919-671
401-949-2442
ralpheiannitelli@aol.com
www.lions4sight.org

William J. Poole, 1st VP
Steven Kreiger, President
Domingos Branco, Secretary
William Scot Narragansett, Treasurer
Camp serving those who are blind/visually impaired. Campers enjoy developing and maintaining friendships with fellow campers. Some of the activities include boating and other water sports, as well as hiking and nature studies.

1362 Camp Ruggles
PO Box 353
Chepachet, RI 02814
401-567-8914
info@ricamps.org
www.ricamps.org

Peter Swain, President
Camp Ruggles is located in Glocester, RI, and is a summer day camp for emotionally handicapped children. The Camp offers a 6 week co-ed summer session for 60 children ages 6-12.

1363 Canonicus Camp
American Baptist Churches Rhode Island
54 Exeter Road
Exeter, RI 02822-503
401-294-6318
800-294-6318
FAX: 401-294-7780
camp@canonicus.org
www.canonicus.org

Colleen Tolhurst, Office Manager
Shyral Wallis, Hospitality
Jason Clark, Food Service Manager
Matt Black, Facilities Manager
Summer sessions for children with asthma/respiratory ailments. Coed, ages 4-18.

1364 Hasbro Children's Hospital Asthma Camp
593 Eddy Street
Providence, RI 02903
401-444-4000
webteam@lifespan.org.
www.hasbrochildrenshospital.org/services/asth

Timothy J. Babineau,MD, President & CEO
Fred Macri, Executive Vice President
Mamie Wakefield, Executive Vice President
Myra Edens, RN, Administrative Director
Camp for children with asthma. Children learn about asthma and asthma management through interactive, educational and fun activities. The camp also offers activities such as swimming, canoeing and arts & crafts.

South Carolina

1365 Burnt Gin Camp
SC Department of Health and Environmental Control
P.O.Box 101106
Mills-Jarrett Complex
Columbia, SC 29011
803-898-0784
FAX: 803-898-0613
aimonemi@dhec.sc.gov
www.scdhec.gov

Marie I Aimone, Camp Director
A residential camp for children who have physical disabilities and/or chronic illnesses. Camper/staff ratio is 2:1. Five seven-day sessions for 7-15 year olds and one six-day session for 16-19 year olds. Limited to residents of South Carolina.

1366 Camp Adam Fisher
P.O. Box 5226
Columbia, SC 29250
803-434-2442
scottm14@earthlink.net
www.campadamfisher.com

Elizabeth Todd-Heckel, Program Director
Scott McFarland, Camp Director
For children with diabetes and their siblings. Campers enjoy swimming, horseback riding, tubing, basketball, volleyball and arts & crafts, while also learning how to manage their diabetes so they can live longer, healthier lives.

1367 Camp Debbie Lou
726 Lucky Run
Latta, SC 29565
843-752-5416
info@campdebbielou.com
www.campdebbielou.com

1368 Camp Gravatt
1006 Camp Gravatt Rd
Aiken, SC 29805-8730
803-648-1817
FAX: 803-648-7453
development@campgravatt.org
www.bishopgravatt.org

Lauri SoJourner Yeargin, Executive Director
Ellen Grbic, Office Manager
Thomas K. Coleman, Program Director
Scott McNeely, Camp Director
Project adventure includes swimming, fishing, music and art and more in which disabled campers participate. Enjoy the fun and adventure of exploring a river in a canoe in the new canoe program. Title: Gravatt Camp and Conference Center

1369 Camp Spearhead
Greenville County Recreation District
4806 Old Spartanburg Road
Taylors, SC 29687
864-288-6470
FAX: 864-288-6499
randy@gcrd.org
www.campspearhead.org

Gene Smith, Executive Director
Chanell Moore, Deputy Director/ CFO
Stacey Bechtold, HR Director
Don Shuman, Parks Director
Camp for children with disabilities age 8 years and up. The mission of Camp Spearhead is to provide an environment of unconditional acceptance for children and adults with disabilities. A caring staff, creative programming, and a state-of-the-art campsite all combine to offer a safe and nurturing camp experience for every camper.

South Dakota

1370 Camp Friendship
P.O. Box 1986
Rapid City, SD 57709
campfriendshipdirector@hotmail.com
www.campfriendship.org

Kristi Berg, Camp Director
Nancy Clary, Camp Historian
Stacie Kellogg, Assistant Director in Training
Kathleen Haibeck
Held in the Black Hills of South Dakota, Camp Friendship is for individuals with physical and developmental disabilities. Campers go fishing, swimming, have cook outs and sing-a-longs, and just have fun!

1371 Camp Gilbert
Sanford Children's Specialty Clinic
P.O. Box 89406
Sioux Falls, SD 57109-9406
605-212-6027
800-850-0064
campgilbertinfo@gmail.com
www.campgilbert.com

Kay Schroeder, Pediatric Dietician
Nancy Hartung, Staffing/Treasurer

For children ages 8-18 with diabetes. Campers can enjoy a week of canoeing, swimming, sing-a-longs, crafts, and games, while also attending educational programs covering nutrition, exercise and lifestyle management.

1372 NeSoDak
Lutherans Outdoors in South Dakota
3285 Camp Dakota Dr.
Waubay, SD 57273
605-947-4440
800-888-1464
nesodak@losd.org
www.losd.org/

Rev. Layne Nelson, Executive Director
Karen Kraus, Development Director
Mara Stillson, Marketing Coordinator
Laura Eiesland, Executive Asst.
Camp is located in Waubay, South Dakota. Sessions for children with diabetes. Coed, ages 8-18.

Tennessee

1373 ACM Lifting Lives Music Camp
Vanderbilt Kennedy Center
110 Magnolia Circle
Nashville, TN 37203
615-322-8240
kc@vanderbilt.edu
www.kc.vanderbilt.edu/site/services/page.aspx
Tracy P. Beard, Assistant Director
Cole Beck, Biostatistics Programmer
Tammy Day, Program Director
Kyle Jonas, Media Specialist
A camp for individuals with developmental disabilities where they can come to celebrate music by participating in songwriting workshops, recording sessions and live performances.

1374 All Days Are Happy Days Summer Camp
Boling Center
711 Jefferson Avenue
Memphis, TN 38105
901-448-6511
888-572-2249
FAX: 901-448-7097
TTY:901-448-4677
annested@uthsc.edu
www.uthsc.edu
Frederick B. Palmer, MD, Director
Bruce Keisling, PhD, Associate Director
Elizabeth Bishop, M.S., LEND Training Coordinator
Vanessa Baker, Business Manager
Week long camp for children ages 6-11 years of age who have been diagnosed with ADHD. The primary goal is to educate campers and their parents about the diagnosis, treatment, and self-management of ADHD and related behaviors.

1375 Bill Rice Ranch
627 Bill Rice Ranch Road
Murfreesboro, TN 37128
615-893-2767
800-253-7423
FAX: 615-898-0656
info@billriceranch.org
www.billriceranch.org
Wil Rice IV, President
Troy Carlson, Director
Nathan McConnell, Deaf Ministries Director
Camping for hearing impaired children and youths ages 9-19.

1376 Camp Discovery
Tennessee Jaycees and Tennessee Jaycee Foundation
400 Camp Discovery Ln
Gainsboro, TN 38562
931-704-0107
FAX: 931-268-6737
director@jayceecamp.org
www.jayceecamp.org
Dawn Hickman, PhD., Vice President of Camp Operation
Faith Henshaw, Camp Director
Chester Lowe, Vice President of Camp Operation
Millie Dawkins, Camp Off Season Rentals

Serves children with skin conditions including: Epidermolysis Bullosa, Psoriasis, Alopecia, Vitiligo, Eczema, Scleroderma, Congenital Nevus, Ehlers-Danlos, Ichthyosis, Ectodermal Dysplasia and more. The Camp is located at 400 Camp Discovery Lane in Gainsboro, TN.

1377 Camp Koinonia
University Of Tennessee
1914 Andy Holt Avenue
HPER Building 362
Knoxville, TN 37996
865-974-1289
FAX: 865-974-8981
thecampkoinonia@gmail.com
www.thecampkoinonia.com
Joseph L. Ortiz, President
J.D. King, Vice President
Carlene LeCompte, Treasurer
Dr. Angela Wozencroft, Secretary
Outdoor education program for children and young adults ages 7-22 who have multiple disabilities. The camp offers recreational activities such as canoeing, music and games.

1378 Camp Okawehna
1633 Church Street
Suite 500
Nashville, TN 37203
615-327-3061
877-326-1109
FAX: 605-329-2513
CampO@dciinc.org
www.dciinc.org/camp_info.php
Andy Parker, Camp Director
Week-long summer camp for critically ill children ages 6-18 years suffering from kidney disease. Children who have had kidney transplants as well as children on hemodialysis and peritoneal dialysis are welcome. The camp focuses on the critically ill child who needs to have fun and be in the company of other children who suffer from the same disease.

1379 Camp Sugar Falls
American Diabetes Association
4205 Hillsboro Road
Suite 200
Nashville, TN 37215-3339
615-298-3066
888-342-2383
FAX: 615-292-5357
dbradford@diabetes.org
www.childrenwithdiabetes.com/camps/campsugarf
Devin Anna Bradford, Camp Coordinator
Week long camp for children ages 6-12 who have diabetes and their siblings. Activities include education sessions, athletics and exercise.

1380 Easter Seals Tennessee Camping Program
Easter Seals Tennessee - State Headquarters
3011 Armory Drive
Suite 100
Nashville, TN 37204
615-292-6640
FAX: 615-251-0994
TTY:615-385-3485
www.easterseals.com
Mike Campbell, Chairman
John Pfeiffer, Vice Chairman
Jeff Bridges, Treasurer
Gay Bruner, Camp Director
Offers a variety of services to people with disabilities.

1381 Indian Creek Camp
Kentucky Tennessee Conference
150 Cabin Circle Dr.
Liberty, TN 37095
615-548-4411
FAX: 615-548-4029
info@indiancreekcamp.com
www.indiancreekcamp.com
Ken Wetmore, Summer Camp Director
Stephanie Rufo, Assistant Director & PR
Morgan Aumack, Activity Director
Kaity Clements, Program Director

Camp is located in Liberty, Tennessee. Summer sessions for children and adults who are blind/visually impaired. Coed, ages 7-17, families and seniors.

1382   LeBonheur Cardiac Kids Camp
LeBonheur Children's Hospital
848 Adams Ave.
Memphis, TN 38103
901-287-5437
FAX: 901-287-4646
info@lebonheur.org
www.lebonheur.org

Meri Armour, M.S.N., M.B.A., Camp Director
Bill May, M.D., M.B.A, Camp Administrator
Larry Spratlin, M.B.A
Dave Rosenbaum
Camp for children and young adults ages 8-16 with cardiac-related diagnoses. Children enjoy a fun-filled week at camp where they learn about their heart conditions and meet other children just like them.

1383   Paddy Rossbach Youth Camp
Amputee Coalition Of America
900 East Hill Avenue
Suite 290
Knoxville, TN 37915
888-267-5669
TTY:865-525-4512
www.amputee-coalition.org

Dan Berschinski, Chairman
Gregory D. Gadson, Vice Chair
Susan Stout, President/CEO
Carole Folta, Chief Financial Officer
Georgia camp for youths ages 10-17 years of age who have limb loss or limb difference. Activities include sports, swimming, fishing, arts and crafts.

Texas

1384   Camp Be An Angel
2003 Aldine-Bender Rd.
Houston, TX 77032
281-219-3313
FAX: 281-219-7746
www.beanangel.org/prog_camp.html#.VZAxuvmqqko
Bill Shank, Chairman
Marti Boone, Executive Director
Russ Massey, Program Director
Katie Kasprzak, Development Director
Camp Be An Angel is designed to be a retreat for special needs children under the age of 22 and their immediate families (Mom, Dad, Brothers and Sisters).

1385   Camp CAMP
P.O.Box 27086
San Antonio, TX 78227
210-671-5411
FAX: 210-671-5225
campmail@campcamp.org
www.campcamp.org

Mike Zerda, Chairman
Susan Osborne, Executive Director
Jean Magargee, Treasurer
Toni Hill, Ph.D, Secretary
Camping for children and young adults with a variety of disabilities. Coed, ages 5-21. Respite services throughout calendar year. Adult camp ages 22-45.

1386   Camp Cpals
5501A Balcones #160
Austin, TX 78731
866-74C-PATH
?info@cpathtexas.com
www.cpathtexas.com

Laura Romero, President
Victoria Polega, Vice President
Marielle Deckard, Secretary
Jamie L. Eppele, Director of Fundraising

CPals is a social group designed to give children with cerebral palsy the opportunity to meet others as well as bring parents and siblings together.

1387   Camp John Marc
Special Camps for Special Kids
2929 Carlisle Street
Suite 355
Dallas, TX 75204
214-360-0056
FAX: 214-368-2003
mail@campjohnmarc.org
www.campjohnmarc.org

Vance Gilmore, Executive Director
Kevin Randles, Camp Director
Megan White, Associate Camp Director
Bre Loveless, Assistant Camp Director
Camp is located in Meridian, Texas. Year-round camping for children with a variety of disabilities. Coed, ages 6-16 and families.

1388   Camp Neuron
1411 Amarillo Boulevard East
Amarillo, TX 79107
806-352-5426
888-548-9716
FAX: 806-352-6249
info@eftx.org
eftx.org

Donna Stahlhut, Founder/ CEO
Donna Stahlhut, Chief Executive Officer
Shannon Robbins, Assistant Director
Jeanette Hartshorn, Clinic Services Director
Camp Neuron offers a safe and fun residential camping experience for children and teens living with epilepsy. The Epilepsy Foundation Texas provides this unique opportunity at no cost to families of children with epilepsy. At Camp Neuron campers build self-esteem, create life-long friendships, participate in team building, and learn more about living with epilepsy.

1389   Camp Quality Texas
26302 Fieldhaven Court
Cypress, TX 77433
330-671-0167
FAX: 866-285-5208
texas@campqualityusa.org
www.campqualityusa.org/TX
Anneliese Kulakofsky, Camp Director
Falyne Perrin, Secretary
Sherri Scott, Personnel Committee Chair
Stephanie Weber, Financial Committee Chair
Camp Quality is for children with cancer and their siblings. The camp offers a stress-free environment that offers exciting activities and fosters new friendships, while helping to give the children courage, motivation and emotional strength.

1390   Camp Spike 'n' Wave
1411 Amarillo Boulevard East
Amarillo, TX 79107
806-352-5426
888-548-9716
FAX: 806-352-6249
info@eftx.org
eftx.org

Donna Stahlhut, Founder/ CEO
Donna Stahlhut, Chief Executive Officer
Shannon Robbins, Assistant Director
Jeanette Hartshorn, Clinic Services Director
Camp Spike 'n' Waver offers a safe and fun residential camping experience for children and teens living with epilepsy. The Epilepsy Foundation Texas provides this unique opportunity at no cost to families of children with epilepsy.

1391 **Camp Summit**
17210 Campbell Road
Suite 180-W
Dallas, TX 75252

972-484-8900
FAX: 972-620-1945
camp@campsummittx.org
www.campsummittx.org

Lee Hines, Chair
Cole Ballweg, Vice Chair
Carla R. Weiland, President/CEO
Lisa Braziel, Camp Director
Camp is located in Argyle, Texas. Camping for children and adults with a variety of disabilities. Coed, ages 6-99.

1392 **Camp Sweeney**
Southwestern Diabetic Fund
P.O. Box 918
Gainesville, TX 76241

940-665-2011
FAX: 940-665-9467
info@campsweeney.org
www.campsweeney.org

T. Milton Dickson, Jr. DDS, Chair
Robert D. Vandermeer, MD, Vice Chair
Ernie Fernandez, M.D., Camp Director
Skip Rigsby, Program Director
Teaches self-care and self-reliance to children ages 7-18 with diabetes. Campers participate in such activities such as swimming, fishing, horseback riding and arts and crafts while learning about how to self manage their diabetes.

1393 **Camp for All**
Camp for All Foundation
6301 Rehburg Rd
Burton, TX 77835

979-289-3752
FAX: 979-289-5046
campsite@campforall.org
www.campforall.org

Liz Rigney, Chairman
Rogers L. Crain, Vice Chair
Pat Prior Sorrells, President and CEO
Kurt R. Podeszwa, Camp Director
Fully-accessible year round camp facility is located in Burton, Texas. Camping for children and adults with a variety of disabilities. Coed, ages 5-35 and up and families.

1394 **Children's Association for Maximum Potential Summer Camp**
2525 Ladd Street
Lackland AFB, TX 78236

210-671-5411
FAX: 210-671-5225
campmail@campcamp.org
www.campcamp.org

Susan Osborne, Executive Director
Laura Leach, CFRE, Chief Development Officer
Ben Elble, Camp Director
Michelle Elble, Director of Family Support
Summer Camp is a series of six-day, five-night sessions for children and adults, aged 5 to 50 years, with a variety of special needs and their siblings.

1395 **Dallas Academy**
950 Tiffany Way
Dallas, TX 75218

214-324-1481
FAX: 214-327-8537
mail@dallas-academy.com
www.dallas-academy.com

Troy Sturrock, Chair
Terrence S. Welch, Vice Chair
Dallas Cothrum, Secretary
Redonna Higgins, Treasurer
7-week summer session for students who are having difficulty in regular school classes.

1396 **Growing Together Diabetes Camp**
1000 S. Beckham
P.O. Box 6400
Tyler, TX 75711-6400

903-596-3645
800-232-8318
www.etmc.org/diabetes_day_camp.htm

Anjani Upponi, Camp Director
Vicki Jowell, Director
Dr. Stella Hecker, Medical Director
A summer camp for youths ages 6 to 15 with Type 1 or Type 2 diabetes.

1397 **Hill School of Fort Worth**
4817 Odessa Avenue
Fort Worth, TX 76133

817-923-9482
FAX: 817-923-4894
hillschool@hillschool.org
www.hillschool.org

John W. Wright, Chairman
Randall Connelly, Vice Chair
Audrey Boda-Davis, Executive Director
Roxam Breyer, Principal
Provides an alternative learning environment for students having average or above-average intelligence with learning differences. Hill school is an established leader in North Texas with a 25 year history of effectively serving LD children. Beginning in 1961 as a tutorial service, Hill became a formal school in 1973. Our mission is to help those who learn differently develop skills and strategies to succeed. We do this by developing academic/study skills, and self-discipline.

1398 **Kamp Kaleidoscope**
1411 Amarillo Boulevard East
Amarillo, TX 79107

806-352-5426
888-548-9716
FAX: 806-352-6249
info@eftx.org
eftx.org

Donna Stahlhut, Founder/ CEO
Donna Stahlhut, Chief Executive Officer
Shannon Robbins, Assistant Director
Jeanette Hartshorn, Clinic Services Director
Kamp Kaleidoscoper offers a safe and fun residential camping experience for teens living with epilepsy. The Epilepsy Foundation Texas provides this unique opportunity at no cost to families of teens with epilepsy.

1399 **Texas Lions Camp**
Lions Club Of Texas
P.O. Box 290247
Kerrville, TX 78029

830-896-8500
FAX: 830-896-3666
tlc@ktc.com
www.lionscamp.com

Stephen Mabry, Executive Director
The primary purpose of the League shall be to provide, without charge, a camp for physically disabled, hearing/vision impaired and diabetic children from the State of Texas, regardless of race, religion, or national origin. Our goal is to create an atmosphere wherein campers will learn the can do philosophy and be allowed to achieve maximum personal growth and self-esteem. The camp welcomes boys and girls ages 7-16.

Utah

1400 **Camp Giddy-Up**
National Ability Center
PO Box 682799
Park City, UT 84068

435-649-3991
FAX: 435-658-3992
info@DiscoverNAC.org
www.discovernac.org

Alan Mciver, President
Sean Carroll, VP, People
Andy Dahmen, VP, Facilities & Capital
Shawn Fojtik, VP, Programs

Camp Giddy Up is for individuals of all abilities ages 8 - 18 who are interested in a horsemanship-focused camp designed to facilitate shared experiences for people both with and without disabilities. Campers will start the day with grooming, riding and barn activities in the morning and then enjoy a variety of outdoor recreational activities in the afternoon. This is a great opportunity to learn more about horses and riding, while making new friends.

1401 Camp Hobe
P.O. Box 520755
Salt Lake City, UT 84152-755   801-631-2742
wapitimama@camphobekids.org
www.camphobekids.org

Christina Beckwith, PharmD, President
Phillip Barnette, MD, Medical Director, Vice President
Christina Beckwith, Executive Director
Jamie Seale, Medical Co-Director
A special summer camp for children with cancer and their siblings.

1402 Camp Kostopulos
Kostopulos Dream Foundation
4180 Emigration Canyon Road
Salt Lake City, UT 84108   801-582-0700
FAX: 801-583-5176
kdf@campk.org
www.campk.org

John Miller, Chairman
Rick Lifferth, Vice Chair
Layne Smith, Vice Chair
Mircea Divricean, President & CEO
Summer camping for children and adults ages 7-65 with a variety of disabilities. Year round recreation on site and community based activities.

1403 Camp Nah-Nah-Mah
University Health Care Burn Camp Programs
50 N. Medical Drive
Salt Lake City, UT 84132   801-581-2700
healthcare.utah.edu/burncenter/
Brad Wiggins, Burn Camp Director
For children ages 6-12 years of age that are burn survivors. Some of the activities include canoeing, rock climbing and archery.

1404 Camp Vision
National Ability Center
PO Box 682799
Park City, UT 84068   435-649-3991
FAX: 435-658-3992
info@DiscoverNAC.org
www.discovernac.org

Alan Mciver, President
Sean Carroll, VP, People
Andy Dahmen, VP, Facilities & Capital
Shawn Fojtik, VP, Programs
Camp Vision is specifically designed for teens and young adults with visual impairments. Participants experience the thrill of recreation during this week long overnight camp. Campers can experience everything from horseback riding to cycling, pedaling on tandem bikes or with experienced guides. Camp Vision is a great match for all levels and abilities.

1405 Camp X-Treme
National Ability Center
PO Box 682799
Park City, UT 84068   435-649-3991
FAX: 435-658-3992
info@DiscoverNAC.org
www.discovernac.org

Alan Mciver, President
Sean Carroll, VP, People
Andy Dahmen, VP, Facilities & Capital
Shawn Fojtik, VP, Programs
This is an outdoor overnight camp for teens with physical disabilities. Campers can fly down the mountains of Park City on a zip line, ride the alpine slide, ski or snowboard, rock climb and more. This week-long overnight camp is designed to build confidence

and self-esteem. Camps are offered in both the summer and winter.

1406 Discovery Camps
National Ability Center
PO Box 682799
Park City, UT 84068   435-649-3991
FAX: 435-658-3992
info@DiscoverNAC.org
www.discovernac.org

Alan Mciver, President
Sean Carroll, VP, People
Andy Dahmen, VP, Facilities & Capital
Shawn Fojtik, VP, Programs
Discovery Camps are available for youth ages 8 - 18 with physical disabilities (Pathfinders), intellectual disabilities (Crusaders) and Autism Spectrum Disorders (Adventurers). Other Discovery Camps include Intro to Camp (ages 6-8) and Siblings Camp, where brothers and sisters have an opportunity to experience everything camp has to offer together. Discovery Camps are primarily day camps, with a few overnight experiences included during specific weeks.

1407 FCYD Camp
Foundation for Children and Youth with Diabetes
1995 West 9000 South
West Jordan, UT 84088   801-566-6913
www.fcydcamp.org

David Okubo, MD, Co-Founder, Trustee
Elizabeth Elmer, Co-Founder, Trustee
Nathan Gedge, Co-Founder, Trustee
Camping for children with diabetes. Coed, ages 1-18 and families.

1408 Overnight Camps
National Ability Center
PO Box 682799
Park City, UT 84068   435-649-3991
FAX: 435-658-3992
info@DiscoverNAC.org
www.discovernac.org

Alan Mciver, President
Sean Carroll, VP, People
Andy Dahmen, VP, Facilities & Capital
Shawn Fojtik, VP, Programs
Overnight Camps are available for teens and young adults ages 15 - 24 depending on specific camps. Overnight campers stay in our lodge and sometimes get to sleep under the stars in tents on-site. Each room has two twin beds and a private accessible bathroom. Days and evenings are full of fun activities and campers often end the day around the campfire singing songs and playing games.

Vermont

1409 Camp Betsey Cox
140 Betsey Cox Lane
Pittsford, VT 05763   802-483-6611
info@campbetseycox.com
www.campbetseycox.com

Lorrie Byrom, Director and Co-Owner
Mike Byrom, Co-owner and Associate Director
Devri Byrom, Associate Director
Camp is located in Pittsford, Vermont. Summer sessions for girls aged 9-15 with ADD.

1410 Camp Thorpe
680 Capen Hill Road
Goshen, VT 05733   802-247-6611
info@campthorpe.org
www.campthorpe.org

Lyle Jepson, Director
Elizabeth Giard, Board of Trustee
Richard Giard, Board of Trustee
Ralph O. Hathaway, Board of Trustee
Focuses on meeting the needs of each individual camper; showing each of them that they have the ability and potential. Also pro-

vides positive camping experience for children challenged with handicapping conditions.

1411 Silver Towers Camp
56 Silver Towers Rd
Ripton, VT 5766

802-388-6446
FAX: 877-417-7661
info@vtelks.org
www.vtelks.org/programs/silver-towers/

Frederick Dusablon, President
Brian Gaura, 1st Vice President
Carolyn Ravenna, Camp Director
Robert Campo, Camp Committee

Two-week residential camp for ages 6-75 who are physically or mentally challenged. Campers gain the social skills and personal enrichment they seek. Activities include swimming, horseback riding, music, sing-a-longs, dancing, nature studies and more.

Virginia

1412 ADA Camp Grenada
American Diabetes Association
1701 N. Beauregard St.
Alexandria, VA 22311

312-346-1805
888-342-2383
FAX: 317-594-0748
wwallace@diabetes.org
www.diabetes.org

Dwight Holing, Chair
Larry Hausner, CEO
Debbie Johnson, CFO
Greg Elfers, Chief Field Development Officer

Camp Granada is an American Diabetes Association resident Camp located in Monticello, Illinois at the 4H Memorial Camp owned by the University of Illinois. For children with diabetes, ages 8-16. Activities include swimming, canoeing, wall climbing, tie-dying shirts, arts & crafts and fun filled evening programs.

1413 Adventure Camp
Amputee Coalition Of America
P.O. Box 485
Lovingston, VA 22949

434-263-5432
meh8f@virginia.edu
www.adventurecampinc.org

Mary Grant, President
Dwayne Strong, Vice President
Ed Hicks, Treasurer
Jennifer Puskaric, Secretary

Adventure Camp is held each summer for children and adolescents with limb loss. Activities include swimming, ropes course, canoeing, fishing, golf , scavenger hunts, karaoke and much more.

1414 Adventure Day Camp
3480 Commission Ct
Lake Ridge, VA 22192

703-491-1444
office@princewilliamacademy.com
www.princewilliamacademy.com

Dr. Samia Harris, Founder, Executive Director
Dr. Shiree Slade, Principal
Dr. Rebecca Nykwest, PhD, Director of Communications
Lindsay Chickering, Office Manager

Camping for children with asthma/respiratory ailments and cancer. Coed, ages 2-13.

1415 Camp Dickenson
Holston Conference of United Methodist Church
801 Camp Dickson Ln
Fries, VA 24330-4348

276-744-7241
campdickenson@centurylink.net
www.campdickenson.com

Michael Snow, Manager

Camp is located in Fries, Virginia. Camping for children and adults with developmental disabilities. Coed, ages 5-18, families, seniors and single adults.

1416 Camp Easter Seals Virginia
Easter Seals: Virginia
900 Camp Easter Seals Rd.
New Castle, VA 24127

540-777-7325
800-365-1656
FAX: 540-777-2194
camp@eastersealsucp.com
www.easterseals.com

Alex Barge, Camp Director
Luanne Welch, President & CEO
Tristan Robertson, Executive Director
Gayle M. Rose, Executive Director

Summer camp sessions for children and adults ages 5-99 with physical disabilities, cognitive disabilities and sensory impairments. Therapeutic recreation activities including swimming, fishing, sports, horseback riding, rock climbing, and more. Twenty-six-day speech therapy camp children with disabilities ages 8-16. Twelve-day Spina Bifida Self Help Skills Camp.

1417 Camp Holiday Trails
400 Holiday Trails Lane
Charlottesville, VA 22903

434-977-3781
FAX: 434-977-8814
info@campholidaytrails.org
www.campholidaytrails.org

Joe Cashman, President
Kellie Sauls, Vice President
Tina La Roche, Executive Director
Heather Mott, Development Director

Private, nonprofit camp for children with special health needs and various chronic illnesses. Residential, 2-week sessions are open June - August; camperships are available. Coed 7-17, nationwide and international. Canoeing, swimming, horseback riding, arts and crafts, drama, ropes course, etc. 24-hr. medical supervision by doctor and nursing staff. Air conditioned cabins.

1418 Camp Loud And Clear
Holiday Lake 4-H Educational Center
1267 4-H Camp Road
Appomattox, VA 24522

434-248-5444
FAX: 434-248-6749
heathern@vt.edu
holidaylake4h.com/camploud.php

Preston Willson, President/ CEO
Heather Benningrove, Program Director
Bryan Branch, Center Director
Rich Hilbers, Facilities Manager

No other summer camp in Virginia is staffed or equipped to accept children with hearing loss regardless of their communication means. This camp will offer deaf/hard of hearing children the environment with staff and programming to augment healthy, satisfying socialization experiences.

1419 Camp Virginia Jaycee
2494 Camp Jaycee Road
P.O. Box 648
Blue Ridge, VA 24064

540-947-2972
800-865-0092
FAX: 540-947-2043
info@campvajc.org
www.campvajc.org

Tom King, Chair
Kathleen King, Vice Chair
Lisa Parrish, Treasurer
William B Robertson, Founder

Summer camping for children and adults with developmental disabilities. Coed, ages 7-70. Weekend respite camps for children and adults with mental retardation.

1420 Camps for Children & Teens with Diabetes
Diabetes Society
1701 N. Beauregard St.
Alexandria, VA 22311
408-287-3785
800-DIA-ETES
FAX: 408-287-2701
camp@diabetessociety.org
www.diabetessociety.org

Dwight Holing, Chair
Larry Hausner, CEO
Debbie Johnson, CFO
Greg Elfers, Chief Field Development Officer
Since 1974, sponsors up to 20 day camps, family camps and resident camps for children 4 through 17. These camps provide an opportunity for children with diabetes to go to camp, meet other children and gain a better understanding of their diabetes. The total experience can help campers develop more confidence in their abilities to control their diabetes effectively while enjoying the traditional camp experience. Camps are located throughout CA and parts of Nevada.

1421 Civitan Acres for the Disabled
Eggleston Services
1161 Ingleside Road
Norfolk, VA 23502-5608
757-858-8011
866-386-GIVE
FAX: 757-627-4760
TTY: 757-852-9310
info@egglestonservices.org
www.egglestonservices.org

Paul Atkinson, President and CEO
Rick Biggs, SVP/ CFO
Thomas L. Redmond, VP, Marketing & Development
Chris Hoagland, VP, Government Contracts
Offers a summer camp for adult and children with disabilities. Participants can choose from day or overnight packages.

1422 Loudoun County Special Recreation Programs
Loudoun County Local Government
P.O. Box 7000
Leesburg, VA 20177
703-777-0100
FAX: 703-771-5354
TTY:703-711-0343
prcs@loudoun.gov
www.loudoun.gov

Scott K. York, Chairman At-Large
Shawn M. Williams, Vice Chairman
Kenneth D. Reid, Board Member
Ralph M. Buona, Board Member
Offers and promotes integration opportunities for individuals with disabilities. Coordinates ADA issues and Very Special Arts and Special Olympics for Loudoun County. Summer camps, sports, socials and community trips.

1423 Makemie Woods Camp
Presbytery of Eastern Virginia
3700 Ropers Church Road
Lanexa, VA 23089
757-566-1496
800-566-1496
FAX: 757-566-8803
admin@makwoods.org
www.makwoods.org

Chad Rockett, Operations Manager
Beth Martin, Office Assistant
Anthony Burcher, Storyteller in Residence
Fran Parkhurst, Food Services Manager
Residential Christian camp that tailors each group and individual goals. Counselors serve as teachers, friends and activity leaders. For children 8-18 with diabetes.

1424 Oakland School & Camp
128 Oakland Farm Way
Troy, VA 22974
434-293-9059
FAX: 434-296-8930
information@oaklandschool.net
www.oaklandschool.net

Carol Williams, Head of School
Jamie Cato, Admissions Director
Amanda Baber, Admissions Director
Pete Cormons, Operations Director
A highly individualized program stresses improving reading ability. Subjects taught are reading, English composition, math and word analysis. Recreational activities include horseback riding, sports, swimming, tennis, crafts, archery and camping. For girls and boys, ages 8-14.

Washington

1425 Camp Fun in the Sun
Inland NorthWest Health Services
501 N. Riverpoint Blvd.
Suite 245
Spokane, WA 99202
509-232-8138
FAX: 509-232-8145
randalll@cherspokane.org
wellness.inhs.org

Tom Fritz, CEO
Nicole Stewart, Dir. of Mktg & Communications
Jerrie Heyamoto, Communication Coordinator
Tamitha Anderson, Communication Coordinator
Summer camping for children with diabetes. Coed, ages 6-18.

1426 Camp Killoqua
Camp Fire USA
4312 Rucker Ave
Everett, WA 98203
425-258-KIDS
FAX: 425-252-2267
killoqua@campfiresnoco.org
www.campfireusasnohomish.org

Terri Vail, President
Elizabeth Johnson, Vice President
Dave Surface, Executive Director
Michael Deal, Operations Director
Camp is located in Stanwood, Washington. Camping for children with developmental disabilities. Coed, ages 6-17.

1427 Camp Prime Time
6 S. 2nd Street
Suite 815
Yakima, WA 98901
509-248-2854
FAX: 509-248-5505
families@campprimetime.org
www.campprimetime.org

Ralph Berthon, Co-Founder
Dave Berthon, Co-Founder
Dick Haapala, President
Mike Burnam, Vice President
Prime Time serves children and adults with disabilities or have terminal or serious illnesses.

1428 Camp Volasuca
Volunteers of America: Western Washington
2802 Broadway
Everett, WA 98201
425-259-3191
888-216-5459
FAX: 425-258-2838
info@voaww.org
www.voaww.org

Phil Smith, President/CEO
Kim Conant, Vice President - Human Resource
Mark Johnson, Vice President of Development &
Bruce Keller, Chief Financial Officer
Camp is located in Sultan, Washington. Summer sessions for children and adults with a variety of disabilities. Coed, ages 6-13, families and single adults.

1429 Easter Seals Camp Stand by Me
Easter Seal Society of Washington
17809 S. Vaughn Road KPN
PO Box 289
Vaughn, WA 98394- 0313

253-884-2722
800-678-5708
FAX: 253-590-0594
mayer@wa.easterseals.com
www.easterseals.com

Kristopher Kohl, Board Chair
Stephanie Nelson, Vice Chair
Cathy Bisaillon, President/ CEO
Steve Rummel, Treasurer
Camp is located in Vaughn, Washington. Summer camping for adults and children with developmental disabilities and mobility limitation. Coed, ages 7-65, seniors. Respite weekends October thru May.

1430 Northwest Kiwanis Camp
P.O.Box 1227
Port Hadlock, WA 98339

360-732-7222
nwkc@earthlink.net
weareugn.org

Kim Hammers, President
Steve Rafoth, Vice President
Joyce Cardinal, Chief Nurse Executive
Joan Williams, Senior Services Consultant
Campers range from 6-60 in age, and includes those with developmental disabilities, cerebral palsy, autism, downs syndrome, and other physical and/or mental handicaps.

1431 YMCA Camp Orkila
YMCA of Greater Seattle
909 4th Ave
Seattle, WA 98104

206-382-5000
FAX: 203-382-4920
websiteadmin@seattleymca.org
www.seattleymca.org

Mark N. Tabbutt, Chair
Carolyn S Kelly, Vice Chair
John F. Vynne, Vice Chair
Robert B. Gilbertson, Jr., President/CEO
Camping for children with blood disorders and diabetes, ages 8-18.

West Virginia

1432 Mountaineer Spina Bifida Camp
534 New Goff Mountain Road
Charleston, WV 25313

304-776-7513
800-642-9704
info@drewsday.org
www.drewsday.org/

Susan Nelsen, 5K Coordinator
Stephanie Gregory, 5K run/walk/stroll coordinator
Suzie Humphreys, 5K run/walk/stroll coordinator
Is a non profit organization which pursues education and training and focuses on activities that promote independence and those that facilitate everyday life. The objectives are to build self esteem, promote independence and enhance the development of social skills.

1433 YMCA Camp Horseshoe
Ohio-West Virginia YMCA
Horseshoe Leadership Center
3309 Horseshoe Run Road
Parsons, WV 26287-9029

304-478-2481
FAX: 304-478-4446
Horseshoe@YLA-youthleadership.org
www.yla-youthleadership.org/Horseshoe.html

David King, Director
Tom Starr, Executive Director
Sharon Cassidy, Administrative Coordinator
Stacie Pearson, Program Coordinator
Summer camping for children with cancer, ages 7-18.

Wisconsin

1434 Camp Kee-B-Waw
101 Nob Hill Road
Suite 301
Madison, WI 53713

608-277-8288
800-422-2324
FAX: 608-277-8333
camp@eastersealswisconsin.com
camp.eastersealswisconsin.com

1435 Camp Needlepoint
American Diabetes Association
YMCA Camp St. Croix
532 County Road F
Hudson, WI 54016

763-593-5333
800-342-2383
FAX: 952-582-9000
rbarnett@diabetes.org
www.diabetes.org

Kevin L. Hagan, CEO
Debbie Johnson, CFO
Greg Elfers, Chief Field Development Officer
Shereen Arent, EVP
Camping for children who have type 1 diabetes. Coed, ages 5-16.

1436 Easter Seal Camp Wawbeek
Easter Seals: Wisconsin
1450 Highway 13
Wisconsin Dells, WI 53965

608-254-8319
800-422-2324
FAX: 608-254-8310
wawbeek@eastersealswisconsin.com
camp.eastersealswisconsin.com

Carissa Miller, Director
Nanc Howard, Executive Assistant
Brian Schuetz, Director
Pam Ganser, Chief Financial Officer
Hundreds of people with mild to severe disabilities attend Easter Seals Wisconsin camps. The camp offers adventure programs, camp sessions for other health agencies, family camp opportunities and year round respite sessions. Coed, ages 8-99.

1437 Lutherdale Bible Camp
Lutherdale Ministries
N7891 US Highway 12 Elkhorn
Elkhorn, WI 53121

262-742-2352
FAX: 888-248-4551
info@lutherdale.org
www.lutherdale.org

Jeff Bluhm, Executive Director
David Box, Program Director
Maggie Atkinson, Program Director
Matt Coddington, Program Asst.
Summer camping for people with developmental disabilities. Coed, ages 9-18 and families, seniors.

1438 Phantom Lake YMCA Camp
S110W30240 YMCA Camp Road
Mukwonago, WI 53149

262-363-4386
FAX: 262-363-4351
office@phantomlakeymca.org
www.phantomlakeymca.org

Ray Gooden, Chair of the Board
Walter Stewart, Vice Chair
James Scharine, Vice Chair
Mike Hase, Treasurer
Summer camping for children with epilepsy, ages 7-15.

1439 **Timbertop Nature Adventure Camp**
YMCA Camp Glacier Hollow
1000 Division Street
Stevens Point, WI 54481

715-342-2980
FAX: 715-342-2987
pmatthai@spymca.org
www.glacierhollow.com

Pete Matthai, Camp Director
Tiffany Gecko Praeger, Summer Camp Program Director
For children who can benefit from an individualized program of
learning in a non-competitive outdoor setting under the skilled
leadership of people who understand the environment and the
unique potential of these children.

1440 **Wisconsin Badger Camp**
11815 Munz Lane
Prairie Du Chien, WI 53821

608-988-4558
FAX: 608-988-4586
wiscbadgercamp@centurytel.net
www.badgercamp.org

Carol Beals, Chair
Gerry O'Rourke, Vice Chair
Michelle Eno, Treasurer
Kim Martens, Secretary
Wisconsin Badger Camp, established in 1966, is a summer camp
that serves individuals with developmental disabilities. Badger
camp offers eight one-week camps and one two-week camp for
ages 3-93. One week is for ages 14-25, one week for ages 3-13 and
all other weeks for ages 18 and older.

1441 **Wisconsin Elks/Easter Seals Respite Camp**
1550 Waubeek Road
Wisconsin Dells, WI 53965

608-254-2502
800-422-2324
FAX: 608-253-3027
dfourness@eastersealswisconsin.com
camp.eastersealswisconsin.com

Dan Fourness, Director, Respite Services

1442 **Wisconsin Lions Camp**
Wisconsin Lions Foundation
3834 County Road A
Rosholt, WI 54473

715-677-4969
FAX: 715-677-3297
TTY:715-677-6999
info@wisconsinlionscamp.com
www.wisconsinlionscamp.com

Evett J. Hartvig, Executive Director
Andrea Yenter, Camp Director
Jamie Jannusch, Assistant Camp Director
Dale Schroeder, Facility Director
Serves children who have either a visual, hearing or mild cognitive disability, as well as diabetes types I and II. Program activities include sailing, ropes course, hiking and canoe trips,
environmental education, swimming, camping, canoeing, outdoor living skills and handicrafts. ACA accredited, located in
central Wisconsin, near Stevens Point.

1443 **Wisconson Badger Camp**
P.O. Box 723
Platteville, WI 53818

608-348-9689
FAX: 608-348-9737
bbowers@badgercamp.org
www.badgercamp.org

Carol Beals, Chair
Bruce Rathe, Vice Chair
Michelle Eno, Treasurer
Kim Martens, Secretary
Badger Camp gives individuals with developmental disabilities a
chance to experience camp and enjoy themselves in an outdoor
setting.

Wyoming

1444 **Camp Hope**
3920 West 45th Street
Casper, WY 82604

307-265-5865
FAX: 307-472-5008
camphope@bresnan.net
www.camphopewy.com

Mary Barbato, VP, Marketing
Todd Colowell, Chief Financial Officer
Monica Dennis, Managing Editor
Sid Fein, EVP, Technology
Camp Hope is a camp for children and young adults with diabetes.
Some of the activities include biking, swimming, sports and
games.

1445 **Eagle View Ranch**
SOAR
184 Uphill Road
P.O. Box 584
Dubois, WY 82513

307-455-3084
FAX: 801-820-3050
evr@soarnc.org
www.soarnc.org

John Willson, M.S., Executive Director
Jonathan Jones, Founder, Director Emeritus
Laura Pate, Operations Director
Wandajean Jones, Director Emeritus
Camp for youths with learning disabilities and attention deficit
disorder. Campers enjoy a broad range of wilderness adventure
experiences that help to empower them to overcome challenges,
while helping them to learn how to develop problem solving
skills, effective communication strategies and social skills.

Clothing

Dresses & Skirts

1446 Budget Cotton/Poly Open Back Gown
Buck & Buck
3111 27th Ave S
Seattle, WA 98144-6502
206-722-4196
800-458-0600
FAX: 800-317-2182
info@buckandbuck.com
www.buckandbuck.com

Julie Buck, Owner
Short raglan sleeves, lace at neck and bodice over lapping snapback closure. *$14.00*

1447 Budget Flannel Open Back Gown
Buck & Buck
3111 27th Ave S
Seattle, WA 98144-6502
206-722-4196
800-458-0600
info@buckandbuck.com
www.buckandbuck.com

Julie Buck, Owner
3/4 raglan sleeve, lace at neck and bodice. *$17.00*

1448 Cotton/Poly House Dress
Buck & Buck
3111 27th Ave S
Seattle, WA 98144-6502
206-722-4196
800-458-0600
info@buckandbuck.com
www.buckandbuck.com

Julie Buck, Owner
Comes in short and long sleeves, assorted florals and plaids. *$36.00*

1449 Dusters
Buck & Buck
3111 27th Ave S
Seattle, WA 98144-6502
206-722-4196
800-458-0600
info@buckandbuck.com
www.buckandbuck.com

Julie Buck, Owner
Three types: Floral, Budget Better. Snap front styles and gathered yokes, flannel $16.00-$24.00. *$36.00*

1450 Flannel Gowns
Buck & Buck
3111 27th Ave S
Seattle, WA 98144-6502
206-722-4196
800-458-0600
info@buckandbuck.com
www.buckandbuck.com

Julie Buck, Owner
Comes in long or short with a deep button-front opening for ease of slipping on. Shorter long length. *$21.00*

1451 Float Dress
Buck & Buck
3111 27th Ave S
Seattle, WA 98144-6502
206-722-4196
800-458-0600
info@buckandbuck.com
www.buckandbuck.com

Julie Buck, Owner
A safe bet for everyone from a size medium to a 3X. Gathered yoke front and back and literally yards of fabric for fullness. Comes in cotton or polyester. *$32.00*

1452 Muu Muu
Buck & Buck
3111 27th Ave S
Seattle, WA 98144-6502
206-722-4196
800-458-0600
info@buckandbuck.com
www.buckandbuck.com

Julie Buck, Owner
Comes in long and short styles, assorted bright floral prints. $20.00-$22.00. *$31.00*

1453 Polyester House Dress
Buck & Buck
3111 27th Ave S
Seattle, WA 98144-6502
206-722-4196
800-458-0600
info@buckandbuck.com
www.buckandbuck.com

Julie Buck, Owner
Comes in short and long sleeves, assorted florals. *$ 36.00*

Footwear

1454 Booties with Non-Skid Soles
Buck & Buck
3111 27th Ave S
Seattle, WA 98144-6502
206-722-4196
800-458-0600
FAX: 800-317-2182
info@buckandbuck.com
www.buckandbuck.com

Julie Buck, Owner
Acrylic knit or quilted cotton/poly and shearling inner. *$17.00*

1455 Foot Snugglers
Buck & Buck
3111 27th Ave S
Seattle, WA 98144-6502
206-722-4196
800-458-0600
FAX: 800-317-2182
info@buckandbuck.com
www.buckandbuck.com

Julie Buck, Owner
Quilted poly/cotton outers lined with plush shearling pile, provide a thick, comfortable cushion which helps minimize the pressure points on tender areas. *$.30*

1456 Propet Leather Walking Shoes
Buck & Buck
3111 27th Ave S
Seattle, WA 98144-6502
206-722-4196
800-458-0600
FAX: 800-317-2182
info@buckandbuck.com
www.buckandbuck.com

Julie Buck, Owner
Two velcro straps, leather upper, shock-absorbing sole. *$58.00*

1457 TRU-Mold Shoes
42 Breckenridge St
Buffalo, NY 14213-1555
716-881-4484
800-843-6653
FAX: 716-881-0406
www.trumold.com

Husain Syed, Production Manager
Custom made, fully molded shoes, relieve pressure in sensitive areas by taking all of the weight off the painful areas.

1458 Velcro Booties
Buck & Buck
3111 27th Ave S
Seattle, WA 98144-6502
206-722-4196
800-458-0600
FAX: 800-317-2182
info@buckandbuck.com
www.buckandbuck.com

Julie Buck, Owner
The high-domed toe, and extra-wide, non-skid sole design accommodates virtually every foot related problem. *$20.00*

1459 Washable Shoes
Buck & Buck
3111 27th Ave S
Seattle, WA 98144-6502
206-722-4196
800-458-0600
FAX: 800-317-2182
info@buckandbuck.com
www.buckandbuck.com

Julie Buck, Owner
Vinyl upper with velcro closure, nonskid sole. *$20.00*

Miscellaneous & Catalogs

1460 Adaptations by Adrian
PO Box 7
San Marcos, CA 92079-0007
760-744-3565
888-214-8372
FAX: 760-471-7560
adrians1@sbcglobal.net
www.adaptationsbyadrian.com

1461 Adaptive Clothing: Adults
Special Clothes
P.O.Box 333
E Harwich, MA 02645-333
508-430-2410
FAX: 508-430-2410
specialclo@aol.com
www.special-clothes.com

Judith Sweeney, President
Special Clothes produces a catalogue of garments for adults with disabilities and/or incontinence. Offerings include: undergarments, snap-crotch tee shirts, jumpsuits, and denim travel cath. The catalogue is available without charge. Comparable to department store prices. Special Clothes produces a catalog of adaptive clothing for children in sizes from toddler through young adults. A full line of clothing is included from undergarments through wheelchair jackets and ponchos.

1462 Adult Short Jumpsuit
Special Clothes
P.O.Box 333
E Harwich, MA 02645-333
508-430-2410
FAX: 508-430-2410
specialclo@aol.com
www.special-clothes.com

Judith Sweeney, President
This pull-on jumpsuit provides comfort and full coverage without bulk. Wide leg ribbing ends at mid-thigh, with snaps at the crotch. We use fine quality, comfortable cotton knit. 100% cotton knit. Made in USA. Option: long sleeves - add $3.00. Colors: white, navy, teal, light blue, light pink, red, royal blue, black, khaki and juvenile print. S,M & L $43.00; XL & XXL $45.00

1463 Body Suits
Special Clothes
P.O.Box 333
E Harwich, MA 02645-333
508-430-2410
FAX: 508-430-2410
specialclo@aol.com
www.special-clothes.com

Judith Sweeney, President
These are one piece garments that can be used to protect skin under braces, to add warmth and to shield incisions. S,M & L $42.00; XL & XXL $44.00.

1464 Buck and Buck Clothing
3111 27th Ave S
Seattle, WA 98144-6502
206-722-4196
800-458-0600
FAX: 800-317-2182
info@buckandbuck.com
www.buckandbuck.com

Julie Buck, Owner
Clothing for the disabled and elderly.
88 pages Yearly

1465 Carolyn's Catalog
3938 S Tamiami Trl
Sarasota, FL 34231-3622
941-373-9100
800-648-2266
FAX: 941-739-5503
support@carolynscatalog.com
www.carolynscatalog.com

John Colton, Owner
Free, mail-order catalog of items for visually impaired people.

1466 Exquisite Egronomic Protective Wear
Plum Enterprises
P.O.Box 85
Valley Forge, PA 19481-85
610-783-7377
800-321-7586
FAX: 610-783-7577
info@plument.com
www.plument.com

Janice Carrington, President/CEO
Egronomic Protective Wear; ProtectaCap custom-fitting headgear has earned an unparalleled reputation for quality, safety, and comfort. ProtectaCap+Plus technologically-advanced protective headgear closes the gap between hard and soft helmets. Comes with optional ProtectaChin Guard and new sporty design. Protectahip protective undergarment is the intelligent, innovative solution to the problem of hip injuries for both men and women. Ladies' styles are covered with attractive stretch lace.

1467 Headliner Hats
Designs for Comfort
PO Box 671044
Marietta, GA 30066-2429
770-565-8246
800-443-9226
FAX: 770-565-8425
headliner@mindspring.com
www.headlinerhats.com

Curt Maurer, President
A patented cap and hairpiece combination, the Headliner is both a quick, stylish coverup and an upbeat wig alternative for women experiencing hair care problems or hair loss. Ideal for social gatherings and outdoor activities as well as for sleeping and hospital stays. *$ 25.00*

1468 Knee Socks
Buck & Buck
3111 27th Ave S
Seattle, WA 98144-6502
206-722-4196
800-458-0600
FAX: 800-317-2182
info@buckandbuck.com
www.buckandbuck.com

Julie Buck, Owner
Comes in regular and large size. $3.00 - $8.00

1469 M&M Health Care Apparel Company
Fashion Collection
1541 60th St
Brooklyn, NY 11219-5023
718-871-8188
800-221-8929
FAX: 718-436-2067
info@fashionease.com
www.fashionease.com

Abraham Klein, Owner
Specialized clothing for disabled people.

1470 Professional Fit Clothing
Ste 1
831 N Lake St
Burbank, CA 91502-1600
818-563-1975
800-422-2348
FAX: 818-563-1834
sales@professionalfit.com
www.professionalfit.com

Kurt Rieback, Owner
Professional fit clothing caters to homes that care for people with developmental disabilities and individuals who are physically challenged. Our clothing is fashionable, affordable and can be adapted to each person's special needs.

1471 Spec-L Clothing Solutions
849 Performance Drive
Stockton, CA 95206
714-427-0781
800-445-1981
FAX: 800-683-6510
rlfortun@clothingsolutions.com
www.clothingsolutions.com

Jim Lechner, Owner
The nation's leading designer and manufacturer of assistive clothing for men and women. Free 56 page catalog available.

1472 Special Clothes Adult Catalogue
Special Clothes
P.O.Box 333
E Harwich, MA 02645-333
508-430-2410
FAX: 508-430-2410
specialclo@aol.com
www.special-clothes.com

Judith Sweeney, President
Produces a catalogue of adaptive clothing for adults with disabilities. Offers include undergarments, casual bottoms, jumpsuits, swimwear, footwear and bibs. Prices are comparable to deparment store prices. The catalogue is free.

1473 Special Clothes for Special Children
Special Clothes
P.O.Box 333
E Harwich, MA 02645-333
508-430-2410
FAX: 508-430-2410
specialclo@aol.com
www.special-clothes.com

Judith Sweeney, President
All special adaptations, such as velcro closures, snap crotches, bib fronts and G-tube access openings. Every item is fully washable. Offering optional features to customize each item to meet the needs of your child.

1474 Specialty Care Shoppe
16126 E 161st St S
Bixby, OK 74008-7325
918-366-2901
FAX: 918-366-9445
deb@specialtycareshoppe.com
www.specialtycareshoppe.com

K J Marshall, Owner
Catalog of attractive, affordable clothing and accessories for adults with special needs. Includes items for edema, incontinence, alzheimers, limited mobility, and hand impairment.

1475 Super Stretch Socks
Buck & Buck
3111 27th Ave S
Seattle, WA 98144-6502
206-722-4196
800-458-0600
FAX: 800-317-2182
info@buckandbuck.com
www.buckandbuck.com

Julie Buck, Owner
This sock has been improved to stretch laterally throughout the foot area as well as at the top. *$3.75*

1476 Thigh-Hi Nylon Stockings
Buck & Buck
3111 27th Ave S
Seattle, WA 98144-6502
206-722-4196
800-458-0600
FAX: 800-317-2182
info@buckandbuck.com
www.buckandbuck.com

Julie Buck, Owner
A sheer, full length stocking. *$4.50*

1477 Waterproof Bib
Buck & Buck
3111 27th Ave S
Seattle, WA 98144-6502
206-722-4196
800-458-0600
FAX: 800-317-2182
info@buckandbuck.com
www.buckandbuck.com

Julie Buck, Owner
Made with 3 layers of fabric including waterproof backing, these attractive bibs will not soak through like most others, protecting clothing from stains. *$18.00*

1478 Wishing Wells Collection
Ste 965
11684 Ventura Blvd
Studio City, CA 91604-2699
818-840-6919
FAX: 818-760-3878
wishingwells@dawn-wells.com
www.dawn-wells.com

Dawn Wells, Owner
Lorraine Parker, General Manager
Features designs full of back overlap construction and all velcro closures clothing.

Robes & Sleepwear

1479 Creative Designs
3704 Carlisle Ct
Modesto, CA 95356-924
209-523-3166
800-335-4852
robes4you@aol.com
www.robes4you.com

Barbara Arnold, Owner
Designer of the original Change-A-Robe and the new Handi-Robe, which allows the wearer to put it on without having to stand up. Robes are designed especially for physically challenged, disabled individuals, and wheelchair users. *$69.95*

1480 Flannel Pajamas
Buck & Buck
3111 27th Ave S
Seattle, WA 98144-6502
206-722-4196
800-458-0600
FAX: 800-317-2182
info@buckandbuck.com
www.buckandbuck.com

Julie Buck, Owner
$25.00

1481 His & Hers
Wishing Wells Collection
Ste 965
11684 Ventura Blvd
Studio City, CA 91604-2699
818-840-6919
FAX: 818-760-3878
wishingwells@dawn-wells.com
www.dawnwells.com

Dawn Wells, Owner
This sleep shirt is designed for him or her. *$21.99*

1482 Nightshirts
Buck & Buck
3111 27th Ave S
Seattle, WA 98144-6502
　206-722-4196
　800-458-0600
　FAX: 800-317-2182
　info@buckandbuck.com
　www.buckandbuck.com

Julie Buck, Owner
Come in flannel or cotton patterns and prints in sizes S/M, 4XL, 2XL/3XL $29.00

1483 Open Back Nightgowns
Buck & Buck
3111 27th Ave S
Seattle, WA 98144-6502
　206-722-4196
　800-458-0600
　FAX: 800-317-2182
　info@buckandbuck.com
　www.buckandbuck.com

Julie Buck, Owner
Come in cotton (sizes S-4X) or flannel (sizes S-3X). $20.00

1484 Seersucker Shower Robe
Buck & Buck
3111 27th Ave S
Seattle, WA 98144-6502
　206-722-4196
　800-458-0600
　FAX: 800-317-2182
　info@buckandbuck.com
　www.buckandbuck.com

Julie Buck, Owner
Totally covers a man or woman being wheeled to and from the shower or bath. A crisp, light weight shower robe. $34.00

Shirts & Tops

1485 Basic Rear Closure Sweat Top
Buck & Buck
3111 27th Ave S
Seattle, WA 98144-6502
　206-722-4196
　800-458-0600
　FAX: 800-317-2182
　info@buckandbuck.com
　www.buckandbuck.com

Julie Buck, Owner
Top opens completely down the back for ease of dressing with snaps. $19.00

1486 Cotton Full-Back Vest
Buck & Buck
3111 27th Ave S
Seattle, WA 98144-6502
　206-722-4196
　800-458-0600
　FAX: 800-317-2182
　info@buckandbuck.com
　www.buckandbuck.com

Julie Buck, Owner
Wide shoulder straps that don't slide off shoulders. $5.00

1487 Dutch Neck T-Shirt
Buck & Buck
3111 27th Ave S
Seattle, WA 98144-6502
　206-722-4196
　800-458-0600
　FAX: 800-317-2182
　info@buckandbuck.com
　www.buckandbuck.com

Julie Buck, Owner
Stretchy neck makes it easy to get over the head. $ 5.50

1488 Printed Rear Closure Sweat Top
Buck & Buck
3111 27th Ave S
Seattle, WA 98144-6502
　206-722-4196
　800-458-0600
　FAX: 800-317-2182
　info@buckandbuck.com
　www.buckandbuck.com

Julie Buck, Owner
Comes in assorted colors, plain or with animal motifs and snaps all the way down the back. $28.00

1489 Rear Closure Shirts
Buck & Buck
3111 27th Ave S
Seattle, WA 98144-6502
　206-722-4196
　800-458-0600
　FAX: 206-722-1144
　info@buckandbuck.com
　www.buckandbuck.com

Julie Buck, Owner
Snaps down the back on T-shirts and dress shirts. $ 33.00

1490 Rear Closure T-Shirt
Buck & Buck
3111 27th Ave S
Seattle, WA 98144-6502
　206-722-4196
　800-458-0600
　FAX: 800-317-2182
　info@buckandbuck.com
　www.buckandbuck.com

Julie Buck, Owner
Closes down the back with velcro snaps. $10.00

Slacks & Pants

1491 Jumpsuits
Special Clothes
PO Box 333
E Harwich, MA 02645-333
　508-430-2410
　FAX: 508-430-2410
　lou@lnrmusic.com
　www.special-clothes.com

Judith Sweeney, President
Several styles of one-piece garments are available for dressing ease. Front opening styles are designed for easy access. Prices range from $32.20-$44.00. $55.00

1492 Side Velcro Slacks
Buck & Buck
3111 27th Ave S
Seattle, WA 98144-6502
　206-722-4196
　800-458-0600
　FAX: 800-317-2182
　info@buckandbuck.com
　www.buckandbuck.com

Julie Buck, Owner
Slacks open down both sides from waist to hip with snap closures at sides. $36.00

1493 Side-Zip Sweat Pants
Buck & Buck
3111 27th Ave S
Seattle, WA 98144-6502
　206-722-4196
　800-458-0600
　FAX: 800-317-2182
　info@buckandbuck.com
　www.buckandbuck.com

Julie Buck, Owner
Out-seam zippers un-zip 22-inch zippers down both sides to enable dressing a resident with severe leg contractures. $25.00

1494 Trunks
Buck & Buck
3111 27th Ave S
Seattle, WA 98144-6502   206-722-4196
                                      800-458-0600
                                 FAX: 800-317-2118
                              info@buckandbuck.com
                               www.buckandbuck.com

Julie Buck, Owner
Come in cotton or nylon, flare leg, full cut. *$5.00*

Undergarments

1495 Adult Absorbent Briefs
Special Clothes
PO Box 333
E Harwich, MA 02645-333   508-430-2410
                                 FAX: 508-430-2410
                                  lou@lnrmusic.com
                              www.special-clothes.com

Judith Sweeney, President
Soft, comfortable, 100% cotton knit brief is seven layers thick at the crotch. Sides of the brief are a non-bulky single layer. The waistband elastic is enclosed in a soft cotton knit casing and does not touch the skin. Comfortable cotton rib knit bands circle the leg. This brief will not replace a diaper, but provides absorbency for light incontinence. *$18.50*

1496 Adult Lap Shoulder Bodysuit
Special Clothes
PO Box 334
E Harwich, MA 02645-333   508-430-2410
                                 FAX: 508-430-2410
                                 TTY: 508-430-2410
                                  lou@lnrmusic.com
                              www.special-clothes.com

1497 Adult Sleeveless Bodysuit
Special Clothes
PO Box 335
E Harwich, MA 02645-333   508-430-2410
                                 FAX: 508-430-2410
                                  lou@lnrmusic.com
                              www.special-clothes.com

Judith Sweeney, President
Bodysuit styles fasten at the crotch with sturdy snaps to stay neatly tucked. All are made of soft, absorbent 100% cotton knit for maximum comfort. They are cut wide at the hip and seat for full coverage, and will accomodate a diaper if necessary. Soft knit rib circles the neck and leg. This cool tank style slips on easily. Deep armholes are banded with rib knit. All styles: S,M,L $42, XL,XXL $44. A choice of 12 colors.

1498 Adult Swim Diaper
Special Clothes
PO Box 336
E Harwich, MA 02645-333   508-430-2410
                                 FAX: 508-430-2410
                                  lou@lnrmusic.com
                              www.special-clothes.com

Judith Sweeney, President
This pant is made of soft, silent, light-weight, impermeable fabric- waterproof and secure. It is a containment brief, designed to be used in the pool in place of cloth or disposable diapers, which can become waterlogged or disintegrate in the water. Waist and legbands should be snug for proper fit, so please consult sizing chart before ordering. Darlex with lining of 100% cotton knit. Lycra waist and legbands. Made in USA. *$40.00*

1499 Adult Tee Shoulder Bodysuit
Special Clothes
PO Box 337
E Harwich, MA 02645-333   508-430-2410
                                 FAX: 508-430-2410
                                 TTY: 508-430-2410
                                  lou@lnrmusic.com
                               www.special-clothes.com

1500 Adult Waterproof Overpant
Special Clothes
PO Box 338
E Harwich, MA 02645-333   508-430-2410
                                 FAX: 508-430-2410
                                  lou@lnrmusic.com
                               www.special-clothes.com

Judith Sweeney, President
Overpants are made of a soft, silent, lightweight fabric which is waterproof and very secure. It is designed to be used over our Adult Absorbent Brief, or cloth diapers. It is completely latex-free and is an excellent non-allergenic substitute for rubber or vinyl pants. Waist and legbands should be snug to minimize leakage, so please consult the sizing chart before ordering. Lycra waist and legbands. Made in USA. *$40.00*

1501 Briefs
Special Clothes
P.O.Box 333
E Harwich, MA 02645   508-430-2410
                                 FAX: 508-430-2410
                                 specialclo@aol.com
                               www.special-clothes.com

Judith Sweeney, President
A variety of unique brief styles available for easy access and practicality.

1502 Panties
Buck & Buck
3111 27th Ave S
Seattle, WA 98144-6502   206-722-4196
                                      800-458-0600
                                 FAX: 800-317-2182
                              info@buckandbuck.com
                               www.buckandbuck.com

Julie Buck, Owner
Come in nylon or cotton, band leg for comfort. *$5.00*

1503 Support Plus
5581 Hudson Industrial Parkway
PO Box 2599
Hudson, OH 44236-0099   508-359-2910
                                      866-229-2910
                                 FAX: 800-950-9569
                                 www.supportplus.com

Ed Janos, President
Offers a selection of support undergarments, braces and shoes for the physically challenged and medical professionals.

Computers

Assistive Devices

1504 Ability Research
PO Box 1721
Minnetonka, MN 55345-721

952-939-0121
FAX: 952-227-5809
info@abilityresearch.net
www.abilityresearch.net

Suzanne Severson, Administrator
Manufacturers and marketers of assistive technology equipment.

1505 Academic Software Inc
3504 Tates Creek Rd
Lexington, KY 40517-2601

859-552-1020
FAX: 253-799-4012
asistaff@acsw.com
www.acsw.com

Warren E Lacefield PhD, President
Penelope Ellis, Marketing Director
Sylvia P Lacefield, Graphic Artist
Employs a unique, goal-oriented approach to aid individuals in identifying adaptive devices with potential to support various physical limitations. Devices are categorized in seven databases: Existence, Travel, In-situ Motion, Environmental Adaptation, Communication, and Sports & recreation. ADLS provides its users with device descriptions, pictures and lists of sources for locating products and product information.

1506 Adaptivation
Ste 100
2225 W 50th St
Sioux Falls, SD 57105-6536

605-335-4445
800-723-2783
FAX: 605-335-4446
info@adaptivation.com
www.adaptivation.com

Jonathan Eckrich, President
Manufacturers of switches, voice output devices and enviromental controls.

1507 Analog Switch Pad
Academic Software
331 W 2nd St
Lexington, KY 40507-1113

859-233-2332
800-842-2357
FAX: 859-231-0725

Warren E Lacefield PhD, President
Penelope Ellis, Marketing Director
A touch-activated, force-adjustable, low-voltage DC, electronic switch designed to control battery-operated toys, environmental controls, and computer access interfaces. This device features a large activation area that is soft and compliant to the touch. Force sensitivity is adjusted by a small dial from approximately 1 ounce to 32 ounces activation pressure, applied over an area ranging from the size of a fingertip to the size of the entire switch surface.

1508 Arkenstone: The Benetech Initiative
480 S California Ave
Palo Alto, CA 94306-1609

650-644-3400
FAX: 650-475-1066
hrdag@benetech.org
www.hrdag.org

Jim Fruthterman, CEO
Roberta G Brosnaha, General Manager/VP
Patrick Ball, Executive Director
Offers various models of ready-to-read personal computers for the disabled.

1509 Augmentative Communication Systems (AAC)
ZYGO-USA
48834 Kato Road
Suite 101A
Freemont, CA 94538

510-249-9660
800-234-6006
FAX: 510-770-4930
zygo@zygo-usa.com
www.zygo-usa.com

Lawrence Weiss, President
Full range of AAC systems and assistive technology including computer-based systems and computer access programs and devices.

1510 Away We Ride IntelliKeys Overlay
Soft Touch Inc
12301 Central Ave NE
Ste 205
Blaine, NE 55434

763-755-1402
888-755-1402
sales@marblesoft.com
www.softtouch.com

Joyce Meyer, President
Four full color preprinted overlays to use with Away We Ride. Just put them on an IntelliKeys keyboard and you are ready to go.

1511 BIGmack Communication Aid
AbleNet
2625 Patton Road
Roseville, MN 55113

651-294-2200
800-322-0956
FAX: 651-294-2222
customerservice@ablenetinc.com
www.ablenetinc.com

Jen Thalhuber, CEO
A single message communication aid, BIGmack has 2 minutes of memory and has a 5 inches in diameter switch surface. *$86.00*

1512 Close-Up 6.5
Norton- Lambert Corporation
PO Box 4085
Santa Barbara, CA 93140-4085

805-964-6767
sales@norton-lambert.com
www.norton-lambert.com

Jeannie Vesely, Marketing Coordinator
Remotely controls PC's via modem. Telecommute from your home or laptop PC to your office PC. Run applications, update spreadsheets, print documents remotely and access networks on remote PCs. Features: fast screen and file transfers, synchronize files, unattended transfers, multi-level security, transaction logs, automated installation. *$99.95*

1513 Concepts on the Move Advanced Overlay CD
Soft Touch Inc
12301 Central Ave NE
Ste 205
Blaine, MN 55434

763-755-1402
888-755-1402
FAX: 763-862-2920
sales@marblesoft.com
www.softtouch.com

Joyce Myer, President
Use this overlay CD with Concepts on the Move Advanced Preacademics. Overlays match the concepts and graphics in the program. Includes standard overlays with all the choices and SoftTouch's changeable format overlays. Print and laminate the blank templates. Then print and laminate the picture keys in all three sizes - small, medium and large. Includes Overlay Printer by IntelliTools for easy printing. *$115.00*

1514 Concepts on the Move Basic Overlay CD
Soft Touch Inc
12301 Central Ave NE
Ste 205
Blaine, MN 55434   763-755-1402
                                             888-755-1403
                                        FAX: 763-862-2920
                                        sales@marblesoft.com
                                        www.softtouch.com

Joyce Meyer, President
Use this Overlay CD with Concepts on the Move Basic
Preacademics. Overlays match the conepts and graphics in the
program. Includes standard overlays with all the choices and
SoftTouch's changeable format overlays. Print and laminate the
blank templates. Then print and laminate the picture keys in all
three sizes - small, medium and large. It is easy and fast to place
the images on the blank templates. *$115.00*

1515 Darci Too
WesTest Engineering Corporation
810 Shepard Ln
Farmington, UT 84025-3846   801-451-9191
                                        FAX: 801-451-9393
                                        larryk@westest.com
                                        westest.com

Robert Lessmann, President
A universal device which allows people with physical disabilities
to replace the keyboard and mouse on a personal computer with a
device that matches their physical capabilities. DARCI TOO
works with almost any personal computer and provides access to
all computer functions. *$995.00*

1516 Eyegaze Computer System
LC Technologies Inc
10363A Democracy Lane
Fairfax, VA 22030   703-385-7133
                                             800-393-4293
                                        FAX: 703-385-7137
                                        info0309@eyegaze.com
                                        www.eyegaze.com

Nancy Cleveland, Medical Coordinator
Enables people with physical disabilities to do many things with
their eyes that they would otherwise do with their hands.

1517 Five Green & Speckled Frogs IntelliKeys Overlay
Soft Touch Inc
12301 Central Ave NE
Ste 205
Blaine, MN 55434   763-755-1402
                                             888-755-1403
                                        FAX: 763-862-2920
                                        sales@marblesoft.com
                                        www.softtouch.com

Joyce Meyer, President
Seven full color preprinted overlays to use with Five Green and
Speckled Frogs. Just put them on an IntelliKeys keyboard and
you are ready to go. *$49.00*

1518 GW Micro
725 Airport North Office Park
Fort Wayne, IN 46825-6707   260-489-3671
                                        FAX: 260-489-2608
                                        sales@gwmicro.com
                                        www.gwmicro.com

Dan Weirich, Sales Executive
Marty Hord, Sales Manager
Computer hardware and software products for people with dis-
abilities.

1519 InvoTek, Inc.
1026 Riverview Dr
Alma, AR 72921   479-632-4166
                                        FAX: 479-632-6457
                                        invotek.org

Thomas Jakobs, President
Diane Jakobs, Vice President, Operations
John Riggins, Chief Marketing Officer

InvoTek, Inc. is a research and development company that improves the quality of life for people who find it difficult or impossible to use their hands by giving them new, efficient ways to
access computers.

1520 Jelly Bean Switch
AbleNet
2625 Patton Road
Roseville, MN 55113-1308   651-294-2200
                                             800-322-0956
                                        FAX: 651-294-2259
                                        customerservice@ablenetinc.com
                                        www.ablenetinc.com

Jen Thalhuber, CEO
A momentary touch switch made of shatterproof plastic, small
and sensitive to 2-3 ounces of pressure, this switch is provided
audible feedback when activated and is a compact version of the
Big Red Switch. Choice of colors: red, blue, green and yellow.

1521 Large Print Keyboard Labels
Hooleon Corp
P.O.Box 589
Melrose, NM 88124-589   575-253-4503
                                             800-937-1337
                                        FAX: 928-634-4620
                                        sales@hooleon.com
                                        www.hooleon.com

Shannen Aikman, Admin Manager/Sales
Joan Crozier, President/Sales
Pressure sensitive labels for computer keyboards.

1522 MessageMate
Words+ Inc
42505 10th Street W
Lancaster, CA 93534-7059   661-723-6523
                                             800-869-8521
                                        FAX: 661-723-2114
                                        www.prentrom.com
                                        www.words-plus.com

Jeff Dahlan, President
Ginger Woltosz, General Manager
Lightweight, hand-held communicator providing high-quality
analog recording capability using either direct select keyboards
or 1 to 2 switch access. Price ranges from $549.00 to $999.00.
$1550.00

1523 Mouthsticks
Sammons Preston Rolyan
1000 Remington Blvd
Suite 210
Bolingbrook, IL 60440-5117   630-378-6000
                                             800-323-5547
                                        FAX: 630-378-6010
                                        sp@patterson-medical.com
                                        www.pattersonmedical.com

Sandra Brown, Customer Service Director
Wide offering of mouthsticks featuring various functions (BK
5380, 5381, 5383, 5385, 6002, or BK 5370 series).

1524 Old MacDonald's Farm IntelliKeys Overlay
Soft Touch Inc
12301 Central Ave NE
Ste 205
Blaine, MN 55434   763-755-1402
                                             888-755-1403
                                        FAX: 763-862-2920
                                        sales@marblesoft.com
                                        www.softtouch.com

Joyce Meyer, President
Extend your students' learning with more than 45 pre-made overlays that support all of the skills learned at the farm. Use with the
IntelliKeys keyboard. Simply print and use. Print an extra set to
make off computer activities, too. Note: Requires Overlay Maker
or Overlay Printer by IntelliTools.

1525 Origin Instruments Corporation
854 Greenview Dr
Grand Prairie, TX 75050
972-606-8740
FAX: 972-606-8741
support@orin.com
www.orin.com

1526 Perfect Solutions
2685 Treanor Ter
Wellington, FL 33414-6460
561-790-1070
800-726-7086
FAX: 561-790-0108
perfect@gate.net
www.perfectsolutions.com

Andrew Kramer, President
A computer for every student and it speaks! Wireless laptop computers starting at $299.00 are ideal for students to carry with them all day. Text-to-speech and web browsing are available. *$299.00*

1527 Phillip Roy
13064 Indian Rocks Road
PO Box 130
Indian Rocks Beach, FL 33785-130
727-593-2700
800-255-9085
FAX: 877-595-2685
info@philliproy.com
www.philliproy.com

Ruth Bragman PhD, President
Phil Padol, VP
Offers multimedia materials appropriate for use with individuals with disabilities. Programs range from preschool through the adult level. Many of the programs are high interest topics/low vocabulary, ideal for transition and employability skills. Materials are also available which focus on social and personal development. Call for a free catalog.

1528 SS-Access Single Switch Interface for PC'swith MS-DOS
Academic Software
3504 Tates Creek Road
Lexington, KY 40517-2601
859-552-1020
800-842-2357
FAX: 253-799-4012
asistaff@acsw.com
www.acsw.com

Warren E Lacefield PhD, President
Penelope Ellis, Marketing Director
A general purpose single switch hardware and software interface for DOS and the IBM and compatible PC family. It is designed to be easy to install, simple to use, and compatible with the widest possible range of computers and application software programs. SS-ACCESS! connects to one of the PC serial ports and provides a jack to connect an external switch. The DOS version of the software works by sending a user defined keystroke to the PC keyboard buffer whenever the switch is pressed. *$ 90.00*

1529 Simplicity
Words+
42505 10th Street W
Lancaster, CA 93534-7059
661-723-6523
800-869-8521
FAX: 661-723-2114
info@words-plus.com
www.words-plus.com

Jeff Dahlan, President
Ginger Wolosz, General Manager
Swing-down mount for portable computers and other devices is made from high-quality aircraft aluminum. Simplicity contains very few moving parts and installs in minutes, providing a positive, secure support for computer/device in both the stored and overlap position. *$1199.00*

1530 Slim Armstrong Mounting System
AbleNet
2625 Patton Road
Roseville, MN 55113-1308
612-379-0956
800-322-0956
FAX: 651-294-2259
customerservice@ablenetinc.com
www.ablenetinc.com

Jen Thalhuber, CEO
Slim Armstrong is a mounting system strong enough to hold up to five pounds in any position. Mix and match parts to create the system length you desire. *$188.00*

1531 Songs I Sing at Preschool IntelliKeys Overlay
Soft Touch
12301 Central Ave NE
Ste 205
Blaine, MN 55434
763-755-1402
888-755-1403
FAX: 763-862-2920
sales@marblesoft.com
www.softtouch.com

Joyce Meyer, President
Pre-made overlays for use with Songs I Sing at Preschool. Simply print and use with an IntelliKeys keyboard. Print an extra set to make off computer activities, too.

1532 Switch Basics IntelliKeys Overlay
Soft Touch
12301 Central Ave NE
Ste 205
Blaine, MN 55434
763-755-1402
888-755-1403
FAX: 763-862-2920
sales@marblesoft.com
www.softtouch.com

Joyce Meyer, President
Four preprinted overlays to use with Switch Basics. Just put them on an IntelliKeys keyboard and you're ready to go.

1533 Teach Me Phonemics Blends Overlay CDSoftTouch Inc.
12301 Central Ave NE
Ste 205
Blaine, MN 55434
763-755-1402
888-755-1403
FAX: 763-862-2920
sales@marblesoft.com
www.softtouch.com

Roxanne Butterfield, Marketing
Joyce Meyer, President
Teach Me Phonemics Blends Overlay CD contains over 40 IntelliKeys overlays for use with Teach Me Phonemics - Blends program. Choose either 4-item or 9-item layout to match the presentation you use in the program. Print extra copies of the overlays for off computer activites, too.

1534 Teach Me Phonemics Medial Overlay CD
SoftTouch Incorporated
Ste C
17117 Oak Dr
Omaha, NE 68130-2193
402-330-1301
877-763-8868
FAX: 402-334-8478
support@softtouch.com
www.softtouch.com

Kip Fisher, Manager
Roxanne Butterfield, Marketing
Teach Me Phonemics Medial Overlay CD contains over 40 IntelliKeys overlays for use with Teach Me Phonemics - Medial program. Choose either 4-item or 9-item layout to match the presentation you use in the program. Print extra copies of the overlays for off computer activites, too.

1535 Teach Me Phonemics Overlay Series Bundle
SoftTouch
Ste 401
4300 Stine Rd
Bakersfield, CA 93313-2352
661-396-8676
877-763-8868
FAX: 661-396-8760
softtouch@funsoftware.com
www.softtouch.com

Roxanne Butterfield, Marketing
Joyce Meyer, President
Teach Me Phonemics Overlay Series Bundle includes one copy of each Teach Me Phonemics Overlay CD - Initial, Medial, Final and - four CD's in all.

1536 Teach Me to Talk Overlay CD
Soft Touch
12301 Central Ave NE
Ste 205
Blaine, MN 55434
763-755-1402
888-755-1403
FAX: 763-862-2920
sales@marblesoft.com
www.softtouch.com

Joyce Meyer, President
For older version of Teach Me to Talk. Mac only version with red label and PC only version with yellow label. More than 48 pre-made overlays that match the activities on Teach Me to Talk. Simply print and use with an IntelliKeys keyboard. Print an extra set to make off computer activities, too.

1537 Teach Me to Talk: USB-Overlay CD
Soft Touch
12301 Central Ave NE
Ste 205
Blaine, MN 55434
763-755-1402
888-755-1403
FAX: 763-862-2920
sales@marblesoft.com
www.softtouch.com

Joyce Meyer, President
Revised version of Teach Me to Talk Overlays for the newest version that is USB IntelliKeys compatible. This CD contains more than 48 overlays that match the activities and updated graphics of Teach Me to Talk. Includes Overlay Printer by IntelliTools for easy printing.

1538 Teen Tunes Plus IntelliKeys Overlay
Soft Touch
12301 Central Ave NE
Ste 205
Blaine, MN 55434
763-755-1402
888-755-1403
FAX: 763-862-2920
sales@marblesoft.com
www.softtouch.com

Joyce Meyer, President
Seven full color, preprinted overlays to use with Teen Tunes Plus. Just put them on an IntelliKeys keyboard and you're ready to go. *$49.00*

1539 U-Control III
Words+
42505 10th St W
Lancaster, CA 93534-7059
575-253-4503
800-869-8521
FAX: 661-723-2114
www.prentrom.com
www.words-plus.com

Jeff Dahlan, President
Ginger Wolosz, General Manager
Works with the Words+ system (EX Keys, Morse WSKE, Scanning WSKE, Talking Screen) to provide wireless, portable control of items which are already infrared-controlled such as a TV, VCR, CD player, etc. *$499.00*

1540 Universal Switch Mounting System
AbleNet
2625 Patton Road
Roseville, MN 55113-1308
612-379-0956
800-322-0956
FAX: 651-294-2259
customerservice@ablenetinc.com
www.ablenetinc.com

Jen Thalhuber, CEO
Mounting system that allows switch placement in any position. A single lever locks all joints securely in place. Extends to 20 1/2 inches and holds up to five pounds. A mounting system for quick and easy positioning. *$210.00*

1541 WinSCAN: The Single Switch Interface for PC's with Windows
Academic Software
3504 Tates Creek Rd
Lexington, KY 40517-2601
859-522-1020
FAX: 253-799-4012
asistaff@acsw.com
www.acsw.com

Warren E Lacefield, President
Penelope Ellis, Marketing Director/COO
A general purpose single-switch control interface for Windows. It provides single-switch users independent control access to educational and productivity software, multimedia programs, and recreational activities that run under Windows 3.1 and higher versions on IBM and compatible PC's. The user can navigate through Windows; choose program icons and run programs, games, and CD's; even surf the Internet with WinSCAN and his or her adaptive switch. *$349.00*

1542 Words+ IST (Infrared, Sound, Touch)
Words+
42505 10th St W
Lancaster, CA 93534-7059
575-253-4503
800-869-8521
FAX: 661-723-2114
www.prentrom.com
www.words-plus.com

Jeff Dahlan, President
Ginger Wolosz, General Manager
A unique switch that is activated by slight movement or faint sound. The switch provides user control when connected to a device driven by a single switch. Individuals are currently accessing a wide variety of communication and computer systems with movement using the IST switch. *$395.00*

Braille Products

1543 Braille Keyboard Labels
Hooleon Corporation
PO Box 589
Melrose, NM 88124-589
928-634-7515
800-937-1337
FAX: 928-634-4620
sales@hooleon.com
www.hooleon.com

Barry Green, Sales Manager
Joan Crozier, President/Sales
Also large print keyboard labels and large print with Braille.

1544 Brailon Thermoform Duplicator
American Thermoform Corporation
1758 Brackett St
La Verne, CA 91750-5855
909-593-6711
800-331-3676
FAX: 909-593-8001
pnunnelly@americanthermoform.com
www.americanthermoform.com

Patrick Nunnelly, VP
Gary Nunnelly, Owner
This copy machine, for producing tactile images, copies any brailled or embossed original, by a vacuum forming process. This model is for the reproduction of teaching aids and mobility maps.

1545   Computer Paper for Brailling
Maxi Aids
42 Executive Blvd
Farmingdale, NY 11735-4710   631-752-0521
                                    800-522-6294
                                    FAX: 631-752-0689
                                    TTY: 631-752-0738
                                    sales@maxiaids.com
                                    www.maxiaids.com

Elliot Zaretsky, President
Specially made paper for braille printing. 1,500 sheets/case
$85.99

1546   Duxbury Braille Translator
Duxbury Systems
Ste 6
270 Littleton Rd
Westford, MA 01886-3523   978-692-3000
                                    FAX: 978-692-7912
                                    info@duxsys.com
                                    www.duxburysystems.com

Joe Sullivan, President
A complete line of easy to use word processing and Braille translation software available for Windows (including 64 bit windows. Applications for anyone wanting to produce or
communicate with Braille; signs, note cards, textbooks, business
communications and forms, telephone bills, etc. Simple to use,
FREE technical support. Free one year upgrades. DBT is for producing Braille in English, Spanish, French, Portuguese, Italian,
Latin, Greek, German and 125 other languages. *$600.00*

1547   Enabling Technologies Company
1601 NE Braille Pl
Jensen Beach, FL 34957-5345   772-225-3687
                                    800-777-3687
                                    FAX: 772-225-3299
                                    info@brailler.com
                                    www.brailler.com

Tony Schenk, President
Kate Schenk, Product Manager Western US
Greg Schenk, Sales & Marketing
Manufactures the most complete line of American made Braille
embossers, including desktop or portable models capable of producing high quality single sided or interpoint Braille. Also carries a complete line of adaptive technology aids for the blind
community at affordable prices.

1548   Freedom Scientific Blind/Low Vision Group
11800 31st Ct N
St Petersburg, FL 33716-1805   727-803-8000
                                    800-444-4443
                                    FAX: 727-803-8001
                                    info@freedomscientific.com
                                    www.freedomscientific.com

Brad Davis, VP Hardware Product Management
Dr Lee Hamilton, President/CEO
Developer and manufacturer of assistive technology products for
people who are blind or who have low vision. Innovative blindness products include: JAWS® screen reading software; the PAC
Mate Omni™, an accessible Pocket PC; the SARA™ scanning
and reading appliance; OpenBook™ scanning and reading software; FSReader™ DAISY player; FaceToFace™ deaf-blind
communications solution; and PAC Mate and Focus Braille Displays. *$16.95*

1549   Hooleon Corporation
PO Box 589
Melrose, NM 88124-589   928-634-7515
                                    800-937-1337
                                    FAX: 928-634-4620
                                    sales@hooleon.com
                                    www.hooleon.com

Kim Green, Manager
Joan Crozier, President/Sales
Large print and combination Braille adhesive keytop labels for
computer keyboards. Helps visually impaired computer users access correct key strokes either by sight or by touch. Raised Braille
meets ADA specifications and large print fills key top surface.

1550   Infogrip: Large Print/Braille Keyboard Labels
1899 E. Main Street
Ventura, CA 93001   805-652-0770
                                    800-397-0921
                                    FAX: 805-652-0880
                                    sales@infogrip.com
                                    www.infogrip.com

Liza Jacobs, President
Aaron Gaston, VP
Makes a standard keyboard more accessible for visually impaired
individuals with large print or Braille keyboard labels. Characters on the large print labels are .5 by .25 inches, about 3 times
larger than standard keyboard characters. Braille labels are available as clear labels with Braille dots or large print with Braille.
Each set includes all the keys used on a standard Windows keyboard. *$29.00*

1551   Raised Dot Computing
Duxbury Systems Incorporated
270 Littleton Rd.
Unit 6
Westford, MA 01886-3523   978-692-3000
                                    FAX: 978-692-7912
                                    info@duxsys.com
                                    www.duxburysystems.com

Joe Sullivan, President
Peter Sullivan, VP of Software Development
Genevieve Sullivan, Treasurer
Dana Winikates, Software Engineer
Software for the visually impaired.

1552   Touchdown Keytop/Keyfront Kits
Hooleon Corporation
P.O.Box 589
304 West Denby Ave
Melrose, NM 88124   575-253-4503
                                    800-937-1337
                                    FAX: 575-253-4299
                                    Sales@Hooleon.com
                                    www.hooleon.com

Bob Crozier, Founder
Joan Crozier, President
Barry Green, Sales Manager
These kits enlarge the key legends of a computer and include
Braille for easy recognition.

Information Centers & Databases

1553   ABLEDATA
103 West Broad St.
Suite 400
Falls Church, VA 22046   703-356-8035
                                    800-227-0216
                                    FAX: 703-356-8314
                                    TTY: 703-992-8313
                                    abledata@neweditions.net
                                    www.abledata.com

Katherine Belknap, Project Director
David Johnson, Publications Director
Juanita Hardy, Information Specialist
David Johnson, Publications Director
ABLEDATA is an electronic database of assistive technology and
rehabilitation equipment products for children and adults with
physical, cognitive and sensory disabilities. ABLEDATA staff
can perform database searches or the database can be searched on
the ABLEDATA website, database printouts, informed consumer
guides and fact sheets are available at cost from the office or free
from the website.

1554 ATTAIN
Division of Disability Aging & Rehab Services
Ste 1400
32 E Washington St
Indianapolis, IN 46204-3552   317-232-1147
800-528-8246
FAX: 317-486-8809
attain@attaininc.org
www.attaininc.org

Gary R Hand, Executive Director
Peter Bisbecos, Manager
Nonprofit organization that creates system change by expanding the availability of community-based technology-related activities, outreach services, empowerment and advocacy activities through the development of a comprehensive, consumer-responsive, statewide program to serve individuals with disabilities, of all ages and all disabilities, their families, caregivers, educators and service providers. Provides training, information and referrals, system change and assessments for equipment needs.

1555 Aloha Special Technology Access Center
710 Green St
Honolulu, HI 96813-2119   808-523-5547
FAX: 808-536-3765
astachi@yahoo.com
www.alohastac.org

Ali Silvert, President
Ms. Jacquely Brand, Founder
Computer technology center.

1556 Audiogram/Clinical Records Manager
19 State Route 10 E
Ste 25
Succasunna, NJ 7876   862-251-4637
FAX: 862-251-4642
npdunn@thedaviscenter.com
www.thedaviscenter.com

Dorinne.S Davis,MA, CCC-A, FAAA, Director
Elizabeth Meade, Head Sound Therapist
Nancy Puckett-Dunn, Office Manager
Donna Warr, Office Assistant
Sound-based therapy—Uses sound vibration with special equipment, specific programs, modified music, and/or specific tones/beats, the need for which is identified with appropriate testing. Sound-based therapy fits under the term sound therapy so The Davis Center is considered a sound therapy center. *$414.75*

1557 Birmingham Alliance for Technology Access Center
Birmingham Independent Living Center
206 13th St S.
Birmingham, AL 35233-1317   205-251-2223
FAX: 205-251-0605
TTY:205-251-2223
judy.roy@drradvocates.org
www.drradvocates.org

Kathy Lovell, President
Phil Klebine, Vice President
Daniel Kessler, Executive Director
Judy Roy, Programs Coordinator
Computer technology center.

1558 Bluegrass Technology Center
409 Southland Drive
Lexington, KY 40503   859-294-4343
800-209-7767
FAX: 866-576-9625
office@bluegrass-tech.org
www.bluegrass-tech.org

Debbie Sharon, Acting Executive Director
Linnie Lee, Assistive Technology Specialist
Jean Isaacs, Assistive Technology Consultant
Linda Gassaway, PhD, Assistive Technology Consultant
Provides assistive technology information, consulting and training for education, health professionals, consumers and parents of consumers. Maintains extensive lending library of assistive devices and adapted toys. Statewide training such as; AAC, how to obtain funding for assistive technology, augmentative and alter-

nate communication, equipment implementation strategies, specific to hardware and software, etc.

1559 CITE: Lighthouse for Central Florida
215 East New Hampshire Street
Orlando, FL 32804   407-898-2483
FAX: 407-898-0236
csacca@lcf-fl.org
www.lighthousecentralflorida.org/Default.asp

Lee Nasehi, MSW, President/CEO
Donna Esbensen CPA,MBA, VP/CFO
Jeff Whitehead, MPA, MS, Director of Program Services
Casey Mathews, Access Technology Specialist
CITE promotes the independence of adults and children with blindness, low vision and other disabilities through technology, education, support and advocacy.

1560 Carolina Computer Access Center
P.O.Box 247
Cramerton, NC 28032   704-342-3004
FAX: 704-342-1513
bellsluth.net
www.ccac.ataccess.org

Linda Schilling, Executive Director
Nonprofit, community-based technology resource center for people with disabilities, providing information about and demonstration of the technology tools that enable individuals with disabilities to control and direct their own lives. Services and programs include: assessments, demonstrations, resource information, lending library, workshops and outreach.

1561 Center for Accessible Technology
3075 Adeline
Suite 220
Berkeley, CA 94703   510-841-3224
FAX: 510-841-7956
info@cforat.org
www.cforat.org

Dmitri Belser, Executive Director
Eric Smith, Associate Director
A consumer-based technology resource and demonstration center for adults and children with disabilities, families, teachers, and professionals. The primary focus is on assistive technology for computer access. Seen by appointment only.

1562 Center for Applied Special Technology
40 Harvard Mills Square
Suite 3
Wakefield, MA 01880-3233   781-245-2212
FAX: 781-245-5212
cast@cast.org
www.cast.org/

Anne Meyer, Founder
David H. Rose, Founder
Lisa Poller, Co-President
Gabrielle Rappolt-Schlichtmann, Co-President
Expands opportunities for individuals with special needs through innovative use of computers and related technology. We pursue this mission through research and product development that further universal design for learning.

1563 Center for Assistive Technology & Inclusive Education Studies
2000 Pennington Rd.
P.O.Box 7718
Ewing, NJ 08628-0718   609-771-3016
FAX: 609-637-5179
caties@tcnj.edu
caties.pages.tcnj.edu

Amanda Norvell, President
Matt Bender, VP
Regina Morin, Parliamentarian
Laurie Wanat, Secretary
Computer technology center offering resource time, workshops, technology, training and evaluations.

1564   Center on Evaluation of Assistive Technology
National Rehabilitation Hospital
102 Irving St NW
Washington, DC 20010   202-877-1000
                                        TTY:202-726-3996
                                justin.m.carter@medstar.net
                                    www.medstarhealth.org

Kenneth A. Samet, FACHE, President, CEO
Michael J. Curran, EVP, Chief Administrative and Financial Officer
Christine Swearingen, EVP, Planning, Marketing and Community Relations
Stephen R.T. Evans, MD, EVP, Medical Affairs and Chief Medical Officer
The center develops ways of collecting, producing and distributing information to help users, prescribers and third-party payers make intelligent selections of devices.

1565   Compuserve: Handicapped Users' Database
5000 Arlington Centre Blvd
Columbus, OH 43220-2913   614-326-1002
                                           800-848-8990
                                       FAX: 614-538-4023
                        webcenters.netscape.compuserve.com

1566   Computer & Web Resources for People With Disabilities
Alliance for Technology Access
Ste 240
1304 Southpoint Blvd
Petaluma, CA 94954-7464   707-778-3011
                                       FAX: 707-765-2080
                                       TTY:707-778-3015
                                   atainfo@ataaccess.org
                                       www.ataaccess.org

Sharon Hall, Manager
A guide to maneuvering the growing world of computers, both the mainstream and the assistive technology.

ISBN 0-897933-00-1

1567   Computer Access Center
P.O. Box 12464
Albuquerque, NM 87195   505-242-9588
                                           info@cac.org
                                           www.cac.org

Richard Barlow, Board of Director
Richard Rohr, Board of Director
Michael Poffenberger, Board of Director
Damien Faughnan, Board of Director
Computer technology center.

1568   Computer Center for Visually Impaired People: Division of Continuing Studies
Baruch College
1 Bernard Baruch Way
Box H-648
New York, NY 10010   646-312-1420
                                       FAX: 646-312-5101
                              judith.gerber@baruch.cuny.edu
                                 www.baruch.cuny.edu/ccvip

Karen Gourgey, Director
Judith Gerber, Operations Manager
Lynette Tatum, Training Specialist
William Reed, Assistant Director
Offers courses, tutors, equipment and assistance.

1569   Computer Resources for People with Disabilities
Hunter House Publishers, Inc
424 Church Street
Suite 2240
Nashville, TN 37219   615-255-BOOK
                                 info@turnerpublishing.com
                                      www.hunterhouse.com

Kiran Rana, Publisher
Chris Alexander, Author
Sheila Alson, Author
Peter Axt, Author

Part One describes conventional and assistive technologies and gives strategies for accessing the Internet. Part Two features easy-to-use charts organized by key access concerns, and provides detailed descriptions of software, hardware, and communication aids. Part Three is a gold mine of Web resources, publications, support organizations, government programs, and technology vendors.

1570   Computer-Enabling Drafting for People with Physical Disabilities
County College of Morris
214 Center Grove Road
Randolph, NJ 07869-2086   973-328-5000
                                           888-226-8001
                                       FAX: 973-328-5067
                                           www.ccm.edu

Edward J Yaw, President
Dr. Dwight Smith, Vice President of Academic Affairs
Karen VanDerhoof, Vice President for Business and Finance
Dr. Bette M. Simmons, VP of Student Development & Enrollment Management
Since they opened in 1968, more than 40,000 graduates have passed through their halls. Many have become teachers, nurses, police officers, doctors and engineers. CCM has also been a community resource for those seeking to enhance their careers through additional education. They drafted a newsletter on Computer-Enabling Drafting for People with Physical Disabilities

1571   DIRLINE
National Library of Medicine
8600 Rockville Pike
Bethesda, MD 20894   301-594-5983
                                           888-346-3656
                                       FAX: 301-402-1384
                                       TTY:800-735-2258
                                    custserv@nml.nih.gov
                                       www.nlm.nih.gov/

Dr. Donald A B. Lindberg, Director
Milton Corn, Deputy Director
Betsy Humphreys, Deputy Director
Todd Danielson, Office of Administration
18,000 listings of organizations that serve as information resources, including libraries, professional associations and government agencies.

1572   Developmental Disabilities Council
626 Main Street, Suite A
P.O.Box 3455
Baton Rouge, LA 70821-3455   225-342-6804
                                           800-450-8108
                                       FAX: 225-342-1970
                                    shawn.fleming@la.gov
                                           www.laddc.org

Sandee Winchell, Executive Director
Shawn Fleming, Deputy Director
Derek White, Program Manager
Robbie Gray, Program Monitor
The Louisiana Developmental Disabilities Council is made up of people from every region of the state who are appointed by the governor to develop and implement a five year plan to address the needs of persons with disabilities. Membership includes persons with developmental disabilities, parents, advocates, professionals, and representatives from public and private agencies.

1573   Employment Resources Program
330 South Grand Avenue West
Springfield, IL 62704   217-523-2587
                                           800-447-4221
                                       FAX: 217-523-0427
                                       TTY: 217-523-2587
                                           scil@scil.org
                                           www.scil.org

Pete Roberts, Executive Director
Susanne Cooper, Program Director
Robin Ashton- Hale, Reintegration Coordinator
Kathryn Cline, Business Manager
An information and referral service that encourages inquiries from professionals, individuals with disabilities, family mem-

bers, organizations or anyone requesting information pertaining to disabilities. The staff at DRN uses both computer listings and in-house library files to provide the programs services. The DRN program is funded by a grant from the Illinois Department of Rehabilitation Services.

1574 Functional Skills Screening Inventory
Functional Resources
3905 Huntington Dr
Amarillo, TX 79019-4047   806-353-1114
                                        FAX: 806-353-1114
                                        info@winfssi.com
                                        www.winfssi.com

Ed Hammer, Owner
Heather Becker PhD, Owner
Assesses the individual's level of functional skills and identifies supports needed by educational, rehabilitation and residential programs serving moderately and severely disabled persons. Includes environmental assessments as well as profiles of jobs and training sites.

1575 High Tech Center
Sacremento State
6000 J Street
Sacramento, CA 95819   916-278-6011
                                        sswd@csus.edu
                                        www.csus.edu

Alexander Gonzalez, President
Judy Dean, Co-Director
Melissa Repa, Co-Director
Terry Gomez, Office Manager
The Center offers assessment and training in adaptive hardware/software for eligible students with disabilities at Sacramento State upon referral from the Office of Services to Students with Disabilities.

1576 Idaho Assistive Technology Project
121 W 3rd St
Moscow, ID 83843-2268   208-885-3557
                                        FAX: 208-885-3628
                                        rseiler@uidaho.edu
                                        www.idahoat.org

Ron Seiler, Project Director
Sue House, Information Specialist
A federally funded program managed by the center on disabilities and human development at the university of Idaho. The goal of the IATP is to increase the availability of assistive technology devices and services for Idahoans with disabilities. The IATP offers free trainings and technical assistance, a low-interest loan program, assistive technology assessments for children and agriculture workers, and free informational materials.

1577 Increasing Capabilities Access Network
525 W.Capitol
Little Rock, AR 72201   501-666-8868
                                        800-828-2799
                                        FAX: 501-666-5319
                                        TTY:501-666-8868
                                        nfo@ar-ican.org
                                        www.arkansas-ican.org

Bryen Ayres, Member of Advisory Council
Billy Altom, Member of Advisory Council
Adrienne Brown, Member of Advisory Council
Carolyn Boyles, Member of Advisory Council
A consumer responsive statewide systems change program promoting assistive technology for persons of all ages with disabilities. The program provides information on new and existing technology and maintains an equipment exchange free of charge. Training on assistive technology is also provided.

1578 International Center for the Disabled
340 E 24th St
New York, NY 10010-4019   212-585-6000
                                        FAX: 212-585-6161
                                        info@icdnyc.org
                                        www.icdnyc.org

Jill Bowman, Manager
Les Halpert, CEO

The ICD is a comprehensive outpatient rehabilitation facility, providing medical rehabilitation, behavioral health and vocational services to children and adults with a broad range of physical, communication, emotional and cognitive disabilities.

1579 Kentucky Assistive Technology Service Network
200 Juneau Dr.
Suite 200
Louisville, KY 40243   502-429-4484
                                        800-327-5287
                                        FAX: 502-429-7114
                                        www.katsnet.org

Derrick Cox, Manager
Statewide network of four regional assistive technology centers with a central coordinating office in Louisville and two regional centers in eastern Kentucky. Network services include but are not limited to assistive technology of services, loan of assistive devices, funding information and referral, assessment and evaluations, consultations on appropriate technologies, training, and technical assistance.

1580 Learning Independence Through Computers
2301 Argonne Drive
Baltimore, MD 21218   410-554-9134
                                        FAX: 410-261-2907
                                        info@linc.org
                                        www.linc.org

Theo Pinette, Executive Director
Sandy Fishman, Office and Computer Center Coordinator
Angela Tyler, Volunteer Services Manager
Christy Wooden, AT Learning Specialist
V-LINC creates technological solutions to improve the independence and quality of life for individuals of all ages with disabilities in Maryland. We do this through a mix of off-the-shelf computer software and equipment, and one-of-a-kind, customized assistive technology.

1581 MEDLINE
Dialog Corporation
2250 Perimeter Park Drive
Suite 300
Morrisville, NC 27560
                                        800-334-2564
                                        919-804-6400
                                        FAX: 919-804-6410
                                        www.dialog.com

Tim Wahlberg, Genral Manager
Morten Nicholaisen, VP Global Sales and Account Mana
Libby Trudell, VP Strategic Initiatives
Tim Hall, Director Integration and Busines
Bibliographic citations to biomedical literature.

1582 Maine CITE
University of Maine at Augusta
46 University Avenue
Augusta, ME 04330   207-621-3195
                                        FAX: 207-629-5429
                                        TTY:877-475-4800
                                        iweb@mainecite.org
                                        www.mainecite.org

Robert McPhee, Member of Advisory Council
Deborah Gardner, Member of Advisory Council
Anita Dunham, Member of Advisory Council
Sandra Jaeger, Member of Advisory Council
Computer technology center.

1583   Maryland Technology Assistance Program
Maryland Department of Disabilities
2301 Argonne Drive
Rm T-17
Baltimore, MD 21218   410-554-9361
                                            800-832-4827
                                        FAX: 410-554-9237
                                        TTY: 866-881-7488
                                     MDOD@mdod.state.md.us
                                             www.mdtap.org

James McCarthy, Executive Director
Denise Schuler, Assistive Technology Specialist
Tanya Goodman, Loan Program Assistant Director
Lori Markland, Director of Communications, Outreach &Program Development
Assistive technology center. Information and referral, equipment display loans and demonstration, funding sources, alternative media, training, workshops and seminars. Rural outreach for individuals with disability in Maryland.

1584   Minnesota STAR Program
358 Centennial Office Building 658
Saint Paul, MN 55155- 1402   651-201-2640
                                            800-627-3529
                                            888-234-1267
                                        FAX: 651-282-6671
                                    star.program@state.mn.us
                          www.admin.state.mn.us/assistivetechnology
Chuck Rassbach, Program Director
Jennis Delisi, Program Staff
Jaoan Gillum, Program Staff
Kim Moccia, Program Staff
STAR's mission is to help all Minnesotans with disabilities gain access to and acquire the assistive technology they need to live, learn, work and lay. The Minnesota STAR program is federally funded by the Rehabilitation Services Administration.

1585   Mississippi Project START
2550 Peachtree Street
Jackson, MS 39216   601-987-4872
                                            800-852-8328
                                        FAX: 601-364-2349
                                    pgaltelli@mdrs.ms.gov
                                     www.msprojectstart.org
Patsy Galtelli, Executive Director
Dorothy Young, Project Director
Nekeba Simmons, Administrative Assistant
Jason Mac McMaster, Repair Specialist
Project START is a Tech Act project established to bring about systems change in the field of assistive technology in the State of Mississippi. Activities include providing training opportunities for consumers and service providers on subjects such as state-of-the-art AT devices, their application and funding resources; referral information on AT evaluation centers; technical assistance to AT users; establishment of an AT equipment loan program and an Information and Referral Service.

1586   National Technology Database
American Foundation for the Blind/ AF B Press
2 Penn Plaza
Suite 1102
New York, NY 10121   212-502-7600
                                            800-232-5463
                                        FAX: 888-545-8331
                                        afbinfo@afb.net
                                            www.afb.org
Carl.R Augusto, President and CEO
Robin Vogel, Vice President, Resource Development
Kelly Bleach, Chief Administrative Officer
Rick Bozeman, Chief Financial Officer
This database includes resources for visually impaired persons.
$99.00

1587   New Jersey Department of Labor & Workforce Development
Office of the Commissioner
1 John Fitch Plaza
P.O.Box 110
Trenton, NJ 08625-0110   609-292-7060
                                        FAX: 609-633-1359
                                   cmycoff@dol.state.nj.us
                                     www.state.nj.us/labor
Harold J. Wirths, Commissioner
Aaron R. Fichtner, Ph.D., Deputy Commissioner
Frederick J. Zavaglia, Chief of Staff
David Ramsay, Director
Oversees various federal and state vocational rehabilitation services including sheltered workshops and independent living centers; adjudication of permanent disability claims filed with the Social Security Administration; oversees New Jersey's temporary disability program covering non-work related illnesses and injuries

1588   New Mexico Technology Assistance Program
435 Saint Michaels Drive
Ste D
Santa Fe, NM 87505-7679   505-827-8535
                                            800-866-2253
                                        FAX: 505-954-8608
                                   julie.martinez1@state.nm.us
                                            www.nmtap.com
Julie Martinez, Program Director
Examines and works to eliminate barriers to obtaining assistive technology in New Mexico. Has established a statewide program for coordinating assistive technology services; is designed to assist people with disabilities to locate, secure, and maintain assistive technology.

1589   Northern Illinois Center for Adaptive Technology
3615 Louisiana Rd
Rockford, IL 61108   815-229-2163
                                    davegrass@eartlink.net
                                     www.nicat.ataccess.org
Dave Grass, President
Computer technology center.

1590   OCCK
1710 W. Schilling Road
Salina, KS 67402-1160   785-827-9383
                                            800-526-9731
                                        FAX: 785-823-2015
                                        TTY: 785-827-9383
                                        occk@occk.com
                                            www.occk.com
Shelia Nelson Stout, President, CEO
Carolee Miner, CEO
Computer technology center; training center for employment and independent living for people with disabilities; family support center. Kansas AgrAbility program coordinator, Kansas equipment exchange site.

1591   Parents, Let's Unite for Kids
516 N 32nd St
Billings, MT 59101-6003   406-255-0540
                                            800-222-7585
                                        FAX: 406-255-0523
                                        TTY: 406-657-2055
                                        info@pluk.org
                                            www.pluk.org
Roger Holt, Executive Director
Computer technology center. Parents, Let's Unite for Kids offers an assistive technology lab that is open to people of all ages. The lab is a computer and assistive technology demonstration site. There is no charge for services.

1592 Pennsylvania's Initiative on Assistive Technology
Temple University
1755 N. 13th St
Student Center, Room 4115
Philadelphia, PA 19122-6024

215-204-1356
800-204-7428
FAX: 215-204-6336
TTY: 866-268-0579
ATinfo@temple.edu
www.disabilities.temple.edu

Amy S Goldman, Director
Pennsylvania's Initiative on Assistive Technology (PIAT) offers information and referral about assistive Technology (AT), device demonstrations, and awareness-level presentations. PIAT also operates Pennsylvania's AT Lending Library, a free, state-supported program that loans AT devices to Pennsylvanians of all ages. This program allows you to try a device for a limited time to be sure it meets your needs.

1593 Rehabilitation Engineering & Assistive Technology Society of North America (RESNA)
1700 North Moore Street
Suite 1540
Arlington, VA 22209

703-524-6686
FAX: 703-524-6630
TTY:703-524-6639
membership@resna.org
www.resna.org

Alex Mihailidis, PhD, P.Eng, President
Ray Grott, ATP, RET, President-Elect
Paul J. Schwartz, Treasurer
Michael J. Brogioli, Executive Director
Improves the potential of people with disabilities to achieve their goals through the use of technology and disability. Promotes research, development, education, advocacy and provision of technology, and by supporting the people engaged in theses activities.

1594 Resource Center for Independent Living(RCIL)
409 Columbia St.
PO Box 210
Utica, NY 13503-210

315-797-4642
FAX: 315-797-4747
TTY:315-797-5837
burt.danovitz@rcil.com
www.rcil.com

Burt Danovitz, Executive Director
The RCIL aggressively advocates for and defends the rights of persons with disabilities. RCIL believes in integration adn assisting people to reach their full potential, encouraging a culture of risk-taking, creativity and innovation through our programs and services. They monitor and assess the current legal climate around rights for persons with disabilities on an ongoing bases and are committed and deliberate in speaking about the problems and obstacles faced by persons with disabilities.

1595 SACC Assistive Technoloy Center
P.O.Box 1325
Simi Valley, CA 93062-1325

805-582-1881
www.semel.ucla.edu

Debi Schultze, CEO
SACC connects children, adults and seniors with special needs to computers, technologies and resources. We provide information and referral, assessments, tutoring, presentations and outreach awareness.

1596 South Dakota Department of Human Services: Computer Technology Services
Properties Plaza
500 East Capitol Avenue
Pierre, SD 57501

605-773-5990
800-265-9684
FAX: 605-773-5483
TTY: 605-773-6412
infodhs@state.sd.us
dhs.sd.gov

Dan Lusk, Division Director
Ted Williams, Director
Eric Weiss, Director
Gaye Mattke, Director
Computer technology center.

1597 Star Center
1119 Old Humboldt Rd
Jackson, TN 38305-1752

731-668-3888
888-398-5619
FAX: 731-668-1666
TTY: 731-668-9664
information@starcenter.tn.org
www.starcenter.tn.org

John Borden, CEO
Nation's largest assistive technology center dedicated to helping children and adults with disabilities achieve their goals for competitive employment, effective learning, returning to or starting school and independent living. Programs include: high-tech training, music therapy, art therapy, low vision evaluation, orientation and mobility evaluation and training, augmentative communication evaluation, vocational evaluations, assistive technology, job placement services and job skills training.

1598 Students with Disabilities Office
University of Texas at Austin
100 West Dean Keeton A5800
Austin, TX 78712-1100

512-471-5017
FAX: 512-471-7833
deanofstudents@austin.utexas.edu
deanofstudents.utexas.edu

Soncia Reagins-Lilly, Ed.D., Senior Associate VP for Student Affairs & Dean of Students
Douglas Garrard, Ed.D., Senior Associate Dean of Students
Wanda Brune, Administrative Associate
Sara LeStrange, Manager of Communications

1599 TASK Team of Advocates for Special Kids
100 W Cerritos Ave
Anaheim, CA 92805

714-533-8275
866-828-8275
FAX: 714-533-2533
task@taskca.org
www.taskca.org

Marta Anchondo, Executive Director
Tom Bratkovich, Treasurer
Leana Way, Director
Computer technology center.

1600 Tech Connection
35 Haddon Avenue
Shrewsbury, NJ 07702

732-747-5310
FAX: 732-747-1896
info@frainc.org
www.frainc.org

Bill Sheeser, President
Nancy Phalanukom, Executive Director
Sue Levine, Program Administrator
Vicky Butler, EI Program Coordinator
Offers a noncommercial center to examine and try computers, adapted equipment, alternative input devices, and a variety of software. Program of Family Resource Associates and a member of the Alliance for Technology Access (ATA), a growing national coalition of computer resource centers, professionals, technology developers and vendors, interacting with new technology to enrich the lives of people with disabilities. Tech Connection offers evaluations, for computer technology.

1601 Tech-Able
1451 Klondike Road, Suite D
Conyers, GA 30094

770-922-6768
FAX: 770-922-6769
c.b.wright@techable.org
www.techable.org

Cassandra Baker, Executive Director
Pat Hanus, Program Assistant
Erika Ruffin-Mosley, Assistive Technology Trainer
Jason Chadwell, AT & Blind / Low Vision Trainer
Provide assistive technology to individuals with disabilities, toy-lending and software libraries, product demonstration, access to technology devices and fabrication of keyguards for keyboards. Low vision consultant on Thursdays; computer training for persons with disabilities.

1602 Technology Access Center of Tucson
P.O.Box 13178
Tucson, AZ 85732-3178

520-638-2733
FAX: 520-519-7954
tact1@qwestoffice.net
http://www.uacoe.arizona.edu/tact/

1603 Technology Assistance for Special Consumers
1856 Keats Dr NW.
Huntsville, AL 35810

256-859-8300
FAX: 256-859-4332
tasc@ucphuntsville.org
ucphuntsville.org/what-we-do/t-a-s-c/
Cheryl Smith, Chief Executive Officer
T.A.S.C. is a computer resource center with 10 computers, which are equipped with special adaptations for those who are blind, visually impaired, or severely physically disabled. The staff demonstrates and trains individuals on this equipment so that they can become more independent at home, school, and work. Over 2,500 pieces of educational software are available for individuals who are learning disabled, mentally retarded or who have developmental delays.

1604 Tidewater Center for Technology Access Special Education Annex
1415 Laskin Rd
Virginia Beach, VA 23451

757-424-2672
FAX: 757-263-2801
tcta@aol.com
www.tcta.access.org

Pat Mc Gee, Manager
Myra Jessie Flint, Designee
Nonprofit organization providing persons with disabilities access, support, and knowledge—re: technology; organization contracts for consultations, workshops and training, or conventional and assistive technologies including computers, augmented communication devices and software; resources: extensive lending library of educational software; books and videotape library; yearly individual membership and corporate membership fees; working/presentation and evaluation fees available upon request.

1605 Vermont Assistive Technology Project: Department of Aging & Disabilities
Agency of Human Services
103 South Main Street
Weeks Building
Waterbury, VT 05671-2305

802-871-3353
800-750-6355
FAX: 802-871-3048
TTY: 802-241-1464
amber.fulcher@state.vt.us
atp.vermont.gov

Amber Fulcher, Program Director
Sharon Alderman, Assistive Technology Reuse Coordinator
Emma Cobb, Assistive Technology Services Coordinator
Increase the awareness and change policies to insure assistive technology is available to all Vermonters with disabilities.

Keyboards, Mouses & Joysticks

1606 A4 Tech (USA) Corporation
5585 Brooks St
Montclair, CA 91763-4547

909-988-9633
info@a4tech.com
www.a4tech.com

Robert C
Manufacturers of a cordless mouse, trackballs and joysticks that emulate mouse controls, flatbed scanners, modified keyboards, and other specialty mouses.

1607 Abacus
3150 Patterson Ave SE
Grand Rapids, MI 49512

616-698-0330
800-451-4319
FAX: 616-698-0325
info@abacuspub.com
www.abacuspub.com

Arnie Lee, President
Designs a mouse software program that permits programs written for one computer to be run on another computer.

1608 Ability Center of Greater Toledo
5605 Monroe Street
Sylvania, OH 43560

419-885-5733
FAX: 419-882-4813
www.abilitycenter.org

Tim Harrington, Executive Director
Dale Abell, Director of Program Development
Debbie Andriette, Director of Human Resources
Kimberley Arnett, Director of Community Services
Manufactures keyboard wrist supports to help prevent repetitive motion disorders.

1609 Dreamer
TS Micro Tech
17109 Gale Ave
City of Industry, CA 91745-1810

626-939-8998
FAX: 626-839-8516
sales@fancard.com
www.fancard.com

Steve Heung, Owner
An intelligent, add-on function keyboard providing single-keystroke access to multiple-keystroke functions.

1610 FlexShield Keyboard Protectors
Hooleon Corporation
P.O.Box 589
Melrose, NM 88124-589

928-634-7515
800-937-1337
FAX: 928-634-4620
sales@hooleon.com
www.hooleon.com

Barry Green, Sales Manager
Joan Crozier, President
Transparent keyboard protectors allowing instant recognition of keytop legends. They have a matte finish to reduce glare. Also available are large print and braille keyboard labels and large print/braille combo labels.

1611 Infogrip: King Keyboard
1899 E. Main Street
Ventura, CA 93001

805-652-0770
800-397-0921
FAX: 805-652-0880
support@infogrip.com
www.infogrip.com

Lisa Jacobs, President
Giant alternative keyboard that plugs directly into a computer—no special interface is required. The keys are 1.25 inches in diameter, slightly recessed, and provide both tactile and auditory feedback. The King has a built-in keyboard so that you can rest on its surface without activating keys. This keyboard allows you to control both keyboard and mouse functions, so it's great for people who have difficulty maneuvering a standard mouse. *$130.00*

1612 Infogrip: Large Print Keyboard
1899 E. Main Street
Ventura, CA 93001
805-652-0770
800-397-0921
FAX: 805-652-0880
support@infogrip.com
www.infogrip.com

Lisa Jacobs, President
Standard Windows keyboard with large print keys. The keyboard and its keys are the same size as a standard keyboard; however, the print has been enhanced. The characters measure .5 by .25 inches, about 3 times larger than standard keyboard characters. *$130.00*

1613 Infogrip: OnScreen
1899 E. Main Street
Ventura, CA 93001
805-652-0770
800-397-0921
FAX: 805-652-0880
support@infogrip.com
www.infogrip.com

Lisa Jacobs, President
OnScreen features word prediction/completion (with an editable dictionary), Key Dwell Timer (a timer that selects a key under the cursor), integrated Verbal Keys Feedback, Show and Hide Keys (turns on/off keys to prevent access and minimize confusion) a Smart Window (automatically re-positions the keyboard or panels off of the area in use). On Screen also offers edit, numeric, macro, calculator and Windows enhancement capabilities. *$200.00*

1614 IntelliKeys
Intelli Tools
1720 Corporate Circle
Petaluma, CA 94954
707-773-2000
800-899-6687
FAX: 707-773-2001
info@intellitools.com
www.intellitools.com

Dayton Johnson, VP, Sales
Arjan Khalsa, CEO
Alternative, touch-sensitive keyboards; plugs into any Macintosh or Windows computer. *$395.00*

1615 IntelliKeys USB
Intelli Tools
1720 Corporate Circle
Petaluma, CA 94954
707-773-2000
800-899-6687
FAX: 707-773-2001
info@intellitools.com
www.intellitools.com

Dayton Johnson, VP, Sales
Arjan Khalsa, CEO
IntelliKeys alternative keyboard for USB computers and Windows 2000, Mac OSX. *$69.95*

1616 Key Tronic KB 5153 Touch Pad Keyboard
KeyTronic
N. 4424 Sullivan Road
Spokane Valley, WA 99216
509-928-8000
FAX: 509-927-5555
EMSsales@keytronicems.com
www.keytronic.com

Craig.D Gates, President/CEO
Ronald.F Klawitter, EVP of Administration and Chief Financial Officer
Douglas G. Burkhardt, Executive Vice President of Worldwide Operations
Philip S. Hochberg, Executive Vice President of Business Development
Integrates a regular full-function keyboard, a numeric keypad with a cursor key capability and a touch pad into one unit.

1617 Magic Wand Keyboard
In Touch Systems
11 Westview Road
Spring Valley, NY 10977
845-354-7431
800-332-6244
sc@magicwandkeyboard.com
www.magicwandkeyboard.com

Jerry Crouch, President
Susan Crouch, VP
The magic wand keyboard allows your child to use a keyboard and mouse easily-no light beams, microphones, or sensors to wear of position. This miniature computer keyboard has zero-force keys that work with the slightest touch of a wand (hand-held of mouthstick). No strength required.

1618 McKey Mouse
In Touch Systems
11 Westview Road
Spring Valley, NY 10977
845-354-7431
800-332-6244
sc@magicwandkeyboard.com
www.magicwandkeyboard.com

Jerry Crouch, President
Susan Crouch, VP
Microsoft compatible mouse for persons with little or no hand/arm movement; it's an option for the Magic Wand Keyboard and adds full mouse function without adding any extra devices.

1619 PortaPower Plus
Words+
42505 10th Street West
Lancaster, CA 93534-7059
661-723-7723
800-869-8521
FAX: 661-723-5524
info@simulations-plus.com
www.simulations-plus.com

Walter S Woltosz, M.S., M.A.S., President, CEO
John A. DiBella, Vice President, Marketing & Sales
John R. Kneisel, Chief Financial Officer
Robert D. Clark, Ph.D., Director, Life Sciences
Rechargeable battery pack designed to give longer life and remote usage time to laptop computers and other portable battery-operated devices and accessories. Requires a 12 volt auto adapter. *$149.00*

1620 Unicorn Keyboards
Intelli Tools
1720 Corporate Circle
Petaluma, CA 94954
707-773-2000
800-899-6687
FAX: 707-773-2001
info@intellitools.com
www.intellitools.com

Dayton Johnson, VP, Sales
Arjan Khalsa, CEO
Alternative keyboards with membrane surface and large, user-defined keys. Large and small sizes are available. *$250.00*

Scanners

1621 Scanning WSKE
Words+
42505 10th Street West
Lancaster, CA 93534-7059
661-723-7723
888-266-9294
FAX: 661-723-5524
info@simulations-plus.com
www.simulations-plus.com

Walter S Woltosz, M.S., M.A.S., President, CEO
John A. DiBella, Vice President, Marketing & Sales
John R. Kneisel, Chief Financial Officer
Robert D. Clark, Ph.D., Director, Life Sciences
A software and a hardware product designed to operate on an IBM compatible PC. The software provides dual word prediction, abbreviation expansion, five different methods of voice output, and access to commercial software applications.

1622 System 2000/Versa
Words+
42505 10th Street West
Lancaster, CA 93534-7059

661-723-7723
800-869-8521
FAX: 661-723-5524
info@simulations-plus.com
www.simulations-plus.com

Walter S Woltosz, M.S., M.A.S., President, CEO
John A. DiBella, Vice President, Marketing & Sales
John R. Kneisel, Chief Financial Officer
Robert D. Clark, Ph.D., Director, Life Sciences
Provides all of the strategies currently being used in AAC, from dynamic display color pictographic language, to dual-word prediction text language, in a single system.

1623 Zygo-UsaSvc Corporation
48834 Kato Road Suite 101-A
Fremont, CA 94538

510-249-9660
800-234-6006
FAX: 510-770-4930
zygo@zygo-usa.com
www.zygo-usa.com

Adam Weiss, Vp Sales & Marketing
ZYGO-USA has been involved in manufacturing and distributing assistive technologies since 1974. They specialize in augmentative and alternative computer access. They offer a wide range of technology products to our clients so they can achieve a greater independence and to enhance the quality of their lives. These soloutins improve and individual's ability to learn, work, and interact with family and friends.

Screen Enhancement

1624 Boxlight
Boxlight Corporation
151 State Highway 300, Suite A
P.O. Box 2609
Belfair, WA 98528

360-464-2119
866-972-1549
sales@boxlight.com
www.boxlight.com

Herb Myers, CEO/Founder
Sloan Myers, Founder
Hank Nance, President
BOXLIGHT is a global presentation solutions partner for trainers, educators and professional speakers. Solutions include projector sales, national rental service, technical support, repair, and presentation peripherals. For more information visit us online.

1625 FDR Series of Low Vision Reading Aids
Optelec U S
Breslau 4
Barendrecht, LT 92081-8358

886-783-444
800-826-4200
FAX: 886-783-400
info@optelec.com
in.optelec.com

Stephan Terwolbeck, President
Michiel van Schaik, VP
Janet Lennex, Director of Customer Excellence
Jade Arbelo, Director of Human Resources
The Low Vision Reading Aids features; high resolution, positive and negative display, a high-quality zoom lens, versatile swivel and a 12 inch or 19 inch high-resolution monitor, color or black and white, computer compatible, or portable.

1626 InFocus
AI Squared
130 Taconic Business Park Road
Manchester Center, VT 05255

802-362-3612
800-859-0270
FAX: 802-362-1670
sales@aisquared.com
www.aisquared.com

David Wu, CEO
Jost Eckhardt, VP of Engineering
Scott Moore, VP of Marketing
Shawn Warren, VP of Product Support
A memory-resident program that magnifies text and graphics - the entire screen, a single line or a portion of the screen.

1627 Portable Large Print Computer
Human Ware
1800, Michaud street
Drummondville, CA 94520-1213

819-471-4818
888-723-7273
FAX: 925-681-4630
ca.info@humanware.com
www.humanware.com/en-australia/home

Real Goulet, Chairman
Gilles Pepin, CEO
Michel Cote, Corporate Director
Georges Morin, Corporate Director
A portable large print computer which magnifies up to 64 times. It is linked to a PC and has a hand-held camera.

1628 ZoomText
A I Squared
130 Taconic Business Park Road
Manchester Center, VT 05255

802-362-3612
800-859-0270
FAX: 802-362-1670
sales@aisquared.com
www.aisquared.com

David Wu, CEO
Jost Eckhardt, VP of Engineering
Scott Moore, VP of Marketing
Shawn Warren, VP of Product Support
A RAM-resident program that enlarges screen characters up to eight times. It runs on IBM PC, XT, AT and PS/2.

Speech Synthesizers

1629 Artic Business Vision (for DOS) and Artic WinVision (for Windows 95)
Artic Technologies
3456 Rodchester Road
Troy, MI 48083

248-689-9883
FAX: 248-588-2650
info@ablezone.com
www.articannex.ws/artictec.htm

Dale McDaniel, Founder
Kathy Gargagliano, Founder
A speech processor for blind computer users featuring true interactive speech with spread sheets, word processors, database managers, etc. Now available with both Windows 3.1 and Windows 95 access. $ 495.00

1630 Computerized Speech Lab
Kay Elemetrics Corporation
3 Paragon Drive
Montvale, NJ 07645

973-628-6200
800-289-5297
FAX: 201-391-2063
www.kaypentax.com

John Crump, President
Hardware/software for the acquisition, analysis/display, playback and storage of speech signals.

1631   DynaVox Technologies Speech Communication Devices
Dyna Vox Technologies
2100 Wharton St
Suite 400
Pittsburgh, PA 15203-1945   412-381-4883
                                             866-396-2869
                                        FAX: 412-381-5241
                                  Ray.Merk@dynavoxtech.com
                                        www.dynavoxtech.com

Ed Donnelly, CEO
Michelle Heying, President and COO
Kenneth Misch, CFO
Ray Merk, VP Finance
Develops and manufactures speech communication devices that
help individuals who are unable to speak due to speech, language
and/or learning disabilities to communicate quickly and easily.

1632   Electronic Speech Assistance Devices
Luminaud
8688 Tyler Blvd
Mentor, OH 44060-4348   440-255-9082
                                             800-255-3408
                                        FAX: 440-255-2250
                                        info@luminaud.com
                                          www.luminaud.com

Thomas M Lennox, President
Dorothy Lennox, VP
Offers a full line of speech aids, voice amplifiers, mini-vox am-
plifiers, laryngectomec products.

1633   Keywi
Hoffmann + Krippner Inc.
200 Westpark Drive
Suite 270
Peachtree City, GA 30269   770-487-1950
                                        FAX: 770-487-1945
                                        www.keywi-usa.com

1634   Little Mack Communicator
AbleNet
2625 Patton Road
Roseville, MN 55113-1308   651-294-2200
                                             800-322-0956
                                        FAX: 651-294-2259
                              customerservice@ablenetinc.com
                                         www.ablenetinc.com

Bill Sproull, Chairman
Jennifer Thalhuber, President/CEO
Paul Sugden, Former Vice President of Finance
William Mills, Board of Directors
The Little Mack Communicator has 2 minutes of memory and has
an angled switch surface making it easy to see and access. The
switch surface is 2 1/2 inches in diameter. Detachable mounting
base makes it easy to position a single unit in a variety of locations. *$129.00*

1635   Mega Wolf Communication Device
Wayne County Regional Educational Service Agency
33500 Van Born Rd
Wayne, MI 48184-2474   734-334-1300
                                        FAX: 734-334-1620
                                              www.resa.net

Lynda S. Jackson, President
Kenneth E. Berlinn, Vice President
James Petrie, Secretary
Mary E. Blackmon, Treasurer
A low cost voice output communication device which is primarily
intended to provide the power of speech to those individuals who
are most severely challenged mentally and/or physically. The
WOLF device is User programmable and uses the Texas Instruments' Touch and Tell case and touch panel; ADAMLAB electronics with synthesized (robotic) voice. For users able to point
with approximately 6 ounces of pressure. *$400.00*

1636   Talking Screen
Words+
42505 10th St W
Lancaster, CA 93534-7059   661-723-7723
                                             888-266-9294
                                        FAX: 661-723-5524
                                   info@simulations-plus.com
                                     www.simulations-plus.com

Walter S Woltosz, M.S., M.A.S., Chairman, President and Chief Ex
John R. Kneisel, Chief Financial Officer
John DiBella, Vice President, Marketing and Sales
Robert D. Clark, Ph.D, Director, Life Sciences
An augmentative communication program that allows the user to
select graphic symbols on the display to produce speech output.
Symbols can be used either singly or in sequence as picture abbre-
viations. *$ 1395.00*

**1637   Turnkey Computer Systems for the Visually, Physically, and
Hearing Impaired**
E VA S
39 Canal St P.O. Box 371
Westerly, RI 02891-1511   401-596-3155
                                             800-872-3827
                                        FAX: 401-596-3979
                                        TTY: 401-596-3500
                                          contact@evas.com
                                              www.evas.com

Gerald Swerdlick, Owner
Jerry Swerdlick, CEO
Offers clear speech with pleasant inflection and tonal quality as
well as variable pitch, intonation and voices.

1638   Voice-It
V XI Corporation Incorporated
271 Locust Street
Denver, NH 03820   603-742-2888
                                             800-742-8588
                                        FAX: 603-742-5065
                                          info@vxicorp.com
                                            www.vxicorp.com

Michael Ferguson, President
Tom Manero, Chief Financial Officer
Phil Pane, Vice President Operations
Brian Cole, Vice President Engineering
Adds voice to popular spreadsheet and word processing applica-
tions on IBM PCs and compatibles, turning spreadsheets and
word processing documents into talking documents.

1639   Window-Eyes
G W Micro
725 Airport North Office Park
Fort Wayne, IN 46825   260-489-3671
                                        FAX: 260-489-2608
                                         sales@gwmicro.com
                                           www.gwmicro.com

Dan Weirich, Owner/Vice President of Sales an
Doug Geoffray, Owner
Provides access to available software automatically reading information important to the user while ignoring the rest. A screen
reader for the windows operative system.

Software: Math

1640   AIMS Multimedia
Discovery Education
8145 Holton Dr
Florence, KY 41042-3009   859-342-7200
                                        FAX: 877-324-6830
                                       info@multimedia.com
                                      www.aimsmultimedia.com

Mike Wright, Director
Lynn Fassett, Administrative Assistant
Cindy Vogt, Human Resources Executive
AIMS Multimedia is a leader in the production and distribution of
training and educational programs for the business and K-12

communities via YHS, interactive CD-ROM, DVD and Internet streaming video.

1641 Basic Math: Detecting Special Needs
Allyn & Bacon
One Liberty Square
Suite 1200
Boston, MA 02109-3988
617-261-0040
800-852-8024
FAX: 617-944-7273
samplingdept@pearson.com
www.greenellp.com

Thomas M Greene, Attorney at Law
Michael Tabb, Attorney at Law
Describes special mathematics needs of special learners.
180 pages
ISBN 0-205116-35-3

1642 Campaign Math
Mindplay
4400 E. Broadway Blvd
Suite 400
Tucson, AZ 85711-1726
520-888-1800
800-221-7911
FAX: 520-888-7904
mail@mindplay.com
www.mindplay.com

Judith Bliss, CEO
Brian Williams, Development Manager
Lisa Garcia, Director of Educational Services
Chris Coleman, Vice President of Business Development
A complete program on the electoral process as well as a math package which teaches ratios, fractions and percentages.

1643 Educational Activities Software
5600 W 83rd Street
Suite 300, 8200 Tower
Bloomington, MN 55437
866-243-8464
FAX: 239-225-9299
jwest@orchardlng.com
www.edmentum.com

Vin Riera, President & Chief Executive Officer
Rob Rueckl, Chief Financial Officer
Dave Adams, Chief Academic Officer
Paul Johansen, Chief Technology Officer
Comprehensive MATH SKILLS software tutorials teach concepts ranging from rounding and tables to measuring area. MAC/WIN compatible. *$369.00*
Per Unit

1644 Fraction Factory
Queue
80 Hathaway Drive
Stratford, CT 06615
800-232-2224
FAX: 800-775-2729
jdk@queueinc.com
qworkbooks.com

Anna Christopoulos, General Manager
Peter Uhrynowski, Comptroller
Steve Pernett, Director of Printing and Graphic
Ann Pleszko, Shipping Manager
In 1980, Jonathan Kantrowitz started Queue, Inc. as an educational software company. After twenty thriving years publishing and distributing high-quality software to educators, Queue began transitioning from software to workbooks, focusing on state-specific test preparation.

1645 Information & Referral Services
Information + Referral Services
2590 N. Alvernon Way
Tucson, AZ 85712
520-323-1708
FAX: 520-325-8841
inform@azinfo.org
www.azinfo.org

Patti Caldwell, Executive Director
Chuck Palm, Treasurer
Ben Rensvold, Vice President
Tom DeSollar, President
Provides information about health and human services for people in Arizona over the telephone. Information specialists help callers clarify their needs, and provide referrals to the appropriate service agency.

1646 King's Rule
WINGS for Learning
1600 Green Hills Rd
Scotts Valley, CA 95066-4981
831-426-2228
FAX: 831-464-3600

Ani Stocks, Owner
A software mathematical problem solving game. Students discover mathematical rules as they work their way through a castle and generate and test a working hypothesis by asking questions.

1647 Learning About Numbers
C&C Software
5713 Kentford Cir
Wichita, KS 67220-3131
316-683-6056
800-752-2086

Carol Clark, President
Three programs use the power of computer graphics to provide young children with a variety of experiences in working with numbers. *$50.00*

1648 Math Rabbit
Learning Company
Ste 1900
100 Pine St
San Francisco, CA 94111-5205
415-659-2000
800-825-4420
FAX: 415-659-2020
thelearningco@hmhpub.com
www.hmhco.com

Linda K. Zecher, President, Chief Executive Officer and Director
Eric Shuman, Chief Financial Officer
William Bayers, Executive Vice President and General Counsel
Dr. Tim Cannon, Executive Vice President,
Teaches early math concepts by matching objects to numbers, then adding and subtracting up to 18.

1649 Math for Everyday Living
Educational Activities Software
5600 W 83rd Street
Suite 300, 8200 Tower
Bloomington, MN 55437
866-243-8464
FAX: 239-225-9299
jwest@orchardlng.com
www.edmentum.com

Vin Riera, President & Chief Executive Officer
Rob Rueckl, Chief Financial Officer
Dave Adams, Chief Academic Officer
Paul Johansen, Chief Technology Officer
Real life math skills are taught with this tutorial and practice software program. Examples include Paying for a Meal (addition and subtraction), Working with Sales Slips (multiplication), Unit Pricing (division), Sales Tax (percent), Earning with Overtime (fractions) plus more. Software: CD-ROM, Windows, MAC, and DOS. *$159.00*

1650 Math for Successful Living
Siboney Learning Group
5600 W 83rd Street
Suite 300, 8200 Tower
Bloomington, MN 55437

866-243-8464
FAX: 239-225-9299
jwest@orchardlng.com
www.edmentum.com

Vin Riera, President & Chief Executive Officer
Rob Rueckl, Chief Financial Officer
Dave Adams, Chief Academic Officer
Paul Johansen, Chief Technology Officer
These programs include managing a checking account, budgeting, shopping strategies and buying on credit.

1651 Piece of Cake Math
Queue Inc
80 Hathaway Drive
Stratford, CT 06615

800-232-2224
FAX: 800-775-2729
jdk@queueinc.com
www.qworkbooks.com

Anna Christopoulos, General Manager
Peter Uhrynowski, Comptroller
Steve Pernett, Director of Printing and Graphic
Ann Pleszko, Shipping Manager
In 1980, Jonathan Kantrowitz started Queue, Inc. as an educational software company. After twenty thriving years publishing and distributing high-quality software to educators, Queue began transitioning from software to workbooks, focusing on state-specific test preparation.

1652 Puzzle Tanks
WINGS for Learning
1600 Green Hills Rd
Scotts Valley, CA 95066-4981

831-426-2228
FAX: 831-464-3600

Ani Stocks, Owner
A mathematical problem solving game that involves multi-step problems.

1653 Right Turn
WINGS for Learning
1600 Green Hills Rd
Scotts Valley, CA 95066-4981

831-426-2228
FAX: 831-464-3600

Ani Stocks, Owner
Requires students to predict, experiment and learn about the mathematical concepts of rotation and transformation.

1654 RoboMath
4400 E. Broadway Blvd
Suite 400
Tucson, AZ 85711-1726

520-888-1800
800-221-7911
FAX: 520-888-7904
mail@mindplay.com
www.mindplay.com

Judith Bliss, CEO
Brian Williams, Development Manager
Lisa Garcia, Director of Educational Services
Chris Coleman, Vice President of Business Development
A complete program on the electoral process as well as a math package which teaches ratios, fractions and percentages.

1655 Stickybear Math I Deluxe
Optimum Resource
1 Mathews Drive
Suite 107
Hilton Head Island, SC 29926- 3689

843-689-8000
FAX: 843-689-8008
info@stickybear.com
www.stickybear.com

Richard Hefter, President

Sharpen basic addition and subtraction skills with this captivating series of math exercises. Grades Pre-K to 2. Available in as single edition with sizing up to 30 users at a site. English/Spanish. *$59.95*

1656 Stickybear Math II Deluxe
Optimum Resource
1 Mathews Drive
Suite 107
Hilton Head Island, SC 29926- 3689

843-689-8000
FAX: 843-689-8008
info@stickybear.com
www.stickybear.com

Richard Hefter, President
Multiplication and division, beginning with the elementary problems and developing into the more complex problems with regrouping. Grades 2-4. Available for single user through the 30 user site package. English/Spanish. *$59.95*

1657 Stickybear Math Splash
Optimum Resource
1 Mathews Drive
Suite 107
Hilton Head Island, SC 29926- 3689

843-689-8000
FAX: 843-689-8008
info@stickybear.com
www.stickybear.com

Richard Hefter, President
Unique multiple activities keep the learning level high while children acquire skills in addition, subtraction, multiplication and division. K-5th grade. Available as single edition up to 30 user site package. English/Spanish. *$59.95*

1658 Stickybear Math Word Problems
Optimum Resource
1 Mathews Drive
Suite 107
Hilton Head Island, SC 29926- 3689

843-689-8000
FAX: 843-689-8008
info@stickybear.com
www.stickybear.com

Richard Hefter, President
Hundreds of different word problems make it easy for students to practice basic math skills around analyzing and solving word problems. Grades 1-5. Available as single edition up to 30 user site package. English/Spanish. *$59.95*

1659 Stickybear Money
Optimum Resource
1 Mathews Drive
Suite 107
Hilton Head Island, SC 29926- 3667

843-689-8000
FAX: 843-689-8008
info@stickybear.com
www.stickybear.com

Chris Gintz, President
Teaches children to recognize US coins and paper money and introduces simple counting. K to 3rd grade. Bilingual. *$59.95*

1660 Stickybear Numbers Deluxe
Optimum Resource
1 Mathews Drive
Suite 107
Hilton Head Island, SC 29926- 3689

843-689-8000
FAX: 843-689-8008
info@stickybear.com
www.stickybear.com

Richard Hefter, President
Counting and number recognition are as easy as 1-2-3 with this award-winning program. Teaches number recognition of numbers 0-9 and 0-30. Pre-K to 2nd grade. Available as single edition up to 30 user site package. *$59.95*

1661   Tomorrow's Promise: Mathematics
Compass Learning
203 Colorado Street
Austin, TX 78701

512-478-9600
800-678-1412
866-586-7387
www.compasslearning.com

Eric Loeffel, President
Trey Chambers, Chief Financial Officer
ARTHUR VANDERVEEN, Vice President, Business Strategy and
Development
CHIPP WALTERS, Chief Designer Officer
By integrating interdisciplinary content and real-world application of skills, this product emphasizes the practical value of fundamental math skills. It helps your students develop a problem-solving aptitude for ongoing mathematics achievement.

Software: Miscellaneous

1662   Adventures in Musicland
Electronic Courseware Systems
1713 S State St
Champaign, IL 61820-7258

217-359-7099
800-832-4965
FAX: 217-359-6578
support@ecsmedia.com
http://ecsmedia.com.np/

G Peters, President
Jodie Varner, Marketing Manager
This unique set of music games features characters from Lewis Carroll's, Alice in Wonderland. Players learn through pictures, sounds, and animation which help develop understanding of musical tones, composers, and musical symbols. Games include MusicMatch, Melody Mixup, Picture Perfect and Sound Concentration. *$49.95*

1663   Ai Squared
130 Taconic Business Park Road
Manchester Center, VT 05255-669

802-362-3612
800-859-0270
FAX: 802-362-1670
sales@aisquared.com
http://www.aisquared.com

David Wu, CEO
Jost Eckhardt, VP of Engineering
Scott Moore, VP of Marketing
Shawn Warren, VP of Product Support
Developers of software for the visually impaired.

1664   All About You: Appropriate Special Interactions and Self-Esteem
P CI Educational Publishing
P.O. Box 34270
San Antonio, TX 78265-4270

210-377-1999
800-594-4263
800-471-3000
FAX: 888-259-8284
submissions@pcieducation.com
www.pcicatalog.com

Lee Wilson, President and CEO
Randy Pennington, Executive VP
Jeff McLane, Founder
David Keith, Vice President of IT
This game offers parents and game players a new line of communication when discussing various issues such as learning to be thoughtful, respecting the rights and feelings of others, how to make and keep friends and more. *$49.95*

1665   All Star Review
Tom Snyder Productions
100 Talcott Ave
Watertown, MA 02472-5703

800-342-0236
dealer@tomsnyder.com.
www.tomsnyder.com

Rick Abrams, Manager
Tom Synder, Founder
Bridget Dalton, Ed.D., Author
Peggy Healy Stearns, Ph.D., Author
This package turns group review into a baseball game for small and large groups.

1666   Attainment Company
I ET Resources
P.O. Box 930160
Verona, WI 53593-160

608-845-7880
800-327-4269
FAX: 608-845-8040
info@attainmentcompany.com
www.attainmentcompany.com

Don Bastian, President
Julie Denu, Technical Support
Theresa O'Connor, Office Manager
Augmentative/alternative communication, software, videos, print and hands-on functional life skills and basic acdemics materials for developmental and cognitive disabilities.

1667   Attention Getter
Soft Touch
12301 Central Ave NE Ste 205
4300 Stine Rd
Blaine, MN 55434

763-755-1402
888-755-1402
FAX: 763-862-2920
support@marblesoft.com
www.softtouch.com

Joyce Meyer, President
The whimsical photos morph to another photo and then to a third photo in categories. Paired with interesting sounds and music, the photo animations are so engaging that the student is motivated to activate the computer to see and hear the next one. This is a perfect vehicle to achieve goals aimed at attention getting, activating a switch or intentionally. Compatible with USB IntelliKeys keyboards.

1668   Attention Teens
Soft Touch
12301 Central Ave NE Ste 205
Blaine, MN 55434

763-755-1403
888-755-1403
FAX: 763-862-2921
support@marblesoft.com
www.softtouch.com

Joyce Meyer, President
Attention Teens (formerly known as Loony Teens) is a program for teens with disabilities who need powerful input to get their attention. Attention Teens is a computer program to do just this. Paired with interesting sounds and music, the photo animations are so engaging that the student is motivated to activate the computer to see and hear the next one. Compatible with USB IntelliKeys keyboards.

1669   Away We Ride
Soft Touch
12301 Central Ave NE Ste 205
4300 Stine Rd
Blaine, MN 55434

763-755-1404
888-755-1404
FAX: 763-862-2922
support@marblesoft.com
www.softtouch.com

Joyce Meyer, President
Software for children and teens. For Macintosh and PC.

1670 Battenberg & Associates
11135 Rolling Springs Dr
Carmel, IN 46033-3629   317-843-2208

Jan Battenberg, Owner
Offers various software programs that develop the user's visual memory, sequencing skills, word recognition, hand-eye coordination and more.

1671 Behavior Skills: Learning How People Should Act
PCI Education Publishing
P.O.Box 34270
San Antonio, TX 78265-4270   210-377-1999
                                        800-471-3000
                                        FAX: 888-828-
                                        www.pcieducation.com

Jeff Clain, CEO
Erin Kinard, VP Product Development/Publisher
Helps players learn what behavior is acceptable and what behavior is not acceptable in the real world. *$49.95*

1672 Blocks in Motion
Don Johnston
26799 W Commerce Dr
Volo, IL 60073-9675   847-740-0749
                                        800-999-4660
                                        FAX: 847-740-7326
                                        info@donjohnston.com
                                        www.donjohnston.com

Ruth Ziolkowski, President
Don Jhonson, Founder
This unique art and motion program makes drawing, creating and animating fun and educational for all users. Based on the Piagetian Theory for motor-sensory development, this program promotes the concept that the process is as educational and as much fun as the end result. *$79.00*

1673 CINTEX: Speak to Your Appliances
NanoPac
4823 S Sheridan Rd
Suite 302
Tulsa, OK 74145-5717   918-665-0329
                                        800-580-6086
                                        FAX: 918-665-0361
                                        TTY: 918-665-2310
                                        info@nanopac.com
                                        www.nanopac.com

Silvio Cianfrone, President
CINTEX, with a voice recognition program, will control up to 256 off/on appliances, dial and answer the phone, flash for call waiting, dial from a directory, control TV's, VCR's, stereos and more — all with your voice. CINTEX2 includes the necessary hardware and voice macros which you can use to immediately control your environment. You can tailor these macros to your personal needs and add new macros. Pops-up over current application allowing instant access. $695-$2,000.

1674 Car Builder Deluxe
Optimum Resource
1 Mathews Drive
Suite 107
Hilton Head Island, SC 29926- 3689   843-689-8000
                                        FAX: 843-689-8008
                                        info@stickybear.com
                                        www.stickybear.com

Richard Hefter, President
As design engineers, users build cars on screen, specifying chassis length, wheelbase, engine type, transmission, fuel tank size, suspension, steering, tires and brakes. All functional choices are interrelated and will affect the performance of the final design. Grades 3 & up. *$59.99*

1675 Center for Best Practices in Early Childhood
Horrabin Hall 32
Macomb, IL 61455   309-298-1634
                                        FAX: 309-298-2305
                                        jk-johanson@wiu.edu
                                        www.wiu.edu/thecenter/

Linda Robinson, Assistant Director
The Center, part of the College of Education and Human Services at Western Illinois University, provides products, training materials, and information related to best practices for educators and families of young children with disabilities.

1676 Clock
Compass Learning
203 Colorado Street
Austin, TX 78701-3922   512-478-9600
                                        800-678-1412
                                        866-586-7387
                                        www.compasslearning.com

Eric Loeffel, President
Trey Chambers, Chief Financial Officer
Arthur Vanderveen, Vice President, Business Strategy and Development
Chipp Walters, Chief Designer Officer
An extremely simple, easy-to-use program for children who are learning how to read the time of day from clocks and digital displays. Apple and MS-DOS and Mac available. *$39.95*

1677 Community Skills: Learning to Function in Your Neighborhood
Programming Concepts
8700 Shoal Creek Boulevard
Austin, TX 78757-6897   210-377-1999
                                        800-594-4263
                                        800-471-3000
                                        FAX: 888-259-8284
                                        submissions@pcieducation.com
                                        www.proedinc.com

Lee Wilson, President and CEO
Randy Pennington, Executive VP
Jeff McLane, Founder
David Keith, Vice President of IT
Offers parents and educators a functional way to teach community life skills. *$49.95*

1678 Companion Activities
Soft Touch
12301 Central Ave NE Ste 205
4300 Stine Rd
Blaine, MN 55434   763-755-1404
                                        888-755-1404
                                        FAX: 763-862-2922
                                        support@marblesoft.com
                                        www.softouch.com

Joyce Meyer, President
Print your own books, worksheets, flash cards, board games, matching games, bingo games, card games and many more. This CD offers numerous companion activities to different SoftTouch software titles. Activities range from very easy to difficult. Companion activities are great tools to reinforce learning. Use the work sheets - black and white and color - in the inclusion class for students with special needs.

1679 Concepts on the Move Advanced Preacademics
Soft Touch
12301 Central Ave NE Ste 205
P.O.Box 490215
Blaine, MN 55449   763-862-2920
                                        888-755-1402
                                        FAX: 763-862-2922
                                        support@marblesoft.com
                                        www.marblesoft.com

Joyce Meyer, President
Choose from five concepts groups: categories, occupations, functions, goes with and prepositions. Use our Steps to Learning Design to choose how many concepts to present at one time and where to place each one in the scan array, on screen keyboard or IntelliKeys keyboard. Watch and listen as the concept morphs or

changes and music plays. The words are also shown to reinforce emerging literacy skills. Compatible with USB IntelliKeys.

1680 Cooking Class: Learning About Food Preparation
Programming Concepts
8700 Shoal Creek Boulevard
Austin, TX 78757-6897
512-451-3246
800-897-3202
800-471-3000
FAX: 800-397-7633
general@proedinc.com
www.proedinc.com

Jeff McLane, Founder
Lee Wilson, President and CEO
Randy Pennington, Executive VP
David Keith, Vice President of IT
This game offers parents and educators a new way to teach basic preparation skills. Kitchen safety and sanitation are stressed throughout the game. *$49.95*

1681 Dilemma
Educational Activities Software
5600 West 83rd Street
Suite 300, 8200 Tower
Bloomington, MN 55437
800-447-5286
FAX: 239-225-9299
info@edmentum.com
www.edmentum.com

Vin Riera, President/CEO
Dan Juckniess, SVP, Sales & Professional Services
Stacey Herteux, VP, Human Resources
Rob Rueckl, Chief Financial Officer
Realistic stories with a choice of different gripping endings, color graphics, a built-in dictionary and a user controlled reading rate make these computer programs compelling enough to interest all students. Comprehension and vocabulary questions follow each story. *$159.00*

1682 Dino-Games
Academic Software
3504 Tates Creek Road
Lexington, KY 40517-2601
859-552-1020
859-552-1040
FAX: 253-799-4012
asistaff@acsw.com
www.acsw.com

Dr. Warren E Lacefield PhD, President
Penelope D. Ellis, COO, Sales & Marketing Director
Sylvia B. Lacefield, Graphic Artist
Cindy L George, Author
Dino-Games are single switch software programs for early switch practice. Dinosaur games provide practice in pattern recognition, cause and effect demonstration, directionality training, number concepts and problem solving. They are compatible with most popular switch interfaces and alternate keyboards. For Macintosh, IBM and compatibles. DINO-LINK is a matching game; DINO-MAZE is a series of maze games; DINO-FIND is a game of concentration; and DINO-DOT is a collection of dot-to-dot games.
$39.95 per game

1683 Directions: Technology in Special Education
DREAMMS for Kids
273 Ringwood Road
Freeville, NY 13068-5606
607-539-3027
FAX: 607-539-9930
janet@dreamms.org
www.dreamms.org

Janet P. Hosmer, Editor/Publisher
Chester D. Hosmer, Jr., Technical Editor
Susan Lait, Regular Contributor
Lorianne Hoenninger, Regular Contributor
A CD containing all of 'Directions' past articles and information gathered from their newsletter which lists resources for assistive and adaptive computer ethnologies in the home, school and community. *$24.95*

1684 ESI Master Resource Guide
Educational Software Institute
4213 S 94th St
Omaha, NE 68127-1223
402-592-3300
800-955-5570
FAX: 402-592-2017
info@edsoft.com
www.edsoft.com

Lee Myers, President
Kathy Cavanaugh, Catalog Manager
Educational Software Institute (ESI) provides a one-stop shop to purchase software titles by all of the best publishers. The ESI Master Gold Book catalog and CD-ROM represents more than 400 software publishers, with information on more than 8,000 software titles. Take the confusion out of software selection by calling ESI for all of your software needs - including competitive prices, software previews, knowledgeable assistance, and the largest selection available all in one place.
Yearly

1685 EZ Keys
Words+
42505 10th Street West
Suite 109
Lancaster, CA 93534- 7059
661-723-7723
888-266-9294
FAX: 661-723-5524
info@simulations-plus.com
www.simulations-plus.com

Walter S Woltosz, M.S., M.A.S., Chairman, President and Chief Executive Officer
John A. Dibella, VP, Marketing & Sales
Virginia E. Woltosz. M.B.A., Secretary & Treasurer
John R. Kneisel, Chief Financial Officer
A software and hardware product designed to operate on an IBM compatible PC. The software provides dual word prediction, abbreviation expansion, five different methods of voice output and access to commercial software applications. *$1395.00*

1686 Early Games for Young Children
Queue Incorporated
80 Hathaway Drive
Stratford, CT 06615
800-232-2224
FAX: 800-775-2729
jdk@queueinc.com
www.qworkbooks.com

Anna Christopoulos, General Manager
Peter Uhrynowski, Comptroller
Steve Perrett, Director of Printing and Graphics
Ann Pleszko, Shipping Manager
Software that includes nine activities that entertain preschoolers in honing basic math and language skills.

1687 Early Music Skills
Electronic Courseware Systems
1713 S State St
Champaign, IL 61820-7258
217-359-7099
800-832-4965
FAX: 217-359-6578
support@ecsmedia.com
www.ecsmedia.com

G Peters, President
Jodie Varner, Marketing Manager
A tutorial and drill program designed for the beginning music student. It covers four basic music reading skills: recognition of line and space notes; comprehension of the numbering system for the musical staff; visual and aural identification of notes moving up and down; and recognition of notes stepping and skipping up and down. *$ 39.95*

1688 Eating Skills: Learning Basic Table Manners
PCI Education Publishing
P.O.Box 34270
San Antonio, TX 78265-4270   210-377-1999
                                    800-594-4263
                              FAX: 210-377-1121
                           pciinfo@pcieducation.com
                           www.pcieducation.com

Erin Kinard, VP Product Development/Publisher
Jeff Clain, CEO
Offers parents and educators a functional way to teach and rein-force basic table manners. *$49.95*

1689 Electronic Courseware Systems
1713 S State St
Champaign, IL 61820-7258   217-359-7099
                                  800-832-4965
                            FAX: 217-359-6578
                         support@ecsmedia.com
                         www.ecsmedia.com

Jodie Varner, Manager
G Peters, President
Offers a complete library of instructional software for music, math, science and social studies.

1690 Fall Fun
Soft Touch
12301 Central Ave NE Ste 205
P.O.Box 490215
Blaine, MN 55449   763-862-2920
                                  888-755-1402
                            FAX: 763-862-2922
                         support@marblesoft.com
                         www.marblesoft.com

Joyce Meyer, President
Your students can begin their day with the Pledge of Allegiance, Pumpkins, Owls, and Cats. Witches adorn Five Pumpkins Sitting on the Gate. Five Fat Turkeys out smart the pilgrims with song and antics. The owl and cat have songs of their own. A variety of activities reinforce concepts such as short, tall, first, second, third, same and different. Fall Fun includes cause and effect and easy to more difficult levels. Eight songs in all.

1691 Five Green & Speckled Frogs
Soft Touch
12301 Central Ave NE Ste 205
P.O.Box 490215
Blaine, MN 55449   763-862-2920
                                  888-755-1402
                            FAX: 763-862-2922
                         support@marblesoft.com
                         www.marblesoft.com

Joyce Meyer, President
Laugh, learn and sing with Five Humorous Frogs. Activities start with cause and effect and progress to teach directionality and simple subtraction. This classic song makes learning numbers and number worlds easy. Selections can be set to 2, 3, 4, 5, or 6 on-screen choices. Two games are included. One teaches direction on a number line. If the child moves the frog in the correct direction, the frog gets a point. The other game teaches beginning subtraction.

1692 Free and User Supported Software for the IBM PC: A Resource Guide
McFarland & Company
960 NC Highway 88 W
P.O.Box 611
Jefferson, NC 28640-8813   336-246-4460
                                  800-253-2187
                            FAX: 336-246-5018
                         info@mcfarlandpub.com
                         www.mcfarlandpub.com

Robert McFarland Franklin, Founder
Kenneth.J Ansley, Author
Victor.D Lopez, Author
A selection of word processing, database management, spread-sheets, and graphics programs are described and evaluated. Describes how the program works and its strengths and weaknesses.

Rating charts cover such aspects as ease of use, ease of learning, documentation, and general utility. *$27.50*
224 pages Paperback
ISBN 0-89950-99-0

1693 GoalView: Special Education and RTI Student Management Information System
Learning Tools International
2391 Circadian Way
Santa Rosa, CA 95407-5439   707-521-3530
                                   800-333-9954
                             info@goalview.com
                             www.ltools.com

Cathy Zier, President/CEO
Natalie Sipes, VP
Michael R. Paul, Director of IT/Senior Web Engine
A Web Based information system for students, educators and parents that enables accountability and achievement tracking; prepares IDEA compliant IEP's in minutes; provides over 250,000 education standards and special education goals and objectives in English and Spanish; generates Federal compliance reports; and creates IDEA GoalCard progress reports for students, schools and districts for every reporting period.

1694 HELP
V OR T Corporation
P.O.Box G (George)
Menlo Park, CA 94026   650-322-8282
                                  888-757-8678
                            FAX: 650-327-0747
                         custserv@vort.com
                         vort.com

Tom Holt, Owner
A software version of HELP, covers over 650 skills in 6 developmental areas; cognitive, motor skills, language, gross motor, social and self-help.

1695 Handbook of Adaptive Switches and Augmentative Communication Devices
Academic Software
3504 Tates Creek Road
Lexington, KY 40517-2601   859-552-1020
                                  859-552-1040
                            FAX: 253-799-4012
                         asistaff@acsw.com
                         www.acsw.com

Dr. Warren E Lacefield PhD, President
Penelope D. Ellis, COO, Sales & Marketing Director
Cindy L George, Author
Sylvia B. Lacefield, Graphic Artist
This second edition contains physical descriptions and laboratory test data for a variety of commercially available pressure switches and augmentative communication devices and chapters on physical interaction, seating and positioning, and control access. It is an essential tool for assistive technology professionals and therapists who make decisions concerning physical access. *$60.00*
300 pages Hardcover

1696 HandiWARE
Microsystems Software
600 Worcester Rd
Framingham, MA 01702-5303   508-626-8511
                                   800-828-2600
                             FAX: 508-879-1069
                          infor@microsys.com
                          www.handiware.com

Terri McGrath, Sales/Marketing
Bill Kilroy, Product Manager
Adapted access software, assists persons with physical, hearing and visual impairments in accessing computers running DOS and Windows. HandiWARE is a suite of 8 software programs which provide users with screen magnification, alternate keyboard access, word prediction, augmentative communication, hands free telephone access, a visual beep. $20.00-$595.00.

1697 How to Write for Everyday Living
Educational Activities Software
5600 West 83rd Street
Suite 300, 8200 Tower
Bloomington, MN 55437-585

800-447-5286
FAX: 239-225-9299
info@edmentum.com
www.edmentum.com

Vin Riera, President/CEO
Dan Juckniess, SVP, Sales & Professional Services
Stacey Herteux, VP, Human Resources
Rob Rueckl, Chief Financial Officer
An individualized Life Skills WRITING Software program emphasizing the reading, writing, communication and reference skills needed for real-life tasks: preparing a resume, an employment form, a business letter and envelope, a learner's permit, a social security application and banking forms. *$159.00*

1698 I KNOW American History
Soft Touch
12301 Central Ave NE Ste 205
P.O.Box 490215
Blaine, MN 55449-2352

763-862-2920
888-755-1402
FAX: 763-862-2922
support@marblesoft.com
www.marblesoft.com

Joyce Meyer, President
The new I KNOW programs is the way students practice attending, choice making and turn-taking while uncovering learning puzzles. Each press reveals more of the image while the narrator reads the text on the screen. Offers three levels of language: short phrases, short sentences and longer sentences to match the student's learning level. Choose from the five topic areas: American Symbols, Westward Movement, Early Colonial Americans, Industrial Revolution and Biographies.

1699 I KNOW American History Overlay CD
Soft Touch
12301 Central Ave NE Ste 205
P.O.Box 490215
Blaine, MN 55449-2352

763-862-2920
888-755-1402
FAX: 763-862-2922
support@marblesoft.com
www.marblesoft.com

Joyce Meyer, President
Use this Overlay CD with I KNOW American History program. Includes standard overlays and SoftTouch's changeable overlays. Includes Overlay Printer by IntelliTools. Use Overlay Maker by IntelliTools (not included) to modify the overlays or to make additional learning materials.

1700 Incite Learning Series
Don Johnston
26799 West Commerce Drive
Volo, IL 60073

847-740-0749
800-999-4660
FAX: 847-740-7326
info@donjohnston.com
www.donjohnston.com

Don Johnston, Founder
Ruth Ziolkowski, President
A collection of original short films and a thought-provoking instruction model to engage every student in the critical thinking and feeling process. This research-based program was developed around the science of how students learn best using the theory of 'anchored instruction' and 'front-loading' standards-based curriculum. *$79.00*

1701 Innovation Management Group
179 Niblick Rd
Ste 454
Paso Robles, CA 93446

818-701-1579
800-889-0987
FAX: 818-936-0200
cs@imgpresents.com
www.imgpresents.com

Jerry Hussong, VP of Marketing
Publisher of the Assistive Technology Suite. The ultimate set of general purpose, adaptive computer access available today. Site License includes ALL computers and ALL active students and teachers at a single or multi-site location.

1702 IntelliPics Studio 3
Intelli Tools
1720 Corporate Cir
Petaluma, CA 94954-6924

707-773-2000
800-547-6747
FAX: 707-773-2001
info@intellitools.com
www.intellitools.com

Arjan Khalsa, CEO
Multimedia authoring tool for both students and teachers to create activities, games, quizzes, slide shows, reports and presentations. *$395.00*

1703 KIDS (Keyboard Introductory Development Series)
Electronic Courseware Systems
1713 S State St
Champaign, IL 61820-7258

217-359-7099
800-832-4965
FAX: 217-359-6578
support@ecsmedia.com
www.ecsmedia.com

G Peters, President
Jodie Varner, Marketing Manager
A four disk series for the very young. Zoo Puppet Theater reinforces learning correct finger numbers for piano playing; Race Car Keys teaches keyboard geography by recognizing syllables or note names; Dinosaurs Lunch teaches placement of the notes on the treble staff; and Follow Me asks the student to play notes that have been presented aurally. *$49.95*

1704 Keyboard Tutor, Music Software
Electronic Courseware Systems
1713 S State St
Champaign, IL 61820-7258

217-359-7099
800-832-4965
FAX: 217-359-6578
support@ecsmedia.com
www.ecsmedia.com

G Peters, President
Jodie Varner, Marketing Manager
Presents exercises for learning elementary keyboard skills including knowledge of names of the keys, piano keys matched to notes, notes matched to piano keys, whole steps and half steps. Each lesson allows unlimited practice of the skills. The program may be used with or without a midi keyboard attached to the computer. *$39.95*

1705 Keyboarding by Ability
Teachers Institute for Special Education
9933 NW 45th St
Sunrise, FL 33351-4744

954-235-7940
FAX: 866-843-0765
Support@Special-Education-Soft.com
www.special-education-soft.com

Gary Byowitz, President
Allows the learning disabled or dyslexic student to acquire keyboarding skills through visually cued alphabetical approach designed and tested to meet the specific learning style needs of this unique population at every grade level. Package contains: IBM software, a set of lesson plans and instructional goals; supplemental graded data input exercises. *$369.00*

1706 Keyboarding for the Physically Handicapped
Teachers Institute for Special Education
9933 NW 45th Street
Sunrise, FL 33351
954-235-7940
FAX: 866-843-0765
Support@Special-Education-Soft.com
www.special-education-soft.com

Jack Heller, Director/Owner
Gary Byowitz, President
Custom designed touch typing programs for any student. A person needs order by the number of usable fingers on each hand (not counting the thumb), and whether or not a one finger or a head-pointer edition is wanted. Package includes IBM software; a complete set of lesson plans and instructional goals. *$149.95*

1707 Keyboarding with One Hand
Teachers Institute for Special Education
P.O.Box 2300
Wantagh, NY 11793-140
FAX: 516-781-4070
jackheller@aol.com
www.users.aol.com/jackheller

Jack Heller, Director
This 22 lesson tutorial developed through 25 years of research, testing and teaching allows a student with one hand to acquire employable keyboarding skills using a touch system designed for the standard IBM PC keyboard. *$79.95*

1708 LPDOS Deluxe
Optelec U S
3030 Enterprise Court
STE C
Vista, CA 92081-8358
800-826-4200
FAX: 800-368-4111
info@optelec.com
us.optelec.com

Stephan Terwolbeck, President
Michiel van Schaik, VP
Janet Lennex, Director of Customer Excellence
Jade Arbelo, Director of Human Resources
Large print software programs. *$595.00*

1709 Large Print DOS
Optelec U S
3030 Enterprise Court
STE C
Vista, CA 92081-8358
800-826-4200
FAX: 800-368-4111
info@optelec.com
us.optelec.com

Stephan Terwolbeck, President
Michiel van Schaik, VP
Janet Lennex, Director of Customer Excellence
Jade Arbelo, Director of Human Resources

1710 Laureate Learning Systems
110 E Spring St
Winooski, VT 05404-1898
802-655-4755
800-562-6801
FAX: 802-655-4757
info@llsys.com
www.laureatelearning.com

Mary Wilson, Owner
Kathy Hollandsworth, Office Manager
Laureate publishes award-winning talking software for children and adults with disabilities. Programs cover cause and effect, language development, cognitive processing, and reading. High-quality speech, colorful graphics and amusing animation make learning fun. Accessible with touchscreen, single switch, keyboard and mouse. No reading required. Available on a hybrid CD-ROM for Windows and Macintosh. Visit our website for more information or call for a free catalog.

1711 Learning Company
Ste 400
222 3rd Ave SE
Cedar Rapids, IA 52401-1542
319-395-9626
888-242-6747
FAX: 319-395-0217
info@riverdeep.net
http://web.riverdeep.net

Barry O'Callaghan, Executive Chairman & Chief Executive Officer
Tony Mulderry, Executive Vice President, Corporate Development
Ciara Smyth, Executive Vice President, Global Business Operations
Scott Campbell, Executive Vice President, Strategic Sales
Software for children. For Macintosh or Windows (3.1 DOS or Windows 95, Windows 98 required). The Learning Company has been added to Riverdeep.

1712 Little Red Hen
Compass Learning
203 Colorado Street
Austin, TX 78701
512-478-9600
800-678-1412
866-586-7387
FAX: 619-622-7873
support@compasslearning.com
www.compasslearning.com

Eric Loeffel, President, CEO
Tammy Deal, VP, Human Resources
Eric Wasser, VP, Sales
Eileen Shihadeh, VP, Marketing
Children learn about the rewards of hard work when they discover who the Little Red Hen's friends miss out on freshly baked bread. Puzzles, rhymes, story writing and other interactive exercises enhance the creative learning process. *$34.95*

1713 Looking Good: Learning to Improve Your Appearance
Programming Concepts
8700 Shoal Creek Boulevard
Austin, TX 78757-6897
512-451-3246
800-897-3202
800-471-3000
FAX: 800-397-7633
general@proedinc.com
www.proedinc.com

Jeff McLane, Founder
Lee Wilson, President and CEO
Randy Pennington, Executive VP
David Keith, Vice President of IT
This game offers a creative way to discuss all areas of grooming. *$49.95*

1714 Monkeys Jumping on the Bed
Soft Touch
12301 Central Ave NE Ste 205
P.O.Box 490215
Blaine, MN 55449-2352
763-862-2920
888-755-1402
FAX: 763-862-2922
support@marblesoft.com
www.marblesoft.com

Joyce Meyer, President
This program combines a favorite preschool song with number and color activities. Children and adults will enjoy engaging music and delightful animation. Students with cognitive delays respond to upbeat music and interesting sounds. Large graphics help learners focus on the action. Several important concepts are presented in enjoyable activity formats. Students learn cause and effect in Let's Play and Just for Fun.

1715 Morse Code WSKE
Words+
42505 10th Street West
Suite 109
Lancaster, CA 93534- 7059
661-723-7723
888-266-9294
FAX: 661-723-5524
info@simulations-plus.com
www.simulations-plus.com

Walter S Woltosz, M.S., M.A.S., Chairman, President and Chief Executive Officer
John A. Dibella, VP, Marketing & Sales
Virginia E. Woltosz. M.B.A., Secretary & Treasurer
John R. Kneisel, Chief Financial Officer
A software and hardware product designed to operate on an IBM compatible PC.

1716 Multi-Scan Single Switch Activity Center
Academic Software
3504 Tates Creek Road
Lexington, KY 40517-2601
859-552-1020
859-552-1040
FAX: 253-799-4012
asistaff@acsw.com
www.acsw.com

Dr. Warren E Lacefield PhD, President
Penelope D. Ellis, COO, Sales & Marketing Director
Cindy L George, Author
Sylvia B. Lacefield, Graphic Artist
A single switch activity center containing four educational games: Match, Maze, Dot-to-Dot, and Concentration, along with six graphics libraries; Dinosaurs, Sports, Animals, Independent Living, Vocations, and Cosmetology. MULTI-SCAN allows you to select a graphic library, choose games for each user, and adjust the difficulty level and other settings for each game. Other features allow you to save the game setups under each user's name and print out individual performance reports after sessions.
$154.00

1717 Muppet Learning Keys
WINGS for Learning
1600 Green Hills Rd
Scotts Valley, CA 95066-4981
831-426-2228
FAX: 831-464-3600

Ani Stocks, Owner
Designed to introduce children to the world of the computer as they become familiar with letters, numbers and colors.

1718 My Own Pain
Soft Touch
12301 Central Ave NE Ste 205
P.O.Box 490215
Blaine, MN 55449-2352
763-862-2920
888-755-1402
FAX: 763-862-2922
support@marblesoft.com
www.marblesoft.com

Joyce Meyer, President
Three activities - three levels. Press the switch and the paint brush chooses the color and paints the vehicle. Music reinforces the sounds when the picture is complete. A second activity allows the student to choose the color and paint the vehicle parts any color he or she wants. The third activity is a blueprint. Print the color that matches the one in the wire drawing. Color the drawing to complete the picture.

1719 Old MacDonald's Farm Deluxe
Soft Touch
12301 Central Ave NE Ste 205
P.O.Box 490215
Blaine, MN 55449-2352
763-862-2920
888-755-1402
FAX: 763-862-2922
support@marblesoft.com
www.marblesoft.com

Joyce Meyer, President
Toddlers, preschoolers and early elementary students will be entertained and captivated by the six major activities and animations in the delightful program. Includes 18 real animation images or 9 cartoon like characters. The teacher or child can choose which animals they want to sing about. Some activities are designed for children within the normal population, others are designed for students with moderate and severe disabilities.

1720 Optimum Resource Educational Software
Optimum Resource
1 Mathews Drive
Suite 107
Hilton Head Island, SC 29926
843-689-8000
FAX: 843-689-8008
info@stickybear.com
www.stickybear.com

Richard Hefter, President
A complete topical curriculum of reading, math, keyboard skills and science programs that are age and skill specific. Programs include: Early Learning for Pre-K to 1st grade with introductions to numbers, language, shapes, and time; Language Arts from Pre-K to 12; Math for Pre-K to 12; two distinct Science programs; Tools for Educators provides Spelling and Math generators; and Bilingual programs for Pre-K through 9th grade. All are available as single user up to 30 user site packages.

1721 Optimum Resources/Stickybear Software
1 Mathews Drive
Suite 107
Hilton Head Island, SC 29926
843-689-8000
FAX: 843-689-8008
info@stickybear.com
www.stickybear.com

Richard Hefter, President
Publisher of award-winning educational software for thirty years. Programs in use by millions of students nationwide.
$59.95

1722 Please Understand Me: Software Program and Books
Cambridge Educational
132 West 31st Street
17th Floor
New York, NY 10001
800-322-8755
FAX: 800-678-3633
custserv@films.com
www.films.com

209 pages BiAnnual
ISBN 0-927368-56-x

1723 Pond
WINGS for Learning
1600 Green Hills Rd
Scotts Valley, CA 95066-4981
831-426-2228
FAX: 831-464-3600

Ani Stocks, Owner
Software game that teaches pattern recognition and encourages observation, trial and error and the interpretation of data.

1724 Print, Play & Learn #1 Old Mac's Farm
Soft Touch Incorporated
12301 Central Ave NE Ste 205
P.O.Box 490215
Blaine, MN 55449-2352
763-862-2920
888-755-1402
FAX: 763-862-2922
support@marblesoft.com
www.marblesoft.com

Joyce Meyer, President
Once your students have completed Old Mac's Farm, let them use the fun off-computer activities to continue learning. Over 25 activities with 250 sheets you print. Board games, dot-to-dot drawings, word puzzles, make a scene, flash cards. Concentration, sentence strips, worksheets and much more are available for teachers to expand their teaching goals. This CD is full of activities to print and use.

1725 Print, Play & Learn #7: Sampler
Soft Touch
12301 Central Ave NE Ste 205
P.O.Box 490215
Blaine, MN 55449-2352
763-862-2920
888-755-1402
FAX: 763-862-2922
support@marblesoft.com
www.marblesoft.com

Joyce Meyer, President
Print, Play and Learn Sampler gives you over 200 activities organized by training, easy, medium and hard levels so you can ready to help your student advance. Activities cover a wide range of basic knowledge, including colors, shapes, numbers, letters and much, much more. Note: Requires Overlay Maker or Overlay Printer by IntelliTools and a color printer.

1726 Puzzle Power: Sampler
Soft Touch
12301 Central Ave NE Ste 205
P.O.Box 490215
Blaine, MN 55449-2352
763-862-2920
888-755-1402
FAX: 763-862-2922
support@marblesoft.com
www.marblesoft.com

Joyce Meyer, President
Puzzle Power - Sampler offers a variety of puzzles in different themes. Each theme puzzle is followed by a puzzle of one item in this category. For example, first solve a puzzle for occupations. Then, solve a puzzle that is a baker. The pictures are large, clear and easily identifiable.

1727 Puzzle Power: Zoo & School Days
Soft Touch
12301 Central Ave NE Ste 205
P.O.Box 490215
Blaine, MN 55449-2352
763-862-2920
888-755-1402
FAX: 763-862-2922
support@marblesoft.com
www.marblesoft.com

Joyce Meyer, President
Here is a program for all of our students who need puzzle skills, but cannot access commercial puzzles. Puzzle Power puzzles start with just two pieces and progress to 16 pieces. The pictures are large, clear and easily identifiable. Four different activities enable all students to be successful. Automatic Placement: the student just presses the switch or keyboard to place the pieces. Magnet Mouse: all the student needs to do is move the mouse and it drops into place.

1728 Rodeo
Soft Touch
12301 Central Ave NE Ste 205
P.O.Box 490215
Blaine, MN 55449-2352
763-862-2920
888-755-1402
FAX: 763-862-2922
support@marblesoft.com
www.marblesoft.com

Joyce Meyer, President
Rodeo action and familiar tunes for teens and preteens. Four activities invite students to learn, laugh, and sing as they go to the rodeo with up to six age-peer friends. Age-appropriate graphics with surprising animations reinforce the learning. The graphics are large and colorful, the melodies familiar, and the words descriptive of the action on the screen.

1729 Shop Til You Drop
Soft Touch
12301 Central Ave NE Ste 205
P.O.Box 490215
Blaine, MN 55449-2352
763-862-2920
888-755-1402
FAX: 763-862-2922
support@marblesoft.com
www.marblesoft.com

Joyce Meyer, President
Designed specifically for preteens and teens with moderate and severe disabilities, this program will become a staple for the classroom. The student goes shopping and can choose which outfits to put together. They may choose to purchase the outfit - of course, with mom's credit card. Another activity is a video arcade game about money. Shop 'Til You Drop can be adjusted from a single switch cause-and-effect program to row-and-column scanning to direct choice.

1730 Songs I Sing at Preschool
Soft Touch
12301 Central Ave NE Ste 205
P.O.Box 490215
Blaine, MN 55449-2352
763-862-2920
888-755-1402
FAX: 763-862-2922
support@marblesoft.com
www.marblesoft.com

Joyce Meyer, President
Songs I Sing at Preschool offers many options for the teacher and the student. Over the years, our software has used music because our students really respond to the sounds and rhythms of songs. Teachers select which songs to present, how many to present at one time and where to place each song on the overlay, keyboard or scan array.

1731 Stickybear Early Learning Activities
Optimum Resource
1 Mathews Drive
Suite 107
Hilton Head Island, SC 29926
843-689-8000
FAX: 843-689-8008
info@stickybear.com
www.stickybear.com

Richard Hefter, President
Two modes of play allow youngsters to learn through prompted direction or by the discovery method. Lively animation and sound keep attention levels high as children learn writing, counting, shapes, opposites and colors. Stickybear Early Learning Activities is bilingual, so youngsters can build skills in both English and Spanish. Pre-K to 1st grade. *$59.95*

1732 Stickybear Kindergarden Activities
Optimum Resource
1 Mathews Drive
Suite 107
Hilton Head Island, SC 29926
843-689-8000
FAX: 843-689-8008
info@stickybear.com
www.stickybear.com

Richard Hefter, President
This dynamic new multifaceted program covers a wide range of preschool skills that go far beyond the strictly academic. At Stickybear's house, children discover the alphabet, numbers, shapes, colors, plus - social skills, important safety messages and delightful off-screen activities that foster creativity. Over three hours of original music can be composed by a child and saved for future use. *$59.95*

1733 Stickybear Science Fair Light
Optimum Resource
1 Mathews Drive
Suite 107
Hilton Head Island, SC 29926
843-689-8000
FAX: 843-689-8008
info@stickybear.com
www.stickybear.com

Richard Hefter, President

The first in the new series of science-based programs Stickybear Science Fair Light presents a content rich environment which allows students in grades 7-12 to explore, experiment with and understand light and it's properties. The program presents experiments, both structured and free-form, which allow users to work with prisms, lenses, color mixing, optical illusions and more. *$59.95*

1734 Stickybear Town Builder
Optimum Resource
1 Mathews Drive
Suite 107
Hilton Head Island, SC 29926
843-689-8000
FAX: 843-689-8008
info@stickybear.com
www.stickybear.com
Richard Hefter, President
Children learn to read maps, build towns, take trips and use a compass in this simulation program. *$59.95*

1735 Stickybear Typing
Optimum Resource
1 Mathews Drive
Suite 107
Hilton Head Island, SC 29926
843-689-8000
FAX: 843-689-8008
info@stickybear.com
www.stickybear.com
Richard Hefter, President
Sharpen typing skills with three challenging activities: Stickybear Keypress, Stickybear Thump and Stickybear Stories. Pre-K to 5th. *$59.95*

1736 Storybook Maker Deluxe
Compass Learning
203 Colorado Street
Austin, TX 78701
512-478-9600
800-678-1412
866-586-7387
FAX: 619-622-7873
support@compasslearning.com
www.compasslearning.com
Eric Loeffel, President, CEO
Tammy Deal, VP, Human Resources
Eric Wasser, VP, Sales
Eileen Shihadeh, VP, Marketing
Using Storybook Maker Deluxe and their imaginations, students can create and publish stories filled with exciting graphics. Students can write stories and watch as the text appears in the setting they've chosen. Engaging sounds and music, plus lively animations, provide positive learning reinforcement throughout the program. *$44.95*

1737 Super Challenger
Electronic Courseware Systems
1713 S State St
Champaign, IL 61820-7258
217-359-7099
800-832-4965
FAX: 217-359-6578
support@ecsmedia.com
www.ecsmedia.com
Jodie Varner, Manager
G Peters, President
An aural-visual musical game that increases the player's ability to remember a series of pitches as they are played by the computer. The game is based on a 12-note chromatic scale, a major scale, and a minor scale. Each pitch is reinforced visually with a color representation of a keyboard on the display screen. Computer/software. *$39.95*

1738 Switch Basics
Soft Touch
12301 Central Ave NE Ste 205
P.O.Box 490215
Blaine, MN 55449-2352
763-862-2920
888-755-1402
FAX: 763-862-2922
support@marblesoft.com
www.marblesoft.com
Joyce Meyer, President
Discover whimsical animations and real life pictures while learning switch operations. Intriguing and humorous, nine different programs offer a multitude of learning experiences for all ages. Program options include: cause and effect, scanning, step scanning, row and column activities for one or two players. Watch the clouds roll away revealing African animals; visit the beauty salon or barber shop; work two to sixteen piece puzzles; or add swimming fish to a huge aquarium.

1739 Switch Interface Pro 5.0
Don Johnston
26799 West Commerce Drive
Volo, IL 60073
847-740-0749
800-999-4660
FAX: 847-740-7326
info@donjohnston.com
www.donjohnston.com
Don Johnston, Founder
Ruth Ziolkowski, President
Allows individuals with physical disabilities to access the computer. Five ports accommodate multiple switches and emulate everything from a single-click to a return. Consequently, individuals gain access to the widest variety of switch-accessible software available. It requires no software and can be used with both Windows and Macintosh computers. *$79.00*

1740 Teach Me Phonemics Series Bundle
SoftTouch
Ste 401
4300 Stine Rd
Bakersfield, CA 93313-2352
661-396-8676
877-763-8868
FAX: 661-396-8760
support@softtouch.com
www.funsoftware.com
Joyce Meyer, President
Roxanne Butterfield, Marketing
The Teach Me Phonemics Series Bundle includes one copy of each Teach Me Phonemics program - Initial, Medial, Final and Blends - four CD's in all.

1741 Teach Me Phonemics Super Bundle
SoftTouch
Ste 401
4300 Stine Rd
Bakersfield, CA 93313-2352
661-396-8676
877-763-8868
FAX: 661-396-8760
softtouch@funsoftware.com
www.funsoftware.com
Roxanne Butterfield, Marketing
Joyce Meyer, President
Teach Me Phonemics Super Bundle includes all 4 Teach Me Phonemics programs and all 4 Teach Me Phonemics overlay CD's - eight CD's in all.

1742 Teach Me Phonemics: Blends
SoftTouch
Ste 401
4300 Stine Rd
Bakersfield, CA 93313-2352
661-396-8676
877-763-8868
FAX: 661-396-8760
softtouch@funsoftware.com
www.funsoftware.com
Roxanne Butterfield, Marketing
Joyce Meyer, President

Teach Me Phonemics - Blends helps students explore words and hear the initial blend sounds. It features musical interludes and movement to engage the student. Teachers select the best combination options to motivate and engage the student. Options turn off and on the fly so you can quickly make changes to keep the student engaged.

1743   Teach Me Phonemics: Final
SoftTouch
Ste 401
4300 Stine Rd
Bakersfield, CA 93313-2352

661-396-8676
877-763-8868
FAX: 661-396-8760
softtouch@funsoftware.com
www.funsoftware.com

Roxanne Butterfield
Joyce Meyer, President
Teach me Phonemics - Final helps students explore words and hear the final sounds. It features musical interludes and movement to engage the student. Options turn off and on the fly so you can quickly make changes to keep the student engaged.

1744   Teach Me Phonemics: Initial
SoftTouch
12301 Central Ave NE
Ste 205
Blaine, MN 55434

763-755-1402
888-755-1403
FAX: 763-862-2920
sales@marblesoft.com
www.softtouch.com

Roxanne Butterfield, Marketing
Joyce Meyer, President
Teach Me Phonemics - Initial helps students explore the words and hear the initial sounds. It features musical interludes and movement to engage the student. Teachers select the best combination options to motivate and engage the student. Options turn off and on the fly so you can quickly make changes to keep the student engaged.

1745   Teach Me Phonemics: Medial
SoftTouch
12301 Central Ave NE
Ste 205
Blaine, MN 55434

763-755-1402
888-755-1403
FAX: 763-862-2920
sales@marblesoft.com
www.softtouch.com

Roxanne Butterfield, Marketing
Joyce Meyer, President
Teach Me Phonemics - Medial helps students explore the words and hear the medial sounds. It features musical interludes and movement to engage the student. Teachers select the best combination options to motivate and engage the student. Options turn off and on the fly so you can quickly make changes to keep the student engaged.

1746   Teach Me to Talk
Soft Touch
12301 Central Ave NE Ste 205
P.O.Box 490215
Blaine, MN 55449-2352

763-862-2920
888-755-1402
FAX: 763-862-2922
support@marblesoft.com
www.marblesoft.com

Joyce Meyer, President
The first activity Teach Me to Talk is used as a springboard for the student to learn to speak the word. There are 150 real pictures. When a picture is chosen, it appears on a clear background with musical interludes, movement, written word and spoken word. It culminates by morphing to the corresponding black and white Mayer-Johnson symbol. The second activity Story Time, takes some of these nouns and puts them in four line poetry. This helps students hear the word in the midst of a sentence.

1747   Teen Tunes Plus
Soft Touch
12301 Central Ave NE Ste 205
P.O.Box 490215
Blaine, MN 55449-2352

763-862-2920
888-755-1402
FAX: 763-862-2922
support@marblesoft.com
www.marblesoft.com

Joyce Meyer, President
Introduce switch use to older students with disabilities. Large interesting graphics, a variety of musical interludes, and surprising animations are combined with calm soothing music and beautiful pictures in the software specifically designed for preteens and teens with severe cognitive delays and/or physical disabilities, and older students learning to use a switch.

1748   There are Tyrannosaurs Trying on Pants in My Bedroom
Compass Learning
203 Colorado Street
Austin, TX 78701-3922

512-478-9600
800-678-1412
866-586-7387
FAX: 619-622-7873
support@compasslearning.com
www.compasslearning.com

Eric Loeffel, President, CEO
Tammy Deal, VP, Human Resources
Eric Wasser, VP, Sales
Eileen Shihadeh, VP, Marketing
In this popular story, Saturday chores turn into fun-filled frolicking when dinosaurs come for a visit. Sounds, music and animation make learning about phonics and vocabulary dyno-mite. *$34.95*

1749   Three Billy Goats Gruff
Compass Learning
203 Colorado Street
Austin, TX 78701-3922

512-478-9600
800-678-1412
866-586-7387
FAX: 619-622-7873
support@compasslearning.com
www.compasslearning.com

Eric Loeffel, President, CEO
Tammy Deal, VP, Human Resources
Eric Wasser, VP, Sales
Eileen Shihadeh, VP, Marketing
Motivating exercises and creative activities provide hours of learning fun while young students follow the adventure of The Three Billy Goats Gruff in this animated version of the timeless tale. *$ 34.95*

1750   Three Little Pigs
Compass Learning
203 Colorado Street
Austin, TX 78701-3922

512-478-9600
800-678-1412
866-586-7387
FAX: 619-622-7873
support@compasslearning.com
www.compasslearning.com

Eric Loeffel, President, CEO
Tammy Deal, VP, Human Resources
Eric Wasser, VP, Sales
Eileen Shihadeh, VP, Marketing
Help young students build reading comprehension and writing skills with this interactive version of the children's classic, The Three Little Pigs. Animated storytelling and creative activities inspire children to read, write and rhyme. *$34.95*

1751 TouchCorders
Soft Touch
12301 Central Ave NE Ste 205
P.O.Box 490215
Blaine, MN 55449-2352   763-862-2920
888-755-1402
FAX: 763-862-2922
support@marblesoft.com
www.marblesoft.com

Joyce Meyer, President
TouchCorders are the flexible and easy-to-use communicator designed by Jo Meyer and Linda Bidabe for reach classroom use. TouchCorders are sensitive to touch at every angle and give the student kinesthetic feedback. With the unique Add 'n Touch system, Jo connects the puzzles bases of 2 or more TouchCorders on the fly to present vocabulary, sequencing, story telling, social stories, concepts and other curriculum and communication opportunities.

1752 TouchWindow Touch Screen
Riverdeep Incorporated
100 Pine Street
Suite 1900
San Francisco, CA 94111   415-659-2000
800-542-4222
FAX: 415-659-2020
info@riverdeep.net
www.riverdeep.net

Barry O'Callaghan, Executive Chairman & Chief Executive Officer
Tony Mulderry, Executive Vice President, Corporate Development
Ciara Smyth, Executive Vice President, Global Business Operations
Scott Campbell, Executive Vice President, Strategic Sales
Software for children. *$335.00*

1753 Turtle Teasers
Soft Touch
12301 Central Ave NE Ste 205
P.O.Box 490215
Blaine, MN 55449-2352   763-862-2920
888-755-1402
FAX: 763-862-2922
support@marblesoft.com
www.marblesoft.com

Joyce Meyer, President
Three Games, Three Levels from Easy, Medium to Hard. The Shell Game - easy: Watch one of the three turtles get the tomato. Then watch carefully as they switch positions and pop shut. Choose incorrectly and the frog disappears until the correct one is displayed. The Pond - medium: Watch the tomato disappear somewhere in the pond scene. Tomato Dump - hard: Hit the shell and it turns into the tomato, giving a score. There are different difficulty levels to equalize all students.

1754 What Was That!
Compass Learning
203 Colorado Street
Austin, TX 78701-3922   512-478-9600
800-678-1412
866-586-7387
FAX: 619-622-7873
support@compasslearning.com
www.compasslearning.com

Eric Loeffel, President, CEO
Tammy Deal, VP, Human Resources
Eric Wasser, VP, Sales
Eileen Shihadeh, VP, Marketing
In this bedtime story, noises in the night send three brother bears scurrying out of bed. Thoughtful questions test young readers' comprehension, while games, voice recording, writing practice and other playful activities stimulate their creativity.

1755 Wivik 3
Prentke Romich Company
1022 Heyl Road
Wooster, OH 44691   330-262-1984
800-262-1984
FAX: 330-263-4829
info@prentrom.com
www.prentrom.com

David L Moffatt, President
On-screen keyboard provides access to any application in the latest Windows operating systems. Selections are made by clicking, dwelling or switch scanning. Enhancements include word prediction and abbreviation expansion.

1756 WordMaker
Don Johnston
26799 West Commerce Drive
Volo, IL 60073   847-740-0749
800-999-4660
FAX: 847-740-7326
info@donjohnston.com
www.donjohnston.com

Don Johnston, Founder
Ruth Ziolkowski, President
The computer version of Dr Patricia Cunningham's book 'Systematic Sequential Phonics They Use.' The program systematically builds spelling and word decoding skills for struggling readers and writers. *$79.00*

1757 Write: Out Loud
Don Johnston
26799 West Commerce Drive
Volo, IL 60073   847-740-0749
800-999-4660
FAX: 847-740-7326
info@donjohnston.com
www.donjohnston.com

Don Johnston, Founder
Ruth Ziolkowski, President
Write: Out Loud is an easy-to-use talking word processor that uses text-to-speech and revision and editing supports to help students write more effectively, more often and with more enthusiasm as they share creative thoughts on paper. *$79.00*

1758 You Tell Me: Learning Basic Information
Programming Concepts
8700 Shoal Creek Boulevard
Austin, TX 78757-6897   512-451-3246
800-897-3202
800-471-3000
FAX: 800-397-7633
general@proedinc.com
www.proedinc.com

Jeff McLane, Founder
Lee Wilson, President and CEO
Randy Pennington, Executive VP
David Keith, Vice President of IT
This game teaches and reinforces basic information all individuals need to know. Questions asked in this game help prepare people to communicate personal identification information important to community survival. *$49.95*

Software: Professional

1759 Acrontech International
5500 Main St
Williamsville, NY 14221-6755

FAX: 716-854-4014

1760 DPS with BCP
V OR T Corporation
P.O.Box G (George)
Menlo Park, CA 94026

650-322-8282
888-757-8678
FAX: 650-327-0747
custserv@vort.com
vort.com

Tom Holt, Owner
This program uses unique DPS branching techniques to access goals and objectives.

1761 Diagnostic Report Writer
Parrot Software
P.O. Box 250755
West Bloomfield, MI 48325

248-788-3223
800-727-7681
FAX: 248-788-3224
support@parrotsoftware.com
www.parrotsoftware.com

Dr. Frederic Weiner, Ph. D., CCC-SP, President, Owner
Creates a three page single-spaced diagnostic report for a child with a communication disorder from a list of questions; sections of the report include developmental and background history, oral peripheral exam, speech and language analysis, summary and recommendations.

1762 Discriptive Language Arts Development
Educational Activities Software
5600 West 83rd Street
Suite 300, 8200 Tower
Bloomington, MN 55437

888-351-4199
800-447-5286
FAX: 239-225-9299
info@edmentum.com
www.edmentum.com

Vin Riera, President/CEO
Dan Juckniess, SVP, Sales & Professional Services
Stacey Herteux, VP, Human Resources
Rob Rueckl, Chief Financial Officer
This multimedia language arts development program provides instruction and application of fundamental English skills and concepts. *$395.00*

1763 Draft: Builder
Don Johnston
26799 West Commerce Drive
Volo, IL 60073

847-740-0749
800-999-4660
FAX: 847-740-7326
info@donjohnston.com
www.donjohnston.com

Don Johnston, Founder
Ruth Ziolkowski, President
A software-based graphic organizer that breaks down the writing process into manageable chunks to structure planning, organizing, and draft-writing. *$79.00*

1764 EZ Dot
CAPCO Capability Corporation
3910 S. Union Court
Spokane Valley, WA 99206-6345

509-927-8195
800-827-2182
FAX: 800-827-2182
info@skilltran.com
www.skilltran.com

Jeff Truthan, President
A critical software tool used in vocational counseling, job restructuring, recruitment and placement, better utilization of workers, and safety issues. This software offers occupational data by title, code, industry, GEO, DPT, or OGA. *$295.00*

1765 EZ Keys for Windows
Words+
Ste 109
42505 10th St W
Lancaster, CA 93534-7059

661-723-6523
800-869-8521
FAX: 661-723-2114
info@words-plus.com
www.words-plus.com

Jean Dobbs, Editorial Director
Tim Gilmer, Editor
Josie Byzek, Managing Editor
Doug Lathrop, Senior Correspondent
A software and hardware product designed to operate on an IBM compatible PC. The software provides dual word prediction, abbreviation expansion, five different methods of voice output and access to commercial software applications. *$1395.00*

1766 Goals and Objectives
JE Stewart Teaching Tools
P.O.Box 15308
Seattle, WA 98115-308

206-262-9538
FAX: 206-262-9538

Jeff Stewart, Owner
Goals and Objectives software helps teachers make student plans including IEP's, IPP's and IHP's. The system provides curricula for all students and programs to develop and evaluate plans, print reports and make data forms. Systems are available for Windows and Macintosh for $139.

1767 Goals and Objectives IEP Program Curriculum Associates LLC
153 Rangeway Road
P.O.Box 2001
North Billerica, MA 01862-0901

978-667-8000
800-225-0248
FAX: 800-366-1158
www.curriculumassociates.com

Frank E. Ferguson, Chairman
Renee Foster, President & Publisher
Woody Palk, Senior Vice President, Sales
Robert Waldron, CEO
BRIGANCE CIBS-R standardized scoring conversion software, is a teacher's tool that prints goal and objective pages of the IEP. In less than two minutes per student, a teacher types student data into the computer.

1768 Nasometer
Kay Elemetrics Corporation
3 Paragon Drive
Montvale, NJ 07645

973-628-6200
800-289-5297
FAX: 201-391-2063
sales@kaypentax.com
www.kaypentax.com

John Crump, President
Steve Crump, Direct Sales
Measures the ratio of acoustic energy for the nasal and real-time visual cueing during therapy. Used clinically in the areas of cleft palate, motor speech disorders, hearing impairment and palatal prosthetic fittings.

1769 PSS CogRehab Software
Psychological Software Services
3304 W 75th St
Indianapolis, IN 46268-1664

317-257-9672
FAX: 317-257-9674
nsc@neuroscience.cnter.com
www.neuroscience.cnter.com

Odie L Bracy, Executive Director
PSS CogRehab Software is a comprehensive and easy-to-use multimedia cognitive rehabilitation software available, for clinical and educational use with head injury, stroke LD/ADD and other brain compromises. The packages include 64 computerized therapy tasks which contain modifiable parameters that will accommodate most requirements. Exercises include attention and

executive skills, multiple modalities of visuosatial and memory skills, simple, complex, problem-solving skills.
$260 - $2500

1770 Parrot Easy Language Simple Anaylsis
Parrot Software
P.O.Box 250755
West Bloomfield, MI 48325
248-788-3223
800-727-7681
FAX: 248-788-3224
support@parrotsoftware.com
www.parrotsoftware.com
Dr. Frederic Weiner, Ph. D., CCC-SP, President, Owner
Designed for grammatical analysis of language samples. The user types and translates language samples of up to 100 utterances.

1771 SOLO Literacy Suite
Don Johnston
26799 West Commerce Drive
Volo, IL 60073
847-740-0749
800-999-4660
FAX: 847-740-7326
info@donjohnston.com
www.donjohnston.com
Don Johnston, Founder
Ruth Ziolkowski, President
Places all of the right tools, and a wide-range of embedded learning supports, at their fingertips. SOLO includes word prediction, a text reader, graphic organizer and talking word processor, putting students in charge of their own learning and accommodations. Students of varying ages and abilities have access to, and make progress in, the general education curriculum. *$79.00*

1772 TOVA
Universal Attention Disorders
3321 Cerritos Avenue
Los Alamitos, CA 90720
562-594-7700
800-729-2886
FAX: 800-452-6919
info@tovatest.com
www.tovatest.com
Lawrence M. Greenberg, MD
A computerized assessment which, in conjunction with classroom behavior ratings, is a highly effective screening tool for ADD. TOVA includes software, complete instructions, and supporting data including norms.

1773 Visi-Pitch III
Kayelemetrics Corporation
3 Paragon Drive
Montvale, NJ 07645
973-628-6200
800-289-5297
FAX: 201-391-2063
sales@kaypentax.com
www.kaypentax.com
John Crump, President
Steve Crump, Direct Sales
Assists the speech/voice clinician in assessment and treatment tasks across an expansive range of disorders.

Software: Reading & Language Arts

1774 Choices, Choices 5.0
Tom Snyder Productions
100 Talcott Avenue
Watertown, MA 02472-5703
800-342-0236
Ask@tomsnyder.com
www.tomsnyder.com
Tom Snyder, Founder
Bridget Dalton, Ed.D, Author
Peggy Healy Stearns, Ph.D., Author
David Dockterman, Ed.D., Author
Teaches students to take responsibility for their behavior. Helps students develop the skills and awareness they need to make wise choices and to think through the consequences of their actions.

1775 Co: Writer
Don Johnston
26799 West Commerce Drive
Volo, IL 60073
847-740-0749
800-999-4660
FAX: 847-740-7326
info@donjohnston.com
www.donjohnston.com
Don Johnston, Founder
Ruth Ziolkowski, President
A software-based writing assistant that uses word prediction to cut through writing barriers and improve written expression. It is intended for students who struggle to write because of difficulty with spelling, syntax, and translating thoughts into writing. As students type, Co: Writer learns the context of the sentence and accurately 'predicts' words even when spelled phonetically or inventively. *$79.00*

1776 Community Exploration
Compass Learning
203 Colorado Street
Austin, TX 78701-3922
512-478-9600
800-678-1412
866-586-7387
FAX: 619-622-7873
support@compasslearning.com
www.compasslearning.com
Eric Loeffel, President, CEO
Tammy Deal, VP, Human Resources
Eric Wasser, VP, Sales
Eileen Shihadeh, VP, Marketing
An award-winning learning adventure takes students who are learning English as a second language on a field trip to the make-believe town of Cornerstone. More than 50 community locations come to life with sound and animation. While exploring places in this typical American community where people live, work and play, students also enhance important English language skills. Offers an exciting approach for any age student who needs to improve their English language proficiency. 4-12. *$19.95*

1777 Conversations
Educational Activities Software
5600 West 83rd Street
Suite 300, 8200 Tower
Bloomington, MN 55437
888-351-4199
800-447-5286
FAX: 239-225-9299
info@edmentum.com
www.edmentum.com
Vin Riera, President/CEO
Dan Juckniess, SVP, Sales & Professional Services
Stacey Herteux, VP, Human Resources
Rob Rueckl, Chief Financial Officer
Using American digitized voices, CONVERSATIONS provides 14 different dialogues in which the student can participate. The topics offer learners important information about American culture and the workplace. Available for DOS. *$195.00*

1778 Core-Reading and Vocabulary Development
Educational Activities
P.O.Box 87
Baldwin, NY 11510
516-223-4666
800-797-3223
FAX: 516-623-9282
learn@edact.com
www.edact.com
Alfred Harris, President
Carol Stern, VP
Students begin with 36 basic words and progress to more than 200. Reading and writing activities are coordinated and integrated throughout the program for more substantial permanent learning. Five units covering readability levels from pre-primer to grade three.
Full Program

1779 Friday Afternoon
203 Colorado Street
Austin, TX 78701-3922

512-478-9600
800-678-1412
866-586-7387
FAX: 619-622-7873
support@compasslearning.com
www.compasslearning.com

Eric Loeffel, President, CEO
Tammy Deal, VP, Human Resources
Eric Wasser, VP, Sales
Eileen Shihadeh, VP, Marketing

Save hours of preparation time and dazzle your students with interesting new activities to supplement their classroom learning. With Friday afternoon, you'll produce flash cards, word puzzles, even customized bingo cards and more, all at the click of a mouse. MacIntosh diskette. *$99.95*

1780 How to Read for Everyday Living
Educational Activities Software
5600 West 83rd Street
Suite 300, 8200 Tower
Bloomington, MN 55437

888-351-4199
800-447-5286
FAX: 239-225-9299
info@edmentum.com
www.edmentum.com

Vin Riera, President/CEO
Dan Juckniess, SVP, Sales & Professional Services
Stacey Herteux, VP, Human Resources
Rob Rueckl, Chief Financial Officer

Basic vocabulary and key words are taught and, when need, retaught using alternative teaching strategies. Passages that students read help put the vocabulary into context. Each lesson is followed by crossword and other puzzles check comprehension.

1781 Learning English: Primary
203 Colorado Street
Austin, TX 78701-3922

512-478-9600
800-678-1412
866-586-7387
FAX: 619-622-7873
support@compasslearning.com
www.compasslearning.com

Eric Loeffel, President, CEO
Tammy Deal, VP, Human Resources
Eric Wasser, VP, Sales
Eileen Shihadeh, VP, Marketing

Four stories and rhymes help students familiarize themselves with essential English language concepts, recognize patterns in language and associate words with objects. *$49.95*

1782 Learning English: Rhyme Time
Compass Learning
203 Colorado Street
Austin, TX 78701-3922

512-478-9600
800-678-1412
866-586-7387
FAX: 619-622-7873
support@compasslearning.com
www.compasslearning.com

Eric Loeffel, President, CEO
Tammy Deal, VP, Human Resources
Eric Wasser, VP, Sales
Eileen Shihadeh, VP, Marketing

Using classic children's rhymes in an animated multimedia program, students work on language skills, vocabulary and comprehension.

1783 Lexia I, II and III Reading Series
Lexia Learning Systems
200 Baker Ave Ext.
Concord, MA 01742

978-405-6200
800-435-3942
800-507-2772
FAX: 978-287-0062
info@lexialearning.com
www.lexialearning.com

Nick Gaehde, President and CEO
Paul More, Vice President, Finance
Collin Earnst, Vice President of Marketing
Peter Koso, Vice President of Operations

Lexia's software helps children and adults with learning disabilities master their core reading skills. Based on the Orton Gillingham method, Lexia Early Reading, Phonics Based Reading and SOS (Strategies for Older Students) apply phonics principles to help students learn essential sound-symbol correspondence and decoding skills. The Quick Reading Tests generate detailed skill reports in only 5-8 minutes per student to provide data for further instruction. Price: $40-400 per workstation.

1784 Memory Castle
WINGS for Learning
1600 Green Hills Rd
Scotts Valley, CA 95066-4981

831-426-2228
FAX: 831-464-3600

Ani Stocks, Owner

Introduces a strategy to increase memory skills via an adventure Q198game. Set in a castle, the game requires memory, reading, spelling skills and more to win.

1785 On a Green Bus: A UKanDu Little Book
Don Johnston
26799 West Commerce Drive
Volo, IL 60073

847-740-0749
800-999-4660
FAX: 847-740-7326
info@donjohnston.com
www.donjohnston.com

Don Johnston, Founder
Ruth Ziolkowski, President

This early literacy program that consists of several create-your-own 4-page animated stories that help build language experience on each page and then watch the page come alive with animation and sound. After completing the story, students can print it out to make a book which can be read over and over again. Because there are no wrong answers, all children can have a successful literacy experience. *$ 45.00*

1786 Open Book
Freedom Scientific
11800 31st Court North
St Petersburg, FL 33716

727-803-8000
800-444-4443
FAX: 727-803-8001
info@freedomscientific.com
www.freedomscientific.com

Lee Hamilton, President, CEO, and Chairman of
Mike Self, Sales Representative (Alabama)
Joseph McDaniel, Sales Representative (Alaska and
Bobby Lakey, Sales Representative (Arkansas)

Software that reads scanned text allowed and includes other features that aid the vision-impaired. *$995.00*

1787 Optimum Resource Software
1 Mathews Drive
Suite 107
Hilton Head Island, SC 29926

843-689-8000
FAX: 843-689-8008
info@stickybear.com
www.stickybear.com

Richard Hefter, President

Optimum Resource publishes over 100 K-12 education curriculum software titles under its varietal brands, StickyBear, MiddleWare, High School and Tools for Teachers. Most programs are available in Bilingual English/Spanish, and are offered with options for the single user through 30 users.

1788 Parts of Speech
Optimum Resource
1 Mathews Drive
Suite 107
Hilton Head Island, SC 29926
843-689-8000
FAX: 843-689-8008
info@stickybear.com
www.stickybear.com

Richard Hefter, President
Designed to help students build grammar and vocabulary as they strengthen reading and writing ability. Grades 3 to 9. *$59.95*

1789 Programs for Aphasia and Cognitive Disorders
Parrot Software
P.O.Box 250755
West Bloomfield, MI 48325
248-788-3223
800-727-7681
FAX: 248-788-3224
support@parrotsoftware.com
www.parrotsoftware.com

Dr. Frederic Weiner, Ph. D., CCC-SP, President, Owner
Over 50 different computer programs that facilitate language, memory and attention training. Programs are available for MS DOS, WINDOWS and Apple II.

1790 Punctuation Rules
Optimum Resource
1 Mathews Drive
Suite 107
Hilton Head Island, SC 29926
843-689-8000
FAX: 843-689-8008
info@stickybear.com
www.stickybear.com

Richard Hefter, President
Punctuation Rules is designed to help students improve their punctuation skills. Students work with appropriate level sentences which follow common rules of punctuation. The program covers material ranging from categories of sentences to forming possessives and allows students to gain strength in their ability to correctly use periods, commas, apostrophes, question marks, colons, hyphens, quotation marks, exclamation points and more. Grades 3-9. Bilingual. *$59.95*

1791 Quick Reading Test, Phonics Based Reading, Reading SOS (Strategies for Older Students)
Lexia Learning Systems
200 Baker Ave. Ext.
Concord, MA 01742
978-405-6200
800-435-3942
800-507-2772
FAX: 978-287-0062
info@lexialearning.com
www.lexialearning.com

Nick Gaehde, President and CEO
Paul More, Vice President, Finance
Collin Earnst, Vice President of Marketing
Peter Koso, Vice President of Operations
Lexia's software helps children and adults with learning disabilities master their core reading skills. Based on the Orton Gillingham method, Phonics Based Reading and S.O.S. (Strategies for the Older Student) apply phonics principles to help students learn essential sound-symbol correspondence and decoding skills. The Quick Reading Tests generate detailed phonemic skills reports in only 5-8 minutes per student to provide teachers with accurate data to focus their instruction. Price: $67-$500.

1792 Quick Talk
Educational Activities Software
5600 West 83rd Street
Suite 300, 8200 Tower
Bloomington, MN 55437
888-351-4199
800-447-5286
FAX: 239-225-9299
info@edmentum.com
www.edmentum.com

Vin Riera, President/CEO
Dan Juckniess, SVP, Sales & Professional Services
Stacey Herteux, VP, Human Resources
Rob Rueckl, Chief Financial Officer
Students will learn and use new vocabulary immediately: high-frequency, everyday vocabulary words are introduced and used contextually using human speech, graphics and text. Voice-interactive program (MS-DOS). *$65.00*

1793 Race the Clock
Mindplay
4400 E. Broadway Blvd
Suite 400
Tucson, AZ 85711
520-888-1800
800-221-7911
FAX: 520-888-7904
mail@mindplay.com
www.mindplay.com

Dan Figurski, Senior Vice President of Business
Chris Coleman, VP, Business Development
Judith Bliss, CEO
Brian Williams, Development Manager
A matching game, uses the animation capabilities to teach verbs. The player chooses a matching game from a menu.

1794 Read: Out Loud
Don Johnston
26799 West Commerce Drive
Volo, IL 60073
847-740-0749
800-999-4660
FAX: 847-740-7326
info@donjohnston.com
www.donjohnston.com

Don Johnston, Founder
Ruth Ziolkowski, President
An accessible text reader that provides access to the curriculum. It features high-quality text to speech and study tools that help students read with comprehension. *$79.00*

1795 Reader Rabbit
Learning Company
Ste 1900
100 Pine St
San Francisco, CA 94111-5205
415-659-2000
800-825-4420
FAX: 415-659-2020
thelearningco@hmhpub.com
www.thelearningcompany.com

Linda K. Zecher, President and CEO
Eric Shuman, Chief Financial Officer
John K. Dragoon, Executive Vice President and Chi
William Bayers, Executive Vice President and Gen
Supports young students in building fundamental reading readiness skills in a playful, multi-sensory environment.

1796 Reading Comprehension Series
Optimum Resource
1 Mathews Drive
Suite 107
Hilton Head Island, SC 29926- 3765
843-689-8000
FAX: 843-689-8008
info@stickybear.com
www.stickybear.com

Richard Hefter, President
The Reading Comprehension Series, includes seven volumes packed with intriguing multi-level stories. Each volume will capture the interest of children ages 8-14 while teaching them crucial reading comprehension skills. These open-ended programs are versatile and easy to use, and Bilingual. *$59.95*

1797 Simon SIO
Don Johnston
26799 West Commerce Drive
Volo, IL 60073
847-740-0749
800-999-4660
FAX: 847-740-7326
info@donjohnston.com
www.donjohnston.com

Don Johnston, Founder
Ruth Ziolkowski, President
A researched and widely field-tested phonics program for beginning readers, developed in collaboration with Dr. Ted Hasselbring of Vanderbilt University. The program uses a personal tutor to deliver individualized instruction and corrective feedback. *$79.00*

1798 Sound Sentences
Educational Activities Software
5600 West 83rd Street
Suite 300, 8200 Tower
Bloomington, MN 55437
888-351-4199
800-447-5286
FAX: 239-225-9299
info@edmentum.com
www.edmentum.com

Vin Riera, President/CEO
Dan Juckniess, SVP, Sales & Professional Services
Stacey Herteux, VP, Human Resources
Rob Rueckl, Chief Financial Officer
This sound-interactive program breaks away from traditional language instruction. Instead of formal concentration on verb and basic vocabulary, students meet everyday English with colloquialisms they will hear in real life situations. They reinforce their knowledge of sentence structure while acquiring the ability to communicate in daily settings. (For MAC, MS-DOS and Windows). *$65.00*

1799 Spelling Rules
Optimum Resource
1 Mathews Drive
Suite 107
Hilton Head Island, SC 29926- 3765
843-689-8000
FAX: 843-689-8008
info@stickybear.com
www.stickybear.com

Richard Hefter, President
A curriculum based, easy-to-use program that provides students with the practice they need to build strong spelling skills. Concepts discussed include plurals, compounds, i-before-e, capitalization, and more. Grades 3 to 9. Bilingual. *$59.95*

1800 Start-to-Finish Library
Don Johnston
26799 West Commerce Drive
Volo, IL 60073
847-740-0749
800-999-4660
FAX: 847-740-7326
info@donjohnston.com
www.donjohnston.com

Don Johnston, Founder
Ruth Ziolkowski, President
Offers struggling readers a wide selection of engaging narrative chapter books written at two readability levels (2-3rd and 4-5th grade) and delivered in three media formats. Professionally-narrated audio and computer supports help scaffold reading to ensure success. *$79.00*

1801 Start-to-Finish Literacy Starters
Don Johnston
26799 West Commerce Drive
Volo, IL 60073
847-740-0749
800-999-4660
FAX: 847-740-7326
info@donjohnston.com
www.donjohnston.com

Don Johnston, Founder
Ruth Ziolkowski, President
A reading series intended for students with multiple disabilities who are in 3-12th grade, but reading at a beginning level. Dr. Karen Erickson developed this series, which combines switch-accessible software with three types of text. *$79.00*

1802 Stickybear Reading Comprehension
Optimum Resource
1 Mathews Drive
Suite 107
Hilton Head Island, SC 29926- 3765
843-689-8000
FAX: 843-689-8008
info@stickybear.com
www.stickybear.com

Richard Hefter, President
This multi-level reading comprehension program helps children improve reading skills with 30 high-interest stories and question sets created by the Weekly Reader editors. Children learn to recognize main ideas, define sequence, using context to identify words, and more. Grades 2 to 4. Bilingual. *$59.95*

1803 Stickybear Reading Fun Park
Optimum Resource
1 Mathews Drive
Suite 107
Hilton Head Island, SC 29926- 3765
843-689-8000
FAX: 843-689-8008
info@stickybear.com
www.stickybear.com

Richard Hefter, President
Children discover and practice critical reading skills as the Stickybear family guides users through unique, action-packed activities, each with multiple levels of difficulty and skills that address both the auditory and visual needs of budding readers. Pre-K through 3rd grade. *$59.95*

1804 Stickybear Reading Room Deluxe
Optimum Resource
1 Mathews Drive
Suite 107
Hilton Head Island, SC 29926- 3765
843-689-8000
FAX: 843-689-8008
info@stickybear.com
www.stickybear.com

Richard Hefter, President
Children build vocabulary and reading comprehension skills using hundreds of word/picture sets and thousands of put-together sentence parts. K-3rd grade. Bilingual, English/Spanish. *$59.95*

1805 Stickybear Spelling
Optimum Resource
1 Mathews Drive
Suite 107
Hilton Head Island, SC 29926- 3765
843-689-8000
FAX: 843-689-8008
info@stickybear.com
www.stickybear.com

Richard Hefter, President
Children discover and practice critical spelling skills as they work with three unique action-packed activities, each with four graded levels of difficulty. The program is open-ended and teachers may add, change and modify the word lists for each individual. Stickybear Spelling contains more than 2000 recorded words. Levels may be set to allow students of different ages or abilities to compete effectively. Grades 2 through 4. *$59.95*

1806 Tomorrow's Promise: Language Arts
Compass Learning
13500 Evening Creek Drive North
Suite 600
San Diego, CA 92128
858-668-2586
866-475-0317
FAX: 858-408-2903
info@bridgepointeducation.com
www.bridgepointeducation.com

Andrew S. Clark, Founder, Chief Executive Officer
Diane Thompson, SVP, General Counsel
Charlene Dackerman, SVP, Human Resources
Daniel J. Devine, Executive Vice President & CFO

You'll strengthen students' grammar, usage and vocabulary skills and promote higher order thinking skills with this comprehensive Language Arts curriculum. It utilizes cross-curricular, thematic instruction engaging multimedia learning exercises that encourage writing, speaking and listening proficiency. Promotes higher order thinking skills. *$279.95*

1807 Tomorrow's Promise: Reading
Compass Learning
203 Colorado Street
Austin, TX 78701-3922   512-478-9600
                              800-678-1412
                              866-586-7387
                        FAX: 619-622-7873
              support@compasslearning.com
              www.compasslearning.com

Eric Loeffel, President, CEO
Tammy Deal, VP, Human Resources
Eric Wasser, VP, Sales
Eileen Shihadeh, VP, Marketing
This multimedia curriculum balances thematic, interactive exploration with core skills development, increasing your students' early reading proficiency, building a solid literacy foundation and fostering a lifelong love for reading. *$279.95*

1808 Tomorrow's Promise: Spelling
Compass Learning
203 Colorado Street
Austin, TX 78701-3922   512-478-9600
                              800-678-1412
                              866-586-7387
                        FAX: 619-622-7873
              support@compasslearning.com
              www.compasslearning.com

Eric Loeffel, President, CEO
Tammy Deal, VP, Human Resources
Eric Wasser, VP, Sales
Eileen Shihadeh, VP, Marketing
Lovable characters and engaging multimedia effects put young students on a fast-track to early spelling proficiency with fourteen activities and three games. A full year's instruction on each CD includes 30 world lists per grade, in story context, or create word lists to suit your needs. This program addresses students' multiple learning styles and rewards students as they progress through each stage of spelling skill acquisition. *$99.95*

1809 Vocabulary Development
Optimum Resource
1 Mathews Drive
Suite 107
Hilton Head Island, SC 29926- 3765   843-689-8000
                                      FAX: 843-689-8008
                                      info@stickybear.com
                                      www.stickybear.com

Richard Hefter, President
A featured program in the middle school series. Vocabulary Development is designed to help students increase vocabulary as they strengthen reading skills. Students relate their current knowledge of vocabulary to the context in which they discover an unfamiliar word. Utilizing a variety of contextual aids, this program illustrates synonyms, antonyms, prefixes, suffixes, homophones, multiple meanings and context clues, allowing students to apply experience and context. *$59.95*

1810 Whoops
Cornucopia Software
P.O.Box 6111
Albany, CA 94706   510-528-7000
                    supportstaff@practicemagic.com
                    www.practicemagic.com

Christina Morua, Manager
Checks spelling three ways. It checks words as they are typed, it checks an entire screen and highlights the errors and it reads ASCII text files from a disk and lists errors.

Software: Vocational

1811 Films Media Group
Infobase Publishing
132 W 31st St, 17th Floor
New York, NY 10001
                              800-322-8755
                        FAX: 800-678-3633
              custserv@factsonfile.com
              www.infobaselearning.com

Melinda Gallo, Senior Account Executive
Educational publisher of DVD programming for schools and libraries. *$64.86*

ISBN 0-927368-59-5

1812 Functional Literacy System
Conover Company
4 Brookwood Court
Appleton, WI 54914   920-231-4667
                              800-933-1933
                        FAX: 800-933-1943
              support@conovercompany.com
              www.conovercompany.com

Terry Schmitz, Founder and Owner
Mike , Vice President of Operations
Art Janowiak, Vice President of Sales
Assessment and skill building for basic functional literacy. This multimedia software program is adult in format and uses live action video taken in actual community settings to help learners become more capable of functioning independently. Twenty different programs are currently available. *$99.00*

1813 Learning Activity Packets
4 Brookwood Court
Appleton, WI 54914   920-231-4667
                              800-933-1933
                        FAX: 800-933-1943
              support@conovercompany.com
              www.conovercompany.com

Terry Schmitz, Founder and Owner
Mike , Vice President of Operations
Art Janowiak, Vice President of Sales
Demonstrates how basic academic skills relate to 30 major career areas. LAPs provide valuable diagnostics in applied academic applications and demonstrates to users the importance of academics as they relate to the workplace. Software. *$99.00*

1814 Microcomputer Evaluation of Careers & Academics (MECA)
Conover Company
4 Brookwood Court
Appleton, WI 54914   920-231-4667
                              800-933-1933
                        FAX: 800-933-1943
              support@conovercompany.com
              www.conovercompany.com

Terry Schmitz, Founder and Owner
Mike , Vice President of Operations
Art Janowiak, Vice President of Sales
A cost-effective, technology-based, career development system which provides users with opportunities to get their hands dirty. The MECA system utilizes work simulations and is built around common occupational clusters. Each cluster, or career area, consists of hands-on WORK SAMPLES which provide a variety of career exploration and assessment experiences, linked to LEARNING ACTIVITY PACKETS, which integrate basic academic skills into the career planning and placement process. $580-$1,070.

1815 OASYS
Vertek
12835 Bellevue-Redmond Road
Suite 310
Bellevue, WA 98005
425-455-9921
800-220-4409
FAX: 425-454-7264
sales@vertekinc.com
www.vertekinc.com

Debra Callahan, Sales Representative, Northern California
Tim Whitney, Sales Representative, Ohio, Michigan
Beverly Duncan, Sales Representative, Florida
Debbie Gordon, Sales Representative, Illinois
A software system that matches a person's skills and abilities to occupations and employers.

1816 Reading in the Workplace
Educational Activities Software
5600 West 83rd Street
Suite 300, 8200 Tower
Bloomington, MN 55437-585
888-351-4199
800-447-5286
FAX: 239-225-9299
info@edmentum.com
www.edmentum.com

Vin Riera, President/CEO
Dan Juckniess, SVP, Sales & Professional Services
Stacey Herteux, VP, Human Resources
Rob Rueckl, Chief Financial Officer
A job-based, reading software program using real-life problems and solutions to capture students' attention and improve their vocabulary and comprehension skills. Units include: automotive, clerical, health care and construction. *$295.00*

1817 Stickybear Typing
Optimum Resource
1 Mathews Drive
Suite 107
Hilton Head Island, SC 29926- 3765
843-689-8000
FAX: 843-689-8008
info@stickybear.com
www.stickybear.com

Richard Hefter, President
The award winning Stickybear Typing program allows users to sharpen typing skills and achieve keyboard mastery with three engaging and amusing multi-level activities. *$59.95*

1818 Work-Related Vocational Assessment Systems: Computer Based
Valpar International
P.O.Box 5767
Tucson, AZ 85703-767
262-797-0840
800-633-3321
FAX: 262-797-8488
sales@valparint.com
www.valparint.com

Neal Gunderson, President
Criterion-referenced to Department of Labor standards. Evaluate academic levels for reading, spelling, math and language, interests, personalities, cognitive and physical aptitudes.

1819 Workplace Skills: Learning How to Function on the Job
Programming Concepts
8700 Shoal Creek Boulevard
Austin, TX 78757-6897
512-451-3246
800-897-3202
FAX: 800-397-7633
general@proedinc.com
www.proedinc.com

Jeff McLane, Founder
Lee Wilson, President and CEO
Randy Pennington, Executive VP
David Keith, Vice President of IT
Offers parents and educators a functional means by which to discuss all aspects of finding and keeping a job. *$49.95*

Word Processors

1820 DARCI
Wes Test Engineering Corporation
810 Shepard Lane
Farmington, UT 84025
801-451-9191
FAX: 801-451-9393
webmail@westest.com
westest.com

Robert Lessmann, President
James Lynds
Provides transparent access to all computer functions by replacing the computer's keyboard with a smart joystick. *$975.00*

1821 Eye Relief Word Processing Software
SkiSoft Publishing Corporation
P.O.Box 364
Lexington, MA 02420-4
781-863-1876
info@skisoft.com
www.skisoft.com

Ken Skier, President
Cynthia Skier, CFO
Large-type word processing program for visually-impaired PC users. *$295.00*

1822 IntelliTalk
Intelli Tools
24 Prime Parkway
Natick, MA 01760
707-773-2000
800-547-6747
FAX: 707-773-2001
customerservice@cambiumtech.com
www.intellitools.com

Beth Davis, Director Sales Operations
Lori Castle, Supervisor
Arjan Khalsa, CEO
Talking word-processing program available for MacIntosh, Apple IIe, IBM compatible and Windows computers. *$39.95*

1823 Large Type
P.O.Box T
Hewitt, NJ 07421-2088
973-853-6585
800-736-2216
FAX: 928-832-2894
nire@theoffice.net
http://www.angelfire.com

Don Selwyn, Vice President
Rev. Tom Schwanda, President & Chairman
Robt. Fondiller, Ph.D., P.E, Vice President
Everett G. Ball, Treasurer
Display enlargement programs for visually impaired users. Consist of a variety of programs for different needs, ranging from basic to full-featured.

1824 Pegasus LITE
Words+
Ste 109
42505 10th St W
Lancaster, CA 93534-7059
661-723-6523
800-869-8521
FAX: 661-723-2114
info@words-plus.com
www.words-plus.com

Phil Lawrence, VP
Provides all of the strategies currently being used in AAC, from dynamic display color pictographic language, to dual-word prediction text language, in a single system. *$6995.00*

1825   Up and Running
Intelli Tools
24 Prime Parkway
Natick, MA 01760

707-773-2000
800-547-6747
FAX: 707-773-2001
customerservice@cambiumtech.com
www.intellitools.com

Beth Davis, Director Sales Operations
Lori Castle, Supervisor
Arjan Khalsa, CEO
Instantly use hundreds of popular commercial software programs with this custom collection of setups and overlays. *$69.95*

1826   Write: OutLoud
Don Johnston
26799 West Commerce Drive
Volo, IL 60073-9675

847-740-0749
800-999-4660
FAX: 847-740-7326
info@donjohnston.com
www.donjohnston.com

Don Johnston, Founder
Ruth Ziolkowski, President
The award-winning feasible and user friendly talking word processor with talking spell checker. Text-to-speech technology provides multi-sensory learning and positive reinforcements for writers of all ages and ability levels. *$99.00*

Conferences & Shows

General

1827 AACRC Annual Meeting
American Assn. of Children's Residential Centers
11700 W Lake Park Drive
Milwaukee, WI 53224-3021

877-332-2272
FAX: 877-362-2272
info@aacrc-dc.org
www.aacrc-dc.org

Christopher Bellonci, M.D., Past President
Laurah Currey, MA, LSW, LPC, President Elect
Gayle Wiler, Director
Joseph Whalen, Director
One-day program that addresses accreditation as it relates to current behavioral health care challenges held in Pasadena, CA.
October

1828 AADB National Conference
American Association of the Deaf-Blind
PO Box 8064
Silver Spring, MD 20907-8064

301-563-9064
FAX: 301-495-4404
TTY:301-495-4402
aadb-info@aadb.org
www.aadb.org

Jill Gaus, President
Randall Pope, President, Maryland
Lynn Jansen, Vice President
Adam Drake, Treasurer
A week of general meetings, workshops, tours and evening recreational activities.

1829 AAIDD Annual Meeting
American Association on Mental Retardation
501 3rd Street
NW Suite 200
Washington, DC 20001

202-387-1968
800-424-3688
FAX: 202-387-2193
maria@aaidd.org
www.aamr.org

James R. Thompson, PhD, President
Amy S. Hewitt, PhD, President Elect
Susan B. Palmer, PhD, Vice President
Patti N. Martin, Secretary, Treasurer
At The Crossroads: Ethics, Genetics, Leadership and self-determination, this annual meeting offers a full compliment of workshops, symposia, and multiperspective sessions that fill four days including social events.
May/June

1830 AAO Annual Meeting
American Academy Of Opthamology
655 Beach Street
San Francisco, CA 94109-1336

415-561-8500
FAX: 415-561-8567
faao@aao.org
www.faao.org

Brad A. Wong, Executive Director
Shawn C. Fallon, Director, Administration
Todd Lyckberg, Director of Development
Jenny E. Benjamin, Director
Offers the most comprehensive program with more than 2000 scientific presentations and six subspecialty day programs
October

1831 ABD Winter Conference
American Board of Disability Analysts
Belle Meade Office Park, 4525 Hardi
Second Floor
Nashville, TN 37205

615-327-2984
FAX: 615-327-9235
americanbd@aol.com
www.americandisability.org

Alexander Horowitz, MD, ABDA, Executive Officer Emeritus
Kenneth Anchor, Ph.D., ABPP, Administrative Offices
Dana Adair, MS, RN, C (ABDA, Professional Advisory Council
Francella W. Betancourt, MA, CRC (A, Professional Advisory Council
Joint Conference: American Board of Disability.
February

1832 ACA Annual Conference
American Counseling Association
5999 Stevenson Ave
Alexandria, VA 22304

703-823-9800
800-347-6647
FAX: 800-473-2329
webmaster@counseling.org
www.counseling.org

Robert L. Smith, President
Thelma Duffey, President Elect
Brian Canfield, Treasurer
Richard Yep, CEO
Promotes the development of professional counselors, advancing the counseling profession, and using the profession and practice of counseling to promote respect for human dignity and diversity.
March/April

1833 ACB Annual Convention
American Council for the Blind
2200 Wilson Boulevard
Suite 650
Arlington, VA 22201-3354

202-467-5081
800-424-8666
FAX: 703-465-5085
info@acb.org
www.acb.org

Kim Charlson, President
Mitch Pomerantz, Immediate Past President
Jeff Thom, First Vice President
Marlaina Lieberg, Second Vice President
Offers 50-75 booths of information for the blind.
June/July

1834 ADA Annual Scientific Sessions
American Diabetes Association
1701 North Beauregard St
Alexandria, VA 22311

703-549-1500
800-342-2383
FAX: 703-836-7439
webmaster@diabetes.org
www.diabetes.org

Don Laing, Senior Vice President, Human Resources
Rodney Sampson, Senior Vice President, Chief Technology Officer
Lois A. Witkop, MBA, Senior Vice President, Marketing Communications
Shereen Arent, Executive Vice President, Government Affairs & Advocacy
Trade show featuring exhibits of equipment and supplies used by professionals involved in the treatment of diabetes.

1835 AER Annual International Conference
Assoc. for Educ. & Rehab of the Blind/Vis. Imp.
1703 N Beauregard Street
Suite 440
Alexandria, VA 22311
703-671-4500
877-492-2708
FAX: 703-671-6391
aer@aerbvi.org
www.aerbvi.org

Jim Adams, President
Lou Tutt, Executive Director
Ginger Croce, Senior Director, Marketing & Office Operations
Barbara James, Director, Membership & Office Operations
Dedicated to rendering support and assistance to the professionals who work in all phases of education and rehabilitation of blind and visually impaired children and adults.
July

1836 AG Bell Convention
Alexander Graham Bell Association
3417 Volta Place, NW
Washington, DC 20007
202-337-5220
FAX: 202-337-8314
TTY:202-337-5221
info@agbell.org
www.listeningandspokenlanguage.org

Meredith K. Sugar, Esq. (OH), President
Donald M. Goldberg, Immediate Past President
Ted A. Meyer, President-Elect, Secretary, Treasurer
Emilio Alonso Mendoza (DC), Chief Executive Officer
Over 60 booths offering information on resources and technology for the deaf and hard of hearing.
June

1837 AHEAD
Association on Higher Education And Disability
107 Commerce Centre Drive
Suite 204
Huntersville, NC 28078
704-947-7779
FAX: 704-948-7779
information@ahead.org
www.ahead.org

Stephan J. Smith, Executive Director
Richard Allegra, Director, Professional Development
Jeremy Jarrell, Director, Innovation & Development
Oanh Huynh, Associate Executive Director
AHEAD is a professional membership organization for individuals involved in the development of policy and in the provision of quality services to meet the needs of persons with disabilities involved in all areas of higher education.
July

1838 APSE Conference: Revitalizing Supported Employment, Climbing to the Future
Association for Persons in Supported Employment
416 Hungerford Dr.
Suite 418
Rockville, MD 20850
301-279-0060
FAX: 301-279-0075
jenny@apse.org
www.apse.org

David Hoff, President
Laura A. Owens, Ph.D., Executive Director
Jenny Levet, Communications/Membership Director
Boshia McRoy, Administrative Associate
A major conference on Supported Employment. The conference includes 130 sessions presented by nationally recognized leaders in the field. Conference attendees come from all 50 states, Canada and several foreign countries and include professionals in supported employment, occupational therapy, rehabilitation technology and other related fields.
July

1839 ASHA Convention
American Speech-Language-Hearing Association
2275 Research Blvd
Suite 500
Rockville, MD 20850
646-328-2552
800-638-8255
FAX: 301-296-8580
TTY: 301-897-5700
convention@asha.org
www.synutra.com

Liang Zhang, Chairman of the Board and Chief Executive Officer
Weiguo Zhang, President
Ning Clare Cai, Chief Financial Officer
Lei Lin, Director
Exhibits by companies specializing in alternative and augmentative communication products, publishers, software and hardware companies, and hearing aid testing equipment manufacturers. Speech-Language Pathologists are professionals who identify, assess, and treat speech and language problems. Audiologists are hearing health care professionals who specialize in preventing, identifying and assessing hearing disorders as well as providing audiologic treatment including hearing aids and more.
November

1840 ASIA Annual Scientific Meeting
American Spinal Injury Association
2020 Peachtree Rd NW
Atlanta, GA 30309-1426
404-355-9772
FAX: 404-355-1826
ASIA_Office@shepherd.org
www.asia-spinalinjury.org

Lesley M Hudson MA, Executive Director
Patricia Duncan, Administrative Coordinator
Professional association for physicans and other health professionals working in all aspects of spinal cord injury. Also holds an annual scientific that surveys the latest advancements in the field.
May

1841 ATIA Conference
Assistive Technology Industry Association
330 N Wabash Ave
Ste 2000
Chicago, IL 60611-4267
312-321-5172
877-687-2842
FAX: 312-673-6659
info@atia.org
atia.org

Daniel Hubbell, Board President
David Wu, Treasurer
Tara Rudnicki, Secretary
The ATIA Conference is the largest international conference showcasing excellence in assistive technology.

1842 Abilities Expo
16501 Ventura Blvd
Ste 1510
Encino, CA 91436
310-405-1317
FAX: 424-238-6358
info@abilities.com
abilities.com/expos

David Korse, President & CEO
Abilities Expo is a national event for people with disabilities, their families, caregivers, and healthcare professionals. Meets in Chicago, Houston, Boston, Bay Area, Los Angeles, New York, and Toronto.

1843 American Academy for Cerebral Palsy and Developmental Medicine Annual Conference
555 East Wells
Suite 1100
Milwaukee, WI 53202
414-918-3014
FAX: 414-276-2146
info@aacpdm.org
www.aacpdm.org

Richard Stevenson, MD, President
Darcy Fehlings, MD MSc FRCPC, First Vice President
Eileen Fowler, PhD PT, Second Vice President
Joshua Hyman, MD, Treasurer

The Annual Meeting is a 3-day event, held in the Fall, designed to provide targeted opportunities for dissemination of information in the basic sciences, prevention, diagnosis, treatment, and technical advances as applied to persons with cerebral palsy and development disorders.
September

1844   American Board of Disability Analysts Annual Conference
Disability Analyst
Belle Meade Office Park, 4525 Hardi
Second Floor
Nashville, TN 37205
615-327-2984
FAX: 615-327-9235
americanbd@aol.com
www.americandisability.org
Alexander Horowitz, MD, ABDA, Executive Officer Emeritus
Kenneth Anchor, Ph.D., ABPP, Administrative Offices
Dana Adair, MS, RN, C (ABDA, Professional Advisory Council
Francella W. Betancourt, MA, CRC (A, Professional Advisory Council
Annual conference held for members to meet and discuss current events and attend seminars.

1845   Annual Conference on Dyslexia and Related Learning Disabilities
New York Branch International Dyslexia Association
71 West 23rd Street
Suite 1527
New York, NY 10010
212-691-1930
FAX: 212-633-1620
info@everyonereading.org
www.everyonereading.org
Jo Anne Simon, P.C., President
Leonard Gubar, Esq., Treasurer
Lavinia Mancuso, Interim Administrative Director
Jo Anne Lense, Director, Professional Development
Provides educational support services to people concerned and affected by dyslexia and related learning disabilities.
March

1846   Annual TASH Conference, The
TASH
2013 H Street NW
Washington, DC 20006
202-540-9020
FAX: 202-540-9019
info@tash.org
tash.org/conferences-events
Ruthie Marie Beckwith, Executive Director
Dawn Brown, Development Director
Edwin Canizalez, Director, Operations & Change Management
Bethany Alvar,, Advocacy Communications Manager
Each year, the TASH Conference strengthens the disability field by connecting attendees to innovative information and resources, facilitating connections between stakeholders within the disability movement, and helping attendees reignite their passion for an inclusive world.

1847   Arc National Convention, The
The Arc
1825 K Street NW
Ste 1200
Washington, DC 20006
202-534-3700
800-433-5255
FAX: 202-534-3731
info@thearc.org
convention.thearc.org
Laura Schroeder, Sponsorship
Dawn Cooper, Program
C.T. Turner, Accessibility
Join the global conversation as people from all over the world share best practices, struggles, successes and hopes for the future, and continue the conversation about protecting and promoting the human and civil rights for individuals with intellectual and developmental disabilities - both in the U.S. and internationally.

1848   Attention Deficit Disorders Association, Southern Region: Annual Conference
12345 Jones Road
Suite 287-7
Houston, TX 77070
281-897-0982
FAX: 281-894-6883
addaoffice@sbcglobal.net
www.adda-sr.org
Laura Peddicord, President
Pam Esser, Executive Director
Opal Harris, Secretary
Tina Peden, Office Manager
Mission is to: provide a resource network; to support individuals impacted by attention deficit disorders; and to advocate for the development of community resources and services that meet the educational, social, and health care needs of all individuals with ADD/ADHD.
February

1849   Believable Hope Conference
United Cerebral Palsy Association
Ste 700
1660 L St NW
Washington, DC 20036-5638
202-776-0414
800-872-5827
FAX: 202-776-0414
TTY: 202-973-7197
info@ucp.org
www.ucpa.org
Stephen Bennett, CEO
National, not-for-profit self-help organization dedicated to providing information and support to individuals with cerebral palsy and other disabilities, and their families. Supports more than 160 local affiliates; these affiliates provide a variety of programs and services for affected families, including support groups. Offers several educational and support materials, including a quarterly magazine, regular newsletters, and research reports.

1850   Blazing Toward a Cure Annual Conference
National Parkinson Foundation
1150 NW 72 Ave.
Suite 760
Miami, FL 33126
305-592-9954
800-327-4545
FAX: 305-477-7379
info@acfm-cpa.com
www.acfm-cpa.com
Daniel Arty, Partner
Joel L. Moskowits, Partner
Julia Alemany, Audit Manager
Lester Feuer
Purpose is to find the cause and cure for Parkinson's Disease and related neurodegenerative disorders through research, education and dissemination of current information to patients, caregivers and families.
July/August

1851   Blind Childrens Center Annual Meeting
Blind Childrens Center
4120 Marathon Street
Los Angeles, CA 90029-3584
323-664-2153
800-222-3567
FAX: 323-665-3828
Info@blindchildrenscenter.org
www.blindchildrenscenter.org
Midge Horton, Executive Director
Muriel Scharf, Director of Development
Jennifer Brown, President
Kristin Dark, Director
A family-centered agency which serves children with visual impairments from birth to school-age. The center-based and home-based services help the children to acquire skills and build their independence. The Center utilizes its expertise and experience to serve families and professionals worldwide through support services, education and research.
September

1852 Blinded Veterans Association National Convention
Blinded Veterans Association
477 H Street
Northwest Washington, DC 20001-2694
                                    202-371-8880
                                    800-669-7079
                                    FAX: 202-371-8258
                                    bva@bva.org
                                    www.bva.org

Mark Cornell, National President
Robert Dale Stamper, National Vice President
Paul Mimms, National Treasurer
Joe Parker, National Secretary
Conventions have a three-fold purpose, to conduct Association business, to educate blinded veterans about the resources available to them, and to provide a means whereby blinded veterans can better strengthen and help one another.
August

1853 CQL Accreditation
Council on Quality and Leadership
100 West Road
Suite 300
Towson, MD 21204
                                    410-583-0060
                                    FAX: 410-583-0063
                                    info@thecouncil.org
                                    www.c-q-l.org

Cathy Ficker Terrill, President and CEO
Tammi Watkins, Vice President, Operations
Kerri Melda, Vice President, Research & Product Development
Becky Hansen, Vice President, Accreditation & Training
Prepares you for CQL Accreditation, addressing Shared Values, Basic Assurances®, Personal Outcomes, Service Responsiveness and Commitment to Community Life.

1854 Closing the Gap's Annual Conference
Assist. Tech. Resources for Children & Adults
526 Main Street
P.O.Box 68
Henderson, MN 56044
                                    507-248-3294
                                    FAX: 507-248-3810
                                    info@closingthegap.com
                                    www.closingthegap.com

Dolores Hagen, Co-Founder
Budd Hagen, Co-Founder
Connie Kneip, Vice President/General Manager
Megan Turek, Managing Editor/Advertising and Exhibit Sales
Topics cover a broad spectrum of technology as it is being applied to all disabilities and age groups in education, rehabilitation, vocation and independent living. People with disabilities, special educators, rehabilitation professionals, administrators, service/care providers, personnel managers, government officials, and hardware/software developers share their experiences and insights at this significant networking experience.
October

1855 Council for Exceptional Children Annual Convention and Expo
2900 Crystal Drive
Suite 1000
Arlington, VA 22202-3557
                                    703-620-3660
                                    866-509-0218
                                    888-232-7733
                                    FAX: 703-264-9494
                                    TTY:866-915-5000
                                    service@cec.sped.org
                                    www.cec.sped.org

Robin D. Brewer, President
James P. Heiden, President Elect
Christy A. Chambers, Immediate Past President
Mikki Garcia, Executive Director
Works to improve the educational success of children with disabilities and/or gifts and talents.
April

1856 Disability Matters
Springboard Consulting
14 Glenbrook Dr
Mendham, NJ 07945
                                    973-813-7260
                                    FAX: 973-813-7261
                                    info@consultspringboard.com
                                    www.consultspringboard.com

Nadine Vogel, Chief Executive Officer
Ivette Lopez, Chief of Staff & Chief Operations Officer
Troy Balthazor, Manager, Physical Accessibility
Rubiana Duerte, Manager, Global Events
Features outstanding content as delivered by leading disability experts from corporations, academia, national non-profits and governments across North America. Conferences also take place in Europe and Asia-Pacific.

1857 Eye Bank Association of America Annual Meeting
Eye Bank Association of America
1015 18th Street, NW
Suite 1010
Washington, DC 20036
                                    202-775-4999
                                    FAX: 202-429-6036
                                    malene@restoresight.org
                                    www.restoresight.org

Kevin Corcoran, CAE, President / CEO
Molly Georgakis, Vice-President of Member Services
Bernie Dellario, Director of Finance
Jennifer DeMatteo, Director of Regulations and Standards
A four day program, which includes a series of presentations in administrative, hospital development, scientific and technical fields that are relative to eye banking.
June

1858 IDF National Conference
Immune Deficiency Foundation
40 West Chesapeake Avenue
Suite 308
Towson, MD 21204
                                    410-321-6647
                                    800-296-4433
                                    FAX: 410-321-9165
                                    idf@primaryimmune.org
                                    www.primaryimmune.org

Marcia Boyle, President & Founder
Katherine Antilla, Vice President, Education & Volunteers
Christine Belser, Vice President, Programs & Communications
Lawrence A. LaMotte, Vice President, Public Policy
World-renowned immunologists will share their time and expertise with families. Attendees will learn about scientific advancements in the diagnosis and treatment of these diseases and gain skills needed to manage their healthcare.
June

1859 Joint Conference with ABMPP Annual Conference
American Board of Disability Analysts
Belle Meade Office Park, 4525 Hardi
Second Floor
Nashville, TN 37205
                                    615-327-2984
                                    FAX: 615-327-9235
                                    americanbd@aol.com
                                    www.americandisability.org

Alexander Horowitz, MD, ABDA, Executive Officer Emeritus
Kenneth Anchor, Ph.D., ABPP, Administrative Offices
Dana Adair, MS, RN, C (ABDA, Professional Advisory Council
Francella W. Betancourt, MA, CRC (A, Professional Advisory Council
Joint Conference with ABMPP Annual Conference Charleston, South Carolina.
May

1860 Lowe's Syndrome Conference
Lowe's Syndrome Association
PO Box 864346
Plano, TX 75086-4346   972-733-1338
                                          FAX: 612-866-3222
                                          info@lowesyndrome.org
                                          www.lowesyndrome.org

Debbie Jacobs, President
Jane Gallery, Treasurer
Fiona Fisher, Secretary
Christine Knight, Board Member and Director
An international conference held approximately every two years
where family, friends, medical and other professionals gather to
exchange ideas and information.
June

1861 NACDD Annual Conference
1825 K Street NW
Suite 600
Washington, DC 20006   202-506-5813
                                          info@nacdd.org
                                          www.nacdd.org

1862 NADD
National Association for the Dually Diagnosed
132 Fair St
Kingston, NY 12401-4802   845-331-4336
                                          800-331-5362
                                          FAX: 845-331-4569
                                          info@thenadd.org
                                          www.thenadd.org

Robert Fletcher, CEO
NADD is a non-for-profit membership organization designed to
promote awareness of, and services for, individuals who have
co-occuring intellectual disability and mental illness. NADD
provides training, consultation services, and publishes journals
and books.
November

1863 NADR Conference
PO Box 96503 #30550
Washington, DC 20090-6503   202-822-2155
                                          800-747-6131
                                          FAX: 972-245-6701
                                          www.nadr.org

Robert McDowell, President
Steven Skinner, Vice President
Philip Litteral, Secretary
Michael Wener, Treasurer
For many years, Professional Social Security Claimants Repre-
sentatives have wanted to have an organization that would be in-
terested in their issues, educational opportunities, and interests.
In March of 2000, 35 Professional Social Security Claimants
Representatives met in St. Louis, MO and formed NADR, Inc.

**1864 NASPAC Annual Conference Association Annual
Convention/Expo**
National Assoc. of Subacute and Post Acute Care
P.O.Box 65085
Washington, DC 20035-5085   202-429-2700
                                          FAX: 202-429-2701
                                          www.naspac.net

Lyle Williams, President
Totally dedicated to servicing the subacute arena and its major en-
tities. Features 100+ booths and over 75 exhibitors.
March

1865 NASW-NYS Chapter
NASW
188 Washington Ave
Albany, NY 12210   518-463-4741
                                          800-724-6279
                                          FAX: 518-463-6446
                                          info@naswnys.org
                                          www.naswnys.org

Peter Chernack, DSW, LCSW-R, President
Diane Bessel Matteson, Ph.D., Vice President
Brian Masciadrelli, Ph.D., Treasurer
Karen Rich, PhD, LCSW, Secretary
Workshops, keynote speakers, and presentations offered at this
event will develop and enhance practice skills and knowledge in
the provision of quality mental health and community services.
March

1866 National Council on the Aging Conference
Conference Department
1901 L Street, NW
4th Floor
Washington, DC 20036   202-479-1200
                                          800-424-9046
                                          800-677-1116
                                          FAX: 202-479-0735
                                          TTY:202-479-6674
                                          membership@ncoa.org
                                          www.ncoa.org

James P Firman, EdD, President and CEO
Donna Whitt, Senior Vice President, Chief Financial Officer
Wendy Zenker, Vice President, Public and Private Partnerships
Ramsey Alwin, Vice President, Economic Security
Offers ideas and programs to increase program and administra-
tive skills through NCOA's professional development tracks and
offering of continuing education units.
May

1867 PVA Summit & Expo
Paralyzed Veterans Of America
801 Eighteenth St NW
Washington, DC 20006-3517
                                          800-424-8200
                                          TTY:8007954327
                                          summit@pva.org
                                          summitpva.org

1868 PWSA (USA) Conference
Prader-Willi Alliance Of New York
244 5th Avenue
Suite D-110
New York, NY 10001   718-846-6606
                                          800-442-1655
                                          FAX: 914-312-0142
                                          alliance@prader-willi.org
                                          www.prader-willi.org

Amy McDougall, President, Fulton
Hon. Daniel Angiolillo, President Emeritus, Director, W. Harrison
Rachel Johnson, Vice President, Endicott
Nancy Finegold, Vice President, W. Hempstead
Through conferences, publications, electronic communication
and networking (parent-to-parent, parent-to professional, and
professional-to-professional), the Prader-Willi Alliance pro-
vides a valuable resource for individuals and families sharing the
same concerns.
July

**1869 Pacific Rim International Conference onDisability And
Diversity**
171F - 1410 Lower Campus Rd
Honolulu, HI 96822   808-956-7539
                                          FAX: 808-956-4437
                                          cccrocke@hawaii.edu
                                          www.pacrim.hawaii.edu

Charmaine Crockett, Conference Organizer
Leslie Dorman, Registration Support
The Pacific Rim International Conference on Disability and Diversity, considered one of the most diverse gatherings in the
world, encourages and respects voices from diverse perspective

across numerous areas including voices from persons representing all disability areas, and experiences of family members and supporters across all disability and diversity areas.

1870   RESNA Annual Conference
Rehab Engineering & Assistive Tech. North America
1700 North Moore Street
Suite 1540
Arlington, VA 22209
703-524-6686
FAX: 703-524-6630
TTY:703-524-6639
conference@resna.org
www.resna.org

Alex Mihailidis, Ph.D, P.En, President
Jerry Weisman, Immediate Past-President
Ray Grott, ATP, RET, President Elect
Paul J. Schwartz, Treasurer
Sponsored by a multidisciplinary association for the advancement of rehabilitation and assistive technologies, this annual conference brings together a large number of rehabilitation professionals, products and services from around the world and has something to offer for both professionals and consumers. The conference provides an informative and thought provoking forum for anyone with interests in rehabilitation technology.
June

1871   Rehabilitation International
25 East 21st Street,
4th floor
New York, NY 10010-6207
212-420-1500
FAX: 212-505-0871
ri@riglobal.org
riglobal.org

Venus Ilagan, Manager
RI is a global network of people with disabilities, service providers, researchers, government agencies, and advocates protecting and promoting the rights and inclusion of people with disabilities. RI has over 1,000 member organizations in all regions on the world.

1872   Rehabilitation Technology Association Conference
PO Box 1004
Institute, WV 25112-1004
304-766-4602
800-624-8284
FAX: 304-766-2689

Betty Jo Tyler, RTA Coordinator
Dave Whipp, Information Manager
RTA holds this annual conference for the rehab technology community. It also publishes a quarterly newsletter and houses the Project Enable computerized bulletin board system.
Spring

1873   Source-APTA Audio Conference
American Physical Therapy Association
1111 North Fairfax Street
Alexandria, VA 22314-1488
703-684-2782
800-999-2782
FAX: 703-706-8536
TTY: 703-683-6748
consumer@apta.org
apta.org

Paul Rockar, Jr, PT, DPT, M, President
Sharon L. Dunn, PT, PhD, OCS, Vice President
Laurita M. Hack, Secretary
Elmer Platz, PT, Treasurer
The American Physical Therapy Association (APTA), a national professional organization representing more than 66,000 members, sponsors this annual conference. The goal is to foster advancements in physical therapy practice, research, and education.

1874   Southwest Conference On Disability
University of New Mexico
2300 Menaul Blvd NE
Albuquerque, NM 87107
505-272-2990
FAX: 505-272-9594
hsc-swdisabilityconference@salud.unm.edu
cdd.unm.edu/swconf/

Dr. Anthony Cahill, Conference Director
Bev Nagy, Disability & the Arts Program
Reducing disparities for people with disparities through systems change.

1875   TSA National Conference
Tourette Syndrome Association
42-40 Bell Boulevard
Bayside, NY 11361
718-224-2999
800-237-0717
FAX: 718-279-9596
ts@tsa-usa.org
www.tsa-usa.org

Judit Unger, President
Gary Frank, Executive VP
More than 400 attendees come together for this biennial conference that includes members of the TS community and their families, educators, TS advocates, physicians, researchers, allied professionals, and TSA staff members. Attendees interact, socialize, share ideas, discuss issues of concern, learn from experts, and in many instances meet face to face for the first time.
Spring

1876   Young Onset Parkinson Conference
National Parkinson Foundation & ADPF
200 SE 1st Street
Suite 800
Miami, FL 33131
305-243-6666
800-473-4636
FAX: 305-537-9901
contact@parkinson.org
www.parkinson.org

Joyce Oberdorf, President and CEO
Amy Gray, Vice President, Chapter Relations & Community Partnerships
Jill Davidson, Vice President, Finance & Administration
Peter Schmidt, PhD, Vice President, Programs, Chief Information Officer
Purpose is to find the cause and cure for Parkinson's Disease and related neurodegenerative disorders through research, education and dissemination of current information to patients, care-givers and families.
Annual

Construction & Architecture

Associations

1877 Adaptive Environments Center
200 Portland Street
Suite 1
Boston, MA 02114
617-695-1225
FAX: 617-482-8099
info@HumanCenteredDesign.org
www.humancentereddesign.org

Ralph Jackson, FAIA, President
Chris Pilkington, Vice President
Nancy Jenner, Treasurer
Valerie Fletcher, Executive Director
Develops educational programs and materials on universal design, Americans with Disabilities Act, home adaptation, and more. Central Adaptive Environments publication list also available.

1878 Building Owners and Managers Association International
1101 15th St., NW
Suite 800
Washington, DC 20005
202-408-2662
FAX: 202-326-6377
info@boma.org
www.boma.org

John G. Oliver, Chair and Chief Elected Officer
Kent C. Gibson, CPM, Chair-Elect
Henry H. Chamberlain, President, COO
Brian Harnetiaux, Vice Chair
Conducts seminars nationwide and publishes resource guidebooks for building owners and managers on ADA requirements for commercial facilities and places of public accommodation.

1879 Institute for Human Centered Design
Formerly Adaptive Environments
200 Portland St
Ste 1
Boston, MA 02214
617-695-1225
FAX: 617-482-8099
TTY:617-695-1225
info@humancentereddesign.org
humancentereddesign.org

Valerie Fletcher, Executive Director
Gabriela Bonome-Sims, Director, Administration
Institute focused on collaborating and working with citizens to design communal places to be accessible for all, including those with disabilities.

1880 Mark Elmore Associates Architects
Ste 104
42 East St
Crystal Lake, IL 60014-4400
815-455-7260
800-801-7766
FAX: 815-455-2238
mark@elmore-architects.com
www.elmore-architects.com

Mark A Elmore, Owner
Architectural designs for accessible residential and commercial buildings. ADA compliance reviews.

1881 National Conference on Building Codes and Standards
505 Huntmar Park Drive
Suite 210
Herndon, VA 20170
703-437-0100
FAX: 703-481-3596
membership@ncsbcs.org
www.ncsbcs.org

Cynthia Wilk, President
Robert C. Wible, Executive Director
Debbie Becker, Administrative Assistant
Kevin Egilmez, Project Manager
Serves as a forum in the interchange of information and provides technical services, education and training to our members to enhance the public's social and economic well being through safe, durable, affordable, accessible and efficient buildings.

1882 National Council of Architectural Registration Boards (NCARB)
1801 K Street NW
Suite 700K
Washington, DC 20006
202-879-0520
FAX: 202-783-0290
customerservice@ncarb.org
ncarb.org

Michael J. Armstrong, Chief Executive Officer
Mary S. de Sousa, CAE, Chief Operating Officer
Stephen Nutt, AIA, NCARB, CAE, Senior Architect and advisor to the CEO
Sandy Vasan, Director, Marketing & Communications
Research service in print and online information. Large collection of books and periodicals on the building/architectural environments.

1883 Overcoming Mobility Barriers International
1022 S 4st St
Omaha, NE 68105
402-342-5731
FAX: 402-342-5731

Kay Neil, Executive Director
Members are government officials, service consumers and providers, and other persons interested in removing mobility barriers for elderly, handicapped and disadvantaged persons. Advises and works in conjunction with other groups and government agencies to establish safety standards for special equipment used in retrofitting vehicles and works to retrain drivers in the use of nonconventional driving controls.

1884 Paradigm Design Group
Paralyzed Veterans of America
801 Eighteenth Street, NW
Washington, DC 20006-3517
202-872-1300
800-424-8200
FAX: 202-785-4432
info@pva.org
www.pva.org

Bill Lawson, National President
Homer S. Townsend Jr., Executive Director
Al F. Kovach Jr., National Senior Vice Presedent
Craig F. Enenbach, National Treasurer
Specialized firm providing architectural consulting services related to accessible designs. Experience includes product design and building codes and standards.

1885 United States Access Board
Ste 1000
1331 F St NW
Washington, DC 20004-1111
202-272-0080
800-872-2253
FAX: 202-272-0081
TTY: 800-993-2822
info@access-board.gov
www.access-board.gov

Dave Yanchulis, Public Affairs Specialist
Offers information and technical assistance to the public on accessible design under the Americans with Disabilities Act and other laws. Guidance and publications are available free that address access to facilities, transit vehicles and information technology.

Publications & Videos

1886 Access Currents
United States Access Board
1331 F Street, NW
Suite 1000
Washington, DC 20004-1111   202-272-0080
                                        800-872-2253
                                   FAX: 202-272-0081
                                   TTY: 800-993-2822
                                   info@access-board.gov
                                   www.access-board.gov
Michael K. Yudin, Chair, Department of Education
Sachin Dev Pavithran, Vice Chair, Logan, Utah
Regina Blye, Public Member
Patrick D. Cannon, Public Member
Offers information and referrals on architectural accessibility for architects, designers, government agencies, building owners and consumers. A list of free publications is available on request.
bi-monthly

1887 Access Equals Opportunity
Council of B BB s Foundation
3033 Wilson Blvd
Suite 600
Arlington, VA 22201   703-276-0100
                                   media@cbbb.bbb.org
                                   www.bbb.org
Beverly Baskin, Senior VP, Chief Mission Officer
Genie Barton, Vice President and Director, Onl
Rodney L. Davis, Senior VP Enterprise Programs
Joseph E. Dillon, VP and CFO
These six Title III compliance guides for existing small businesses offer creative cheap and easy suggestions for complying with the public accommodations section of the ADA. Each guide is industry specific for: retail stores, car sales/service, restaurants/bars, medical offices and fun/fitness centers. They include suggestions for readily achievable removal of architectural barriers; effective communication; and guidance for nondiscriminatory policies or procedures. *$2.50*

1888 Access for All
Hospital Audiences
548 Broadway
3rd Floor
New York, NY 10012   212-575-7676
                                   FAX: 212-575-7669
                                   info@hostau.org
                                   www.hospitalaudiences.org
David Sweeny, Executive Director
Jane Kleinsinger, Director of Operations
Jill Bernard, Marketing & Outreach Manager
JoAnne Brockways, Chief Financial Officer
Provides physical and program accessibility information for people with disabilities to New York City cultural institutions including theaters, museums, galleries, etc.

1889 Accessible Home of Your Own
Accent Special Publications
Bloomington, IL 61702-700

Raymond C Cheever, Publisher
Betty Garee, Editor
This guide includes 14 articles on the popular subject of how to make a disabled persons home more accessible. *$7.99*
52 pages Paperback 1990
ISBN 0-915708-29-9

1890 Adaptable Housing: A Technical Manual for Implementing Adaptable Dwelling
H UD U SE R
P.O.Box 23268
Washington, DC 20026-3268   202-708-3178
                                        800-245-2691
                                   FAX: 202-708-9981
                                   TTY: 800-927-7589
                                   helpdesk@huduser.org
                                   www.huduser.org
Patrick J. Tewey, Director, Budget, Contracts, and Program Control Division
Jacqueline D Buford, Director, Management and Administrative Services Division
Jean Lin Pao, General Deputy Assistant Secretary
Katherine M. O'Regan, Assistant Secretary for Policy Development and Research
An illustrated manual describing methods for implementing adaptability in housing. *$3.00*

1891 Consumer's Guide to Home Adaptation
Adaptive Environments Center
200 Portland Street
Suite 1
Boston, MA 02114   617-695-1225
                                   FAX: 617-482-8099
                                   info@HumanCenteredDesign.org
                                   www.humancentereddesign.org
Ralph Jackson, FAIA, President
Chris Pilkington, Vice President
Nancy Jenner, Treasurer
Valerie Fletcher, Executive Director
A workbook that enables people with disabilities to plan the modifications necessary to adapt their homes. Describes how to widen doorways, lower countertops, etc. *$12.00*
52 pages Paperback

1892 Design for Acessibility
National Endowment for the Arts Office
400 7th Street, SW
Washington, DC 20506-0001   202-682-5400
                                   FAX: 202-682-5715
                                   webmgr@arts.gov
                                   arts.gov
Jane Chu, Chairman
Joan Shigekawa, Senior Deputy Chairman
Mike Burke, Chief Information Officer
Joseph Smith, Deputy Chief Information Officer
A handbook for compliance with Section 504 of the Rehabilitation Act of 1973 and the Americans with Disabilities Act of 1990 including technical assistance on making arts programs accessible to staff, performers and audience.
101 pages
ISBN 0-160042-83-6

1893 Directory of Accessible Building Products
N AH B Research Center
400 Prince George's Blvd
Upper Marlboro, MD 20774   301-249-4000
                                        800-638-8556
                                   FAX: 301-430-6180
                                   www.homeinnovation.com
Michael Luzier, CEO & President
Michelle Desiderio, Vice President of Innovation Services
Tom Kenney, P.E, Vice President of Engineering & Research
Phil Davis, Senior Economist & Analyst
Contains descriptions of more than 200 commercially available products designed for use by people with disabilities and age-related limitations. Paperback. *$5.00*
104 pages Yearly

1894 Do-Able Renewable Home
A AR P Fulfillment
601 E Street NW
Washington, DC 20049
202-434-3525
888-687-2277
877-342-2277
FAX: 202-434-3443
member@aarp.org
www.aarp.org

John Wider, President, CEO, AARP Services Inc.
Lisa M. Ryerson, President, AARP Foundation
Robert R. Hagans, Jr., Executive Vice President & Chief Financial Officer
Hollis Terry Bradwell III, Executive Vice President & Chief Information Officer
Describes how individuals with disabilities can modify their homes for independent living. Room-by-room modifications are accompanied by illustrations.

1895 ECHO Housing: Recommended Construction and Installation Standards
601 E Street NW
Washington, DC 20049
202-434-3525
888-687-2277
877-342-2277
FAX: 202-434-3443
member@aarp.org
www.aarp.org

John Wider, President, CEO, AARP Services Inc.
Lisa M. Ryerson, President, AARP Foundation
Robert R. Hagans, Jr., Executive Vice President & Chief Financial Officer
Hollis Terry Bradwell III, Executive Vice President & Chief Information Officer
Illustrated design, construction, and installation standards for temporary dwelling units for elderly people on single family residential property.

1896 Electronic House: Enhanced Lifestyles with Electronics
Electronic House
111 Speen Street, Suite 200
P.O. Box 989
Framingham, MA 01701-2000
508-663-1500
800-375-8015
FAX: 508-663-1599
eheditorial@ehpub.com
electronichouse.com

Kenneth D. Moyes, President
Karen Bligh, Marketing Director
John Brillon, Web Creative Director
Guy Caiola, Director of Internet Operations
Dedicated to home automation. Featuring both extravagant and affordable smart homes that can be controlled with one touch. EH covers electronic systems that give homeowners more security, entertainment, convenience, and fun. Articles cover whole house control and subsystems like residential lighting, security, home theater, energy management and telecommunications. *$23.95*
84 pages BiMonthly
ISSN 0886-66 3

1897 Fair Housing Design Guide for Accessibility
National Council on Multifamily Housing Industry
1201 15th Street NW
Washington, DC 20005
202-266-8200
800-368-5242
FAX: 202-266-8400
ggsmith@nahb.org
www.nahb.com

Kevin Kelly, Chairman of the Board
Tom Woods, First Vice Chairman of the Board
Ed Brady, Second Vice Chairman of the Board
Gerald M. Howard, CEO
Specifically tailored to address the needs of architects and builders. The book includes a detailed technical analysis of the legislation's impact on multifamily design, highlights potential construction problems, and identifies possible solutions. *$29.95*

1898 Ideas for Making Your Home Accessible
Accent Books & Products
P.O.Box 700
Bloomington, IL 61702-0700
309-378-2961
800-787-8444
FAX: 309-378-4420
acmtlvng@aol.com
www.accentonliving.com

Raymond C Cheever, Publisher
Betty Garee, Editor
Offers over 100 pages of tips and ideas to help build or remodel a home. Includes many special devices and where to get them. *$7.50*
94 pages Paperback
ISBN 0-91570 -08-6

1899 North Carolina Accessibility Code
North Carolina Department of Insurance
P.O.Box 26387
Raleigh, NC 27611-6387
919-833-2110
FAX: 919-833-1801
lwright@ncdoi.net

Gregory Griggs, Executive VP
Making buildings and facilities accessible to and usable by the physically handicapped. *$20.00*
678 pages Triannually

1900 Removing the Barriers: Accessibility Guidelines and Specifications
A PP A
1643 Prince Street
Alexandria, VA 22314
703-684-1446
FAX: 703-549-2772
webmaster@appa.org
www.appa.org

John F. Bernhards, Associate Vice President
E. Lander Medlin, Executive VP
Steve Glazner, Director of Knowledge Management
Suzanne M. Healy, Director of Professional Development
Offers site accessibility, building entrances, doors, interior circulation, restrooms and bathing facilities, drinking fountains and additional resources. *$45.00*
125 pages
ISBN 0-91335 -59-9

1901 Smart Kitchen/How to Design a Comfortable, Safe & Friendly Workplace
Ceres Press
P.O.Box 87
Woodstock, NY 12498-87
845-679-5573
FAX: 845-679-5573
cem620@aol.com
healthyhighways.com

David Goldbeck, Owner
This book provides information about designing kitchens that may be helpful to people with disabilities as well as safe and energy efficient. *$16.95*
132 pages Paperback

1902 United Spinal Association
75-20 Astoria Blvd
Suite 120
East Elmhurst, NY 11370- 1177
718-803-3782
800-444-0120
FAX: 718-803-0414
mkurtz@unitedspinal.org
www.unitedspinal.org

Paul Tobin, President
Maria Kurtz, Executive Assistant
Information on spinal cord injury and laws and regulations concerning people with disabilities, including veterans.
Monthly

Education

Aids for the Classroom

1903   **AEPS Child Progress Record: For Children Ages Three to Six**
Brookes Publishing
PO Box 10624
Baltimore, MD 21285-624
410-337-9580
800-638-3775
FAX: 800-638-3775
custserv@brookespublishing.com
www.brookespublishing.com

Paul Brooks, President
Melissa Behm, Executive VP
George Stamathis, VP and Publisher
This chart helps monitor change by visually displaying current abilities, intervention targets, and child progress. In packages of 30. *$21.00*
8 pages Gate-fold
ISBN 1-557662-51-7

1904   **AEPS Curriculum for Three to Six Years**
Brookes Publishing
PO Box 10624
Baltimore, MD 21285-0624
410-337-9580
800-638-3775
FAX: 410-337-8539
webmaster@brookespublishing.com
www.brookespublishing.com
Paul H. Brookes, Chairman of the Board
Jeffrey D. Brookes, President
George S. Stamathis, VP/Publisher
Melissa A. Behn, Executive Vice President
Used after the AEPS® Test is completed and scored, this developmentally sequenced curriculum allows professionals to match the child's IFSP/IEP goals and objectives with activity-based interventions — beginning with simple skills and moving on to more advanced skills. *$ 65.00*
304 pages Spiral-bound
ISBN 1-557665-65-6

1905   **AEPS Data Recording Forms: For Children Ages Three to Six**
Brookes Publishing
PO Box 10624
Baltimore, MD 21285-624
410-337-9580
800-638-3775
FAX: 800-638-3775
custserv@brookespublishing.com
www.readplaylearn.com
Paul Brooks, President
These forms can be used by child development professionals on four separate occasions to pinpoint and then monitor a child's strengths and needs in the six key areas of skill development measured by the AEPS Test. Packages of 10. *$24.00*
36 pages Saddle-stiched
ISBN 1-557662-49-5

1906   **AEPS Family Interest Survey**
Brookes Publishing
PO Box 10624
Baltimore, MD 21285-624
410-337-9580
800-638-3775
FAX: 800-638-3775
custserv@brookespublishing.com
www.brookespublishing.com
Paul Brooks, President
Tracy Gracy, Educational Sales Manager
This is a 30-item checklist that helps families to identify interests and concerns to address in a child's IEP/IFSP. Comes in packages of 30. *$15.00*
8 pages Saddle-stiched
ISBN 1-557660-98-0

1907   **Adaptivemall.com**
15 South Second Street
Dolgeville, NY 13329
315-429-7112
800-371-2778
FAX: 315-429-8862
info@adaptivemall.com
www.adaptivemall.com
Katie Bergeron Peglow,PT,MS, COO
Adaptivemall.comr help families find the best equipment to support their children at their highest functioning level.

1908   **Advanced Language Tool Kit**
School Specialty
625 Mt. Auburn Street, 3rd Floor
PO Box 9031
Cambridge, MA 02139-9031
617-547-6706
800-225-5750
FAX: 888-440-2665
Feedback.EPS@schoolspecialty.com
eps.schoolspecialty.com
Rick Holden, President, EPS
Jean S Osman, Co-Author
Paula D Rome, Author
Provides an overview o the structure, organization, and sound units that are needed to develop skills for advanced reading and spelling. The kit contains a teacher's manual and 3 pack of cards, with features similar to the cards in the Language Tool Kit. *$60.00*

ISBN 0-838885-48-9

1909   **All Kinds of Minds**
School Specialty
625 Mt. Auburn Street, 3rd Floor
PO Box 9031
Cambridge, MA 02139-9031
617-547-6706
800-225-5750
FAX: 888-440-2665
Feedback.EPS@schoolspecialty.com
eps.schoolspecialty.com
Rick Holden, President, EPS
Melvin D Levine, Author
A fictitious account of five different students who have learning disabilities. *$33.00*
296 pages
ISBN 0-838820-90-5

1910   **American Sign Language Handshape Cards**
T J Publishers, Distributor
Ste 206
817 Silver Spring Ave
Silver Spring, MD 20910- 4617
301-585-4440
800-999-1168
FAX: 301-585-5930
tjpubinc@aol.com
Angela K Thames, President
Jerald A Murphy, VP
Durable flashcards illustrate basic handshapes, classifiers and the American manual alphabet. An instructional booklet describes games for differing skill levels to improve vocabulary, increase hand and eye coordination, sign recognition and usage. *$16.95*

1911   **Asthma Action Cards: Child Care Asthma/Allergy Action Card**
Asthma and Allergy Foundation of America
8201 Corporate Drive
Suite 1000
Landover, MD 20785
202-466-7643
800-727-8462
FAX: 202-466-8940
info@aafa.org
www.aafa.org
Tom Flanigan, Chariman
William Mclin, President and CEO
Yolanda Miller, VP and CFO

Includes necessary information a provider needs to care for a young child who has asthma and allergies. The card includes a medication plan, a list of the child's specific signs and symptoms that indicate the child is having trouble breathing, and steps on how to handle an emergency situation.

1912   Asthma Action Cards: Student Asthma Action Card
Asthma and Allergy Foundation of America
1233 20th St NW
Suite 610
Washington, DC 20036-2330
202-833-1700
800-727-8462
FAX: 202-833-2351
info@aafa.org
www.swmlaw.com

Bill Mc Lin, Executive Director
Ben C Hadden, VP Finance & Treasurer
Bill Lin, Executive Director
Tool for communicating school aged children's and teen's asthma managment plan to school personnel. Includes sections for asthma triggers, daily medications, and emergency directions.

1913   Auditech: Classroom Amplification System Focus CFM802
PO Box 821105
Vicksburg, MS 39182-1105
800-229-8293
FAX: 800-221-8639
info@auditechusa.com
www.auditechusa.com

1914   Auditech: Personal FM Educational System
PO Box 821105
Vicksburg, MS 39182-1105
800-229-8293
FAX: 800-221-8639
info@auditechusa.com
www.auditechusa.com

1915   Auditory-Verbal Therapy for Parents and Professionals
Alexander Graham Bell Association
3417 Volta Place, NW
Washington, DC 20007
202-337-5220
FAX: 202-337-8314
TTY: 202-337-5221
info@agbell.org
www.listeningandspokenlanguage.org
Meredith K. Sugar, Esq. (OH), President
Donald M. Goldberg, Immediate Past President
Ted A. Meyer, M.D., Ph.D. (SC, President-Elect, Secretary, Treasurer
Emilio Alonso Mendoza (DC), Chief Executive Officer
A must-have for hearing health professionals, students entering hearing health fields and parents who want to explore the theory and practices of auditory-verbal therapy. *$54.95*
313 pages Paperback

1916   Autism Community Store
7800 E. Iliff Ave.
Suite J
Denver, CO 80231
303-309-3647
866-709-4344
FAX: 303-756-2311
support@autismcommunitystore.com
www.autismcommunitystore.com
Shannon Sullivan, Co-Founder
The Autism Community Store is a parent-owned autism and special needs resource, a special little shop helping families, teachers and therapists get hard-to-find products for kids with ASD, PDD-NOS, Aspergers, SPD, ADHD and other special needs at reasonable prices.

1917   Autism-Products.com
8776 E. Shea Blvd.
Suite 106-552
Scottsdale, AZ 85260
FAX: 815-550-1819
Kelly@Autism-Products.com
www.autism-products.com

1918   Barrier Free Education
Center for Assistive Technology & Env Access
490 10th St NW
Atlanta, GA 30332-156
404-894-4960
800-726-9119
FAX: 404-894-9320
catea@coa.gatech.edu
www.catea.org
Elizabeth Bryant, Project Director
Math and science activities pose unique accommodation challenges for students with disabilities. The Barrier Free Education resource on accessible science experiments was developed for high school chemistry and physics students with physical or visual disabilities under the National Science Foundation's Program for Persons with Disabilities.

1919   Beginning Reasoning and Reading
School Specialty
625 Mt. Auburn Street, 3rd Floor
PO Box 9031
Cambridge, MA 02139-9031
617-547-6706
800-225-5750
FAX: 888-440-2665
Feedback.EPS@schoolspecialty.com
eps.schoolspecialty.com
Rick Holden, President, EPS
Joanne Carlisle, Author
This workbook develops basic language and thinking skills that build the foundation for reading comprehension. Workbook exercises reinforce reading as a critical reasoning activity. *$10.45*

ISBN 0-838830-01-3

1920   Buy!
JE Stewart Teaching Tools
PO Box 15308
Seattle, WA 98115-308
206-262-9538
FAX: 206-262-9538
Jeff Stewart, Owner
Teaches 50 words as they appear in commercial and community situations such as clinic, sale, receipt, price and cleaner. These words are functional at school, on the job and shopping. *$32.50*
116 pages
ISBN 1-877866-05-9

1921   Catalog for Teaching Life Skills to Persons with Development Disability
PCI Education Publishing
PO Box 34270
San Antonio, TX 78265-4270
210-377-1999
800-594-4263
FAX: 888-259-8284
www.pcieducation.com
Lee Wilson, President/CEO
Erin Kinard, VP Product Development/Publisher
Randy Pennington, VP, Sales & Marketing
Over 200 educational products that help individuals learn and maintain the life skills they need to succeed in an inclusive society.

1922   Classroom GOAL: Guide for Optimizing Auditory Learning Skills
Alexander Graham Bell Association
3417 Volta Pl NW
Washington, DC 20007-2737
202-337-5220
FAX: 202-337-8314
info@agbell.org
www.agbell.org
Alexander Graham, Executive Director
Judy Harrison, Director of Programs
Susan Boswell, Communications and Marketing
This reader-friendly teacher's guide filled with tips, source materials and sample charts and plans is designed for educators who have yearned for a resource that explains how to incorporate auditory goals into academic learning for students with different degrees of hearing loss. *$34.95*
Paperback

1923 **Classroom Notetaker: How to Organize a Program Serving Students with Hearing Impairments**
Alexander Graham Bell Association
3417 Volta Pl NW
Washington, DC 20007-2737   202-337-5220
                                FAX: 202-337-8314
                                info@agbell.org
                                www.agbell.org
Alexander Graham, Executive Director
Judy Harrison, Director of Programs
Susan Boswell, Communications and Marketing
This detailed manual for instructors, administrators and staff notetakers promotes classroom notetaking within long-term educational programs as absolutely vital for students who are deaf and hard of hearing from elementary school to college. *$24.95*
127 pages Paperback

1924 **Community Services for the Blind and Partially Sighted Store: Sight Connection**
9709 Third Ave NE
Ste 100
Seattle, WA 98115-2027   206-525-5556
                              800-458-4888
                              FAX: 206-525-0422
                              info@sightconnection.org
                              www.sightconnection.org
Miles Otoupal, Chair
Jonathan Avedovech, Vice Chair
David McBride, Treasurer
Mary Lewis, Secretary
Over 400 products specifically designed to make life easier for people with vision loss.

1925 **Community Signs**
JE Stewart Teaching Tools
P.O.Box 15308
Seattle, WA 98115-308   206-262-9538
                             FAX: 206-262-9538
Jeff Stewart, Owner
Teaches 50 words like go, fire, rest room, men, women, danger and walk needed to successfully navigate our environment. *$ 32.50*

1926 **Comprehensive Assessment of Spoken Language (CASL)**
AGS
PO Box 99
Circle Pines, MN 55014-99
                             800-328-2560
                             FAX: 800-471-8457
                             agsmail@agsnet.com
                             www.agsnet.com
Kevin Brueggeman, President
Robert Zaske, Market Manager
CASL is an individually and orally administered research-based, theory-drive oral language assessment battery for ages 3 through 21. Fifteen tests measure language processing skills - comprehension, expression, and retrieval - in four language structure categories: lexical/semantic, syntactic, supralinguistic and pragmatic. *$299.95*

1927 **Creative Arts Therapy Catalogs**
MMB Music
9051 Watson Road
Suite 161
Saint Louis, MO 63126-1019   314-531-9635
                                  800-543-3771
                                  FAX: 314-531-8384
                                  info@mmbmusic.com
                                  www.mmbmusic.com
Marcia Goldberg, President
Catalogs of books, videos, recordings for the creative arts and wellness (music, art, dance, poetry, drama, therapies, photography).

1928 **Cursive Writing Skills**
School Specialty
625 Mt. Auburn Street, 3rd Floor
PO Box 9031
Cambridge, MA 02139-9031   617-547-6706
                                800-225-5750
                                FAX: 888-440-2665
                                Feedback.EPS@schoolspecialty.com
                                eps.schoolspecialty.com
Rick Holden, President, EPS
Diana Hanbury King, Author
Boosts writing achievement through handwriting skills. Handwriting instruction helps students become fluent writers, allowing them to focus on their thoughts and ideas rather than on letter and word formation. *$12.00*

1929 **Different Roads to Learning**
37 East 18th Street
10th Floor
New York, NY 10003   212-604-9637
                          800-853-1057
                          FAX: 212-206-9329
                          info@difflearn.com
                          www.difflearn.com
Julie Azuma, Founder
Its product line supports the social, academic and communicative development of children on the autism spectrum through Applied Behavior Analysis (ABA) and Verbal Behavior interventions

1930 **Discount School Supply**
PO Box 6013
Carol Stream, IL 60197-6013
                          800-627-2829
                          FAX: 800-879-3753
                          customerservice@discountschoolsupply.com
                          www.discountschoolsupply.com
Ron Elliott, Founder
Kelly Crampton, Chief Executive Officer
Discount School Supply offers the highest quality educational products at the lowest possible prices, supported by an extraordinary level of service.

1931 **Do2learn**
3204 Churchill Road
Raleigh, NC 27607   919-755-1809
                         FAX: 919-420-1978
                         www.do2learn.com

1932 **Don Johnston**
26799 West Commerce Drive
Volo, IL 60073-9675   847-740-0749
                           800-999-4660
                           FAX: 847-740-7326
                           info@donjohnston.com
                           www.donjohnston.com
Don Johnston, Founder
Ruth Ziolkowski, President
Kevin Johnston, Director of Product Design
Ben Johnston, Director of Marketing
A provider of quality products and services that enable people with special needs to discover their potential and experience success. Products are developed for the areas of Physical Access, Augmentative Communication and for those who struggle with reading and writing.

1933 **Dyslexia Training Program**
School Specialty
625 Mt. Auburn Street, 3rd Floor
PO Box 9031
Cambridge, MA 02139-9031   617-547-6706
                                800-225-5750
                                FAX: 888-440-2665
                                Feedback.EPS@schoolspecialty.com
                                eps.schoolspecialty.com
Rick Holden, President, EPS
This 2-year, cumulative series of daily 1-hour video lessons and accompanying Student's Books and Teacher's Guides is a structured, multisensory sequence of alphabet, reading, spelling, cur-

sive handwriting, listening, language history, and review activities. Written by the Texas Scottish Rite Hospital for Children.

1934   ESpecial Needs
11704 Lackland Industrial Drive
St. Louis, MO 63146   314-692-2424
                                          877-664-4565
                                     FAX: 314-692-2428
                                     www.especialneeds.com

1935   Encyclopedia of Basic Employment and Daily Living Skills
Phillip Roy, Inc.
13064 Indian Rocks Road
P.O. Box 130
Indian Rocks Beach, FL 33785   727-593-2700
                                          800-255-9085
                                     FAX: 727-595-2685
                                     info@philliproy.com
                                     www.philliproy.com

Ruth Bragman PhD, President
Phil Padol, Consultant
Contains developmental skills for special education students. Contains lessons in 6 curriculum areas covering 80 objects with 541 lessons. Also includes objectives, instructional strategies, and assessment tasks.

1936   Exceptional Teaching Inc
Exceptional Teaching Inc
3994 Oleander Way
PO Box 2330
Castro Valley, CA 94546   510-889-7282
                                          800-549-6999
                                     FAX: 510-889-7382
                                 info@exceptionalteaching.com
                                    www.exceptionalteaching.com

Helene Holman, Owner/manager
Providing educational products for those with special needs via catalog and online store.

1937   Explode the Code
School Specialty
625 Mt. Auburn Street, 3rd Floor
PO Box 9031
Cambridge, MA 02139-9031   617-547-6706
                                          800-225-5750
                                     FAX: 888-440-2665
                              Feedback.EPS@schoolspecialty.com
                                    eps.schoolspecialty.com

Rick Holden, President, EPS
Nancy M Hall, Author
Helps students build the essential literacy skills needed for reading success: phonological awareness, decoding, vocabulary, comprehension, fluency and spelling. *$6.20*

Grades K-4, 1-3

1938   Food!
JE Stewart Teaching Tools
PO Box 15308
Seattle, WA 98115-308   206-262-9538
                                     FAX: 206-262-9538

Jeff Stewart, Owner
Teaches 50 words like salt, pepper, hamburger, fruit, milk and soup, seen commonly on menus, packages and in directions used at home and at play. *$32.50*

1939   Fun for Everyone
AbleNet
2625 Patton Road
Roseville, MN 55113-1308   651-294-2200
                                          800-322-0956
                                     FAX: 651-294-2259
                                 customerservice@ablenetinc.com
                                     www.ablenetinc.com

Jen Thalhuber, CEO
Ann Meyer, Vice President
Paul Sugden, VP Finance
Jason Voiovich, VP Marketing
Today, simple technology allows children and adults with disabilities to participate in leisure activities they were limited or excluded from in the past. *$20.00*

1940   Fundamentals of Autism
Slosson Educational Publications Inc.
538 Buffalo Road
East Aurora, NY 14052-280   716-652-0930
                                          800-655-3840
                                          888-756-7760
                                     FAX: 716-655-3840
                                     slossonprep@gmail.com
                                     www.slosson.com

Steven Slosson, President
John Slosson, VP
David Slosson, VP
The Fundamentals of Autism handbook provides a quick, user friendly, effective and accurate approach to help in identifying and developing educationally related program objectives for children diagnosed as autistic. These materials have been designed to be easily and functionally used by teachers, therapists, special education/learning disability resource specialists, psychologists and others who work with children diagnosed as autistic. *$56.00*

72 pages

1941   GO-MO Articulation Cards- Second Edition
Sage Publications
2455 Teller Road
Thousand Oaks, CA 91320   805-499-9774
                                          800-818-7243
                                     FAX: 800-583-2665
                                     info@sagepub.com
                                     www.sagepub.com

Blaise R Simqu, President & CEO
Tracey Ozmina, VP and COO
Chris Hickok, Senior VP and CFO
Stephen Barr, Managing Director
The most popular system used for remedying defective speech articulation in children and adults. This popular card set was the first and is still the best therapy tool of its kind, as it continues to produce results and maintains the interest of students of all ages.

1942   Gillingham Manaual
School Specialty
625 Mt. Auburn Street, 3rd Floor
PO Box 9031
Cambridge, MA 02139-9031   617-547-6706
                                          800-225-5750
                                     FAX: 888-440-2665
                              Feedback.EPS@schoolspecialty.com
                                    eps.schoolspecialty.com

Rick Holden, President, EPS
Anna Gillingham, Author
Bessie W Stillman, Co-Author
Remedial training for children with specific disability in reading, spelling, and penmanship.
352 pages 69.95
ISBN 0-83880 -00-

1943 **Guide to Teaching Phonics**
School Specialty
625 Mt. Auburn Street, 3rd Floor
PO Box 9031
Cambridge, MA 02139-9031
617-547-6706
800-225-5750
FAX: 888-440-2665
Feedback.EPS@schoolspecialty.com
eps.schoolspecialty.com

Rick Holden, President, EPS
June Lyday Orton, Author
This flexible teacher's guide presents multisensory procedures developed in association with the late Dr. Samuel Orton. They consist of 100 phonograms for teaching phonetic elements and their sequences in words for reading, writing and spelling. Also contains coordinated Phonics Cards. *$19.25*
96 pages
ISBN 0-838802-41-9

1944 **Homemade Battery-Powered Toys**
Special Needs Project
Ste H
324 State St
Santa Barbara, CA 93101-2364
818-718-9900
800-333-6867
FAX: 818-349-2027
editor@specialneeds.com.
www.specialneeds.com

Hod Gray, Owner
Laraine Gray, Coordinator
Describes how to make simple switches and educational devices for severely handicapped children. *$7.50*

1945 **Idaho Assistive Technology Project**
University of Idaho
PO Box 444061
Moscow, ID 83844-4061
208-885-6097
800-432-8324
FAX: 208-885-6145
janicec@uidaho.edu
www.idahoat.org

Janice Carson, Project Director
Sue House, Information/Referral Specialist
A federally funded program managed by the Center on Disabilities and Human Development at the University of Idaho. The goal is to increase the availability of assistive technology devices and services for Idahoans with disabilities. *$15.00*

1946 **If It Is To Be, It Is Up To Me To Do It!**
AVKO Educational Research Foundation
3084 Willard Road
Birch Run, MI 48415-9404
810-686-9283
866-285-6612
FAX: 810-686-1101
webmaster@avko.org
www.avko.org

Don McCabe, President, Research Director Emeritus, Birch Run, Michigan
Linda Heck, VP, Clio, Michigan
Michael Lane, Treasurer, Clio, Michigan
Amy Messer, Board Member, Flint, Michigan
A student and tutor's text, for use on dyslexics and non-dyslexics, by parents, spouses, or friends. *$29.95*
206 pages
ISBN 1-564007-42-1

1947 **Inclusive Play People**
Educational Equity Concepts
Fl 8
100 5th Ave
New York, NY 10011-6903
212-243-1110
FAX: 212-627-0407
TTY:212-725-1803
information@edequity.org
www.iconcapital.com

Jacqueline Johnson, Manager

Six sturdy multiracial wooden figures that provide a unique variety of nonstereotyped work and family roles and are inclusive of disabled and nondisabled people of various ages. For block building and dramatic play. *$25.00*

1948 **Individualized Keyboarding**
AVKO Educational Research Foundation
3084 Willard Road
Birch Run, MI 48415-9404
810-686-9283
866-285-6612
FAX: 810-686-1101
webmaster@avko.org
www.avko.org

Don McCabe, President, Research Director Emeritus, Birch Run, Michigan
Linda Heck, VP, Clio, Michigan
Michael Lane, Treasurer, Clio, Michigan
Amy Messer, Board Member, Flint, Michigan
Utilizes a multi-sensory approach to teach typing skills. It not only teaches typing skills, it also reinforces the reading patterns that are necessary for typing proficiency. *$14.95*
96 pages
ISBN 1-654004-01-5

1949 **Instruction of Persons with Severe Handicaps**
McGraw-Hill School Publishing
PO Box 182604
Columbus, OH 43272
877-833-5524
FAX: 614-759-3749
customer.service@mcgraw-hill.com
www.mcgraw-hill.com

Harold McGraw, President and CEO
Jack Callahan, Executive VP
John Berisford, Executive VP of HR
A complete introduction to the status of education as it pertains to people with severe handicaps.

1950 **Kaplan Early Learning Company**
1310 Lewisville Clemmons Rd
Lewisville, NC 27023
336-766-7374
800-334-2014
FAX: 800-452-7526
info@kaplanco.com
www.kaplanco.com

Hal Kaplan, President & CEO
Kaplan Early Learning Company is a international provider of products and services that enhance children's learning.

1951 **Keeping Ahead in School**
Educators Publishing Service
PO Box 9031
Cambridge, MA 2139-9031
617-547-6706
800-225-5750
FAX: 888-440-2665
feedback@epsbooks.com
www.epsbooks.com

Charles H Heinle, VP
Alexandra S Bigelow, Author
Gunnar Voltz, President
This book helps students not only understand their own strengths and weaknesses but also more fully appreciate their individuality. He suggests specific ways to approach work, bypass or overcome learning disorders, and manage other struggles that may beset students in school. *$24.75*
320 pages Paperback
ISBN 0-838820-69-7

1952   KeyMath Teach and Practice
AGS
P.O.Box 99
Circle Pines, MN 55014-99

800-328-2560
FAX: 800-471-8457
agsmail@agsnet.com
www.agsnet.com

Kevin Brueggeman, President
Robert Zaske, Market Manager
This set of materials provides all the tools needed to assess students' math skills...and the strategies to deal with problem areas. Three sets are available: Basic Concepts Package; Operations Package; and Applications Package. $219.95 each or $599.95 for whole set.

1953   Lakeshore Learning Materials
2695 E. Dominguez Street
Carson, CA 90895

310-537-8600
800-421-5354
FAX: 800-537-5403
lakeshore@lakeshorelearning.com
www.lakeshorelearning.com

Bo Kaplan, President/CEO
Josh Kaplan, VP Merchandising
Mat , Vice President of Operations
Offers books, resources, testing materials, assessment information and special education materials for the professional in the field of special education.
190 pages

1954   Language Parts Catalog
School Specialty
625 Mt. Auburn Street, 3rd Floor
PO Box 9031
Cambridge, MA 02139-9031

617-547-6706
800-225-5750
FAX: 888-440-2665
Feedback.EPS@schoolspecialty.com
eps.schoolspecialty.com

Rick Holden, President, EPS
Melvin D Levine, Author
Offers a humorous and informative explanation of the various aspects of language and how they operate. Laid out in the form of a catalog, the book presents various parts that can help students improve their language abilities. *$12.65*

ISBN 0-838819-80-X

1955   Language Tool Kit
School Specialty
625 Mt. Auburn Street, 3rd Floor
PO Box 9031
Cambridge, MA 02139-9031

617-547-6706
800-225-5750
FAX: 888-440-2665
Feedback.EPS@schoolspecialty.com
eps.schoolspecialty.com

Rick Holden, President, EPS
Paula D Rome, Author
Jean S Osman, Co-Author
Designed for use by a teacher or parents, teaches reading and spelling to students with specific language disability. *$43.25*
32 pages English Edition
ISBN 0-838885-20-3

1956   Language, Speech and Hearing Services in School
American Speech-Language-Hearing Association
10801 Rockville Pike
Rockville, MD 20852-3226

301-296-5700
800-638-8255
FAX: 301-296-8580
actioncenter@asha.org
www.asha.org

Paul Rao, President
Robert Augustine, VP of Finance
Arlene Pietranton, Executive Director

Professional journal for clinicians, audiologists and speech-language pathologists. *$30.00*

1957   Learning American Sign Language
Harris Communications
15155 Technology Dr
Eden Prairie, MN 55344-2273

952-906-1180
800-825-6758
FAX: 952-906-1099
info@harriscomm.com
www.harriscomm.com

Robert Harris, President
Kevin Horsky, Business Director
Offers over 700 titles on ASL including books, videotapes, CDs & DVDs. Free catalog available. *$78.95*
350 pages Video & Book

1958   Learning Resources
380 N. Fairway Drive
Vernon Hills, IL 60061

800-333-8281
FAX: 888-892-8731
info@learningresources.com
www.learningresources.com

1959   Learning to Sign in My Neighborhood
T J Publishers
2544 Tarpley Rd
Suite 108
Carrollton, TX 75006-2288

972-416-0800
800-999-1168
FAX: 301-585-5930
tjpubinc@aol.com

Angela K Thames, President
Jerald A Murphy, VP
Beautifully illustrated coloring book lets children learn signs from kids just like themselves! Recommended for ages 4 and up, let children have fun while they learn signs for words typically used in day-to-day activities. *$3.50*
32 pages Softcover
ISBN 0-93266 -36-1

1960   Literacy Program
School Specialty
625 Mt. Auburn Street, 3rd Floor
PO Box 9031
Cambridge, MA 02139-9031

617-547-6706
800-225-5750
FAX: 888-440-2665
Feedback.EPS@schoolspecialty.com
eps.schoolspecialty.com

Rick Holden, President, EPS
Paula D Rome, Author
Jean S Osman, Co-Author
Written by the Texas Scottish Rite Hospital for Children. A one-year course that consists of 160 one-hour videotaped lessons accompanied by student workbooks, designed for high school students and adults who read below sixth grade level.

1961   Literature Based Reading
Oryx Press
4041 N Central Ave
Phoenix, AZ 85012-3330

602-265-2651
800-279-6799
FAX: 800-279-4663

1962   Living an Idea: Empowerment and the Evolution of an Alternative School
Brookline Books
8 Trumbull Rd, Suite B-001
Northampton, MA 1060-4533

413-584-0184
800-666-2665
FAX: 413-584-6184
brbooks@yahoo.com
www.brooklinebooks.com

William H Walters, Author
Esther Wilder, Co-Author

This book is about the creation and 14 year evolution of a public alternative inner-city high school. The school lived an idea - empowerment. Students were encouraged to participate in shaping many aspects of their education, teachers were responsible for running the school, and parents invited to help govern. *$27.95*

ISBN 0-91479-68-9

1963 Low Tech Assistive Devices: A Handbook for the School Setting
Therapro, Inc.
225 Arlington Street
Framingham, MA 02139-8723
508-872-9494
800-257-5376
800-268-6624
FAX: 508-875-2062
info@therapro.com
www.therapro.com

Karen Conrad, Owner
A how-to book with step by step directions and detailed illustrations for fabrication of frequently requested low-tech assistive devices. *$45.00*
320 pages Paperback

1964 MTA Readers
Educators Publishing Service
625 Mt. Auburn Street, 3rd Floor
PO Box 9031
Cambridge, MA 02139-9031
617-547-6706
800-225-5750
FAX: 888-440-2665
Feedback.EPS@schoolspecialty.com
www.epsbooks.com

Rick Holden, President, EPS
Illustrated readers for grades 1-3 that accompany the MTA Reading and Spelling Program (Multisensory Teaching Approach). Phonetic elements in a structured, but entertaining context.
48+ pages $4.65 - $11.65
ISBN 0-83882-33-3

1965 Making School Inclusion Work: A Guide to Everyday Practice
Brookline Books
8 Trumbull Rd, Suite B-001
Northampton, MA 2445-4533
413-584-0184
800-666-2665
FAX: 413-584-6184
brbooks@yahoo.com
www.brooklinebooks.com

William H Walters, Author
Esther Wilder, Co-Author
This book tells the reader how to conduct a truly inclusive program, regardless of ethnic or racial background, economic level and physical or cognitive ability. *$24.95*
254 pages
ISBN 0-914791-96-4

1966 Making the Writing Process Work: Strategies for Composition and Self-Regulation
Brookline Books
8 Trumbull Rd, Suite B-001
Northampton, MA 2445-4533
413-584-0184
800-666-2665
FAX: 413-584-6184
brbooks@yahoo.com
www.brooklinebooks.com

William H Walters, Author
Esther Wilder, Co-Author
This book is geared toward students who have difficulty organizing their thoughts and developing their writing. The specific stategies teach students how to approach, organize, and produce a final written product.. *$24.95*
240 pages Paperback
ISBN 1-571290-10-9

1967 Manual Alphabet Poster
TJ Publishers
Ste 108
2544 Tarpley Rd
Carrollton, TX 75006-2288
972-416-0800
800-999-1168
FAX: 972-416-0944
TJPubinc@aol.com
www.TJpublishers.com

Pat O'Rourke, President
Poster presents the manual alphabet. *$4.50*

1968 Many Faces of Dyslexia
40 York Rd
4th Floor
Baltimore, MD 21204-5243
410-296-0232
FAX: 410-321-5069
www.interdys.org

Nancy Hennessy, President
Sandra Soper, Vice President
Thoman Viall, Executive Director
Gives information on the teaching and rehabilitation techniques for people with dyslexia. *$16.50*
Paperback

1969 Match-Sort-Assemble Job Cards
Exceptional Education
PO Box 15308
Seattle, WA 98115-308
206-262-9538

Jeff Stewart, Owner
Teaches workers to use a series of symbolic cues to control their own production cycles. *$565.00*
Class Set

1970 Match-Sort-Assemble Pictures
Exceptional Education
PO Box 15308
Seattle, WA 98115-308
206-262-9538

Jeff Stewart, Owner
People with profound, severe and moderate mental retardation have immediate access with MSA Pictures. Students work with pictures (and if necessary a template) to match, sort, assemble and disassemble parts that vary in shape, length and diameter. *$426.00*
Class Set

1971 Match-Sort-Assemble SCHEMATICS
Exceptional Education
PO Box 15308
Seattle, WA 98115-308
206-262-9538

Jeff Stewart, Owner
Students with moderate and mild mental retardation and those who have completed MSA Pictures are ready for MSA Schematics. It increases abstraction and displacement of instruction from the work clearly and simply. *$495.00*
Class Set

1972 Match-Sort-Assemble TOOLS
Exceptional Education
PO Box 15308
Seattle, WA 98115-308
206-262-9538
FAX: 475-486-4510

Jeff Stewart, Owner
Students and clients learn to use the tools required for many jobs in light industry. Mastery of the production cycle with independence, endurance and the ability to learn new tasks through pictures and schematics and basic hand functions will help clients acquire and maintain employment in a competitive field. *$595.00*
Class Set

1973 Meeting-in-a-Box
Asthma and Allergy Foundation of America
1233 20th St NW
Suite 610
Washington, DC 20036-7322
202-833-1700
800-7AS-THMA
FAX: 202-833-2351
info@aafa.org
www.swmlaw.com

Bill Mc Lin, Executive Director
Bill Mclin, Executive Director
A series of self-contained, comprehensive kits that contain all the necessary components for a successful asthma presentation.

1974 More Food!
JE Stewart Teaching Tools
PO Box 15308
Seattle, WA 98115-308
206-262-9538
FAX: 206-262-9538

Jeff Stewart, Owner
Teaches 50 more words found in restaurants, grocery stores, cookbooks such as pizza, carrot, tacos, oysters and pineapple. These words are functional at home, going shopping and during leisure. *$32.50*

1975 More Work!
J E Stewart Teaching Tools
PO Box 15308
Seattle, WA 98115-308
206-262-9538
FAX: 206-262-9538

Jeff Stewart, Owner
Teaches 50 words as they appear on parts, tools, job instructions, signs and labels, such as fill, grasp, release, lock, search, position and select. These words are functional in school and on-the-job. *$32.50*

1976 Multisensory Teaching Approach
Educators Publishing Service
PO Box 9031
Cambridge, MA 2139-9031
617-367-2700
800-225-5750
FAX: 617-547-0412
www.epsbooks.com

$110 - $140
ISBN 0-83888 -10-9

1977 National Autism Resources
6240 Goodyear Rd.
Benicia, CA 94510
707-745-3308
877-249-2393
FAX: 877-259-9419
customerservice@nationalautismresources.com
www.nationalautismresources. com

1978 Peabody Articulation Decks
AGS
PO Box 99
Circle Pines, MN 55014-99
651-287-7220
800-328-2560
FAX: 763-786-9007
agsmail@agsnet.com
www.agsnet.com

Keith Powel, Special Education Transition Coo
Robert Zaske, Marketing Manager
Complete kit of playing-card sized PAD decks let students focus on the 18 most commonly misarticulated English consonants and blends. *$115.95*

ISBN 0-88671 -75-4

1979 Phonemic Awareness in Young Children: A Classroom Curriculum
Brookes Publishing
PO Box 10624
Baltimore, MD 21285-624
410-337-9580
custserv@brookespublishing.com
www.brookespublishing.com

Clary Creighton, Exhibits Coordinator
Tracy Gray, Educational Sales Manager
Paul Brooks, Owner
This is a supplemental, whole-class curriculum for improving pre-literacy listening skills. It contains activities that are fun, easy to use, and proven to work in any kindergarten classroom - general, bilingual, inclusive, or special education. This program takes only 15-20 minutes a day. *$24.95*
208 pages Spiral-bound
ISBN 1-557663-21-1

1980 Phonics for Thought
Educators Publishing Service
PO Box 9031
Cambridge, MA 2139-9031
617-367-2700
800-225-5750
FAX: 617-547-0412
www.epsbooks.com

Paperback

1981 Phonological Awareness Training for Reading
Sage Publications
2455 Teller Road
Thousand Oaks, CA 91320
805-499-9774
800-818-7243
FAX: 800-583-2665
info@sagepub.com
www.sagepub.com

Blaise R Simqu, President & CEO
Tracey Ozmina, Executive VP
Chris Hickok, Executive VP and CFO
Stephen Barr, Managing Director
Designed to increase the level of phonological awareness in young children. Can be taught individually or in small groups and takes about 12 to 14 weeks to complete if children are taught in short sessions three or four times a week. *$129.00*

1982 Play!
JE Stewart Teaching Tools
PO Box 15308
Seattle, WA 98115-308
206-262-9538
FAX: 206-262-9538

Jeff Stewart, Owner
Teaches 50 more words as they appear at recreation sites, on signs and labels and in newspapers and magazines, such as movie, visitor, ticket, gallery and zoo. These words are functional in school and at leisure. *$32.50*

1983 Power Breathing Program
Asthma and Allergy Foundation of America
8201 Corporate Drive
Suite 1000
Landover, MD 20785
202-466-7643
800-727-8462
FAX: 202-466-8940
info@aafa.org
www.aafa.org

Bill McLin, Executive Director
Devoloped the only asthma education program specifically designed for and pre-tested with teens. Teens with asthma have special challenges. This interactive program covers everything from the basics of asthma to dealing with their asthma in social situations, in college, and on the job. Includes everything you need to present this three-four session program. *$295.00*

1984 Primary Phonics
School Specialty
625 Mt. Auburn Street, 3rd Floor
PO Box 9031
Cambridge, MA 02139-9031
617-547-6706
800-225-5750
FAX: 888-440-2665
Feedback.EPS@schoolspecialty.com
eps.schoolspecialty.com

Rick Holden, President, EPS
Barbara W Makar, Author
A program of storybooks and coordinated workbooks that teaches reading for grades K-2. A structured phonetic approach. Contains 8 student workbooks, with 8 sets of 10 coordinated storybooks; consonant workbooks; initial consonant blend workbooks; picture dictionary, and coloring book.

ISSN 0838-83 0

1985 Reading for Content
School Specialty
625 Mt. Auburn Street, 3rd Floor
PO Box 9031
Cambridge, MA 02139-9031
617-547-6706
800-225-5750
FAX: 888-440-2665
Feedback.EPS@schoolspecialty.com
eps.schoolspecialty.com

Rick Holden, President, EPS
Carol Einstein, Author
A series of 4 books designed to help students improve their reading comprehension skills. Each book contains 43 reading passages followed by 4 questions. Two questions as for a recall of main ideas, and two ask the student to draw conclusions from what they have read. *$ 11.45*
96 pages

1986 Reading from Scratch
Educators Publishing Service
P.O.Box 9031
Cambridge, MA 2139-9031
617-367-2700
800-225-5750
FAX: 617-547-0412
www.epsbooks.com

$6.25 - $49.30
ISBN 0-83888 -75-5

1987 Recipe for Reading
School Specialty
625 Mt. Auburn Street, 3rd Floor
PO Box 9031
Cambridge, MA 02139-9031
617-367-2700
800-225-5750
FAX: 888-440-2665
Feedback.EPS@schoolspecialty.com
eps.schoolspecialty.com

Rick Holden, President, EPS
Nina Traub, Author
Frances Bloom, Co-Author
Contains comprehensive, multisensory, phonics-based reading program presents a skill sequence and lesson structured designed for beginning, at-risk, or struggling readers.

1988 Rewarding Speech
Speech Bin
PO Box 1579
Appleton, WI 54912-1579
772-770-0007
888-388-3224
FAX: 888-388-6344
customercare@schoolspecialty.com
www.speechbin.com

Jan J Binney, Senior Editor
Reproducible reward certificates for children. *$12.95*
32 pages

1989 SAYdee Posters
Speech Bin
PO Box 1579
Appleton, WI 54912-1579
772-770-0007
888-388-3224
FAX: 888-388-6344
customercare@schoolspecialty.com
www.speechbin.com

Jan J Binney, Senior Editor
Colorful speech and language posters. *$20.00*
24 pages
ISBN 0-93785 -47-5

1990 Sensation Products
74 Cotton Mill Hill
Unit A-350
Brattleboro, VT 5301
802-254-4480
FAX: 802-254-4481
www.sensationproducts.com

1991 Sensory University Toy Company, The
4992 Bristol Industrial Hwy
Buford, GA 30518
888-831-4701
FAX: 770-904-6418
sales@sensoryuniversity.com
sensoryuniversity.com

1992 Sequential Spelling: 1-7 with 7 Student Response Books
AVKO Educational Research Foundation
3084 Willard Rd
Birch Run, MI 48415-9404
810-686-9283
866-285-6612
FAX: 810-686-1101
webmaster@avko.org
www.avko.org

Deborah Wolf, President
Aaron Miller, Vice President
Sequential Spelling uses immediate student self-correction. It builds from easier words of a word family such as all and then builds on them to teach; all, tall, stall, install, call, fall, ball, and their inflected forms such as: stalls, stalled, stalling, installing, installment. *$89.95*
72 pages $8.95 each
ISBN 1-56400 -11-6

1993 Signing Naturally Curriculum
Harris Communications
15155 Technology Dr
Eden Prairie, MN 55344-2273
952-906-1180
800-825-6758
FAX: 952-906-1099
info@harriscomm.com
www.harriscomm.com

Robert Harris, President
Kevin Horsky, Business Director
A series based on the functional approach that is the most popular and widely used sign language curriculum designed for teaching American Sign Language. Book and videotape set for level 1 & 2. Teacher's curriculum is also available. *$59.95*

1994 Small Wonder
AGS
PO Box 99
Circle Pines, MN 55014-99
651-287-7220
800-328-2560
FAX: 763-786-9007
agsmail@agsnet.com
www.agsnet.com

Kevin Brueggeman, President
Robert Zaske, Marketing Manager
This infant through toddler program offers a delightful array of activities to teach babies about themselves, others, their surroundings and the world outside. Level One - zero to 18 months;

Level Two 18-36 months. Discount price of $389.95 when both levels ordered. *$229.95*

ISBN 0-91347 -62-5

1995   Solving Language Difficulties
School Specialty
625 Mt. Auburn Street, 3rd Floor
PO Box 9031
Cambridge, MA 02139-9031
617-547-6706
800-225-5750
FAX: 888-440-2665
Feedback.EPS@schoolspecialty.com
eps.schoolspecialty.com

Rick Holden, President, EPS
Amey Steere, Author
Caroline Z Peck, Co-Author
This basic workbook can be used in any corrective reading program. It deals extensively with syllables, syllable division, prefixes, suffixes and accent. *$9.75*
176 pages
ISBN 0-838803-26-1

1996   Speech Bin
Abilitations
PO Box 1579
Appleton, WI 54912-1579
772-770-0007
800-513-2465
FAX: 80- 51- 246
onlinehelp@schoolspecialty.com
www.speechbin.com

Jan J Binney, Senior Editor
Activities, worksheets and games to encourage practice of speech and language skills. *$25.00*
128 pages
ISBN 0-93785 -42-4

1997   Speech-Language Delights
1965 25th Ave
Vero Beach, FL 32960-3062
772-770-0007

1998   Spell of Words
School Specialty
625 Mt. Auburn Street, 3rd Floor
PO Box 9031
Cambridge, MA 02139-9031
617-547-6706
800-225-5750
FAX: 888-440-2665
Feedback.EPS@schoolspecialty.com
eps.schoolspecialty.com

Rick Holden, President, EPS
Elsie T Rak, Author
Covers syllabication, word building along with prefixes, phonograms, word patterns, suffixes, plurals, and possessives. *$14.70*
128 pages Grades 7-Adult

1999   Spellbound
School Specialty
625 Mt. Auburn Street, 3rd Floor
PO Box 9031
Cambridge, MA 02139-9031
617-547-6706
800-225-5750
FAX: 888-440-2665
Feedback.EPS@schoolspecialty.com
eps.schoolspecialty.com

Rick Holden, President, EPS
Elsie T Rak, Author
This workbook begins with teaching simple, consistent rules and then moves on to those that are more difficult. By an inductive process, students use their own observations to confirm the spelling rules they learn. Each portion of the text is followed by exercises for drill and kinesthetic reinforcement. *$12.85*
144 pages Grades 7-Adult
ISBN 0-838801-65-X

2000   Spelling Dictionary
School Specialty
625 Mt. Auburn Street, 3rd Floor
PO Box 9031
Cambridge, MA 02139-9031
617-547-6706
800-225-5750
FAX: 888-440-2665
Feedback.EPS@schoolspecialty.com
eps.schoolspecialty.com

Rick Holden, President, EPS
Gregory Hurray, Author
Contains the most frequently used and misspelled words for students at these grade levels. Designed to be useable and reliable, to build research and writing skills, and to help teachers promote independent learning in a classroom setting *$6.35*

ISBN 0-838820-56-5

2001   Starting Over
School Specialty
625 Mt. Auburn Street, 3rd Floor
PO Box 9031
Cambridge, MA 02139-9031
617-547-6706
800-225-5750
FAX: 888-440-2665
Feedback.EPS@schoolspecialty.com
eps.schoolspecialty.com

Rick Holden, President, EPS
Joan Knight, Author
For students who are ready to try to learn to read again, or for those who are learning English as a second language. *$38.40*

ISBN 0-838881-65-5

2002   Studio 49 Catalog
MMB Music
9051 Watson Road
Suite 161
Saint Louis, MO 63126-1019
314-531-9635
800-543-3771
FAX: 314-531-8384
info@mmbmusic.com
www.mmbmusic.com

Marcia Goldberg, President
Michelle Greenlaw, VP
Percussion instruments for school, therapy, church and family.

2003   Syracuse Community-Referenced Curriculum Guide for Students with Disabilties
Brookes Publishing
PO Box 10624
Baltimore, MD 21285-624
410-337-9580
800-638-3775
FAX: 410-337-8539
custserv@brookespublishing.com
www.readplaylearn.com

Paul Brooks, President
Serving learners from kindergarten through age 21, this field-tested curriculum is a for professionals and parents devoted to directly preparing a student to function in the world. it examines the role of community living domains, functional academics, and embedded skills and includes practical implementation strategies and information for preparing students whose learning needs go beyond the scope of traditional academic programs. *$54.95*
416 pages Spiral-bound
ISBN 1-557660-27-1

2004 Teaching Individuals with Physical and Multiple Disabilities
McGraw-Hill, School Publishing
PO Box 182604
Columbus, OH 43272

877-833-5524
FAX: 614-759-3749
customer.service@mcgraw-hill.com
www.mcgraw-hill.com

Harold McGraw, President and CEO
Jack Callahan, Executive VP
John Berisford, Executive VP of HR
Focuses on the functional needs of the handicapped and the teaching skills of background teachers that they need to help them reach the highest possible level of self-sufficiency.
410 pages

2005 Teaching Students Ways to Remember
Brookline Books
8 Trumbull Rd, Suite B-001
Northampton, MA 1060

60- 66- 703
800-666-2665
FAX: 413-584-6184
brbooks@yahoo.com
www.brooklinebooks.com

ISBN 0-914797-67-0

2006 Teaching Test-Taking Skills: Helping Students Show What They Know
Brookline Books
8 Trumbull Rd, Suite B-001
Northampton, MA 1060

60- 66- 703
800-666-2665
FAX: 414-584-6184
brbooks@yahoo.com
www.brooklinebooks.com

ISBN 0-914797-76-X

2007 Therapy Shoppe
PO Box 8875
Grand Rapids, MI 49518

616-696-7441
800-261-5590
FAX: 616-696-7471
info@therapyshoppe.com
www.therapyshoppe.com

2008 To Teach a Dyslexic
AVKO Educational Research Foundation
3084 Willard Rd
Birch Run, MI 48415-9404

810-686-9283
866-686-9283
FAX: 810-686-1101
webmaster@avko.org
www.avko.org

Deborah Wolf, President
Aaron Miller, Vice President
A video available in DVD or video CD that shows Don McCabe working with a dyslexic teenager. The video helps teachers learn more about dyslexia and how to go about teaching a dyslexic student using the AVKO methodology and philosophy. This is a free video.
288 pages Paperback

2009 Tools for Transition
AGS
PO Box 99
Circle Pines, MN 55014-99

651-287-7220
800-328-2560
FAX: 763-786-9007
agsmail@agsnet.com
www.agsnet.com

Kevin Brueggeman, President
Robert Zaske, Marketing Manager
This program prepares students with learning disabilities for postsecondary education. *$129.95*

2010 United Art and Education
PO Box 9219
Fort Wayne, IN 46899-9219

260-478-1121
800-322-3247
FAX: 800-858-3247
www.unitednow.com

2011 VAK Tasks Workbook: Visual, Auditory and Kinesthetic
Educational Tutorial Consortium
4400 S 44th St
Lincoln, NE 68516-1109

402-489-8133
FAX: 402-489-8160
etc@altel.net
www.etc-ne.com

T Elli Cross, Owner
A workbook emphasizing the multisensory approach to teaching vocabulary and spelling. It is intended for middle-grade and older students working with prefixes, roots, suffixes, homonyms, and the spelling of easily confused endings. Includes spelling posters. *$7.00*
96 pages Paperback

2012 Volunteer Transcribing Services
Ste 200
205 E 3rd Ave
San Mateo, CA 94401-4028

650-357-1571
FAX: 650-632-3510

Alanah Hoffman, Coordinator
VTS is a nonprofit California corporation that produces large print school books for visually impaired students in grades K-12.

2013 Wordly Wise 3000
School Specialty
625 Mt. Auburn Street, 3rd Floor
PO Box 9031
Cambridge, MA 02139-9031

617-547-6706
800-225-5750
FAX: 888-440-2665
Feedback.EPS@schoolspecialty.com
eps.schoolspecialty.com

Rick Holden, President, EPS
Kenneth Hodkinson, Author
Sandra Adams, Co-Author
Cheryl Dressler, Co-Author
Begins with a word list of 8-12 words, followed by clear, brief definitions and sentences that illustrate the meaning of the word. Books B and C often present more than one meaning of a word. Throughout all three books, drawings illustrate the meanings.

ISSN 0838-84 8

2014 Work!
JE Stewart Teaching Tools
PO Box 15308
Seattle, WA 98115-308

206-328-7664
FAX: 206-262-9538

Jan Gleason, Executive Director
Teaches 50 words as they appear on parts, tools, job instructions, signs, labels such as: hard hat, assembly, clamp, cut, drill, package and schedule. These words are functional in school and on-the-job. *$32.50*

2015 Working Together & Taking Part
A GS
PO Box 99
Circle Pines, MN 55014-99

651-287-7220
800-328-2560
FAX: 763-786-9007
agsmail@agsnet.com
www.agsnet.com

Kevin Brueggeman, President
Robert Zaske, Market Manager
Two programs to build children's social skills in grades 3-6 through folk literature. Has 31 activity-rich lessons, teaching skills like: following rules, accepting differences, speaking assertively and helping others. Discount price of $279.00 when ordering both. *$149.95*

Associations

2016 **AVKO Educational Research Foundation**
3084 Willard Rd
Birch Run, MI 48415-9404
810-686-9283
866-686-9283
FAX: 810-686-1101
webmaster@avko.org
www.avko.org

Deborah Wolf, President
Aaron Miller, Vice President
Comprised of individuals interested in helping others learn to read and spell. Develops and sells materials for teaching dyslexics or others with learning disabilities using a method involving audio, visual, kinesthetic and oral (multi-sensory) techniques.

2017 **Alliance for Parental Involvement in Education**
PO Box 59
East Chatham, NY 12060-59
518-392-6900
FAX: 518-392-6900
allpie@taconic.net
www.croton.com/allpie

2018 **Alternative Work Concepts**
PO Box 11452
Eugene, OR 97440-3652
541-345-3043
FAX: 541-345-9669
awc@efn.com
www.alternativeworkconcepts.org

Liz Fox, Executive Director
To promote individualized, integrated, and meaningful employment opportunities in the community for adults with multiple disabilities; to improve the quality of life and provide continuous opportunities for personal growth for these individuals; and to assist businesses with workforce diversification.

2019 **American Council for Headache Education(ACHE)**
19 Mantua Rd
Mount Royal, NJ 8061-1006
856-423-0043
FAX: 856-423-0082
achehq@talley.com
www.achenet.org

Fred Sheftell, Chairman
Nonprofit, patient-health, professional partnership dedicated to advancing the treatment and management of headaches and to raising the public awareness of headache as valid, biologically based illness.

2020 **American School Counselor Association**
American Counselling Association
1101 King St
Suite 625
Alexandria, VA 22314-2957
703-683-2722
800-306-4722
FAX: 703-683-1619
asca@schoolcounselor.org
www.schoolcounselor.org

Richard Wong, Executive Director
Kathleen Rakestraw, Director of Communications
Carolyn Stone, Board President
ASCA focuses on providing professional devleopment, enhancing school counseling programs, and research effective school counseling practices. Mission is to promote excellence in professional school counseling and the development of all students.

2021 **Association for Driver Rehabilitation Specialists**
200 First Ave NW
Suite 505
Hickory, NC 28601
866-672-9466
FAX: 828-855-1672
info@aded.net
www.aded.net

Jenny Nordine, President
Elizabeth Green, Executive Director
Beth Gibson, Secretary
Robert Dan, Office Manager

The Association for Driver Rehabilitation Specialists was established in 1977 to support professionals working in the field of driver education / driver training and transportation equipment modifications for persons with disabilities through education and information dissemination.

2022 **Association on Higher Education and Disability**
107 Commerce Centre Dr
Suite 204
Huntersville, NC 28078-5870
704-947-7779
FAX: 704-948-7779
TTY:617-287-3882
ahead@ahead.org
www.ahead.org

Jean Ashmore, President
Michael Johnson, Treasurer
Stephan Smith, Executive Director
Higher education for people with disabilities. A vital resource, promoting excellence through education, communication and training.

2023 **CARF International (Commission on Accreditation of Rehabilitation Facilities)**
CARF International
6951East Southpoint Road
Tucson, AZ 8575-9407
520-325-1044
888-281-6531
FAX: 520-318-1129
info @carf.org
carf.org

Brian J Boon, CEO
An independent, nonprofit accreditor of human service providers in the areas of aging services, behavioral health, child and youth services, DMEPOS, employment and community services, medical rehabilitation, and opioid treatment programs.

2024 **CEC-Division for Early Childhood**
Council for Exceptional Children
27 Fort Missoula Road
Suite 2
Missoula, MT 59804
406-543-0872
888-232-7733
FAX: 406-543-0887
dec@dec-sped.org
www.dec-sped.org

Sarah Mulligan, Executive Director
Cynthia Wood, Associate Executive Director
Natalie Forcier, Program/Accounting Assistant
Marina Zaleski, Program Assistant
Promotes policies and advances evidence-based practices that support families and enhance the optimal development of young children who have or are at risk for developmental delays and disabilities.

2025 **Council for Exceptional Children**
2900 Crystal Drive
Suite 1000
Arlington, VA 22202-3557
703-620-3660
866-509-0218
888-232-7733
FAX: 703-264-9494
TTY:866-915-5000
service@cec.sped.org
www.cec.sped.org

Robin D. Brewer, President
James P. Heiden, President Elect
Christy A. Chambers, Immediate Past President
Mikki Garcia, Executive Director
The largest international professional organization dedicated to improving the educational success of individuals with disabilities and/or gifts and talents. Advocates for appropriate governmental policies, sets professional standards, provides professional development, advocates for individuals with exceptionalities, and helps professionals obtain conditions and resources necessary for effective professional practice

2026 Division for Physical, Health & Multiple Disabilities
Council for Exceptional Children (CEC)
2900 Crystal Drive,
Suite 1000
Arlington, VA 22202

888-232-7733
FAX: 703-264-9494
TTY:866-915-5000
service@cec.sped.org
www.cec.sped.org

Linda Thomas, President of DPHMD
Juliet Hart, Vice President

The DPHD is the official division of the CEC that advocates for quality education for all individuals with physical disabilities, multiple disabilities, and special health care needs served in schools, hospitals, or home settings. The goals of DPHD include: promoting the continued development adequate resources and programs; disseminating relevant and timely information on issues, instructional strategies, and research through meetings and publications; and many more services and activities.

2027 Educational Referral Service
Doctor Yvonne Jones and Associates
2222 Eastlake Ave E
Seattle, WA 98102-3419

206-325-2600
FAX: 206-328-9172

Yvonne Jones

Specializes in matching children with the learning environments that are best for them and works with families to help them identify concerns and establish priorities about their child's education.

2028 HEAL: Health Education AIDS Liaison
New York, NY

347-867-4497
michaelellner2@gmail.com
www.healaids.com

Michael Ellner, President
Barnett J. Weiss, Board Member
Roberto Giraldo, Board Member

Nonprofit, community-based educational organization providing information, hope, and support to people who are HIV positive or living with AIDS. The men and women at HEAL are health professionals, people living with life threatening diseases, and concerned volunteers.

2029 International Association of Parents and Professionals for Safe Alternatives in Childbirth
Box 646
Rr 4
Marble Hill, MO 63764-9418

573-238-4273
FAX: 573-238-2010
napsac@clas.org
www.napsac.org

Lee Stewart, Publisher
David Stewart, Executive Director

Dedicated to exploring, implementing, and establishing safe, family-centered childbirth programs that meet the social and emotional needs of families as well as provide the safe, appropriate aspects of medical science.

2030 International Childbirth Education Association
1500 Sunday Drive
Suite 102
Raleigh, NC 27607-48

919-863-9487
800-624-4934
FAX: 919-787-4916
info@icea.org
www.icea.org

Denise Wheatley, President
Nancy Lantz, President- Elect
Deborah Codde, Treasurer
Debra Tolson, Secretary

Offer teaching certificates, seminars, continuing education workshops, and a mail order center.

2031 International Dyslexia Association
40 York Road
4th Floor
Baltimore, MD 21204-5243

410-296-0232
800-222-3123
FAX: 410-321-5069
info@interdys.org
www.interdys.org

Guinevere Eden, President
Stephen Peregoy, Executive Director
Sandra Soper, Vice President

IDA is a clearinghouse of scientific data and practice-based information related to dyslexia. We also provide community-based referrals and information fact sheets in response to thousands of emails, calls & letters. Our annual conference attracts thousands of researchers, clinicians, parents, teachers, psychologist, educational therapists and people with dyslexia.

2032 International Organization for the Education of the Hearing Impaired
Alexander Graham Bell Association
3417 Volta Pl NW
Washington, DC 20007-2737

202-337-5220
FAX: 202-337-8314
TTY:202-337-5221
info@agbell.org
www.agbell.org

Kathleen Treni, President
Meredith Knueve, Secretary Treasurer
Alexander Graham, Executive Director/CEO

Professional educators of the hearing impaired make up the members of this organization which promotes the excellence in teaching the hearing impaired child.

2033 Jewish Guild for the Blind
15 W 65th St
New York, NY 10023-6601

212-769-6200
800-284-4422
FAX: 212-769-6266
info@guildhealth.org
www.jgb.org

Pauline Raiff, Chairman
Aaron Kesselman, President
Eileen Hanley, Senior VP
Barbara Klein, Director of Development

Full service vision care agency for children, adults and elderly people who are blind or visually impaired.

2034 Job Accommodation Network
Office of Disability and Employment Policy
PO Box 6080
Morgantown, WV 26506-6080

800-232-9675
800-526-7234
FAX: 304-093-5407
TTY: 877-781-9403
jan@jan.wvu.edu
www.jan.wvu.edu

DJ Hendricks, Director

International toll-free consulting service that provides information about job accommodations and the employability of people with disabilities. Also provides information regarding the Americans with Disabilities Act (ADA).

2035 Michigan Psychological Association
124 W Allegan St
Suite 1900
Lansing, MI 48933-1768

517-347-1885
FAX: 517-484-4442
office@michiganpsychologicalassociation.org
www.michiganpsychologicalass ociation.org

William Nicholson, President
Judith Kovach, Executive Director

Nonprofit organization of over 1000 psychologists, working to advance psychology as a science and a profession and to promote the public welfare by encouraging the highest professional standards, offering public education and providing a public service, and by participating in the public policy process on behalf of the profession and health care consumers.

2036   National Association for Adults with Special Learning Needs
PO Box 716
Bryn Mawr, PA 19010

naasln.org

2037   National Association for the Education of African American Children with LD
PO Box 09521
Columbus, OH 43209

614-237-6021
FAX: 614-238-0929
info@aacld.org
www.aacld.org

Linda James Myers, Ph.D., Chairman
Nancy R. Tidwell, Founder & President
Donald W. Tidwell, Jr, Co-Founder
Nicholas S. Tidwell, Co-Founder
The AACLD is a non profit organization founded in 2000 for the purpose of increasing awareness in minority communities about learning differences and promoting parent advocacy.

2038   National Association of Colleges and Employers
62 Highland Ave
Bethlehem, PA 18017-9481

610-868-1421
800-544-5272
FAX: 610-868-0208
naceweb.org

Vanessa Strauss, President
Donnie Brown, VP of Human Resources
A national association with services for career planning, placement and recruitment professionals.

2039   National Association of Parents with Children in Special Education
3642 E Sunnydale Drive
Chandler Heights, AZ 85142

800-754-4421
FAX: 800-424-0371
contact@napcse.org
www.napcse.org

Dr. George Giuliani, President
(NAPCSE)is a national membership organization dedicated to rendering all possible support and assistance to parents whose children receive special education services, both in and outside of school

2040   National Association of Private Special Education Centers
601 Pennsylvania Avenue
Suite 900, South Building
Washington, DC 20004-1202

202-434-8225
FAX: 202-434-8224
napsec@aol.com
napsec.org

Sherry Kolbe, Executive Director
Membership directory offering information on NAPSEC member schools nationwide available.

2041   National Association of State Directors of Special Education
225 Reinekers Lane
Suite 420
Alexandria, VA 22314

703-519-3800
FAX: 703-519-3808
www.nasdse.org

Frank Podobnik, President
Bill East, Executive Director
Nancy Deputy Exe Dir/Gov Rel
Eileen Ahearn, Director
NASDSE focuses on improving educational services and outcomes for children and youth with disabilities throughout the United States, the Department of Defense, the federated territories and the Freely Associated States of Palau, Micronesia and the Marshall Islands.

2042   National Center for Homeopathy
101 S Whiting St
Alexandria, VA 22304-3418

703-548-7790
FAX: 703-548-7792
info@homeopathic.org
nationalcenterforhomeopathy.org

Sharon Stevenson, Executive Director
Provides information, referral lists, online webinars to members, and an annual homeopathic conference.

2043   National Clearinghouse for Professions
2900 Crystal Drive
Suite 1000
Arlington, VA 22202

703-264-9454
888-232-7733
FAX: 703-264-1637
service@cec.sped.org
www.cec.sped.org

Bruce Ramirez, Executive Director

2044   National Council on Rehabilitation Education (NCRE)
1099 E. Champlain Drive, Suite A
PMB # 137
Fresno, CA 93720

559-906-0787
FAX: 559-412-2550
info@ncre.org
www.rehabeducators.org

Charles Degeneffe, President
Ken Hergenrather, First VP
Jared Schultz, Second VP
Members include academic institutions and organizations, professional educators, researchers, and students. Assists in the documentation of the effect of education in improving services to persons with disabilities; determines the skills and training necessary for effective rehabilitation services; develops role models, standards and uniform licensure and certification requirements for rehabilitation personnel.

2045   National Education Association of the United States
1201 16th St NW
Washington, DC 20036-3290

202-833-4000
FAX: 202-822-7974
www.nea.org

Dennis Van Roekel, President
Lily Eskelsen, Vice President
Rebecca Pringle, VP and Secretary
John Wilson, Executive Director
Offers information to educational professionals.

2046   National Society for Experiential Education
19 Mantua Rd
Mount Royal, NJ 8061-1006

856-423-3427
FAX: 856-423-3420
nsee@talley.com
www.nsee.org

James Walters, President
Mary King, Vice President
Haley Brust, Executive Director
National nonprofit organization which advocates experiential learning and works with college administrators and high school and college internship programs.

2047   President's Committee for People with Intellectual Disabilities
Administration for Children & Families
370 L Enfant Promenade SW
Washington, DC 20447-1

202-619-0634
FAX: 202-205-9519
www.acf.hhs.gov/programs/pcpid

Sally Atwater, Executive Director
Dalls Rob Sweezy, Chairperson
MJ Karimi, Executive Director Assistant
Prepares an annual report to the president of the United States addressing issues concerning citizens with intellectual disabilities.

2048 Rifin Family/Daughters of Israel
JGB Audio Library for the Blind
15 W 65th St
New York, NY 10023-6601   212-769-6200
800-284-4422
FAX: 212-769-6266
info@JGB.org
www.JGB.org
Pauline Raiff, Chairman
Aaron Kesselman, President
Eileen Hanley, Senior VP

2049 SSD (Services for Students with Disabilities)
College Board
45 Columbus Ave
New York, NY 10023-6917   212-713-8000
866-630-9305
FAX: 212-713-8255
help@cssprofile.org
www.collegeboard.com
Gaston Caperton, President
National, nonprofit membership association dedicated to preparing, inspiring and connecting students to college and opportunity. Founded in 1900, the association is composed of more than 3,800 schools, colleges, universities and other educational organizations. Services for Students with Disabilities (SSD) provides special arrangements to minimize the possible effects of disabilities on test performance through it's Admissions Testing Program (ATP).

2050 Society for Disability Studies
538 Park Hall
University at Buffalo
Buffalo, NY 14260- 4130   716-645-0276
FAX: 716-645-5954
info@disstudies.org
www.disstudies.org
Mike Rembis, President
SDS is a lively scholarly association of more than 400 artists, scholars and activists who promote Disability Studies, recognizing disability as a complex and valuable aspect of human experience.

2051 Society for the Study of Disability in the Middle Ages
One Brookings Drive
St. Louis, MO 63130-4899
jesinger@wustl.edu
pages.wustl.edu/ssdma

2052 Target Teach
Evans Newton
Ste 1
15941 N 77th St
Scottsdale, AZ 85260-1217   480-998-2777
800-443-0544
FAX: 480-951-2895
info@evansnewton.com
www.target.com
Jamie Piotti, CEO
Gary Davis, Director of Curriculum and Instr
Aligns and monitors Special Education Instructional Materials to tests that are used to measure the effectiveness of Special Education Instructional Programs.

2053 United Cerebral Palsy
1825 K Street NW
Suite 600
Washington, DC 20006-5638   202-776-0406
800-872-5827
FAX: 202-776-0414
info@ucp.org
www.ucp.org
Stephen Bennett, CEO
Bruce Fried, Chariman
Keith Green, Vice Chair
Grants are awarded to institutions or organizations on behalf of a principal investigator in support of biomedical and bioengineering research in areas which have a significant relationship to cerebral palsy. While most research on central nervous system structure, function and disorder may be useful, the Foundation requires that research proposals address issues of relevance to cerebral palsy.

Directories

2054 ADDitude Directory
108 West 39th St.
Suite 805
New York, NY 10018   646-366-0830
FAX: 646-366-0842
customerservice@additudemag.com
directory.additudemag.com

2055 BOSC: Directory of Facilities for People with Learning Disabilities
Books on Special Children
PO Box 3378
Amherst, MA 1004-3378   413-256-8164
FAX: 413-256-8896
irene@boscbooks.com
www.boscbooks.com
Michael Young, President
Directory of schools, independent living programs, clinics and centers, colleges and vocational programs, agencies and commercial products. Five sections in special post binder that can be updated annually. Hardcover. *$70.00*
300+ pages Yearly
ISSN 0961-3888

2056 Community Resource Directory
5300 Hiatus Road
Sunrise, FL 33351   954-745-9779
800-963-5337
webmaster@adrcbroward.org
www.adrcbroward.org

2057 Complete Directory for Pediatric Disorders
Sedgwick Press/Grey House Publishing
4919 Route 22
P.O. Box 56
Amenia, NY 12501   518-789-8700
800-562-2139
FAX: 518-789-0556
books@greyhouse.com
www.greyhouse.com
Leslie Mackenzie, Publisher
Laura Mars, Editorial Director
Jessica Moody, Marketing Director
Diana Delgado, Editorial Assistant
An annual directory for professionals, parents and caregivers. Provides valuable information on more than 200 pediatric conditions, disorders, diseases and disabilities, including informative descriptions and a wide variety of resources, from associations to publications. *$165.00*
1000 pages Annual
ISBN 1-592374-30-1

2058 Complete Directory for People with Chronic Illness
Sedgwick Press/Grey House Publishing
4919 Route 22
P.O. Box 56
Amenia, NY 12501   518-789-8700
800-562-2139
FAX: 518-789-0556
books@greyhouse.com
www.greyhouse.com
Leslie Mackenzie, Publisher
Laura Mars, Editorial Director
Jessica Moody, Marketing Director
Diana Delgado, Editorial Assistant
This directory is structured around the ninety most prevalent chronic illnesses. Each chronic illness chapter includes an informative description, plus a comprehensive listing of resources and

support services available for people diagnosed with chronic illness and their network of supportive individuals. *$165.00*
1000 pages Annual
ISBN 1-592374-15-8

2059   Complete Learning Disabilities Directory
Sedgwick Press/Grey House Publishing
4919 Route 22
P.O. Box 56
Amenia, NY 12501   518-789-8700
                                    800-562-2139
                                    FAX: 518-789-0556
                                    books@greyhouse.com
                                    www.greyhouse.com

Leslie Mackenzie, Publisher
Laura Mars, Editorial Director
Jessica Moody, Marketing Director
Diana Delgado, Editorial Assistant
A comprehensive educational guide offering over 6,500 listings on associations and organizations, schools, government agencies, testing materials, camps, products, books, newsletters, legal information, classroom materials and more. Includes separate chapters on ADD and Literacy, as well as informative articles. *$150.00*
800 pages Annual
ISBN 1-592375-86-3

2060   Complete Mental Health Directory
Sedgwick Press/Grey House Publishing
4919 Route 22
P.O. Box 56
Amenia, NY 12501   518-789-8700
                                    800-562-2139
                                    FAX: 518-789-0556
                                    books@greyhouse.com
                                    www.greyhouse.com

Leslie Mackenzie, Publisher
Laura Mars, Editorial Director
Jessica Moody, Marketing Director
Diana Delgado, Editorial Assistant
This directory offers comprehensive information covering the field of behavioral health, with critical information for both the layman and the mental health professional. It covers, in depth, 25 specific mental disorders, and includes informative descriptions and a complete list of resources. *$165.00*
800 pages Annual
ISBN 1-592375-44-8

2061   Directory Of Services For People With Disabilities
117 W. Duval St.
Suite 205
Jacksonville, FL 32202-4111   904-630-4940
                                    FAX: 904-630-3476
                                    TTY:904-630-4933
                                    disabledservices@coj.net
                                    www.coj.net

2062   Directory for Exceptional Children
Prorter Sargent
2 LAN Drive
Suite 100
Westford, MA 01886   978-692-5092
                                    800-342-7470
                                    FAX: 978-692-4714
                                    info@carnegiecomm.com
                                    www.carnegiecomm.com

Joe Moore, President, CEO
Mark Cunningham, SVP, Enrollment Marketing
Melissa Rekos, SVP, Digital Services
Gary Allen Williams, VP, Special Projects
Supports parents and professionals seeking the optimal educational, therapeutic or clinical environment for special-needs youth. *$75.00*
1120 pages Trienniel
ISBN 0-875581-50-1

2063   Educators Resource Directory
Sedgwick Press/Grey House Publishing
4919 Route 22
PO Box 55
Amenia, NY 12501   518-789-8700
                                    800-562-2139
                                    FAX: 845-373-6390
                                    books@greyhouse.com
                                    www.greyhouse.com

Leslie Mackenzie, Publisher
Laura Mars, Editorial Director
Jessica Moody, Marketing Director
Kristen Thatcher, Production Manager
Gives education professionals immediate access to Associations and Organizations, Conferences and Trade Shows, Educational Research Centers, Employment Opportunities and Teaching Abroad, School Library Services, Scholarships, Financial Resources and much more. *$ 145.00*
650 pages Annual
ISBN 1-592377-43-5

2064   Greater Milwaukee Area Health Care Guide for Older Adults
PO Box 285
Germantown, WI 53022   262-253-0901
                                    FAX: 262-253-0903
                                    info@seniorresourcesonline.com
                                    www.seniorresourcesonline.com

Gary Knippen, President
This directory is designed for older adults, family members and professionals looking for health care options in Milwaukee, Ozaukee, Washington and Waukesha counties. The directory is comprehensive with all providers included at no charge.

2065   Greater Milwaukee Area Senior Housing Options
PO Box 285
Germantown, WI 53022   262-253-0901
                                    FAX: 262-253-0903
                                    info@seniorresourcesonline.com
                                    www.seniorresourcesonline.com

Gary Knippen, President
This directory is designed for older adults, family members and professionals looking for senior housing options in Milwaukee, Ozaukee, Washington and Waukesha counties. The directory is comprehensive with all providers included at no charge.

2066   Increasing and Decreasing Behaviors of Persons with Severe Retardation and Autism
Research Press
P.O. Box 7886
Champaign, IL 61826   217-352-3273
                                    800-519-2707
                                    FAX: 217-352-1221
                                    orders@researchpress.com
                                    www.researchpress.com

Robert W. Parkinson, Founder
Dr Richard M Foxx, Author
Shows how to increase desirable behaviors by using techniques such as shaping, prompting, fading, modeling, backward chaining and graduated guidance. Offers specific guidelines for arranging and managing the learning environment as well as standards for evaluating and maintaining success. *$21.95*
230 pages
ISBN 0-878222-65-0

2067   Indiana Directory of Disability Resources
225 S. University Street
ABE Bldg.
West Lafayette, IN 47907-2093   765-494-5013
                                    800-825-4264
                                    bng@ecn.purdue.edu%20
                                    engineering.purdue.edu/~bng/IDDR/

2068 Nevada's Care Connection
3416 Goni Road
Suite D-132
Carson City, NV 89706　　　702-486-3600
cpasquale@adsd.nv.gov
www.nevadaadrc.com

Cheyenne Pasquale, ADRC Project Manager
Nevada's Care Connection: Aging and Disability Resource Center (ADRC) program provides information and access to programs and services that benefit Nevada's seniors, people with disabilities and caregivers.

2069 Northeast Wisconsin Directory of Servicesfor Older Adults
PO Box 285
Germantown, WI 53022　　　262-253-0901
FAX: 262-253-0903
info@seniorresourcesonline.com
www.seniorresourcesonline.com

Gary Knippen, President
This directory is designed for older adults, family members and professionals looking for housing and health care options in Brown, Calumet, Door, Fond du Lac, Green Lake, Kewaunee, Manitowoc, Marinette, Marquette, Oconto, Outagamie, Shawano, Sheboygan, Waupaca, Waushara and Winnebago counties.

2070 ODHH Directory of Resources and Services
1521 N. 6th Street
Harrisburg, PA 17102　　　717-783-4912
TTY:717-783-4912
RA-LI-OVR-ODHH@pa.gov
www.portal.state.pa.us

2071 Responding to Crime Victims with Disabilities
2000 M Street NW
Suite 480
Washington, DC 20036　　　202-467-8700
FAX: 202-467-8701
webmaster@ncvc.org
www.victimsofcrime.org

Philip M. Gerson, Chair
G. Morris Gurley, Vice-Chair
Mai Fernandez, Executive Director
Jeffrey R. Dion, Deputy Executive Director
The mission of the National Center for Victims of Crime is to forge a national commitment to help victims of crime rebuild their lives. It is dedicated to serving individuals, families, and communities harmed by crime.

2072 Selective Placement Program Coordinator Directory
1900 E Street, NW
Washington, DC 20415-1000　　　202-606-1800
www.opm.gov

2073 South Central Wisconsin Directory of Services for Older Adults
PO Box 285
Germantown, WI 53022　　　262-253-0901
www.seniorresourcesonline.com

Gary Knippen, President
This directory is designed for older adults, family members and professionals looking for housing and health care options in Columbia, Dane, Dodge, Grant, Green, Iowa, Jefferson, Juneau, Lafayette, Richland, Rock, Sauk, and Walworth counties.

2074 Southeast Wisconsin Directory of Servicesfor Older Adults
PO Box 285
Germantown, WI 53022　　　262-253-0901
www.seniorresourcesonline.com

Gary Knippen, President
This directory is designed for older adults, family members and professionals looking for housing and health care options in Kenosha, Racine and Walworth counties.

2075 Teaching Special Students in Mainstream
Books on Special Children
P.O.Box 305
Congers, NY 10920-305　　　845-638-1236
FAX: 845-638-0847
irene@boscbooks.com

515 pages Softcover

Educational Publishers

2076 AFB Press
American Foundation for the Blind / AFB Press
2 Penn Plaza
Suite 1102
New York, NY 10121　　　212-502-7600
FAX: 888-545-8331
afbinfo@afb.net
www.afb.org

Carl R. Augusto, President and CEO
Paul Schroeder, Vice President, Programs and Policy
Rick Bozeman, Chief Financial Officer
Kelly Bleach, Chief Administrative Officer
Develops, publishes, and sells a wide variety of informative books, pamphlets, periodicals, and videos for students, professionals, and researchers in the blindness and visual impairment fields, for people professionally involved in making the mainstream community accessible, and for blind and visually impaired people and their families; publication and video orders.

2077 Academic Therapy Publications
20 Leveroni Court
Novato, CA 94949-5746　　　415-883-3314
800-422-7249
FAX: 415-883-3720
sales@academictherapy.com
www.academictherapy.com

2078 AccessText Network
512 Means Street NW
Suite 250
Atlanta, GA 30318　　　866-271-4968
FAX: 404-894-7565
membership@accesstext.org
www.accesstext.org

2079 American Association of University Affiliated Programs for Persons with Dev Disabilities
1100 Wayne Ave.
Suite 1000
Silver Spring, MD 20910　　　301-588-8252
FAX: 301-588-2842
aucdinfo@aucd.org
www.aucd.org/

Andrew J. Imparato, JD, Executive Director
Abigail Alberico, MPH, Project Manager
Leon Barnett, MSEd, Program Specialist
Anna Costalas, MPA, Program Specialist
The Association of University Centers on Disabilities (AUCD) is a membership organization that supports and promotes a national network of university-based interdisciplinary programs

2080 American Counseling Association
5999 Stevenson Ave
Alexandria, VA 22304　　　703-823-0252
800-347-6647
FAX: 800-473-2329
webmaster@counseling.org
www.counseling.org

Robert L. Smith, President
Thelma Duffey, President Elect
Brian Canfield, Treasurer
Richard Yep, CEO
Offers tools and books for the professional.

2081 Brookes Publishing Company
PO Box 10624
Baltimore, MD 21285-0624   410-337-9580
                                            800-638-3775
                                       FAX: 410-337-8539
                    webmaster@brookespublishing.com
                         www.brookespublishing.com

Paul H. Brookes, Chairman of the Board
Jeffrey D. Brookes, President
George S. Stamathis, VP/Publisher
Melissa A. Behn, Executive Vice President
Publishes highly respected resources in early childhood, early intervention, inclusive and special education, developmental disabilities, learning disabilities, communication and language, behavior and mental health.

2082 Brookline Books
8 Trumbull Rd
B-001
Northampton, MA 01060   413-584-0184
                                            800-666-2665
                                       FAX: 413-584-6184
                              brbooks@yahoo.com
                            www.brooklinebks.com

2083 Brooks/Cole Publishing Company
511 Forest Lodge Rd
Pacific Grove, CA 93950-5040   831-373-0728
                                            800-354-9706
                                       FAX: 831-375-6414

2084 BurnsBooks Publishing
680 Ridge Road
Middletown, CT 6457   860-344-0233
                                       FAX: 860-344-0233
                         burnsbookspub@aol.com
                    www.burnsbookspublishing.com

2085 Charles C Thomas Publisher LTD
2600 S 1st Street
Springfield, IL 62704-4730   217-789-8980
                                            800-258-8980
                                       FAX: 217-789-9130
                            books@ccthomas.com
                             www.ccthomas.com

Michael P. Thomas, President
Publishes specialty titles and textbooks in medicine, dentistry, nursing, and veterinary medicine, as well as a complete line in the behavioral sciences, criminal justice, education, special education, and rehabilitation. Aims to accommodate the current needs for information.

2086 Dolphin Computer Access
231 Clarksville Road
Suite 7
Princeton Junction, NJ 8550
                                            866-797-5921
                                       FAX: 609-799-0475
                             info@dolphinusa.com
                            www.yourdolphin.com

Noel Duffy, Managing Director
Dolphin helps vision and print impairments

2087 ERIC Clearinghouse on Disabilities and Gifted Education
2900 Crystal Drive
Suite 1000
Arlington, VA 22202-3557   703-264-9454
                                            888-232-7733
                                       FAX: 703-264-1637
                             service@cec.sped.org
                               www.cec.sped.org

Bruce Ramirez, Executive Director

2088 Eric Clearinghouse on Disabilities and Gifted Education
Council for Exceptional Children
2900 Crystal Drive
Suite 1000
Arlington, VA 22202-3557   703-264-9454
                                            888-232-7733
                                       FAX: 703-264-1637
                             service@cec.sped.org
                               www.cec.sped.org

Bruce Ramirez, Executive Director
Provides information on special and gifted education. Provides referrals, offers patient networking services and provides information on current research programs. Focuses its efforts on prevention, identification, assessment, intervention and enrichment both in special settings and within mainstream communities. Offers a variety of materials including brochures and Spanish language matereials.

2089 Gallaudet University Press
800 Florida Avenue, NE
Washington, DC 20002-3695   202-651-5488
                                       FAX: 202-651-5489
                              gupress@gallaudet.edu
                             gupress.gallaudet.edu

David F Armstrong, Executive Director
Publishes scholarly trade books and journals about deaf people and their language, history, and culture for deaf people, parents of deaf children, professionals, educators and the general public. Produces spring and fall catalogs.

2090 Greenwood Publishing Group
88 Post Rd W
Westport, CT 06880-4208   203-226-3571
                                       FAX: 203-222-1502
                         webmaster@greenwood.com
                                    greenwood.com

Wayne Smith, President
Kirstin Olsen, Author
ABC-CLIO and Greenwood Press are recognized as industry-leading providers of the highest-quality reference materials. These imprints offer authoritative reference scholarship and innovative coverage of history and humanities topics across the secondary and higher education curriculum.

2091 Grey House Publishing
4919 Route 22
P.O. Box 56
Amenia, NY 12501   518-789-8700
                                            800-562-2139
                                       FAX: 518-789-0556
                             books@greyhouse.com
                             www.greyhouse.com

Leslie Mackenzie, Publisher
Laura Mars, Editorial Director
Jessica Moody, Marketing Director
Kristen Thatcher, Production Manager
Grey House Publishing publishes directories, handbooks and reference works for public, high school and academic libraries and the business and health communities. Most titles are available as online databases.

2092 Hammill Institute on Disabilities
8700 Shoal Creek Blvd.
Austin, TX 78757-6897   512-451-3521
                                       FAX: 512-451-3728
                           info@hammill-institute.org
                           www.hammill-institute.org

Donald D. Hammill, Board Director
Robert K. Lum, Board Director
Herbert J. Reith, Board Director
Katherine O. Synatschk, Board Director
The Institute was organized in 2005 exclusively for charitable, scientific, and educational purposes to enhance the well-being of people with disabilities, their parents, and the professionals who are devoted to their interests.

2093 Harbor House Law Press
PO Box 480
Hartfield, VA 23071
804-758-8400
FAX: 202-318-3239
webmaster@wrightslaw.com
www.harborhouselaw.com

2094 Information from HEATH Resource Center
National Clearinghouse on Postsecondary Education
2134 G Street, N.W.
Washington, DC 20052
202-939-9320
800-544-3284
FAX: 202-833-5696
heath@ace.nche.edu
www.HEATH-resource-center.org

2095 Lynne Rienner Publishers
1800 30th St.
Ste. 314
Boulder, CO 80301
303-444-6684
FAX: 303-444-0824
questions@rienner.com
www.rienner.com

2096 MAPCON Technologies
8191 Birchwood Court
Suite A
Johnston, IA 50131-2930
515-331-3358
800-223-4791
FAX: 515-331-3373
www.mapcon.com

Joel Tesdall, President/CEO
Diane Wiand, Client Solutions Advocate
Lora Whicker, Accounting
Bailey Merritt, Administrative Assistant
MAPCON is a computerized maintainance management software.

2097 McGraw-Hill Company
PO Box 182605
Columbus, OH 43218
800-338-3987
FAX: 609-308-4480
customer.service@mheducation.com
www.mcgraw-hill.com

David Levin, President, CEO
Ellen Haley, President, CTB
Peter Cohen, President, School Education
Mark Dorman, President, International
Offers a catalog of testing resources and materials for the special educator.

2098 National Association of School Psychologists
4340 East West Highway
Suite 402
Bethesda, MD 20814
301-657-0270
866-311-6277
FAX: 301-657-0275
TTY: 301-657-4155
webmaster@naspweb.org
www.nasponline.org

Stephen E. Brock, President
Todd A. Savage, President-Elect
Laura Benson, Chief Operating Officer
Susan Gorin, Executive Director
Represents over 22,500 school psychologists and related professionals. It serves its members and society by advancing the profession of school psychology and advocating for the rights, welfare, education and mental health of children, youth and their families.

2099 PEAK Parent Center
611 N Weber
Suite 200
Colorado Springs, CO 80903-1072
719-531-9400
800-284-0251
FAX: 719-531-9452
info@peakparent.org
www.peakparent.org

Barbara Buswell, Executive Director
PEAK Parent Center is a federally-designated Parent Training and Information Center (PTI). As a PTI, PEAK supports and empowers parents, providing them with information and strategies to use when advocating for their children with disabilities. PEAK works one-on-one with families and educators helping them realize new possibilities for children with disabilities by expanding knowledge of special education and offering new strategies for success.

2100 PRO-ED
8700 Shoal Creek Boulevard
Austin, TX 78757-6897
512-451-3246
800-897-3202
FAX: 512-451-8542
info@proedinc.com
www.proedinc.com

2101 Peytral Publications
P.O. Box 1162
Minnetonka, MN 55345
952-949-8707
TTY: 952-906-9777
help@peytral.com
www.peytral.com

2102 Prufrock Press
PO Box 8813
Waco, TX 76714-8813
254-756-3337
800-998-2208
FAX: 800-240-0333
jmcintosh@prufrock.com
www.prufrock.com

Joel McIntosh, Publisher & Marketing Director
Lacy Compton, Senior Editor
Rachel Taliaferro, Editor
Raquel Trevino, Graphic Designer and Production Coordinator
Publishes books, textbooks, teaching aids, journals, and magazines supporting gifted education and gifted children.

2103 Research Press
P.O. Box 7886
Champaign, IL 61826
217-352-3273
800-519-2707
FAX: 217-352-1221
orders@researchpress.com
www.researchpress.com

Robert W. Parkinson, Founder
Dr Richard M Foxx, Author
Jeffrey S. Allen, Author
Bryce Alvord, Author
Research Press is an independent, family-owned business founded in 1968 by Robert W. Parkinson (1920-2001). During the past 40 years, the company has earned a solid reputation for publishing practical and effective educational and mental health resources. Authors from the early years include well-known names in the field of psychology, such as B.F. Skinner, Albert Ellis, Gerald Patterson, Wesley Becker, John Guttmann, Richard Foxx, Arnold Lazarus, and Joseph Cautela.

2104 Research Press Company
2612 N. Mattis Ave.
Champaign, IL 61822
217-352-3273
800-519-2707
FAX: 217-352-1221
www.researchpress.com

2105   Sage Publications
2455 Teller Road
Thousand Oaks, CA 91320   805-499-0721
                                 800-818-7243
                                 FAX: 800-583-2665
                                 info@sagepub.com
                                 www.sagepub.com
Sara Miller McCune, Founder, Publisher & Executive Chairman
Blaise R Simqu, President/CEO
Chris Hickok, Senior Vice President & Chief Financial Officer
Stephen Barr, Managing Director/SAGE London, President of SAGE Internation
Publishes books, text books, journals, reference books, and databases mainly related to psychology, special education and speech, language and hearing.

2106   Special Needs Project
324 State St
Ste H
Santa Barbara, CA 93101
                                 818-718-9900
                                 FAX: 818-349-2027
                                 hgray@specialneeds.com
                                 www.specialneeds.com
Hod Gray, Owner
Publishes child development textbooks, books about aspergers syndrome, autism, and other disabilities.

2107   Supporting Success for Children with Hearing Loss
15619 Premiere Drive
Suite 101
Tampa, FL 33624   850-363-9909
                                 FAX: 480-393-4331
                   accounting@successforkidswithhearingloss.com
                              successforkidswithhearinglo ss.com
Karen Anderson, PhD, Director
Improving the Outcomes of Children with Hearing Loss

2108   Woodbine House
6510 Bells Mill Road
Bethesda, MD 20817
                                 800-843-7323
                                 info@woodbinehouse.com
                                 www.woodbinehouse.com

State Agencies: Alabama

2109   Alabama Department of Education: Division of Special Education Services
50 North Ripley St
P.O. Box 302101
Montgomery, AL 36104   334-242-9700
                                 FAX: 334-262-2677
                                 speced@alsde.edu
                                 www.alsde.edu
Crystal Richardson, Program Coordinator
Provides technical assistance to all education agencies serving Alabama's gifted children as well as children with disabilities.

State Agencies: Alaska

2110   Alaska Department of Education: SpecialEducation
State of Alaska
801 West 10th St
Ste 200, P.O.Box 110500
Juneau, AK 99811-0500   907-465-8693
                                 FAX: 907-465-2806
                                 TTY:907-465-2815
                                 sped@alaska.gov
                           www.education.alaska.gov/TLS/SPED
Dr. Susan McCauley, Division Director
Paul Prussing, Deputy Director
Cassidy Jones, Special Education Programs Manager

Administers special educational programs to the disabled residents of Alaska, through the Division of Teaching & Learning Support.

State Agencies: Arkansas

2111   Arkansas Department of Special Education
1401 West Capitol Ave, Victory Bldg
Suite 450
Little Rock, AR 72201   501-682-4221
                                 FAX: 501-682-3456
                                 TTY:501-682-4222
                                 spedsupport@arkansas.gov
                                 arksped.k12.ar.us
Tom Hicks, Interim Associate Director
Ella Albert, Management Project Analyst
Howie Knoff, Director
Tony Boaz, Director
Provides oversight of all educational programs for children and youth with disabilities, ages 3 to 21. Provides technical assistance to all public agencies providing educational services to this population.

State Agencies: California

2112   California Department of Education: Special Education Division
1430 N Street
Sacramento, CA 95814-5901   916-319-0800
                                 FAX: 916-327-3516
                                 scheduler@cde.ca.gov
                                 www.cde.ca.gov
Tom Torlakson, State Superintendent of Public Instruction and Director of E
Fred Balcom, Director
Gordon Jackson, Director
Phyllis Bramson, Director
Information and resources to serve the unique needs of persons with disabilities so that each person will meet or exceed high standards of achievement in academic and nonacademic skills.

State Agencies: Colorado

2113   Colorado Department of Education: Special Education Service Unit
Colorado Department of Education
201 E Colfax Ave
Denver, CO 80203-1704   303-866-6600
                                 FAX: 303-830-0793
                                 steinberg_c@cde.state.co.us
                                 www.cde.state.co.us
Ed Steinberg, Commissioner
Provides consultation on materials and educational services for visually handicapped children, supervises volunteer services, transcribes textbooks for visually handicapped students.

State Agencies: Connecticut

2114   Connecticut Department of Education: Bureau of Special Education
165 Capitol Avenue
Hartford, CT 06106   860-713-6543
                                 FAX: 860-713-7014
                                 annelouise.thompson@ct.gov
                                 www.sde.ct.gov
Anne Louise Thompson, Bureau Chief
Lisa Spooner, Administrative Assistant
Regina Gaunichaux, Secretary
Carol Leddy, Secretary, Due Process Unit

The State Board of Education believes each student is unique and needs an educational environment that provides for, and accommodates, his or her strengths and areas of needed improvement.

2115 Department of Rehabilitation Services &Bureau of Education And Services for the Blind
State of Connecticut Agency
184 Windsor Ave
Windsor, CT 06095-4536   860-602-4000
800-842-4510
FAX: 860-602-4020
TTY: 860-602-4221
brian.sigman@ct.gov
www.ct.gov/besb

State Agencies: Delaware

2116 Department of Public Instruction: Exceptional Children & Special Programs Division
Department of Education
Ste 2
401 Federal St
Dover, DE 19901-3639   302-739-5471
FAX: 302-739-2388
www.doe.k12.de.us

Martha Toomey, Executive Director

State Agencies: DC

2117 Administration for Community Living
One Massachusetts Avenue NW
Washington, DC 20001   202-401-4634
800-677-1116
FAX: 202-357-3555
aclinfo@acl.hhs.gov
www.acl.gov

Kathy Greenlee, Administrator
Sharon Lewis, Principal Deputy Administrator
Edwin Walker, Deputy Assis Secretary for Aging
Aaron Bishop, Comm., Admin on Disabilities
ACL brings together the efforts and achievements of the Administration on Aging, the Administration on Intellectual and Developmental Disabilities, and the HHS Office on Disability to serve as the Federal agency responsible for increasing access to community supports, while focusing attention and resources on the unique needs of older Americans and people with disabilities across the lifespan.

2118 District of Columbia Public Schools: Special Education Division
1200 First Street, NE
Washington, DC 20002-4210   202-442-5885
202-442-5517
FAX: 202-442-5026
www.dcps.dc.gov

Paul L Vance MD, Superintendent
Committed to providing a continuum of services that offers students with disabilities the opportunity to actively participate in the learning environment of their neighborhood school.

2119 Federal Emergency Management Agency
500 C Street S.W.
Washington, DC 20472   202-646-2500
800-621-3362
TTY:800-427-5593
www.fema.gov

W. Craig Fugate, Administrator
Michael Coen, Jr., Chief of Staff
Joseph Nimmich, Deputy Administrator
Alyson Vert, Director
FEMA's mission is to support the citizens and first responders to ensure that as a nation we work together to build, sustain and im-

prove our capability to prepare for, protect against, respond to, recover from and mitigate all hazards.

2120 National Clearinghouse on Family Support and Children's Mental Health
Ste 800
1 Dupont Cir NW
Washington, DC 20036-1149   202-939-9320
800-544-3284
FAX: 202-833-4760
heatah@ace.nche.edu
ncfy.acf.hhs.gov/

State Agencies: Florida

2121 Florida Department of Education: Bureau of Exceptional Education And Student Services
325 West Gaines Street
Turlington Building, Suite 1514
Tallahassee, FL 32399   850-245-0505
FAX: 850-245-9667
Monica.Verra-Tirado@fldoe.org
www.fldoe.org/ese

Monica Verra-Tirado, Ed.D., Bureau Chief
Gerard Robinson, Commissioner
Randy Hanna, Chancellor
Pam Stewart, Chancellor
Administers programs for students with disabilities and for gifted students. Coordinates student services throughout the state and participates in multiple inter-agency efforts designed to strengthen the quality and variety of services to students with special needs.

State Agencies: Hawaii

2122 Hawaii Department of Education: Special Needs
Hawaii Department of Education
3430 Leahi Ave
Honolulu, HI 96815-4246   808-941-3894
FAX: 808-941-3894

Margaret Donovan MD, State Administrator
Provides consultation on educational services for local schools, offers psychological testing and evaluation, maintains resource rooms in district schools and more for the blind and handicapped throughout the state.

State Agencies: Illinois

2123 Illinois State Board of Education: Department of Special Education
100 N 1st St
Springfield, IL 62777   217-782-5589
FAX: 217-782-0372
www.isbe.net

Elizabeth Hanselman, Asst Superintendent Special Ed.
Mission is to advance the human and civil rights of people with disabilities in Illinois. Statewide advocacy organization providing self-advocacy assistance, legal services, education and public policy initiatives. Designated to implement the federal protection and advocacy system; has broad statutory power to enforce the rights of people with physical and mental disabilities, including developmental disabilities and mental illnesses.

State Agencies: Indiana

2124   Indiana Department of Education: Special Education Division
Indiana Department of Education
South Tower, Suite 600
115 W. Washington Street
Indianapolis, IN 46204-2731   317- 23- 661
                                                877-851-4106
                                           FAX: 317- 23- 800
                                    webmaster@doe.in.gov
                                           www.doe.in.gov/

Robert A Marra, Manager
Tony Bennett, Chair
Provides consultation on educational services for local schools, offers psychological testing and evaluation, maintains resource rooms in district schools and more for the blind and handicapped throughout the state.

State Agencies: Iowa

2125   Iowa Department of Public Instruction: Bureau of Special Education
400 E 14th St
Des Moines, IA 50319-9000   515-457-2000
                                           FAX: 515-242-6019
                                           www.educateiowa.gov/

Tom Kuehl, CEO
Jason Glass, Director
Jeff Berger, Administrative Services

State Agencies: Kansas

2126   Kansas State Board of Education: Special Education Services
900 SW Jackson Street
Topeka, KS 66612-1212   785-296-3201
                                                800-203-9462
                                           FAX: 785-296-7933
                                           TTY: 785-296-6338
                                         contact@ksde.org
                                                www.ksde.org
Ethan Erickson, Director
Kathy Gosa, Director
Denise Kahler, Director
Scott Myers, Director
Provides leadership and support for exceptional learners receiving special education services throughout Kansas schools and communities.

State Agencies: Kentucky

2127   Kentucky Department of Education: Divisionof Exceptional Children's Services
500 Mero St
Capital Tower Plaza
Frankfort, KY 40601   502-564-4770
                                           FAX: 502-564-7749
                                darlene.jesse@kde.state.ky.us
                                           www.education.ky.gov

Darlene Jesse, Director
Provides consultation on educational services for local schools, offers psychological testing and evaluation, maintains resource rooms in district schools and more for the blind and handicapped throughout the state.

State Agencies: Louisiana

2128   Louisiana Department of Education: Office of Special Education Services
Louisiana Department of Education
1201 North Third Street
Baton Rouge, LA 70802   225-342-0090
                                                877-453-2721
                                           FAX: 225-342-0193
                                           www.doe.state.la.us

David Elder, Manager
Kim Fitch, Director Human Resources
George Nelson, President

State Agencies: Massachusetts

2129   Getting Ready for the Outside World (G.R.O.W.)
Riverview School
551 Route 6A East Sandwich
Cape Cod, MA 2537-1448   508-888-0489
                                           FAX: 508-833-7001
                                admissions@riverviewschool.org
                                           www.riverviewschool.org

Janice James, Vice Chairman
Deborah Cowan, Vice Chair
James Shallcross, Treasurer
Kathleen Yazbak, Secretary
Riverview School's G.R.O.W. Program is a unique ten month transitional prgoram (1-3 years) for young adults with complex language, learning and cognitive disabilities. This post secondary program is designed to further develop academic, vocational and independent living skills, to enable students to function as independently as possible.

2130   Massachusetts Department of Education: Program Quality Assurance
Massachusetts Department of Education
75 Pleasant Street
Malden, MA 2148-4906   781-388-3300
                                           FAX: 617-388-3476
                                        boe@doe.mass.edu
                                           www.doe.mass.edu/pqa/

Pamela Kaufamann, Administrator

State Agencies: Maryland

2131   Agency for Healthcare Research and Quality
540 Gaither Road
Rockville, MD 20850   301-427-1364
                                                www.ahrq.gov

Richard G. Kronick, PhD, Director, Director
Sharon B. Arnold, PhD, Deputy Director
The Agency for Healthcare Research and Quality's (AHRQ) mission is to produce evidence to make health care safer, higher quality, more accessible, equitable, and affordable, and to work within the U.S. Department of Health and Human Services and with other partners to make sure that the evidence is understood and used.

2132   Center for Mental Health Services
Room 6-1057
1 Choke Cherry Road
Rockville, MD 20857   240-276-1310
                                           FAX: 240-276-1320
                                                www.samhsa.gov

Paolo del Vecchio, M.S.W., Director
Elizabeth Lopez, Ph.D., Deputy Director
Elizabeth Lopez, Ph.D., Acting Director
Anne Mathews-Younes, Ed.D., Director
The Center for Mental Health Services leads federal efforts to promote the prevention and treatment of mental disorders. Con-

gress created CMHS to bring new hope to adults who have serious mental illness and children with emotional disorders.

2133   Centers for Medicare & Medicaid Services
7500 Security Boulevard
Baltimore, MD 21244
410-786-3000
877-267-2323
TTY:866-226-1819
Mandy.Cohen@cms.hhs.gov
www.cms.gov

Dr. Mandy Cohen, M.D., MPH, Chief of Staff
Deborah Taylor, Acting Chief Operating Officer
Andy Slavitt, Acting Administrator
Patrick Conway, MD, MSc, Acting Principal Deputy Admin
US federal agency which administers Medicare, Medicaid, and the State Children's Health Insurance Program.

2134   Maryland State Department of Education: Division of Special Education
200 West Baltimore Street
Baltimore, MD 21201-2595
410-767-0100
888-246-0016
FAX: 410-333-8165
dmcmicha@msde.state.md.us
www.marylandpublicschools.org

Nancy S Grasmick, State Supertintendent
Dr. Lillian Lowery, Superintendent of Schools
James V. Foran, Assistant State Superintendent
Katharine Oliver, Assistant State Superintendent
Collaborates with families, local early intervention systems, and local school systems to ensure that all children and youth with disabilities have access to appropriate services and educational opportunities to which they are entitled under federal and state laws.

2135   National Human Genome Research Institute
National Institutes of Health
Building 31, Room 4B09
31 Center Drive, MSC 2152
Bethesda, MD 20892-2152
301-402-0911
FAX: 301-402-2218
lbrody@mail.nih.gov
www.genome.gov

Eric D. Green, M.D., Ph.D., Director
Lawrence Brody, Ph.D., Director
Bettie Graham, Ph.D., Director
Ellen Rolfes, M.A., Director, Division of Management
The National Human Genome Research Institute began as the National Center for Human Genome Research (NCHGR), which was established in 1989 to carry out the role of the National Institutes of Health (NIH) in the International Human Genome Project (HGP).

2136   National Institute of General Medical Sciences
45 Center Drive MSC 6200
Bethesda, MD 20892-6200
301-496-7301
info@nigms.nih.gov
www.nigms.nih.gov

Jon R. Lorsch, Ph.D., Director
Judith H. Greenberg, Ph.D., Deputy Director
Ann Hagan, Ph.D., Associate Director
Sally Lee, Executive Officer
The National Institute of General Medical Sciences (NIGMS) supports basic research that increases understanding of biological processes and lays the foundation for advances in disease diagnosis, treatment and prevention.

State Agencies: Michigan

2137   Michigan Department of Education: Special Education Services
608 W. Allegan Street
PO Box 30008
Lansing, MI 48909
517-373-3324
FAX: 517-373-7504
DHS-OCS-PEP@michigan.gov
www.michigan.gov/mde

John C. Austin, President
Kathleen N. Straus, President of the State Board
Michelle Fecteau, Executive Director
Daniel Varner, Chief Executive Officer of Excellent Schools Detroit
Oversees the administrative funding of education and early intervention programs and services for young children and students with disabilities.

2138   Services for Students with Disabilities
University of Michigan
G-664 Haven Hall
505 South State St.
Ann Arbor, MI 48109-1045
734-763-3000
FAX: 734-936-3947
TTY:734-615-4461
ssdoffice@umich.edu
www.ssd.umich.edu

Stuart Segal, Director
Offers information to students of the University of Michigan and their parents.

State Agencies: Minnesota

2139   Community Supports for People with Disabilities (CSP)
South Central Technical College (SCTC)
1920 Lee Blvd
North Mankato, MN 56003-2504
507-389-7200
800-722-9359
online@southcentral.edu
www.southcentral.edu

Christensen Tami, Executive Director
Keith Stover, President
Human services program available as a physical or online program, designed for those wanting to earn a certificate, diploma or associate degree as a Direct Support Professional for use in the health and human services industries. The program comprises eight courses relating to professional services and support for people with disabilities.

2140   Professional Development Programs
6303 Osgood Ave. N.
Ste 104
Stillwater, MN 55082
651-439-8865
877-439-8865
FAX: 877-259-5906
programs@pdppro.com
www.pdppro.com

Cindy Lacosse, VP
Lori Lacrosse, President
Sponsors cutting edge and popular continuing education workshops and symposia of interest to professionals who provide services to children and adults with special needs.

State Agencies: Missouri

2141   Missouri Department of Elementary and Secondary Education: Special Education Programs
205 Jefferson St
PO Box 480
Jefferson City, MO 65102   573-751-5739
FAX: 573-526-4404
TTY:800-735-2966
www.dese.mo.gov

Stephen Barr, Assistant Commissioner
The Office of Special Education administers state and federal funds to support services for students and adults with disabilities.

State Agencies: Mississippi

2142   Mississippi Department of Education: Office of Special Services
359 North West Street
P.O. Box 771
Jackson, MS 39201   601-359-3513
FAX: 601-987-3892
www.mde.k12.ms.us

Dr Tom Burnham, Superintendent
Key priorities are: reading, early literacy, student achievement, teachers/teaching, leadership/principals, safe and orderly schools, parent relations/community involvement, and technology.

State Agencies: Montana

2143   Department of Public Health Human Services
PO Box 4210
Helena, MT 59604-4210   406-444-5622
FAX: 406-444-1970
hhsea@mt.gov
www.dphhs.mt.gov

Anna Whitin Sorrell, Director
Bernie Jacobs, Chief Legal Counsel
Deb Sloat, Human Resources Office
Jon Ebelt, Public Information Office
Provides consultation on educational services for local schools, offers psychological testing and evaluation, maintains resource rooms in district schools and more for the blind and handicapped throughout the state.

State Agencies: North Carolina

2144   National Institute of Environmental Health Sciences
111 T.W. Alexander Drive
Research Triangle Park, NC 27709   919-541-4580
birnbaumls@niehs.nih.gov
www.niehs.nih.gov
Linda S. Birnbaum, Ph.D., Director
Richard Woychik, Ph.D., Deputy Director
Sheila A. Newton, Ph.D., Policy, Planning, and Evaluation
Ericka Reid, Ph.D., Science Education & Diversity
The mission of the NIEHS is to discover how the environment affects people in order to promote healthier lives.

2145   North Carolina Department of Public Instruction: Exceptional Children Division
301 N Wilmington St
Raleigh, NC 27601   919-807-3300
FAX: 919-715-1569
lharris@dpi.state.nc.us
www.ncpublicschools.org
June St. Clair Atkinson, Ed.D, State Superintendent of Public Instruction
Mike McLaughlin, Senior Policy Advisor to the State Superintendent
Rachel Beaulieu, Legislative & Community Affairs Director
Jeani Allen, Director of Internal Auditing
The mission is to assure that students with disabilities develop mentally, physically, emotionally, and vocationally through the provision of an appropriate individualized education in the least restrictive environment.

State Agencies: North Dakota

2146   North Dakota Department of Education: Special Education
600 E. Boulevard Avenue, Dept. 201
Floors 9, 10, and 11
Bismarck, ND 58505-0440   701-328-2260
866-741-3519
FAX: 701-328-2461
TTY: 701-328-4920
mdanderson@nd.gov
www.dpi.state.nd.us
Kirsten Baesler, State Superintendent
Jerry Coleman, Director, School Finance & Organization
Linda Schloer, Child Nutrition & Food Distribution, Director
Gerry Teevens, Director, Special Education
Provides consultation on educational services for local schools, offers psychological testing and evaluation, maintains resource rooms in district schools and more for the blind and handicapped throughout the state.

State Agencies: Nebraska

2147   Nebraska Department of Education: Special Populations Office
1200 N Street, Suite 400
PO Box 98922
Lincoln, NE 68509   402-471-2186
877-253-2603
FAX: 402-471-2909
NDEQ.moreinfo@Nebraska.gov
deq.ne.gov
Rod Gangwish Shelton, Council Member
Douglas Anderson Aurora, Council Member
Mark Whitehead Lincoln, Council Member
Mark Czaplewski Grand Islan, Council Member
Assists school districts in establishing and maintaining effective special education programs for children with disabilities (date of diagnosis through the school year when a child reaches 21). Major function: provide technical assistance to school districts and to parents of children with disabilities, assist programs in meeting state and federal special education regulations. Also responsible for assuring that the rights of children with disabilities and their parents are protected.

State Agencies: New Hampshire

2148 Institute on Disability
University of New Hampshire
10 West Edge Drive
Suite 101
Durham, NH 03824 603-862-4320
FAX: 603-862-0555
contact.iod@unh.edu
www.iod.unh.edu

Charles E. Drum, Director & Professor
Andrew Houtenville, Director of Research
Matthew Gianino, Director of Communications
Mary Schuh, Director of Development and Consumer Affairs
Provides coherent university-based focus for the improvement of knowledge, policies, and practices related to the lives of persons with disabilities and their families.

2149 New Hampshire Department of Education: Bureau for Special Education Services
101 Pleasant Street
Concord, NH 03301-3860 603-271-3494
FAX: 603-271-1953
Lori.Temple@doe.nh.gov
www.education.nh.gov

Santina Thibedeau, Administrator
Virginia Barry, Commissioner
Linda Breden, Secretary
Traci Biron, Secretary
The mission of Special Education is to improve educational outcomes for children and youth with disabilities by providing and promoting leadership, technical assistance and collaboration statewide. Provides oversight and implementation of federal and state laws that ensure a free appropriate public education for all children and youth with disabilities in New Hampshire.

State Agencies: New Jersey

2150 New Jersey Department of Education: Office of Special Education Program
New Jersey Department of Education
PO Box 500
Trenton, NJ 8625-500 609-292-0147
FAX: 609-984-8422
www.nj.gov/education/specialed/info/

Barbara Gantwerk, Director
Alfred Murray, Executive Director

State Agencies: New Mexico

2151 New Mexico State Department of Education
300 Don Gaspar Ave
Santa Fe, NM 87501-2744 505-827-6508
FAX: 505-827-6696
www.sde.state.nm.us

Bill Trant, Assistant Director
Judy Parks, Assistant Director
Provides consultation on educational services for local schools, offers psychological testing and evaluation, maintains resource rooms in district schools and more for the blind and handicapped throughout the state.

State Agencies: Nevada

2152 Nevada Department of Education: Special Eduction Branch
700 E Fifth St
Carson City, NV 89701-5096 775-687-9800
FAX: 775-687-9101
www.doe.nv.gov

Nick Gakalatos, Manager

The Office of Special Ed and School Improvement Program of the Nevada State Department of Education is responsible for management of state and federal programs providing educational opportunities for students with diverse learning needs. Included are such programs as: special education/disabled (IDEA); disadvantaged/at-risk programs (Title I/IASA); early childhood programs (Title I/ESEA); early childhood programs; migrant education; English language learners; NRS 395 student placement program.

State Agencies: New York

2153 New York State Education Department
1606 One Commerce Plz
Albany, NY 12234 518-474-5930
FAX: 518-486-6880
nysed@mail.gov
www.nysed.gov

Bernard Margolis, Manager
Provides vocational rehabilitation and educational services for eligible individuals with disabilities throughout New York State. Services include evaluation, counseling, job placement, and referral to other agencies.

State Agencies: Ohio

2154 Ohio Department of Education: Division of Special Education
Ohio Department of Education
25 S Front St
Columbus, OH 43215-4183 614-995-1545
877-644-6338
FAX: 614-728-1097
TTY: 888-886-0181
www.ode.state.oh.us

Mike Armstrong, Manager
Provides technical assistance to educational agencies for the development and implementation of educational services to meet the needs of students with disabilities and/or those who are gifted. Provides information to parents. Administers state and federal funds allocated to educational agencies for the provision of services to students with disabilities and/or those who are gifted.

State Agencies: Oklahoma

2155 Oklahoma State Department of Education
2500 N Lincoln Blvd
Oklahoma City, OK 73105-4599 405-521-3301
FAX: 405-521-6205
www.sde.state.ok.us

Misty Kimbrough, Manager
Sandy Garrett, Administrator
Janet Barresi, State Superintendent
Provides consultation on educational services for local schools, offers psychological testing and evaluation, maintains resource rooms in district schools and more for the blind and handicapped throughout the state.

State Agencies: Oregon

2156 Oregon Department of Education: Office of Special Education
Oregon Department of Education:
255 Capitol St NE
Salem, OR 97310-1300 503-945-5600
FAX: 503-378-2897
www.dpeducation.com

Bruce Goldberg, Manager
Heidi Cockrell, Executive Assistant
Katy Coba, Executive Director

State agency ensuring provision of special education services to children with disabilities from birth to age 21.

State Agencies: Pennsylvania

2157 Pennsylvania Department of Education: Bureau of Special Education
333 Market St
Harrisburg, PA 17126-333
717-783-6788
FAX: 717-783-6139
TTY:717-783-8445
00specialed@psupen.psu.edu
www.pde.state.pa.us

Linda Rhen, Administrator
John Tommasini, Assistant Director
Provides effective and efficient administration of the Commonwealth of Pennsylvania's resources dedicated to enabling school districts to maintain high standards in the delivery of special education services and programs for all exceptional students.

State Agencies: Rhode Island

2158 Rhode Island Department of Education: Office of Special Needs
255 Westminster St
Providence, RI 2903
401-222-4600
FAX: 401-784-9513
www.ride.ri.gov

Al Moscola, Manager
Alfred Moscola, Manager
Provides consultation on educational services for local schools, offers psychological testing and evaluation, maintains resource rooms in district schools and more for the blind and handicapped throughout the state.

State Agencies: South Carolina

2159 South Carolina Assistive Technology Program (SCATP)
Center for Disability Resources
8301 Farrow Rd
Columbia, SC 29208-3245
803-935-5263
800-915-4522
FAX: 800-935-5342
evelyne@cdd.sc.edu
www.sc.edu/scatp

Carol Page, Program Director
Mary Bechter, Program Coordinator
SCATP is a federally funded project concerned with getting technology into th hands of people with disabilities so that they might live, work, learn and be a more independent part of the community.

2160 South Carolina Department of Education: Office of Exceptional Children
1429 Senate St
Suite 808
Columbia, SC 29201-3730
803-734-8224
FAX: 803-734-4824
sdeservicedesk@sde.ok.gov
www.scschools.com

Susan Durant, State Director
Provides consultation on educational services for local schools, offers psychological testing and evaluation, maintains resource rooms in district schools and more for the blind and handicapped throughout the state.

State Agencies: South Dakota

2161 South Dakota Department of Education & Cultural Affairs: Office of Special Education
700 Governors Dr
Pierre, SD 57501-2291
605-773-3804
FAX: 605-773-6041

Chelle Somsen, Manager
Dorothy Liegl, Manager

State Agencies: Tennessee

2162 Tennessee Department of Education
710 James Robertson Pkwy
Nashville, TN 37243-1219
615-741-2731
888-212-3162
FAX: 615-741-1791
www.state.tn.us/education

Ruth S Letson, Manager
Kevin Huffman, Commissioner
Provides consultation on educational services for local schools, offers psychological testing and evaluation, maintains resource rooms in district schools and more for the blind and handicapped throughout the state.

State Agencies: Texas

2163 Texas Education Agency
1701 N Congress Ave
Austin, TX 78701-1494
512-463-8532
FAX: 512-463-8057
www.tealighthouse.org

Shirley J Neeley, Commissioner of Education
Provides consultation on educational services for local schools, offers psychological testing and evaluation, maintains resource rooms in district schools and more for the blind and handicapped throughout the state.

2164 Texas Education Agency: Special Education Unit
1701 Congress Ave
PO Box 420637
Austin, TX 77242-637
512-463-8532
FAX: 512-463-8057
info@tdea.org
www.tdea.org

Gene Lenz, Deputy Associate Commissioner
Shirley Neeley, Administrator

2165 Texas School of the Deaf
1102 S Congress Ave
Austin, TX 78704-1791
512-462-5353
800-332-3873
FAX: 512-462-5424
ercod@tsd.state.tx.us
tsd.state.tx.us

Claire Bugen, Superintendent
Russell West, Residential Services Director
Gary Bego, Business and Operations Director
Brenda Fraenkel, Special Education Director
Ensures that students excel in an environment where they learn, grow and belong. Supports deaf students, families and professionals in Texas by providing resources through outreach services.

State Agencies: Utah

2166 **Utah State Office of Education: At-Risk and Special Education Service Unit**
Utah State Office of Education
250 East 500 South
P.O.Box 144200
Salt Lake City, UT 84114-4200
801-538-7500
FAX: 801-538-7521
webmaster@schools.utah.gov
schools.utah.gov

Sandra Cox, Financial Analyst
Mark Peterson, Director
Glenna Gallo, State Director of Special Educat
Rebecca Donovan, Administrative Secretary
Provides consultation on educational services for local schools, offers psychological testing and evaluation, maintains resource rooms in district schools and more for the blind and handicapped throughout the state.

State Agencies: Virginia

2167 **National Science Foundation**
4201 Wilson Blvd
Arlington, VA 22230
703-292-5111
TTY:703-292-5090
info@nsf.gov
www.nsf.gov

France A. Córdova, Director
Richard O. Buckius, Chief Operating Officer
Michael Van Woert, Executive Officer/Director
Dr. James L. Olds, Assistant Director
NSF is the only federal agency whose mission includes support for all fields of fundamental science and engineering, except for medical sciences.

2168 **Virginia Department of Education: Divisionof Pre & Early Adolescent Education**
Virginia Department Of Education
James Monroe Building, 101, N. 14th
P.O.Box 2120
Richmond, VA 23219
804-236-3631
FAX: 804-236-3635
webmaster@doe.virginia.gov
www.pen.k12.va.us

Dr. Steven R Staples, Superintendent of Public Instruction
Kent Dickey, Deputy Superintendent, Finance & Operations
Chris Sorensen, Director, Budget
Becky Marable, Director, Human Resources
Provides consultation on educational services for local schools, offers psychological testing and evaluation, maintains resource rooms in district schools and more for the blind and handicapped throughout the state.

State Agencies: Washington

2169 **Superintendent of Public Instruction: Special Education Section**
Old Capitol Building, 600 Washingto
P.O. Box 47200
Olympia, WA 98504-7200
360-725-6000
FAX: 360-586-0247
TTY:360-664-3631
webmaster@k12.wa.us
www.k12.wa.us

Randy I. Dorn, State Superintendent of Public I
Alan Burke, Deputy Superintendent
Robert Butts, Assistant Superintendent
Bob Harmon, Assistant Superintendent
Provides leadership, service and support for the development and implementation of research-based curriculum to assure that all learners achieve at all levels.

State Agencies: West Virginia

2170 **West Virginia Department of Education: Office of Special Education**
Rm 6
1900 Kanawha Blvd E
Charleston, WV 25305-0001
304-558-3660
FAX: 304-558-3741
http://wvde.state.wv.us/boe/
wvde.state.wv.us

Liza Cordeiro, Executive Director
Mary Nunn, Assistant Director
Marshall Patton, Executive Director
Brenda Williams, Executive Director
Provides consultation on educational services for local schools, offers psychological testing and evaluation, maintains resource rooms in district schools and more for the blind and handicapped throughout the state.

State Agencies: Wyoming

2171 **Wyoming Department of Education**
2300 Capitol Avenue
Hathaway Building, 2nd Floor
Cheyenne, WY 82002-2060
307-777-7690
FAX: 307-777-6234
edu.wyoming.gov

Cindy Hill, WDE Superintendent
Deb Lindsey, Division Administrator, Assessment
Teri Wigert, Division Administrator, Support Systems & Resources
Dianne Bailey, Division Administrator, Finance & Data
Mission is to lead, model, and support continuous improvement of education for everyone in Wyoming.

Magazines & Journals

2172 **Adapted Physical Activity Programs**
Human Kinetics
1607 N. Market Street
P.O.Box 5076
Champaign, IL 61820
800-747-4457
FAX: 217-351-1549
info@hkusa.com
www.humankinetics.com

Patty Lehn, Publicity Manager
Lori Cooper, Marketing Manager
Bill Dobrik, Sales Associate
Dan Stebel, Sales Associate
Human Kinetics produces a variety of resources for adapted physical education practitioners, including books on activities, a research journal and higher education references. *$24.00*
Quarterly
ISSN 0736-58 9

2173 **Advance for Providers of Post-Acute Care**
Merion Publications
2900 Horizon Drive
King of Prussia, PA 19406
610-278-1400
800-355-5627
FAX: 610-278-1421
webmaster@advanceweb.com
advanceweb.com

Timothy Baum, MS, CRNP, Author
A free magazine for providers of post-acute care.

2174 **American Journal on Intellectual and Developmental Disabilities**
501 3rd Street, NW
Suite 200
Washington, DC 20001
202-387-1968
FAX: 202-387-2193
mnygren@aaidd.org
aaidd.org

Deborah Fidler,PhD, Editor
Glenn T. Fujiura, PhD, Editor
Michael L. Wehmeyer, PhD, Co-Editor
Karrie A. Shogren, PhD, Co-Editor
American Journal on Intellectual and Developmental Disabilities (AJIDD)is a scientific, scholarly, and archival multidisciplinary journal for reporting original contributions of the highest quality to knowledge of intellectual disability, its causes, treatment, and prevention.

2175 **CEC Catalog**
Council for Exceptional Children
2900 Crystal Drive
Suite 1000
Arlington, VA 22202-3557
703-620-3660
866-509-0218
888-232-7733
FAX: 703-264-9494
TTY:866-915-5000
service@ccc.spcd.org
www.cec.sped.org

Robin D. Brewer, President
James P. Heiden, President Elect
Christy A. Chambers, Immediate Past President
Mikki Garcia, Executive Director
Semi-annual catalog from the Council for Exceptional Children offering books, guides, materials, products and services for the special educator.
18 pages

2176 **Career Development and Transition for Exceptional Individuals**
2455 Teller Road
Thousand Oaks, CA 91320
800-818-7243
FAX: 800-583-2665
journals@sagepub.com
cde.sagepub.com

Blaise R. Simqu, President/ CEO
Tracey A. Ozmina, EVP/ COO
Chris Hickok, SVP/ CFO
Phil Denvir, Global Chief Information Officer
Career Development and Transition for Exceptional Individuals (CDTEI) specializes in the fields of secondary education, transition, and career development for persons with documented disabilities and special needs.

2177 **Case Manager Magazine**
Elsevier Health
3251 Riverport Lane
Maryland Heights, MO 63043
314-447-8070
800-222-9570
textbook@elsevier.com
journals.elsevierhealth.com

Thomas Reller, Vice President Global Corporate
Harald Boersma, Senior Manager Corporate Relatio
Ylann Schemm, Corporate Relations Manager
Sacha Boucherie, Press Officer
This national magazine is for medical case managers, social workers, counselors and home health professionals who work with people with serious injury or illness. It is a membership benefit of CMSA, the national association for case managers. *$55.00*
84 pages BiMonthly

2178 **Catalyst**
The Catalyst
Ste 275
1259 El Camino Real
Menlo Park, CA 94025-4208
800-647-0314
info@thecatalyst.us
www.thecatalyst.us

Sue Swezey, Editor
Digest of news and information on the use of computers in special education. *$15.00*
20 pages Quarterly

2179 **Challenge Magazine**
451 Hungerford Drive
Suite 100
Rockville, MD 20850
301-217-0960
FAX: 301-217-0968
Info@dsusa.org
www.disabledsportsusa.org

Kirk Bauer, Executive Director
Claire Duffy, Program Coordinator
Orlando Gill, Field Representative
Huarya Gomez-Garcia, Program Manager
Challenge Magazine is a publication of Disabled Sports USA, providing adaptive sports information to adults and children with disabilities, including those who are visually impaired, amputees, spinal cord injured (paraplegic and quadriplegic), and those who have multiple sclerosis, head injury, cerebral palsy, autism and other related intellectual disabilities.

2180 **Clinical Connection**
American Advertising Dist of Northern Virginia
708 Pendleton St
Alexandria, VA 22314-1819
703-549-5126
FAX: 703-548-5563
www.onlineceus.com

Kathie Harrington, M.A., CCC, Author
Covers speech language pathology.

2181 **College and University**
AACRAO
One Dupont Circle NW
Suite 520
Washington, DC 20036
202-293-9161
FAX: 202-872-8857
reillym@aacrao.org
aacrao.org

Brad Myers, President
Dan Garcia, President Elect
Adrienne McDay, Past President
Stan DeMerritt, VP, Finance
Scholarly research journal. American Association of Collegiate Registrars and Admissions Offers (AACRAO) is a nonprofit, voluntary, professional, educational association of degree-granting, postsecondary institutions, government agencies, private educational organizations and education-oriented businesses in the United States and abroad. $80 per year US; $90 per year international.
30 pages Quarterly
ISSN 0010-0889

2182 **Communication Disorders Quarterly**
2455 Teller Road
Thousand Oaks, CA 91320
800-818-7243
FAX: 800-583-2665
journals@sagepub.com
cde.sagepub.com

Blaise R. Simqu, President/ CEO
Tracey A. Ozmina, EVP/ COO
Chris Hickok, SVP/ CFO
Phil Denvir, Global Chief Information Officer
Communication Disorders Quarterly (CDQ) presents cutting edge information on typical and atypical communication — from oral language development to literacy.

2183 Continuing Care
Stevens Publishing Corporation
14901 Quorum Dr,
Suite 425
Dallas, TX 75254

972-687-6700
FAX: 972-687-6750
info@1105media.com
1105media.com

Neal Vitale, President & Chief Executive Officer
Richard Vitale, Senior Vice President & Chief Financial Officer
Mike Valenti, Executive Vice President
Jeff Klein, Non-Executive Chairman of the Board
A national magazine for case management and discharge planning professionals published monthly except for December. $119.00
34 pages Monthly

2184 Counseling Psychologist
American Psychological Association
2455 Teller Road
Thousand Oaks, CA 91320

805-499-0721
800-818-7243
FAX: 800-583-2665
info@sagepub.com
www.sagepub.com

Sara Miller McCune, Founder, Publisher & Executive Chairman
Blaise R Simqu, President/CEO
Chris Hickok, Senior Vice President & Chief Financial Officer
Stephen Barr, Managing Director/SAGE London
Thematic issues in the theory, research and practice of counseling psychology. $78.00
Bi-Monthly

2185 Counseling and Values
American Counseling Association
5999 Stevenson Ave
Alexandria, VA 22304

703-823-0252
800-347-6647
FAX: 800-473-2329
webmaster@counseling.org
counseling.org

Robert L. Smith, President
Thelma Duffey, President Elect
Brian Canfield, Treasurer
Richard Yep, CEO
Counseling and Values is the official journal of the Association for Spiritual, Ethical, and Religious Values in Counseling (ASERVIC), a member association of the American Counseling Association. Counseling and Values s a professional journal of theory, research, and informed opinion concerned with the relationships among psychology, philosophy, religion, social values, and counseling. $12.00
TriAnnual

2186 Disability & Society
711 3rd Avenue
8th Floor
New York, NY 10017

212-216-7800
800-634-7064
FAX: 212-564-7854
www.routledge.com

Len Barton, Author
The study of disability has traditionally been influenced mainly by medical and psychological models. The aim of this new text, Disability and Society, is to open up the debate by introducing alternative perspectives reflecting the increasing sociological interest in this important topic.

2187 Disability Studies Quarterly
552 Park Hall
Buffalo, NY 14260-4130

marembis@buffalo.edu
dsq-sds.org

Michael Rembis, Interim Editor-in-Chief
Tanja Aho, Interim Managing Editor
Disability Studies Quarterly (DSQ) is the journal of the Society for Disability Studies (SDS). It is a multidisciplinary and international journal of interest to social scientists, scholars in the humanities, disability rights advocates, creative writers, and others concerned with the issues of people with disabilities.

2188 Disability and Health Journal
110 N. Washington Street
Suite 328-J
Rockville, MD 20850

301-545-6140
FAX: 301-545-6144
www.aahd.us

Ronald G. Blankenbaker, President
Roberta Carlin, Executive Director
E. Clarke Ross, Public Policy Director
Wanda C. Smith, Program Associate
Disability and Health Journal is a scientific, scholarly and multidisciplinary journal for reporting original contributions that advance knowledge in disability and health.

2189 Early Intervention
Early Childhood Intervention Clearinghouse
51 Gerty Drive
Room 20
Champaign, IL 61820-7469

217-333-1386
877-275-3227
FAX: 217-244-7732
Illinois-eic@illinois.edu
www.eiclearinghouse.org

Susan Fowler, Director
Features articles, conference calendar, material reviews and news concerning early childhood intervention and disability.
4 pages Quarterly

2190 Emerging Horizon
PO Box 278
Ripon, CA 95366-0278

209-599-9409
emerginghorizons.com

2191 Exceptional Children
Council for Exceptional Children
2900 Crystal Drive
Suite 1000
Arlington, VA 22202-3557

703-620-3660
866-509-0218
888-232-7733
FAX: 703-264-9494
TTY:866-915-5000
service@cec.sped.org
cec.sped.org

Robin D. Brewer, President
James P. Heiden, President Elect
Christy A. Chambers, Immediate Past President
Mikki Garcia, Executive Director
Articles include research, literature surveys and position papers concerning exceptional children, special education and mainstreaming. $58.00
96 pages BiMonthly

2192 Focus on Autism and Other Developmental Disabilities
Sage Publications
2455 Teller Road
Thousand Oaks, CA 91320

805-499-0721
800-818-7243
FAX: 800-583-2665
info@sagepub.com
www.sagepub.com

Sara Miller McCune, Founder, Publisher & Executive Chairman
Blaise R. Simqu, President & CEO
Chris Hickok, Senior Vice President & Chief Financial Officer
Stephen Barr, Managing Director/SAGE London
Practical management, treatment and planning strategies; a must for persons working with individuals with autism and other developmental disabilities. $43.00
64 pages Quarterly

2193 **Focus on Exceptional Children**
Love Publishing Company
9101 East Kenyon Avenue
Suite 2200
Denver, CO 80237

303-221-7333
FAX: 303-221-7444
lpc@lovepublishing.com
www.lovepublishing.com

Steve Graham, Consulting Editor
Ron Nelson, Consulting Editor
Eva Horn, Consulting Editor
Contains research and theory-based articles on special education topics, with an emphasis on application and intervention, of interest to teachers, professors and administrators. *$36.00*
Monthly

2194 **HomeCare Magazine**
Cahaba Media Group
1900-28th Ave S.
Ste 200
Birmingham, AL 35209

205-212-9402
cahabamedia.com

Wally Evans, Publisher
Greg Meineke, Vice President, Sales
Stephanie Gibson Lepore, Editor
The business magazine of the home medical equipment industry offering information on legislation and regulations affecting the homecare industry, monthly profiles of suppliers, operational tips, newest products in the industry, advice on sales, government regulations. *$ 65.00*
120 pages Monthly

2195 **I Wonder Who Else Can Help**
AARP
601 E Street NW
Washington, DC 20049

202-434-3525
888-687-2277
877-342-2277
FAX: 202-434-3443
member@aarp.org
www.aarp.org

John Wider, President, CEO, AARP Services Inc.
Lisa M. Ryerson, President, AARP Foundation
Robert R. Hagans, Jr., Executive Vice President & Chief Financial Officer
Hollis Terry Bradwell III, Executive Vice President & Chief Information Officer
Contains information about crisis counseling, needs and resources, written in lay terms.

2196 **Inclusion**
501 3rd Street, NW
Suite 200
Washington, DC 20001

202-387-1968
FAX: 202-387-2193
mnygren@aaidd.org
aaidd.org

Deborah Fidler,PhD, Editor
Glenn T. Fujiura, PhD, Editor
Michael L. Wehmeyer, PhD, Co-Editor
Karrie A. Shogren, PhD, Co-Editor
Inclusionis an open submission ejournal. Inclusion is published quarterly in an online-only format, enabling timely dissemination of emerging and promising research, policy, and practices.

2197 **Intellectual and Developmental Disabilities**
501 3rd Street, NW
Suite 200
Washington, DC 20001

202-387-1968
FAX: 202-387-2193
mnygren@aaidd.org
aaidd.org

Deborah Fidler,PhD, Editor
Glenn T. Fujiura, PhD, Editor
Michael L. Wehmeyer, PhD, Co-Editor
Karrie A. Shogren, PhD, Co-Editor

Intellectual and Developmental Disabilities (IDD) is a peer reviewed multidisciplinary journal of policy, practices, and perspectives.

2198 **International Rehabilitation Review**
Rehabilitation International
41 Madison Avenue
Office 3141
New York, NY 10010

212-420-1500
FAX: 212-505-0871
info@riglobal.org
riglobal.org

Anne Hawker, President
Patric Fougeyrollas, Deputy Vice President for the No
Marca Bristo, Vice President for the North Ame
Martin Grabois, Treasurer
International overview of activities and programs in vocational and medical rehabilitation, prosthesis and orthotics and special education. *$30.00*
TriAnnual

2199 **Intervention in School and Clinic**
Sage Publications
2455 Teller Road
Thousand Oaks, CA 91320

805-499-0721
800-818-7243
FAX: 800-583-2665
info@sagepub.com
www.sagepub.com

Sara Miller McCune, Founder, Publisher & Executive Chairman
Blaise R. Simqu, President & CEO
Chris Hickok, Senior Vice President & Chief Financial Officer
Stephen Barr, Managing Director/SAGE London
A hands-on, how-to resource for teachers and clinicians working with students for whom minor curriculum and environmental modifications are ineffective. *$35.00*
64 pages

2200 **Journal for Vocational Special Needs Education**
University of Wisconsin
1025 W Johnson St
Madison, WI 53706-1706

608-263-9250
FAX: 608-262-3050
jgugerty@education.wisc.edu
www.cew.wisc.edu/jvsne/

John Gugerty, Co-Editor
Articles on vocational education for special needs population, including persons with physical and mental disabilities. *$16.00*

2201 **Journal of Applied School Psychology**
Haworth Press
711 Third Avenue
New York, NY 10017

212-216-7800
800-354-1420
FAX: 212-244-1563
subscriptions@tandf.co.uk
www.haworthpress.com

BiAnnually

2202 **Journal of Counseling & Development**
American Counseling Association
5999 Stevenson Ave
Alexandria, VA 22304-3304

703-823-0252
800-347-6647
FAX: 800-473-2329
webmaster@counseling.org
counseling.org

Robert L. Smith, President
Thelma Duffey, President Elect
Brian Canfield, Treasurer
Richard Yep, CEO
Publishes archival material, also publishes articles that have broad interest for a readership composed mostly of counselors and other mental health professionals who work in private practice, schools, colleges, community agencies, hospitals, and government. An appropriate outlet for articles that: critically integrate published research; examine current professional and

scientific issues; report research, new techniques, innovative programs and practices; and examine ACA as an organization. *$140.00*
128 pages Quarterly

2203 Journal of Disability Policy Studies
2455 Teller Road
Thousand Oaks, CA 91320

800-818-7243
FAX: 800-583-2665
journals@sagepub.com
cde.sagepub.com

Blaise R. Simqu, President/ CEO
Tracey A. Ozmina, EVP/ COO
Chris Hickok, SVP/ CFO
Phil Denvir, Global Chief Information Officer
Journal of Disability Policy Studies (DPS) addresses compelling variable issues in ethics, policy and law related to individuals with disabilities.

2204 Journal of Emotional and Behavioral Disorders
Sage Publications
2455 Teller Road
Thousand Oaks, CA 91320

805-499-0721
800-818-7243
FAX: 800-583-2665
info@sagepub.com
www.sagepub.com

Sara Miller McCune, Founder, Publisher & Executive Chairman
Blaise R. Simqu, President & CEO
Chris Hickok, Senior Vice President & Chief Financial Officer
Stephen Barr, Managing Director/SAGE London
An international, multidisciplinary journal featuring articles on research, practice and theory related to individuals with emotional and behavioral disorders and to the professionals who serve them. *$39.00*
64 pages Quarterly

2205 Journal of Learning Disabilities
Sage Publications
2455 Teller Road
Thousand Oaks, CA 91320

805-499-0721
800-818-7243
FAX: 800-583-2665
info@sagepub.com
www.sagepub.com

Sara Miller McCune, Founder, Publisher & Executive Chairman
Blaise R. Simqu, President & CEO
Chris Hickok, Senior Vice President & Chief Financial Officer
Stephen Barr, Managing Director/SAGE London
An international, multidisciplinary publication containing articles on practice, research and theory related to learning disabilities. Published bi-monthly. *$49.00*
Magazine

2206 Journal of Motor Behavior
Heldref Publications
325 Chestnut Street
Suite 800
Philadelphia, PA 19106

215-625-8900
800-354-1420
FAX: 215-625-2940
customer.service@taylorandfrancis.com
www.heldref.org

Emilli Pawlowsky, Marketing Manager
Laura Rosse, Assistant Marketing Manager
Douglas Kirkpatrick, Publisher
A professional journal aimed at psychologists, therapists and educators who work in the areas of motor behavior, psychology, neurophysiology, kinesiology, and biomechanics. Offers up-to-date information on the latest techniques, theories and developments concerning motor control. Titles previously published by Heldref Publications will be joining the T&F portfolio. *$77.00*
115 pages Quarterly

2207 Journal of Musculoskeletal Pain
Haworth Press
711 Third Avenue
New York, NY 10017

212-216-7800
800-354-1420
FAX: 212-244-1563
subscriptions@tandf.co.uk
www.haworthpress.com

110 pages Quarterly

2208 Journal of Positive Behavior Interventions
2455 Teller Road
Thousand Oaks, CA 91320

800-818-7243
FAX: 800-583-2665
journals@sagepub.com
cde.sagepub.com

Blaise R. Simqu, President/ CEO
Tracey A. Ozmina, EVP/ COO
Chris Hickok, SVP/ CFO
Phil Denvir, Global Chief Information Officer
Journal of Positive Behavior Interventions (PBI) offers sound, research-based principles of positive behavior support for use in school, home and community settings with people with challenges in behavioral adaptation.

2209 Journal of Postsecondary Education & Disability
AHEAD
107 Commerce Centre Drive
Suite 204
Huntersville, NC 28078

704-947-7779
FAX: 704-948-7779
information@ahead.org
www.ahead.org/publications/jped

Stephan J. Smith, Executive Director
Richard Allegra, Director, Professional Development
Jeremy Jarrell, Director, Innovation & Development
Oanh Huynh, Associate Executive Director
Provides in-depth examination of research, issues, policies and programs in postsecondary education.

2210 Journal of Prosthetics and Orthotics
330 John Carlyle Street
Suite 210
Alexandria, VA 22314

703-836-7114
FAX: 703-836-0838
info@abcop.org
www.abcop.org

Catherine Carter, Executive Director
Debbie Ayres, Director, Marketing & Public Relations
Stephen Fletcher, CPO, LPO, Director, Clinical Resources
Heather Harris, Director, Continuing Education Programs
Provides the latest research and clinical thinking in orthotics and prosthetics, including information on new devices, fitting techniques and patient management experiences. Each issue contains research-based information and articles reviewed and approved by a highly qualified editorial board. *$60.00*
64 pages Quarterly
ISSN 1040-88 0

2211 Journal of Reading, Writing and Learning Disabled International
Hemisphere Publishing Corporation
7625 Empire Drive
Florence, KY 41042-2919

800-634-7064
FAX: 800-248-4724
orders@taylorandfrancis.com
www.taylorandfrancis.com

2212   Journal of School Health Association
Suite 403
4340 East West Highway
Bethesda, MD 20814

301-652-8072
FAX: 301-652-8077
info@ashaweb.org
ashaweb.org

Jeffrey K. Clark, President
Stephen Conley, Executive Director
Julie Greenfield, Marketing and Conferences Direct
Beverly Samek, Chair of Advocacy

This is a monthly journal which offers information to professionals and parents on school health. Membership dues, $95.00.

2213   Journal of Special Education
Sage Publications
2455 Teller Road
Thousand Oaks, CA 91320

805-499-0721
800-818-7243
FAX: 800-583-2665
info@sagepub.com
www.sagepub.com

Sara Miller McCune, Founder, Publisher & Executive Chairman
Blaise R. Simqu, President & CEO
Chris Hickok, Senior Vice President & Chief Financial Officer
Stephen Barr, Managing Director/SAGE London

Internationally known as the prime research journal in special education. JSE provides research articles of special education for individuals with disabilities, ranging from mild to severe. Published quarterly. *$39.00*

Magazine

2214   Journal of Vocational Behavior
Academic Press, Journals Division

www.academicpress.com/jvb

2215   Learning Disabilities: A Contemporary Journal
14 Nason St.
Maynard, MA 1754

978-897-5399
FAX: 978-897-5355
info@ldworldwide.org
www.ldworldwide.org

Matthias Grunke, Editor
Teresa Allissa Citro, Editor
Bruce Saddler, Associate Editor
Juan E. Jim,nez, Associate Editor

Learning Disabilities: A Contemporary Journal (LDCJ), distributed to over 24,000 subscribers, is a peer-reviewed forum for research, practice, and opinion regarding learning disabilities (LD) and associated disorders.

2216   Learning Disabilities: A Multidisciplinary Journal
Learning Disabilities Association of America
4156 Library Road
Pittsburgh, PA 15234-1349

412-341-1515
FAX: 412-344-0224
info@ldaamerica.org
ldaamerica.org

Nancie Payne, President
Allen Broyles, First Vice President
Evalynne W. Lindberg, Secretary
Myrna Soule, Treasurer

The journal is a vehicle for disseminating the most current thinking on learning disabilities and to provide information on research, practice, theory, issues, and trends regarding learning disabilities from the perspectives of varied disciplines involved in broadening the understanding of learning disabilities.

2217   Learning Disability Quarterly
2455 Teller Road
Thousand Oaks, CA 91320

800-818-7243
FAX: 800-583-2665
journals@sagepub.com
ldq.sagepub.com

Blaise R. Simqu, President/ CEO
Tracey A. Ozmina, EVP/ COO
Chris Hickok, SVP/ CFO
Phil Denvir, Global Chief Information Officer

Learning Disability Quarterly (LDQ) publishes high-quality research and scholarship concerning children, youth, and adults with learning disabilities.

2218   MDA Newsmagazine
Muscular Dystrophy Association
3300 E. Sunrise Drive
Tucson, AZ 85718

520-529-2000
800-572-1717
FAX: 520-795-3989
tusconservices@mdausa.org
alsn.mda.org

Danielle Trzyna, Manager

Presents news related to muscular dystrophy and other neuromuscular diseases including research, personal profiles, fundraising activities and patient services.

2219   Measurement and Evaluation in Counseling
5999 Stevenson Ave
Alexandria, VA 22304-3304

703-823-0252
800-347-6647
FAX: 800-473-2329
webmaster@counseling.org
www.counseling.org

Robert L. Smith, President
Thelma Duffey, President Elect
Brian Canfield, Treasurer
Richard Yep, CEO

The American Counseling Association is a not-for-profit, professional and educational organization that is dedicated to the growth and enhancement of the counseling profession

2220   Movement Disorders
555 East Wells Street
Suite 1100
Milwaukee, WI 53202- 3823

414-276-2145
FAX: 414-276-3349
info@movementdisorders.org
www.movementdisorders.org

Matthew B. Stern, President
Oscar S. Gershanik, President-Elect
Francisco Cardoso, Secretary
Christopher Goetz, Treasurer

Movement Disorders, the official Journal of the International Parkinson and Movement Disorder Society (MDS), is a highly read and referenced journal covering all topics of the field - both clinical and basic science.

2221   Our World
National Center for Learning Disabilities
381 Park Avenue South
Suite 1401
New York, NY 10016

212-545-7510
800-575-7373
888-575-7373
FAX: 212-545-9665
help@ncld.org
ncld.org

Frederic M. Poses, Chairman, CEO
Mary Kalikow, Vice Chairman
John R. Langeler, Treasurer
William Haney, Secretary

Contains features, articles, human interest news and information and information, and other practical material to benefit the millions of children and adults with learning disabilities and their

families, as well as educators and other helping professionals.
Magazine.
Quarterly

2222   People & Families
PO Box 700
Trenton, NJ 8625-700

609-292-345
800-792-8858
FAX: 609-292-7114
TTY: 609-777-3238
njcdd@njcdd.org
www.njcdd.org

*Kevin T. Jonathan, Waller
Editor*
People & Families, the NJCDD's nationally recognized magazine, focuses on issues of importance to the developmental disabilities community in New Jersey.

2223   Psychiatric Staffing Crisis in Community Mental Health
Nat l Council for Community Behavioral Healthcare
76 Ninth Avenue
New York, NY 10011

201-559-3882
800-THE-BOOK
amilevoj@bn.com
www.barnesandnoble.com

*Andy Milevoj, Vice President, Investor Relations
Mary Ellen Keating, SVP, Corporate Communications & Public Affairs
Carolyn Brown, Director of Corporate Communications*
Find out some of the simple, low-cost ways you can increase workplace satisfaction among staff psychiatrists and compete successfully for their talents. *$20.00*

2224   Readings: A Journal of Reviews and Commentary in Mental Health
American Orthopsychiatric Association
3524 Washington Avenue
P.O. Box 1048
Sheboygan, WI 53081-1048

920-457-5051
800-558-7687
FAX: 920-457-1485
info@americanortho.com
www.americanortho.com

*Michael Bogenschuetz, President
Randy Benz, Chief Executive Officer
Charles Achter, Assistant Controller
Deb Schmidt, Administrative Manager*
Reviews of recent books in mental health and allied disciplines.
Includes essay reviews and brief reviews. *$25.00*
32 pages Quarterly

2225   Rehab Pro
1926 Waukegan Rd
Suite 1
Glenview, IL 60025-1770

847-657-6964
FAX: 847-657-6963
carlw@tcag.com
www.rehabpro.org

Carl Wangman, Executive Director
The magazine is to promote the profession and to inform the public about the activities of the national organization, its state chapter affiliates, and the work of its special interest sections.
38 pages BiMonthly

2226   Remedial and Special Education
Sage Publications
2455 Teller Road
Thousand Oaks, CA 91320

805-499-0721
800-818-7243
FAX: 800-583-2665
info@sagepub.com
www.sagepub.com

*Sara Miller McCune, Founder, Publisher & Executive Chairman
Blaise R. Simqu, President & CEO
Chris Hickok, Senior Vice President & Chief Financial Officer
Stephen Barr, Managing Director/SAGE London*

A professional journal that bridges the gap between theory and practice. Emphasis is on topical reviews, syntheses of research, field evaluation studies and recommendations for the practice of remedial and special education. Published six times a year.
$39.00
64 pages

2227   Teaching Exceptional Children
Council for Exceptional Children
2900 Crystal Drive
Suite 1000
Arlington, VA 22202-3557

703-620-3660
866-509-0218
888-232-7733
FAX: 703-264-9494
TTY:866-915-5000
service@cec.sped.org
www.cec.sped.org

*Robin D. Brewer, President
James P. Heiden, President Elect
Christy A. Chambers, Immediate Past President
Mikki Garcia, Executive Director*
Journal designed for teachers of gifted students and students with disabilities, featuring practical methods and materials for classroom use. *$58.00*
96 pages BiMonthly

Newsletters

2228   APA Access
750 First Street, NE
Washington, DC 20002-4242

202-336-5500
800-374-2721
rllowman@gmail.com
www.apa.org

*Rodney L. Lowman, PhD, Chair
Barry Anton, PhD, President
Bonnie Markham, PhD, PsyD, Treasurer
Norman Anderson, PhD, CEO, EVP*
Exclusively for APA members, APA Access provides a helpful insider's view of the latest APA news. Each monthly issue highlights an array of current topics, such as advocacy updates, continuing education opportunities, press releases, previews of Monitor on Psychology articles, APA publishing news, new APA products and a calendar of events.

2229   Alert
Association on Handicapped Student Service Program
P.O.Box 21192
Columbus, OH 43221

614-365-5216
FAX: 614-365-6718

2230   Camp Virginia Jaycee Newsletter
Dare Care Charity
2494 Camp Jaycee Rd
P.O. Box 648
Blue Ridge, VA 24064

540-947-2972
info@campvajc.org
www.campvajc.org

*Tom King, Chairman
Kathleen King, Vice Chair
Lisa Parrish, Treasurer
William Hartz, Past Chair*
Summer camping for children and adults with developmental disabilities. Coed, ages 7-70. Weekend respite camps for children and adults with mental retardation.
8 pages quarterly

2231   Children's Mental Health and EBD E-news
8161 Normandale Blvd.
Bloomington, MN 55437

952-838-9000
800-537-2237
888-248-0822
FAX: 952-838-0199
www.pacer.org

Paula F. Goldberg, Executive Director

It can be quite difficult to address children's mental health and emotional or behavioral issues. From multiple diagnoses and co-occurring conditions to the confusion of navigating often overlapping systems of care, it is often overwhelming for parents. PACER's goal is to provide family friendly, culturally competent resources to help parents be effective advocates for their child.

2232   Counseling Today
American Counseling Association
5999 Stevenson Ave
Alexandria, VA 22304-3304   703-823-0252
                                  800-347-6647
                             FAX: 800-473-2329
                          webmaster@counseling.org
                                  counseling.org

Robert L. Smith, President
Thelma Duffey, President Elect
Brian Canfield, Treasurer
Richard Yep, CEO
Aims to serve individuals active in professional counseling, in the school and university, in the workplace and the marketplace, as well as other citizens, community leaders and policy makers who appreciate the importance of the role of professional counselors in today's society.
Monthly

2233   Counselor Education and Supervision
American Counseling Association
5999 Stevenson Ave
Alexandria, VA 22304-3304   703-823-0252
                                  800-347-6647
                             FAX: 800-473-2329
                          webmaster@counseling.org
                               www.counseling.org

Robert L. Smith, President
Thelma Duffey, President Elect
Brian Canfield, Treasurer
Richard Yep, CEO
Dedicated to the growth and development of the counseling profession and those who are served. *$18.00*
Quarterly

2234   Disability Compliance for Higher Education
LRP Publications
P.O. Box 24668
West Palm Beach, FL 33416-4668   561-622-2423
                                  800-341-7874
                             FAX: 561-622-1375
                              custserve@lrp.com
                                    lrp.com

Kenneth F. Kahn, Owner and President
Ed Chase, Vice President
The only newsletter that is dedicated to the exclusive coverage of disability issues that affect colleges and universities. *$195.00*
8 pages Monthly

2235   Disability Pride Newsletter
900 Rebecca Avenue
Pittsburgh, PA 15221

                                  800-633-4588
                             FAX: 412-371-9430
                               lgray@trcil.org
                             trcil.myfastsite.net

Rachel Rogan, CEO
Gregory Daigle, Chief Financial Officer
Lisa Wilson, HR Program Manager
Victoria Johnson, Human Resources Assistant
Three Rivers Center for Independent Living (TRCIL) is a non-residential, non-profit, community-based human service organization. There purpose is to assist people with disabilities to lead self-directed and productive lives within the community.

2236   Disability Resources Monthly
Disability Resources
4 Glatter Ln
South Setauket, NY 11720-1032   631-585-0290
                            FAX: 631-585-0290
                       pubs@disabilityresources.org
                          disabilityresources.org

Avery Klauber, Executive Director
A newsletter that monitors, reviews and reports on resources for independent living. A monthly newsletter that features short topical articles, news items and reviews of books, pamphlets, periodicals, videotapes, on-line services, organizations and other resources for and about people with disabilities. It is intended primarily for librarians, social workers, educators, rehabilitation specialists, disability advocates, ADA coordinators and other health and social service professionals. *$33.00*
4 pages Monthly
ISSN 1070-72 0

2237   Early Childhood Connection
8161 Normandale Blvd.
Bloomington, MN 55437   952-838-9000
                                 800-537-2237
                                 888-248-0822
                            FAX: 952-838-0199
                               www.pacer.org

Paula F. Goldberg, Executive Director
PACER's Early Childhood Family Information and Resources Project gives parents of children ages birth through 5 years the confidence, knowledge, and skills they need to help their children obtain the education, health care, and other services they deserve.

2238   Early Childhood E-News
8161 Normandale Blvd.
Bloomington, MN 55437   952-838-9000
                                 800-537-2237
                                 888-248-0822
                            FAX: 952-838-0199
                               www.pacer.org

Paula F. Goldberg, Executive Director
Highlights early childhood news and information. Published quarterly.

2239   Early Childhood Reporter
LRP Publications
P.O. Box 24668
West Palm Beach, FL 33416-4668   561-622-2423
                                  800-341-7874
                             FAX: 561-622-1375
                              custserve@lrp.com
                                  www.lrp.com

Kenneth F. Kahn, Owner and President
Ed Chase, Vice President
Monthly reports with information on federal, state, and local legislation affecting the implementation of early intervention and preschool programs for children with disabilities. *$145.00*
12-16 pages $10 shipping

2240   FYI
501 3rd Street, NW
Suite 200
Washington, DC 20001   202-387-1968
                            FAX: 202-387-2193
                            mnygren@aaidd.org
                                  aaidd.org

Deborah Fidler,PhD, Editor
Glenn T. Fujiura, PhD, Editor
Michael L. Wehmeyer, PhD, Co-Editor
Karrie A. Shogren, PhD, Co-Editor
This monthly eblast provides news and information about AAIDD resources, educational opportunities, and other activities.

2241 Fellow Insider
501 3rd Street, NW
Suite 200
Washington, DC 20001
202-387-1968
FAX: 202-387-2193
mnygren@aaidd.org
aaidd.org

Deborah Fidler,PhD, Editor
Glenn T. Fujiura, PhD, Editor
Michael L. Wehmeyer, PhD, Co-Editor
Karrie A. Shogren, PhD, Co-Editor
Published quarterly.

2242 Field Notes
501 3rd Street, NW
Suite 200
Washington, DC 20001
202-387-1968
FAX: 202-387-2193
mnygren@aaidd.org
aaidd.org

Deborah Fidler,PhD, Editor
Glenn T. Fujiura, PhD, Editor
Michael L. Wehmeyer, PhD, Co-Editor
Karrie A. Shogren, PhD, Co-Editor
This monthly eblast promotes the translation of research to practice by providing a brief summary of approximately 10 studies recently published in peer reviewed journals with links to the original articles.

2243 Gram Newsletter, The
PO Box 1114
Claremont, CA 91711
909-621-1494
contact@ldaca.org
www.ldaca.org

Arline Krieger, President
Pam Hamilton, 1st Vice-President
EunMi Cho, 3rd Vice-President
William McKinley, Treasurer
The Learning Disabilities Association of California's (LDA-CA's) quarterly newsletter, The GRAM, provides LDA-CA members with timely information.

2244 Growing Readers
2775 S. Quincy St.
Arlington, VA
FAX: 703-998-2060
www.ldonline.org

Noel Gunther, Executive Director
Bridget Brady, Web Assistant
Lydia Breiseth, Manager
Tina Chovanec, Director
Monthly tips for raising strong readers and writers, written especially for parents. Used by schools and PTAs in parent newsletters, and by libraries and community literacy organizations.

2245 HEALTH E-News
8161 Normandale Blvd.
Bloomington, MN 55437
952-838-9000
800-537-2237
888-248-0822
FAX: 952-838-0199
www.pacer.org

Paula F. Goldberg, Executive Director
If you need information or individual assistance about navigating the health care system, PACER's F2F HICcan help. It provides a central source for Minnesota families of children and youth with special health care needs and/or disabilities and the professionals who serve them to obtain support, advocacy, and information about the health care system.

2246 Healthline
CV Mosby Company
1600 John F. Kennedy Boulevard
Suite 1800
Philadelphia, PA 19103-2822
215-239-3900
800-523-1649
FAX: 215-239-3990
www.us.elsevierhealth.com

Monthly

2247 Help Newsletter
Learning Disabilities Association of Arkansas
P.O. Box 23514
Little Rock, AR 72221
501-666-8777
FAX: 501-666-8777
info@ldaarkansas.org
www.ldaarkansas.org

Nathan Green, President
Rebecca Walker, VP
Becca Green, Past President, Treasurer
Doris Pierce, Secretary
Information on how to overcome obstacles and to achieve in spite of learning disabilities. *$30.00*
8 pages Quarterly

2248 Insights
135 Parkinson Avenue
Staten Island, NY 10305
800-223-2732
FAX: 718-981-4399
apda@apdaparkinson.org
www.apdaparkinson.org

Fred Greene, Chairman
Patrick McDermott, 1st Vice Chairman
Jerry Wells, Esq., Secretary
Elena Imperato, Treasurer
APDA was founded in 1961 with the dual purpose to Ease the Burden - Find the Cure for Parkinson's disease.

2249 International Rolf Institute
5055 Chaparral Ct.
Suite 103
Boulder, CO 80301
303-449-5903
800-530-8875
FAX: 303-449-5978
dyourell@rolf.org
rolf.org

Kevin McCoy, Chairperson
Diana Yourell, Executive Director
Jim Jones, Director of Education
Carah Wertheimer, Admissions Advisor
Information, practitioner training and certification.

2250 LD Monthly Report
2775 S. Quincy St.
Arlington, VA
FAX: 703-998-2060
www.ldonline.org

Noel Gunther, Executive Director
Bridget Brady, Web Assistant
Lydia Breiseth, Manager
Tina Chovanec, Director
LD OnLine seeks to help children and adults reach their full potential by providing accurate and up-to-date information and advice about learning disabilities and ADHD.

2251 Learning Disabilities Consultants Newsletter
Learning Disabilities Consultants
P.O.Box 716
Bryn Mawr, PA 19010
610-446-6126
800-869-8336
FAX: 610-446-6129
rcooper-ldr@comcast.net
www.thebrookhospitals.com/Resources/Childrens

Richard Cooper, Director
Newsletter providing information about learning disabilities and differences. It contains both local and national news items and in-

cludes in each issue articles about various aspects of learning problems encountered in both children and adults. *$10.00*
6 pages 5x Year

2252 MA Report
National Allergy and Asthma Network
Ste 200
3554 Chain Bridge Rd
Fairfax, VA 22030-2709
703-385-4403
FAX: 703-352-4354

Monthly

2253 Member Update
501 3rd Street, NW
Suite 200
Washington, DC 20001
202-387-1968
FAX: 202-387-2193
mnygren@aaidd.org
aaidd.org

Deborah Fidler,PhD, Editor
Glenn T. Fujiura, PhD, Editor
Michael L. Wehmeyer, PhD, Co-Editor
Karrie A. Shogren, PhD, Co-Editor
This weekly eblast updates readers on time-sensitive professional development opportunities, such as conferences and webinars, job postings, calls for papers, and opportunities to join advisory committees and provide comments on federal initiatives.

2254 O&P Almanac
American Orthotic & Prosthetic Association
330 John Carlyle Street
Suite 200
Alexandria, VA 22314
571-431-0876
FAX: 571-431-0899
info@aopanet.org
www.aopanet.org

Anita Liberman-Lampear, MA, President
Charles H. Dankmeyer, Jr, CPO, President-Elect
James Campbell, CO, Ph.D., Vice President
Jim Weber, MBA, Treasurer
Offers in-depth coverage on orthotics and prosthetics to current professional, government, business and reimbursement activities affecting the orthotics and prosthetics industry. *$59.00*
80 pages Monthly

2255 Occupational Therapy in Health Care
Haworth Press
711 Third Avenue
New York, NY 10017
212-216-7800
800-354-1420
FAX: 212-244-1563
subscriptions@tandf.co.uk
www.haworthpress.com

2256 Ohio Coalition for the Education of Children with Disabilities
165 W Center St, 3rd Floor, Chase B
Suite 302
Marion, OH 43302
740-382-5452
800-374-2806
FAX: 740-383-6421
ocecd@ocecd.org
www.ocecd.org

Martha Lause, Manager
Lee Ann Derugen, Co-Director
Margaret Burley, Executive Director
Lee Ann Derugen, Co-Director
Forum is a newsletter reporting on educational, legislative and other developments affecting persons with disabilities.
8 pages

2257 PACER E-News
8161 Normandale Blvd.
Bloomington, MN 55437
952-838-9000
800-537-2237
888-248-0822
FAX: 952-838-0199
www.pacer.org

Paula F. Goldberg, Executive Director
Published monthly, it provides resources and information for children with disabilities and their families.

2258 PACER Partners
8161 Normandale Blvd.
Bloomington, MN 55437
952-838-9000
800-537-2237
888-248-0822
FAX: 952-838-0199
www.pacer.org

Paula F. Goldberg, Executive Director
Connecting families, friends, donors, and staff of PACER. Published by the Development Office at PACER.

2259 PACESETTER
8161 Normandale Blvd.
Bloomington, MN 55437
952-838-9000
800-537-2237
888-248-0822
FAX: 952-838-0199
www.pacer.org

Paula F. Goldberg, Executive Director
PACER's main newsletter; information on special education, PACER programs, and resources.

2260 SAMHSA News
U S Department of Health and Human Services
1 Choke Cherry Road
Rockville, MD 20857
202-690-7650
877-SAM-SA 7
TTY:800-487-4889
www.samhsa.gov

Pamela S. Hyde, J.D., Administrator
Kana Enomoto, M.A., Principal Deputy Administrator
Daryl W. Kade, M.A., Chief Financial Officer and Director,OFR
Marla Hendriksson, M.P.M., Director, Office of Communications
This quarterly agency newsletter reports on information on substance abuse, mental health treatment and prevention programs of the Substance Abuse and Mental Health Services Administration.
Quarterly

2261 Sibling Information Network Newsletter
AJ Pappanikou Center
270 Farmington Avenue
Suite 181
Farmington, CT 06030
860-679-1500
866-623-1315
FAX: 860-679-1571
TTY: 860-679-1502
contact.us.ucedd@uchc.edu
www.uconnucedd.org

Mary Beth Bruder, PhD, UCEDD/LEND Director
Gerarda Hanna, J.D., M.Ed., Associate UCEDD Director
Gabriela Freyre-Calish, MSW, Coordinator, Director, Cultural Diversity
Linda Procko, Program Coordinator
Contains information aimed at the varying interested of our membership. Program descriptions, requests for assistance, conference announcements, literature summaries and research reports.
$8.50

2262 Sibpage
AJ Pappanikou Center
270 Farmington Avenue
Suite 181
Farmington, CT 06030 860-679-1500
866-623-1315
FAX: 860-679-1571
TTY: 860-679-1502
contact.us.ucedd@uchc.edu
www.uconnucedd.org
Mary Beth Bruder, PhD, UCEDD/LEND Director
Gerarda Hanna, J.D., M.Ed., Associate UCEDD Director
Gabriela Freyre-Calish, MSW, Coordinator, Director, Cultural Diversity
Linda Procko, Program Coordinator
Developed specifically for children containing games, recipes, pen pals, and articles written by siblings relating to developmental disabilities.
4 pages

2263 Special Edge
Resources in Special Education
Fl 4
1107 9th St
Sacramento, CA 95814-3616 916-492-9999
877-493-7833
FAX: 916-492-4004
rise@wested.org
Virigina Reynolds, President
Provides education news, collaborative programs, amendments to the laws, tools for accommodations, resource information, a calendar of events, and more.
BiMonthly

2264 Special Education Report
LRP Publications
360 Hiatt Dr
Dept. 150F
Palm BeachGardens, FL 33418 800-341-7874
FAX: 561-622-2423
custserve@lrp.com
lrp.com
Current, pertinent information about federal legislation, regulations, programs and funding for educating children with disabilities. Covers federal and state litigation on the Individuals with Disabilities Education Act and other relevant laws. Looks at innovations and research in the field.

2265 Tech Notes
8161 Normandale Blvd.
Bloomington, MN 55437 952-838-9000
800-537-2237
888-248-0822
FAX: 952-838-0199
www.pacer.org
Paula F. Goldberg, Executive Director
Events, resources and more for families and professionals interested in assistive technology, published quarterly.

2266 Tiny Tech
8161 Normandale Blvd.
Bloomington, MN 55437 952-838-9000
800-537-2237
888-248-0822
FAX: 952-838-0199
www.pacer.org
Paula F. Goldberg, Executive Director
Highlights technology and resources of interest to parents and professionals of children age 0 - 5, published monthly.

2267 Topics in Early Childhood Special Education
Sage Publications
2455 Teller Road
Thousand Oaks, CA 91320 805-499-0721
800-818-7243
FAX: 800-583-2665
info@sagepub.com
www.sagepub.com
Sara Miller McCune, Founder, Publisher & Executive Chairman
Blaise R. Simqu, President & CEO
Chris Hickok, Senior Vice President & Chief Financial Officer
Stephen Barr, Managing Director/SAGE London
Designed for professionals helping young children with special needs in areas such as assessment, special programs, social policies and developmental aids. *$43.00*
Quarterly

2268 Treatment Review
AIDS Treatment Data Network
57 Willoughby St.
2nd Floor
Brooklyn, NY 11201 347-473-7400
800-734-7104
TTY:212-925-9560
info@housingworks.org
www.housingworks.org
Charles King, Chair
Linney Smith, Vice Chair
Earl Ward, Vice Chair
Andrew Coarney, Secretary
Individual members receive treatment education, counseling, referrals and case management support. Services are available in both English and Spanish. The Treatment Review newsletter includes descriptions of approved, alternative and experimental treatments, as well as announcements of seminars and forums on treatments and clinical trials.
Quarterly

2269 VIP Newsletter
Blind Children's Fund
6761 West US 12
P.O. Box 363
Three Oaks, MI 49128 989-779-9966
FAX: 269-756-3133
BCF@blindchildrensfund.org
www.blindchildrensfund.org
Karla B. Kwast, Executive Director
Jeremy Murphy, President
Robert R. Storrer Jr., Vice President
Carrie L. Owens, Director
Provides parents and professionals with information, materials and resources that help them successfully teach and nurture blind, visually and multi-impaired infants and preschoolers. *$10.00*

Professional Texts

2270 7 Steps for Success
2900 Crystal Drive
Suite 1000
Arlington, VA 22202-3557 888-232-7733
alisonh@cec.sped.org
www.cec.sped.org
Elizabeth C. Hamblet, Author
The transition from high school is challenging for any student, but for young adults with disabilities, it can be even more difficult. In addition to adjusting to increased academic demands in an environment where there is less structure and support, students have to navigate a disability services system that is very different from the one they knew in high school. But with the proper preparation, students can enjoy success.

2271 A Guide to Teaching Students With Autism Spectrum Disorders
2900 Crystal Drive
Suite 1000
Arlington, VA 22202-3557

888-232-7733
alisonh@cec.sped.org
www.cec.sped.org

Monica E. Delano, Co-Author
Darlene E. Perner, Co-Author
This book is a must-have resource for all special educators and general educators who work with students with autism spectrum disorders (ASD). The strategies and teaching techniques discussed here are those that have shown great promise in helping students with ASD to succeed. The underlying premise is that students with ASD should be explicitly taught a full range of social, self-help, language, reading, writing and math skills, as are their typically developing classmates.

2272 A Teacher's Guide to Isovaleric Acidemia
150 North 18th Avenue
Phoenix, AZ 85007

602-542-1025
FAX: 602-542-0883
www.azdhs.gov

Will Humble, Director
Thomas Salow, Manager
Resource book for preschool teachers and school staff on isovaleric academia basics and classroom activities. *$2.50*

2273 A Teacher's Guide to Methylmalonic Acidemia
Arizona State Department of Health Services
150 North 18th Avenue
Phoenix, AZ 85007

602-542-1025
FAX: 602-542-0883
www.azdhs.gov

Will Humble, Director
Thomas Salow, Manager
Resource book for preschool teachers and school staff on methylmalonic academia basics and classroom activities. *$2.50*

2274 A Teacher's Guide to PKU
Arizona Department of Health Services
150 North 18th Avenue
Phoenix, AZ 85007

602-542-1025
FAX: 602-542-0883
www.azdhs.gov

Will Humble, Director
Thomas Salow, Manager
Resource book for preschool teachers and school staff on PKU basics, NutraSweet warning, and classroom activities. *$2.50*
13 pages

2275 AD/HD and the College Student: The Everything Guide to Your Most Urgent Questions
750 First Street, NE
Washington, DC 20002-4242

202-336-5500
800-374-2721
rllowman@gmail.com
www.apa.org

Patricia O. Quinn, MD, Author
Whether you are looking for information or facing an urgent situation, AD/HD and the College Student provides answers to your most pressing questions. Organized in a question-and-answer format, this guide is loaded with helpful information, practical tips, and resources.

2276 ADD Challenge: A Practical Guide for Teachers
2612 N. Mattis Ave.
P.O. Box 7886
Champaign, IL 61822

217-352-3273
800-519-2707
FAX: 217-352-1221
orders@researchpress.com
www.researchpress.com

Robert W. Parkinson, Founder
Steven B. Gordon, Author
Dr Richard M Foxx, Author
Michael J. Asher, Author
Research Press is an independent, family-owned business founded in 1968 by Robert W. Parkinson (1920-2001).

2277 ADHD Coaching: A Guide for Mental Health Professionals
750 First Street, NE
Washington, DC 20002-4242

202-336-5500
800-374-2721
rllowman@gmail.com
www.apa.org

Frances Prevatt, PhD, Co-Author
Abigail Levrini, PhD, Co-Author
This book describes the underlying principles as well as the nuts and bolts of ADHD coaching. Step-by-step details for gathering information, conducting the intake, establishing goals and objectives, and working through all stages of coaching are included, along with helpful forms and a detailed list of additional resources.

2278 ADHD in the Classroom: Strategies for Teachers
Guilford Publication
72 Spring Street
New York, NY 10012

212-431-9800
800-365-7006
FAX: 212-966-6708
info@guilford.com
www.guilford.com

Bob Matloff, President
Seymour Weingarten, Editor-in-Chief
Russell A. Barkley, Author
Gary Stoner, Author
Designed specifically to help teachers with their ADHD students, thereby providing a better learning environment for the entire class. *$95.00*

ISBN 0-898629-85-3

2279 ADHD in the Schools: Assessment and Intervention Strategies
72 Spring Street
New York, NY 10012

212-431-9800
800-365-7006
FAX: 212-966-6708
info@guilford.com
www.guilford.com

Bob Matloff, President
Seymour Weingarten, Editor-in-Chief
George J. DuPaul, Author
Gary Stoner, Author
The landmark volume emphasizes the need for a team effort among parents, community-based professionals, and educators. Provides practical information for educators that is based on empirical findings. Chapters Focus on how to identify and assess students who might have ADHD, the relationship between ADHD and learning disabilities; how to develop and supplement classroom-based programs. Communication strategies to assist physicians and the need for community-based treatments *$36.00*
269 pages Paperback
ISBN 0-898622-45-X

2280 AEPS Curriculum for Birth to Three Years
Brookes Publishing
P.O.Box 10624
Baltimore, MD 21285-0624

410-337-9580
800-638-3775
FAX: 410-337-8539
custserv@brookespublishing.com
readplaylearn.com

496 pages
ISBN 1-557660-96-4

2281 Access to Health Care: Number 3&4
World Institute on Disability
3075 Adeline Street
Suite 155
Berkeley, CA 94703

510-225-6400
FAX: 510-225-0477
TTY:510-225-0478
wid@wid.org
www.wid.org

Paul W. Schroeder, Chairman
Linda M. Dardarian, Vice Chairman
Anita Shafer Aaron, Executive Director
Mary Brooner, Treasurer
These policy bulletins focus on the capacity of the private and public health insurance systems to respond to the health care needs of persons with disabilities or chronic illness. *$6.50*
91 pages Paperback

2282 Activity-Based Approach to Early Intervention, 2nd Edition
Brookes Publishing
P.O.Box 10624
Baltimore, MD 21285-0624

410-337-9580
800-638-3775
FAX: 410-337-8539
webmaster@brookespublishing.com
www.brookespublishing.com

Paul H. Brookes, Chairman of the Board
Jeffrey D. Brookes, President
George S. Stamathis, VP/Publisher
Melissa A. Behn, Executive Vice President
Activity-based intervention shows how to use natural and relevant events to teach infants and young children, of all abilities, effectively and efficiently. *$24.00*
240 pages
ISBN 1-55766-87-5

2283 Adapted Physical Education for Students with Autism
Charles C. Thomas
2600 S First St
Springfield, IL 62704-4730

217-789-8980
800-258-8980
FAX: 217-789-9130
books@ccthomas.com
www.ccthomas.com

Kimberly Davis, Author
Focuses on the physical education needs and curriculum for autistic children. Available in cloth, paperback and hardcover. *$27.95*
142 pages Paper
ISBN 0-398060-85-1

2284 Adapting Early Childhood Curricula for Children with Special Needs (9th Edition)
Pearson Higher Education
330 Hudson St
New York, NY 10013

212-641-2400
www.pearsonhighered.com

Ruth E. Cook, Author
M. Diane Klein, Author
Deborah Chen, Author
This highly readable, well researched, and current resource uses a developmental focus, rather than a disability orientation, to discuss typical and atypical child development and curricular adap-

tations, and encourage the treatment of students as children first, without regard to their learning differences. *$102.67*
528 pages Loose-Leaf or Access Code Card 1915
ISBN 0-134019-41-3

2285 Adapting Instruction for the Mainstream: A Sequential Approach to Teaching
McGraw-Hill School Publishing
P.O. Box 182605
Columbus, OH 43218

800-338-3987
FAX: 609-308-4480
customer.service@mheducation.com
mcgraw-hill.com

David Levin, President, CEO
Ellen Haley, President, CTB
Peter Cohen, President, School Education
Mark Dorman, President, International
This text gives both regular and special education teachers everything they need to help mildly handicapped students succeed in the mainstream.
226 pages

2286 Adaptive Education Strategies Building on Diversity
Brookes Publishing Company
P.O.Box 10624
Baltimore, MD 21285-0624

410-337-9580
800-638-3775
FAX: 410-337-8539
webmaster@brookespublishing.com
www.brookespublishing.com

Paul H. Brookes, Chairman of the Board
Jeffrey D. Brookes, President
George S. Stamathis, VP/Publisher
Melissa A. Behn, Executive Vice President
Based on more than two decades of systematic research, this comprehensive manual provides a road map to the effective implementation of adaptive education. *$35.00*
304 pages Paperback
ISBN 1-557880-84-0

2287 Adolescents and Adults with Learning Disabilities and ADHD
370 Seventh Avenue
Suite 1200
New York, NY 10001-1020

800-365-7006
FAX: 212-966-6708
info@guilford.com
www.guilford.com

No%ol Gregg, PhD, Author
Most of the literature on learning disabilities and attention-deficit/hyperactivity disorder (ADHD) focuses on the needs of elementary school-age children, but older students with these conditions also require significant support.

2288 Advanced Sign Language Vocabulary: A Resource Text for Educators
Charles C. Thomas
2600 S First St
Springfield, IL 62704-4730

217-789-8980
800-258-8980
FAX: 217-789-9130
books@ccthomas.com
www.ccthomas.com

Elizabeth E. Wolf, Author
Janet R. Coleman, Author
This book is a collection of advanced sign language vocabulary for use by educators, interpreters, parents or anyone wishing to enlarge their sign vocabulary. *$53.95*
202 pages Spiralbound
ISBN 0-398057-22-2

2289 Advances in Cardiac and Pulmonary Rehabilitation
Haworth Press
711 Third Avenue
New York, NY 10017
212-216-7800
800-354-1420
FAX: 212-244-1563
subscriptions@tandf.co.uk.
www.haworthpress.com
74 pages Hardcover
ISBN 0-866869-86-3

2290 Aging Brain
Taylor & Francis Group
Ste 800
325 Chestnut St
Philadelphia, PA 19106-2608
215-625-8900
800-354-1420
FAX: 215-625-2940
www.taylorandfrancisgroup.com
225 pages Paperback
ISBN 0-85066 -78-0

2291 Aging and Disability: Crossing Network Lines
Springer Publishing
11 West 42nd Street
15th Floor
New York, NY 10036
212-431-4370
877-687-7476
FAX: 212-941-7842
marketing@springerpub.com
springerpub.com
Theodore C. Nardin, CEO/Publisher
Jason Roth, VP/Marketing Director
Annette Imperati, Marketing/Sales Director
Stephanie Drew, Acquisitions Editor,Social Work
Michelle Putnam has set forth this volume to reflect the current research, facilitate collaboration across service networks, and encourage movement toward more effective service policies. Professional stakeholders evaluate the bridges and barriers to crossing network lines, and chapter on current websites, agencies, and coalitions provides the much needed tools to bring collaboration into practice.

2292 Aging and Rehabilitation II: The State ofthe Practice
Springer Publishing Company
11 W 42nd St
15th Fl
New York, NY 10036-8002
212-431-4370
877-687-7476
FAX: 212-941-7842
cs@springerpub.com
www.springerpub.com
Ted Nardin, chief Executive Officer
Jason Roth, Vice President, Marketing & Sales
Kathy Weiss, Senior Sales Director
Annette Imperati, Sales Director, Corporate, Government, & Associations
Current, multidisciplinary investigations of various practice issues. Leading experts in the field use a practical perspective to provide specific comments on interventions. The scope of this work encompasses the autonomy of elderly disabled, mobility, mental health and value issues, as well as basic aspects in rehabilitation of the elderly. *$8.95*
348 pages Hardcover 1990
ISBN 0-826170-80-3

2293 Alphabetic Phonics Curriculum
Educators Publishing Service
625 Mount Auburn Street
3rd Floor
Cambridge, MA 02138- 3039
617-547-6706
800-225-5750
Feedback.EPS@schoolspecialty.com
www.epsbooks.com
Rick Holden, President, EPS
Ungraded multisensory curriculum for teaching phonics and the structure of language. Uses Orton-Gillingham approach to teach handwriting, spelling, reading, reading comprehension, and oral and written expression. program includes basic manual, workbooks, tests, teachers' guides, drill cards and all cards. *$28.15*
ISSN 8388-42

2294 Alternative Educational Delivery Systems
National Association of School Psychologists
4340 East West Highway
Suite 402
Bethesda, MD 20814
301-657-0270
866-331-NASP
FAX: 301-657-0275
TTY: 301-657-4155
webmaster@naspweb.org
nasponline.org
Stephen E. Brock, President
Todd A. Savage, President-Elect
Laura Benson, Chief Operating Officer
Susan Gorin, Executive Director
A book offering information to the professional on how to enhance educational options for all students.

2295 Alternative Teaching Strategies
Special Needs Project
324 State St
Ste H
Santa Barbara, CA 93101
818-718-9900
FAX: 818-349-2027
hgray@specialneeds.com
www.specialneeds.com
Hod Gray, Owner
Offers help for teachers who teach behaviorally troubled students.

2296 Antecedent Control: Innovative Approaches to Behavioral Support
Brookes Publishing
P.O.Box 10624
Baltimore, MD 21285-0624
410-337-9580
800-638-3775
FAX: 410-337-8539
webmaster@brookespublishing.com
www.brookespublishing.com
Paul H. Brookes, Chairman of the Board
Jeffrey D. Brookes, President
George S. Stamathis, VP/Publisher
Melissa A. Behn, Executive Vice President
This book explains the theory and methodology of antecedent control. The treatment techniques in this book are effective for both children and adults.
416 pages Paperback
ISBN 1-55766 -34-3

2297 Anxiety-Free Kids: An Interactive Guide for Parents and Children
Prufrock Press
PO Box 8813
Waco, TX 76714-8813
800-998-2208
FAX: 800-240-0333
info@prufrock.com
www.prufrock.com
Joel McIntosh, Publisher & Marketing Director
Lacy Compton, Senior Editor
Rachel Taliaferro, Editor
Raquel Trevino, Graphic Designer and Production Coordinator
Offers parents strategies that help children happy and worry-free, methods that relieve a child's excessive anxieties and phobias, and tools for fostering interaction and family-oriented solutions. *$19.95*
280 pages Paperback
ISBN 1-593633-43-1

2298 Applied Rehabilitation Counseling (Springer Series on Rehabilitation)

Springer Publishing Company
11 W 42nd St
15th Fl
New York, NY 10036-8002 212-431-4370
877-687-7476
FAX: 212-941-7842
cs@springerpub.com
www.springerpub.com

Ted Nardin, Chief Executive Officer
Jason Roth, Vice President, Marketing & Sales
Kathy Weiss, Senior Sales Director
Annette Imperati, Sales Director, Corporate, Government, & Associations

This comprehensive text describes current theories, techniques, and their applications to specific disabled populations. Perspectives on varying counseling approaches such as psychodynamic, existential, gestalt, behavioral and psychoeducational orientations are systematically outlined in an easy-to-follow format. Practical applications for counseling are emphasized with attention given to strategies, goal-setting and on-going evaluations. *$43.95*
404 pages Paperback 1986
ISBN 0-826153-71-2

2299 Art-Centered Education and Therapy for Children with Disabilities

Charles C. Thomas
2600 S First St
Springfield, IL 62704-4730 217-789-8980
800-258-8980
FAX: 217-789-9130
books@ccthomas.com
www.ccthomas.com

Frances E. Anderson, Author

This book has been written to help both the regular education, and art and special education teachers, both pre- and in-service, better understand some of the issues and realities of providing education and remediation to children with disabilities. The book is also offered as model concept that has govern the author's personal and professional career of over thirty years. *$41.95*
284 pages Paperback
ISBN 0-398060-06-1

2300 Assessing the Handicaps/Needs of Children

Books on Special Children
P.O.Box 3378
Amherst, MA 01004-3378 413-256-8164
FAX: 413-256-8896
irene@boscbooks.com
www.boscbooks.com

260 pages Hardcover
ISBN 0-12218 -02-0

2301 Assessment & Management of Mainstreamed Hearing-Impaired Children

Sage Publications
2455 Teller Road
Thousand Oaks, CA 91320 805-499-0721
800-818-7243
FAX: 800-583-2665
info@sagepub.com
www.sagepub.com

Sara Miller McCune, Founder, Publisher & Executive Chairman
Blaise R. Simqu, President & CEO
Chris Hickok, Senior Vice President & Chief Financial Officer
Stephen Barr, Managing Director/SAGE London

The theoretical and practical considerations of developing appropriate programming for hearing-impaired children who are being educated in mainstream educational settings are presented in this book.

2302 Assessment Log & Developmental Progress Charts for the Carolina Curriculum

Brookes Publishing
P.O.Box 10624
Baltimore, MD 21285-0624 410-337-9580
800-638-3775
FAX: 410-337-8539
webmaster@brookespublishing.com
www.brookespublishing.com

Paul H. Brookes, Chairman of the Board
Jeffrey D. Brookes, President
George S. Stamathis, VP/Publisher
Melissa A. Behn, Executive Vice President

This 28-page booklet allows the progress of children with skills in the 12-36 month development range to be easily recorded. Available in packages of 10. *$23.00*
28 pages Saddle-stiched
ISBN 1-557662-21-5

2303 Assessment and Remediation of Articulatoryand Phonological Disorders

McGraw-Hill School Publishing
PO Box 182604
Columbus, OH 43218 877-833-5524
800-338-3987
FAX: 609-308-4480
customer.service@mheducation.com
www.mcgraw-hill.com

David Levin, President/Chief Executive Officer
David Stafford, Senior Vice President/General Counsel
Maryellen Valaitis, Senior Vice President Human Resources
Patrick Milano, Chief Financial Officer/Chief Administrative Officer

Offers comprehensive coverage of articulation disorders.

2304 Assessment in Mental Handicap: A Guide to Assessment Practices & Tests

Brookline Books
8 Trumbull Rd
Suite B-001
Northampton, MA 01060 413-584-0184
800-666-2665
FAX: 413-584-6184
brbooks@yahoo.com
www.brooklinebooks.com

Esther Wilder, Co-Author

Helps professionals understand the rationale and uses for assessment practices, and provides details of appropriate instruments within each type: adaptive behavior scales, assessment of behavioral disturbances, early development and Plagetian tests. *$20.00*
Hardcover
ISBN 0-91479 -31-X

2305 Assessment of Children and Youth

Longman Education/Addison Wesley
1185 Avenue of the Americas
New York, NY 10036-2601 212-997-8500
866-203-6215
TTY:800-231-5469
www.hess.com

Dr. Mark R. Williams, Chairman of the Board
Gregory P. Hill, President/COO
John B. Hess, Chief Executive Officer
Gary Boubel, Senior Vice President-Developments

Introductory text for preservice and in-service special educators on assessment, based on the principle that every child is unique. Comprehensive coverage of both formal and informal assessment instruments. *$50.00*
640 pages Paperback
ISBN 0-80131 -02-5

2306 Assessment of Individuals with Severe Disabilities
Brookes Publishing Company
PO Box 10624
Baltimore, MD 21285-0624
410-337-9580
800-638-3775
FAX: 410-337-8539
custserv@brookespublishing.com
www.brookespublishing.com

Paul H. Brookes, Chairman
Jeffrey D. Brookes, President
Melissa A. Behm, ExecutiveVice President
George S. Stamathis, Vice President & Publisher
This expanded text offers instructors guidelines to design a comprehensive educational assessment for individuals with severe disabilities. *$34.00*
432 pages Paperback
ISBN 1-557660-67-0

2307 Assessment of the Technology Needs of Vending Facilitiy Managers In Tennessee
Mississippi State University
108 Herbert - South
Room 150/PO Drawer 6189
Mississippi State Univers, MS 39762-6189
662-325-2001
800-675-7782
FAX: 662-325-8989
TTY: 662-325-2694
nrtc@colled.msstate.edu
www.blind.msstate.edu

Jacqui Bybee, Research and Training Coordinato
Michele Capella McDonnall, Ph.D., Research Professor/Interim Director
Jessica Thornton, Business Manager
Marty Giesen, Ph.D., Senior Research Scientist
This report summarizes the results and recommendations of a survey conducted of vending facility managers throughout the state of Tennessee who participate in the Randolph-Sheppard program. *$15.00*
39 pages Paperback

2308 Assessment: The Special Educator's Role
Brookes Publishing Company
PO Box 10624
Baltimore, MD 21285-0624
410-337-9580
800-638-3775
FAX: 410-337-8539
custserv@brookespublishing.com
www.brookespublishing.com

Paul H. Brooks, Chairman
Jeffrey D. Brookes, President
Melissa A. Behm, ExecutiveVice President
George S. Stamathis, Vice President & Publisher
Aimed at students with little or no classroom experience in assessment, the book focuses on the integration of dynamic, curriculum-based and norm-referenced data for diagnostic decisions and program planning.
580 pages Casebound
ISBN 0-53421 -32-1

2309 Assistive Technology in the Schools: AGuide for Idaho Educators
Idaho Assistive Technology Project
University of Idaho
1187 Alturas Dr.
Moscow, ID 83843- 8331
205-885-3557
800-432-8324
FAX: 208-885-6102
idahoat@uidaho.edu
www.idahoat.org

LaRhae Rhoads, Author
Ron Seiler, Author
Michelle Doty, Author
This manual is designed to provide educators, parents, students with disabilities and related service providers with assistance in identifying, selecting, and acquiring assistive technology (AT) devices and services.

2310 Asthma Management and Education
Asthma and Allergy Foundation of America
8201 Corporate Drive
Suite 1000
Landover, MD 20785
202-466-7643
800-727-8462
info@aafa.org
www.aafa.org

Lynn Hanessian, Chair
Mitchell Grayson, MD, Chair, Research
Barbara Corn, Chair, Governance
Calvin Anderson, Chair/Finance/Treasurer
One session, two hour program developed to educate allied health professionals about up-to-date asthma care and patient education, information and materials. Includes hands on experience with peak flow meters and demonstrations of medical devices.

2311 Aston-Patterning
PO Box 3568
Incline Village, NV 89450-3568
775-831-8228
FAX: 775-831-8955
office@astonkinetics.com
www.astonkinetics.com

J Aston, Owner
Angelina Calafiore, Office Manager
Integrated system of movement education, body assessment, environmental modification and fitness training.

2312 Attention Deficit Disorder in Children
Charles C. Thomas
2600 S First St
Springfield, IL 62704-4730
217-789-8980
800-258-8980
FAX: 217-789-9130
books@ccthomas.com
www.ccthomas.com

2313 Aural Habilitation
Alexander Graham Bell Association
3417 Volta Pl NW
Washington, DC 20007-2737
202-337-5220
FAX: 202-337-8314
TTY:202-337-5221
info@agbell.org
www.listeningandspokenlanguage.org

Meredith K. Sugar, Esq. (OH), President
Ted A. Meyer, M.D., Ph.D, President-Elect/Secretary-Treasurer
Emilio Alonso-Mendoza, Chief Executive Officer
Susan Boswell, Director of Communications and Marketing
This classic text for professionals, educators and parents discusses verbal learning and aural habilitation of young children with hearing losses to ensure that each child is educated in the best setting. It discusses communication, normal development of spoken language, speech audiologic assessment, hearing aids and use of residual hearing, and program designs for individualized needs, including the assessment and planning of IEPs. *$26.95*
324 pages

2314 Behavior Analysis in Education: Focus on Measurably Superior Instruction
Brookes Publishing Company
PO Box 10624
Baltimore, MD 21285-0624
410-337-9580
800-638-3775
FAX: 410-337-8539
custserv@brookespublishing.com
www.brookespublishing.com

Paul H. Brookes, Chairman
Jeffrey D. Brookes, President
Melissa A. Behm, ExecutiveVice President
George S. Stamathis, Vice President & Publisher
Designed to disseminate measurably superior instructional strategies to those interested in advancing sound, pedagogically effective, field-tested educational practices, this book is intended for graduate-level courses and seminars in special education and/or psychology focusing on behavior analysis and instruction.
512 pages Casebound
ISBN 0-53422 -60-9

2315 Behavior Modification

Sage Publications
2455 Teller Rd
Thousand Oaks, CA 91320-2218

805-499-0721
800-818-7243
FAX: 800-583-2665
info@sagepub.com
www.sagepub.com

Sara Miller McCune, Founder, Publisher and Executive Chairman
Blaise R. Simqu, President & CEO
Chris Hickok, Senior Vice President & Chief Financial Officer
Stephen Barr, Managing Director/SAGE London

Describes in detail for replication purposes assessment and modification techniques for problems in psychiatric, clinical, educational and rehabilitation settings. *$53.00*

640 pages Quarterly

2316 Behavioral Disorders

Council for Exceptional Children
2900 Crystal Drive
Suite 1000
Arlington, VA 22202-3557

703-620-3660
866-509-0218
888-232-7733
FAX: 703-264-9494
TTY:866-915-5000
services@cec.sped.org
www.cec.sped.org

Robin D. Brewer, President
James P. Heiden, President Elect
Joni L. Baldwin, Director
Christy A. Chambers, Immediate Past President

Provides professionals with a means to exchange information and share ideas related to research, empirically tested educational innovations and issues and concerns relevant to students with behavioral disorders. Individual, $20; Institution, $50.

Quarterly

2317 Behind Special Education

Love Publishing Company
9101 E Kenyon Ave
Suite 2200
Denver, CO 80237-1854

303-221-7333
FAX: 303-221-7444
lpc@lovepublishing.com
www.lovepublishing.com

ISBN 0-89108-17-4

2318 Biomedical Concerns in Persons with Down's Syndrome

Paul H Brookes Publishing Company
PO Box 10624
Baltimore, MD 21285-0624

410-337-9580
800-638-3775
FAX: 410-337-8539
custserv@brookespublishing.com
www.brookespublishing.com

Paul H. Brookes, Chairman
Jeffrey D. Brookes, President
Melissa A. Behm, ExecutiveVice President
George S. Stamathis, Vice President & Publisher

Written by leading authorities and spanning many disciplines and specialties, this comprehensive resource provides vital information on biomedical issues concerning individuals with Down's Syndrome. *$45.00*

336 pages Hardcover
ISBN 1-557660-89-1

2319 Breaking Barriers

AbleNet
2625 Patton Road
Roseville, MN 55113-5423

651-294-2200
800-322-0956
FAX: 651-294-2259
customerservice@ablenetinc.com
www.ablenetinc.com

Bill Sproull, Chairman of the Board
William Mills, Board of Directors, Chair
Jennifer Thalhuber, President/CEO
Paul Sugden, Vice President of Finance, IT & CFO, Trustee

A practical resource for parents, caregivers, teachers and therapists. *$15.00*

2320 Building Skills for Independence in the Mainstream

15619 Premiere Drive
Suite 101
Tampa, FL 33624

850-363-9909
FAX: 480-393-4331
accounting@successforkidswithhearingloss.com
successforkidswithhearinglo ss.com

Karen L. Anderson, Director/ Co-Author
Gale Wright, Co-Author

Building Skills for Independence in the Mainstream was developed as a Guide for DHH professionals to support their work with classroom teachers and with students to develop the skills needed for independence with hearing aids and self-advocacy.

2321 Building Skills for Success in the Fast-Paced Classroom

15619 Premiere Drive
Suite 101
Tampa, FL 33624

850-363-9909
FAX: 480-393-4331
accounting@successforkidswithhearingloss.com
successforkidswithhearinglo ss.com

Karen L. Anderson, PhD, Co-Author
Kathleen A. Arnoldi, MA

The purpose of this book is to provide resources that will assist these students in optimizing their achievement through improved access and self-advocacy. The information contained in this book targets the expanded core curriculum, or those skills that must be mastered in order to benefit from the core curriculum. This book is meant to be a practical ready-to-go resource for professionals who work with school-age children with hearing loss.

2322 Building the Healing Partnership: Parents, Professionals and Children with Chronic Illnesses

Brookline Books
8 Trumbull Rd
Ste B-001
Northampton, MA 01060

413-584-0184
800-666-2665
FAX: 413-584-6184
brbooks@yahoo.com
www.brooklinebks.com

Patricia Tanner Leff, Author
Elaine H. Walizer, Author

Successful programs understand that the disabled child's needs must be considered in the context of a family. This book was specifically written for practitioner's who must work with families but who have insufficient training in family systems assessment and intervention. It is a valuable blend of theory and practice with pointers for applying the principles. *$24.95*

312 pages Paperback 1992
ISBN 0-914797-60-3

2323 CAI, Career Assessment Inventories for theLearning Disabled

Academic Therapy Publications
20 Leveroni Crt
Novato, CA 94949-5746

415-883-3314
800-422-7249
FAX: 888-287-9975
sales@academictherapy.com
www.academictherapy.com

Carol Weller, Author
Mary Buchanan, Author

Takes personality, ability and interest into account in pointing learning disabled students of all ages toward intelligent and realistic career choices. Contains binder with paperback teaching guide plus 50 interest inventories and 50 abilities inventories.
64 pages 1983
ISBN 0-878793-50-X

2324 Caring for Children with Chronic Illness
11 W 42nd St
15th Floor
New York, NY 10036-8002   212-431-4370
    877-687-7476
    FAX: 212-941-7842
    cs@springerpub.com
    www.springerpub.com

Ursula Springer, President
Theodore C. Nardin, CEO/Publisher
Jason Roth, VP/Marketing Director
James C. Costello, Vice President, Journal Publishing
A critical look at the current medical, social, and psychological framework for providing care to children with chronic illnesses. Emphasizing the need to create integrated, interdisciplinary approaches, it discusses issues such as the roles of families, professionals, and institutions in providing health care, the impact of a child's illness on various family structures, financing care, the special problems of chronically ill children as they become adolescents and more. *$36.95*
320 pages Hardcover
ISBN 0-82615-00-1

2325 Carolina Curriculum for Infants and Toddlers with Special Needs (3rd Edition)
Brookes Publishing
P.O. Box 10624
Baltimore, MD 21285-0624   410-337-9580
    800-638-3775
    FAX: 410-337-8539
    custserv@brookespublishing.com
    www.brookespublishing.com

Nancy M. Johnson-Martin, Author
Susan M. Attermeier, Author
Bonnie J. Hacker, Author
This book includes detailed assessment and intervention sequences, daily routine integration strategies, sensorimotor adaptations, and a sample 24-page assessment log that shows readers how to chart a child's individual progress.
504 pages Spiral-bound

2326 Carolina Curriculum for Preschoolers with Special Needs
Brookes Publishing
PO Box 10624
Baltimore, MD 21285-0624   410-337-9580
    800-638-3775
    FAX: 410-337-8539
    custserv@brookespublishing.com
    www.brookespublishing.com

Paul H. Brookes, Chairman
Jeffrey D. Brookes, President
Melissa A. Behm, ExecutiveVice President
George S. Stamathis, Vice President & Publisher
This curriculum provides detailed teaching and assessment techniques, plus a sample 28-page assessment log that shows readers how to chart a child's individual progress. This guide is for children between 2 and 5 in their developmental stages who are considered at risk for developmental delay or who exhibit special needs. *$34.00*
352 pages Spiral-bound
ISBN 1-55766-32-8

2327 Challenge of Educating Together Deaf and Hearing Youth: Making Manistreaming Work
Charles C. Thomas
2600 S First St
Springfield, IL 62704-4730   217-789-8980
    800-258-8980
    FAX: 217-789-9130
    books@ccthomas.com
    www.ccthomas.com

198 pages Hardcover
ISBN 0-398063-91-5

2328 Challenged Scientists: Disabilities and the Triumph of Excellence
Greenwood Publishing Group
130 Cremona Drive
Santa Barbara, CA 93117   805-968-1911
    800-368-6868
    FAX: 866-270-3856
    CustomerService@abc-clio.com
    www.abc-clio.com

208 pages
ISBN 0-275938-73-5

2329 Child Care and the ADA: A Handbook for Inclusive Programs
Brookes Publishing
PO Box 10624
Baltimore, MD 21285-0624   410-337-9580
    800-638-3775
    FAX: 410-337-8539
    custserv@brookespublishing.com
    www.brookespublishing.com

Paul H. Brookes, Chairman
Jeffrey D. Brookes, President
Melissa A. Behm, ExecutiveVice President
George S. Stamathis, Vice President & Publisher
This book is designed for educators and administrators in child care settings. It offers a straightforward discussion of the Americans with Disabilities Act including children with disabilities in community programs. *$25.95*
240 pages Paperback
ISBN 1-55766-85-5

2330 Child with Disabling Illness
Lippincott, Williams & Wilkins
16522 Hunters Green Pkwy
Hagerstown, MD 21740   301-223-2300
    800-638-3030
    FAX: 301-223-2400
    orders@lww.com
    www.lww.com

700 pages

2331 Childhood Behavior Disorders: Applied Research & Educational Practice
Sage Publications
2455 Teller Road
Thousand Oaks, CA 91320-2218   805-499-0721
    800-818-7243
    FAX: 800-583-2665
    info@sagepub.com
    www.sagepub.com

Sara Miller McCune, Founder, Publisher, Chairperson
Blaise R. Simqu, President/CEO
Chris Hickok, Senior Vice President & Chief Fi
Stephen Barr, Managing Director/SAGE London, P
The only comprehensive overview of childhood behavior disorders. This book gives you the how and why for helping children with behavior disorders.

2332 Childhood Disablity and Family Systems(Routledge Library Editions) (Volume 5)
Routledge (Taylor & Francis Group)
711 Third Ave
New York, NY 10017 212-216-7800
800-634-7064
FAX: 202-564-7854
enquiries@taylorandfrancis.com
www.routledge.com

Michael Ferrari, Editor
Marvin B. Sussman, Editor
Focuses on what the presence of a disabled child means to a family. Those professionals involved in teaching, research, and direct care with families having disabled children will value the coverage of such topics as the contemporary context of disability, ethical issues, family effects, and care systems. First published in 1987 by Haworth Press, the book is now published under Routledge. *$140.00*
256 pages Hardcover 1916
ISBN 1-138101-55-9

2333 Children and Youth Assisted by Medical Technology in Educational Settings, 2nd Edition
Brookes Publishing
PO Box 10624
Baltimore, MD 21285-0624 410-337-9580
800-638-3775
FAX: 410-337-8539
custserv@brookespublishing.com
www.brookespublishing.com

Paul H. Brookes, Chairman
Jeffrey D. Brookes, President
Melissa A. Behm, ExecutiveVice President
George S. Stamathis, Vice President & Publisher
Contains detailed daily care guidelines and emergency-response techniques, including information on working with a range of students who have the HIV infection, that rely on ventilators, that utilize tube feeding, or require catheterization. Also covers every aspect of planning for inclusive classrooms, including information on personnel training, entrance planning and transition, legal requirements, and transportation issues. *$52.00*
432 pages Spiral-bound
ISBN 1-55766 -36-3

2334 Children's Needs Psychological Perspective
National Association of School Psychologists
8455 Colesville Rd
Suite 1000
Silver Spring, MD 20910- 3392 301-589-3300
FAX: 301-589-5175
www.musictherapy.org
637 pages

2335 Choices: A Guide to Sex Counseling with Physically Disabled Adults
Krieger Publishing Company
1725 Krieger Dr
Malabar, FL 32950 321-724-9542
800-724-0025
FAX: 321-951-3671
info@krieger-publishing.com
www.krieger-publishing.com

Maureen E. Neistadt, Author
Provides rehabilitation professionals with the basic information necessary for limited sexuality counseling of physically disabled adults. *$20.90*
132 pages
ISBN 0-898749-03-4

2336 Choosing Options and Accommodations for Children
Brookes Publishing
PO Box 10624
Baltimore, MD 21285-0624 410-337-9580
800-638-3775
FAX: 410-337-8539
custserv@brookespublishing.com
www.brookespublishing.com

192 pages
ISBN 1-55766 -06-5

2337 Cirriculum Development for Students with Mild Disabilities
Charles C. Thomas
2600 S First St
Springfield, IL 62704-4730 217-789-8980
800-258-8980
FAX: 217-789-9130
books@ccthomas.com
www.ccthomas.com

Carroll J. Jones, Author
This book was designed to provide the foundation from which to write cirrocumuli that will provide academic and social skills for Individual Education Programs (IEPs). *$38.95*
258 pages Spiral-Paper
ISBN 0-398070-18-2

2338 Classroom Success for the LD and ADHD Child
John F. Blair Publishing
1406 Plaza Dr
Winston Salem, NC 27103-1470 336-768-1374
800-222-9796
FAX: 336-768-9194
sparrow@blairpub.com
www.blairpub.com

Steve Kirk, Editor-In-Chief
Anna Sutton, Vice President, Sales & Marketing
Artie Sparrow, Office Manager & Customer Service
Suzanne H. Stevens, Author
This book offers suggestions on teaching techniques, adapting texts, recognition of children with disabilities and testing, grading and mainstreaming the learning disabled and ADHD child. *$13.95*
333 pages Paperback 1997
ISBN 0-895871-59-9

2339 Clinical Alzheimer Rehabilitation
Springer Publishing
11 W 42nd St
15th Floor
New York, NY 10036-8002 212-431-4370
877-687-7476
FAX: 212-941-7842
cs@springerpub.com
www.springerpub.com

Theodore C. Nardin, CEO/Publisher
Jason Roth, VP/Marketing Director
Annette Imperati, Marketing/Sales Director
James C. Costello, Vice President, Journal Publishing
This comprehensive and easy-to-read guidebook contains the latest research on dementia and AD in the elderly population, including the causes and risk factors of AD, diagnosis information, and symptoms and progressions of the disease. Significant emphasis is given to the physical, mental, and verbal rehabilitation challenges of patients with AD. The authors outline specific rehabilitation goals for the physical therapist, speech-language pathologist, and general caregiver.

2340 Clinical Management of Childhood Stuttering, 2nd Edition
Sage Publications
2455 Teller Road
Thousand Oaks, CA 91320-2218   805-499-0721
                                             800-818-7243
                                        FAX: 800-583-2665
                                        info@sagepub.com
                                        www.sagepub.com

Sara Miller McCune, Founder, Publisher, Chairperson
Blaise R. Simqu, President/CEO
Chris Hickok, Senior Vice President/CFO
Stephen Barr, Managing Director/SAGE London
Updates and integrates recent findings in childhood stuttering into a broad range of therapeutic strategies for assessing and treating the young dysfluent child. *$38.00*
336 pages

2341 Cognitive Approaches to Learning Disabilities
Sage Publications
2455 Teller Road
Thousand Oaks, CA 91320-2218   805-499-0721
                                             800-818-7243
                                        FAX: 800-583-2665
                                        info@sagepub.com
                                        www.sagepub.com

Sara Miller McCune, Founder, Publisher, Chairperson
Blaise R. Simqu, President/CEO
Chris Hickok, Senior Vice President/CFO
Stephen Barr, Managing Director/SAGE London
The first to bridge the gap between cognitive psychology and information processing theory in understanding learning disabilities. *$39.00*
495 pages Hardcover

2342 Cognitive Strategy Instruction That Really Improves Children's Academic Skills
Brookline Books
8 Trumbull Rd
Suite B-001
Northampton, MA 01060   413-584-0184
                                             800-666-2665
                                        FAX: 413-584-6184
                                        brbooks@yahoo.com
                                        www.brooklinebooks.com

Esther Isabe Wilder, Author
A concise and focused work that summarily presents the few procedures for teaching strategies that aid academic subject matter learning: decoding reading comprehension, vocabulary, math, spelling and writing. Learning unrelated facts and science. Completely revised in 1995. *$27.95*
Paperback
ISBN 1-571290-07-9

2343 Collaborating for Comprehensive Services for Young Children and Families
Brookes Publishing Company
PO Box 10624
Baltimore, MD 21285-0624   410-337-9580
                                             800-638-3775
                                        FAX: 410-337-8539
                                        custserv@brookespublishing.com
                                        www.brookespublishing.com

Paul H. Brookes, Chairman
Jeffrey D. Brookes, President
Melissa A. Behm, ExecutiveVice President
George S. Stamathis, Vice President & Publisher
Taking collaboration a step beyond basic implementation, this useful book shows agency and school leaders how to coordinate their efforts to stretch human services dollars while still providing quality programs. Provides the building blocks needed to establish a local interagency coordinating council. *$37.00*
272 pages
ISBN 1-557661-03-0

2344 Collaborative Teams for Students with Severe Disabilities
Brookes Publishing
PO Box 10624
Baltimore, MD 21285-0624   410-337-9580
                                             800-638-3775
                                        FAX: 410-337-8539
                                        custserv@brookespublishing.com
                                        www.brookespublishing.com

Paul H. Brookes, Chairman
Jeffrey D. Brookes, President
Melissa A. Behm, ExecutiveVice President
George S. Stamathis, Vice President & Publisher
How can educators, parents and therapists work together to ensure the best possible educational experience for students with severe disabilities? This resource describes how a collaborative team can successfully create exciting learning opportunities for students, while teaching them to participate fully at home, school, work and play. *$ 30.00*
304 pages
ISBN 1-55766 -88-3

2345 Communicating with Parents of Exceptional Children
Love Publishing Company
9101 E Kenyon Ave
Suite 2200
Denver, CO 80237-1854   303-221-7333
                                        FAX: 303-221-7444
                                        lpc@lovepublishing.com
                                        www.lovepublishing.com

Roger L. Kroth, Author
Denzil Denzil Edge, Author
This book shows how teachers can facilitate parent involvement with children's education. It presents the mirror model of parent involvement, family, dynamics, how to listen actively to parents, values and perceptions, problem-solving, parent conferences and training groups. *$19.95*

ISBN 0-89108 -67-4

2346 Communication & Language Acquisition: Discoveries from Atypical Development
Brookes Publishing
PO Box 10624
Baltimore, MD 21285-0624   410-337-9580
                                             800-638-3775
                                        FAX: 410-337-8539
                                        custserv@brookespublishing.com
                                        www.brookespublishing.com

Paul H. Brookes, Chairman
Jeffrey D. Brookes, President
Melissa A. Behm, ExecutiveVice President
George S. Stamathis, Vice President & Publisher
This text demonstrates how the study of language acquisition in children with atypical development promotes advances in basic theory. *$44.00*
352 pages Hardcover
ISBN 1-557662-79-7

2347 Communication Skills for Working with Elders
Springer Publishing Company
11 W 42nd St
15th Floor
New York, NY 10036-8002   212-431-4370
                                             877-687-7476
                                        FAX: 212-941-7842
                                        cs@springerpub.com
                                        www.springerpub.com

Ursula Springer, President
Theodore C. Nardin, CEO/Publisher
Jason Roth, VP/Marketing Director
James C. Costello, Vice President, Journal Publishing
How aging and illness affects communication. *$17.95*
160 pages Softcover
ISBN 0-82615 -20-7

2348 Communication Unbound
Teachers College Press
Ste 2115
14781 Memorial Dr
Houston, TX 77079-5210

415-738-4323
FAX: 415-738-4329
tcc.orders@aidcvt.com
www.pearsonhighered.com

240 pages Paperback
ISBN 0-087737-21-4

2349 Complete Handbook of Children's Reading Disorders: You Can Prevent or Correct LDs
Gallery Bookshop
319 Kasten Street
PO Box 270
Mendocino, CA 95460-270

707-937-2215
FAX: 707-937-3737
info@gallerybookshop.com
www.gallerybooks.com

Tony Miksak, Owner
The complete handbook of children's reading disorders. *$34.95*
732 pages Paperback
ISBN 0-80772 -83-3

2350 Computer Access/Computer Learning
Special Needs Project
324 State St
Suite H
Santa Barbara, CA 93101-2364

805-962-8087
800-333-6867
FAX: 805-962-5087
editor@specialneeds.com
www.specialneeds.com

Mark Darrow, Founder, The Prolotherapy Institu
A resource manual in adaptive technology and computer training. *$22.50*

2351 Consulting Psychologists Press
1055 Joaquin Rd
Suite. 200
Mountain View, CA 94043-1243

650-969-8901
800-624-1765
FAX: 650-969-8608
custserv@cpp.com
www.cpp-db.com

Carl E. Thoresen, Chairman
Jeffrey Hayes, President and Chief Executive Officer
Andrew Bell, Vice President of International
Catey DeBalko, Vice President of Marketing
Catalog offering job assessment software, career development reports, educational assessment information and books for the professional.

2352 Counseling Persons with Communication Disorders and Their Families
Sage Publications
2455 Teller Road
Thousand Oaks, CA 91320-2218

805-499-0721
800-818-7243
FAX: 800-583-2665
info@sagepub.com
www.sagepub.com

Sara Miller McCune, Founder, Publisher, Chairperson
Blaise R. Simqu, President & CEO
Chris Hickok, Senior Vice President & Chief Fi
Stephen Barr, Managing Director/SAGE London, P
A learning manual for speech-language pathologists and audiologists on how to deal with the emotional issues facing them in their work with clients with communication disorders and their families. *$ 29.00*
187 pages

2353 Counseling in the Rehabilitation Process
Charles C. Thomas
2600 S First St
Springfield, IL 62704-4730

217-789-8980
800-258-8980
FAX: 217-789-9130
books@ccthomas.com
www.ccthomas.com

Gerald L. Gandy, Author
E. Davis Martin Jr, Author
Richard E. Hardy, Author
This text provides the reader with a comprehensive overview and introduction to the field of rehabilitation counseling and services, and also has applicability in the growing field of community counseling. *$51.95*
358 pages paper 1999
ISBN 0-398069-70-4

2354 Creating Positive Classroom Environments: Strategies for Behavior Management
Brooks / Cole Publishing Company
511 Forest Lodge Rd
Pacific Grove, CA 93950-5040

831-373-0728
800-354-9706
FAX: 831-375-6414
bc-info@brookscole.com
www.cengage.com

448 pages Paperbound
ISBN 0-53422 -54-4

2355 Critical Voices on Special Education: Problems & Progress Concerning the Mildly Handicapped
State University of New York Press
22 Corporate Woods Boulevard
3rd Floor
Albany, NY 12211-2504

518-472-5000
866-430-7869
FAX: 518-472-5038
info@sunypress.edu
www.sunypress.edu

James Peltz, Associate Director
Janice Vunk, Assistant to the Director
Scott B Sigmon, Editor
Problems and progress concerning the mildly handicapped. *$24.95*
265 pages Paperback 1990
ISBN 0-79140 -20-3

2356 Cultural Diversity, Families and the Special Education System
Teachers College Press
1234 Amsterdam Ave
New York, NY 10027-6602

212-678-3929
800-575-6566
FAX: 212-678-4149
tcpress@tc.columbia.edu
www.teacherscollegepress.com

Beth Harry, Author
This timely and thought-provoking book explores the quadruple disadvantage faced by the parents of poor, minority, handicapped children whose first language is not that of the school they attend. *$22.95*
296 pages Paperback
ISBN 0-807731-19-6

2357 Curriculum Decision Making for Students with Severe Handicaps
Teachers College Press
1234 Amsterdam Ave
New York, NY 10027-6602

212-678-3929
800-575-6566
FAX: 212-678-4149
tspress@ts.columbia.edu.
www.teacherscollegepress.com

192 pages Paperback
ISBN 0-807728-61-6

2358 Deciphering the System: A Guide for Families of Young Disabled Children
Brookline Books
8 Trumbull Rd
Ste B-001
Northampton, MA 01060

413-584-0184
800-666-2665
FAX: 413-584-6184
brbooks@yahoo.com
www.brooklinebks.com

Paula Beckman, Author
This book informs parents of disabled children (0-5) of their rights and the service system, e.g., ways to manage the cumulating information, tips on IEP and IFSP meetings and the educational assessment process, and how parents can work with multiple service providers. It includes contributions from both parents and professionals who have experience with the service system. *$21.95*
208 pages Paperback 1999
ISBN 0-914797-87-5

2359 Defining Rehabilitation Agency Types
Mississippi State University
108 Herbert - South
Room 150 Industrial Education Depar
Mississippi State, MS 39762-6189

662-325-2001
800-675-7782
FAX: 662-325-8989
TTY: 662-325-2694
nrtc@colled.msstate.edu
www.blind.msstate.edu

Jacqui Bybee, Research Associate II
Michele Capella McDonnall, Ph.D., Research Professor/Interim Director
Jessica Thornton, Business Manager
Marty Giesen, Ph.D., Senior Research Scientist
Relationships of participant selection and cost factors of service delivery across rehabilitation agency types. A national survey of state agencies for the blind was conducted to examine factors that define the characteristics of different agencies; similar programs were grouped together. Classification criteria were developed to distinguish agencies into logical groups based on line of authority, funding and operating procedures. *$10.00*
15 pages Paperback

2360 Designing and Using Assistive Technology: The Human Perspective
Brookes Publishing
PO Box 10624
Baltimore, MD 21285-0624

410-337-9580
800-638-3775
FAX: 410-337-8539
custserv@brookespublishing.com
www.brookespublishing.com

Paul H. Brookes, Chairman
Jeffrey D. Brookes, President
Melissa A. Behm, ExecutiveVice President
George S. Stamathis, Vice President & Publisher
Presented here is a holistic perspective on how and why people choose and use AT. Features personal insights and the latest research on design and development. *$31.00*
352 pages Paperback
ISBN 1-55766-14-9

2361 Developing Cross-Cultural Competence:Guideto Working with Young Children & Their Families
Brookes Publishing
PO Box 10624
Baltimore, MD 21285-0624

410-337-9580
800-638-3775
FAX: 410-337-8539
custserv@brookespublishing.com
www.brookespublishing.com

Paul H. Brookes, Chairman
Jeffrey D. Brookes, President
Melissa A. Behm, ExecutiveVice President
George S. Stamathis, Vice President & Publisher

This enlightening book perceptively and sensitively explores cultural, ethnic, and language diversity in human services. For those who work with families whose infants and young children may have or be at risk for a disability or chronic illness. (Second Edition) *$ 32.00*
448 pages Paperback
ISBN 1-55766 -31-9

2362 Developing Individualized Family Support Plans: A Training Manual
Brookline Books
Suite B-001
8 Trumbull Rd
Northampton, MA 01060

413-584-0184
800-666-2665
FAX: 413-584-6184
brbooks@yahoo.com
www.brooklinebooks.com

Esther Wilder, Co-Author
This manual provides in-service training coordinators, administrators, supervisors and university personnel with a compact package of functional and practical methods to train professionals about implementing family-centered individualized family support plans (IFSP'S). Also, case studies provide concrete examples to aid in learning to write IFSP's. *$24.95*

ISBN 0-914797-69-7

2363 Developing Staff Competencies for Supporting People with Disabilities
Brookes Publishing
PO Box 10624
Baltimore, MD 21285-0624

410-337-9580
800-638-3775
FAX: 410-337-8539
custserv@brookespublishing.com
www.brookespublishing.com

Paul H. Brookes, Chairman
Jeffrey D. Brookes, President
Melissa A. Behm, ExecutiveVice President
George S. Stamathis, Vice President & Publisher
This timely second edition, now in a new easier to read format, gives service providers helpful strategies for increasing effectiveness and maintaining well-being while working in the rewarding yet challenging field of human services. *$34.00*
480 pages Paperback
ISBN 1-55766 -07-3

2364 Development of Language
McGraw-Hill, School Publishing
220 E Danieldale Rd
Desoto, TX 75115-2490

800-648-2970
FAX: 800-593-4418
www.mhschool.com

464 pages

2365 Developmental Disabilities of Learning
Gallery Bookshop
319 Kasten Street
PO Box 270
Mendocino, CA 95460-270

707-937-2215
FAX: 707-937-3737
info@gallerybookshop.com
www.gallerybooks.com

Tony Miksak, Owner
Manual for professionals on developmental and learning disabilities in the growing child. *$25.00*
224 pages Illustrated

2366 Developmental Disabilities: A Handbook for Occupational Therapists
Haworth Press
711 Third Avenue
New York, NY 10017
212-216-7800
800-354-1420
FAX: 212-244-1563
subscriptions@tandf.co.uk.
www.haworthpress.com

268 pages Hardcover
ISBN 0-866569-59-6

2367 Developmental Disabilities: A Handbook for Interdisciplinary Practice
Brookline Books
8 Trumbull Rd
Suite B-001
Northampton, MA 01060
413-584-0184
800-666-2665
FAX: 413-584-6184
brbooks@yahoo.com
www.brooklinebooks.com

Esther Wilder, Co-Author
Successful interdisciplinary team practice for persons with developmental disabilities that require each team member to understand and respect the contributions of the others. This handbook explains the professions most often represented on interdisciplinary teams: their natures, concerns and roles in the interdisciplinary context. *$29.95*
256 pages
ISBN 1-571290-03-6

2368 Developmental Variation and Learning Disorders
Educators Publishing Service
PO Box 9031
Cambridge, MA 02139-9031
617-367-2700
800-225-5750
FAX: 617-547-0412
eps@schoolspecialty.com
www.epsbooks.com

Rick Holden, President
Discusses seven major areas of development and four major areas of academic proficiency and then ties this information together by examining factors that predispose a child to dysfunction and disability, offering guidelines to assessment and management, and analyzing long-range outcomes and factors that promote resiliency for parents, educators and clinicians. *$69.00*
640 pages Cloth
ISBN 0-838819-92-3

2369 Digest of Neurology and Psychiatry
Institute of Living: Hartford Hospital
80 Seymour Street
Hartford, CT 06106-3309
860-545-5000
800-673-2411
FAX: 860-545-5066
Fishe@harthosp.org
www.harthosp.org

Douglas Elliot, Chair of the Board
Stuart K. Markowitz, MD, FACR, President/SVP
Gerald J. Boisvert, HHC Regional Vice President / Chief Financial Officer,
Peter Q. Fraser, Regional Vice President Human Resources
Abstracts and reviews of selected current literature in psychiatry, neurology and related fields.

2370 Disability Funding News
8204 Fenton St
Silver Spring, MD 20910-4502
301-588-6380
800-666-6380
FAX: 301-588-6385
info@cdpublications.com,
www.cdpublications.com

Mike Gerecht, Publisher

2371 Disability Studies and the Inclusive Classroom
711 3rd Avenue
8th Floor
New York, NY 10017
212-216-7800
800-634-7064
FAX: 212-564-7854
www.routledge.com

Susan Baglieri, Co-Author
Arthur Shapiro, Co-Author
This book's mission is to integrate knowledge and practice from the fields of disability studies and special education. Parts I & II focus on the broad, foundational topics that comprise disability studies (culture, language, and history) and Parts III & IV move into practical topics (curriculum, co-teaching, collaboration, classroom organization, disability-specific teaching strategies, etc.) associated with inclusive education.

2372 Disability and Rehabilitation
Taylor & Francis
7625 Empire Dr
Florence, KY 41042-2919
800-634-7064
FAX: 800-248-4724
orders@taylorandfrancis.com
www.taylorandfrancis.com

Monthly
ISSN 0963-82 8

2373 Disability, Sport and Society
711 3rd Avenue
8th Floor
New York, NY 10017
212-216-7800
800-634-7064
FAX: 212-564-7854
www.routledge.com

Nigel Thomas, Co-Author
Andy Smith, Co-Author
Disability sport is a relatively recent phenomenon, yet it is also one that, particularly in the context of social inclusion, is attracting increasing political and academic interest. The purpose of this important new text - the first of its kind - is to introduce the reader to key concepts in disability and disability sport and to examine the complex relationships between modern sport, disability and other aspects of wider society.

2374 Disabled Rights: American Disability Policy and the Fight for Equality
3240 Prospect Street, NW
Suite 250
Washington, DC 20007
202-687-5889
FAX: 202-687-6340
gupress@georgetown.edu
press.georgetown.edu/

Jacqueline Vaughn Switzer, Author
Disabled Rights explains how people with disabilities have been treated from a social, legal, and political perspective in the United States.

2375 Divided Legacy: A History of the Schism in Medical Thought, The Bacteriological Era
North Atlantic Books
2526 Martin Luther King Jr. Way
Berkeley, CA 94704
510-549-4270
800-337-2665
FAX: 510-549-4276
orders@northatlanticbooks.com
www.northatlanticbooks.com

Alla Spector, Director of Finance & Office Operations
Doug Reil, Executive Director/Associate Publisher
Ed Angel, Director of Office Administration
Janet Levin, Senior Director of Sales & Distribution
Concluding volume of Coulter's history of medical philosophy, from ancient times to today. Covers the origins of bacteriology and immunology in world medicine; describes the clash between orthodox and alternative medicine.

2376 Dual Relationships in Counseling
5999 Stevenson Ave
Alexandria, VA 22304-3304 703-823-0252
800-347-6647
FAX: 800-473-2329
webmaster@counseling.org
www.counseling.org

Robert L. Smith, President
Thelma Duffey, President-Elect
Brian Canfield, Treasurer
Catherine Roland, Representative
Publishes archival material, also publishes articles that have broad interest for a readership composed mostly of counselors and other mental health professionals who work in private practice, schools, colleges, community agencies, hospitals, and government. An appropriate outlet for articles that: critically integrate published research; examine current professional and scientific issues; report research, new techniques, innovative programs and practices; and examine ACA as an organization.

2377 Early Communication Skills for Children with Down Syndrome
Woodbine House
6510 Bells Mill Rd
Bethesda, MD 20817-1636 301-897-3570
800-843-7323
FAX: 301-897-5838
info@woodbinehouse.com
www.woodbinehouse.com

Nancy Gray Paul, Acquisitions Editor
Libby Kumin, Author
An expert shares her knowledge of speech and language development in young children with Down syndrome. Intelligibility, hearing loss, apraxia and other factors that affect communications are discussed. It also covers speech-language assessments and alternative communication options and literacy. *$19.95*
368 pages
ISBN 1-890627-27-5

2378 Early Intervention: Implementing Child & Family Services for At-Risk Infants and Toddlers
PRO-ED Inc.
8700 Shoal Creek Blvd
Austin, TX 78757-6897 512-451-3246
800-897-3202
FAX: 800-397-7633
general@proedinc.com
www.proedinc.com

Marci J. Hanson, Author
Eleanor W. Lynch, Author
New directions and recent legislation have produced a need for this guide which is designed for professionals facing the challenge of program development for disabled and at-risk infants, toddlers and their families. *$68.20*
394 pages Paperback 1995
ISBN 0-890796-21-1

2379 Ecology of Troubled Children
Brookline Books Publications
8 Trumbull Rd
Suite B-001
Northampton, MA 01060 413-584-0184
800-666-2665
FAX: 413-584-6184
brbooks@yahoo.com
www.brooklinebooks.com

Esther Isabe Wilder, Author
Designed for frontline mental health clinicians working with children with serious emotional disturbances; shows how to make children's' worlds more supportive by changing the places, activities and people in their lives. *$15.95*
256 pages
ISBN 1-571290-57-5

2380 Educating Children with Disabilities: A Transdisciplinary Approach
Brookes Publishing
PO Box 10624
Baltimore, MD 21285-0624 410-337-9580
800-638-3775
FAX: 410-337-8539
custserv@brookespublishing.com
www.brookespublishing.com

Paul H. Brookes, Chairman
Jeffrey D. Brookes, President
Melissa A. Behm, ExecutiveVice President
George S. Stamathis, Vice President & Publisher
Widely respected textbook presents you with the strategies you need for developing an inclusive curriculum, integrating health care and educational programs and addressing needs and concerns. *$38.00*
512 pages
ISBN 1-557662-46-0

2381 Educating Children with Multiple Disabilities: A Transdisciplinary Approach
Brookes Publishing
PO Box 10624
Baltimore, MD 21285-0624 410-337-9580
800-638-3775
FAX: 410-337-8539
custserv@brookespublishing.com
www.brookespublishing.com

Paul H. Brookes, Chairman
Jeffrey D. Brookes, President
Melissa A. Behm, ExecutiveVice President
George S. Stamathis, Vice President & Publisher
Emphasizing transdisciplinary cooperation between teachers, therapists, nurses and parents, this book describes a general model and specific techniques for effectively educating children with multiple disabilities. *$29.00*
496 pages Paperback
ISBN 1-557662-46-0

2382 Educating Individuals with Disabilities:IDEIA 2004 and Beyond (1st Edition)
Springer Publishing Company
11 W 42nd St
15th Fl
New York, NY 10036-8002 212-431-4370
877-687-7476
FAX: 212-941-7842
cs@springerpub.com
www.springerpub.com

Ted Nardin, Chief Executive Officer
Jason Roth, Vice President, Marketing & Sales
Kathy Weiss, Director, Sales
Elena L. Grigorenko, Editor
Discusses how learning-disabled students are identified and assessed today, in light of the 2004 Individuals with Disabilities Education Improvement Act. Grigorenko's interdisciplinary collection is the first to comprehensively review the IDEIA 2004 Act and distill the changes professionals working with learning-disabled students face. The text takes an overarching perspective, first discussing the IDEIA in its historical, political, and legal context. *$100.00*
512 pages Hardcover 1908
ISBN 0-826103-56-1

2383 Educating Students Who Have Visual Impairments with Other Disabilities
Brookes Publishing
PO Box 10624
Baltimore, MD 21285-0624 410-337-9580
800-638-3775
FAX: 410-337-8539
custserv@brookespublishing.com
www.brookespublishing.com

Paul H. Brookes, Chairman
Jeffrey D. Brookes, President
Melissa A. Behm, ExecutiveVice President
George S. Stamathis, Vice President & Publisher

This introductory text provides techniques for facilitating functional learning in students with a wide range of visual impairments and multiple disabilities. With a concentration on educational needs and learning styles, the authors of this multidisciplinary volume demonstrate functional assessment and teaching adaptations that will improve students' inclusive learning experiences. *$49.95*

552 pages Paperback
ISBN 1-557662-80-0

2384 Educating all Students in the Mainstream
Brookes Publishing Company
PO Box 10624
Baltimore, MD 21285-0624
410-337-9580
800-638-3775
FAX: 410-337-8539
custserv@brookespublishing.com
www.brookespublishng.com

Paul H. Brookes, Chairman
Jeff Brookes, President
Melissa A. Behm, ExecutiveVice President
Cary Gold, Educational Sales Representative
Incorporating the research and viewpoints of both regular and special educators, this textbook provides an effective approach for modifying, expanding, and adjusting regular education to meet the needs of all students. *$34.00*

304 pages
ISBN 1-557660-22-0

2385 Educational Audiology for the Limited Hearing Infant and Preschooler
Charles C. Thomas
2600 S First St
Springfield, IL 62704-4730
217-789-8980
800-258-8980
FAX: 217-789-9130
books@ccthomas.com
www.ccthomas.com

Donald Goldberg, Author
Nancy Coleffe-Schenck, Author
Doreen Pollack, Author
Offers information on current concepts and practices in audio-logic screening and evaluation, development of the listening function, development of speech, development of language, the role of parents, parent education, mainstreaming of the limited-hearing child, and program modifications for the severely learning disabled child. Also includes information on auditory assessment, sensory aides, cochlear implants, acoupedics and auditory verbal programs. *$79.95*

430 pages Paperback
ISBN 0-398067-51-1

2386 Educational Care
Educators Publishing Service
625 Mount Auburn St
3rd Floor
Cambridge, MA 02138-3039
617-547-6706
800-225-5750
Feedback.EPS@schoolspecialty.com
www.eps.schoolspecialty.com

Paula Fabbro, Sales Consultant
Leo Micale, Sales Consultant
Kristen Colson, Sales Consultant
Flora Francis, Sales Consultant
This book, written for both parents and teachers, is based on the view that education should be a system of care that is able to look after the specific needs of individual students. Using case studies, it analyzes various types of learning disorders and then suggests ways to help students with these problems. *$31.50*

325 pages
ISBN 0-838819-87-7

2387 Educational Intervention for the Student
Charles C. Thomas
2600 S First St
Springfield, IL 62704-4730
217-789-8980
800-258-8980
FAX: 217-789-9130
books@ccthomas.com
www.ccthomas.com

2388 Educational Prescriptions
Educators Publishing Service
625 Mount Auburn St
3RD Floor
Cambridge, MA 02138-3039
617-547-6706
800-225-5750
Feedback.EPS@schoolspecialty.com
www.eps.schoolspecialty.com

Paula Fabbro, Sales Consultant
Leo Micale, Sales Consultant
Kristen Colson, Sales Consultant
Flora Francis, Sales Consultant
This book provides specific recommendations for the classroom management of students who are experiencing subtle developmental and/or learning difficulties. Intended for regular classroom teachers, specific examples of accommodations teachers can make are provided for grades 1-3 and 4-6. *$13.50*

64 pages
ISBN 0-838819-90-7

2389 Effective Instruction for Special Education
Sage Publications
2455 Teller Road
Thousand Oaks, CA 91320-2218
805-499-0721
800-818-7243
FAX: 805-583-2665
info@sagepub.com
www.sagepub.com

Sara Miller McCune, Founder, Publisher, Chairperson
Blaise R. Simqu, President/CEO
Chris Hickok, Senior Vice President/CFO
Stephen Barr, Managing Director/SAGE London, P
This exciting and wide-ranging book provides special educators with effective methods for teaching students with mild and moderate learning and behavioral problems, as well as for teaching remedial students in general. *$37.00*

419 pages Paperback

2390 Effectively Educating Handicapped Students
Longman Publishing Group
9th Fl
Upper Saddle River, NJ 07458-1813
201-236-3281
800-922-0579
FAX: 201-236-3290
www.pearsoned.com

468 pages Paperback
ISBN 0-801303-17-6

2391 Emotional Problems of Childhood and Adolescence
McGraw-Hill School Publishing
PO Box 182604
Columbus, OH 43218
877-833-5524
800-338-3987
FAX: 609-308-4480
customer.service@mheducation.com
www.mcgraw-hill.com

David Levin, President/Chief Ex
David Stafford, Senior Vice President/General Counsel
Maryellen Valaitis, Senior Vice President Human Resources
Patrick Milano, Chief Financial Officer Chief Administrative Officer
For future special educators, psychologists and others who work with emotionally disturbed children and adolescents.

2392 Enabling & Empowering Families: Principles & Guidelines for Practice
Brookline Books
8 Trumbull Rd
Suite B-001
Northampton, MA 01060   413-584-0184
                          800-666-2665
                          FAX: 413-584-6184
                          brbooks@yahoo.com
                          www.brooklinebooks.com

Esther Wilder, Co-Author
This book was written for practitioners who must work with families but who have insufficient training in family systems assessment and intervention. The authors' system enables professionals to help the family identify its needs, locate the formal and informal resources to meet these needs and develop the abilities to effectively access these resources. *$24.95*
220 pages
ISBN 0-914797-59-X

2393 Evaluation and Educational Programming of Students with Deafblindness & Severe Disabilities
Charles C. Thomas
2600 S First St
Springfield, IL 62704-4730   217-789-8980
                               800-258-8980
                               FAX: 217-789-9130
                               books@ccthomas.com
                               www.ccthomas.com

Carroll J. Jones, Author
Subtitle: Sensorimotor Stage. This second edition offers a very complete package of information on the special education of deaf-blind students; including detailed diagnostic information to assist the instructor in evaluating the physical, social, mental status of the student, as well as the educational progress. *$50.95*
265 pages Spiral-Paper 2001
ISBN 0-398072-16-2

2394 Evaluation and Treatment of the Psychogeriatric Patient
Haworth Press
711 Third Avenue
New York, NY 10017   212-216-7800
                       800-354-1420
                       FAX: 212-244-1563
                       subscriptions@tandf.co.uk.
                       www.haworthpress.com

111 pages Hardcover
ISBN 1-560240-52-0

2395 Exceptional Children in Focus
McGraw-Hill School Publishing
PO Box 182604
Columbus, OH 43218   877-833-5524
                       800-338-3987
                       FAX: 609-308-4480
                       customer.service@mheducation.com
                       www.mcgraw-hill.com

David Levin, President/Chief Ex
David Stafford, Senior Vice President/General Counsel
Maryellen Valaitis, Senior Vice President Human Resources
Patrick Milano, Chief Financial Officer Chief Administrative Officer
Combines a light, personal look at the problems of special educators experiences with the basic facts of exceptionality.
288 pages

2396 Exceptional Lives: Special Education in Today's Schools, 4th Edition
Pearson Education
1 Lake St
Upper Saddle River, NJ 07458-1813   201-236-3281
                                      800-922-0579
                                      FAX: 201-236-3290
                                      www.pearsoned.com

592 pages
ISBN 0-131126-00-8

2397 Facilitating Self-Care Practices in the Elderly
Haworth Press
711 Third Avenue
New York, NY 10017   212-216-7800
                       800-354-1420
                       FAX: 212-244-1563
                       subscriptions@tandf.co.uk.
                       www.haworthpress.com

185 pages Hardcover
ISBN 1-560240-13-X

2398 Family-Centered Early Intervention with Infants and Toddlers
Brookes Publishing
PO Box 10624
Baltimore, MD 21285-0624   410-337-9580
                             800-638-3775
                             FAX: 410-337-8539
                             custserv@brookespublishing.com
                             www.brookespublishing.com

Paul H. Brookes, Chairman
Jeffrey D. Brookes, President
Melissa A. Behm, ExecutiveVice President
George S. Stamathis, Vice President & Publisher
This informative text provides professionals with insight and practical guidelines to help fulfill the federal requirements for provision of early intervention services. *$37.00*
368 pages Hardcover
ISBN 1-557661-24-3

2399 Feeding Children with Special Needs
Arizona Department of Health Services
150 North 18th Avenue
Phoenix, AZ 85007-2607   602-542-1025
                           FAX: 602-542-0883
                           www.azdhs.gov

Will Humble, Director
Jeff Bloomberg, J.D., Manager
Robert Lane, Esq., Administrative Counsel
Lynn Golder, Esq., Administrative Counsel & HIPAA Privacy Officer
Guide designed to help develop a greater awareness of the special challenges involved in the nutrition and feeding concerns for children with special health care needs, and ways to approach the issues. *$5.00*

2400 Focal Group Psychotherapy
New Harbinger Publications
5674 Shattuck Ave
Oakland, CA 94609-1662   510-652-0215
                           800-748-6273
                           FAX: 800-652-1613
                           customerservice@newharbinger.com
                           www.newharbinger.com

Matthew McKay, Founder
Patrick Fanning, Co-Founder/Writer
Guide to leading brief, theme-based groups. This book offers an extensive week-by-week description of the basic concepts and interventions for 14 theme or focal groups for: codependency, rape victims, shyness, survivors of incest, agoraphobia, survivors of toxic parents, depression, child molesters, anger control, domestic violence offenders, assertiveness, alcohol and drug abuse, eating disorders, and parent training. *$59.95*
544 pages Cloth
ISBN 1-879237-18-0

2401 Free Hand: Enfranchising the Education of Deaf Children
TJ Publishers
                           www.amazon.com

Margaret Walworth, Author
Donald F. Moores, Author
Terrence J. O'Rourke, Author
A select group of nationally prominent educators, linguists and researchers met at Hofstra University to consider the most vital and controversial question in education of the deaf: what role

should ASL play in the classroom? Become part of that discussion with A Free Hand. *$16.95*
204 pages Softcover
ISBN 0-93266 -40-X

2402 Friendship 101
2900 Crystal Drive
Suite 1000
Arlington, VA 22202-3557

888-232-7733
alisonh@cec.sped.org
www.cec.sped.org

Juliet E. Hart Barnett, Co-Author/ Editor
Kelly J. Whalon, Co-Author/ Editor
An essential characteristic of autism spectrum disorder (ASD) is difficulty acquiring the social skills needed to develop social competence, including the ability to form and maintain friendships and relationships with others. This webinar, designed for general and special educators who work with children with ASD, presents evidence-based practices shown to enhance social competence in children and youth with ASD.

2403 Functional Assessment Inventory Manual
Stout Vocational Rehab Institute
655 15th St. NW
Suite 800
Washington, DC 20005

715-232-1411
800-538-3742
FAX: 715-232-2356
botterbuschd@uwstout.edu
www2.epa.gov

Gina McCarthy, Administrator
Gwen Keyes Fleming, Chief of Staff
Bob Perciasepe, Deputy Administrator
Craig E. Hooks, Office of Administration and Resource Management (OARM)
The Functional Assessment is a systematic enumeration of a client's vocationally relevant strengths and limitations. *$12.00*
96 pages Paperback
ISBN 0-916671-53-4

2404 Get Ready for Jetty!: My Journal About ADHD and Me
750 First Street, NE
Washington, DC 20002-4242

202-336-5500
800-374-2721
rllowman@gmail.com
www.apa.org

Jeanne Kraus, Author
Jetty writes about these things as well as her recent ADHD diagnosis in her journal.

2405 Getting Around Town
2900 Crystal Drive
Suite 1000
Arlington, VA 22202-3557

888-232-7733
alisonh@cec.sped.org
www.cec.sped.org

M. Sherril Moon, Co-Author
Emily M. Luedtke, Co-Author
Elizabeth Halloran-Tornquist, Co-Author
Getting Around Town: Teaching Community Mobility Skills to Students with Disabilitiesprovides examples of possible IEP goals and field-tested lesson plans for individual students or entire classes across all age and grade levels.

2406 Global Perspectives on Disability: A Curriculum
Mobility International U SA
132 E Broadway
Suite 343
Eugene, OR 97401-3155

541-343-1284
FAX: 541-343-6812
TTY:541-343-1284
info@miusa.org
www.miusa.org

Susan Sygall, CEO/Founder
Cerise Roth-Vinson, Chief Operating Officer
Cindy Lewis, Director of Programs
Stephanie Gray, Program Managers
Designed for secondary and higher education instructors. Includes five lesson plans covering disability awareness, disability rights and international perspectives on disability. Available in alternative formats. *$40.00*

2407 Glossary of Terminology for Vocational Assessment/Evaluation/Work
Rehabilitation Resource University
University of Wisconsin-Stou
Menomonie, WI 54751

715-232-2236
FAX: 715-232-2356
gundlachj@uwstout.edu

Ronald Fry, Manager
Jennifer Gundlach Klatt, Program Assistant
This glossary contains 254 terms and their definitions. Primary focus is on the terminology related to the practice and professionals of vocational assessment, vocational evaluation and work adjustment. *$9.50*
40 pages Softcover

2408 Graduate Technological Education and the Human Experience of Disability
Haworth Press
711 Third Avenue
New York, NY 10017

212-216-7800
800-354-1420
FAX: 212-244-1563
subscriptions@tandf.co.uk.
www.haworthpress.com

115 pages Hardcover
ISBN 0-789060-08-6

2409 HIV Infection and Developmental Disabilities
Brookes Publishing
PO Box 10624
Baltimore, MD 21285-0624

410-337-9580
800-638-3775
FAX: 410-337-8539
custserv@brookespublishing.com
www.brookespublishing.com

Paul H. Brookes, Chairman
Jeffrey D. Brookes, President
Melissa A. Behm, ExecutiveVice President
George S. Stamathis, Vice President & Publisher
A resource for service providers pinpointing the most crucial medical, legal and educational issues to control HIV infection. *$47.00*
320 pages
ISBN 1-557660-83-2

2410 Handbook for Implementing Workshops for Siblings of Special Children
Special Needs Project
324 State St
Suite H
Santa Barbara, CA 93101-2364

805-962-8087
800-333-6867
FAX: 805-962-5087
editor@specialneeds.com
www.specialneeds.com

Mark Darrow, Founder,The Prolotherapy Institu
Based on three years of professional experience, this handbook provides guidelines and techniques for those who wish to start and conduct workshops for siblings. *$40.00*

2411 Handbook for Speech Therapy
Psychological & Educational Publications
PO Box 520
Hydesville, CA 95547

800-523-5775
FAX: 800-447-0907
psych-edpublications@suddenlink.net
www.psych-edpublications.com

143 pages paperback

2412 Handbook for the Special Education Administrator
Edwin Mellen Press
PO Box 450
Lewiston, NY 14092-1205

716-754-2266
FAX: 716-754-4056
jrupnow@mellenpress.com
www.mellenpress.com

Arthur R. Crowell, Author
Bonnie Crogan, Marketing
Irene Miller, Accounting
Patricia Schultz, Production
Organization and procedures for special education. *$ 49.95*
96 pages Hardcover
ISBN 0-88946 -22-9

2413 Handbook of Acoustic Accessibility
15619 Premiere Drive
Suite 101
Tampa, FL 33624

850-363-9909
FAX: 480-393-4331
accounting@successforkidswithhearingloss.com
successforkidswithhearinglo ss.com

Joseph J. Smaldino, Co-Author
Carol Flexer, Co-Author
Most students with hearing loss are educated in mainstream education classrooms the majority of each school day.Communication - between peers and with teachers - is the coin of education and upon which a wealth of knowledge is built.Unfortunately for students with hearing loss, the typical classroom environment is hazardous for listening and interferes with access to all classroom communication.

2414 Handbook of Developmental Education
Greenwood Publishing Group
130 Cremona Drive
Santa Barbara, CA 93117

805-968-1911
800-368-6868
FAX: 866-270-3856
CustomerService@abc-clio.com
www.abc-clio.com

This comprehensive handbook has brought together the leading practitioners and researchers in the field of developmental education to focus on the developmental learning agenda. Hardcover.
400 pages $65 - $75
ISBN 0-275932-97-4

2415 Handbook on Supported Education for Peoplewith Mental Illness
Brookes Publishing
PO Box 10624
Baltimore, MD 21285-0624

410-337-9580
800-638-3775
FAX: 410-337-8539
custserv@brookespublishing.com
www.brookespublishing.com

Paul H. Brookes, Chairman
Jeffrey D. Brookes, President
Melissa A. Behm, ExecutiveVice President
George S. Stamathis, Vice President & Publisher
Here you will find all necessary information that mental health professionals need in order to provide supported education services. There are specific suggestions on how to help people with mental illness return to or remain in college, trade school, or GED

programs. Also addressed are funding and legal issues, accommodations, and specific interventions.
208 pages Paperback
ISBN 1-55766 -52-1

2416 Head Injury Rehabilitation: Children
Taylor & Francis
47 Runway Dr
Ste G
Levittown, PA 19057-4738

267-580-2622
FAX: 215-785-5515

460 pages Cloth
ISBN 0-85066 -67-1

2417 Health Care Management in Physical Therapy
Charles C. Thomas
2600 S First St
Springfield, IL 62704-4730

217-789-8980
800-258-8980
FAX: 217-789-9130
books@ccthomas.com
www.ccthomas.com

2418 Health Care for Students with Disabilities
Brookes Publishing Company
PO Box 10624
Baltimore, MD 21285-0624

410-337-9580
800-638-3775
FAX: 410-337-8539
custserv@brookespublishing.com
www.brookespublishing.com

Paul H. Brookes, Chairman
Jeffrey D. Brookes, President
Melissa A. Behm, ExecutiveVice President
George S. Stamathis, Vice President & Publisher
This practical guidebook provides detailed descriptions of the 16 health-related procedures most likely to be needed in the classroom by students with disabilities. *$25.00*
304 pages Paperback
ISBN 1-557660-37-9

2419 Helping Learning- Disabled Gifted ChildrenLearn Through Compensatory Active Play
Charles C. Thomas
2600 S First St
Springfield, IL 62704-4730

217-789-8980
800-258-8980
FAX: 217-789-9130
books@ccthomas.com
www.ccthomas.com

James Harry Humphrey, Author
$36.95
156 pages Hardcover 1990
ISBN 0-398056-95-1

2420 Helping Students Grow
American College Testing Program
500 ACT Drive
PO Box 168
Iowa City, IA 52243-0168

319-337-1000
info@keytrain.com
www.act.org

Jon Whitmore, Chief Executive Officer
Tom J. Goedken, Chief Financial Officer/Senior Vice President
Patricia C. Steinbrech, Chief Information Officer
Janet E. Godwin, Chief of Staff/Accountability Officer
Designed to assist counselors in using the wealth of information generated by the ACT Assessment.

2421 Home Health Care Provider: A Guide to Essential Skills
Springer Publishing
11 W 42nd St
15th Floor
New York, NY 10036-8002
212-431-4370
877-687-7476
FAX: 212-941-7842
cs@springerpub.com
www.springerpub.com

Theodore C. Nardin, CEO/Publisher
Jason Roth, VP/Marketing Director
Annette Imperati, Marketing/Sales Director
James C. Costello, Vice President, Journal Publishing

This book is designed to foster quality care to home care recipients. Prieto provides information, tips, and techniques on personal care routines as well as additional responsibilities, including home safety and maintenance, meal planning, errand running, caring for couples, and making use of recreational time. The book focuses on the psycho-social needs of home care recipients, stressing the need to maintain the house as a home, and sustaining the recipient's way of life throughout caregiving.

2422 How to Teach Spelling/How to Spell
Educators Publishing Service
625 Mount Auburn St
3rd Floor
Cambridge, MA 02138-3039
617-547-6706
800-225-5750
Feedback.EPS@schoolspecialty.com
www.eps.schoolspecialty.com

Paula Fabbro, Sales Consultant
Leo Micale, Sales Consultant
Kristen Colson, Sales Consultant
Flora Francis, Sales Consultant

This is a comprehensive resource manual based on the Orton-Gillingham approach to reading and spelling. It recommends what and how much to teach at each grade level at the beginning of each lesson or section. There are four student manuals that accompany this. *$22.50*
Teachers Manual
ISBN 0-838818-47-1

2423 Human Exceptionality: School, Community, and Family (12th Edition)
Cengage Learning
20 Channel Center St
Boston, MA 02210
617-289-7700
617-289-7844
www.cengage.com/us

Michael L. Hardman, Author
M. Winston Egan, Author
Clifford J. Drew, Author

An evidence-based testament to the critical role of cross-professional collaboration in enhancing the lives of exceptional individuals and their families. This text's unique lifespan approach combines powerful research, evidence-based practices, and inspiring stories, engendering passion and empathy and enhancing the lives of individuals with exceptionalities.
544 pages Hardcover

2424 I Can't Hear You in the Dark: How to Lean and Teach Lipreading
Charles C. Thomas
2600 S First St
Springfield, IL 62704-4730
217-789-8980
800-258-8980
FAX: 217-789-9130
books@ccthomas.com
www.ccthomas.com

Betty Woerner Carter, Author

The goal of this text is to improve communication and strengthen relationships with others. *$40.95*
226 pages Spiral-Paper 1997
ISBN 0-398067-89-2

2425 I Heard That!
3417 Volta Pl NW
Washington, DC 20007-2737
202-337-5220
FAX: 202-337-8314
TTY:202-337-5221
info@agbell.org
www.listeningandspokenlanguage.org

Meredith K. Sugar, Esq. (OH), President
Ted A. Meyer, M.D., Ph.D, President-Elect/Secretary-Treasurer
Emilio Alonso-Mendoza, Chief Executive Officer
Susan Boswell, Director of Communications and Marketing

Provides a framework for teachers, clinicians and parents when writing objectives and designing activities to develop listening skills in children with hearing loss from newborn to 3 years. *$7.95*
36 pages

2426 I Heard That!2
Alexander Graham Bell Association
3417 Volta Pl NW
Washington, DC 20007-2737
202-337-5220
FAX: 202-337-8314
TTY:202-337-5221
info@agbell.org
www.listeningandspokenlanguage.org

Meredith K. Sugar, Esq. (OH), President
Ted A. Meyer, M.D., Ph.D, President-Elect/Secretary-Treasurer
Emilio Alonso-Mendoza, Chief Executive Officer
Susan Boswell, Director of Communications and Marketing

Provides a framework for teachers, clinicians and parents when writing objectives and designing activities to develop listening skills in children who are deaf or hard of hearing. *$7.95*
36 pages

2427 If It Is To Be, It Is Up To Us To Help!
AVKO Educational Research Foundation
3084 Willard Rd
Ste W
Birch Run, MI 48415-9404
810-686-9283
866-285-6612
FAX: 810-686-1101
webmaster@avko.org
www.avko.org

Don Mc Cabe, President
Ted A. Meyer, M.D., Ph.D, Vice-President
Michael Lane, Treasurer
Birch Run, Research Director Emeritus

A book of lesson plans for an Adult Community Education Course for Volunteer Tutors. Contains information on how to go about establishing such a course and how to secure cooperation from local and national organizations. Free as an e-book for Foundation members. *$ 14.95*

ISBN 1-56400 -42-1

2428 Images of the Disabled, Disabling Images
ABC-CLIO
130 Cremona Dr
Santa Barbara, CA 93117
805-968-1911
800-368-6868
FAX: 866-270-3856
customerservice@abc-clio.com
www.abc-clio.com

Alan Gartner, Author

Combines an examination of the presentation of persons with disabilities in literature, film and the media with an analysis of the ways in which these images are expressed in public policy concerning the disabled. *$84.00*
227 pages Hardcover 1986
ISBN 0-275921-78-6

2429 **Implementing Family-Centered Services in Early Intervention**
Brookline Books
8 Trumbull Rd
Suite B-001
Northampton, MA 01060

413-584-0184
800-666-2665
FAX: 413-584-6184
brbooks@yahoo.com
www.brooklinebooks.com

180 pages Paperback
ISBN 0-91479 -62-

2430 **Including All of Us: An Early Childhood Curriculum About Disability**
Educational Equity Concepts
71 Fifth Avenue
6th Floor
New York, NY 10003

212-243-1110
FAX: 212-627-0407
lcolon@fhi360.org
www.edequity.org

Frank Schneiger, President
Antonia Cottrell Martin, Founder and President
Merle Froschl, Co-director
Barbara Sprung, Co-director
The first nonsexist, multicultural, mainstreamed curriculum. Step-by-step activities incorporate disability into three curriculum areas: Same/Different (hearing impairment), Body Parts (visual impairment), and Transportation (mobility impairment). *$14.95*
144 pages
ISBN 0-93162 -00-4

2431 **Including Students with Severe and Multiple Disabilites in Typical Classrooms**
Brookes Publishing
PO Box 10624
Baltimore, MD 21285-0624

410-337-9580
800-638-3775
FAX: 410-337-8539
custserv@brookespublishing.com
www.brookespublishing.com

Paul H. Brookes, Chairman
Jeffrey D. Brookes, President
Melissa A. Behm, ExecutiveVice President
George S. Stamathis, Vice President & Publisher
This straightforward and jargon free resource gives instructors the guidance needed to educate learners who have one or more sensory impairments in addition to cognitive and physical disabilities. *$32.95*
224 pages Paperback
ISBN 1-55766 -39-8

2432 **Including Students with Special Needs: A Practical Guide for Classroom Teachers**
Allyn & Bacon
75 Arlington St
Suite 300
Boston, MA 02116-3988

ab_webmaster@abacon.com
www.home.pearsonhighered.com

544 pages
ISBN 0-20528 -85-4

2433 **Inclusive & Heterogeneous Schooling: Assessment, Curriculum, and Instruction**
Brookes Publishing
PO Box 10624
Baltimore, MD 21285-0624

410-337-9580
800-638-3775
FAX: 410-337-8539
custserv@brookespublishing.com
www.brookespublishing.com

Paul H. Brookes, Chairman
Jeff Brookes, President
Melissa A. Behm, ExecutiveVice President
Cary Gold, Educational Sales Representative
Presents methods for successfully restructuring classrooms to enable all students, particularly those with disabilities, to flourish. Provides specific strategies for assessment, collaboration, classroom management, and age-specific instruction. *$34.95*
448 pages Paperback
ISBN 1-55766 -02-9

2434 **Independent Living Approach to Disability Policy Studies**
World Institute on Disability
3075 Adeline Street
Suite 155
Berkeley, CA 94703

510-225-6400
FAX: 510-225-0477
TTY:510-225-0478
wid@wid.org
www.wid.org

Paul W. Schroeder, Chairman
Linda M. Dardarian, Vice Chairman
Mary Brooner, Treasurer
Cassandra Malry, Secretary
This collection of essays and bibliographies attempts to build a framework for understanding how the relationship between public policy, disability studies and disability policy studies will impact us in the future. *$17.50*
240 pages Paperback

2435 **Information & Referral Center**
Mississippi State University
108 Herbert - South
Room 150/PO Drawer 6189
Mississippi State Univers, MS 39762-6189

662-325-2001
800-675-7782
FAX: 662-325-8989
TTY: 662-325-2694
nrtc@colled.msstate.edu
www.blind.msstate.edu

Jacqui Bybee, Research and Training Coordinato
Michele Capella McDonnall, Ph.D., Research Professor/Interim Director
Jessica Thornton, Business Manager
Marty Giesen, Ph.D., Senior Research Scientist
A comprehensive website that includes information about client assistance programs, vocational rehabilitation agencies, low vision clinics and information about blindness and low vision. *$25.00*
150 pages

2436 **Instructional Methods for Students**
Allyn & Bacon
75 Arlington St
Suite 300
Boston, MA 02116-3988

ab_webmaster@abacon.com
www.home.pearsonhighered.com

450 pages
ISBN 0-205087-35-3

2437 **Interactions: Collaboration Skills for School Professionals**
Longman Education/Addison Wesley
75 Arlington St
Suite 300
Boston, MA 02116-3988
ab_webmaster@abacon.com
www.longman.awl.com

270 pages Paperback
ISBN 0-80131-21-2

2438 **International Journal of Arts Medicine**
MMB Music
9051 Watson Road
Suite 161
Saint Louis, MO 63126
314-531-9635
800-543-3771
FAX: 314-531-8384
info@mmbmusic.com
www.mmbmusic.com

Norm Goldberg, Founder/chairman
Exploration of the creative arts and healing. Presents peer-reviewed articles clearly written by educators in the creative arts, as well as internationally prominent physicians, therapists and health care professionals.

2439 **Interpreting Disability: A Qualitative Reader**
Teachers College Press
1234 Amsterdam Avenue
New York, NY 10027
212-678-3929
800-575-6566
FAX: 212-678-4149
tcpress@tc.columbia.edu
www.tcpress.com

Brian Ellerbeck, Executive Acquisitions Editor
Marie Ellen Larcada, Senior Acquisitions Editor
Emily Spangler, Acquisitions Editor
Meg Hartmann, Acquisitions Assistant
This book offers a collection of exemplary qualitative research affecting people with disabilities and their families. Instead of focusing upon methodological details, the chapters illustrate the variety of styles and formats that interpretive research can adopt in reporting its results. $24.95
328 pages Paperback
ISBN 0-807731-21-8

2440 **Intervention Research in Learning Disabilities**
Gallery Bookshop
319 Kasten Street
PO Box 270
Mendocino, CA 95460-270
707-937-2215
FAX: 707-937-3737
info@gallerybookshop.com
www.gallerybooks.com

Tony Miksak, Owner
Based on the Symposium on Intervention Research, this volume presents 12 papers addressing issues in intervention research, academic interventions, social and behavioral interventions, and postsecondary interventions. $30.00
347 pages

2441 **Introduction to Learning Disabilities**
Allyn & Bacon
75 Arlington St
Suite 300
Boston, MA 02116-3988
ab_webmaster@abacon.com
www.pearsonhighered.com

608 pages
ISBN 0-20529-43-4

2442 **Introduction to Mental Retardation**
Allyn & Bacon
75 Arlington St
Suite 300
Boston, MA 02116-3988
ab_webmaster@abacon.com
www.pearsonhighered.com

350 pages Casebound
ISBN 0-134879-27-9

2443 **Introduction to Special Education: Teaching in an Age of Challenge, 4th Edition**
Allyn & Bacon
75 Arlington St
Suite 300
Boston, MA 02116-3988
ab_webmaster@abacon.com
www.pearsonhighered.com

640 pages cloth
ISBN 0-20526-94-4

2444 **Introduction to the Profession of Counseling**
McGraw-Hill School Publishing
PO Box 182604
Columbus, OH 43218
877-833-5524
800-338-3987
FAX: 609-308-4480
customer.service@mheducation.com
www.mcgraw-hill.com

David Levin, President/Chief Executive Officer
David Stafford, Senior Vice President/General Counsel
Maryellen Valaitis, Senior Vice President Human Resources
Patrick Milano, Chief Financial Officer/Chief Administrative Officer
Offers information, theories and techniques for counseling numerous cases from drug addiction to special populations.
464 pages

2445 **Issues and Research in Special Education**
Teachers College Press
PO Box 20
Williston, VT 05495-0020
800-575-6566
FAX: 802-664-7626
tcp.orders@aidcvt.com
www.teacherscollegepress.com

264 pages Hardcover
ISBN 0-807731-95-1

2446 **Kendall Demonstration Elementary School Curriculum Guides**
Gallaudet University Bookstore
800 Florida Ave NE
Washington, DC 20002-3695
202-651-5488
800-621-2736
FAX: 202-651-5489
TTY: 888-630-9347
gupress@gallaudet.edu
www.gupress.gallaudet.edu

Dr. T Alan Hurwitz, President
Edward Bosso, Vice President for Administration
Dr. Lynne Murray, Vice President for Development
Donald Beil, Chief of Staff
KDES is a day school serving students from birth through age 15, beginning with the Parent-Infant Program and ending in grade 8. Students come from the Washington, D.C., metropolitan area.

2447 **Language Arts: Detecting Special Needs**
Allyn & Bacon
75 Arlington St
Suite 300
Boston, MA 02116-3988
617-848-7500
800-852-8024
FAX: 617-944-7273
www.home.pearsonhighered.com
Bill Barke, Chairman/CEO
Nancy Forfyth, President
Kevin Stone, Vice President, National Sales M
Thomas A. Rakes, Author
Describes special language arts needs of special learners.
180 pages paperback
ISBN 0-205116-36-1

2448 **Language Learning Practices with Deaf Children**
Sage Publications
2455 Teller Road
Thousand Oaks, CA 91320
805-499-9774
800-818-7243
FAX: 800-583-2665
books.claim@sagepub.com
www.sagepub.com
Sara Miller McCune, Founder, Publisher, Chairperson
Stephen P. Quigley, Co-Author
Susan Rose, Co-Author
Patricia L. McAnally, Co-Author
This new edition describes the variety of language-development theories and practices used with deaf children without advocating anyone. *$38.00*
321 pages Hardcover

2449 **Language and Communication Disorders in Children**
McGraw-Hill School Publishn
PO Box 182604
Columbus, OH 43218
877-833-5524
800-338-3987
FAX: 609-308-4480
customer.service@mheducation.com
www.mcgraw-hill.com
David Levin, President/Chief Executive Officer
David Stafford, Senior Vice President/General Counsel
Maryellen Valaitis, Senior Vice President Human Resources
Patrick Milano, Chief Financial Officer/Chief Administrative Officer
Comprehensive coverage encompassing all aspects of children's language disorders.
512 pages

2450 **Learning Disabilities, Literacy, and Adult Education**
Brookes Publishing
PO Box 10624
Baltimore, MD 21285-0624
410-337-9580
800-638-3775
FAX: 410-337-8539
custserv@brookespublishing.com
www.brookespublishing.com
Paul H. Brookes, Chairman
Jeffrey D. Brookes, President
Melissa A. Behm, ExecutiveVice President
George S. Stamathis, Vice President & Publisher
This book focuses on adults with severe learning disabilities and the educators who work with them. Described are the characteristics, demographics, and educational and employment status of adults with LD and the laws that protect them in the workplace and in educational settings.
450 pages Paperback
ISBN 1-55766 -47-5

2451 **Learning Disabilities: Concepts and Characteristics**
McGraw-Hill School Publishing
220 E Danieldale Rd
Desoto, TX 75115-2490
972-224-4772
800-442-9685
FAX: 972-228-1982
www.mhschool.com
Harold McGraw III, Chairman/ President/ Chief Ex
Jack F. Callahan, Executive Vice President, Chief
James A. McLoughlin, Co-Author
Gerald Wallace, Co-Author
Covers the conceptual basis of learning disabilities, identification, etiology and diagnosis.
448 pages

2452 **Learning Disability: Social Class and the Cons of Inequality In American Education**
Greenwood Publishing Group
130 Cremona Drive
Santa Barbara, CA 93117
805-968-1911
800-368-6868
FAX: 866-270-3856
CustomerService@abc-clio.com
www.abc-clio.com
James Carrier, Author
Presents a detailed historical description of the social and educational assumptions integral to the idea of learning disability.
167 pages $43.95 - $47.95
ISBN 0-313253-96-X

2453 **Learning and Individual Differences**
National Association of School Psychologists
8455 Colesville Rd
Suite 1000
Silver Spring, MD 20910- 3392
301-589-3300
FAX: 301-589-5175
info@musictherapy.org
www.musictherapy.org
Andrea Farbman, EdD, Executive Director
Judy Simpson, MT-BC, Director of Government Relations
Jane Creagan, MME, MT-BC, Director of Professional Program
E.L. Grigorenko, Editor
A multidisciplinary journal in education.

2454 **Learning to Feel Good and Stay Cool: Emotional Regulation Tools for Kids With AD/HD**
750 First Street, NE
Washington, DC 20002-4242
202-336-5500
800-374-2721
rllowman@gmail.com
www.apa.org
Judith M. Glasser, PhD, Co-Author
Kathleen G. Nadeau, PhD, Co-Author
Packed with practical advice and fun activities, this book will show you how to Understand your emotions, Practice healthy habits to stay in your Feel Good Zone, Feel better when you get upset, Know the warning signs that you are heading into your Upset Zone, Problem-solve so upsets come less often

2455 **Learning to See: American Sign Language asa Second Language**
Gallaudet University Press
800 Florida Ave NE
Washington, DC 20002-3695
202-651-5206
800-621-2736
FAX: 800-621-8476
TTY: 888-630-9347
clerc.center@gallaudet.edu.
www.gupress.gallaudet.edu
Dr. T Alan Hurwitz, President
Edward Bosso, Vice President for Administration
Phyliss Wilcox, Co-Author
Sherman Wilcox, Co-Author
This important book has been updated to help teachers teach American Sign Language as a second language, including infor-

mation on Deaf culture, the history and structure of ASL, teaching methods and issues facing educators. *$19.95*
160 pages Softcover

2456 Let's Write Right: Teacher's Edition
AVKO Educational Research Foundation
3084 Willard Rd
Ste W
Birch Run, MI 48415-9404   810-686-9283
866-285-6612
FAX: 810-686-1101
webmaster@avko.org
www.avko.org

Barry Chute, President
Julie Guyette, Vice President
Don Mc Cabe, Research Director
Clifford Schroeder, Treasurer
A manuscript and cursive writing program designed not only to teach handwriting but help with reading and spelling patterns as well. Teaches students to learn to read cursive as manuscript is being taught and ease the transition to cursive by using a D'Nealian-like script. Exercises involve phoically consistent patterns to help reinforce fluency with spelling and handwriting. *$39.95*
164 pages

2457 Library Manager's Guide to Hiring and Serving Disabled Persons
McFarland & Company
960 NC Hwy 88 W
Jefferson, NC 28640   336-246-4460
800-253-2187
FAX: 336-246-5018
infoinso@mcfarlandpub.com
www.mcfarlandbooks.com

Kieth C. Wright, Author
Judith F. Davie, Author
Information for library staff on hiring and serving disabled persons. *$27.50*
171 pages Library binding 1990
ISBN 0-899505-16-3

2458 Life-Span Approach to Nursing Care for Individuals with Developmental Disabilities
Brookes Publishing
PO Box 10624
Baltimore, MD 21285-0624   410-337-9580
800-638-3775
FAX: 410-337-8539
custserv@brookespublishing.com
www.brookespublishing.com

Paul H. Brookes, Chairman
Jeffrey D. Brookes, President
Melissa A. Behm, ExecutiveVice President
George S. Stamathis, Vice President & Publisher
This reference book was written by and for nurses. This guide addresses fundamental nursing issues such as health promotion, infection control, seizure management, adaptive and assistive technology, and sexuality. Also offered are in-depth case studies, helpful charts and tables, and problem-solving strategies. *$49.95*
464 pages Hardcover
ISBN 1-557661-51-0

2459 Mainstreaming Deaf and Hard of Hearing Students: Questions and Answers
Gallaudet University Bookstore
800 Florida Ave NE
Washington, DC 20002-3600   202-651-5000
800-451-1073
FAX: 202-651-5489
TTY: 888-630-9347
clerc.center@gallaudet.edu
www.gupress.gallaudet.edu

Dr. T Alan Hurwitz, President
Debra S. Lipkey, University Budget Director
Donald Beil, Chief of Staff
Edward Bosso, Vice President for Administratio

This booklet presents mainstreaming as one educational option and suggests some considerations for parents, teachers and administrators. *$6.00*
40 pages

2460 Mainstreaming Exceptional Students: A Guide for Classroom Teachers
Allyn & Bacon
75 Arlington St
Suite 300
Boston, MA 02116-3988   617-848-7500
800-852-8024
FAX: 617-944-7273
www.home.pearsonhighered.com

Nancy Forfyth, President
Bill Barke, CEO
Jane B. Schulz, Co-Author
C. Dale Carpenter, Co-Author
Covers the various categories of exceptional students and discusses educational strategies and classroom management.
464 pages paperback
ISBN 0-20515 -24-6

2461 Mainstreaming: A Practical Approach for Teachers
McGraw-Hill School Publishing
PO Box 182604
Columbus, OH 43218   877-833-5524
800-338-3987
FAX: 609-308-4480
customer.service@mheducation.com
www.mcgraw-hill.com

David Levin, President/Chief Executive Officer
David Stafford, Senior Vice President/General Counsel
Maryellen Valaitis, Senior Vice President Human Resources
Patrick Milano, Chief Financial Officer/Chief Administrative Officer
Provides teachers, administrators and school psychologists with the background, techniques and strategies they need to offer appropriate services for mildly handicapped students in the mainstream classroom.

2462 Managing Diagnostic Tool of Visual Perception
Gallery Bookshop
319 Kasten Street
PO Box 270
Mendocino, CA 95460-270   707-937-2215
FAX: 707-937-3737
info@gallerybookshop.com
www.gallerybooks.com

Constantine Mangina, Author
For diagnosing specific perceptual learning abilities and disabilities. *$14.00*

ISBN 0-80580 -83-4

2463 Medical Rehabilitation
Lippincott, Williams & Wilkins
227 S 6th St
Suite 227
Philadelphia, PA 19106-3713   215-545-5630
800-777-2295
FAX: 215-732-9988
www.lpub.com

Cheryl Murkey, Manager
Information for the professional on new techniques and treatments in the medical rehabilitation fields. *$80.50*
368 pages Illustrated
ISBN 0-88167 -85-5

2464 Meeting the ADD Challenge: A Practical Guide for Teachers
Research Press
PO Box 7886
Champaign, IL 61826-9177
217-352-3273
800-519-2707
FAX: 217-352-1221
rp@researchpress.com
www.researchpress.com

Robert W. Parkinson, Founder
Dr. Michael Asher, Co-Author
Dr. Steven B Gordon, Co-Author
$24.95

ISBN 0-878223-45-9

2465 Mental & Physical Disability Law Digest
A BA Commission on Mental and Physical Disability
1050 Connecticut Ave. N.W.
Suite 400
Washington, DC 20036-1019
202-662-1000
800-285-2221
FAX: 202-442-3439
cmpdl@abanet.org
www.americanbar.org

Robert M. Carlson, Chair, House of Delegates:
James R. Silkenat, President
William C. Hubbard, President-Elect
Cara Lee, Secretary
Provides comprehensive, summary and analysis of federal and state disability and state disability laws from mental disability law and disability discrimination law perspectives. *$60.00*
376 pages
ISBN 1-590310-05-5

2466 Mental Health Concepts and Techniques for the Occupational Therapy Assistant
Lippincott, Williams & Wilkins
227 S 6th St
Suite 227
Philadelphia, PA 19106-3713
215-521-8300
800-777-2295
FAX: 301-824-7390
www.lpub.com

J Lippincott, CEO
This text offers clear and easily understood explanations of the various theoretical and practiced health models. *$36.00*
344 pages
ISBN 0-88167 -53-X

2467 Mental Health and Mental Illness
Lippincott, Williams & Wilkins
227 S 6th St
Suite 227
Philadelphia, PA 19106-3713
215-592-5400
800-777-2295
FAX: 301-824-7390
www.lpub.com

Kathy Sykes, Manager
Concise, comprehensive and completely up to date, this book presents the most current theory in mental health nursing for the student and the new practitioner. *$28.95*
480 pages
ISBN 0-39755 -73-7

2468 Mentally Ill Individuals
Mainstream
Ste 830
3 Bethesda Metro Ctr
Bethesda, MD 20814-6301
301-961-9299
800-247-1380
FAX: 301-654-6714
info@mainstreaminc.org

Charles Moster
Mainstreaming mentally ill individuals into the workplace. *$2.50*
12 pages

2469 Midland Treatment Furniture
Sammons Preston Rolyan
W68 N158 Evergreen Blvd
Cedarburg, WI 53012-2637
262-387-8720
800-228-3693
FAX: 262-387-8748
CustomerSupport@PattersonMedical.com
www.pattersonmedical.com

Free

2470 Multidisciplinary Assessment of Children With Learning Disabilities and Mental Retardation
Gallery Bookshop
319 Kasten Street
PO Box 270
Mendocino, CA 95460-270
707-937-2215
FAX: 707-937-3737
info@gallerybookshop.com
www.gallerybooks.com

David L. Wodrich, Author
James E. Joy, Editor
Assessment of children with learning disabilities and mental retardation. *$24.00*
346 pages Illustrated
ISBN 0-93371 -62-1

2471 Multisensory Teaching of Basic Language Skills: Theory and Practice
Brookes Publishing
PO Box 10624
Baltimore, MD 21285-0624
410-337-9580
800-638-3775
FAX: 410-337-8539
custserv@brookespublishing.com
www.brookespublishing.com

Paul H. Brookes, Chairman
Jeffrey D. Brookes, President
Melissa A. Behm, ExecutiveVice President
George S. Stamathis, Vice President & Publisher
This book presents specific multisensory methods for helping students who are having trouble learning to read due to dyslexia or other learning disabilities. Recommended techniques are offered for teaching alphabet skills, composition, comprehension, handwriting, math, organization and study skills, phonological awareness, reading and spelling. *$59.00*
608 pages Hardcover
ISBN 1-557663-49-1

2472 Music, Disability, and Society
1852 North 10th Street
Philadelphia, PA 19122
215-926-2140
800-621-2736
www.temple.edu/tempress

Alex Lubet, Author
In Music, Disability, and Society, Alex Lubet challenges the rigid view of technical skill and writes about music in relation to disability studies. He addresses the ways in which people with disabilities are denied the opportunity to participate in music.

2473 No Longer Immune: A Counselor's Guide to AIDS
American Counceling Association
5999 Stevenson Ave
Alexandria, VA 22304-3304
703-823-9800
800-347-6647
FAX: 703-823-0252
membership@counseling.org
www.counseling.org

Robert L. Smith, President
Thelma Duffey, President-Elect
Cirecie A. West-Olatunji, Past-President
Brian Canfield, Treasurer
Covers a broad range of issues such as working with specific populations, handling pre and post testing situations, coping with fear, grief and survivor guilt, struggling with spiritual issues and dealing with counter transference. *$26.95*
295 pages
ISBN 1-55620 -64-1

2474 Occupational Therapy Across Cultural Boundaries
Haworth Press
711 Third Avenue
New York, NY 10017
212-216-7800
800-354-1420
FAX: 212-244-1563
subscriptions@tandf.co.uk.
www.taylorandfrancisgroup.com

Derek Mapp, Non-Executive Chairman
Roger Horton, CEO
Emma Blaney, Group HR Director - Head of Corporate Responsibility
Isobel Peck, Group Chief Marketing Officer

Examines the concept of culture from a unique perspective, that of individual occupational therapists who have worked in environments very different from those in which they were educated or had worked previously. Journal publications formerly published by Haworth Press are now listed on the Taylor & Francis Journals website. *$74.95*
107 pages Hardcover
ISBN 1-560242-23-X

2475 Occupational Therapy Approaches to Traumatic Brain Injury
Routledge (Taylor & Francis Group)
711 Third Ave
New York, NY 10017
212-216-7800
800-634-7064
FAX: 212-564-7854
enquiries@taylorandfrancis.com
www.routledge.com

Laura H. Krefting, Author
Jerry A. Johnson, Author

Focusing on the disabled individual, the family, and the societal responses to the injured, this comprehensive book covers the spectrum of available services from intensive care to transitional and community living. Formerly published by Haworth Press, titles are now listed on Routledge/Taylor Francis Group. *$140.00*
137 pages Hardcover
ISBN 1-560240-64-4

2476 Overcoming Dyslexia in Children, Adolescents and Adults
Sage Publications
2455 Teller Road
Thousand Oaks, CA 91320
805-499-9774
800-818-7243
FAX: 800-583-2665
books.claim@sagepub.com
www.sagepub.com

Sara Miller McCune, Founder, Publisher, Chairperson
Blaise R Simqu, President/CEO
Tracey A. Ozmina, Executive Vice President & Chief
Dale R. Jordan, Author

This book describes some forms of dyslexia in detail and then relates those problems to the social, emotional and personal development of dyslexic individuals. *$34.00*
350 pages Paperback

2477 Oxford Textbook of Geriatric Medicine
Oxford University Press
198 Madison Ave
New York, NY 10016-4308
212-726-6000
800-445-9714
FAX: 919-677-1303
custserv.us@oup.com
www.global.oup.com

Rebecca Seger, Director, Institutional Sales, Americas
Lesa Moran Owen, Library Sales Operations Manager
Lenny Allen, Director, Institutional Accounts
Nancy Roy, Library Sales Manager

This comprehensive text brings together extensive experience in clinical geriatrics with a strong scientific base in research. *$125.00*
784 pages

2478 PKU for Children: Learning to Measure
University of Washington PKU Clinic
PO Box 357920
University of Washington
Seattle, WA 98195-7920
206-598-1800
877-685-3015
FAX: 206-598-1915
pku@u.washington.edu
www.depts.washington.edu/pku

C. Ronald Scott, MD, Professor, Pediatrics, Division
Michael J. Bamshad, MD, Division Chief and Professor
Eileen Chin, BA (Acc), Division Administrator
Susanna Ngai, BS, Fiscal Specialist 2 - Administra

Lesson format for parents and teachers.

2479 Pain Centers: A Revolution in Health Care
Lippincott Williams And Wilkins
227
227 S 6th St
Philadelphia, PA 19106-3713
215-521-8300
800-777-2295
FAX: 301-824-7390
www.lpub.com

J Lippincott, CEO
$103.00
280 pages

2480 Parental Concerns in College Student Mental Health
Haworth Press
711 Third Avenue
New York, NY 10017
212-216-7800
800-354-1420
FAX: 212-244-1563
subscriptions@tandf.co.uk.
www.taylorandfrancisgroup.com

Derek Mapp, Non-Executive Chairman
Roger Horton, CEO
Emma Blaney, Group HR Director - Head of Corporate Responsibility
Isobel Peck, Group Chief Marketing Officer

An instructive guide for parents and mental health professionals regarding the most important issues about psychological development in college students. Journal publications formerly published by Haworth Press are now listed on the Taylor & Francis Journals website. *$74.95*
204 pages Hardcover
ISBN 0-866567-20-8

2481 Parents and Teachers
Alexander Graham Bell Association
3417 Volta Pl NW
Washington, DC 20007-2737
202-337-5220
866-337-5220
FAX: 202-337-8314
TTY: 202-337-5221
info@agbell.org
www.listeningandspokenlanguage.org

Kathleen S. Treni, M.Ed., M.A., President
Meredith K. Knueve, Esq., Secretary-Treasurer
Alexander T. Graham, Executive Director/CEO
Corrine Altman, Director

This excellent book offers in-depth guidance to parents and teachers whose partnership can foster language in school-aged children with hearing impairments. The first section examines roles of parents, teachers, professionals and children in language acquisition, residual hearing and audiological management, language development stages and readying children for preschool. The second portion of the book presents specific objectives and teaching strategies to use at school and at home. *$27.95*
386 pages

2482 **Patient and Family Education**
Springer Publishing Company
11 W 42nd St
15th Floor
New York, NY 10036-8002 212-431-4370
877-687-7476
FAX: 212-941-7842
cs@springerpub.com
www.springerpub.com

Dr. Ursula Springer, President
Ted Nardin, CEO
James C. Costello, Vice President, Journal Publishi
James C. Costello, Vice President, Journal Publishing
This guide outlines the actual clinical content needed to develop, implement and maintain patient education programs. Conveniently arranged in one-hour long lesson plans, each disease or condition is organized in an easy-to-follow format. *$26.95*
272 pages Softcover
ISBN 0-82615-41-7

2483 **Person to Person: Guide for Professionals Working with the Disabled**
Paul H Brookes Publishing Company
PO Box 10624
Baltimore, MD 21285-0624 410-337-9580
800-638-3775
FAX: 410-337-8539
custserv@brookespublishing.com
www.brookespublishing.com

Paul H. Brookes, Chairman
Jeffrey D. Brookes, President
Melissa A. Behm, ExecutiveVice President
George S. Stamathis, Vice President & Publisher
This second edition of an already-popular book helps professionals approach interactions with a people-first, disability second attitude. *$29.00*
288 pages Paperback
ISBN 1-557661-00-6

2484 **Personality and Emotional Disturbance**
Taylor & Francis
Ste G
47 Runway Dr
Levittown, PA 19057-4738 267-580-2622
FAX: 215-785-5515

Richard Roberts, CEO
The brain injured person has unique needs. Recent findings have highlighted that it is the personality, behavioral and emotional problems which most prohibit a return to work, create the greatest burden for the long-term care and rehabilitation of physical and cognitive functions. *$72.00*
260 pages Cloth
ISBN 0-85066-71-3

2485 **Phenomenology of Depressive Illness**
Human Sciences Press
233 Spring St
New York, NY 10013-1522 212-229-2859
877-283-3229
FAX: 212-463-0742
ainy@aveda.com
www.aveda.edu

263 pages Cloth
ISBN 0-89885-69-9

2486 **Physical Disabilities and Health Impairments: An Introduction**
McGraw-Hill School Publishing
PO Box 182604
Columbus, OH 43218 877-833-5524
800-338-3987
FAX: 609-308-4480
customer.service@mheducation.com
www.mcgraw-hill.com

David Levin, President/Chief Executive Officer
David Stafford, Senior Vice President/General Counsel
Maryellen Valaitis, Senior Vice President Human Resources
Patrick Milano, Chief Financial Officer/Chief Administrative Officer
A comprehensive text which presents a wealth of up-to-date medical information for teachers.

2487 **Physical Education and Sports for Exceptional Students**
McGraw-Hill Company
2460 Kerper Blvd
Dubuque, IA 52001-2224 800-338-3987
FAX: 614-755-5654
customer.service@mcgraw-hill.com
www.mhhe.com/hper/physed

Michael Horvat, Author
Harold McGraw III, Chairman, President and Chief Ex
Jack F. Callahan, Executive Vice President, Chief
John Berisford, Executive Vice President, Human
Physical education for exceptional students and teaching students with learning and behavior exceptionalities.
Cloth

2488 **Physical Management of Multiple Handicaps: A Professional's Guide**
Brookes Publishing Company
PO Box 10624
Baltimore, MD 21285-0624 410-337-9580
800-638-3775
FAX: 410-337-8539
custserv@brookespublishing.com
www.brookespublishing.com

Paul H. Brookes, Chairman
Jeffrey D. Brookes, President
Melissa A. Behm, ExecutiveVice President
George S. Stamathis, Vice President & Publisher
Comprehensive guide, takes a transdisciplinary approach to therapeutic/technological management of persons with multiple handicaps. *$36.00*
352 pages Hardcover
ISBN 1-557660-47-6

2489 **Physically Handicapped in Society**
Ayer Company Publishers
Ste 322
400 Bedford St
Manchester, NH 03101-1195 603-669-9307
888-267-7323
FAX: 603-669-7945
stg@ncia.net
www.ayerpub.com

Kathy Train, Office Manager
Ellie Phipps, Customer Service
A group of 39 books. Biographies that offer studies on attitudes, sociological and psychological. Please write or call for catalog. *$965.00*
Hardcover
ISBN 0-40513-00-3

2490 Practicing Rehabilitation with Geriatric Clients
Springer Publishing Company
11 W 42nd St
15th Floor
New York, NY 10036-8002

212-431-4370
877-687-7476
FAX: 212-941-7842
cs@springerpub.com
www.springerpub.com

Dr. Ursula Springer, President
Ted Nardin, CEO
James C. Costello, Vice President, Journal Publishi
James C. Costello, Vice President, Journal Publishing
Physical therapy in the geriatric client, psychological and psychiatric considerations in the rehabilitation of the elderly. *$32.95*
256 pages Hardcover
ISBN 0-82616 -80-5

2491 Pragmatic Approach
Educators Publishing Service
625 Mount Auburn St
3RD Floor
Cambridge, MA 02138-3039

617-547-6706
800-225-5750
FAX: 617-547-0285
www.eps.schoolspecialty.com

Paula Fabbro, Sales Consultant
Leo Micale, Sales Consultant
Kristen Colson, Sales Consultant
Flora Francis, Sales Consultant
Monograph on evaluation of children's performances on Slingerland Pre-Reading Screening Procedures to Identify First Grade Academic Needs. *$6.00*
56 pages
ISBN 0-838816-85-1

2492 Preschoolers with Special Needs: Children At-Risk, Children with Disabilities
Allyn & Bacon
75 Arlington St
Suite 300
Boston, MA 02116-3988

617-848-7500
800-852-8024
FAX: 617-944-7273
www.home.pearsonhighered.com

Bill Barke, CEO
Janet W. Lerner, Co-Author
Barbara Lowenthal, Co-Author
Rosemary W. Egan, Co-Author
Explores ways of providing preschool children with special needs and their families with a learning environment that will help them develop and learn. Emphasizes the needs of preschoolers age three to six and provides information to teachers and others who work with young children in all settings. Current models of curricula, which incorporate new features from research and practical expreiences with children who have special needs, are described and discussed. *$59.00*
336 pages cloth
ISBN 0-205358-79-9

2493 Preventing Academic Failure - TeachersHandbook
Educators Publishing Service
625 Mount Auburn St
3rd Fl
Cambridge, MA 02138-3039

617-547-6706
800-225-5750
FAX: 617-547-0285
eps.schoolspecialty.com

Paperback
ISBN 0-838852-71-8

2494 Preventing School Dropouts
Sage Publications
2455 Teller Road
Thousand Oaks, CA 91320

805-499-9774
800-818-7243
FAX: 800-583-2665
books.claim@sagepub.com
www.sagepub.com

Sara Miller McCune, Founder, Publisher, Chairperson
Blaise R Simqu, President/ CEO
Tracey A. Ozmina, Executive Vice President & Chief
Thomas C. Lovitt, Author
For secondary teachers, special education and regular, who have difficulty teaching youth in their classes. Presented are 120 tactics, specific instructional techniques, for helping adolescents to stay in school. Each tactic is written in a format that includes five sections. *$38.00*
509 pages

2495 Prevocational Assessment
Exceptional Education
P.O.Box 15308
Seattle, WA 98115-308

206-262-9538
FAX: 475-486-4510

Jeff Stewart, Owner
Use the PACG to assess your students in nine areas (attendance and endurance, learning and behavior, communication skills, social skills, grooming and eating and toileting) covering 46 specific workshop experiences. *$12.00*
16 pages Complete Set
ISBN 1-87786 -23-7

2496 Primary Special Needs and the National Curriculum
7625 Empire Drive
Florence, KN 41042-2919

800-634-4724
orders@taylorandfrancis.com
www.psypress.com

Ann Lewis, Author
This new edition of Ann Lewis's widely acclaimed text has been substantially revised and updated to take into account the recent revisions to the National Curriculum and the guidance of the Code of Practice.

2497 Progress Without Punishment: Approaches for Learners with Behavior Problems
Teachers College Press
1234 Amsterdam Ave
New York, NY 10027-6602

212-678-3929
800-575-6566
FAX: 212-678-4149
tcpress@tc.columbia.edu
www.teacherscollegepress.com

Anne M. Donnellan, Author
In this volume, the authors argue against the use of punishment, and instead advocate the use of alternative intervention procedures. *$17.95*
184 pages Paperback
ISBN 0-807729-11-6

2498 Promoting Postsecondary Education for Students with Learning Disabilities
Sage Publications
2455 Teller Road
Thousand Oaks, CA 91320

805-499-9774
800-818-7243
FAX: 800-583-2665
books.claim@sagepub.com
www.sagepub.com

Sara Miller McCune, Founder, Publisher, Chairperson
Stan F. Shaw, Co-Author
Joan M. McGuire, Co-Author
Loring Cowles Brinckerhoff, Co-Author
Primarily designed for postsecondary service providers who are responsible for serving college students with learning disabilities. *$41.00*
440 pages

2499 **Psychiatric Mental Health Nursing**
Lippincott, Williams & Wilkins
227 S 6th St
Suite 227
Philadelphia, PA 19106-3713   215-521-8300
800-777-2295
FAX: 301-824-7390
www.lpub.com

J Lippincott, CEO
This text emphasizes and contrasts the roles of the generalist nurse and the psychiatric nurse specialist. *$52.00*
1120 pages Illustrated

2500 **Psychoeducational Assessment of Visually Impaired and Blind Students**
Sage Publications
2455 Teller Road
Thousand Oaks, CA 91320   805-499-9774
800-818-7243
FAX: 800-583-2665
books.claim@sagepub.com
www.sagepub.com

Sara Miller McCune, Founder, Publisher, Chairperson
Blaise R Simqu, President/CEO
Tracey A. Ozmina, Executive Vice President & Chief
Sharon Bradley-Johnson, Author
Professional reference book that addresses the problems specific to assessment of visually impaired and blind children. Of particular value to the practitioner are the extensive reviews of available tests, including ways to adapt those not designed for use with the visually handicapped. *$29.00*
140 pages Paperback
ISBN 0-890791-08-2

2501 **Psychological and Social Impact of Illness and Disability**
Springer Publishing
11 W 42nd St
15th Floor
New York, NY 10036-8002   212-431-4370
877-687-7476
FAX: 212-941-7842
cs@springerpub.com
www.springerpub.com

Dr. Ursula Springer, President
Ted Nardin, CEO
Ph.D. Orto Arthur E. Dell, Editor
James C. Costello, Vice President, Journal Publishing
The newest edition of Psychological and Social Impact of Illness and Disability continues the tradition of presenting a realistic perspective on life with disabilics and then improves upon its predecessors with the inclusion of illness as a major influence on client care needs. Further broadening the scope of this edition is the inclusion of personal perspectives and stories from those living with illness or disabilities. These stories offer a look into what it is like to cope with these issues.

2502 **Reading and Deafness**
Sage Publications
2455 Teller Road
Thousand Oaks, CA 91320   805-499-9774
800-818-7243
FAX: 800-583-2665
books.claim@sagepub.com
www.sagepub.com

Sara Miller McCune, Founder, Publisher, Chairperson
Beverly J Trezek, Co-Author
Peter V. Paul, Co-Author
Ye Wang, Co-Author
Three areas are looked at in this book: deaf children's prereading development of real-world knowledge, cognitive abilities and linguistic skills. *$39.00*
422 pages

2503 **Readings on Research in Stuttering**
Longman Publishing Group
1 Penn Plaza
Suite 2222
New York, NY 10119   646-556-8401
FAX: 646-556-8415
coffee@rothfos.com
www.rothfos.com

Dan Dwyer, CEO
Thomas Minogue, CFO
Maria Tanpinco-Queyquep, Traffic Manager
Joseph P. Thomas, Traffic Coordinator
Collection of the key journal articles published on stuttering over the past decade, addressing trends in recent research in the field.
231 pages Paperback
ISBN 0-801304-10-5

2504 **Recreation Activities for the Elderly**
Springer Publishing Company
11 W 42nd St
15th Floor
New York, NY 10036-8002   212-431-4370
877-687-7476
FAX: 212-941-7842
cs@springerpub.com
www.springerpub.com

Dr. Ursula Springer, President
Ted Nardin, CEO
James C. Costello, Vice President, Journal Publishi
James C. Costello, Vice President, Journal Publishing
Included in this volume are simple crafts that utilize easily obtainable, inexpensive materials, hobbies focusing on collections, nature, and the arts' and games emphasizing both mental and physical activity. *$23.95*
240 pages Softcover
ISBN 0-82616 -30-1

2505 **Reference Manual for Communicative Sciences and Disorders**
Pro- Ed Publications
8700 Shoal Creek Blvd
Austin, TX 78757-6897   512-451-3246
800-897-3202
FAX: 512-451-8542
info@proedinc.com
www.proedinc.com

Raymond D. Kent, Author
An indispensable guide to standards and values essential in the assessment of communication disorders. *$54.00*
393 pages

2506 **Rehabilitation Interventions for the Institutionalized Elderly**
Haworth Press
711 Third Avenue
Floor 8th
New York, NY 10017   212-216-7800
800-354-1420
FAX: 212-564-7854
subscriptions@tandf.co.uk.
www.taylorandfrancisgroup.com

Derek Mapp, Non-Executive Chairman
Roger Horton, CEO
Emma Blaney, Group HR Director - Head of Corporate Responsibility
Isobel Peck, Group Chief Marketing Officer
Gerontology professionals offer suggestions to enrich the quality of rehabilitation services offered to the institutionalized elderly. This volume examines up to the minute ideas, some that would have been unlikely even a few years ago, that focus exclusively on rehabilitation services for the institutionalized elderly. Journal publications formerly published by Haworth Press are now listed on the Taylor & Franc *$44.95*
77 pages Hardcover
ISBN 0-866568-33-6

2507 Rehabilitation Nursing for the Neurological Patient
Springer Publishing Company
11 W 42nd St
15th Fl
New York, NY 10036-8002 212-431-4370
877-687-7476
FAX: 212-941-7842
cs@springerpub.com
www.springerpub.com

Ted Nardin, Chief Executive Officer
Jason Roth, Vice President, Sales & Marketing
Kathy Weiss, Director, Sales
Marcia Hanak, Author
Reviews the physiology, pathophysiology, & nursing management of problems frequently encountered in neuro- rehabilitation and reviews the pathphysiology of specific disabilities & the related nursing interventions. *$32.95*
229 pages Hardcover 1992
ISBN 0-826176-60-7

2508 Rehabilitation Resource Manual: VISION
Resources for Rehabilitation
22 Bonad Rd
Winchester, MA 01890-1302 781-368-9094
FAX: 781-368-9096
info@rfr.org
www.rfr.org

Marshall E. Flax, MS, Author
A desk reference that enables service providers, librarians and others to make effective referrals. Includes guidelines on establishing self-help groups, information on research and service organizations, and chapters on assistive technology, for special population groups and by eye condition. *$44.95*
Biennial

2509 Rehabilitation Technology
CRC Press
6000 Broken Sound Pkwy NW
Ste 300
Boca Raton, FL 33487
800-634-7064
FAX: 800-374-3401
orders@crcpress.com
www.crcpress.com

Glenn E. Hedman, Author
Learn how the use of technological devices can enhance the lives of disabled children. Informs physical therapists, occupational therapists, and rehabilitation technologists about the devices that are available today and provides important background information on these devices. CRC Press is part of the Taylor & Francis Group. *$39.95*
173 pages Hardcover 1990
ISBN 1-560240-33-4

2510 Report Writing in Assessment and Evaluation
Stout Vocational Rehab Institute
University of Wisconsin-Stout
712 South Broadway
Menomonie, WI 54751 715-232-1478
FAX: 715-232-2356
giffordj@uwstout.edu
www.uwstout.edu

Charles W. Sorensen, Chancellor
Judy Gifford, Director
Stephen W. Thomas, Author
Linda Vanderloop, CFSC Office
This examines questions of who are you writing for and what does the referral source want. Defines characteristics of good reports, common problems, writing in different settings, types of reports, getting ready to write, and writing prescriptive recommendations. *$ 17.75*
188 pages Softcover

2511 Resource Room, The
State University of New York Press
22 Corporate Woods Boulevard
3rd Floor
Albany, NY 12210-2314 518-472-5000
866-430-7869
FAX: 518-472-5038
info@sunypress.edu
www.sunypress.edu

Barry Edwards McNamara, Author
Provides teachers and administrators with helpful, practical information and explores the role of the resource room teacher as it relates to three major functions: assessment, instruction and consultation. It will also assist supervisors and administrators in evaluating their resource programs. *$28.95*
148 pages Paperback
ISBN 0-887069-84-0

2512 Resources for Rehabilitation
22 Bonad Rd
Winchester, MA 01890-1302 781-368-9094
FAX: 781-368-9096
info@rfr.org
www.rfr.org

2513 Restructuring High Schools for All Students: Taking Inclusion to the Next Level
Brookes Publishing
PO Box 10624
Baltimore, MD 21285-0624 410-337-9580
800-638-3775
FAX: 410-337-8539
custserv@brookespublishing.com
www.brookespublishing.com

Paul H. Brookes, Chairman
Jeffrey D. Brookes, President
Melissa A. Behm, ExecutiveVice President
George S. Stamathis, Vice President & Publisher
Details the process of creating an inclusive, collaborate community of learners and teachers at the secondary level. *$29.95*
304 pages Paperback
ISBN 1-557663-13-0

2514 Restructuring for Caring and Effective Education: Administrative Guide
Brookes Publishing
PO Box 10624
Baltimore, MD 21285-0624 410-337-9580
800-638-3775
FAX: 410-337-8539
custserv@brookespublishing.com
www.brookespublishing.com

Paul H. Brookes, Chairman
Jeffrey D. Brookes, President
Melissa A. Behm, ExecutiveVice President
George S. Stamathis, Vice President & Publisher
In this empowering book, leading general and special education schools reform experts synthesize the major school restructuring initiatives and describe the processes and rationale for changing the organizational structure and instructional practices of schools. *$ 29.00*
384 pages Paperback
ISBN 1-55766 -91-3

2515 Scoffolding Student Learning
Brookline Books
8 Trumbull Rd
Suite B-001
Northampton, MA 01060 413-584-0184
800-666-2665
FAX: 413-584-6184
brbooks@yahoo.com
www.brooklinebooks.com

Paul H. Brookes, Chairman
Jeffrey D. Brookes, President
Melissa A. Behm, ExecutiveVice President
George S. Stamathis, Vice President & Publisher

Collection of papers on the theory and practice of scaffolding—an interactive style of instructions that helps students develop more powerful thinking tools. *$21.95*
180 pages Paperback
ISBN 1-571290-36-2

2516   Selective Nontreatment of Handicapped
Oxford University Press
2001 Evans Rd
Cary, NC 27513-2009   919-677-0977
                                    800-445-9714
                                FAX: 919-677-1303
                            custserv.us@oup.com
                            www.global.oup.com

Lesa Moran Owen, Library Sales Operations Manager
Rebecca Seger, Director, Institutional Sales, Americas
Lenny Allen, Director, Institutional Accounts
Nancy Roy, Library Sales Manager
Information on selective nontreatment of handicapped newborns, moral dilemmas in neonatal medicine. *$17.95*
304 pages Paperback

2517   Semiotics and Dis/ability: Interogating Categories of Difference
State University of New York Press
22 Corporate Woods Boulevard
3rd Floor
Albany, NY 12210-2314   518-472-5000
                                    866-430-7869
                                FAX: 518-472-5038
                            info@sunypress.edu
                            www.sunypress.edu

James Peltz, Associate Director
Linda Rogers, Editor
Beth Blue Swadener, Editor
Examines the ways the words disability and difference and socially and culturally constructed. *$25.95*
265 pages Paperback 1990
ISBN 0-791449-06-6

2518   Service Coordination for Early Intervention: Parents and Friends
Brookline Books
8 Trumbull Rd
Suite B-001
Northampton, MA 01060   413-584-0184
                                    800-666-2665
                                FAX: 413-584-6184
                            brbooks@yahoo.com
                            www.brooklinebooks.com

Deborah D. Hatton, Co-Author
R. A. McWilliam, Co-Author
P. J. Winton, Co-Author
This book helps administrators and professionals to structure early intervention and ongoing services so that professionals work collaboratively with parents to promote the health, well being and development of children with special needs. *$19.95*
110 pages Paperback
ISBN 0-91479-91-3

2519   Services for the Seriously Mentally Ill: A Survey of Mental Health Centers
Nat'l Council for Community Behavioral Healthcare
12300 Twinbrook Pkwy
Ste 320
Rockville, MD 20852-1606   301-984-6200
                                FAX: 301-881-7159
                            www.nccbh.org

Linda Rosenberg, CEO
Dale K Klatzker, Board Chair
This ground-breaking report documents what administrators and practitioners have maintained for many years: community mental health organizations devote a significant percentage of the human and financial resources to serving the seriously mentally ill. *$30.00*

2520   Sexuality and Disability
Springer Publishing
11 W 42nd St
15th Fl
New York, NY 10036-8002   212-431-4370
                                FAX: 212-460-1575
                            www.springer.com

Sigmund Hough, Editor-in-Chief
A journal devoted to the psychological and medical aspects of sexuality in rehabilitation and community settings. The journal features original scholarly articles that address the psychological and medical aspects of sexuality in the field of rehabilitation, case studies, clinical practice reports, and guidelines for clinical practice.
Quarterly

2521   Shop Talk
PO Box 7886
Champaign, IL 61826-9177   217-352-3273
                                    800-519-2707
                                FAX: 217-352-1221
                            rp@researchpress.com
                            www.researchpress.com

Robert W. Parkinson, Founder
Philip Roth, Author

2522   Signed English Schoolbook
Gallaudet University Press
800 Florida Ave NE
Washington, DC 20002-3600   202-651-5488
                                    800-451-1073
                                FAX: 202-651-5489
                                TTY: 888-630-9347
                            clerc.center@gallaudet.edu
                            www.gupress.gallaudet.edu

Harry Bornstein, Co-Author
Karen L. Saulnier, Co-Author
Dr. T Alan Hurwitz, President
Edward Bosso, Vice President for Administratio
The Signed English Schoolbook provides vocabulary for teachers and others who serve school-age children and adolescents and covers the full range of school activities. *$13.95*
184 pages Softcover

2523   Social Skills for Students With Autism Spectrum Disorders and Other Dev Disabilities
2900 Crystal Drive
Suite 1000
Arlington, VA 22202-3557   888-232-7733
                            alisonh@cec.sped.org
                            www.cec.sped.org

Laurence R. Sargent, Co-Author
Toni Cook, Co-Author
Darlene E. Perner, Co-Author
Know the warning signs that you are heading into your Upset Zone.

2524   Social Studies: Detecting and Correcting Special Needs
Allyn & Bacon
75 Arlington St
Suite 300
Boston, MA 02116-3988   617-848-7500
                                    800-852-8024
                                FAX: 617-944-7273
                            www.home.pearsonhighered.com

Harry Bornst Barke, CEO
Nancy Forfyth, President
Lana J. Smith, Co-Author
Dennie L. Smith, Co-Author
Describes social studies and special needs for special learners.
180 pages
ISBN 0-205121-51-9

2525   **Social and Emotional Development of Exceptional Students: Handicapped**
Charles C. Thomas
2600 S First St
Springfield, IL 62704-4730   217-789-8980
     800-258-8980
     FAX: 217-789-9130
     books@ccthomas.com
     www.ccthomas.com

Michael P. Thomas, President
Carroll J. Jones, Author
Sixteen years after the passage of P.L. 94-142, the dream of special educators to educate the handicapped and nonhandicapped children and youth together resulting in increased academic gains and age-appropriate school skills for handicapped children and youth has not yet materialized. This book helps eliminate an existing void by providing teachers with understandable information regarding the social and emotional development of exceptional students. Also in cloth at $41.95 (ISBN# 0-398-05781-8) *$29.95*
218 pages Softcover
ISBN 0-398061-94-7

2526   **Special Education Today**
LifeWay Christian Resources Southern Baptist Conv.
One LifeWay Plaza
Nashville, TN 37234   615-251-2000
     800-458-2772
     FAX: 615-532-9412
     specialed@lifeway.com
     www.lifeway.com

Thom S. Rainer, President/CEO
Brad Waggoner, Executive Vice President
Eric Geiger, Vice President, Church Resources Division
Tim Hill, Vice President/Chief Information Officer
This unique quarterly publications ministers to people with special education needs and to their families, the church, and other caregivers. It offers a variety of helps and encouragement, including: What's working in churches, Suggestions for adapting teaching techniques, inspirational stories about people who have disabilities, Parenting and family issues, Ideas for reaching, witnessing, worship, and recreation. *$4.25*
36 pages Quarterly

2527   **Special Education for Today**
Allyn & Bacon
75 Arlington St
Suite 300
Boston, MA 02116-3988   617-848-7500
     800-852-8024
     FAX: 617-944-7273
     www.home.pearsonhighered.com

See search r Barke, CEO
Michael S. Rosenberg, Co-Author
David L. Westling, Co-Author
James McLeskey, Co-Author
An undergraduate introduction to special education covering all major areas of exceptionality. Contains pedagogical features designed to make the book accessible to the undergraduate.
576 pages hardcover
ISBN 0-138264-53-8

2528   **Speech and the Hearing-Impaired Child**
Alexander Graham Bell Association
3417 Volta Pl NW
Washington, DC 20007-2737   202-337-5220
     866-337-5220
     FAX: 202-337-8314
     TTY: 202-337-5221
     info@agbell.org
     www.listeningandspokenlanguage.org

Meredith K. Sugar, Esq. (OH), President
Ted A. Meyer, M.D., Ph.D, President-Elect/Secretary-Treasurer
Emilio Alonso-Mendoza, Chief Executive Officer
Susan Boswell, Director of Communications and Marketing
This textbook for professionals deals with basic theoretical issues in the acquisition of speech and the form of language (phonetics and phonology) in children with hearing losses. It provides a systematic framework to develop and evaluate speech target behaviors and their underlying subskills. *$29.95*
402 pages Paperback

2529   **Speech-Language Pathology and Audiology: An Introduction**
McGraw-Hill School Publishing
PO Box 182604
Columbus, OH 43218   877-833-5524
     800-338-3987
     FAX: 609-308-4480
     customer.service@mheducation.com
     www.mcgraw-hill.com

David Levin, President/Chief Executive Officer
David Stafford, Senior Vice President/General Counsel
Maryellen Valaitis, Senior Vice President Human Resources
Patrick Milano, Chief Financial Officer & Chief Administrative Officer
Offers classroom-tested coverage of clinical objectives and functioning.
301 pages

2530   **Spinal Cord Dysfunction**
Oxford University Press
2001 Evans Rd
Cary, NC 27513-2009   919-677-0977
     800-451-7556
     FAX: 919-677-1303
     humanres@oup-usa.org
     www.global.oup.com

Lesa Moran Owen, Library Sales Operations Manager
Rebecca Seger, Director, Institutional Sales, Americas
Lenny Allen, Director, Institutional Accounts
Nancy Roy, Library Sales Manager
Offers information on restoration of function after spinal cord damage as seen from the point of view of identification of impaired or absent function in the nerve cells and processes which survive after the initial insult, intact but with impaired functions. *$95.00*
368 pages

2531   **Steps to Success: Scope & Sequence for Skill Development**
15619 Premiere Drive
Suite 101
Tampa, FL 33624   850-363-9909
     FAX: 480-393-4331
     accounting@successforkidswithhearingloss.com
     successforkidswithhearinglo ss.com

Lynne H. Price, Author
Steps to Success is a curriculum for students who are deaf or hard of hearing in grades kindergarten through 12.

2532   **Strategies for Teaching Learners with Special Needs**
McGraw-Hill School Publishing
PO Box 182604
Columbus, OH 43218   877-833-5524
     800-338-3987
     FAX: 609-308-4480
     customer.service@mheducation.com
     www.mcgraw-hill.com

David Levin, President/Chief Executive Officer
David Stafford, Senior Vice President/General Counsel
Maryellen Valaitis, Senior Vice President Human Resources
Patrick Milano, Chief Financial Officer & Chief Administrative Officer
This is a text that helps special educators develop the full range of teaching competencies needed to be effective.
560 pages

2533 **Strategies for Teaching Students with Learning and Behavior Problems**
Allyn & Bacon
75 Arlington St
Suite 300
Boston, MA 02116-3988   617-848-7500
800-852-8024
FAX: 617-944-7273
www.home.pearsonhighered.com

Bill Barke, CEO
Nancy Forfyth, President
Sharon R. Vaughn, Co-Author
Candace S. Bos, Co-Author
Provides descriptions of methods and strategies for teaching students with learning and behvior problems, managing professional roles, and collaborating with families, professionals, and paraprofessionals.
544 pages
ISBN 0-205113-89-3

2534 **Students with Acquired Brain Injury: The School's Response**
Brookes Publishing
PO Box 10624
Baltimore, MD 21285-0624   410-337-9580
800-638-3775
FAX: 410-337-8539
custserv@brookespublishing.com
www.brookespublishing.com

Ann Glang, Editor
Bonnie Todis, Editor
Paul H. Brooks, Chairman of the Board
Cary Gold, Educational Sales Representative
This book is designed for school professionals and describes a range of issues that this population faces and presents proven means of addressing them in ways that benefit all students. Included topics are hospital-to-school transitions, effective assessment strategies, model programs in public schools, interventions to assist classroom teachers, and ways to involve family members in the educational program. *$29.95*
424 pages Paperback
ISBN 1-55766 -85-1

2535 **Students with Mild Disabilities in the Secondary School**
Longman Group
75 Arlington St
Suite 300
New York, NY 10036-2601   212-782-3300
800-852-8024
www.home.pearsonhighered.com

William Hitchings, Co-Author
Michael Horvath, Co-Author
Bonnie Schmalle, Co-Author
Paul Retish, Co-Author, Editor
Provides methods and strategies for curriculum delivery to students with mild disabilities at the secondary school level.
2313G pages Paperback
ISBN 0-801301-66-1

2536 **Supporting and Strengthening Families**
Brookline Books
8 Trumbull Rd
Suite B-001
Northampton, MA 01060   413-584-0184
800-666-2665
FAX: 413-584-6184
brbooks@yahoo.com
www.brooklinebooks.com

Carl J Dunst, Author
A collection of papers addressing the theory, methods, strategies, and practices involved in adopting an empowerment and family-centered resources approach to supporting families and strengthening individual and family functioning. *$30.00*
252 pages Paperback
ISBN 0-91479 -94-8

2537 **TESTS**
Slosson Educational Publications
538 Buffalo rd
PO Box 280
East Aurora, NY 14052   716-652-0930
888-756-7766
FAX: 800-665-3840
slossonprep@gmail.com
www.slosson.com

Steven W. Slosson, President
Dr. Georgina Moynihan, Office Personnel
Slosson Educational Publications, Inc. offers educators an extensive selection of testing products, along with books on autism. ADED and other special needs materials. Our catalog includes 30 pages of speech-language testing and language rehabilitation products. The behavioral conduct. Special needs section includes checklist and scales on aberrant/disruptive behavior, tapes on ADD, as well as products for dyslexia and remediation of reversals.

2538 **Teacher's Guide to Including Students with Disabilities in Regular Physical Education**
Brookes Publishing
PO Box 10624
Baltimore, MD 21285-0624   410-337-9580
800-638-3775
FAX: 410-337-8539
custserv@brookespublishing.com
www.brookespublishing.com

Martin E. Block, Author
Melissa A. Behm, Executive Vice President
Paul H. Brooks, Chairman of the Board
Cary Gold, Educational Sales Representative
Provides simple and creative strategies for meaningfully including children with disabilities in regular physical education programs. *$39.00*
288 pages Paperback
ISBN 1-557661-56-1

2539 **Teachers Working Together**
Brookline Books
8 Trumbull Rd
Suite B-001
Northampton, MA 01060   413-584-0184
800-666-2665
FAX: 413-584-6184
brbooks@yahoo.com
www.brooklinebooks.com

Carol Davis, Co-Author
Alice Yang, Co-Author
This collection of papers describes collaborabrative efforts for such classroom settings as preschools, elementary, middle and high schools, for content area teaching and into the transition to work. Each chapter describes actual practice and analyzes what is required to accomplish this collaboration. *$19.95*
Paperback
ISBN 1-57139 -66-4

2540 **Teachig Students with Special Needs inInclusive Classrooms**
SAGE Publications
2455 Teller Rd
Thousand Oaks, CA 91320   800-818-7243
FAX: 800-583-2665
orders@sagepub.com
us.sagepub.com

Diane P. Bryant, Author
Brian P. Bryant, Author
Deborah D. Smith, Author
Using the research-validated ADAPT framework, Teaching Students with Special Needs in Inclusive Classrooms helps future teachers determine how, when, and with whom to use proven academic and behavioral interventions to obtain the best outcomes for students with disabilities. This book will provide the skills and inspiration that teachers need to make a positive difference in the educational lives of struggling learners.

2541 Teaching Adults with Learning Disabilities
Krieger Publishing Company
1725 Krieger Drive
Malabar, FL 32902   321-724-9542
     800-724-0025
     FAX: 321-951-3671
     info@krieger-publishing.com
     www.krieger-publishing.com

Dale R. Jordan, Author
R Krieger, Owner
Designed to teach literacy providers and classroom instructors how to recognize specific learning disability (LD) patterns and block reading, spelling, writing and arithmetic skills in students of all ages. One of the major problems faced by literary providers is keeping low-skill adults involved in basic education programs long enough to increase their literacy skills to the level of success. Shows instructors in adult education how to modify teaching strategies. *$25.50*
160 pages
ISBN 0-894649-10-8

2542 Teaching Children With Autism in the General Classroom
Prufrock Press
PO Box 8813
Waco, TX 76714-8813   254-756-3337
     800-998-2208
     FAX: 254-756-3339
     gbates@prufrock.com
     www.prufrock.com

Joel McIntosh, Publisher & Marketing Director
Ginny Bates, Customer Service and Office Manager
Lacy Compton, Senior Editor
Rachel Taliaferro, Editor
Provides an introduction to inclusionary practices that serve children with autism, giving teachers the practical advice they need to ensure each students receives the quality education he or she deserves. *$39.95*
350 pages Paperback
ISBN 1-593633-64-6

2543 Teaching Disturbed and Disturbing Students: An Integrative Approach
Sage Publications
2455 Teller Road
Thousand Oaks, CA 91320   805-499-9774
     800-818-7243
     FAX: 800-583-2665
     books.claim@sagepub.com
     www.sagepub.com

Sara Miller McCune, Founder, Publisher, Chairperson
Blaise R Simqu, President & CEO
Tracey A. Ozmina, Executive Vice President & Chief
Paul Zionts, Author
Using an integrative approach, this text provides teachers with step-by-step details of how to implement and use the methods and theories discussed in each chapter. *$37.00*
465 pages

2544 Teaching Every Child Every Day: Integrated Learning in Diverse Classrooms
Brookline Books
8 Trumbull Rd
Suite B-001
Northampton, MA 01060   413-584-0184
     800-666-2665
     FAX: 413-584-6184
     brbooks@yahoo.com
     www.brooklinebooks.com

Karen R. Harris, Editor
Steve Graham, Editor
Don Deshler, Editor
Collection of articles addressing various issues in teaching to diverse classrooms—varied in need for special educational services, English proficiency, and socioeconomic and racial backgrounds. *$19.95*
224 pages Paperback
ISBN 0-57129 -40-0

2545 Teaching Infants and Preschoolers with Handicaps
Mc Graw- Hill, School Publishing
PO Box 182604
Columbus, OH 43218   877-833-5524
     800-338-3987
     FAX: 609-308-4480
     customer.service@mheducation.com
     www.mcgraw-hill.com

David Levin, President/Chief Executive Officer
David Stafford, Senior Vice President/General Counsel
Maryellen Valaitis, Senior Vice President Human Resources
Patrick Milano, Chief Financial Officer & Chief Administrative Officer
Builds a solid background in early childhood special education.
380 pages

2546 Teaching Language-Disabled Children: A Communication/Games Intervention
Brookline Books
8 Trumbull Rd
Ste B-001
Northampton, MA 01060   413-584-0184
     800-666-2665
     FAX: 413-584-6184
     brbooks@yahoo.com
     www.brooklinebks.com

Susan Conant, Author
Offers practitioners specific teaching methods for helping students play communication games. *$22.95*
185 pages Hardcover 1983
ISBN 0-914797-38-7

2547 Teaching Learners with Mild Disabilities: Integrating Research and Practice
Brooke Publishing
PO Box 10624
Baltimore, MD 21285-0624   410-337-9580
     800-638-3775
     FAX: 410-337-8539
     custserv@brookespublishing.com
     www.brookespublishing.com

Ruth Lyn Meese, Author
Melissa A. Behm, Executive Vice President
Paul H. Brooks, Chairman of the Board
Cary Gold, Educational Sales Representative
The authors illustrate interactions among regular teachers, special education teachers and students with mild disabilities through the use of hypothetical case studies of students and teachers.
496 pages Paperbound
ISBN 0-53421 -02-0

2548 Teaching Mathematics to Students with Learning Disabilities
Sage Publications
2455 Teller Road
Thousand Oaks, CA 91320   805-499-9774
     800-818-7243
     FAX: 800-583-2665
     books.claim@sagepub.com
     www.sagepub.com

Sara Miller McCune, Founder, Publisher, Chairperson
Blaise R Simqu, President & CEO
Nancy S. Bley, Co-Author
Carol A. Thornton, Co-Author
New trends in school mathematics have surfaced in the teaching world. Problem-solving, estimation and the use of computers are receiving considerably greater emphasis than in the past and these areas are included in the new text. *$38.00*
486 pages Paperback

2549 Teaching Mildly and Moderately Handicapped Students
Allyn & Bacon
75 Arlington St
Suite 300
Boston, MA 02116-3988 617-848-7500
800-852-8024
FAX: 617-944-7273
www.home.pearsonhighered.com

Bill Barke, CEO
Nancy Forfyth, President
B. R. Gearheart, Author
Kevin Stone, Vice President, National Sales M
A cross-categorical text providing teaching ideas and techniques. Focuses on the theme of learning as a constructive process in which the learner interacts with the environment, constructing new systems of knowledge, Behavioral techniques and research are also presented.
hardcover
ISBN 0-138939-00-4

2550 Teaching Reading to Children with Down Syndrome: A Guide for Parents and Teachers
Woodbine House
6510 Bells Mill Rd
Bethesda, MD 20817-1636 301-897-3570
800-843-7323
FAX: 301-897-5838
info@woodbinehouse.com
www.woodbinehouse.com

Irvin Shapell, Publisher
Patricia Logan Oelwein, Author
Beth Binns, Special Marketing Manage
Fran Marinaccio, Marketing Manager
Guide includes lessons customized to meet the unique interests and learning style of each child. *$16.95*
371 pages Paperback
ISBN 0-933149-55-7

2551 Teaching Reading to Disabled and Handicapped Learners
Charles C. Thomas
2600 S First St
Springfield, IL 62704-4730 217-789-8980
800-258-8980
FAX: 217-789-9130
books@ccthomas.com
www.ccthomas.com

Michael P. Thomas, President
Freddie W. Litton, Author
Harold D. Love, Author
Designed as a text for undergraduate and graduate students, this resource aims to help the many children, adolescents, and adults who encounter difficulty with reading. It guides prospective and present special education teachers in assisting and teaching handicapped learners to read. The text integrates traditional methods with newer perspectives to provide and effective reading program in special education. *$43.95*
252 pages Paperback 1996
ISBN 0-398062-48-X

2552 Teaching Reading to Handicapped Children
Love Publishing Company
9101 E Kenyon Ave
Suite 2200
Denver, CO 80237-1854 303-221-7333
FAX: 303-221-7444
lpc@lovepublishing.com
www.lovepublishing.com

Charles H. Hargis, Author
The author covers skills teaching through letter sound association, word identification, synthetic and analytic methods and others, plus testing and assessment. *$24.95*

ISBN 0-89108-13-5

2553 Teaching Self-Determination to Students with Disabilities
Brookes Publishing
PO Box 10624
Baltimore, MD 21285-0624 410-337-9580
800-638-3775
FAX: 410-337-8539
custserv@brookespublishing.com
www.brookespublishing.com

Michael L. Wehmeyer, Co-Author
Martin Agran, Co-Author
Paul H. Brooks, Chairman of the Board
Cary Gold, Educational Sales Representative
Basic skills for successful transition. This teacher-friendly source will help educators prepare students with disabilities with the specific skills they need for a satisfactory, self-directed life once they leave school. *$34.95*
384 pages Paperback
ISBN 1-55766 -02-5

2554 Teaching Students with Learning Problems
McGraw-Hill School Publishing
PO Box 182604
Columbus, OH 43218 877-833-5524
800-338-3987
FAX: 609-308-4480
customer.service@mheducation.com
www.mcgraw-hill.com

David Levin, President/Chief Executive Officer
David Stafford, Senior Vice President/General Counsel
Maryellen Valaitis, Senior Vice President Human Resources
Patrick Milano, Chief Financial Officer & Chief Administrative Officer
Expanded coverage of learning strategies, generalization training, self-monitoring techniques, and techniques for increasing the time students spend on academic tasks.
608 pages

2555 Teaching Students with Learning and Behavior Problems
Sage Publications
2455 Teller Road
Thousand Oaks, CA 91320 805-499-9774
800-818-7243
FAX: 800-583-2665
books.claim@sagepub.com
www.sagepub.com

Sara Miller McCune, Founder, Publisher, Chairperson
Blaise R Simqu, President & CEO
Sharon R. Vaughn, Co-Author
Candace S. Bos, Co-Author
$65.00
444 pages Paperback
ISBN 0-890799-28-4

2556 Teaching Students with Mild and Moderate Learning Problems
Allyn & Bacon Longman College Faculty
75 Arlington St
Suite 300
Boston, MA 02116-3988 617-367-0025
800-852-8024
FAX: 617-367-2155
www.home.pearsonhighered.com

Bill Barke, CEO
John Langone, Author
Kevin Stone, Vice President, National Sales M
Kevin Stone, Vice President, National Sales M
Provides teachers with skills for assisting students with mild to moderate handicaps in making successful transitions in school and community environments.
496 pages
ISBN 0-205123-62-7

2557 Teaching Students with Moderate/Severe Disabilities, Including Autism
Charles C. Thomas
2600 S First St
Springfield, IL 62704-4730   217-789-8980
                                              800-258-8980
                                         FAX: 217-789-9130
                                       books@ccthomas.com
                                          www.ccthomas.com
Michael P. Thomas, President
Elva Duran, Author
This resource and guide was written to help teachers, parents, and other caregivers provide the best educational opportunities for their students with moderate and severe disabilities. The author addresses functional language and other language intervention strategies, vocational training, community based instruction, transition and postsecondary programming, the adolescent student with autism, students with multiple disabilities, parent and family issues, and legal concerns. *$58.95*
416 pages Paperback
ISBN 0-398067-01-5

2558 Teaching Students with Special Needs in Inclusive Settings
Allyn & Bacon
75 Arlington St
Suite 300
Boston, MA 02116-3988   617-848-7500
                                              800-852-8024
                                         FAX: 617-944-7273
                                  www.home.pearsonhighered.com
Tom E.C. Smith, Co-Author
Edward A. Polloway, Co-Author
James Patton, Co-Author
Carol A. Dowdy, Co-Author
This text is intended to be a survey text providing practical guidance to general education teachers. It will help them to meet the diverse needs of students with disabilities.
544 pages
ISBN 0-20527-16-6

2559 Teaching Young Children to Read
Brookline Books
8 Trumbull Rd
Suite B-001
Northampton, MA 01060   413-584-0184
                                              800-666-2665
                                         FAX: 413-584-6184
                                       brbooks@yahoo.com
                                      www.brooklinebooks.com
Dolores Durkin, Author
John P.
Detailed instructions on teaching reading to preschoolers. Gradually develops full fluency. *$16.95*
192 pages Paperback
ISBN 0-57129-48-6

2560 Teaching the Bilingual Special Education Student
Ablex Publishing Corporation
P.O.Box 811
Stamford, CT 06904-811
                                         FAX: 201-767-6717

ISBN 0-89391-23-4

2561 Teaching the Learning Disabled Adolescent: Strategies and Methods
Love Publishing Company
9101 E Kenyon Ave
Ste 2200
Denver, CO 80237-1813   303-221-7333
                                         FAX: 303-221-7444
                                      lpc@lovepublishing.com
                                      www.lovepublishing.com
Gordon R. Alley, Author

This book gives expert strategies and methods for teaching learning disabled adolescents how, rather than what, to learn. *$39.95*
360 pages Hardcover 1979
ISBN 0-891080-94-5

2562 Teaching the Mentally Retarded Student: Curriculum, Methods, and Strategies
Allyn & Bacon
75 Arlington St
Suite 300
Boston, MA 02116-3988   617-367-0025
                                              800-852-8024
                                         FAX: 617-367-2155
                                  www.home.pearsonhighered.com
Bill Barke, CEO
Richard L. Luftig, Author
Nancy Forfyth, President
Kevin Stone, Vice President, National Sales M
Represents a comprehensive approach to curriculum, methods and strategies for teaching the mildly mentally retarded student.
640 pages hardcover
ISBN 0-205102-62-X

2563 Technology and Handicapped People
Springer Publishing Company
11 W 42nd St
15th Floor
New York, NY 10036-8002   212-431-4370
                                              877-687-7476
                                         FAX: 212-941-7842
                                       cs@springerpub.com
                                        www.springerpub.com
Dr. Ursula Springer, President
Ted Nardin, CEO
James C. Costello, Vice President, Journal Publishi
James C. Costello, Vice President, Journal Publishing
Important information for concerned professionals about new rehabilitation techniques and treatments for handicapped people. *$29.95*
224 pages Hardcover
ISBN 0-82614-10-8

2564 Textbooks and the Student Who Can't Read Them: A Guide for Teaching Content
Brookline Books
8 Trumbull Rd
Suite B-001
Northampton, MA 01060   413-584-0184
                                              800-666-2665
                                         FAX: 413-584-6184
                                       brbooks@yahoo.com
                                      www.brooklinebooks.com
Paperback
ISBN 0-91479-57-3

2565 The Education of Children with Acquired Brain Injury
David Fulton Publishers (Routledge)
711 Third Ave
New York, NY 10017   212-216-7800
                                         FAX: 212-564-7854
                                  orders@taylorandfrancis.com
                                         www.routledge.com
Sue Walker, Author
Beth Wicks, Author
Teachers have to be aware of their pupils' special educational needs. Find out what an acquired brain injury is and how to maximize learning opportunities for those with the condition with this book.
128 pages

2566 The Fundamentals of Special Education: APractical Guide for Every Teacher
Corwin Press Inc.
2455 Teller Rd
Thousand Oaks, CA 91320
805-499-9734
800-233-9936
FAX: 805-499-5323
order@corwin.com
us.corwin.com

Bob Algozzine, Author
Jim Ysseldyke, Author
This guide highlights major concepts in special education-from disability categories, identification issues, and IEPs to appropriate learning environments and the roles general and special educators play.
104 pages

2567 The K&W Guide to Colleges for Studentswith Learning Disabilties (13th Edition)
The Princeton Review - Penguin Random House
1745 Broadway
New York, NY 10019
212-782-9000
customerservice@penguinrandomhouse.com
www.penguinrandomhouse.com

848 pages Paperback 1916
ISBN 1-101920-38-6

2568 There's a Hearing Impaired Child in My Class
Gallaudet University Bookstore
800 Florida Ave NE
Washington, DC 20002-3600
202-651-5000
800-451-1073
FAX: 202-651-5489
TTY: 888-630-9347
clerc.center@gallaudet.edu.
www.bookstore.gallaudette.edu

Debra Nussbaum, Author
Dr. T Alan Hurwitz, President
Edward Bosso, Vice President for Administratio
Donald Beil, Chief of Staff
This complete package provides basic facts about deafness, practical strategies for teaching hearing impaired children, and the question-and-answer information for all students. *$16.95*
44 pages

2569 Toward Effective Public School Program for Deaf Students
Teachers College Press
525 W 120th St
New York, NY 10027-6605
212-678-3000
800-575-6566
FAX: 212-678-4149
webcomments@tc.columbia.edu
www.tc.columbia.edu

Susan H. Fuhrman, Ph.D., President of the College
Harvey Spector, Vice President for Finance and Administration
Suzanne M. Murphy, Vice President for Development and External Affairs
Janice S. Robinson, Vice President for Diversity and Community Affairs
This book translates research and data into useable recommendations and possible courses of action for organizing effective public school programs for deaf students. *$22.95*
272 pages Paperback
ISBN 0-807731-59-5

2570 Treating Adults with Disabilities: Access and Communication
World Institute on Disability
3075 Adeline Street
Suite 155
Berkeley, CA 94703
510-225-6400
FAX: 510-225-0477
TTY:510-225-0478
wid@wid.org
www.wid.org

Paul W. Schroeder, Chairman
Linda M. Dardarian, Vice Chairman
Mary Brooner, Treasurer
Cassandra Malry, Secretary
This training curriculum is for medical professionals who want to improve the quality of care for people with disabilities and chronic illnesses. Also covers architectural, communication, attitudinal and economic policy barriers to quality health care and specific skills to increase good communication and rapport. *$6.50*
63 pages Paperback

2571 Treating Cerebral Palsy for Clinicians by Clinicians
Sage Publications
2455 Teller Road
Thousand Oaks, CA 91320
805-499-9774
800-818-7243
FAX: 800-583-2665
books.claim@sagepub.com
www.sagepub.com

Sara Miller McCune, Founder, Publisher, Chairperson
Blaise R Simqu, President & CEO
Tracey A. Ozmina, Executive Vice President & Chief
Eugene T. McDonald, Editor
A clinical manual for professionals beginning to work with persons who have cerebral palsy. *$31.00*
312 pages

2572 Treating Disordered Speech Motor Control
Sage Publications
2455 Teller Road
Thousand Oaks, CA 91320
805-499-9774
800-818-7243
FAX: 800-583-2665
books.claim@sagepub.com
www.sagepub.com

Sara Miller McCune, Founder, Publisher, Chairperson
Blaise R Simqu, President & CEO
Deanie Vogel, Author
Michael Cannito, Editor
This book about neuromotor disturbances of speech production is aimed at practicing professionals and advanced graduate students interested in the neuropathologies of communication. *$36.00*
410 pages

2573 Treating Families of Brain Injury Survivors
Springer Publishing Company
11 W 42nd St
15th Floor
New York, NY 10036-8002
212-431-4370
877-687-7476
FAX: 212-941-7842
cs@springerpub.com
www.springerpub.com

Dr. Ursula Springer, President
Ted Nardin, CEO
James C. Costello, Vice President, Journal Publishi
James C. Costello, Vice President, Journal Publishing
Provides the mental health practitioner with a comprehensive program for helping families of head injury survivors cope with the change in their lives. Includes background on medical aspects of head injury, family structure functioning and special needs of various family members.
220 pages
ISBN 0-82616 -20-1

2574 **Understanding and Teaching Emotionally Disturbed Children & Adolescents**
Sage Publications
2455 Teller Road
Thousand Oaks, CA 91320
805-499-9774
800-818-7243
FAX: 800-583-2665
books.claim@sagepub.com
www.sagepub.com

Sara Miller McCune, Founder, Publisher, Chairperson
Blaise R Simqu, President & CEO
Tracey A. Ozmina, Executive Vice President & Chief
Phyllis L. Newcomer, Author

The teacher's handbook provides information that will change misconceptions about children who are frequently labeled as emotionally disturbed. It also gives information about a wide variety of intervention methods and approaches for use in educational settings. *$41.00*
620 pages Hardover

2575 **Using the Dictionary of Occupational Titles in Career Decision Making**
Stout Vocational Rehab Institute
University of Wisconsin Stou
Menomonie, WI 54751
715-232-2470
FAX: 715-232-5008
luij@uwstout.edu
www.svri.uwstout.edu

John Lui, Contact Person

This is a self-study manual for learning how to use the 1991 U.S. Department of Labor's Dictionary of Occupational Titles. It gives the DOT user a tool to understand the DOT and then put its information to work. Shows how to quickly obtain information about the work performed in 12,741 occupations listed and described in the DOT and the worker requirements for those occupations. *$24.00*
142 pages Softcover

2576 **VBS Special Education Teaching Guide**
Life Way Christian Resources Southern Baptist Conv
1 Lifeway Plz
Nashville, TN 37234-1001
615-251-2000
specialed@lifeway.com
www.lifeway.com

Tom Hellam, VP of Executive Communications a
Thom Rainer, President & CEO

This book contains teaching plans for five bible study sessions with reproducible handouts for learners. The plans use multisensory, experiential-based learning activities designed for adults and older youth who have mental retardation. Suggestions for Bible learning, crafts, recreation, snacks and theme interpretation are included. Designed primarily for Vacation Bible School, but may be used in camp/retreat settings. *$9.95*
56 pages Yearly

2577 **Vermont Interdependent Services Team Approach (VISTA)**
Brookes Publishing
PO Box 10624
Baltimore, MD 21285-624
410-337-9580
800-638-3775
FAX: 410-337-8539
custserv@brookespublishing.com
www.brookespublishing.com

Paul Kelly, National Textbook Sales Manager
Tracy Gray, Educational Sales Manager
Paul Brooks, President

A guide to coordinating educational support services. This manual enables IEP team members to fulfill the related services provisions of IDEA as they make effective support services decisions using a collaborative team approach. *$27.95*
176 pages Spiral bound
ISBN 1-55766-30-4

2578 **What School Counselors Need to Know**
2900 Crystal Drive
Suite 1000
Arlington, VA 22202-3557
888-232-7733
alisonh@cec.sped.org
www.cec.sped.org

Barbara E. Baditoi, Co-Author
Pamelia E. Brott, Co-Author

What School Counselors Need to Know About Special Education provides counselors (and school administrators) with essential information to make the most of their participation in providing special education services.

2579 **When You Have a Visually Impaired Student in Your Classroom: A Guide for Teachers**
American Foundation for the Blind
2 Penn Plaza
Suite1102
New York, NY 10121
212-502-7600
800-232-5463
FAX: 888-545-8331
afbinfo@afb.net
afb.org

Carl Augusto, President

This guide provides information on students' abilities and needs, resources and educational team members, federal special education requirements, and technology materials used by students. *$9.95*
84 pages
ISBN 0-891283-93-5

2580 **Working Bibliography on Behavioral and Emotional Disorders**
Natl. Clearinghouse for Alcohol & Drug Information
1 Choke Cherry Road
Rockville, MD 20857
301-468-2600
877-SAM-SA 7
FAX: 301-468-6433
info@health.org
www.health.org

Lizabeth J Foster, Librarian/Info. Resource Manager
Pamela S. Hyde, Administrator

NCADI is a service of the U.S. Substance Abuse and Mental Health Services Administration. As the national focal point for information on alcohol and other drugs, NCADI collects, prepares, classifies, and distributes information about alcohol, tobacco and other drugs, prevention strategies and materials, research, treatment, etc.
40 pages

2581 **Working Together with Children and Families: Case Studies**
Brookes Publishing Company
PO Box 10624
Baltimore, MD 21285-624
410-337-9580
800-638-3775
FAX: 410-337-8539
custerv@brookespublishing.com
www.brookespublishing.com

Paul Kelly, National Textbook Sales Manager
Tracy Gray, Educational Sales Manager
Paul Brooks, Owner

Early interventionists will be able to bridge the gap between theory and practice with this edited collection of case studies. *$23.00*
336 pages
ISBN 1-557661-23-5

2582 **Working with Visually Impaired Young Students: A Curriculum Guide for 3 to 5 Year Olds**
Charles C. Thomas
2600 S First St
Springfield, IL 62704-4730   217-789-8980
                                    800-258-8980
                               FAX: 217-789-9130
                                books@ccthomas.com
                                 www.ccthomas.com

Michael P. Thomas, President
Ellen Trief, Editor
The first step in the education process of a visually impaired child is the early identification and treatment by an eye care specialist. This book is geared to the age of birth through 3-years. Available in cloth, paperback and hardcover. *$42.95*
194 pages Paperback
ISBN 0-398068-75-2

Testing Resources

2583 **ADD-SOI Center, The**
2007 Cedar Avenue
Manhattan Beach, CA 90266   310-546-6500
                               FAX: 310-546-9068
                                 ADDSOI@aol.com
                                  www.addsoi.com

2584 **AEPS Child Progress Report: For Children Ages Birth to Three**
Brookes Publishing
PO Box 10624
Baltimore, MD 21285-624   410-337-9580
                                    800-638-3775
                               FAX: 410-337-8539
                        custserv@brookespublishing.com
                           www.brookespublishing.com

Paul Kelly, National Textbook Sales Manager
Tracy Gray, Educational Sales Manager
Paul Brooks, Owner
This chart helps monitor change by visually displaying current abilities, intervention targets, and child progress. In packages of 30. *$18.00*
6 pages Gate-fold
ISBN 1-55766-65-0

2585 **AEPS Data Recording Forms: For Children Ages Birth to Three**
Brookes Publishing
PO Box 10624
Baltimore, MD 21285-624   410-337-9580
                                    800-638-3775
                               FAX: 410-337-8539
                        custserv@brookespublishing.com
                              readplaylearn.com

Paul Brooks, Owner
Melissa Behm, Executive Vice President
These forms can be used by child development professionals on four separate occasions to pinpoint and then monitor a child's strengths and needs in the six key areas of skill development measured by the AEPS Test. Packages of 10. *$23.00*
36 pages Saddle-stiched
ISBN 1-55766-97-2

2586 **AEPS Measurement for Birth to Three Years**
Brookes Publishing
PO Box 10624
Baltimore, MD 21285-624   410-337-9580
                                    800-638-3775
                               FAX: 410-337-8539
                        custserv@brookespublishing.com
                           www.brookespublishing.com

Paul Kelly, National Textbook Sales Manager
Tracy Gray, Educational Sales Manager
Paul Brooks, Owner

This dynamic volume explains the Assessment, Evaluation and Programming System, provides the complete AEPS Test and parallel assessment/evaluation tools for families and includes the forms and plans needed for implementation. *$39.00*
352 pages

2587 **AEPS Measurement for Three to Six Years**
Brookes Publishing
PO Box 10624
Baltimore, MD 21285-624   410-337-9580
                                    800-638-3775
                               FAX: 410-337-8539
                        custserv@brookespublishing.com
                           www.brookespublishing.com

Paul Kelly, National Textbook Sales Manager
Tracy Gray, Educational Sales Manager
Paul Brooks, Owner
Resources in early childhood, early intervention, inclusive and special education, developmental disabilities, learning disabilities, communication and language, behavior, and mental health. *$57.00*
400 pages Spiral-bound
ISBN 1-55766-87-1

2588 **AIR: Assessment of Interpersonal Relations**
Sage Publications
2455 Teller Road
Thousand Oaks, CA 91320   805-499-0721
                                    800-818-7243
                               FAX: 800-583-2665
                                 info@sagepub.com
                                  www.sagepub.com

Sara Miller McCune, Founder, Publisher, Chairperson
Blaise R Simqu, President & CEO
A thoroughly researched and standardized clinical instrument assessing the quality of adolescents' interpersonal relationships in a hierarchical fashion, including global relationship quality and relationship quality with three domains: Family, Social and Academic. *$89.00*

2589 **ALST: Adolescent Language Screening Test**
Sage Publications
2455 Teller Road
Thousand Oaks, CA 91320   805-499-0721
                                    800-818-7243
                               FAX: 800-583-2665
                                 info@sagepub.com
                                  www.sagepub.com

Sara Miller McCune, Founder, Publisher, Chairperson
Blaise R Simqu, President & CEO
Provides speech/language pathologists and other interested professionals with a rapid thorough method for screening adolescents (ages 11-17). *$119.00*

2590 **Adaptive Mainstreaming: A Primer for Teachers and Principals, 3rd Edition**
Longman Publishing Group
1330 Avenue of the Americas
New York, NY 10019   212-641-2400
                                    800-745-8489
                          wendy.spiegel@pearsoned.com
                                  www.pearson.com

Glen Moreno, Chairman
Marjorie Scardino, Chief Executive Officer
An introduction to education for handicapped and gifted students. Presents research-based rationales for teaching exceptional students in the least restrictive environment. Provides historical perspectives, offers realistic descriptions of prevailing practices in the field, and reviews trends and new directions.
366 pages Paperback
ISBN 0-582285-04-6

2591 Ages & Stages Questionnaires
Brookes Publishing
PO Box 10624
Baltimore, MD 21285-624
410-337-9580
800-638-3775
FAX: 410-337-8539
custserv@brookespublishing.com
www.brookespublishing.com

Paul Kelly, National Textbook Sales Manager
Tracy Gray, Educational Sales Manager
Paul Brooks, Owner
ASQ is an economical and field-tested system for identifying whether infants and young children may require further developmental evaluation and offers a screening and tracking program that helps early intervention professionals, service coordinators, and administrators maximize financial resources while promoting the health and growth of the children they serve. Set includes 11 color-coded, reproducible questionnaires, 11 reproducible, age appropriate scoring sheets. *$135.00*

2592 American College Testing Program
500 Act Drive
PO Box 168
Iowa City, IA 52243-168
319-337-1000
FAX: 319-339-3021
act.org

John Whitmore, CEO
Mark D Musik, President Emeritus
An independent, nonprofit organization that provides a variety of educational services to students and their parents, to high schools and colleges, and to professional associations and government agencies.

2593 Assessing Students with Special Needs
Longman Publishing Group
10 Bank Street
9th Floor
White Plains, NY 10606-1933
914-993-5000
www.ablongman.com

Joanne Dresner, President
Step-by-step guide to informal, classroom assessment of students with special needs.
174 pages Paperback
ISBN 0-801301-77-7

2594 Assessment Log & Developmental Progress Charts for the CCPSN
Brookes Publishing
P.O.Box 10624
Baltimore, MD 21285-624
410-337-9580
800-638-3775
FAX: 410-337-8539
custserv@brookespublishing.com
www.brookespublishing.com

Paul Kelly, National Textbook Sales Manager
Tracy Gray, Educational Sales Manager
Paul Brooks, Owner
This 28-page booklet allows readers to actually chart the ongoing progress of each preschool child. Available in packages of 10. *$22.00*
28 pages Saddle-stiched
ISBN 1-55766 -39-5

2595 Assessment of Learners with Special Needs
Allyn & Bacon
75 Arlinton Street
Ste 300
Boston, MA 2116-3988
617-848-7500
800-852-8024
FAX: 617-944-7273
www.ablongman.com

Bill Barke, CEO
Thomas Longman, Founder
The central goal of this book is to help teachers become sophisticated, informed test consumers in terms of choosing, using and interpreting commercially prepared tests for their special needs students.
508 pages Casebound
ISBN 0-205227-33-3

2596 Benchmark Measures
Educators Publishing Service
PO Box 9031
Cambridge, MA 2139
617-547-6706
800-225-5750
FAX: 888-440-2665
feedback@epsbooks.com
www.epsbooks.com

Charles H Heinle, VP
Alexandra S Bigelow, Author
Gunnar Voltz, President
Ungraded test containing three sequential levels that assess alphabet and dictionary skills, reading, handwriting and spelling, and correspond to the first three schedules of the Alphabetic Phonics curriculum. The tests can be used at any level to measure a student's general knowledge of phonics. *$64.40*
Kit

2597 Brain Clinic, The
19 West 34th Street
Penthouse
New York, NY 10001
212-268-8900
nurosvcs@aol.com
thebrainclinic.com

Dr. James Lawrence Thomas, Director
The brain clinic offers diagnosis and Treatment of ADD, Learning Disabilities, Migraines, and Traumatic Brain Injury.

2598 CREVT: Comprehensive Receptive and Expressive Vocabulary Test
Sage Publications
2455 Teller Road
Thousand Oaks, CA 91320
805-499-0721
800-818-7243
FAX: 800-583-2665
info@sagepub.com
www.sagepub.com

Sara Miller McCune, Founder, Publisher, Chairperson
Blaise R Simqu, President & CEO
A new, innovative, efficient measure of both receptive and expressive oral vocabulary. The CREVT has two subtests and is based on the most current theories of vocabulary development, suitable for ages 4 through 17. *$174.00*
Complete Kit

2599 Carolina Curriculum for Preschoolers with Special Needs
Brookes Publishing
P.O.Box 10624
Baltimore, MD 21285-624
410-337-9580
800-638-3775
FAX: 410-337-8539
custserv@brookespublishing.com
www.brookespublishing.com

Paul Kelly, National Textbook Sales Manager
Tracy Gray, Educational Sales Manager
Paul Brooks, Owner
This curriculum provides detailed teaching and assessment techniques, plus a sample 28-page Assessment Log that shows readers how to chart a child's individual progress. This guide is for children between 2 and 5 in their developmental stages who are considered at risk for developmental delay or who exhibit special needs. *$35.95*
352 pages Spiral-bound
ISBN 1-557660-32-8

2600   **Center For Personal Development**
405 North Wabash Ave.
Suite 208 & 1114
Chicago, IL 60611   312-755-7000
                                  FAX: 312-755-7001
                          info@chicagotherapist.com
                          www.chicagotherapist.com

Steven Nakisher, Licensed Clinical Psychologist
Cara McCanse, Licensed Clinical Psychologist
Sarah Krcmarik, Staff Psychotherapist
Amy Zurawic, Staff Psychotherapist
The Center for Personal Development was founded in 1998 to provide a diverse range of high-quality mental health services.

2601   **Center for Human Potential**
525 East 100 South
Suite 120
Salt Lake City, UT 84102   801-483-2447
                                      801-486-8705
                                      www.c4hp.com

C. Brendan Hallett Psy.D., Clinical Director
Michael DeCaria, Ph.D., Licensed Clinical Psychologist
Annice Julian, Psy.D., Licensed Clinical Psychologist
Stephanie Voigt, Psy.D., Licensed Clinical Psychologist
Center for Human Potentialis a human services company that helps individuals, businesses and organizations reach their potential by achieving balance in the fundamental areas of life: Emotional, Physical, Mental, Spiritual and Financial. We offer individual, couples, and family counseling to help with a number of issues.

2602   **Center for Neuropsychology, Learning & Development**
1955 Pauline Blvd
Suite 100A
Ann Arbor, MI 48103   734-994-9466
                                  FAX: 734-994-9465
                                      www.cnld.org

Roger E. Lauer, Clinical Director
Jodene Goldenring Fine, Ph.D., Licensed Psychologist
CNLD was founded over 20 years ago to serve Southeast Michigan and the greater Ann Arbor community by providing quality mental health care for children, adolescents, adults and families.

2603   **Center for Student Health and Counseling**
1825 SW Broadway
Portland, OR 97201   503-725-3000
                                      800-547-8887
                                  FAX: 503-725-4882
                                  askadm@pdx.edu
                          www.pdx.edu/shac/ldadhd

2604   **Children's Assessment Center, The**
2500 Bolsover St.
Houston, TX 77005   713-986-3300
                                  FAX: 713-986-3553
                                  info@cac.hctx.net
                                  cachouston.org

Brady E. Crosswell, Chairman
Gail Prather, President
Elaine Stolte, Executive Director
Mark Anderson, Treasurer
The Children's Assessment Center (CAC)provides a safe haven to sexually abused children and their families.

2605   **Cognitive Solutions Learning Center**
2409 N. Clybourn Ave.
Chicago, IL 60614   773-755-1775
                                  FAX: 773-439-5499
                                  info@helpforld.com
                          www.helpforld.com/index.php/about-us/

Dr. Ari Goldstein, Founder
Jason Almodovar, M.S.Ed., Office Manager
Cognitive Solution offers a broad range of services, including learning disability and attention deficit disorder assessment and remediation, executive functions training, and the latest neurofeedback technologies.

2606   **DAYS: Depression and Anxiety in Youth Scale**
Sage Publications
2455 Teller Road
Thousand Oaks, CA 91320   805-499-0721
                                      800-818-7243
                                  FAX: 805-376-9443
                                  info@sagepub.com
                                  www.sagepub.com

Sara Miller McCune, Founder, Publisher, Chairperson
Blaise R Simqu, President & CEO
A unique battery of three norm-references scales useful in identifying major depressive disorder and overanxious disorders in children and adolescents. *$129.00*
Complete Kit

2607   **DOCS: Developmental Observation Checklist System**
Pro- Ed Publications
8700 Shoal Creek Blvd
Austin, TX 78757-6897   512-451-3246
                                      800-897-3202
                                  FAX: 800-397-7633
                                  general@proedinc.com
                                  www.proedinc.com

Donald D Hammill, Owner
Courtney King, Marketing Coordinator
A three-part system for the assessment of very young children with respect to general development, adjustment behavior and parent stress and support. *$124.00*

2608   **Dennis Developmental Center**
1 Children's Way
Little Rock, AR 72202-3591   501-364-1100
                                  TTY:501-364-1184
                                  www.archildrens.org

2609   **Developmental Services Center**
Therapeutic Nursery Program
4525 Lee St NE
Washington, DC 20019   202-388-3216
                                  FAX: 202-576-8799

Alice Anderson
Offers assessment information and evaluation for developmentally delayed students.

2610   **Frames of Reference for the Assessment of Learning Disabilities**
Brookes Publishing
P.O.Box 10624
Baltimore, MD 21285-624   410-337-9580
                                      800-638-3775
                                  FAX: 410-337-8539
                          custserv@brookespublishing.com
                          www.brookespublishing.com

Paul Kelly, National Textbook Sales Manager
Tracy Gray, Educational Sales Manager
Paul Brooks, Owner
New views on measurement issues. Here you'll find an in=depth look at the fundamental concerns facing those who work with children with learning disabilities - assessment and identification. *$55.00*
672 pages Hardcover
ISBN 1-55766 -38-3

2611   **How to Conduct an Assessment**
FSSI
3905 Huntington Dr
Amarillo, TX 79109-4047   806-353-1114
                                  FAX: 806-353-1114
                                  webmaster@winfssi.com
                                  www.winfssi.com

Ed Hammer, Owner
The Functional Skills Screening Inventory,this behavioral checklist allows for parents and professionals to observe critical behaviors in individuals with multiple disabilities (7 years to adult years).

2612 Inclusive & Heterogeneous Schooling: Assessment, Curriculum, and Instruction
Brookes Publishing
P.O.Box 10624
Baltimore, MD 21285-624

410-337-9580
800-638-3775
FAX: 410-337-8539
custserv@brookespublishing.com
www.brookespublishing.com

Paul Kelly, National Textbook Sales Manager
Tracy Gray, Educational Sales Manager
Paul Brooks, Owner
Presents methods for successfully restructuring classrooms to enable all students, particularly those with disabilities, to flourish. Provides specific strategies for assessment, collaboration, classroom management, and age-specific instruction. *$34.95*
448 pages Paperback
ISBN 1-557662-02-9

2613 Infant & Toddler Convection of Fairfield: Falls Church
Joseph Willard Health Center
3750 Old Lee Hwy
Fairfax, VA 22030-1806

703-246-7180
FAX: 703-246-7307

Susan Sigler, Program Coordinator
Allan Phillips, Director Early Intervention
Offers assessments, evaluations and educational/therapeutic infant programs for parents infants and toddlers birth to age 3.
Sliding Scale

2614 K-BIT: Kaufman Brief Intelligence Test
AGS
Ste 1000
5910 Rice Creek Pkwy
Shoreview, MN 55126-5023

651-287-7220
800-328-2560
FAX: 800-471-8457
agsmail@agsnet.com
www.agsnet.com

Kevin Brueggeman, President
Robert Zaske, Market Manager
Quick and easy-to-use, KBIT assesses verbal and non-verbal abilities through two reliable subtests - vocabulary and matricies.
$ 124.95
Ages 4-90

2615 K-FAST: Kaufman Functional Academic Skills Test
AGS
Ste 1000
5910 Rice Creek Pkwy
Shoreview, MN 55126-5023

651-287-7220
800-328-2560
FAX: 800-471-8457
agsmail@agsnet.com
www.agsnet.com

Robert Zaske, Market Manager
Helps assess a person's capacity to function effectively in society regarding functional reading and math skills. *$99.95*
Ages 15-85+

2616 K-SEALS: Kaufman Survey of Early Academic and Language Skills
AGS
5910 Rice Creek Pkwy
Shoreview, MN 55126-5025

651-287-7220
800-328-2560
FAX: 800-471-8457
agsmail@agsnet.com
www.agsnet.com

Kevin Brueggeman, President
Robert Zaske, Market Manager
An individually administered test of children's of both expressive and receptive skills, pre-academic skills and articulation. K-SEALS offers reliable scores usually in less than 25 minutes. *$ 179.95*
Ages 3-0; 6-11

2617 KLST-2: Kindergarten Language Screening Test Edition, 2nd Edition
Sage Publications
2455 Teller Road
Thousand Oaks, CA 91320

805-499-9774
800-818-7243
FAX: 800-583-2665
info@sagepub.com
www.sagepub.com

Paul Kelly, National Textbook Sales Manager
Blaise R Simqu, President & CEO
Identifies children who need further diagnostic testing to determine whether or not they have language deficits that will accelerate academic failure. *$94.00*

2618 Kaufman Test of Educational Achievement(K-TEA)
AGS
PO Box 99
Circle Pines, MN 55014-99

800-328-2560
FAX: 800-471-8457
agsmail@agsnet.com
www.agsnet.com

Robert Zaske, Marketing Manager
Kevin Brueggeman, President
K-TEA is an individually administered diagnostic battery that measures reading, mathematics, and spelling skills. Setting the standards in achievement testing today, K-TEA Comprehensive provides the complete diagnostic information you need for educational assessment and program planning. The Brief Forum is indispensable for school and clinical psychologists, special education teachers when a quick a measure of achievement is needed. *$249.95*

2619 Learning House
264 Church Street
Guilford, CT 6437

203-453-3691
www.learninghouse-ct.com

Susan Santora, Founder and Director
Learning House is a professional community committed to enhancing the lives of individuals with dyslexia and other learning disabilities in safe and supportive surroundings.

2620 LearningRx
5085 List Drive
Suite 200
Colorado Springs, CO 80919

719-264-8808
www.learningrx.com

Dr. Ken Gibson, Founder
LearningRx is a brain training program.

2621 Life Centered Career Education: A Contemporary Based Approach, 4th Edition
Council for Exceptional Children
2900 Crystal Drive
Suite1000
Arlington, VA 22202-3557

703-264-9454
888-232-7733
FAX: 703-264-1637
president@cec.sped.org
www.cec.sped.org

Marilyn Friend, President
Provides a framework for building 97 functional skill competencies appropriate for preparing for adult life and special education students. *$28.00*
175 pages

2622 Measure of Cognitive-Linguistic Abilities(MCLA)
Speech Bin
PO Box 1579
Appleton, VA 54912-1579

772-770-0007
888-388-3224
FAX: 888-388-6344
onlinehelp@schoolspecialty.com
www.speechbin.com

Jan J Binney, Senior Editor

A diagnostic test of cognitive-linguistic abilities of adolescents and adults with traumatically induced brain injuries. High level. Normed. *$89.00*
100 pages
ISBN 0-93785 -72-

2623 Miriam

501 Bacon Avenue
St. Louis, MO 63119-1512

314-968-3893
FAX: 314-962-0482
athorp@miriamstl.org
www.miriamstl.org/learning-center

Andrew Thorp, Executive Director
Sarah Scott, Development Director
Carol Faust, Business Manager
Tam Nguyen, Facilities Manager
Miriam improves the quality of life for children with learning disabilities and their families through innovative and comprehensive programs.

2624 Neuropsychology Assessment Center

One University Place
Chester, PA 19013

610-499-4273
www.widenernac.org

Mary F. Lazar, PsyD, Director
Wendy M. Sarkisian, PsyD, Assistant Director
Located in the Philadelphia area, the Neuropsychology Assessment Center (NAC) specializes in neuropsychological evaluations for the investigation of a variety of psychological conditions.

2625 ONLINE

West Virginia Research and Training Center
P.O. Box 1004
Institute, WV 25112-1004

304-766-9495
800-624-8284
FAX: 304-766-2689
info@icdi.wvu.edu
www.icdi.wvu.edu

Clifford Lantz, President
A quarterly newsletter offering information about hardware technology, software (commercial and home grown); applications that work and bonuses such as an exchange program for copyright-free software. *$25.00*
Quarterly

2626 OWLS: Oral and Written Language Scales LC/OE & WE

AGS
P.O. Box 99
Circle Pines, MN 55014-99

800-328-2560
FAX: 800-471-8457
agsmail@agsnet.com
www.agsnet.com

Kevin Brueggeman, President
Robert Zaske, Market Manager
One kit provides an assessment of listening comprehension while the other assesses oral expression tasks: semantic, syntactic, pragmatic, and supralinguistic aspects of language. Written Expression may be administered individually or in small groups. *$249.95*

2627 PAT-3: Photo Articulation Test

Sage Publications
2455 Teller Road
Thousand Oaks, CA 91320

805-499-9774
800-818-7243
FAX: 800-583-2665
info@sagepub.com
www.sagepub.com

Paul Kelly, National Textbook Sales Manager
Blaise R Simqu, President & CEO
This test consists of 72 color photographs. The first 69 photos test consonants and all but one vowel and one diphthong. The remaining pictures test connected speech and the remaining vowel and diphthong. *$144.00*
Complete Kit

2628 Peabody Early Experiences Kit (PEEK)

AGS
P.O. Box 99
Circle Pines, MN 55014-99

800-328-2560
FAX: 800-471-8457
agsmail@agsnet.com
www.agsnet.com

Kevin Brueggeman, President
Robert Zaske, Market Manager
1,000 activities and all the materials you need to build youngsters' cognitive, social and language skills. Manuals, puppets, manipulatives, picture card deck, picture mini decks and more to teach early development concepts. *$789.95*

2629 Peabody Individual Achievement Test-Revised Normative Update (PIAT-R-NU)

AGS
P.O. Box 99
Circle Pines, MN 55014-99

800-328-2560
FAX: 800-471-8457
agsmail@agsnet.com
www.agsnet.com

Kevin Brueggeman, President
Robert Zaske, Market Manager
PIAT-R-NU is an efficient individual measure of academic achievement. Reading, mathematics, and spelling are assessed in a simple, non-threatening format that requires only a pointing response for most items. This multiple choice format makes the PIAT-R ideal for assessing individuals who hesitate to give a spoken response, or have limited expressive abilities. *$289.98*

2630 Peabody Language Development Kits (PLDK)

AGS
P.O. Box 99
Circle Pines, MN 55014-99

800-328-2560
FAX: 800-471-8457
agsmail@agsnet.com
www.agsnet.com

Kevin Brueggeman, President
Robert Zaske, Market Manager
The main goals of the Peabody Kit language program are to stimulate overall language skills in Standard English and, for each level of the program, advance children's cognitive skills about a year. *$ 649.95*
Level P
ISBN 0-88671 -25-1

2631 Pediatric Early Elementary (PEEX II) Examination

Educators Publishing Service
625 Mount Auburn Street
3rd Floor
Cambridge, MA 2138- 3039

617-547-6706
800-225-5750
FAX: 888-440-2665
feedback@epsbooks.com
www.epsbooks.com

Charles H Heinle, VP
Alexandra S Bigelow, Author
Gunnar Voltz, President
Assesses the second-fourth grade child's performance on thirty-two tasks in six specific areas of development: fine-motor function, language, gross-motor function, memory, visual processing, and delayed recall. At three points during the exam, the child is rated on selective attention and behavior and effect.
$15.40 - $93
ISBN 0-83888 -80-6

2632 Pediatric Exam of Educational-PEERAMID Readiness at Middle Childhood
Educators Publishing Service
625 Mount Auburn Street
3rd Floor
Cambridge, MA 2138- 3039 617-547-6706
800-225-5750
FAX: 888-440-2665
feedback@epsbooks.com
www.epsbooks.com

Charles H Heinle, VP
Alexandra S Bigelow, Author
Gunnar Voltz, President
Assesses the 4th-10th grade child's performance on thirty-one tasks in six specific areas: minor neurological indicators, fine-motor function, language, gross-motor function, temporal-sequential organization, and visual processing. Complete set.
$15.40 - $109
ISBN 0-83888 -99-3

2633 Pediatric Examination of Educational Readiness
Educators Publishing Service
625 Mount Auburn Street
3rd Floor
Cambridge, MA 2139- 3039 617-547-6706
800-225-5750
FAX: 888-440-2665
feedback@epsbooks.com
www.epsbooks.com

Charles H Heinle, VP
Alexandra S Bigelow, Author
Gunnar Voltz, President
Assesses the Pre-1st grade child's performance on twenty-nine tasks in six specific areas of development: orientation, gross-motor, visual-fine motor, sequential, linguistic and preacademic learning. The child is rated on ten dimensions of selective attention/activity processing efficiency and adaptation. Complete set.
$12.85 - $86.40
ISBN 0-83888 -80-1

2634 Pediatric Extended Examination at-PEET Three
Educators Publishing Service
625 Mount Auburn Street
3rd Floor
Cambridge, MA 2138- 3039 617-547-6706
800-225-5750
FAX: 888-440-2665
feedback@epsbooks.com
www.epsbooks.com

Charles H Heinle, VP
Alexandra S Bigelow, Author
Gunnar Volta, President
Assesses the preschool-age child's performance on twenty-eight tasks in five basic areas of development: gross-motor, language, visual-fine motor, memory, and intersensory integration. Complete set.
$13.75 - $126
ISBN 0-83888 -79-4

2635 Pre-Reading Screening Procedures
Educators Publishing Service
625 Mount Auburn Street
3rd Floor
Cambridge, MA 2138- 3039 617-547-6706
800-225-5750
FAX: 888-440-2665
feedback@epsbooks.com
www.epsbooks.com

Charles H Heinle, VP
Alexandra S Bigelow, Author
Gunnar Voltz, President
This revised group test, for grades K-1, evaluates auditory, visual and kinesthetic strengths in order to identify children who may have some form of dyslexia or specific language disability. *$18.00*
Grades K-1
ISBN 0-83885 -23-4

2636 Preparing for ACT Assessment
American College Testing Program
500 Act Drive
PO Box 168
Iowa City, IA 52243-168 319-337-1000
FAX: 319-339-3021
act.org

Richard L Ferguson, CEO
Designed to help high school students ready themselves for the ACT Assessment's subject area tests, explains the purposes of the four tests, describes their content and format, provides tips and exercises to improve student's test-taking skills and includes a complete sample text with scoring key.

2637 Psycho-Educational Assessment of Preschool Children
National Association of School Psychologists
Ste 105
4340 East West Hwy
Bethesda, MD 20814-4468 301-657-0270
866-331-NASP
FAX: 301-657-0275
ADMIN@SOELIN.COM
soelin.com

Susan Gorin, Executive Director
This is a contributed text on assessing specific skills of preschool children.
592 pages

2638 RULES: Revised
Speech Bin
PO Box 1579
Appleton, VA 54912-1579 772-770-0007
888-388-3224
FAX: 888-388-6344
customercare@schoolspecialty.com
www.speechbin.com

Jan J Binney, Senior Editor
Treatment program for young children who have phonological disorders. *$43.95*
280 pages
ISBN 0-93785 -51-3

2639 Receptive-Expressive Emergent-REEL-2 Language Test, 2nd Edition
Sage Publications
2455 Teller Road
Thousand Oaks, CA 91320 805-499-9774
800-818-7243
FAX: 800-583-2665
info@sagepub.com
www.sagepub.com

Paul Kelly, National Textbook Sales Manager
Blaise R Simqu, President & CEO
A revision of the popular scale used for the multidimensional analysis of emergent language. The REEL-2 is specifically designed for use with a broad range of at risk infants and toddlers in the new multidisciplinary programs developing under P.L. 99-457. *$79.00*

2640 Regents' Center for Learning Disorders
103 Hooper Street
Athens, GA 30602 706-542-4589
FAX: 706-583-0001
rcld@uga.edu
rcld.uga.edu

Tasha Falkingham, Office Manage
Karen Myers, Budget Analyst
Trish Foels, Staff Clinician, Psychologist
Lisa McLain, Staff Clinician
Provide assessment, training, research, andresources related to students who have learning disorders (e.g., Attention-Deficit/Hyperactivity Disorder, Autism Spectrum Disorders, Learning Disabilities, Emotional Disorders, and Traumatic Brain Injury) that impact their functioning in the academic environment.

2641 Schmieding Developmental Center
519 Latham Drive
Lowell, AR 72745
479-750-0125
FAX: 479-750-0323
www.archildrens.org

Mary Ann Scott, PhD, Program Director
Damon Lipinski, PhD, Program Director
Jerie Beth Karkos, MD, Medical Director
Arkansas Children's Hospital (ACH) is the a pediatric medical center in Arkansas.

2642 Slingerland Screening Tests
Educators Publishing Service
625 Mount Auburn Street
3rd Floor
Cambridge, MA 2138- 3039
617-547-6706
800-435-7728
FAX: 888-440-2665
feedback@epsbooks.com
www.epsbooks.com

Charles H Heinle, VP
Alexandra S Bigelow, Author
Gunnar Voltz, President
These tests, by Beth Slingerland, for individuals or groups of children, grades 1-6, identify children who show indications of having specific language disability in reading, handwriting, spelling or speaking. Form D evaluates personal orientation in time and space as well as the ability to express ideas in writing.
$14.80 - $27.45
ISBN 0-83882 -02-2

2643 Special Needs Advocacy Resource Book
Prufrock Press
PO Box 8813
Waco, TX 76714-8813
800-998-2208
FAX: 800-240-0333
info@prufrock.com
www.prufrock.com

Joel McIntosh, Publisher & Marketing Director
Rich Weinfield, Author
Michelle Davis, Author
Subtitle: What You Can Do Now to Advocate for Your Exceptional Child's Education. This is a unique hadnbook that teaches parents how to work with schools to achieve optimal learning situations and accommodations for their child's needs. *$19.95*
328 pages
ISBN 1-593633-09-7

2644 Speech Bin
PO Box 1579
Appleton, VA 54912-1579
772-770-0007
888-388-3224
FAX: 888-388-6344
customercare@schoolspecialty.com
www.speechbin.com

Jan J Binney, Senior Editor
Catalog offering test materials, assessment information, books and special education resources for speech-language pathologists, occupational and physical therapists, audiologists, and other rehabilitation professionals in schools, hospitals, clinics and private practices.

ISSN 4773-324

2645 Stuttering Severity Instrument for Children and Adults
Psychological & Educational Publications
P.O.Box 520
Hydesville, CA 95547-520
707-768-1807
800-523-5775
FAX: 800-447-0907
psych-edpublications@cox.net
www.psych-edpublications.com

Morrison Gardner, President
With this tool teachers can determine whether to schedule a child for therapy or to evaluate the effects of treatment.

2646 Taking Part: Introducing Social Skills to Young Children
AGS
P.O.Box 99
Circle Pines, MN 55014-99
800-328-2560
FAX: 800-471-8457
agsmail@agsnet.com
www.agsnet.com

Kevin Brueggeman, President
Robert Zaske, Market Manager
The first social skills curriculum to be linked directly to an assessment tool. More than 30 lessons correlate with the skills assessed by the Social Skills Rating System, a multirater approach to assessing prosocial and problem behaviors. *$149.95*

2647 Teaching of Reading: A Continuum from Kindergarten through College, The
AVKO Educational Research Foundation
3084 Willard Rd
Birch Run, MI 48415-9404
810-686-9283
866-285-6612
FAX: 810-686-1101
webmaster@avko.org
avko.org

Don Mc Cabe, Executive Director
A textbook for teaching teachers how to teach language arts with lessons about dyslexia, phonics, learning to write, the connection between reading and spelling, and diagnostic and prescriptive tests. Free as an e-book for Foundation members. *$49.95*
364 pages

2648 Test Critiques: Volumes I-X
Sage Publications
2455 Teller Road
Thousand Oaks, CA 91320
805-499-9774
800-818-7243
FAX: 800-583-2665
info@sagepub.com
www.sagepub.com

Paul Kelly, National Textbook Sales Manager
Blaise R Simqu, President & CEO
Provides the professional and nonprofessional with in-depth, evaluative studies of more than 800 of the most widely used of these assessment instruments. *$649.00*

2649 Test of Early Reading Ability Deaf or Hard of Hearing
Pro- Ed Publications
8700 Shoal Creek Blvd
Austin, TX 78757-6816
512-451-3246
800-897-3202
FAX: 800-397-7633
general@proedinc.com
www.proedinc.com

Donald D Hammill, Owner
Courtney King, Marketing Coordinator
This adaptation of the TERA-2 for simultaneous communication of American Sign Language is the ONLY individually administered test of reading designed for children with moderate to profound sensory hearing loss. *$169.00*
Complete Kit

2650 Test of Language Development: Primary
Sage Publications
2455 Teller Road
Thousand Oaks, CA 91320
805-499-9774
800-818-7243
FAX: 800-583-2665
info@sagepub.com
www.sagepub.com

Paul Kelly, National Textbook Sales Manager
Blaise R Simqu, President & CEO
TOLD P:2 and TOLD 1:2 are the most popular tests of spoken language used by clinicians today. They are used to identify children who have language disorders and to isolate the particular types of disorders they have. Primary Edition for ages 1-4 to 8-11: Intermediate Edition for ages 8-6 to 12-11.

2651 Test of Mathematical Abilities, 2nd Edition
Sage Publications
2455 Teller Road
Thousand Oaks, CA 91320
805-499-9774
800-818-7243
FAX: 800-583-2665
info@sagepub.com
www.sagepub.com

Paul Kelly, National Textbook Sales Manager
Blaise R Simqu, President & CEO
The latest version was developed for use in grades 3 through 12. It measures math performance on the two traditional major skill areas in math as well as attitude, vocabulary and general application of math concepts in real life. *$84.00*

2652 Test of Nonverbal Intelligence, 3rd Edition
Sage Publications
2455 Teller Road
Thousand Oaks, CA 91320
805-499-9774
800-818-7243
FAX: 800-583-2665
info@sagepub.com
www.sagepub.com

Paul Kelly, National Textbook Sales Manager
Blaise R Simqu, President & CEO
A language-free measure of intelligence, aptitude and reasoning. The administration of the test requires no reading, writing, speaking or listening on the part of the test subject. The items included in this test are problem-solving tasks that increase in difficulty. Each item presents a set of figures in which one or more components is missing. The test items include one or more of the characteristics of shape, position, direction, rotation, contiguity, shading, size, movement or pattern. *$229.00*
Complete Kit

2653 Test of Phonological Awareness
Sage Publications
2455 Teller Road
Thousand Oaks, CA 91320
805-499-9774
800-818-7243
FAX: 800-583-2665
info@sagepub.com
www.sagepub.com

Paul Kelly, National Textbook Sales Manager
Blaise R Simqu, President & CEO
Measures young children's awareness of the individual sounds in words. Children who are sensitive to the phonological structure of words in oral language have a much easier time learning to read than children who are not. *$143.00*

2654 Test of Written Spelling, 3rd Edition
Pro- Ed Publications
8700 Shoal Creek Blvd
Austin, TX 78757-6897
512-451-3246
800-897-3202
FAX: 800-397-7633
general@proedinc.com
www.proedinc.com

Donald D Hammill, Owner
Courtney King, Marketing Coordinator
This revised edition assesses the student's ability to spell words whose spellings are readily predictable in sound-letter patterns, words whose spellings are less predictable and both types of words considered together. *$74.00*

2655 Texas Scottish Rite Hospital for Children
2222 Welborn Street
Dallas, TX 75219
214-559-5000
FAX: 800-421-1121
tsrhdv@tsrh.org
www.tsrhc.org

Robert L. Walker, President/ CEO
Mark G. Bateman, SVP, Public Relations
Leslie A. Clonch, Jr., Vice President/ CIO
Stephanie Brigger, Vice President, Development
TSRHC treats children with orthopedic conditions, such as scoliosis, clubfoot, hand disorders, hip disorders and limb length differences, as well as certain related neurological disorders and learning disorders, such as dyslexia.

2656 Treatment and Learning Centers
2092 Gaither Road
Suite 100
Rockville, MD 20850
301-424-5200
FAX: 301-424-8063
TTY:301-424-5203
info@ttlc.org
www.ttlc.org

Dr Lisa Lenhart, Tutoring/Testing Services Dir
Diagnostic evaluations are provided on an individual basis to identify the learning differences and needs of students who may have learning disabilities, or who are struggling with the academic environment.

2657 Woodcock Reading Mastery Tests
Pearson
5601 Green Valley Dr
Bloomington, MN 55437-1099
800-627-7271
FAX: 800-232-1223
pearsonassessments@pearson.com
www.pearsonassessments.com

Christine Carlson, Product Manager
Doug Kubach, President & CEO
The Woodcock Reading Mastery Tests - Revised provides an interpretive system and age range to help you assess reading skills of children and adults. Two forms, G and II, make it easy to test and retest, or you can combine the results of both forms for a more comprehensive assessment. Revised with recent updates. *$329.95*

2658 Young Children with Special Needs: A Developmentally Appropriate Approach
Allyn & Bacon
75 Arlington Street
Ste 300
Boston, MA 2116-3988
617-848-7500
800-852-8024
FAX: 617-944-7273
www.ablongman.com

Bill Barke, CEO
Thomas Longman, Founder
This book is designed to prepare students in making curriculum decisions in order to care for and foster the development of young children with special needs in normal early childhood settings.
270 pages
ISBN 0-20518 -94-X

Treatment & Training

2659 ABLE Program MCC-Longview
3200 Broadway
Kansas City, MO 64111-2105
816-604-1000
FAX: 816-672-2719
joan.bergstrom@mcckc.edu
mcckc.edu/ABLE

Joan Bergstrom, Director
Kay Owens, Administrative Assistant
Intensive support services program for post secondary students with neurological disabilities. The ABLE Program can be reached at http://mcckc.edu/ABLE

2660 Academy for Guided Imagery
30765 Pacific Coast Hwy
Ste 355
Malibu, CA 90265-3643
800-726-2070
FAX: 800-727-2070
info@acadgi.com
www.acadgi.com

David E Bresler, President
The Academy aims to teach people to access and use the power of the mind/body connection for healing, and to further understand-

ing of the imagery process in human life and development. They provide systematic training and guidance to health professionals who are interested in the use of Guided Imagery in their practice. The Academy's Imagery Store offers guided imagery CDs, DVDs and books for self-healing.

2661 Adventist HealthCare
820 West Diamond Avenue
Suite 600
Gaithersburg, MD 20878
301-315-3030
FAX: 301-315-3000
www.adventisthealthcare.com

David E. Weigley, M.B.A., Chairman
Robert T. Vandeman, Vice-Chair
Terry Forde, Secretary
dventist HealthCare, based in Gaithersburg, Md., is a not-for-profit organization of dedicated professionals who work together to provide excellent wellness, disease management and health-care services to the community.

2662 Asthma & Allergy Education for Worksite Clinicians
Asthma and Allergy Foundation of America
8201 Corporate Drive
Suite 1000
Landover, VA 20785
202-466-7643
800-727-8462
FAX: 202-466-8940
info@aafa.org
aafa.org

Bill Mc Lin, President & CEO
Helen Taylor, Information Specialist
Developed to teach health professionals in the worksite about asthma and allergies and ultimately improve the health of the employees who have theses de\iseases. The program gives worksite clinicians the knowledge and tools they need to give employees guidance on how to control environmental factors both in the home and in the workplace, self-manage thier asthma and/or allergies and to determaine if ti is necessary for employees to see an allergist if symptoms persist.

2663 Asthma & Allergy Essentials for Children's Care Provider
Asthma and Allergy Foundation of America
8201 Corporate Drive
Suite 1000
Landover, VA 20785
202-466-7643
800-727-8462
FAX: 202-466-8940
info@aafa.org
aafa.org

Bill Mc Lin, President & CEO
Helen Taylor, Information Specialist
Course gives child care providers the tools and knowledge they need to care for children with asthma and allergies. During the interactive, three hour program, a trained health professional teaches providers how to recognize the signs and symptoms of an asthma or allergy episode, how to institute environmental control measures to prevent these episodes, and how to properly use medication and the tools for asthma management. In areas of the country serviced by AAFA's 14 chapters.

2664 Asthma Care Training for Kids (ACT)
Asthma and Allergy Foundation of America
8201 Corporate Drive
Suite 1000
Landover, VA 20785
202-466-7643
FAX: 202-466-8940
info@aafa.org
www.aafa.org

Bill Mc Lin, President & CEO
Helen Taylor, Information Specialist
Interactive program for children ages seven to 12 and their families. Children and their families attend three group sessions seperately to learn their own unique styles and then come together at the end of each session to share their knowledge.

2665 Ayurvedic Institute
PO Box 23445
Albuquerque, NM 87292-1445
505-291-9698
800-863-7721
FAX: 505-294-7572
registrar@ayurveds.com
ayurveda.com

Wynn Werner, Administrator
Directed by Dr. Vasant Lad, trains people in Ayurveda.

2666 Brooks Rehabilitation Hospital
3599 University Blvd S
Jacksonville, FL 32216
904-345-7600
FAX: 904-345-7619
www.brookshealth.org

Gary W. Sneed, Chairman
Michael Spigel, President/ COO
Douglas M. Baer, Chief Executive Officer
Bruce M. Johnson, Vice-Chair
Brooks Rehabilitation provides the most advanced therapy and medical care.

2667 Center for Parent Information and Resources
35 Halsey St.
Fourth Floor
Newark, NJ 7102
malizo@spannj.org
www.parentcenterhub.org

Myriam Alizo, Project Assistant
Debra Jennings, Project Director
Lisa K▢pper, Product Development Coordinator
Idira Medina, Coordinator
The Center for Parent Information and Resources (CPIR) serves as a central resource of information and products to the community of Parent Training Information (PTI) Centers and the Community Parent Resource Centers (CPRCs), so that they can focus their efforts on serving families of children with disabilities.

2668 Center for Spinal Cord Injury Recovery
261 Mack
Detroit, MI 48201
866-724-2368
FAX: 313-745-9064
krodgers@dmc.org
www.centerforscirecovery.org

Krystal Rodgers, Administrative Assistant
The Center for SCI Recoveryr (CSCIR)provides long-term, high intensity, non-traditional, activity based therapy to maximize recovery.

2669 Cottage Rehabilitation Hospital
400 W. Pueblo Street
Santa Barbara, CA 93105
805-682-7111
mzate@sbch.org
www.cottagehealth.org

2670 Courage Kenny Rehabilitation Institute
800 E. 28th St.
Minneapolis, MN 55407
612-863-4200
866-880-3550
couragekenny@allina.com
www.couragecenter.org

2671 Harriet & Robert Heilbrunn Guild School
JGB Audio Library for the Blind
15 W 65th St
New York, NY 10023-6601
212-769-6200
800-284-4422
FAX: 212-769-6266
info@JGB.org
www.JGB.org

Allen R Morse, JD, PhD, President & CEO
Ken Stanley, Manager
A Jewish Guild for the blind.

2672 Howard School, The
1192 Foster St NW
Atlanta, GA 30318-4329 404-377-7436
FAX: 404-377-0884
admissions@howardschool.org
howardschool.org
Marifred Cilella, Head Of School
The Howard School educates students 5 years old through 12th grade with language learning disabilities and learning differences. Small student/teacher ratios allow for instruction that is personalized to complement the individual learning styles and to help each student understand his/her learning process. Students gain the tools and strategies needed to become independent, life-long learners.

2673 Kennedy Krieger Institute
707 North Broadway
Baltimore, MD 21205 443-923-9200
800-873-3377
888-554-2080
www.kennedykrieger.org
Jennifer Accardo, M.D., Neurologist
Adrianna Amari, Ph.D., Training & Research Coordinator
Roberta L. Babbitt, Ph.D, Program Director
Amy J. Bastian, Ph.D., P.T., Chief Science Officer
Kennedy Krieger Institute is an internationally recognized institution dedicated to improving the lives of children and young adults with pediatric developmental disabilities and disorders of the brain, spinal cord and musculoskeletal system, through patient care, special education, research, and professional training.

2674 Kessler Rehabilitation Corporation
1199 Pleasant Valley Way
West Orange, NJ 7052 973-731-3600
FAX: 973-243-6819
www.kessler-rehab.com
Robert Brehm, President
Bruce M. Gans, MD, Executive VP and CMO
Sue Kida, PT, MHA, VP and COO
Steven Kirshblum, MD, Medical Director
Provides physical medicine and rehabilitation by delivering an exceptional patient experience through the integration of quality care, technology, education, research, and advocacy.

2675 Lake Michigan Academy
West Michigan Learning Disabilities Foundation
2428 Burton St SE
Grand Rapids, MI 49546-4806 616-464-3330
FAX: 616-285-1935
info@wmldf.org
www.wmldf.org
Amy Barto, Executive Director
Is a private day school for children with learning disabilities.

2676 Levinson Medical Center
98 Cutter Mill Road
Suite 90
Great Neck, NY 11021 516-482-2888
800-334-7323
FAX: 516-482-2480
drlevinson@aol.com
www.dyslexiaonline.com
Dr. Harold Levinson, Psychiatrist, Neurologist
Carolyn Malman, Office Manager
Lisa Danziger, Patient Coordinator
Dr. Margaret , Neurological Test & Evaluations
Medical center groundbreaking medical treatment offers rapid and often dramatic help to suffering dyslexic/ADHD children and adults

2677 Mad Hatters: Theatre That Makes a World of Difference
P.O.Box 50002
Kalamazoo, MI 49005-2
FAX: 269-385-5868
Bobbe A Luce, Executive Director
A nationally-known theater which has presented effective and innovative programs to more than 175,000 people in over 1,150 performances in the past 15 years. Our presentations and training programs are a proven method of changing attitudes and behaviors. The Mad Hatters is a leader in the field of sensitivity training to build community and foster the inclusion of all people in society. Fees: $500-$4000 per program, depending on topic and audience.

2678 MedStar National Rehabilitation Network
102 Irving Street NW
Washington, DC 20010 202-877-1000
www.medstarnrh.org

2679 Missouri Rehabilitation Center
One Hospital Drive
Columbia, MO 65212 573-882-4141
www.muhealth.org

2680 Neuroxcel
401 Northlake Blvd.
North Palm Beach, FL 33048
866-391-6247
www.neuroxcel.com

2681 Ramapo Training
Ramapo for Children
Route 52/Salisbury Turnpike
PO Box 266
Rhinebeck, NY 12572 845-876-8403
FAX: 845-876-8414
office@ramapoforchildren.org
www.ramapoforchildren.org
Richard Rosenthal, President
Teri Goldberg Horowitz, First Vice President
Claude Ann Mellins, Ph.D., Vice President
Deusdedi Merced, Esq., Vice President
Ramapo Training was established to provide staff training and program support for educational and recreational programs, especially those that serve children-at-risk and those with special needs.

2682 Sandhills School
1500 Hallbrook Dr
Columbia, SC 29209-4021 803-695-1400
FAX: 803-695-1214
info@sandhillsschool.org
www.sandhillsschool.org
Anne Vickers, Head of School
Erika Senneseth, Asst Head of School
Angela Daniel, Director of Development
Carmen Kennedy, Business Manager
Exists to provide educational programs and intellectual development for average to above average students, six to 15, who learn differently and to promote the development of self-awareness, joy in learning and a vision of themselves as life-long learners.

2683 Senior Program for Teens and Young Adults with Special Needs
Camp J CC
6125 Montrose Rd
Rockville, MD 20852-4860 301-881-0100
FAX: 301-881-6549
jcccamp@jccgw.org
www.jccgw.org
Scott Cohen, President
Mindy Burger, Vice President for Development
The senior Program is a transitional program for teens and young adults with mental retardation, severe learning disabilities and multiple disabilities. Socialization, recreation and independent living skills are enhanced ina fun enviroment. Activities include art, music, recreational swim and more.

2684 Spinal Cord Injury Center
132 S. 10th Street
375 Main Building
Philadelphia, PA 19107   215-955-6579
                                      FAX: 215-955-5152
                                www.spinalcordcenter.org
Marilyn P. Owens, RN, BSN, Project Coordinator
Brittany Hayes, Research Coordinator
Jacqueline Robinson, Administrative Assistant
Susan Sakers Sammartino, BS, Data Coordinator
SCI provides medical care for their injuries, along with emotional, social, vocational and psychological rehabilitation to cope with the changes in their bodies and in their lifestyles that often result from the injury.

2685 Stanford Health Care
300 Pasteur Drive
Stanford, CA 94304   650-498-3333
                                         800-756-9000
                                  stanfordhealthcare.org
Amir Dan Rubin, President and CEO
Raj Behal, MD, Chief Quality Officer
James Hereford, Chief Operating Officer
Daniel J. Morissette, Chief Financial Officer
Stanford Health Care provides patients with the very best in diagnosis and treatment.

2686 Teacher of Students with Visual Impairments
3635 Coal Mountain Rd.
Cumming, GA 30028
                  c.willings@teachingvisuallyimpaired.com
                      www.teachingvisuallyimpaired.com

2687 The Glenholme School
Devereux Advanced Behavioral Health Connecticut
81 Sabbaday Ln.
Washington, CT 06793   860-868-7377
                                      FAX: 860-868-7894
                        info@theglenholmeschool.org
                          www.theglenholmeschool.org

2688 UAB Spain Rehabilitation Center
1720 2nd Ave South
Birmingham, AL 35294   205-934-4011
                                     TTY:205-934-4642
                                          www.uab.edu
Ray L. Watts, M.D., President
G. Allen Bolton Jr., VP, Financial Affairs
UAB's missionis to be a research university and academic health center that discovers, teaches and applies knowledge for the intellectual, cultural, social and economic benefit of Birmingham, the state and beyond.

2689 University of Maryland Rehabilitation andOrthopaedic Institute
Uni of MD Rehab & Ortho Institute
2200 Kernan Drive
Baltimore, MD 21207   410-448-2500
                                         888-453-7626
                                    TTY:800-735-2258
                                   www.umrehabortho.org
Cynthia A. Kelleher, MPH, MBA, Interim President and CEO
John P. Straumanis, VP, Medical Affairs
W. Walter Augustin, III, CPA, VP of Financial Services
Cheryl D. Lee, RN, MSN, CRRN, VP, Patient Care Services
University of Maryland Rehabilitation & Orthopaedic Institute (formerly Kernan Hospital), a committed provider of orthopaedic surgery and the largest inpatient rehabilitation hospital and provider of rehabilitation services in the state of Maryland, has been serving the Baltimore community for over 100 years.

2690 Vanguard School, The
Valley Forge Specialized Educational Services
1777 N Valley Rd
Paoli, PA 19301   610-296-6700
                                      FAX: 610-640-0132
                          info@vanguardschool_pa.org
                           www.vanguardschool-pa.org
Tim Lanshe, Director of Education
James Kirkpatrick, CFO
Peg Osborne, Admissions Director
An Approved Private School (APS) for students aged 4-21 years with exceptionalities including autism spectrum disorder, mild emotional disturbances and/or neurological impairments.

2691 Worthmore Academy
3535 Kessler Boulevard East Dr
Indianapolis, IN 46220-5154   317-902-9896
                                        877-700-6516
                                     FAX: 317-251-6516
                       bjackson@worthmoreacademy.org
                          www.worthmoreacademy.org
Brenda Jackson, Director
Alyssa Blaire Cook, Assistant Director
A place where children with learning disabilities receive individualized instruction to help remediate his or her condition. The most common learning disabilities we work with are Dyslexic, A.D.D, A.D.H.D, Autism Spectrum (including Asperger's Syndrome), and communication disorders.

Exchange Programs

General

2692 A Guide to International Educational Exchange
Mobility International USA
132 E. Broadway
Suite 343
Eugene, OR 97401-2767

541-343-1284
FAX: 541-343-6812
info@miusa.org
www.miusa.org

Susan Sygall, CEO
A Guide to International Educational Exchange, Community Service and Travel for People with Disabilities includes information travel and international programs, as well as personal experience stories from people with disabilities who have had successful international experiences. *$45.00*
600 pages
ISBN 1-880034-24-7

2693 American Institute for Foreign Study
River Plaza 9 W Broad St
Stamford, CT 6902-3788

203-399-5000
866-906-2437
FAX: 203-399-5590
info@aifs.com
www.aifs.com

William L Gertz, CEO
Organizes cultural exchange programs throughout the world for more than 50,000 students each year and arranges insurance coverage for our own participants as well as participants of other organizations. Also provides summer travel programs overseas and in the US ranging from one week to a full academic year.

2694 American Universities International Programs
307 S College Ave
Fort Collins, CO 80524-2801

970-495-0084
888-730-2847
FAX: 970-495-0114
info@auip.com
www.auip.com

Laurie Klith, Executive Director
Study abroad organization sending students to universities in Australia and New Zealand.

2695 American-Scandinavian Foundation
58 Park Ave
38 Street
New York, NY 10016-3007

212-779-3587
FAX: 212-686-1157
info@amscan.org
scandinaviahouse.org

Edward Gallagher, President
Promotes international understanding through educational and cultural exchange between the United States and Denmark, Finland, Iceland, Norway and Sweden.

2696 Antioch College
One Morgan Place
Yellow Springs, OH 45387-1635

937-319-6082
FAX: 937-319-6085
aea@antioch-college.edu
www.antioch-college.edu

Mark Roosevelt, President
Thomas Brookley, CFO & COO
Gariot Louima, Chief Communications Officer
Education abroad offers numerous programs which can be included in undergraduate and graduate study programs.

2697 Army and Air Force Exchange Services
PO Box 660202
Dallas, TX 75266-202

214-312-2011
800-527-2345
FAX: 800-446-0163
TTY: 800-423-2011
www.aafes.com

James Moore, Senior VP
MG Bruce Casella, Commander/CEO
Brings a tradition of value, service, and support to its 11.5 million authorized customers at military installations in the United States, Europe and in the Pacific.

2698 Association for International Practical Training
10400 Little Patuxent Pkwy
Suite 250
Columbia, MD 21044-3519

410-997-2200
FAX: 410-992-3924
aipt@aipt.org
aipt.org

Elizabeth Chazottes, CEO
Nonprofit organization dedicated to encouraging and facilitating the exchange of qualified individuals between the US and other countries so they may gain practical work experience and improve international understanding.

2699 Basic Facts on Study Abroad
International Education
809 United Nations Plz
New York, NY 10017-3503

212-883-8200
FAX: 212-984-5452
publications@un.org
iie.org

Allen E Goodman, CEO
Peggy Blumenthal, Executive Vice President
Information book including foreign study planning, educational choices, finances and study abroad programs. *$35.00*
30 pages

2700 Beaver College
Arcadia University
450 S Easton Rd
Glenside, PA 19038-3215

215-572-2901
888-232-8379
FAX: 215-572-2174
cea@beaver.edu
www.beaver.edu/cea

Lorna Stern, Deputy Director
One of the largest college-based study abroad programs in the country. Prices from $8000.00 semester to $22000.00 a year.

2701 Buffalo State (SUNY)
1300 Elmwood Ave
South Wing 410
Buffalo, NY 14222-1095

716-878-4620
FAX: 716-878-3054
intleduc@buffalostate.edu
www.buffalostate.edu/studyabroad

Lee Ann Grace, Asst Dean Int'l/Exchange Program
Provides international educational exchange opportunities for students of university age and older through its Office of International Education.

2702 Building Bridges: Including People with Disabilities in International Programs
Mobility International USA
132 E Broadway
Suite 343
Eugene, OR 97401-3155

541-343-1284
FAX: 541-343-6812
info@miusa.org
miusa.org

Susan Sygall, CEO
Michele Scheib, Project Specialist
Melissa Mitchell, Public Relations Coordinator
Empowers people with disabilities around the world through international exhange and international development to achieve

their human rights. The international exchange programs usually last two-four weeks and are held throughout the year in the US and abroad. Activities include living with homestay families, leadership seminars, disability rights workshops, cross cultural learning and teambuilding activities such as river rafting and challenging courses.

2703 Davidson College, Office of Study Abroad
Davidson College
PO Box 7171
Davidson, NC 28035-7171
704-894-2000
FAX: 704-894-2005
kocampbell@davidson.edu
www3.davidson.edu

Carol Quillen, President
Recognizes the value of study abroad for both the devlopment of worl understanding and the development of the student as a broadminded, objective and mature individual.

2704 High School Students Guide to Study, Travel, and Adventure Abroad
300 Fore Street
Portland, ME 4101
207-553-4000
FAX: 207-553-4299
contact@ciee.org
www.ciee.org

Robert E. Fallon, CEO & President
Kenton Keith, Senior Vice President for Progra
This guide provides high school students with all the information they need for a successful trip abroad. Included are sections to help students find out if they're ready for a trip abroad, make the necessary preparations and get the most from their experience. Over 200 programs are described including language study, summer camps, homestays, study tours and work camps. The program descriptions include information for people with disabilities.

ISSN 0312-11

2705 International Christian Youth Exchange
134 W 26th St
New York, NY 10001-6803
212-206-7307
FAX: 212-633-9085

Ed Gragert
Offers participants a unique experience to learn about another culture and make friends from different countries.

2706 International Partnership for Service-Learning and Leadership
1515 SW 5th Avenue
Suite 606
Portland, OR 97201
503-954-1812
FAX: 503-954-1881
info@ipsl.org
ipsl.org

Nevin Brown, President
A not for profit educational organization incorporated in New York State serving students, colleges, universities, service agenices and related organizations around the world by fostering programs that link volunteer service to the community and academic study.

2707 International Student Exchange Programs (I SEP)
1655 N Fort Myer Drive
Suite 400
Arlington, VA 22209
703-504-9960
FAX: 703-243-8070
info@isep.org
www.isep.org

Dr. Thomas Hochstettler, Chair
Dr. Tony Atwater, President
ISEP is a network of 275 post-secondary institutions in the United States and 38 other countries cooperating to provide affordable international educational experiences for a diverse student population.

2708 International University Partnerships
University of Pennsylvania
1011 South Dr
Indiana, PA 15705-1046
724-357-2100
FAX: 724-357-6213
iup.edu

David Werner, President
Offers a variety of international educational exchange programs to students who wish to study overseas.

2709 Lake Erie College
391 W. Washington St.
Painesville, OH 44077
440-296-1856
800-533-4996
FAX: 440-375-7005
admissions@lec.edu
www.lec.edu

Michael Victor, President
Michael Keresman lll, Director
Sends students abroad for a term or longer to develop intellectual awareness and individual maturity.

2710 Lane Community College
4000 E 30th Ave
Eugene, OR 97405-640
541-463-3000
FAX: 541-463-5201
asklane@lanecc.edu
www.lanecc.edu

Mary Spilde, President
Lane Community Colloege offers a wide variety of instructional programs including transfer credit programs, career and technical degree and certificate programs, continuing education noncredit courses, programs in English as a Second Language and International ESL, GED programs, and customized training for local businesses.

2711 Lions Clubs International
300 W 22nd St
Oak Brook, IL 60523-8842
630-571-5466
FAX: 630-571-8890
lions@lionsclub.org
www.lionsclubs.org

Joe Preston, International President
Jitsuhiro Yamada, First Vice President
Robert E. Corlew, Second Vice President
Eric R. Carter, First Year Directors
Over 46,000 individual clubs in over 194 countries and geographical areas which provide community service and promote better international relations. Clubs work with local communities to provide needed and useful programs for sight, diabetes and hearing, and aid in study abroad.

2712 Lisle
900 County Road 269
Leander, TX 78641-1633
512-259-4404
lisle2@io.com
www.lisle.utoledo.edu

Barbara E Bratton, Owner
Educational organization which works toward world peace and better quality of human life through increased understanding between persons of similar and different cultures.

2713 National 4-H Council
7100 Connecticut Ave
Chevy Chase, MD 20815-4934
301-961-2800
FAX: 301-961-2894
www.4-h.org

Donald Floyd, President
Jennifer Sirangelo, Executive Vice President
4-H opened the door for young people to learn leadership skills and explore ways to give back. 4-H revolutionized how youth connected to practical, hands-on learning experiences while outside of the classroom.

2714 New Directions for People with Disabilities
5276 Hollister Avenue
Suite 207
Santa Barbara, CA 93111-3068   805-967-2841
                                       888-967-2841
                              FAX: 805-964-7344
                        hello@newdirectionstravel.org
                        www.newdirectionstravel.org

Dee Duncan, Executive Director
Jeanne Mohle, Director of Operations
Danna Mead, Program Director
Colette Piacentini, Business Manager
Provides high quality local, national, and international travel vacations and holiday programs for people with mild to moderate developmental disabilities. Through these programs, people with disabilities are increasingly understood, appreciated and more accepted as important and contributing members of our world.

2715 People to People International
911 Main Street
Suite 2110
Kansas City, MO 64105-2246   816-531-4701
                              FAX: 816-561-7502
                                    ptpi@ptpi.org
                                    www.ptpi.org

Mary Eisenhower, CEO
Roseanne Rosen, Senior Vice President of Operati
Brian Hueben, Senior Director, Administration
Stacey Chance, Director, Publications
Exchanges international understanding and friendship through educational, cultural and humantarian activities involving the exchange of ideas and experiences directly among people of different countries and diverse cultures. Is also dedicated to enhancing cross cultural communication within each communityand across communities and nations.

2716 Rotary Youth Exchange
Rotary International
1560 Sherman Ave
Evanston, IL 60201-4818   847-866-3000
                                   866-976-8279
                              FAX: 847-328-4101
                        youthexchange@rotary.org
                               www.rotary.org

Kalyan Banerjee, International President
Noel A Bajat, Vice President
Kenneth R Boyd, Director
Elizabeth Demaray, Director
This worldwide organization of business and professional leaders provides humanitarian service, encourages high ethical standards in all vocations, and helps build goodwill and peace in the world. Approximately 1.2 million Rotarians belong to more than 31,000 Rotary clubs located in 167 countries for exchange opportunities.

2717 Scandinavian Exchange
24 Dickinson Street
Amherst, MA 1002   413-253-9737
                     FAX: 413-253-5282
                 howery@scandinavianseminar.org
                 www.scandinavianseminar.org

Jacqueline D Waldman, CEO
William Kaufmann, Chair
Student exchange program founded in 1949.

2718 Sister Cities International
915 15th Street, NW
4th Floor
Washington, DC 20005   202-347-8630
                         FAX: 202-393-6524
                            info@sister-cities.org
                               sister-cities.org

Patrick Madden, President
Jim Doumas, Executive Vice President, & Inte
A non profit citizen diplomacy network creating and strengthening partnerships between US and international communities in an effort to increase global cooperation at the municipal level, to promote cultural understnading and to stimulate economic development. Encourages local community development and volunteer action by motivating and empowering private citizens, municipal officials and business leaders to conduct long term programs of mutual benefits including exchange situations.

2719 State University of New York
1400 Washington Ave
Albany, NY 12222-100   518-442-3300
                          FAX: 518-442-5383
                          ugadmissions@albany.edu
                               www.albany.edu

George Philip, President
Alain Kaloyeros, Senior Vice President & CEO
Susan Phillips, Provost & VP for Academic Affai
James Dias, VP for Research
Offers over 150 international educational exchange programs in 37 different countries. Broad mission of excellence in undergraduate and graduate education, research and public service engages 17,000 diverse students in nine schools and colleges across three campuses.

2720 University of Minnesota at Crookston
2900 University Ave
Crookston, MN 56716-5000   218-281-6510
                                    800-862-6466
                              FAX: 218-281-8050
                               UMCinfo@umn.edu
                               www.crk.umn.edu

Charles Casey, CEO
Eric Kaler, President
The University of Minnesota, Crookston (UMC) is a public, baccalaureate, coeducational institution and a coordinate campus of the University of Minnesota

2721 University of Oregon
5000 N Willamette Blvd
Portland, OR 97203-5798   503-943-8000
                            FAX: 503-725-3067
                                webmaster@up.edu
                                         up.edu

Patricia Esley, Manager
Rev.E.Willia Beauchamp, President
James Lyons, VP University Relations
Jim Ravelli, VP for University Research
Study/cultural experience is available in Tokyo and other Japanese cities as part of the Japan Studies Program at the University.

2722 Western Washington University
516 High St
Bellingham, WA 98225-5996   360-650-3000
                              FAX: 360-650-3022
                                   www.wwu.edu

Bruce Shepard, President
Paul Dunn, Senior Executive Asst. to the Pr
Barbara Stoneberg, Assistant to the President
Mary Lacher, Receptionist, President & Provis

2723 World Experience Teenage Exchange Program
2440 S Hacienda Blvd
Suite 116
Hacienda Heights, CA 91745-4763   626-330-5719
                                            800-633-6653
                                       FAX: 626-333-4914
                                    info@worldexperience.org
                                       worldexperience.org

Kerry Gonzales, President
Marge Archaumbault, President
Offers a quality and affordable program for over two decades and continues to provide students and host families a youth exchange program based on individual attention, with the help of an international network of overseas directors and USA coordinators.

2724   World of Options
Mobility International USA
132 E Broadway
Suite 343
Eugene, OR 97401-3155

541-343-1284
FAX: 541-343-6812
info@miusa.org
miusa.org

Susan Sygall, CEO
Cerise Roth-Vinson, COO
Susan Dunn, Executive Asst. to the CEO
Alison Eker, Project Assistant

Empowering people with disabilities around the world through international exchange and international development to achieve their human rights. *$16.00*

338 pages
ISBN 1-880034-01-8

2725   Youth for Understanding International Exchange
6400 Goldsboro Road
Suite 100
Bethesda, MD 20817-5841

240-235-2100
800-833-6243
FAX: 240-352-2104
admissions@yfu.org
yfu.org

Rachel Andreson, Founder
Samantha Brizzolara, Chair

Youth for Understanding (YFU) International Exchange, an educational, nonprofit organization, prepares young people for the opportunities and responsabilities in a changing, independent world. With YFU, students can choose a year, semenster, or summer program in one or more than 35 countries worldwide. More than 200,000 young people from more than 50 nations in Asia, Europe, North and South America, Africa and the Pacific have participated in YFU exchanges.

Foundations & Funding Resources

Alabama

2726 Alabama Power Foundation
PO Box 2641
Birmingham, AL 35291-11
205-257-2508
800-245-2244
FAX: 205-257-1860
rsking@southernco.com
powerofgood.com

John O. Hudson III, President
Richard King, Director of Charitable Giving
Alisa Summerville, Manager of Charitable Giving
Kim Thrift, Program Manager
Honoring its mission to strengthen the communities the company serves, the foundation focuses its efforts on organizations that support education, civic activities, health services, the environment and the arts. By supporting the state's educational system ☐ from pre-K to universities ☐ the foundation is investing in Alabama's future and the well-being of its residents.

2727 Andalusia Health Services
700 River Falls Street
PO Box 667
Andalusia, AL 36420
334-222-2030
FAX: 334-222-7844
chrissie@andalusiachamber.com
www.andalusiachamber.com

Janna McGlamory, President
Debbie Marcum, Vice President
Ashley Eiland, Executive Vice President
Gail Hayes, Treasurer
Only offers grants to the residents of Covington County in Alabama who are pursuing a degree in a medical field.

2728 Arc Of Alabama, The
557 S Lawrence St
Montgomery, AL 36104-4611
334-262-7688
866-243-9557
FAX: 334-834-9737
info@thearcofAl.org
www.thearcofal.org/#!contact/c1d94

Larry Bailey, President
Sherron Culpepper, 1st Vice President
Bruce Koppenhoeffer, 2nd Vice President
Jack Knight, Treasurer
The Arc of Alabama, Inc. is a volunteer-based membership organization made up of individuals with intellectual (such as mental retardation, an old and outdated term seldom used anymore), developmental and other disabilities, their families, friends, interested citizens, and professionals in the disability field.

Alaska

2729 Arc of Alaska
The Arc of Anchorage
2211 Arca Dr
Anchorage, AK 99508-3462
907-277-6677
800-258-2232
FAX: 907-272-2161
TTY: 907-277-0735
info@thearcofanchorage.org
www.thearcofanchorage.com

Rod Shipley, President
Dave Falsey, Vice President
Meredith Parham, Secretary
Sharon Purkis, Treasurer
The Arc helps Alaskans who experience developmental disabilities, behavioral health concerns or deafness achieve lives of dignity and independence as valued members of our community.

2730 Rasmuson Foundation
301 West Northern Lights Blvd.
Suite 400
Anchorage, AK 99503
907-297-2700
877-366-2700
FAX: 907-297-2770
rasmusonfdn@rasmuson.org
www.rasmuson.org

Edward B. Rasmuson, Chairman
Cathryn Rasmuson, Vice Chair
Diane Kaplan, President & CEO
Chris Perez, Program Officer
The Rasmuson Foundation invests both in individuals and well managed organizations dedicated to improving the quality of life for Alaskans.

Arizona

2731 Arizona Autism Resources
The Arc of Arizona
PO Box 90714
Phoenix, AZ 85066
602-234-2721
800-433-5255
FAX: 602-234-5959
arc@arcarizona.org
www.arcarizona.org

Robert Snyder, President
Michael Leyva, Vice President
Jon Meyers, Executive Director
Kim Dorshaw, Secretary
The Arc, a national organization on mental retardaion, is committed to securing for all people with developmental disabilities the opportunity to choose and realize their goals in regard to where they live, learn, work and play.

2732 Arizona Community Foundation
2201 E Camelback Road
Suite 405B
Phoenix, AZ 85016
602-381-1400
800-222-8221
FAX: 602-381-1575
info@azfoundation.org
www.azfoundation.org

Ron Butler, Chair
Shelly Cohn, Vice Chair
Steven G. Seleznow, President & CEO
John Gogolak, Treasurer
The mission of the Arizona Community Foundation is to empower and align philanthropic interests with community needs and build a legacy of living.

2733 Arizona Instructional Resource Center for Students who are Blind or Visually Impaired, The
Foundation For Blind Children
1235 E. Harmont Drive
Phoenix, AZ 85020
602-678-5800
800-322-4870
FAX: 602-678-5819
mashton@SeeItOurWay.org
www.seeitourway.org

Dee Nortman, CFO
Marc Ashton, Chief Executive Officer
Barbra Smith, Chief of Staff
Alexander Pushman, Director, Mark & Dev
The Foundation for Blind Children contracts with the Arizona Department of Education to provide statewide media services for students between pre-kindergarten and 12th grade who have a visual impairment or are blind andEneed their instructional materials in a specialized medium such as braille, large print, or electronic files as well as adaptive equipment.

2734 Margaret T Morris Foundation
PO Box 592
Prescott, AZ 86302-592
928-445-6633
FAX: 928-445-6633
www.archive.naccho.org

Susan Rheem, Executive Director

Arkansas

2735 Arc of Arkansas
2004 Main St
Little Rock, AR 72206-1526
501-375-7770
FAX: 501-372-4621
shitt@arcark.org
www.arcark.org

Willie Jones, President
Steve Hitt, Chief Executive Officer
Roger Williams, Chief Financial Officer
Cynthia Stone, Chief Operating Officer
Serving people with disabilites and their families for over forty years.

2736 Winthrop Rockefeller Foundation
225 East Markham Street
Suite 200
Little Rock, AR 72201
501-376-6854
FAX: 501-374-4797
webfeedback@wrfoundation.org
www.wrfoundation.org

Phillip N. Baldwin, Chair
David Rainey, Ed.D., Vice chair
Sherece Y. West-Scantlebury, Ph.D, President & CEO
Andrea M. Dobson, CPA, COO & CFO
Mission is to improve the quality of life in Arkansas. It focuses its grantmaking efforts in three areas: education, economic development and civic affairs. Education projects funded in the past have included grants to schools that are working to involve teachers and parents in making decisions about what happens at their schools, projects that work to remove prejudice from the educational process and more. Major grants are made to support the development of new programs.

California

2737 Ahmanson Foundation
9215 Wilshire Blvd
Beverly Hills, CA 90210
310-278-0770
info@theahmansonfoundation.org
www.theahmansonfoundation.org

William H. Ahmanson, President
Karen Ahmanson Hoffman, Managing Director & Secretary
Kristen K. O'Connor, CFO & Treasurer
Jennie H. Chin, Senior Accountant
The Foundation primarily gives in Southern California with major emphasis in Los Angeles County. The Foundation focuses on the arts and humanities, education, mental health and support for a broad range of social welfare programs.

2738 Alice Tweed Touhy Foundation
205 E Carrillo Street
Suite 219
Santa Barbara, CA 93101-7186
805-962-6430

Jeanne Mc Kay, Manager
Rehabilitation, recreation and building funds are given to organizations only within the Santa Barbara area.

2739 Alternating Hemiplegia of Childhood Foundation
2000 Town Center
Suite 1900
Livonia, MI 48075
313-663-7772
FAX: 313-733-8987
sharon@ahckids.org
www.ahckids.org

Lynn Egan, President
Gene Andrasco, Vice President
Vicky Platt, Development Chair
Mollie Erpenbeck, Major Giving Officer
Voluntary not-for-profit organizations dedicated to promoting professional and public awareness of Alternating Hemiplegia of Childhood (AHC) and providing current information to affected individuals and their families. Supports ongoing medical research into the cause, treatment and potential cure of AHC. Disseminates information about this disorder to promote proper diagnosis and maintains a registry of families, affected chidren and physicians who are familiar with AHC.

2740 Arc of California
1225 8th Street
Suite 350
Sacramento, CA 95815
916-552-6619
800-698-6619
FAX: 916-441-3494
arcca@arccalifornia.org
www.thearcca.org

Tony Anderson, Executive Director
Richard Fitzmaurice, President
Betsy Katz, Secretary
Bruce MacKenzie, Treasurer
Advocates for people with intellectual and all developmental disabilities since 1953. The ARC of California is committed to securing for all people with developmental disabilities, in partnership with thier families, legal guardians or conservators the opportunity to choose and realize their goals of where and how they learn, live, work and play.

2741 Atkinson Foundation
1660 Bush Street
Suite 300
San Mateo, CA 94109
415-561-6540
FAX: 650-357-1101
sangeles@pfs-llc.net
www.atkinsonfdn.org

Elizabeth Curtis, Administrator
Stacey Angels, Grants Manager
The Foundation focuses and awards grants to community service and civic organizations serving the residents of San Mateo County, California through programs that benefit children, youth, seniors, the disadvantaged and those in need of rehabilitation. Grants are also made to local churches and schools, and overseas for sustainable development, health education and family planning. No grants to individuals or for research, travel, special events, annual campaigns, media and publications.

2742 Baker Commodities Corporate Giving Program
4020 Bandini Blvd
Vernon, CA 90058
323-268-2801
FAX: 323-268-5166
info@bakercommodities.com
www.bakercommodities.com

Jim Andreoli, President
Baker Commodities has been one of the nation's leading providers of rendering, and grease removal services. Baker Commodities, Inc. is a completely sustainable company, recycling animal by-products and kitchen waste into valuable products that can be used to feed livestock, power vehicles, and act as a base for everyday items.

2743 Bank of America Foundation
315 Montgomery St
Fl 8
San Francisco, CA 94104-1803
415-622-8248
888-488-9802
FAX: 704-386-6444
www.bankamerica.com/foundation
Ilana Orin, Manager
The Foundation will consider grants in four categories including: Health & Human Services, which provides support to health & human service organizations primarily through grants to the United Way campaigns; Education, with the focus on preparing people to become productive employees and participating citizens; Conservation & Environment, the improvement of California communities for the benefit of their citizens; and Culture & The Arts, supporting the leading performing and visual arts groups.

2744 Blind Babies Foundation
1814 Franklin Street
Suite 300
Oakland, CA 94612
510-446-2229
FAX: 510-446-2262
bbfinfo@blindbabies.org
www.blindbabies.org
Dottie Bridge, President
Sharon Sacks, PhD, 1st Vice President
Clare Friedman, PhD, 2nd Vice President
Deborah Orel-Bixler, PhD, OD, Secretary
Founded in 1949, the foundation provides home-based early intervention services to families with young children with vision impairment in the Northern and Central regions of California.

2745 Bothin Foundation
1660 Bush Street
Suite 300
San Francisco, CA 94109
415-561-6540
FAX: 415-561-6477
ccasey@pfs-llc.net
www.pfs-llc.net/bothin/index.html
Lyman H. Casey, President
A. Michael Casey, Vice President & Treasurer
Devon Laycox, Vice President
Charlie Casey, Program Officer
The Bothin Foundation makes grants for capital, building, and equipment needs to organizations providing direct services to low-income, at risk children, youth and families, the elderly, and the disabled in San Francisco, Marin, Sonoma, and San Mateo counties.

2746 Briggs Foundation
1969 Lancewood Ln
Carlsbad, CA 92009-6826
760-704-6481
FAX: 760-704-6483
Blaine A Briggs, President
Private non-operating foundation.

2747 Burns-Dunphy Foundation
5 3rd Street
Suite 528
San Francisco, CA 94103-3213
415-421-6995
FAX: 415-882-7774
Walter Gleason
Cressey Nakagawa
Grants are given to promote wellness for the visually impaired, physically and mentally disabled and to promote research in these areas.

2748 California Community Foundation
221 S. Figueroa Street
Suite 400
Los Angeles, CA 90012
213-413-4130
FAX: 213-383-2046
info@ccf-la.org
www.calfund.org
Cynthia A. Telles, Chairman
Antonia Hernandez, President & CEO
John E. Kobara, EVP & COO
Stephen J. Cobb, VP & CFO
Areas of funding priority include grants for the disabled, child welfare, rehabilitation, developmentally disabled, employment projects, research and computer projects. Giving is limited to the greater Los Angeles area.

2749 California Endowment
1000 N Alameda St
Los Angeles, CA 90012
213-628-1001
800-449-4149
FAX: 213-703-4193
questions@calendow.org
www.calendow.org
Zac Guevara, Vice Chair
Robert Ross, President & CEO
Martha Jimenez, EVP/ Counsel
Anthony Iton, SVP
California Endowment's mission is to expand access to affordable, quality health care for underserved individuals and communities, and to promote fundamental improvements in the health status of all Californians.

2750 Carrie Estelle Doheny Foundation
707 Wilshire Boulevard
Suite 4960
Los Angeles, CA 90017
213-488-1122
FAX: 213-488-1544
doheny@dohenyfoundation.org
www.dohenyfoundation.org
Robert A. Smith, III, President
Nina Shepherd, CAO/ CFO
Pam Thomas, Grants Administrator
Lisa Rogers, Grants Administrator
The Foundation primarily funds local, not-for-profit organizations endeavoring to advance education, medicine and religion, to improve the health and welfare of the sick, aged, incapacitated, and to aid the needy.

2751 Coeta and Donald Barker Foundation
3740 Cahuenga Blvd
Studio City, CA 91604
760-340-1162
818-980-3630
FAX: 818-980-2709
info@scga.org
www.scga.org
Nancy Harris, President
Kevin Heaney, Executive Director
Andrea Fredlin, Admin Asst., Club Services
Evan Belfi, Asst. Director, Marketing
It is an independent organization that gives its attention to organizations that are charitable or nonprofit under the laws of the state of Oregon or California.

2752 Crescent Porter Hale Foundation
1660 Bush Street
Suite 300
San Francisco, CA 94109
415-561-6540
FAX: 415-561-5477
evalentine@pfs-llc.net
www.crescentporterhale.org
E. William Swanson, President
Sr. Estela Morales, MSW, Vice President
Eunice Valentine, Executive Director
Patricia Fata, Secretary/Treasurer
Serves organizations in the San Francisco Bay Area who are involved in the following areas of concern: education in the fields of art and music; private elementary, high school and university education; capital funding; and other worthwhile programs

which can be demonstrated as serving broad community purposes, leading toward the improvement of the quality of life.

2753   David and Lucile Packard Foundation
343 Second Street
Los Altos, CA 94022   650-917-7142
                                              FAX: 650-948-5793
                                    communications@packard.org
                                               www.packard.org

Susan Packard Orr, Chairman
Julie E. Packard, Vice Chairman
Nancy Packard Burnett, Vice Chairman
Carol S Larson, President & CEO
This foundation provides grants to nonprofit organizations in the following areas: conservation; population; science; children, familes, and communities; arts and organizational effectiveness; and philanthropy. It provides national and international grants and also has a special focus on the Northern California Counties.

2754   Deutsch Foundation
5454 Beethoven St
Los Angeles, CA 90066   310-862-3000
                                                   877-340-7700
                                              FAX: 310-862-3100
                                                   deutschinc.com

Linda Sawyer, Chairman
Kim Getty, President, North America
Val Difebo, CEO, Deutsch NY
Mike Sheldon, CEO, North America
Learning disabled, visually impaired, mental health, eye research, child welfare, speech and hearing impaired, physically disabled and independence projects are funded through this Foundation. Giving is limited to California.

2755   East Bay Community Foundation
De Domenico Building
200 Frank H Ogawa Plaza
Oakland, CA 94612   510-836-3223
                                              FAX: 510-836-7418
                                           jwhead@eastbaycf.org
                                                  www.ebcf.org

Sherry M. Hirota, Chair
Ingrid Lamirault, Vice Chair
Peter Garcia, Vice Chair
James W. Head, President & CEO
A collection of funds created by many people, organizations and businesses, the Foundation helps those people and groups to support effective nonprofit organizations to the East Bay and beyond.

2756   Evelyn and Walter Hans JrHaas Jr
114 Sansome Street
Suite 600
San Francisco, CA 94104   415-856-1400
                                              FAX: 415-856-1500
                                                  www.haasjr.org

Walter J. Haas, Chair
Ira S. Hirschfield, President & Trustee
Michael Blake, VP of Finance
Robert D. Haas, Treasurer
A private foundation interested in programs which assist people who are hungry, homeless, or at risk of homelessness; enable older adults to maintain independent lives in the community and support Hispanic community development in San Francisco's Mission District. The Foundation also encourages proposals for corporate social responsibility efforts within the business community.

2757   Family Caregiver Alliance
785 Market St.
Suite 750
San Francisco, CA 94103   415-434-3388
                                                   800-445-8106
                                              FAX: 415-434-3508
                                               info@caregiver.org
                                               www.caregiver.org

Ping Hao, MBA, President
Jacquelyn Kung, Vice President
Kathleen Kelly,MPA, Executive Director
Deborah Wolter, Secetary
To improve the quality of life for caregivers and those they care for through information, services, and advocacy.

2758   Financial Aid for the Disabled and Their Families
Reference Service Press
2310 Homestead Rd.
Suite C1 #219
Los Altos, CA 94024   650-861-3170
                                              FAX: 650-861-3171
                                            info@rspfunding.com
                                              www.rspfunding.com

Gail Schlachter, President
R David Weber, Editor-in-Chief
Mike Fields, Database and Website Manager
Sandy Perez, Online and Print Sales
This directory, which Children's Bookwatch calls invaluable describes more than 1,100 financial aid opportunities available to support persons with disabilities and members of their families. Updated ever 2 years. *$39.50*
300 pages
ISBN 1-588410-31-5

2759   Firemans Fund Foundation
Firemans Fund Insurance Companies
777 San Marin Dr
Novato, CA 94998   415-899-2000
                                                   800-227-1700
                                              FAX: 415-899-3600
                                         customerrelations@ffic.com
                                             www.firemansfund.com

Lori Dickerson Fouche, President & CEO
Jill Paterson, Chief Financial Officer
Eleanor Barnard, Chief Distribution & Sales
Sally Narey, Chief Counsel, Corp. Secretary
Provides discretionary grants to the disabled only in Marin and Sonoma counties in the San Francisco Bay area.

2760   Fred Gellert Foundation
1038 Redwood Highway
Building B, Suite 2
Mill Valley, CA 94941   415-381-7575
                                              FAX: 415-381-8526
                                           patty@fgffoundation.com
                              foundationcenter.org/grantmaker/fredgellert/

Fred Gellert, Founder
Patty Oday, Administrator
Focuses on organizations and programs serving residents of San Mateo and San Francisco and Marin counties in California, with the exception of environmentally concerned organizations.

2761   Gallo Foundation
P.O. Box 1130
Modesto, CA 95353-1130   209-579-3204
                                                   877-687-9463
                                              FAX: 209-341-3307
                                                  www.ejgallo.com

John Gallo, Senior VP Operations
Physically and mentally disabled, child welfare, Special Olympics, United Cerebral Palsy and Easter Seal Society are among the grants provided by this foundation.

2762   Glaucoma Research Foundation
251 Post Street
Suite 600
San Francisco, CA 94108   415-986-3162
                                           800-826-6693
                                    FAX: 415-986-3763
                              question@glaucoma.org
                                   www.glaucoma.org

Andrew Iwach, MD, Board Chair
Robert L. Stamper, MD, Vice Chair
Thomas M. Brunner, President/CEO
Fred H. Brinkmann, Treasurer
A national organization dedicated to protecting the sight of people with glaucoma through research and education. The Foundation conducts and supports research that contributes to improved patient care and a better understanding of the disease process. Provides education, advocacy and emotional support to patients and their families.

2763   Harden Foundation
1636 Ercia Street
Salinas, CA 93906   831-442-3005
                                    FAX: 831-443-1429
                              joe@hardenfoundation.org
                                www.hardenfoundation.org

Patricia Tynan Chapman, President
C. Bill Elliott, Vice President/Treasurer
Joseph C. Grainger, Executive Director
Linda Taylor, Secretary
Founded to assist charitable organizations in the Salinas Valley.

2764   Henry J Kaiser Family Foundation
2400 Sand Hill Rd
Menlo Park, CA 94025-6941   650-854-9400
                                    FAX: 650-854-4800
                                          www.kff.org

Drew Altman, President/CEO
Gary Claxton, Vice President
Esther Dicks, Vice President
Mollyann Brodie, SVP for Executive Operations
A non-profit, private operating foundation focusing on the major health care issues facing the US, with a growing role in global health. Kaiser develops and runs its own research and communications programs, sometimes in partnership with other non-profit research organizations or major media companies.

2765   Henry W Bull Foundation
Santa Barbara Bank & Trust
P.O. Box 2340
Santa Barbara, CA 93120   202-720-7871
                                    FAX: 805-884-1404
                              info@coreprojects.com
                          www.activistfacts.com/about/

Janice Gibbons, VP/Senior Trust Officer
Grant given to a wide range of organizations that include those which provide services for the disabled; arts, education, services for elderly and youth grants awarded two times a year. Grant size ranges from $500 to $5,000. Proposal deadlines April 1, Sept 1.

2766   Irvine Health Foundation
18301 Von Karman Avenue
Suite 440
Irvine, CA 92612-0120   949-253-2959
                                    FAX: 949-253-2962
                                          info@ihf.org
                                          www.ihf.org

Timothy L. Strader, Sr., Chairman
Carol Mentor McDermott, Vice Chairman
Edward B. Kacic, President
Ptricia A. Meredith, VP, Administration & Programs
Mission is to improve the physical, mental and emotional well-being of all Orange County residents.

2767   Joseph Drown Foundation
1999 Avenue of the Stars
Suite 2330
Los Angeles, CA 90067   310-277-4488
                                    FAX: 310-277-4573
                                    staff@jdrown.org
                                      www.jdrown.org

Norman C Obrow, President
Giving is focused primarily in California. No support for religious purposes or to individuals. Goal is to assist individuals in becoming successful, self-sustaining, contributing citizens.

2768   Junior Blind of America
5300 Angeles Vista Blvd
Los Angeles, CA 90043   323-295-4555
                                           800-352-2290
                                    FAX: 323-296-0424
                              info@juniorblind.org
                                   www.juniorblind.org

Harold A. Davidson, DBA, Chair
Robert D. Held, Vice Chair
Miki Jordan, President/CEO
Scott Farkas, Treasurer
Junior Blind provides programs and services for children and adults who are blind or visually impaired and their families to achieve independence and self-esteem. Programs include; Camp Bloomfield, Visions: Adventures in Learning, Infant-Family Program, Early Childhood Program, Special Education School, Children's Residential Program, Davidson Program for Independence, and Student Transition and Enrichment Program, Vision Screening and After School enrichment.

2769   Kenneth T and Eileen L Norris Foundation
11 Golden Shore
Suite 450
Long Beach, CA 90802   562-435-8444
                                    FAX: 562-436-0584
                                    grants@ktn.org
                               www.norrisfoundation.org

Lisa D Hanson, Chairman
Ronald R Barnes, Executive Director & Trustee
Walter J Zanino, Controller
William G Corey, Medical Advisor
The Foundation is primarily focused on medicine and education. To a lesser extent the foundation contributes to community programs including visually impaired, autism, mentally and physically disabled, deaf and mental health in the Southern California area. Average grant size in this area is $5,000-$10,000. Grants are also given in the area of culture and youth.

2770   Koret Foundation
33 New Montgomery Street
Suite 1090
San Francisco, CA 94105-4526   415-882-7740
                                    FAX: 415-882-7775
                              info@koretfoundation.org
                                www.koretfoundation.org

Susan Koret, Board Chair
Anita L. Friedman, President
Michael J. Boskin, President
Jeffery A. Farber, CEO
Koret seeks to fund outstanding examples of innovative approaches to community challenges and opportunities.

2771   LA84 Foundation
2141 W Adams Blvd
Los Angeles, CA 90018   323-730-4600
                                    FAX: 323-730-9637
                                        info@la84.org
                                          www.la84.org

Frank M. Sanchez, Chair
Anita L. DeFrantz, President
F. Patrick Escobar, VP, Grants & Programs
Robert Wagner, Vice President, Partnerships
The LA84 Foundation was established to manage Southern California's share of the surplus from the highly successful 1984 Olympic Games in Los Angeles and offers sports programs, a premier sports library and meeting facilities. The foundation cur-

rently serves two million youth in eight Southern California counties.

2772 LJ Skaggs and Mary C Skaggs Foundation
1221 Broadway
21st Floor
Oakland, CA 94612-1837   510-451-3300
                                     FAX: 510-451-1527
                                     skaggs@fablaw.com
                                     www.skaggs.org

Philip M Jelley, President
Jayne C Davis, Vice President
Robert N Janopaul, Director
Joseph W Martin, Jr., Secretary, Treasurer
The Foundation presently makes grants under four program categories: performing arts, social concerns, projects of historic interest and special projects.

2773 LK Whittier Foundation
Whittier Trust Company Foundations Office
1600 Huntington Dr
S Pasadena, CA 91030   626-441-5111
                                     FAX: 626-441-0420
                                     hrdept@whittiertrust.com
                                     www.whittiertrust.com
Michael J Casey, Chairman & CEO
David A. Dahl, President
James A. Jeffs, Managing Dir.
Andrew S. Gabo, Director
Giving is primarily offered to preselected organizations. No grants are given to individuals.

2774 Legler Benbough Foundation
2550 Fifth Avenue
Suite 132
San Diego, CA 92103   619-235-8099
                                     FAX: 619-235-8077
                                     peter@benboughfoundation.org
                                     www.benbough.org
Peter K. Elsworth, President
John G. Rebelo, Jr., Treasurer
Nbob Kelly, Director
Peter K. Ellsworth, Director
The mission of the foundation is to improve the quality of life of the people of San Diego. The foundation focuses on three target areas for funding, one in the area of providing economic opportunity, one in the area of enhancing cultural opportunity, and one that provides focus for health, education and welfare funding.

2775 Levi Strauss Foundation
1155 Battery St
San Francisco, CA 94111-1264   415-501-7208
                                     800-872-5384
                                     FAX: 415-544-3490
                                     www.levistrauss.com/levi-strauss-foundation
Chip Bergh, President & CEO
Roy Bagattini, EVP/President
Lisa Collier, EVP/President
James Curleigh, EVP/President
Has a funding initiative to support organizations which provide services for people with AIDS, and/or educational programs which help prevent the further spread of the HIV virus. The Foundation will assist in the development and enhancement of such services only in those communities where Levi Strauss & Co. has plants and distribution centers.

2776 Louis R Lurie Foundation
555 California Street
Suite 5100
San Francisco, CA 94104-1707   415-392-2470
                                     FAX: 415-421-8669
                                     www.foundationcenter.org/grantmaker/lurie
Nancy Terry, Foundation Administrator
Visually impaired, hard-of-hearing and physically disabled in the San Francisco Bay Area and Metropolitan Chicago areas only.

2777 Luke B Hancock Foundation
360 Bryant St
Palo Alto, CA 94301-1409   650-321-5536
                                     FAX: 650-321-0697
Ruth Ramel, Director
Has concentrated its resources over the past year on programs which provide job training and employment for at-risk youth. Consortium funding with other foundations in areas where there is unmet need; emergency and transitional funding; and selected funding for music education. .

2778 Marin Community Foundation
5 Hamilton Landing
Suite 200
Novato, CA 94949   415-464-2500
                                     FAX: 415-464-2555
                                     info@marincf.org
                                     www.marincf.org
Cleveland Justis, Chair
Thomas Peters, Ph.D., President & CEO
Sid Hartman, CFO/COO
Aileen Sweeney, VP Of Finance
Mission is to encourage and apply philanthropic contributions to help improve the human condition, embrace diversity, promote a humane and democratic society, and enhance the communities quality of life, now and for future generations.

2779 Mary A Crocker Trust
57 Post Street
Suite 610
San Francisco, CA 94104-5023   650-576-3384
                                     FAX: 415-982-0141
                                     staff@mactrust.org
                                     www.mactrust.org

2780 National Center on Caregiving at Family Caregiver Alliance (FCA)
785 Market Street
Suite 750
San Francisco, CA 94103   415-434-3388
                                     800-445-8106
                                     FAX: 415-434-3508
                                     info@caregiver.org
                                     www.caregiver.org
Ping Hao, MBA, President
Jacquelyn Kung, Vice President
Kathleen Kelly, MPA, Executive Director
Jeff Kumataka, CPA, MBA, Treasurer
FCA offers programs at national, state and local levels to support and sustain caregivers. The National Center on Caregiving (NCC) program works to advance the development of high-quality, cost-effective policies and programs for caregivers in every state of the country. Uniting research, public policy and services, the NCC serves as a central source of information on caregiving and long term care issues for policy makers, service providers, media, funders and family caregivers.

2781 National Foundation of Wheelchair Tennis
940 Calle Amanecer
Suite B
San Clemente, CA 92673-6218   714-361-3663
                                     FAX: 714-361-6603
                                     nfwt@aol.com
                                     www.nfwt.org
Bill Butler
Founded in January of 1980, the intention of this foundation is to assist the newly physically disabled individual to realize his full potential in society by enhancing his esteem, independence productivity and physical capabilities regardless of age, sex, creed or disability extent.

2782 Parker Foundation
2604-B El Camino Real
Suite 244
Carlsbad, CA 92008
760-720-0630
FAX: 760-720-1239
mail@theparkerfoundation.org
www.theparkerfoundation.org

Judy McDonald, President
Gordon Swanson, Vice President
Ann Davies, Secretary
Raymond Ellis, Treasurer
The assets are directed to projects which will contribute to the betterment of any aspect of the people of San Diego County, California and solely to entities which, among other things, are organized exclusively for charitable purposes and are operating in San Diego County, California.

2783 Pasadena Foundation
301 East Colorado Boulevard
Suite 810
Pasadena, CA 91101-2824
626-796-2097
FAX: 626-583-4738
pcfstaff@pasadenacf.org
www.pasadenacf.org

David M. Davis, Chair
Judy Gain, Vice Chair
Jennifer Fleming DeVoll, Executive Director
Mariver Copeland, Director of Finance
The mission of the Pasadena Foundation is to improve the quality of life for citizens of the Pasadena area through support of nonprofit organizations that provide services beneficial to the community.

2784 RC Baker Foundation
P.O. Box 6150
Orange, CA 92863-6150
714-750-8987

F L Scott, Manager
Established in 1952, for general philanthropic purposes. The bulk of assistance and support has been to religious, scientific, educational institutions and youth organizations.

2785 Ralph M Parsons Foundation
888 West Sixth Street
Suite 700
Los Angeles, CA 90017
213-362-7600
FAX: 213-482-8878
www.rmpf.org

James A. Thomas, Chairman
Elizabeth Lowe, Vice Chairman
Wendy Garen, President & CEO
Astra Anderson Galang, CFO
The Foundation is concerned with the encouragement and support of projects and programs deemed beneficial to mankind in several major areas of interest such as: education; social impact; civic and cultural; health and special products. Only funds in Los Angeles County.

2786 Robert Ellis Simon Foundation
312 S Canyon View Drive
Los Angeles, CA 90049-3812
310-275-7335

Joan Willens
Mental health and visually impaired grants are the main concerns of this organization.

2787 San Francisco Foundation
One Embarcadero Cente
Suite 1400
San Francisco, CA 94111
415-733-8500
FAX: 415-477-2783
info@sff.org
www.sff.org

Sandra R Hernandez, CEO
Nick Hodges, VP for Philanthropic Services
Bobbie Chapman, Director of Business Development
Shona Carter, Donor Relations Officer

The Foundation's purpose is to improve life, promote greater equality of opportunity and assist those in need or at risk in the San Francisco Bay Area. The Foundation strives to protect and enhance the unique resources of the Bay Area, committed to equality of opportunity for all and the elimination of any injustice, seeks to enhance human dignity and seeks to establish mutual trust, respect and communication among the Foundation.

2788 Santa Barbara Foundation
1111 Chapala Street
Suite 200
Santa Barbara, CA 93101
805-963-1873
FAX: 805-966-2345
info@sbfoundation.org
www.sbfoundation.org

Eileen Sheridan, Chair
James Morouse, Vice Chair
Ronald Gallo, President & CEO
Maria Caudillo, Exec. Asst. to President & CEO
The Foundations mission is to enrich the lives of the people of Santa Barbara County through philanthropy. The Foundation awards grants to nonprofits within the County in the areas of education, health, human services, personal development, cluture, recreation, community enhancement and environment. No support is given to individuals except through student aid.

2789 Sidney Stern Memorial Trust
860 Via de la Paz
PO Box 457
Pacific Palisades, CA 90272
310-459-2117
info@sidneysternmemorialtrust.org
www.sidneysternmemorialtrust.org

Betty Hoffenberg, Director
A Southern California-based foundation providing grants to nonprofit organizations for various projects. The foundation gives priority to the following areas of interest: education, health and science, community service projects, youth, services to the mentally and emotionally disabled, the arts, organizations and activities serving California. The Board prefers to make contributions to organizations that use the funds directly in the furtherance of their charitable and public purposes.

2790 Sierra Health Foundation
1321 Garden Hwy
Sacramento, CA 95833
916-922-4755
FAX: 916-922-4024
info@sierrahealth.org
www.sierrahealth.org

Jose Hermocillo, Chair
David W. Gordon, Vice Chair
Chet P. Hewitt, President & CEO
Gil Alvarado, VP of Administration/CFO
The Foundation strives to establish a collaborative relationship with its grantees, and with other funders and foundations, through an open dialogue. The Foundation approaches each grant as a partnership, with opportunities for the grantee and grantor to work cooperatively to enhance the effectiveness of the grant project.

2791 Silicon Valley Community Foundation
2400 West El Camino Real
Suite 300
Mountain View, CA 94040-1498
650-450-5400
FAX: 650-450-5401
info@siliconvalleycf.org
www.siliconvalleycf.org

C.S. Parker, Chair
Samuel Johnson,Jr., Vice Chair
Emmitt D. Carson, Ph.D, President & CEO
George Dallas, Administrative Asst.
Serving all of San Mateo & Santa Clara counties, Silicon Valley Foundation has more than $1.5B in assets under management and 1500 philanthropic funds. The community provides grants through donor advised and corporate funds in addition to its own Community Endowment Fund. In addition, the community foundation serves as a regional center for philanthropy, providing donors simple and effective ways to give locally & globally.

2792 Sonora Area Foundation
362 S Stewart Street
Sonora, CA 95370
209-533-2596
FAX: 209-533-2412
edwyllie@sonora-area.org
www.sonora-area.org

Jim Johnson, President SAF
Roger Francis, Vice President
Edward B. Wyllie, Executive Director
Lin Freer, Program Manager
The Sonora Area Foundation strengthens its community through assisting donors, making grants, and providing leadership.

2793 Stella B Gross Charitable Trust C/O Bank of The West Trust Department
PO Box 1121
San Jose, CA 95108-1121
408-947-5203
gpadilla@bankofthewest.com

Gabe Padilla, Trust Admin
Organization must be federal and state tax-exempt and reside within the bounds of Santa Clara County, California to be eligible.

2794 Teichert Foundation
3500 American River Dr
Sacramento, CA 95864
916-484-3011
FAX: 916-484-6506
www.teichert.com

Frederick Teichert, LHD, Executive Director
Awards grants to community organizations and provides employee matching grants. Teichert Foundation expresses the companie's commitment to build and preserve a healthy and prosperous region.

2795 WM Keck Foundation
550 South Hope Street
Suite 2500
Los Angeles, CA 90071- 2617
213-680-3833
FAX: 213-614-0934
info@wmkeck.org
www.wmkeck.org

Allison Keller, Executive Director & CFO
Maria Pellegrini, Ph.D, Executive Director of Programs
Thomas Everhart, Ph.D, Senior Scientific Advisor
Matesh Varma, Ph.D, Senior Program Director
Created to support accredited colleges and universities with particular emphasis on the sciences, engineering and medical research. The Foundation also maintains a Southern California Grant Program that provides support for non-profit organizations in the field of civic and community services, health care, precollegiate education and the arts.

2796 Willam G Gilmore Foundation
1660 Bush Street
Suite 300
San Francisco, CA 94109
415-561-0650
FAX: 415-561-5477
www.pfs-llc.net/gilmore/index.html

William N Hancock, Owner

Colorado

2797 AV Hunter Trust
650 South Cherry Street
Suite 535
Glendale, CO 80246- 1897
303-399-5450
FAX: 303-399-5499
afreeman@pfs-llc.net
www.avhuntertrust.org

Mary K. Anstine, President
George C. Gibson, Vice President
Barbara L. Howie, Executive Director
Jessica Sutton, Grants Manager
Donated nearly $50 million to nonprofit organizations serving those who captured Mr. Hunter's attention and sparked his compassion. Trust gives aid, comfort, support, or assistance to children or aged people or indigent adults.

2798 Adolph Coors Foundation
215 St. Paul Street
Suite 300
Denver, CO 80206
303-388-1636
FAX: 303-388-1684
generalinfo@acoorsfdn.org
www.coorsfoundation.org

John W. Jackson, Executive Director
Jeanne L. Bistranin, Senior Program Officer
Carrie C. Tynan, Program Officer
Carol S. Strathman, Financial/Special Projects Coord
Applicant organizations must be classified as 501 and must operate within the United States. The areas covered by the Foundation are health, education, youth, community services, civic and cultural and public affairs.

2799 Arc of Colorado
1580 Logan Street
Suite 730
Denver, CO 80203
303-864-9334
800-333-7690
FAX: 303-864-9330
mrymer@thearcofco.org
www.thearcofco.org

Randy Patrick, President
Tonna Kelly, Vice President
Marijo Rymer, Executive Director
Lynnelle Zackroff, Secretary
A private not-for-profit, membership-based, grassroots association. The Arc of Colorado is the state office whith local units located in various areas throughout the state.

2800 Bonfils-Stanton Foundation
Daniels and Fisher Tower
1601 Arapahoe Street
Suite 500
Denver, CO 80202
303-825-3774
FAX: 303-825-0802
webinfo@bonfils-stanton.org
bonfils-stantonfoundation.org

Gary P. Steuer, President & CEO
Gina A. Ferrari, Director, Grants Program
Ann M. Hovland, CFO/Treasurer
Monique M. Loseke, Executive Asst.
Grants limited to Colorado 501 (c) (3) organizations. Grants are for general, charitable philanthropic activities within the State. Major categories include education, scientific (including hospital and health services), civic and cultural, community and human services. Organizations should request foundation guidelines before submitting a proposal.

2801 Comprecare Foundation
PO Box 740610
Arvada, CO 80006
303-432-2808
FAX: 303-432-2808
www.comprecarefoundation.org

Milton W. Bollman, Chairman of the Board
Dr. Ellen Mangione, MD, MPH, Vice Chairman
James R. Gilsdorf, Executive Director
Dennis E. Baldwin, Secretar/Treasurer
The purpose of the Comprecare Foundation is to encourage, aid or assist specific health related programs and to make grants to support the activities of organizations which are designed to advance and promote health care education, the delivery of health care services, and the improvement of community health and welfare.

2802 **Denver Foundation**
55 Madison Street
8th Floor
Denver, CO 80206 303-300-1790
FAX: 303-300-6547
information@denverfoundation.org
www.denverfoundation.org

Sandra Shreve, Chair
Ginny Bayless, Vice Chair and Chair-Elect
David M Miller, President & CEO
Sarah Bock, Secretary

Neighbors helping neighbors, that's what the foundation is for. As Denver's only community foundation we've been accepting charitable donations since 1925. Those funds have been given back to the community in ongoing grants to nonprofit organizations - organizations that touch nearly every meaningful artistic, cultural, civic, health and human services interest of metro Denver's citizens.

2803 **El Pomar Foundation**
10 Lake Circle
Colorado Springs, CO 80906 719-633-7733
800-554-7711
FAX: 719-577-5702
grants@elpomar.org
www.elpomar.org

William J. Hybl, Chairman/CEO
William Ward, Vice Chair
R. Thayer Tutt, Jr., President/CIO
Kyle Hybl, COO/General Counsel

Mission of El Pomar is to enhance, encourage and promote the current and future well being of the people of Colorado through grantmaking and community stewardship.

2804 **Helen K and Arthur E Johnson Foundation**
1700 Broadway
Suite 1100
Denver, CO 80290-1718 303-861-4127
800-232-9931
FAX: 303-861-0607
info@www.johnsonfoundation.org
www.johnsonfoundation.org

Ms. Lynn H. Campion, Chairman
Ms. Berit K. Campion, Vice Chair
John H Alexander Jr, President
Jacque Beaty, Finance Director

A nonprofit, grantmaking private foundation incorporated under the laws of the State of Colorado in 1948. The Foundation is a general purpose foundation whose grant program consists of a wide variety of creative efforts to solve problems and to enrich the quality of life. The areas of interest are: education, youth, health, community services, civic and culture and senior citizens. Grants limited to the state of Colorado.

Connecticut

2805 **Aetna Foundation**
151 Farmington Ave
Hartford, CT 06156 860-273-0123
800-872-3862
www.aetnahealthinsurance.com

Mark T Bertolini, Chairman/CEO
Karen S. Rohan, President
William J. Casazza, EVP & General Counsel
Richard di Benedetto, EVP, Aetna International

The Aetna Foundation is the independent charitable and philanthropic arm of Aetna Inc. The Foundation helps build healthy communities by promoting volunteerism, forming partnerships and funding initiatives that improve the quality of life where our employees and customers live and work.

2806 **Arc of Connecticut**
43 Woodland Street
Suite 260
Hartford, CT 6105-2300 860-246-6400
FAX: 860-246-6406
arcct@aol.com
www.arcct.com

Leslie Simoes, Interim Executive Director

The Arc of Connecticut is an advocacy organization committed to protecting the rights of people with intellectual, cognitive, and developmental disabilities and to promoting opportunities for their full inclusion in the life of thier communities.

2807 **Community Foundation of Southeastern Connecticut**
68 FederalStreet
PO Box 769
New London, CT 06320 860-442-3572
877-442-3572
FAX: 860-442-0584
maryam@cfect.org
www.cfect.org

Susan Pochal, Chair
Dianne E. Williams, Vice Chair
Maryam Elahi, President & CEO
Alison Woods, Vice President & COO

Provides donors with an easy and convenient way to give back to our community with joy and impact. We make grants to nonprofit organizations and support their efforts to strengthen our community.

2808 **Connecticut Mutual Life Foundation**
140 Garden St
Hartford, CT 6154 860-727-3000

Astrida Olds, Executive Director

Distinguished throughout its long history by unusual commitment to high principles of corporate purpose and business ethics. That commitment has been reflected not only in the firm belief that normal business functions must be carried out with a sense of responsibility beyond that required by the marketplace. Maintains an ongoing program of corporate contributions, a nationwide matching gifts plan for all employees on behalf of private and public education, skills training programs, and more.

2809 **Cornelia de Lange Syndrome Foundation**
302 West Main Street
#100
Avon, CT 06001 860-676-8166
800-753-2357
FAX: 860-676-8337
info@cdlsusa.org
www.cdlsusa.org

Robert Boneberg, Esq., President
Richard Haaland, Ph.D., Vice President
David Harvey, Vice President
Wendy Miller, Esq., Secretary

Provides information about birth defects caused by Cornelia de Lange Syndrome.

2810 **Fidelco Guide Dog Foundation**
103 Vision Way
Bloomfield, CT 06002 860-243-5200
FAX: 860-769-0567
admissions@fidelco.org
www.fidelco.org

Karen C. Tripp, Chair
G. Kenneth Bernhard, Esq., Vice Chair
Diane R. Lindeland, VP, Director of Finance
Eliot D. Russman, CEO

The Fidelco Guide Dog Foundation, located in Bloomfield, Conn., is dedicated to providing increased freedom and independence to men and women who are blind by providing them with the highest quality guide dogs. We rely solely on the gifts and the generosity of individuals, foundations, corporations and organizations that partner with Fidelco to 'Share the Vision.'

2811 GE Foundation
General Electric Company
3135 Easton Tpke
Fairfield, CT 6828
203-373-3216
FAX: 203-373-3029
gefoundation@ge.com
www.ge.com

Jeffrey R. Immelt, Chairman/ CEO
Daniel C. Heintzelman, Vice Chair
Jeffrey S. Bornstein, SVP & CFO, GE
Shane Fitzsimons, SVP Global Operations
Believes that our greatest national resource is the work force. If we are to successfully compete in the global arena, then we become involved in improving the education of all of our citizens. The Foundation sets examples for others to emulate helping people with their international grant program to higher education and to health care for children in developing countries.

2812 Hartford Foundation for Public Giving
10 Columbus Blvd
8th Floor
Hartford, CT 06106
860-548-1888
FAX: 860-524-8346
lindakelly@hfpg.org
www.hfpg.org

Yvette Melendez, Chair
Bonnie J. Malley, Vice Chair
Linda J. Kelly, President
Julie Feidner, Exec. Asst. to the President
Developmentally disabled, housing, deaf, recreation and education grants.

2813 Hartford Insurance Group
1 Hartford Plz
Hartford, CT 6155-1708
860-547-5000
www.thehartford.com

Christopher Swift, Chairman/ CEO
Doug Elliot, President
Beth Bombara, Chief Financial Officer
Kathy Bromage, Chief Marketing Officer
Giving is primarily in the Hartford, CT area and in communities where the company has a regional office. No support is available for political or religious purposes. Grants are given in the areas of education, health and United Way organizations.

2814 Henry Nias Foundation
20 Carmen Rd
Milford, CT 6460-7508
203-874-2787

Charles D Fleischman, President
Giving limited to NY metropolitan area. Arts, cultural programs, medical school/education, and children and youth.

2815 Jane Coffin Childs Memorial Fund for Medical Research
333 Cedar St, SHM
L300
New Haven, CT 6510-3206
203-785-4612
FAX: 203-785-3301
jccfund@yal.edu
www.jccfund.org

Dr Randy Schekman, Director
The Fund awards fellowships to suitably qualified individuals for full time postdoctoral studies in the medical and related sciences bearing on cancer.

2816 John H and Ethel G Nobel Charitable Trust
Bankers Trust Company
1 Fawcett Pl
PO Box 1297
New York, NY 1008-1297
203-629-7120
FAX: 203-629-7170
john-h-ethel-g-noble-charitable-trust.idilogi

Paul J Bisset, VP

2817 Scheuer Associates Foundation
960 Lake Ave
Greenwich, CT 6831-3032
203-622-5002
FAX: 203-622-5002
scheuer-associates-foundation-inc.idilogic.ai

Thomas Scheuer, President

2818 Swindells Charitable Foundation Trust
Shawmut Bank
1221SW YamhillStreet
Suite 100
Portland, OR 97205-2303
503-222-0689
FAX: 503-222-0726
dwecker@swindellstrust.org
www.swindellstrust.org

Maggie Willard, President
Grants made to charitable organizations or societies incorporated for the relief of sick and suffering poor children and/or the relief of sick suffering and indigent aged men and women and/or the support of public charitable hospitals. Geographic area includes Hartford, CT area primarily. Application is required, deadlines are Feb. 1 and Aug. 1.

Delaware

2819 Arc of Delaware
2 S Augustine Street
Suite B
Wilmington, DE 19804-2504
302-996-9400
FAX: 302-996-0683
TTY:800-232-5460
craign@arcde.org
www.thearcofdelaware.org

Bill Seufert, President
Becky Hill, Vice President
Merry Jones, Vice President
Barbara Robeleto, Vice President
The Arc of Delaware is a non-profit organization of volunteers and staff who work together to improve the quality of life for people with disabilitiesand their families. We strive to include all children and adults with cognitive, intellectual and developmental disabilities in every community.

2820 Longwood Foundation
100 W 10th St
Suite 1109
Wilmington, DE 19801-1694
302-683-8200
FAX: 302-654-2323
www.longwoodfoundation.com

ThŚre du Pont, President
Peter Morrow, Executive Director
Offers grants to the mentally and physically disabled - capital, program, education and housing grants in the state of Delaware.

District of Columbia

2821 Alexander and Margaret Stewart Trust
Brawner Building
888 17th Street NW
Suite 1250
Washington, DC 20006-3321
202-333-1277
FAX: 202-333-3128
aplatt@projectsinternational.com
www.projectsinternational.com

Chas W. Freeman, Chairman
Peter J.C, Young, President
Imtiaz T. Ladak, Chief Financial Officer
Landon K. Thorne, Managing Director
Grants are given only to the Washington, DC area organizations providing care or treatment to cancer patients or those with childhood afflictions.

2822 Arc of the District of Columbia
415 Michigan Avenue, NE
Suite 150
Washington, DC 20017- 2144   202-636-2950
FAX: 202-635-7086
arcdc@arcdc.net
www.arcdc.net

Robert A. Anderson, President
Mary Lou Meccariello, Executive Director
Michael Gonzales, Chief Operating Officer
Ed Cabatic, Director of Finance
Advocating for and providing services to persons with mental re-
tardation. Mission is to improve the quality of life of all persons
with mental retardation and their families through supports and
advocacy.

2823 Eugene and Agnes E Meyer Foundation
The Meyer Foundation
1250 Connecticut Ave NW
Suite 800
Washington, DC 20036- 2620   202-483-8294
FAX: 202-328-6850
meyer@meyerfdn.org
www.meyerfoundation.org

Joshua Bernstein, Chair
Deborah Ratner Salzberg, Vice Chair
Nicky Goren, President & CEO
Barbara Lang, Secretary-Treasurer
Awards grants to projects dealing with the learning disabled,
blind, mental health and vocational training in the Washington
metropolitan area.

2824 Federal Student Aid Information Center
US Department of Education
400 Maryland Ave SW
Washington, DC 20202   202-275-5446
800-872-5327
www.ed.gov

Arne Duncan, Secretary of Education
Tony Miller, Deputy Secretary
Martha Kanter, Under Secretary
Answers questions about Federal student aid from students, par-
ents and Members of Congress, as well as financial aid adminis-
trators.

2825 GEICO Philanthropic Foundation
1 Geico Plz
Washington, DC 20076   301-986-3000
800-841-3000
FAX: 301-986-2851
www.geico.com

Tony M Nicely, CEO
Hospitals, physically disabled and Special Olympics.

2826 Jacob and Charlotte Lehrman Foundation
1836 Columbia Rd NW
Washington, DC 20009-2002   202-328-8400
FAX: 202-338-8405
www.lehrmanfoundation.org

Elizabeth Berry, Director
Robert Lehrman, Trustee
Samuel Lehrman, Trustee
Barbara Ferguson, Administrative/Program assistant
The Jacob & Charlotte Lehrman Foundation supports and seeks
to enrich Jewish life in Washington DC, Israel and around the
world. It is committed to making Washington a better place for all
people and supports the arts, education and undeserved children,
the environment, and healthcare.

2827 John Edward Fowler Memorial Foundation
79 Fifth Avenue
16th Street
New York, NY 10003-3076   212-620-4230
800-424-9836
FAX: 212-807-3677
www.foundationcenter.org

Bradforth K. Smith, President
Lisa Philp, Vice President
Lawrence T. McGill, Vice President
Jen Bokoff, Director
Although not a program priority, the foundation does offer grants
to the physically disabled in the Washington, DC area only.

2828 Joseph P Kennedy Jr Foundation
1133 19th Street NW
12th Floor
Washington, DC 20036-3604   202-393-1250
FAX: 202-824-0351
jpkf@jpkf.org
www.jpkf.org

Rebecca Salon, President
Steven Eidelman, Executive Director
Has two firm objectives: to seek the prevention of mental retardation, and to improve the way society deals with its citizens who
are already mentally retarded. The Foundation uses its funds in
areas where a multiplier effect can be achieved through development of innovative models for the prevention and amelioration of
mental retardation, through provision of seed money that encourages new researchers, and thorough use of the Foundation's
influence to promote public awareness.

2829 Kiplinger Foundation
1100 13th Street, NW
Suite 750
Washington, DC 20005-3938   202-887-6400
800-544-0155
FAX: 202-778-8976
foundation@kiplinger.com
www.kiplinger.com

Knight Kiplinger, VP
Limited to the greater Washington, DC area, the grants focus primarily on education, social welfare, cultural activities and community programs. Matching grants to eligible secondary or
higher education institutions are provided on behalf of employees and retirees of Kiplinger Washington Editors, Inc. The
Foundation does not fund scholarships.

2830 Morris and Gwendolyn Cafritz Foundation
1825 K St NW
Ste 1400
Washington, DC 20006-1271   202-223-3100
800-544-0155
FAX: 202-296-7567
info@cafritzfoundation.org
www.cafritzfoundation.org

Calvin Cafritz, Chairman/President/ CEO
John E. Chapoton, Vice Chairman and Treasurer
Ed McGeogh, Vice President - Asset Managemen
Rohan Rodrigo, Vice President - Finance
Grants are awarded to only 501(c)(3) organizations that are in the
DC area. Grants are not awarded for capitol purposes, special
events, endowments, or to individuals.

2831 Paul and Annetta Himmelfarb Foundation
4545 42nd St NW
Ste 203
Washington, DC 20016-4623   202-966-3796

M Preston, Executive Director
Primary areas of interest include health, children, human need,
and Israel.

2832   Public Welfare Foundation
1200 U St NW
Washington, DC 20009-4443
202-965-1800
info@publicwelfare.org
www.publicwelfare.org

Lydia M. Marshall, Chair
Mary E. McClymont, President
Phillipa Taylor, Chief Financial and Administrati
Alyssa Piccirilli, Manager of Administration
The foundation's funding is specifically targeted to economically disadvantaged populations. Proposals must fall within one of the following categories: criminal justice, disadvantaged elderly, disadvantaged youth, environment, health and population and reproductive health, human rights and global security, and community economic developmental and participation. Proposals should be addressed to the Review Committee.

Florida

2833   Able Trust
3320 Thomasville Road
Suite 200
Tallahassee, FL 32308
850-224-4493
FAX: 850-224-4496
TTY:850-224-4493
info@abletrust.org
www.abletrust.org

Susanne Homant, President
Guenevere Crum, Senior Vice President
Kathryn McManus, MA, Chief Development Director
Allison Chase, MS, State Director, Florida High Sch
The Able Trust is a non-profit, public/private partnership that supports non-profit vocational rehabilitation programs throughout Florida with fundraising, grant making and public awareness of disability issues.

2834   Arc of Florida
2898 Mahan Dr
Ste 1
Tallahassee, FL 32308-5462
850-921-0460
800-226-1155
info@arcflorida.org
www.arcflorida.org

Pat Young, President
Dick Bradley, Vice President Administration
Linda Bloom, Vice President Advocacy
Greg Roe, Treasurer
Promotes, for all people with mental retardation and other developmental disabilities, through education, awareness, research, advocacy and the support of families, friends and community.

2835   Bank of America Client Foundation
50 Central Avenue
Suite 750
Sarasota, FL 34236-5900
941-951-4103
maryann.l.smith@ustrust.com
www.fdnweb.org/boacf/

Maryann L. Smith, Vice President, Senior Trust Off
Committed to creating meaningful change in the communities we serve through our philanthropic efforts, associate volunteerism, community development activities and investing, support of arts and culture programming and environmental initiatives.

2836   Barron Collier Jr Foundation
2600 Golden Gate Pkwy
Naples, FL 34105-3227
239-262-2600
FAX: 239-262-1840
ContactUs@BarronCollier.com
www.barroncollier.com

Karen V. Triplett, Director of Property Management
Jose Medina, Facilities Manager
Barron Collier Companies - dedicated to the responsible development, management and stewardship of its extensive land holdings and other assets in the businesses of agriculture, real estate, and mineral management.

2837   Camiccia-Arnautou Charitable Foundation
Ste 402
980 N Federal Hwy
Boca Raton, FL 33432-2712
561-368-5757
FAX: 561-368-8505

Ronda Gluck, President

2838   Chatlos Foundation
PO Box 915048
Longwood, FL 32791-5048
407-862-5077
info@chatlos.org
www.chatlos.org

Bill Chatlos, Trustee
Funds nonprofit organizations in the USA and around the globe. Funding is provided in the following areas of giving: Bible Colleges/Seminaries, Religious Causes, Medical Concerns, Liberal Arts Colleges and Social Concerns. Category of placement is determined by the organizations overall mission rather than the project under consideration. The Foundation does not make scholarship grants directly to individuals but rather to educational institutions which in turn select recipients.

2839   Edyth Bush Charitable Foundation
199 E Welbourne Ave
Ste 100
Winter Park, FL 32789-4365
407-647-4322
888-647-4322
FAX: 407-647-7716
dodahowski@edythbush.org
www.edythbush.org

Gerald F. Hilbrich, Chairman
Herbert W. Holm, Vice Chairman
David A. Odahowski, President/CEO
Mary Ellen Hutcheson, Vice-President/Treasurer
Funding is resrticted to 501c3 nonprofit organizations located and operating in Orange, Osceola, Seminole and Lake Counties, Florida. Visit www.edythbush.org for a list of funding policies.

2840   FPL Group Foundation
700 Universe Blvd
Juno Beach, FL 33408-2657
561-694-4000
888-488-7703
FAX: 561-694-4620
PoweringFlorida@FPL.com
www.fpl.com

Maria V. Fogarty, Senior Vice President, Internal
James L. Robo, President and Chief Operating Of
Joseph T. Kelliher, Executive Vice President, Federa
Antonio Rodriguez, Executive Vice President, Power
The company consistently outperforms national averages for service reliability while customer bills are below the national average. A clean energy leader, FPL has one of the lowest emissions profiles and one of the leading energy efficiency programs among utilities nationwide. FPL is a subsidiary of Juno Beach, Fla.-based NextEra Energy, Inc.

2841   Jefferson Lee Ford III Memorial Foundation
9600 Collins Ave
Bal Harbour, FL 33154-2202
305-868-2609
FAX: 305-868-2640

Sanford L King, Director
Yvonne Quatrale, President
Disabled children, hearing and speech center. Grants are only given to tax exempt organizations, no individual grants are offered.

2842 **Jessie Ball duPont Fund**
40 East Adams Street
Ste 300
Jacksonville, FL 32202-3302
904-353-0890
800-252-3452
FAX: 904-353-3870
contactus@dupontfund.org
www.dupontfund.org

Sherry P. Magill, President
Mark D. Constantine, Vice President for Strategy, Pol
Barbara Roole, Senior Program Officer
Katie Ensign, Senior Program Officer

Established under the terms of the will of the late Jessie Ball duPont. The fund is a national foundation having a special though not exclusive interest in issues affecting the South. The Fund works with the approximately 325 individual institutions to which Mrs. duPont personally contributed during the five-year period, 1960 through 1964.

2843 **Lost Tree Village Charitable Foundation**
8 Church Lane
North Palm Beach, FL 33408-2908
561-622-3780
FAX: 561-841-6773
info@losttreefoundation.org
www.losttreefoundation.org

Pam Rue, Executive Director
Teresa Elu, Executive Assistant
Bob Heon, Controller

The Lost Tree Village Charitable Foundation is dedicated to building a stronger community and improving the quality of life for all local residents. Grants are awarded annually to local non-profit health and human service organizations providing information, expertise and assistance to those in need. Applications are only accepted from organizations located in Palm Beach and Southern Martin Counties. Visit the website for guidelines and further information.

2844 **Miami Foundation, The**
40 NW 3rd Street
Suite 405
Miami, FL 33128
305-371-2711
FAX: 305-371-5342
info@miamifoundation.org
www.miamifoundation.com

Javier Alberto Soto, President and CEO
Rebecca Mandelman, VP for Strategy and Engagement

The Foundation approaches all of its program activities with a focus on building the community. We conduct acticvities and support efforts that build community assets and relationships among individuals, organizations, and communities that connect people with resources and opportunities to improve their quality of life.

2845 **National Parkinson Foundation**
200 SE 1st Street
Suite 800
Miami, FL 33131-1494
305-243-6666
800-473-4636
FAX: 305-537-9901
contact@parkinson.org
www.parkinson.org

John W. Kozyak, Chairman
Joyce Oberdorf, President/CEO
Amy Gray, Vice President, Chapter and Comm
Peter Schmidt, PhD, Vice President, Programs, Chief

The mission of the NPF is to improve the quality of care for people with Parkinson's disease through research, education, and outreach.

2846 **Publix Super Markets Charities**
Publix Super Market Corporation Office
PO Box 407
Lakeland, FL 33802-0407
800-242-1227
www.publix.com

Gino DiGrazia, Vice President of Finance
Maria Brous, Director of Media & Community R
Kimberly Reynolds, Media & Community Relations

In addition to giving to thousands of local projects, Publix annually supports five organizations in companywide campaigns: Special Olympics, March of Dimes, Children's Miracle Network, United Way and Food for All

Georgia

2847 **Arc Of Georgia**
100 Edgewood Ave NE
Ste 1675
Atlanta, GA 30303-3068
678-733-8969
888-401-1581
FAX: 678-733-8970
info@thearcofgeorgia.org
www.thearcofgeorgia.org

Torin Togut, President
David Glass, Vice President
Julie Lee, Secretary
Will Hudson, Treasurer

The Arc of Georgia advocates for the rights and full participation of all children and adults with intellectual and developmental disabilities. Together with our network of members and other local Chapters, we improve systems of supports and services, connect families, inspire communities, and influence public policy.

2848 **Community Foundation for Greater Atlanta**
50 Hurt Plz SE
Ste 449
Atlanta, GA 30303-2915
404-688-5525
FAX: 404-688-3060
info@cfgreateratlanta.org
www.cfgreateratlanta.org

Suzanne Boas, Board Chair
Alicia Philipp, President
Robert Smulian, Vice President of Philanthropic
Lesley Grady, Senior Vice President of Communi

The Community Foundation for Greater Atlanta is a creative, cost-effective and tax-efficient way for people to invest in our community. We help donors and their families meet their charitable goals by educating them or critical issues and by matching them with organizations that serve their interests. By working with donors and the community, we improve the quality of life for residents in our region.

2849 **Florence C and Harry L English Memorial Fund**
Sun Trust Bank Atlanta
PO Box 4418
Mail Code 041
Atlanta, GA 30302
404-588-8250
FAX: 404-724-3082
raymond.king@suntrust.com
www.suntrustatlantafoundation.org

Anil T. Cheriyan, Chief Information Officer
Kenneth J. Carrig, Chief Human Resources Officer
Rilla S. Delorier, Chief Marketing and Client Exper
Thomas E. Freeman, Chief Risk Officer

Grants only made to Metro Atlanta non-profit organizations; no grants to churches or individuals.

2850 **Georgia Power**
96 Annex
Atlanta, GA 30308-3374
404-506-6526
888-655-5888
www.georgiapower.com

W. Paul Bowers, Chairman/ President/ CEO
John L. Pemberton, Senior VP/SPO,

Georgia Power is an investor-owned, tax-paying utility that serves 2.25 million customers in all but four of Georgia's 159 counties.

2851 Grayson Foundation
1701 Willa Place Drive
Kernersville, NC 2728
336-650-9914
graysonfoundation@gmail.com
www.graysonfoundation.net

Donna Sherrell, Finance- Public Relations
Tricia Gladstone, Behavior Analyst-Finance Public
Roger Sherrell, Information Technology-Web Manag
Bob Sherrell, Finance
Grayson Foundation enhances the quality of public education for the students of the Grayson cluster of schools by providing funds which enrich and extend educational oppurtunities.

2852 Harriet McDaniel Marshall Trust in Memory of Sanders McDaniel
Sun Trust Bank Atlanta
96 Annex
PO Box 4418
Atlanta, GA 30396
404-588-8250
888-891-0938
FAX: 404-724-3082
raymond.king@suntrust.com
www.suntrustatlantafoundation.org

Anil T. Cheriyan, Chief Information Officer
Kenneth J. Carrig, Chief Human Resources Officer
Rilla S. Delorier, Chief Marketing and Client Exper
Thomas E. Freeman, Chief Risk Officer
Grants only made to Metro Atlanta non-profit organizations, no grants to churches or individuals.

2853 IBM Corporation
1 New Orchard Rd
Armonk, NY 10504-1772
914-499-1900
800-425-3333
TTY:804-068-4225
response@in.ibm.com
www.ibm.com

Samuel J Palmisano, Chairman
Virginia M. Rometty, President and Chief Executive Of
Rodney C. Adkins, Senior Vice President
Michael E. Daniels, Senior Vice President and Group
Manages disability programs (which leverage IBM resources through partnerships) designed to train persons with disabilities and assist them in gaining employment. Also, disseminates information regarding products and resources for persons with disabilities with those of other companies and organizations.

2854 John H and Wilhelmina D Harland Charitable Foundation
3565 Piedmont Road, NE
Two Piedmont Center, Suite 710
Atlanta, GA 30305-1502
404-264-9912
FAX: 404-266-8834
info@harlandfoundation.org
www.harlandfoundation.org

Margaret C. Reiser, President
Winifred S. Davis, Vice President/Treasurer
Robert E. Reiser, Secretary
Jane G. Hardesty, Executive Director
The Harland Charitable Foundation was established in 1972 by John H. and Wilhelmina D. Harland to support worthy local causes in Atlanta, with a particular interest in improving the welfare of children and youth as well as support of community services and arts and culture.

2855 Lettie Pate Whitehead Foundation
191 Peachtree Street NE
Suite 3540
Atlanta, GA 30303- 2951
404-522-6755
FAX: 404-522-7026
fdns@woodruff.org
www.woodruff.org

James B. Williams, Chairman
James M. Sibley, Vice Chairman
Lawrence L. Gellerstedt, President /CEO
J. Lee Tribble, Treasurer
Non-profit organization dedicated to the support of needy women in nine southeastern states.

2856 Rich Foundation
222 Summer Street
Stamford, CT 06901
203-359-2900
FAX: 203-328-7980
info@fdrich.com
www.fdrich.com

2857 SunTrust Bank, Atlanta Foundation
Sun Trust Bank Atlanta
PO Box 4418
Mail Code 041
Atlanta, GA 30302
404-588-8250
FAX: 404-724-3082
raymond.king@suntrust.com
www.suntrust.com

Anil T. Cheriyan, Chief Information Officer
Kenneth J. Carrig, Chief Human Resources Officer
Rilla S. Delorier, Chief Marketing and Client Exper
Thomas E. Freeman, Chief Risk Officer

Hawaii

2858 Arc of Hawaii
3989 Diamond Head Rd
Honolulu, HI 96816-4413
808-737-7995
FAX: 808-732-9531
info@thearcinhawaii.org
www.thearcinhawaii.org

Thomas Huber, President
Lee Moriwaki, Vice President
Duane Bartholomew, Secretary
Kevin Dooley, Treasurer
The Arc is a national, grassroots organization of and for people with intellectual and related developmental disabilities. With more then 140,000 members in 1000 local and state chapters. The Arc is the largest volunteer organization devoted soley to working on behalf of people with intellectual disabilities.

2859 Atherton Family Foundation
827 Fort Street Mall
Honolulu, HI 96813-2817
808-566-5524
888-731-3863
FAX: 808-521-6286
foundations@hcf-hawaii.org
www.atherton.hawaiicommunityfoundation.org

Patricia R. Giles, Vice President
Judith M. Dawson, President
Frank C. Atherton, Vice President and Treasurer
Paul F. Morgan, Vice President
Supports educational projects, programs and institutions as the highest priority, with the enterprises of a religious nature and those concerned with health and social services given careful attention. The Foundation is one of the largest private resources in the State devoted exclusively to the support of activities of a charitable nature.

2860 GN Wilcox Trust
Bank of Hawaii
PO Box 3170
Honolulu, HI 96802-3170
808-649-8580
800-272-7262
FAX: 808-538-4006
stafford.kiguchi@boh.com
www.boh.com

Paul Boyce, AVP and Grants Administrator
Elaine Moniz, Trust Specialist
William L. Carpenter, Senior Vice President
Diane W. Murakami, Senior Vice President
Benefits the people of Hawaii by funding programs that support social services, education, culture, the arts, youth services, religion, health and rehabilitation.

2861 Hawaii Community Foundation
827 Fort Street Mall
Honolulu, HI 96813-2817
                              808-537-6333
                              888-731-3863
                         FAX: 808-521-6286
                         info@hcf-hawaii.org
                         www.hawaiicommunityfoundation.org

Kelvin Taketa, President/CEO
Chris van Bergeijk, Vice President/Chief Operating O
Joseph Martyak, Vice President of Communications
Tom Kelly, Vice President for Knowledge, Ev
The Hawaii Community Foundation is a public, statewide, charitable services and grantmaking organization supported by donor contributions for the benefit of Hawaii's people.

2862 McInerny Foundation Bank Of Hawaii, Corporate Trustee
PO Box 3170
Honolulu, HI 96802-3170
                              808-649-8580
                              800-272-7262
                         FAX: 808-538-4006
                         stafford.kiguchi@boh.com
                         www.boh.com

Paula Boyce, Avp And Grants Administrator
Elaine Moniz, Trust Specialist
William L. Carpenter, Senior Vice President
Diane W. Murakami, Senior Vice President
Although the Trust is broad-purposed, it does not make grants to churches or individuals, nor for endowments, reserve purposes, deficit financing, or for the purchase of real estate.

2863 Sophie Russell Testamentary Trust Bank Of Hawaii
PO Box 3170
Honolulu, HI 96802-3170
                              808-649-8580
                              800-272-7262
                         FAX: 808-538-4006
                         stafford.kiguchi@boh.com
                         www.boh.com

Paula Boyce, Asst. Vice President
Elaine Moniz, Trust Specialist
William L. Carpenter, Senior Vice President
Diane W. Murakami, Senior Vice President
Supports qualified tax-exempt charitable organizations, in the State of Hawaii only. Offers grants to the Humane Society and institutions giving nursing care and serving the physically and mentally handicapped.

Illinois

2864 Alzheimer's Association
225 N Michigan Ave
Fl 17
Chicago, IL 60601-7633
                              312-335-8700
                              800-272-3900
                         FAX: 866-699-1246
                         TTY: 312-335-5886
                         info@alz.org
                         www.alz.org

Stewart Putnam, Chair
Christopher Binkley, Vice Chair
Harry Johns, President /CEO
Deborah Jones, Secretary
Mission is to eliminate Alzheimer's disease through the advancement of research, to provide and enhance care and support for all affected, and to reduce the risk of dementia through the promotion of brain health.

2865 American National Bank and Trust Company
33 N La Salle St
PO Box 191
Danville, VA 24543-0191
                              312-661-6000
                              800-240-8190
                         FAX: 815-961-7745
                         www.amnb.com

Charles H. Majors, Chairman/ CEO
Jeffrey V. Haley, President
Charles T. Canaday, Jr., Senior Vice President
R. Helm Dobbins, Senior Vice President
Supports the endeavors of organizations working to meet the critical needs of the city and its surrounding communities. Success is greatly affected by the well-being of the communities the company serves, thus the foundation seeks to fulfill the social obligations both through financial funding and human resources. The Foundation funding categories include organizations and programs involved in economic development, education, community and social services, healthcare and culture and the arts.

2866 Amerock Corporation
P.O.Box 7018
Rockford, IL 61125-7018
                              815-963-9631
                              800-435-6959
                         FAX: 800-618-6733
                         www.amerock.com

Robert Bailey, President
Grants are given to organizations promoting wellness, health and rehabilitation of the visually impaired and physically disabled.

2867 Arc of Illinois
The Illinois Life Span Project
20901 S La Grange Rd
Ste 209
Frankfort, IL 60423-3213
                              815-464-1832
                              800-588-7002
                         FAX: 815-464-5292
                         mike@illinoislifespan.org
                         www.thearcofil.org

Brain Rubin, President
Therese Devine, Vice President
Tony Paulauski, Executive Director
Janet Donahue, Director of Development
The Arc of Illinois is committed to empowering persons with disabilities to achieve full participation in community life thru informed choices.

2868 Benjamin Benedict Green-Field Foundation
18313 Greenleaf Ct
Tinley Park, IL 60487-2176
                              708-444-4241
                         FAX: 708-614-0496
                         kathy@greenfieldfoundation.org
                         www.greenfieldfoundation.org

Colin Fisher, Chairman of the Board
Kathryn Groenendal, President
Dan Jarke, Vice President
Sheldon K. Rachman, Secretary
A privately endowed grantmaking organization trying to improve the qaulity of life for children and the elderly in the city of chicago.

2869 Blowitz-Ridgeway Foundation
1701 E Woodfield Rd
Suite 201
Schaumburg, IL 60173-5127
                              847-330-1020
                         FAX: 847-330-1028
                         laura@blowitzridgeway.org
                         www.blowitzridgeway.org

Daniel L Kline, President
Pierre R. LeBreton, Ph.D., Vice-President
Thomas P. Fitzgibbon, Treasurer
Sandra Swantek, M.D., Secretary
Provides limited program, capital and research grants to organizations aiding the physically and mentally disabled, and agencies serving children and youth. Grants generally limited to Illinois.

2870 Chaddick Institute for Metropolitan Development
2352 N. Clifton Ave.
Suite 130
Chicago, IL 60614-2302   773-325-7310
                                   FAX: 312-362-5506
                                   lasadvising@depaul.edu
                                   www.las.depaul.edu

Joseph P Scwieterman PhD, Director
Marisa Schulz, LEED AP, Assistant Director
Justin Kohls, Program Manager
Susan Aaron, Civic Program Design
Advances the principals of effective land use, transportation, and
community planning. Offers planners, attorneys, developers, and
entrepreneurs a forum to share expertise on difficult land-use is-
sues through workshops, conferences, and policy studies.

2871 Chicago Community Trust
225 North Michigan Avenue
Suite 2200
Chicago, IL 60601- 4501   312-616-8000
                                   FAX: 312-616-7955
                                   alla@cct.org
                                   www.cct.org

Frank M. Clark, Chairman
Terry Mazany, President /CEO
Jamie Phillippe, Vice President-Development and D
Chae Dawning, Sr. Director of Human Resources
A community foundation established in 1915, which receives
gifts and bequests from individuals, families or organizations interested in providing through the community foundation, financial support for the charitable agencies or institutions which
serve the residents of metropolitan Chicago.

2872 Chicago Community Trust and Affiliates
225 North Michigan Avenue
Suite 2200
Chicago, IL 60601- 4501   312-616-8000
                                   FAX: 312-616-7955
                                   TTY:312-853-0394
                                   alla@cct.org
                                   www.cct.org

Frank M. Clark, Chairman
Terry Mazany, President /CEO
Jamie Phillippe, Vice President-Development and D
Chae Dawning, Sr. Director of Human Resources
Provides critical charitable resources in the arts, community and
economic development, education, health and wellness, hunger
and homeless alleviation, legal services, programs for youth, the
elderly, and people with disabilities, and services to assure that
basic human needs are met for all members of our community.

2873 Community Foundation of Champaign County
307 W University Ave
Champaign, IL 61820-3411   217-359-0125
                                   FAX: 217-352-6494
                                   cfcc@soltec.net
                                   www.cfeci.org

Brooke Didier Starks, Chair
Tom Costello, Vice-Chair
Joan M. Dixon, President /CEO
Bradley Uken, Treasurer
A network of cultural resource providers and educational organi-
zations who collaborate in the creation, coordination, and promo-
tion of cultural resource programs for Champaign County
Schools.

2874 Dr Scholl Foundation
1033 Skokie Blvd
Ste 230
Northbrook, IL 60062-4109   847-559-7430
                                   www.drschollfoundation.com

Pamela Scholl, President
The Foundation is dedicated to providing financial assistance to
organizations committed to improving our world. Grants are
made annually after an executive review by the staff and all the
directors.

2875 Duchossois Foundation
Chamberlain Group
845 N Larch Ave
Elmhurst, IL 60126-1114   630-279-3600
                                   FAX: 630-530-6091
                                   employment@duch.com
                                   www.duch.com

Richard L. Duchossois, Chairman
Robert L. Fealy, President /COO
Craig J. Duchossois, Chief Executive Officer
Michael E. Flannery, Executive Vice President/Chief F
Established in 1984, the foundation returns dollars to the commu-
nities supporting its facilities and employees. Within these fol-
lowing areas, organizations are carefully selected on the basis of
community needs and the organization's value and performance.
Areas aimed at include: medical research, children/youth
programs and cultural institutions.

2876 Evenston Community Foundation
1560 Sherman Ave
Suite 535
Evanston, IL 60201-5910   847-492-0990
                                   FAX: 847-492-0904
                                   info@evanstonforever.org
                                   www.evanstonforever.org

Sara Schastok, Phd., President and CEO
Gwen Jessen, Vice President for Philanthropy
Marybeth Schroeder, Vice President for Programs
Jan Fischer, Chief Financial Officer
The Foundation is a publicly supported plilanthropic organization dedicated to enriching Evanston and the lives of its people,
now and in the future. The Foundation builds and manages its
own and other community endowments, addresses Evanston's
changing needs through grant making, and provides leadership
on important community needs.

2877 Field Foundation of Illinois
200 S Wacker Dr
Ste 3860
Chicago, IL 60606-5848   312-831-0910
                                   FAX: 312-831-0961
                                   byoung@fieldfoundation.org
                                   www.fieldfoundation.org

Lyle Logan, Board Chair
Aurie A. Pennick, Executive Director and Treasurer
Sarah M. Linsley, Secretary
Mark C. Murray, Program Director
The Field Foundation seeks to provide support for community,
civic and cultural organizations in the Chicago area, enabling
both new and established programs to test innovations, to expand
proven strengths or to address specific, time-limited operational
needs.

2878 Francis Beidler Charitable Trust
53 W Jackson Blvd
Ste 530
Chicago, IL 60604-3422   312-922-3792
                                   FAX: 312-922-3799

Francis Beidler, Owner
Children/youth, services. Community development, business
promotion, crime and violence prevention. Federated giving programs, higher education, human services and family planning.

2879 Fred J Brunner Foundation
9300 King St
Franklin Park, IL 60131-2114   847-678-3232
                                   FAX: 847-678-0642
                                   www.fjbfoundation.com

Fred J Brunner, CEO
General disability grants.

2880 George M Eisenberg Foundation for Charities
Ste 480
2340 S Arlington Heights Rd
Arlington Heights, IL 60005-4507   847-981-0545
                                   FAX: 847-941-0548

James Marousis, Manager

2881 Grover Hermann Foundation
233 S Wacker Dr
Suite 6600
Chicago, IL 60606-6473   312-258-5500
FAX: 312-258-5600
rsafer@schiffhardin.com
www.schiffhardin.com

Ronald S. Safer, Managing Partner, Executive Comm
Provides funds for educational, health, public policy, community and religious organizations throughout the United States. Its major interests are in higher education and health.

2882 John D and Catherine T MacArthur Foundation
Office of Grants Management
140 S Dearborn St
Chicago, IL 60603-5285   312-726-8000
FAX: 312-920-6258
TTY:312-920-6285
4answers@macfound.org
www.macfound.org

Marjorie M. Scardino, Chair
Julia Statch, Interim President
Cecilia A. Conrad, Vice President-MacArthur Fellows
Susan E. Manske, Vice President/Chief Investment
The Foundation supports creative people and effective institutions committed to building a more just, verdant, and peaceful world. In addition, we work to defend human rights, advance global conservation, & security, make cities better places, and understand how technology is affecting children and society.

2883 Les Turne Amyotrophic Laterial Sclerosis Foundation
5550 Touhy Ave
Ste 302
Skokie, IL 60077-3254   847-679-3311
888-257-1107
FAX: 847-679-9109
info@lesturnerals.org
www.lesturnerals.org

Ken Hoffman, President
Andrea Paul Backman, Executive Director
Shari Diamond, RN, BSN, Director of Patient Services
Kim McIver, Director
Voluntary health organization dedicated to raising funds for ALS research, patient services and public awareness. Provides educational materials for affected individuals and family members, health care professionals, and the general public. Program services include referrals and counseling; audio-visual aids and periodic newsletters. Offers support groups and patient networking to affected individuals, family members, and caregivers.

2884 Little City Foundation
1760 W Algonquin Rd
Palatine, IL 60067-4799   847-358-5510
FAX: 847-358-3291
info@littlecity.org
www.littlecity.org

Matthew B. Schubert, President
B. Timothy Desmond, Executive Vice President
David Rose, Vice President
Douglas A. Wilson, Vice President
We offer innovative and personalized programs to fully assist and empower children & adults with autism and other intellectual and developmental disabilities. With a commitment to attaining a greater quality of life for Illinois most vulnerable citizens, we actively promote choice, person-centered planning and a holistic approach to health and wellness. 'ChildBridge' services include in-home personal & family supports, clinical behavior intervention, 24/7 residential services and much more.

2885 MAGIC Foundation for Children's Growth
6645 North Ave
Oak Park, IL 60302-1057   708-383-0808
800-362-4423
FAX: 708-383-0899
ContactUs@magicfoundation.org
www.magicfoundation.org

Rich Buckley, Chairman
Ken Dickard, Vice Chairman
Mary Andrews, CEO and Co-Founder
Dianne Kremidas, Executive Director
This is a national nonprofit organization providing support and education regarding growth disorders in children and related adult disorders, including adult GHD. Dedicated to helping children whose physical growth is affected by a medical problem by assisting families of afflicted children through local support groups, public education/awareness, newsletters, specialty divisions and programs for the children.

2886 McDonald's Corporation Contributions Program
2111 McDonalds Dr
Oak Brook, IL 60523-5500   630-623-3000
800-244-6227
FAX: 630-623-5700
www.mcdonalds.com

Don Thompson, President and Chief Executive Of
Tim Fenton, Chief Operating Officer
Peter J. Bensen, Executive Vice President and Chi
Jose Armario, Corporate Executive Vice Preside

2887 Michael Reese Health Trust
150 N Wacker Dr
Ste 2320
Chicago, IL 60606-1608   312-726-1008
FAX: 312-726-2797
wpalmer@healthtrust.net
www.healthtrust.net

Herbert S. Wander, Chairman
The Hon. How Carroll, Vice Chairman
Walter R. Nathan, Secretary
Gregory S. Gross, EdD, President
The trust seeks to improve the health of people in Chicago's metropolitan communities through effective grantmaking in health care, health education, and health research.

2888 National Eye Research Foundation
910 Skokie Blvd
Ste 207a
Northbrook, IL 60062-4033   847-564-9400
800-621-2258
FAX: 847-564-0807
info@nerf.org
www.subway.com

Joel Tenner, Manager
Dedicated to improving eye care for the public and meeting the professional needs of eye care practitioners; sponsors eye research projects on contact lens applications and eye care problems. Special study sections in such fields as orthokertology, primary eyecare, pediatrics, and through continuing education programs. Provides eye care information for the public and professionals. Educational materials including pamphlets. Program activities include education and referrals.

2889 National Foundation for Ectodermal Dysplasias
6 Executive Dr
Suite 2
Fairview Heights, IL 62208-1360   618-566-2020
FAX: 618-566-4718
info@nfed.org
www.nfed.org

Anil Vora, President
George Barbar, Vice President
Mary Fete, Executive Director
Kelley Atchison, Director
To empower and connect people touched by ectodermal dysplasias through education, support, and research.

2890   National Headache Foundation
820 N Orleans St
Ste 411
Chicago, IL 60610-3131   312-274-2650
                                           888-643-5552
                                      FAX: 312-640-9049
                                      info@headaches.org
                                      www.headaches.org

Seymour Diamond, M.D., Executive Chairman
Roger K. Cady, M.D., Associate Executive Chairman
Arthur H. Elkind, M.D., President
Vincent Martin, M.D., Vice President
Foundation exists to enhance the healthcare of headache suffer-
ers. It is a source of help to sufferers' families, physicians who
treat headache sufferers, allied healthcare professionals and to
the public.

2891   OMRON Foundation OMRON Electronics
1 Commerce Dr
Schaumburg, IL 60173-5330   847-843-7900
                                           800-556-6766
                                      FAX: 847-884-1866
                                      aoisales@omron.com
                                      www.omron247.com

Tastu Goto, CEO
Supports local community projects through direct donations and
matching employee-directed contributions.

2892   Parkinson's Disease Foundation
1359 Broadway
Suite 1509
New York, NY 10018-2331   212-923-4700
                                           800-457-667
                                      FAX: 212-923-4778
                                      info@pdf.org
                                      www.pdf.org

Howard D. Morgan, Chair
Constance Woodruff Atwell, Ph.D., Vice Chair
Robin Anthony Elliott, President
James Beck, Ph.D., Vice President
International voluntary not-for-profit organization dedicated to
patient services; education of affected individuals, family members, and healthcare professionals; and promotion and support of
research for Parkinson's Disease and related disorders. Offers an
extensive referral service to guide affected individuals to proper
diagnosis and clinical care. Provides referrals to genetic counseling and support groups; promotes patient advocacy; and offers a
variety of educational and support materials
Quarterly

2893   Peoria Area Community Foundation
331 Fulton St
Ste 310
Peoria, IL 61602-1449   309-674-8730
                                      FAX: 309-674-8754
                                      jim@communityfoundationci.org
                                      www.communityfoundationci.org

Donna Maracci, Chair
David Wynn, Vice Chair
Mark Roberts, CEO
Jessica Dillon, Program Manager
Established to meet a wide variety of social, cultural, educational
and other charitable needs throughout Central Illinois.

2894   Polk Brothers Foundation
20 W Kinzie St
Ste 1110
Chicago, IL 60654-5815   312-527-4684
                                      FAX: 312-527-4681
                                      questions@polkbrosfdn.org
                                      www.polkbrosfdn.org

Sandra P. Guthman, Chair
Raymond F. Simon, Vice Chair
Gordon S. Prussian, Secretary
Gillian Darlow, CEO
The Polk Brothers Foundation seeks to improve the quality of life
for the people of Chicago. We partner with local nonprofit organi-
zations that work to reduce the impact of poverty and provide area

residents with better access to quality education, preventive
health care and basic human services.

2895   Retirement Research Foundation
8765 W Higgins Rd
Ste 430
Chicago, IL 60631-4170   773-714-8080
                                      FAX: 773-714-8089
                                      info@rrf.org
                                      www.rrf.org

Nathaniel P. McParland, M.D., Chairman
Ruth Ann Watkins, Secretary
Downey R. Varey, Treasurer
Irene Frye, Executive Director
A private philanthropy with primary interest in improving the
quality of life of older persons in the United States.

2896   Sears-Roebuck Foundation
3333 Beverly Rd
Hoffman Estates, IL 60179   847-286-2500
                                           800-932-3188
                                      FAX: 800-326-0485
                                      www.sears.com

W Bruce Johnson, CEO
Has a special interest in projects that address women, families,
and diversity, but awards most of its funding to disease-specific
charities and United Way in the Chicago area.

2897   Siragusa Foundation
1 E Wacker Dr
Ste 2910
Chicago, IL 60601-1912   312-755-0064
                                      FAX: 312-755-0069
                                      www.siragusa.org

John E. Hicks, Chair & President
Ross D. Siragusa, Vice Chair
John R. Siragusa, Treasurer
Sharmila Rao Thakkar, Executive Director
The Siragusa Foundation, is a private family foundation that is
committed to honoring its founder by sustaining and developing
Chicago's extraordinary nonprofit resources.

2898   Square D Foundation
1415 S Roselle Rd
Palatine, IL 60067-7337   847-397-2600
                                      FAX: 847-925-7500
                                      www.schneider-electric.com/site/home/i

2899   WP and HB White Foundation
540 W Frontage Rd
Ste 3240
Northfield, IL 60093-1232   847-446-1441

Margaret Blandford, Executive Director
The Foundation's funds are allocated on a continuing basis
within the metropolitan area of Chicago where our founder's
business prospered. The Foundation helps organizations specializing in the visually impaired, mental health, youth and
recreation.

2900   Washington Square Health Foundation
875 N Michigan Ave
Ste 3516
Chicago, IL 60611-1957   312-664-6488
                                      FAX: 312-664-7787
                                      washington@wshf.org
                                      www.wshf.org

William N. Werner, MD, MPH, Board Chair
Howard Nochumson, Executive Director/President
William B. Friedeman, Secretary
James M. Snyder, Treasurer
Grants funds in order to promote and maintain access to adequate
healthcare for all people in the Chicagoland area regardless of
race, sex, creed or financial need.

2901 Wheat Ridge Ministries
1 Pierce Pl
Ste 250 E
Itasca, IL 60143-2634 630-766-9066
800-762-6748
FAX: 630-766-9622
wrmail@weatridge.org
www.wheatridge.org

Kevin Boettcher, Chair
Richard Herman, President
Brain Becker, Senior Vice President
Holly Harrison Fiala, Vice President of Advancement
Weat Ridge supports more then 100 new health-related ministries
each year through a variety of grant programs

Indiana

2902 Arc of Indiana
107 N Pennsylvania St
Suite 800
Indianapolis, IN 46204- 2423 317-977-2375
800-382-9100
FAX: 317-977-2385
thearc@arcind.org
www.arcind.org

Kerry Fletcher, President
Marlene Lu, Vice President
Mike Foddrill, Treasurer
Erika Steuterman, Secretary
Arc of Indiana is commited to people with cognitive and develop-
mental disabilities realizing their goals of learning, living, work-
ing, and playing in the community.

2903 Ball Brothers Foundation
222 S Mulberry St
Muncie, IN 47305-2802 765-741-5500
FAX: 765-741-5518
info@ballfdn.org
www.ballfdn.org

James A. Fisher, Chairman/ CEO
Jud Fisher, President/Chief Operating Office
Frank B. Petty, Vice Chairman
Tammy Phillips, Treasurer, ex-officio
The Ball Brothers Foundation is dedicated to the stewardship leg-
acy of the Ball brothers and to the pursuit of improving the quality
of the Muncie, Delaware County, east Central Indiana and Indi-
ana, through philanthropy and leadership.

2904 Community Foundation of Boone County
102 N. Lebanon
Suite 200
Lebanon, IN 46052 317-873-0210
FAX: 317-873-0219
info@communityfoundationbc.org
www.communityfoundationbc.org

Marc Applegate, Chairman of the Board
Ray Ingham, Vice Chair
Mike Harlos, Treasurer
Suzy Rich, Secretary
The Community Foundation of Boone County provides pathways
for connecting people who care with causes that matter for now
and in the future.

2905 John W Anderson Foundation
402 Wall St
Valparaiso, IN 46383-2562 219-462-4611
FAX: 219-531-8954
andersonfnd@aol.com

Bruce Wargo, Manager
Physically and mentally disabled, recreation and youth agencies
in Northwest Indiana area.

Iowa

2906 Arc of Iowa
114 S. 11th Street
Ste 302
West Des Moines, IA 50265- 3259 515-402-1618
800-362-2927
FAX: 515-330-2195
casey@thearcofiowa.org
www.thearcofiowa.org

Casey Westhoff, Executive Director
The Arc of Iowa exists to ensure that people with intellectual disabilities and developmental disabilities receive the services, supports and opportunities necessary to fully realize their right to
live, work and enjoy life in the community without
discrimination.

2907 Hall-Perrine Foundation
115 3rd St SE
Ste 803
Cedar Rapids, IA 52401-1222 319-362-9079
FAX: 319-362-7220
kristin@hallperrine.org
www.hallperrine.org

William Whipple, Chairman
Jack Evans, President
Darrel Morf, Vice President
Iris Muchmore, Secretary
This foundation is dedicated tio improving the quality of life for
peole in Linn County, IA by responding to the changing social,
economic, and cultural needs of the community.

2908 Mid-Iowa Health Foundation
3900 Ingersoll Ave
Ste 104
Des Moines, IA 50312-3535 515-277-6411
FAX: 515-271-7579
info@midiowahealth.org
www.midiowahealth.org

Becky Miles-Polka, Chairman
Rob Hayes, Vice Chair
Suzanne Mineck, President
Cheryl Harding, Secretary/Treasurer
Mission is to serve as a partner and catalyst for improving the
health of vulnerable people in greater Des Moines.

2909 Principal Financial Group Foundation
711 High St
Des Moines, IA 50392 515-247-5111
800-986-3343
FAX: 515-235-5724
www.principalfinancialgroup.com

Larry Zimpleman, Chairman/ President/ CEO
Daniel J. Houston, President - Retirement, Insuranc
James P. McCaughan, President - Principal Global Inv
Luis Valdes, President - Principal Internatio
The Principal Financial Group is a leading global financial com-
pany offering businesses, individuals and industrial clients a
wide range of financial products and services.

2910 Siouxland Community Foundation
505 5th St
Suite 412
Sioux City, IA 51101-1507 712-293-3303
FAX: 712-293-3303
office@siouxlandcommunityfoundation.org
www.siouxlandcommunityfoundation .org

Richard J. Dehner, President
Robert F. Meis, Vice President
Marilyn J. Hagberg, Secretary
Mary E. Anderson, Treasurer
The Siouxland Community Foundation strives to enhance the
quality of life in the greater Siouxland tri-state area by seeking
charitable gifts to build permanent endowments as charitable
capital for the community, providing a flexable vehicle to receive
and distribute gifts of any size, making grants in response to com-

munity needs, and providing services that will help shape the well-being of Siouxland.

Kansas

2911   Arc of Kansas
2701 SW Randolph Ave
Topeka, KS 66611-1536

785-232-0597
FAX: 785-232-3770
info@tarcinc.org
www.tarcinc.org

Barbara Duncan, President
Matthew Bergman, Vice President
Travis Stryker, Secretary
Kim Savage, Treasurer
Organzation works to ensure that the estimated 7.2 million Americans with intellectual and developmental disabilities have the services and supports they need to grow, develop, and live in communities across the nation.

2912   Hutchinson Community Foundation
1 North Main, Suite 501
PO Box 298
Hutchinson, KS 67504-0298

620-663-5293
FAX: 620-663-9277
info@hutchcf.org
www.hutchcf.org

Aubrey Abbot Patterson, President and Executive Director
Terri L. Eisiminger, Vice President of Administration
Janet Hamilton, Community Investment Officer
Maria G. Kicklighter, Finance Assistant
Connects donors to community needs and opportunities, increases philanthropy and provides community leadership.

2913   Richard W Higgins Charitable Foundation
Marshall & Ilsley Trust of Florida
2520 South Iowa
Ste 100
Lawrence, KS 66046-2713

877-202-9234
www.applebees.com

Ken Krei, President
Jessica James, Executive Chef
Patrick Humphrey, Executive Chef
Michael Slavin, Executive Chef
Gives primarily for medical research with geographical focus on New York and Florida.

Kentucky

2914   Arc of Kentucky
706 E. Main Street
Suite A
Frankfort, KY 40601-2408

502-875-5225
800-281-1272
FAX: 502-875-5226
arcofky@aol.com
arcofky.org

James Cheely, President
Patty Dempsey, Executive Director
Ellen Nicholson, Secretary
Bob Gray, Treasurer
The Arc of Kentucky works to ensure a quality of life for children and adults with intellectual and developmental disabilities to help in securing a positive future. The Arc values services and supports that enhance the quality of life through independence, friendship, choice and respect for individuals with intellectual and developmental disabilities.

Louisiana

2915   Arc of Louisiana
606 Colonial Dr
Ste G
Baton Rouge, LA 70714-6535

225-383-1033
866-966-6260
FAX: 225-383-1092
info@thearcla.org
www.thearcla.org

Larry Pete, President
Henry Friloux, Vice President
Kelly Serrett, Executive Director
Ashley Courville, Project Director
The Arc of Louisiana advocates for and with individuals with intellectual and developmental disabilities and their families that they shall live to their fullest potential.

2916   Baton Rouge Area Foundation
402 N 4th St
Baton Rouge, LA 70802-5506

225-387-6126
877-387-6126
FAX: 225-387-6153
mverma@braf.org
www.braf.org

C. Kris Kirkpatrick, Chair
S. Dennis Blunt, Vice Chair
John G. Davies, President/CEO
Annette D. Barton, Secretary
The Foundation provides grants to nonprofits to make lives better in the region. It also takes on projects, often with parters, to remake Baton Rouge.

2917   Community Foundation of Shreveport-Bossier
401 Edwards St
Ste 105
Shreveport, LA 71101-5551

318-221-0582
FAX: 318-221-7463
info@cfnla.org
www.cfnla.org

Janie D. Richardson, Chairman
Thomas H. Murphy, Vice Chairman
Terry C. Davis, Ph.D, Secretary
Rand Falbaum, Treasurer
Provides a variety of charitable funds and gift options to help our partners achieve their vision for a stronger, more vibrant community. By bringing together fund donors, their financial advisors and non profit agencies, the Foundation is a powerful catalyst for building charitable giving and effecting positive change in our area

Maine

2918   BCR Foundation
83 Mussey Rd.
Scarborough, ME 04074

207-883-8000
800-227-6111
FAX: 207-883-0100
solutions@bcr.net
www.bcr.net

2919   UNUM Charitable Foundation
Maine Association of Non Profits
565 Congress St
Ste 301
Portland, ME 04101-3308

207-871-1885
FAX: 207-780-0346
Manp@NonprofitMaine.org
www.nonprofitmaine.org

Doug Woodbury, Board President
Ted Scontras, Board Vice President
Joan Smith, Board Treasurer
Stephanie Eglinton, Board Secretary
The Foundation encourages projects that: stimulate others in the private or public sector to participate in problem solving; ad-

vance innovative and cost-effective approaches for addressing defined, recognized needs; and demonstrate ability to obtain future project funding, if needed. The foundation generally limits its consideration of capital campaign requests to the Greater Portland, Maine area.

Maryland

2920 American Health Assistance Foundation
22512 Gateway Center Dr
Clarksburg, MD 20871-2005

301-948-3244
800-437-2423
FAX: 301-258-9454
info@brightfocus.org
www.brightfocus.org

Stacy Pagos Haller, President / CEO
Donna Callison, Vice President of Development
Michael Buckley, Vice President of Public Affairs
Guy Eakin, Ph.D., Vice President of Scientific Aff

The American Health Assistance Foundation (AHAF) is a registered non-profit organization that funds research into cures for Alzheimer's disease, macular degeneration and glaucoma, and provides the public with informantion about risk factors, preventative lifestyles, availiable treatments and coping strategies.

2921 American Occupational Therapy Foundation
4720 Montgomery Lane
Suite 202
Bethesda, MD 20814-3449

240-292-1079
FAX: 240-396-6188
aotf@aotf.org
aotf.org

Diana L. Ramsay, Chair
Wendy J. Coster, Vice Chair
Scott Campbell, CEO
Emily Kringle, President

AOFT provides advanced research, education and public awareness for occupational therapy, so that all people may participate fully in life regardless of their physical, social, mental or developmental circumstances.

2922 Arc of Maryland
121 Cathedral St, 2B
PO Box 1747
Annapolis, MD 21401- 1747

410-571-9320
888-272-3449
FAX: 410-974-6021
info@thearcmd.org
www.thearcmd.org

Richard Dean, President
Aileen O'Hare, Vice President
Annette Hinkle, Treasurer
Adam Vanderhook, Secretary

The Arc of Maryland works to create a world where children and adults with cognitive and developmental disabilities have and enjoy equal rights and opportunities.

2923 Baltimore Community Foundation
2 E Read Street
Floor 9
Baltimore, MD 21202-6903

410-332-4171
FAX: 410-837-4701
questions@bcf.org
www.bcf.org

Raymond L. Bank, Chair
Tedd Alexander, Vice Chair
Laura L. Gamble, Vice Chair
Thomas E. Wilcox, President

Makes grants in Baltimore City and Baltimore County; see website for how to apply. BCF is governed by a 30-member board of trustees, made up of a cross section of Baltimore.

2924 Candlelighters Childhood Cancer Foundation
10920 Connecticut Ave.
PO Box 498
Kensington, MD 20895- 0498

301-962-3520
855-858-2226
FAX: 301-962-3521
staff@acco.org
www.acco.org

Naomi Bartley, President
Janine Lynne, Vice President
Ken Phillips, Treasurer
Judy Mendoza, Secretary

An international organization providing information and support, and advocacy to parents of children with cancer and survivors of childhood cancer.Health and Education professionals also welcome as members.Network of local support groups. Information on disabilities related to treatment of childhood cancer. Publications.

2925 Children's Fresh Air Society Fund
Baltimore Community Foundation
2 E Read St
Baltimore, MD 21202-2470

410-332-4171
FAX: 410-837-4701
grants@bcf.org
bcf.org

Tom E. Wilcox, President
Danista Hunte, Vice President, Community Invest
Ralph M. Serpe, CFRE, Vice President, Development
Amy T. Seto, CPA, Vice President, Finance and Admi

Makes grants to nonprofit camps to provide tuition for disadvantaged and disabled Maryland children to attend summer camp. See website for how to apply.

2926 Clark-Winchcole Foundation
3 Bethesda Metro Ctr
Suite 550
Bethesda, MD 20814-5358

301-654-3607

Laura Phillips, President

Supported tax-exempt charitable organizations operating in the metropolitan area of Washington, DC in the following areas: deaf, higher education and physically disabled.

2927 Columbia Foundation
10630 Little Patuxent Parkway
Century Plaza, Suite 315
Columbia, MD 21044

410-730-7840
FAX: 410-997-6021
info@columbiafoundation.org
www.cfhoco.org

Bruce Harvey, Chair
Joseph Maranto, Vice Chair
Barb Van Winkle, Secretary
Lynne Schaefer, Treasurer

The Columbia Foundation serves as a catalyst for building a more caring, creative and effective community in Howard County by promoting and creating opportunities for personal and corporate philanthropy, managing endowments, anticipating and responding to community needs, and strategically granting funds.

2928 Corporate Giving Program
Ryland Group
11000 Broken Land Pkwy
Columbia, MD 21044

410-715-7022
800-267-0998
FAX: 410-715-7909

Bruce N Haas, President

Contributions of equipment, volunteers and financial support to organizations working to meet the challenges and needs of modern society.

2929 Cystic Fibrosis Foundation
6931 Arlington Rd
2nd floor
Bethesda, MD 20814-5200
301-951-4422
800-344-4823
FAX: 301-951-6378
info@cff.org
www.cff.org

Catherine C. McLoud, Board Chair
Robert J. Beall, Ph.D., President/Chief Executive Office
C. Richard Mattingly, Executive Vice President/Chief O
Preston W. Campbell, III, M.D., Executive Vice President for Med
The mission of the Cystic Fibrosis Foundation, a nonprofit donor-supported organization is to assure the development of the means to cure and control cystic fibrosis and to improve the quality of life for those with the disease.

2930 Foundation Fighting Blindness
7168 Columbia Gateway Dr.
Ste 100
Columbia, MD 21046
410-423-0600
800-683-5555
FAX: 410-363-2393
TTY: 800-683-5551
info@fightblindness.org
www.blindness.org

William T. Schmidt, Chief Executive Officer
Valerie Navy-Daniels, Chief Development Officer
Stephen M. Rose, Chief Research Officer
Rhea K. Farberman, Senior Director, Communications & Marketing
The foundation's mission is to drive the research that will provide preventions, treatments, and cures for people affected by retinitis pigmentosa, macular degeneration, Usher syndrome and the entire spectrum of retinal degenerative diseases.

2931 George Wasserman Family Foundation
Grossberg Company
6707 Democracy Blvd
Suite 300
Bethesda, MD 20817-1176
301-571-4977
FAX: 301-571-6250

Helen Salud, Manager
Anthony Cpa, Partner

2932 Giant Food Foundation
8301 Professional Pl
Ste 115
Landover, MD 20785-2351
301-341-4100
888-469-4426
jmiller@giantfood.com
www.giantfood.com

Anthony Hucker, President
Brian Beatty, Md. Director of Marketing and Ex
Stefanie Cain, Md. District Director
Bob Haas, Md. District Director
Offers grants in the areas of mental health, recreation, community and cultural programs, art, and educational programs for the health and prosperity of the greater Washington area.

2933 Harry and Jeanette Weinberg Foundation
7 Park Center Ct
Owings Mills, MD 21117-4200
410-654-8500
FAX: 410-654-4900
cdemchak@hjweinberg.org
hjweinbergfoundation.org

Ellen M. Heller, Chair
Barry I. Schloss, Treasurer
Alvin Awaya, Vice-President
Rachel Garbow Monroe, President and Chief Executive Of
The Harry & Jeanette Weinberg Foundation, Inc. is dedicated to assisting the poor, primarily through operating and capital grants to direct service organizations located in Baltimore, Hawaii, Northeastern Pennsylvania, New York, Israel and the Former Soviet Union. These grants are focused on meeting basic needs such as shelter, nutrition, health & socialization & on enhancing an individual's ability to meet those needs. Within that focus, emphasis is placed on the elderly & Jewish community.

2934 Kennedy Krieger Institute
707 North Broadway
Baltimore, MD 21205
443-923-9200
800-873-3377
888-554-9400
TTY:443-923-2645
findaspecialist@kennedykrieger.org
www.kennedykrieger.org

Gary W. Goldstein, MD
Internationally recognized for improving the lives of children and adolescents with disorders and injuries of the brain, spinal cord and musculoskeletal system, the Kennedy Krieger Institute serves more than 20,000 individuals each year through inpatient and outpatient clincs, home and community services and school-based programs. Kennedy Krieger provides a wide range of services for children and young adults with developmental concerns mid to severe, and is home to a team of investigators.

2935 Miracle-Ear Children's Foundation
5000 Cheshire Ln N
Minneapolis, MN 55446-3706
763-268-4000
800-464-8002
FAX: 763-268-4365
www.miracle-ear.com/en-us/

2936 National Federation of the Blind
200 E. Wells St.
at Jernigan Place
Baltimore, MD 21230- 4998
410-659-9314
FAX: 410-685-5653
nfb@nfb.org
nfb.org

John Berggren, Executive Director, Operations
John G. Par, Jr., Executive Director, Advocacy & Policy
Anil Lewis, Executive Director, NFB Jernigan Institute
The National Federation of the Blind (NFB) is the largest organization of the blind in the world. The Federation's purpose is to help blind people achieve self-confidence, self-respect, and self-determination. Their goal is the complete integration of the blind into society on a basis of equality.

2937 Optometric Extension Program Foundation
2300 York Road
Suite 113
Timonium, MD 21093
410-561-3791
FAX: 949-250-8157
Kelin.Kushin@oep.org
www.oepf.org

Paul A. Harris, OD, President
Robin Lewis, OD, Vice President
Kelin Kushin, Executive Director
Eric Ikeda, Secretary-Treasurer
Vision care for learning disabilities and head trauma patients.

2938 Sjogren's Syndrome Foundation
6707 Democracy Blvd
Suite 325
Bethesda, MD 20817-1164
301-530-4420
800-475-6473
FAX: 301-530-4415
tms@sjogrens.org
www.sjogrens.org

Kenneth Economou, Chairman of the Board
Stephen Cohen, OD, Chairman-Elect
Vidya Sankar, DMD, MHS, Treasurer
Janet Ee. Church, Secretary
Provides patients practical information and coping strategies that minimize the effects of Sjogren's syndrome. In addition, the Foundation is the clearinghouse for medical information and is the recognized national advocate for Sjogren's syndrome. *$25.00 Monthly*

Massachusetts

2939 Abbot and Dorothy H Stevens Foundation
P.O. Box 111
North Andover, MA 01845
                                        978-688-7211
                                    FAX: 978-686-1620

Josh Miner, Executive Director
Established in 1953, Purpose is giving primarily to the arts, education, conservation, and health and human services.

2940 Arc of Massachusetts, The
217 South St
Waltham, MA 02453-2710
                                        781-891-6270
                                    FAX: 781-891-6271
                                    arcmass@arcmass.org
                                    www.arcmass.org

Leo Sarkissian, Executive Director
Joshua Komyerox, Government Affairs Director
Brenda Asis, Development Director
Quarterly newsletter for The Arc of Massachusetts is Advocate.

2941 Arc of Northern Bristol County
141 Park St
Attleboro, MA 02703-3020
                                        508-226-1445
                                        888-343-3301
                                    FAX: 508-226-1476
                                    info@arcnbc.org
                                    arcnbc.org

Richard Harwood, Chairperson
Valerie Zagami, Vice Chairperson
Paul Oliveira, Treasurer
D. Randall Hays, III, Secretary/Clerk
Mission is to strive for the right of all people with developmental disabilities to be valued as individuals, to experience choice, and to be fully included in all aspects of community life

2942 Boston Foundation
75 Arlington St
10th Fl
Boston, MA 02116-3992
                                        617-338-1700
                                    FAX: 617-338-1604
                                    info@tbf.org
                                    tbf.org

Michael Keating, Esq., Chair
Catherine D'Amato, Vice Chair
Paul S. Grogan, President & CEO
Alfred F. Van Ranst, Jr., CFO and Treasurer
The Foundation's grantmaking, special initiatives and civic leadership promote innovation across a broad range of compelling community issues, from educational excellence to affordable housing to workforce development and the arts.

2943 Boston Globe Foundation
P.O. Box 55819
Boston, MA 02205-5819
                                        617-929-2000
                                    lbailey@globe.com
                                    bostonglobe.com

Mary Jacobus, President
The mission of the Boston Globe Foundation is to empower community-based organizations to effect real change in the ares of greatest need, where the Globe is uniquely postioned to add the most value. Priority focus areas: strengthen the reading, writing and critical thinking of young people, while fostering their inherent love of learning. Strengthen the roads that link people to culture. Strengthen the civic fabric of the city. Be responsive to the needs of our immediate community.

2944 Bushrod H Campbell and Ada F Hall Charity Fund
Palmer & Dodge
111 Huntington Ave
Boston, MA 02199-7610
                                        617-239-0540
                                    FAX: 617-227-4420

Brenda Taylor, Foundation Administrator
The fund's areas of interest include organizations and/or their projects supporting aid to the elderly, healthcare and population control. Medical research grants are administered through the Medical Foundation. No grants are awarded to individuals and the geographical area of support is limited to organizations located in Massachusetts within the area of Boston and Route 128.

2945 Clipper Ship Foundation
77 Summer St
8th Floor
Boston, MA 02110-1006
                                        617-391-3088
                                    FAX: 617-426-7087
                                    hblaisdell@gmafoundations.com
                                    clippershipfoundation.org

Ron Ancrum, President
Makes grants to federally tax-qualified non-profit organizations offering human services to individuals living in Greater Boston and the cities of Lawrence and Brockton.

2946 Community Foundation of Western Massachusetts
1500 Main Street, Suite 2300
P.O. Box 15769
Springfield, MA 01115-5769
                                        413-732-2858
                                    FAX: 413-733-8565
                                    wmass@communityfoundation.org
                                    www.communityfoundation.org

Katie Allan Zobel, President and CEO
Nancy Reiche, M.S.W., Vice President for Programs
Donna Roseman David, Chief Financial Officer/Chief Ad
Kristin Leutz, Vice President of Philanthropic
Provides a simple way to achieve the charitable objectives of donors most effectively; supports nonprofit organizations that offer programs in the arts, education, human services, healthcare, housing, and the environment; and works to improve the quality of life in our region.

2947 Frank R and Elizabeth Simoni Foundation
1401 Boston Providence Tpke
Norwood, MA 02062-5053
                                        781-762-3449
                                    FAX: 781-769-6166

Matthew Mac Donald, President
Ann Mac Donald, Secretary
Robert Mac Donald, Clerk

2948 Frank Stanley Beveridge Foundation
3 Upland Lane
West Newbury, MA 01985
                                        800-229-9667
                                    administrator@beveridge.org
                                    www.beveridge.org

Ward Slocum Caswell, President
Philip Caswell, Chairman and Vice President
Ruth S. DuPont, Treasurer
Leah Beveridge Richardson, Clerk
The mission of The Frank Stanley Beveridge Foundation, Inc. is to preserve and enhance the quality of life by embracing and perpetuating Frank Stanley Beveridge's philanthropic vision through grantmaking initiatives in support of The Stanley Park of Westfield, Inc. and programs in youth development, health, education, religion, art and environment primarily in Hampden and Hampshire Counties, Massachusetts.

2949 Friendly Ice Cream Corp Contributions Program
1855 Boston Rd
Wilbraham, MA 01095-1002
                                        413-543-3544
                                        800-966-9970
                                    FAX: 413-731-4467
                                    friendlys.com

John Maguire, Chief Financial Officer
Steve Weigel, EVP, Chief Operating Officer
Pat Hickey, EVP, Chief Financial Officer
Tim Hopkins, EVP, Retail and Manufacturing

2950 Greater Worcester Community Foundation
370 Main St
Ste 650
Worcester, MA 01608-1738
508-755-0980
FAX: 508-755-3406
info@greaterworcester.org
greaterworcester.org

Gerald Gaudette III, Chair
Warner S. Fletcher, Vice Chair
Thomas J. Bartholomew, Treasurer
Carolyn Stempler, Clerk
By focusing on the entire community rather then on any specific issue, the community foundation is able to address matters of greater importance to the people of the region. The Foundation has built a permanent, flexable endowment and has distributed grants and awards to a broad range of organizations and people throughout the region.

2951 Hyams Foundation
50 Federal St
Fl 9
Boston, MA 02110-2241
617-426-5600
FAX: 617-426-5696
info@hyamsfoundation.org
hyamsfoundation.org

Martella Wilson-Taylor, Chair
Adam D. Seitchik, Treasurer
Roslyn M. Watson, Assistant Treasurer
Iris Gomez, Clerk
Mission is to increase economic and social justice and power within low-income communities in Boston and Chelsea, Massachusetts.

2952 Raytheon Company Contributions Program
870 Winter St
Waltham, MA 02451-1449
781-522-3000
FAX: 781-860-2172
raytheon.com

Thomas A. Kennedy, Chief Financial Officer
David C. Wajsgras, Senior Vice President and Chief
Keith J. Peden, Senior Vice President - Human Re
Jay B. Stephens, Senior Vice President - General
Industry leader in defense and government electronics, space, information technology, technical services, and business aviation and special mission aircraft.

2953 TJX Foundation
TJX Companies
770 Cochituate Rd
Framingham, MA 01701-4666
508-390-1000
FAX: 508-390-2091
www.tjx.com

Carol Meyrowitz, CEO
The purpose of the TJX Foundation's Giving Program is to support qualified, tax-exempt nonprofit organizations that provide services which promote and improve the quality of life for children, women and families in need.

2954 Vision Foundation
8901 Strafford Cir
Knoxville, TN 37923-1500
865-357-4603
FAX: 865-690-9322
gordon@visionfoundation.net
www.visionfoundation.net

Gordon Adams, President
Offers counseling, support groups, seminars and transportation for the blind providing 600 members.

Michigan

2955 Ann Arbor Area Community Foundation
301 N Main St
Ste 300
Ann Arbor, MI 48104-1296
734-663-0401
FAX: 734-663-3514
info@aaacf.org
aaacf.org

Michelle Crumm, Chair
Tim Wadhams, Vice Chair
Neel Hajra, President & CEO
Shelley Strickland, Vice President
Interested in funding projects which will improve the quality of life for citizens of the Ann Arbor area. Eligible projects generally fall within these categories: education, culture, social service, community development, environmental awareness and health and wellness. The Foundation aims to support creative approaches to community needs and problems by making grants which will benefit the widest possible range of people.

2956 Arc of Michigan
State of Michigan
1325 S Washington Ave
Lansing, MI 48910-1652
517-487-5426
800-292-7851
FAX: 517-487-0303
dhoyle@arcmi.org
arcmi.org

Shari Fitzpatrick, President
Kim Brown, Vice President
Bob Altizer, Secretary
Laurel Robb, Treasurer
The Arc Michigan empowers local chapters to assure that citizens with disabilities are valued and that they and their families participate fully in and contribute to the life of their community.

2957 Berrien Community Foundation
2900 S State St
Ste 2e
Saint Joseph, MI 49085-2467
269-983-3304
FAX: 269-983-4939
bcf@BerrienCommunity.org
berriencommunity.org

Hillary Bubb, Chair
Mabel Mayfield, Vice Chair
Lisa Cripps-Downey, President
Sandra Tardi, Finance Director
The Foundation is a union of numerous gifts, bequests and other contributions that form permanent endowments and other funds.

2958 Blind Children's Fund
6761 West 45-12
P.O. Box 363
Three Oaks, MI 49128
989-779-9966
FAX: 269-756-3133
bcf@blindchildrensfund.org
www.blindchildrensfund.org

Karla B. Kwast, Executive Director
Provides parents and profesionsals informaion materials and resources that help them scuccesfullly teach and nurture blind, visually and multi-impaired infants and preschoolers.

2959 Community Foundation of Monroe County
P.O. Box 627
28 S. Macomb St.
Monroe, MI 48161-627
734-242-1976
FAX: 734-242-1234
info@cfmonroe.org
cfmonroe.org

Kathleen Russeau, MBA, Executive Director
Michele Sandiefer, Office Manager
Julie Rhinehart, YAC Coordinator
Doug Redding, Project Manager
The mission of the Community Foundation of Monroe County is to encourage and facilitate philanthropy in Monroe County.

2960 Cowan Slavin Foundation
7881 Dell Rd
Saline, MI 48176-9744   734-944-1439
                          FAX: 734-944-3529

David Bovee, Owner

2961 Daimler Chrysler
Automobility Program
P.O. Box 5080
Troy, MI 48007-5080

                          800-255-9877
                     FAX: 855-409-0475
                  rebates@chrysler.com
               www.chryslerautomobility.com

2962 Frank & Mollie S VanDervoort Memorial Foundation
4646 Okemos Rd
Okemos, MI 48864-1795   517-349-7232

Ann L Gessert, Secretary

2963 Fremont Area Community Foundation
4424 W. 48th Street
PO Box B
Fremont, MI 49412-176   231-924-5350
                          FAX: 231-924-5351
                              info@tfacf.org
                                     tfacf.org

Robert Zeldenrust, Chair
William Johnson, Vice Chair
Carla Roberts, President & CEO
Cathy Kissinger, Secretary
A local nonprofit organization serving the residence of Newaygo County. We connect the needs of the community with those who have the conviction to make a lasting impact. Our mission is to improve the quality of life for the people of Newaygo County. Zeldenrust

2964 Grand Rapids Foundation
185 Oakes St SW
Grand Rapids, MI 49503-4008   616-454-1751
                          FAX: 616-454-6455
                     grfound@grfoundation.org
                              grfoundation.org

Paul M. Keep, Chair
Laurie Finney Beard, Vice Chair
Diana R. Sieger, President
Ren Guttrich, Executive Assistant
Grand Rapids Community Foundation leads the community in making positive, sustainable change. Through our grantmaking and leadership initiatives we help foster academic achievement, build economic prosperity, achieve healthy ecosystems, encourage healthy people, support social enrichment, and create vibrant neighborhoods.

2965 Granger Foundation
6267 Aurelius Rd
Lansing, MI 48911-2187   517-393-1670
                          FAX: 517-393-1382
                  elee@grangerconstruction.com
                       grangerconstruction.com

Alton Granger, Chairman
Glenn D. Granger, President & CEO
The primary purpose of the Granger Foundation is to enhance the quality of life within the Greater Lansing, Michigan Area. Our mission is to support Christ-centered activities. We also support efforts that enhance the lives of youth in our community.

2966 Harvey Randall Wickes Foundation
4800 Fashion Square Blvd
Suite 472
Saginaw, MI 48604- 2677   989-799-1850
                          FAX: 989-799-3327
                                  www.tgci.com

James Finkbeiner

Grants for rehabilitation.

2967 Havirmill Foundation
3505 Greenleaf Blvd
Ste 203
Kalamazoo, MI 49008-2580   269-375-1193
                          millenniumrestaurants.com

Ken Miller, CEO, Principal Partner
Matthew Burian, President
Bob Lewis, Operating Partner
Shelly Pastor, Operating Partner

2968 Kelly Services Foundation
999 W Big Beaver Rd
Troy, MI 48084-4782   248-362-4444
                          FAX: 248-244-4588
                     kfirst@kellyservices.com
                              kellyservices.com

George S. Corona, Chief Operating Officer
Carl T. Camden, President & CEO
Terence E. Adderley, Executive Chairman
Olivier Thirot, Acting Chief Financial Officer

2969 Kresge Foundation
3215 W Big Beaver Rd
Troy, MI 48084-2818   248-643-9630
                          FAX: 248-643-0588
                              info@kresge.org
                                    kresge.org

Rip Rapson, President and CEO
Amy B. Coleman, VP/CFO
Ariel H. Simon, Vice President, Chief Program
Marcus L. McGrew, Director of Grants Management
This foundation offers challenge grants for capital projects, most often for construction or renovation of buildings, but also for the purchase of major equipment and real estate. As challenge grants, they are intended to stimulate new, private gifts in the midst of an organized fund raising effort. Offers special opportunities to build capacity, both in providing enhanced facilities in which to present programs and in generating private support. Only charitable organizations may apply.

2970 Lanting Foundation
1575 S Shore Dr
Holland, MI 49423-4436   616-335-2033

Arlyn Lanting, Partner

2971 Rollin M Gerstacker Foundation
PO Box 1945
Midland, MI 48641-1945   989-631-6097
                       www.gerstackerfoundation.org

Gail E. Lanphear, Chairperson
Lisa J. Gerstacker, President
E. N. Brandt, Vice President /Secretary
Alan W Ott, Vice President /Treasurer
The Rollin M. Gerstacker Foundation was founded by Mrs. Eda U. Gerstacker in 1957, in memory of her husband. Its primary purpose is to carry on, indefinitely, financial aid to charities of all types supported by Mr. and Mrs. R.M. Gerstacker during their lifetimes. These charities are concentrated in the states of Michigan and Ohio.

2972 Steelcase Foundation
PO Box 1967
GH-4E
Grand Rapids, MI 49501-1967   616-246-4695
                          FAX: 616-475-2200
                     pgebben@steelcase.com
                              steelcase.com

Phyllis Gebben, Coordinator of Donations
James P. Hackett, President & CEO
Established in 1951, the Foundation focuses on the areas of human service, health, education, community development, the arts

and the environment - giving particular concern to people who are disadvantaged, disabled, young and elderly as they attempt to improve the quality of their lives.

Minnesota

2973   Arc of Minnesota
800 Transfer Road
Suite 7A
St. Paul, MN 55114   651-523-0823
     800-582-5256
     FAX: 651-523-0829
     mail@arcmn.org
     www.arcmn.org

John Rentschler, President
Lisa Schoneman, Vice President
Amy Hewitt, Secretary
Rob Wolf, Treasurer
Your membership in The Arc of Minnesotta benefits persons with developmental disabilities and their families as they live, learn, work and play. Please join today!

2974   Deluxe Corporation Foundation
Deluxe Corporation
3680 Victoria St N
Shoreview, MN 55126-2966   651-483-7111
     800-328-0304
     FAX: 651-483-7270
     feedback@deluxe.com
     ww.deluxe.com

Lee J Schram, CEO
Terry D. Peterson, CFO /Senior VP
Malcolm J. McRoberts, Senior Vice President, Small Bus
John D. Filby, Senior Vice President, Financial
Funds programs such as schools, museums, programs for the disadvantaged. We believe programs and services like these represent the heart and soul of our communities.

2975   General Mills Foundation
P.O. Box 9452
Minneapolis, MN 55440-9452
     800-248-7310
     FAX: 763-764-8330
     corporate.response@genmills.com
     generalmills.com
Kendall J. Powell, Chairman / CEO
Ann W.H. Simonds, Senior Vice President/ Chief Mar
Keith A Woodward, Vice President, Treasurer
Gary Chu, Senior Vice President

2976   Hugh J Andersen Foundation
342 5th Ave N
Suite 200
Bayport, MN 55003-4502   651-439-1557
     888-439-9508
     FAX: 651-439-9480
     contact@srinc.biz
     www.srinc.biz
Brad Kruse, Program Director
Established in 1962, this fund is a nonprofit charitable corporation classified as a private foundation. The Foundation was established as a general charitable fund, but now identifies projects that build individual and community capacity to be a priority. Giving is focused primarily in the counties of Washington, Minnesota, & St, Croix, Polk and Pierce of Wl. Grants are given in the areas of human services, health, education, arts and culture, community services and the environment.

2977   James R Thorpe Foundation
5866 Oakland Avenue
Minneapolis, MN 55417-5418   763-250-9304
     info@jamesrthorpefoundation.org
     www.jamesrthorpefoundation.org

Tim Thorpe, President
Robert C. Cote, Treasurer
Kerrie Blevins, Foundation Manager
S. Ruggles Cote, Board Member
Foundation based on values of respect and compassion, and is dedicated to making the greater Minneapolis area better for all its citizens.

2978   Jay and Rose Phillips Family Foundation
615 First Ave. NE
Ste. 330
Minneapolis, MN 55413   612-623-1654
     FAX: 612-623-1653
     info@phillipsfamilyfoundationmn.org
     www.phillipsfnd.org

Patrick Troska, Executive Director
Joel Luedtke, Senior Program Officer
Tracy Lamparty, Grants and Operations Manager
Salena Acox, Vista Program Manager

2979   Minneapolis Foundation
80 S 8th St
800 IDS Center
Minneapolis, MN 55402-2100   612-672-3878
     866-305-0543
     FAX: 612-672-3846
     email@mplsfoundation.org
     www.mplsfoundation.org

Sandra L. Vargus, President and CEO
Jean M. Adams, Chief Operating Officer/Chief Fi
Teresa Morrow, Vice President, External Relatio
Luz Maria Frias, Vice President, Community Impact
Provides a variety of charitable fund and gift options to help Minnesotans make a difference.

2980   Ordean Foundation
424 W Superior St
Duluth, MN 55802-1591   218-726-4785

Steve Mangan, Executive Director
Grants are given for a variety of purposes including: treatment and rehabilitation for persons who are chronically or temporarily mentally ill, persons whose physical capacity is impaired by injury or illness, promotes mental and physical health of the elderly, provides for youth guidance programs designed to avoid delinquency, and provides relief, aid and charity to people with no or low incomes. Grants are only offered to certain cities and townships near and around St. Louis County/Duluth.

2981   Otto Bremer Foundation
445 Minnesota St
Ste 2250
Saint Paul, MN 55101-2161   651-227-8036
     888-291-1123
     FAX: 651-312-3665
     obf@ottobremer.org
     www.ottobremer.org

Kari Suzuki, Director of Operations
Diane Benjamin, Executive Director
Danielle Cheslog, Grants Manager
Rose Carr, Program Officer
Mission is to assist people in achieving full economic, civic and social participation in and for the betterment of their communities.

303

2982 **Rochester Area Foundation**
400 South Broadway
Suite 300
Rochester, MN 55904

507-282-0203
FAX: 507-282-4938
info@rochesterarea.org
rochesterarea.org

JoAnn Stormer, President
Max Evans, Administration/Communications
Ann Fahy-Gust, Grants and Impact Officer
Paul Harkess, Development Officer

The mission of the Rochester Area Foundation is to strengthen community philanthropy by promoting responsible and informed giving and to assist donors in meeting their charitable objectives.

Mississippi

2983 **Arc of Mississippi**
704 North President Street
Jackson, MS 39202

601-355-0220
800-717-1180
FAX: 601-355-0221
info@arcms.org
www.arcms.org

Kim Duffy, President
Ronnie Raggio, Senior Vice-President
Shirley Miller, Secretary
Cherri Hedglin, Treasurer

The Arc is Committed to securing for all people with developmental disabilities the opportunity to choose and realize their goals of where and how they learn live work and play.

Missouri

2984 **Allen P & Josephine B Green Foundation**
1055 Broadway
Suite 130
Kansas City, MO 64105

816-627-3420
FAX: 816-268-3420
greenfoundation@gkccf.org
www.greenfdn.org

Matthew Fuller, Manager of Community Investment

While the Foundation makes grants in a variety of fields, in the past its major support was in the field of medical research. During a 20-year period, 1951-71, it contributed over $900,000 to research in Parkinson's and related diseases of the nervous system; $600,000 for research in pediatric neurology and lesser amounts in other areas of medical research, but the board is now trending in other directions. Grants are limited to Missouri and none are offered to individuals.

2985 **Anheuser-Busch**
1 Busch Pl
Saint Louis, MO 63118-1852

314-577-2000
800-342-5283
FAX: 314-577-2900
anheuser-busch.com

August A Busch Iv, President

Supports education, helped fund health and human services organizations, provided disaster relief, and worked to preserve the environment.

2986 **Arc of the US Missouri Chapter**
PO Box 7823
Columbia, MO 65205

573-552-7648
arcmoinfo@arcofmissouri.org
www.arcofmissouri.org

2987 **Greater Kansas City Community Foundation & Affiliated Trusts**
1055 Broadway Blvd
Suite 130
Kansas City, MO 64105-1595

816-842-0944
866-719-7886
FAX: 816-842-8079
info@gkccf.org
www.growyourgiving.org

William S. Berkley, Past Chair
Dr. Jim Hinson, Vice Chair
William H. Coughlin, President
Mary Bloch, Community Volunteer

Mission is to improve the quality of life in Greater Kansas City by increasing charitable giving, connecting donors to community needs they care about, and providing leadership on critical community issues.

2988 **Greater St Louis Community Foundation**
319 N 4th St
Ste 300
Saint Louis, MO 63102-1906

314-588-8200
FAX: 314-588-8088
dluckes@gstlcf.org
gstlcf.org

Stephen J. Rafferty, Chair
Thomas R. Collins, Vice Chair & Secretary
Amelia A.J. Bond, President & CEO
Mara Mitch Meyers, Treasurer

To improve the quality of life across the region by helping individuals, families and businesses make a difference through charitable giving.

2989 **H&R Block Foundation**
1 H and R Block Way
Kansas City, MO 64105-1905

816-854-4363
FAX: 816-854-8025
foundation@hrblock.com
www.blockfoundation.org

Henry W. Bloch, Chairman/ Treasurer/ Director
Thomas M. Bloch, Vice Chairman & Director
David P. Miles, President
Carey Wilker Looney, Vice President and Secretary

A charitable organization under the not-for-profit corporation law of the state of Missouri. Grants are made only to organizations which are tax exempt from Federal Income taxation and which are not classified as private foundations. Major emphasis is placed in the metropolitan areas of Kansas City, Missouri: and Columbus, Ohio. The goal is to provide proportionately significant support of relatively few activities, as opposed to minor support for a great many.

2990 **James S McDonnell Foundation**
1034 S Brentwood Blvd
Suite 1850
Saint Louis, MO 63117- 1284

314-721-1532
FAX: 314-721-7421
info@jsmf.org
jsmf.org

Susan M Fitzpatrick, President
John T. Bruer, President Emeritus
Cheryl A. Washington, Grants Manager
M. Brent Dolezalek, Senior Program Associate

The Foundation supports scientific, educational, and charitable causes locally, nationally and internationally.

2991 **Lutheran Charities Foundation of St Louis**
8860 Ladue Road
Suite 200
Saint Louis, MO 63124

314-231-2244
FAX: 314-727-7688
info@lutheranfoundation.org
www.lutheranfoundation.org

Karl A. Dunajcik, Chairperson of the Board
Ann L. Vazquez, President/ CEO
Melinda K. McAliney, Program Director
Donna Luker, Office/Grants Manager

Seeks the improved care of people in the greater St. Louis metropolitan region. Lutheran Foundation of St. Louis manages the endowment established upon the sale of the Lutheran Medical Center and provides grant awards for health, human care, Lutheran congregations' community service programs, and Lutheran education.

2992   RA Bloch Cancer Foundation
1 H and R Block Way
Kansas City, MO 64105-1905   816-854-5050
                                         800-433-0464
                                    FAX: 816-854-8024
                              hotline@blochcancer.org
                                   www.blochcancer.org

Vangie Rich, Executive Director
Rosanne Wickman, Hotline Director
Provides a hotline that matches newly diagnosed cancer patients with someone who has survived the same kind of cancer. Offers free infomration, resources and support groups, and distributes lists of multidisciplinary second opinion centers. Also supplies three books at no charge: Fighting Cancer; Cancer... There's Hope; and A Guide for Cancer Supporters. All services and books are free of charge.

2993   Victor E Speas Foundation
10434 Indiana Ave
Kansas City, MO 64137-1532   816-868-9300
                          mo.grantmaking@ustrust.com
                                   www.bankofamerica.com

Latricia Scott Adams, President
VCC is a membership-based organization that brings together area volunteer managers and others interested in volunteerism for mutual support, exchange of ideas and information, and educational programs of timely interest.

Nebraska

2994   Arc of Nebraska
215 Centennial Mall South
Suite 508
Lincoln, NE 68508   402-475-4407
                                         888-519-6524
                                    FAX: 402-475-0214
                                 info@arc-nebraska.org
                                   www.arc-nebraska.org

Debbie Salomon, President
David Rowe, 1st Vice President
Kadi Holmberg, 2nd Vice President
Michael Chittenden, Executive Director
Arc of Nebraska is commited to helping children and adults with disabilities secure the oppurtunity to choose and realize their goals of where and how they learn, live, work, and play.

2995   Cooper Foundation
1248 O St
Suite 870
Lincoln, NE 68508-1493   402-476-7571
                                    FAX: 402-476-2356
                                info@cooperfoundation.org
                                   cooperfoundation.org

Jack Campbell, Chair
Brad Korell, VP Business Development
Art Thompson, President
Robert Nefsky, Attorney & Partner
Serves only Nebraska with the primary interest in education, arts and humanities and the human services area.

2996   Mosaic
4980 S 118th St
Omaha, NE 68137-2200   402-896-9988
                                         877-366-7242
                                    FAX: 402-896-1511
                                   info@mosaicinfo.org
                                     www.mosaicinfo.org

Linda Timmons, President / CEO
Cindy Schroeder, Chief Financial Officer
Raul Saldivar, Chief Operating Officer
Scott Hoffman, Senior Vice President of Finance
Headquarters for the faith-based organization providing services to people with disabilities in communities nationwide, and in conjunction with international partners. Mosaic was born of a merger of these two Lutheran organizations: Bethpage and Martin Luther Homes Society.

2997   Slosburg Family Charitable Trust
10040 Regency Cir
Ste 200
Omaha, NE 68114-3734   402-391-7900
                                    FAX: 402-391-2991
                                         richdale.com

David Slosburg, Owner

2998   Union Pacific Foundation
1400 Douglas Street
Omaha, NE 68179   402-544-5000
                                         888-870-8777
                                         888-877-7267
                                    FAX: 402-501-0021
                                         www.up.com

John J. Koraleski, Executive Chairman
Lance M. Fritz, President & COO of Union Pacific
Eric L. Butler, EVP, Marketing and Sales
Diane K. Duren, EVP/ Corporate Secretary
The Union Pacific Foundation is the philanthropic arm of the Union Pacific Corporation and Union Pacific Railroad. Union Pacific believes that the quality of life in the commuinities in which its employees live and work is an integral part of its own success.

Nevada

2999   Conrad N Hilton Foundation
30440 Agoura Road
Agoura Hills, CA 91301   818-851-3700
                                    FAX: 310-694-9051
                               cnhf@hiltonfoundation.org
                                   hiltonfoundation.org

Steven M. Hilton, Chairman, President & CEO
Barron Hilton, Chairman Emeritus
Donald H Hubbs, Director Emeritus
Katherine Miller, Facilities and Office Services M
Our grant-making style is to initiate and develop major long-term projects and then seek out the organizations to implement them. As a consequence of this proactive approach, the Foundation does not generally consider unsolicited proposals. Our major projects currently include: blindness prevention and treatment, support the work of the Catholic Sisters, drug abuse prevention among youth, support of the Conrad N. Hilton College of Hotel and Restaurant Management, and much more.

3000   EL Wiegand Foundation
165 W Liberty St
Suite 200
Reno, NV 89501-1955   775-333-0310
                                    FAX: 775-333-0314
                               www.thewiegandfoundationinc.com

Kristen A Avansino, President/Executive Director

3001 Nell J Redfield Foundation
PO Box 61
Reno, NV 89504-0061
775-323-1373
FAX: 775-323-4476
redfieldfoundation@yahoo.com

Jerry Smith, Manager
Gerald C. Smith, V.P. and Secy

3002 William N Pennington Foundation
441 W Plumb Ln
Reno, NV 89509-3766
775-333-9100
FAX: 775-333-9111

William Pennington, Owner

New Hampshire

3003 Agnes M Lindsay Trust
660 Chestnut St
Manchester, NH 03104-3550
603-669-1366
866-669-1366
FAX: 603-665-8114
admin@lindsaytrust.org
lindsaytrust.org

Susan E. Bouchard, Administrative Director
Ernest E. Dion, CPA, Trustee
Alan G. Lampert, Esq., Trustee
Michael S. Delucia, Esq., Trustee

Funding for health and wefare organizations, special needs, mental health, blind, deaf and cultural programs to organizations, specifically for capital needs, not operating funds, located in the New England states of Maine, Massachusetts, New Hampshire and Vermont. We highly recommend you visit our web site.

3004 Foundation for Seacoast Health
100 Campus Dr
Ste 1
Portsmouth, NH 03801-5892
603-422-8200
FAX: 603-422-8206
ffsh@communitycampus.org
ffsh.org

Debra S. Grabowski, Executive Director
Kathleen Taylor, Finance Director
Eligio Santana, Facility Manager
Noreen Hodgdon, Executive Assistant

Giving limited to Portsmouth, Rye, New Castle, Greenland, Newington, North Hampton, NH; and Kittery, Eliot, and York, ME.

New Jersey

3005 Arc of New Jersey
985 Livingston Ave
N Brunswick, NJ 08902-1843
732-246-2525
FAX: 732-214-1834
info@arcnj.org
arcnj.org

Robert Hage, President
Joanne Bergin, First Vice President
Kevin Sturges, Second Vice President
Elspeth Moore, Secretary

The Arc of New Jersey is committed to enhancing the quality of life of children and adults with intellectual and developmental disabilities and their families, through advocacy, empowerment, education and prevention.

3006 Arnold A Schwartz Foundation
15 Mountain Blvd
Warren, NJ 7059-5611
908-757-7800
FAX: 908-757-8039
skunzmannewjerseylaw.net

Steven A Kunzman, President

3007 Campbell Soup Foundation
1 Campbell Pl
Camden, NJ 08103-1701
800-257-8443
media@campbellsoup.com
campbellsoup.com

Denise M. Morrison, President/ CEO
Anthony P. DiSilvestro, Senior Vice President and Chief
Mark Alexander, President
Carlos J. Barraso, Senior Vice President - Global R

Goal of this foundation is to match the company's assets with community needs in order to help forge solutions to community challenges. The Foundation believes that involvement at the community level can play a catalytic role in improving the quality of life. Giving is located in the areas of education, nutrition and health, cultural and youth related programs. The major focus of the foundation is on nutrition and health related matters, and places a high priority on Camden, New Jersey areas.

3008 Children's Hopes & Dreams Wish Fulfillment Foundation
280 US Highway 46
Dover, NJ 07801-2084
706-482-2248
FAX: 706-482-2289
info@chddover.org
www.helpingnow.org

3009 Community Foundation of New Jersey
35 Knox Hill Road Morristown
PO Box 338
Morristown, NJ 07963-0388
973-267-5533
800-659-5533
FAX: 973-267-2903
info@cfnj.org
www.cfnj.org

Hans Dekker, President
Madeline Rivera, Program Officer
Susan I. Soldivieri, Chief Financial Officer
Faith Krueger, Chief Operating Officer

The Community Foundation of New Jersey is an alliance of families, businesses, and foundations that work together to create lasting differences in lives and communities today and tomorrow.

3010 FM Kirby Foundation
17 DeHart Street
PO Box 151
Morristown, NJ 07963-0151
973-538-4800
www.fdncenter.org/grantmaker/kirby

S. Dillard Kirby, President and Director
Jefferson W Kirby, Vice President and Director
Alice Kirby Horton, Assistant Secretary and Director
Walker D. Kirby, Director

Family foundation, grants made to a wide range of nonprofit organizations in education, health and medicine, the arts and humanities, civic and public affairs, as well as religious, welfare and youth organizations.

3011 Fannie E Rippel Foundation
14 Maple Avenue
Suite 200
Morristown, NJ 07960
973-540-0101
FAX: 973-540-0404
info@rippelfoundation.org
www.rippelfoundation.org

Laura K Landy, President/ CEO
Chana Fitton, Chief Operating Officer
John D. Campbell, Chairman
Elizabeth G. Christopherson, Secretary

Core purposes: research and treatment related to cancer and heart disease, the health of women and the elderly, and the quality of our nation's hospitals.

3012 Fund for New Jersey
One Palmer Square East
Suite 303
Princeton, NJ 08542   609-356-0421
                          lmandell@fundfornj.org
                                  fundfornj.org

Kiki Jamieson, President
Lucy Vandenberg, Senior Program Officer
Laura Mandell, Office Manager
Ami Kachalia, Program Associate
Our grants promote projects that share a high purpose of further-
ing effective democracy through a range of methods encompass-
ing education, advocacy, public policy analysis, and community
problem-solving.

3013 Merck Company Foundation
2000 Galloping Hill Road
Kenilworth, NJ 07033   908-740-4000
                                       merck.com

Kenneth C. Frazier, Chairman
Robert M. Davis, Executive Vice President and Chi
Willie A. Deese, EVP and President, Merck Manufac
Clark Golestani, Executive Vice President and Chi
Mission of the foundation is to support organizations and innovative programs in alignment with four strategic profiles: Improving access to quality health care and the appropriate use of
medicines and vaccines, building capacity in the biomedical and
health sciences, promoting environments that support innovation, economic growth and development in and ethical and fair
context, and supporting communities where Merck employees
work and live.

3014 Nabisco Foundation
7 Campus Dr
Parsippany, NJ 07054-4413   973-682-7096
                             FAX: 973-503-3018

Henry Sandbach, Director

3015 Ostberg Foundation
PO Box 1098
Alpine, NJ 07620-1098   201-569-6800
                             FAX: 201-767-8006

3016 Prudential Foundation
Prudential Financial
751 Broad St
15th Floor
Newark, NJ 07102-3714   973-802-6000
                             FAX: 973-802-7486
               community.resources@prudential.com
                                  prudential.com

John R Strangfeld, Chairman and CEO
Mark B. Grier, Vice Chairman
Charles Lowrey, Executive Vice President, Chief
Sharon C. Taylor, Senior Vice President, Corporate
Gives priority to national programs that further our objectives
and programs serving areas where The Prudential has a substan-
tial employee presence. Places special emphasis on the home
state of New Jersey and the headquarters city, Newark.

3017 Robert Wood Johnson Foundation
Route 1 and College Road East
P.O. Box 2316
Princeton, NJ 08543-2316   609-452-8701
                                   877-843-7953
                             FAX: 888-727-1966
                                 mail@rwjf.org
                                       rwjf.org

Roger S. Fine, Chairman
Risa Lavizzo-Mourey, President and CEO
Robin E. Mockenhaupt, Chief of Staff
Joan F. McKay, Executive Assistant, Executive O
Our mission is to assure that all Americans have access to basic
health care at reasonable cost, improve care and support for peo-
ple with chronic health conditions, promote healthy communities

and lifestyles and also, reduce the personal, social and economic
harm caused by substance abuse.

3018 Victoria Foundation
31 Mulberry Street
5th Floor
Newark, NJ 07102-1397   973-792-9200
                             FAX: 973-792-1300
                        info@victoriafoundation.org
                        www.victoriafoundation.org

Frank Alvarez, President
Margaret H. Parker, Vice President
Gary M. Wingens, Treasurer
Irene Cooper-Basch, Executive Officer
Desire is to help individuals in need reach their potential remains.
Provides emergency coal for needy families and treated rheu-
matic fever in children.

New Mexico

3019 Arc of New Mexico
3655 Carlisle NE
Albuquerque, NM 87110-1644   505-883-4630
                                   800-358-6493
                             FAX: 505-883-5564
                             rcostales@arcnm.org
                                      arcnm.org

John Hall, President
Dolores Harden, Senior Vice President
Elaine Palma, Secretary
Randy Costales, Executive Director
Our mission is to improve the quality of life for individuals with
developmental disabilities of all ages by advocating for equal opportunities and choices in where and how they learn, live, work,
play and socialize. The Arc of New Mexico promotes self-determination, healthy families, effective community support systems
and partnerships.

3020 Frost Foundation
511 Armijo St
Suite A
Santa Fe, NM 87501-2899   505-986-0208
                              info@frostfound.org
                                   frostfound.org

Mary Amelia Whited-Howell, President
Philip B. Howell, Executive Vice President
Taylor F. Moore, Secretary/Treasurer
Ann Rogers Gerber, Board Member
The Frost Foundation was created to be operated excusively for
educational, charitable, and religious purposes.

3021 McCune Charitable Foundation
345 E Alameda St
Santa Fe, NM 87501-2229   505-983-8300
                             FAX: 505-983-7887
                            mccune@nmmccune.org
                                   nmmccune.org

Sarah McCune Losinger, Chair
Wendy Lewis, Executive Director
Henry Rael, Program Officer
Carla Romero, Administrative Director
Dedicated to enriching the health, education, environment, and
cultural and spiritual life of New Mexicans.

3022 Santa Fe Community Foundation
501 Halona Street
Santa Fe, NM 87505   505-988-9715
                             FAX: 505-988-1829
                         foundation@santafecf.org
                            www.santafecf.org

Suzanne Ortega Cisneros, Chair
Barry Herskowitz, Vice Chair
Kenneth Romero, Secretary
Stephen G. Gaber, Treasurer

New York

3023 AT&T Foundation
32 Avenue of the Americas
24th Floor
New York, NY 10013-2473 212-226-2216
FAX: 212-387-5097
info@att.com
www.att.com

Randall L Stephenson, Chairman, Chief Executive Office
John T. Stanky, Group President and Chief Strate
Wayne Watts, Senior Executive Vice President
John Stephens, Senior Executive Vice President
Committed to advancing education, strengthening communities and improving lives.

3024 Altman Foundation
521 5th Ave
Fl 35
New York, NY 10175-3500 212-682-0970
FAX: 212-682-1648
info@altman.org
altmanfoundation.org

Karen L. Rosa, President
Jeremy Tennenbaum, Chief Financial Officer
Ann E. Maldonado, Office Manager
Megan McAllister, Program Officer
For the benefit of such charitable and educational institutions in the City of New York as said directors shall approve. Foundation grants support programs and institutions that enrich the quality of life in the city, with a particular focus on initiatives that help individuals, families and communities benefit from the services and opportunities that will enable them to achieve their full potential.

3025 Ambrose Monell Foundation
1 Rockefeller Plz
Suite 301
New York, NY 10020-2002 212-586-0700
FAX: 212-245-1863
info@monellvetlesen.org
www.monellvetlesen.org

Ambrose K. Monell,, President and Treasurer
Eugene P. Grisanti, Vice-President
George Rowe, Vice-President
Kristen G. Pemberton, Secretary
Voluntary aiding and contributing to religious, charitable, scientific, literary, and educational uses and purposes, in New York, elsewhere in the US and throughout the world.

3026 American Chai Trust
41 Madison Ave
Suite 400
New York, NY 10010-2202 212-889-0575
FAX: 212-743-8120
info@perlmanandperlman.com
www.perlmanandperlman.com

3027 American Express Foundation
P.O. Box 981540
El Paso, TX 79998-1540

800-528-4800
TTY:800-221-9950
americanexpress.com
Kenneth I Chenault, Chairman and Chief Executive Off
L. Kevin Cox, Chief Human Resources Officer
Marc D. Gordon, Executive Vice President and Chi
John D. Hayes, Executive Vice President and Chi
Grants are awarded in the three program areas: Community Service, Cultural Heritage, and Economic Independence. Most grants are made for projects operating where the company has a major employee or market presence.

3028 American Foundation for the Blind
2 Penn Plaza
Suite 1102
New York, NY 10001-2018 212-502-7600
200-232-5463
FAX: 888-545-8331
afbinfo@afb.net
afb.org

Carl R Augusto, President/ CEO
Kelly Bleach, Chief Administrative Officer
Rick Bozeman, Chief Financial Officer
Adrianna Montague-Devaud, Chief Communications and Marketi
Dedicated to addressing issues of literacy, independent living, employment, and access through technology for the ten million Americans who are blind or visually impaired.

3029 Arthur Ross Foundation
20 E 74th St
Ste 4c
New York, NY 10021-2654 212-737-7311
FAX: 212-650-0332

Arthur Ross, President

3030 Artists Fellowship
47 5th Ave
New York, NY 10003-4303 212-255-7740
info@artistsfellowship.org
www.artistsfellowship.org
Babette Bloch, President
Private, charitable foundation that assists professional fine arts and their families in times of emergency, disability, or bereavement.

3031 Bodman Foundation
767 3rd Ave
4th Floor
New York, NY 10017-2023 212-644-0322
FAX: 212-759-6510
main@achelis-bodman-fnds.org
www.achelis-bodman-fnds.org

John N. Irwin III, Chairman
Russell P. Pennoyer, President
Peter Frelinghuysen, Vice President
John B. Krieger, Executive Director
Foundation concentrates their grant programs in New York City, but foundation also makes some grants in Northern New Jersey. Funding is concentrated in six program areas: Arts & Culture, Education, Employment, Health, Public Policy and Youth and Families.

3032 Brooklyn Home for Aged Men
P.O.Box 280062
Brooklyn, NY 11228 718-745-1638
FAX: 718-745-0813
www.brooklynhome.org

Catherine M. Birdseye, Co-President
William E. Spaulding, Co-President
Andelusia Wheeler, Co-President
Edwin A. Ames, Co-President
The Brooklyn Home For Aged Men has served the community for more than one hundred years. Although originally set up as a residence for men, it later accepted women and couples as well.

3033 Cancer Care
275 7th Avenue
22nd Floor
New York, NY 10001-6754 212-712-8400
800-813-4673
FAX: 212-712-8495
info@cancercare.org
www.cancercare.org

Patricia J. Goldsmith, Chief Executive Officer
John Rutigliano, Chief Operating Officer
Sue Lee, Senior Director of Development
Ann Navarria, Director of Human Resources

A national non-profit organization that provides free, professional support services to anyone affected by cancer: people with cancer, caregivers, children, loved ones, and the bereaved.

3034 Children's Tumor Foundation
120 Wall Street
16th Floor
New York, NY 10005-3904

212-344-6633
800-323-7938
FAX: 212-747-0004
info@ctf.org
ctf.org

Linda Halliday Martin, Chairperson
Colin Bryar, Vice Chairperson
Annette Bakker, PhD, President and Chief Scientific Officer
Tracy Galloway, Secretary

A nonprofit 501 (c)(3) medical foundation, dedicated to improving the health and well-being of individuals and families affected by neurofibromatosis. The Foundation sponsors medical research, clinical services, public education programs and patient support services. It is the central source for up-to-date and accurate information about NF. It also assists patients and families with referrals to NF clinics and healthcare professionals specializing in NF. The goal is to find a cure for NF.

3035 Commonwealth Fund
1 E 75th St
New York, NY 10021-2692

212-606-3800
FAX: 212-606-3500
info@cmwf.org
www.commonwealthfund.org

Benjamin K. Chu, Chairman
Cristine Russell, Vice Chairman
Donald Moulds, Executive Vice President for Pro
Barry Scholl, Senior Vice President for Commun

A private foundation with the broad charge to enhance the common good. Carries out this mandate by supporting efforts that help people live healthy and productive lives, and by assisting certain groups with serious and neglected problems. Supports independent research on health and social issues and makes grants to improve heathcare practice and policy.

3036 Community Foundation for Greater Buffalo
726 Exchange Street,
Suite 525
Buffalo, NY 14210

716-852-2857
FAX: 716-852-2861
mail@cfgb.org
cfgb.org

Marsha Joy Sullivan, Chair
William Joyce, Vice Chair
Gary L. Mucci,, Secretary
Ross Eckert, Treasurer

Mission is connecting people, ideas, and resources to improve lives in Western New York

3037 Community Foundation of Herkimer & Oneida Counties
2608 Genesee Street
Utica, NY 13502-4728

315-735-8212
FAX: 315-735-9363
info@foundationhoc.org
foundationhoc.org

Alicia Dicks, President/CEO
Gilles Lauzon, Director of Finance
Elayne Johnson, Director of Fund Administration
Laura Cohen, Program Officer

Mission of the foundation is to improve the lives of the residents of Herkimer and Oneida Counties.

3038 Community Foundation of the Capitol Region
Six Tower Place
Albany, NY 12203-3749

518-446-9638
FAX: 518-446-9708
info@cfgcr.org
www.cfgcr.org

Karen Bilowith, President/CEO
Mindy Derosia, Development Officer
Shelly Connolly, Program Assistant
Jackie Mahoney, Vice President of Programs

Mission is to strengthen our community by attracting charitable endowments both large and small, maximizing benefits to donors, making effective gtants, and providing leadership to address community needs.

3039 Comsearch: Broad Topics
Foundation Center
79 5th Ave
New York, NY 10003-3034

212-620-4230
800-424-9836
FAX: 212-807-3677
communications@foundationcenter.org
www.fdncenter.org

Bradford K. Smith, President
Lisa Philip, Vice President for Strategic Phi
Jen Bokoff, Director of GrantCraft
Steven Lawrence, Director of Research

Subset publications of The Foundation Grants Index, are print-outs of actual foundation grants, covering 26 key areas of grantmaking. This tool is designed for fundraisers who wish to examine grantmaking activities in a broad field of interest. *$55.00*

3040 DE French Foundation
Ste 503
120 Genesee St
Auburn, NY 13021-3672

315-252-3634

Walter Lowe, Owner

3041 Dana Foundation
Dana Alliance for Brain Initiatives
505 Fifth Avenue
6th floor
New York, NY 10017

212-223-4040
FAX: 212-317-8721
danainfo@dana.org
www.dana.org

Edward F Rover, President /Chairman
Burton M. Mirsky, Executive Vice President, Financ
Barbara Rich, Ed.D., EVP, Communications; Assistant S
Barbara E Gill, Executive Vice President

A private philanthropy with principal interests in brain science, immunology, and arts education.

3042 David J Green Foundation
Ste 12
599 Lexington Ave
New York, NY 10022-6030

212-317-8820
FAX: 212-371-5099
www.djgreenc.com

Valerie Ventolora, Manager
Michael Greene, Manager

3043 Easter Seals New York
40 W 37th St
Suite 503
New York, NY 10018-7907

212-220-2290
800-727-8785
FAX: 212-695-4807
jmcgrath@eastersealsny.org
www.easterseals.com/newyork

John W. McGrath, MPA, Chief Executive Director
Aris Pavlides, Senior Vice President Developmen
Thomas Renart, M.A., M.S., Senior Vice-President Program Se
Kevin Carey, Director of Finance

Offers resources and expertise that allow children and adults with disabilities to live with dignity and independence. A long standing commitment to serve those for whom no other resources exist. Statewide, provides innovative solutions that enhance the lives of people with disabilities, while heightening community awareness and acceptance.

3044 Edna McConnel Clark Foundation
415 Madison Ave
Tenth Floor
New York, NY 10017-7949 212-551-9100
FAX: 212-421-9325
info@emcf.org
emcf.org

Nancy Roob, President
Woodrow C. McCutchen, Vice President, Senior Portfolio
Kelly Fitzsimmons, Vice President, Chief Program an
Charles Harris, Portfolio Manager
Helps young people, ages 9-24, from low-income backgrounds become independent, productive adults.

3045 Edward John Noble Foundation
Fl 19
32 E 57th St
New York, NY 10022-8562 212-759-4212
FAX: 212-888-4531

June Noble Larkin, Owner
June Larkin, Owner

3046 Epilepsy Foundation of Long Island
1500 Hempstead Turnpike
East Meadow, NY 11554 516-739-7733
888-672-7154
FAX: 516-739-1860
jlpsky@epil.org
efli.org

Thomas Hopkins, President & CEO
Paul Giotis, Chief Operating Officer
Lawrence Boord, Chief Financial Officer
Gladys Brown, Director of Intake Coordination
Provides education, counseling and residential care to Long Island residents with epilepsy and related conditions.

3047 Episcopal Charities
1047 Amsterdam Avenue
New York, NY 10025-1747 212-316-7575
episcopalcharities@dioceseny.org
episcopalcharities-newyork.org

John Talty, President
Lorraine A. LaHuta, Vice President
Evan A. Davis, Secretary
John P Banning, Treasurer
Provides funding and support to a broad range of community-based human service programs throughout the Diocese of New York. These programs, sponsored by Episcopal congregations, serve disadvantaged individuals, youth and families on a non-sectarian basis.

3048 Esther A & Joseph Klingenstein Fund
125 Park Avenue
Suite 1700
New York, NY 10017-5529 212-492-6195
kathleen.pomerantz@klingenstein.com
www.klingfund.org

Charles D. Gilbert, Chairman
Andrew D. Klingenstein, President
Kathleen Pomerantz, Vice President
Supports young investigators engaged in basic or clinical research that may lead to a better understanding of epilepsy

3049 Fay J Lindner Foundation
189 Wheatley Road
Brookville, NY 11545 516-686-4440
www.fayjlindnercenter.org

Terrence Ullrich, President
Dr. Robert Steinberger, Vice President
Thomas F. Moore, Treasurer
Frederick Sterbenz, Secretary

3050 Ford Foundation
320 E 43rd St
New York, NY 10017-4890 212-573-5000
FAX: 212-351-3677
office-of-communications@fordfoundation.org
www.fordfound.org

Darren Walker, President
Kenneth T Monterio, Vice President, Secretary and Ge
Alfred Ironside, Vice President/Communications
Nicholas M. Gabriel, Vice President, Treasurer and Ch
A resource for innovative people and institutions worldwide. Goals are to: strenghthen democratic values; reduce poverty and injustice; promote international cooperation; and advance human achievement. While not specific to disabilities, the Ford Foundation operates on several levels that indirectly assist and support those with disabilities through human and civil rights issues, social justice support, economic fairness and opportunity, and access to education involvements.

3051 Fortis Foundation
28 Liberty Street
New York, NY 10005-1401 212-859-7197
FAX: 212-859-7010
Investor.Relations@assurant.com
ir.assurant.com

Elaine D. Rosen, Chair
Howard L. Carver, Director
Melissa Kivett, Senior Vice President, Investor
Suzanne Shepherd, Director, Investor Relations

3052 Foundation Center
79 5th Ave
16th Street
New York, NY 10003-3076 212-620-4230
800-424-9836
FAX: 212-807-3677
communications@foundationcenter.org
foundationcenter.org

Bradford K Smith, President
Lisa Philip, VP, Strategic Philanthropy
Jen Bokoff, Director of GrantCraft
Steven Lawrence, Director of Research
The Foundation Center publishes Foundation Directory Online, with key facts on the US grantmakers and their grants.

3053 Foundation Center Library Services
Foundation Center
79 5th Ave
16th Street
New York, NY 10003-3076 212-620-4230
800-424-9836
FAX: 212-807-3677
communications@foundationcenter.org
foundationcenter.org

Bradford K Smith, President
Lisa Philip, VP, Strategic Philanthropy
Jen Bokoff, Director of GrantCraft
Steven Lawrence, Director of Research
The Center disseminates current information on foundation and corporate giving through our national collections in New York City and Washington D.C., our field offices in San Francisco and our network of over 180 cooperating libraries in all 50 states and abroad.

3054 Foundation for Advancement in Cancer Therapy
P.O.Box 1242
Old Chelsea Station
New York, NY 10113-1242   212-741-2790
                                    info@rethinkingcancer.org
                                    www.rethinkingcancer.org
Ruth Sackman, Founder
A clearinghouse for information regarding alternative cancer
therapies, emphasizing nutritional and metabolic approaches.

3055 Gebbie Foundation
215 Cherry St
Jamestown, NY 14701-5207   716-487-1062
                                    FAX: 716-484-6401
                                    info@gebbie.org
                                    www.gebbie.org
Gregory J Edwards, CEO
Daniel Kathman, President
Jonathan Taber, Vice President
Nancy Gleason, Secretary
Giving in Chautauqua County, and secondly, in neighboring ar-
eas of western New York. Giving is offered in other areas only
when the project is consonant with program objectives that can-
not be developed locally.

3056 Gladys Brooks Foundation
1055 Franklin Avenue
Suite 208
Garden City, NY 11530
                    kathy@gladysbrooksfoundation.org
                    www.gladysbrooksfoundation.org
Jessica L Rutledge, Director
The purpose of this Foundation is to provide for the intellectual,
moral and physical welfare of the people of this country by establishing and supporting nonprofit libraries, educational institutions, hospitals and clinics. The Foundation will make grants
only to private, publicly supported, nonprofit, tax-exempt
organizations.

3057 Glickenhaus Foundation
546 5th Ave
New York, NY 10036-5000   212-953-7800
                                    info@glickenhaus.com
                                    glickenhaus.com
Seth M. Glickenhaus, Senior Partner and Chief Investm

3058 Guide Dog Foundation for the Blind
371 East Jericho Turnpike
Smithtown, NY 11787-2976   631-930-9000
                                    800-548-4337
                                    FAX: 631-930-9009
                                    info@guidedog.org
                                    guidedog.org
James C. Bingham, Chair
Alphonce J. Brown, Vice Chair
Barbara J. Kelly, Secretary
Donald Dea, Treasurer
Providing mobility through the use of trained guide or service
dogs to individuals who are blind or with other special needs.

3059 Hearst Foundations
300 W 57th St
Fl 26
New York, NY 10019-3741   212-649-2000
                                    FAX: 212-887-6855
                                    hearst.com
Steven R. Swartz, President and Chief Executive Of
National philanthropic resources for organziations and institutions working in the fields of education, health, culture and social
services. Our goal is to ensure that people of all backgrounds
have the opportunity to build healthy, productive and inspiring
lives.

3060 Henry and Lucy Moses Fund
405 Lexington Ave
New York, NY 10174-1299   212-554-7800
                                    FAX: 212-554-7700
                                    klinhardt@mosessinger.com
                                    www.mosessinger.com
Irving Sitnick, President
Provides legal services to many prominent industries, individuals
and families in the New York City area.

3061 Herman Goldman Foundation
Fl 18
61 Broadway
New York, NY 10006-2708   212-797-9090
                                    nlnfoundation.org
Alan Nisselson, President
A private nonoperating foundation.

3062 Kenneth & Evelyn Lipper Foundation
Fl 6
101 Park Ave
New York, NY 10178   212-883-6333
Kenneth Lipper, Director

3063 Long Island Alzheimer's Foundation
5 Channel Drive
Port Washington, NY 11050-2216   516-767-6856
                                    FAX: 516-767-6864
                                    info@liaf.org
                                    www.liaf.org
Paul Eibeler, Chairman
Fred Jenny, Executive Director
Sean Phillips, Director of Development
Tiffany Ewald, Program Assistant

3064 Louis and Anne Abrons Foundation
First Manhattan Company
399 Park Avenue
New York, NY 10022-7001   212-756-3300
                                    FAX: 212-223-4175
                                    info@firstmanhattan.com
                                    firstmanhattan.com
David Manischewitz, CEO
Sam Colin, Senior Managing Director
Allan Glick, Senior Managing Director
Neal Sterns, Senior Managing Director

3065 Margaret L Wendt Foundation
Ste 277
40 Fountain Plz
Buffalo, NY 14202-2200   716-855-2146
                                    FAX: 716-855-2149
Robert J Kresse, Manager

3066 Merrill Lynch & Company Foundation
250 Vesey St
New York, NY 10080   212-449-1000
                                    800-637-7455
                                    FAX: 212-449-7969
                                    ml.com
Brian T Moynihan, CEO
John Theil, Head
Andy M Sieg, Managing Director
John Hogarty, Chief Operating Officer
Ongoing support for the arts, health, human services, and civic is-
sues. Merrill Lynch's philanthropic priority is a sustained invest-
ment in education. Q992

3067 Metzger-Price Fund
Ste 2300
230 Park Ave
New York, NY 10169
212-867-9500
FAX: 212-599-1759

Isaac A Saufer, Secretary/Treasurer

3068 Milbank Foundation for Rehabilitation
116 Village Boulevard
Suite 200
New York, NY 08540
609-951-2283
FAX: 609-951-2281
fdnweb.org/milbank

Jeremiah M. Bogert, Chairman & Secretary
Jeremiah Milbank III, President and Treasurer
Carl Helstrom, Executive Director
Carmel Mazzola, Administrative Assistant

Awarding grants from trust funds based on a competitive selection process or the preferences of the foundation managers and granters. The foundations mission is to integrate people with disabilities into all aspects of american life. Current priorities include, but are not limited to: consumer-focused initiatives that enable people with disablities to lead fulfilling,independent lives; innovative policy research and education on market-based approaches to health care and rehabilitation...

3069 Morgan Stanley Foundation
1585 Broadway
New York, NY 10036-8293
212-761-4000
FAX: 212-761-0086
mediainquiries@morganstanley.com
morganstanley.com

James P. Gorman, Chairman and Chief Executive Off
Thomas Nides, Vice Chairman
Jeff Brodsky, Chief Human Resources Officer
Jim Rosenthal, Chief Operating Officer

Our overachieving mission is threefold: build the potential of individuals and families, encourage and support our employees charitable efforts, and strengthen relationships with our communities.

3070 Mount Sinai Medical Center
4300 Alton Road
Miami Beach, FL 33140-6574
305-674-2121
305-674-2777
www.msmc.com/foundation

Wayne Chaplin, Chairman
Steven D. Sonenreich, President & CEO
Jason Loeb, Foundation President
Kenneth L. Davis, MD, Chief Executive Officer and Pres

Autism Research

3071 National Foundation for Facial Reconstruction
333 East 30th Street
Lobby Unit
New York, NY 10016-4974
212-263-6656
FAX: 212-263-7534
info@nffr.org
nffr.org

Carolyn Spector, J.D., LLM., Executive Director
Erin Johnson, Director of Development
Kirsten Selert, Development and Events Manager
Dina Zuckerberg, Director of Family Programs

A nonprofit organization whose major purposes are to provide facilities for the treatment and assistance of individuals who are unable to afford private reconstructive surgical care, to train and educate professionals in this surgery, to encourage research in the field and to carry on public education.

3072 National Hemophilia Foundation
7 Penn Plaza
Suite 1204
New York, NY 10001-3212
212-328-3700
800-424-2634
FAX: 212-328-3799
handi@hemophilia.org
hemophilia.org

Jorge de la Riva, Chair
Carol Simonetti, Vice Chair
Mark Borreliz, Secretary
Brian Andrew, Treasurer

Dedicated to finding better treatments and cures for bleeding and clotting disorders to preventing the complications of these disorders through education, advocacy and research.

3073 Neisloss Family Foundation
Ste 7
1737 Veterans Hwy
Central Islip, NY 11749-1533
631-234-1600
FAX: 631-234-1066

Stanley Neisloss, President/Owner

3074 New York Community Trust
909 3rd Ave
22nd Floor
New York, NY 10022-4752
212-686-0010
FAX: 212-532-8528
aw@nyct-cfi.org
nycommunitytrust.org

Lorie A Slutsky, President
Carolyn M Weiss, CFO
Mary Z. Greenebaum, Chief Investment Officer
Eileen Casey, Director of Investment Reporting

Our goal is to out charitable money to work, making grants to the city's nonprofit community and building an endowment to tackle future problems.

3075 New York Foundation
10 E 34th St
10th Floor
New York, NY 10016-4327
212-594-8009
info@nyf.org
nyf.org

Marlene Provizer, Chair
Roger Schwed, Vice Chair
Sue A Kaplan, Secretary
Gail Gordon, Treasurer

Grants are given that involve New York City or a particular neighborhood of the city. Emphasize advocacy and community organizing. Address a critical need or disadvantaged population, particularly youth or the elderly. Are strongly identified with a particular community. Require an amount of funding to which a Foundation grant would make a substantial contribution. And can show a clear role for the Foundation's funds.

3076 Northern New York Community Foundation
120 Washington St
Suite 400
Watertown, NY 13601-3376
315-782-7110
FAX: 315-782-0047
info@nnycf.org
www.nnycf.org

Joseph W. Russell, President
Linda S. Merrell, Vice President
Jacquelyn A. Schell, Secretary
Rande S. Richardson, Executive Director

Raises, manages and administers an endowment and collection of funds for the benefit of the community

3077 Parkinson's Disease Foundation
1359 Broadway
Room 1509
New York, NY 10018-7867   212-923-4700
                                 800-457-6676
                           FAX: 212-923-4778
                                 info@pdf.org
                                 www.pdf.org

Howard D Morgan, Chair
Constance Atwell, Vice Chair
Isobel Konecky, Secretary
Stephen Ackerman, Treasurer
The Parkinson's Disease Foundation is a leading national presence in Parkinson's disease research, education and public advocacy. We are working for the nearly one million people in the US who live with Parkinson's by funding promising scientific research to find the causes of and a cure for Parkinson's while supporting people with Parkinson's, their families and caregivers through educational programs and support services.

3078 Reader's Digest Foundation
Readers Digest Association
Readers Digest Rd
Pleasantville, NY 10570   914-238-1000
                            FAX: 914-238-4559
                                 letters@rd.com
                                 rd.com

Mary G Berner, CEO
Dedicated to creating opportunities and promoting efforts that encourage individuals to make a positive difference in their communities, and to supporting programs designed to help young people learn, grow and enrich their lives.

3079 Research to Prevent Blindness
645 Madison Ave
Floor 21
New York, NY 10022-1010   212-752-4333
                                 800-621-0026
                           FAX: 212-688-6231
                           inforequest@rpbusa.org
                                 www.rpbusa.org

Diane S. Swift, Chair
Brian F. Hofland PhD, President
David H Brenner, Vice President and Secretary
Richard E. Baker, Treasurer and Assistant Secretar
National voluntary health foundation supported by foundations, corporations and voluntary gifts and bequests from individuals. Established to stimulate basic and applied research into the causes, prevention and treatment of blinding eye diseases.

3080 Rita J and Stanley H Kaplan Foundation
Rm 306
866 United Nations Plz
New York, NY 10017-1822   212-688-1047
                           FAX: 212-688-6907
                           www.kaplanfoundation.org

Nancy Kaplan Belsky, President
Susan B. Kaplan, Vice President
Scott Kaplan Belsky, Secretary & Treasurer
Rebecca Tobin, Executive Director

3081 Robert Sterling Clark Foundation
135 E 64th St
New York, NY 10065-7045   212-288-8900
                           FAX: 212-288-1033
                                 rscf@rsclark.org
                                 rsclark.org

James Allen Smith, Chairman
Vincent McGee, President
Clara Miller, Treasurer
Julie Muraco, Secretary
Giving primarily in New York with emphasis on advocacy, research, and public education aimed at informing New York City of state policies.

3082 Skadden Fellowship Foundation
4 Times Sq
New York, NY 10036-6518   212-735-3000
                           FAX: 212-735-2000
                                 info@skadden.com
                                 www.skadden.com

Alan C Myers, Director
William Schumann, Legal Assistant
The aim of the Foundation is to give Fellows the freedom to pursue public intrest work, thus the Fellows create their own projects at public interest organizations with at least 2 lawyers on staff before they apply.

3083 St George's Society of New York
216 E 45th St
Suite 901
New York, NY 10017-3304   212-682-6110
                           FAX: 212-682-3465
                           info@stgeorgessociety.org
                                 stgeorgessociety.org

John Shannon, Almoner
Anna Titley, Director of Operations and Commu
Samantha Hamilton, Director of Development and Memb
Daisy Rowan, Operations Executive
St George's Society provides monthly stipends to the elderly and the handicapped.

3084 Stanley W Metcalf Foundation
Ste 503
120 Genesee St
Auburn, NY 13021-3672   315-252-3634

Walter Lowe, Owner

3085 Stonewall Community Foundation
446 West 33rd Street
New York, NY 10001-1913   212-367-1155
                           FAX: 212-367-1157
                           stonewall@stonewallfoundation.org
                                 www.stonewallfoundation.org

Dante Mastri, President
Neill Coleman, Vice President
Chris Davis, Secretary
Tina Salandra, Treasurer
Mission is to promote the well being of lesbian, gay, bisexual, and transgender (LGBT) individuals and strengthen the LGBT community. We do this by increasing resources; targeting those resources strategically to areas of greatest need; and by serving as a catalyst and clearinghouse for ideas and solutions. Through grant-making donor-advised funds, endowment funds and charitable education, Stonewall supports LGBT organizations and helps donors realize their philanthropic goals.

3086 Surdna Foundation
330 Madison Ave
30th Floor
New York, NY 10017-5016   212-557-0010
                                 grants@surdna.org
                                 surdna.org

Jocelyn Downie, Chairperson
Peter B Benedict, Vice Chairperson
Lawrence S.C Griffth, Secretary & Treasurer
Jonathan Goldberg, Director of Grants Management, L
The Foundation makes grants in the areas of environment, community revitalization, effective citizenry, the arts and the nonprofit sector.

3087 Tisch Foundation
Fl 19
655 Madison Ave
New York, NY 10065-8043   212-521-2930
                           FAX: 212-521-2983

Mark J Krinsky, VP

3088 Van Ameringen Foundation
509 Madison Avenue
New York, NY 10022-5501 212-758-6221
FAX: 212-688-2105
info@vanamfound.org
www.vanamfound.org

Kenneth A. Kind, President / Treasurer
Steadman Westergaard, Vice President and Secretary
Eleanor Sypher, Executive Director
Helaine Williams, Office Manager

From its beginning the Foundation has sought to stimulate prevention, education, and direct care in the mental health field with an emphasis on those individuals and populations having an impoverished background and few opportunities, for whom appropriate intervention would produce positive change.

3089 Verizon Foundation
1 Verizon Way
Basking Ridge, NJ 07920-1097 866-247-2687
FAX: 908-630-2660
verizonfoundation@verizon.com
www.verizon.com

Lowell C McAdam, Chairman & CEO
Roy H Chestnutt, Executive Vice President
James J Gerace, Chief Communications Officer
Craig Silliman, Executive Vice President

Mission is to improve education, literacy, family safety and healthcare by supporting Verizon's commitment to deliver technology that touches life. We focus our philanthropic efforts on 3 areas: Education, Safety and Health. & Volunteerism.

3090 Western New York Foundation
11 Summer St
Third Floor
Buffalo, NY 14209-2256 716-839-4225
FAX: 716-883-1107
bgosch@wnyfoundation.org
www.wnyfoundation.org

Jennifer S. Johnson, Chairman
James A. W. McLeod, President
John N. W. Walsh III, Vice President
Theodore V. Buerger, Treasurer

The Western New York Foundation makes grants in the seven counties of Western New York State: Erie, Niagra, Genesee, Wyoming, Allegany, Cattaraugus and Chautauqua

3091 William T Grant Foundation
570 Lexington Avenue
18th Floor
New York, NY 10022-6837 212-752-0071
FAX: 212-752-1398
info@wtgrantfdn.org
wtgrantfoundation.org

Adam Gamoran, President
Vivian Tseng, Vice President, Program
Deborah McGinn, Vice President, Finance and Admi
Vivian Louie, Program Officer

Purpose is to further the understanding of human behavior through research. The mission focuses on improving the lives of youth ages 8 to 25 in the United States.

North Carolina

3092 Arc of North Carolina
343 East Six Forks Rd.
Suite 320
Raleigh, NC 27609 919-782-4632
800-662-8706
FAX: 919-782-4634
info@arcnc.org
www.arcnc.org

Adonis Brown, President
Robert Rusty Bradstock, Senior Vice President
Rhonda Schandevel, Secretary
Ed McShane, Treasurer

Committed to securing for all people with mental retardation and other developmental disabilities the opportunity to choose and realize their goals of where and how they learn, live, work, and play.

3093 Bob & Kay Timberlake Foundation
1660 E Center Street Ext
Lexington, NC 27292-1309 336-243-7777
800-776-0822
FAX: 336-249-2469
bobtimberlake.com

Daniel Timberlake, President

3094 Duke Endowment
800 East Morehead Street
Charlotte, NC 28202-4012 704-376-0291
FAX: 704-376-9336
info@tde.org
dukeendowment.org

Eugene W. Cochrane Jr., President
Arthur E. Morehead IV, Vice President/General Counsel
Susan L. McConnell, Director of Higher Education
Terri W. Honeycutt, Corporate Secretary

Mission is to serve the people of North Carolina and South Carolina by supporting selected programs of higher education, health care, children's welfare, and spiritual life.

3095 First Union Foundation
301 S College St
Charlotte, NC 28288 704-383-0525
FAX: 704-374-2484

Judy Allison, Director

3096 Foundation for the Carolinas
220 N. Tryon Street
Charlotte, NC 28202 704-973-4500
800-973-7244
FAX: 704-973-4599
mmarsicano@fftc.org
fftc.org

Michael Marsicano, Ph.D., President & CEO
Brian Collier, Executive Vice President
Debra S. Watt, SVP, Information Technology
Laura Smith, Executive Vice President

Giving primarily to organizations serving the citizens of North and South Carolina.

3097 Kate B Reynolds Charitable Trust
128 Reynolda Village
Winston Salem, NC 27106-5123 336-397-5500
800-485-9080
FAX: 336-723-7765
joyce@kbr.org
kbr.org

Karen McNeil-Miller,, President
Lori Fuller, Director, Evaluation and Learnin
Joel Beeson, Director, Operations
Nora Ferrell, Director, Communications

Mission is to improve the quality of life and quality of health for the financially needy of North Carolina. Grants resricted to the state of North Carolina only.

3098 Mary Reynolds Babcock Foundation
2920 Reynolda Rd
Winston Salem, NC 27106-3016 336-748-9222
FAX: 336-777-0095
info@mrbf.org
mrbf.org

Jennifer Barksdale, Finance Officer
Toshawia Bruner, Office Assistant
Lavastian Glenn, Network Officer
Justin Maxson, Executive Director

For 1994, this foundation is committed to an extensive educational and planning process to better understand the Southeast and to articulate the role the foundation seeks to play in the region into the twenty-first century.

3099 Triangle Community Foundation
324 Blackwell St
Suite 1220
Durham, NC 27701-3690
919-474-8370
FAX: 919-941-9208
info@trianglecf.org
trianglecf.org

Lacy M. Presnell, Chair
Pat Nathan, Secretary
C. Perry Colwell, Assistant Secretary
James A. Stewart, Treasurer
Triangle Community Foundation connects philanthropic resources with community needs, creates opportunity for enlightned change and encourages philanthropy as a way of life.

North Dakota

3100 Alex Stern Family Foundation
4141 28th South Avenue
Suite 102
Fargo, ND 58104-8403
701-271-0263
FAX: 701-271-0408
alexsternfamilyfoundation.org

Don Scott, Executive Director
Rondi McGovern, Trustee
Dan Carey, Trustee
The Foundation supports the arts, social welfare/human services, education, youth recreation, civic projects and health issues for the benefit of the greater Fargo-Moorhead area.

3101 Arc of North Dakota
2500 DeMers Avenue
Grand Forks, ND 58201-2420
701-772-6191
877-250-2022
FAX: 701-772-2195
thearc@arcuv.com
www.thearcuppervalley.com

Peggy Johnson, President
Joan Karpenko, First Vice President
Ruth Jenny, Secretary
Pam Heyd, Treasurer
Mission is to work in partnership with our constituents, members and affiliated chapters to ensure that children and adults with intellectual and developmental disabilities have the supports, benefits, and services they need, and are accepted, respected and fully included in their communities.

3102 North Dakota Community Foundation
309 N Mandan Street
309 N Mandan Street, Suite 2
P.O.Box 387
Bismarck, ND 58502-0387
701-222-8349
kdvorak@ndcf.net
www.ndcf.net

Kevin J Dvorak, CFP, President & CEO
Amy N. Warnke, CFRE, Development Director East
Kara L. Geiger, Development Director West
Cynthia Kaip, Accountant/Administrator
The mission of the North Dakota Community Foundation is to improve the quality of life for North Dakota's citizens through charitable giving and promoting philanthropy.

Ohio

3103 Akron Community Foundation
345 W Cedar St
Akron, OH 44307-2407
330-376-8522
FAX: 330-376-0202
jpetures@akroncf.org
www.akroncommunityfdn.org

Mark Alio, Chair
Steven Cox, Vice Chair
Dr. Sandra Selby, Secretary
Paul Belair, Treasurer
Mission is to improve the quality of life in the Greater Akron area by building permanent endowments, and providing philanthropic leadership that enables donors to make lasting investments in the community.

3104 Albert G and Olive H Schlink Foundation
49 Benedict Avenue, Suite C
Norwalk, OH 44857
curtis@hwak.com
www.schlinkfoundation.org

3105 American Foundation Corporation
4518 North 32nd Street
Phoenix, AZ 85018
602-955-4770
FAX: 602-955-4700
info@americanfoundation.org
www.americanfoundation.org

Ben L. Schaub, Founder and CEO
The American Foundation can be your sponsor, and help your company set up a corporate foundation in a public charity or support organization format.

3106 Arc of Ohio
1335 Dublin Rd
Suite 100-A
Columbus, OH 43215-7037
614-487-4720
800-875-2723
FAX: 614-487-4725
info@thearcofohio.org
thearcofohio.org

Gary Tonks, Executive Director
John Hannah, President
Connie Calhoun, Vice President
Josh Ebling, Treasurer
The mission of The Arc of Ohio is to advocacte for human rights, personal dignity and community participation of individuals with mental retardation and other developmental disabilities, through legislative and social action, information and education, local chapter support and family involvement.

3107 Bahmann Foundation
8041 Hosbrook Rd
Suite 210
Cincinnati, OH 45236-2909
513-891-3799
FAX: 513-891-3722
info@bahmann.org
www.bahmann.org

John Gatch, Executive Director
The mission of the Bahmann Foundation is to reduce isolation of low-income older adults through technology.

3108 Cleveland Foundation
1422 Euclid Ave
Suite 1300
Cleveland, OH 44115-2063
216-861-3810
FAX: 216-861-1729
Hello@CleveFdn.org
clevelandfoundation.org

James A. Ratner, Chairman
Paul J. Dolan, Vice Chairman
Ronald B. Richard, President and CEO
Robert E. Eckardt, Executive Vice President
In general, grants are made in (but not restriced to) the areas of arts and culture, community development, economic development, education, environment, health and human services.

3109 Columbus Foundation and Affiliated Organizations
1234 E Broad St
Columbus, OH 43205-1453
614-251-4000
FAX: 614-251-4009
info@columbusfoundation.org
columbusfoundation.org

Doug F. Kridler, President & CEO
Raymond J. Biddiscombe, CPA, Senior Vice President - Finance
Lisa Schweitzer Courtice, P, EVP - Community Research and Gra
Alicia Szempruch, Scholarship Manager
The Columbus Foundation offers a range of charitable fund types that can be used for individuals, families and businesses.

3110 Eleanora CU Alms Trust
Fifth Third Bank
Department 00864
9990 Montgomery Rd
Cincinnati, OH 45263
513-793-2200

Robert W Laclair, President
Giving is limited to Cincinnati, OH.

3111 Eva L And Joseph M Bruening Foundation
Foundation Management Services
1422 Euclid Ave
Suite 966
Cleveland, OH 44115-1952
216-621-2901
FAX: 216-621-8198
cstarkey@fmscleveland.com
www.fmscleveland.com

Janet E. Narten, Founder
Cristin N. Slesh, President
Valerie Schramm, Operations Assistant
Kara L. McCullough, Manager, Grants and Office Opera
Charitable foundation providing grants to nonprofit organizations located inCuyahoga county Ohio. No grant are awarded to inviduals.

3112 Fred & Lillian Deeks Memorial Foundation
P.O.Box 1118
Cincinnati, OH 45201-1118
937-339-2329
FAX: 937-339-1861

3113 GAR Foundation
277 East Mill Street
Akron, OH 44308
330-576-2926
FAX: 330-294-5315
info@garfdn.org
www.garfdn.org

Christine Amer Mayer, President
Kirstin S. Toth, Senior Vice President
Candace Campbell Jackson, Consulting Program Officer
Brittany G. Zaehringer, Senior Program Officer
The mission of the Foundation is to strengthen communities in our region through discerning and creative support of worthy organizations.

3114 George Gund Foundation
1845 Guildhall Building
45 Prospect Avenue, West
Cleveland, OH 44115-1008
216-241-3114
FAX: 216-241-6560
info@gundfdn.org
gundfoundation.org

Geoffrey Gund, President & Treasurer
Ann L. Gund, Vice President
David T. Abbott, Executive Director
Catherine Gund, Secretary
The George Gund Foundation was established in 1952 as a private, nonprofit institution with the sole purpose of contributing to human well-being and the progress of society.

3115 Greater Cincinnati Foundation
200 West Fourth St.
Cincinnati, OH 45202-2775
513-241-2880
FAX: 513-852-6886
info@gcfdn.org
www.gcfdn.org

Kathryn e. Merchant, President/CEO
Terri Masur, Executive Assistant
Elizabeth Reiter Benson, APR, Vice President for Communic
Shiloh Turner, Vice President for Community Inv
Offers a wide variety of giving tools to help people achieve their charitable goals and create lasting good work in their communities.

3116 HCR Manor Care Foundation
333 N. Summit St.
P.O.Box 10086
Toledo, OH 43699-0086
419-252-5500
FAX: 419-252-6404
foundation@hcr-manorcare.com
hcr-manorcare.com

Paul A Ormond, Chairman, President and CEO
An independent, not-for-profit corporation that provides funding for organizations and programs that address the needs of the elderly and individuals requiring post-acute care services.

3117 Harry C Moores Foundation
100 South Third Street
Columbus, OH 43215-4291
614-227-2300
FAX: 614-227-2390
info@bricker.com
bricker.com

Kurtis A Tunnell, Managing Partner
Ahmad Sino, Chief Information Officer
Steve P Odum, Chief Financial Officer
Angela M Gelst, Chief Human Resources Officer

3118 Helen Steiner Rice Foundation
1301 Western Ave.
Cincinnati, OH 45203
513-287-7022
800-877-2665
hrice@cincymuseum.org
helensteinerrice.com

Virginia J. Ruehlmann, Creative Consultant
Dorothy C. Lingg, Office Manager
Willis D. Gradison, Jr., Board of Trustee
Gregory Ionna, Board of Trustee
Non-profit corporation whose purpose is to award grants to worthy charitable programs that aid the poor, the needy, and the elderly.

3119 Herbert W Hoover Foundation
220 Market Ave S
Canton, OH 44702-2180
330-818-1300
FAX: 330-453-5622
contacthwh@hwhfoundation.org
www.hwhfoundation.org

Mark Butterworth, Ohio Director
Lynn Davidson, Program Director
Elizabeth Lacey Hoover, Chair
Colton Hoover Chase, Member of Trust Committee
The Herbert W Hoover Foundation will take a leadership role in funding unique opportunities that provide solutions to issues relater to the Community, Education, and the Environment.

3120 Nationwide Foundation
One Nationwide Plaza
Columbus, OH 43215-2220
614-249-7111
800-882-2822
FAX: 614-249-5721
www.nationwide.com

Kirt A. Walker, President and COO Nationwide Fin
Mark A. Pizzi, President and Chief Operating Of
Stephen S. Rasmussen, Chief Executive Officer, Nationw
W. Kim Austen, President and COO, Allied Group,

The Nationwide Foundation is an independent corporation funded by Nationwide Companies to help positively impact the quality of life in communities where our associates, agents and their families live and work.

3121　Nordson Corporate Giving Program
28601 Clemens Rd
Westlake, OH 44145-1148　　440-892-1580
FAX: 440-892-9507
kladiner@nordson.com
nordson.com

Michael F. Hilton, President and Chief Executive O
Gregory A. Thaxton, Senior Vice President, Chief Fin
John J. Keane, Senior Vice President, Advanced
Gregory P. Merk, Senior Vice President, Adhesive
Nordson Corporation encourages individual financial support of nonprofit organizations, colleges, and universities

3122　Parker-Hannifin Foundation
6035 Parkland Blvd
Cleveland, OH 44124-4141　　216-896-3000
800-272-7537
FAX: 216-896-4000
parker.com

Donald E. Washkewicz, Chairman, Chief Executive Office
Lee C. Banks, Executive Vice President and Ope
Robert P. Barker, Executive Vice President, Operat
Jon P. Marten, Executive Vice President - Finan
To be a leading worldwide manufacturer of components and systems for the builders and users of durable goods.

3123　Reinberger Foundation
30000 Chagrin Blvd.
Suite 300
Cleveland, OH 44124-4439　　216-292-2790
FAX: 216-292-4466
info@reinbergerfoundation.org
www.reinbergerfoundation.org

Karen R. Hooser, President
Sally R. Dyer, Trustee
Richard H. Oman, Trustee
William C. Reinberger, Trustee
Committed to enhancing the quality of life for individuals from all walks of life. To achieve this goal, proposals in the areas of the arts, education, healthcare, and social service are favored.

3124　Robert Campeau Family Foundation
7 West Seventh Street
Cincinnati, OH 45202-2424　　513-579-7000
FAX: 513-579-7555
federated-fds.com

Terry J Lundgren, Chairman and Chief Executive Officer

3125　Sisler McFawn Foundation
P.O.Box 149
Akron, OH 44309　　330-849-8887
FAX: 330-996-6215

Charlotte M Stanley, Grants Manager
Our trust restricts giving to certain programs and types of organizations. You can see recent giving has been by referring to the list of grants approved and paid during the past year. Call foundation office to request a guidelines brochure and list.

3126　Stark Community Foundation
400 Market Ave North
Suite 200
Canton, OH 44702-1557　　330-454-3426
FAX: 330-454-5855
info@starkcf.org
www.starkcommunityfoundation.org

Mark Samolczyk, President
Patricia Quick, VP/ CFO
Chris Decker, Finance and Systems Officer
Bridgette Neisel, Vice President of Advancement

Stark Community Foundation is dedicated to promoting the betterment of Stark County and enhancing the quality of life of all its citizens.

3127　Stocker Foundation
201 Burns Road
Elyria, OH 44035　　440-366-4884
FAX: 440-366-4656
contact@stockerfoundation.org
stockerfoundation.org

Brenda Norton, President
Dawn Dobras, Treasurer
Patricia O'Brien, Executive Director
Melanie R Wilson, Office Manager
The Stocker Foundation seeks creative ideas and projects that are catalysts for constructive change in the community through arts and culture, community needs, education, health social services and women's issues.

3128　Toledo Community Foundation
300 Madison Avenue
Suite 1300
Toledo, OH 43604-1583　　419-241-5049
FAX: 419-242-5549
toledocf@toledocf.org
www.toledocf.org

David F. Waterman, Chair
Dr. Anthony Armstrong, Vice Chair
Rita N.A. Mansour, Secretary
Scott A Estes, Treasurer
The Toledo Community Foundation is a public, charitable foundation which exists to improve the quality of life in the region.

3129　William J and Dorothy K O'Neill Foundation
7575 Northcliff Ave.
Suite 205
Cleveland, OH 44144　　216-831-4134
FAX: 216-378-0594
info@oneill-foundation.org
www.oneillfdn.org

Leah S Gary, President & CEO
Symone R McClain, Manager of Grants & Office Opera
Timothy M. McCue, MPH, Senior Program Officer

3130　Youngstown Foundation
100 Federal Plaza East, Suite 101
P.O.Box 1162
Youngstown, OH 44503-1162　　330-744-0320
FAX: 330-744-0344
Jan@youngstownfoundation.org
www.youngstownfoundation.org

Jan Strasfeld, Executive Director
Crissi Jenkins, Program Coordinator
Rena Colarossi, Admin. Assistant
Funds proposals that provide direct services to children with medically diagnosed disabilities. Grants are awarded to Ohio non-profit agencies that are qualified under the Internal Revenue Service Code 501 (c) (3) for the care of such children in the greater Youngstown Area.

Oklahoma

3131　Anne and Henry Zarrow Foundation
401 S Boston Ave
Suite 900
Tulsa, OK 74103-4012　　918-295-8004
FAX: 918-295-8049
bmajor@zarrow.com
www.zarrow.com

3132 Sarkeys Foundation
530 East Main St
Norman, OK 73071-5823

405-364-3703
FAX: 405-364-8191
angela@sarkeys.org
sarkeys.org

Kim Henry, Executive Director
Lori Sutton, Facilities Manager
Angella Holladay, Director of Grants Management
Susan C. Frantz, Senior Program Officer
Improves the quality of life in Oklahoma. Offers contributions in the areas of social services, arts and cultural programs, educational funding and health care and medical research. Funding only in agencies in the state of Oklahoma.

Oregon

3133 Arc of Oregon
2405 Front Street NE
Suite 120
Salem, OR 97301-4342

503-581-2726
877-581-2726
FAX: 503-363-7168
info@arcoregon.org
www.thearcoregon.org

Marcie Ingledue, Executive Director
Tiffany Tombleson, Administrative Assistant
Paula Boga, OSNT Program Director
Cici Gaynor, OSNT Administrative Assistant
Guardianship, Advocacy and Planning Services. Oregon special needs trust; information and referral.

3134 Chiles Foundation
1614 Mahan Center Boulevard
Suite 104
Tallahassee, Fl 32308

805-385-7800
FAX: 805-385-7808
kchiles@lawtonchiles.org
chilesfoundation.org

Kitty Chiles, Executive Director
Bud Chiles, President
Dr. Wil J. Blechman, Board Member
Todd Abernethy, Chief Financial Officer
Giving in Oregon, with emphasis on Portland, and the Pacific Northwest.

3135 Jackson Foundation
P.O.Box 3168
Portland, OR 97208-3168

503-275-4414
march.voyles@usbank.com
www.thejacksonfoundation.com

Robert H Depew, Vice President & Senior Trust Of
Libby Voyles, Trust Relationship Associate
Purpose is to respond to the requests deemed appropriate to promote the welfare of the public of the city of Portland or the State of Oregon or both.

3136 Leslie G Ehmann Trust
P.O.Box 3168
Portland, OR 97208-3168

503-275-5929
800-522-9100
FAX: 503-275-4117
william.dollan@usbank.com

William Dolan, Trustee

Pennsylvania

3137 Air Products Foundation
7201 Hamilton Blvd
Allentown, PA 18195-9642

610-481-4911
FAX: 610-481-5900
gigmrktg@airproducts.com
www.airproducts.com

Seifi Ghasemi, Chairman & CEO
M. Scott Crocco, Senior Vice President and Chief
Guillermo Novo, Senior Vice President
Corning F. Painter, Executive Vice President
Giving primarily in areas of company operations throughout the US.

3138 Arc of Pennsylvania
301 Chestnut Street
Suite 403
Harrisburg, PA 17101-2535

717-234-2621
800-692-7258
FAX: 717-234-2622
info@thearcpa.org
thearcpa.org

Maureen Cronin, Executive Director
Pam Klipa, Government Relations Director
Gwen Adams, Operations Director
Ashlinn Masland-Sarani, Policy and Development Director
The Arc's mission is to work to include all children and adults with cognitive, intellectual, and developmental disabilities in every community. We promote active citizenship and inclusion in every community.

3139 Arcadia Foundation
105 E Logan St
Norristown, PA 19401-3058

202-747-0876
arcadiafoundation.org

Marilyn L Steinbright, President
Robert Carmona-Borjas, Founder

3140 Brachial Plexus Palsy Foundation
210 Springhaven Cir
Royersford, PA 19468-1178

contact@brachialplexuspalsyfoundation.org
www.brachialplexuspalsyfoundation.org

3141 Columbia Gas of Pennsylvania Corporate Giving
650 Washington Rd
Pittsburgh, PA 15228-2702

412-572-7104
FAX: 412-572-7140
info@columbiaenergygroup.com
www.columbiagaspamd.com/html/

Rosemary Martinelli, Manager Corporation

3142 Connelly Foundation
100 Front Street,
Suite 1450
West Conshohocken, PA 19428-2873

610-834-3222
FAX: 610-834-0866
info@connellyfdn.org
connellyfdn.org

Josephine C. Mandeville, Chair & President
Emily C Riley, Executive Vice President
Lewis W Bluemle, Senior Vice President
Carol L. Cromie, Executive Assistant
Seeks to foster learning and to improve the quality of life in the Greater Philadelphia area. The Foundation supports local non-profit organizations in the fields of education, health and human services, arts and culture and civic enterprise.

3143   Dolfinger-McMahon Foundation
30 South 17th Street
Philadelphia, PA 19103-4196   215-979-1768
www.dolfingermcmahonfoundation.org

Sheldon M. Bonovitz, Trustee
David E. Loder, Trustee
Frank G. Cooper, Counsel
Sharon M. Renz, Executive Secretary

3144   Heinz Endowments
Howard Heinz Endowment
625 Liberty Ave
30 Dominion Tower
Pittsburgh, PA 15222- 3115   412-281-5777
FAX: 412-281-5788
bobbyvagt@heinz.org
heinz.org

Grant Oliphant, President
Edward Kolano, Vice President Finance and Admin
Ann C. Plunkett, Director, Human Resources
Donna Evans Sebastian, Executive Assistant
Mission is to help our region thrive as a whole community-economically, ecologically, educationaly, and culturaly while advancing the state of knowledge and practice in the fields in which we work.

3145   Henry L Hillman Foundation
310 Grant Street
Suite 2000
Pittsburgh, PA 15219   412-338-3466
foundation@hillmanfo.com
hillmanfamilyfoundations.org

David K Roger, President
Lisa R Johns, Treasurer and Senior Program Off
Lauri K. Fink, Senior Program Officer
D.Tyler Gourley, Program Officer
Established with a broad purpose to improve the quality of life in Pittsburgh and southwestern Pennsylvania.

3146   Jewish Healthcare Foundation of Pittsburgh
650 Smithfield Street
Suite 2400
Pittsburgh, PA 15222- 3915   412-594-2550
FAX: 412-232-6240
info@jhf.org
jhf.org

Karen Wolk Feinstein, PhD, President and Chief Executive Of
Carla Barricella, Communications Director
Lindsey Kirstatter Hartle, Accounting Manager
Millie Greene, Executive Assistant
The mission of the JHF is to support and foster the provision of healthcare services, healthcare education, and, when appropriate, medical and scientific research, and to respond to the health-related needs of elderly, underprivileged, indigent, and undeserved persons in both the Jewish and general community throughout Western Pennsylvania. .

3147   Juliet L Hillman Simonds Foundation
310 Grant Street
Suite 2000
Pittsburgh, PA 15219   412-338-3466
FAX: 412-338-3520
foundation@hillmanfo.com
hillmanfamilyfoundations.org/foundations/juli

David K. Roger, President
Lisa R. Johns, Treasurer and Senior Program Off
Lauri K. Fink, Senior Program Officer
D.Tyler Gourley, Program Officer

3148   Oberkotter Foundation
1600 Market St
Suite 3600
Philadelphia, PA 19103-7212   215-751-2601
FAX: 215-751-2678
info@oberkotterfoundation.org
oberkotterfoundation.org

George H Nofer, Executive Director
Mildred L. Oberkotter, M.S.W., Trustee
Bruce A. Rosenfield, J.D., Trustee
David A. Pierson, Ph.D., Trustee
The Oberkotter Foundation focuses its efforts on supporting families who have chosen listening and spoken language for their child and on opportunities for children learning listening and spoken language to develop their social, emotional, language and educational skills.

3149   PECO Energy Company Contributions Program
Fl 7toorh
2301 Market St
Philadelphia, PA 19103-1338   215-841-4000
800-494-4000
FAX: 215-841-6830
www.peco.com

Denis P O'Brien, SVP/ CEO
Michael A. Innocenzo, SVP/ COO
Phillip S. Barnett, SVP/ CFO/ Treasurer
Scott A. Bailey, VP/ Controller

3150   PNC Bank Foundation
249 5th Ave
Pittsburgh, PA 15222-2707   412-762-2000
FAX: 412-762-7829
marianna.hallett@pnc.com
www.pncbank.com

Samuel R Patterson, Senior VP
The PNC Foundation's priority is to form partnerships with community-based nonprofit organizations within the markets PNC serves in order to enhance educational opportunities for children, particularly underserved pre-K children though our signature, PNC Grow Uo Great Program, and to promote the growth of targeted communities through economic development initiatives.

3151   Philadelphia Foundation
1234 Market St
Suite 1800
Philadelphia, PA 19107-3704   215-563-6417
FAX: 215-563-6882
EOConnell@philafound.org
philafound.org

R Andrew Swinney, President
Pat Meller, Vice President for Finance & Adm
Andrea Congo, Executive Assistant
Betsy Anderson, Communications Director
The Philadelphia Foundation improves our community by advancing change, leading on issues of importance, forging meaningful relationships and providing knowledge, resources and stewardship.

3152   Pittsburgh Foundation
Five PPG Place
Suite 250
Pittsburgh, PA 15222-5405   412-391-5122
FAX: 412-391-7259
oliphantg@pghfdn.org
pittsburghfoundation.org

Maxwell King, President and CEO
Jonathan Brelsford, Vice President of Investments
Jay Donato, Senior Investment Analyst
Marianne Cola, Special Assistant
The Pittsburgh Foundation works to improve the quality of life in the Pittsburgh region by evaluating and addressing community issues, promoting responsible philanthropy, and connecting donors to the critical needs of the community.

3153 Shenango Valley Foundation
7 West State Street
Suite 301
Sharon, PA 16146-2713
724-981-5882
866-901-7204
FAX: 724-983-9044
info@comm-foundation.com
comm-foundation.org

Lawrence E. Haynes, Executive Director
Amy Atkinson, Associate Director
Shelly Mason, Chief Financial Officer
Tristan Rice, Development Coordinator
Mission is to promote the betterment of our region and enhancement of the quality of life for all of its citizens.

3154 Staunton Farm Foundation
650 Smithfield Street
Suite 210
Pittsburgh, PA 15222- 3907
412-281-8020
FAX: 844-281-8020
office@stauntonfarm.org
stauntonfarm.org

Joni S. Schwager, Executive Director
Bethany Hemingway, Program Officer
Jason Fate, Office Manager
Robert Musca, Financial Manager
Dedicated to improving the lives of people who live with mental illness.

3155 Stewart Huston Charitable Trust
50 South First Avenue
Coatesville, PA 19320-3418
610-384-2666
FAX: 610-384-3396
admin@stewarthuston.org
stewarthuston.org

Scott G. Huston, Executive Director
Charles L. Huston III, Trustee
Shelton P Sanford, Trustee
Elinor Lashley, Trustee
The purpose of the Trust is to provide funds, technical assistance and collaboration on behalf of non-profit organizations engaged exclusively in religious, charitable or educational work; to extend opportunities to deserving needs persons and, in general, to promote any of the above causes.

3156 Teleflex Foundation
155 S Limerick Rd
Limerick, PA 19468-1603
610-948-5100
FAX: 610-948-5101
teleflex.com

Jeffrey P Black, CEO
The Teleflex Foundation strives to create an impact on the quality of life in Teleflex communities and build supportive relationships among our stakeholders. The Foundation places a priority on progrmas that have the commitmenet and volunteer involvement of Teleflex communities.

3157 USX Foundation
600 Grant St
Pittsburgh, PA 15219-2702
412-433-1121
FAX: 412-433-6847
www.ussteel.com

CD Mallick, General Manager
Patricia Funaro, Program Manager
Giving primarily in areas of company operations located within the United States.

3158 William B Dietrich Foundation
Duane Morrs Llt
30 S 17th St
Philadelphia, PA 19103-4001
215-979-1000
FAX: 215-979-1020
www.duanemorris.com

William B Dietrich, President

3159 William Talbott Hillman Foundation
310 Grant Street
Suite 2000
Pittsburgh, PA 15219
412-338-3466
FAX: 212-792-2677
foundation@hillmanfo.com
hillmanfamilyfoundations.org/foundations/will

David K. Roger, President
Lisa R. Johns, Treasurer and Senior Program Off
Lauri K. Fink, Senior Program Officer
D.Tyler Gourley, Program Officer

3160 William V and Catherine A McKinney Charitable Foundation
20 Stanwix St
Pittsburgh, PA 15222-4802
412-644-8332
FAX: 412-644-6058
verizon.com

William M Schmidt, Senior Vice President

Rhode Island

3161 Arc South County Chapter
2 Barber Avenue
Warwick, RI 02886-3549
401-480-9355
paul@pence.com
www.riroads.com

3162 Arc of Blackstone Valley
500 Prospect St.
Wing B, Suite 203
Pawtucket, RI 02860- 4332
401-727-0150
800-257-6092
FAX: 401-727-1545
contact@bvcriarc.org
www.bvcriarc.org

Kathleen O'Neill, President
Thomas E. Hodge, Vice President
John J. Padien III, Chief Executive Officer
Katherine S. Hunt, Chief Operating Officer
A private nonprofit organization providing residential, developmental, employment and recreational programs and services to more then 400 individuals with intellectual and related disabilities

3163 Arc of Northern Rhode Island
The Homestead Group Administrative Offices
68 Cumberland St
Suite 200
Woonsocket, RI 02895-3323
401-765-3700
FAX: 401-765-1124
info@thgri.org
arcofnri.org

3164 Champlin Foundations
2000 Chapel View Boulevard
Suite 350
Cranston, RI 02920
401-944-9200
FAX: 401-944-9299
www.champlinfoundations.org

Jonathan K. Farnum, Distribution Committee
John Gorham, Distribution Committee
Dione D. Kenyon, Distribution Committee
Lisa P. Koelle, Distribution Committee
Giving in the Rhode Island area. Champlin does not give grants to individuals, only to RI tax-exempt organizations.

3165 **CranstonArc**
The Keystone Group
PO Box 20130
Cranston, RI 02920-942

401-941-1112
FAX: 401-383-8751
info@accesspointri.org
www.accesspointri.org

Thomas Kane, President & CEO
Kevin McHale, Chief Operating Officer
Maureen Russo, Director of Human Resources
Gary Paulhus, Director of Clinical Services
Mission is to empower persons with differing abilites to claim and enjoy their right to dignity and respect through their lives.

3166 **Down Syndrome Society of Rhode Island**
4635 Post Road
Warwick, RI 02818

401-463-5751
FAX: 401-463-5337
TTY:800-745-5555
coordinatordssri@verizon.net
www.dssri.org

Claudia M. Lowe, Coordinator
Marilyn Blanche
Jeff DiMillio
Gail Doyle
The Down Syndrome Society of Rhode Island (DSSRI) is dedicated to promoting the rights, dignity and potential of all individuals with Down syndrome through advocacy, education, public awareness, and support.

3167 **Frank Olean Center**
93 Airport Rd
Westerly, RI 02891-3420

401-596-2091
FAX: 401-596-3945
info@oleancenter.org
oleancenter.org

Joan Gradilone, President
Tony Vellucci, Executive Director
Rick Harley, Vice President
Christine Martone, Secretary
A non-profit organization representing and providing services and supports to persons with developmental disabilities and their families throughout Southern Rhode Island and Southeastern Connecticut.

3168 **Horace A Kimball and S Ella Kimball Foundation**
23 Broad Street
Westerly, RI 02891-1879

401-348-1238
FAX: 401-364-3565
www.hkimballfoundation.org

Thomas F Black III, President
Norman D. Baker, Jr., Secretary and Treasurer
Edward C. Marth, Foundation Trustees
Makes grants almost exclusively to Rhode Island operatives (charities) or those benefitting Rhode Island residents and causes.

3169 **James L. Maher Center**
120 Hillside Avenue
Newport, RI 02840

401-846-0340
FAX: 401-849-4267
www.mahercenter.org

Jack Casey, President
William Maraziti, Executive Director
Barbara Burns, President
John S Dugan, Secretary
The mission is to advance independence and opportunity for children and adults with developmental disabilities and their families.

3170 **Kent County Arc**
2922 Fuller Ave. NE
Ste 201
Grand Rapids, MI 49505

616-459-3339
FAX: 401-737-8907
info@arckent.org
www.arckent.org

Pam Cross, President
Tim Lundgren, Vice-President
Tammy Finn, Executive Director
Maggie Kolk, Advocate/WIPA Benefits Counselor
Providing individuals with disabilties meaningful opportunities throughout their communities.

3171 **Rhode Island Arc**
99 Bald Hill Rd
Cranston, RI 02920-2647

401-463-9191
FAX: 401-463-9244
riarc@compuserve.com
riarc@compuserve.com

Mary Lou Mc Caffray, Executive Director

3172 **Rhode Island Foundation**
One Union Station
Providence, RI 02903-1758

401-274-4564
FAX: 401-331-8085
info@rifoundation.org
rifoundation.org

Neil Steinberg, President & CEO
Wendi DeClercq, Executive Assistant
James S. Sanzi, Esq., Vice President of Development
Pamela Tesler Howitt, Senior Development Officer
The Rhode Island Foundation works to build a better Rhode Island as a philanthropic resource, for people, communities, organizations, and programs.

South Carolina

3173 **Arc of South Carolina**
1202 12th Street
Cayce, SC 29033

803-748-5020
FAX: 803-445-1026
TheArc@ArcSC.org
www.arcsc.org

Margie Williamson, Executive Director
Caroline Kistler, Project Director
Carly Prince, Case Manager
Hilary Bell, Case Manager
The Arc of South Carolina advocates for and alongside people with cognitive, intellectual and developmental disabilities and their families.

3174 **Center for Disability Resources**
University of South Carolina
8301 Farrow Rd
Columbia, SC 29208-1

803-935-5231
FAX: 803-935-5059
David.Rotholz@uscmed.sc.edu
uscm.med.sc.edu

Dr. David A. Rotholz, Director
A University Affiliated Program which develops model programs designed to serve persons with disabilities and to train students in fields related to disabilities.

3175 **Colonial Life and Accident Insurance Company Contributions Program**
1200 Colonial Life Blvd W
Columbia, SC 29210-7670

803-798-7000
FAX: 803-731-2618

Randy Horn, President and Chief Executive Of
Bill Deeham, Senior Vice President of Sales
Tim Arnold, Senior Vice President of Sales a
John Garrison, Vice President, General Counsel

Tennessee

3176 Arc of Anderson County
728 Emory Valley Road, Suite 42
P.O.Box 4823
Oak Ridge, TN 37831-4823
865-481-0550
arc@arcaid.org
www.thearcandersoncounty.com

Sally Browning, President
Dargie Arwood, Executive Director
Ginny Miceli, President
Elizabeth Bonner, Vice President
The Arc of Anderson County provides support and advocacy to people with cognitive, intellectual and developmental disabilities. The Arc provides support, information and training for families and caregivers of adults and children with these disabilities.

3177 Arc of Davidson County
111 N Wilson Blvd
Nashville, TN 37205-2411
615-248-4112
FAX: 615-322-9184
arc@arcdc.org
arcdc.org

Kate Deitzer, President
Cynthia Gardner, Vice President
Thom Druffel, Treasurer
Elizabeth Ralph, Secretary
Provides services to adults and children with intellectual and developmental disabilities through a contract with the Tennessee Departmant of Mental Retardation Services Medicaid Waiver Program.

3178 Arc of Hamilton County
4613 Brainerd Rd
Chattanooga, TN 37411-3826
423-624-6887
800-624-6887
FAX: 423-624-3974
arcofhamilton@aol.com
thearchc.org

Shawn Ellis, Executive Director
Provides assistance to individuals and families with mental retardation and related disabilities, in the form of advocacy, information, and support coordination

3179 Arc of Tennessee
151 Athens Way
Suite 100
Nashville, TN 37228-1367
615-248-5878
800-835-7077
FAX: 615-248-5879
info@thearctn.org
thearctn.org

John Lewis, President
John Shouse, Vice President
Donna Lankford, Secretary
Ann Curl, Treasurer
Advocacy, information, referral and support for people with intellectual and developmental disabilities and their families.

3180 Arc of Washington County
110 East Mountcastle Drive
Johnson City, TN 37601-7557
423-928-9362
FAX: 423-928-7431
kim@arcwc.org
www.arcwc.org

Malessa Fleenor, Executive Director
Kim Reid, Human Resources, Quality Assuran
Kim Wheeler, Respite Coordinator
Linda Tilson, Family Support Program Manager
Is a non-profit organization that serves individuals with disabilities and their families. They have an independent support coordination service, as well as, early intervention, family support and respite services.

3181 Arc of Williamson County
129 W Fowlkes St
Suite 151
Franklin, TN 37064-3562
615-790-5815
FAX: 615-790-5891
sbbarc@thearcwc.org
thearcwc.org

Donna Isbell, President
Steve Cassidy, Vice President
Ashley Coulter, Secretary
Jan Lincoln, Treasurer
The Arc is a family-based organization committed to securing for all people with intellectual, developmental, or other disabilities the opportunity to choose and realize their goals of where and how they live, learn, work, and play.

3182 Arc-Diversified
453 Gould Dr
Cookeville, TN 38506
931-432-5981
800-239-9029
FAX: 931-432-5987
www.arcdiversified.com

3183 Benwood Foundation
736 Market St
Suite 1600
Chattanooga, TN 37402-4812
423-267-4311
FAX: 423-267-9049
info@benwood.org
benwood.org

Sarah Morgan, President
Kristy Huntley, Program & Financial Officer
Connie Perrin, Accounting & Grants Manager
Jeff Pfitzer, Program Officer
Benwood Foundation seeks to stimulate creative and innovative efforts to build and strengthen the Chattanooga community.

3184 Community Foundation of Greater Chattanooga
1270 Market St
Chattanooga, TN 37402-2713
423-265-0586
FAX: 423-265-0587
info2@cfgc.org
cfgc.org

Peter T. Cooper, President
Rebecca Underwood, Vice President, Finance & Admini
Marty Robinson, Vice President, Donor Relations
Rebecca Smith, Director of Scholarships
A non-profit organization which receives, holds, invests and distributes assets contributed by individuals and organizations for the benefit of Chattanooga, its citizens and its institutions.

3185 Education and Auditory Research Foundation
PO Box 330867
Nashville, TN 37203-7506
615-627-2724
800-545-4327
FAX: 615-627-2728
info@earfoundation.org
www.earfoundation.org

Michael Glasscock, President
Provides the general public support services promoting the integration of the hearing and balance impaired into mainstream society; to provide practicing ear specialists continuing medical education courses and related programs specifically regarding rehabilitation and hearing preservation; to educate young people and adults about hearing preservation and early detection of hearing loss, enabling them to prevent at an early age hearing and balance disorders.

3186 International Paper Company Foundation
6400 Poplar Ave
Memphis, TN 38197
901-419-9000
800-207-4003
FAX: 901-419-4439
internationalpaper.comm@ipaper.com
internationalpaper.com

Mark S Sutton, Chairman & CEO
David J Bronczek, President & CEO
C. Cato Ealy, Senior Vice President, Corporate
William P. Hoel, Senior Vice President
The Foundation's primary focus is education-specifically environmental education, iliteracy programs for young children and minority career development opportunities for college bound youth.

3187 Montgomery County Arc
1825 K Street
NW, Suite 1200
Washington, DC 20006-2145
202-534-3700
800-433-5255
FAX: 202-534-3731
info@thearc.org
www.thearc.org

Ronald Brown, President
Elise McMillan, Vice President
Peter V Berns, Chief Executive Officer
M.J. Bartelmay, Secretary
Organization works to ensure that the estimated 7.2 million Americans with intellectual and developmental disabilities have the services and supports they need to grow, develop and live in communities across the nation.

Texas

3188 AFB Center on Vision Loss
American Foundation for the Blind
2 Penn Plaza
Suite 1102
New York, NY 10121-4524
212-502-7600
FAX: 888-545-8331
afbinfo@afb.net
afb.org

Carl R Augusto, President & CEO
Kelly Bleach, Chief Administrative Officer
Rick Bozeman, Chief Financial Officer
Paul Schroeder, Vice President
National nonprofit organization that expands possibilities for people with vision loss.

3189 Abell-Hangar Foundation
P.O.Box 430
Midland, TX 79702-0430
432-684-6655
FAX: 432-684-4474
abell-hanger.org

David L Smith, Executive Director
The Foundation makes grants to nonprofit organizations, which are involved in such undertakings for public welfare, including but not limited to, education, health services, human services, arts and cultural activities and community or social benefit.

3190 Albert & Bessie Mae Kronkosky Charitable Foundation
112 East Pecan
Suite 830
San Antonio, TX 78205-1574
210-475-9000
888-309-9001
FAX: 210-354-2204
kronfndn@kronkosky.org
kronkosky.org

Palmer Moe, Managing Director
Mission is to produce profound good that is tangible and measurable in Bandera, Bexar, Comal, and Kendall counties in Texas by implimenting the Kronkosky's charitable purposes.

3191 Arc of Texas, The
8001 Centre Park Dr
Suite 100
Austin, TX 78754-5118
512-454-6694
800-252-9729
FAX: 512-454-4956
www.thearcoftexas.org

Charlie Huber, President
John Schneider, Vice President
Amy Mizcles, Executive Director
Terri Schonfeld, Secretary
The Arc of Texas creates opportunities for all people with intellectual and developmental disabilities to actively participate in their communities and make the choices that affect their lives in a positive manner.

3192 BA and Elinor Steinhagen Benevolent Trust
Chase Bank of Texas
700 North St.
Suite D
Beaumont, TX 77701-3928
409-832-6565
FAX: 409-832-7532
cjourdan@setxnonprofit.org
www.setxnonprofit.org

Jean Moncla, CTFA, President
Ivy Pate, Treasurer
Chester Jourdan, Executive Director
Kristi Stott, Administrative Assistant

3193 Brown Foundation
P.O.Box 130646
Houston, TX 77219-0646
713-523-6867
FAX: 713-523-2917
bfi@brownfoundation.org
brownfoundation.org

Nancy Pittman, Executive Director
The purpose of the Brown Foundation is to distribute funds for public charitable purposes, principally for support, encouragement and assistance to education, the arts and community service.

3194 Burnett Foundation
P.O. Box 633
Northfield, MN 55057-6881
817-877-3344
tomburnettfamilyfoundation@msn.com
www.tomburnettfoundation.org

V Neils Agather, Executive Director

3195 CH Foundation
P.O.Box 94038
Lubbock, TX 79493-4038
806-792-0448
FAX: 806-792-7824
ksanford@chfoundation.com
www.chfoundationlubbock.com

Kay Sanford, Executive Director
Heather Hocker, Grants Administrator
Cheryl Sanford, Administrative Assistant
Mission of the CH foundation is to significantly improve human services and cultural and educational opportunities for the residents of the South Plain of Texas.

3196 Cockrell Foundation
1000 Main St
Suite 3250
Houston, TX 77002-6338
713-209-7500
foundation@cockrell.com
www.cockrell.com

Ernest H. Cockrell, President
Nancy Williams, Executive Vice President
Purpose is for giving for higher education at the University of Texas at Austin; support also for cultural programs, social services, youth services and health care. Limitations are giving in Houston, Texas and no grants are awarded to individuals.

3197 Communities Foundation of Texas
5500 Caruth Haven Ln
Dallas, TX 75225-8146
214-750-4222
FAX: 214-750-4210
jsmith@cftexas.org
cftexas.org

Brent E. Chrisopher, President and Chief Executive Of
Elizabeth W. Bull, Senior Vice President and Chief
Jeverley R. Cook, Ph.D., Executive Director, W.W. Caruth,
John Fitzpatrick, Executive Director
Mission is to improve lives, we serve the community by investing wisely and making effective charitable grants.

3198 Community Foundation of North Texas
306 West 7th
Suite 1045
Fort Worth, TX 76102-4906
817-877-0702
FAX: 817-632-8711
cfntx.org

Nancy E. Jones, President
Rob Miller, Director of Finance
Vicki Andrews, Director of Operations/Donor Ser
Rose Bradshaw, Executive Vice President
Community Foundation is a tax exempt organization that provides stewardship for many individual charitable funds. With its specialized services, Community Foundation of North Texas gives donors efficient charitable fund administration.

3199 Cullen Foundation
601 Jefferson St
40th Floor
Houston, TX 77002-7900
713-651-8837
FAX: 713-651-2374
cullenfdn.org

Isaac Arnold, Jr, President
Wilhelmina E Robertson, Vice President and Secretary
Meredith T Cullen, Assistant Secretary
Bert L. Campbell, Director
Grants are restricted to Texas-based organizations for programs in Texas, primarily in the Houston area.

3200 Curtis & Doris K Hankamer Foundation
Ste 530
9039 Katy Fwy
Houston, TX 77024-1656
713-461-8140

Gregory A Herbst, Manager

3201 Dallas Foundation
3963 Maple Avenue
Ste. 390
Dallas, TX 75219-4447
214-741-9898
FAX: 214-741-9848
info@dallasfoundation.org
dallasfoundation.org

Mary M Jalonick, President & CEO
Gary W. Garcia, Senior Director of Development
Dawn Townsend, Director of Marketing & Communic
William T. Solomon, Jr., Chief Financial Officer
Serves as a leader, catalyst and resource for philanthropy by providing donors with a flexible means of making gifts to charitable causes that enhance our community.

3202 David D & Nona S Payne Foundation
P.O.Box 174
Pampa, TX 79066-174
806-665-0063
www.davidandnonapaynefoundation.com
Vanessa G Buzzard, Director
The David & Nona S Payne Foundation was established in August 1980. Mrs Payne established the foundation and did much of her charitable giving in honor of her late husband.

3203 El Paso Natural Gas Foundation
P.O.Box 2511
Houston, TX 77252-2511
713-420-2600
FAX: 713-420-5312
foundation@elpaso.com
www.kindermorgan.com

Douglas Foshee, CEO
Focuses on the areas in locations where we have significant facilities or concentrated employees. Primary area of focus is Civic and Community, Education and Health and Human Services. Secondary area of focus is Arts and Culture and Environment.

3204 Epilepsy Foundation of Southeast Texas
8301 Professional Place
Suite 200
Landover, MD 20785- 2353
866-330-2718
800-332-1000
FAX: 301-459-1569
ContactUs@efa.org
www.epilepsyfoundation.org

Warren Lammert, Chair
Roger Heldman, Treasurer
May J. Liang, Secretary
Joyce A. Bender, Chief Executive Officer
The Epilepsy Foundation of Southeast Texas is a non-profit organization to improve the lives of almost 100,000 adultsand children with epilepsy in the counties of north and southeast Texas.

3205 Epilepsy Foundation: Central and South Texas
10615 Perrin Beitel Rd
Ste 602
San Antonio, TX 78217- 3142
210-653-5353
888-606-5353
FAX: 210-653-5355
staff@efcst.org
www.efcst.org

Anna Amos, President
Todd Drexler, Vice President
The Epilepsy Foundation of Central & South Texas is a voluntary health organization. We value all people with epilepsy. We commit our resources to empowering their independence and inspiring productive lives.

3206 Harris and Eliza Kempner Fund
2201 Market St
12th Floor
Galveston, TX 77553-1529
409-765-6671
FAX: 409-765-9098
information@kemperfund.org
kempnercapital.com

Diana L. Bartula, Vice President, Chief Compliance
V. Delynn Greene, Vice President, Head Trader, Ope
Mission is to further the vision and heritage of the Kemper Family's commitment to philanthropy and sense of responsibility to society.

3207 Hillcrest Foundation
Bank of America
P.O.Box 830241
Dallas, TX 75283
214-209-1965

Daniel Kelly, VP

3208 Hoblitzelle Foundation
5556 Caruth Haven Lane
Suite 200
Dallas, TX 75225-8020
214-373-0462
kstone@hoblitzelle.org
www.hoblitzelle.org

William T Solomon, Chairman
Caren H. Prothro, Vice Chairman
J. McDonald Williams, Treasurer
Karl Hoblitzelle, Founder
Grants made by the directors are usually focused on specific, non-recurring needs of the educational, social service, medical,

cultural, and civic organizations in Texas, particularly in the Dallas area.

3209   Houston Endowment
600 Travis St
Suite 6400
Houston, TX 77002-3003   713-238-8100
                                     FAX: 713-238-8101
                              info@houstonendowment.org
                                  houstonendowment.org

Ann B Stern, President
Sheryl L Johns, Vice President for Admin
F. Xavier Pena, Vice President for Finance and G
Lisa A. Hall, Vice President for-Programs
A private philanthropic foundation that improves life for people of the greater Houston area through its contributions to charitable organizations and educational institutions.

3210   John G & Marie Stella Kennedy Memorial Foundation
555 N Carancahua
Suite 1700, Tower II
Corpus Christi, TX 78401-0851   361-887-6565
                                     FAX: 361-887-6582
                                          www.kenedy.org

Judge J. A. Garcia, President and Director
Marc A. Cisneros, Chief Executive Officer
Sylvia Whitmore, Chief Operating Officer
Gloria Hicks, Secretary and Director
To advance and nurture activities that contribute to the foundation's core, Catholic values.

3211   John S Dunn Research Foundation
3355 West Alabama
Suite 990
Houston, TX 77098-1722   713-626-0368
                                     FAX: 713-626-3866
                                         jsdrf@swbell.net
                                   johnsdunnfoundation.org

J. Dickson Rogers, President
Dan S. Wilford, Vice President
John R. Wallace, Secretary and Treasurer
John S. Dunn, Trustee

3212   Lola Wright Foundation
515 Congress Avenue
10th Floor
Austin, TX 78701   512-397-2001
                             amber.carden@ustrust.com
                                  fdnweb.org/lolawright

Wilford Flowers, President and Director
Paul Hilgers, Vice-President and Director
Ron Oliveira, Secretary and Director
Jay Stewart, Director

3213   Meadows Foundation
3003 Swiss Ave
Dallas, TX 75204-6049   214-826-9431
                                          800-826-9431
                                     FAX: 214-827-7042
                                          grants@mfi.org
                                              www.mfi.org

Linda P Evans, President and CEO
Tom Gale, Vice President and Chief Investm
Paula Herring, Vice President and Treasurer
Laura Bowers, Corporate Secretary
The Meadows Foundation exists to assist people and institutions of Texas improve the quality and circumstances of life for themselves and future generations.

3214   Moody Foundation
2302 Post Office St
Suite 704
Galveston, TX 77550-1994   409-797-1500
                                    colleen@moodyf.org
                                             moodyf.org

Frances Moody-Dahlderg, Executive Director
Jamie G. Williams, Human Resources Director
Garrik Addison, Chief Financial Officer
Samantha Seale, Scholarship Administrator
Created for the perpetual benefit of present and future generations.

3215   Pearle Vision Foundation
2534 Royal Ln
Dallas, TX 75229-3884   214-821-7770
                                   www.pearlevision.com

Leo Priolo Jr, Owner
Organization dedicated to sight preservation through vision research and education.

3216   San Antonio Area Foundation
303 Pearl Parkway
Suite 114
San Antonio, TX 78215   210-225-2243
                                     FAX: 210-225-1980
                                         info@saafdn.org
                                              saafdn.org

Marie Smith, Chair
G.P. Singh, Vice Chair
Michelle R. Scarver, Secretary
Luis de la Garza, Treasurer
The San Antionio Area Foundation aspires to significantly enhance the quality of life in our community by providing outstanding service to donors, producing significant asset growth, strengthning community collaboration and managing an exemplary grants program.

3217   Shell Oil Company Foundation
40 Bank Street
London, TX 77252-2463   281-544-7171
                                     FAX: 713-241-3329
                                  info@shellfoundation.org
                                   www.shellfoundation.org

Malcolm Brinded, Chairman
Ben van Beurden, Trustee
William Kalema, Trustee
Hugh Mitchell, Trustee
A not-for-profit foundation funded by donations from Shell Oil Company and other participating Shell companies and subsidiaries.

3218   South Texas Charitable Foundation
P.O.Box 2459
Victoria, TX 77902   512-573-4383

Rayford L Keller, Secretary

3219   Sterling-Turner Foundation
5850 San Felipe Street
Suite 125
Houston, TX 77057-3292   713-237-1117
                                     FAX: 713-223-4638
                            jeannie.arnold@stfdn.org
                          www.sterlingturnerfoundation.org

T. R. Reckling, President
Isla C. Reckling, Treasurer
Patricia Stilley, Executive Director
Christiana R McConn, Secretary
Sterling Turner Foundation is a private trust which can assist any Section 501 (c) (3) organization in the state of Texas. The Foundation is not permitted to assist any individuals

3220 **TLL Temple Foundation**
109 Temple Blvd
Lufkin, TX 75901-7321
936-639-5197
wcorley@tlltf.com

Wayne Corley, Executive Director

3221 **William Stamps Farish Fund**
Ste 1250
1100 Louisiana St
Houston, TX 77002-5232
713-757-7313

Terry Ward, Manager

Utah

3222 **Arc of Utah**
18585 Coastal Hwy # 19
Rehoboth Beach, DE 19971
801-364-5060
800-371-3060
FAX: 801-364-6030
gacosta@dunndunn.com
www.bewitchedtattoos.com

Kathy Scott, Executive Director
The Arc of Utah advocates for and with cognitive, intellectual and developmental disabilities and their families through awareness, outreach, education, support and public policy.

3223 **Marriner S Eccles Foundation**
79 S Main St
Salt Lake City, UT 84111-1929
801-532-0934

Shannon K Toronto

3224 **Questar Corporation Contributions Program**
333 South State Street
P.O. Box 45433
Salt Lake City, UT 84145-0433
801-324-5000
www.questar.com

Ronald W Jibson, President & CEO
Craig C Wagstaff, Executive vice president
Micheal Dunn, Executive vice president
Brady Rasmussen, Executive Vice President
Focuses on promoting a healthy environment by investing in and fulfilling its corporate responsibility to support the well-being of communitites where Questar and its subsidiaries conduct business.

Vermont

3225 **Vermont Community Foundation**
3 Court Street
Middlebury, VT 05753
802-388-3355
FAX: 802-388-3398
info@vermontcf.org
www.vermontcf.org

Stuart Comstock-Gay, President
Nina McDonnell, Grants Administrator
Janet McLaughlin, Special Projects Director
Jen Peterson, Vice President for Program and G
Helps build and manage charitable funds created by individuals, families, groups, organizations, and institutions to improve the quality of life in Vermont.

Virginia

3226 **Arc of Virginia**
2147 Staples Mill Road
Richmond, VA 23230
804-649-8481
FAX: 804-649-3585
info@thearcofva.org
www.thearcofva.org

Howard Cullum, President
Shareen Young-Chavez, President-Elect
Marisa Laios, Vice President
Donalda Lovelace, Secretary
The Arc of Virginia advocactes for individuals with mental retardation and developmental disabilities and their families, so they may all lead productive and fulfilling lives.

3227 **Camp Foundation**
P.O.Box 813
Franklin, VA 23851
757-562-3439

Bobby B Worrell, CEO

3228 **Community Foundation of Richmond & Central Virginia**
7501 Boulder View Drive
Suite 110
Richmond, VA 23225- 4047
804-330-7400
FAX: 804-330-5992
info@tcfrichmond.org
tcfrichmond.org

Darcy Oman, President
Bobby Thalhimer, Senior Advisor
Molly Dean Bittner, Vice President
Lisa Pratt O'Mara, Vice President
The Community Foundation provides effective stewardship of philanthropic assets entrusted to its care by donors who wish to enhance the quality of community life.

3229 **John Randolph Foundation**
112 North Main Street
P.O.Box 1606
Hopewell, VA 23860- 1161
804-458-2239
FAX: 804-458-3754
lsharpe@johnrandolphfoundation.org
www.johnrandolphfoundation.org

Lisa H. Sharpe, Executive Director
M. Stephen Cates, Director of Finance and Accounti
Kiffy Werkheiser, Development Program Officer
Tammy E. McCollum, Administrative Associate
The John Randolph Foundation is a community-based Foundation working to improve the health and quality of life for residents of Hopewell and surrounding areas through Grants and Scholarships.

3230 **Norfolk Foundation**
101 W. Main Street,
Suite 4500
Norfolk, VA 23510-2103
757-622-7951
FAX: 757-622-1751
mbrunson@hamptonroadscf.org
www.hamptonroadscf.org

Deborah M DiCroce, Ed.D., President and CEO
Tim McCarthy, Chief Financial Officer
Kay A. Stine, CFRE, Vice President for Development
Lynn Watson Neumann, Director of Gift Planning
The mission of the Norfolk Foundation is to inspire philanthropy and transform the quality of life in southeastern Virginia.

3231 **Robey W Estes Family Foundation**
Robey W Estes Jr
3901 West Broad Street
P.O. Box 25612
Richmond, VA 23230-5612
866-378-3748
estes-express.com

Robey W Estes Jr, President and CEO

3232   Virginia Beach Foundation
Suite 4500
101 W. Main Street,
Virginia Beach, VA 23454   757-422-5249
                                        FAX: 757-422-1849
                            mbrunson@hamptonroadscf.org
                                www.hamptonroadscf.org

Deborah M DiCroce, President
Tim McCarthy, Chief Financial Officer
Mission is to stimulate the establishment of endowments to serve the people of Virgina Beach now and in the future. Respond to changing, emerging, community needs. Provide a vehicle and a service for donors with varied interests. Serve as a resource, broker, catalyst and leader in the community.

Washington

3233   Arc of Washington State
2638 State Avenue NE
Olympia, WA 98506-4880   360-357-5596
                                        FAX: 360-357-3279
                                          info@arcwa.org
                                             arcwa.org

Cindy O'Neill, President
Nancy Stark, Vice President
Angie Ziska, Secretary
Martha Schulte, Treasurer
Mission is to advocacte for the rights and full participation of all people with developmental disabilities.

3234   Ben B Cheney Foundation
3110 Ruston Way
Suite A
Tacoma, WA 98402-5308   253-572-2442
                            Info@benbcheneyfoundation.org
                                benbcheneyfoundation.org

Bradbury F. Cheney, President
Piper Cheney, Vice President
Carolyn J. Cheney, Secretary Treasurer
Allan L. Undem, Board Member
The Foundation makes grants in communities where the Cheney Lumber Company was active. The Foundation's goal is to improve the quality of life in those communities by making grants to a wide range of activities.

3235   Community Foundation of North Central Washington
9 South Wenatchee Ave
Wenatchee, WA 98801-3332   509-663-7716
                                        FAX: 888-317-8314
                                           info@cfncw.org
                                          www.cfncw.org

Beth Stipe, Executive Director
Kristy Harris, Chief Financial Officer
Lila R. Edlund, Director of Administration
Jennifer Dolge, Director of Donor Services and C
Assists donors by helping identify their specific charitable and goals and provide grants and scholarships that help groups and people address critical issues in North Central Washington

3236   Glaser Progress Foundation
1601 Second Avenue
Suite 1080
Seattle, WA 98101-9223   206-728-1050
                                        FAX: 206-728-1123
                                martin@glaserfoundation.org
                                  www.glaserfoundation.org

Martin Collier, Executive Director
Mitchell Fox, Program Officer
Melessa Rogers, Operations Manager
The Glaser Prograss Foundation focuses on four program areas: measuring progress, animal advocacy, independent media and global HIV/AIDS.

3237   Greater Tacoma Community Foundation
950 Pacific Avenue
Suite 1100
Tacoma, WA 98402-4423   253-383-5622
                                        FAX: 253-272-8099
                                            info@gtcf.org
                                            www.gtcf.org

Rose Lincoln Hamilton, President and CEO
Shirley Brockmann, CPA, Vice President Finance & Adminis
Elyse Rowe, Chief of Strategy and Community
Gina Anstey, Vice President, Grants
Mission is fostering generosity by connecting people who care with causes that matter, forever enriching our community.

3238   Inland Northwest Community Foundation
421 West Riverside Avenue
Suite 606
Spokane, WA 99201- 0405   509-624-2606
                                            888-267-5606
                                        FAX: 509-624-2608
                                           admin@inwcf.org
                                            www.inwcf.org

Mark Hurtubise, Ph.D., J.D., President and CEO
Troy Braga, CPA, Controller
P J Watters, Director of Gift Planning
Molly Sanchez, Director of Community Engagement
Serving 20 counties throughout Eastern Washington and Northern Idaho, mission is to foster vibrant and sustainable communities in the Inland Northwest.

3239   Medina Foundation
801 2nd Ave
Suite 1300
Seattle, WA 98104-1517   206-652-8783
                                        FAX: 206-652-8791
                                  info@medinafoundation.org
                                    www.medinafoundation.org

Jennifer Teunon, Executive Director
Jessica Case, Program Officer
Aana Lauckhart, Program Officer
Alexia Cameron, Grants Administrator
A family foundation that works to foster positive change in the Greater Puget Sound area. The Foundation strives to improve the human condition by supporting organizations that provide critical services to those in need.

3240   Norcliffe Foundation
999 3rd Ave
Suite 1006
Seattle, WA 98104-4001   206-682-4820
                                        FAX: 206-682-4821
                          arline@thenorcliffefoundation.com
                            www.thenorcliffefoundation.com

Arline Hefferline, Foundation Manager
Nora P. Kenway, President
Geographic area of funding limited to the Puget Sound Region in and around Seattle, Washington.

3241   Stewardship Foundation
1145 Broadway
Suite 1500
Tacoma, WA 98402-1278   253-620-1340
                                        FAX: 253-572-2721
                                    info@stewardshipfdn.org
                                    www.stewardshipfdn.org

William T. Weyerhaeuser, Chair
Gail T. Weyerhaeuser, Vice Chair and Treasurer
Chi- Dooh, Director
J. Derek McNeil, Director
Christian, evangelical organizations - national or international impact.

3242 **Weyerhaeuser Company Foundation**
33663 Weyerhaeuser Way South
Federal Way, WA 98003   253-924-2345
                          800-525-5440
                   www.weyerhaeuser.com

Daniel S Fulton, President & CEO
Patricia M Bedient, EVP & CFO
Sandy D McDade, SVP & General Counsel
John A Hooper, SVP, Human Resources
Although the foundation does fund programs for disabled persons from time to time, it is not a specific priority for the foundation. Since it was formed in 1948, the foundation has given more than $81.1 million to nonprofit organizations and is one of the oldest funds for corporate philanthropy in the country. Nearly all of its contributions have been made within the communities where Weyerhaeuser employees live and work and awards approximately 600 grants annually.

West Virginia

3243 **Arc Of West Virginia, The**
912 Market Street
Parkersburg, WV 26101-4737   304-422-3151
                 christina.smith@arcwd.org
                       www.thearcwv.org

3244 **Bernard McDonough Foundation**
311 Fourth Street
Parkersburg, WV 26101-5315   304-424-6280
                          FAX: 304-424-6281
              www.mcdonoughfoundation.org

Robert W Stephens, Ed.D., President
Mary Riccobene, Vice President
Francis C. McCusker, Treasurer
Katrina Valentine, Corporate Secretary
Directors and officers continue the legacy of the McDonoughs by providing grants that create a healthier, more educated and culturally appreciative citizenry.

Wisconsin

3245 **Arc of Dunn County**
2602 Hils Court
Menomonie, WI 54751-4160   715-235-7373
                          FAX: 715-233-3565
              rebecca@arcofdunncounty.org
                  www.arcofdunncounty.org

Rebecca Cooper, Executive Director
Kathy Lausted, Guardianship Director
Advocating for the rights of citizens with disabilities.

3246 **Arc of Eau Claire**
4800 Golf Road
Suite 450
Eau Claire, WI 54701-6130   715-833-1735
                          FAX: 715-833-1215
                          frcec@frcec.org
                          www.frcec.org

Brook Steele, President
Melanie Koehler, Vice President
Dr. Jennifer Eddy, Secretary
Dr. Emily Smith-Nguyen, Treasurer
Mission is to provide programs and services that build on family strengths through prevention, education, support and networking in collaboration with other resources in the community.

3247 **Arc of Fox Cities**
211 E. Franklin St.
Suite A
Appleton, WI 54911   920-735-0943
                   FAX: 920-725-1531
                   info@arcfoxcities.com
                       arcfoxcities.com

Laura McCormick, President
Todd Klauer, Vice President
Bryan Mueller, Secretary
Rico Tomasi, Treasurer
Mission statement is to utilize advocacy, respect and concern to empower all people with disabilities to have the opportunity to choose and realize their goal of a full life and a secure future.

3248 **Arc of Racine County**
6214 Washington Ave
Suite C-6
Racine, WI 53404-3350   262-634-6303
                 info@thearcofracine.org
                 www.thearcofracine.org

Peggy Foreman, Executive Director
Alison Henry, Program Manager
Ross Gietzel, Program Assistant
The Arc of Racine's mission is to advocate for and provide information and services to improve lives.

3249 **Arc of Wisconsin Disability Association**
2800 Royal Ave
Suite 202
Monona, WI 53713-1518   608-222-8907
                          877-272-8400
                   FAX: 608-222-8908
                       arcw@att.net
                   www.arc-wisconsin.org

John Beisbier, President
Donna Auchue, Vice President
Tina Beauprey, Secretary
The Arc-Wisconsin strives to be a major force in advocating and promoting self-determined quality of life opportunities for poeple with developmental and related disabilities and their families.

3250 **Arc-Dane County**
6602 Grand Teton Plz
Madison, WI 53719-1091   608-833-1199
                          FAX: 608-833-1307
                       arcdane@chorus.net
                       arcdanecounty.org

Ken Hobbs, President
John Leemkuil, Vice President
Mark Lederer, Secretary
Todd Grundahl, Treasurer
The Arc-Dane County is a non-profit organization whose primary objective is to support children and adults with developmental disabilities and their families through advocacy to assure these individuals are offered the same opportunities and have the rights due all people. The Arc-Dane County provides numerous services through education, overall support, and legislation that assists those individuals with developmental disabilities be it within their homes, communities, or at work.

3251 **Faye McBeath Foundation**
101 W. Pleasant Street
Suite 210
Milwaukee, WI 53212- 3157   414-272-2626
                          FAX: 414-272-6235
                       info@fayemcbeath.org
                       www.fayemcbeath.org

P. Michael Mahoney, Chair
Mary T. Kellner, Vice Chair
Gregory M. Wesley, Secretary
Scott E. Gelzer, Executive Director
A private independent foundation providing grants to tax exempt nonprofit organizations principally the metropolitan Milwaukee area.

3252   Helen Bader Foundation
233 North Water Street
4th Floor
Milwaukee, WI 53202- 5761   414-224-6464
                                         FAX: 414-224-1441
                                             info@hbf.org
                                              www.hbf.org

Daniel J. Bader, President/CEO
Lisa G. Hiller, VP, Administration
Maria Lopez Vento, VP, Programs and Partnerships
Robert Tobon, Director, Foundation Relations
Strives to be a philanthropic leader in improving the quality of
life of the diverse communities in which it works. The Founda-
tion makes grants, convenes partners, and shares knowledge to
affect emerging issues in key areas.

3253   Johnson Controls Foundation
5757 N Green Bay Ave
P.O. Box 591
Milwaukee, WI 53201- 4408   414-524-1200
                                             800-333-2222
                                         FAX: 414-524-2077
                                        johnsoncontrols.com

Stephen A Molinaroli, Chairman, President and CEO
Dr. Breda Bolzenius, Vice President, Vice Chairman
Kim Metcalf-Kupres, Vice President and Chief Marketi
R. Bruce McDonald, Executive Vice President and CF
Organized and directed to be operated for charitable purposes
which include the distribution and application of financial sup-
port to soundly managed and operated organizations or causes
which are fundamentally philanthropic.

3254   Lynde and Harry Bradley Foundation
1241 N Franklin Pl
Milwaukee, WI 53202-2901   414-291-9915
                                         FAX: 414-291-9991
                                           www.bradleyfdn.org

Dennis J. Kuester, Chairman
David V. Uihlein, Vice Chairman
Michael W. Grebbe, President and CEO
Patrick J. English, Chief Investment Officer
The Foundation's programs support limited, competent government; a dynamic marketplace for economic, intellectual and cultural activity; a vigorus defense at home and abroad, of American
ideas and institutions; and scholarly studies and academic
achievement.

3255   Milwaukee Foundation
101 W Pleasant St
Suite 210
Milwaukee, WI 53212-3963   414-272-5805
                                         FAX: 414-272-6235
                             info@greatermilwaukeefoundation.org
                             www.greatermilwaukeefoundation.org

Ellen M Gilligan, President and CEO
Marcus White, Vice President
Kathryn J. Dunn, Vice President
Danae Davis, Executive Director
Guided by three tenets- helping donors create personal legacies
of giving that last beyond their lifetimes, investing donor funds
for maximum return with minimal risk, and playing a leadership
role tackling the communities most challenging needs.

3256   Northwestern Mutual Life Foundation
720 E Wisconsin Ave
Milwaukee, WI 53202-4703   414-271-1444
                                       www.northwesternmutual.com

John E Schlifske, Chairman and CEO
Gregory C. Oberland, President
Michael G. Carter, Executive Vice President and CFO
Joann M. Eisenhart, Senior Vice President - Human Re

3257   Patrick and Anna M Cudahy Fund
70 E. Lake St.,
Suite 1120
Chicago, Il 60601   312-422-1442
                                         FAX: 312-641-5736
                                      laurenkrieg@cudahyfund.org
                                             cudahyfund.org

Janet S Cudahy MD, President
Lauren Krieg, Executive Director
A general purpose foundation which primarily supports organizations in Wisconsin and the metropolitan Chicago area. Interests
are social service, youth, and education with some giving for the
arts, and other areas.

3258   SB Waterman & E Blade Charitable Foundation
Marshall & Ilsley Trust Company
111 E. Kilbourn Ave.,
Milwaukee, WI 53202-2980   414-287-8700
                                         FAX: 414-765-8200
                                             www.mitrust.com

Thomas C Boettcher, Director
Giving primarily to health associations. Geographical focus is
Wisconsin.

Wyoming

3259   Arc of Natrona County
314 W. Midwest Ave
P.O. Box 393
Casper, WY 82601   307-577-4913
                                             800-433-5255
                                         FAX: 307-577-4014
                                             info@thearc.org
                                         arcofnatronacounty.org

Beau Covert, President
Dr. Nathan Edwards, Vice President
Kelley Reimer, Treasurer
Colbi Maddox, Secretary
Organization works to ensure that the estimated 7.2 million
Americans with intellectual and developmental disabilities have
the services and supports they need to grow, develop and live in
communities across the nation.

Funding Directories

3260   Chronicle Guide to Grants
318 S. Lee Street
Alexandria, DC 20037-1146   202-466-1200
                                             800-287-6072
                                         FAX: 202-452-1033
                                        help@philanthropy.com
                                             heideninc.com

Phil Semas, Manager
Edward J. Heiden, President
A computerized research tool, on floppy disks or a CD-ROM, for
immediate use on any IBM compatible personal computer. Offers
electronic listings of 10,000 grants from hundreds of foundations, with a subscription that offers 1,000 plus new listings every
two months. Each listing offers grant information as well as
names, addresses and phone numbers of the grant-making organizations. *$295.00*

3261 College Student's Guide to Merit and Other No-Need Funding

Reference Service Press
5000 Windplay Dr
Suite 4
El Dorado Hills, CA 95762-9319   916-939-9620
                                        FAX: 916-939-9626
                                        info@rspfunding.com
                                        www.rspfunding.com

Gail Schlachter, Founder
R. David Weber, Editor
Sandy Hirsh, Editor
Sandy Perez, Funding Finder
More than 1,200 funding opportunities for currently-enrolled or returning college students are described in this directory. *$32.50*
450 pages
ISBN 1-588410-41-2

3262 Community Health Funding Report

CD Publications
8204 Fenton St
Silver Spring, MD 20910-4502   301-588-6380
                                           800-666-6380
                                      FAX: 301-588-6385
                                   subscriptions@cdpublications.com
                                      www.cdpublications.com

Michael Gerecht, President
The once twice-monthly report is now web-based to allow for breaking news updates and up the the minute information about funding, including: public and private grant announcements; reports on successful health programs nationwide; interviews with grant officials; plus national news on health policy topics affecting various organizations. *$439.00*
Web-based

3263 Directory of Financial Aids for Women

Reference Service Press
2310 Homestead Rd
Suite C1 #219
Los Altos, CA 94024   650-861-3170
                                      FAX: 650-861-3171
                                      info@rspfunding.com
                                      www.rspfunding.com

Gail Schlachter, Founder
R. David Weber, Editor
Sandy Hirsh, Editor
Sandy Perez, Funding Finder
Funding programs listed support study, research, travel, training, career development, or innovative effort at any level; descriptions of more than 1,700 funding programs - representing billions of dollars in financial aid set aside for women; also an annotated bibliography of 60 key directories that identify even more financial aid opportunities and a set of indexes that let you search the directory by title, sponser, researching, tenability, subject, and deadline. *$45.00*
578 pages Biennial
ISBN 1-588410-00-5

3264 Disability Funding News

8204 Fenton St
Silver Spring, MD 20910-4502   301-588-6380
                                           800-666-6380
                                      FAX: 301-588-6385
                                   subscriptions@cdpublications.com
                                      www.cdpublications.com

Michael Gerecht, President

3265 FC Search

Foundation Center
79 fifth Avenue
New York, NY 10003-3034   212-620-4230
                                           800-424-9836
                                      FAX: 212-807-3677
                                   order@foundationcenter.org
                                      foundationcenter.org

Bradford K Smith, President
Lisa Philip, Vice President for Strategic Phi
Jen Bokoff, Director of GrantCraft
Lawrence T. McGill, Vice President for Research
Provides access to the Foundation Center's comprehensive database of funders in a convenient CD-ROM format. *$1845.00*

3266 Federal Grants & Contracts Weekly

LRP Publications
360 Hiatt Drive
Palm Beach Gardens, FL 33418-1718   800-341-7874
                                      FAX: 561-622-2423
                                      custserve@lrp.com
                                      www.lrp.com

Kelly Sullivan, Editor
Kenneth F. Kahn, President
The latest funding announcements of federal grants for project opportunities in research, training and services. Provides profiles of key programs, tips on seeking grants, updates on legislation and regulations, budget developments and early alerts to upcoming funding opportunities. *$340.00*
Weekly

3267 Financial Aid for Asian Americans

Reference Service Press
2310 Homestead Rd
Suite C1 #219
Los Altos, CA 94024   650-861-3170
                                      FAX: 650-861-3171
                                      info@rspfunding.com
                                      www.rspfunding.com

Gail Schlachter, Founder
R. David Weber, Editor
Sandy Hirsh, Editor
Sandy Perez, Funding Finder
This is the source to use if you are looking for financial aid for Asian Americans; nearly 1,000 funding opportunities are described. *$35.00*
336 pages
ISBN 1-588410-02-1

3268 Financial Aid for Hispanic Americans

Reference Service Press
2310 Homestead Rd
Suite C1 #219
Los Altos, CA 94024   650-861-3170
                                      FAX: 650-861-3171
                                      info@rspfunding.com
                                      www.rspfunding.com

Gail Schlachter, Founder
R. David Weber, Editor
Sandy Hirsh, Editor
Sandy Perez, Funding Finder
Nearly 1,300 funding programs open to Americans of Mexican, Puerto Rican, Central American, or other Latin American heritage are described here. *$37.50*
472 pages
ISBN 1-588410-03-X

3269   Financial Aid for Native Americans
Reference Service Press
2310 Homestead Rd
Suite C1 #219
Los Altos, CA 94024
650-861-3170
FAX: 650-861-3171
info@rspfunding.com
www.rspfunding.com

Gail Schlachter, Founder
R. David Weber, Editor
Sandy Hirsh, Editor
Sandy Perez, Funding Finder
Detailed information is provided on 1,500 funding opportunities open to American Indians, Native Alaskans, and Native Pacific Islanders. *$37.50*
562 pages
ISBN 1-588410-04-8

3270   Financial Aid for Research and Creative Activities Abroad
Reference Service Press
2310 Homestead Rd
Suite C1 #219
Los Altos, CA 94024
650-861-3170
FAX: 650-861-3171
info@rspfunding.com
www.rspfunding.com

Gail Schlachter, Founder
R. David Weber, Editor
Sandy Hirsh, Editor
Sandy Perez, Funding Finder
Described here are 1,200 funding programs (scholarships, fellowships, grants, etc.) available to support research, professional, or creative activities abroad. *$45.00*
378 pages
ISBN 1-588410-82-5

3271   Financial Aid for Veterans, Military Personnel and their Dependents
Reference Service Press
2310 Homestead Rd
Suite C1 #219
Los Altos, CA 94024
650-861-3170
FAX: 650-861-3171
info@rspfunding.com
www.rspfunding.com

Gail Schlachter, Founder
R. David Weber, Editor
Sandy Hirsh, Editor
Sandy Perez, Funding Finder
According to Reference Book Review, this directory (with its 1,100 entries) is the most comprehensive guide available on the subject. *$40.00*
392 pages
ISBN 1-588410-43-9

3272   Financial Aid for the Disabled and Their Families
Reference Service Press
2310 Homestead Rd
Suite C1 #219
Los Altos, CA 94024
650-861-3170
FAX: 650-861-3171
info@rspfunding.com
www.rspfunding.com

Gail Schlachter, Founder
R. David Weber, Editor
This directory, which Children's Bookwatch calls invaluable describes more than 1,100 financial aid opportunities available to support persons with disabilities and members of their families. Updated every 2 years. *$37.50*
508 pages Every other yr.
ISBN 1-588410-01-3

3273   Foundation & Corporate Grants Alert
LRP Publications
360 Hiatt Drive
Palm Beach Gardens, FL 33418-1718
800-341-7874
FAX: 561-622-2423
custserve@lrp.com
www.lrp.com

Kelly Sullivan, Editor
Kenneth F. Kahn, President
A complete guide to foundation and corporate grant opportunities for nonprofit organizations. Tracks developments and trends in funding and provides notification of changes in foundations' funding priorities. *$245.00*
Monthly
ISSN 1062-46 6

3274   Foundation 1000
Foundation Center
79 fifth Avenue
New York, NY 10003-3076
212-620-4230
800-424-9836
FAX: 212-807-3691
order@foundationcenter.org
www.foundationcenter.org

Bradford K Smith, President
Lisa Philip, Vice President for Strategic Phi
Jen Bokoff, Director of GrantCraft
Lawrence T. McGill, Vice President for Research
Offers comprehensive information on the 1000 largest foundations in the US. *$195.00*

3275   Foundation Directories
Foundation Center
79 fifth Avenue
New York, NY 10003-3034
212-620-4230
800-424-9836
FAX: 212-807-3677
order@foundationcenter.org
foundationcenter.org

Bradford K Smith, President
Lisa Philip, Vice President for Strategic Phi
Jen Bokoff, Director of GrantCraft
Lawrence T. McGill, Vice President for Research
Lists key facts on the top 20,000 US foundations. *$ 125.00*

ISBN 0-87954 -36-1

3276   Foundation Grants to Individuals
Foundation Center
79 fifth Avenue
New York, NY 10003-3034
212-620-4230
800-424-9836
FAX: 212-807-3677
order@foundationcenter.org
foundationcenter.org

Bradford K Smith, President
Lisa Philip, Vice President for Strategic Phi
Jen Bokoff, Director of GrantCraft
Lawrence T. McGill, Vice President for Research
The only publication that provides extensive coverage of foundation funding prospects for individual grantseekers. *$40.00*
Biennially

3277   From the State Capitals: Public Health
Wakeman/Walworth
P.O.Box 7376
Alexandria, VA 22307-376
703-768-9600
FAX: 703-768-9690
newsletters@statecapitals.com
www.statecapitals.com

Mark Willen, Editor
Digest of state and municipal health care financing and cost containment measures, includes medical legislation, disease control, etc. *$245.00*
6 pages

331

3278 Grant Guides
Foundation Center
79 fifth Avenue
New York, NY 10003-3034   212-620-4230; 800-424-9836
FAX: 212-807-3677
order@foundationcenter.org
foundationcenter.org

Bradford K Smith, President
Lisa Philip, Vice President for Strategic Phi
Jen Bokoff, Director of GrantCraft
Lawrence T. McGill, Vice President for Research
Provides descriptions of actual foundation grants awarded in various subject fields. $35.00

ISBN 0-87954-90-6

3279 Guide to Funding for International and Foreign Programs
79 fifth Avenue
New York, NY 10003-3034   212-620-4230; 800-424-9836
FAX: 212-807-3677
order@foundationcenter.org
foundationcenter.org

Bradford K Smith, President
Lisa Philip, Vice President for Strategic Phi
Jen Bokoff, Director of GrantCraft
Lawrence T. McGill, Vice President for Research
Grantmakers featured in this guide provide funding for international relief, disaster assistance, human rights, civil liberties, community development, conferences, and education. $190.00

3280 Guide to US Foundations their Trustees, Officers and Donors
Foundation Center
79 fifth Avenue
New York, NY 10003-3034   212-620-4230; 800-424-9836
FAX: 212-807-3677
order@foundationcenter.org
foundationcenter.org

Bradford K Smith, President
Lisa Philip, Vice President for Strategic Phi
Jen Bokoff, Director of GrantCraft
Lawrence T. McGill, Vice President for Research
Provides crucial facts on grantmaking. Each entry includes contact information, current assets, annual contributions, officers, donors and more. $135.00

3281 High School Senior's Guide to Merit and Other No-Need Funding
Reference Service Press
2310 Homestead Rd
Suite C1 #219
Los Altos, CA 94024   650-861-3170
FAX: 650-861-3171
info@rspfunding.com
www.rspfunding.com

Gail Schlachter, Founder
R. David Weber, Editor
Sandy Hirsh, Editor
Sandy Perez, Funding Finder
Here's your guide to 1,100 funding programs that never look at income level when making awards to college bound high school seniors. $29.95
400 pages
ISBN 1-588410-44-X

3282 How to Pay for Your Degree in Business & Related Fields
Reference Service Press
2310 Homestead Rd
Suite C1 #219
Los Altos, CA 94024   650-861-3170
FAX: 650-861-3171
info@rspfunding.com
www.rspfunding.com

Gail Schlachter, Founder
R. David Weber, Editor
Sandy Hirsh, Editor
Sandy Perez, Funding Finder

If you need funding for an undergraduate or graduate degree in business or related fields, this is the directory to use (500+ funding programs described). $30.00
290 pages
ISBN 1-588411-45-1

3283 How to Pay for Your Degree in Education& Related Fields
Reference Service Press
2310 Homestead Rd
Suite C1 #219
Los Altos, CA 94024   650-861-3170
FAX: 650-861-3171
info@rspfunding.com
www.rspfunding.com

Gail Schlachter, Founder
R. David Weber, Editor
Sandy Hirsh, Editor
Sandy Perez, Funding Finder
Here's hundreds of funding opportunities available to support undergraduate and graduate students preparing for a career in education, guidance etc. $30.00
250 pages
ISBN 1-588411-46-x

3284 National Directory of Corporate Giving
Foundation Center
79 fifth Avenue
New York, NY 10003-3034   212-620-4230; 800-424-9836
FAX: 212-807-3677
order@foundationcenter.org
foundationcenter.org

Bradford K Smith, President
Lisa Philip, Vice President for Strategic Phi
Jen Bokoff, Director of GrantCraft
Lawrence T. McGill, Vice President for Research
Offers over 2,000 corporate funders, current giving reviews and profiles of sponsoring companies. $195.00

3285 Older Americans Report
Business Publishers
2222 Sedwick Drive
Durham, NC 27713-1995   240-514-0600; 800-223-8720
FAX: 800-508-2592
custserv@bpinews.com
www.bpinews.com

Leonard Eiser, Publisher
Follows all programs and funding sources in education, housing, job training, therapy, Social Security Supplemental Security Income, Medicare, Medicaid and more of importance to persons with disabilities. Also covers the latest on the Americans with Disabilities Act. Publishes a newsletter. $327.00

3286 Student Guide
US Department of Education
400 Maryland Avenue SW
Washington, DC 20202   202-401-2000; 800-872-5327
FAX: 202-401-0689
TTY: 800-437-0833
customerservice@inet.ed.gov
ed.gov

Arne Duncan, Secretary of Education
Jim Shelton, Deputy Secretary
Ted Mitchell, Under Secretary
Describes the major student aid programs the US Department of Education administers and gives detailed information about program procedures.
74 pages

Government Agencies

Federal

3287   Administration on Aging
One Massachusetts Ave NW
Washington, DC 20001   202-401-4634
                                     FAX: 202-357-3555
                                     aclinfo@acl.hhs.gov
                                                aoa.gov

Kathy Greenlee, Administrator
Sharon Lewis, Principal Deputy Administrator
Aaron Bishop, Commissioner
John Wren, Deputy Administrator
Administers the Older Americans Act of 1965 to assist states and local communities to develop programs for older persons.

3288   Administration on Children, Youth and Families
370 L Enfant Promenade SW
Washington, DC 20447   202-401-4634
                                          800-422-4453
                                     TTY:800-787-3224
                                          www.acf.hhs.gov

William H. Bentley, Associate Commissioner
Jeannie Chaffin, Director
Naomi Goldstein, Director
Mathew McKearn, Director
Responsible for federal programs that promote the economic and social well-being of families, children, individuals and communities.

3289   Administration on Developmental Disabilities
U S Department of Health and Human Services
One Massachusetts Ave NW
Washington, DC 20001   202-401-4634
                                          800-422-4453
                                     TTY:800-787-3224
                                     aclinfo@acl.hhs.gov
                              www.acf.hhs.gov/programs/add

William H. Bentley, Associate Commissioner
Jeannie Chaffin, Director
Eskinder Negash?, Director
Mathew McKearn?, Director
Ensures that individuals with developmental disabilities and their families participate in the design of and have access to culturally competent services, supports, and other assistance and opportunities that promote independence, productivity, and integration and inclusion into the community.

3290   Americans with Disabilities Act Informationn
US Department of Justice
950 Pennsylvania Avenue NW
Washington, DC 20530   202-282-8000
                                          800-514-0301
                                     FAX: 202-307-1197
                                     TTY: 800-514-0383
                                          www.ada.gov

Gregory B. Friel, Chief
The ADA assures that Americans with disabilities have the same opportunities as all Americans. To this end, the Justice Department produces publications and conducts programs to increase compliance of the ADA nationwide.

3291   Civil Rights Division/Disability Rights Section
US Department Of Justice
950 Pennsylvania Avenue NW
Washington, DC 20530   202-282-8000
                                          800-514-0301
                                     FAX: 202-307-1197
                                     TTY: 800-514-0383
                                          www.ada.gov

Gregory B. Friel, Chief
The US Department of Justice answers questions about the American Disabilities Act (ADA) and provides free publications by mail and fax through its ADA Information Line.

3292   Committee for Purchase from People Who Are Blind or Severely Disabled
1401 S. Clark Street
Suite 715
Arlington, VA 22202-3259   703-603-7740
                                          800-999-5963
                                     FAX: 703-603-0655
                                     info@abilityone.gov
                                          www.abilityone.gov

Tina Ballard, Executive Director & CEO
J Anthony Poleo, Chairperson
Kimberly Zeich, Deputy Executive Director & Chie
Angela Phifer, Chief of Staff
A federal agency that administers the Javits-Wagner-O'Day Program, directing federal agencies to purchase products and services from nonprofit agencies that employ people who are blind or have other severe disabilities. Provides a wide range of vocational options to individuals with severe disabilities.

3293   Equal Opportunity Employment Commission
131 M Street NE
Washington, DC 20507-100   202-663-4599
                                          800-669-4000
                                     FAX: 202-419-0739
                                     info@eeoc.gov
                                          www.eeoc.gov

Jenny R Yang, Chair
Constance S Barker, Commissioner
Chai R Feldblum, Commissioner
David Lopez, General Counsel
This agency is responsible for drafting and implementing the regulations of Title I of the ADA.

3294   Federal Communications Commission
445 12th Street SW
Washington, DC 20554   888-225-5322
                                          888-835-5322
                                     FAX: 866-418-0232
                                     fccinfo@fcc.gov
                                          fcc.gov

Tom Wheeler, Chairman
Mignon Clyburn, Commissioner
Jessica Rosenworcel, Commissioner
Ajit Pai, Commissioner
Enforces ADA telecommunications provisions which require that companies offering telephone service to the general public must offer telephone relay services to individuals who use text telephones or similar devices. Also enforces closed captioning rules, hearing compatibility and access to equipment and services for people with disabilities.

3295   Health Care Financing Administration
200 Independence Ave SW
Washington, DC 20201-4   202-690-6726
                                     FAX: 202-690-6262
                              www.federalregister.gov/agencies/

William Roper, Administrator
Thomas Scully, President
Through the Social Security administration, it administers the Medicare program under Title XVIII of the Social Security Act. Administers grants to the states for Medicaid under Title XIX of the Social Security Act for individuals who are medically indigent.

3296   National Coalition of Federal Aviation Employees with Disabilities
Federal Aviation Administration
800 Independence Avenue, SW
Washington, DC 20591   405-954-4709
                                          866-835-5322
                                     FAX: 405-954-4490
                                     TTY: 405-954-4587
                              www.faa.gov/acr/ncfaed.htm

Becky Pritchett, Treasurer
Alan Jones, President of Aeronautical Center
NCFAED is working on: 1) improvement of work conditions for employees; 2) expansion on National Coalition to serve all FAA employees; 3) promote equal opportunity for people with disabil-

ities in the FAA workplace; 4) assist the FAA in its commitment to remove physical and attudinal barriers which inhibit opportunities for people with disabilities; 5) align with internal and external organizations to attract future generations of people with disabilities to the FAA as employees.

3297 National Council on Disability
1331 F Street Northwest
Suite 850
Washington, DC 20004- 1138   202-272-2004
                                          FAX: 202-272-2022
                                          TTY:202-272-2074
                                          www.ncd.gov

Jeff Rosen, Chairperson
Kartherine D Seelman, Co Vice Chair
Rebecca Cokley, Executive Director
Joan M Durocher, General Counsel
Federal agency led by 15 members appointed by the President of the United States and confirmed by the United States Senate. The overall purpose of the National Council is to promote policies, programs, practices and procedures that guarantee equal opportunities to persons with disabilities.

3298 National Division of the Blind and Visually Impaired
330 C St NW
Washington, DC 20001   202-205-8520

Chester Avery, Director
Develops methods, standards and procedures to assist state agencies in the rehabilitation of blind persons. Administers the Randolph-Sheppard Act, which assures priority for blind persons in the operation of vending facilities on federal property and serves as a program manager for the Helen Keller National Center for Youth who are deaf-blind.

3299 National Institutes of Health: National Eye Institute
31 Center Drive MSC 2510
Bethesda, MD 20892-2510   301-496-5248
                                          2020@nei.nih.gov
                                          www.nei.nih.gov

Paul A Sieving MD PhD, Director
Finances intramural and extramural research on eye diseases and vision disorders. Supports training of eye researchers.

3300 Office of Policy
Social Security Administration
1100 West High Rise
6401 Security Blvd
Baltimore, MD 21235   202-293-9138
                                          800-772-1213
                                          TTY:800-325-0778
                                          concepcion.mcneace@ssa.gov
                                          www.ssa.gov/policy

Michael J Astrue, Commissioner
Edward Demarco, Assitant Deputy Commissioner
Serge Harrison, Executive Officer
Administers grants to the states for social services under Title XX of the Social Security Act to welfare recipients and others likely to become them.

3301 Office of Special Education Programs: Department of Education
400 Maryland Avenue SW
Washington, DC 20202-7100   202-401-2000
                                          800-872-5327
                                          FAX: 202-401-0689
                                          TTY: 800-437-0833
                                          customerservice@inet.ed.gov
                                          www2.ed.gov/about/offices/list/osers/osep

Arne Duncan, Secretary of Education
Jim Shelton, Deputy Secretary
Ted Mitchell, Under Secretary
The Office of Special Education Programs (OSEP) is dedicated to improving results for infants, toddlers, children and youth with disabilities ages birth through 21 by providing leadership and financial support to assist states and local districts.

3302 President's Committee on People with Intellecutual Disabilities
370 L Enfant Promenade SW
Washington, DC 20447   202-619-0364
                                          800-422-4453
                                          TTY:800-787-3224
                                          www.acf.hhs.gov

George Sheldon, Acting Assistant Secretary
Laverdia Roach, Acting Executive Director
Formerly the President's Committee on Mental Retardation, a federal advisory committee, estalished by the presidential executive order to adivse the President of the United States and the Secretary of the Department of Health and Human Services on issues concerning citizens with intellectual disabilities, coordinate activities between different federal agencies and assess the impact of their policies upon the lives of citizens with intellectual disabilities and their families.

3303 Rehabilitative Services Administration
400 Maryland Ave SW
Washington, DC 20202-7100   202-401-2000
                                          800-872-5327
                                          FAX: 202-401-0689
                                          TTY: 800-437-0833
                                          customerservice@inet.ed.gov
                                          www2.ed.gov

Arne Duncan, Secretary of Education
Jim Shelton, Deputy Secretary
Ted Mitchell, Under Secretary
The Rehabilitation Services Administration (RSA) oversees formula and discretionary grant programs that help individuals with physical or mental disabilities to obtain employment and live more independently through the provision of such supports as counseling, medical and psychological services, job training and other individualized services.

3304 Social Security Administration
5 Park Center Court
Suite 100
Owing Mills, MD 21117   410-965-6114
                                          800-772-1213
                                          FAX: 410-966-2027
                                          www.ssa.gov

Bill Vitek, Manager
Administers old age, survivors, and disability insurance programs under Title II of the Social Security Act. Also administers the federal income maintenance program under Title XVI of the Social Security Act. Maintains network of local/regional offices nationwide.

3305 US Department of Education: Office of Civil Rights
400 Maryland Avenue SW
Washington, DC 20202-1100   800-421-3481
                                          800-877-8339
                                          FAX: 202-453-601
                                          TTY: 800-437-0833
                                          OCR@ed.gov
                                          www2.ed/gov/about/offices/list/ocr/index.html

Catherine E Lhamon, Assistant Secretary
Seth Galanter, Principal Deputy Asst Secretary
Sandra Battle, Deputy Assistant Secretary
James Ferg Cadima, Senior Counsel
Prohibits discrimination on the basis of disability in programs and activities funded by the Department of Education. Investigates complaints and provides technical assistance to individuals and entities with rights and responsibilities under Section 504.

3306 **US Department of Labor: Office of Federal Contract Programs**
200 Constitution Ave NW
Washington, DC 20210

866-487-2365
TTY:877-889-5627
webmaster@dol.gov
www.dol.gov/ofccp

Thomas E. Perez, Secretary of Labor
Christopher Lu, Deputy Secretary of Labor
Mathew Colangelo, Chief of Staff
James Moore, Deputy Assistant Secretary
Prohibits discrimination on the basis of disability and requires federal contractors and sub-contractors with contracts of $2,500 or more to take affirmative action to employ and advance individuals with disabilities.

3307 **US Department of Transportation**
1200 New Jersey Ave SE
Washington, DC 20590

202-366-4000
855-368-4200
TTY:800-877-8339
www.dot.gov

Anthony Foxx, Secretary of Transportation
Peter Rogoff, Secretary for Police
Kathryn Thomson, General Counsel
Greg Winfree, Assistant Secretary for Research
Enforces ADA provisions that require nondiscrimination in public and private mass transportation systems and services.

3308 **US Office of Personnel Management**
1900 E St NW
Washington, DC 20415-1000

202-606-1800
FAX: 202-606-0909
TTY:202-606-2532
Informationquality@opm.gov
opm.gov

Katherine Archuleta, Director
Ann Marie Habershaw, Chief of Staff & Director Extern
Angela Bailey, Chief Operating Officer
Jen Mason, Director, Office of Public Engag
Establishes policies for employment of the handicapped within the federal service. Administers a merit system for the federal employment that includes recruiting, examining, training, and promoting people on the basis of knowledge and skills, regardless of sex, race, religion or other factors.

Alabama

3309 **Alabama Council For Developmental Disabilities**
RSA Union Building
RSA Union Building
PO Box 301410
Montgomery, AL 36130- 1410

334-242-3973
800-232-2158
FAX: 334-242-0797
Myra.Jones@mh.alabama.gov
www.acdd.org

Stefan Eisen, Jr., Chair, Parent Advocate
Sophia Whitted, Fiscal Manager
Elmyra Jones-Banks, Executive Director
Shungulla Moorey, Office Manager
Serves as an advocate for Alabama's citizens with developmental disabilities and their families; to empower them with the knowledge and opportunity to make informed choices and exercise control over their own lives; and to create a climate for positive socialchange to enable them to be respected, independent and productive integrated members of society.

3310 **Alabama Department of Public Health**
The RSA Tower, 201 Monroe Street
PO Box 303017
Montgomery, AL 36130-3017

334-206-5300
800-ALA-1818
www.adph.org

Kathy Vincent, Staff Assistant
Donald E Williamson, Administrator
Provides professional services for the improvement and protection of the public's health through disease prevention and the assurance of public health services to resident and transient populations of the state regardless of social circumstances or the ability to pay.

3311 **Alabama Department of Rehabilitation Services**
602 S Lawrence St
Montgomery, AL 36104

334-293-7500
800-441-7607
FAX: 334-293-7383
cary.boswell@rehab.alabama.gov
www.rehab.alabama.gov

Cary F Boswell, Commissioner
Jim Carden, Deputy Commissioner
Jim Harris Iii, Assistant Commissioner
Winona Nelson, Cheif Financial Officer
To enable Alabama's children and adults with disabilities to achieve their maximum potential.

3312 **Alabama Department of Senior Services**
201 Monroe Street
RSA Tower Suite 350
Montgomery, AL 36140

334-242-5743
877-425-2243
FAX: 334-242-5594
Ageline@adss.alabama.gov
www.adss.alabama.gov

Irene Collins, Executive Director
Thomas Ray Edwards, Board Chairman
Dr. Horace Patterson, Vice-Chair
The mission of the Alabama Department of Senior Services is to promote the independence and dignity of those we serve through a comprehensive and coordinated system of quality services

3313 **Alabama Disabilities Advocacy Program**
University of Alabama
P.O.Box 870395
Tuscaloosa, AL 35487-0395

205-348-4928
800-826-1675
FAX: 205-348-3909
adap@adap.ua.edu
www.adap.net

Anita Davidson, Legal Assistant
Janet Owens, Accounting Specialist
James Tucker, Director
Rosemary Beck, Information Systems Administrato
The federally mandate statewide protection and advocacy system serving eligible individuals with disabilities in Alabama. ADAP has five program components: Protection and Advocacy for persons with developmental disabilities (PADD), Protection and Advocacy for Individuals with Mental Illness (PAIMT), Protection and Advocacy of Individual Rights (PAIR), Protection and Advocacy for Assistive Technology (PAAT) and Protection & Advocacy For Beneficiaries of Social Security (PABSS).

3314 **Alabama Division of Rehabilitation and Crippled Children**
602 S Lawrence Street
Montgomery, AL 36104

334-293-7500
800-441-7607
FAX: 334-293-7383
sshiver@rehab.state.al.us
www.rehab.state.al.us

Cary F Boswell, Commissioner
Steven Kayes, Board Member
Jimmie Varnado, Board Member

3315 Alabama Governor's Committee on Employment of Persons with Disabilities
602 S Lawrence St
Montgomery, AL 36104 334-293-7500
800-441-7607
FAX: 334-293-7383
www.rehab.alabama.gov

Jimmie Varnado, Board Chairperson
Stacy Mitchell, Board Member
Stephen G Keys, Board Member
Andrea Collett, Board Member
The Alabama Governor's Committee on Employment of People with Disabilities (AGCEPD) is a program of the Alabama Department of Rehabilitation Services (ADRS).

3316 Alabama State Department of Human Resources
Childcare Services Division
50 North Ripley Street
Montgomery, AL 36130 334-242-1310
FAX: 334-353-1115
barry.spear@dhr.alabama.gov
www.dhr.state.al.us

Nancy T. Buckner, Commissioner
Nancy Jinright, Chief of Staff/Ethics Officer
John Hardy, Communications
Conitha King, Finance
Partners with communities to promtoe family stability and provide for the safety and self-sufficiency of vulnerable Alabamians.

3317 Client Assistance Program: Alabama
400 South Union Street
Suite 465
Montgomery, AL 36104 334-263-2749
800-288-3231
FAX: 334-230-9765
rachel.hughes@rehab.alabama.gov
www.sacap.alabama.gov

Rachel Hughes, Director/Advocate

3318 Disability Determination Service: Birmingham
P.O.Box 830300
Birmingham, AL 35283-0300 205-989-2100
800-292-8106
FAX: 205-989-2295
ssa.gov

Tommy Warren, Executive Director
Janet Cox, Owner

3319 Social Security: Mobile Disability Determination Services
PO Box 2371
Mobile, AL 36652-2371 251-433-2820
800-292-6743
FAX: 251-436-0599
www.ssa.gov

Tommy Warren, Executive Director
Jack Miller, Office Manager

3320 Workers Compensation Board Alabama
649 Monroe Street
Montgomery, AL 36131 334-242-2868
800-528-5166
FAX: 334-353-8262
webmaster@labor.alabama.gov
labor.alabama.gov/wc

Charles DeLamar, Director
Al Pelham, Supervisor
Sandy Hallmark, Supervisor
Peggy Barton, Supervisor
The Workers' Compensation Division is responsible for the administration of the Alabama Workers' Compensation Law to ensure proper payment of benefits to employees injured on the job and encourage safety in the work place

Alaska

3321 ATLA
2217 E Tudor Rd
Ste 4
Anchorage, AK 99507-1068 907-563-2599
800-723-2852
FAX: 907-563-0699
atla@atla.biz
www.atla.biz

Kathy Privratsky, Executive Director
Mystie Rail, Commissioner
Margaret Cisco, AT Specialist
Assistive Technology sales and services. ATLA is Alaska's only assistive technology resource center.

3322 Alaska Commission on Aging
150 Third Street #103
PO Box 110693
Juneau, AK 99811- 0693 907-465-3250
FAX: 907-465-1398
denise.daniello@alaska.gov
dhss.alaska.gov/acoa

Mary Shields, Chair
Rolf Numme, Vice Chair
Denise Daniello, Executive Director
Sherice Cole, Admin Assistant II
Works to promote and protect the health and well-being of Alaskans.

3323 Alaska Department of Handicapped Children
Ste 314
1231 Gambell St
Anchorage, AK 99501-4664 907-346-1995

Gregory Lee, CEO

3324 Alaska Division of Vocational Rehabilitation:
801 W. 10th Street,
Suite A
Juneau, AK 99801-1878 907-465-2814
800-478-2815
FAX: 907-465-2856
dawn.duval@alaska.gov
labor.alaska.gov

Dianne Blummer, Commissioner
David G Stone, Deputy commissioner
John Cannon, Director
Provides comprehensive services to people with disabilities to assist in achieving an employment outcome.

3325 Client Assistance Program: Alaska
2900 Boniface Pkwy
Ste 100
Anchorage, AK 99504-3195 907-333-2211
800-478-0047
FAX: 907-333-1186
akcap@alaska.com
www.icdri.org/legal/AlaskaCAP.htm

Pam Stratton, Executive Director
We provide informatory referral to other programs in Alaska that are funded under the Rehabilitation Act of 1973 as amended; Individual assistance or advocacy, if an individual with disability has applied for or received services from an agency funded under the Rehabilitation Act and has concerns or questions we will work with them to help resolve their concerns with the agency.

3326 Department Of Health& Social ServicesDivision Of Behaviorial Health
350 Main Street
Suite 214
Juneau, AK 99801-1149
907-465-3370
800-465-4828
FAX: 907-465-2668
albert.wall@alaska.gov
www.alaska.gov

Albert E. Wall, Director
Stacy Toner, Division Operations Manager
Liz Clement, Program Coordinator
The division plans for and provides appropriate prevention, treatment and support for families impacted by mental disorders or developmental disabilities while maximizing self-determination. Community based services are provided by grantees. Inpatient services are provided in two division operated facilities.

3327 Governor's Committee on Employment and Rehabilitation of People with Disabilities
Division of Vocational Rehabilitation (DVR)
801 W 10th Street
Suite A
Juneau, AK 99801-1878
907-465-2814
800-478-2815
FAX: 907-465-2815
dawn.duval@alaska.gov
www.labor.state.ak.us/dvr

Cheryl Walsh, Executive Director
Carries on a continuing program to promote the employment and rehabilitation of citizens with disabilities in the State of Alaska. Advocates for a comprehensive statewide system for access to assistive technology. Obtains and maintains cooperation with public and private groups and individuals in this field.

3328 Governor's Council on Disabilities and Special Education
3601 C Street
Suite 740
Anchorage, AK 99524-0249
907-269-8990
888-269-8990
FAX: 907-269-8995
GCDSE@alaska.gov
www.hss.state.ak.us/gcdse/

Patrick Reinhart, Executive Director
Rich Sanders, Planner III
Britteny M Howell, M.A., ABD, Research Analyst III
Lanny Mommsen, Health Program Manager
The Governor's Council on Disabilities & Special Education was created to meet Alaska's diverse needs.

3329 Protection & Advocacy System: Alaska
Disability Law Center of Alaska
3330 Arctic Blvd
Ste 103
Anchorage, AK 99503-4580
907-565-1002
800-478-1234
FAX: 907-565-1000
akpa@dlcak.org
dlcak.org

Deborah Smith, President
James M Shine Sr
Deals with rights of the disabled. Works in conjunction with agencies, law offices and family members.

3330 Protection & Advocacy for Persons with Developmental Disabilities: Alaska
Advocacy Services of Alaska
Ste 101
615 E 82nd Ave
Anchorage, AK 99518-3100
907-222-2652
866-275-7273
FAX: 907-677-8777
TTY: 866-232-4525
rtessardore@dlcakelcak.org

Greg Schomaker, Manager

3331 Workers Compensation Division
Department of Labor & Workforce Development
PO Box 115512
Juneau, AK 99811-5512
907-465-2790
FAX: 907-465-2797
workerscomp@alaska.gov
www.labor.state.ak.us/wc

Clark Bishop, Commissioner
Trena Heikes, Division Director
Michael Monagle, Director
The Division of Workers' Compensation is the agency charged with the administration of the Alaska Workers' Compensation Act (Act). The Act provides for the payment by employers or their insurance carriers of medical, disability and reemployment benefits to injured workers

Arizona

3332 Arizona Department of Economic Security
1717 W Jefferson Room 119
Site Code 050Z-1
Phoenix, AZ 85007-3295
602-542-4791
FAX: 602-542-5320
www.azdes.gov

Neal Young, Director
Lynne Smith, Chief Executive Officer
Will Humble, Director
Rex Critchfield, Manager
The Department of Economic Security is a human service agency providing services in six areas: Aging and Community Services, Benefits and Medical Eligibility, Child Support Enforcement, Children and Family Services, Developmental Disabilities and Employment and Rehabilitation Services.

3333 Arizona Department of Health Services
150 North 18th Avenue
Ste 330
Phoenix, AZ 85007-3243
602-542-1025
FAX: 602-542-0883
www.azdhs.gov

Will Humble, Director
Neal Young, Director
Lynne Smith, Chief Executive Officer
Rex Critchfield, Manager
The mission of Children's Rehabilitative Services is to improve the quality of life for children by providing family-centered medical treatment, rehabilitation, and related support services to enrolled individuals who have certain medical, handicapping, or potentially handicapping conditions.

3334 Arizona Division of Aging and Adult Services
1789 West Jefferson Street
Site Code 950A
Phoenix, AZ 85007-3202
602-542-4446
FAX: 602-542-6655
www.azdes.gov

Rex Critchfield, Manager
Neal Young, Director
Lynne Smith, Chief Executive Officer
Will Humble, Director
The Division supports at-risk Arizonans to meet their basic needs and to live safely, with dignity and independence.

3335 Arizona Rehabilitation State Services for the Blind and Visually Impaired
4620 N 16th St, B-106
Ste 100
Phoenix, AZ 85016-5121
602-266-9579
FAX: 602-264-7819
www.azdes.gov

Paul Howell, Vocational Rehab Supervisor
Suzanne Sayre f, Rehab Counselor for Blind
Offers clients a conservation program, eye examinations, treatments, counseling, social work, psychological testing and evaluation, professional training, computer training and more for the visually impaired. The staff includes 56 full time employees.

3336 Developmental Disability Council: Arizona
2828 N Country Club Rd
Ste 100
Tucson, AZ 85716-3202
602-542-4049
800-889-5893
FAX: 602-542-5320
valeria.hill@mail.de.state.az.us
www.cpes.com

David A Berns, *Manager*
Nebal Chavez, *Executive Director*
Susan Madison, *Manager*
The mission of the GovernorOs Council on Developmental Disabilities is to bring together persons with disabilities representing Arizona cultural diversity and their families and other community members, to protect rights, eliminate barriers, and jointly promote equal opportunities

3337 Governor's Council on Developmental Disabilities
1700 West Wasington Street
Suite 420
Phoenix, AZ 85007
520-325-9688
877-665-3176
FAX: 520-325-3561
lclausen@azdes.gov
azgovernor.gov/DDPC/

Larry Clausen, *Executive Director*
Shelly Adams, *Executive Secretary*
The purpose of the council is to advocate for and assure that individuals with developmental disabilities and their families participate in the design of and have access to culturally competent services, supports and provides opportunities to become integrated and included in the community.

3338 International Dyslexia Association: Arizona Branch
Meredith Puls AZ-IDA
985 W. Silver Spring Place
Oro Valley, AZ 85755-6548
480-941-0308
arizona.ida@gmail.com
www.dyslexia-az.org

Meredith Puls, *President*
Rebekah Dyer, *Vice President*
Melissa A. L. Pallister, *Treasurer*
Sue Noel, *Secretary*
Provides free information and referral services for diagnosis and tutoring for parents, educators, physicians, and individuals with dyslexia. The voice of our membership is heard in 48 countries. Membership includes yearly journal and quarterly newsletter. Call for conference dates.

3339 Protection & Advocacy for Persons with Disabilities: Arizona
Arizona Center for Disability Law
5025 E Washington St
Suite 202
Phoenix, AZ 85034
602-274-6287
800-927-2260
FAX: 602-274-6779
TTY: 602-274-6287
center@azdisabilitylaw.org
www.azdisabilitylaw.org

Anthony DiRienzi, *President*
Art Gode, *Vice President*
J. J. Rico, *Executive Director*
John Chalmers, *Treasurer*
The Center provides disability-related legal information and advice to individuals who need their services and assistance. In addition to limited legal representation, their goal is to provide efficient, streamlined services to educate people with disabilities and their support on how to enforce their legal rights through self-advocacy. Guides and documents are available online by selecting Self-Advocacy Materials button on the homepage.

3340 Social Security: Phoenix Disability Determination Services
Social Security Admission
4000 North Central Avenue
Suite 1800
Phoenix, AZ 85714
520-638-2000
800-772-1213
TTY:800-325-0778
www.ssa.gov

3341 Social Security: Tucson Disability Determination Services
4710 South Palo Verde Road
Tucson, AZ 85714-2030
520-638-2000
800-772-1213
TTY:800-325-0778
www.ssa.gov

Arkansas

3342 Arkansas Assistive Technology Projects
Increasing Capabilities Access
900 W.7th Street
Little Rock, AR 72201-4538
501-666-8868
800-828-2799
FAX: 501-666-5319
info@ar-ican.org
www.arkansas-ican.org

Eddie Schmeckenbecher, *Supervisor*
Essie Hardin, *Secretary*
Bryan Ayres, *Advisory Counsel*
Billy Altom, *Advisory Counsil*
A consumer responsive ,statewide program promoting assistive technology devices and sources for persons of all ages with all disabilities. Referral and information services provide information about devices, where to obtain them and their cost.

3343 Arkansas Division of Aging & Adult Services
Department of Human Services
PO Box 1437
Slot-S-530
Little Rock, AR 72203-1437
501-682-2441
FAX: 501-682-8155
aging.services@arkansas.gov
www.state.ar.us/dhs/aging

Craig Cloud, *Director*
Stephenie Blocker, *Assistant Director*
Brad Nye, *Assistant Director*
Brian Bowen, *Assistant Director*
The division provides services geared for adults and the elderly including supervised living, home delivered meals, adult day care, senior centers, personal care, household chores, and adult protective services.

3344 Arkansas Division of Developmental Disabilities Services
Donaghey Plaza
PO Box 1437
Little Rock, AR 72203-1437
501-682-1001
FAX: 501-682-8820
humanservices.arkansas.gov/ddds/Pages/default

Charlie Green, *Manager*
State agency to assist persons with developmental disabilities and their family in obtaining appropriate assistance and services.

3345 Arkansas Division of Services for the Blind
Department Of Health and Human Services
700 Main St
Little Rock, AR 72203-4608
501-682-5463
800-960-9270
FAX: 501-682-0366
TTY: 800-285-1131
donnabirdwell@arkansas.gov
humanservices.arkansas.gov/dsb

Terry Sheeler, *Chairman*
Dickie Walker, *Vice Chairman*
Sandy Edwards, *Secretary*
Harold Brewer, *Ex-Officio Member*

State program which offers services in the areas of health, counseling, social work, self help and education for the visually and multihandicapped. The staff includes 4 full time and 13 part time members including mobility specialists and rehabilitation teachers.

3346 Arkansas Governor's Developmental Disabilities Council
5800 West 10th Street
Suite 805
Little Rock, AR 72204- 1763

501-661-2589
855-627-7580
FAX: 501-661-2399
Regina.L.Wilson@arkansas.gov
ddcouncil.org

Regina Wilson, Executive Director
Teresa Sandar, Family Services Coordinator
Lee Russell, Information Oficer
Michelle Boyd, Administrative Assistant

A federally-funded state agency established to bring the perspective of individuals with developmental disabilities and his or her family or natural support system to policy makers and make improvements to the service system.

3347 Baptist Health Rehabilitation Institute
Baptist Heath
9601 Interstate 630 Exit 7
Little Rock, AR 72205-7299

501-202-2000
800-991-0888
FAX: 501-202-1115
www.baptist-health.com

Ellen Callaway, Director, Rehabilition Therapy
Jerry Baugh, Vice President
Russell Harrington, President

Acute rehab facility serving patients with ortho, spinal cord injury, brain injury, CVA, arthritis, cardiac and generalized weakness; JCAHO and CARF accredited; 17 outpatient therapy centers throughout central Arkansas.

3348 Children's Medical Services
P.O.Box 1437
Little Rock, AR 72203-1437

501-682-8207
800-482-5850
FAX: 501-682-8247
www.cms-kids.com

Nancy Holder, Program Director
Iris Fehr, Nursing Director
Rodney Farley, Parent Activities Coordinator

A collection of programs for eligible children with special needs. Each one of our programs and services are family-centered and designed to help children with a variety of conditions and needs.

3349 President's Committee on People with Disabilities: Arkansas
7th & Main St
Little Rock, AR 72203

3350 Social Security: Arkansas Disability Determination Services
701 Pulaski Street
Little Rock, AR 72201-3990

501-682-3030
800-772-1213
FAX: 501-682-7553
www.socialsecurity.gov

Arthur Boutiette, COO

California

3351 California Department of Aging
1300 National Drive
Suite 200
Sacramento, CA 95834-1992

916-419-7500
FAX: 916-928-2267
TTY:800-735-2929
webmaster@aging.ca.gov
aging.ca.gov

Lora Connoly, Director
Diane Paulsen, Chief Deputy Director
Anna Esparza, Executive Assistant
Chisorom Okwuosa, Chief Counsel

The Department contracts with the network of Area Agencies on Aging, who directly manage a wide array of federal and state-funded services that help older adults find employment; support older and disabled individuals to live as independently as possible in the community; promote healthy aging and community involvement; and assist family members in their vital care giving role

3352 California Department of Handicapped Children
714 P Street
Rm 323
Sacramento, CA 95814-6401

916-445-4171

Maridee Gregory
Diana Bonta, Chief Executive Officer

3353 California Department of Rehabilitation
721 Capitol Mall
Sacramento, CA 95814-3510

916-324-1313
800-952-5544
TTY:916-558-5807
externalaffairs@dor.ca.gov
www.rehab.cahwnet.gov

Joe Xavier, Director
David Supkofl, Manager

Assists people with disabilities, particularly those with severe disabilities, in obtaining and retaining meaningful employment and living independently in their communities. The department develops, purchases, provides and advocates for programs and services in vocational rehabilitation, habilitation and independent living with a priority on serving persons with all disabilities, especially those with the most severe disabilities.

3354 California Governor's Committee on Employment of People with Disabilities
Employment Development Department
800 Capitol Mall
PO Box 826880
Sacramento, CA 94280-0001

916-654-8055
800-695-0350
FAX: 916-654-9821
TTY: 916-654-9820
www.edd.ca.gov

Charlie Kaplan, Staff Director

GCEPD works to eliminate the barriers that preclude equal consideration for employment opportunities for people with disabilities. The Governor's Committee is responsible for providing leadership to increase the numbers of people with disabilities in the California workforce.

3355   California Protection & Advocacy: (PAI) A Nonprofit Organization
Protection and Advocacy (PA I)
1831 K Street
Sacramento, CA 95811-4114   916-504-5800
                                             800-776-5746
                                        FAX: 916-504-5802
            SERVICES@DISABILITYRIGHTSCA.ORG
                      www.disabilityrightsca.org

Catherine Blakemore, Executive Director
Andrew Mudryk, Deputy Director
Alan Gildestein, Managing Attorney
Sujatha Branch, Associate Managing Attorney
Advancing the human and legal rights of people with disabilities.

3356   California State Council on Developmental Disabilities
1507 21st Street
Suite 210
Sacramento, CA 95811-5297   916-322-8481
                                             866-802-0514
                                        FAX: 916-443-4957
                                        council@scdd.ca.gov
                                          www.scdd.ca.gov

April Lopez, Chairperson
Jenny Ning Yang, Interim Vice-Chairperson
Tammy Eudy, Office Assistant
Robin Maitino, Executive Assistant
The State Council on Developmental Disabilities (SCDD) is established by state and federal law as an independent state agency to ensure that people with developmental disabilities and their families receive the services and supports they need.

3357   Client Assistance Program: California
CA Health and Human Services Agency Dept of Rehab
721 Capitol Mall
PO Box 944222
Sacramento, CA 95814   916-324-1313
                                             800-952-5544
                                        FAX: 916-558-5391
                                        TTY:916- 558-580
                                        capinfo@dor.ca.gov
                                          www.dor.ca.gov

Tony P Sauer, Director
We have a three-pronged mission to provide services and advocacy that assist people with disabilities to live independently, become employed and have equality in the communities in which they live and work.

3358   International Dyslexia Association: Central California Branch
4594 E Michigan Ave
Fresno, CA 93703-1556   559-251-9385
                                             800-222-3123
                                        FAX: 599-252-1216
                                        dyslexias@attbi.com
                                          www.interdys.org

Joy Moody, President
Provides free information and referral services for diagnosis and tutoring for parents, educators, physicians, and individuals with dyslexia. The voice of our membership is heard in 48 countries. Membership includes yearly journal and quarterly newsletter. Call for conference dates. Other locations also available in California.

3359   Long Beach Department of Health and Human Services
2525 Grand Avenue
Long Beach, CA 90815-1765   562-570-4000
                                        FAX: 562-570-4049
            info@ci.long-beach.ca.us/health
                      www.longbeach.gov/health/

Ron Arias, Executive Director
Michael Johnson, Manager
The Long Beach Department of Health and Human Services (Health Department) has been improving the health of the Long Beach community for over a century.

3360   Los Angeles County Department of Health Services
313 N Figueroa Street
Los Angeles, CA 90012-2602   213-240-8101
                                             800-427-8700
                                        FAX: 213-250-4013
                                        webmaster@adhs.org
                                          www.ladhs.org

Mitchell H Katz, MD, Director
Hal F. Yee, Jr., M.D., Ph.D., Chief Medical Officer
Allan Wecker, Chief Financial Officer
Alexander Li, M.D., Deputy Director
Los Angeles County Department of Health Services is one of the US's largest publicly supported health systems. The system is the main provider of health care for the area's poor and uninsured. It provides general medical and surgical care and is affiliated with the medical school at USC. The system also manages the Emergency Medical Services (EMS) Agency and the Community Health Plan HMO, a low-cost managed care plan for members of Medicaid and other state-funded programs.

3361   Social Security: California Disability Determination Services
3164 Garrity Way
Richmond, CA 94806-1983
                                             800-772-1213
                                        TTY:800-325-0778
                                          www.ssa.gov

Sally Keen, San Francisco Regional PDF Coord

3362   Social Security: Fresno Disability Determination Services
Social Security
1052 C St
Fresno, CA 93706-3245   559-487-5391
                                             800-772-1213
                                        FAX: 510-970-2947
                                        TTY: 800-325-0778
                                        sally.keen@ssa.gov
                                          www.ssa.gov

Sally Keen, Regional PDF Coordinator

3363   Social Security: Oakland Disability Determination Services
P.O. Box 24225
Oakland, CA 94623-1225   510-622-3506
                                             800-772-1213
                                        TTY:800-325-0778
                                          www.ssa.gov

3364   Social Security: Sacramento Disability Determination Services
P.O. Box 997121
Suite A
Sacramento, CA 95899-7121   916-515-4400
                                             800-772-1213
                                        FAX: 916-263-5310
                                        TTY: 916-381-9445
                                          ssa.gov

3365   Social Security: San Diego Disability Determination Services
P.O. Box 85326
San Diego, CA 92186-5326   619-278-4300
                                             800-772-1213
                                        FAX: 619-278-4303
                                        TTY: 800-325-0778
                                        josesanbria@ssa.gov
                                          www.ssa.gov

Colorado

3366 Colorado Department of Aging & Adult Services
1575 Sherman St
10th Floor
Denver, CO 80203-1702
303-866-5700
FAX: 303-620-2696
cdhs.communications@state.co.us
www.cdhs.state.co.us/ADRS/AAS

Reggie Bicha, Executive Director
A department providing services to the elderly.

3367 Colorado Developmental Disabilities Council
1120 Lincoln
Suite 706
Denver, CO 80203
720-941-0176
FAX: 720-941-8490
cddpc.email@state.co.us
coddc.org

Katherine Carol, Chairperson
Irene Aguilar, Colorado Senate
Marcia Tewell, Executive Director
Lionel Llewellyn, Administrative Assistant
The mission is to advocate in collaboration with and on behalf of people with developmental disabilities for the establishment and implementation of public policy which will further their independence, productivity and integration.

3368 Colorado Division of Mental Health
3824 W. Princeton Circle
Denver, CO 80236-3111
303-866-7400
FAX: 303-866-7428
colorado.gov

Patrick K. Fox, Director
Administration of public health program

3369 Colorado Health Care Program for Children with Special Needs
4300 Cherry Creek Drive south
Denver, CO 80246-1530
303-692-2370
800-886-7689
FAX: 303-753-9249
cdphe.psdrequests@state.co.us
www.colorado.gov/cdphe/hcp

Christopher Stanley, Board member
Angie Goodger, HCP Consultant
Kelsey Minor, HCP Consultant
Jennie Munthali, HCP Section Manager
Provides information and state aid to children with disabilities.

3370 Division of Workers' Compensation Dapartment of Labor & Employment
633 17th Street
Suite 201
Denver, CO 80202-3660
303-318-8700
800-388-5515
888-390-7936
FAX: 303-575-8882
cdle_workers_compensation@state.co.us
www.coworkforce.com/dwc/

Ellen Golombek, Executive Director
Infomation regarding Division Rules and procedures for Claimants, Employers, Adjusters, and parties to claim.

3371 Eastern Colorado Services for the Disabled
P. O. Box 1682
617 South 10th Avenue
Sterling, CO 80751-3168
970-522-7121
FAX: 970-522-1173
rhonda@ecsdd.org
www.easterncoloradoservices.org

Rhonda Roth, Executive Director
Traci Schrade, Finance Director
Melissa Dassaro, Case Management Director
Dave Fast, PHR, Human Resources

Case coordination, infant stimulation, family support, residential and vocational programs.

3372 International Dyslexia Association: Rocky Mountain Branch
740 Yale Road
Boulder, CO 80305-5010
303-721-9425
855-5ID- RMB
FAX: 303-721-9425
ida_rmb@yahoo.com
www.dyslexia-rmbida.org

Karen Leopold, President
Lynn Kuhn, Secretary
Yona Sammartino, Administrative Director
Julie Bottom, Board of Director
Provides free information and referral services for diagnosis and tutoring for parents, educators, physicians, and individuals with dyslexia in Utah, Colorado and Wyoming. The voice of our membership is heard in 48 countries. Membership includes yearly journal and quarterly newsletter. Call for conference dates.

3373 Legal Center for People with Disabilities& Older People
455 Sherman St
Ste 130
Denver, CO 80203-4403
303-722-0300
800-288-1376
FAX: 303-722-0720
TTY: 303-722-3619
tlcmail@thelegalcenter.org
thelegalcenter.org

John R. Posthumus, President
Stephen P. Rickles, Vice President
Nancy Tucker, Secretary
John Paul Anderson, Treasurer
Uses the legal system to protect and promote the rights of people with disabilities and older people in Colorado through direct legal representation, advocacy, education and legislative analysis. The Legal Center is Colorado's Protection and Advocacy System. We are also the State Ombudsman for nursing homes and assisted living facilities. Call for a free publications and products list.

Connecticut

3374 Connecticut Board of Education and Servicefor the Blind
184 Windsor Avenue
Windsor, CT 06095-4536
860-602-4000
800-842-4510
FAX: 860-602-4020
TTY: 860-602-4221
brian.sigman@CT.GOV
www.ct.gov/besb/site/default.asp

Amy Porter, Commissioner
Offers rehabilitative services and information for persons with legal blindness and childrenwhoare visually impaired that are residents of Connecticut.

3375 Connecticut Commission on Aging
210 Capitol Avenue
Hartford, CT 06106
860-240-5200
FAX: 860-240-5204
coa@cga.ct.gov
www.cga.ct.gov/coa

Julia Evans Starr, Executive Director
Deborah Migneault, Senior Policy Analyst
Alyssa Norwood, Project Manager
Christianne Kovel, Communications Specialist
Advocates on beha;f of elderly persons in Connecticut by regularly monitoring their status, assessing the impact of current and propsed initiatives, and conducting activities which promote the interests of these individuals and report to the Governor and the Legislature.

3376 **Connecticut Department of Children and Youth Services**
505 Hudson Street
Hartford, CT 06106   860-550-6300
FAX: 860-724-2001
Commissioner.dcf@ct.gov
www.ct.gov

Gary Scappini, Manager
Bruce Douglas, Executive Director

3377 **Connecticut Developmental Disabilities Council**
263 Farmington Avenue
Farmington, CT 6030   860-679-1561
800-653-1134
FAX: 860-679-1571
TTY: 860-679-1502
ctkasa.org

Ed Preneta, Executive Director
Kids As Self Advocates (KASA) is a national grassroots network that helps youth with special needs and their friends become self-advocates, helps other people in the community understand what it's like to live with special health care needs.

3378 **Connecticut Office of Protection and Advocacy for Persons with Disabilities**
60B Weston Street
Suite B
Hartford, CT 06120-1551   860-297-4300
800-842-7303
FAX: 860-566-8714
TTY: 860-297-4320
OPA-Information@po.state.ct.us
www.ct.gov/opapd

Craig B Henrici, Executive Director
Alexandria Bode, Board Member
Thomas Behrendt, Board Member
John Clausen, Board Member
Provides information, referrals, advocacy assistance & limited legal services to people with disabilities in the state of Connecticut whose civil rights have been violated or who are experiencing the difficulty securing relevant support services. P & A supports the development of community advocacy groups by providing training & technical assistance. P & A is responsible for investigating abuse & neglect of all individuals with intellectual disability ages 18-59.

3379 **Social Security: Hartford Area Office**
960 Main Street
2nd Floor
Hartford, CT 06103-1228   877-619-2851
800-772-1213
FAX: 860-566-1795
TTY: 860-525-4967
www.ssa.gov

Jan Gilbert, Professional Relations Coord.

Delaware

3380 **Delaware Assistive Technology Initiative(DATI)**
461 Wyoming Road
Newark, DE 19716-0269   302-831-0354
FAX: 302-831-4690
TTY:800-870-3284
dati@asel.udel.edu
www.dati.org

Beth Mineo, Project Director
Joann McCafferty, Staff Assistant
The Delaware Assistive Technology Initiative (DATI) connects Delawareans who have disabilities with the tools they need in order to learn, work, play and participate in community life safely and independently. DATI services include: Equipment demonstration centers in each county; no-cost, short-term equipment loans that let you try before you buy; Equipment Exchange Program; AT workshops and other training sessions; advocacy for improved AT access policies and funing and several more.

3381 **Delaware Client Assistance Program**
United Cerebral Palsy Association
254 E Camden Wyoming Ave
Camden, DE 19934-1303   302-698-9336
800-640-9336
FAX: 302-698-9338
capucp@magpage.com
icdri.org/legal/DelawareCAP.htm

Melissa Shahan, Executive Director
Provides advocacy services for persons involved with programs covered under the Rehabilitation Act of 1973 as amended, information and referrals on ADA, Title I.

3382 **Delaware Department of Health and Social Services**
Administration Building D HS S Campus
1901 N Du pont Highway
Main Building
New Castle, DE 19720-1160   302-255-9040
800-464-4357
FAX: 302-255-4429
TTY: 302-744-4556
dhssinfo@state.de.us
www.dhss.delaware.gov

Rita Landgraf, Cabinet Secretary
Henry Smith III, Deputy secretary
Provides most of the human services available through Delaware State Government, including Medicaid, the Children's Health Insurance Program, food stamps, welfare-to-work, vaccines for children, child support enforcement, public health programs, and general services for the aging. Also for individuals with developmental and physical disabilities, visual impairments, mental illness and other vulnerable populations.

3383 **Delaware Department of Public Instructing**
Townsend Building
401 Federal Street
Dover, DE 19901- 1402   302-735-4000
800-433-5292
FAX: 302-739-4654
deeds@doe.k12.de.us
http://www.doe.k12.de.us

Mark T. Murphy, Secretary of Education
David J. Blowman, Deputy Secretary
Mary Kate McLaughlin, Chief of Staff
Penny Schwinn, Chief Accountability Officer
A publicly funded, state agency that gives information about local facilities and administers supplemental funds for visually handicapped students in local schools. It also maintains special teachers of sight conservation and braille programs for both children and adults.

3384 **Delaware Developmental Disability Council**
410 Federal Street 2nd Floor
Suite 2
Dover, DE 19901- 3640   302-739-3333
800-464-4357
FAX: 302-739-2015
pat.maichle@state.de.us
www.ddc.delaware.gov

Barbara Monaghan, Council Chair
Patricia L. Maichle, Senior Administrator
Kristin Cosden, Social Service Administrator
Stefanie Lancaster, Administrative Officer
Working to ensure that people with developmental disabilities enjoy the same quality of life as the rest of society.

3385 **Delaware Division for the Visually Impaired**
1901 North Dupont Highway
New Castle, DE 19720-1160   302-255-9800
FAX: 302-255-4441
dhssinfo@state.de.us
www.dhss.delaware.gov/dvi/

Rita Landgraf, Secretary
Henry Smith, Deputy Secretary
Betsy Deldeo, Office Manager
State agency serving the visually impaired persons from birth, with or without other handicaps. Services offered include voca-

tional rehabilitation, independent living, orientation and mobility, technology assessment, transition from school to work.

3386 Delaware Industries for the Blind
1901 North Dupont Highway
New Castle, DE 19720-1160
302-255-9855
FAX: 302-255-4485
DIBcustomerservice@state.de.us
www.promoplace.com/dib

Andy Kloepfer, General Manager
Romy Mikhail, Customer Service Manager
Malvern Slawter, Plant Production Manager
Delaware Industries for the Blind is a multi-faceted company that specializes in creating employment opportunities for Delaware citizens who are blind and visually impaired. DIB accomplishes this by providing quality goods and guaranteed services under contracts from Federal, State and Local Agencies and Industries.

3387 Delaware Protection & Advocacy for Persons with Disabilities
Arc of Delaware
144 E Market St
Georgetown, DE 19947-1411
302-856-6019
FAX: 302-856-6133
challdover@aol.com

Becky Allen, Executive Director

3388 Delaware Workers Compensation Board
Industrial Accident Board de dept
4425 North Market Street
Wilmington, DE 19802-1307
302-761-8085
FAX: 302-761-6601
www.delawareworks.com

James Cagle, Manager
The Office of Workers' Compensation administers and enforces state laws, rules and regulations regarding industrial accidents and illnesses.

3389 Social Security: Wilmington Disability Determination
U S Department of Health and Human Services
1528 S 16th Street
Wilmington, NC 28401-3908
866-964-6227
800-772-1213
FAX: 910-254-3444
TTY: 910-815-4695
www.socialsecurity.gov

J Allen Murphy, Founder
Vickie O'Brien, Manager

District of Columbia

3390 District of Columbia Department of Handicapped Children
D C General Hospital
Bldg 10
1900 Massachusetts Ave SE
Washington, DC 20003- 2542
202-541-6337
FAX: 202-675-7694

Jacqueline Mcmorris, Acting Chief
Nayab Ali, MD

3391 District of Columbia Office on Aging
500 K Street NE
Washington, DC 20002-2714
202-724-5622
FAX: 202-724-4979
TTY:202-724-8925
dcoa@dc.gov
dcoa.dc.gov

John M Thompson, Executive Director
Deborah Royster, General Counsel
Tanya Reid, Executive Assistant
Camile Williams, Chief of Staff

Serves the District of Columbia residents 60 years of age and older. Contact the Information and Assistance Unit for more information about innovative programs and services offered by the Office.

3392 Information, Protection & Advocacy for Persons with Disabilities
IPACHI
220 I Street, N.E.
Suite 130
Washington, DC 20002
202-547-0198
FAX: 202-547-2083
jbrown@uls-dc.org
www.acf.hhs.gov/programs/add/states/pas.html

Jane Brown, Executive Director
Ronald Tyson, Information/Referral
Offers services and support for persons with disabilities in the Washington, DC area.

3393 Information, Protection and Advocacy Center for Handicapped Individuals
220 I Street, N.E.
Suite 130
Washington, DC 20002-2340
202-547-0198
FAX: 202-547-2083
jbrown@uls-dc.org
www.acf.hhs.gov/programs/add/states/pas.html

Jane Brown, Executive Director
Serves all persons with disabilities in the DC, Maryland and Virginia areas offering them legal representation and advocacy, information and referrals and several publications.

3394 International Dyslexia Association of DC
40 York Rd., 4th Floor
Baltimore, MD 21204-1016
410-296-0232
800-222-3123
FAX: 410-321-5069
info@interdys.org
www.interdys.org

Ruth R Tifford LCSW, President
The DC Capital Area Branch, provides support for individuals with dyslexia and their families in the Washington, DC metropolitan area, including parts of Maryland, Virginia and West Virginia. Our conferences, book sales and online information resources are designed to further the understanding of dyslexia and encourage the use of systematic, multisensory teaching methods enabling children and adults to reach their educational potential.

3395 Wage and Hour Division of the Employment Standards Administration
US Department of Labor
200 Constitution Ave NW
Washington, DC 20210-1
202-693-5000
866-487-2365
FAX: 202-219-8822
TTY: 877-889-5627
webmaster@dol.gov
www.dol.gov

Hilda Solis, Secretary of Labor
Seth Harris, Deputy Secretary
Elizabeth Kim, Executive Secretariat Director
Betsey Stevenson, Chief Economist
Administers regulations governing the employment of individuals with disabilities in sheltered workshops and the disabled workers industries.

3396 Washington Hearing and Speech Society
2150 N 107th St, Suite 205
Seattle, WA 98133-2633
206-209-5271
FAX: 206-367-8777
office@wslha.org
www.wslha.org

Paul Diez, President
Judith Bernier, Secretary
Julie Leonardo, Treasurer
Lesley Stephens, Clinical SLP

Offers individuals with hearing or speech impairments, in the DC area, speech, reading classes, audiological services and new aids.

3397 Well Mind Association of Greater Washington
18606 New Hampshire Ave
Ashton, MD 20861-9789
301-774-6617
FAX: 301-946-1402

3398 Workers Compensation Board: District of Columbia
4058 Minnesota Avenue, NE,
Washington, DC 20019-5626
202-724-7000
202-698-4817
FAX: 202-673-6993
does@dc.gov
Deborah A Carroll, Director
The Workers' Compensation Program processes claims and monitors the payment of benefits to injured private-sector employees in the District of Columbia

Florida

3399 ARC Gateway
3932 North 10th Avenue
Pensacola, FL 32503-2807
850-434-2638
FAX: 850-438-2180
info@arc-gateway.org
www.arc-gateway.org

Peter Mougey, President
Patricia Young, Vice President
Lynn Erickson, Secretary
Donna Fassett, Executive Director
ARC Gateway is a non-profit organization that serves children who have or are at risk of developmental disabilities as well as adults with developmental disabilitie

3400 Advocacy Center for Persons with Disabilities
2473 Care Drive
Suite 200
Tallahassee, FL 32308-5020
850-488-9071
800-342-0823
FAX: 850-488-8640
TTY: 800-346-4127
info@advocacy.org
www.disabilityrightsflorida.org
Catherine Piecora, Chair
Maryellen McDonald, Executive Director
Carol Stachurski, Program Operations Manage
Paige Morgan, Executive Assistant
Disability Rights Florida is the designated protection and advocacy system for individuals with disabilities in the State of Florida.

3401 Assistive Technology Educational Network of Florida
1207 S Mellonville Avenue
Sanford, FL 32771-2240
800-558-6580
FAX: 407-320-2379
Diane_Penn@scps.k12.fl.us
www.icdri.org/Assistive%20Technology/aten.htm
Dee Wright, Executive Secretary
Diane Penn, MA, Technology Specialist
Provides state-wide information, awareness and training for students, family members, teachers and other professionals in the area of assisted technology; a quarterly newsletter and a network of specialists (Local Assistive Technology Specialists) trained by ATEN to provide support at the district level.

3402 Bureau Of Exceptional Education And Student Services
325 West Gaines Street Suite 614
Tallahassee, FL 32399
850-245-0475
FAX: 850-245-0953
Monica.Verra-Tirado@fldoe.org
www.fldoe.org
Pam Stewart, Education Commissioner
Monica Verra Tirado, Bureau Chief
Chatherine Aponte Gray, Administrative Assistant
Tonya Milton, Program Planner
Provides consultative services for the establishment and operation of school programs for visually impaired students. Provides assistance for in-service teacher training through state or regional workshops or technical assistance to individual programs.

3403 Department of Health & Rehabilitative Services
1317 Winewood Blvd
Building 1
Tallahassee, FL 32399-700
850-487-1111
FAX: 850-922-2993
www.dcf.state.fl.us
David Wilkins, Secretary
Ramin Kouzehkanani, Deputy Secretary
John Bryant, Manager
The Florida Department of Children and Families has adopted an integrated approach to programs and services as we work to help improve the lives of individuals and families.

3404 Division of Workers Compensation
200 East Gaines Street
Tallahassee, FL 32399-0318
850-413-3089
877-693-5236
FAX: 850-413-2950
Tanner.Holloman@myfloridacfo.com
www.fldfs.com
Tanner Holloman, Division Director
Andrew Sabolic, Assistant Director
Terry Kester, Chief Information Officer
Robin Delaney, Bureau Chief of Compliance
To actively ensure the self-execution of the workers' compensation system through education and informing all stakeholders of their rights and responsibilities, leveraging data to deliver exceptional value to our customers and stakeholders, and holding parties accountable for meeting their obligations.

3405 Florida Adult Services
1317 Winewood Boulevard
Building 1, Room 202
Tallahassee, FL 32399-700
850-488-2881
800-962-2873
800-273-8255
FAX: 850-922-4193
www.myflfamilies.com
Robert Anderson, State Director
Jan Chaney, Administrative Assistant
Roy Car, Data/Systems
Lindsay Conrad, HCDA and CCDA
The Florida Department of Children and Families has adopted an integrated approach to programs and services as we work to help improve the lives of individuals and families.

3406 Florida Department of Handicapped Children
4030 Esplanade Way
Suite 380
Tallahassee, FL 32399-7016
850-488-4257
866-273-2273
FAX: 850-245-1075
apd_info@apd.state.fl.us
www.apd.myflorida.com
Mike Gresham, Executive Director
John Bryant, Manager
The APD works in partnership with local communities and private providers to assist people who have developmental disabilities and their families.

3407 Florida Department of Mental Health and Rehabilitative Services
1317 Winewood Blvd
Building 1
Tallahassee, FL 32399-700
850-487-1111
FAX: 850-922-2993
www.dcf.state.fl.us

David Wilkins, Secretary
Ramin Kouzehkanani, Deputy Secretary

3408 Florida Developmental Disabilities Council
124 Marriott Drive
Suite 203
Tallahassee, FL 32301-2981
850-488-4180
800-580-7801
FAX: 850-922-6702
TTY: 888-488-863
fddc@fddc.org
fddc.org

Sylvia James Miller, Council Chair & Parent Advocate
Tricia Riccardi, Council Vice-Chair
Debra Dowds, Executive Director
Vanda Bowman, Staff Assistant
To advocate and promote meaningful participation in all aspects of life for Floridians with developmental disabilities.

3409 Florida Division of Vocational Rehabilitation
4070 Esplanade Way
Building 1
Tallahassee, FL 32399- 7016
850-245-3399
800-451-4327
FAX: 850-245-3316
TTY: 850-488-2867
costin@vr.doe.state.fl.us
rehabworks.org

Bill Palmer, Manager
Linda Parnell, Manager
Aleisa Mckinlay, Director
Don Chester, Counsil Member
State agency serving individuals with physical or mental disabilities that interfere with them keeping or maintaining employment.

3410 Florida's Protection and Advocacy Programs for Persons with Disabilities
2473 Care Drive
Suite 200
Tallahassee, FL 32308
850-488-9071
800-342-0823
FAX: 850-488-8640
TTY: 800-346-4127
www.disabilityrightsflorida.org

Catherine Piecora, Chair
Maryellen McDonald, Executive Director
Carol Stachurski, Program Operations Manager
Paige Morgan, Executive Assistant
The Center is a non-profit organization providing protection and advocacy services in the State of Florida. The Center's mission is to advance the dignity, equality, self-determination and expressed choices of individuals with disabilities.

3411 International Dyslexia Association: Florida Branch
40 York Rd., 4th Floor
Baltimore, MD 21204-3896
410-296-0232
800-222-3123
FAX: 410-321-5069
ear228@aol.com
www.interdys.org

Kristen Penczek, Executive Director
David Holste, Director Of Operations
Stacy Friedman, Manager of Operation
Cyndi Powers, Office Manager
The Florida Branch is a non-p;rofit, scientific, educational organization committed to the study, prevention and treatment of language-based learning disabilities (dyslexia) for those in Florida and Puerto Rico. It is specifically concerned with the many children and adults with average or superior intelligence who experi-

ence difficulty in learning skills such as speaking, reading, writing, spelling and math.

3412 Social Security Administration
2002 Old Saint Augustine Rd
Suite B12
Tallahassee, FL 32301-4861
850-942-8978
800-772-1213
FAX: 850-942-8980
ssa.gov

Carrie Tucker, Operations Supervisor
Sheila Lee, Management Support Specialist
Administers the Title II and Title XVII disability programs. To be insured for Title II benefits, applicants must have worked in covered employment for at least five of the last ten years prior to becoming disabled. To be eligible for Title XVII disability benefits, applicants must meet an income and resource test.

3413 Social Security: Miami Disability Determination
Social Security
11401 W Flagler St
Miami, FL 33174-1023
305-226-0449
800-772-1213
TTY:800-325-0778
www.ssa.gov

Robert L Meekins, Deputy General for Executive Ope

3414 Social Security: Orlando Disability Determination
Social Security
P.O. Box 144040
Orlando, FL 32814-2231
407-648-6673
800-342-2065
TTY:407-245-7057
www.ssa.gov

John C Massolio Jr, Founder
Neil Bush, President

3415 Social Security: Tampa Disability Determination
Social Security Administration
PO Box 340572
Tampa, FL 33694-572
813-878-2906
800-772-1213
info@dbstampabay.org
www.dbsatampabay.org

John Balcomb, President
Carol Yaros, 1st Vice President
Cheryl McGhan , 2nd Vice President
Neil Bush, Treasurer
The Depression and Bipolar Support Alliance Tampa Bay , is a nonprofit and all volunteer organization for individuals, family and friends of those who have been diagnosed with bipolar disorder, depression and other affective disorders.

Georgia

3416 ADA Technical Assistance Program
Southeast Disability & Business Technical Assist.
1419 Mayson Street NE
Atlanta, GA 30324
404-541-9001
800-949-4232
FAX: 404-541-9002
ADAsoutheast@law.syr.edu
www.sedbtac.org

Pamela Williamson, Project Director
Cheri Hofmann, Information Specialist
Cyndi Smith, Office Assistant
Marsha Schwanke, Web Manager
One of ten regional centers funded by NIDRR, to provide information and technical assistance to assist in voluntary compliance with the Americans with Disabilities Act, and accessible education-based information technology.

3417   Division of Birth Defects and Developmental Disabilities
1600 Clifton Road
Atlanta, GA 30333-4027   404-498-3800
                                                 800-232-4636
                                          TTY:888-232-6348
                                          cdcinfo@cdc.gov
                                                www.cdc.gov

Coleen A Boyle, Director
The mission of CDC's National Center on Birth Defects and Developmental Disabilities (NCBDDD) is to promote the health of babies, children and adults and to enhance the potential for full, productive living.

3418   Georgia Advocacy Office
150 East Ponce De Leon Avenue
Suite 430
Decatur, GA 30030-2547   404-885-1234
                                                 800-537-2329
                                          FAX: 404-378-0031
                                          info@thegao.org
                                                thegao.org

Ruby Moore, Executive Director
Crystal Rasa, Program Manager
Mona Givens, Director of Investigation
Olwyn Mayer, Chief Operating Officer
Protection and advocacy services for Georgians with disabilities.

3419   Georgia Client Assistance Program
Division of Rehabilitation Services
2 Peachtree Street NW
Suite 29-250
Atlanta, GA 30303- 3141   404-656-4507
                                                 800-822-9727
                                          FAX: 404-651-6880
                                          connect.georgia.gov
                                                dhs.georgia.gov/

Mark Trail, Manager
Robertiena Fletcher, Chair
Franklin G Auman, Vice Chair
Monica Walters, Secretary
Helps eligible persons with complaints, appeals and understanding available benefits under the 1992 Rehabilitation Act Amendments and Title I of the Americans with Disabilities Act. CAP investigates complaints, mediates conflict, represents complainants in appeals, provides legal services if warranted, advocates for due process, identifies and recommends solutions to system problems, advises of benefits available under the 1992 Rehab Act Amendments and Americans with Disabilities Act.

3420   Georgia Council On Developmental Disabilities
2 Peachtree St N.W.
26th Floor, Suite 246
Atlanta, GA 30303-3141   404-657-2126
                                                 888-275-4233
                                          FAX: 404-657-2132
                                          TTY:404-657-2133
                                          eric.jacobson@gcdd.ga.gov
                                                www.gcdd.org

Eric E. Jacobson, Executive Director
Caitlin Childs, Organizing Director
Dottie Adams, Family/Individual Support Dir.
Valerie Meadows Suber, Public Information Director
The Georgia Council on Developmental Disabilities collaborates with Georgia's citizens, public and private advocacy organizations and policymakers to positively influence public policies that enhance the quality of life for people with disabilities and their families. GCDD provides this through education and advocacy activities, program implementation, funding and public policy analysis and research.
Quartlery

3421   Georgia Department of Aging
2 Peachtree Street NW
33rd Floor
Atlanta, GA 30303-3142   404-657-5258
                                                 866-552-4464
                                          FAX: 404-657-5285
                                          connect.georgia.gov
                                                dhs.georgia.gov/

Stephen Dolinger, President
Andrea Fuller-Ruffin, Administrator
The Division of Aging Services (DAS) works to continuously improve the effectiveness and efficiency of services.

3422   Georgia Department of Handicapped Children
2600 Skyland Dr NE
Atlanta, GA 30319-3640   404-679-1625
                                          FAX: 404-679-1630

Ron Jackson, Manager
Frank Koues, Auditor

3423   Georgia Division of Mental Health, Developmental Disabilities & Addictive Diseases
Two Peachtree Drive NW
24th Floor
Atlanta, GA 30303-3142   404-657-2252
                                                 800-715-4225
                                          FAX: 404-657-2310
                                          srhall1@dhr.ga.gov
                                                mhddad.dhr.georgia.gov

Kimberly Ryan, Board Member
David Glass, Board member
Ellice P. Martin, Board Member
Kimberly Carroll-Hawkins, Board Member
MHDDAD provides treatment and support services to people with mental illnesses and addictive diseases, and support to people with mental retardation and related developmental disabilities. MHDDAD serves people of all ages with the most severe and likely to be long-term conditions.

3424   Georgia State Board of Workers' Compensation
270 Peachtree St NW
Atlanta, GA 30303-1299   404-656-3875
                                                 800-533-0682
                                          FAX: 404-657-1767
                                                sbwc.georgia.gov

Frank McKay, Chairman
Elizabeth Gobeil, Director
Delece A. Brooks, Executive Director
Martine Schweitzer, Administrative Assistant
To provide superior access to the Georgia Workers' Compensation program for injured workers and employers in a manner that is sensitive, responsive, and effective and to insure efficient processing and swift, fair resolution of claims, while encouraging workplace safety and return to work.

3425   International Dyslexia Association: Georgia Branch
1951 Greystone Rd.
Atlanta, GA 30318   404-256-1232
                                          info@idaga.org
                                                www.idaga.org

Jennifer Kopp, President
jennings Miller, Vice-President
Robert Moore, Treasurer
Susie McDaniel, Corresponding Secretary
The Georgi Branch was formed to increase public awareness about dyslexia in the State of Georgia. In addition, the Branch encourages teachers to train in multisensory language instruction. The Branch also provides a network for individuals with dyslexia, their families and professionals in the educational and medical fields.

3426 **Social Security: Atlanta Disability Determination**
401 W Peachtree St NW
Suite 2860 Flr 28
Atlanta, GA 30308-3538

800-772-1213
TTY:800-325-0778
www.socialsecurity.gov

3427 **Social Security: Decatur Disability Determination**
2853 Candler Rd
Suite 8
Decatur, GA 30034-1421

800-772-1213
TTY:800-325-0778
ssa.gov

Hawaii

3428 **Assistive Technology Resource Centers of Hawaii**
200 North Vineyard Boulevard
Suite 430
Honolulu, HI 96817-5362

808-532-7110
800-645-3007
FAX: 808-532-7120
TTY: 808-532-7113
atrc-info@atrc.org
www.atrc.org

Barbara Fischlowitz-Leong, Executive Director
Jodi Asato, Deputy Director
Edna Kaahaaina, Office Manager
Joseph Go, Assistive Technology Trainer
Provides information and referral to anyone interested in assistive technology devices and services. Operates equipment loan. Bank Provides training to consumer and professional groups including self-advocacy skills for consumers and family members. Works to ensure that schools, vocational rehabilitation agencies and health insurers provide assessments, funding and training in the use of assistive technology devices and services for their clients. Low-interest loan programs available.

3429 **Diabetes Network of East Hawaii**
1221 Kilauea Ave
Suite 70
Hilo, HI 96720-4264

808-935-1673
FAX: 808-935-6760

Steve Fukunada, Manager

3430 **Disability and Communication Access Board**
919 Ala Moana Blvd
Room 101
Honolulu, HI 96814-4920

808-586-8121
FAX: 808-586-8129
dcab@doh.hawaii.gov
hawaii.gov/health/dcab

Michael Okamoto, Chairperson
Jodi Asato, Deputy Director
Edna Kaahaaina, Office Manager
Joseph Go, Assistive Technology Trainer
Provides ADA coordination for state & county government; reviews state & county construction documents to appropriate federal & state accessibility guidelines; credentials american sign language interpreters; coordinates parking for persons with disabilites; coordinates information & referral for consumers, parents and others seeking disability related information.

3431 **Hawaii Assistive Technology Training and**
200 North Vineyard Boulevard
Suite 430
Honolulu, HI 96817-5362

808-532-7110
800-645-3007
FAX: 808-532-7120
atrc-info@atrc.org
www.atrc.org

Barbara Fischlowitz-Leong, Executive Director

3432 **Hawaii Department for Children With Special Needs**
Department of Health
741 Sunset Avenue
Honolulu, HI 96816-2343

808-733-9070
FAX: 808-733-9068
patricia.heu@doh.hawaii.gov
health.hawaii.gov

Patricia Heu, Manager
Karen Mak, Manager
Children with Special Health Needs Branch(CSHNB) is working to assure that all children and youth with special health care needs (CSHCN) will reach optimal health, growth, and development, by improving access to a coordinated system of family-centered health care services and improving outcomes, through systems development, assessment, assurance, education, collaborative partnerships, and family support.

3433 **Hawaii Department of Health, Adult Mental Health Division**
P.O.Box 3378
Honolulu, HI 96801-3378

808-586-4686
FAX: 808-586-4745
www.amhd.org

3434 **Hawaii Department of Human Services**
Hawaii Department of Human Serv
P.O. Box 339
Honolulu, HI 96813

808-586-4892
FAX: 808-586-4890
dhs@dhs.hawaii.gov
humanservices.hawaii.gov

Rachael Wong, Director
Pankaj Bhanot, Deputy Director
Lisa Nakao, Admin Assis. & Legislative Coor.
Scott Nakasone, Acting Administrator
To provide timely, efficient and effective programs, services and benefits for the purpose of achieving the outcome of empowering Hawaii's most vulnerable people; and to expand their capacity for self-sufficiency, self-determination, independence, healthy choices, quality of life, and personal dignity.

3435 **Hawaii Disability Compensation Division Department of Labor and Industrial Relations**
830 Punchbowl Street
Room 209
Honolulu, HI 96813-5095

808-586-9200
FAX: 808-586-9219
dlir.director@hawaii.gov
hawaii.gov/labor

Walter Kawamura, Administrator
Clyde Imada, Workers Comp Chief
The Disability Compensation Division (DCD) administers the Workers' Compensation (WC) law, the Temporary Disability Insurance (TDI) law, and the Prepaid Health Care (PHC) law. All employers with one or more employees, whether working full-time or part-time, are directly affected.

3436 **Hawaii Disability Rights Center**
1132 Bishop Street
Suite 2102
Honolulu, HI 96813-3701

808-949-2922
800-882-1057
FAX: 808-949-2928
info@hawaiidisabilityrights.org
hawaiidisabilityrights.org

John Dellera, Executive Director
Ann Collins, Director Of Operations
IT IS THE POLICY OF HDRCto advocate for as many people with disabilities in the State of Hawaii, on as wide a range of disability rights issues, as our resources allow; and to resolve rights violations with the lowest feasible level of intervention; but, if necessary, to also provide full legal representation to protect the rights of people with disabilities, consistent with authorizing statutes and Center priorities.

3437   Hawaii Executive Office on Aging
250 South Hotel Street
Suite 406
Honolulu, HI 96813-2831   808-586-0100
     800-468-4644
FAX: 808-586-0185
eoa@mail.health.state.hi.us
hawaii.gov/health/eoa

Noemi Pendleton, Manager
Virginia Pressler, Director
Keith Y. Yamamoto, Deputy Director
Danette Wong Tomiyasu, Deputy Director
State unit on aging responsible for policy formulation, program development, planning, information dissemination, advocacy and other activities, for persons age 60 and over.

3438   Hawaii State Council on Developmental Disabilities
919 Ala Moana Blvd
Suite113
Honolulu, HI 96814-4920   808-586-8100
FAX: 808-586-7543
council@hiddc.org
www.hiddc.org

Waynette K Y Cabral, Executive Administrator
Joe Shacter, Planner
Debbie Miyasaka Gushiken, Community & Legislative Liaison
Susan Kawano, Secretary
The mission of the council is to support people with developmental disabilities to control their own destiny and determine the quality of life they desire. The Council: engages in analysis and policy development; provides training in legislative advocacy and leadership development for individuals with disabilities and their families; demonstrates new approaches to services and supports; informs policymakers about developmental disability issues; and fosters interagency collaboration.

3439   International Dyslexia Association: Hawaii Branch
913 Alewa Drive
Honolulu, HI 96817-1610   808-538-7007
FAX: 808-566-6837
HIDA@dyslexia-hawaii.org
dyslexia-hawaii.org

Charles Bering, President
Deborah Knight, Vice President
Laurie Moore, Executive Director
Margaret J Higa, Executive Director
Provides free information and referral services for diagnosis and tutoring for parents, educators, physicians, and individuals with dyslexia. The voice of our membership is heard in 48 countries. Membership includes yearly journal and quarterly newsletter. Call for conference dates.

3440   Social Security: Honolulu Disability Determination
Social Security
300 Ala Moana Blvd
Honolulu, HI 96850-1   808-541-3600
     800-772-1213
TTY:800-825-0778
hivrsbd@kestrok.com
www.ssa.gov
Neil Shim, Administrator

3441   State Planning Council on Developmental Disabilities
919 Ala Moana Blvd
Room 101
Honolulu, HI 96814-4920   808-586-8121
FAX: 808-586-8129
TTY:808-586-8121
dcab@doh.hawaii.gov
hawaii.gov/health/dcab

Michael Okamoto, Chairperson
Peter Fritz, Vice Chairperson
Francine Wai, Executive Director
Debbra Jackson, Planning and ADA Cooordinator
Consists of 25 Hawaii residents appointed by the governor. The council addresses the needs of the people with developmental

disabilities: specifically, develops a state plan that sets the priorities for persons with developmental disabilities.

Idaho

3442   Idaho Commission on Aging
341 W Washington
Boise, ID 83702-1   208-334-3833
     800-926-2588
FAX: 208-334-3033
ICOA@aging.idaho.gov
www.idahoaging.com

Sam Haws, Administrator
Cathy Hart, State Ombudsman
Jeff Weller, Deputy Administrator
Raul Enriquez, Program Specialist
There number one priority is to provide the best possible service through this single point of entry website where people of all incomes and ages can obtain information on a full range of long-term care support programs and services.

3443   Idaho Council on Developmental Disabilities
Health and Wellfare
700 W. State Street
Suite 119
Boise, ID 83702-5868   208-334-2178
     800-544-2433
FAX: 208-334-3417
info@icdd.idaho.gov
icdd.idaho.gov

Jim Baugh, Council Member
Christine Pisani, Executive Director
Tracy Warren, Program Specialist/Planner
Deborah Daniels, Management Assistant
The mission of the Idaho Council on Developmental Disabilities is to promote the capacity of people with developmental disabilities and their families to determine, access, and direct the services and/or support they need to live the lives they choose, and to build the communities ability to support their choices.

3444   Idaho Department of Handicapped Children
Statehouse
Boise, ID 83720-1   208-334-8000

Thomas Bruck, Chief
Sandy Frazier, Manager

3445   Idaho Disability Determinations Service
PO Box 21
Boise, ID 83707-0021   208-327-7333
     800-626-2681
FAX: 208-327-7331
TTY: 800-377-3529
labor.idaho.gov

Roger B Madsen, Director
Rogelio Valdez, Executive Director
Under contract with the Social Security Administration, makes determinations of medical eligibility for disability benefits.

3446   Idaho Industrial Commission
P.O. Box 83720
Boise, ID 83720-0041   208-334-6000
     800-950-2110
FAX: 208-334-2321
mholbrook@iic.idaho.gov
www.iic.idaho.gov

Mindy Montgomery, Manager
Beth Kilian, Commission Secretary
Free rehabilitation services to workers' who have suffered on the job injuries in Idaho. Field offices throughout the state.

3447   Idaho Mental Health Center
1720 Westgate Dr
Boise, ID 83704-7164   208-334-0808
                                                   800-926-2588
                                              FAX: 208-334-0828
                                        healthandwelfare.idaho.gov

Richard Armstrong, Director
Darrell Kerby, Chairperson
Tom Stroschein, Vice Chair
Stephen Weeg, Board Member
The State of Idaho provides state funded and operated community based mental health care services through Regional Behavioral Health Centers (RBHC) located in each of the seven geographical regions of the state. Each RBHC provides mental health services through a system of care that is both community-based and consumer-guided.

Illinois

3448   Attorney General's Office: Disability Rights Bureau & Health Care Bureau
100 W Randolph Street
Chicago, IL 60601-3218   312-814-3000
                                                   877-305-5145
                                              FAX: 312-793-0802
                                              TTY: 800-964-3013
                                       illinoisattorneygeneral.gov

Lisa Madigan, Manager
Raymond Throlkeld, Chief Health Care Bureau
Information on Illinois' Comprehensive Health Insurance Plan and architectural accessibility. Enforcement of Illinois' access law and standards and other disability rights laws. Information on initiatives such as: Opening the Courthouse Doors to People with Disabilities; the abuse, neglect or financial exploitation of people with disabilities and voter accessibility. Other information and referrals.

3449   Client Assistance Program (CAP)
Illinois State Board of Education
100 N 1st St
1st Floor West
Springfield, IL 62702-1   217-782-4321
                                                   800-641-3929
                                                   866-262-6663
                                              FAX: 217-524-1790
                                              TTY: 217-782-1900
                                            dhs.cap@illinois.gov
                                             www.dhs.state.il.us

Dr. Christop Koch, State Superintendent
The Client Assistance Program (CAP) helps people with disabilities receive quality services by advocating for their interests and helping them identify resources, understand procedures, resolve problems, and protect their rights in the rehabilitation process, employment, and home services.

3450   Equip for Equality
20 North Michigan Avenue
Suite 300
Chicago, IL 60602- 4861   312-341-0022
                                                   800-537-2632
                                              FAX: 312-541-7544
                                              TTY: 800-610-2779
                                     contactus@equipforequality.org
                                              equipforequality.org

Zena Naiditch, President/CEO
Barry C Taylor, Vice President
Lia Burkey, Administrative Assistant
Thomas Fischer, Special Assistant to President
Equip for equality is an independent, private, not-for-profit organization designated by the Governor in 1985 to implement the federally mandated Protection and Advocacy (P&A) System in Illinois. The mission of Equip for Equality is to advance the human and civil rights of children and adults with disabilities in Illinois.

3451   Equip for Equality - Carbondale Office
300 East Main St
Suite 18
Carbondale, IL 62901   618-457-7930
                                                   800-758-0559
                                              FAX: 618-457-7985
                                              TTY: 800-610-2779
                                     contactus@equipforequality.org
                                              equipforequality.org

Zena Naiditch, President/CEO
Barry C Taylor, Vice President
Lia Burkey, Administrative Assistant
Thomas Fischer, Special Assistant to President
Equip for equality is an independent, private, not-for-profit organization designated by the Governor in 1985 to implement the federally mandated Protection and Advocacy (P&A) System in Illinois. The mission of Equip for Equality is to advance the human and civil rights of children and adults with disabilities in Illinois.

3452   Equip for Equality - Moline Office
1515 Fifth Ave
Suite 420
Moline, IL 61265   309-786-6868
                                                   800-758-6869
                                              FAX: 309-797-8710
                                              TTY: 800-610-2779
                                     contactus@equipforequality.org
                                              equipforequality.org

Zena Naiditch, President/CEO
Barry C Taylor, Vice President
Lia Burkey, Administrative Assistant
Thomas Fischer, Special Assistant to President
Equip for equality is an independent, private, not-for-profit organization designated by the Governor in 1985 to implement the federally mandated Protection and Advocacy (P&A) System in Illinois. The mission of Equip for Equality is to advance the human and civil rights of children and adults with disabilities in Illinois.

3453   Equip for Equality - Springfield Office
1 West Old State Capitol Plaza
Suite 816
Springfield, IL 62701   217-544-0464
                                                   800-758-0464
                                              FAX: 217-523-0720
                                              TTY: 800-610-2779
                                     contactus@equipforequality.org
                                              equipforequality.org

Zena Naiditch, President/CEO
Barry C Taylor, Vice President
Lia Burkey, Administrative Assistant
Thomas Fischer, Special Assistant to President
Equip for equality is an independent, private, not-for-profit organization designated by the Governor in 1985 to implement the federally mandated Protection and Advocacy (P&A) System in Illinois. The mission of Equip for Equality is to advance the human and civil rights of children and adults with disabilities in Illinois.

3454   Illinois Assistive Technology Project
1 West Old State Capitol Plaza
Suite 100
Springfield, IL 62701-1200   217-522-7985
                                                   800-852-5110
                                              FAX: 217-522-8067
                                              TTY: 217-522-9966
                                                   iatp@iltech.org
                                                   iltech.org

Wilhelmina Gunther, Executive Director
Shelly Lowe, Finance/Personnel Manager
Yvonne Miller, Administrative Assistant
Barbara Howell, Administration
Directed by and for people with disabilities and their family members. As a federally mandated program, IATP strives to break down barriers and change policies that make getting and using technology difficult. IATP offers solutions to help people find

what is available in products and services that will best meet their needs, where to find it, and how to get it.

3455 Illinois Council on Developmental Disability
State of Illinois Center
100 W Randolph St
16-100
Chicago, IL 60601-3218
312-814-2121
800-843-6154
FAX: 312-814-7441
drs@dhs.state.il.us
www.state.il.us/agency/icdd/

Sheila T. Romano, Executive Director
Dennis Sienko, Manager
The Illinois Council on Developmental Disabilities (ICDD) is dedicated to leading change in Illinois so that all people with developmental disabilities are able to exercise their rights to freedom and equal opportunity.

3456 Illinois Department of Mental Health and Developmental Disabilities
Suite 3b
314 E Madison
Springfield, IL 62701
217-782-6680
FAX: 217-524-3834

Karen Perrin, Manager
Lori Stone, Director

3457 Illinois Department of Rehabilitation
100 South Grand Avenue East
Springfield, IL 62762-1304
217-782-6680
800-843-6154
FAX: 217-524-3834
TTY: 800-447-6404
DHS.WEBBITS@ILLINOIS.GOV
www.dhs.state.il.us/page.aspx?item=29736

Robert Kilbury, Director
Timothy Martin, Manager
DHS's Division of Rehabilitation Services is the state's lead agency serving individuals with disabilities. DRS works in partnership with people with disabilities and their families to assist them in making informed choices to achieve full community participation through employment, education, and independent living opportunities.

3458 Illinois Department on Aging
One Natural Resources Way
Suite 100
Springfield, IL 62702-1271
217-785-2870
800-252-8966
FAX: 217-785-4477
TTY: 888-206-1327
ilsenior@illinois.gov
www.state.il.us/aging

John K. Holton, Director
Jennifer Reif, Deputy Director
Matthew Ryan, Chief of Staff
Bradley A. Rightnowar, General Counsil
The MISSION of the Illinois Department on Aging is to serve and advocate for older Illinoisans and their caregivers by administering quality and culturally appropriate programs that promote partnerships and encourage independence, dignity, and quality of life.

3459 International Dyslexia Association: Illinois Branch
751 Roosevelt Road
Suite 116
Glen Ellyn, IL 60137
630-469-6900
800-222-3123
FAX: 630-469-6810
info@readibida.org
www.readibida.org

Jo Ann Paldo, President
Foley Burckardt, Vice President
Joan Budovec, Treasurer
Sherry Grobe, Secretary

Provides free information and referral services for diagnosis and tutoring for parents, educators, physicians, and individuals with dyslexia in Illinois and Missouri. The voice of our membership is heard in 48 countries. Membership includes yearly journal and quarterly newsletter. Call for conference dates.

3460 Social Security: Springfield Disability Determination
3112 CONSTITUTION DR
Springfield, IL 62704-1323
877-279-9504
800-772-1213
TTY:800-325-0778
ssa.gov

3461 Workers Compensation Board Illinois
100 W Randolph St
Ste 8-200
Chicago, IL 60601-3227
312-814-6611
866-352-3033
FAX: 312-814-6523
infoquestions.wcc@illinois.gov
www.state.il.us/agency/iic/

Joann Fratianni, Chairman
The Illinois Workers' Compensation Commission resolves disputes between employees and employers regarding work-related injuries and illnesses.

Indiana

3462 Indiana Client Assistance Program
4701 N. Keystone Avenue
Suite 222
Indianapolis, IN 46204-1191
317-722-5555
800-622-4845
FAX: 317-722-5564
TTY: 317-722-5555
tgallagher@ipas.state.in.us
www.icdri.org/legal/IndianaCAP.htm

Michael Burks, Chairman
Wen Lu, Secretary and Treasurer

3463 Indiana Developmental Disability Council
402 West Washington Street
Room E145
Indianapolis, IN 46204-2801
317-232-7770
FAX: 317-233-3712
GPCPD@gpcpd.org
www.in.gov

Katrina Gossett, Chair
Dawn Adams JD, Agency representative
Suellen Jackson-Boner, Executive Director
Christine Dahlberg, Deputy Director
The Indiana Governor's Council is an independent state agency that facilitates change. Our mission is to promote public policy which leads to the independence, productivity and inclusion of people with disabilities in all aspects of society

3464 Indiana Protection & Advocacy Services Commission
4701 N. Keystone Avenue
Suite 222
Indianapolis, IN 46205-1561
317-722-5555
800-622-4845
FAX: 317-722-5564
ExecutiveDirector@ipas.in.gov
www.in.gov/ipas

Dawn Adams, Executive Director
Milo Gray, Client & Legal Services Director
Gary Richter, Support Services Director
Karen Pedevilla, Education/Training Director
An independent state agency established to protect and promote the rights of individuals with disabilities through empowerment and advocacy.

3465 Indiana State Commission for the Handicapped
P.O.Box 1964
Indianapolis, IN 46206   317-233-1292

3466 International Dyslexia Association: Indiana Branch
7944 Destry Place
Fisher, IN 46038   317-926-1450
                                          800-222-3123
                                          FAX: 317-926-1450
                                          gcrahen@sbcglobal.net
                                          www.ida-indiana.org

Merry Binnion, President
Tracy Brazda, Vice President
Ginger Lentz, Secretary
Therese Rooney, Treasurer
The Indiana Branch was formed to help the members of the learning disabilities community in Indiana. Promotes understanding and facilitate treatment of the Specific Language Disability (Dyslexia) in children and adults, promotes teacher training and educational intervention strategies for dyslexic students and to foster effective teaching, supports research in the field and early identification of dyslexia, serves as a clearinghouse for information and to actively disseminate knowledge.

Iowa

3467 Governor's Developmental Disability Council
617 East Second Street
Des Moines, IA 50309-1831   515-281-9082
                                          800-452-1936
                                          FAX: 515-281-9087
                                          fmorris@dhs.state.ia.us
                                          http://idaction.com/

Becky Harker, Executive Director
Rik Shannon, Public Policy Manager
Janet Shoeman, Program Planner/Contract Manager
Fran Morris, Council Secretary
The Council identifies, develops and promotes public policy and support practices through capacity building, advocacy, and systems change activities. The purpose is to ensure that people with developmental disabilities and their families are included in planning, decision making, and development of policy related to services and supports that affect their quality of life and full participation in communities of their choice.

3468 International Dyslexia Association: Iowa Branch
P.O. Box 11188
Cedar Rapids, IA 52410-1188   765-507-9432
                                          800-222-3123
                                          FAX: 410-321-5069
                                          info@iowaida.org
                                          www.ida-ia.org

Denise Little, President
Tricia Krsek, Vice President
Genevieve Monthie, Secretary
Wayne Wunschel, Treasurer
The purpose of the Iowa Branch of IDA (IDA-IA) is to increase awareness of dyslexia and promote services that address the importance of diagnosis and remediation for those not meeting their reading potential. Our goal is to provide services and assistance in a way that promotes unity, support, and cooperation among those who work with these individuals so that all communities in Iowa benefit from the skills and talents of its citizens.

3469 Iowa Child Health Specialty Clinics
100 Hawkins Drive
Room 247 CDD
Iowa City, IA 52242-1016   319-356-1117
                                          866-219-9119
                                          FAX: 319-356-3715
                                          kathy-colbert@uiowa.edu
                                          www.chsciowa.org

Jeffrey Lobas, Director
Brian Wilkes, Director Of Operations

Child Health Specialty Clinics has a mission to improve the health, development, and well-being of Iowa's children and youth with special health care needs in partnership with families, service providers, and communities.

3470 Iowa Commission of Persons with Disabilities
Department of Human Rights
Lucas State Office Bldg, 2nd Floor
Des Moines, IA 50319- 2006   515-242-6171
                                          888-219-0471
                                          FAX: 515-242-6119
                                          TTY: 888-219-0471
                                          dhr.disabilities@dhr.state.ia.us
                                          www.state.ia.us/dhr/pd

Jill Fulitano-Avery, Administrator
To equalize opportunities for full participation in employment and other areas of the state's economic, educational, social and political life for Iowans with disabilities.

3471 Iowa Compass
Center for Disabilities and Development
100 Hawkins Dr
#S295
Iowa City, IA 52242-1011   319-353-6900
                                          800-779-2001
                                          FAX: 319-356-1343
                                          TTY: 877-686-0032
                                          iowa-compass@uiowa.edu
                                          www.iowacompass.org/

Jane Gay, Project Director
David Sorton, President
Mark Moser, Administrator
A statewide program provides free information and referral about disability related services and resources: advocacy, assistive technology, community services, early intervention, education, financial support, healthcare, legal aid, residential services and transportation.
BiMonthly

3472 Iowa Department for the Blind
State Of Iowa
524 4th Street
Des Moines, IA 50309-2364   515-281-1333
                                          800-362-2587
                                          FAX: 515-281-1263
                                          TTY: 515-281-1355
                                          information@blind.state.ia.us
                                          www.IDBonline.org

Richard Sorey, Director
Jodi Aldini, Library Support Staff
Julie Aufdenkamp, Transition Specialist, Transitio
Jessica Badding, Vocational Rehabilitation Counse
Mission is to be the means for persons who are blind to obtain univeral access and full participation as citizens in whatever roles they may choose.

3473 Iowa Department of Human Services
1305 E Walnut St
Des Moines, IA 50319-114   515-242-6510
                                          800-972-2017
                                          FAX: 515-281-4597
                                          mfinkel@dhs.state.ia.us
                                          www.dhs.state.ia.us

Terry E Branstad, Governor
Charles M Palmer, Director
Sally Titus, Deputy Director
Richard Shults, Division Administrator
Help individuals and families to achieve stable and healthy lives.

3474 Iowa Department on Aging
510 E 12th Street
Suite 2
Des Moines, IA 50319-9025   515-725-3333
                                   800-532-3213
                                   FAX: 866-236-1430
                                   www.aging.iowa.gov

Donna K. Harvey, Director
Danika Welch, Executive Secretary
Joel Wulf, Administrator
Jeanne Yordi, State Long Term Care Ombudsman

3475 Iowa Protection & Advocacy for the Disabled
400 East Court Avenue
Suite 300
Des Moines, IA 50309   515-278-2502
                              800-779-2502
                              FAX: 515-278-0539
                              info@DRIowa.org
                              disabilityrightsiowa.org

Christine Glosser, President
Todd Lantz, Vice President
Jane Hudson, Executive Director
Cyndy Miller, Senior Staff Attorney
Disability Rights IOWA aims to defend and promote the human and legal rights of Iowans who have disabilities and mental illness.

3476 Social Security: Des Moines Disability Determination
Social Security Administration
Riverpoint Office Complex
455 SW 5TH ST STE F
Des Moines, IA 50309-2115   515-284-4260
                                   800-772-1213
                                   FAX: 515-284-4394
                                   TTY: 800-325-0778
                                   ssa.gov

Leroy Brown, Manager

3477 Workers Compensation Board Iowa
1000 East Grand Avenue
Des Moines, IA 50319-0209   515-281-5387
                                   FAX: 515-281-6501
                                   IWD.DWC@iwd.iowa.gov
                                   www.iowaworkforce.org

Joseph S Cortese II, Commissioner
Janna E. Martin, Commissioner
Sandy Breckenridge, Administrative Secretary
Jolene Doll, Support Staff
The Workers' Compensation Act is a part of the Iowa Code designed to provide certain benefits to employees who receive injury (85), occupational disease (85A) or occupational hearing loss (85B) arising out of and during the course of their employment.

Kansas

3478 Beach Center on Families and Disability
University of Kansas
1200 Sunnyside Ave
Room 3136
Lawrence, KS 66045-7600   785-864-7600
                                 866-783-3378
                                 FAX: 785-864-7605
                                 beachcenter@ku.edu
                                 www.beachcenter.org

Michael Wehmeyer, Co-Director
Ann Turnbull, Co-Founder
Shonda Anderson, Project Coordinator
Peter Griggs, Evaluation Coordinator
A federally funded center that conducts research and training in the factors that contribute to the successful functioning of families with members who have disabilities.

3479 International Dyslexia Association: Kansas/West Missouri Branch
430 East Blue Ridge Blvd
Kansas City, MO 64145-1422   816-838-7323
                                    FAX: 816-942-6898
                                    info@ksmoida.org
                                    www.ksmoida.org

Angie Schreiber, President
Pamela Taylor, Vice President
Joseph Cowin, Treasurer
Ann Marie Corry, Secretary
IDA members in Kansas and Missouri work to establish and maintain a presence for IDA with parents, schools, and teachers in order to help individuals with dyslexia. We maintain a list of individuals in Kansas and Missouri who have specialized training and who are available for diagnosis and remediation of reading, writing, and spelling problems, information for parents, information for teachers, an annual spring conference, newsletter dealing with state and local issues.

3480 Kansas Advocacy and Protective Services
214 SW 6th Ave.,
Ste 100
Topeka, KS 66603-3726   785-273-9661
                               877-776-1541
                               FAX: 785-273-9414
                               TTY: 877-335-3725
                               www.drckansas.org/

Rocky Nichols, Executive Director
Debbie White, Deputy Director
Lane Williams, Deputy Director
Catherine Johnson, Disability Rights Attorney
Protection and advocacy for persons with disabilities.

3481 Kansas Client Assistance Program
635 SW Harrison
Suite 100
Topeka, KS 66603   785-273-9661
                          877-776-1541
                          FAX: 785-273-9414
                          TTY: 877-335-3725
                          rocky@drckansas.org
                          www.icdri.org/legal/KansasCAP.htm

3482 Kansas Commission on Disability Concerns
900 SW Jackson
Suite 100
Topeka, KS 66612-1246   785-296-1722
                               800-295-5232
                               FAX: 785-296-1795
                               KCDCoffice@ks.gov
                               kcdcinfo.ks.gov

Martha Gabehart, Executive Director
Kerrie Bacon, Employment/Training Liaison
Kerrie Bacon, Legislative Liaison
KCDC believes that all people with disabilities are entitled to be equal citizens and partners in Kansas society. The purpose is to involve all segments of the Kansas Community through legislative advocacy, education and resource networking to ensure full and equal citizenship for all Kansans with disabilities.

3483 Kansas Department on Aging
503 S Kansas Ave
New England Building
Topeka, KS 66603- 3404   785-296-4986
                                800-432-3535
                                FAX: 785-296-0256
                                TTY: 785-291-3167
                                wwwmail@kdads.ks.gov
                                www.kdads.ks.gov

Kathy Greenlee, Manager
Barbara Conant, Public Information Officer
Kari Bruffett, Secretary
Services and information for Kansas seniors, over age 60.

3484   Kansas Developmental Disability Council
Disability Rights Center of Kansas
915 SW Harrison
DSOB Rm 141
Topeka, KS 66612-3726   785-296-2608
                                         877-431-4604
                              FAX: 785-296-2861
                              TTY: 877-335-3725
                                   sgieber@kcdd.org
                                      www.kcdd.org/

Steve Gieber, Executive Director
Craig Knutson, Public Policy Coordinator
Charline Cobbs, Senior Administrative Assistant
The purpose of the Kansas Council on Developmental Disabilities (KCDD) is to support people of all ages with developmental disabilities so they have the opportunity to make choices regarding both their participation in society, and their quality of life.

Kentucky

3485   Kentucky Council on Developmental Disability
1151 So. Fourth Street
Louisville, KY 40203   502-584-1239
                                         800-372-2973
                              FAX: 502-584-1261
                                 info@councilondd.org
                                      councilondd.org

Richard Bush, President
Dave Fowler, Treasurer
Missy Kinnaird, Secretary
Donovan Fornwalt, Chief Executive Officer
Implementation of Developmental Disabilities Planning Council responsible under P.L. 101-496.

3486   Kentucky Department for Mental Health and Mental Retardation Services
275 E. Main St.,
1E-B
Frankfort, KY 40621   502-564-4527
                              FAX: 502-564-5478
                                        chfs.ky.gov

Deborah Anderson, Commissioner
Chris Harbeck, Executive Secretary
Marnie Mountjoy, Staff Assistant
Kristi Gentry, Executive Staff Advisor
The Department for Mental Health and Mental Retardation Services contracts with fourteen regional community mental health and mental broads to provide an array of community based mental health services; operates three psychiatric hospitals and contracts with two additional hospitals; operates or contracts for 10 ICFs/MR; also operates two nursing facilities.

3487   Kentucky Department for Mental Health:
275 E. Main St.,
1E-B
Frankfort, KY 40621   502-564-4527
                              FAX: 502-564-5478
                                        chfs.ky.gov

Deborah Anderson, Commissioner
Chris Harbeck, Executive Secretary
Marnie Mountjoy, Staff Assistant
Kristi Gentry, Executive Staff Advisor
The Department for Mental Health and Mental Retardation Services contracts with fourteen regional community mental health and mental broads to provide an array of community based mental health services; operates three psychiatric hospitals and contracts with two additional hospitals; operates or contracts for 10 ICFs/MR; also operates two nursing facilities.

3488   Kentucky Department for the Blind
275 East Main Street
Frankfort, KY 40621   502-564-4754
                                         800-321-6668
                              FAX: 502-564-2951
                              TTY: 502-564-2929
                                Wayne.Thompson@ky.gov
                                     http://blind.ky.gov

Beth Cross, Executive Director
Provides career services and assistance to adults with severe visual handicaps who want to become productive in the home or work force. Also provides the Client Assistance Program established to provide advice, assistance and information available from rehabilitation programs to persons with handicaps.

3489   Kentucky Office of Aging Services
Cabinet for Health Services
275 East Main Street
Suite 1E-B
Frankfort, KY 40621   502-564-6930
                              FAX: 502-564-4595
                              TTY: 888-642-1137
                                 David.Boswell@ky.gov
                                     www.kcdd.ky.gov

Deborah Anderson, Commissioner
Chris Harbeck, Executive Secretary
Marnie Mountjoy, Staff Assistant
Kristi Gentry, Executive Staff Advisor
The Kentucky Office of Aging Services is the state agency directly responsible for programs and services for people with disabilities. Efforts are made to fully integrate the service response information that considers broad farmiliar implications.

3490   Kentucky Protection & Advocacy
100 Fair Oaks Ln 3rd Fl
Frankfort, KY 40601-1108   502-564-2967
                                         800-372-2988
                              FAX: 502-564-0848
                                         info@kypa.net
                                            kypa.net

Marsha Hockensmith, Executive Director
Protection and advocacy, Kentucky's federally-mandated protection and advocacy system, protects & promotes the disability rights of individuals through free legally-based advocacy, technical assistance, and education.

3491   Social Security: Frankfort Disability Determination
Social Security
140 Flynn Avenue
Frankfort, KY 40601   866-964-1724
                                         800-772-1213
                              FAX: 502-226-4519
                              TTY: 502-226-4519
                                         www.ssa.gov

Stephen Jones, Director
Burton Sisk, Manager

3492   Social Security: Louisville Disability Determination
Social Security
601 W Broadway
Room 101
Louisville, KY 40202-2227   866-716-9671
                                         800-772-1213
                              TTY: 502-582-5238
                                          ssa.gov

Louisiana

3493 Advocacy Center
8325 Oak Street
New Orleans, LA 70118
504-237-2337
800-960-7705
FAX: 504-522-5507
TTY: 855-861-3577
advocacycenter@advocacyla.org
advocacyla.org

Lois Simpson, Executive Director
Susan Gibbens, Volunteer
Laurie Peller, Attorney
John Felt, Chief Information Officer
The Advocacy Center is Louisiana's protection and advocacy system. AC provides free legal services to people with disabilities in designated priority areas. In addition, AC also provides legal assistance to people residing in nursing homes in Louisiana and people over 60 in Orleans, Plaquemines and St. Tammany parishes. AC ombudsmen advocate for the rights of group home and nursing home residents. Benefits specialists help people who receive public benefits to return to work or go to work.

3494 Louisiana Assistive Technology Access Network
3042 Old Forge Dr.
P O Box 14115
Baton Rouge, LA 70898
225-925-9500
800-270-6185
FAX: 225-925-9560
cporciau@latan.org
www.latan.org/

Jim Parks, President & CEO
Sandee Winchell, Executive Director
An information and training resource on Assistive Technology for the State of Louisiana. LATAN operates three regional centers to provide better access for consumers.

3495 Louisiana Center for Dyslexia and Related Learning Disorders
PO Box 2050
Thibodaux, LA 70310-1
985-448-4214
FAX: 985-448-4423
karen.chauvin@nicholls.edu
www.nicholls.edu

Karen Chauvin, Director
Jason Talbot, Assessment & Research Coor
Ashley D Munson, Senior Program Coordinator
Sue Benoit, Administrative Coordinator 3
Provides free information and referral services for diagnosis and tutoring for parents, educators, physicians and individuals with dyslexia. The voice of our membership is heard in 48 countries. Membership includes yearly journal and quarterly newsletter. Call for conference dates.

3496 Louisiana Department of Aging
Office of Elderly Affairs
PO Box 629
Baton Rouge, LA 70821-0629
225-342-9500
FAX: 225-342-5568
robin.wagner@la.gov
new.dhh.louisiana.gov/

Tara LeBlanc, Assistant Secretary
Robin Wagner, Deputy Assistant Secretary
Kirsten Clebart, Director
Annie Olivier, Director-Program Operation
Serves as a focal point for Louisiana's senior citizens and administers a broad range of home and community based services through a network of 37 Area Agencies on Aging. Serve as the focal point for the development, implementation, and administration of the public policy for the state of Louisiana, and address the needs of the state's elderly citizens.

3497 Louisiana Developmental Disability Council
PO Box 3455
626 Main Street, Suite A
Baton Rouge, LA 70821-3455
225-342-6804
800-450-8108
FAX: 225-342-1970
shawn.fleming@la.gov
www.laddc.org

Sandra Sam Beech, Chairperson
Brenda Cosse, Vice Chairperson
Sandee Winchell, Executive Director
Shawn Fleming, Deputy Director
The Council's mission is to lead and promote advocacy, capacity building, and systemic change toimprove the quality of life for individualswith developmental disabilities and their families.

3498 Louisiana Division of Mental Health
PO Box 629
Baton Rouge, LA 70821-0629
225-342-9500
FAX: 225-342-5568
rochelle.dunham@la.gov
new.dhh.louisiana.gov/index.cfm/directory/det

Dr. Rochelle Head-Dunham, Medical Director
Janice Petersen, Deputy Assistant Secretary
Cindy Rives, Deputy Assistant Secretary
Karen Stubbs, Deputy Assistant Secretary
The Office of Behavioral Health's mental health services provide a variety of treatments for people who have different types of mental illnesses.

3499 Louisiana Learning Resources System
2525 Wyandotte St
Baton Rouge, LA 70805-6464
225-355-6197
FAX: 225-357-3508

Bobbie Robertson, Administrator
Provides consultation on educational seOrvices for local schools, offers psychological testing and evaluation, maintains resource rooms in district schools and more for the blind and handicapped throughout the state.

3500 Social Security: Baton Rouge Disability Determination
Department of Social Services
5455 Bankers Ave
Baton Rouge, LA 70808
866-613-3070
800-772-1213
FAX: 225-219-9399
TTY: 225-382-2090
adren.wilson@dss.state.la.us
www.ssa.gov

Shirley Williams, Director
Ann Williamson, Manager

3501 Workers Compensation Board Louisiana
1001 North 23rd Street
Post Office Box 94094
Baton Rouge, LA 70804-9094
225-342-3111
800-259-5154
FAX: 225-342-7960
owd@lwc.la.gov
www.laworks.net

Curt Eysink, Executive Director
Carey Foy, Deputy Executive Director
Renee Ellender Roberie, Chief Financial Officer
Bryan Moore, Director
The Louisiana Workforce Commission's vision is to make Louisiana the best place in the country to get a job or grow a business, and our goal is to be the country's best workforce agency.

Maine

3502 Maine Assistive Technology Projects
University of Maine at Augusta
Georgia Institute of Technology
490 Tenth Street
Atlanta, GA 30332-0156
404-894-4960
FAX: 404-894-9320
catea@coa.gatech.edu
assistivetech.net

3503 Maine Bureau of Elder and Adult Services
11 State House Station
41 Anthony Avenue
Augusta, ME 04333
207-287-9200
800-262-2232
FAX: 207-287-9229
www.maine.gov

Ricker Hamilton, Director
AnnMarie Stevens, Administrative Assistant
Lois Emerson, Office Specialist I
Maureen Hill, Office Associate II
Adult Protective Services (APS), is responsible for providing or arranging for services to protect incapacitated and/or dependent adults in danger.

3504 Maine Department of Health and Human Services
221 State Street
Augusta, ME 04333-0040
207-287-3707
FAX: 207-287-3005
brenda.harvey@maine.gov
www.maine.gov/dhhs

Mary C. Mayhew, Commissioner
Sam Adolphsen, Chief Operating Officer
Ricker Hamilton, Deputy Commissioner of Programs
Alec Porteous, Deputy Commissioner of Finance
Provision of an array of services to people with nental illness, substance abuse issues, children with special needs and people with developmental disabilities.

3505 Maine Developmental Disabilities Council
225 Western Avenue
Suite 4
Augusta, ME 04330
207-287-4213
800-244-3990
FAX: 207-287-8001
nancy.e.cronin@maine.gov
www.maineddc.org

Nancy Cronin, Executive Director
Rachel Dyer, Associate Director
Erin Howes, Office Manager
The MDDC is a partnership of people with disabilities, their families, and agencies which identifies barriers to community inclusion, self-determination, and independence, and acts to effect positive change.

3506 Maine Division for the Blind and Visually Impaired
21 Enterprise Dr
Suite 2
Augusta, ME 04333-0073
207-624-5120
800-760-1573
FAX: 207-624-5133
TTY: 800-633-0770
mdol@maine.gov
www.maine.gov/rehab/dbvi

Harold Lewis, Director
Sandra Cavanaugh, Executive Director
Works to bring about full access to employment, independence and community integration for people with disabilities in Maine.

3507 Maine Office of Elder Services
State of Maine
11 State House Station
41 Anthony Avenue
Augusta, ME 04333
207-287-9200
800-262-2232
FAX: 207-287-9229
TTY: 800-606-0215
mdol@maine.gov
www.maine.gov/dhhs/oads/aging

James Martin, Director
Gary Wolcott, Associate Director
Romaine Turyn, Aging Service Manager
Elizabeth Gattine, Long Term Care Service Manager
The Office of Elder Services (OES), an Office within the Maine Department of Health and Human Services, promotes programs and services for older adults, their families and for people with disabilities.

3508 Maine Workers' Compensation Board
27 State House Station
Augusta, ME 04333
207-287-3751
888-801-9087
FAX: 207-287-7198
TTY:877-832-5525
www.maine.gov/wcb

Paul H Sighinolfi, Executive Director
Lindsay Lizzotte, Secretary Specialist
Gary Koocher, Management Representative
Ron Green, Labor Representative
The general mission of the Maine Workers' Compensation Board is to serve the employees and employers of the State fairly and expeditiously by ensuring compliance with the workers' compensation laws, ensuring the prompt delivery of benefits legally due, promoting the prevention of disputes, utilizing dispute resolution to reduce litigation and facilitating labor-management cooperation.

3509 Social Security: Maine Disability Determination
330 Civic Center Dr
Suite 4
Augusta, ME 04330-6325
866-882-5422
800-772-1213
TTY:207-623-4190
ssa.gov

Louis Tepin, Manager
This office makes the medical determination about whether a consumer is disabled and, therefore, medically eligible for Social Security benefits. Legally, an individual is considered disabled if he or she is unable to do any substantial gainful work activity because of a medical condition (or conditions), that has lasted, or can be expected to last for at least 12 months, or that is expected to result in death.

Maryland

3510 Health Resources & Services Administration: State Bureau of Health
Federal Government
5600 Fishers Lane
Rockville, MD 20857
301-443-2216
888-275-4772
ask@hrsa.gov
www.hrsa.gov

Diana Espinosa, Deputy Administrator
Jim Macrae, Acting Administrator
Deborah Parham Hopson, Senior Advisor
Sarah Linde, Chief Public Health Officer
Through appropriated funds, supports education programs, credentialing analysis, and development of human resources needed to staff the U.S. health care system.

3511 International Dyslexia Association: Maryland Branch
International Dyslexia Association
40 York Rd 4th floor
Baltimore, MD 21204
410-296-0232
800-222-3123
FAX: 410-321-5069
info@interdys.org
www.interdys.org

Hal Malchow, President
Eric Q. Tridas, M.D., Immediate Past President
Suzanne Carreker, Ph.D., CALT, Secretary
Ben Shifrin, M.Ed., Vice President
Nonprofit organization providing free information and referral services for diagnosis and tutoring for parents, educators, physicians, and individuals with dyslexia. The voice of our membership is heard in 48 countries. Membership includes yearly journal and quarterly newsletter. Call for conference dates.

3512 Maryland Client Assistance Program Division of Rehabilitation Services
2301 Argonne Drive
Baltimore, MD 21218-1628
410-554-9442
888-554-0334
FAX: 410-554-9362
TTY: 443-798-2840
dors@maryland.gov
dors.maryland.gov

Suzanne R. Page, DORS Director
Helps individuals with disabilities understand the rehabilitation process and receives appropriate and quality services from the Division of Rehabilitation Services and other programs and facilities providing services under the Rehabilitation Act of 1973.

3513 Maryland Department of Aging
State Office Building
301 West Preston Street
Suite 1007
Baltimore, MD 21201- 2393
410-767-1100
800-243-3425
FAX: 410-333-7943
drb@mail.ooa.state.md.us
www.mdoa.state.md.us/

Stuart Rosenthal, Chair
Sharonlee J. Vogel, Vice-Chair
Rona E. Kramer, Secretary
Sandie Callis, Commissiom Member
The Department of Aging protects the rights and quality of life of older persons in Maryland. To meet the needs of senior citizens, the Department administers programs throughout the State, primarily through local area agencies on aging.

3514 Maryland Department of Handicapped Children
201 W Preston St
Unit 50
Baltimore, MD 21201-2301
410-335-6470
www.msa.md.gov

Judson Force, Director
Children's Medical Services is a joint federal/state/local program which assists in obtaining specialized medical, surgical and related habilitative/rehabilitative evaluation and treatment services for children with special health care needs and their families. To be eligible for the program's services, an individual must be a resident of Maryland, younger than 22 years, have or be suspected of having an eligible medical condition and meet both medical and financial criteria.

3515 Maryland Developmental Disabilities Council
217 E Redwood Street
Suite 1300
Baltimore, MD 21202-3313
410-767-3670
800-305-6441
FAX: 410-333-3686
BrianC@md-council.org
www.md-council.org

Brian Cox, Executive Director
Catherine Lyle, Deputy Director
Rachel London, Director, Children & Family Poli
Kelley Malone, Director of Communications

A public policy organization comprised of people with disabilities and family members who are joined by state officials, service providers and other designated partners. The Council is an independent, self-governing organization that represents the interests of people with developmental disabilities and their families.

3516 Maryland Division of Mental Health
201 W. Preston Street
Baltimore, MD 21201
410-767-6500
877-463-3464
dhmh.healthmd@maryland.gov
www.dors.state.md.us/dors

Norma Pinette, Executive Director
Van T. Mitchell, Secretary
Our Public Health Services Division oversees vital public services to Maryland residents including infectious disease and environmental health concerns, family health services and emergency preparedness and response activities.

3517 National Maternal and Child Health Bureau
Rm 1805
5600 Fishers Ln
Rockville, MD 20852-1750
301-443-2216
888-275-4772
ask@hrsa.gov
hrsa.gov

Michael C. Lu, Associate Administrator
Laura Kavanagh, Deputy Associate Administrator
Natasha Coulouris, Senior Advisor
Angela Hooten, Executive Officer
Offers information, books and pamphlets to professionals, parents and children facing health issues or disabilities.

3518 Social Security: Baltimore Disability Determination
711 West 40th Street
Ste 415 Rotunda Mall
Baltimore, MD 21211-2120
800-772-1213
TTY:800-325-0778
ssa.gov

3519 Workers Compensation Board Maryland
10 East Baltimore Street
Baltimore, MD 21202-1641
410-864-5100
800-492-0479
FAX: 410-333-8122
info@wcc.state.md.us
www.wcc.state.md.us

R. Karl Aumann, Chairperson
Mary K. Ahearn, Chief Executive Officer
David E. Jones, Chief Financial Officer
Joyce McNemar, Chief Information Officer

Massachusetts

3520 Center for Public Representation
22 Green Street
Northampton, MA 01060-3708
413-586-6024
FAX: 413-586-5711
info@cpr-ma.org
centerforpublicrep.org

Bob Agoglia, President
Nickie Chandler, Clerk/Treasurer
Bob Riedel, Director
Neal Rosen, Esq., Director
The Center seeks to improve the quality of lives of people with mental illness and other disabilities through the systemic enforcement of their legal rights while promoting improvements in services for citizens with disabilities

3521 International Dyslexia Association of New England
40 York Rd 4th floor
Baltimore, MD 21204
410-296-0232
800-222-3123
FAX: 410-321-5069
info@interdys.org
www.interdys.org

Hal Malchow, President
Eric Q. Tridas, M.D., Immediate Past President
Suzanne Carreker, Ph.D., CALT, Secretary
Ben Shifrin, M.Ed., Vice President

Provides free information and referral services for diagnosis and tutoring for parents, educators, physicians, and individuals with dyslexia in Connecticut, Maine, New Hampshire, Rhode Island, and Vermont. The voice of our membership is heard in 48 countries. Membership includes yearly journal and quarterly newsletter. Call for conference dates.

3522 Massachusetts Assistive Technology Partnership
Children s Hospital Boston
1295 Boylston St
Suite 310
Boston, MA 02215-3407
617-355-7820
800-848-8867
FAX: 617-355-6345
info@matp.org
www.mass.gov/eohhs/gov/departments/dds/assist

Marylyn Howe, Project Director
Pat Hill, Training Coordinator

A statewide program promoting assistive technology devices and services for persons with all disabilities.

3523 Massachusetts Client Assistance Program
Massachusetts Office on Disability
1 Ashburton Pl
Suite 1305
Boston, MA 02108-1518
617-727-7440
800-322-2020
james.aprea@state.ma.us
www.mass.gov/anf/employment-equal-access-disa

Barbara Lybarger, Assistant Director
Myra Berloff, Director
Michael Dumont, Assistant Director
Jeffrey Dougan, Assistant Director

Provides advocacy and information services.

3524 Massachusetts Department of Mental Health
25 Staniford St
Boston, MA 02114-2503
617-626-8000
800-221-0053
FAX: 617-727-9842
TTY:617-727-9842
dmhinfo@dmh.state.ma.us
http://www.mass.gov/eohhs/gov/departments/dmh

Eileen Elias, Commissioner
Michele Anzaldi, Site Director

The Massachusetts Department of Mental Health (DMH) sets the standards for the operation of mental health facilities and community residential programs and provides clinical, rehabilitative and supportive services for adults with serious mental illness, and children and adolescents with serious mental illness or serious emotional disturbance.

3525 Massachusetts Developmental Disabilities Council
100 Hancock Street
Second Floor, Suite 201
Quincy, MA 02169-4398
617-770-7676
FAX: 617-770-1987
TTY:617-770-9499
adelia.deltrecco@state.ma.us
www.state.ma.us/mddc/

Daniel Shannon, Executive Director
Faith Behum, Disability Policy Specialist
Kristin Britton, Director of Public Policy
Adelia DelTrecco, Member Services Coordinator

Group of citizens which analyzes needs of people with severe, lifelong disabilities and works to improve public policy. MDDC

produces several publications and has committees and a grants program to study and advocate for changes in the service system.

3526 Social Security: Boston Disability Determination
110 Chauncy Street
Boston, MA 02111
617-727-7600
800-772-1213
TTY:800-882-2040
www.socialsecurity.gov

Michael F. Bertrand, Commissioner

3527 Workers Compensation Board Massachusetts
Rm 211
1 Ashburton Pl
Boston, MA 02108-1518
617-626-7122
FAX: 617-727-1090
www.state.ma.us/dia

Russell Gilfus, Manager

The Massachusetts Workers' Compensation system is in place to make sure that workers are protected by insurance if they are injured on the job or contract a work-related illness. Under this system, employers are required by Massachusetts General Laws c. 152, 25A to provide workers' compensation (WC) insurance coverage to all their employees.

Michigan

3528 Department of Blind Rehabilitation
Western Michigan University
1903 W Michigan Ave
Kalamazoo, MI 49008-5218
269-387-3455
FAX: 269-387-3567
g.dennis@wmich.edu
www.wmich.edu/visionstudies

James Leja, Chair
Charles Adams, Faculty Specialist I
Gayla Dennis, Office Coordinator
Jeannyne Depoian, Office Associate

The Department of Blindness and Low Vision Studies at Western Michigan University is recognized internationally as the oldest, largest and best program of its kind. It originated in 1961 with a graduate degree in Orientation and Mobility, responding to the need for professionals to rehabilitate the many military personnel blinded during World War Two and the Korean War.

3529 Michigan Association for Deaf and Hard of Hearing
5236 Dumond Court
Suite C
Lansing, MI 48917-6001
517-487-0066
800-968-7327
FAX: 517-487-0202
TTY: 517-487-2586
info@madhh.org
www.madhh.org

Nancy Asher, Executive Director
Pat Walton, Office Manager

MADHH is a statewide collaboration agency dedicated to improving the lives of people who are deaf and hard of hearing through leadership in education, advocacy & services. Interpreter IC print-out, assistive devices available.

3530 Michigan Association for Deaf, and Hard of Hearing
5236 Dumond Court
Suite C
Lansing, MI 48917-6001
517-487-0066
800-968-7327
FAX: 517-487-2586
info@madhh.org
www.madhh.org

Nancy Asher, Executive Director
Pat Walton, Office Manager

MADHH is a statewide collaboration agency dedicated to improving the lives of people who are deaf and hard of hearing through leadership in education, advocacy and services.

3531 **Michigan Client Assistance Program**
4095 Legacy Pkwy
Ste 500
Lansing, MI 48911-4264

517-487-1755
800-288-5923
FAX: 517-487-0827
TTY: 800-288-5923
molson@mpas.org
www.mpas.org

Kate Pew Wolters, President
Thomas Landry, 1st Vice President
John McCulloch, 2nd Vice President
Elmer L. Cerano, Executive Director

The Client Assistance Program (CAP) assists people who are seeking or receiving services from Michigan Rehabilitation Services, Consumer Choice Programs, Michigan Commission for the Blind, Centers for Independent Living, and Supported Employment and Transition Programs. The CAP program is part of Michigan Protection and Advocacy Service, Inc.

3532 **Michigan Coalition for Staff Development and School Improvement**
12236 6 1/2 Mile Road
MCES
Battle Creek, MI 49014-1062

269-967-2086
800-444-2014
FAX: 517-371-1170
michigances.org

3533 **Michigan Commission for the Blind - Gaylord**
Ste 102
209 W 1st St
Gaylord, MI 49735-1386

989-732-2448
800-292-4200
FAX: 989-731-3587
www.michigan.gov

Judy Terwilliger, Manager

The mission of the Michigan Commission for the Blind (MCB) is to provide opportunity to individuals who are blind or visually impaired to achieve employability and/or function independently in society. The MCB vision is that someday it will be said that Michigan is a great place for blind people to live, learn, work, raise a family, and enjoy life

3534 **Michigan Commission for the Blind**
Michigan Dept Of Energy, Labor & Economic Growth
PO Box 30652
Lansing, MI 48909-8152

517-373-2062
800-292-4200
FAX: 517-335-5140
TTY: 517-373-4025
turneys@michigan.gov
www.michigan.gov/mcb

Patrick Cannon, State Director

The Michigan Commision for the blind is a state government agency that provides state and federally funded training and other services to individuals who are legally blind (blind and visually impaired). Services are provided to people of all ages throughout the state of Michigan toward the goal of employment and/or independence.

3535 **Michigan Commission for the Blind Training Center**
PO Box 30652
Lansing, MI 48909

517-373-2062
800-292-4200
FAX: 517-335-5140
TTY: 517-373-4025
mossc@michigan.gov
www.michigan.gov/mcb

Cheryl L Heibeck, Director
Bruce Schultz, Assistant Director

Residential facility that provides instruction to legally blind adults in braille, computer operation and assistive technology, handwriting, cane travel, cooking, personal management, industrial arts and also crafts. During training students will develop career plans which may include work experience, internships, volunteer opprtunities and even part-time paid employment.

3536 **Michigan Commission for the Blind: Escanaba**
305 Ludington St
State Office Bldg., 1st Floor
Escanaba, MI 49829-4029

906-786-8602
800-323-2535
FAX: 906-786-4638
michigan.gov/mcb

Bernie Kramer, Manager

The mission of the Michigan Commission for the Blind (MCB) is to provide opportunity to individuals who are blind or visually impaired to achieve employability and/or function independently in society. The MCB vision is that someday it will be said that Michigan is a great place for blind people to live, learn, work, raise a family, and enjoy life

3537 **Michigan Commission for the Blind: Flint**
125 E Union St
Seventh Floor
Flint, MI 48502-2041

810-760-2030
800-292-4200
FAX: 810-760-2032
www.dlcq.state.mi.us

Debbie Wilson, Manager

Vocational and Independent living skills training for individuals who are legally blind.

3538 **Michigan Commission for the Blind: Grand Rapids**
250 Ottawa Avenue
Grand Rapids, MI 49503-4029

906-786-8602
800-323-2535
FAX: 906-786-4638
michigan.gov/mcb

Bernie Kramer, Manager

The mission of the Michigan Commission for the Blind (MCB) is to provide opportunity to individuals who are blind or visually impaired to achieve employability and/or function independently in society. The MCB vision is that someday it will be said that Michigan is a great place for blind people to live, learn, work, raise a family, and enjoy life

3539 **Michigan Council of the Blind and Visually Impaired (MCBVI)**
Neal Freeling
350 Ottawa Ave NW
Grand Rapids, MI 49503-2316

616-356-0180
800-292-4200
FAX: 616-356-0199
michigan.gov/mcb

Bernie Kramer, Manager

MCBVI is a diverse group of very friendly people from around the state working together to improve the lives of all citizens who are blind or visually impaired.

3540 **Michigan Department of Handicapped Children**
3423 N Martin Luther King Jr Blvd
Lansing, MI 48906-2934

517-484-9312
FAX: 517-484-9836

Alan Curtiss, President
Bobbie Butler, Manager

3541 **Michigan Developmental Disabilies Council**
201 Townsend Street
Suite 120
Lansing, MI 48910-1646

517-335-3158
FAX: 517-335-2751
TTY:517-335-3171
mdch-dd-council@michigan.gov
www.michigan.gov/ddcouncil

Nick Lyon, Director
Nancy Grijalva, Assistant
Tim Becker, Chief Deputy Director
Trish Ray, Assistant

The Michigan DD Council is a group of citizens from across the state. Its membership is made up of: people with developmental disabilities; people from families who have, among their members, people with developmental disabilities; and professionals from state and local agencies charged with assisting people with developmental disabilities.

3542   Michigan Office of Services to the Aging
P.O. Box 30676
Lansing, MI 48909-8176
517-373-8230
FAX: 517-373-4092
OSAInfo@michigan.gov
www.michigan.gov/osa

Wendi Middleton, Division Director
Kari Sederburg, Director
Carol Dye, Senior Executive Assistant
Annette Gamez, Executive Assistant
State unit on aging; allocates and monitors state and federal funds for the Older American Act services: nutrition, community services, administers home and community based waiver, develops programs through Area Agencies on Aging, advocates on behalf of seniors with legislature, governor, state departments, federal government, responsible for state planning of aging services, develops formula for distribution of state and federal funds.

3543   Michigan Protection & Advocacy Service
4095 Legacy Pkwy
Ste 500
Lansing, MI 48911-4264
517-487-1755
800-288-5923
FAX: 517-487-0827
molson@mpas.org
www.mpas.org

Kate Pew Wolters, President
Thomas Landry, 1st Vice President
John McCulloch, 2nd Vice President
Elmer L. Cerano, Executive Director
People with disabilities have to deal with a wide variety of issues. TThey try to answer any questions you may have relating to disability. They have experience in the following areas: discrimination in education, employment, housing, and public places; abuse and neglect; Social Security benefits; Medicaid, Medicare and other insurance; housing; Vocational Rehabilitation; HIV/AIDS issues; and many other disability-related topics

3544   Michigan Rehabilitation Services
300 N. Washington Sq.
Lansing, MI 48913
517-335-4590
888-784-7328
FAX: 517-373-0059
TTY: 517-373-4035
zimmermanng@michigan.org
www.michigan.org

George Zimmermann, Vice President
Michelle Begnoche, Communications Specialist
Bonnie Fink, Travel Consultant Coordinator
David Lorenz, Public and Industry Relations Ma
A state and federally funded program that helps persons with disabilities prepare for and fund a job that matches their interests and abilities. Assistance is also available to workers with disabilities who are having difficulty keeping a job. A person is eligible for MRS services if he or she has a disability, is unemployed and needs vocational rehabilitation services to prepare for and find a job or independent living services.

3545   Social Security Administration
1100 West High Rise
6401 Security Blvd.
Baltimore, MD 21235-3878
517-393-3876
800-772-1213
FAX: 517-393-4686
TTY: 800-325-0778
jennifer.bower@ssa.gov
ssa.gov

Tiffany L. Flick, Executive Secretary
Michael J. Astrue, Commissioner
Carolyn W. Colvin, Deputy Commissioner
We deliver services through a nationwide network of over 1,400 offices that include regional offices, field offices, card centers, teleservice centers, processing centers, hearing offices, the Appeals Council, and our State and territorial partners, the Disability Determination Services. We also have a presence in U.S.

embassies around the globe. For the public, we are the face of the government. The rich diversity of our employees mirrors the public we serve.

3546   State of Michigan Workers' Compensation Agency
PO Box 30016
Lansing, MI 48909-7516
888-396-5041
FAX: 517-322-1808
wcinfo@michigan.gov
www.michigan.gov/wca/

Mark C. Long, Director
Jack A. Nolish, Deputy Director
Julie Lenneman, Administrative Assistant
Ted Day, Division Manager
Michigan's injured workers and their employers are governed by the Workers' Disability Compensation Act. This Act was first adopted in 1912 and provides compensation to workers who suffer an injury on the job and protects employers' liability. The mission of the Workers' Compensation Agency is to efficiently administer the Act and provide prompt, courteous and impartial service to all customers.

Minnesota

3547   International Dyslexia Association: Minnesota Branch
International Dyslexia Association
5021 Vernon Avenue South
#159
Minneapolis, MN 55436-2102
612-486-4242
800-222-3123
FAX: 410-321-5069
info@ida-umb.org
www.ida-umb.org

Tom Strewler, President
Susan Hegland, First Vice President
Colee Bean, Second Vice President
Brian Pittenger, Treasurer
UMBIDA-the Upper Midwest Branch of the International Dyslexia Association (IDA-serves the residents of Minnesota, North Dakota, South Dakota, and Winnipeg, Canada and offers: local educational conferences about dyslexia and related subjects, Orton-Gillingham training for teachers, tutors, and parents, Quarterly speaker series, member discounts on conferences, information line, and tutor referral.

3548   Minnesota Assistive Technology Project
STAR
358 Centennial Office Building
658 Cedar Street
Saint Paul, MN 55155-1402
651-201-2640
888-234-1267
800-627-3529
FAX: 651-282-6671
star.program@state.mn.us
mn.gov/star/about.htm

Chuck Rassbach, Program Director
Kim Moccia, Program Coordinator
Jennie Delisi, Resource Specialist
Joan Gillum, Contracts Coordinator
A statewide program promoting assistive technology devices and services for persons of all ages with all disabilities.

3549   Minnesota Board on Aging
P.O. Box 64976
Saint Paul, MN 55164-0976
651-431-2500
800-882-6262
800-333-2433
FAX: 651-431-7453
TTY: 800-627-3529
mba@sate.mn.us
www.mnaging.org

Don Samuelson, Chair
Jean Wood, Executive Director
Leonard Axelrod, Board Member
Tracy Keibler, Board Member

A state unit on aging for the state of Minnesota. Funds 14 area agencies on aging throughout the state that provide services at the local level. The mission is to keep older people in the homes or places of residence for as long as possible.

3550 Minnesota Children with Special Needs, Minnesota Department of Health
P.O.Box 64882
Saint Paul, MN 55164-0882
651-201-3650
800-728-5420
FAX: 651-201-3655
TTY: 651-201-5797
health.cyshn@state.mn.us
www.health.state.mn.us/mcshn
Dr. Edward Ehlinger, Commissioner
Daniel L. Pollock, Deputy Commissioner
Jeanne F. Ayers, Assistant Commissioner
Barb Dalbec, Director
Minnesota Children with Special Health Needs (MCSHN) provides leadership through partnerships with families and other key stakeholders to improve the access and quality of all systems impacting children and youth with special health care needs and their families.

3551 Minnesota Department of Labor & Industry Workers Compensation Division
443 Lafayette Rd N
Saint Paul, MN 55155-4301
651-284-5005
800-342-5354
TTY:651-297-4198
dli.communications@state.mn.us
doli.state.mn.us
Ken Petersom, Commissioner
Jessica Looman, Deputy Commissioner
James Honerman, Communications
Wendy Legge, General Counsil
To reduce the impact of work related injuries for employees and employers. Advice is given and questions answered on the toll-free number.

3552 Minnesota Disability Law Center
430 1st Avenue North
Suite 300
Minneapolis, MN 55401- 1780
612-334-5970
800-292-4150
FAX: 612-334-5755
TTY: 612-332-4668
website@mylegalaid.org
mylegalaid.org/about/our-work/disability-law
Mary L. Knoblauch, Chair
Cathy Haukedahl, Executive Director
Andrea Kaufman, Director of Development
Lisa Cohen, Deputy Director of Operations
Provides free, civil, legal assistance to Minnesotans with disabilities on issues related to their disability.

3553 Minnesota Governor's Council on Developmental Disabilities GCDD
370 Centennial Office Building
658 Cedar Street
Saint Paul, MN 55155-1603
651-296-4018
877-348-0505
FAX: 651-297-7200
TTY: 800-627-3529
admin.dd@state.mn.us
www.mncdd.org
David R. Johnson, Chair
Dawn D. Bly, Council Member
Mary Hauff, Council Member
Ashley Bailey, Council Member
The mission of the Minnesota Governor's Council on Developmental Disabilities is to provide information, education, and training to build knowledge, develop skills, and change attitudes that will lead to increased independence, productivity, self determination, integration and inclusion (IPSII) for people with developmental disabilities and their families.

3554 Minnesota Mental Health Division
Human Services Building
PO Box 64981
Saint Paul, MN 55164-0981
651-431-2225
800-366-5411
FAX: 651-431-7418
TTY: 800-627-3529
dhs.info@state.mn.us
www.dhs.state.mn.us
Lucinda Jesson, Commissioner
Anne M. Barry, Deputy Commissioner
Jennifer DeCubellis, Assistant Commissioner
Loren Colman, Assistant Commissioner
Oversees the provision of services to people with mental illness in the state of Minnesota. Services are provided on the local level through a network of 87 county social service departments.

3555 Minnesota Protection & Advocacy for Persons with Disabilities
Minnesota Disability Law Center
2324 University Avenue West
Suite 101B
Saint Paul, MN 55114-1742
651-228-9105
800-292-4150
FAX: 651-222-0745
statesupport@mnlegalservices.org
www.mnlegalservices.org/mdlc
Mary Kaczorek, Supervising Attorney
Ann Conroy, Office Manager
Elsa Marshall, Education for Justice Coordinato
Emily Good, Legal Project Manager
Provide public legal information on legal issues impacting the rights of low-income Minnesotans

3556 Minnesota State Council on Disability(MSCOD)
121 E 7th Place
Suite 107
Saint Paul, MN 55101-2114
651-361-7800
800-945-8913
FAX: 651-296-5935
council.disability@state.mn.us
www.disability.state.mn.us
Joan Willshire, Executive Director
Linda Gremillion, Business Operations Manager
Margot Imdieke Cross, Accessibility Specialist
David Fenley, Legislative Coordinator
The MSCOD collaborates, advocates, advises and provide technical information to expand opportunities, increase the quality of life and empower all persons with disabilities. This mission is accomplished by: providing information, referral and technical assistance to thousands of individuals every year via email, letter or telephone; through trainings on a variety of disability related topics; through publications and its web site; and through its advocacy and advisory work.

3557 Minnesota State Services for the Blind
2200 University Avenue West
Suite 240
Saint Paul, MN 55114-1840
651-539-2300
800-652-9000
FAX: 651-649-5927
TTY: 651-642-0506
star.program@state.mn.us
http://mn.gov/deed/job-seekers/blind-visual-i
Richard Strong, Executive Director
Kenneth Trebelhorn, Council Member
Jan Bailey, Chair
Steve Jacobson, Council Member
State agency serving blind and visually impaired persons with rehabilitation, information access, assistive technology, training and job placement services. Extensive older blind program.

3558 **Social Security: St. Paul Disability Determination**
5210 Perry Robinson
Lansing, MI 48911-3878
877-512-5944
800-772-1213
FAX: 517-393-4686
TTY: 800-325-0778
jennifer.bower@ssa.gov
www.ssa.gov

Karena L. Kilgore, Executive Secretary
Carolyn W. Colvin, Commissioner
Carolyn W. Colvin, Deputy Commissioner
James A. Kissko, Chief of Staff
We deliver services through a nationwide network of over 1,400 offices that include regional offices, field offices, card centers, teleservice centers, processing centers, hearing offices, the Appeals Council, and our State and territorial partners, the Disability Determination Services. We also have a presence in U.S. embassies around the globe. For the public, we are the face of the government. The rich diversity of our employees mirrors the public we serve.

Mississippi

3559 **International Dyslexia Association: Mississippi Branch**
1997 Atkins Rd.
Ruston, LA 71270
985-414-2575
800-222-3123
FAX: 410-321-5069
alicehiginbotham@hotmail.com
http://www.ladyslexia.com/LaBIDA/Welcome.ht ml
Alice Higginbotham, President
Maureen Landry, Vice President/Chair of Public
Becky Clingman, Branch Council Rep
Dawn Amy, Director/Chair Education
It is the mission of the Louisiana Branch to provide information and resources to parents, educators, students and the community in a way that creates a clear and positive understanding of dyslexia and related language learning needs so that every individual has the opportunity to lead a productive and fulfilling life for the benefit of society.

3560 **Mississippi Assistive Technology Division**
1281 Highway 51
PO Box 1698
Jackson, MS 39215-1698
601-853-5160
800-443-1000
FAX: 601-853-5158
www.mdrs.ms.gov
Jean Massey, Superintendent of Education
Carey Wright, Superintendent of Education
Jack Virden, Chairman
Diana Mikula, Executive Director
A statewide program promoting assistive technology devices and services for persons of all ages with all disabilities.

3561 **Mississippi Bureau of Mental Retardation**
1101 Robert E. Lee Bulding
239 North Lamar Street
Jackson, MS 39201
601-359-1288
877-210-8513
FAX: 601-359-6295
TTY: 601-359-6230
ed.legrand@dmh.state.ms.us
www.dmh.state.ms.us
Sampat Shivangi, M.D., Chair
George Harrison, Vice Chair
Edwin C. Legrand, Executive Director
Kris Jones, Bureau Director of Quality Manag
Since its inception in 1974, the Mississippi Department of Mental Health has endeavored to provide services of the highest quality through a statewide service delivery system. As one of the major state agencies in Mississippi, the Department of Mental Health provides a network of services to persons who experience problems with mental illness, alcohol and/or drug abuse/dependence, or who have intellectual and developmental disabilities. Services are provided through an array of facilities and ag

3562 **Mississippi Client Assistance Program**
Mississippi Department of Rehabilitation Services
500-G East Woodrow Wilson Drive
P.O. Box 4958
Jackson, MS 39296
601-982-7051
FAX: 601-982-1951
www.msdisabilities.com
Dr. Ken Cleveland, President
Presley Posey, Executive Director
Dr. Michael Ogburn, Executive Director
David Cleland, Executive Director
Advocacy program for clients/client applicants for state of MS vocational services.

3563 **Mississippi Department of Mental Health**
1101 Robert E Lee Bldg
239 North Lamar Street
Jackson, MS 39201
601-359-1288
877-240-8513
FAX: 601-359-6295
TTY: 601-359-6230
ed.legrand@dmh.state.ms.us
dmh.state.ms.us
Sampat Shivengi, M.D., Chair
George N. Harrison, Vice Chair
Edwin C. Legrand, Executive Director
Kris Jones, Bureau Director of Quality Manag
Administers Mississippi's public programs of serving persons with mental illness, mental retardation, alcohol and substance abuse problems, and alzheimer's disease and related dementia.

3564 **Mississippi Division of Aging and Adult Services**
Mississippi Department Of Human Services
750 North State Street
Jackson, MS 39202-3033
601-355-5536
800-345-6347
877-882-4916
FAX: 601-359-3664
webspinner@mdhs.state.ms.us
www.mdhs.state.ms.us/
Donald R. Taylor, Executive Director
Julia M. Todd, Director
Judy Collins, Director
Mary Scott, Director
Protects the rights of older citizens while expanding their opportunities and access to quality services.

3565 **Mississippi State Department of Health**
Children s Medical Program
570 East Woodrow Wilson Drive
Post Office Box 1700
Jackson, MS 39216-1700
601-576-7400
866-458-4948
FAX: 601-364-7447
web@HealthyMS.com
www.msdh.state.ms.us
Larry Clark, Director
Vickey Berryman, Director, Bureau of Licensure
Jim Craig, Director, Office of Health Pro
Tim Darnell, Director, MSDH Field Services
Financial assistance to families of children with physical handicaps. Rehabilitative in nature and has as its goal the correction or reduction of physical handicaps. Eligibility determined by diagnosis and provided to children from birth to age twenty-one. Financial eligibility is determined by factors of family income, family size, estimated cost of treatment and family liabilities. Categories include, but are not limited to: orthopedic, congenital heart defects, cerebral palsy, etc.

3566 Mississippi: Workers Compensation Commission
1428 Lakeland Dr
P.O. Box 5300, 39296-5300
Jackson, MS 39216-4718
601-987-4200
866-473-6922
FAX: 601-987-4220
mwcc.state.ms.us
www.mwcc.state.ms.us

Liles Williams, Chairman
John Junkin, Commissioner
Debra Gibbs, Commissioner
Cindy Polk Wilson, Administrative Judge
Our goal is to provide the public with useful information regarding Workers' Compensation in the state of Mississippi.

Missouri

3567 Institute for Human Development
University of Missouri-Kansas City
215 W. Pershing Road
6th floor
Kansas City, MO 64108- 2639
816-235-1770
800-444-0821
FAX: 888-503-3107
TTY: 800-452-1185
beckmanncc@umkc.edu
www.ihd.umkc.edu

Carl F. Calkins, Ph.D., Director
Kay Conklin, Training Director
Cindy Beckmann, Assistant to the Director
Kathy Fuger, Director, Early Childhood and Yo
A statewide program promoting person-centered planning and services for persons of all ages with all disabilities.

3568 Missouri Division Of Developmental Disabilities
Missouri Department Of Mental Health
1706 E. Elm St.
P.O.Box 687
Jefferson City, MO 65102
573-751-4122
800-364-9687
FAX: 573-751-8224
ddmail@dmh.mo.gov
www.dmh.mo.gov

Jay Nixon, Governor
Keith Schafer, Ed.D., Director
Bob Bax, Deputy Director
Rikki J. Wright, J.D., General Counsel
The Missouri Department of Mental Health was first established as a cabinet-level state agency by the Omnibus State Government Reorganization Act, effective July 1, 1974. State law provides three principal missions for the department: (1) the prevention of mental disorders, developmental disabilities, substance abuse, and compulsive gambling; (2) the treatment, habilitation, and rehabilitation of Missourians who have those conditions; and (3) the improvement of public understanding and attitudes

3569 Missouri Protection & Advocacy Services
925 S Country Club Dr
Jefferson City, MO 65109-4510
573-893-3333
866-777-7199
FAX: 573-893-4231
TTY: 800-735-2966
mopasjc@embarqmail.com
moadvocacy.org

Joe Wrinkle, Chair
Barbara H. French, Vice Chair
Shawn De Loyola, Executive Director
Susan Pritchard-Green, Secretary/Treasurer
MO P&A potects the rights of individuals with disabilities by providing advocacy and legal services for disability related issues. As Missouri's Protection and Advocacy system, Mo P&A investigates allegations of abuse, neglect, death, and violations of rights against individuals with disabilities. Those who contact Mo P&A can receive information, referrals, advocacy services or legal counsel provided through one of nine federally-funded programs.

3570 Missouri Rehabilitation Services for the Blind
615 Howerton Court
PO Box 2320
Jefferson City, MO 65102-2320
573-751-3221
800-592-6004
FAX: 573-751-3091
askrsb@dss.mo.gov
www.dss.mo.gov/fsd/rsb/

Mark Laird, Executive Director
Ronald J. Levy, Director
Brian Kinkade, Deputy Director
Jennifer Tidball, Division Director
Offers services for the totally blind, legally blind, visually impaired, including counseling, educational, recreational, rehabilitation, computer training and professional training services.

3571 Social Security: Jefferson City Disability Determination
129 SCOTT STATION ROAD
Jefferson City, MO 65101-4421
877-405-9803
800-772-1213
FAX: 517-393-4686
TTY: 800-325-0778
jennifer.bower@ssa.gov
www.ssa.gov

Karena L. Kilgore, Executive Secretary
Carolyn W. Colvin, Commissioner
Carolyn W. Colvin, Deputy Commissioner
James A. Kissko, Chief of Staff
We deliver services through a nationwide network of over 1,400 offices that include regional offices, field offices, card centers, teleservice centers, processing centers, hearing offices, the Appeals Council, and our State and territorial partners, the Disability Determination Services. We also have a presence in U.S. embassies around the globe. For the public, we are the face of the government. The rich diversity of our employees mirrors the public we serve.

3572 Workers Compensation Board Missouri
Department of Labor and Industrial Realtions
421 East Dunkin Street
P.O. Box 58
Jefferson City, MO 65102-0058
573-751-4231
800-775-2667
800-320-2519
FAX: 573-751-4945
workerscomp@labor.mo.gov
labor.mo.gov/DWC/

Butch Albert, Chairman
James Avery, Commissioner
Curtis E. Chick, Commissioner
Ryan McKenna, Department Director
The Missouri Division of Workers' Compensation administers the programs providing services to all stake holders including workers who have been injured on the job or been exposed to occupational disease arising out of and in the course of employment. The Division makes sure that an injured worker receives benefits that he/she is entitled to under the Missouri Workers' Compensation law. The Division's Administrative Law Judges have the authority to approve settlements or issue awards after a hear

Montana

3573 Addictive & Mental Disorders Division
555 Fuller Ave
PO Box 202905
Helena, MT 59620-2905
406-444-3964
FAX: 406-444-4435
lothompson@mt.gov
http://www.dphhs.mt.gov/amdd/

Lou Thompson, Administrator
Joan Cassidy, Chemical Dependency Bureau Chief
E. Lee Simes, Medical Director
Deb Matteucci, Behavioral Health Program Facili
The mission of the Addictive and Mental Disorders Division (AMDD) of the Montana Department of Public Health and Hu-

man Services is to implement and improve an appropriate state-wide system of prevention, treatment, care, and rehabilitation for Montanans with mental disorders or addictions to drugs or alcohol.

3574 Disability Rights Montana
1022 Chestnut Street
Helena, MT 59601-890
    406-449-2344
    800-245-4743
    FAX: 406-449-2418
    TTY: 406-449-2344
    advocate@disabilityrightsmt.org
    www.disabilityrightsmt.org/janda3/
Bernadette Franks-Ongoy, Executive Director
Kelli Kaufman, Director of Finance & Administra
Steve Heaverlo, Director of Programs/Advocacy Sp
Laurie t Danforth, Paralegal/Executive Suppor
Protects and advocates the human and legal rights of Montanans with mental and physical disabilities while advancing dignity, equality, and self-determination. Designated federal P&A, with AT, CAP, PADD, PAIMI and PAIR programs. Advocacy and legal services for abuse, neglect, rights violations, access, discrimination in employment, accommodations and housing, and assistance with vocational rehabilitation/visual services.

3575 MonTECH
700 SW Higgins Ave.
Suite 250
Missoula, MT 59803
    406-243-5751
    877-243-5511
    FAX: 406-243-4730
    montech@ruralinstitute.umt.edu
    www.montech.ruralinstitute.umt.edu
Kathleen Laurin, Program Director
Chris Clasby, Program Coordinator
Leslie Mullette
Specialzing in Assistive Technology and oversee a variety of AT related grants and contracts. The overall goal is to develop a comprehensive, statewide system of assistive technology related assistance. Striving to ensure that all people in Montana with disabilities have equitable access to assistive technology devices and services in order to enhance their independence, productivity and quality of life.

3576 Montana Blind & Low Vision Services
111 N Last Chance Gulch, Suite 4C
PO Box 4210
Helena, MT 59604-4210
    406-444-2590
    877-296-1197
    FAX: 406-444-3632
    lothompson@mt.gov
    http://www.dphhs.mt.gov/vocrehab/blvs/
Lou Thompson, Administrator
Joan Cassidy, Chemical Dependency Bureau Chief
E. Lee Simes, Medical Director
Deb Matteucci, Behavioral Health Program Facili
Mission: promoting work and independence for Montanans with disabilities.

3577 Montana Council on Developmental Disabilities
2714 Billings Ave
Helena, MT 59601-9767
    406-443-4332
    866-443-4332
    FAX: 406-443-4192
    deborah@mtcdd.or
    www.mtcdd.org
Deborah Swingley, CEO/Executive Director
Dee Burrell, Contract Manager
The Council is made up of Montanans both with and without developmental disabilities, who believe in improving the lives of Montana's citizens who have a disability. We concentrate on issues related to self-determination, education, employment, transportation, housing, recreation, health care, community inclusion and the overall quality of life of people with developmental disabilities. As a Council we are committed to both question, and action as we work to discover and promote creative ways t

3578 Montana Department of Aging
Room 210
111 Sanders
Helena, MT 59604
    406-444-7734
    FAX: 406-444-3465
    www.agingcare.com
Keith Messmer, Manager
Jeff Sturm, President

3579 Montana Department of Handicapped Children
111 North Sanders Street
Helena, MT 59620
    406-444-7734
    FAX: 406-444-3465
    dphhs.mt.gov
Keith Messmer, Manager

3580 Montana Protection & Advocacy for Persons with Disabilities
1022 Chestnut Street
Helena, MT 59601-820
    406-449-2344
    800-245-4743
    FAX: 406-449-2418
    TTY: 406-449-2344
    advocate@disabilityrightsmt.org
    www.disabilityrightsmt.org/janda3/
Susie McIntyre, President
Will Warberg, Sales and Marketing Manager
Bernadette Franks-Ongoy, Executive Director
Kelli Kaufman, Director of Finance & Administra
Disability Rights Montana is the federally-mandated civil rights protection and advocacy system for Montana. We have the legal authority to represent almost any person with a disability.

3581 Montana State Fund
P.O.Box 4759
Helena, MT 59604-4759
    406-495-5000
    800-332-6102
    FAX: 406-495-5020
    TTY: 406-495-5030
    www.montanastatefund.com
Elizabeth Best, Chairman
Montana State Fund is committed to the health and economic prosperity of Montana through superior service, leadership and caring individuals, working in an environment of teamwork, creativity and trust.

3582 Social Security: Helena Disability Determination
10 W 15th St
Ste 1600
Helena, MT 59626-9704
    406-441-1270
    800-772-1213
    TTY:406-441-1278
    www.socialsecurity.gov
Karena L. Kilgore, Executive Secretary
Carolyn W. Colvin, Commissioner
Carolyn W. Colvin, Deputy Commissioner
James A. Kissko, Chief of Staff
Social Security offers online information and services to third parties who do business with them.

Nebraska

3583 International Dyslexia Association: Nebraska Branch
40 York Rd.
4th Floor
Baltimore, MD 21204
    410-296-0232
    800-222-3123
    FAX: 410-321-5069
    carolyn.brandle@ne-ida.com
    www.interdys.org
Hal Malchow, President
Elsa Cardenas-Hagan, Vice President
Ben Shifrin, Vice President
Kristen Penczek, Interim Executive Director

The Nebraska Branch of the International Dyslexia Association is a 501(c)(3), non-profit organization dedicated to the study and treatment of dyslexia and related learning differences. This Branch was formed in 1981 to increase public awareness of dyslexia throughout Nebraska, and to serve individuals with dyslexia and their families. The organization includes professionals in the area of learning disabilities education, counseling and medicine as well as dylexics and their families and friends.

3584 Nebraska Advocacy Services
134 S 13th St
Suite 600
Lincoln, NE 68508-1930   402-474-3183
                                          800-422-6691
                                  FAX: 402-474-3274
                  info@disabilityrightsnebraska.org
                  www.disabilityrightsnebraska.org

Jill Flagel, Chairperson
Mary Angus, Vice-Chairperson
Timothy F. Shaw, Chief Executive Officer
Eric Evans, Chief Operating Officer
Offers protection and advocacy services to people with developmental disabilities or mental illness. Direct assistance provided if issue within broad case priorities. Sliding scale fee. Information and referral at no cost.

3585 Nebraska Client Assistance Program
301 Centennial Mall South
P. O. Box 94987
Lincoln, NE 68509-4987   402-471-3656
                                          800-742-7594
                                  FAX: 402-471-3656
                  victoria.rasmussen@nebraska.gov
                  www.cap.state.ne.us/

3586 Nebraska Commission for the Blind & Visually Impaired
4600 Valley Rd
Suite 100
Lincoln, NE 68510-4844   402-471-2891
                                          877-809-2419
                                  FAX: 402-471-3009
                  kathy.stephens@nebraska.gov
                  ncbvi.state.ne.us

Pearl Van zandt, Executive Director
Carlos Servan, Deputy Director
Bob Deaton, Deputy Director
Barbara Loos, Chairman
Offers services for the totally blind, legally blind, visually impaired, mentally retarded blind and more with health, counseling, educational, recreational, rehabilitation, computer training and professional training services.

3587 Nebraska Department of Health & Human Services of Medically Handicapped Children's Prgm
301 Centennial Mall S
5TH Floor
Lincoln, NE 68508-2529   402-471-3121
                                          800-383-4278
                                  FAX: 402-471-3577
                  mary.gordon@nebraska.gov
                  dhhs.ne.gov

Kerry Winterer, Chief Executive Officer
Amy Borer, Admininstrative Assistant,Divisi
Dan Howell, CEO,Beatrice State Developmental
Maternal and child health, Title V, children with special health care needs; community based, statewide programs to facilitate diagnoses and care of children with disabilities and chronic medical conditions.

3588 Nebraska Department of Health and Human Services, Division of Aging Services
P.O.Box 95026
301 Centennial Mall South
Lincoln, NE 68509-5026   402-471-2115
                                          800-942-7830
                                  FAX: 402-471-3577
                  mary.gordon@nebraska.gov
                  dhhs.ne.gov

Kerry Winterer, Chief Executive Officer
Amy Borer, Admininstrative Assistant,Divisi
Dan Howell, CEO,Beatrice State Developmental
The Council focuses on persons who experience a severe disability that occurs before the individual attains the age of 22, which includes persons with physical disabilities, mental/behavioral health conditions and persons that are served by the current state developmental disabilities system.

3589 Nebraska Department of Mental Health
4545 South 86th Street
Lincoln, NE 68526-2529   402-483-6990
                                          888-210-8064
                                  FAX: 402-483-7045
                  www.nmhc-clinics.com

Jill Zlomke McPherson, Executive Director
Thomas I. McPherson, Technical Coordinator
Lee Zlomke, Clinical Director
Lisa Logsden, Staff Psychologist
Nebraska Mental Health Centers is a family mental health clinic for people from all walks of life. Among the many services we provide are psychological evaluations, individual and group counseling, substance abuse care, neuropsychological services, domestic violence group intervention and help for victims of domestic violence, treatment for eating disorders, an ADHD clinic, Women's Counseling and much more.

3590 Nebraska Planning Council on Developmental Disabilities
Department of Health and Human Services
P.O.Box 95026
Lincoln, NE 68509-5026   402-471-2115
                                  FAX: 402-471-3577
                                  TTY:402-471-9570
                  mary.gordon@nebraska.gov
                  dhhs.ne.gov/developmental_disabilities/Pages/

Mary Gordon, Executive Director
Kerry Winterer, Chief Executive Officer
Amy Borer, Admininstrative Assistant,Divisi
Dan Howell, CEO,Beatrice State Developmental
The Council focuses on persons who experience a severe disability that occurs before the individual attains the age of 22, which includes persons with physical disabilities, mental/behavioral health conditions and persons that are served by the current state developmental disabilities system.

3591 Nebraska Workers' Compensation Court
State of Nebraska
P.O.Box 98908
Lincoln, NE 68509-8908   402-471-6468
                                          800-599-5155
                                  FAX: 402-471-8231
                  www.wcc.ne.gov/

Glenn W. Morton, Administrator
Susan K. Davis, Public Information Manager
Jacqueline J Boesen, General Counsel
Randall Cecrle, Information Technology Manager
It is the web site of the Nebraska Workers' Compensation Court. The court maintains this web site to enhance public access and provide general information regarding workers' compensation in Nebraska.

3592   **Social Security: Lincoln Disability Determination**
Department of Education
P.O.Box 94987
Lincoln, NE 68509-4987   402-471-2295
800-772-1213
TTY:402-471-3659
flloyd@nde4.nde.state.ne.us
www.socialsecurity.gov

Karena L. Kilgore, Executive Secretary
Carolyn W. Colvin, Commissioner
Carolyn W. Colvin, Deputy Commissioner
James A. Kissko, Chief of Staff
Social Security offers online information and services to third parties who do business with them.

Nevada

3593   **Aging and Disability Services Division**
3416 Goni Rd
Suite D 132
Carson City, NV 89706-8008   775-687-4210
800-992-0900
FAX: 775-687-0574
adsd@adsd.nv.gov
adsd.nv.gov

Jane Gruner, Administrator
Tina Gerber-Winn, Deputy Administrator
Michele Ferral, Deputy Administrator
Jill Berntson, Deputy Administrator
Provides services for seniors in Nevada including community based care. advocacy and volunteer programs. Call write or e-mail for more information.

3594   **Nevada Assistive Technology Project**
Ste 32
3656 Research Way
Carson City, NV 89706-7932   775-687-4452
888-337-3839
FAX: 775-687-3292
www.hr.state.nv.us

Todd Butterworth, Manager
Serves all ages and all disabilities through partnerships with community organizations. The NATP provides training, advocacy, funding, information and referral services, a newsletter and weekly television show.

3595   **Nevada Bureau of Vocational Rehabilitation**
500 East Third Street
Carson City, NV 89713   775-684-0400
FAX: 775-684-4184
TTY:775-684-0360
detr.state.nv.us

Maureen Cole, Administrator
Melaine Mason, Deputy Administrator, Operations
Janice John, Deputy Administrator, Programs
Mechelle Merrill, Rehabilitation Chief II
Bureau of Vocational Rehabilitation is a state and federally funded program designed to help people with disabilities become employed and to help those already employed perform more successfully through training, counseling and other support methods.

3596   **Nevada Community Enrichment Program (NCEP)**
2550 University Avenue
Suite 330N
Saint Paul, MN 55114   651-645-7271
800-466-7722
FAX: 651-645-0541
TTY: 800-627-352
info@accessiblespace.org
accessiblespace.org

Mark E. Hamel, Esq., Chair
Kay Knutson, Vice Chair
John W. Adams, MBA, Secretary
Mary Lindgren, Board Member

Comprehensive neurological rehabilitation and life skills training.

3597   **Nevada Developmental Disability Council**
896 W. Nye Ln.
Suite 202
Carson City, NV 89703   775-687-8619
FAX: 775-684-8626
smanning@dhhs.nv.gov
www.nevadaddcouncil.org

Jodi Thornley, Chairman
Santa Perez, Vice Chairman
Sherry Manning, Executive Director
Kari Horn, Project Manager
The mission of the Nevada Developmental Disabilities Council is to provide resources at the community level which promote equal opportunity and life choices for people with disabilities through which they may positively contribute to Nevada society.

3598   **Nevada Disability Advocacy and Law Center -Sparks/Reno Office**
2820 West Charleston
Boulevard #11
Las Vegas, NV 89102   702-257-8150
888-349-3843
FAX: 702-257-8170
lasvegas@ndalc.org
www.ndalc.org

Reggie Bennettr, Secretary/Treasurer
Jana Spoor, President
John Miller, Vice President
Bob Bennett, Chairman
Nevada's protection and advocacy system for the human legal and service rights of individuals with disabilities. NDALC has offices in Reno/Sparks and Las Vegas, with services provided statewide.

3599   **Nevada Division for Aging: Las Vegas**
175 Berkeley Street
Boston, MA 02116   888-398-8924
libertymutual.com

Michael J. Babcockrs, Director
Marian L. Heard, Director
Martn P. Slark, Director
Develops, coordinates and delivers a comprehensive support service system in order for Nevada' senior citizens to lead independent, meaningful and dignified lives.

3600   **Nevada Division of Mental Health and Developmental Services**
5865 Lakeshore Road
Buford, GA 30518   770-945-4441
FAX: 678-482-1965
info@mhds.net
mhds.com

Keith Mixon, CEO/President
Offers treatment, prevention, education, habitation and rehabilitation for mental disorders. Works with advocacy groups, families, agencies and the community.

3601   **Social Security: Carson City Disability Determination**
1170 Harvard Way
Reno, NV 89502-2107   775-784-5221
800-772-1213
FAX: 775-784-5501
TTY: 800-325-0778
www.socialsecurity.gov

Karena L. Kilgore, Executive Secretary
Carolyn W. Colvin, Commissioner
Carolyn W. Colvin, Deputy Commissioner
James A. Kissko, Chief of Staff
Social Security offers online information and services to third parties who do business with them.

3602 State of Nevada Client Assistance Program
1631 W. Craig Rd.
Suite # 9-162
North Las Vegas, NV 89032-3767
702-635-4020
800-633-9879
800-633-9879
FAX: 702-642-7020
TTY:800-633-9879
info@eelders.org
www.eelders.org

3603 Workers Compensation Board Nevada
1301 North Green Valley Parkway
Suite 200
Henderson, NV 89074
702-486-9000
FAX: 775-687-6305
dirweb.state.nv.us

New Hampshire

3604 New Hampshire Workers Compensation Board
46 Donovan St
Concord, NH 03301-2624
603-225-2841
800-698-2364
FAX: 603-226-6903
www.nhprimex.org

Ty Gagne, CEO
Jonathan Kipp, Operations Manager
Julie Converse, Director of Finance
Carl Weber, Director of Member Services
Primex3 stands ready to provide our school, municipal, and county government members with the most comprehensive coverages and services available to New Hampshire local government.

3605 New Hampshire Assistive Technology Partnership Project
Department of Education
10 West Edge Drive
Suite 101
Durham, NH 03824
603-862-4320
FAX: 603-862-0555
atinnh.org

Jan Nisbet, Director
Mary Schuh, Associate Director
Eve Fralick, Associate Director
The goal of the New Hampshire Assistive Technology Partnership Project is to increase access to assistive technology through the creation and support of consumer driven systems for the provision of state-of-the-art assistive technology products and services for citizens with disabilities in the state of New Hampshire.

3606 New Hampshire Bureau of Developmental Services
Department of Health and Human Services
129 Pleasant St
Concord, NH 03301-3852
603-271-5034
FAX: 603-271-5166
mertas@dhhs.state.nh.us
www.dhhs.nh.gov

Matthew Ertas, Director
Peggy Sue Greenwood, Administrative Assistant
Developmental Services promotes opportunities for normal life experiences for persons with developmental disabilities and aquired brain disorders in all areas of community life: employment, housing, recreation, social relationships and community association. Services and supports are organized throught a central state office and ten private nonprofit community area agencies. Family support is provided to families of children with chronic health conditions or are developmentally disabled.

3607 New Hampshire Client Assistance Program
121 South Fruit Street
Suite 101
Concord, NH 03301-8518
603-271-2773
800-852-3405
FAX: 603-271-2837
Disability@nh.gov
www.state.nh.us/disability/caphomepage.html

Bill Hagy, Ombudsman
John Richards, Executive Director
Jillian Shedd, Accessibility Coordinator
Gayle Baird, Accountant
The Commission's goal is to remove the barriers, architectural, attitudinal or programmatic, that bar persons with disabilities from participating in the mainstream of society.

3608 New Hampshire Commission for Human Rights
64 South Street
Concord, NH 03301-8501
603-225-3431
800-735-2964
FAX: 603-224-3766
webmaster@nh.gov
www.nh.gov

Peggy Mc Allister, Executive Director
Enforces New Hampshire law against discrimination in housing, employment or public accomodations. Disability discrimination is prohibited under New Hampshire law. Takes formal charges and investigates them.

3609 New Hampshire Department of Mental Health
129 Pleasant Street
Concord, NH 03301-3852
603-226-0111
FAX: 603-271-5058
www.dhhs.nh.gov

Donald Shumway, Director
Paul Garmon
Tim Rourke, Religious Leader

3610 New Hampshire Developmental Disabilities Council
2 1/2 Beacon Street
21 Fruit Street
Concord, NH 03301- 4447
603-271-3236
800-852-3345
800-852-3236
FAX: 603-271-1156
TTY:800-735-2964
nhddc.org

Kristen McGraw, Chairman
Katherine Epstein, Vice-Chair
Carol Stamatakis, Executive Director
David Ouellette, Project Director
Offers information, referral and support services to disabled persons. A federally funded state agency.

3611 New Hampshire Division of Elderly and Adult Services
Bureau of Elderly & Adult Services
129 Pleasant St
Concord, NH 03301-3852
603-271-4680
800-351-1888
FAX: 603-271-4643
pio@dhhs.state.nh.us
www.dhhs.state.nh.us

Nicholas A. Toumpas, Comissioner
Mary Maggioncaida, Administrator
Marilee Nihan, Deputy Commissioner
Sheri Rockburn, Chief Financial Officer
The Bureau of Elderly and Adult Services provides a variety of social and long-term supports to adults age 60 and older and to adults between the ages of 18 and 60 who have a chronic illness or disability. These services range from home care, meals on wheels, care management, transportation assistance and assisted living to nursing home care.

3612 New Hampshire Governor's Commission on Disability
121 South Fruit Street
Suite 101
Concord, NH 03301-8518

603-271-2773
800-852-3405
FAX: 603-271-2837
Disability@nh.gov
www.nh.gov/disability

Paul Van Blarigan, Chairman
Charles J. Saia, Executive Director
Michael Coe, Accessibility Coordinator
Carol Conforti-Adams, Information and Referral Special
The Commission's goal is to remove the barriers, architectural, attitudinal or programmatic, that bar persons with disabilities from participating in the mainstream of socie

3613 New Hampshire Protection & Advocacy for Persons with Disabilities
Disabilities Rights Center, Inc
64 North Main Street
Suite 2, 3rd Floor
Concord, NH 03301-4913

603-228-0432
800-834-1721
FAX: 603-225-2077
TTY: 800-834-1721
advocacy@drcnh.org
drcnh.org

Paul Levy, President
Joanne Malloy, Vice President
Richard Cohen, Executive Director
Aaron Ginsberg, Staff Attorney
Legal services for individuals with disabilities; I & R.

3614 Social Security: Concord Disability Determination
Ste 100
70 Commercial St
Concord, NH 03301-5005

603-224-1939
800-772-1213
TTY:800-325-0778
www.ssa.gov

Karena L. Kilgore, Executive Secretary
Carolyn W. Colvin, Commissioner
Carolyn W. Colvin, Deputy Commissioner
James A. Kissko, Chief of Staff
Social Security offers online information and services to third parties who do business with them.

3615 Workers Compensation Board New Hampshire
PO Box 2076
95 Pleasant Street
Concord, NH 03301

603-271-3176
800-272-4353
FAX: 603-271-2668
workerscomp@labor.state.nh.us
www.nh.gov/labor

Kathryn J. Barger, Director, Workers' Compensation
George N. Copadis, Commissioner of Labor
David M. Wihby, Deputy Commissioner
The Department of Labor monitors Employers, Workers Compensation, and Insurance Carriers to insure that they are in compliance with NH Labor laws. These laws range from minimum wage, overtime, safety issues and workers compensation.

New Jersey

3616 Division of Developmental Disabilities
210 South Broad Street
3rd Floor
Trenton, NJ 08608

609-292-9742
800-922-7233
FAX: 609-777-0187
TTY: 609-633-7106
advocate@drnj.org
www.njpanda.org

James W Smith Jr, Executive Director

New Jersey's designated protection and advocacy system for poeple with disabilities and provides legal, nonlegal individual and systems advocacy.

3617 International Dyslexia Association: New Jersey Branch
40 York Rd.
4th Floor
Baltimore, MD 21204

410-296-0232
FAX: 410-321-5069
njida@msn.com
www.interdys.org

Hal Malchow, President
Elsa Cardenas-Hagan, Ed.D.,, Vice President
Ben Shifrin, M.Ed., Vice President
Kristen Penczek, Interim Executive Director
The New Jersey Branch of The International Dyslexia Association is a 501(c)(3) non-profit, scientific and educational organization which was formed to increase public awareness of dyslexia in New Jersey. We have been serving individuals with dyslexia, their families, and professionals in the field in this community for more than 25 years.

3618 New Jersey Commission for the Blind and Visually Impaired
153 Halsey St, Fl 6
PO Box 47017
Newark, NJ 7101-4701

973-648-3333
877-685-8878
FAX: 973-693-5046
Vito.DeSantis@dhs.state.nj.us
www.state.nj.us/humanservices/cbvi

Daniel B. Frye, J.D., Executive Director
Bernice Davis, Executive Assistant
Edward Szajdecki, Manager
John Walsh, Chief of Program Administration
The mission of the New Jersey Commission for the Blind and Visually Impaired is to promote and provide services in the areas of education, employment, independence and eye health through informed choice and partnership with persons who are blind or visually impaired, their families and the community. Serves Bergen, Essex, Hudson, Morris, Passaic, Sussex and Warren Counties.

3619 New Jersey Department of Aging
210 South Broad Street
3rd Floor
Trenton, NJ 08608

609-292-9742
800-922-7233
FAX: 609-777-0187
TTY: 609-633-7106
advocate@drnj.org
www.drnj.org

Walter Anthony Woodberry, Chairman
Andrew McGeady, Vice Chairman
Linda K. Soley, Treasurer
Leah Ziskin, Secretary

3620 New Jersey Department of Health/Special Child Health Services
New Jersey Department of Health and Senior Service
P.O.Box 360
Trenton, NJ 08625-0360

609-777-7778
FAX: 609-292-3580
plisciotto@doh.state.nj.us
www.nj.gov/health/fhs/sch/

Jennifer Velez, ESQ, Commissioner
Provides services for New Jersey children that will prevent or reduce the effects of a developmental delay, chronic illness or behavioral disorder.

3621 New Jersey Division of Mental Health Services
Department Human Services
222 South Warren Street
P.O. Box 700
Trenton, NJ 8625- 700   609-292-3717
                                               800-382-6717
                                          FAX: 609-341-3333
                              www.state.nj.us/humanservices

Jennifer Velez, ESQ, Commissioner
Lynn A. Kovich, Assistant Commissioner
Oversees the public mental health system for the state of New Jersey. Operates six regional and specialty psychiatric hospitals, and contracts with over 125 not-for-profit agencies to provide a comprehensive system of community mental health services throughout all counties in the state.

3622 New Jersey Governor's Liaison to the Office of Disability Employment Policy
1 John Fitch Plaza
P. O.Box 110
Trenton, NJ 08625-110   609-659-9045
                                          FAX: 609-633-9271
                     Constituent.Relations@dol.state.nj.us
                                          lwd.state.nj.us/labor

Harold J. Wriths, Commissioner
Frederick J. Zavaglia, Chief of Staff
Aaron R. Fichtner, Ph.D., Deputy Commissioner
Brian T. Murray, Director of Communications & Mar
The Division of Vocational Rehabilitation Services provides vocational rehabilitation services to prepare and place in employment eligilbe individuals with disabilities who, because of their disabling conditions, would otherwise be unable to secure and/or mantain employment

3623 New Jersey Protection & Advocacy for Persons with Disabilities
210 South Broad Street
3rd Floor
Trenton, NJ 08608   609-292-9742
                                               800-922-7233
                                          FAX: 609-777-0187
                                          TTY: 609-633-7106
                                          advocate@drnj.org
                                               www.drnj.org

Walter Anthony Woodberry, Chairman
Andrew McGeady, Vice Chairman
Linda K. Soley, Treasurer
Leah Ziskin, Secretary

3624 Regional ADA Technical Assistance Center
United Cerebral Palsy Associations of New Jersey
201 Dolgen Hall
Ithaca, NY 14853   607-255-6686
                                               800-949-4232
                                          FAX: 607-255-2763
                               northeastada@cornell.edu
                                     www.northeastada.org

LaWanda H. Cook, Ph.D., Extension Associate/Training Spe
Hannah Rudstam, Ph.D., Director of Training
Erin Sember-Chase, Project Coordinator and Technic
Luz Semeah, Technical Assistance

3625 Social Security Administration
1100 West High Rise
6401 Security Blvd.
Baltimore, MD 21235
                                               800-772-1213
                                          TTY:800-325-0778
                                               www.ssa.gov

Karena L. Kilgore, Executive Secretary
Carolyn W. Colvin, Commissioner
Carolyn W. Colvin, Deputy Commissioner
James A. Kissko, Chief of Staff
Social Security disability is a social insurance program that workers and employers pay for with their Social Security taxes. Eligibility is based on your work history, and the amount of your

benefit is based on your earnings. Social Security also has a disability program for people with limited income and resources- the Supplemental Security Income (SSI) program. For more information on these federal programs, please call our nationwide toll-free number.

New Mexico

3626 New Mexico Aging and Long-Term Services Department
2550 Cerrillos Rd
P.O. Box 27118
Santa Fe, NM 87505-3260   505-476-4799
                                               866-451-2901
                                          FAX: 505-476-4836
                               www.nmaging.state.nm.us

Miles Copeland, Deputy Secretary
Retta Ward, Secretary
Jason Sanchez, Administrative Services Division
Greg Rockstroh, IT Manager
Information and services for seniors, people with disabilities and their families.

3627 New Mexico Client Assistance Program
1720 Louisiana Blvd NE
Site 204
Albuquerque, NM 87110- 7070   505-256-3100
                                               800-432-4682
                                          FAX: 505-256-3184
                                               info@drnm.org
                                               www.drnm.org

Katie Toledo, Chairperson
Cyndy Costanza, Vice Chairperson
Jeanne A. Hamrick, President
Larry Rodriguez, Vice President
The mission of Disability Rights New Mexico (DRNM) is to protect, promote and expand the legal and civil rights of persons with disabilities. DRNM is an independent, private nonprofit agency operating federally mandated and other advocacy programs in pursuit of this mission.

3628 New Mexico Commission for the Blind
2905 Rodeo Park Dr E
Bldg 4, Suite 100
Santa Fe, NM 87505-6342   505-476-4479
                                               888-513-7968
                                          FAX: 505-476-4475
                               greg.trapp@state.nm.us
                               www.cfb.state.nm.us/

Arthur A. Schreiber, Chairman
Jim Babb, Commissioner
Dallas Allen, Commissioner
Greg Trapp, Executive Director
Offers services for the totally blind, legally blind, visually impaired, mentally retarded blind and more with health, counseling, educational, recreational, rehabilitation, computer training and professional training services.

3629 New Mexico Department of Health: Children's Medical Services
1190 S Saint Francis Dr
Santa Fe, NM 87505-4173   505-841-6100
                                               800-797-3260
                                          FAX: 505-827-2530
                               lchristiansen@doh.state.nm
                               nmhealth.org/phd/cms.shtml

Gloria Bonner, Program Manager
Susan Baum, Medical Director
Freida Adams, Nurse Coordinator
Kim Love, Operations Manager
Title V MCH Program for children with special health care needs from birth to age 21 years. Services provided include: diagnosis, medical intervention, clinics and service coordination.

3630 New Mexico Governor's Committee on Concerns of the Handicapped
491 Old Santa Fe Trl
Santa Fe, NM 87501-2753

505-476-0412
877-696-1470
FAX: 505-827-6328
gcd@state.nm.us
www.gcd.state.nm.us/

Susan Gray, Chair
Curtiss Wilson, Vice Chair
Jim Parker, Director
Karen Courtney-Peterson, Chief Financial Officer

3631 New Mexico Protection & Advocacy for Persons with Disabilities
1720 Louisiana Blvd NE
Site 204
Albuquerque, NM 87110- 7070

505-256-3100
800-432-4682
FAX: 505-256-3184
info@drnm.org
www.drnm.org

Katie Toledo, Chairperson
Cyndy Costanza, Vice Chairperson
Jeanne A. Hamrick, President
Larry Rodriguez, Vice President
The mission of Disability Rights New Mexico (DRNM) is to protect, promote and expand the legal and civil rights of persons with disabilities. DRNM is an independent, private nonprofit agency operating federally mandated and other advocacy programs in pursuit of this mission.

3632 New Mexico Technology Assistance Program
435 Saint Michaels Dr
Ste D
Santa Fe, NM 87505-7679

505-827-8535
800-866-2253
FAX: 505-954-8608
TTY: 800-659-4915
julie.martinez@state.nm.us
www.nmtap.com

Julie Martinez, Program Director
Examines and works to eliminate barriers to obtaining assistive technology in New Mexico. Has established a statewide program for coordinating assistive technology services; is designed to assist people with disabilities to locate, secure, and maintain assistive technology.

3633 New Mexico Workers Compensation Administration
2410 Centre Avenue SE
P.O.Box 27198
Albuquerque, NM 87125-7198

505-841-6000
800-255-7965
FAX: 505-841-6009
www.workerscomp.state.nm.us/

Ned S. Fuller, Director
Robert E. Doucette, Executive Deputy Director
Darin A. Childers, General Counsel
Thomas E. Dow, Executive Deputy Director
Regulates workers' compensation in New Mexico.

3634 Social Security: Santa Fe Disability Determination
6401 Security Blvd.
Baltimore, MD 21235

800-772-1213
TTY:800-325-0778
www.socialsecurity.gov

Karena L. Kilgore, Executive Secretary
Carolyn W. Colvin, Commissioner
Carolyn W. Colvin, Deputy Commissioner
James A. Kissko, Chief of Staff

3635 Southwest Branch of the International Dyslexia Association
International Dyslexia Association
3915 Carlisle Blvd. NE
Albuquerque, NM 87107

505-255-8234
800-222-3123
FAX: 505-262-8547
swida@southwestida.org
southwestida.com

Carolee Dean, President
Claudia Gutierrez, Vice President
Michelle Wick, Recording Secretary
Erin Brown, Corresponding Secretary
Provides free information and referral services for diagnosis and tutoring for parents, educators, physicians, and individuals with dyslexia. The voice of our membership is heard in 48 countries. Membership includes yearly journal and quarterly newsletter. Call for conference dates.

3636 Workers Compensation Board New Mexico
2410 Centre Avenue SE
P.O.Box 27198
Albuquerque, NM 87125-7198

505-841-6000
800-255-7965
FAX: 505-841-6009
www.workerscomp.state.nm.us/

Ned S. Fuller, Director
Robert E. Doucette, Executive Deputy Director
Darin A. Childers, General Counsel
Thomas E. Dow, Executive Deputy Director
Regulates workers' compensation in New Mexico.

New York

3637 Albany County Department for Aging and Albany Social Services
112 State Street
Room 900
Albany, NY 12207-2304

518-447-7000
FAX: 518-447-7188
aging@albanycounty.com
albanycounty.com

George Brown, Commissioner
Judy L. Coyne, Commissioner
Kathleen M. Dalton, Ph.D., Commissioner
The Point of Entry access line provides information and assistance and comprehensive referrals, and or assessments for the elderly, adults and children with disabilities, their family, or service providers.

3638 International Dyslexia Association of NY: Buffalo Branch
40 York Rd
4th Floor
Baltimore, MD 21204-9408

410-296-0232
800-222-3123
FAX: 410-321-5069
bufida@gow.org
www.interdys.org

Hal Malchow, President
Elsa Cardenas-Hagan, Vice President
Ben Shifrin, Vice President
Kristen Penczek, Interim Executive Director

3639 Jawonio
260 N Little Tor Road
New City, NY 10956-2627

845-708-2000
FAX: 845-634-7731
TTY:845-639-3521
www.jawonio.org

Jill A. Warner, Executive Director & CEO
Matthew Shelly, Chief Program Officer
Diana Hess, Chief Communications Officer
Joseph Bloss, Chief Financial Officer
A dedicated community resource providing services to more than 500 children and adults annually. Provide early intervention, day care and pre-school special ed to our children. Job training, day

habilitation, recreation, medical and service coordination for adults.

3640 Jawonio Vocational Center
260 N Little Tor Rd
New City, NY 10956-2627   845-708-2000
FAX: 845-634-7731
TTY: 845-639-3521
jawonio.org

Jill A. Warner, Executive Director & CEO
Matthew Shelly, Chief Program Officer
Diana Hess, Chief Communications Officer
Joseph Bloss, Chief Financial Officer
A dedicated community resource providing services to more than 500 children and adults annually. Provide early intervention, day care and pre-school special ed to our children. Job training, day habilitation, recreation, medical and service coordination for adults.

3641 NYS Commission on Quality of Care & Advocacy for Persons with Disabilities
401 State St
Schenectady, NY 12305-2300   518-388-2892
FAX: 518-388-2890
marcelc@cqc.state.ny.us
www.cqcapd.state.ny.us

Andrew M. Cuomo, Governor
Roger Bearden, Chair
Bruce Blower, Member
Patricia Okoniewski, Member

3642 NYSARC
393 Delaware Ave
Delmar, NY 12054-3094   518-439-8311
800-724-2094
FAX: 518-439-1893
info@nysarc.org
nysarc.org

Laura J. Kennedy, President
Patricia Campanella, Senior Vice President
Joseph M. Bognanno, Vice President
Lori Martindale, Treasurer

3643 National Alliance on Mental Illness of New York State
99 Pine Street
Suite 302
Albany, NY 12207-1336   518-462-2000
800-950-3228
FAX: 518-462-3811
info@naminys.org
www.naminys.org

Sherry Grenz, President
Wend Burch, Executive Director
Sharon Clairmont, Finance & Business Office Dir.
Matthew Shapiro, Development/Events Coordinator

3644 New State Office of Mental Health Agency
Office of Mental Health
44 Holland Ave
Albany, NY 12229   518-474-4403
800-597-8481
FAX: 518-474-2149
www.omh.ny.gov

Mike Hogan, Commissioner
Promoting the mental health of all New Yorkers with a particular focus on providing hope and recovery for adults with serious mental illness and children with serious emotional disturbances.

3645 New York Client Assistance Program
855 Central Avenue
Suite 110
Albany, NY 12206   518-459-6422
FAX: 518-459-7847
TTY: 518-459-6422
www.nls.org/caplist.htm

3646 New York Department of Handicapped Children
Department of Heath Education
Corning Tower
Empire State Plaza
Albany, NY 12237   518-456-0665
866-881-2809
FAX: 518-456-1126
jcrucetti@albanycounty.com
www.health.ny.gov

Andrew M. Cuomo, Governor
Dr James B. Crucetti, MD, MPH, Commissioner
Howard Zucker, Acting Commissioner

3647 New York State Commission for the Blind
52 Washington St
Rensselaer, NY 12144-2796   518-473-7793
866-871-3000
FAX: 518-486-7550
www.ocfs.state.ny.us

Madeline Raciti, Manager
Offers services for the totally blind, legally blind, visually impaired, mentally retarded blind and more with health, counseling, educational, recreational, rehabilitation, computer training and professional training services.

3648 New York State Commission on Quality of Care
401 State St
Schenectady, NY 12305-2300   518-388-2892
FAX: 518-388-2890
marcelc@cqc.state.ny.us
www.cqc.state.ny.us

Andrew M. Cuomo, Governor
Roger Bearden, Chair
Bruce Blower, Member
Patricia Okoniewski, Member

3649 New York State Congress of Parents and Teachers
1 Wembley Ct
Albany, NY 12205-6258   518-452-8808
877-569-7782
FAX: 518-452-8105
pta.office@nyspta.org
nyspta.org

Bonnie Russell, President
Gracemarie Rozea, First Vice President
Judy Van Harren, Secretary
Penny Hollister, Vice President
Parent Teacher Association and PTA are registered service marks of the National Congress of Parents and Teachers (National PTA). Only those groups chartered by the New York State PTA are entitled to use the name PTA. Any other use constitutes trademark infringement.

3650 New York State Office of Advocates for Persons with Disabilities
Ste 1001
1 Empire State Plz
Albany, NY 12223-1100   518-449-7860
800-522-4369
FAX: 518-473-6005
oapwdinfo@oapwd.org
www.oapwd.org

Gary O'Brien, Chair Commissioner
Provides information and referral services; administers NYS Tech Art Project; promotes implementation of disability-related laws.

3651 **New York State Office of Mental Health**
44 Holland Ave
Albany, NY 12229-1
518-474-4403
800-597-8481
FAX: 518-474-2149
www.omh.state.ny.gov in

Michael Hogan, Ph.D.
Promoting the mental health of all New Yorkers with a particular focus on providing hope and recovery for adults with serious mental illness and children with serious emotional disturbances.

3652 **New York State TRAID Project**
New York State Commisionon Qualityof Careand Advoc
Ste 1001
1 Empire State Plz
Albany, NY 12223-1100
518-449-7860
800-522-4369
FAX: 518-473-6005
www.oatwd.org

Cliff Sigfride, Manager

3653 **Parent to Parent of New York State**
500 Balltown Rd
Schenectady, NY 12304-2247
518-381-4350
800-305-8817
FAX: 518-393-9607
mjuda@ptopnys.org
parenttoparentnys.org

Louise Nitto, President
Jim Costello, Vice President
Elizabeth Smithmeyer, Secretary
Michele Juda, Executive Director
Parent to Parent of NYS, which began in 1994, is a statewide not for profit organization established to support and connect families of individuals with special needs. The 13 offices, located throughout NYS, are staffed by Regional Coordinators, who are parents or close relatives of individuals with special needs.

3654 **Protection and Advocacy Agency of NY**
401 State St
Schenectady, NY 12305-2303
518-388-2892
FAX: 518-388-2890
marcelc@cqc.state.ny.us
www.cqc.state.ny.us

Andrew M. Cuomo, Governor
Roger Bearden, Chair
Bruce Blower, Member
Patricia Okoniewski, Member

3655 **Regional Early Childhood Director Center**
89 Washington Ave.
Room 580 EBA
Albany, NY 12234
518-474-2925
800-222-5627
accesadm@mail.nysed.gov
www.acces.nysed.gov

3656 **Schools And Services For Children With Autism Spectrum Disorders.**
116 E 16th St
5th Floor
New York, NY 10003-2164
212-677-4650
FAX: 212-254-4070
info@resourcesnyc.org
www.resourcesnyc.org

Ellen Miller-Wachtel, Chairman
Shon E. Glusky, President
Owen P. J. King, Treasurer
Rachel Howard, Executive Director
This publication fun resource for children provides extreme coverage of services for children with autism, asbergez syndrome, and/or PDD.

3657 **Singeria/Metropolitan Parent Center**
2082 Lexington Ave.
4th Floor
New York, NY 10035
212-643-2840
866-867-9665
FAX: 212-496-5608
intake@sinergiany.org
sinergiany.org

Len Torres, President
Johnny C. Rivera, Vice President
Paola Jordan, Treasurer
Donald Lash, Executive Director

3658 **Social Security: Albany Disability Determination**
1 Clinton Ave
Albany, NY 12207
518-431-4051
800-772-1213
TTY:518-431-4050
www.ssa.gov

Karena L. Kilgore, Executive Secretary
Carolyn W. Colvin, Commissioner
Carolyn W. Colvin, Deputy Commissioner
James A. Kissko, Chief of Staff

3659 **State Agency for the Blind and Visually Impaired**
52 Washington St
Rensselaer, NY 12144-2834
518-473-7793
866-871-3000
FAX: 518-486-7550
info@ocfs.state.ny.us
www.ocfs.state.ny.us

3660 **State Education Agency Rural Representative**
89 Washington Avenue
Albany, NY 12234
518-474-3852
FAX: 518-473-2860
RegentsOffice@mail.nysed.gov
www.nysed.gov

Merryl H. Tisch, Chancellor
Anthony S. Bottar, Vice Chancellor

3661 **State Mental Health Representative for Children and Youth**
44 Holland Ave
Albany, NY 12229
518-473-6328
cocompz@omh.state.ny.us
www.rcybc.ca

David Woodlock, Deputy Commissioner

3662 **State Mental Retardation Program**
44 Holland Ave
Albany, NY 12229
518-474-6601
FAX: 518-473-1271
omr.state.ny.us

Diana Ritter, Manager

3663 **United We Stand of New York**
98 Moore St
Brooklyn, NY 11206-3326
718-302-4313
FAX: 718-302-4315
uwsofny@aol.com
www.uwsony.org

Lourdes Rivera-Putz, Executive Director
Lourdes Figueroa, Intake/Receptionist
Carmen Soltero, Outreach/Trainer
Martha Vizcarrondo, Family Support Associate
Assists families with improving the quality of life for all individuals with disabilities.

3664 University Afiliated Program/Rose F Kennedy Center
1971
1300 Morris Park Avenue
Bronx, NY 10461

718-430-2000
information@einstein.yu.edu
www.einstein.yu.edu

Maris D. Rosenberg, Interim Director
Christine M. Baric, Assistant Director
John J. Foxe, Director
Robert W. Marion, Director

3665 University of Rochester Medical Center
601 Elmwood Ave
Rochester, NY 14642

585-275-8762
FAX: 585-275-3366
phil_davidson@urmc.rochester.edu
www.rochester.edu

Brad Berk, MD, PhD, CEO

3666 VESID
New York State Education Department
89 Washington Ave.
Room 580 EBA
Albany, NY 12234

800-222-5627
FAX: 518-474-8802
accesadm@mail.nysed.gov
www.acces.nysed.gov/vr/

Dr Rebecca Cort, Deputy Commissioner
Vocational and educational services for individuals with disabilities.

3667 VSA Arts of New York City
2700 F Street, NW
Washington, DC 20566

202-467-4600
800-444-1324
FAX: 717-225-6305
bbvsanyc@msn.com
www.vsarts.org

David M. Rubenstein, Chairman
Deborah F. Rutter, President
Christoph Eschenbach, Music Director
Roger L. Stevens, Founding Chairman
Provides art, educational and creative expression experiences to thousands of children, youth, and adults with disabilities who reside in the five boroughs of New York City. It provides opportunities for people with disabilities to demonstrate their accomplishments in the arts and foster increased understanding and acceptance.

3668 Westchester Institute for Human Development
Cedarwood Hall
Valhalla, NY 10595

914-493-8150
info@WIHD.org
www.wihd.org

William H. Bave, Chairman
Pamela Thornton, Vice Chairman
Ansley Bacon PhD, President/CEO
David M.C. Stern, Treasurer
WIHD advances policies and practices that foster the healthy development and ensure the safety of all children, strengthen families and communities, and promote health and well-being among people of all ages with disabilities and special health care needs.

3669 Workers Compensation Board New York
PO Box 5205
328 State Street
Schenectady, NY 12305-2318

518-462-8880
877-632-4996
FAX: 518-473-1415
general_information@wcb.ny.gov
www.wcb.ny.gov

Andrew M. Cuomo, Governor
Robert E. Beloten, Chairman
Richard A. Bell, Commissioner

North Carolina

3670 Developmental Disability Services Section
Building 325n
Albemarle
Raleigh, NC 27699

919-420-7901
FAX: 919-420-7917
www.dhhs.state.nc.us/mhddsas/

Diana Simmons, Human Resources Manager
Ureh N. Lekwauwa, Chief, Clinical Policy
Courtney Cantrell, Acting Director
Jim Jarrard, Deputy Director
Makes policies and monitors public services and supports to people with mental illness, developmental disabilities and substance abuse throughout North Carolina.

3671 International Dyslexia Association: North Carolina Branch
40 York Rd.
4th Floor
Baltimore, MD 21204

410-296-0232
FAX: 410-321-5069
www.interdys.org

Hal Malchow, President
Elsa Cardenas-Hagan, Vice President
Ben Shifrin, Vice President
Kristen Penczek, Interim Executive Director
The North Carolina Branch of The International Dyslexia Association (NCIDA) is a 501 (c)(3) non-profit, scientific and organization dedicated to educating the public about the learning disability, dyslexia. The North Carolina Branch has four objectives: to increase awareness in the dyslexic and general community; to network with other learning disability groups and legislators in education;to increase membership and provide services that will strengthen members presence in their communities

3672 North Carolina Workers Compensation Board
4340 Mail Service Center
Raleigh, NC 27699-4340

919-807-2501
800-688-8349
FAX: 919-508-8210
infospec@ic.nc.gov
www.ic.nc.gov

Julian Bunn, Owner

3673 North Carolina Assistive Technology Project
1110 Navaho Dr
Suite 101
Raleigh, NC 27609-7322

919-872-2298
FAX: 919-850-2792
ncatp@minespring.com
ncatp.org

Ricki Cook, Project Director
Annette Lauber, Funding Specialist
Jacquelyne Gordon, Consumer Resource Specialist
Tony Hiatt, Executive Director
The North Carolina Assistive Technology Project exists to create a statewide, consumer-responsive system of assistive technology services for all North Carolinians with disabilities. The project's activities impact children and adults with disabilities across all aspects of their lives.

3674 North Carolina Children & Youth Branch
North Carolina Publc of Health
1928 Mail Service Ctr
Raleigh, NC 27699-1900

919-839-6262
FAX: 919-733-8034
cathy.kluttz@nemail.net
www.nchealthychildren.com

Lawrence J Wheeler, Manager
Cathy Kluttz, Unit Manager Special Service
Dianne Tyson, Help Line Manager
Ran Coble, Executive Director

3675 **North Carolina Client Assistance Program**
2806 Mail Service Ctr
Raleigh, NC 27699-2806
919-855-3600
800-215-7227
FAX: 919-715-2456
nccap@dhhs.nc.gov
cap.state.nc.us

John Marens, Director
Diane Rawdarowicz, Client Advocate
Sharon Wisner, Client Advocate
Tami Andrews, Processing Assistant

A federally funded program designed to assist individuals with disabilities in understanding and using rehabilitation services. CAP serves as an integral part of the rehabilitation system by advising and informing individuals of all services and benefits available to them through programs authorized under both the Rehabilitation Act and Title 1 of the Americans with Disabilities Act.

3676 **North Carolina Developmental Disabilities**
3125 Poplarwood Court
Suite 200
Raleigh, NC 27604-7368
919-850-2901
800-357-6916
FAX: 919-850-2915
Info@nccdd.org
www.nc-ddc.org

Caroline Valand, Executive Director

A planning council established to assure that individuals with developmental disabilities and their families participate in the planning of and have access to culturally competent services, supports, and other assistance and opportunities that promote independence, productivity, and integration and inclusion into the community; and to promote, through systemic change, capacity building and advocacy activities, a consumer and family-centered comprehensive system.

3677 **North Carolina Division of Aging**
2101 Mail Service Ctr
Raleigh, NC 27699-2001
919-855-4800
FAX: 919-733-0443
ncdhhs.gov

Dennis Streets, Manager
Jim Slate, Director
Laketha Miller, Controller
Emery Edwards Milliken, General Counsel

3678 **North Carolina Industrial Commission**
4340 Mail Service Center
Raleigh, NC 27699-4340
919-807-2501
800-688-8349
FAX: 919-508-5420
infospec@ic.nc.gov
www.ic.nc.gov

J Howard Bunn Jr, Chairman
Peg Dorer, Executive Director

3679 **Social Security Administration**
4701 Old Wake Forest Rd
Raleigh, NC 27609-4919
877-803-6311
800-772-1213
800-325-0778
FAX: 919-790-2860
TTY:919-790-2773
www.socialsecurity.gov
www.socialsecurity.gov

Karena L. Kilgore, Executive Secretary
Carolyn W. Colvin, Commissioner
Carolyn W. Colvin, Deputy Commissioner
James A. Kissko, Chief of Staff

Provides information on how to obtain social security through a disability.

North Dakota

3680 **Division of Mental Health and Substance Abuse**
600 East Boulevard Avenue
Dept 325
Bismarck, ND 58505- 0250
701-328-2310
800-472-2622
FAX: 701-328-2359
dhseo@nd.gov
www.nd.gov/humanservices

Dennis Goetz, Executive Director
Kerry Wicks, Executive Director
Andrew J. McLean, Medical Director
Alex Schweitzer, Superintendent

The Department of Human Services' Mental Health and Substance Abuse Services Division provides leadership for the planning, development, and oversight of a system of care for children, adults, and families with severe emotional disorders, mental illness, and/or substance abuse issues.

3681 **North Dakota Workers Compensation Board**
50 E Front Ave
Bismarck, ND 58504
701-328-3800
800-777-5033
FAX: 701-329-9911
TTY: 701-328-3786
www.ndworkerscomp.com

Brent Edison, Director

3682 **North Dakota Client Assistance Program**
400 East Broadway
Suite 409
Bismarck, ND 58501-4071
701-328-2950
800-472-2670
FAX: 701-328-3934
panda@nd.gov
www.ndpanda.org/cap

Dennis Lyon, CEO
Janelle Olson, Advocate
Paula Rustad, Office Assistant
Angie Dubovoy, Advocate

CAP assists clients and client applicants of North Dakota Vocational Rehabilitation services, Tribal Vocational Rehabilitation, or Independent Living services.

3683 **North Dakota Department of Human Resources**
1237 W Divide Ave
Suite 6
Bismarck, ND 58501-1208
701-328-5300
800-451-8693
FAX: 701-328-5320
dhsaging@nd.gov
www.nd.gov

Shane Goettle, Manager

3684 **North Dakota Department of Human Services**
600 E Boulevard Ave
Dept 325
Bismarck, ND 58505-0250
701-328-2310
800-472-2622
FAX: 701-328-2359
dhseo@nd.gov
www.nd.gov/dhs

Carol K Olson, Executive Director
Dennis Goetz, Executive Director
Kerry Wicks, Executive Director
Andrew J. McLean, Medical Director

Provides services that help vulnerable North Dakotans of all ages to maintain or enhance their quality of life, which may be threatened by lack of financial resources, emotional crises, disabling conditions, or an inability to protect themselves.

3685 Protection & Advocacy Project
1984
400 East Broadway
Suite 409
Bismarck, ND 58501-4071

701-328-2950
800-472-2670
FAX: 701-328-3934
panda@nd.gov
ndpanda.org

Teresa Larsen, Executive Director
Janelle Olson, Advocate
Paula Rustad, Office Assistant
Angie Dubovoy, Advocate
The Protection and Advocacy is a state agency whose purpose is to advocate for and protect the rights of people with disabilities. The Protection and Advocacy Project has programs to serve people with developmental disabilities, mental illnesses and other types of disabilities. The projects programs and services are free to eligible individuals.

3686 Social Security: Bismarck Disability Determination
1680 E Capitol Ave
Bismarck, ND 58501-5603

701-250-4200
800-772-1213
TTY:701-250-4620
ssa.gov

Karena L. Kilgore, Executive Secretary
Carolyn W. Colvin, Commissioner
Carolyn W. Colvin, Deputy Commissioner
James A. Kissko, Chief of Staff

3687 Workers Compensation Board North Dakota
1600EastCenturyAvenue
Suite1
Bismarck, ND 58503-649

701-328-3800
800-777-5033
FAX: 701-328-3820
www.workforcesafety.com

Sandy Blunt, CEO

Ohio

3688 Epilepsy Council of Greater Cincinnati
Ste 550
895 Central Ave
Cincinnati, OH 45202-5700

513-721-2905
877-804-2241
FAX: 513-721-0799
ecgc@fuse.net
ecgc-ohnky.net

Kathy Stewart, Executive Director

3689 International Dyslexia Association: Central Ohio Branch
40 York Rd.
4th Floor
Baltimore, MD 21204

410-296-0232
FAX: 410-321-5069
cybdischultz@columbus.rr.com
www.interdys.org

Hal Malchow, President
Elsa Cardenas-Hagan, Vice President
Ben Shifrin, Vice President
Lee Grossman, Executive Director
Provides free information and referral services for diagnosis and tutoring for parents, educators, physicians, and individuals with dyslexia. The voice of our membership is heard in 48 countries. Membership includes yearly journal and quarterly newsletter. Call for conference dates. Other locations available in Ohio state.

3690 Ohio Bureau for Children with Medical Handicaps
Ohio Department of Health
246 N. High St
P.O.Box 1603
Columbus, OH 43215-1603

614-466-3543
800-755-4769
FAX: 614-728-3616
bcmh@odh.ohio.gov
www.odh.ohio.gov

John R. Kasich, Governor
James Bryant Md, Bureau Chief
Alvin Jackson, MD, Director
Lance D. Himes, Interim Director
Provides funding for the diagnosis, treatment and coordination of services for eligible Ohio children, under age 21, with medical handicaps; conducts quality assurance activities to establish standards of care and determine unmet needs of children with handicaps and their families; collaborates with public health nurses to increase access to care; and assists families to access and use third party resources. Conducts a separate program for adults with cystic fibrosis.

3691 Ohio Bureau of Worker's Compensation
30 W Spring St
Columbus, OH 43215-2256

800-335-0996
FAX: 877-321-9481
TTY:800-292-4833
ombudsperson@bwc.state.oh.us
ohiobwc.com

Stephen Buehrer, Administrator/CEO
Dale Hamilton, Chief Operating Officer (COO)
Kevin Abrams, Chief of Employers Services
Toni Brokaw, Chief of Human Resources
To provide a quality, customer-focused workers' compensation insurance system for Ohio's employers and employees.

3692 Ohio Client Assistance Program
50 W. Broad St.
Suite 1400
Columbus, OH 43215-5923

614-466-7264
800-282-9181
FAX: 614-752-4197
TTY: 614-728-2553
www.olrs.ohio.gov

Donald Bishop, Executive Director

3693 Ohio Department of Aging
1982
50 W Broad St
Fl 9
Columbus, OH 43215-3363

614-466-5500
866-243-5678
888-243-5678
FAX: 614-466-5741
TTY:614-466-6191
www.aging.ohio.gov

Bonnie Kantor-Burman, Director
John Ratliff, Public Information Officer
The department serves and represents about 2 million Ohioans age 60 & older. They advocate for the needs of all older citizens with emphasis on improving the quality of life, helping senior citizens live active, healthy, & independent lives, & promoting positive attitudes toward aging & older people. Committed to helping the frail elderly who choose to remain at home by providing home & community based services, their goal is to promote the level of choice, independence & self-care.

3694 Ohio Department of Mental Health
30 E Broad St
8th Floor
Columbus, OH 43215-3414
614-466-4775
877-275-6364
FAX: 614-752-8410
uhricks@mh.state.oh.us
mh.state.oh.us

Michael Hogan, Director
Christine Vincenty, Manager

3695 Ohio Developmental Disabilities Council
899 E Broad St, Ste 203
Columbus, OH 43205
614-466-5205
800-766-7426
FAX: 614-466-0298
carla.sykes@dmr.state.oh.us
www.ddc.ohio.gov

Carolyn Knight, Executive Director
Mark Seifarth, Chair
Robert Shuemak, Vice Chair
Kimberly Stults, Secretary
The Ohio Developmental Disabilities Council is one of 55 councils found in all states and territories which provides funding for systems change grant projects. The DD Council is a planning and advocacy agency that seeks to improve the lives of Ohioans with disabilities.

3696 Ohio Developmental Disability Council (ODDC)
899 E Broad St, Ste 203
Columbus, OH 43205
614-466-5205
800-766-7426
FAX: 614-466-0298
www.ddc.ohio.gov

Carolyn Knight, Executive Director
Mark Seifarth, Chair
Robert Shuemak, Vice Chair
Kimberly Stults, Secretary

3697 Ohio Governor's Council on People with Disabilities
400 E Campus View Blvd
Columbus, OH 43235-4685
614-438-1200
800-282-4536
RSC.Webmaster@rsc.state.oh.us
gcpd.ohio.gov

Jacqueline Romer-Sensky, Chairman
Jack Licate, Vice Chairman
Kevin Miller, Executive Director
Bill Bishilany, Assistant Executive Director
The Governor's Council on People with Disabilities exists to: Advise the Governor and General Assembly on statewide disability issues, promote the value of diversity, dignity and the quality of life for people with disabilities, be a catalyst to create systemic change promoting awareness of disability-related issues that will ultimately benefit all citizens of Ohio, Educate and advocate for: partnerships at the local, state and national level, promotion of equality, access and independence.

3698 Ohio Rehabilitation Services Commission
400 E Campus View Blvd
Columbus, OH 43235-4604
614-438-1200
800-282-4536
RSC.Webmaster@rsc.state.oh.us
ohio.gov

Kevin Miller, Executive Director
RSC is Ohio's state agency that provides vocational rehabilitation (VR) services to help people with disabilities become employed and independent. We also offer a variety of services to Ohio businesses, resulting in quality jobs for individuals who have disabilities.

3699 Ohio Women, Infants, & Children ProgramOhio Department of Health
246 N High St
Columbus, OH 43215-2406
614-644-8006
FAX: 614-564-2470
odh.ohio.gov

Michele Frizzell, Chief, Bureau of Nutrition Svcs.

3700 Social Security: Columbus Disability Determination
90 E Washington Bridge Rd
Suite 140
Worthington, OH 43085
614-888-5339
800-772-1213
TTY:614-288-0226
www.socialsecurity.gov

Karena L. Kilgore, Executive Secretary
Carolyn W. Colvin, Commissioner
Carolyn W. Colvin, Deputy Commissioner
James A. Kissko, Chief of Staff

Oklahoma

3701 Oklahoma Workers Compensation Board
Department of Labor
3017 N. Stiles, Suite 100
Oklahoma City, OK 73105
405-521-6100
888-269-5353
FAX: 405-521-6018
labor.info@labor.ok.gov
www.ok.gov/odol

Jim Marshall, Chief of Staff
Mark Costello, Commissioner of Labor
Lizzette McNeill, Communications Director
Stacy Bonner, Deputy Commissioner

3702 Oklahoma Client Assistance Program/Office of Disability Concerns
2401 NW 23rd Street
Suite 90
Oklahoma City, OK 73107- 2431
405-521-3756
800-522-8224
FAX: 405-522-6695
www.ok.gov

Todd Lamb, Governor
Gary Jones, Auditor and Inspector
E. Scott Pruitt, Attorney General
Ken Miller, Treasurer
CAP informs and advises applicants and consumers about the vocational rehabilitation process and services available under the Federal Rehabilitation Act, including services provided by DVR and DVS. CAP staff can help you communicate concerns to the DVR/DVS and assist you with administrative, mediation, fair hearing, legal and other solutions

3703 Oklahoma Department of Human Services Aging Services Division
25 Sigourney Street, 10th Floor
Hartford, CT 06106
405-521-3646
866-218-6621
800-522-7233
FAX: 860-424-5301
okdhs.org

Margaret Ger Murkette, MSW, Director
Ed Lake, Director

3704 Oklahoma Department of Labor
3017 N. Stiles
Suite 100
Oklahoma City, OK 73105-5206   405-521-6100
                                       888-269-5353
                                  FAX: 405-521-6018
                                  www.labor.ok.gov

Mark Castello, Commissioner
Jim Marshall, Chief of Staff
Stacy Bonner, Deputy Commissioner
Don Schooler, General Counsel

3705 Oklahoma Department of Mental Health & Substance Abuse Services
1200 NE 13th Street
P.O.Box 53277
Oklahoma City, OK 73152-3277   405-522-3908
                                       800-522-9054
                                  FAX: 405-522-3650
                                  TTY: 405-522-3851
                                  www.odmhsas.org

J. Andy Sullivan, Chairperson
Gail Henderson, Vice-Chair
Terri White, Commissioner
Durand Crosby, Chief Operating Officer
State agency providing mental helath , substance abuse and domestic violence services.

3706 Oklahoma Department of Rehabilitation Services
3535 NW 58th St
Suite 500
Oklahoma City, OK 73112-4824   405-951-3400
                                       800-845-8476
                                  FAX: 405-951-3529
                                  TTY: 405-951-3400
                                  info@okdrs.gov
                                  www.okdrs.gov

Michael O'Brien, Director
Jody Harlan, Public Information Administrator
David Ligon, Chief Of Staff
The Oklahoma Department of Rehabilitation Services (DRS) provides assistance to Oklahomans with disabilities through vocational rehabilitation, employment, independent living, residential and outreach programs, and the determination of medical eligibility for disability benefits.

3707 Workers Compensation Board Oklahoma
1915 N Stiles Ave
Oklahoma City, OK 73105-4918   405-522-8600
                                       800-522-8210
                                  owcc.state.ok.us

Leroy E Young, D.O., Chairman
Joyce Sanders, Supervisor
Michael J. Harkey, Vice Presiding Judge
Katrina Stephenson, Assistant Court Clerk

Oregon

3708 International Dyslexia Association: Oregon Branch
International Dyslexia Association
PO Box 2609
Portland, OR 97208-2609   503-228-4455
                                      800-530-2234
                                 FAX: 410-321-5609
                                 info@orbida.org
                                 www.orbida.org

Karen Brown, President
Provides free information and referral services for diagnosis and tutoring for parents, educators, physicians, and individuals with dyslexia. The voice of our membership is heard in 48 countries. Membership includes yearly journal and quarterly newsletter. Call for conference dates.

3709 Office of Vocational Rehabilitation Services (OVRS)
500 Summer St NE
Salem, OR 97301-1063   503-945-5944
                                 FAX: 503-378-2897
                                 TTY:503-945-6214
                                 www.oregon.gov/dhs/index.shtml

Erinn Kelley-Siel, Director
Gene Evans, Communication Director
Eric Moore, Chief Financial Officer
Jim Scherzinger, Chief Operating Officer
The mission of OVRS to assist Oregonians with disabilities to achieve and maintain employment and independence.

3710 Oregon Advocacy Center
620 SW 5th Ave
5th Floor
Portland, OR 97204-1428   503-243-2081
                                       800-452-6094
                                 FAX: 503-243-1738
                                 TTY: 800-556-5351
                                 welcome@oradvocacy.org
                                 oradvocacy.org

Robert Joondeph, Executive Director
Barbara Herget, Operations Director
The protection and advocacy system for Oregon.

3711 Oregon Client Assistance Program
620 SW 5th Ave
5th Floor
Portland, OR 97204-1420   503-243-2081
                                 FAX: 503-243-1738
                                 TTY:800-556-5351
                                 welcome@oradvocacy.org
                                 oradvocacy.org

Robert Joondeph, Executive Director

3712 Oregon Commission for the Blind
535 SE 12th Ave
Portland, OR 97214-2408   971-673-1588
                                       888-202-5463
                                 FAX: 503-234-7468
                                 TTY: 971-673-1577
                                 ocb.mail@state.or.us
                                 www.oregon.gov/blind

Jodi C. Roth, Chairman
Dacia Johnson, Executive Director
Angel Hale, Director of Rehabilitation Servi
Richard Turner, Director

3713 Oregon Department of Mental Health
500 Summer St NE
Salem, OR 97301-1063   503-945-5944
                                 FAX: 503-378-2897
                                 TTY:503-945-6214
                                 www.oregon.gov/DHS

Erinn Kelley-Siel, Director
Gene Evans, Communication Director
Eric Moore, Chief Financial Officer
Jim Scherzinger, Chief Operating Officer
Sets out the purpose and guides the activities of our large, complex organization. Vision is for better outcomes for clients and communities through collaboration, integration and shared responsibility.

3714 Oregon Technology Access for Life
2225 Lancaster Drive NE
Salem, OR 97305-1396   503-361-1201
                                       800-677-7512
                                 FAX: 503-370-4530
                                 TTY: 503-361-1201
                                 info@accesstechnologiesinc.com
                                 www.accesstechnologiesinc.org

Laurie Brooks, President
A statewide program promoting assistive technology devices and services for persons of all ages with all disabilities.

3715 Social Security: Salem Disability Determination
90 E Washington Bridge Rd
Suite 140
Worthington, OH 43085-3772
614-888-5339
800-722-1213
TTY:614-288-0226
www.socialsecurity.gov

Karena L. Kilgore, Executive Secretary
Carolyn W. Colvin, Commissioner
Carolyn W. Colvin, Deputy Commissioner
James A. Kissko, Chief of Staff

3716 Washington County Disability, Aging and Veteran Services
Ste 208
180 E Main St
Hillsboro, OR 97123-4054
503-640-3489
FAX: 503-693-6124
www.co.washington.or.us/aging

Jeff Hill, Director
Janet Long, Support Staff
Provides services to individuals through the Older Americans Act, state in home care services and represent, veterans in benefit claims process with Federal VA.

Pennsylvania

3717 International Dyslexia Association: Pennsylvania Branch
1062 E. Lancaster Avenue
Suite 15A
Rosemont, PA 19010- 251
610-527-1548
FAX: 610-527-5011
dyslexia@pbida.org
www.pbida.org

Eugenie Flaherty PhD, President
Tracy Bowes, Office Manager
Provides free information and referral services for diagnosis and tutoring for parents, educators, physicians, and individuals with dyslexia. The voice of membership is heard in 48 countries. Membership includes yearly journal and quarterly newsletter, and Pennsylvania newsletter; discounts to conferences and events.

3718 Mental Health Association in Pennysylvania
1414 N Cameron St
1st Floor
Harrisburg, PA 17103-1049
717-346-0549
855-220-8885
FAX: 717-236-0192
mfo@mhapa.org
www.mhapa.org

Julia Sadtler, President
Sue Waither, Executive Director
Madelyn Roman-Scott, Youth Advocate
Carl Onufer, Treasurer

3719 Pennsylvania Workers Compensation Board
651 Boas Street
Room 1700
Harrisburg, PA 17121-2510
717-787-5279
FAX: 717-772-0342
dli.state.pa.us

Joseph Brimmeier, CEO

3720 Pennsylvania Bureau of Blindness & VisualServices
Department of Pennsylvania
1521 N 6th St
Harrisburg, PA 17102
717-787-3201
800-622-2842
FAX: 717-787-3210
www.dli.state.pa.us

David Denotaris, Director
Jennifer Cave, Clerk Typist 3
Offers services for the totally blind, legally blind, visually impaired, mentally retarded blind and more with health, counseling, educational, recreational, rehabilitation, computer training and professional training services.

3721 Pennsylvania Client Assistance Program
1515 Market Street
Suite 1300
Philadelphia, PA 19102- 1819
215-557-7112
888-745-2357
FAX: 215-557-7602
info@equalemployment.org
www.equalemployment.org

Stephen S. Pennington, Executive Director
Jamie C Ray, Assistant Director
Margaret Passio-McKenna, Senior Advocate
Lee Lippi, Advocate
The Pennsylvania Client Assistance Program is dedicated to ensuring that the rehabilitation system in Pennsylvania is open and responsive to your needs. CAP help is provided to you at no charge, regardless of income. CAP helps people who are seeking services from the Office of Vocational Rehabilitation, Blindness and Visual Services, Centers for Independent Living and other programs funded under federal law.

3722 Pennsylvania Department of Aging
555 Walnut St
5th Floor
Harrisburg, PA 17101-1919
717-783-1550
FAX: 717-783-6842
aging@pa.gov
www.aging.state.pa.us

Nora Eisenhower, Manager

3723 Pennsylvania Department of Children with Disabilities
P.O. Box 2675
Harrisburg, PA 17105-2675
717-787-2600
FAX: 717-772-0323
www.pachildren.state.pa.US

Tom Corbett, Governor
Shelly Yanoff, Commission Chair

3724 Pennsylvania Developmental Disabilities Council
605 South Drive
Room 561
Harrisburg, PA 17120
717-789-6057
877-685-4452
TTY:717-705-0819
www.paddc.org

Amy High, Vice Chairperson
Graham Mulholland, Executive Director
Sandra Amador Dusek, Deputy Director

3725 Pennsylvania Protection & Advocacy for Persons with Disabilities
1414 N Cameron St
2nd Floor
Harrisburg, PA 17103-1049
717-236-8110
800-692-7443
FAX: 717-236-0192
TTY: 877-375-7139
ldo@drnpa.org
drnpa.org

Ken Oakes, Chairman
Nicole Turman, Vice Chairman
Peri Jude Radecic, CEO
Suzanne Erb, Secretary
Provide advocacy, information and referral for persons with disabilities and mental illness issues.

3726 Public Interest Law Center of Philadelphia
United Way Building, 2nd Floor
1709 Benjamin Franklin Parkway
Philadelphia, PA 19103-5153
215-627-7100
FAX: 215-627-3183
general@pilcop.org
pilcop.org

Eric J. Rothschild, Chair
Brian T. Feeney, Vice Chair
Jennifer R. Clarke, Executive Director
Latrice Brooks, Director of Administration
A non-profit, public interest law firm with a Disabilities Project specializing in class action suits brought by individuals and organizations.

3727 Social Security: Harrisburg Disability Determination
Suite 160
90 E Washington Bridge Rd
Worthington, OH 17101-1925
614-888-5339
800-722-1213
TTY:614-288-0226
ssa.gov

Karena L. Kilgore, Executive Secretary
Carolyn W. Colvin, Commissioner
Carolyn W. Colvin, Deputy Commissioner
James A. Kissko, Chief of Staff

3728 Workers Compensation Board Pennsylvania
651 Boas Street
Room 1700
Harrisburg, PA 17121-2510
717-787-5279
FAX: 717-772-0342
www.dli.state.pa.us

Tom Corbett, Governor
Julia K. Hearthway, Secretary
Joseph Brimmeier, CEO

Rhode Island

3729 Department of Mental Health, Retardation and Hospitals of Rhode Island
Goverment of Rhode Isalnd
14 Harrington Rd
Cranston, RI 02920-3080
401-462-2339
FAX: 401-462-3204
Craig.Stenning@bhddh.ri.gov
www.bhddh.ri.gov/

Craig S. Stenning, Director
Ellen Nelson, Manager
Kathleen Spangler, Manager
State department responsible for creating and administering systems of care for individuals with disabilities, specifically focused on mental health and mental illness; developmental disabilities, substance abuse and long term hospital care.

3730 Rhode Island Department Health
3 Capitol Hl
Providence, RI 02908-5097
401-222-3855
FAX: 401-222-6548
library@doh.state.ri.us
gotasthma.com

Mary Salerno, Manager
Patricia Nolan, Executive Director
Pamela Corcoran, Disability Health Program

3731 Rhode Island Department of Elderly Affairs
74 West Road
Hazard Bldg, 2nd Floor
Cranston, RI 02920- 3001
401-462-3000
FAX: 401-462-0740
larry@dea.state.ri.us
www.dea.state.ri.us

Corrine Russo, Manager

3732 Rhode Island Department of Mental Health
Cottage 405 Court B
Cranston, RI 02920
401-462-2003
FAX: 401-462-2008
www.butler.org

George W. Shuster, Chairman
Dennis D. Keefe, President & CEO
Reed Cosper, Manager

3733 Rhode Island Developmental Disabilities Council
400 Bald Hill Rd
Suite 515
Warwick, RI 02886-1692
401-737-1238
FAX: 401-737-3395
TTY:401-737-1238
riddc@riddc.org
www.riddc.org

Charles Zawacki, Chairperson, Individual & Family
John Susa, Chairperson, Executive Committee
Anne Frank, Chairperson, Individual & Family
Mary Okero, Executive Director
The Rhode Island Developmental Disabilities Council works to make Rhode Island a better place for people with developmental disabilities to live, work, go to school, and be part of their community.

3734 Rhode Island Governor's Commission on Disabilities
John O Pastore Center
Warwick City Hall
3275 Post Road
Warwick, RI 02920-3049
401-738-2000
FAX: 401-462-0106
disabilities@gcd.state.ri.gov
www.warwickri.gov

Bob Cooper, Executive Secretary
The Commision is responsible for: coordinating compliance by state agencies with federal and state disablty right laws; approving or modifying state and local goverment agency's open meeting accessibility for persons with disabilities transition plans; assisting local boards of canvassers to ensure accessible polling places locations; aproving or rejecting requests to waive the state building code's standards for accessibility at facilities to be leased by state agencies...

3735 Rhode Island Parent Information Network
1210 Pontiac Avenue
Cranston, RI 02920
401-270-0101
800-464-3399
FAX: 401-270-7049
info@ripin.org
ripin.org

Kathleen DiChiara, Chairman
Ammala Douangsavanh, Vice Chairman
Stephen Brunero, Executive Director
Matthew Cox, Associate Exeutive Director
A nonprofit organization established by parents and concerned professionals providing culturally appropriate information, training and support for families and professionals designed to improve educational and life outcomes for all children. Serving the State of Rhode Island.

3736 Rhode Island Protection & Advocacy for Persons with Disabilities
Rhode Island Disability Law Center
275 Westminster Street
Suite 401
Providence, RI 02903- 3434
401-831-3150
800-733-5332
FAX: 401-274-5568
TTY: 401-831-5335
info@ridlc.org
www.ridlc.org

Raymond Bandusky, Executive Director
Rhode Island Disability Law Center (RIDLC) provides free legal assistance to persons with disabilities. Services include individ-

ual representation to protect rights or to secure benefits and services; self-help information; educational programs; and administrative and legislative advocacy. The agency administers eight federally funded advocacy programs, each of which has its own eligibility criteria.

3737 Rhode Island Services for the Blind and Visually Impaired
40 Fountain St
Providence, RI 02903-1830
401-421-7005
800-752-8088
FAX: 401-421-9259
TTY: 401-421-7016
thompson@ors.state.ri.us
www.ors.ri.gov

Kathleen Grygiel, Administrator
Ronald Racine, Associate Director
Laurie DiOrio, Acting Associate Director
JoAnn Nannig, Assistant Administrator of VR
Offers services for the totally blind, legally blind, visually impaired, mentally retarded blind and more with health, counseling, educational, recreational, rehabilitation, computer training and professional training services.

3738 Services for the Blind and Visually Impaired
40 Fountain St
Providence, RI 02903-1830
401-421-7005
FAX: 401-222-1328
TTY:401-421-7016
www.ors.ri.gov

Kathleen Grygiel, Administrator
Ronald Racine, Associate Director
Laurie DiOrio, Acting Associate Director
JoAnn Nannig, Assistant Administrator of VR
Offers services for the blind and visually impaired.

3739 Social Security: Providence Disability Determination
Social Security
40 Fountain Street
6th Floor
Providence, RI 02903-3246
401-222-3182
800-772-1213
FAX: 401-222-3868
TTY: 401-273-6648
Deborah.A.Cannon@ssa.gov
www.ssa.gov

Karena L. Kilgore, Executive Secretary
Carolyn W. Colvin, Commissioner
Carolyn W. Colvin, Deputy Commissioner
James A. Kissko, Chief of Staff
We deliver services through a nationwide network of over 1,400 offices that include regional offices, field offices, card centers, teleservice centers, processing centers, hearing offices, the Appeals Council, and our State and territorial partners, the Disability Determination Services. We also have a presence in U.S. embassies around the globe. For the public, we are the face of the government. The rich diversity of our employees mirrors the public we serve.

3740 Workers Compensation Board Rhode Island
1 Dorrance Plz
Providence, RI 02903-3973
401-458-5000
FAX: 401-222-3121
courts.ri.gov

George E Healy Jr, Manager
George Healy Jr, Manager

South Carolina

3741 Protection & Advocacy for People with Disabilities
Ste 208
3710 Landmark Dr
Columbia, SC 29204-4034
803-782-0639
866-275-7273
FAX: 803-790-1946
TTY: 866-232-4525
info@pandasc.org
protectionandadvocacy-sc.org

Gloria Prevost, Executive Director
Anne Trice, Director of Administration
J. Ashley Twombley, Chair
Sherry Williams, Vice-Chair
An independent, nonprofit organization responsible for safe guarding rights of South Carolinians with disabilities and other handicapped individuals without regard to age, income, severity of disability, sex, race, or religion.

3742 Social Security: West Columbia Disability Determination
P.O. Box 60
Columbia, SC 29171-0060
803-896-6400
800-772-1213
FAX: 803-822-4318
TTY: 800-325-0078
Kenneth.Norris@ssa.gov
www.socialsecurity.gov

Karena L. Kilgore, Executive Secretary
Carolyn W. Colvin, Commissioner
Carolyn W. Colvin, Deputy Commissioner
James A. Kissko, Chief of Staff
We deliver services through a nationwide network of over 1,400 offices that include regional offices, field offices, card centers, teleservice centers, processing centers, hearing offices, the Appeals Council, and our State and territorial partners, the Disability Determination Services. We also have a presence in U.S. embassies around the globe. For the public, we are the face of the government. The rich diversity of our employees mirrors the public we serve.

3743 South Carolina Assistive Technology Project
Midlands Center
8301 Farrow Road
Columbia, SC 29203
803-935-5263
800-915-4522
FAX: 803-935-5342
TTY: 803-935-5263
jjendron@usit.net
www.sc.edu/scatp/

Carol Page, Ph.D, CCC-SLP, A, Program Director
Janet Jendron, Program Coordinator
Mary Alice Bechtler, Program Coordinator
Lydia Durham, Administrative Assistant
A statewide program promoting assistive technology devices and services for persons of all ages with all disabilities. Recently a statewide AT resource, demonstrations and equipment loan center and lab annual expo and training and workshops on a variety of disabilities and technology topics.

3744 South Carolina Client Assistance Program
Governor's Office oe Executive Policy & Programs
1205 Pendleton St
Columbia, SC 29201-3756
803-734-0285
800-868-0040
FAX: 803-734-0546
TTY: 803-734-1147
cap@oepp.sc.gov
www.govoepp.state.sc.us/cap

Denise Riley Pensmith, MSW, Executive Director
Cindy Popenhagen, Administrative Assistant
The Client Assistance Program (CAP) helps citizens of the State by acting as advocates regarding services provided by the Vocational Rehabilitation Department (VR), Commission for the Blind, and all Independent Living programs and projects funded under the Rehabilitation Act of 1973. As advocates, CAP staff

can investigate, negotiate, mediate, and pursue administrative, and other remedies to ensure that clients' rights are protected.

3745 South Carolina Commission for the Blind
1430 Confederate Avenue
P. O. Box 2467
Columbia, SC 29202-79
803-898-8731
800-922-2222
888-335-5951
FAX: 803-898-8800
publicinfo@sccb.sc.gov
www.sccb.state.sc.us

James Kirby, Commissioner
Peter Smith, Board Member
Dr. Julianne Kleckley, Board Member
Dr. Julia Barnes, Board Member

Offers services for the totally blind, legally blind, visually impaired, mentally retarded blind and more with health, counseling, educational, recreational, rehabilitation, computer training and professional training services.

3746 South Carolina Department of Children with Disabilities
2600 Bull St
Columbia, SC 29201-1708
803-434-4260

Miroslav Cuturic, Director
Peter Getz, Administrator

3747 South Carolina Department of Mental Healthand Mental Retardation
Administration Building
2414 Bull Streets
Columbia, SC 29202-485
803-898-8581
800-273-8255
FAX: 864-297-5130
webmaster@scdmh.org
www.state.sc.us/dmh

John H. Magill, State Director
Mark Binkley, Deputy Director
David Schaefer, Director
Eleanor Odom, Director

The S.C. Department of Mental Health gives priority to adults, children, and their families affected by serious mental illnesses and significant emotional disorders. We are committed to eliminating stigma and promoting the philosophy of recovery, to achieving our goals in collaboration with all stakeholders, and to assuring the highest quality of culturally competent services possible.

3748 South Carolina Developmental Disabilities Council
Office of the Governor
1205 Pendleton St
Suite 461
Columbia, SC 29201-3756
803-734-0465
FAX: 803-734-1409
TTY:803-734-1147
jvancleave@oepp.sc.gov
www.scddc.state.sc.us

Valarie Bishop, Executive Director
Cheryl English, Program Information Coordinator
Kimberly Johnson Fontanez, Grants Administrator
Esther Williams, Administrative Support Specialis

The mission of the South Carolina Developmental Disabilities Council is to provide leadership in advocating, funding and implementing initiatives which recognize the inherent dignity of each individual, and promote independence, productivity, respect and inclusion for all persons with disabilities and their families.

3749 Workers Compensation Board: South Carolina
PO Box 1715
Columbia, SC 29202-1715
803-737-5700
FAX: 803-737-5768
www.state.sc.us/wcc

Gary Cannon, Executive Director
Kim Balleutine, Admin. Assistant

3750 Children's Special Health Services Program
600 E Capitol Ave
Pierre, SD 57501-2536
605-773-3361
800-738-2301
FAX: 605-773-5683
DOH.info@state.sd.us
www.doh.sd.gov

Dianne Weyer, Manager
Barb Hemmelman, Program Manager

Health KiCC is a program, funded through federal and state monies, that provides financial assistance for medical appointments, procedures, treatments, medications and travel reimbursement for children with certain chronic health conditions.

3751 Division of Labor and Management
South Dakota Department of Labor
700 Governors Dr
Pierre, SD 57501-2291
605-773-3101
FAX: 605-773-6184
jamesmarsh@state.sd.us
dlr.sd.gov

Sara Minton, Executive Director
Pamela S Roberts, Secretary
Marcia Hultman, Deputy Secretary of Labor and D
Lyle Harter, Director of Administrative Servi

Our mission is to promote economic opportunity and financial security for individuals and businesses through quality, responsive and expert services; fair and equitable employment solutions; and safe and sound business practices.

3752 Health KiCC
South Dakota Department of Health
600 E Capitol Ave
Pierre, SD 57501-2536
605-773-3361
800-738-2301
FAX: 605-773-5683
DOH.info@state.sd.us
www.doh.sd.gov

Dianne Weyer, Manager

Health KiCC is a program, funded through federal and state monies, that provides financial assistance for medical appointments, procedures, treatments, medications and travel reimbursement for children with certain chronic health conditions.

3753 South Dakota Advocacy Services
221 S Central Ave
Ste. 38
Pierre, SD 57501-2479
605-224-8294
800-658-4782
FAX: 605-224-5125
sdas@sdadvocacy.com
sdadvocacy.com

Sandy Stocklin Hook, Partners Coordinator

Designated protection and advocacy progam for South Dakota providing legal, administrative, mediation and other services to elgible persons with disabilities in the state.

3754 South Dakota Department of Aging
700 Governors Dr
Pierre, SD 57501-2291
605-773-3656
866-854-5465
FAX: 605-773-4085
ASA@state.sd.us
pierre.sd.welfareinfo.org

Marilyn Kinsman, Division Director
Lynne Valenti, Deputy Secretary
Amy Iversen-Pollreisz, Deputy Secretary
Kristin Kellar, Communications Director

The Division of Adult Services and Aging (ASA) provides home and community service options to individuals 60 years of age and older and 18 years of age and older with physical disabilities, regardless of income.

3755 South Dakota Department of Human Services Division of Community Behavioral Health
South Dakota of Human Services
700 Governors Drive
Hillsview Properties Plaza
Pierre, SD 57501-5007

605-773-3165
800-265-9684
FAX: 605-773-7076
infoMH@state.sd.us
http://dss.sd.gov/behavioralhealthservices

Shawna Fullerton, Division Director
South Dakota's state mental health authority.

3756 South Dakota Developmental Disability Council
Hillsview Plaza 3800 E Highway 34
c/o 500 East Capital Avenue
Pierre, SD 57501

605-773-5990
800-265-9684
FAX: 605-773-5483
TTY: 605-773-6412
infodhs@state.sd.us
www.state.sd.us/dhs/ddc

Dan Lusk, Director
Laurie R. Gill, Secretary
Carol Ruen, Assistant Director
Lindsay Dummer, Program Specialist II
To assist individuals with developmental disabilities to control their own destiny and to achieve the quality of life they desire.

3757 South Dakota Division of Rehabilitation
700 Governors Dr
Pierre, SD 57501-2291

605-773-3101
FAX: 605-773-6184
jamesmarsh@state.sd.us
www.sdjobs.org

Sara Minton, Executive Director
Pamela S Roberts, Secretary
Marcia Hultman, Deputy Secretary of Labor and D
Lyle Harter, Director of Administrative Servi
Offers diagnosis, evaluation and physical restoration services, counseling, social work, educational and professional training, employment and rehabilitation services for the disabled.

3758 Workers Compensation Board: South Dakota
700 Governors Dr
Pierre, SD 57501-2291

605-773-3101
FAX: 605-773-6184
jamesmarsh@state.sd.us
www.sdjobs.org

Sara Minton, Executive Director
Marcia Hultman, Secretary
Lyle Harter, Director of Administrative Servi
Bret Afdahi, Director of the Division of Bank
Our mission is to promote economic opportunity and financial security for individuals and businesses through quality, responsive and expert services; fair and equitable employment solutions; and safe and sound business practices.

Tennessee

3759 International Dyslexia Association: Tennessee Branch
TTU Box 5074
Cookeville, TN 37931-2311

800-222-3123
877-836-6432
FAX: 865-693-3653
htdainty@gmail.com.
www.tnida.org

Emily Dempster, President
Erin Alexander, Senior Vice President
Shannon Polk, Secretary
Jean Hutchinson, Treasurer
The Tennessee Branch of the International Dyslexia Association (TN-IDA) was formed to increase awareness about Dyslexia in the state of Tennessee. TN-IDA supports efforts to provide information regarding appropriate language arts instruction to those involved with language-based learning differences and to encourage the identity of these individuals at-risk for such disorders as soon as possible.

3760 Social Security: Nashville Disability Determination
Social Security
P.O. Box 77
Nashville, TN 37202-4732

615-743-7774
800-772-1213
800-342-1117
FAX: 615-253-1840
Betty.J.Hood@ssa.gov
ssa.gov

Karena L. Kilgore, Executive Secretary
Carolyn W. Colvin, Commissioner
Carolyn W. Colvin, Deputy Commissioner
James A. Kissko, Chief of Staff
We deliver services through a nationwide network of over 1,400 offices that include regional offices, field offices, card centers, teleservice centers, processing centers, hearing offices, the Appeals Council, and our State and territorial partners, the Disability Determination Services. We also have a presence in U.S. embassies around the globe. For the public, we are the face of the government. The rich diversity of our employees mirrors the public we serve.

3761 Tennessee Assistive Technology Projects
Citizens Plaza State Office Buildin
511 Union St.
Nashville, TN 37219-1403

615-313-5183
800-732-5059
TTY: 615-313-5695
TN.TTAP@tn.gov
www.tn.gov

Bill Haslam, Governor
Raquel Hatter, Commissioner
Beth White, Manager
Julie Oden, Manager
A statewide program promoting assistive technology devices and services for persons of all ages with all disabilities.

3762 Tennessee Client Assistance Program
Tennessee Protection and Advocacy
P.O. Box 121257
Nashville, TN 37212-1257

615-298-1080
800-342-1660
FAX: 615-298-2046
gethelp@tpainc.org
www.tpainc.org

Shirley Shea, Executive Director
Doris Lopez, Assistant Executive Director

3763 Tennessee Commission on Aging and Disability
502 Deaderick Street
9th Floor
Nashville, TN 37243-860

615-741-2056
FAX: 615-741-3309
cindy.warf@tn.gov
www.tn.gov/comaging

Richard M. Honn, Executive Director
Ryan Ellis, Aging Info. & Data Director
Kathy Zamata, Aging Program Director
Richard Presler, Fiscal Director

3764 Tennessee Council on Developmental Disabilities
404 James Robertson Pkwy
Parkway Towers, Suite 130
Nashville, TN 37243

615-532-6615
FAX: 615-532-6964
tnddc@tn.gov
www.state.tn.us/odd

Wanda Willis, Executive Director
Bill Haslam, Governor
Alicia Cone, Coordinator, Project Research an
William Edington, Public Policy Director

Provides leadership to ensure independence, productivity, integration and inclusion of individuals with disabilities in the community through promotion of systems change. The council works with members of the community, including public and private aenqies, business, legislators and policymakers, to create a future in which; people with disabilities are full included in the community and experience no barriers related to attitudes about their disabilities as they persue their goals.

3765 Tennessee Department of Children with Disabilities
511 Union St.
Nashville, TN 37219-9004
615-741-9701
800-861-1935
FAX: 615-253-5216
dcs.email@tn.gov
www.tn.gov

Ruth S Letson, Manager
Haticile Buchanan, Manager
Mary Beth Franklyn, CS Program Director
Kristi Faulkner, Special Counsel to the Commissio
Tennessee's children thrive in safe, healthy and stable families. Families thrive in healthy, safe and strong communities. Tennessee's citizens benefit from the best child welfare and juvenile justice agency in the country.

3766 Tennessee Department of Mental Health
500 Deaderick Street
Nashville, TN 37243-3400
615-532-6597
800-560-5767
FAX: 615-532-6514
oc.tdmh@tn.gov
www.state.tn.us/mental

Doug Varney, Commissioner
Grant Lawrence, Director Office of Communication
Bob Grunow, Deputy Commissioner
Howard Burley, Asst Commissioner Clinical Ldrsp
TDMH is the state's mental health and substance abuse authority. Its mission is to plan for and promote the availability of a comprehensive array of quality prevention, early intervention, treatment, habilitation, and rehabilitation services and supports based on the needs and choices of individuals and families served. Responsible for policy, and oversight, and for advocacy of the consumer within the state.

3767 Tennessee Division of Rehabilitation
400 Deaderick St
Nashville, TN 37243-1403
615-313-4700
800-270-1349
TTY:615-313-5695
connie.phillips@tn.gov
http://www.tn.gov

Patsy Matthews, Commissioner
Randall Beasley, Manager
Raquel Hatter, Commissioner
Bill Haslam, Givernor
Offers rehabilitation, medical and therapeutic information and referrals to the disabled.

3768 Workers Compensation Division Tennessee
Dept of Labor & Workforce Development
220 French Landing Drive
1st Floor
Nashville, TN 37243- 1002
615-741-6642
800-332-2667
FAX: 615-532-1468
wc.info@tn.gov
www.tn.gov/labor-wfd/wcomp.html

Karla Davis, Commissioner
Alisa Malone, Deputy Commissioner
Stephanie Mitchell, General Counsel
Ron Jones, Administrator of Fiscal Services
We administer the workers' compensation system and promote a better understanding of the program's benefits by informing employees and employers of their rights and responsibilities. Workers' Compensation administers a mediation program for disputed claims, encourage workplace safety, participate in a public awareness campaign concerning fraud, and oversee an information awareness program for educating the public on laws

and regulations which define workers' compensation requirements. We ensure

Texas

3769 Disability Policy Consortium
2222 West Braker Lane
Austin, TX 78758-1024
512-454-4816
800-252-9108
FAX: 512-323-0902
dpctexas@advocacyinc.org
www.disabilityrightstx.org

Mary Faithful, Executive Director
Roberta Rosenberg-Roque, Manager
An independent group of statewide advocacy organizations that strives to achieve the development and full implementation of public policy that promotes and supports the rights, inclusion, integration and independence of Texans with disabilities.

3770 Division of Special Education
1701 Congress Ave
Austin, TX 78701-1402
512-463-9734
FAX: 512-463-9838
teainfo@tea.state.tx.us
www.tea.state.tx.us

Bill Abasolo, Federal & State Education Policy
Robert Scott, Commissioner of Education
Lizzette Gonzalez Reynolds, Deputy Commissioner, Policy & Pr
Anita Givens, Associate Commissioner, Standard
The Texas public school system is a $46 billion a year enterprise. Running a school district requires superintendents to operate one of the largest, if not the largest, business in their community. This website attempts to provide administrators with easy access to information they need to successfully carry out their duties.

3771 Easter Seal of Greater Dallas, TX
233 South Wacker Drive
Suite 2400
Chicago, IL 60606-4743
972-394-8900
800-580-4718
800-221-6827
FAX: 972-394-6266
wjohnson@dallas.easterseals.com
easterseals.com

Richard W. Davidson, Chairman
Sandra L. Bouwman, 1st Vice Chairman
Joseph G. Kern, 2nd Vice Chairman
Bennett Leventhal, M.D., President
Easter Seals has a longstanding history in our community of providing a wealth of unique programs and services for individual with a wide variety of disabilities, including Autism Spectrum Disorder, Alzheimer's disease, Down syndrome, Cerebral Palsy, Mental and Developmental Delays, and a wealth of other disabilities. We provide programs and services, education, outreach, and advocacy so that people living with disabilities can live, learn, work and play in our communities.

3772 Easter Seals Greater NW Texas
1424 Hemphill Street
Fort Worth, TX 76104-8130
817-332-717
888-617-7171
FAX: 817-332-7601
wjohnson@dallas.easterseals.com
www.easterseals.com/northtexas

Donna Dempsey, President and Chief Executive Of
Nancy Robinson, Executive Vice President & Chief
Nancy Swartz, Vice President of Development an
Lenee Bassham, Vice President Community Living
Easter Seals has a longstanding history in our community of providing a wealth of unique programs and services for individual with a wide variety of disabilities, including Autism Spectrum Disorder, Alzheimer's disease, Down syndrome, Cerebral Palsy, Mental and Developmental Delays, and a wealth of other disabilities. We provide programs and services, education, outreach, and advocacy so that people living with disabilities can live, learn, work and play in our communities.

3773 El Valle Community Parent Resource Center
Ste J
530 S Texas Blvd
Weslaco, TX 78596-6262   956-969-0215
                                      800-680-0255
                                  FAX: 956-968-7102
                                   texasfiestaedu.org
                                    www.tfepodder.org

Robert Garza, Owner

3774 Grassroots Consortium
Greenroots Consortium
6202 Belmark St
Houston, TX 77087-6324   713-643-9576
                                  FAX: 713-643-6291
                                    Speckids@aol.com

Agnes A Johnson, Director

3775 International Dyslexia Association: Austin Branch
40 York Rd.
4th Floor
Baltimore, MD 21204-2604   410-296-0232
                                      800-222-3123
                                  FAX: 410-321-5069
                                     info@interdys.org
                                      www.interdys.org

Hal Malchow, President
Elsa Cardenas-Hagan, Vice President
Ben Shifrin, Vice President
Lee Grossman, Executive Director
The Austin Area Branch of the International Dyslexia Association is a 501(c)(3) non profit organization dedicated to promoting reading excellence for all children through early identification of dyslexia, effective literacy education for adults and children with dyslexia, and teacher training.

3776 NAMI Texas
FOUNTAIN Park Plaza III
P.O. Box 300817
Austin, TX 78703-5700   512-693-2000
                                      800-633-3760
                                  FAX: 512-693-8000
                                 namitexas@texami.org
                                      namitexas.org

Andrea Hazlitt, President
Ed Dickey, Vice President
Chris Scroggin, Executive Director
Kelly Jeschke, Membership Coordinator
NAMI Texas has a variety of programs directed to mental health consumers, family members, friends, professionals, other stake holders and the community at large to address the mental health needs of Texans. NAMI Texas works to inform the public about mental illness by distributing information about mental illness through every means of communication. Interviews are produced on television, stories are featured in newspapers, brochures are distributed, referrals are provided and more.

3777 Parent Connection
1020 Riverwood Ct
Conroe, TX 77304-2811   936-756-8321
                                      800-839-8876
                                 parentCNCT@aol.com
                  http://www.parentingaspergerscommunity.com/pu
Dave Angel, Founder
Includes parenting help and Aspergers advice, including parenting tips, tricks and techniques to help your child with Aspergers. Our worldwide membership base is helping parents to understand their child with Aspergers better and make their home & family life a better place to be.

3778 Parents Supporting Parents Network
8001 Centre Park Drive
Suite 100
Austin, TX 78754   512-454-6694
                                      800-252-9729
                                  FAX: 512-454-4956
                             secretary@thearcoftexas.org
                                  www.thearcoftexas.org

Charlie Huber, President
John Schneider, Vice-President
Nancy Lepley, Treasurer
Terri Schonfeld, Secretary
Since our founding in 1950 by a group of parents of children with intellectual and developmental disabilities, The Arc at the local, state and national level has been instrumental in the creation of virtually every program, service, right, and benefit that is now available to more than half a million Texans with intellectual and developmental disabilities. Today, The Arc continues to advocate for including people with intellectual and developmental disabilities in all aspects of society.

3779 Partners Resource Network
Ste B
1090 Longfellow Dr
Beaumont, TX 77706-4819   409-898-4684
                                      800-866-4726
                                  FAX: 409-898-4869
                           partnersresource@sbcglobal.net
                                      partnerstx.org

Janice Meyer, Executive Director
Statewide network of three parent training and information centers.

3780 Social Security: Austin Disability Determination
P.O. Box 149198
Austin, TX 78714-9198   512-437-8311
                                      800-772-1213
                                      800-252-9627
                                  FAX: 512-437-8595
                                   TTY:512-916-5958
                                   dan.tippit@ssa.gov
                                      www.ssa.gov

Karena L. Kilgore, Executive Secretary
Carolyn W. Colvin, Commissioner
Carolyn W. Colvin, Deputy Commissioner
James A. Kissko, Chief of Staff
We deliver services through a nationwide network of over 1,400 offices that include regional offices, field offices, card centers, teleservice centers, processing centers, hearing offices, the Appeals Council, and our State and territorial partners, the Disability Determination Services. We also have a presence in U.S. embassies around the globe. The rich diversity of our employees mirrors the public we serve.

3781 Statewide Information at Texas School for the Deaf
1102 S Congress Ave
Austin, TX 78704-1728   512-462-5353
                                  FAX: 512-462-5353
                             webmaster@tsd.state.tx.us
                                   www.tsd.state.tx.us

Sonia Karimi Bridges, Video Communication Specialist
Avonne Brooker-Rutowski, Program Specialist
David Coco, Program Specialist
Lisa Crawford, Parent Liason
Welcome to Texas School for the Deaf, a place where students who are deaf or hard of hearing including those with additional disabilities, have the opportunity to learn, grow and belong in a culture that optimizes individual potential and provides accessible language and communication across the curriculum. Our educational philosophy is grounded in the belief that all children who are deaf and hard of hearing deserve a quality language and communication-driven program that provides education tog

3782 **Texas Advocates Supporting Kids with Disabilities**
P.O. Box 162685
Austin, TX 78716-2685

512-310-2102
FAX: 512-310-2102
ASKTASK@aol.com
www.main.org/task/

3783 **Texas Commission for the Blind**
P.O. Box 149198
Austin, TX 78714-9198

512-459-8575
800-252-5204
FAX: 512-424-4730
DARS.Inquiries@dars.state.tx.us
www.dars.state.tx.us

Canzata Crowder, Manager
Offers services for the totally blind, legally blind, and visually impaired, with counseling, educational, recreational, rehabilitation, computer training and professional training services.

3784 **Texas Commission for the Deaf and Hard of Hearing**
D AR S
P.O. Box 149198
Austin, TX 78714-9198

512-407-3250
800-628-5115
FAX: 512-424-4730
TTY: 512-407-3251
DARS.Inquiries@dars.state.tx.us
www.dars.state.tx.us

Veronda L. Durden, Commissioner
Glenn Neal, Deputy Commissioner
David Myers, Executive Director
Daniel Bravo, Chief Operating Officer

3785 **Texas Council for Developmental Disabilities**
6201 E Oltorf St
Suite 600
Austin, TX 78741-7509

512-437-5432
800-262-0334
FAX: 512-437-5434
TTY: 512-437-5431
tcdd@tcdd.texas.gov
txddc.state.tx.us

Mary Durheim, Chairman
Andrew D. Crim, Vice Chairman
Roger Webb, Executive Director
Koren Vogel, Executive Assistant
The Texas Council for Developmental Disabilities is a 27-member board dedicated to ensuring that all Texans with developmental disabilities, about 411,479 individuals, have the opportunity to be independent, productive and valued members of their communities. The mission of the Texas Council for Developmental Disabilities is to create change so that all people with disabilities are fully included in their communities and exercise control over their own lives.

3786 **Texas Department of Human Services**
701 W 51st St
P.O. Box 149030
Austin, TX 78751-2312

512-438-3011
888-834-7406
FAX: 512-472-0603
TTY: 888-425-6889
mail@dads.state.tx.us
www.dads.state.tx.us

Jon Weizenbaum, Commissioner
Kristi Jordan, Associate Commissioner
Chris Adams, Deputy Commissioner
Elisa J. Garza, Assistant Commissioner for Acces

3787 **Texas Department of Mental Health & Mental Retardation**
P.O. Box 12668
Austin, TX 78711-2668

512-472-4138
FAX: 512-472-0603
www.mhmr.state.tx.us

Bill West, Manager
Randy Fritz, Chief Operating Officer

3788 **Texas Department on Aging**
701 W 51st St
P.O. Box 149030
Austin, TX 78751-2312

512-438-3011
800-252-9240
mail@tdoa.state.tx.us
www.dads.state.tx.us

Jon Weizenbaum, Commissioner
Kristi Jordan, Associate Commissioner
Chris Adams, Deputy Commissioner
Elisa J. Garza, Assistant Commissioner for Acces

3789 **Texas Federation of Families for Children's Mental Health**
Ste 505
7701 N Lamar Blvd
Austin, TX 78752-1000

512-407-8844
866-893-3264
FAX: 512-407-8266
info@txffcmh.org
www.txffcmh.org

Patti Derr, Executive Director
Pat Calley, Chairperson
S Barron, Operations Director

3790 **Texas Governor's Committee on People with Disabilities**
1100 San Jacinto Blvd
P.O. Box 12428
Austin, TX 78701- 1935

512-463-2000
FAX: 513-463-5745
CPD@gov.texas.gov
www.governor.state.tx.us/disabilities

Angela English, LPC, LMFT, Executive Director
Erin Lawler, JD, MS, Accessibility and Disability Rig
Nancy Van Loan, Executive Assistant
Jo Virgil, MS, Community Outreach and Informati
The Governor's Committee on People with Disabilities is within the office of the Governor. The committee's mission is to further opportunities for persons with disabilities to enjoy full and equal access to lives of independence, productivity, and self-determination. The committee is composed of 12 members appointed by the governor and of nonvoting ex officio members.

3791 **Texas Protection & Advocacy Services for Disabled Persons**
Advocacy
2222 West Braker Lane
Austin, TX 78758-1024

512-454-4816
800-252-9108
800-315-3876
FAX: 512-323-0902
dpctexas@advocacyinc.org
www.disabilityrightstx.org

Mary Faithful, Executive Director
Roberta Rosenberg-Roque, Manager
A federally funded, independent, nonprofit agency that advocates for the legal, human and service rights of persons with disabilities. Publishes 'Special Edition' newsletter, at a small fee and 'It's a Good Idea!' a parent manual for $10, plus many other handouts free of charge.

3792 **Texas Respite Resource Network**
P.O. Box 149030
710 West 51st Street
Austin, TX 78714- 9030

512-438-5555
FAX: 512-438-4374
elizabethnewhouse@srhcc.org
archrespite.org

Jill Kagan, Program Director
Liz Newhouse, Assistant Director
Mike Mathers, Executive Director
Maggie Edgar, Senior Consultant
A state clearinghouse and technical assistance network for respite in Texas. TRRN identifies, initiates and improves respite options for families caring for individuals with disabilities on the local, state and national levels. TRRN provides training/techni-

cal assistance to programs/groups wanting to establish respite services.

3793 Texas Technology Access Project
Center for Disabilities Studies
10100 Burnet Rd
Austin, TX 78758-4445

512-232-0740
800-828-7839
FAX: 512-232-0761
TTY: 512-232-0762
rogerlevy@austin.utexas.edu
techaccess.edb.utexas.edu

Roger Levy, Program Director
Darlene West, Assistive Technology Coordinator
Steve Thomas, Operations and External Relation
Darlene West, Assistive Technology Specialist

Their mission is to increase access for people with disabilities to assistive technology that provides them more control over their immediate environments and an enhanced ability to function independently.

3794 Texas UAP for Developmental Disabilities
University of Texas
1 University Station
Austin, TX 78712

512-471-3434
800-828-7839
hello@utexas.edu
www.utexas.edu

Gregory L. Fences, President
Judith H. Langlois, Executive Vice President and Pr
Gregory J. Vincent, Vice President
Patricia C. Ohlendorf, Vice President

Welcome to The University of Texas at Austin. Founded in 1883, UT is one of the largest and most respected universities in the nation. Ours is a diverse learning community, with students from every state and more than 100 countries. We're a university with world talent and Texas traditions. Discover more about us online and come visit our beautiful campus in person.

3795 Texas Workers Compensation Commission
333 Guadalupe
P.O. Box 149104
Austin, TX 78701-1645

512-676-6000
800-578-4677
800-252-3439
FAX: 512-804-4401
TTY:512-322-4238
WebStaff@tdi.state.tx.us
www.tdi.texas.gov

Robert Shipe, Executive Director
Rod Bordelon, Commissioner

Workers' compensation is a state-regulated insurance program that pays medical bills and replaces some lost wages for employees who are injured at work or who have work-related diseases or illnesses.

3796 United Cerebral Palsy of Texas
National Cerebral Palsy of American
Ste 145
1016 La Posada Dr
Austin, TX 78752-3828

512-472-8696
800-798-1492
FAX: 512-472-8026
info@ucptexas.org
ucptexas.org

Jean Langendorf, Executive Director

Offers a unique array of programs and services designed for one specific purpose: to ensure that people with cerebral palsy and similar disabilities have the opportunity to participate fully and equally in every aspect of our society.

Utah

3797 Access Utah Network
Ste 100
155 S 300 W
Salt Lake City, UT 84101-1288

801-533-4636
800-333-8824
FAX: 801-533-3968
access@utah.gov
accessut.org

Mark L. Smith, Information Specialist

Access Utah Network is Utah's prime source for information and referral for individuals with disabilities and their caregivers since 1990. Our operators can provide you with the information you need to find accessible housing, assistive technology and financial and social supports needed to live independently with a disability. Call us or explore our web site today to see how Access Utah Network can help you become more independent.

3798 Social Security: Salt Lake City Disability Determination
Social Security
P.O. Box 144032
Salt Lake City, UT 84111-4032

801-321-6500
800-772-1213
800-221-3493
FAX: 801-321-6599
TTY:801-524-5047
Dave.Carlson@ssa.gov
www.ssa.gov

Karena L. Kilgore, Executive Secretary
Carolyn W. Colvin, Commissioner
Carolyn W. Colvin, Deputy Commissioner
James A. Kissko, Chief of Staff

We deliver services through a nationwide network of over 1,400 offices that include regional offices, field offices, card centers, teleservice centers, processing centers, hearing offices, the Appeals Council, and our State and territorial partners, the Disability Determination Services. We also have a presence in U.S. embassies around the globe. The rich diversity of our employees mirrors the public we serve.

3799 Utah Assistive Technology Projects
Utah State University
6855 Old Main Hl
Logan, UT 84322-6855

435-797-3824
800-524-5152
TTY:435-797-2355
www.uatpat.org

Sachin Pavithran, Program Director
Alma Burgess, UATP Data Collection Coordinator
Clay Christensen, Lab Coordinator
Marilyn ' Hammond, Executive Director

A statewide program promoting assistive technology devices and services for persons of all ages with all disabilities.

3800 Utah Client Assistance Program
205 N 400 W
Salt Lake City, UT 84103-1125

801-363-1347
800-662-9080
FAX: 801-363-1437
www.disabilitylawcenter.org

Bryce Fifield Ph.D, President
Jared Fields, Vice President
Barbara M. Campbell, Treasurer
Kevin Murphy, Board Member

Since 1979, the Disability Law Center (DLC) has helped thousands of Utahns with disabilities and their families. The DLC has broad statutory powers to safeguard the human and civil rights of persons with disabilities. We provide self-advocacy assistance, legal services, disability rights education, and public policy advocacy on behalf of the more than 400,000 Utah residents with disabilities. Our services are available statewide and without regard for ability to pay.

3801 Utah Department of Aging
195 North 1950 West
Salt Lake City, UT 84116

801-538-3910
877-424-4640
FAX: 801-538-4395
debooth@utah.gov
www.hsdaas.utah.gov

Nels Holmgren, Director
Michael S. Styles, Assistant Director
Michelle Benson, Director
Sarah Brenna, Director
We administer a wide variety of home and community-based services for Utah residents who are 60 or older. Programs and services are primarily delivered by a network of 12 Area Agencies on Aging which reach all geographic areas of the state. Our goal is to provide services that allow people to remain independent.

3802 Utah Department of Human Services: Division of Services for People with Disabilities
Utah Department of Human Services
195 North 1950 West
Salt Lake City, UT 84116

801-538-3910
877-424-4640
FAX: 801-538-4395
debooth@utah.gov
www.hsdspd.utah.gov

Paul T. Smith, Division Director
Clay Hiatt, Fiscal Management
Information and referral services for people with disabilities, including DD/MR, brain injury and physical disabilities throughout the state of Utah.

3803 Utah Division Of Substance Abuse & MentalHealth
Utah Department of Human Services
195 No. 1950 West
Salt Lake City, UT 84116-1550

801-538-4171
FAX: 801-538-4016
WWW.DHS.UTAH.GOV

Lana Stohl, Executive Director

3804 Utah Division of Services for the Disabled
195 North 1950 West
Salt Lake City, UT 84116

801-538-3910
877-424-4640
FAX: 801-538-4395
dirdhs@utah.gov
www.hsdspd.utah.gov

Paul T. Smith, Division Director
Clay Hiatt, Fiscal Management
Offers services for the totally blind, legally blind, visually impaired, mentally retarded blind and more with health, counseling, educational, recreational, rehabilitation, computer training and professional training services.

3805 Utah Governor's Council for People with Disabilities
155 S 300 W
Suite 100
Salt Lake City, UT 84101-1288

801-533-4636
FAX: 801-533-3968
alozano@utah.gov
www.gcpd.org/

Mark Smith, Manager
Angela Allen, Administrative Secretary

3806 Utah Labor Commission
160 East 300 South, 3rd Floor
P.O.Box 146630
Salt Lake City, UT 84114-6600

801-530-6800
800-222-1238
FAX: 801-530-6390
laborcom@utah.gov
www.laborcommission.utah.gov

Sherrie Hayashi, Commissioner and Department Dire
Jaceson Maughan, Deputy Commissioner
Pete Hackford, Director
Ron Dressler, Director

Problems with employers not paying employees, employers not paying the minimum wage, the employment of minors and retaliation for wage complaints filed are handled by the Wage Claim Unit.

3807 Utah Protection & Advocacy Services for Persons with Disabilities
Disability Law Center
205 N 400 W
Salt Lake City, UT 84103-1125

801-363-1347
800-662-9080
FAX: 801-363-1437
www.disabilitylawcenter.org

Bryce Fifield Ph.D, President
Jared Fields, Vice President
Barbara M. Campbell, Treasurer
Kevin Murphy, Board Member
Since 1979, the Disability Law Center (DLC) has helped thousands of Utahns with disabilities and their families. The DLC has broad statutory powers to safeguard the human and civil rights of persons with disabilities. We provide self-advocacy assistance, legal services, disability rights education, and public policy advocacy on behalf of the more than 400,000 Utah residents with disabilities. Our services are available statewide and without regard for ability to pay.

Vermont

3808 Disability Law Project
57 N Main St
Rutland, VT 05701-3246

800-889-2047
FAX: 802-775-0022
nbreiden@vtlegalaid.org
vtlegalaid.org

Nanci Smith, President
Jessica Porter, Vice President/Secretary
John Holme, Treasurer
Eric Avildsen, Executive Director
Legal services (protection and advocacy) for people with disabilities on legal issues arising from disability. Statewide. Adults and children. Employment, education, discrimination, housing, public benefits, health care.

3809 Disability Rights Vermont
141 Main Street
Suite 7
Montpelier, VT 05602-2916

802-229-1355
800-834-7890
FAX: 802-229-1359
TTY: 800-889-2047
info@disabilityrightsvt.org
www.disabilityrightsvt.org

Sarah Wendell-Launderville, President
David Gallagher, Vice president
Crocker Paquin, Treasurer
Michael Sabourin, Secretary
Advocacy and legal services for people with mental illness on legal issues arising, out of disabilities. Children and adults.

3810 Social Security: Vermont Disability Determination Services
Ste 6
93 Pilgrim Park Rd
Waterbury, VT 05676-1729

802-241-2463
800-734-2463
800-772-1213
FAX: 802-241-2492
Deborah.Fennell@ssa.gov
www.ssa.gov

Karena L. Kilgore, Executive Secretary
Carolyn W. Colvin, Commissioner
Carolyn W. Colvin, Deputy Commissioner
James A. Kissko, Chief of Staff
We deliver services through a nationwide network of over 1,400 offices that include regional offices, field offices, card centers, teleservice centers, processing centers, hearing offices, the Ap-

peals Council, and our State and territorial partners, the Disability Determination Services. We also have a presence in U.S. embassies around the globe. The rich diversity of our employees mirrors the public we serve.

3811   Vermont Assistive Technology Projects
103 S Main St
Weeks Building
Waterbury, VT 05671-2305   800-750-6355
                                            800-750-6355
                                            FAX: 802-871-3048
                                            TTY: 802-241-1464
                                            amber.fulcher@state.vt.us
                                            atp.vermont.gov

Amber Fulcher, Program Director
Sharon Alderman, Assistive Technology Reuse Coord
Emma Cobb, Assistive Technology Services Co
Dan Gilman, ATP, Assistive Technology Access Spec
Increase awareness and change policies to insure assistive technology (AT) is available to all Vermonters with disabilities. Our Commitment is to enable Vermonters with disabilities to have greater independence, productivity, and confidence. To provide them with a clear and direct avenue toward integration and inclusion within the work force and community.

3812   Vermont Client Assistance Program
57 N Main St
Rutland, VT 05701-3246   802-775-0021
                                            800-769-7459
                www.vocrehabvermont.org/html/clientassistance
Patrick Flood, Commissioner
The Client Assistance Program (CAP) is an independent advocacy program to help if you are applying for or receiving services from one of the following sources: Division of Vocational Rehabilitation (VR); Vermont Center for Independent Living (VCIL); Division for the Blind and Visually Impaired (DBVI); Vermont Association of Business, Industry & Rehabilitation (VABIR); Vermont Association for the Blind and Visually Impaired (VABVI); Supported Employment Programs; Transition Programs.

3813   Vermont Department of Aging
103 S Main St
Weeks Building
Waterbury, VT 05671-1601   802-241-2401
                                            FAX: 802-871-3281
                                            TTY: 802-241-3557
                        AHS-DAIL-DeptWebMaster@state.vt.us
                                            dail.vermont.gov

Susan Wehry, Commissioner
Marybeth McCaffrey, Director
Linda Henzel, Executive Staff Assistant
Adele Edelman, Assistant Division Director

3814   Vermont Department of Developmental and
103 S Main St
Weeks Building
Waterbury, VT 05671-1601   802-241-2401
                                            FAX: 802-871-3281
                                            TTY: 802-241-3557
                                            dail.vermont.gov

Jonathan Wood, Manager

3815   Vermont Department of Disabilities, Aging and Independent Living
Aging and Disabilities
103 S Main St
Waterbury, VT 05671-1601   802-241-2401
                                            FAX: 802-241-2325
                                            dail.vermont.gov

Susan Wehry, Commissioner
Camille George, Deputy Commissioner

3816   Vermont Department of Health: Children with Special Health Needs
Vermont Department Of Health
108 Cherry Street
Burlington, VT 05402-70   802-863-7200
                                            800-464-4343
                                            FAX: 802-865-7754
                                            healthvermont.gov

Harry Chen, M.D., Commissioner
Barbara Cimaglio, Deputy Commissioner for Alcohol
Tracy Dolan, Deputy Commissioner for Public H
Dixie Henry, Esq., Senior Policy and Legal Advisor
Multidisciplinary clinics and family support for children with chronic conditions, birth to age 21 years.

3817   Vermont Developmental Disabilities Council
103 S Main St
Waterbury, VT 05671-9800   082-241-2220
                                            vtddc@upgate1.ahs.state.vt.us
                                            www.ahs.state.vt.us/vtddc

Cynthia D LaWare, Secretary
The mission of VTDDC is to facilitate connections and to promote supports that bring people with developmental disabilities into the heart of Vermont Communities.

3818   Vermont Division for the Blind & Visually Impaired
Agency of Human Svcs Dept Disabilities, Aging & IL
103 S Main St
Weeks Building
Waterbury, VT 5671-2304   802-871-3038
                                            800-405-5005
                                            888-405-5005
                                            FAX: 802-871-3048
                                            DBVI-Info@state.vt.us
                                            www.dbvi.vermont.gov

Fred Jones, Director
Scott Langley, Counselor
Heather Allen, Administrative Assistant
Paul Putnam, Rehabilitation Associate
Offers services for the totally blind, legally blind, visually impaired, mentally retarded blind and more with health, counseling, educational, recreational, rehabilitation, computer training and professional training services.

3819   Vermont Division of Disability & Aging Services
103 S Main St
Weeks Building
Waterbury, VT 05671-1601   802-241-2401
                                            FAX: 802-871-3281
                                            TTY: 802-241-3557
                        AHS-DAIL-DeptWebMaster@state.vt.us
                                            www.dail.vermont.gov

Susan Wehry, Commissioner
Marybeth McCaffrey, Director
Linda Henzel, Executive Staff Assistant
Adele Edelman, Assistant Division Director
Provides services to adults and children with developmental disabilities all to the aging.

3820   Workers Compensation Board Vermont
Department of Labor
5 Green Mountain Drive
PO Box 488
Montpelier, VT 05601- 0488   802-828-4000
                                            FAX: 802-828-4022
                                            labor-wccomp@state.vt.us
                                            labor.vermont.gov

Deborah Bruce, Human Resource Administrator
Allen Evans, Executive Director Workforce Dev
Annie Noonan, Commissioner
Erika Wolf?ng, Principal Assistant
Welcome to the Vermont Department of Labor's website. VDOL's primary focus is to provide services that assist businesses, workers, and job seekers.

Virginia

3821 International Dyslexia Association: Virginia Branch
40 York Rd.
4th Floor
Baltimore, MD 21204   410-296-0232
                                              800-988-8336
                                       FAX: 410-321-5069
                                            info@vbida.org
                                          www.interdys.org

Hal Malchow, President
Elsa Cardenas-Hagan, Vice President
Ben Shifrin, Vice President
Rick Smith, Executive Director

The Virginia Branch of The International Dyslexia Association
(VBIDA) is a 501(c)(3) non-profit, scientific and educational organization dedicated to the study and treatment of the learning
disability, dyslexia. This Branch was formed to increase public
awareness of dyslexia in the State of Virginia. We serve the entire
state, with the exception of Northern Virginia, which is part of the
DC-Capital Branch in Washington, DC. We have been serving individuals with dyslexia, their families.

3822 Virginia Department for the Blind and Vision Impaired
397 Azalea Ave
Richmond, VA 23227-3623   804-371-3140
                                              800-622-2155
                                       FAX: 804-371-3157
                       Kimberley.Jennings@dbvi.virginia.gov
                                             www.vdbvi.org

Robert S. Dendy, Chair
Raymond E. Hopkins, Commissioner
Dr. Rick L. Mitchell, Deputy Commissioner
James R. Meehan, Deputy Commissioner

Offers services for the totally blind, legally blind, visually impaired, mentally retarded blind and more with health, counseling,
educational, recreational, rehabilitation, computer training and
professional training services.

3823 Virginia Department of Mental Health
P.O.Box 1797
Richmond, VA 23218-1797   804-786-3921
                                       FAX: 804-371-6638
                                       TTY:804-371-8977
               jim.stewart@dbhds.virginia.gov?subject=(E-mai
                                      www.dbhds.virginia.gov

Debra Ferquson, Commissioner
John Pezzoli, Deputy Commissioner
Daniel Herr, Assistant Commissioner of Behavi
Connie Cochran, Assistant Commissioner of Develo

Available to citizens statewide, Virginia's public mental health,
intellectual disability and substance abuse services system is
comprised of 16 state facilities and 40 locally-run community services boards (CSBs) The CSBs and facilities serve children and
adults who have or who are at risk of mental illness, serious emotional disturbance, intellectual disabilities, or substance abuse
disorders.

3824 Virginia Developmental Disability Council
103 S Main St
Waterbury, VT 05671-9800   082-241-2220
                                   vtddc@upgate1.ahs.state.vt.us
                                   www.ahs.state.vt.us/vtddc

Cynthia D LaWare, Secretary

The mission of VTDDC is to facilitate connections and to promote supports that bring people with developmental disabilities
into the heart of Vermont Communities.

**3825 Virginia Office Protection and Advocacy for People with
Disabilities**
1512 Willow Lawn
Suite 100
Richmond, VA 23230-3034   804-225-2042
                                              800-552-3962
                                       FAX: 804-662-7057
                                            info@dLCV.org
                                        disabilitylawva.org

Coleen Miller, Executive Director
LaToya Blizzard, Deputy Director
Mickie Chapman, IT Specialist
Melissa Charnes-Gibson, Staff Attorney

Through zealous and effective advocacy and legal representation
to: protect and advance legal, human, and civil rights of persons
with disabilities; combat and prevent abuse, neglect, and discrimination; and promote independence, choice, and self-determination by persons with disabilities.

3826 Virginia Office for Protection & Advocacy
5005 Mitchelldale
Suite #100
Houston, TX 77092-3034   713-574-5287
                                              866-964-2867
                                       FAX: 281-476-7800
                                            info@dLCV.org
                                         vopa.state.va.us

V Coleen Miller, Executive Director
Rusty Hill, Administrative Assistant
LaToya Blizzard, Deputy Director for Fiscal and O
Mickie Chapman, Information Technology Specialis

An independent state agency that helps ensure that the rights of
persons with disabiltiies in the Commonwealth are protected.
The mission of DRVD is to provide zealous and effective advocacy and legal representation to protect and advance legal, human
and civil rights of persons with disabilities, combat and prevent
abuse, neglect and discrimination, and promote independence,
choice and self-determination by persons with disabilities.

3827 Virginia Office for Protection and Advocacy
5005 Mitchelldale
Suite #100
Houston, TX 77092-3034   713-574-5287
                                              866-964-2867
                                       FAX: 281-476-7800
                                            info@dLCV.org
                                         vopa.state.va.us

V Coleen Miller, Executive Director
Rusty Hill, Administrative Assistant
LaToya Blizzard, Deputy Director for Fiscal and O
Mickie Chapman, Information Technology Specialis

An independent state agency that helps ensure that the rights of
persons with disabiltiies in the Commonwealth are protected.
The mission of DRVD is to provide zealous and effective advocacy and legal representation to protect and advance legal, human
and civil rights of persons with disabilities, combat and prevent
abuse, neglect and discrimination, and promote independence,
choice and self-determination by persons with disabilities.

3828 Virginia's Developmental Disabilities Planning Council
Stae Agency
1100 Bank Street
7th Floor
Richmond, VA 23219-3426   804-786-0016
                                              800-846-4464
                                       FAX: 804-662-7662
                                       TTY: 800-811-7893
                                     info@vbpd.virginia.gov
                                           www.vaboard.org

Korinda Rusinyak, Chairman
Charles Meacham, Vice Chairman
Dennis Manning, Secretary
Heidi L. Lawyer, Executive Director

To create a Commonwealth that advances opportunities for independence, personal decision-making and full participation in
community life for individuals with developmental disabilities.

Washington

3829 DSHS/Aging & Adult Disability Services Administration
P.O.Box 45130
Olympia, WA 98504-5130
360-902-7797
800-737-0617
FAX: 360-902-7848
TTY: 800-737-7931
aasa.dshs.wa.gov

Dan Murphy, Director
Bea Rector, Project Director
Tamarra Paradee, Executive Secretary
Bill Moss, Director
The Aging and Disability Services Administration assists children and adults with developmental delays or disabilities, cognitive impairment, chronic illness and related functional disabilities to gain access to needed services and supports by managing a system of long-term care and supportive services that are high quality, cost effective, and responsive to individual needs and preferences.

3830 Disability Rights: Washington
315 5th Avenue South
Suite 850
Seattle, WA 98104-2691
206-324-1521
800-562-2702
FAX: 206-957-0729
TTY: 206-957-0728
info@dr-wa.org
www.disabilityrightswa.org

Mark Stroh, Executive Director
David Carison, Director of Legal Advocacy
Emily Cooper, Staff Attorney
Charlotte Cunningham, Staff Attorney
WPAS is a private, non-profit right protection agency for persons with disabilities residin in Washington state. Our advocacy services include information referral, technical assistance, training, publications and systemic advocacy.

3831 International Dyslexia Association: Washington State Branch
P.O.Box 27435
Seattle, WA 98165
206-382-1020
800-222-3123
info@wabida.org
www.wabita.org

Kay Nelson, President
Kathleen Conklin, Secretary
Bev Wolf, Treasurer
Janet Miller, Managing Director
Provides free information and referral services for diagnosis and tutoring for parents, educators, physicians, and individuals with dyslexia in Arkansas, Idaho, Montana and Washington state. The voice of our membership is heard in 48 countries. Membership includes yearly journal and quarterly newsletter. Call for conference dates.

3832 Social Security: Olympia Disability Determination
Social Security
P.O. Box 9303-MS-45550
Olympia, WA 98507
360-664-7356
800-772-1213
800-562-6074
FAX: 360-586-0851
TTY:800-325-0778
Jennifer.Elsen@ssa.gov
www.ssa.gov

Karena L. Kilgore, Executive Secretary
Carolyn W. Colvin, Commissioner
Carolyn W. Colvin, Deputy Commissioner
James A. Kissko, Chief of Staff
We deliver services through a nationwide network of over 1,400 offices that include regional offices, field offices, card centers, teleservice centers, processing centers, hearing offices, the Appeals Council, and our State and territorial partners, the Disability Determination Services. We also have a presence in U.S. embassies around the globe. The rich diversity of our employees mirrors the public we serve.

3833 WA Department of Services for the Blind
4565 7th Avenue SE
PO Box 40933
Lacey, WA 98503
360-725-3830
800-552-7103
FAX: 360-407-0679
info@dsb.wa.gov
www.dsb.wa.gov

Sue Ammeter, council chair
Nancy Kim
Veronica Baca, Council Member
Michael Cunningham, Council Member
Vocational rehabilitation for the blind.

3834 Washington Client Assistance Program
2531 Rainier Ave S
Seattle, WA 98144-5328
206-721-5999
800-544-2121
888-721-6072
FAX: 206-721-4537
TTY:206-721-6072
info@washingtoncap.org
www.washingtoncap.org

Jerry Johnson, Executive Director
Bob Huven, rehabilitation coordinator
Advocacy and information assistance for persons of disability seeking services through vocational rehabilitation or other program under the 1973 Rehabilitation Act as commented. We provide counseling.

3835 Washington Department of Mental Health
Department of Social and Health Services
PO Box 45130
Olympia, WA 98504-5130
360-725-3700
800-446-0259
FAX: 360-902-7691
TTY: 800-833-6384
adsahelpdesk@dshs.wa.gov
www.dshs.wa.gov

Chris Imhoff, DBHR Director
David Albert, Sr. Planner and Policy Analyst,
Debbie Arthur, Fiscal Program Manager
Stephanie Atherton,, Prevention Systems Manager
In July 2009 the DSHS Division of Alcohol and Substance Abuse and the Mental Health Division merged to become the Division of Behavioral Health and Recovery (DBHR). Through this integration, we are in a better position to both assess and treat patients with co-occurring mental health and substance use disorders. Our longer term vision calls for the fullest possible integration of behavioral health and primary care services under health reform, creating a person-centered health care home for al

3836 Washington Developmental Disability
2600 Martin Way E
Suite F
Olympia, WA 98506-4974
360-586-3560
800-634-4473
FAX: 360-586-2424
Ed.Holen@ddc.wa.gov
www.ddc.wa.gov

Diana Zottman, Chairman
Ed Holen, Executive Director
Brain Dahl, Support Coordinator
Aziz Aladin, Budget & Fiscal Director
Developmental Disabilities Council members are appointed by the Governor to plan comprehensive services for the State of Washington's citizens with developmental disabilities.

3837   Washington Governor's Committee on Disability Issues & Employment
605 Woodland Square Loop SE
Lacey, WA 98503
                                    360-438-3168
                              FAX: 928-447-6579
                              gcdetz@gmail.com
                              www.gcde.org

Martin Haule, Director
Toby Olson, Manager

3838   Washington Office of Superintendent of Public Instruction
600 Washington St. S.E.
P. O. Box 47200
Olympia, WA 98504-7200
                                    360-725-6000
                              TTY:360-644-3631
                              webmaster@ospi.wednet.edu
                              www.k12.wa.us

Randy Dorn, State Superintendent
Gil Mendoza, Deputy Superintendent
JoLynn Berge, Assistant Superintendent
Ken Kanikeberg, Chief of Staff
The Office of Superintendent of Public Instruction (OSPI) is the primary agency charged with overseeing K-12 education in Washington state. OSPI works with the state's 296 school districts to administer basic education programs and implement education reform on behalf of more than one million public school students.

3839   Washington State Developmental Disabilities Council
2600 Martin Way E
Suite F
Olympia, WA 98506-4974
                                    360-586-3560
                                    800-634-4473
                              FAX: 360-586-2424
                              Ed.Holen@ddc.wa.gov
                              www.ddc.wa.gov

Diana Zottman, Chairman
Ed Holen, Executive Director
Brain Dahl, Support Coordinator
Aziz Aladin, Budget & Fiscal Director
Developmental Disabilities Council members are appointed by the Governor to plan comprehensive services for the State of Washington's citizens with developmental disabilities.

3840   Workers Compensation Board Washington
State of Washington
7273 Linderson Way SW
Tumwater, WA 98501-5414
                                    360-902-5800
                                    800-547-8367
                              FAX: 360-902-5798
                              TTY: 360-902-5797
                              www.lni.wa.gov

Judy Schurke, Director
Lisa Rodriguez, Executive Assistant
Vickie Kennedy, Special Assistant
Tamara Jones, Dir of Government Relations
&I is a diverse state agency dedicated to the safety, health and security of Washington's 3.2 million workers. We help employers meet safety and health standards and we inspect workplaces when alerted to hazards. As administrators of the state's workers' compensation system, we are similar to a large insurance company, providing medical and limited wage-replacement coverage to workers who suffer job-related injuries and illness. Our rules and enforcement programs also help ensure workers are pai

West Virginia

3841   Bureau of Employment Programs Division of Workers' Compensation
State of West Virginia
407 Virginia Street East
Charleston, WV 25301-2531
                                    304-357-0101
                                    800-628-4265
                              FAX: 304-357-0788
                              helpdesk@kanawha.us
                              kanawha.us

Patricia Starkey, Manager
Vern Cormick, Manager
Michael ' Campbell, Director of IT
Larry McDonnell, Chief Webmaster
Kanawha County today is an exciting technology center that is earning recognition in information technology, medical research, chemical synthesis research, and telecommunications.

3842   Disability Determination Section
Ste 500
500 Quarrier St
Charleston, WV 25301-2913
                                    304-343-5055
                                    800-772-1213
                                    800-344-5033
                              FAX: 304-353-4212
                              Kenneth.Lim@ssa.gov
                              www.ssa.gov

Karena L. Kilgore, Executive Secretary
Carolyn W. Colvin, Commissioner
Carolyn W. Colvin, Deputy Commissioner
James A. Kissko, Chief of Staff
We deliver services through a nationwide network of over 1,400 offices that include regional offices, field offices, card centers, teleservice centers, processing centers, hearing offices, the Appeals Council, and our State and territorial partners, the Disability Determination Services. We also have a presence in U.S. embassies around the globe. The rich diversity of our employees mirrors the public we serve.

3843   Social Security: Charleston Disability Determination
Social Security
500 Quarrier Street
Suite 500
Charleston, WV 25301-2913
                                    304-343-5055
                                    800-772-1213
                                    800-344-5033
                              FAX: 304-353-4212
                              Kenneth.Lim@ssa.gov
                              www.ssa.gov

Karena L. Kilgore, Executive Secretary
Carolyn W. Colvin, Commissioner
Carolyn W. Colvin, Deputy Commissioner
James A. Kissko, Chief of Staff
We deliver services through a nationwide network of over 1,400 offices that include regional offices, field offices, card centers, teleservice centers, processing centers, hearing offices, the Appeals Council, and our State and territorial partners, the Disability Determination Services. We also have a presence in U.S. embassies around the globe. The rich diversity of our employees mirrors the public we serve.

3844   West Virginia Advocates
1207 Quarrier St
Suite 400
Charleston, WV 25301-1826
                                    304-346-0847
                                    800-950-5250
                              FAX: 304-346-0867
                              kellie.l.aikman@wv.gov
                              wvadvocates.org

Terry Dilcher, President
John Galloway, Treasurer
Don Neurman, Secretary
Clarice Hausch, Executive Director
West Virginia Advocates, Inc. (WVA) is the federally mandated protection and advocacy system for people with disabilities in

West Virginia. WVA is a private, nonprofit agency. Our services are confidential and free of charge.

3845 West Virginia Client Assistance Program
West Virginia Advocates
1900 Kanawha Blvd E
Room 9
Charleston, WV 25305-1   304-558-3780
FAX: 304-558-4092
vhuffman@access.k12.wv.us
legis.state.wv.us

Clarice Hausch, Executive Director

3846 West Virginia Department of Aging
1900 Kanawha Blvd. East
Charleston, WV 25305   304-558-3317
877-987-3646
FAX: 304-558-5609
hollygrove@juno.com
www.wvseniorservices.gov

Robert E. Roswall, Commissioner
Nel Kimble
The information we offer is tailored to those who are seeking to locate programs and services for themselves or their loved ones and also for professionals who may be looking for up-to-date information relating to the field of aging.

3847 West Virginia Department of Children with Disabilities
Children with Special Health Care Needs
One Davis Square
Suite 100 East
Charleston, WV 25301- 1757   304-558-0684
FAX: 304-558-1130
DHHRSecretary@wv.gov
www.dhhr.wv.gov

Douglas M. Robinson, Deputy Commissioner
Virginia Mahan, Executive Secretary
Karen Villanueva-Matkovich, General Counsel
Melissa Rosen, CFO
The Bureau for Public Health directs public health activities at all levels within the state to fulfill the core functions of public health: the assessment of community health status and available resources; policy development resulting in proposals to support and encourage better health; and assurance that needed services are available, accessible, and of acceptable quality.

3848 West Virginia Department of Health
One Davis Square
Suite 100 East
Charleston, WV 25301   304-558-0684
FAX: 304-558-1130
DHHRSecretary@wv.gov
www.dhhr.wv.gov

Douglas M. Robinson, Deputy Commissioner
Virginia Mahan, Executive Secretary
Karen Villanueva-Matkovich, General Counsel
Melissa Rosen, CFO
The Bureau for Public Health directs public health activities at all levels within the state to fulfill the core functions of public health: the assessment of community health status and available resources; policy development resulting in proposals to support and encourage better health; and assurance that needed services are available, accessible, and of acceptable quality.

3849 West Virginia Developmental Disabilities Council
110 Stockton St
Charleston, WV 25387   304-558-0416
FAX: 304-558-0941
TTY:304-558-2376
dhhrwvddc@wv.gov
www.ddc.wv.gov

Diana Zottman, Chairman
Ed Holen, Executive Director
Brain Dahl, Support Coordinator
Laurie Bahr, Budget & Fiscal Director
Working to assure that West Virginians with developmental disabilities receive the services, supports, and other forms of assis-

tance they need to exercise self-determination and achieve independence, productivity, integration, and inclusion in the community.
6-8 pages Quarterly Newsl

3850 West Virginia Division of Rehabilitation Services
107 Capitol Street
Charleston, WV 25301-2609   304-356-2060
800-642-8207
www.wvdrs.org

Donna L. Ashworth, Acting Director
Kay Goodwin, Cabinet Secretary
DRS' mission is to enable and empower individuals with disabilities to work and to live independently.

Wisconsin

3851 Disability Rights Wisconsin: Milwaukee Office
Ste 3230
6737 W Washington St
Milwaukee, WI 53214-5651   414-773-4646
800-708-3034
FAX: 414-773-4647
TTY: 888-758-6049
info@drwi.org
disabilityrightswi.org

Ted Skemp, President
Beth Moss, Vice President
Susan Gramling, Secretary
Dan Idzikowski, Executive Director
The protection and advocacy agency for people with disabilities in Wisconsin. DRW provides guidance, advice, investigation, negotiation and in some cases legal representation to people with disabilities and their families. Local and state level systems advocacy and training are also provided.

3852 International Dyslexia Association: Wisconsin Branch
133 W. Ellsworth Lane Bayside
Baraboo, WI 53217   608-355-0911
800-222-3123
wibida@gmail.com.
www.wibida.org

Tammy Tillotson, President
Kimberly Chan, Treasurer
Connie Day, Director
Darlene Larson, Director
The International Dyslexia Association actively promotes effective teaching approaches and related clinical educational intervention strategies for dyslexics. We support and encourage interdisciplinary study and research. We facilitate the exploration of the causes and early identification of dyslexia and are committed to the responsible and wide dissemination of research-based knowledge.

3853 Social Security: Madison Field Office
6011 Odana Rd
Madison, WI 53719-1101   866-770-2262
800-772-1213
FAX: 608-270-1021
TTY: 800-325-0778
wi.fo.madison@ssa.gov
www.ssa.gov

3854 West Virginia Department of Health
One Davis Square
Suite 100 East
Charleston, WV 25301   304-558-0684
800-441-4576
FAX: 304-558-1130
DHHRSecretary@wv.gov
www.dhhr.wv.gov

Rocco S. Fucillo, Cabinet Secretary
Susan Shelton Perry, Deputy Secretary for Legal Servi
Ellen Cannon, Privacy Officer
Virginia Mahan, Executive Secretary

The Department of Health and Family Services operates the federal Title V Maternal and Child Health Block Grant Program for Children with Special Health Care Needs. The program provides program monitoring, consultation and technical assistance to five regional CSHCN centers throughout Wisconsin; a Birth Defects Monitoring and Surveillance Program and a Universal Newborn Hearing Screening Program.

3855 Wisconsin Board for People with Developmental Disabilities (WBPDD)
201 W Washington Ave
Suite 111
Madison, WI 53703-2796
608-266-7826
888-332-1677
FAX: 608-267-3906
TTY:608-266-6660
bpddhelp@wcdd.org
wcdd.org

Jennifer Ondrejka, Manager
Joshua Ryf, Office Manager
Statewide systems advocacy group for people with developmental disabilities in Wisconsin.

3856 Wisconsin Bureau of Aging
State Office of Wisconsin
1 West Wilson Street
Madison, WI 53703
608-266-1865
FAX: 608-267-3203
TTY:888-701-1251
DHSwebmaster@wisconsin.gov
www.dhfs.state.wi.us/aging

Donna Mc Dowell, Executive Director
Gail Schwersenska, Section Chief
Dennis G. Smith, Secretary
Keeps and updates information and printed materials on senior housing directories, nursing home listings, and home care agencies.

3857 Wisconsin Coalition for Advocacy: Madison Office
16 N Carroll St
Suite 400
Madison, WI 53703-2762
608-267-0214
800-928-8778
FAX: 608-267-0368
www.w-c-a.org

Kim Hogan, Intake Specialist
Mr Lynn Breedlove, Executive Director
The protection and advocacy agency for people with disabilities in Wisconsin. WCA provides guidance, advice, investigation, negotiation and in some cases legal representation to people with disabilities and their families. Local and state level systems advocacy and training are also provided.

3858 Wisconsin Governor's Committee for People with Disabilities
1 West Wilson Street
Madison, WI 53703
608-266-1865
877-865-3432
FAX: 608-266-3386
TTY: 888-701-1251
DHSwebmaster@wisconsin.gov
www.dhfs.state.wi.us

Donna Mc Dowell, Executive Director
Gail Schwersenska, Section Chief
Dennis G. Smith, Secretary
To advise the Governor and state agencies on problems faced by people with disabilities; to review legislation affecting people with disabilities; to promote effective operation of publicly-administered or supported programs serving people with disabilities; to promote the collection, dissemination and incorporation of adequate information about persons with disabilities for purposes of public planning at all levels of government.

3859 Workers Compensation Board Wisconsin
Room C100, 201 E. Washington Avenue
P. O. Box 7901
Madison, WI 53707-7901
608-266-1340
FAX: 608-267-0394
dwd.wisconsin.gov/wc

Reggie Newson, Secretary
Jonathan Barry, Deputy Secretary
John Metcalf, Division Administrator
Brain Krueger, Deputy Administrator
The Worker's Compensation Division administers programs designed to ensure that injured workers receive required benefits from insurers or self-insured employers; encourage rehabilitation and reemployment for injured workers; and promote the reduction of work-related injuries, illnesses, and deaths.

Wyoming

3860 Social Security: Cheyenne Disability Determination
Social Security
821 W Pershing Blvd
Cheyenne, WY 82002-1
307-777-7341
800-438-5788
FAX: 307-637-0247
Jeff.Graham@ssa.gov
ssa.gov

Karena L. Kilgore, Executive Secretary
Carolyn W. Colvin, Commissioner
Carolyn W. Colvin, Deputy Commissioner
James A. Kissko, Chief of Staff
We deliver services through a nationwide network of over 1,400 offices that include regional offices, field offices, card centers, teleservice centers, processing centers, hearing offices, the Appeals Council, and our State and territorial partners, the Disability Determination Services. We also have a presence in U.S. embassies around the globe. The rich diversity of our employees mirrors the public we serve.

3861 WY Department of Health: Mental Health and Substance Abuse Service Division
401 Hathaway Building
Cheyenne, WY 82002-1
307-777-7656
800-535-4006
FAX: 307-777-7439
TTY: 307-777-5581
wdh@state.wy.us
www.health.wyo.gov

Thomas O. Forslund, Director
Lee Clabots, Deputy Director
Bob Peck, Chief Financial Officer
Heather Babbitt, Senior Administartor
State office responsible for purchase of service and program development policy.

3862 Workers Compensation Board Wyoming
350 South Washington Street
PO Box 1068
Afton, WY 83110-3004
307-886-9260
FAX: 307-886-9269
wyomingworkforce.or

3863 Wyoming Client Assistance Program
Protection and Advocacy System
2nd Fl
320 W 25th St
Cheyenne, WY 82001-3069
307-632-2682
877-854-5041
FAX: 307-638-0815
wypanda@vcn.com
ap.org

Jeanne Thobro, Manager
Jeanne A Thobro, Executive Director

3864   Wyoming Department of Aging
State Department of Wyoming
401 Hathaway Building
Cheyenne, WY 82002-1
307-777-7656
800-442-2766
FAX: 307-777-7439
wyaging@wyo.gov
health.wyo.gov

Thomas O. Forslund, Director
Lee Clabots, Deputy Director
Bob Peck, Chief Financial Officer
Heather Babbitt, Senior Administartor
The Wyoming Department of Health's Aging Division is committed to providing care, ensuring safety and and promoting independent choices for Wyoming's older adults

3865   Wyoming Developmental Disability Council
122 W 25th St
1st. Fl. West, Herschler Building,
Cheyenne, WY 82002
307-777-7230
800-438-5791
FAX: 307-777-5690
wgcdd@wyo.gov
ddcouncil.state.wy.u

Shannon Buller, Executive Director
Von Maul, Administrative Assistant
Sam Janney, Public Information Officer
Calob Taylor, Grants & Policy Analyst
Our purpose is to assure that individuals with developmental disabilities and their families participate in and have access to needed community services, individualized supports and other forms of assistance that promote independence, productivity, integration and inclusion in all facets of community life.

3866   Wyoming Protection & Advocacy for Persons with Disabilities
7344 Stockman Street
Cheyenne, WY 82009
307-632-3496
FAX: 307-638-0815
wypanda@wypanda.com
wypanda.com

Tori Rosenthal, President
Jeanne A Thobro, Executive Director
Wyoming Protection & Advocacy System, Inc. (P&A), established in 1977, is the official non-profit corporation authorized to implement certain mandates of several federal laws. Enacted by Congress, these laws provide various protection and advocacy services.

Independent Living Centers

Alabama

3867 **Birdie Thornton Center**
2350 Hine Street
Athens, AL 35611   256-232-0366
                          FAX: 256-230-9398
                  www.birdiethorntoncenter.com

Kristy Allen King, Program Director
Heather Mereidth, Program Professional, QMRP
Rabieb Clem, Senior Aid
Kay Green, Training Specialist
The Birdie Thornton Center is devoted to providing care, education, and training to adults with developmental delays and disabilities.

3868 **Independent Living Center of Mobile**
5301 Moffett Rd
Suite 110
Mobile, AL 36618-2926   251-460-0301
                               FAX: 251-341-1267
                               TTY:251-460-2872
                          Michaeld@ilcmobile.org
                               ilcmobile.org

Michael Davis, Executive Director
Darmita Flood, Administrative Assistant
Barbara Hattier, ILS/Transportation Coordinator
James Flora, ILS/Outreach Specialist
Helping people with disabilities become independent.

3869 **Independent Living Resources Of Greater Birmingham: Alabaster**
120 Plaza Cir, Suite C
P. O. Box 2048
Alabaster, AL 35007-7034   205-685-0570
                                  FAX: 205-251-0605
                                  TTY:205-685-0570
                       gwen.brown@drradvocates.org
                                  www.ilrgb.org

Kathy Lovell, President
Phil Klebine, Vice President
Susan Parker, Secretary
Milton Moats, Treasurer
The mission of this Independent Living Center is to empower people with disabilities to fully participate in the community.

3870 **Independent Living Resources of Greater Birmingham: Jasper**
300 Birmingham Ave
PO Box 434
Jasper, AL 35502-3811   205-387-0159
                               FAX: 205-387-0162
                               TTY:205-387-0159
                     vickie.stovall@drradvocates.org
                               www.ilrgb.org

Kathy Lovell, President
Phil Klebine, Vice President
Susan Parker, Secretary
Milton Moats, Treasurer
The purpose of this Independent Living Center is to empower people with disabilities to fully participate in the community.

3871 **Independent Living Resources of Greater Birmingham**
1418 6th Avenue North
Birmingham, AL 35203-1317   205-251-2223
                                   FAX: 205-251-0605
                                   TTY:205-251-2223
                          judy.roy@drradvocates.org
                                   www.ilrgb.org

Kathy Lovell, President
Phil Klebine, Vice President
Susan Parker, Secretary
Milton Moats, Treasurer

The mission of this Independent Living Center is to empower people with disabilities to fully participate in the community.

3872 **Montgomery Center for Independent Living**
600 S Court St
Montgomery, AL 36104-4106   334-240-2520
                                   FAX: 334-240-6869
                                   TTY:334-240-2520
                              mcil@bellsouth.net
                          www.cilmontgomery.org

Scott Renner, Executive Director
Barbara F. Crozier, President
Kenneth Marshall, Vice President
Vickie P. FitzGerald, Secretary
Encourgaes people with disabilities to support one another in reaching their own independent living goals.

Alaska

3873 **Access Alaska: ADA Partners Project**
1217 East 10th Ave
Suite 105
Anchorage, AK 99501-2044   907-248-4777
                                  800-770-4488
                                  888-462-1444
                                  FAX: 907-263-1942
                                  TTY:907-248-8799
                            info@accessalaska.org
                                  accessalaska.org

Lorali Simon, President
Mike O'Neill, Vice President
Jim Duffield, Treasurer
Eric Spangler, Member
Assisting Alaskans with disabilities to live independently in the community of their choice.

3874 **Access Alaska: Fairbanks**
526 Gaffney Rd
Suite 100
Fairbanks, AK 99701-4914   907-479-7940
                                  800-770-7940
                                  FAX: 907-474-4052
                                  TTY: 907-474-8619
                            info@accessalaska.org
                                  accessalaska.org

Lorali Simon, President
Mike O'Neill, Vice President
Jim Duffield, Treasurer
Eric Spangler, Member
A local non profit agency using its resources to actively promote a society where persons with disabilities can live and work independently in the community of their choice.

3875 **Access Alaska: Mat-Su**
1075 Check St,
Suite 109
Wasilla, AK 99654-6937   907-357-2588
                                800-770-0228
                                FAX: 907-357-5585
                          info@accessalaska.org
                                accessalaska.org

Lorali Simon, President
Mike O'Neill, Vice President
Jim Duffield, Treasurer
Eric Spangler, Member
Provides independent living services to persons with significant disabilities. Mission is to encourage and promote the total integration of persons with disabilities into the community of their choice. Services include independent living skills training, information and referral, advocacy, peer support, and at home modifications.

3876   Alaska SILC
Ste 206
1217 East 10th Ave
Anchorage, AK 99501-1760
907-248-4777
800-770-4488
888-294-7452
FAX: 907-263-1942
info@accessalaska.org
www.alaskasilc.org

Jim Beck, Executive Director
Lorali Simon, President
Mike O'Neill, Vice President
Jim Duffield, Treasurer
The Alaska Statewide Independent Living is committed to promoting a philosophy of consumer control, peer support, self help, self determination, equal access, and individual and systems advocacy, in order to maximize leadership, empowerment, independence, productivity, and to support full inclusion and integration of individuals with disabilities into the mainstream of American society.

3877   Arctic Access
P.O.Box 930
Kotzebue, AK 99752-930
907-412-0695
877-442-2393
TTY:907-442-2393
arcticaccesskotz@gci.net
arcticaccesscil.org

Roger Wright Jr, Executive Director
Russell Williams, Jr,, Elder & Disability Resource Coor
Audrey Aanes
The Arctic Access Independent Living Center provides services and opportunities for elders and others with disabilities so they may remain in their village and be as active as possible with their families and commuities in the North West Arctic and Bering Straits Regions of Alaska.

3878   Hope Community Resources
540 W Intl Airport Rd
Anchorage, AK 99518-1105
907-561-5335
800-478-0078
FAX: 907-564-7429
info@hopealaska.org
hopealaska.org

Robert Owens, President
John Dittrich, Vice President
Eugene 'Gene' Bates, Treasurer
Stephen P. Lesko, Executive Director
Provider of services to individuals who experience a disability.

3879   Kenai Peninsula Independent Living Center
265 E. Pioneer Suite 201
P.O.Box 2474
Homer, AK 99603- 2474
907-235-7911
800-770-7911
FAX: 907-235-6236
info@peninsulailc.org
peninsulailc.org

Candy Norman, President
Mike Harmer, Vice President
Offers peer counseling, disability education and awareness, attendant care registry and information on accessible housing.

3880   Kenai Peninsula Independent Living Center: Seward
201 Third Avenue, Suite 101Bs
P. O. Box 3523
Seward, AK 99664-3523
907-224-8711
FAX: 907-224-7793
info@peninsulailc.org
www.peninsulailc.org

Candy Norman, President
Mike Harmer, Vice President
Offers peer counseling, disability, education and awareness, attendant care registry and information on accessible housing.

3881   Keni Peninsula Independent Living Center: Central Peninsula
47255 Princeton Avenue
Suite 8
Soldotna, AK 99669
907-262-6333
FAX: 907-260-4495
info@peninsulailc.org
www.peninsulailc.org

Candy Norman, President
Mike Harmer, Vice President
Offers peer counseling, disability education and awareness, attendant care registry and information on accessible housing.

3882   Southeast Alaska Independent Living
3225 Hospital Drive
Suite 300
Juneau, AK 99801-7863
907-586-4920
800-478-7245
FAX: 907-586-4980
TTY: 907-523-5285
info@sailinc.org
sailinc.org

Robert Purvis, President
Jeff Irwin, Vice President
Suzanne Williams, Secretary
Mary Gregg, Treasurer
To empower consumers with disabilities by providing services and information to support them in making choices that will positively affect their independence and productivity in society.

3883   Southeast Alaska Independent Living: Ketchikan
602 Dock St
Suite 107
Ketchikan, AK 99901-6574
907-225-4735
888-452-7245
FAX: 907-247-4735
ketchikan@sailinc.org
www.sailinc.org

Robert Purvis, President
Jeff Irwin, Vice President
Suzanne Williams, Secretary
Mary Gregg, Treasurer
To empower consumers with disabilities by providing services and information to support them in making choices that will positively affect their independence and productivity in society.

3884   Southeast Alaska Independent Living: Sitka
514 Lake St
Suite C
Sitka, AK 99835-7405
907-747-6859
888-500-7245
FAX: 907-747-6783
sitka@sailinc.org
www.sailinc.org

Robert Purvis, President
Jeff Irwin, Vice President
Suzanne Williams, Secretary
Mary Gregg, Treasurer
To empower consumers with disabilities by providing services and information to support them in making choices that will positively affect their independence and productivity in society.

Arizona

3885   ASSIST! to Independence
P.O.Box 4133
Tuba City, AZ 86045-4133
928-283-6261
888-848-1449
FAX: 928-283-6284
TTY: 928-283-6672
assist01@frontiernet.net
www.assisttoindependence.org

Michael Blatchford, Executive Director
Priscilla Lane, IL Services Coordinator/Dep Dir
A community based, American Indian owned and operated non-profit agency that was established by and for people with dis-

abilities and chronic health conditions to help fill some of the gaps in service delivery.

3886 Arizona Bridge to Independent Living
5025 E Washington St
Suite 200
Phoenix, AZ 85034-7439

602-256-2245
800-280-2245
FAX: 602-254-6407
boardofdirectors@abil.org
www.abil.org

Mary Slaughter, Chairman
Brad Wemhaner, Vice Chairman
Michael Somsan, Secretary
Jim Winterton, Treasurer

ABIL offers and promotes programs designed to empower people with disabilities to take personal responsibility so they may achieve or continue independent lifestyles within the community.

3887 Arizona Bridge to Independent Living: Phoenix
1229 E. Washington St.
Suite D405
Phoenix, AZ 85034

602-296-0551
800-280-2245
FAX: 602-256-0184
TTY: 602-296-0591
boardofdirectors@abil.org
www.abil.org

Mary Slaughter, Chairman
Brad Wemhaner, Vice Chairman
Michael Somsan, Secretary
Jim Winterton, Treasurer

ABIL offers and promotes programs designed to empower people with disabilities to take personal responsibility so they may achieve or continue independent lifestyles within the community.

3888 Arizona Bridge to Independent Living: Mesa
2150 S Country Club Dr
Suite 10
Mesa, AZ 85210-6879

480-655-9750
800-280-2245
FAX: 480-655-9751
TTY: 480-655-9750
boardofdirectors@abil.org
www.abil.org

Mary Slaughter, Chairman
Brad Wemhaner, Vice Chairman
Michael Somsan, Secretary
Jim Winterton, Treasurer

ABIL offers and promotes programs designed to empower people with disabilities to take personal responsibility so they may achieve or continue independent lifestyles within the community.

3889 Community Outreach Program for the Deaf
268 W Adams St
Tucson, AZ 85705-6534

520-792-1906
FAX: 520-770-8554
TTY: 520-792-1906
request@copdaz.org
copdaz.org

Anne Levy, Executive Director

A non-profit organization, which has been serving the needs of people in Southern Arizona who are deaf or hard of hearing.

3890 DIRECT Center for Independence
1023 N Tyndall Ave
Tucson, AZ 85719-4446

520-624-6452
800-342-1853
FAX: 520-792-1438
TTY: 520-624-6452
direct@directilc.org
www.directilc.org

Ron Trozzi, President
Marrill Eisenberg, Vice President
Steve Fristoe, Treasurer
Loretta Alvarez, Secretary

A non-consumer directed, community-based advocacy organization, that promotes independent living and offers a variety of programs for all people with disabilities which encourage them to achieve their full potential and to participate in the community.

3891 New Horizons Independent Living Center: Prescott Valley
8085 E Manley Dr
Prescott Valley, AZ 86314-6154

928-772-1266
800-406-2377
FAX: 928-772-3808
TTY: 928-772-1266
ltoone@newhorizonsilc.org
www.newhorizonsilc.org

Deborah Henderson, Office Manager
Liz Toone, Executive Director
Nick Perry, President
Jim Stobbs, Vice President

To provide services and advocacy which empower and enable people with disabilities to self-determine the goals and activities of their lives.

3892 Services Maximizing Independent Living and Empowerment (SMILE)
1931 South Arizona Ave
Suite 4
Yuma, AZ 85364-5721

928-329-6681
855-209-8363
FAX: 928-329-6715
TTY: 928-782-7458
info@smile-az.org
www.smile-az.org

Laura Duval, Executive Director
Brenda Howard, Finance Manager/ Admin Assistant
Shawnnita Miranda, Advocate/ Home modification Mana
Brandon Howard, Outreach Coordinator, Technology

SMILE continually advocates for the Independent Living Philosophy, both individually and system wide. The Board and staff constantly strives to improve the system by writing letters, training staff, providing services, and creating public awareness as to the services and opportunities open to people who have disabilities.

3893 Sterling Ranch: Residence for Special Women
Sterling Ranch
P.O.Box 36
Skull Valley, AZ 86338-36

928-442-3289
FAX: 928-442-9272
director@sterlingranch.info
www.sterlingranch.info

Russell Dryer, Executive Director
Trent Nichel, Manager

A nonprofit residence for women with developmental disabilities which has been in operation since 1947. As a small facility (19 residents) the orientation is personal and family-like. Offers activities that range from gardening, quilting, academics, sign-language, crafts and a myriad of field trips and excursions. Private rooms and spacious living on 4 1/2 acres.

Arkansas

3894 Arkansas Independent Living Council
11324 Arcade Drive
Suite 7
Little Rock, AR 72212

501-372-0607
800-772-0607
FAX: 501-372-0598
arkansasilc@att.net
www.ar-silc.org

Sha Stephens, Executive Director
Cheryl , Director
Brenda Stinebuck, Chair
Liz Adams, Vice Chair

A non-profit organization promoting independent living for people with disabilities.

3895 Delta Resource Center for Independent Living
11324 Arcade Drive
Little Rock, AR 72212-6249
501-372-0607
800-772-0607
FAX: 501-372-0598
drcilar@yahoo.com
www.ar-silc.org

Sha Stephens, Executive Director
Katy Morris, Director
Cheryl , Director
Brenda Stinebuck, Chair
Provides services, support, and advocacy which enables people with severe disabilities to live as independently as possible within their family and community.

3896 Mainstream
300 S Rodney Parham Rd
Suite 5
Little Rock, AR 72205- 4774
501-280-0012
800-371-9026
FAX: 501-280-9267
TTY: 501-280-9262
mainstreamlrc@earthlink.net
mainstreamilrc.com

Rita Byers, Executive Director
Vincent McKinney
Vincent Acklin
Debbie Gillespie
A non residential, consumer driven independent living resource center for persons with disabilities. Mainstream operates with conviction that people with disabilities have the right and responsibility to make choices, to control their lives and to participate fully and equally in the community.

3897 Our Way: The Cottage Apt Homes
9175 Greenback Lane
Orangevale, CA 95662-6616
501-225-5030
888-879-9584
FAX: 501-225-5190
rentthecottages.com

Katrina Williams, Manager
Crystal Brown, Assistant Manager
Advocacy and information services. One bedroom apartments for mobility impaired and elderly 62 years or older persons.
Based on income

3898 Sources for Community IL Services
1918 N Birch Ave
Fayetteville, AR 72703-2408
479-442-5600
888-284-7521
FAX: 479-442-5192
TTY: 479-251-1378
jmather@arsources.org
www.arsources.org

Brent Williams, PhD, President
Elise Burt, Treasurer
Burke Fanari, Secretary
Jim Mather, Executive Director
Provides services, support, and advocacy for individuals with disabilities, their families and the community.

3899 Spa Area Independent Living Services
621 Albert Pike
Hot Springs, AR 71913
501-624-7710
800-255-7549
FAX: 501-624-7003
info@restsearch.com
www.ar-sails.org

Dejan S. Vojnovic, President
Joseph E. Anderson, Vice President - Real Estate
Bryan S. Cox, Vice President - Technology
Brenda Stinebuck, Executive Director
Provides services and advocacy by and for persons with all types of disabilities. The goal is to assist individuals with disabilities to achieve thier maximum potential within their families and communities.

California

3900 Access Center of San Diego
8885 Rio San Diego Dr
Suite 131
San Diego, CA 92108-1625
619-293-3500
800-300-4326
FAX: 619-293-3508
TTY: 619-293-7757
info@a2isd.org
www.a2isd.org

Louis Frick, Executive Director
Derek Parker, Chair
Jacquelyn E. Nash, Vice Chair
Nick Bradley, Treasurer
Access to Independence is an independent living center (ILC), a nonresidential, cross-disability, non-profit corporations that provide services to people with disabilities to help maximize their independence and fully integrate into their communities. Access to Independence is one of 391 ILCs across the country and one of 29 serving Californians. Like all ILCs, Access to Independence offers required federal and state programs and services to people of all disability types and ages at no charge.

3901 Access to Independence
8885 Rio San Diego Drive
Suite 131
San Diego, CA 92108- 1625
619-293-3500
800-300-4326
FAX: 619-293-3508
TTY: 619-293-7757
info@a2isd.org
www.a2isd.org

Louis Frick, Executive Director
Derek Parker, Chair
Jacquelyn E. Nash, Vice Chair
Nick Bradley, Treasurer
A community resource for people with disabilities to lead independent lives.

3902 Access to Independence of Imperial Valley
101 Hacienda Drive
Suite 13
Calexico, CA 92231-2875
760-768-2044
866-976-3515
FAX: 760-768-4977
TTY: 619-293-7757
info@a2isd.org
www.a2sid.org

Louis Frick, Executive Director
Derek Parker, Chair
Jacquelyn E. Nash, Vice Chair
Nick Bradley, Treasurer
A community resource for people with disabilities to lead independent lives.

3903 Access to Independence of North County
209 E Broadway
Vista, CA 92084-6005
760-643-0447
FAX: 760-435-9206
info@a2isd.org
www.a2sid.org

Louis Frick, Executive Director
Derek Parker, Chair
Jacquelyn E. Nash, Vice Chair
Nick Bradley, Treasurer
A community resource for people with disabilities to lead independent lives.

3904 Beaumont Senior Center: Community Access Center
1310 Oak Valley Parkway
Beaumont, CA 92223-2218
951-769-8524
FAX: 951-769-8519
TTY:909-769-2794
ilser5@ilcac.org
www.ci.beaumont.ca.us

Laurie Hoirup, Director

A non profit organization; one of 29 similar programs throughout the state of California CAC is a community resource, advocate, and educator for Riverside County residents with disabilities.

3905 California Foundation For Independent Living Centers
1234 H Street
Suite 100
Sacramento, CA 95814-1912
916-325-1690
FAX: 916-325-1699
TTY:916-325-1695
cfilc@cfilc.org
www.cfilc.org

Robert Hand, Chairperson
Ana Acton, Vice Chairperson
Tink Miller, Executive Director
Kim Cantrell, Program Director
Community Rehabilitation Services, Inc. (CRS) is a private, non-profit agency established in 1974 to assist persons with disabilities within the East/North East areas of Los Angeles County to enhance their options for living independently. Any person who is 18 yrs of age or more with physical, sensory, mental/emotional or developmental disabilities can work with us to become more self-sufficient. Our intake procedures provide an orientation to the staff, facilities and services at CRS.

3906 California Foundation for Independent Living Centers
1235 H Street
Suite 100
Sacramento, CA 95814-1913
916-325-1690
FAX: 916-325-1699
TTY:916-325-1695
cfilc@cfilc.org
www.cfilc.org

Robert Hand, Chairperson
Ana Acton, Vice Chairperson
Tink Miller, Executive Director
Kim Cantrell, Program Director
CFILC's mission is to support independent living centers in their local communities through advocating for systems change and promoting access and integration for people with disabilities.

3907 California State Independent Living Council (SILC)
1235 H Street
Suite 100
Sacramento, CA 95814-4010
916-325-1690
866-866-7452
FAX: 916-325-1699
TTY: 866-745-2889
neal@calsilc.org
www.calsilc.org

Susan M. Madison, Chairman
Eli Gelardin, Vice Chairman
Liz Pazdral, Executive Director
Caroline Kuhn, Staff Services Analyst
To maximize options for independence for persons with disabilities

3908 Center for Independence of the Disabled
Suite 103
2001 Winward Way
San Mateo, CA 94404-3062
650-645-1780
FAX: 650-645-1785
TTY:650-522-9313
info@cidbelmont.org
http://www.cidsanmateo.org

Brad Friedman, Co-President
Laura Whitsitt Hillyard, Co-President
Thomas J. Devine, Vice President
John Horgan, Secretary
Increase the social, educational, and economic participation of persons with disabilities in San Mateo County, and to encourage, support, and provide options for self determination, equal access and freedom of choice.

3909 Center for Independence of the Disabled- Daly City
Ste 256
355 Gellert Blvd
Daly City, CA 94015-2675
650-991-5124
FAX: 650-757-2075
TTY:650-991-5182
dalycity5@aol.com
www.cidbelmont.org

Kent Mickelson, Director
The Daly City Branch office fulfills its mission by serving disabled consumers in Brisbane, Colma, Daly City, El Granada, Half Moon Bay, Montara, Moss Beach, Pacifica, Pescadero, Princeton and South San Francisco. Our mission is to increase the social, educational, economic, social and political participants of persons with disabilities in San Mateo county, California.

3910 Center for Independent Living
Suite 103
2001 Winward Way
San Mateo, CA 94404
650-645-1780
FAX: 650-645-1785
TTY:510-848-3101
ywrong@cilberkeley.org
www.cidsanmateo.org

Yomi Wrong, Executive Director
Makr Burns, Deputy Director
The Center for Independent Living, Inc (CIL) is a national leader in helping people with disabilities live independently and become productive members of society. Founded in 1972, CIL is a pioneer advocating for greater accessibility in communities, designing techniques in independent living and providing direct services to people with disabilities. A partial list of services includes Information and Referral, Personal Assistance Services, Independent Living Skills Training and Peer Counseling.

3911 Center for Independent Living: East Oakland
Suite 100
3075 Adeline Street
Berkeley, CA 94703-2403
510-841-4776
FAX: 510-841-6168
info@cilberkeley.org
www.cilberkeley.org

Melissa Male, Chair
Bea Worthen, Vice-Chair
Paul Hippolitus, Secretary
A national leader in helping people with disabilities live independently and become productive, fully participating members of society.

3912 Center for Independent Living: Oakland
Suite 100
3075 Adeline Street
Berkeley, CA 94703-1285
510-841-4776
FAX: 510-841-6168
TTY:510-444-1837
info@cilberkeley.org
cilberkeley.org

Melissa Male, Chair
Bea Worthen, Vice-Chair
Paul Hippolitus, Secretary
Ted Dienstfrey, Finance Committee
A national leader in supporting disabled people in their efforts to lead independent lives.

3913 Center for Independent Living: Tri-County
2822 Harris Street
Eureka, CA 95503
707-445-8404
877-576-5000
FAX: 707-445-9751
TTY: 707-445-8405
aa@tilinet.org
www.tilinet.org

Gail Pascoe, President
Linda Arnold, Vice President
Kevin O'Brien, Treasurer
Chris Jones, Executive Director

3914 **Center for Independent Living:Fresno**
3475 Wesy Shaw Ave
Suite 101
Fresno, CA 93711 559-276-6777
FAX: 559-276-6778
TTY:559-276-6779
execdirector@cil-fresno.org
www.cil-fresno.org

Bob Hand, Manager

3915 **Center for Independent Living; Oakland**
1904 Franklin Street
Suite 320
Oakland, CA 94612-2324 510-763-9990
FAX: 510-763-4910
TTY:510-536-2271
info@cilberkeley.org
cilberkeley.org

Melissa Male, Chair
Bea Worthen, Vice-Chair
Hank Stratford, Treasurer
Paul Hippolitus, Secretary
Independent living center to maximise the options for independence for persons with disabilities.

3916 **Center of Independent Living: Visalia**
121 E Main
Suite 101
Visalia, CA 93291-6262 559-622-9276
FAX: 559-622-9638
f_phillips@cil-fresno.org
www.cil-fresno.org

Fran Phillips, Executive Directorram Manager
Renee Ezelle, Manager

3917 **Central Coast Center for IL: San Benito**
1234 H Street
Suite 100
Sacramento, CA 95814-1914 916-325-1690
FAX: 916-325-1699
TTY:916-325-1695
cfile@cflc.org
www.cfilc.org

Ana Acton, Chairperson
Larry Grable, Vice Chairperson
Nayana Shah, Treasurer
Jessie Lorenz, Secretary
To advocate for barrier-free access and equal opportunity for people with disabilities to participate in the community life by increasing the capacity of Independent Living Centers to achieve their missions.

3918 **Central Coast Center for Independent Living**
318 Cayuga St.
Suite 208
Salinas, CA 93901-2600 831-757-2968
FAX: 831-757-5549
TTY:831-757-3949
cccil@cccil.org
cccil.org

Jennifer L. Williams, President
Elsa Quezada, Executive Director
Brenda Cardoza, Information and Referral Special
Gabriel Garcia, Independent Living Specialist
CCCIL promotes the independence of people with disabilities by supporting their equal and full participation in community life. CCCIL provides advocacy, education and support to all people with disabilities, their families and the community.

3919 **Central Coast Center: Independent Living - Santa Cruz Office**
1350 - 41st Avenue
Suite 101
Capitola, CA 95010-3930 831-462-8720
FAX: 831-462-8727
TTY:831-462-8729
cccil@cccil.org
www.cccil.org

Jennifer L. Williams, President
Elsa Quezada, Executive Director
Brenda Cardoza, Information and Referral Special
Gabriel Garcia, Independent Living Specialist
CCCIL promotes the independence of people with disabilities by supporting their equal and full participation in community life. CCCIL provides advocacy, education and support to all people with disabilities, their families and the community.

3920 **Central Coast for Independent Living**
1111 San Felipe Rd
Suite 107
Hollister, CA 95023-2814 831-636-5196
FAX: 831-637-0478
TTY:831-637-6235
cccil@cccil.org
www.cccil.org

Jennifer L. Williams, President
Elsa Quezada, Executive Director
Brenda Cardoza, Information and Referral Special
Gabriel Garcia, Independent Living Specialist
CCCIL promotes the independence of people with disabilities by supporting their equal and full particpation in community life. CCCIL provides advocacy, education and support to all people with disabilities, their families and the community.

3921 **Central Coast for Independent Living: Watsonville**
18 W. Beach St.
Suite Y
Watsonville, CA 95076-4371 831-724-2997
FAX: 831-724-2915
TTY:831-786-0915
cccil@cccil.org
www.cccil.org

Jennifer L. Williams, President
Elsa Quezada, Executive Director
Brenda Cardoza, Information and Referral Special
Gabriel Garcia, Independent Living Specialist
An advocacy and information center organized by and for people with disabilities that strives to make our communities more accessible and to empower people with disabilities with information and skills to live fulfilling lives in our communities.

3922 **Communities Actively Living Independent and Free**
634 S Spring St
2nd Floor
Los Angeles, CA 90014-3921 213-627-0477
FAX: 213-627-0535
TTY:213-623-9502
info@calif-ilc.org
califilc.webs.com

Lillibeth Navarro, Founder & Executive Director
Alex San Martin, Temporary Chair
Fernando Roldan, Board Secretary
Ben Rockwell, Temporary Board Treasurer
Envisions a culturally diverse independent living center designed to empower the Disability Community.

3923 Community Access Center
6848 Magnolia Ave
Suite 150
Riverside, CA 92506-2858 951-274-0358
FAX: 951-274-0833
TTY:951-274-0834
execdir@ilcac.org
www.ilcac.org

Mark Dyer, President
Janet Newcomer, Vice President
Perry Halteman, Secretary
Chuck Reutter, Treasurer
A non-profit organization; one of 29 similar programs throughout the state of California. CAC is a community resource, advocate, and educator for Riverside County residents with disabilities.

3924 Community Access Center: Indio Branch
83233 Indio Blvd
Indio, CA 92201-4748 760-347-4888
FAX: 760-347-0722
TTY:760-347-6802
pmgr3@ilcac.org
www.ilcac.org

Mark Dyer, President
Janet Newcomer, Vice President
Perry Halteman, Secretary
Chuck Reutter, Treasurer
To empower persons with disabilities to control their own lives, create an accessible community and advocate to achieve complete social, economic, and political integration. We implement this vision by providing information, supportive services and independent living skills training.

3925 Community Access Center: Perris
371 Wilkerson Ave
Perris, CA 92570-2241 951-443-1158
FAX: 951-443-2608
TTY:951-443-1158
spmgr@ilcac.org
www.ilcac.org

Mark Dyer, President
Janet Newcomer, Vice President
Perry Halteman, Secretary
Chuck Reutter, Treasurer
Community Access Center empowers persons with disabilities to control their own lives, create an accessible community and advocate to achieve complete social, economic, and political integration. CAC also implements this vision by providing information, suportive services and independent living skills training.

3926 Community Rehabilitation Services
844 E. Mission Road
Suite A & B
San Gabriel, CA 91776- 2759 323-266-0453
FAX: 626-614-1590
TTY:323-266-3016
executivedirector@crs-ilc.org
www.crs-ilc.org

Frances Garcia, Executive Director
CRS is an independent living center that provides free services to persons with disabilities in the areas of advocacy, housing and independent living skills; assistive technology, employment, personal assistant services, peer counseling and information and referral.

3927 Community Resources for Independence: Mendocino/Lake Branch
Ste B
415 Talmage Rd
Ukiah, CA 95482-7486 707-463-8875
FAX: 707-463-8878
TTY:707-463-4498
www.cri-dove.org

Tanner Silva, Manager
A non-profit corporation established by a group of disabled and non-disabled individuals to advance the rights of persons with disabilities to equal justice, access, opportunity and participation in the communities.

3928 Community Resources for Independence: Napa
Ste 208
1040 Main St
Napa, CA 94559-2605 707-258-0270
FAX: 707-258-0275
TTY:707-257-0274
cri-dove.org

Tyler Stanley, Manager
Matthew Shultz, Independent Living Advocate
A non-profit corporation established by a group of disabled and non-disabled individuals to advance the rights of persons with disabilities to equal justice, access, opportunity and participation in the communities.

3929 Community Resources for Independent Living: Hayward
3311 Pacific Ave
Livermore, CA 94550-5013 925-371-1531
FAX: 925-373-5034
TTY:925-371-1533
info@cril-online.org
crilhayward.org

Sheri Burns, Executive Director
Michael Galvan, PhD., Program Director
April Monroe, Finance Director
Esperanza Diaz-Alvarez, IL Coor - Travel Trainer & PAS
CRIL offers independent living services at no charge to persons with disabilities living in southern and eastern Alameda county. CRIL is also a resource for disability awareness education and training, advocacy and technical advice.

3930 Community Resources for Independent Living
39155 Liberty St
Suite A100
Fremont, CA 94538-1503 510-794-5735
info@cril-online.org
crilhayward.org

Sheri Burns, Executive Director
Michael Galvan, PhD., Program Director
April Monroe, Finance Director
Esperanza Diaz-Alvarez, PAS Coordinator/Benefits Advocat
Community Resources for Independent Living is a peer-based disability organization that advocates and provides resources for people with disabilities to improve lives and make communities fully accessible.

3931 DRAIL (Disability Resource Agency for Independent Living)
501 W Weber Ave
Ste 200-A
Stockton, CA 95203-6239 209-477-8143
FAX: 209-477-7730
TTY:209-465-5643
barry@drail.org
www.drail.org

Terry Gray, President
Michael Kim Cornelius, Treasurer
Adeline Bagwell, Secretary
Barry Smith, Executive Director
A non-profit corporation that is community based, consumer controlled, consumer choice, cross disability center for independent living.

3932 Dayle McIntosh Center: Laguna Niguel
24031 El Toro Road
Suite 300
Laguna Hills, CA 92653-3632 949-460-7784
800-422-7444
FAX: 949-334-2302
TTY: 800-735-2929
www.daylemc.org

Libby Partain, President
Cindy McLeroy, Vice President
Eva Casas-Sarmiento, Secretary
Michael Ryan, Treasurer
DMC advances empowerment and inclusion of all persons with disabilities. DMC is the largest Independent Living Center in California, and was named in memory of a young woman with a severe physical disability who worked to found the center.

3933   **Disability Resource Agency for Independent Living: Modesto**
920-12th Street
Modesto, CA 95354-543   209-521-7260
                                      FAX: 209-521-4763
                                      TTY:209-576-2409
                                      larry@drail.org
                                      www.drail.org

Terry Gray, President
Michael Kim Cornelius, Treasurer
Adeline Bagwell, Secretary
Barry Smith, Executive Director
A non-profit corporation that is community based, consumer controlled, consumer choice, cross disability center for independent living.

3934   **Disability Services & Legal Center**
521 Mendocino Ave.
Santa Rosa, CA 95401-1649   707-528-2745
                                     FAX: 707-528-9477
                                     TTY:707-528-2151
                                     dawsons@sonic.net
                                     www.disabilityserviceandlegal.org

Adam Brown, Chairman
Shirley Johnson-Foell, Board President
Jack Geary, Board Member
Ben Karpilow, Board Secretary
A non-profit corporation established by a group of disabled and non-disabled individuals to advance the rights of persons with disabilities to equal justice, access, opportunity and participation in the communities.

3935   **Disabled Resources Center**
2750 E Spring St
Suite 100
Long Beach, CA 90806-2263   562-427-1000
                                    FAX: 562-427-2027
                                    TTY:562-427-1366
                                    info@drcinc.org
                                    drcinc.org

C. Timothy Lashlee, President
Dora Hogan, Vice President
Finola Campbell, Treasurer
Dolores Nason, Executive Director
To empower people with disabilities to live independently in the community, to make their own decisions about their lives and to advocate on their own behalf.

3936   **FREED Center for Independent Living**
2059 Nevada City Hwy
Suite 102
Grass Valley, CA 95945- 3227   530-477-3333
                                    800-655-7732
                                    FAX: 530-477-8184
                                    TTY: 530-477-8194
                                    contact-04@freed.org
                                    freed.org

Ana Acton, Executive Director
To eliminate barriers to full equality for people with disabilities through programs which promote independent living.

3937   **FREED Center for Independent Living: Marysville**
508 J St
Marysville, CA 95901-5636   530-742-4476
                                    TTY:530-742-4474
                                    contact-04@freed.org
                                    freed.org

Claudia Hallis, Manager
To eliminate barriers to full equality for people with disabilities through programs which promote independent living.

3938   **First Step Independent Living**
1174 Nevada St
Redlands, CA 92374-2893

                                    800-362-0312
                                    cvsfs@deltanet.com

3939   **Independent Living Center of Kern County**
5251 Office Park Dr
Suite 200
Bakersfield, CA 93309   661-325-1063
                                    877-688-2079
                                    800-529-9541
                                    FAX: 661-325-6702
                                    TTY:661-325-6702
                                    info@ilcofkerncounty.org
                                    www.ilcofkerncounty.org

Jimmie Soto, Executive Director
Tammy Hartsch, Finance Manager
Harvey Clowers, Special Projects and AT Coordina
Olivia Kent, Systems Change Advocate
A consumer-based consumer-directed non-profit agency assisting persons with disabilities to live independently in their community. The ILCKC presently offers a wide range of services to a growing population of persons with disabilities.

3940   **Independent Living Center of Lancaster**
606 East Avenue K4
Lancaster, CA 93535-2844   661-942-9726
                                    FAX: 661-945-5690
                                    TTY:661-723-2509
                                    ilcsclanc@ilcsc.org
                                    www.ilcsc.org

Taura Jacob, Manager
Marcy Hernandez
Niyanta Dave
ILCSC is a non-profit, consumer based, non-residential agency providing a wide range of services to a growing population of people with disabilities. ILCSC is dedicated to empowering persons with disabilities to exercise indpendence-pofessionally, personally and creatively-while striving to educate the community on their needs.

3941   **Independent Living Resource Center**
7425 El Camino Real
Suite R
Atascadero, CA 93422-4656   805-464-3203
                                    FAX: 805-462-1166
                                    TTY:805-462-1162
                                    info@ilrc-trico.org
                                    www.ilrc-trico.org

Kit McMillion, President
Larry Laborde, Vice President
Dani Anderson, Executive Director
Jennifer Griffin, Business Manager
To assist and encourage individuals to achieve their optimal level of self-sufficiency while eliminating the architectural, communication and attitudinal barriers which prevent them from full participation in the community.

3942   **Independent Living Resource Center: Santa Barbara**
423 W Victoria St
Santa Barbara, CA 93101-3619   805-284-9051
                                    FAX: 805-963-1350
                                    TTY:805-963-0595
                                    info@ilrc-trico.org
                                    www.ilrc-trico.org

Kit McMillion, President
Larry Laborde, Vice President
Dani Anderson, Executive Director
Jennifer Griffin, Business Manager
To assist and encourage individuals to achieve their optimal level of self-sufficiency while eliminating the architectural, communication and attitudinal barriers which prevent them from full participation in the community.

3943 Independent Living Resource Center: San Francisco
825 Howard Street
San Francisco, CA 94103-4128   415-543-6222
                                      FAX: 415-543-6318
                                      TTY:415-543-6698
                                      info@ilrcsf.org
                                      ilrcsf.org

Juma Byrd, President
Kolya Kirienko, Vice President
Ben MacMullan, Treasurer
Will Simpson, Secretary
To ensure that people with disabilities are full social and economic partners, both within their families and in a fully accessible community.

3944 Independent Living Resource Center: Santa Maria Office
327 East Plaza Dr
Suite 3A
Santa Maria, CA 93454-6930   805-354-5948
                                    FAX: 805-349-2416
                                    TTY:805-925-0015
                                    info@ilrc-trico.org
                                    www.ilrc-trico.org

Kit McMillion, President
Larry Laborde, Vice President
Dani Anderson, Executive Director
Jennifer Griffin, Business Manager
To assist and encourage individuals to achieve their optimal level of self-sufficiency while eliminating the architectural, communication and attitudinal barriers which prevent them from full participation in the community.

3945 Independent Living Resource Center: Ventura
1802 Eastman Ave
Suite 112
Ventura, CA 93003-5759   805-256-1036
                                FAX: 805-650-9278
                                TTY:805-650-5993
                                info@ilrc-trico.org
                                www.ilrc-trico.org

Kit McMillion, President
Larry Laborde, Vice President
Dani Anderson, Executive Director
Jennifer Griffin, Business Manager
An organization of, by and for persons with disabilities who reside or work in the service area. Purpose is to assist and encourage individuals to achieve their optimal level of self-sufficiency while eliminating the architectural, communication and attitudinal barriers which prevent them from full participation in the community.

3946 Independent Living Resource of Contra Coast
1850 Gateway Blvd
Suite 120
Concord, CA 94520-3293   925-363-7293
                                FAX: 925-363-7296
                                www.ilrscc.org

Sarah BirdwelL, Board President
Kathy Mitsopoulos, Board Vice President
Teri Ruggiero, Board Secretary
Susan Rotchy, Executive Director
Offers workshops, services are accessible to individuals with cognitive disabilities, physical disabilities, deaf and hard of hearing, emotional disabilities, visual impairments, learing disabilities and seniors.

3947 Independent Living Resource of Fairfield
470 Chadbourn Rd
Ste. B
Fairfield, CA 94534   707-435-8174
                             FAX: 707-435-8177
                             susanr@ilrcoco-sol.org
                             www.ilrscc.org

Sarah BirdwelL, Board President
Kathy Mitsopoulos, Board Vice President
Teri Ruggiero, Board Secretary
Susan Rotchy, Executive Director

To empower people with disabilities to: control their own lives, provide advocacy and support for individuals with disabilities to live independently, create an accessible community free of physical and attitudinal barriers.

3948 Independent Living Resource: Antioch
3727 Sunset Lane
#103
Antioch, CA 94509-1761   925-754-0539
                                TTY:925-755-0934
                                www.ilrscc.org

Sarah BirdwelL, Board President
Kathy Mitsopoulos, Board Vice President
Teri Ruggiero, Board Secretary
Susan Rotchy, Executive Director
Non-profit organizations run and controlled by persons with disabilities. They are non-residential, community-based centers where people with disabilities can receive assistance with a variety of daily living issues and learn the skills they need to take controll of their lives from people who have had similar experiences living with a disability.

3949 Independent Living Resource: Concord
1850 Gateway Blvd
Suite 120
Concord, CA 94520-3293   925-363-7293
                                FAX: 925-363-7296
                                gilc@ilrccc.org
                                www.ilrscc.org

Sarah BirdwelL, Board President
Kathy Mitsopoulos, Board Vice President
Teri Ruggiero, Board Secretary
Susan Rotchy, Executive Director
To empower people with disabilities to: control their own lives, provide advocacy and support for individuals with disabilities to live independently, create an accessible community free of physical and attitudinized barriers.

3950 Independent Living Resources (ILR)
Bldg 2a
101 Broadway
Richmond, CA 94804-1945   510-233-7400
                                 info@ilrccc.org

Marvin Dyson, Manager
Provides services to meet the diverse needs of people who have a variety of disabilities in all age groups.

3951 Independent Living Service Northern California: Redding Office
169 Hartnell Ave
Suite 128
Redding, CA 96002-1849   530-242-8550
                                800-464-8527
                                FAX: 530-241-1454
                                TTY: 530-242-8550
                                info@ilsnc.org
                                actionctr.org

Lauri Evans, President
Frank Smith, Vice President
Evan Levang, Executive Director
Tracy Barker, Program Manager
Independent Living Services of Northern California is a private non profit organization that provides support services to help empower community members with disabilities.

3952 Independent Living Services of Northern California
Jennifer Roberts Building
1161 East Ave
Chico, CA 95926-1018   530-893-8527
                              800-464-8527
                              FAX: 530-893-8574
                              TTY: 530-893-8527
                              info@ilsnc.org
                              actionctr.org

Lauri Evans, President
Frank Smith, Vice President
Evan Levang, Executive Director
Tracy Barker, Program Manager

Independent Living Services of Northern California is a private, non profit organization that provides support services to help empower community members with disabilities.

3953 Marin Center for Independent Living
710 4th St
San Rafael, CA 94901-3213
415-459-6245
FAX: 415-459-7047
TTY:415-459-7027
marincil.org

Chris Schultz, President
Joe Brnnett, Vice President
Eli Gelardin, Executive Director
Susan Malardino, Deputy Director
A non-profit organization that provides advocacy and services for seniors and persons with disabilities.

3954 Mother Lode Independent Living Center(DRAIL: Disability Resource Agency for Independent
Living)
67 Linoberg St
Suite A.
Sonora, CA 95370-4646
209-532-0963
FAX: 209-532-1591
TTY:209-288-3309
barry@drail.org
www.drail.org

Terry Gray, President
Michael Kim Cornelius, Treasurer
Adeline Bagwell, Secretary
Barry Smith, Executive Director
DRAIL is a non-profit, community based, consumer controlled, cross disability center for independent living.

3955 Placer Independent Resource Services
11768 Atwood Road
Suite 29wood Rd
Auburn, CA 95603-9074
530-885-6100
800-833-3453
FAX: 530-885-3032
TTY: 530-885-0326
tmiller@pirs.org
pirs.org

Eldon Luce, President
Michael Cummings, Vice President
Dan Roye, Secretary
Dawn Davidson, Treasurer
A non profit independent living center whose mission is to advocate, empower, educate and provide services for people with disabilities enabling them to control their alternatives for independent living.

3956 Resources for Independent Living
420 i St, Level B.
Suite 3
Sacramento, CA 95814-2319
916-446-3074
FAX: 916-446-2443
leonc@ril-sacramento.org
www.ril-sacramento.org

Ramona Garcia, Board Chairperson
Francisco Godoy, Vice Chairperson
Joanne Bodine, Treasurer
Frances Gracechild, Executive Director
Promoting the socio-economic independence of persons with disabilities by providing peer-supported, consumer-directed independent living services and advocacy.

3957 Rolling Start
570 W 4th St
Suite 107
San Bernardino, CA 92401-1438
909-884-2129
FAX: 909-386-7446
TTY:909-884-7396
support@rollingstart.com
www.rollingstart.org

John Anaya, Chairperson
Kathi Pryor, Treasurer
Francis Bates, Executive Director
Tony Chavez, Deputy Director
Empowers and educates people with disabilities to achieve the independent life of their choice.

3958 Rolling Start: Victorville
17330 Bear Valley Road
Suite A102
Victorville, CA 92395
760-843-7959
FAX: 760-843-7977
TTY:760-951-8175
Patty@rollingstart.com
www.rollingstart.org

John Anaya, Chairperson
Kathi Pryor, Treasurer
Francis Bates, Executive Director
Tony Chavez, Deputy Director
Empowers and educates people with disabilities to achieve the independent life of their choice.

3959 Services Center For Independent Living
107 S Spring Street
Claremont, CA 91711-549
909-621-6722
800-491-6722
FAX: 909-445-0727
TTY: 949-445-0726
janice@scil-ilc.org.
www.scil-ilc.org

Larry Grable, Executive Director
Janice Ornelas, Independent Living Specialist
Angela Nwokike, System Change Advocate
Albert Gonzales, Benefits Specialist
Dedicated to expanding access, information and resources to help increase independence and enhance the quality of life for the East San Gabriel Valley residents with disabilities.

3960 Silicon Valley Independent Living Center
2202 N. First St.
San Jose, CA 95131-1115
408-894-9041
FAX: 408-894-9050
TTY:408-894-9012
info@svilc.org
svilc.org

Patricia Kokes, President
Richard A. Wentz, Vice President
Gabe Lopez, Treasurer
Nayana Shah, Executive Director
A private, consumer-driven, nonprofit corporation that offers quality services to individuals with disabilities in Silicon Valley.

3961 Silicon Valley Independent Living Center: South County Branch
7881 Church Street
Suite C
Gilroy, CA 95020-7346
408-843-9100
FAX: 408-842-4791
TTY:408-842-2591
info@svilc.org
svilc.org

Patricia Kokes, President
Richard A. Wentz, Vice President
Gabe Lopez, Treasurer
Nayana Shah, Executive Director
A private, consumer-driven, non-profit corporation that offers quality services to individuals with disabilities in Silicon Valley.

3962 Southern California Rehabilitation Services
7830 Quill Dr
Suite D
Downey, CA 90242-3440

562-862-6531
FAX: 562-923-5274
TTY:562-869-0931
scrs@scrs-ilc.org
scrs-ilc.org

Lisa Hayes, President
Michael Strong, Vice President
Carol Trees, Secretary/Treasurer
Chad Williams, Board Member
Empowers persons with disabilities to achieve their personalized goals through community education and individualized services that provide the knowledge, skills, and confidence building to maximize their quality of life.

3963 Through the Looking Glass
3075 Adeline St.
Ste. 120
Berkeley, CA 94703

510-848-1112
800-644-2666
FAX: 510-848-4445
TTY: 510-848-1005
tlg@lookingglass.org
www.lookingglass.org

Maureen Block, J.D., Board President
Thomas Spalding, Board Treasurer
Alice Nemon, D.S.W., Board Secretary
Karen Fessel, Ph.D., Executive Director
To create, demonstrate and encourage non-pathological and empowering reesources and model early intervention services for families with disability issues in parent or child which integrate expertise derived from personal disability experience and disability culture.

3964 Tri-County Independent Living Center
2822 Harris Street
Eureka, CA 95503

707-445-8404
877-576-5000
FAX: 707-445-9751
TTY: 707-445-8405
aa@tilinet.org
www.tilinet.org

Gail Pascoe, President
Linda Arnold, Vice President
Kevin O'Brien, Treasurer
Chris Jones, Executive Director
Promotes the philosophy of independent living, to connect individuals to services, and to create and accessible community, so that people with disabilities can have control over their lives and full access to the communities in which they live.

3965 Westside Center for Independent Living
12901 Venice Blvd
Los Angeles, CA 90066-3509

310-390-3611
888-851-9245
FAX: 310-390-4906
TTY: 310-398-9204
development@wcil.org
www.wcil.org

David Geffen, President
Chris Knauf, 1st Vice President
Brenda Green, Secretary
Aliza Barzilay, Executive Director
The Westside Center for Independent Living (WCIL) helps people living with disabilities maintain self-sufficient and productive lives through non-residential peer support services and training programs. Independent Living promotes self-determination, community living, full participation in community life and access to the same opportunities and resources available to people without disabilities.

Colorado

3966 Atlantis Community
201 S Cherokee St
Denver, CO 80223-1836

303-733-9324
FAX: 303-733-6211
TTY:303-733-0047
info@atlantiscommunity.org
www.atlantiscommunity.net

David Hays, Manager
Provide direct services, and to empower people with disabilities integrating, with full and equal rights, into all parts of society including employment, affordable, accessible, housing, transportation, recreation, communication, education, and public places while exercising and exerting choice and self determination.

3967 Center for Independence
740 Gunnison Ave
Grand Junction, CO 81501-3222

708-588-0833
FAX: 708-588-0406
center-for-independence.org

Linda Taylor, Executive Director
The Center for Independence works to promote community solutions and to empower individuals with disabilities to live independently.

3968 Center for People with Disabilities
615 Main St
Longmont, CO 80501-4983

303-772-3250
FAX: 303-772-5125
TTY:303-772-3250
info@cpwd.org
www.cpwd-ilc.org

Dale Gaar, Board President
Deborah.A Conley, Board Vice President
Nancy Phares-Zook, Board Secretary
Tony Adams, Board Treasurer
Provides resources, information, and advocacy to assist people with disabilities in overcoming barriers to independent living.

3969 Center for People with Disabilities: Pueblo
1304 Berkley Ave
Pueblo, CO 81004-3002

719-546-1271
800-659-3656
FAX: 719-546-1374
ivaleneamidei@yahoo.com
www.ilcpueblo.org

Larry Williams, Executive Director
One of the 10 centers for independent living in Colorado founded under Title VII of the Rehabilitation Act of 1973 as amended in 1978. All new centers under this Independent Living (CIL) Title of the Act received initial and ongoing grants through this new Federal Program created by the Act.

3970 Center for People with Disabilities: Boulder
1675 Range St
Boulder, CO 80301-2722

303-442-8662
888-929-5519
FAX: 303-442-0502
info@cpwd.org
www.cpwd-ilc.org

Dale Gaar, Board President
Deborah.A Conley, Board Vice President
Nancy Phares-Zook, Board Secretary
Tony Adams, Board Treasurer
Providing resources, information and advocacy to people with disabilities. Assist people with disabilities in transitioning from nursing homes to independent living in the community. Also provide personal assistance services.

3971 Colorado Springs Independence Center
729 South Tejon Street
Colorado Springs, CO 80903
719-471-8181
FAX: 719-471-7829
TTY:719-471-2076
info@csicindliving.org
www.theindependencecenter.org

Billy A. , Chair Elect
Billy B. , Secretary
Dean C. , Treasurer
To empower persons with disabilities to maximize their independence within the community and to remove barriers which impact their quality of life, while encouraging them to live independently in their community.

3972 Connections for Independent Living
1331 8th Avenue
Greeley, CO 80631-4027
970-352-8682
800-887-5828
FAX: 970-353-8058
TTY: 970-352-8682
pattid4z@yahoo.com
www.connectionsforindependentliving.org

Beth Danielson, Executive Director
Michael Stevens, Director of Services
Alicia Garza, Director
Dianna Shmidl, Community Transition Specialist
Certified IL Center, I and R advocacy, peer support, skills training, sign language interpretations, reader services, housing. Cross-disability, all ages.

3973 Denver CIL
Ste 100
777 Grant St
Denver, CO 80203-3501
303-837-1020
FAX: 303-837-0859
www.denverhousing.org

Greg Beran, Owner
Ismael Guerrero, Executive Director
Joshua Crawley, Agency Counsel
Nichole Ford, Chief Financial Officer
Provides resources, information, and advocacy to assist people with disabilities in overcoming barriers to independent living.

3974 Disability Center for Independent Living
4821 East 38th Avenue
Denver, CO 80207-1232
303-320-1345
FAX: 303-320-1345
TTY:303-322-2330
avillasenor.dcil@gmil.com
www.accil.net

Larry Williams, Executive Director
John Wooster, Consultant
Anthony Gonzales, Housing Coordinator
Jenna Emery, OBI Specialist
Independent living center providing quality services for people with disabilities.

3975 Disabled Resource Services
1017 Robertson Street
Unit B
Fort Collins, CO 80524-3915
970-482-2700
FAX: 970-449-6972
TTY:970-407-7060
drs@frii.com
disabledresourceservices.org

George Tremblay, Chairman
John Weins, Vice Chairman
Nancy Jackson, Executive Director
Marj Grell, Office Manager
To empower individuals with disabilities to achieve their maximum level of independence and to gain personal dignity within society. Disabled Resource Services, as a private non-profit state certified center for independent living, is dedicated to working with individuals with all types of disabilities in Larimer County to promote their independence and equality through services

which support advocacy, awareness and access to their community.

3976 Disbled Resource Services
640 E Eisenhower Blvd
Loveland, CO 80537-3954
970-667-0816
FAX: 970-593-6582
drs@frii.com
disabledresourceservices.org

George Tremblay, Chairman
John Weins, Vice Chairman
Nancy Jackson, Executive Director
Marj Grell, Office Manager
To empower individuals with disabilities to achieve their maximum level of independence and to gain personal dignity within society.

3977 Greeley Center for Independence
2780 28th Ave
Greeley, CO 80634-7803
970-339-2444
800-748-1012
FAX: 970-339-0033
gciinc@gciinc.org
www.gciinc.org

Chari Armagost, Chief Financial Officer
Sarita Reddy, PH. D, Executive Director
Rob Rabe, Director of Outpatient Service
Dee Seekamp, Director of Nursing
Provides places of growth, transition and encouragement, where people with temporary and permanent disabilities can reach toward their maximum potential of personal independence and wellness.

3978 Independent Life Center
P.O.Box 612
Craig, CO 81626-612
970-826-0833
888-526-0833
FAX: 970-826-0832
TTY: 970-826-0833
info@indlife.org
www.accil.net

Larry Williams, Executive Director
John Wooster, Consultant
Anthony Gonzales, Housing Coordinator
Jenna Emery, OBI Specialist
Provides resources, information, and advocacy to assist people with disabilities in overcoming barriers to independent living.

3979 Pueblo Goodwill Industries
15810 Indianola Drive
Rockville, MD 20855
240-333-5590
800-GOO-WILL
contactus@goodwill.org
www.goodwill.org

Debi Diaz, CEO
Lauren Lawson-Zilai, Director of Public Relations
Charlene Sarmiento, Senior Specialist, Public Relati
PGoodwill works to enhance the dignity and quality of life of individuals and families by strengthening communities, eliminating barriers to opportunity, and helping people in need reach their full potential through learning and the power of work.

3980 Southwest Center for Independence
3473 Main Avenue
#23
Durango, CO 81301-5474
970-259-1672
866-962-2158
FAX: 970-259-0947
TTY: 970-259-1672
director@swcidur.org
www.swilc.org

Martha Mason, Executive Director
Mariellen Walz, Chair
Patricia Ziegler, Assistant Director
Jason Armstrong, Treasurer
Empowering individuals with disabilities and their families to achieve their maximum level of independence in work, play and other areas of life.

3981 Southwest Center for Independence: Cortez
2409 East Empire Street
PO Box 640
Cortez, CO 81321-9164
970-570-8001
866-962-2158
FAX: 970-565-7169
director@swilc.org
www.swilc.org

Mariellen Walz, Chair
Johnny Bulson, Vice Chair
Jason Armstrong, Treasurer
Martha Mason, Executive Director
Empowers individiuals with disabilities and their families to achieve their maximum level of independence in work, play and other areas of life.

Connecticut

3982 Center for Disability Rights
764-B Campbell Ave
764 Campbell Ave
W Haven, CT 06516- 3786
203-934-7077
FAX: 203-934-7078
TTY:203-934-7079
info@cdr-ct.org
cdr-ct.org

Marc Gallucci, Executive Director
Chris Zurcher, Consumer Relations
Dana Canevari, I&R Specialist
Susan St. John, Administrative Assistant
Resources, information, and advocacy to assist people with disabilities in overcoming barriers to independent living.

3983 Center for Independent Living SC
26 Palmers Hill Rd
Stamford, CT 06902-2113
203-353-8550
FAX: 203-353-1423
TTY:203-353-8550

Dana Canevari, Director
Provides resources, information, and advocacy to assist people with disabilities in overcoming barriers to independent living.

3984 Chapel Haven
1040 Whalley Ave
New Haven, CT 06515-1740
203-397-1714
FAX: 203-937-2466
admissions@chapelhaven.org
chapelhaven.org

Michael Storz, President
The only combined state-accredited special education facility and independent living facility for adults with cognitive disabilities.

3985 Disabilities Network of Eastern Connecticut
19 Ohio Avenue
Suite 2
Norwich, CT 06360-2111
860-823-1898
FAX: 860-886-2316
CFerry@dnec.org
dnec.org

Katherine Pellerin, President
Robert Davidson, Vice President
Jane O'Friel, Secretary/Treasurer
Cathy Ferry, Executive Director
Dedicated to supporting and advancing the rights of individuals with disabilities. The goal is to creat a completely inclusive society where people live together in communities regardless of their abilities.

3986 Disability Resource Center of Fairfield County
80 Ferry Blvd
Suite 205
Stratford, CT 06615-6079
203-378-6977
FAX: 203-375-2748
TTY:203-378-3248
info@drcfc.org
www.accessinct.org

Ethel M R, President
Thomas D, Vice-President
Anthony Lacava, Executive Director
Glenn Calaffin, Program Director
A crosss-disability resource and advocacy organization for people with disabilities that has provided unique, consumer-directed services both for individuals and for the communities of Fairfield County.

3987 Independence Northwest Center for Independent Living
1183 New Haven Rd
Suite 200
Naugatuck, CT 06770-5033
203-729-3299
FAX: 203-729-2839
TTY:203-729-1281
info@independencenorthwest.org
www.independencenorthwest.org

Maureen Mayo, President
Tom Ford, Vice President
Charles Marino, Treasurer
Jaff Laliberte, Secretary
Provides services in such areas as peer counseling, advocacy, independent living skills training and information and referral.

3988 Independence Unlimited
151 New Park Ave
Suite D
Hartford, CT 06106-2170
860-523-0126
FAX: 860-523-5603
info@ctsilc.org
ctsilc.org

Eileen Heall, President
Keith Mullinar, Vice President
Kartherine Pellerin, Secretary
Keith Mullinar, Treasurer
Center for independent living that provides skills training, peer counseling, advocacy, transition from institutions to the community and a variety of other services.

3989 New Horizons Village
37 Bliss Rd
Unionville, CT 06085
860-673-8893
FAX: 860-675-4369
Michael.Shaw@NewHorizonsVillage.com
newhorizonsvillage.com

Carolyn Fields, Administrator
A 68 unit apartment complex designed for people who have severe physical disabilities.

Delaware

3990 Freedom Center for Independent Living
400 N Broad St
Middletown, DE 19709-1089
302-376-4399
866-687-3245
FAX: 302-376-4395
TTY: 302-376-4397
info@fcilde.org
fcilde.org

Hersernest Cole, Executive Director
Lillian Evans, Independent Living Specialist
Protects the Civil Rights and promote the empowerment of persons with disabilities and their families through our independent living philosophy.

3991 **Independent Living**
Apt 210
1800 N Broom St
Wilmington, DE 19802-3854
302-429-6693
FAX: 302-429-8031
TTY:302-429-8034

Susan Cycyk, Executive Director
Providing skilled support and caring guidance to adults with disabilities. Our case management services include: daily living skills training, medical coordination, transportation assistance, financial management, housing assistance, and vocational/educational planning.

3992 **Independent Resource Georgetown**
Ste 37
410 S Bedford St
Georgetown, DE 19947-1850
302-854-9330
FAX: 302-854-9408
TTY:302-854-9340
pboyd@independentresource.org

Larry Henderson, Director
Pat Boyd, Manager
Provides independent living services to persons who experience a significant disability. Offers skills training, individually and in small groups, peer support/peer counseling and information and referral services. Strives to remove the architectural and attitudnal barriers through individual and systems advocacy.

3993 **Independent Resources: Dover**
154 South Governor's Avenue
Dover, DE 19904-7311
302-735-4599
FAX: 302-735-5623
TTY:302-735-5629
lhenderson@independentresources.org
www.iri-de.org

Tes DelTufo, Office Director
Carolyn Miller, IL Specialist
Debbie Justice, IL Specialist
Barty Rochester, Peer Support Coordinator
Private, non-profit, consumer-controlled, community based organization providing services and advocacy by and for persons with all types of disabilities. Their goal is to assist individuals with disabilities to achieve their maximum potential within their families and communities.

3994 **Independent Resources: Wilmington**
6 Denny Rd
Suite 101
Wilmington, DE 19809-3444
302-765-0191
FAX: 302-765-0195
TTY:302-765-0194
fox205007@aol.com
www.iri-de.org

Larry D Henderson, Executive Director
Phyllis Farrare, Director of Operations
Private, non-profit, consumer-controlled, community based organization providing services and advocacy by and for persons with all types of disabilities. Their goal is to assist individuals with disabilities to achieve their maximum potential within their families and communities.

3995 **Mosaic Of De**
4980 S. 118TH ST
Omaha, NE 68137
302-456-5995
877-366-7242
FAX: 402-896-1511
info@mosaicinfo.org
mosaicinfo.org

Terry Olson, Executive Director
Linda Timmons, President and CEO
Raul Saldivar, Chief Operating Officer
Cindy Schroeder, Chief Financial Officer
Provides services to adults with developmental disabilities who reside in homes and apartments. Services are designed to provide them with opportunities for choices and participation in the life of their communities. Supports are geared to assist each individual in becoming more independent in activities of daily living,

vocational skills, community mobility and transportation, and recreation and leisure activities.

District of Columbia

3996 **District of Columbia Center for Independent Living**
1400 Florida Ave NE
Washington, DC 20002-5032
202-388-0033
FAX: 202-398-3018
info@dccil.org
dccil.org

Rev. Patric Hailes Fears, President
Dr. John Thompson, Vice President
Carl Bartels, Treasurer
Angela Washington, Secretary
Mission is to maximize the leadership, empowerment, independence, and productivity of individuals with disabilities, and to integrate these individuals into the mainstream of American society.

3997 **National Council on Independent Living**
2013 H St. NW
6th Floor
Washington, DC 20006-3007
202-207-0334
877-525-3400
FAX: 202-207-0341
TTY: 202-207-0340
ncil@ncil.org
www.ncil.org

Kelly Buckland, Executive Director
Lou Ann Kibbee, President
Mark Derry, Vice President
Roger Howard, Treasurer
As a membership organization, NCIL advances independent living and the rights of people with disabilities through consumer-driven advocacy.

Florida

3998 **Ability 1st**
1300 E. Green Street
Pasadena, CA 91106
626-396-1010
877-768-4600
FAX: 626-396-1021
info@abilityfirst.org
abilityfirst.org

Steve Brockmeyer, Chairman
John Kelly, Vice Chairman
Lori.E Gangemi, President
Kevin Schaffels, CFO
To empower persons with disabilities to live independently and participate actively in their community.

3999 **Adult Day Training**
Goodwill Industries - Suncoast
10596 Gandy Blvd N
St Petersburg, FL 33702-1422
727-523-1512
888-279-1988
FAX: 727-563-9300
TTY:727-579-1068
gw.marketing@goodwill-suncoast.com
www.goodwill-suncoast.org

Oscar J. Horton, Chairman
Martin W. Gladysz, Vice Chairman
Heather Ceresoli, Vice Chairman
Deborah.A Passerini, President
An innovative program which uses job skills to teach self-help, daily living, communication, mobility, travel, decision-making, behavioral and social skills. This focus provides concrete, transferable experiences to help prepare individuals for greater community inclusion by achieving the highest possible degree of independence in their daily life, increasing their confidence and supporting their successful transitions to less structured, self-sufficient environments.

4000 CIL of Central Florida
720 N Denning Dr
Winter Park, FL 32789-3020   407-623-1070
                                   FAX: 407-623-1390
                                   info@cilorlando.org
                                   cilorlando.org

Jason Vennings, Development Director
Kim Byerly, Chair
Cheryl Stone, Secretary
Don Pirozzoli, M.S., Programs Director
A private, non-profit organization dedicated to helping people
with disabilities achieve their self-determined goals for inde-
pendent living.

4001 Caring and Sharing Center for Independent Living
12552 Belcher Rd S
Largo, FL 33773-3014   727-539-7550
                                 866-539-7550
                                 FAX: 727-539-7588
                                 cascil@cascil.org
                                 www.disabilityachievementcenter.org

Barbara Dandro, Treasurer
Mary Bucca, Secretary
Patricia Bell, Director
Dennis Shelt, Director
Empowering people with disabilities.

4002 Caring and Sharing Center: Pasco County
12552 Belcher Rd S
Largo, FL 33773-3014   727-539-7550
                                 866-539-7550
                                 FAX: 727-539-7588
                                 cascil@cascil.org
                                 www.disabilityachievementcenter.org

Barbara Dandro, Treasurer
Mary Bucca, Secretary
Patricia Bell, Director
Dennis Shelt, Director
Empowering people with disabilities.

4003 Center for Independent Living in Central Florida
720 N Denning Dr
Winter Park, FL 32789-3095   407-623-1070
                                   FAX: 407-623-1390
                                   info@cilorlando.org
                                   cilorlando.org

Jason Vennings, Development Director
Kim Byerly, Chair
Cheryl Stone, Secretary
Don Pirozzoli, M.S., Programs Director
In partnership with the community, promotes personal right snad
responsiblities among people with all disabilities.

4004 Center for Independent Living of Broward
4800 N State Road 7
Suite 102
Lauderdale Lakes, FL 33319-5811   954-722-6400
                                   888-722-6400
                                   FAX: 954-735-1958
                                   cilb@cilbroward.org
                                   www.cilbroward.org

Craig Lilienthal, President
Christopher Sharp, VP
Shea Smith, Treasurer
Laurie Menekou, Secretary
Offers assistance to people with disabilities in fulfilling the goals
of independence and self-sufficiency.

4005 Center for Independent Living of Florida Keys
103400 Overseas Hwy
Suite 243
Key Largo, FL 33037-2849   305-453-3491
                                  877-335-0187
                                  FAX: 305-453-3488
                                  TTY: 305-453-3491
                                  cilkeys@cilkeys.org
                                  www.cilofthekeys.org

Brenda K Pierce, Executive Director

Offers assistance to persons with disabilities in acquiring independent living and self-advocacy skills in order to obtain and
maintain independence and self-sufficiency.

4006 Center for Independent Living of N Florida
1823 Buford Ct
Tallahassee, FL 32308-4465   850-575-9621
                                   FAX: 850-575-5740
                                   TTY: 850-575-5245
                                   cilnf@nettally.com
                                   www.ability1st.info/about-us

Judith Barrett, Executive Director
Offers assistance to persons with disabilities in acquiring independent living and self-advocacy skills in order to obtain and
maintain independence and self-sufficiency

4007 Center for Independent Living of NW Florida
3600 N Pace Blvd
Pensacola, FL 32505-4240   850-595-5566
                                   877-245-2457
                                   FAX: 850-595-5560
                                   cil-drc@cil-drc.org
                                   cil-drc.org

James Hicks, President
Kathleen Wilks, Secretary
John Bouchard, Treasurer
Frank Cherry, Executive Director
Provides services such as information and referral, peer counsel-
ing, housing, advocacy, training, independent living skills train-
ing, free wheelchairs, loan locker, assistive technology.

4008 Center for Independent Living of North Central Florida
3445 NE 24th Street
Ocala, FL 34470-9214   352-368-3788
                                   877-232-8261
                                   FAX: 352-629-0098
                                   www.cilncf.org

Joe Dyke, President
Robert Miller, Vice President
David Christie, Treasurer
Jim Gorske, Secretary
Empowers people with disabilities to exert their individual rights
to live as independently as possible, make personal life choices
and achieve full community inclusion.

4009 Center for Independent Living of North Central Florida
222 SW 36th Ter
Gainesville, FL 32607-2863   352-378-7474
                                   800-265-5724
                                   FAX: 352-378-5582
                                   TTY: 352-372-3443
                                   www.cilncf.org

Joe Dyke, President
Robert Miller, Vice President
David Christie, Treasurer
Jim Gorske, Secretary
Empowering people with disabilities to exert their individual
rights to live as independently as possible, make personal life
choices and achieve full community inclusion.

4010 Center for Independent Living of S Florida
6660 Biscayne Blvd
Miami, FL 33138-6285   305-751-8025
                                   FAX: 305-751-8944
                                   TTY: 305-751-8891
                                   info@soflacil.org
                                   soflacil.org

Alvin W. Roberts, President
Gregg Goldfarb, Vice President
Timothy Werner, Ph.D, Secretary
Jay Weiss, M.B.A., Treasurer
A community based non for profit, independent living center
serving people of all ages with any type of disability. Services:
Basic education, GED preperation, American sign language ad-
vocacy, peer support, information and referral, independent liv-
ing skills training, housing assistance, transportation assistance,
home modiifications, transition from nursing facility to the com-

munity assisatnace filing ADA complaints, accessibility surveys, diability awareness traing.

4011 Center for Independent Living of SW Florida
2321 Bruner Ln
Fort Myers, FL 33912-1904   239-277-1447
800-435-7352
FAX: 239-277-1647
www.cilfl.org

Ronald J Muschong, Interim Executive Director
Helping people with disabilities achieve independence and self-determination in their lives.

4012 Coalition for IndependentLiving Options: Okeechobee
1680 SW Bayshore Boulevard
Suite 231
Port St. Lucie, FL 34984   772-878-3500
FAX: 772-878-3344
www.cilo.org

Scott Shoemaker, President
Sharon D'Eusanio, Vice President
Joseph Fields Jr., Esquire, Secretary
Genevieve Cousminer,Esq, Executive Director
Private non-profit promoting independences for people with disabilities in Palm Beach, Martin, St. Lucie & Okeechobee Counties. Services include advocacy, independent living skills & training, peer support, after school & summer programs for teens, crime victim support services, and veterans transition services.

4013 Coalition for Independent Living Options: Fort Pierce
6800 Forest HIll Boulevard
West Palm Beach, FL 33413   561-966-4288
FAX: 561-966-0441
www.cilo.org

Scott Shoemaker, President
Sharon D'Eusanio, Vice President
Joseph Fields Jr., Esquire, Secretary
Genevieve Cousminer,Esq, Executive Director
Private non-profit promoting independences for people with disabilities in Palm Beach, Martin, St. Lucie & Okeechobee Counties. Services include advocacy, independent living skills & training, peer support, after school & summer programs for teens, crime victim support services, and verterans transition services.

4014 Coalition for Independent Living Options
6800 Forest HIll Boulevard
West Palm Beach, FL 33413-3310   561-966-4288
FAX: 561-966-0441
www.cilo.org
Scott Shoemaker, President
Sharon D'Eusanio, Vice President
Joseph Fields Jr., Esquire, Secretary
Genevieve Cousminer,Esq, Executive Director
Private non-profit promoting independences for people with disabilities in Palm Beach, Martin, St. Lucie & Okeechobee Counties. Services include advocacy, independent living skills & training, peer support, after school & summer programs for teens, crime victim support services, and verterans transition services.

4015 Coalition for Independent Living Options: Stuart
1680 SW Bayshore Boulevard
Suite 231
Port St. Lucie, FL 34984   772-878-3500
FAX: 772-878-3344
www.cilo.org

Scott Shoemaker, President
Sharon D'Eusanio, Vice President
Joseph Fields Jr., Esquire, Secretary
Genevieve Cousminer,Esq, Executive Director
Private non-profit promoting independences for people with disabilities in Palm Beach, Martin, St. Lucie & Okeechobee Counties. Services include advocacy, independent living skills & training, peer support, after school & summer programs for teens, crime victim support services, and verterans transition services.

4016 Disability Resource Center
300 W. 5th St.
Panama City, FL 32401-4704   850-769-6890
FAX: 850-769-6891
outreach@drcpc.org
www.drcpc.org

Robert Cox, Executive Director
Becky Cadwell, Independent Living Specialist
They are commiteed to collaborating with other disability/consumer-focused organizations in their community

4017 Lakeland Adult Day Training
3033 Drane Field Rd
Suite 5
Lakeland, FL 33811-3305   863-701-1351
TTY:863-701-1356
gw.marketing@goodwill-suncoast.com
www.goodwill-suncoast.org

Oscar J. Horton, Chairman
Martin W. Gladysz, Vice Chairman
Heather Ceresoli, Vice Chairman
Deborah.A Passerini, President
An innovative program which uses job skills to teach self-help, daily living, communication, mobility, travel, decision-making, behavioral and social skills. This focus provides concrete, transferable experiences to help prepare individuals for greater community inclusion by achieving the highest possible degree of independence in their daily life, increasing their confidence and supporting their successful transitions to less structured, self-sufficient environments.

4018 Lighthouse Central Florida
215 E New Hampshire St
Orlando, FL 32804-6403   407-898-2483
FAX: 407-895-5255
lvaneepoel@lcf-fl.org
www.lighthousecentralflorida.com

Alex B. Hull, Chair
David Stahl, Vice Chair
Paul Prewitt, Secretary
Nancy L. Urbach, Treasurer
Promote the independence and success of people living with vision impairment.

4019 Miami-Dade County Disability Services and Independent Living (DSAIL)
701 NW 1st Court
Miami, FL 33136-1647   786-469-4600
FAX: 305-547-7355
morrina@miamidade.gov
www.miamidade.gov

Michael Moxam, Manager
Lucia Davis-Raiford, Director
Offers information and referral services serving all types of disabilities with the goal of assisting the disabled acquiring independence and control over their lives. Teaches independent living skills, job readiness and placement, home health care, sensitivity training, training in ASL and Braille, counsel people with disabilities or wide range of problems.

4020 Ocala Adult Day Training
2920 W Silver Springs Blvd
Ocala, FL 34475-5654   352-629-0456
TTY:352-629-0874
gw.marketing@goodwill-suncoast.com
www.goodwill-suncoast.org

Oscar J. Horton, Chairman
Martin W. Gladysz, Vice Chairman
Heather Ceresoli, Vice Chairman
Deborah.A Passerini, President
An innovative program which uses job skills to teach self-help, daily living, communication, mobility, travel, decision-making, behavioral and social skills. This focus provides concrete, transferable experiences to help prepare individuals for greater community inclusion by achieving the highest possible degree of independence in their daily life, increasing their confidence and supporting their successful transitions to less structured, self-sufficient environments.

4021 Pinellas Park Adult Day Training
7601 Park Blvd
Pinellas Park, FL 33781-3704
727-541-6205
TTY:727-544-5835
gw.marketing@goodwill-suncoast.com
www.goodwill-suncoast.org

Oscar J. Horton, Chairman
Martin W. Gladysz, Vice Chairman
Heather Ceresoli, Vice Chairman
Deborah.A Passerini, President
An innovative program which uses job skills to teach self-help, daily living, communication, mobility, travel, decision-making, behavioral and social skills. This focus provides concrete, transferable experiences to help prepare individuals for greater community inclusion by achieving the highest possible degree of independence in their daily life, increasing their confidence and supporting their successful transitions to less structured, self-sufficient environments.

4022 SCCIL at Titusville
571-W Haverty Court
Rockledge, FL 32955
321-633-6011
FAX: 321-633-6472
TTY:706-724-6324
jilldunham9@gmail.com
www.virtualcil.net

Jill Dunham-Schuller, Executive Director
Directory of Independent Living Centers throughout the United States.

4023 Self Reliance
8901 N Armenia Ave
Tampa, FL 33604-1041
813-375-3965
FAX: 813-375-3970
TTY:813-375-3972
bruehl@self-reliance.org
www.self-reliance.org

Finn Kavanagh, Executive Director
Michele Pineda, Director of Finance & Operations
Gary Martoccio, Programs Director
Kim Albritton, Chairperson
A cross disability agency providing services to both children and adults with disabilities to identify and overcome barriers to independence in their lives. Self Reliance also promotes independence through empowering persons with disabilities and improving the communities in which they live.

4024 Space Coast Center for Independent Living
571 Haverty Court, Suite W.
Rockledge, FL 32955
321-633-6011
FAX: 321-633-6472
spacecoastcil.org

Michael Lavoie, President
Howard Fetes, VP
Jason Miller, Treasurer/Secretary
Provides overall services for individuals with al types of disabilities. Offers peer support, advocacy, skills training, accessibility surveys, support groups, transportation, specialized equipment and sign language interpreter referral services and home modifications.

4025 Suncoast Center for Independent Living, Inc.
3281 17th Street
Sarasota, FL 34235
941-351-9545
FAX: 941-316-9320
Info@scil4u.org
www.scil4u.org

Kevin Sanderson, Chair
Michael Fluker, Executive Director
Vicke Mack, Treasurer
Scott Biehler, Secretary
Helping people with disabilities live independently.

4026 disAbility Solutions for Independent Living
119 S Palmetto Ave
Suite 180
Daytona Beach, FL 32114- 4369
386-255-1812
866-310-1039
FAX: 386-255-1814
TTY: 386-252-6222
info@dsil.org
www.dsil.org

Julie M Shaw, Executive Director
To maximize the leadership, empowerment, independence and productivity of individuals with disabilities, to promote and attain integration and full inclusion of individuals with disabilities in all aspects of our society; accomplished through consumer control, peer support, education, self-determination, equal access and individual and systems advocacy

Georgia

4027 Arms Wide Open
5036 Snapfinger Woods Drive
Ste 205
Decatur, GA 30035- 1677
678-404-7696
FAX: 770-498-2778
kenmorris@armswideopen.org
www.armswideopen.org

Ken Morris, Director
Arms Wide Open operates a durable medical equipment loan program and a life care program. The mission of Arms Wide Open is to provide support services to the aged, disabled and chronically ill for the purpose of helping them to avoid institutional placement.

4028 Bain, Inc. Center For Independent Living
316 W Shotwell St
Bainbridge, GA 39819-3906
229-246-0150
888-830-1530
FAX: 229-246-1715
TTY: 888-830-1530
bain@surfsouth.com
www.baincil.org

Virginia Harris, Executive Director
Malissa Thompson, Program Manager
Tomonia Becon, Nursing Home Transition Coordina
Julie Harris, Independent Living Specialist
A non-residential Center for Independent Living serving eleven counties throughout Southwest. BAIN is a non-profit, community based resource and advocacy center run by and for individuals with disabilities.

4029 Disability Connections
170 College St
Macon, GA 31201-1656
478-741-1425
800-743-2117
FAX: 478-755-1571
dcinfo@disabilityconnections.com
disabilityconnections.com

Jerilyn Leverett, Executive Director
A private non-profit organization that looks to enable all people with disabilities to attain and have access to all opportunities in life.

4030 Division of Rehabilitation Services
Georgia Department of Labor
410 Mall Blvd
Suite B
Savannah, GA 31406-4869
912-356-2226
FAX: 912-356-2875
TTY:912-356-2940
www.dol.state.ga.us
dol.state.ga.us

Mark Bultler, Commissioner
Jody Lane, Manager
George Foley, Manager
Vocational rehabilitation services.

4031   Living Independence for Everyone (LIFE)
5105 Paulsen Street
Suite 143-B
Savannah, GA 31405

912-920-2414
800-948-4824
FAX: 912-920-0007
info@lifecil.com
www.lifecil.com

Mark Schreiber, President
Stuart Klugler, Vice President
John Paul Berlon, Secretary
Cheryl Brackin, Board Member
The Southeast's Regional disability resource center that offers a wide range of resources, education, and advocacy to the community to help level the playing field for people with disabilities to create a world in which everyone can fully participate.

4032   Multiple Choices Center for Independent Living
145 Barrington Dr.
Athens, GA 30605-3133

706-850-4025
info@multiplechoices.us
www.multiplechoices.us

Doug Hatch, President
Donald Veater, VP
Elllen Des Jardines, Secretary
William Holley, Executive Director
To break down all barriers to inclusion by enhancing the equality of life and empowering people with disabilities through advocacy, education and training.

4033   North District Independent Living Program
Ste 209
311 Green St NW
Gainesville, GA 30501-3364

770-535-5930

Sharon McCurry, Coordinator
Cindy Hanna, Executive Director
Information and referral, advocacy, peer counseling, service coordination and ADA consultation.

4034   Southwest District Independent Living Program
P.O.Box 1606
Albany, GA 31702-1606

229-430-4170
FAX: 229-430-4466

Bill Layton, Director
Diane Davis, Executive Director
Offers peer counseling, disability education and awareness, attendant care registry, and information on accessible home for the disabled.

4035   Statewide Independent Living Council of Georgia
315 West Ponce de Leon Avenue
Suite 600
Decatur, GA 30030-2617

770-270-6860
888-288-9780
FAX: 770-270-5957
shellys5@hotmail.com
silcga.org

Steve Oldaker, President
Angela Denise Davis, Vice President
Mark Schreiber, Treasurer
Scott Osborne, Secretary
Founded to ensure that people with disabilities have opportunities to live as independently as possible.

4036   Walton Options for Independent Living
948 Walton Way
Augusta, GA 30901-519

706-724-6262
877-821-8400
FAX: 706-724-6729
TTY: 706-724-6262
tjohnston@waltonoptions.org
www.waltonoptions.org

Tiffany Cilford, Executive Director
Ann Campbell-Kelly, Special Projects Coordinator
Alyson Schwartz, Special Projects Coordinator
Sam Creech, Director-Information Technology

Services include individual and systems advocacy, peer support, skills training (including basic computer and return to work skills), information and referral services and transition from institutions back to the community.

4037   disABILITY LINK: Rome
1901 Montreal Road
Suite 102
Tucker, GA 30084

404-687-8890
FAX: 404-687-8298
info@disabilitylink.org
disabilitylink.org

Kim Gibson, Executive Director
Travis Evans, Health, Wellness and Resource Sp
Larry Brown, Finance Director
Hillary Elliott, Independent Living Services Prog
Committed to promoting the rights of all people with disabilities.

Hawaii

4038   Center For Independent Living- Kauai
State Office Building 3060 Eiwa Str
Lihue, HI 96766-6529

808-274-3484
FAX: 808-245-3485
kauaiddc@pixi.com
hiddc.org/kauai.htm

Humberto Blanco, Administrator
Teri Yamashiro, IL Specialist
Offers peer counseling, disability education, attendant care registry, outreach services and advocacy.

4039   Hawaii Center For Independent Living
1055 Kinoole Street
Suite 105le St
Hilo, HI 96720-3872

808-935-3777
800-420-6928
TTY:808-935-7888
info@pacificil.org
www.cil-hawaii.org

Gordon Fuller, Executive Director
Provides an array of support services for people with all types of disabilities of any age.

4040   Hawaii Center for Independent Living-Maui
220 Imi Kala Street
Suite 103
Wailuku, HI 96793-1209

808-242-4966
866-303-4245
800-420-6928
FAX: 808-244-6978
TTY:808-242-4968
mcilogg@gte.net/ clytien@pacificil.org
www.cil-hawaii.org

Clytie Nishihara, Manager
T Lay , Administrative Assistant
Offers disability education and awareness, advocacy and counseling.

4041   Hawaii Centers for Independent Living
200 N. Vineyard Blvd Bldg. A501
Honolulu, HI 96817-3950

808-522-5400
800-420-6928
FAX: 808-522-5427
info@pacificil.org
www.cil-hawaii.org

Cheryl Mizusaawa, Executive Director
M.J. (Kimo) Keawe, COO & Executive Director
Our staff and Board of directors are excellent advocates with the disabled community. We will connect you with resources to make your own choices for housing, employment, and personal care and to find assistive devices and technology to improve quality of life. On both the islands of Oahu and Hawaii, we have an independent living specialist who is fluent in American sign language and is well known in the deaf community.

4042 Kauai Center for Independent Living
4340 Nawiliwili Rd.
Lihue, HI 96766-6529

808-246-4800
800-420-6928
FAX: 808-245-7218
kcil@mail.aloha.net
www.cil-hawaii.org

Laurao Tobosa, Program Coordinator
Provides a variety of support services for people with all types of disabilities.

Idaho

4043 American Falls Office: Living Independently for Everyone (LIFE)
250 S. Skyline
Idaho Falls, ID 83402-4508

208-529-8610
FAX: 208-529-6804
diane@idlife.org
www.idlife.org

Dean Nilson, Executive Director
Tina Noreen, Programs Coordinator
Mickey Palmer, Fiscal Intermediary Manager
Enables people with disabilities to manage their own lives, make their own choices, and give information and knowledge to assist in living with dignity and bravado.

4044 Dawn Enterprises
280 Cedar Street P.O.Box 388
Blackfoot, ID 83221-388

208-785-5890
FAX: 208-785-3095
dawnent.org

Donna Butler, Executive Director
Teresa Oakes, Assistant Director/Fiscal Coordi
To assist individuals of Southeastern Idaho with mental, physical or social disabilities in achieving independence through employment training, skill training, social development, or living enhancements up to each individual's maximum capability.

4045 Disability Action Center NW
505 N Main St
Moscow, ID 83843-2615

208-883-0523
800-475-0070
FAX: 208-883-0524
moscow@dacnw.org
www.dacnw.org

Larry Topp, President
Jean Coil, Vice President
Mark Leeper, CEO
Karl Johanson, Treasurer
A non-profit community partnership working to promote the independence and equality of all individuals with disabilities in all aspects of society. $45.00

4046 Disability Action Center NW: Coeur D'Alene
7560 N Government Way
Suite 1
Coeur D Alene, ID 83815- 4069

208-664-9896
800-854-9500
FAX: 208-666-1362
cda@dacnw.org
www.dacnw.org

Larry Topp, President
Jean Coil, Vice President
Mark Leeper, CEO
Karl Johanson, Treasurer
A non-profit community partnership working to promote the independence and equality of all individuals with disabilities in all aspects of society.

4047 Disability Action Center NW: Lewiston
330 5th Street
Suite A1
Lewiston, ID 83501-2086

208-746-9033
800-746-9033
FAX: 208-746-1004
lewiston@dacnw.org
www.dacnw.org

Larry Topp, President
Jean Coil, Vice President
Mark Leeper, CEO
Karl Johanson, Treasurer
A non-profit community partnership working to promote the independence and equality of all individuals with disabilities in all aspects of society.

4048 Idaho Falls Office: Living Independently for Everyone (LIFE)
250 S. Skyline
Idaho Falls, ID 83402-3702

208-529-8610
800-631-2747
FAX: 208-232-2753
diane@idlife.org
www.idlife.org

Dean Nielson, Executive Director
Tina Noreen, Programs Coordinator
Mickey Palmer, Fiscal Intermediary Manager
Enables people with disabilities to manage their own lives, make their own choices, and give information and knowledge to assist in living with dignity and bravado.

4049 LIFE: Fort Hall
1333 Moursund
Houston, TX 77019

713-520-0232
FAX: 713-520-5785
TTY:713-520-0232
ilro@ilro.org
www.ilru.org

Lex Frieden, Director
Linda CoVan, Grant Coordinator
Diego Demaya, Legal Specialist
Marisa Demaya, Training & Information Coor.
Enables people with disabilities to manage their own lives, make thier own choices, and give information and knowledge to assist in living with dignity and bravado.

4050 Living Independence Network Corporation
1878 W Overland Rd
Boise, ID 83705-3142

208-336-3335
FAX: 208-384-5037
info@lincidaho.org
lincidaho.org

Roger Howard, Executive Director
A non-profit organization empowering people with disabilities to achieve their desired level of independence.

4051 Living Independence Network Corporation: Twin Falls
1182 Eastland Dr North
Suite C
Twin Falls, ID 83301-8972

208-733-1712
FAX: 208-733-7711
info@lincidaho.org
www.lincidaho.org

Melva Heinrich, Executive Director
A non-profit organization empowering people with disabilities to achieve their desired level of independence.

4052 Living Independence Network Corporation: Caldwell
1609 Kimball Ave
Ste. 201
Caldwell, ID 83605-6965

208-454-5511
FAX: 208-454-5515
TTY:208-454-5511
info@lincidaho.org
www.lincidaho.org

Heidi Caldwell, Executive Director

A non-profit organization empowering people with disabilities to achieve their desired level of independence.

4053   Living Independent for Everyone (LIFE): Pocatello Office
640 Pershing Ave
PO Box 4185
Pocatello, ID 83201-3702

208-232-2747
800-631-2747
FAX: 208-232-2753
TTY: 208-232-2747
tracy@idlife.org
www.idlife.org

Dean Nielson, Executive Director
Mickey Palmer, Fiscal Intermediary Manager
Tina Noreen, Programs Coordinator
Enables people with disabilities to manage thier own lives, make their own choices, and give information and knowledge to assist in living with dignity and bravado.

4054   Living Independently for Everyone (LIFE): Blackfoot Office
Living Independently for Everyone (LIFE): Pocate
570 W. Pacific
P.O.Box 86
Blackfoot, ID 83221-86

208-785-9648
FAX: 208-785-2398
lori@idlife.org
www.idlife.org

Dean Nielson, Executive Director
Tina Noreen, Programs Coordinator
Mickey Palmer, Fiscal Intermediary Manager
Enable people with disabilities to manage their own lives, make their own choices, and give information and knowledge to assist in living with dignity and bravado.

4055   Living Independently for Everyone: Burley
2311 Park Ave
Suite 7
Burley, ID 83318-2170

208-678-7705
FAX: 208-678-7771
hotwheels@idlife.org
www.idlife.org

Dean Nielson, Executive Director
Mickey Palmer, Fiscal Intermediary Manager
Tina Noreen, Programs Coordinator
Enables people with disabilities to manage their own lives, make their own choices, and give information and knowledge to assist in living with dignity and bravado.

4056   Southwestern Idaho Housing Authority
1108 W Finch Dr
Nampa, ID 83651-1732

208-467-7461
FAX: 208-463-1772

David W Patten, Manager
Offers housing for rent and section/8

Illinois

4057   Access Living of Metropolitan Chicago
115 W Chicago Ave
Chicago, IL 60654-3209

312-640-2100
800-613-8549
FAX: 312-640-2101
TTY: 312-640-2102
info@accessliving.org
accessliving.org

Marca Bristo, CEO
Bhuttu Mathews, Disability Resources Coordinator
Gary Arnold, Public Relations Coordinator
Daisy Feidt, Executive Vice President
Established in 1980,access living is a change agent commited to fostering an incusive society that enables Chicagoans with disabilities to live fully engaged and self-directed lives. Nationally recognized as a leading force in the disability community. Access Living challenges stereotypes, protects civil rights, and champions social reform.

4058   Center on Deafness
3444 Dundee Rd
Northbrook, IL 60062-2258

847-559-0110
FAX: 847-559-8199
TTY:847-559-9493
centerondeafness.org
www.centerondeafness.org

Bonnie Simon, Executive Director
Donna Gomez, Residential Services/ Adult Plac
Brandi Buie, School Intake
David Wood, Coordinator
COD is dedicated to providing quality services for persons who are deaf or hard of hearing and their families, through educational, vocational, and residential services in a therapuetic, community-based environment

4059   Community Residential Alternative
Coleman Tri- County Services
22 Veterans Drive, ST. A
P.O. Box 869
Harrisburg, IL 62946-2017

618-252-0275
FAX: 618-252-2389
TTY:618-269-4211
cts.62946@frontier.com
colemantricounty.tripod.com

Samantha Austin, Executive Director
Six bed group home that provides a residential alternative for the developmentally disabled adult. This program is designed to promote independence in daily living skills, economic self-sufficiency, and integration into the community.

4060   Division of Rehabilitation Services
Department of Human Services
100 South Grand Avenue East
Springfield, IL 62762-2625

217-782-2093
800-843-6154
FAX: 217-524-2471
DHS.WebBits@illinois.gov
www.dhs.state.il.us

Carol Adams, President
Provides medical, therapeutic and counseling services for the disabled, as well as employment services.

4061   DuPage Center for Independent Living
3130 Finley Rd.
Ste. 500
Downers Grove, IL 60515-5877

630-469-2300
FAX: 630-469-2606
TTY:630-469-2300
support@aim-cil.org
www.dupagecil.org

Charles Stack, Board President
Bette Lawrence Water, Vice President
John Lausas, Treasurer
Jeff Gullang, Secretary
A non residential, community based, not for profit agency wich provides advocacy and services to persons with disabilities in DuPage County.

4062   Fite Center for Independent Living
1230 Larkin Ave
Elgin, IL 60123-6200

847-695-5818
FAX: 847-695-5892
info@fitecil.org
www.fitecil.org

Linda Bradford-Foster, Chairman, Board Treasurer
Gracia Bittner, Board Secretary
Provides services to people with disabilities in Kane, Kendall and McHenry counties. Our non-residential agency provides independent living skills training, advocacy, systemic + individual peer counseling, information and referral and housing services. Also provides technical assistance to businesses and agencies to work with people with disabilities. Locations in Elgin and Aurora. Please call for further details.

4063 Illinois Department of Rehab Services
Department of Human Services
100 South Grand Avenue East
Springfield, IL 62762-1   217-782-2093
                                           800-843-6154
                                      FAX: 217-524-2471
                          DHS.WebBits@illinois.gov
                               www.dhs.state.il.us

Carol Adams, President
Karen Perrin, Manager
The state's lead agency serving individuals with disabilities.
DRS works in partnership with people with disabilities and their
families to assist them in making informed choices to achieve full
community participation through employment, education, and
independent living opportunities.

4064 Illinois Valley Center for Independent Living
18 Gunia Dr
La Salle, IL 61301-9780   815-224-3126
                                           800-822-3246
                                      FAX: 815-224-3576
                                        ivcil@ivcil.com
                                             ivcil.com

John Hurst, President
Gary Rydleski, Vice President
Sue Faber, Secretary
Danielle Furar, Treasurer
A nonprofit service and advocacy organization that assists per-
sons with disabilities in opening doors to their independence.

4065 Illinois and Iowa Center for Independent Living
501 11th St.
PO Box 6156
Rock Island, IL 61231-6156   309-793-0090
                                           877-541-2505
                                           855-744-8918
                                      FAX: 309-793-5198
                                        iicil@iicil.com
                                           www.iicil.com

Liz Sherwin, Executive Director
Alfonso Ayew-Ew, Blind Independent Living Skill S
Eddie Williams, CommunityReintegration Advocate
Hershel Jackson, Deaf & Hard of Hearing Advocate
To create and maintain independence options for people with dis-
abilities by advocating for civil rights, providing services, and
promoting full participation of disabled individuals in all aspects
of the community.

4066 Impact Center for Independent Living
2735 E Broadway
Alton, IL 62002-1859   618-462-1411
                                           888-616-4261
                                      FAX: 618-474-5309
                                       staff@impactcil.org
                                           impactcil.org

Susy Woods, President
Judy O'Malley, Vice President
Bishop Samuel White, Treasurer
Cathy Contarino, Executive Director
Promotes pride and respect for people with disabilities by sharing
the tools that are necessary to take control of one's own life.

4067 Jacksonville Area CIL: Havana
220 W Main St
Havana, IL 62644-1138   309-543-6680
                                           877-759-2187
                                      FAX: 309-543-6711
                                        info@jacil.org
                                           www.jacil.org

Phil Foxworth, President
Mark Arnold, Vice President
Ruth Lanier, Secretary
Joe Vieira, Treasurer
Committed to enabling persons with disabilities to gain effective
control and director of their own lives in the home, in the work-
place and in the community.

4068 Jacksonville Area Center for Independent Living
15 Permac Road
Jacksonville, IL 62650-2071   217-245-8371
                                      FAX: 217-245-1872
                                      TTY:217-245-8371
                                        info@jacil.org
                                           www.jacil.org

Phil Foxworth, President
Mark Arnold, Vice President
Ruth Lanier, Secretary
Joe Vieira, Treasurer
Committed to enabling persons with disabilities to gain effective
control and direction of their own lives in the home, in the work-
place and in the community.

4069 LIFE Center for Independent Living
Ste 1
2201 Eastland Dr
Bloomington, IL 61704-7923   309-663-5433
                                           888-543-3245
                                      FAX: 309-663-7024
                                      TTY:309-663-5433
                                        gail@lifecil.org
                                           lifecil.org

Gail Kear, Executive Director
Jill Doran, Associate Director
Brianne Anderson, Office Manager
Rickielee Benecke, Disability Rights Advocate
A community-based, not-for-profit, non-residential organization
that promotes disability rights, equal access, and full community
participation for persons with disabilities.

4070 LINC-Monroe Randolph Center
Ste 4
1514 S Main St
Red Bud, IL 62278-1382   618-282-3700
                                      FAX: 618-282-2740
                                      TTY:618-282-3700

Violete Nast, Manager

4071 Lake County Center for Independent Living
377 N Seymour Ave
Mundelein, IL 60060-2322   847-949-4440
                                      FAX: 847-949-4445
                                      TTY:847-949-0641
                                       lindsey@lccil.org
                                           www.lccil.org

Kelli Brooks, Executive Director
Andy Balint, Director of Finance
Lety Cruz, Bilingual Program Assistant
Jenny Farley, Youth Leadership Advocate
Lake County Center for Independent Living is a disability rights
organization governed and staffed by a majority of people with
disabilities. LCCIL offers services and advocacy that promote a
fully accessible society, which expects participation by persons
with disabilities.

4072 Life Center for Independent Living: Pontiac
318 West Madison Street
Pontiac, IL 61764-1785   815-844-1132
                                      FAX: 815-844-1148
                                        lifecil@lifecil.org
                                           lifecil.org

Gail Kear, Executive Director
Jill Doran, Associate Director
Brianne Anderson, Office Manager
Rickielee Benecke, Disability Rights Advocate
A community-based, not-for-profit, non-residential organization
that promotes disability rights, equal access, and full community
participation for persons with disabilities.

4073 Living Independently Now Center (LINC)
120 E a St
Belleville, IL 62220-1401
618-235-9988
FAX: 618-233-3729
TTY: 618-235-9988
info@lincinc.org
www.lincinc.org

Linda Conley, President
Ron Tialdo, Vice-President
Lynn Jarman, Executive Director
Robert Rahlfs, Treasurer
Empowers persons with disabilities to live independently and to promote accessibility and inclusion in all areas.

4074 Living Independently Now Center: Sparta
Western Egyptian Building
207 West 4th Street
Waterloo, IL 62298
618-317-4028
info@lincinc.org
www.lincinc.org

Linda Conley, President
Ron Tialdo, Vice-President
Lynn Jarman, Executive Director
Robert Rahlfs, Treasurer
Empowers persons with disabilities to live independently and to promote accessibility and inclusion in all areas.

4075 Living Independently Now Center: Waterloo
Western Egyptian Building
207 West 4th Street
Waterloo, IL 62298-1336
618-317-4028
info@lincinc.org
www.lincinc.org

Linda Conley, President
Ron Tialdo, Vice-President
Lynn Jarman, Executive Director
Robert Rahlfs, Treasurer
Empowers persons with disabilities to live independently and to promote accessibility and inclusion in all areas.

4076 Mosaic: Pontiac
4980 S. 118th St.
Omaha, NE 68137
877-366-7242
FAX: 402-896-1511
www.mosaicinfo.org

Max Miller, Chairperson
James Zils, Vice Chairperson
Lisa Negstad, 2nd Vice Chairperson
Kathy Patrick, Secretary
A faith-based organization serving people with developmental disabilities.

4077 Opportunities for Access: A Center for Independent Living
4206 Williamson Pl
Suite 3
Mount Vernon, IL 62864-6705
618-244-9212
FAX: 618-244-9310
TTY: 618-244-9575
spud@ofacil.org
ofacil.org

Michael Egbert, Executive Director
Serves, trains and provides information to persons with disabilities, family members and significant others and service providers. Services include: advocacy, information and referral, peer support, skills training, volunteer programs and other related services. Services are free. A cross disability community based, non-residential, nonprofit organization serving Clay, Clinton, Edwards, Effingham, Fayette, Hamilton, Jasper, Jefferson, Marion, Wabash, Washington, Wayne and White Counties.

4078 Options Center for Independent Living: Bourbonnais
22 Heritage Dr
Suite 107
Bourbonnais, IL 60914-2510
815-936-0100
FAX: 815-936-0117
TTY: 815-936-0132
optionscil@optionscil.com
www.optionscil.org

Mark Mantarian, President
Ronald D. Smith, Vice President
Dina Raymond, Co-Secretary
Daniel Brough, Treasurer
A non-residential, not-for-profit, community-based organization that promotes independent living for people with disabilities.

4079 Options Center for Independent Living: Watseka
103 Laird Ln
Suite 103
Watseka, IL 60970
815-432-1332
FAX: 815-432-1360
TTY: 815-432-1361
optionscil@optionscil.com
www.optionscil.com

Mark Mountain, President
Ronald D. Smith, Vice President
Dina Raymond, Co-Secretary
Daniel Brough, Treasurer
A non-residential, not-for-profit, community-based organization that promotes independent living for people with disabilities.

4080 PACE Center for Independent Living
1317 E Florida Ave
Urbana, IL 61801-6007
217-344-5433
FAX: 217-344-2414
TTY: 217-344-5024
info@pacecil.org
pacecil.org

Evelyn Brown, President
Fred Neubert, Vice President
Nancy McClellan-Hickey, Executive Director
Arland Stratton, Treasurer
Promotes the full participation of people with disabilities in the rights and responsibilities of society. Provides services, which assist people with disabilities in achieving or maintaining independence.

4081 Progress Center for Independent Living
7521 Madison St
Forest Park, IL 60130-1407
708-209-1500
FAX: 708-209-1735
TTY: 708-209-1826
info@progresscil.org
www.progresscil.org

Anne Gunter, Independent Living Advocate
Kim Liddell, Independent Living Advocate
Horacio Esparza, Executive Director
Art Johnson, Home Services Team Coordinator
A community-based, non-profit, non-residential, service and advocacy organization operated for people with disabilities, by people with disabilities.

4082 Progress Center for Independent Living: Blue Island
12940 Western Ave
Blue Island, IL 60406-3766
708-388-5011
FAX: 708-388-5016
TTY: 708-389-8250
info@progresscil.org
www.progresscil.org

Horacio Esparza, Executive Director
Anne Gunter, Independent Living Advocate
Kim Liddell, Independent Living Advocate
Art Johnson, Home Services Team Coordinator
A community-based, non-profit, non residential, service and advocacy organization operated for people with disabilities, by people with disabilities.

4083　**Regional Access & Mobilization Project**
202 Market St
Rockford, IL 61107-3954
　　　　　　　　　　　815-968-7467
　　　　　　　　　　　FAX: 815-968-7612
　　　　　　　　　　　TTY:815-968-2401
　　　　　　　　　　　rampcil.org

Shari Snyder, President
Tina Kaatz, Vice President
Craig Fetty, Secretary
Sharon Wyland, Treasurer
To promote an accessible society that allows and expects full participation by people with disabilities.

4084　**Regional Access & Mobilization Project: Belvidere**
530 S State St
Suite 103
Belvidere, IL 61008-3711
　　　　　　　　　　　815-544-8404
　　　　　　　　　　　FAX: 815-544-1896
　　　　　　　　　　　TTY:815-544-8404
　　　　　　　　　　　rampcil.org

Shari Snyder, President
Tina Kaatz, Vice President
Craig Fetty, Secretary
Sharon Wyland, Treasurer
Promote an accessible society that allows and expects full participation by people with disabilities.

4085　**Regional Access & Mobilization Project: De Kalb**
115 N First Street
Dekalb, IL 60115-3055
　　　　　　　　　　　815-756-3202
　　　　　　　　　　　FAX: 815-756-3556
　　　　　　　　　　　TTY:815-756-4263
　　　　　　　　　　　rampcil.org

Shari Snyder, President
Tina Kaatz, Vice President
Craig Fetty, Secretary
Sharon Wyland, Treasurer
Promotes an accessible society that allows and expects full partiipation by persons with disabilities.

4086　**Regional Access & Mobilization Project: Freeport**
2155 W Galena Ave
Freeport, IL 61032-3013
　　　　　　　　　　　815-233-1128
　　　　　　　　　　　FAX: 815-233-0743
　　　　　　　　　　　TTY:815-233-1128
　　　　　　　　　　　rampcil.org

Shari Snyder, President
Tina Kaatz, Vice President
Craig Fetty, Secretary
Sharon Wyland, Treasurer
Promotes an accessible society that allows and expects full partiipation by persons with disabilities.

4087　**Soyland Access to Independent Living(SAIL)**
2449 E Federal Dr
Decatur, IL 62526-2160
　　　　　　　　　　　217-876-8888
　　　　　　　　　　　800-358-8080
　　　　　　　　　　　FAX: 217-876-7245
　　　　　　　　　　　TTY: 217-876-8888
　　　　　　　　　　　jwooters@decatursail.com
　　　　　　　　　　　www.decatursail.com
Jeri J Wooters, Executive Director
Betty Watkins, Rural Outreach Coordinator
A community-based, non-residential Center for Independent Living whose purpose is to promote and practice independent living for all people with disabilities.

4088　**Soyland Access to Independent Living: Charleston**
757 Windsor Rd
Charleston, IL 61920-7474
　　　　　　　　　　　217-345-7245
　　　　　　　　　　　FAX: 217-345-7226
　　　　　　　　　　　TTY:217-345-7245
　　　　　　　　　　　triplec@consolidated.net
　　　　　　　　　　　www.decatursail.com
Betty Watkins, Rural Outreach Coordinator
Jeri J Wooters, Executive Director

A community-based, non-residential Center for Independent Living whose purpose is to promote and practice independent living for all people iwth disabilities.

4089　**Soyland Access to Independent Living: Shelbyville**
1810 W.S. 3rd ST P.O.Box 650
Shelbyville, IL 62565-650
　　　　　　　　　　　217-774-4322
　　　　　　　　　　　FAX: 217-774-4368
　　　　　　　　　　　TTY:217-774-4322
　　　　　　　　　　　sailsel@consolidated.net
　　　　　　　　　　　www.decatursail.com
Jeri J Wooters, Executive Director
Betty Watkins, Rural Outreach Coordinator
A community-based, non-residential Center for Independent Living whose purpose is to promote and practice independent living for all people with disabilities.

4090　**Soyland Access to Independent Living: Sullivan**
1102 W Jackson St
Sullivan, IL 61951-1067
　　　　　　　　　　　217-728-3186
　　　　　　　　　　　FAX: 217-728-2299
　　　　　　　　　　　TTY:217-728-3186
　　　　　　　　　　　sulsail@wireless111.com
　　　　　　　　　　　www.decatursail.com
Betty Watkins, Rural Outreach Coordinator
Jeri J Wooters, Executive Director
A community-based, non-residential Center for Independent Living whose purpose is to promote and practice independent living for all people with disabilities.

4091　**Springfield Center for Independent Living**
330 South Grand Ave W
Springfield, IL 62704-3716
　　　　　　　　　　　217-523-4032
　　　　　　　　　　　800-447-4221
　　　　　　　　　　　FAX: 217-523-0427
　　　　　　　　　　　TTY: 217-523-4032
　　　　　　　　　　　scil@scil.org
　　　　　　　　　　　scil.org
Pete Roberts, Executive Director
Susan Coopers, Program Director
Denise Groesch, Reintegration Coordinator
Kathryn Cline, Business Manager
To increase opportunities for equality, integration and independence for all persons with disabilities through advocacy, services, and public education.

4092　**Stone-Hayes Center for Independent Living**
39 N Prairie St
Galesburg, IL 61401-4613
　　　　　　　　　　　309-344-1306
　　　　　　　　　　　888-347-4245
　　　　　　　　　　　FAX: 309-344-1305
　　　　　　　　　　　TTY: 309-344-1306
　　　　　　　　　　　stonehayes@misslink.net
　　　　　　　　　　　stone-hayes.org
Vanya Peterson, Executive Director
Michael Bohnenkamp, Associate Director
John Hunigan, Office Manager
Lynn Voeller, Independent Living Associate
The purpose of INCIL is to facilitate the collaboration of all Centers for Independent Living in Illinois for promoting, through the Independent Living Movement, equal opportunities and civil rights for all persons with disabilities.

4093　**West Central Illinois Center for Independent Living**
639 York St.
Suite 204
Quincy, IL 62301-1065
　　　　　　　　　　　217-223-0400
　　　　　　　　　　　FAX: 217-223-0479
　　　　　　　　　　　TTY:217-223-0475
　　　　　　　　　　　info@wcicil.org
　　　　　　　　　　　www.wcicil.org
Glenda Hackemack, Executive Director
Dale Winner, Information & Referral Coordinat
Dustin Gorde Director of Community, Jenny
Kelly Transition Co-Ordinato
A not-for-profit advocacy center funded by state and federal grants to provide services to people with disabilities.

**4094 West Central Illinois Center for Independent Living:
Macomb**
440 N Lafayette St
Macomb, IL 61455-1512

309-833-5766
FAX: 309-833-4690
TTY:217-223-0475
info@wcicil.org
www.wcicil.org

Glenda Hackemack, Executive Director
Dale Winner, Information & Referral Coordinat
Dustin Gorde Director of Community, Jenny
Kelly Transition Co-Ordinato
A not-for-profit advocacy center funded by state and federal
grants to provide services to people with disabilities.

4095 Will Grundy Center for Independent Living
2415 W Jefferson St
Suite A
Joliet, IL 60435-6464

815-729-0162
FAX: 815-729-3697
TTY:815-729-2085
pamwgcil@sbcglobal.net
will-grundycil.org

Elaine Sommer, President
Chris Boyk, Vice President
Dianne Mundle, Treasurer
Rhonda Price, Secretary
A cross-disability, community based organization that strives for
equality and empowerment of persons with disabilities in the Will
and Grundy County areas.

Indiana

**4096 Assistive Technology Training and Information Center
(ATTIC)**
1721 Washington Ave
Vincennes, IN 47591-4823

812-886-0575
877-96A-8842
FAX: 812-886-1128
inbox@atticindiana.org
www.atticindiana.org

Patricia Stewart, Executive Director
Rebecca Anderson, Assistant Director
Mark Schmitt, Fiscal Controller
Jackie Evans, Independent Living Coordinator
ATTIC provides support, information and education for individu-
als with disabilities and for families of children with special
needs, and the professionals who assist these families. All
disabilities, all ages.

4097 DAMAR Services
6067 Decatur Blvd.
Indianapolis, IN 46241

317-856-5201
FAX: 317-856-2333
info@damar.org
damar.org

Gail Shiel, Chairman
Rick Torbeck, Vice Chairman
Jim Dalton, Psy.D., HSPP, President and CEO
Richard L. Harcourt, Vice President & CFO
Builds better futures for children and adults facing life's greatest
developmental and behavioral challenges.

4098 Everybody Counts Center for Independent Living
3616 Elm St
Room 3
East Chicago, IN 46410-7097

219-229-5055
888-769-3636
FAX: 219-769-5326
TTY:219-756-3323
info@everybodycounts.org
everybodycounts.org

Teresa Torres, Executive Director
Emma Lewis Sullivan, On Loan Consultant
Mark Torres, Systems Manager
Jodi Hawn, Administrative Assistant

A nonprofit corporation dedicated to the achievement of maximum independence and enhanced quality of life for persons with
disabilities.

4099 Four Rivers Resource Services
Hwy. 59 South
P.O. Box 249
Linton, IN 47441-249

812-847-2231
FAX: 812-847-8836
fourrivers@frrs.org
frrs.org

Stephen Sacksteder, Executive Director
Robin Duncan, Chief Financial Officer
Dean Dorrell, Information Systems Director
Jessica Davis, Development Coordinator
FRRS is established to enable individuals with disabilities and
other challenges to attain self independence and natural interde-
pendence, inclusion in normal life experiences and opportunities,
and general life enrichment, by working in partnership with them,
their families and the communities in and around Greene,
Sullivan, Daviess, and Martin Counties.

4100 Future Choices Independent Living Center
309 N High St
Muncie, IN 47305-1618

765-741-8332
866-741-3444
FAX: 765-741-8333
futurechoices.org

Beth Y. Quarles, President
Provides unlimited options for minorities, youth, and Hoosiers
with disabilities.

4101 Independent Living Center of Eastern Indiana (ILCEIN)
1818 W Main St
Richmond, IN 47374-3822

765-939-9226
877-939-9226
FAX: 765-935-2215
www.ilcein.org

Jim McCormick, Executive Director
Dean Turner, Administrative Director
Ann Barnhart, Compliance Manager
Michelle Satterfield, Service Coordinator
Serving Fayette, Franklin, Henry, Decatur, Rush, Union and
Wayne Counties.

4102 Indianapolis Resource Center for Independent Living
5302 East Washington Street
Indianapolis, IN 46219

317-926-1660
866-794-7245
FAX: 317-926-1687
info@abilityindiana.org
www.abilityindiana.org

Judy Townsend, President
Dave Trulock, Vice President
Jacqueline Troy, Treasurer
Don Lane, Secretary
Provides services, support and information to people with dis-
abilities to help insure equal access to all aspects of community
life.

4103 League for the Blind and Disabled
5821 S Anthony Blvd
Fort Wayne, IN 46816-3701

260-441-0551
800-889-3443
FAX: 260-441-7760
TTY: 800-889-3443
the-league@the-league.org
the-league.org

David A. Nelson, CEO/President
Catherine Collins, Chair
Anne Palmer, Administrative Assistant
Kevin Showalter, Youth Services Coordinator
To provide and promote opportunities that empower people with
disabilities to achieve their potential.

4104 Martin Luther Homes of Indiana
Mosaic
26 N Brown Ave
Terre Haute, IN 47803-1523
812-235-3399
FAX: 812-235-1590
abean@mlhs.com

4105 Ruben Center for Independent Living
5302 East Washington Street
Indianapolis, IN 46219-3227
317-926-1660
FAX: 317-926-1687
TTY:219-397-6496
info@abilityindiana.org
www.abilityindiana.org

Judy Townsend, President
Dave Trulock, Vice President
Jacqueline Troy, Treasurer
Don Lane, Secretary
An independent living center providing support, information and education.

4106 SILC, Indiana Council on Independent Living (ICOIL)
P.O.Box 7083
Indianapolis, IN 46207-7083
317-232-1303
800-545-7763
FAX: 317-232-6478
nancy.young@fssa.in.gov
www.icoil.org

Nancy Young, Program Director
Richard Simers, SILC Chairperson

4107 Southern Indiana Center for Independent Living
1494 W. Main Street
PO Box 308
Mitchell, IN 47446-1943
812-277-9626
800-845-6914
FAX: 812-277-9628
al@sicilindiana.org
sicilindiana.org

Al Tolbert, Executive Director
Darlene Webster, Independent Living Center Direct
SICIL is a consumer controlled, community based, cross-disability, non-residential and not for profit organization that promotes and practices the philosophy of independent living: consumer control, peer support, self-help, self-determination, equal access, and individual and community advocacy. SICIL also promotes accesible and affordable housing, recreation and transportation.

4108 Wabash Independent Living Center & Learning Center (WILL)
1 Dreiser Square
Terre Haute, IN 47807
812-298-9455
877-915-9455
FAX: 812-299-9061
TTY: 877-915-9455
info@thewillcenter.org
www.thewillcenter.org

Don Rogers, Chairman
Jody Pomfret, Vice Chairman
Kevin Burke, Treasurer
Peter Ciancone, Secretary-Executive Director
To empower people with disabilities to ensure that they have full and complete access to community resources to promote their independence

Iowa

4109 Black Hawk Center for Independent Living
2800 Falls Ave.
P.O. Box 2275
Waterloo, IA 50701-2275
319-291-7755
888-291-7754
FAX: 319-291-7781
TTY:800-735-2942
blackhawkcenter.org

4110 Central Iowa Center for Independent Living
655 Walnut St
Suite 131
Des Moines, IA 50309-3930
515-243-1742
888-503-2287
FAX: 515-243-5385
ctoman@centraliowacil.com
www.centraliowacil.com

Bob Jeppesen, Executive Director
Frank Strong, Associate Director
Crystal Toman, Office Coordinator
Dee Howard, Independent Living Specialist
CICIL is a community based, non-profit, non-residential program serving persons with disabilities. CICIL assists all persons, regardless of disability in making choices about their own lives and in experiencing success in achieving independence.

4111 Evert Conner Rights & Resources CIL
730 S Dubuque St
Iowa City, IA 52240-4202
319-338-3870
800-982-0272
FAX: 319-354-1799
info@ownersvoices.com
www.ownersvoices.com

Scott Gill, Executive Director
Provides community services like disability awareness training and classroom presentations. Individual services include independent living skills training and peer counseling. All services are custom designed to support the independence of people with disabilities in their own community.

4112 Hope Haven
1800 19th St
PO Box 70
Rock Valley, IA 51247-1098
712-476-2737
FAX: 712-476-3110
hopehaven.org

Dr. Kent Eric Eknes, President
Ron Boote, Vice President
David Vanningen, Executive Director
Calvin Helmus, Chief Operating Officer
Unleashes the potential in people through work and life skills so that they may enjoy a productive life in their community.

4113 League of Human Dignity, Center for Independent Living
1520 Avenue M
Council Bluffs, IA 51501-1185
712-323-6863
FAX: 712-323-6811
Cinfo@leagueofhumandignity.com
www.leagueofhumandignity.com
Carrie England, Director
League of Human Dignity actively promotes the full integration of individuals with disabilities into society. To this end, the League will advocate their needs and rights, and provide quality services to involve these persons in becoming and remaining independent citizens.

4114 Martin Luther Homes of Iowa
P.O. Box 2316
Princeton, NJ 08543-2316
877-843-7953
FAX: 563-568-3992
www.rwjf.org

Mary Lynn ReVoir, Project Director
Fred Naumann III, Communications
Richard Wicks, Executive Director

4115 South Central Iowa Center for Independent Living
117 1st Ave W
Oskaloosa, IA 52577-3243
641-672-1867
800-651-7911
FAX: 641-672-1867
brookie43@gmail.com
www.iowasilc.org/cilinfo.html

Deb Philpot, Executive Director

Provides services, support, information and referral to people with disabilities to help insure equal access to all aspects of community life.

4116 Three Rivers Center for Independent Living
900 Rebecca Avenue
Pittsburgh, PA 15221-2938

412-371-7700
800-633-4588
FAX: 412-371-9430
TTY: 412-371-6230
lgray@trcil.org
trcil.myfastsite.net

Stanley A. Holbrook, President & Executive Director
Lisa Wilson, HR Program Manager
Rachel Rogan, Director of Waiver Services
Charles Keenan, TRCIL Real Properties Board
Providing a wide array of services to assist individuals and families in achieving positive life goals.

Kansas

4117 Advocates for Better Living For Everyone(A.B.L.E.)
Ste C
521 Commercial St
Atchison, KS 66002

913-367-1830
888-845-2879
FAX: 913-367-1830
www.ableks.org

Ken Gifford, President & CEO
A not for profit agency providing services within the State of Kansas. ABLE looks to assist people with disabilities as well as any other member of the community to live an integrated, quality life with dignity, respect, and independence.

4118 Center for Independent Living SW Kansas: Liberal
1023 N Kansas Ave
Suite 2
Liberal, KS 67901-2655

620-624-5500
800-327-4048
FAX: 620-624-6576
TTY: 620-624-5500
www.cilswks.org

Victor Otero, Manager
Crystal Tharp, Independent Living Advocate
Dedicated to helping people achieve full participation in society.

4119 Center for Independent Living Southwest Kansas
P.O.Box 2090
Garden City, KS 67846-2090

620-276-1900
800-736-9443
FAX: 620-271-0200
info@cilswks.org
www.cilswks.org

Troy Horton, Executive Director
Dedicated to helping people achieve full participation in society.

4120 Center for Independent Living Southwest Kansas: Dodge City
2601 Central Ave
Dodge City, KS 67801-6200

620-227-6660
800-326-1366
FAX: 620-227-8185
TTY: 620-227-6660
www.cilswks.org

Mary Jane Sandoval, Independent Living Advocate
Dedicated to helping people achieve full participation in society

4121 Coalition for Independence
4911 State Ave
Kansas City, KS 66102-1749

913-321-5140
866-201-3829
FAX: 913-321-5182
TTY: 913-321-5216
cfi-kc.org

Clarence Smith, Executive Director
Laarni Sison, Executive Assistant
Claire Marr, Lead Independent Living Speciali
Shauna Garrett, Lead Accountant
Facilitates positive and responsible independence for all people with disabilities by acting as an advocate for individuals with disabilities, providing services, and promoting accessibility and acceptance.

4122 Cowley County Developmental Services
P.O.Box 618
Arkansas City, KS 67005-618

620-442-5270
866-442-5270
FAX: 620-442-5623
www.ccds-cddo.org

Bill Brooks, Executive Director
Provides services for persons with developmental disabilities in Cowley County..

4123 Independence
2001 Haskell Ave
Lawrence, KS 66046-3249

785-841-0333
888-824-7277
FAX: 785-841-1094
comment@independenceinc.org
independenceinc.org

Karen McGrath, President
Bruce Passman, Vice President
Sandra London, Lieb
Athena Johnson, Secretary
Provides advocacy, services, and education for people with disabilities and our communities.

4124 Independent Connection
1710 W. Schilling Road
P.O.Box 1160
Salina, KS 67402- 1160

785-827-9383
800-526-9731
FAX: 785-823-2015
TTY: 785-827-9383
www.occk.com

Shelia Nelson-Stout, President/CEO
Deanna L. Lamer, Senior Director,Human Resources
Tasha Suppes, Human Resources Coordinator
Dedicated to helping people with physical or mental disabilities remove barriers to employment, independent living, and full participation in their communities.

4125 Independent Connection: Abilene
Suite 221
300 N. Cedar St.
Abilene, KS 67410

785-263-2208
FAX: 785-263-3795
TTY:785-263-2208
www.occk.com

Shelia Nelson-Stout, President/CEO
Deanna L. Lamer, Senior Director,Human Resources
Tasha Suppes, Human Resources Coordinator
Dedicated to helping people with physical or mental disabilities remove barriers to employment, independent living, and full participation in their communities.

4126 Independent Connection: Beloit
501 W 7th St
Beloit, KS 67420-2107

785-738-5423
FAX: 785-738-3320
TTY:785-738-5423
www.occk.com

Shelia Nelson-Stout, President/CEO
Deanna L. Lamer, Senior Director,Human Resources
Tasha Suppes, Human Resources Coordinator

Dedicated to helping people with physical or mental disabilities remove barriers to employment, independent living, and full participation in their communities.

4127 Independent Connection: Concordia
1502 Lincoln St
Concordia, KS 66901-4830

785-243-1977
FAX: 785-243-4524
TTY:785-243-1977
www.occk.com

Shelia Nelson-Stout, President/CEO

Dedicated to helping people with physical or mental disabilities remove barriers to employment, independent living, and full participation in their communities.

4128 Independent Living Resource Center
3033 W 2nd St N
Wichita, KS 67203-5357

316-942-6300
800-479-6861
FAX: 316-942-2078
ilrcks.org

Jean Shuler, President
Angie Schmidt, Vice Chairman
Derrick Prichard, Secretary/Treasurer
James Thayer, Board Member

Empower people with disabilities to lead independent lives by providing advocacy, education and direct services. Serve people with all types of disabilities; permanent or temporary, physical disabilities, mental disabilities, and developmental disabilities.

4129 Kansas Services for the Blind & Visually Impaired
2601 SW East Circle Dr N
Topeka, KS 66606-2445

785-296-3738
800-547-5789
FAX: 785-291-3138
rehab@srskansas.org
srskansas.org

Dennis Ford, Manager
Michael Donnelly, Director

Helps persons who are blind or visually to improve their quality of life. KSBVI provides people with an array of services and experiences aimed at overcoming not only the physical difficulties brought on by the loss of vision, but also the fear of change associated with vision loss. KSBVI can also help with job search and retention activities; life skills training; access to medical services; and technical assistance..

4130 LINK: Colby
505 N Franklin Ave
Suite G
Colby, KS 67701-2342

785-462-7600
800-736-9418
TTY:785-462-7600
brianatwell@linkinc.org
www.linkinc.org

Brian Atwell, Executive Director

Promotes and supports the civil rights of people with disabilities and empowers them to achieve a life of independence and equality..

4131 Living Independently in Northwest Kansas: Hays
2401 E 13th St
Hays, KS 67601-2663

785-625-6942
800-596-5926
FAX: 785-625-2334
TTY: 785-625-6942
brianatwell@linkinc.org
www.linkinc.org

Brian Atwell, Executive Director

Promotes and supports the civil rights of people with disabilities and empowers them to achieve a life of independence and equality.

4132 Prairie IL Resource Center
103 W 2nd St
Pratt, KS 67124-2644

620-672-9600
FAX: 620-672-9601
info@pilr.org
www.pilr.org

Dave Mullins, President
Stephanie Guthrie, Vice President
Chris Owens, Executive Director
Roger Frischenmeyer, Independent Living Specialist

To achieve the full inclusion and acceptance of people with disabilities through education and advocacy

4133 Prairie Independent Living Resource Center
17th S Main St
Hutchinson, KS 67501

620-663-3989
888-715-6818
FAX: 620-663-4711
TTY:620-663-9920
info@pilr.org
www.pilr.org

Dave Mullins, President
Stephanie Guthrie, Vice President
Chris Owens, Executive Director
Roger Frischenmeyer, Independent Living Specialist

To achieve the full conclusion and acceptance of people with disabilities through education and advocacy

4134 Resource Center for Independent Living
104 S. Washington Ave.
Iola, KS 66749-8805

620-365-8144
877-944-8144
FAX: 620-365-7726
rcilinc.org

Chad Wilkins, Executive Director

Committed to working with individuals, families, and communities to promote independent living and individual choice to persons with disabilities.

4135 Resource Center for Independent Living, Inc. (RCIL)
409 Columbia St.
Utica, NY 13503-210

315-797-4642
800-580-7245
FAX: 315-797-4747
TTY: 315-797-5837
rcilinc.org

Chad Wilkins, Executive Director

Committed to working with individuals, families, and communities to promote independent living and individual choice to persons with disabilities. As a center for independent living in Kansas, we provide advocacy, peer counseling, information and referral, independent living skills training and deinstitutionalization. In addition to these services, we also provide HOBS payroll services and a variety of programs benefiting individuals with disabilities.

4136 Resource Center for Independent Living: Emporia
215 West Sixth Avenue
Suite 202
Emporia, KS 66801-2886

620-342-1648
888-261-4024
FAX: 620-342-1821
info@rcilinc.org
rcilinc.org

Deone Wilson, Executive Director
Beth Combes, Information & Outreach Coordinat
Amy Richardson, Targeted Case Manager
Trevor Larson, Office Assistant

Committed to working with individuals, families, and communities to promote independent living and individual choice to persons with disabilities.

4137 Resource Center for Independent Living: Arkansas City
P.O. Box 257
1137 Laing
Osage City, KS 66523 785-528-3105
800-580-7245
FAX: 785-528-3665
TTY: 785-528-3106
info@rcilinc.org
rcilinc.org

Deone Wilson, Executive Director
Tania Harrington, Director of Quality Assurance
Adam Burnett, Director of Core Services
Mike Pitts, Finance Committee Chairperson
Committed to working with individuals, families, and communities to promote independent living and individual choice to persons with disabilities.

4138 Resource Center for Independent Living: Burlington
P.O. Box 257
1137 Laing
Osage City, KS 66523 785-528-3105
800-580-7245
FAX: 785-528-3665
TTY: 785-528-3106
info@rcilinc.org
rcilinc.org

Deone Wilson, Executive Director
Tania Harrington, Director of Quality Assurance
Adam Burnett, Director of Core Services
Mike Pitts, Finance Committee Chairperson
Committed to working with individuals, families, and communities to promote independent living and individual choice to persons with disabilities.

4139 Resource Center for Independent Living: Coffeyville
P.O. Box 257
1137 Laing
Osage City, KS 66523 785-528-3105
800-580-7245
FAX: 785-528-3665
TTY: 785-528-3106
info@rcilinc.org
rcilinc.org

Deone Wilson, Executive Director
Tania Harrington, Director of Quality Assurance
Adam Burnett, Director of Core Services
Mike Pitts, Finance Committee Chairperson
Committed to working with individuals, families, and communities to promote independent living and individual choice to persons with disabilities.

4140 Resource Center for Independent Living: El Dorado
615 1/2 N Main St
El Dorado, KS 67042-2027 316-322-7853
800-960-7853
FAX: 316-322-7888
info@rcilinc.org
rcilinc.org

Macy Gaines, Independent Living Specialist
Doris Hammons, Targeted Case Manager
Shirley Mullin, Targeted Case Manager
Barbara Ehret, Office Assistant
Committed to working with individuals, families, and communities to promote independent living and individual choice to persons with disabilities.

4141 Resource Center for Independent Living: Ft Scott
P.O. Box 257
1137 Laing
Osage City, KS 66523 785-528-3105
800-580-7245
FAX: 785-528-3665
TTY: 785-528-3106
info@rcilinc.org
rcilinc.org

Deone Wilson, Executive Director
Tania Harrington, Director of Quality Assurance
Adam Burnett, Director of Core Services
Mike Pitts, Finance Committee Chairperson
Committed to working with individuals, families, and communities to promote independent living and individual choice to persons with disabilities.

4142 Resource Center for Independent Living: Ottawa
233 W 23rd Street
Ottawa, KS 66067-3533 785-242-1805
800-995-1805
FAX: 785-242-1448
rcilinc.org

Chad Wilkins, Executive Director
Committed to working with individuals, families, and communities to promote independent living and individual choice to persons with disabilities.

4143 Resource Center for Independent Living: Overland Park
Ste 100
10200 W 75th St
Shawnee Mission, KS 66204-2242 913-362-6618
877-439-2847
FAX: 913-677-2742
rcilinc.org

Chad Wilkins, Executive Director
RCIL is committed to working with individuals, families, and communities to promote independent living and individual choice to persons with disabilities.

4144 Resource Center for Independent Living: Topeka
1507 S.W. 21stStreet
Suite 203
Topeka, KS 66604-2356 785-267-1717
877-719-1717
FAX: 785-267-1711
info@rcilinc.org
rcilinc.org

Rosie Cooper, Director of Independent Living S
Stuart Jones, Assistive Technology Specialist
Mikel McCary, Assistive Technology Specialist
Mandy Smith, Finance Committee Chairperson
Committed to working with individuals, families, and communities to promote independent living and individual choice to persons with disabilities.

4145 Southeast Kansas Independent Living (SKIL)
1801 Main
P.O. Box 957
Parsons, KS 67357-957 620-421-5502
800-688-5616
FAX: 620-421-3705
TTY: 620-421-0983
skil@skilonline.com
www.skilonline.com

Nancy Varner, Chairman
Janet Spillman, Vice Chairman
Shari Coatney, CEO/President
Olivia Lyons, Secretary/Treasurer
To empower, integrate and maximize independence for all persons with disabilities.

4146   Southeast Kansas Independent Living: Independence
107 East Main
P.O.Box 944
Independence, KS 67301-944   620-331-1006
                                    866-927-1006
                                    FAX: 620-331-1257
                                    TTY: 620-331-1006
                                    skilindy@skilonline.com
                                    www.skilonline.com

Nancy Varner, Chairman
Janet Spillman, Vice Chairman
Shari Coatney, CEO/President
Olivia Lyons, Secretary/Treasurer
To empower, integrate and maximize independence for all persons with disabilities.

4147   Southeast Kansas Independent Living: Chanute
2 W. Main
P.O.Box 645
Chanute, KS 66720-645   620-431-0757
                                    866-927-0757
                                    FAX: 620-431-7274
                                    TTY: 620-431-0757
                                    skilchanute@skilonline.com
                                    www.skilonline.com

Nancy Varner, Chairman
Janet Spillman, Vice Chairman
Shari Coatney, CEO/President
Olivia Lyons, Secretary/Treasurer
To empower, integrate and maximize independence for all persons with disabilities.

4148   Southeast Kansas Independent Living: Columbus
123 N. Kansas
P.O. Box 478
Columbus, KS 66725-1801   620-429-3600
                                    866-927-3600
                                    FAX: 620-429-1027
                                    skilcolumbus@skilonline.com
                                    www.skilonline.com

Nancy Varner, Chairman
Janet Spillman, Vice Chairman
Shari Coatney, CEO/President
Olivia Lyons, Secretary/Treasurer
To empower, integrate and maximize independence for all persons with disabilities.

4149   Southeast Kansas Independent Living: Fredonia
623 Monroe
P.O.Box 448
Fredonia, KS 66736-448   620-378-4881
                                    866-927-4881
                                    FAX: 620-378-4851
                                    TTY: 620-378-4881
                                    skilfredonia@skilonline.com
                                    www.skilonline.com

Nancy Varner, Chairman
Janet Spillman, Vice Chairman
Shari Coatney, CEO/President
Olivia Lyons, Secretary/Treasurer
To empower, integrate and maximize independence for all persons with disabilities.

4150   Southeast Kansas Independent Living: Hays
510 W. 29thStreet, Suite A
PO Box 366
Hays, KS 67601-366   785-628-8019
                                    800-316-8019
                                    FAX: 785-628-3116
                                    TTY: 785-628-3128
                                    skilhays@skilonline.com
                                    www.skilonline.com

Nancy Varner, Chairman
Janet Spillman, Vice Chairman
Shari Coatney, CEO/President
Olivia Lyons, Secretary/Treasurer
To empower, integrate and maximize independence for all persons with disabilities.

4151   Southeast Kansas Independent Living: Pittsburg
1403 N. Broadway
P.O.Box 1706
Pittsburg, KS 66762-1706   620-231-6780
                                    866-927-6780
                                    FAX: 620-232-9915
                                    TTY: 620-231-6780
                                    skilpittsburg@skilonline.com
                                    www.skilonline.com

Nancy Varner, Chairman
Janet Spillman, Vice Chairman
Shari Coatney, CEO/President
Olivia Lyons, Secretary/Treasurer
To empower, integrate and maximize independence for all persons with disabilities.

4152   Southeast Kansas Independent Living: Sedan
113 West Main
P.O.Box 340
Sedan, KS 67361-340   620-725-3990
                                    866-906-3990
                                    FAX: 620-725-3942
                                    TTY: 620-725-3990
                                    skilsedan@skilonline.com
                                    www.skilonline.com

Nancy Varner, Chairman
Janet Spillman, Vice Chairman
Shari Coatney, CEO/President
Olivia Lyons, Secretary/Treasurer
To empower, integrate and maximize independence for all persons with disabilities.

4153   Southeast Kansas Independent Living: Yates Center
119 W. Butler
P.O.Box 129
Yates Center, KS 66783-129   620-625-2818
                                    866-927-2818
                                    FAX: 620-625-2585
                                    skilyc@skilonline.com
                                    www.skilonline.com

Nancy Varner, Chairman
Janet Spillman, Vice Chairman
Shari Coatney, CEO/President
Olivia Lyons, Secretary/Treasurer
To empower, integrate and maximize independence for all persons with disabilities.

4154   Three Rivers Independent Living Center
504 Miller Drive
P.O.Box 408
Wamego, KS 66547-0408   785-456-9915
                                    800-555-3994
                                    FAX: 785-456-9923
                                    TTY: 785-456-9915
                                    reception@threeriversinc.org
                                    www.threeriversinc.org

Audrey Schremmer-Philips, Executive Director
Keyna Steinbrock, IL Specialist
Erica Christie, Director of Supports & Services
Rebel Eichelberger, Senior Accountant
A nonprofit organization promoting the self reliance of individuals with disabilities through education, advocacy, training and support.

4155   Three Rivers Independent Living Center: Clay
719 5th Street
P.O.Box 33
Clay Center, KS 67432-0033   785-632-6117
                                    FAX: 785-632-6117
                                    TTY:785-632-6117
                                    reception@threeriversinc.org
                                    www.threeriversinc.org

Audrey Schremmer-Philips, Executive Director
Keyna Steinbrock, IL Specialist
Erica Christie, Director of Supports & Services
Rebel Eichelberger, Senior Accountant

A non-profit organization promoting the self reliance of individuals with disabilities through, education, advocacy, training and support.

4156   Three Rivers Independent Living Center: Manhattan
401 Houston St.
Manhattan, KS 66502   785-776-9294
                                                800-432-2703
                                           FAX: 785-776-9479
                                 reception@threeriversinc.org
                                         www.threeriversinc.org

Audrey Schremmer-Philips, Executive Director
Keyna Steinbrock, IL Specialist
Erica Christie, Director of Supports & Services
Rebel Eichelberger, Senior Accountant
A non profit organization promoting the self reliance of individuals with disabilities through education, advocacy, training and support.

4157   Three Rivers Independent Living Center: Seneca
416 Main St
Seneca, KS 66538-1926   785-336-0222
                                           FAX: 785-336-0288
                                 reception@threeriversinc.org
                                         www.threeriversinc.org

Audrey Schremmer-Philips, Executive Director
Keyna Steinbrock, IL Specialist
Erica Christie, Director of Supports & Services
Rebel Eichelberger, Senior Accountant
A non profit organization promoting the self reliance of individuals with disabilities through education, advocacy, training and support.

4158   Three Rivers Independent Living Center: Topeka
P.O.Box 4152
Topeka, KS 66604-4152   785-273-0249
                                           FAX: 785-273-0249
                                 reception@threeriversinc.org
                                         www.threeriversinc.org

Audrey Schremmer-Philips, Executive Director
Keyna Steinbrock, IL Specialist
Erica Christie, Director of Supports & Services
Rebel Eichelberger, Senior Accountant
A non profit organization promoting the self reliance of individuals with disabilities through education, advocacy, training and support.

4159   Topeka Independent Living Resource Center
501 SW Jackson St
Suite 100
Topeka, KS 66603-3300   785-233-4572
                                           FAX: 785-233-1561
                                           TTY:785-233-4572
                                              tilrcweb@tilrc.org
                                                     tilrc.org

Mike Oxford, Executive Director
Evan Korynta, Operations Manager
Angie Harter, Independent Living Advocacy Staf
Carol Doss, Independent Living Advocacy Staf
A civil and human rights organization that advocates for justice, equality and essential services for a fully integrated and accessible society for all people with disabilities.

4160   Whole Person: Nortonville
7301 Mission Road
Suite 135
Prairie Village, KS 66208- 3006   913-262-1294
                                                877-767-8896
                                           FAX: 913-262-2392
                                     info@thewholeperson.org
                                         www.thewholeperson.org

Rick O'Neal, President
Jim Atwater, Vice President
MIchelle Ford, Secretary
Timothy L. Urban, Treasurer
Assists people with disabilities to live independently and encourages change within the community to expand opportunities for independent living.

4161   Whole Person: Nortonville, The
7301 Mission Road
Suite 135
Prairie Village, KS 66208- 3006   913-262-1294
                                                877-767-8896
                                           FAX: 913-262-2392
                                     info@thewholeperson.org
                                         www.thewholeperson.org

Rick O'Neal, President
Jim Atwater, Vice President
MIchelle Ford, Secretary
Timothy L. Urban, Treasurer
Assists people with disabilities to live independently and encourages change within the community to expand opportunities for independent living.

4162   Whole Person: Prairie Village
7301 Mission Rd
Prairie Village, KS 66208-3006   913-262-1294
                                           FAX: 913-262-2392
                                     info@thewholeperson.org
                                         www.thewholeperson.org

Rick O'Neal, President
Jim Atwater, Vice President
MIchelle Ford, Secretary
Timothy L. Urban, Treasurer
Assists people with disabilities to live independently and encourages change within the community to expand opportunities for independent living.

4163   Whole Person: Prairie Village, The
7301 Mission Road
Suite 135
Prairie Village, KS 66208- 3006   913-262-1294
                                                877-767-8896
                                           FAX: 913-262-2392
                                     info@thewholeperson.org
                                         www.thewholeperson.org

Rick O'Neal, President
Jim Atwater, Vice President
MIchelle Ford, Secretary
Timothy L. Urban, Treasurer
Assists people with disabilities to live independently and encourages change within the community to expand opportunities for independent living.

4164   Whole Person: Tonganoxie
7301 Mission Road
Suite 135
Prairie Village, KS 66208- 3006   913-262-1294
                                                877-767-8896
                                           FAX: 913-262-2392
                                     info@thewholeperson.org
                                         www.thewholeperson.org

Rick O'Neal, President
Jim Atwater, Vice President
MIchelle Ford, Secretary
Timothy L. Urban, Treasurer
Assists people with disabilities to live independently and encourages change within the community to expand opportunities for independent living.

Kentucky

4165 Center for Accessible Living
501 S. 2nd Street
Ste 200
Louisville, KY 40202-2121
502-589-6620
888-813-8497
FAX: 502-589-3980
TTY:502-589-6690
info@calky.org
www.calky.org

Jan Day, CEO
Michael Markiewicz, Chief Financial Officer
Jeanne M. Gallimore, Branch Director
Susan Tharpe, Coordinator of Services
To assist the individuals with disabilities who seek to live independently.

4166 Center for Accessible Living: Murray
1051 N 16th St
Suite C
Murray, KY 42071-8511
270-753-7676
888-261-6194
FAX: 270-753-7729
TTY:270-767-0549
info@calky.org
www.calky.org

Jeanne M. Gallimore, Branch Director
Susan Tharpe, Coordinator of Services
Jan Day, CEO
Michael Markiewicz, Chief Financial Officer
To assist the individuals with disabilities who seek to live independently.

4167 Center for Independent Living: Kentucky Department for the Blind
Independent Living Office
Rear
409 N Miles St
Elizabethtown, KY 42701-1834
270-766-5126
buel.stalls@mail.state.ky.us
Buel E Stalls Jr, Office Manager and IL Specialist
Nancy Bachuss, Manager
Offers peer counseling, attendant care registry and other services to the community as they relate to the blind community. The Murray office is an independent living regional office which covers 20 far western counties of Kentucky..

4168 Disability Coalition of Northern Kentucky
Ste 219
525 W 5th St
Covington, KY 41011-1293
859-431-7668
FAX: 859-431-7688
TTY:800-648-6057
dcnky@fuse.net

Kitt Heeg, Executive Director
Empowering people with disabilities through education, networking, and positive attitudes..

4169 Disability Resource Initiative
624 Eastwood St
Bowling Green, KY 42103-1602
270-796-5992
877-437-5045
FAX: 270-796-6630
www.dri-ky.org

Marilyn Mitchell, Executive Director
Tracy Cole, Independent Living Specialist
Steve Burchett, IT Specialist
Jenny McCallister, Administrative Assistant
One of the most important premises in Independent Living is that people with disabilities are the most knowledgable about their own needs. Because of this all of their services are designed to be consumer-driven. Within each service, Center Staff work with both participant and provider to achieve and maintain an Independent Lifestyle.

4170 Independence Place
1093 S. Broadway
Suite 1218
Lexington, KY 40504-1787
859-266-2807
877-266-2807
FAX: 859-335-0627
TTY: 800-648-6056
info@independenceplaceky.org
www.independenceplaceky.org

Michael Fein, Chairman
Carla Webster, Vice Chairwoman
Pamela Roark-Glisson, Executive Director
Orissa Mason, Consumer Services Coordinator
To assist people with disabilities to achieve their full potential for community inclusion through improving access, choice and equal opportunity.

4171 Pathfinders for Independent Living
105 E Mound St
Harlan, KY 40831-2355
606-573-5777
877-340-PATH
FAX: 606-573-5739
TTY: 606-573-5777
www.pahtfindersilc.org

Sandra Goodwyn, Executive Director
Andrew Saylor, Director of IT (Internal) and Fi
Stacy Marple, Director of IT (External)
Ron Walker, Public Affairs Specialist
They publish a newsletter called LifeLine 4-5 times a year. Most articles are written by Sandra Goodwyn. Editor is Andrew Saylor. Serves people with disabilities to maintain as much independence as they desire

4172 SILC Department of Vocational Rehabilitation
209 Saint Clair St
Frankfort, KY 40601-1817
502-564-4440
800-372-7172
FAX: 502-564-6745
sarahf.richardson@ky.gov
www.ovr.ky.org

Sarah Richardson, SILC Liaison
We recognize and respect the contributions of all individuals as a necessary and vital part of a productive society..

Louisiana

4173 New Horizons: Central Louisiana
Ste 18
2406 Ferrand St
Monroe, LA 71201-3236
318-323-4374
800-428-5505
FAX: 318-323-5445
nhilc@nhilc.org
www.nhilc.org

Alan Loosley, President
Sharon Geddes, Vice-President
Clint Snell, Vice-President for Finance
Mary Russell, Secretary
A private, non-profit, non-residential, consumer-controlled, community-based organization that enables people with disabilities to live independently.

4174 New Horizons: Northeast Louisiana
3717 Government Street
Suite 7
Alexandria, LA 71301-4037
318-484-3596
888-361-3596
FAX: 318-484-3640
nhilc@nhilc.org
www.nhilc.org

Alan Loosley, President
Sharon Geddes, Vice-President
Clint Snell, Vice-President for Finance
Mary Russell, Secretary

A private, non-profit, non-residential, consumer controlled, community based organization that enables people with disabilities to live independently.

4175 New Horizons: Northwest Louisiana
1111A Hawn Avenue
Shreveport, LA 71106-6144

318-671-8131
877-219-7327
FAX: 318-688-7823
nhilc@nhilc.org
www.nhilc.org

Alan Loosley, President
Sharon Geddes, Vice-President
Clint Snell, Vice-President for Finance
Mary Russell, Secretary
A private, non-profit, non-residential, consumer-controlled, community based organization that enables people with disabilities to live independently.

4176 Resources for Independent Living: Baton Rouge
New Orleans Resources for Independent Living
3233 South Sherwood Forest Blvd.
Suite 101A
Baton Rouge, LA 70816

225-753-4772
877-505-2260
FAX: 225-753-4831
contact@noril.org
www.noril.org

Yavonka G. Archaga, Executive Director
Alisha S. Hammond, Assistant Director
Rosie Calvin, Program Manager
Deonne T. Bailey, Core Service Manager
RIL provides quality services to individuals with disabilities to assist with living independent. RIL also offers services to inculde information and referral, advocacy, peer support and independent living skills training.

4177 Resources for Independent Living: Metairie
2001 21st Street Kenner
Kenner, LA 70062

504-522-1955
877-505-2260
FAX: 504-522-1954
contact@noril.org
www.noril.org

Yavonka G. Archaga, Executive Director
Alisha S. Hammond, Assistant Director
Rosie Calvin, Program Manager
Deonne T. Bailey, Core Service Manager
RIL provides quality services to individuals with disabilities to assist with living independently. RIL also offers an array of services to include information and referral, advocacy, peer support and independent living skills training.

4178 Southwest Louisiana Independence Center: Lake Charles
2016 Oak Park Boulevard
Lake Charles, LA 70601-5391

337-477-7198
888-403-1062
FAX: 337-477-7198
TTY: 337-477-7198
www.slic-la.org

4179 Southwest Louisians Independence Center: Lafayette
850 Kaliste Saloom Rd
Suite 118
Lafayette, LA 70508-4230

337-269-0027
888-516-5009
FAX: 337-233-7660
www.slic-la.org

4180 Volunteers of America of Greater New Orleans
4152 Canal St.
New Orleans, LA 70119

504-482-2130
FAX: 504-482-1922
voagno.org

Robert C. Rhoden, Chair
Wayne M. Baquet, Chair Elect
James M. Le Blanc, President/CEO
Geoffrey C. Artigues, Treasurer

Volunteers of America Greater New Orleans offers many services that aim to improve the lives of children, youth, and families.

4181 W Troy Cole Independent Living Specialist
Ste H
1900 Lamy Ln
Monroe, LA 71201-9200

318-323-4374

Katherine Carnell, Manager
.

Maine

4182 Alpha One: Bangar
3300 Ponce de Leon Blvd.
Coral Gables, FL 33134

305-567-9888
877-228-7321
FAX: 305-567-1317
info@alpha-1foundation.org
www.alpha1.org

John W. Walsh, President & CEO, Co-founder
Marcia F. Ritchie, Vice President/ COO
Marsha A. Carnes, Director of Program Evaluation
Robert Campbell, Communications Manager
Committed to being a leading enterprise providing the community with information, services and products that create opportunities for people with disabilities to live independently. Provides many services including adaptive and mobility equipment selection, peer support, advocacy, information and referral services, adapted drive evaluation and training, and consumer directed personal assistance.

4183 Alpha One: South Portland
127 Main St
South Portland, ME 04106-2647

207-767-2189
800-640-7200
FAX: 207-799-8346
TTY: 207-767-5387
www.alphaonenow.com

Dennis Stubbs, Chairman
Bob McPhee, Vice-Chairman
Darlene Stewart, Independent Living Specialist
Ketra S Crosson, Aroostook County Coordinator
Committed to being a leading enterprise providing the community with information, services and products that create opportunities for people with disabilities to live independently. Offers adaptive equipment loan program, independent living skills instruction, adapted driver evaluation and training, information and referral services, peer support, advocacy, access design consultation, and more.

4184 Motivational Services
71 Hospital Street
P.O.Box 229
Augusta, ME 04332-0229

207-626-3465
FAX: 207-626-3469
TTY: 207-621-2542
information@mocomaine.com.
www.mocomaine.com

Connie Dunn, President
Grace Leonard, Vice President/Secretary
Faith Madore, Treasurer
Richard Weiss, Executive Director
Improving the lives of people with disabilities through housing, employment and community support.

4185 Shalom House
106 Gilman St
Portland, ME 04102-3034
207-874-1080
FAX: 207-874-1077
TTY: 207-842-6888
generalmail@shalomhouseinc.org
shalomhouseinc.org

Megan Lewis, Human Resources Manager
Mary Haynes-Rodgers, Executive Director
Kristine Lausier, Quality Assurance Administrator
Jane Collette, Accounting Manager
Offers hope for adults living with severe mental illness by providing a choice of quality housing and support services that help people lead stable and fulfilling lives in the community.

Maryland

4186 Broadmead
13801 York Rd
Cockeysville, MD 21030-1899
410-527-1900
877-STA-HOME
www.broadmead.org

Ann H. Heaton, Chair
John E. Howl, Chief Executive Officer
Patricia Gordon, Chief Financial Officer/Treasure
Douglas Bareis, Director of Support Services
To provide continuing care services to a diverse group of seniors in a warm, congenial community founded and operated in the spirit of the Religious Society of Friends.

4187 Eastern Shore Center for Independent Living
309 Sunburst Highway
Suite 13
Cambridge, MD 21613-2050
410-221-7701
800-705-7944
FAX: 410-221-7714
TTY: 410-221-4150
escil@escil.org
www.autismspeaks.org

Liz Feld, President
Alec M. Elbert, Chief Strategy & Dev Officer
Jamitha Fields, VP, Community Affairs
Lisa Goring, EVP, Programs and Services
ESCIL provides services to people with all disabilities regardless of age, religion, gender, ethnicity, race or national origin. In addition to the core services of information and referral, skills training, peer support and advocacy, ESCIL also offers assistance with accessibility modifications, Americans with Disabilities Act education and training, housing referrals and counseling, transportation referral and information, Brailling capabilities, Personal Attendent Services referral, and more.

4188 Freedom Center
14 W. Patrick Street
Suite 10
Frederick, MD 21701
301-846-7811
FAX: 301-846-9070
advocate@thefreedomcenter-md.org
thefreedomcenter-md.org

Jamey George, Executive Director
Russell Holt, President
Patrick Mcmurtray, Vice-President
Craig Shafer, Treasurer
A walk in center for independent living, provides services and supports to empower individuals with disabilities to lead self-directed, independent, and productive lives in a barrier-free community.

4189 Housing Unlimited
Ste G1
1398 Lamberton Dr
Silver Spring, MD 20902-3435
301-592-9314
FAX: 301-592-9318
information@housingunlimited.org
www.housingunlimited.org

Nancy Cohen, President Emerita
Russell Phillips, President
Robyn S. Raysor, Vice President
Johnnie Mae Armstrong, Treasurer
To address the housing crisis for adults with psychiatric disabilities who reside in Montgomery County, Maryland.

4190 Independence Now
Ste 101
12301 Old Columbia Pike
Silver Spring, MD 20904-1656
301-277-2839
FAX: 301-625-9777
info@innow.org
innow.org

Sarah Sorensen, Executive Director
Trish Foley, Director of Community Services
Todd Thorpe, Director of Operations
Robert Watson, President
A nonprofit organization created by people with disabilities and provides services that promote independence and the inclusion of people with disabilities in their communities.

4191 Independence Now: Silver Spring
Ste 101
12301 Old Columbia Pike
Silver Spring, MD 20904-1659
301-277-2839
FAX: 301-625-9777
info@innow.org
innow.org

Sarah Sorensen, Executive Director
Trish Foley, Director of Community Services
Todd Thorpe, Director of Operations
Robert Watson, President
A nonprofit organization created by people with disabilities that provides services that promotes independence and the inclusion of people with disabilities in their communities.

4192 Making Choices for Independent Living
Ste 202
1118 Light St
Baltimore, MD 21230-4152
410-234-8195
888-560-2221
andreab@mcil-md.org
www.mcil-md.org

Jimmie Joku Cooper, Owner
Provides services to help empower people with disabilities to lead self-directed, independent and productive lives in the community and protect their civil rights.OUT OF ORDER.

4193 Resources for Independence
30 N. Mechanic Street
Unit B
Cumberland, MD 21502-2705
301-784-1774
800-371-1986
FAX: 301-784-1776
www.rficil.org

Lori Magruder, Executive Director
John Michaels, Assistant Director
Robert Cannon, Benefits Counselor
Sherry Williams, Finance Director
Private, non-profit, consumer-controlled, community-based organization providing services and advocacy by and for persons with all type of disabilities. Their goal is to create opportunities for independence, and to assist individuals with disabilities to achieve their maximum level of independent functioning within their families and communities.

4194 Southern Maryland Center for LIFE
P.O.Box 657
Charlotte Hall, MD 20622-657
301-884-4498
FAX: 301-884-6099
cflife@eartlink.net
www.somd.com

Marie Robinson, Executive Director
Carrie Lanthier, Administrative Assistant
A non-profit community based organization which provides services to disabled people who live or work in the tri-county area. Our mission is to empower people with disabilities to lead self-directed, independent, and productive lives in their community.

Massachusetts

4195 Adlib
215 North St
Pittsfield, MA 01201-4644
413-442-7047
800-232-7047
FAX: 413-443-4338
adlib@adlibcil.org
adlibcil.org

Linda Febles, President
Michael Hinkley, Vice President
Allison Bedard, Treasurer
Shannon Miller, Secretary/Clerk
Offers information and referral services, independent living skills training, peer counseling, individual and group advocacy services available to all people with disabilities. Access consultation provided to businesses, agencies and institutions in accordance to the Americans with Disabilities Act.

4196 Arc of Cape Cod
P.O.Box 428
171 Main Street
Hyannis, MA 02601-428
508-790-3667
FAX: 508-775-5233
info@arcofcapecod.org
www.arcofcapecod.org

4197 Boston Center for Independent Living
5th Floor
60 Temple Place
Boston, MA 02111-1324
617-338-6665
FAX: 617-338-6661
TTY:617-338-6662
info@bostoncil.org
www.bostoncil.org

Sergio Goncalves, Chairman
Linda Landry, Vice Chairman
Stacey Zelbow, Treasurer
Bill Henning, Executive Director
A frontline civil rights organization led by people with disabilities that advocates to eliminate discrimination, isolation and segregation by providing advocacy, information and referral, peer support, skills training, and PCA services in order to enhance the independence of people with disabilities.

4198 Cape Organization for Rights of the Disabled (CORD)
106 Bassett Lane
Hyannis, MA 2601
508-775-8300
800-541-0282
FAX: 508-775-7022
TTY: 800-541-0282
cordinfo@cilcapecod.org
www.cilcapecod.org
Coreen Brinkerhoff, Executive Director
The Cape Organization for the Rights of the Disabled (CORD) has been aggresively working since 1984 to advance the independence, productivity, and integration of people with disabilities into mainstream society. CORD is the Center for Independent Living (CIL) and is a member of the Aging and Disability Resources Consortium (ADRC) servinf Cape Cod and the Islands.

4199 Center for Living & Working: Fitchburg
76 Summer Street
Suite 110
Fitchburg, MA 01420-5785
978-345-1568
TTY:978-345-1568
centerlwA@centerlw.org
www.centerlw.org

Cindy Purcell, Board President
Mary Ann Donovan, Treasurer
Ed Roth, Secretary
Jim O'Day, Advisor to CLW Board of Director
The Center for Living and Working is a non-profit Independent Living Center which takes its direction from persons with disabilities. The Center advocates to empower persons with disabilities to take active roles in their lives and in their community in which they live. Also provides comprehensive and innovative programs and services in order to maximize individual independence and opportunities.

4200 Center for Living & Working: Framingham
484 Main St
Suite 345
Worcester, MA 01608-1824
508-798-0350
FAX: 508-797-4015
TTY:508-755-1003
opsearch@centerlw.org
www.centerlw.org

Cindy Purcell, Board President
Mary Ann Donovan, Treasurer
Ed Roth, Secretary
Jim O'Day, Advisor to CLW Board of Director
The Center for Living and Working is a non-profit Independent Living Center which takes its direction from persons with disabilities. The Center advocates to empower persons with disabilities to take active roles in their lives and in their community in which they live. Also provides comprehensive and innovative programs and services in order to maximize individual independence and opportunities.

4201 Center for Living & Working: Worcester
484 Main St
Suite 345
Worcester, MA 01608-1824
508-798-0350
FAX: 508-797-4015
TTY:508-755-1003
opsearch@centerlw.org
www.centerlw.org

Cindy Purcell, Board President
Mary Ann Donovan, Treasurer
Ed Roth, Clerk/Secretary
Jim O'Day, Advisor to CLW Board of Director
The Center for Living and Working is a non-profit Independent Living Center which takes its direction from persons with disabilities. The Center advocates to empower persons with disabilities to take active roles in their lives and in their community in which they live. Also provides comprehensive and innovative programs and services in order to maximize individual independence and opportunities.

4202 Developmental Evaluation and Adjustment Facilities
215 Brighton Ave
Allston, MA 02134-2013
617-254-4041
800-886-5195
FAX: 617-254-7091
info@deafinconline.org
deafinconline.org

Sharon L. Applegate, Executive Director
Kelly Kim, President
John Sullivan, Treasurer
Kendra Timko-Hochkeppel, Vice President
Encourages and empowers deaf, hard of hearing, deafblind and late-deafened individuals to lead independent and productive lives.

4203 Independence Associates
100 Laurel Street
1st Suite 122
East Bridgewater, MA 02301-4012   508-583-2166
                                         800-649-5568
                                         FAX: 508-583-2165
                                         info@iacil.org
                                         iacil.org

Mark Lewis, President
James Clark, Treasurer
Anita Ashdon, Secretary
Steven Higgins, Executive Director
Provides comprehensive services which will enhance the range
of acceptable options available to the consumer and improve the
quality of life of persons with disabilities; to work on behalf of
the objective of the disablility rights and independent living
movement.

4204 Independent Living Center of Stavros: Greenfield
55 Federal St
Greenfield, MA 01301-2546   413-774-3001
                                        www.stavros.org

Glenn Hartmann, President
Nancy Bazanchuk, Vice President
Donna M. Bliznak, Treasurer
Greta Biagi, Clerk
Promoting independence and access in the communities for per-
sons with disabilities and deaf people.

4205 Independent Living Center of Stavros: Springfield
210 Old Farm Road
Amherst, MA 01002-2704   413-256-0473
                                        800-804-1899
                                        FAX: 413-256-0190
                                        www.stavros.org

Glenn Hartmann, President
Nancy Bazanchuk, Vice President
Donna M. Bliznak, Treasurer
James Kruidenier, Executive Director
Promoting independence and access in the communities for per-
sons with disabilities and deaf people.

4206 Independent Living Center of the North Shore & Cape Ann
27 Congress St
Suite 107
Salem, MA 01970-5577   978-741-0077
                                        888-751-0077
                                        FAX: 978-741-1133
                                        information@ilcnsca.org
                                        ilcnsca.org

Mary Margaret Moore, Executive Director
Marion A Dawicki, President
Patricia Cox, Vice President
Joe Karaman, Treasurer
A service and advocacy center run by and for people with disabili-
ties that supports the struggle of people who have all types of dis-
abilities to live independently and participate fully in community
life.

4207 MetroWest Center for Independent Living
280 Irving Street
Framingham, MA 01702-7306   508-875-7853
                                        FAX: 508-875-8359
                                        TTY:508-875-7853
                                        info@mwcil.org
                                        mwcil.org

Youcef J. Bellil, President
Michael Kennedy, Vice President
Edward J. Carr, Treasurer
Penny Kelley, Secretary
To help individuals with disabilities become productive and con-
tributing members of the community and to eliminate barriers
within the community that impede this process.

4208 Multi-Cultural Independent Living Center of Boston
329 Centre Street
Jamaica Plain, MA 02130-1232   617-942-8060
                                        FAX: 617-942-8630
                                        TTY:617-288-2707
                                        info@milcb.org
                                        milcb.org

Derrick Dominique, Executive Director
Ana Ortiz, Director of Services
Eleanor Slaughter, Senior IL Advocate
Louise Beach, Community Outreach Coordinator
Seeks to create opportunities for people with disabilities and
their families in unserved/under-served populations and cultures
who reside in Boston's inner city.

4209 Northeast Independent Living Program
20 Ballard Rd
Lawrence, MA 01843-1018   978-687-4288
                                        FAX: 978-689-4488
                                        TTY:978-687-4288
                                        help@nilp.org
                                        nilp.org

June Cowen, Executive Director
Nanette Goodwin, Assistant Director
Lisa DiGiuseppe, Director of Finance
Jim Lyons, Director, Community Development
A consumer controlled Independent Living Center providing Ad-
vocacy and Services to people with all disabilities in the greater
Merrimack Valley who wish to live as independently as possible
in the community.

4210 Renaissance Clubhouse
176 Walker St
2nd Floor
Lowell, MA 01854-3126   978-454-7944
                                        FAX: 978-937-7867
                                        renclub1@gmail.com
                                        www.renclublowell.org

Elaine Walker, Executive Director
Pammy Sadoie, Assistant Director
Offers daily structure, assistance wtih jobs, retirement, and hous-
ing.

4211 Southeast Center for Independent Living
66 Troy Street
Suite 3
Fall River, MA 02720-3023   508-679-9210
                                        FAX: 508-677-2377
                                        TTY:508-679-9210
                                        scil@secil.org
                                        secil.org

Lisa M Pitta, Executive Director
Damase Cote, President
Paul Remy, Vice President
Debbie Pacheco, Treasurer / Secretary
The Philosophy of Independent Living, maintains that individuals with disabilities have the right to choose services and make
decisions for themselves. This belief is the foundation and guiding principle of all of SCIL's policies and operations. SCIL provides training, information and support to help consumers
achieve individual goals, experience personal growth and
participate fully in community life.

**4212 Student Independent Living Experience Massachusetts
Hospital School**
560 Harrison Avenue
Suite 600
Boston, MA 02118-2447   617-338-6409
                                        800-843-5879
                                        TTY:800-328-3202
                                        JurorHelp@jud.state.ma.us.
                                        www.mass.gov

Michigan

4213 Ann Arbor Center for Independent Living
3941 Research Park Drive
Ann Arbor, MI 48108-6852
734-971-0277
FAX: 734-971-0826
www.annarborcil.org

Carolyn Grawi, Executive Director
Chris Baty, Theater Coordinator
Bryan Wilkinson, Director of Operations and Sales
Shirley Coombs, Chief Financial Officer
AACIL assists people with disabilities and their families in living full and productive lives. AACIL assures the equality of opportunity, full participation, independent living and economic self-sufficiency of people with disabilities in the community.

4214 Arc Michigan
1325 S Washington Ave
Lansing, MI 48910-1652
517-487-5426
800-292-7851
FAX: 517-487-0303
dhoyle@arcmi.org
arcmi.org

Donald Teegarden, President
Laurel Robb, Vice President
Dohn Hoyle, Executive Director
Sherri Boyd, Associate Director
Exists to empower local chapters of The ARC to assure that citizens with developmental disabilities are valued and that they and their families can participate fully in and contribute to the life of their community.

4215 Arc/Muskegon
601 Terrace Street
Suite 101
Muskegon, MI 49440-2197
231-777-2006
FAX: 231-777-3507
info@arcmuskegon.org
www.arcmuskegon.org

Tim Michalski, President
Brenda McCarthy Wiener, Vice President
Margaret O'Toole, Executive Director
Janis Milliron, Administrative Assistant
Offers information and referral, advocacy services and peer counseling.

4216 Bad Axe: Blue Water Center for Independent Living
614 N Port Crescent Street
P.O. Box 29
Bad Axe, MI 48413-1207
989-269-5421
810-987-9337
FAX: 989-269-5422
info@bwcil.org
www.bwcil.org

Karen Massaro-Mundt, President
Chuck Wanninger, Treasurer
Jim Whalen, Executive Director
Bill Farris, Administrative Assistant
A non-profit, consumer-based organization that advocates, informs and supports persons with disabilities in the community.

4217 Bay Area Coalition for Independent Living
Ste 17
701 S Elmwood Ave
Traverse City, MI 49684-3185
231-929-4865
FAX: 231-929-4896
steve@bacil.org

Steve Wade, Director

4218 Capital Area Center for Independent Living
2812 N. Martin Luther King Jr. Blvd
Lansing, MI 48906
517-999-2760
877-652-3777
FAX: 517-999-2767
TTY: 800-649-3777
info@cacil.org
www.cacil.org

Mark Pierce, Executive Director
Jeffrey Gass, Financial Manager
Justine Bond, Independent Living Specialist
Jean Harris, Program Coordinator
CACIL provide training, mentoring, and referrals to help people with disabilities and their families live productive lives.

4219 Caro: Blue Water Center for Independent Living
1184 Cleaver Rd
Caro, MI 48723-1143
989-673-3678
810-987-9337
FAX: 989-673-3656
info@bwcil.org
www.bwcil.org

Karen Massaro-Mundt, President
Chuck Wanninger, Treasurer
Jim Whalen, Executive Director
Bill Farris, Administrative Assistant
A non-profit, consumer-based organization that advocates, informs and supports persons with disabilities in the community.

4220 Center for Independent Living of Mid-Michigan
3941 Research Park Drive
Ann Arbor, MI 48108-6832
734-971-0277
FAX: 734-971-0826
www.annarborcil.org

Carolyn Grawi, Executive Director
Chris Baty, Theater Coordinator
Bryan Wilkinson, Director of Operations and Sales
Shirley Coombs, Chief Financial Officer
Comprised of over 51 percent of people with disabilities, and advocates for the rights of people with disabilities in the Mid-Michigan area. Call for information on disability issues or for assistance in obtaining services, within your community..

4221 Community Connections of Southwest Michigan
5671 N. Skeel Ave.
Suite 8
Oscoda, MI 48750
989-569-6001
800-578-4245
FAX: 269-925-7141
kellis@miconnect.org
www.miconnect.org

Kathy Ellis, Director
An advocacy organization that teaches and empowers people with disabilities to make choices about living life to the fullest, controlling and directing their own lives and asserting their rights and responsibilites within their Berrien County communities..

4222 Cristo Rey Handicappers Program
1717 N High St
Lansing, MI 48906-4529
517-372-4700
FAX: 517-372-8499
info@cristo-rey.org
www.cristo-rey.org

Marlene M Berens, Manager
To care for the spiritual and social needs of individuals and families by offering services that encourage self-sufficiency and recognize the dignity of the human person..

4223 **Detroit Center for Independent Living**
1042 Griswold
Suite 2
Port Huron, MI 48060   810-987-9337
810-987-9337
FAX: 810-987-9548
info@bwcil.org
www.bwcil.org

Karen Massaro-Mundt, President
Chuck Wanninger, Treasurer
Jim Whalen, Executive Director
Bill Farris, Administrative Assistant
BWCIL is a consumer-based organization designed to serve persons with disabilities who have physical, psychiatric, sendory, cognitive, and multiple disabilities through the provision of advocacy, information and referral, service provision, and the promotion of needed services so to maximize the individual's optimal level of independence.

4224 **Disability Advocates of Kent County**
3600 Camelot Drive SE
Grand Rapids, MI 49546-8103   616-949-1100
FAX: 616-949-7865
contact@dakc.us
disabilityadvocates.us

David Bulkowski, JD, Executive Director
Denise Borges, Employment Specialist
Jackson Botsford, Accessibility Specialist
Katie Foreman, Independent Living Specialist
Exists to advocate, assist, educate and inform on independent living options for persons with disabilities and to create a barrier-free society for all.

4225 **Disability Connection**
27 E. Clay Avenue
Muskegon, MI 49442   231-722-0088
866-322-4501
FAX: 231-722-0066
dcilmi.org

John Wahlberg, President
Michael Hamm, Vice President
Tamera Collier, Executive Director
Tom Munn, Associate Director
To advocate, educate, empower, and provide resources for persons with disabilities and promote accessible communities.

4226 **Disability Network Southwest Michigan**
517 E Crosstown Pkwy
Kalamazoo, MI 49001-2867   269-345-1516
FAX: 269-345-0229
info@dnswm.org
www.dnswm.org

Cameron J. Lambe, Chair
Cheri Stoltzner, Vice Chair
Joel W Cooper, President
Kevin Klute, Treasurer
To educate and empower people with disabilities to create change intheir own lives, and to advocate for social change to create inclusive communities. As a center for independent living, they are part of the disability rights movement.

4227 **Disability Network of Mid-Michigan**
1705 S. Saginaw Road
Midland, MI 48640-6825   989-835-4041
800-782-4160
FAX: 989-835-8121
info@dnmm.org
dnmm.org

Tom Provoast, President
Dr. Barbara Gibson, Vice President
David Emmel, Executive Director
Steven Locke, Associate Director
To promote and encourage independence for all people with disabilities.

4228 **Disability Network of Oakland & Macomb**
16645 15 Mile Rd
Clinton Township, MI 48035-2206   586-268-4160
800-284-2457
FAX: 586-285-9942
info@dnom.org
dnom.org

Andrew Maurer, Chairperson
Randy Charon, Vice Chairperson
Kellie Boyd, Executive Director
Kelly Winn, Director of Operations
Commited to advancing personal choice, independence, and positive social change for persons with disabilities through advocacy, education and outreach.

4229 **Disability Network/Lakeshore**
426 Century Lane
Holland, MI 49423-2200   616-396-5326
800-656-5245
FAX: 616-396-3220
TTY: 616-396-5326
info@dnlakeshore.org
dnlakeshore.org

Michelle Chaney, President
Amber Marcy, Vice President
Brian Dykhuis, Treasurer
Todd Whiteman, Executive Director
A cross-disability, community-based organization providing advocacy, education, and information and referral to persons with disabilities in Ottawa and Allegan counties.

4230 **Grand Traverse Area Community Living Management Corporation**
935 Barlow St
Traverse City, MI 49686-4250   231-932-9030
mmacy@GTACLMC.com
www.gtaclmc.org

Mary Jean Brick, Administrative Director
We are a training home for individuals with developmental disabilities over the age of 18

4231 **Great Lakes/Macomb Rehabilitation Group**
Apt 104
4 E Alexandrine St
Detroit, MI 48201-2032   313-832-3371
FAX: 313-832-3850
jlcil@home.msen.com

Jeannie Meece-Brooks, Contact
Independent living center. .

4232 **JARC**
30301 Northwestern Hwy
Suite 100
Farmington Hills, MI 48334-3277   248-538-6611
877-767-7781
FAX: 248-538-6615
jarc@jarc.org
jarc.org

Ronald Applebaum, President
Richard A. Loewenstein, Chief Executive Officer
Randy P. Baxter, Chief Financial Officer
Rena Friedberg, CFRE, Chief Development Officer
A nonprofit, nonsecretarian agency dedicated to enabling people with disabilities to live full, dignified lives in the community, and to providing support and advocacy for their families.

4233 **Lapeer: Blue Water Center for Independent Living**
392 West Nepessing Street
Lapeer, MI 48446-2192   810-664-9098
810-987-9337
FAX: 810-664-0937
info@bwcil.org
www.bwcil.org

Karen Massaro-Mundt, President
Chuck Wanninger, Treasurer
Jim Whalen, Executive Director
Bill Farris, Administrative Assistant

A non-profit, consumer-based organization that advocates, informs and supports persons with disabilities in the community.

4234 Livingston Center for Independent Living
3075 E Grand River Ave
Suite 108
Howell, MI 48843-6585   517-545-1741
                                        FAX: 517-548-1751
                                        gsims@aacil.org
                                        www.virtualcil.net

Dan Durci, Director
Independent living skills training and empowerment training for persons with disabilities..

4235 Michigan Commission for the Blind: Independent Living Rehabilitation Program
235 S. Grand Ave.
P.O. Box 30037
Lansing, MI 48909-1254   989-758-1765
                                        800-292-4200
                                        FAX: 989-758-1405
                                        www.michigan.gov

Debbie Wilson, Manager
Patrick Cannon, Agency Director
Rehabilitation teaching, independent living skills for persons over 55 with severe vision loss.

4236 Michigan Commission for the Blind: Detroit
Ste 4-450
3038 W Grand Blvd
Detroit, MI 48202-6012   313-456-1646
                                        FAX: 313-456-1645
                                        mcnealg@michigan.gov

Gwen McNeal, Supervisor
Shawnese Laury-Johnson, Assistant East Region Manager
Promotes the inclusion of people with legal blindness into our communities on a full and equal basis through empowerment, education, participation, and choice..

4237 Monroe Center for Independent Living
1285 N Telegraph Rd
Monroe, MI 48162-3368   734-242-5919
                                        mrawlings@aacil.org
                                        monroecil.tripod.com

Linda Maier, Manager
To act as a catalyst for personal and social change through the empowerment of people with disabilities; and, to replace the perception of disability as tragic with a disability culture promoting pride, power and personal style.

4238 Port Huron: Blue Water Center for Independent Living
1042 Griswold St
Suite 2
Port Huron, MI 48060-5431   810-987-9337
                                        810-987-9337
                                        FAX: 810-987-9548
                                        info@bwcil.org
                                        bwcil.org

Karen Massaro-Mundt, President
Chuck Wanninger, Treasurer
Jim Whalen, Executive Director
Bill Farris, Administrative Assistant
A non-profit, consumer-based organization that advocates, informs and supports persons with disabilities in the community.

4239 Sandusky: Blue Water Center for Independent Living
103 East Sanilac Road
Suite 3
Sandusky, MI 48471-1615   810-648-2555
                                        810-987-9337
                                        FAX: 810-648-2583
                                        info@bwcil.org
                                        www.bwcil.org

Karen Massaro-Mundt, President
Chuck Wanninger, Treasurer
Jim Whalen, Executive Director
Bill Farris, Administrative Assistant

A non-profit, consumer-based organization that advocates, informs and supports persons with disabilities in the community.

4240 Southeastern Michigan Commission for the Blind
4450 Grandy St
Detroit, MI 48207   313-456-0334
                                        877-932-6424
                                        FAX: 313-456-1645
                                        www.michigan.gov

Patrick Cannon, Executive Director
Pat Bragg, Manager
Vocational rehabilitation agency. Personal adjustment vocational assessment and training, job placement and follow-up services. .

4241 Superior Alliance for Independent Living(SAIL)
1200 Wright Street
Suite A
Marquette, MI 49855   906-228-5744
                                        800-379-7245
                                        FAX: 906-228-5573
                                        TTY: 906-228-5744
                                        www.upsail.com

Elgie Dow, President
Aaron Andres, Vice President
Amy Maes, Executive Director
Judy Vivian, Finance Director
Promotes the inclusion of people with disabilities into our communities on a full and equal basis through empowerment, education, participation and choice.

4242 disAbility Connections
409 Linden Ave
Jackson, MI 49203-4065   517-782-6054
                                        FAX: 517-782-3118
                                        lesia@disabilityconnect.org
                                        www.disabilityconnect.org

Michael Jackson, President
James Gorse, Vice President
Lesia Pikaart, Executive Director
Joann Lucas, Associate Director
Supporting Jackson County residents in their efforts to lead independent, fulfilling, productive lives.

Minnesota

4243 Accessible Space, Inc.
2550 University Avenue West
Suite 330N
Saint Paul, MN 55114-1085   651-645-7271
                                        800-466-7722
                                        FAX: 651-645-0541
                                        TTY: 800-627-3529
                                        info@accessiblespace.org
                                        www.accessiblespace.org

Mark E. Hamel, Esq., Chairman
Kay Knutson, Vice Chairman
Steve Schugel, Treasurer
John W. Adams, Secretary
Accessible, rent-subsidized apartments for very low-income adults with qualifying physical disabilities as well as seniors. Accessible Space, Inc., sponsors, develops and manages housing & ASI apartments are rent based on income and are located across the country.

4244 Accessnorth CIL of Northeastern MN: Aitkin
1309 East 40th Street
Hibbing, MN 55746-1821   218-262-6675
                                        800-390-3681
                                        FAX: 218-262-6677
                                        TTY: 218-262-6675
                                        info@accessnorth.net
                                        www.accessnorth.net

Mary Ribich, Chair
David Hohl, Vice-Chair
Donald Brunette, Executive Director
Cathy Baudeck, Program Manager

Assists individuals to live independently, pursue meaningful goals, and have equal opportunities and choices.

4245 Accessnorth CIL of Northeastern MN: Duluth
118 East Superior Street
Duluth, MN 55802-2155
218-625-1400
888-625-1401
FAX: 218-625-1401
info@accessnorth.net
www.accessnorth.net

Mary Ribich, Chair
David Hohl, Vice-Chair
Donald Brunette, Executive Director
Cathy Baudeck, Program Manager
Assisting individuals with disabilities to live independently, puruse meaningful goals, and have equal opportunities and choices.

4246 Center for Independent Living of NE Minnesota
1309 East 40th Street
Hibbing, MN 55746-1821
218-262-6675
800-390-3681
FAX: 218-262-6677
TTY: 218-262-6675
info@accessnorth.net
accessnorth.net

Mary Ribich, Chair
David Hohl, Vice-Chair
Donald Brunette, Executive Director
Cathy Baudeck, Program Manager
Assisting individuals with disabilities to live independently, pursue meaningful goals, and have an equal opportunities and choices

4247 Courage Center
800 E. 28th St.
Minneapolis, MN 55407-4298
612-863-4200
866-880-3550
FAX: 763-520-0577
TTY: 763-520-0245
couragekenny@allina.com
www.allinahealth.org

Jan Malcolm, CEO
Alice Johnson, Chief Financial Officer
Stephen Bariteau, Chief Development Officer
Pamela J. Lindemoen, Executive Vice President of Oper
A nonprofit rehabilitation and resource center that advances the lives of children and adults experiencing barriers to health and independence. Specialize in treating brain injury, spinal cord injury, stroke, chronic pain, autism and disabilities experienced since birth.

4248 Freedom Resource Center for Independent Living: Fergus Falls
125 W Lincoln Avenue
Suite 7
Fergus Falls, MN 56537-2152
218-998-1799
800-450-0459
FAX: 218-998-1798
freedom@freedomrc.org
www.freedomrc.org

Nate Aalgaard, Executive Director
Angie Bosch, Office Coordinator
Mark Mark Bourdon Bourdon, Program Director
Andrea Nelson, Independent Living Advocate
Freedom Resource Center assists people in working towards goals they establish for themselves.

4249 Metropolitan Center for Independent Living
Ste 16
1600 University Ave W
Saint Paul, MN 55104-3825
651-646-8342
FAX: 651-603-2006
TTY:651-603-2001
homeramps@gmail.com
www.klownwerkz.com

4250 Minnesota Association of Centers for Independent Living
215 North Benton Drive
Sauk Rapids, MN 56379
320-529-9000
888-529-0743
FAX: 320-529-0747
ilicil@independentlifestyles.org
independentlifestyles.org

Cara Ruff, Executive Director
Jay Keller, Board Chairman
Pamela Kotzenmacher, Treasurer
Autumn Gould, Attorney
A non-profit organization whose purpose is to advocate for the independent living needs of people with disabilities who are citizens of the State of Minnesota

4251 OPTIONS
Ste B
123 S Main St
Crookston, MN 56716-1970
218-281-5722
FAX: 218-281-5722
TTY:218-281-5722
options3@rrv.net

Gordie Haug, Manager
Provides people with disabilities advocacy, information, skills training and peer mentoring relationships to help them achieve their personal goals of how and where they live their lives.

4252 Options Interstate Resource Center for Independent Living
2200 2nd Street SW
Rochester, MN 55902-1887
507-285-1815
800-726-3692
FAX: 218-773-7119
TTY: 218-773-6100
options@myoptions.info
www.macil.org

Vicki Dalle Molle, President
Randy Sorensen, Executive Director
Located in Minnesota, but also serves North Dakota..

4253 Perry River Home Care
330 High Way Pen S
Saint Cloud, MN 56304
320-255-1882
FAX: 320-255-5137

Berna Florentine, CEO
Ken Figge, President
Courtney Salzi, Administrator
Offers skilled nursing services RN, LPN, TV Therapy, Pediatrics, Rehabilitation Services, PT, OT, ST, Paraprofessional staff, Home Health Aides, Homemakers, Personal Care Attendents, Companions, Live-ins, Sleep overs, Respite care, Extended hours.

4254 SMILES
820 Winnebago Ave
Suite 1
Fairmont, MN 56031-3619
507-345-7139
888-676-6498
FAX: 507-235-3488
www.smilescil.org

Brain Koch, President
Doug Robinson, Vice President
Alan Augustin, Executive Director
Helen Mitchell, Administrative Assistant
A nonprofit organization committed to providing a wide array of services that assist individuals with disabilities that live independently, pursue meaningful goals, and enjoy the same opportunities and choices as all persons.

4255 SMILES: Mankato
709 S. Front Street
Suite 7
Mankato, MN 56001-3887
507-345-7139
888-676-6498
FAX: 507-345-8429
smiles@smilescil.org
smilescil.org

Brain Koch, President
Doug Robinson, Vice President
Alan Augustin, Executive Director
Helen Mitchell, Administrative Assistant
A nonprofit organization committed to providing a wide array of services that assist individuals with disabilities that live independently, pursue meaningful goals, and enjoy the same opportunities and choices as all persons.

4256 Southeastern Minnesota Center for Independent Living: Red Wing
2200 2nd Street SW
Rochester, MN 55902
507-285-1815
888-460-1815
FAX: 507-288-8070
semcil@semcil.org
www.semcil.org

Brian Koch, President
Doug Robinson, Vice President
Alan Augustin, Executive Director
Helen Mitchell, Administrative Assistant
Non profit organization that assists people with disabilities to become independent and productive community members.

4257 Southeastern Minnesota Center for Independent Living: Rochester
2200 Second Street SW
Rochester, MN 55902-3980
507-285-1815
888-460-1815
FAX: 507-288-8070
semcil@semcil.org
www.semcil.org

Brain Koch, President
Doug Robinson, Vice President
Alan Augustin, Executive Director
Helen Mitchell, Administrative Assistant
A non profit organization that assists people with disabilities to become independent and productive community members.

4258 Southwestern Center for Independent Living
2864 S. Nettleton Avenue
SUITE #700
Springfield, MO 65807-1298
507-532-2221
800-422-1485
FAX: 417-886-3619
TTY: 507-532-2221
swcil@swcil.com
www.swcil.org

Amy C. Lewis, President
Mark Grantham, Vice President
Gary Maddox, Chief Executive Officer
Lacee Thompson, Administrative Assistant
SWCIl is a private, non-profit consumer controlled, non-residential, cross-disability, community-based organization providing independent living services to assist people with disabilities in obtaining and maintaining the greatest control over their lives. Services are available in southwestern Minnesota to persons of all ages, with all disability without regard to income.

4259 Vinland Center Lake Independence
3675 Ihduhapi Road
Loretto, MN 55357-308
763-479-3555
866-956-7612
FAX: 763-479-2605
vinland@vinlandcenter.org
www.vinlandcenter.org

Gerald Seck, President
Mary Roehl, Executive Director
Colleen Larson, Operations Manager
Debbie Larson, Accounting Manager
A Minnesota based rehabilitation center which offers services in three distinct service areas: vocational rehabilitation; inclusive community programs; and for people with cognitive disabilities, specially adapted chemical dependency treatment.

Mississippi

4260 Alpha Home Royal Maid Association for the Blind
PO Drawer 30
Hazlehurst, MS 39083-30
601-894-1771
FAX: 601-894-2993
sigworks@teclink.net

Howard Becker, Director
Offers attendant care registry, information on accessible housing and referrals.

4261 Gulf Coast Independent Living Center
18 JM Tatum Industrial Drive
Hattiesburg, MS 39401-8341
601-544-4860
FAX: 601-582-2544

Albert Holifield, Executive Director
Independent living center.

4262 Jackson Independent Living Center
1981 Hollywood Dr
Jackson, TN 38305-2131
731-668-2211
800-848-0298
FAX: 731-668-0406
TTY: 601-351-1585
information@jcil.tn.org
www.j-cil.com/contact-us.html

Denea Smith, Director
Timothy Jackson
Provides services to consumers with severe disabilities.

4263 LIFE of Mississippi
1304 Vine St
Jackson, MS 39202-3429
601-969-4009
800-748-9398
FAX: 601-969-1662
TTY: 800-748-9398
www.lifeofms.com

Augusta Smith, Executive Director
Margie Moore, Project Coordinator
Densie Smith, Assistant
Christine Woodell, ADA Consultant
To empower people wit significant disabilities to be as independent and as fully involved in their communities as they can and want to be.

4264 LIFE of Mississippi: Biloxi
2030 Pass Road
Suite C
Biloxi, MS 39531
228-388-2401
FAX: 228-338-2413
www.lifeofms.com

Augusta Smith, Executive Director
Ruby Jackson, I.L. Specialist
Kim Allison, IL Specialist/ B2I
Christine Woodell, ADA Coordinator
To empower people with significant disabilities to be as independent and as fully involved in their communities as they can and want to be.

4265 LIFE of Mississippi: Greenwood
502a W Park Ave
Greenwood, MS 38930-2906
662-453-9940
FAX: 662-453-9934
www.lifeofms.com

Augusta Smith, Executive Director
Pam Wraggs, I.L. Specialist
Ruth Elliott, IL Specialist Assistant
Christine Woodell, ADA Consultant

To empower people with significant disabilities to be as independent and as fully involved in their communities as they can and want to be.

4266 LIFE of Mississippi: Hattiesburg
710 Katie Ave
Hattiesburg, MS 39401-4377   601-583-2108
                                          www.lifeofms.com

Augusta Smith, Executive Director
Margie Moore, Project Coordinator
Densie Smith, Assistant
Christine Woodell, ADA Consultant
To empower people with significant disabilities to be as independent and as fully involved in their communities as they can and want to be.

4267 LIFE of Mississippi: McComb
915-A S. Locust Street
McComb, MS 39648-4817   601-684-3079
                                          www.lifeofms.com

Augusta Smith, Executive Director
Margie Moore, Project Coordinator
Densie Smith, Assistant
Christine Woodell, ADA Consultant
To empower people with significant disabilities to be as independent and as fully involved in their communities as they can and want to be.

4268 LIFE of Mississippi: Meridian
Ste 103a
2440 N Hills St
Meridian, MS 39305-2653   601-485-7999
                                          www.lifeofms.com

Augusta Smith, Executive Director
Margie Moore, Project Coordinator
Densie Smith, Assistant
Christine Woodell, ADA Consultant
To empower people with significant disabilities to be as independent and as fully involved in their communities as they can and want to be.

4269 LIFE of Mississippi: Oxford
Ste 5
404 Galleria Dr
Oxford, MS 38655-4383   662-234-7010
                                          www.lifeofms.com

Augusta Smith, Executive Director
Margie Moore, Project Coordinator
Densie Smith, Assistant
Christine Woodell, ADA Consultant
To empower people with significant disabilities to be as independent and as fully involved in their communities as they can and want to be.

4270 LIFE of Mississippi: Tupelo
1051 Cliff Gookin Blvd
Tupelo, MS 38801-6739   662-844-6633
                                          FAX: 662-844-6803
                                          www.lifeofms.com

Emily Word, Regional Coordinator
Ronnie Jernigan, I.L. Specialist/HOT
Wayne Lauderdale, I.L. Specialist
Tara Christian, I.L. Specialist Assistant
To empower people with significant disabilities to be as independent and as fully involved in their communities as they can and want to be.

Missouri

4271 Access II Independent Living Center
101 Industrial Parkway
Gallatin, MO 64640-1280   660-663-2423
                                          888-663-2423
                                          FAX: 660-663-2517
                                          access@accessii.org
                                          www.accessii.org

Heather Swymeler, Executive Director
Brandy Gannan, Program Manager
Amber Wells, Financial Director
Dawn Ernat, In-Home Director
The mission of Access II is to remove architectural and attitudinal barriers that limit the independence of persons with disabilities, promote a positive change in attitudes about disability and persons with disabilities, and encourage greater independence for persons with disabilities within our communities. As a Center for Independent Living, Access II is comitted to the provision of a full range of independent living services.

4272 Bootheel Area Independent Living Services
PO Box 326
Kennett, MO 63857-326   573-888-0002
                                          888-449-0949
                                          FAX: 573-888-0708
                                          TTY:573-888-0002
                                          tshaw@bails.org
                                          www.bails.org

Tim Shaw, Executive Director
BAILS goal is to foster an open, barrier free society flor all people regardless of their disability. BAILS service area is predominantly rural and includes the Southeast Missouri counties of: Dunklin, New Madrid, Pemiscot and Stoddard.

4273 Coalition for Independence: Missouri Branch Office
6724 Troost Ave
Ste. 408
Kansas City, MO 66131   816-822-7432
                                          FAX: 816-363-3469
                                          TTY:913-321-5126
                                          csmith@cfi-kc.org
                                          www.cfi-kc.com

Clarenece Smith, Executive Director
Coalition For Independence (CFI) is to facilitate positive and responsible independence for all people with disabilities by acting as an advocate for individuals with disabilities, providing services, and promoting accessibility and acceptance.

4274 Delta Center for Independent Living
PO Box 550
Suite #107
St. Peters, MO 63376-5608   636-926-8761
                                          866-727-3245
                                          FAX: 636-447-0341
                                          info@dcil.org
                                          www.dcil.org

Jennifer Mueller-Sparrow, President
Don Whalen, Vice President
Otis Pitts, Secretary
Bob Zeffert, Treasurer
A non profit corporation which assists people with significant disabilities who want to live more independently.

4275 Disability Resource Association
130 Brandon Wallace Way
Festus, MO 63028-1726   636-931-7696
                                          FAX: 636-931-4863
                                          TTY:636-937-9016
                                          dra@disabilityresourceassociation.org
                                          www.disabilityresourceassociation.org

Craig Henning, Executive Director
Nancy Pope, Assistant Director
Suzan Weller, Director/Resource Developer
Independent Living Cener.

4276 Independent Living Center of Southeast Missouri
511 Cedar St
Poplar Bluff, MO 63901-7301
573-686-2333
888-890-2333
FAX: 573-686-0733
TTY: 573-776-1178
info@ilcsemo.org
www.ilcsemo.org

Bruce Lynch, Executive Director
Debbie Hardin, Independent Living Director
To make Southeast Missouri barrier free for all persons with disabilities, enabling them to live more independently, extending their rights to control and direct their own lives and empowering them to live more producitve lives.

4277 Life Skills Foundation
10176 Corporate Square Drive
Suite #150
Saint Louis, MO 63132-2935
314-432-6200
FAX: 314-432-8894
TTY: 314-802-5299
intake@lifeskills-stl.org
www.eastersealsmidwest.org

Christopher Wittanauer, Chair
Sean Donlin, Vice Chair
Wendy Sullivan, President
Marian Nunn, Secretary
Assists people with disabilities live and work with dignity in the community.

4278 Midland Empire Resources for Independent Living (MERIL)
4420 South 40th St
Saint Joseph, MO 64503-2157
816-279-8558
800-637-4548
FAX: 816-279-1550
TTY: 816-279-4943
www.meril.org

Dr. Robert Bush, Chair
Jaren Pippitt, Vice Chair
Wayne Crawford, Secretary
J. Robert Brown, Treasurer
Designed to promote independent living and to enhance the quality of life for persons with disabilities by empowering them to control and direct their lives.

4279 Northeast Independent Living Services
909 Broadway
Suite 350
Hannibal, MO 63401
573-221-8282
877-713-7900
FAX: 573-221-9445
www.neilscenter.org

Rose McNally, President
Dawn Davis, Vice President
Brooke Kendrick, Executive Director
Tara Fortner, Finance Director
To empower persons with disabilities to live as full and productive members of society.

4280 On My Own
428 E Highland Ave
Nevada, MO 64772-2609
417-667-7007
800-362-8852
FAX: 417-667-6262
onmyowngundy@softnet.net
www.omoinc.org

Jennifer Gundy, Executive Director
A non profit independent living center.

4281 Ozark Independent Living
109 Aid Ave
West Plains, MO 65775-3529
417-257-0038
888-440-7500
FAX: 417-257-2380
TTY: 888-440-7500
info@ozarkcil.com
ozarkcil.com

Michael Conner, Vice Chair
Scott Schneider, Secretary/Treasurer
Cindy Moore, Executive Director
Jane Kramer, Special Education Teacher
OIL?was created to provide independent living services to persons with disabilities who reside in the following counties in Missouri: Oregon Ozark, Shannon, Wright, Howell, Texas, and Douglas. OIL is non-profit, on-residential supported by grants, donations, and volunteers

4282 Paraquad
5240 Oakland Ave
Saint Louis, MO 63110-1436
314-289-4200
FAX: 314-289-4201
TTY: 314-289-4252
contactus@paraquad.org
www.paraquad.org

Robert Funk, Executive Director
Paraquad works to empower people with disabilities to increase their independence through choice and opportunity.

4283 Places for People
4130 Lindell Blvd
Saint Louis, MO 63108-2914
314-535-5600
FAX: 314-535-6037
contact@placesforpeople.org
www.placesforpeople.org

Kevin Kissling, President
Robin Kolker Adkins, Vice President
Joe Yancey, Executive Director
Dennis Wells, Secretary
Places for People provides individualized, high quality and effective services to adults with serious and persistent mental disorders to assist them in living, working and socializing responsibility to serve those individuals who rely on public funding.

4284 RAIL
3024 Dupont Circle
Jefferson City, MO 65109
573-526-7039
877-222-8963
888-667-2117
FAX: 573-751-1441
mo.silc@vr.dese.mo.gov
www.mosilc.org

Chris Camene, Chairperson
Jessica Hatfield, Vice-Chairperson
Barrnie Cooper, Secretary/Treasurer
Teresa Myers, Executive Director
RAIL is an Independent Living Center, one of twenty-two in the State of Missouri, RAIL's Mission is to assist persons with disabilities to live as independently as they choose within the communities of their choice. RAIL offers four core services which are: Advocacy, Peer Support, Information & Referral, and Independent Living Skills Training. RAIL is a Consumer Services Directed Program vendor

4285 SEMO Alliance for Disability Independence
1913 Rusmar St
Cape Girardeau, MO 63701-7623
573-651-6464
800-898-7234
FAX: 573-651-6565
TTY: 573-651-6464
miki@mail.sadi.org
www.sadi.org

Timothy D. Woodard, President
Michelle Spooler, Vice-President
Leemon Priest, Secretary
Janet Wilson, Treasurer

A community based, non-profit, nonresidential center for independent living that is committed to providing services to persons with disabilities to enable them to remain in their own home and community, not an institution.

4286 Services for Independent Living
1401 Hathman Place
Columbia, MO 65201-5552

573-874-1646
800-766-1968
FAX: 573-874-3564
TTY: 573-874-4121
sil@silcolumbia.org
www.silcolumbia.org

Dan Dunham, President
Bonnie Gregg, Vice President
Amy Henderson, Treasurer
Barbara Hammer, Secretary

A non-residential, community-based center for independent living. Provides individualized and group services to persons with severe disabilities in the Mid-Missouri area; works to help people with disabilities achieve their highest potential in independent living and community life.

4287 Southwest Center for Independent Living (S CIL)
2864 S Nettleton Ave
Springfield, MO 65807-5970

417-886-3619
800-676-7245
FAX: 417-886-3619
TTY: 417-886-1188
scil@swcil.org
www.swcil.org

Amy C. Lewis, President
Mark Grantham, Vice President
Gary Maddox, Chief Executive Officer
Lacee Thompson, Administrative Assistant

Provides services, advocacy, and resources for people with any disability in Christian, Dallas, Greene, Lawrence, Polk, Stone, Taney and Webster Counties of Southwest Missouri.

4288 Tri-County Center for Independent Living
1420 HWY 72 East
Rolla, MO 65401

573-368-5933
FAX: 573-368-5991
TTY: 573-368-5933
vevans@fidnet.com
www.tricountycenter.com

Victoria Evans, Executive Director

Mission is to eliminate physical and attitudinal barriers through the power of advocacy, enlightenment, and reformation.

4289 West Central Independent Living Solutions
610 N Ridgeview Dr
Suite B
Warrensburg, MO 64093-9323

660-422-7883
800-236-5175
FAX: 660-422-7895
TTY: 660-422-7894
info@w-ils.org
www.w-ils.org

David De Frain, President
James Piatt, Vice President
Kathy Kay, Executive Director
Julie Steele, Director of Operations

Works to empower people with disabilities to become more independent by providing independent living skills training, peer support, information and referral and advocacy. West Central Independent Living Solutions now has satellite offices in Sedalia, MO and Lexington.

4290 Whole Person, The
3710 Main Street
Kansas City, MO 64111-7501

816-225-0301
800-878-3037
FAX: 816-931-0529
TTY: 816-561-0304
info@thewholeperson.org
www.thewholeperson.org

Rick O'Neal, President
Jim Atwater, Vice President
Julie Dejean, CEO
Mike Wiley, COO

The Whole Person, assists people with disabilities to live independently and encourages change within the community to expand opportunities for independent living.

4291 Whole Person: Kansas City
3710 Main Street
Kansas City, MO 64111-7501

816-561-0304
800-878-3037
FAX: 816-931-0529
TTY: 816-627-2202
info@thewholeperson.org
www.thewholeperson.org

Rick O'Neal, President
Jim Atwater, Vice President
Julie Dejean, CEO
Mike Wiley, COO

Assists people with disabilities to live independently and encourages change within the community to expand opportunities for independent living.

Montana

4292 Living Independently for Today and Tomorrow
1201 Grand Avenue
Suite 1
Billings, MT 59102-2033

406-259-5181
800-669-6319
FAX: 406-259-5259
TTY: 406-245-1225
beckerb@midrivers.com
www.liftt.org

Bobbie Becker, Executive Director
Martha Carstensen, Program Director

LIFTT's Independent living program works with people with disabilities so they can live independently and have access to the community. LIFTT staff, most of whom have disabilities, serve as mentors to people as they work to achieve the goals they have set for themselves.

4293 Montana Independent Living Project, Inc.
825 Great Northern Blvd
Suite 105
Helena, MT 59601-4715

406-442-5755
800-735-6457
FAX: 406-442-1612
TTY: 406-442-5755
bmaffit@milp.us
www.milp.us

Bob Maffit, Executive Director
Les Clark, Independent Living Specialist
Charlene White, Financial Manager
Marie Largent, Office Manager

A not-for-profit agency that provides services that promote independence for people with disabilities.

4294 North Central Independent Living Services
1120 25th Ave
Black Eagle, MT 59414-1037

406-452-9834
800-823-6245
FAX: 406-453-3940
ncils.osborn@sofast.net

Tom Osborn, Executive Director

North Central Independent Living Services is located in Great Falls and provides services from Glacier County across the

Hi-Line to the North Dakota border. A satellite office is set up in Glasgow.

4295   Summit Independent Living Center: Kalispell
1203 Highway 2 W.
Suite #35
Kalispell, MT 59901-6020   406-257-0048
                                      800-995-0029
                                  FAX: 406-257-0634
                                  TTY: 406-257-0048
                                  webmaster@bils.org
                                  www.summitilc.org

Steve Hackler, President
Larry Riley, Vice President
Jenny Montgomery, Secretary
Flo Kiewel, Manager
To promote community awareness, equal access, and the independence of people with disabilities through advocacy, education, and the advancement of civil rights.

4296   Summit Independent Living Center: Hamilton
316 North 3rd St
Suite #113
Hamilton, MT 59840-2479   406-363-5242
                                      800-398-9013
                                  FAX: 406-375-9035
                                  webmaster@bils.org
                                  www.summitilc.org

Steve Hackler, President
Larry Riley, Vice President
Jenny Montgomery, Secretary
Joanne Berwolf, Manager
To promote community awareness, equal access, and the independence of people with disabilities through advocacy, education, and the advancement of civil rights.

4297   Summit Independent Living Center: Missoula
700 SW Higgins Ave
Suite #101
Missoula, MT 59803-1489   406-728-1630
                                      800-398-9002
                                  FAX: 406-829-3309
                                  missoula@summitilc.org
                                  www.summitilc.org

Steve Hackler, President
Larry Riley, Vice President
Jenny Montgomery, Secretary
Mike Mayer, Executive Director
To promote community awareness, equal access, and the independence of people with disabilities through advocacy, education, and the advancement of civil rights.

4298   Summit Independent Living Center: Ronan
124 Main St.
Ronan, MT 59864-2718   406-215-1604
                                      866-230-6936
                                  FAX: 406-552-1028
                                  ronan@summitilc.org
                                  www.summitilc.org

Steve Hackler, President
Larry Riley, Vice President
Jenny Montgomery, Secretary
Gary Stevens, Manager
To promote community awareness, equal access, and the independence of people with disabilities through advocacy, education, and the advancement of civil rights.

Nebraska

4299   Center for Independent Living of Central Nebraska
3335 West Capital Street
Grand Island, NE 68803-1730   308-382-9255
                                      877-400-1004
                                  FAX: 308-384-7832
                                  TTY: 308-382-9255
                                  jthomas@cilne.org
                                  www.cilne.org

Joni Thomas, Executive Director
Irene Britt, Western Program Manager
Lesia Gracia, Independent Living Specialist
Mike Niece, Driving Program Coordinator
Offers independent living skills training, peer sharing, information and referral, housing counseling and referral, accessibility and barrier removal consultation including ADA training and technical assistance, driver education and training, assistive technology services including demonstration and equipment loan, and a free lending library of adapted toys and ability switches for children with severe disabilities. Serves all diabilities and all ages.

4300   League of Human Dignity: Lincoln
1701 P St
Lincoln, NE 68508-1799   402-441-7871
                                      888-508-4758
                                  FAX: 402-441-7650
                                  TTY:402-441-7871
                                  info@leagueofhumandignity.com
                                  www.leagueofhumandignity.com

Mike Schafer, CEO
The mission of the League of Human Dignity is to actively promote the full integration of individuals with disabilities into society. To this end, we will advocate their needs and rights, and provide quality services to involve these persons in becoming and remaining independent citizens.

4301   League of Human Dignity: Norfolk
400 Elm Ave
Norfolk, NE 68701-4033   402-371-4475
                                      800-843-5785
                                  FAX: 402-371-4625
                                  TTY: 402-371-4475
                                  ninfo@leagueofhumandignity.com
                                  leagueofhumandignity.com

Mike Shafer, CEO
Jean M. Kloppenborg, Norfolk CIL Director
The mission of the League of Human Dignity is to actively promote the full integration of individuals with disabilities into society. To this end, we will advocate their needs and rights, and provide quality services to involve these persons in becoming and remaining independent citizens.

4302   League of Human Dignity: Omaha
5513 Center St
Omaha, NE 68106-3001   402-595-1256
                                      800-843-5784
                                  FAX: 402-595-1410
                                  oinfo@leagueofhumandignity.com
                                  www.leagueofhumandignity.com

Mike Schafer, CEO
Bob Gomez, Executive Director
The mission of the League of Human Dignity is to actively promote the full integration of individuals with disabilities into society. To this end, we will advocate their needs and rights, and provide quality services to involve these persons in becoming and remaining independent citizens.

4303 Mosaic of Axtell Bethpage Village
1044 23rd Rd.
PO Box 67
Axtell, NE 68924
308-743-2401
FAX: 308-743-2659
www.mosaicinfo.org/axtell

Max Miller, Chairperson
James Zils, Vice Chairperson
Linda Timmons, President/ CEO
Raul Saldivar, COO

Provides services that respect the human diginity and rights of each person. An interdisciplinary team of family, staffmembers and professional consultatns support individuals served in developing personal goals and programs, helping them to fully participate in Axtell's community life. Mosaic at Axtell offers residential and community services.

4304 Mosaic of Beatrice
722 S. 12th St.
PO Box 607
Beatrice, NE 68310-607
402-223-4066
FAX: 402-223-4951
jerry.campbell@mosaicinfo.org
www.mosaicinfo.org/beatrice

Max Miller, Chairperson
James Zils, Vice Chairperson
Linda Timmons, President/ CEO
Raul Saldivar, COO

Provides individualized services, living options, work choices, spiritual nurture and advocacy to people with disabilities in more than 250 communities across 14 states and Great Britain through the work of 4,800 employees.

4305 Mosiac: York
220 W South 21st St
York, NE 68467-9316
402-362-2180
FAX: 402-362-2961
www.mosaicinfo.org

Max Miller, Chairperson
James Zils, Vice Chairperson
Linda Timmons, President/ CEO
Raul Saldivar, COO

Providing a wide array of services to assist individuals and families in achieving positive life goals. Services to persons with disabilities and other special needs include community living options, training and employment options, spiritual growth and development options, training and counseling support.

Nevada

4306 Carson City Center for Independent Living
900 Mallory Way
Carson City, NV 89701
775-841-2580

Sandra Coyle, Owner

Helps consumers continue to live independently in the community through a variety of individual and community services.

4307 Northern Nevada Center for Independent Living: Fallon
1919 Grimes St
Suite B
Fallon, NV 89406-3100
775-423-4900
800-885-3712
FAX: 775-423-1399
TTY: 775-423-4900
nncilf@cccomm.net
www.nncil.org

Lisa Bonie, Executive Director
Hilda Velasco, Operations Manager
Joni Inglis, Independent Living Advocate
Deb Maijala, Rural Services Coordinator
Independent Living Center.

4308 Rural Center for Independent Living
1895 E Long St
Carson City, NV 89706-3214
775-841-2580
FAX: 775-841-2580
ruralcil@yahoo.com

Dee Dee Foremaster, Executive Director

Advocacy, Benefit Assistance, social security assistance, peer support, housing information and home-less day drop-in center for individuals with disabilities.

4309 Southern Nevada Center for Independent Living: North Las Vegas
3100 E Lake Mead Blvd
North Las Vegas, NV 89030-7380
702-649-3822
800-398-0760
FAX: 702-649-5022
TTY: 702-649-3822
sncilnv@aol.com
www.sncil.org

Connie Kratky, President
Elliot Yug, Vice - President
Pamela Rake, Secretary
William Sheehan, Treasurer
SNCIL is committed to removing barriers preventing indpendent living by providing services designed to empower people with disabilities.

4310 Southern Nevada Center for Independent Living: Las Vegas
2950 S. Rainbow Blvd.
Suite 220
Las Vegas, NV 89146-5611
702-889-4216
800-870-7003
FAX: 702-889-4574
TTY: 702-889-4216
sncil2@aol.com
www.sncil.org

Connie Kratky, President
Elliot Yug, Vice - President
Pamela Rake, Secretary
William Sheehan, Treasurer
SNCIL is committed to removing barriers preventing Independent Living by providing services designed to empower people with disabilities.

New Hampshire

4311 Granite State Independent Living Foundation
21 Chenell Drive
Concord, NH 3301-4079
603-228-9680
800-826-3700
FAX: 603-444-3128
TTY: 603-228-9680
info@gsil.org
www.gsil.org

Ken Traum, Chair
Lorna D. Greer, Vice Chair
Clyde E. Terry, CEO
Deborah Krider, COO

GSIL is a statewide non-profit that recognizes the fact that all of us will need some type of support in the course of the lives. GSIL offers tools and resources so that individuals can participate as fully as the choose in their lives, families and communities. Contact the Independent Living Foundation for referrals to living situations.

New Jersey

4312 Alliance Center for Independance
Alliance for Disabled in Action
629 Amboy Ave, First Floor
Edison, NJ 08837-3579

732-738-4388
FAX: 732-738-4416
TTY:732-738-9644
adacil@adacil.org
www.adacil.org

Colleen Roche, Chair
Bernard Zuckerman, Treasurer
Carole Tonks, Executive Director
Luke Koppisch, Deputy Director
Alliance for Disabled in Action is a private, not-for-profit center for independent living serving people in Middlesex, Somerset and Union Counties of New Jersey. ADA's mission is to support and promote choice, self-direction and independent living in the lives of people with disabilities, with the right of individuals to inclusion in the community as the primary goal.

4313 Camden City Independent Living Center
2600 Mount Ephraim Ave
Camden, NJ 8104-3236

856-966-0800
FAX: 856-966-0832
TTY:856-966-0830
vedasmithccilc@aol.com
www.camdencityilc.org

Bruce Smith, Chairperson
John Quann, Vice Chairperson
Tanya Brown, Treasurer
Veda Smith, Executive Director
Provides services designed to empower people with disabilities. To provide services to individuals with significant disabilities. Services include information referral, advocacy, peer support, and independent living skills training. CCILC services individuals in Camden City

4314 Center for Independent Living: Long Branch
279 Broadway
Suite #201
Long Branch, NJ 7740-6940

732-571-4884
FAX: 732-571-4003
TTY:732-571-4878
www.moceanscil.org

Jennifer Sterner, Vice Chair
Maureen Poling, Secretary
Stan Soden, Director IL Services
Susan Pniewski, IL Transition Specialist
Offers peer support, disability education and personal assistant services. Serving Monmouth and Ocean Counties with information and referrals, advocacy, peer support and independent living instructions.

4315 Center for Independent Living: South Jersey
1150 Delsea Drive
Suite #1
Westville, NJ 8093-2251

856-853-6490
800-413-3791
FAX: 856-853-1466
TTY: 856-853-7602
cilsj@verizon.net
www.cilsj.org

Hazel Lee-Briggs, Executive Director
Danuta Debicki, Program Manager
Terryama Davis, Independent Living Specialist
Dedicated to providing people with disabilities in Gloucester and Camden counties the opportunity to actively participate in society, to provide freedom of choice, to work, to own a home, raise a family and in general, to participate to the fullest extent in day-to-day activities. The center provides information and referrals, advocacy, peer support, and independent living skills training.

4316 DAWN Center for Independent Living
66 Ford Road
Suite 121
Denville, NJ 7834-1235

973-625-1940
888-383-3296
FAX: 973-625-1942
TTY: 973-625-1932
info@dawncil.org
www.dawncil.org

Elizabeth Lehmann, President
Gabrielle Waldman, Vice President
Carmela Slivinski, Executive Director
Caroleen Marano, Independent Living Program
DAWN is the Center for Independent Living serving Morris, Sussex and Warren counties. DAWN empowers people with disabilities to strive for equality and to take control of their own lives by providing the tools that encourage independence and self-advocacy, promoting public awareness of the needs, desires and rights to individuals living with disabilities, and offering community activities that create new experiences and opportunities.

4317 Dial: Disabled Information Awareness & Living
2 Prospect Village Plaza
Floor 1
Clifton, NJ 7013-1918

973-470-8090
866-277-1733
FAX: 973-470-8171
TTY: 973-470-2521
info@dial-cil.org
www.dial-cil.org

Cynthia DeSouza, President
Anthony Gianduso, Vice President
John Petix, Executive Director
Tim Burns, Secretary
Promotes the full inclusion of all people living with disabilities into society and encourage the consumers and the community at large to seek involvement in this self-governing organization to the fullest extent.

4318 Disability Rights New Jersey
New Jersey Protection and Advocacy
210 S. Broad Street
Floor 3
Trenton, NJ 08608-2407

609-292-9742
800-922-7233
FAX: 609-777-0187
TTY: 609-633-7106
advocate@drnj.org
www.drnj.org

Walter Anthony Woodberry, Chair
Andrew McGeady, Vice Chair
Linda K. Soley, Treasurer
Leah Ziskin, Secretary
Assistive Technology Advocacy Center provides assistance to personswith disabilities in helping them to obtain assistive technology devices and/or services.

4319 Family Resource Associates
35 Haddon Ave
Shrewsbury, NJ 7702-4007

732-747-5310
FAX: 732-747-1896
info@frainc.org
www.frainc.org

Allan Proske, President
Bill Sheeser, Vice President
John Feeney, Treasurer
Judy Fuller, Secretary
FRA is dedicated to helping children, adolescents and people of all ages with disabilities to reach their fullest potential. FRA also connects individuals to independence through modern therapies and advanced technology. FRA provides direct services to those in the greater Nonmouth/Ocean County area.

4320 Heightened Independence and Progress: Hackensack
131 Main St
Suite #120
Hackensack, NJ 7601-7182   201-996-9100
FAX: 201-996-9422
TTY:201-966-9424
ber@hipcil.org
www.hipcil.org

Eileen Goff, President/CEO
Trish Carney, Finance and Development Director
Empowers people with disabilities to achieve independent living through outreach, advocacy and education.

4321 Heightened Independence and Progress: Jersey City
35 Journal Square
Suite #703
Jersey City, NJ 7306-4105   201-533-4407
FAX: 201-533-4421
TTY:201-533-4409
hud@hipcil.org
www.hipcil.org

Jean Csaposs, Board Chair
Lottie Esteban, First Vice Chair
Eileen Goff, President/CEO
Trish Carney, Finance and Development Director
Empowering People with Disabilities to Achieve Independent Living through Outreach, Advocacy, and Education.

4322 Progressive Center for Independent Living
3525Quakerbridge Rd.
Suite 904
Hamilton, NJ 8619-3710   609-581-4500
877-917-4500
FAX: 609-581-4555
TTY: 609-581-4550
info@pcil.org
www.pcil.org

Norman Smith, President
John Witman, Vice President
Scott Elliott, Executive Director
Jerry Carbone, Training Coordinator
Advocates for the rights of people with disabilities to achieve and maintain independent lifestyles. The Center has programs to assist with employment, transition from school to adult life, and emergency preparedness.

4323 Progressive Center for Independent Living: Flemington
4 Walter E Foran Blvd
Suite 410
Flemington, NJ 8822-4669   908-782-1055
877-376-9174
FAX: 908-782-6025
TTY: 908-782-1081
info@pcil.org
pcil.org

Norman Smith, President
John Witman, Vice President
Scott Elliott, Executive Director
Jerry Carbone, Training Coordinator
Advocates for the rights of people with disabilities to achieve and maintain independent lifestyles.

4324 Project Freedom
223 Hutchinson Rd
Robbinsville, NJ 8691-3457   609-448-2998
FAX: 609-448-7293
ProjectFreedom1@aol.com
www.projectfreedom.org

Tim Doherty, Executive Director
Norman A. Smith, Assoc Ex Director
Elizabeth Maxwell, Office Manager
Paul Campanella, Property Manager
Dedicated to developing, supporting, and advocating opportunities for independent living persons with disabilities.

4325 Project Freedom: Hamilton
715 Kuser Rd
Hamilton, NJ 8619-3924   609-588-9919
FAX: 609-588-8831
cfunk@projectfreedom.org
www.projectfreedom.org

Cecilia Funk, Social Service Coordinator
Judy Wilkinson, Office Manager
Paul Campanella, Property Manager
Dedicated to developing, supporting, and advocating opportunities for independent living persons with disabilities.

4326 Project Freedom: Lawrence
1 Freedom Blvd
Lawrence, NJ 8648-4531   609-278-0075
FAX: 609-278-1250
jelsowiny@projectfreedom.org
www.projectfreedom.org

Jacklene Elsowiny, Social Serv Coordinator
Tim Doherty, Executive Director
Stephen Schaefer, CFO
Tracee Battis, Director of Housing Development
Dedicated to developing, supporting, and advocating opportunities for independent living persons with disabilities.

4327 Total Living Center
6712 Washington Ave
Egg Harbor Township, NJ 8234-1999   609-645-9547
FAX: 609-813-2318
TTY:609-645-9593
info@tlcenter.org
www.tlcenter.org

Jo Hudson, President
Cliff Anderson, Vice President
Cathy Shaner, Secretary
Julia Bonelli, Executive Director
Total Living Center is a non-profit organization whose mission is to empower individuals with significant disabilities to maximize their potential for independence and productivity, to live as fully as possible within the community, taking responsibility for themselves, and sharing this commitment with others.

New Mexico

4328 Ability Center
715 E. Idaho Ave
Building 3E
Las Cruces, NM 88001-4702   575-526-5016
800-376-4372
FAX: 575-526-1202
TTY: 505-526-5016
freedom@theabilitycenter.org
www.theabilitycenter.org

Vincent Montano, Executive Director
Cesar Rodriguez, Vice-President
C. Neil Gibbs, Treasurer
The Ability Center is a private, nonresidential, nonprofit, New Mexico corporation. As a center for independent living (CIL) TACIL provides a variety of services to promote independence, self-reliance, and community integration. Our professional staff and active board of directors are dedicated to helping our consumers maintain their personal freedom at home, in the community, and throughout the state.

4329 CASA Inc.
116 West Baltimore Street
Hagerstown, MD 21740   301-739-4990
FAX: 301-790-0064
casa4@myactv.net
www.casaabq.com

Sherry Donovan, President
Linda Davis, Vice-President
Melinda Marsden, Treasurer
Laura Allis, Secretary
Offers peer counseling and information and referral services.

4330   CHOICES Center for Independent Living
200 E 4th St.
Suite #200
Roswell, NM 88201-6237   575-627-6727
                                       800-387-4572
                                  FAX: 575-627-6754
                                  TTY: 505-627-6727

Julia Calvert, Executive Director
Offers many core services including independent living skills
training, peer support, information and referral, advocacy and
transition.

4331   New Mexico Technology Assistance Program
625 Silver Ave. SW
Ste. 100 B
Albuquerque, NM 87102   505-841-4464
                                       877-696-1470
                                  FAX: 505-841-4467
                                  TTY: 800-659-4915
                          Tracy.Agiovlasitis@state.nm.us
                               www.tap.gcd.state.nm.us

Julie Martinez, Program Director
Tracy Agiovlasitis, Supervisor
Samuel Castillo, Coordinator
Jesse Armijo, Specialist
Examines and works to eliminate barriers to obtaining assistive
technology in New Mexico. Has established a statewide program
for coordinating assistive technology services; is designed to assist people with disabilities to locate, secure, and maintain
assistive technology.

4332   New Vistas
1205 Parkway Dr.
Suite A
Santa Fe, NM 87501-2483   505-471-1001
                                  FAX: 505-471-4427
                                  info@newvistas.org
                                    www.newvistas.org

Victor Ortega, President
Libby Gonzales, Vice-President
Gay Romero, Secretary/Treasurer
Partners with and supports people with disabilities and families
of children with special needs to enrich their quality of life in
New Mexico.

4333   San Juan Center for Independence
1204 San Juan Blvd
Farmington, NM 87401   505-566-5827
                                       877-484-4500
                                  FAX: 505-566-5842
                                  TTY: 505-566-5827
                                        sjci@sjci.org
                                          www.sjci.org

Patricia Ziegler, Executive Director
Tim Carver, CFO
SJCI is a New Mexico private non residential, nonprofit corporation that serves people with disabilities. The purpose of SJCI is to
provide a variety of community based, consumer driven service
to people with disablities to promote independence, self-resi-
dence and intergration into the community.

New York

4334   AIM Independent Living Center: Corning
271 E 1st St
Corning, NY 14830-2924   607-962-8225
                                  FAX: 607-937-5125
                                  TTY: 607-962-8225
                                   troche@aimcil.com
                                     www.aimcil.com

Rene Snyder, Executive Director
Sabrina Mineo-O'Connell, President
George Spisack, Vice President
Barbara Squires, Treasurer
AIM is a non-profit organization dedicated to people with disabilities, their families, friends, the businesses that serve them
and those with an interest in disabilities. The mission of AIM is to
support the individuals ability to make independent, self-direct-
ing choices through education, advocacy, information and
referral.

4335   AIM Independent Living Center: Elmira
650 Baldwin St.
Elmira, NY 14901-2216   607-733-3718
                                  FAX: 607-733-0180
                                  TTY: 607-733-7764
                                   troche@aimcil.com
                                     www.aimcil.com

Rene Snyder, Executive Director
Sabrina Mineo-O'Connell, President
George Spisack, Vice President
Barbara Squires, Treasurer
AIM's goal is to enable the consumer to live an independent and
comfortable lifestyle in the security of their home environment so
they may feel dignity and pride in their achievements while
controling their own care.

4336   ARISE
635 James St
Syracuse, NY 13203-2661   315-472-3171
                                  FAX: 315-472-9252
                                  TTY: 315-479-6363
                                    info@ariseinc.org
                                     www.ariseinc.org

Tania Anderson, President
Sue Judge, Vice President
Michael Cook, Treasurer
Tom McKeown, Executive Director
Founded in 1979, ARISE's mission is to work with people of all
abilities to create a fair and just community in which everyone
can fully participate. As a center for independent living, ARISE
is a non-profit organization run by and for individuals with disabilities. ARISE serves over 3,000 children and adults with disabilities each year through our programs and services in several
broad areas including advocacy, employment, independent liv-
ing/integrated recreation programs, and much more.

4337   ARISE: Oneida
131 Main St
Suite #107
Oneida, NY 13421-1644   315-363-4672
                                  FAX: 315-363-4675
                                  TTY: 315-363-2364
                                    info@ariseinc.org
                                     www.ariseinc.org

Tania Anderson, President
Sue Judge, Vice President
Michael Cook, Treasurer
Tom McKeown, Executive Director
A consumer controlled, non-profit Independent Living Center
that promotes the full inclusion of people with disabilities in the
community.

4338   ARISE: Oswego
9 Fourth Avenue
Oswego, NY 13126-1803   315-342-4088
                                  FAX: 315-342-4107
                                  TTY: 315-342-8696
                                    info@ariseinc.org
                                     www.ariseinc.org

Tania Anderson, President
Sue Judge, Vice President
Michael Cook, Treasurer
Tom McKeown, Executive Director
A consumer controlled, non-profit Independent Living Center
that promotes the full inclusion of people with disabilities in the
community.

4339 ARISE: Pulaski
2 Broad St
Pulaski, NY 13142-4446   315-298-5726
                                    FAX: 315-298-5729
                                    info@ariseinc.org
                                    www.ariseinc.org

Tania Anderson, President
Sue Judge, Vice President
Michael Cook, Treasurer
Tom McKeown, Executive Director

A consumer controlled, non-profit Independent Living Center
that promotes the full inclusion of people with disabilities in the
community.

4340 Access to Independence of Cortland County, Inc.
26 N Main St
Cortland, NY 13045-2198   607-753-7363
                                    FAX: 607-756-4884
                                    info@aticortland.org
                                    www.aticortland.org

Judy Bentley, Chair
Peter Morse-Ackley, Vice Chair
Chad W. Underwood, CEO
Mary E. Ewing, Program Manager

Access to Independence is Cortland County's foremost disability
resource. It empowers people to lead independent lives in their
community and strives to open doors to full participation and
access for all.

4341 Action Toward Independence: Middletown
130 Dolson Avenue
Suite 35
Middletown, NY 10940-6563   845-343-4284
                                    FAX: 845-342-5269
                                    ati@warwick.net
                                    actiontowardindependence.org
Stephen McLaughlin, Executive Director
Joann Hargabus, Services Director, Orange Cnty.
Gilles Malkine, Services Director, Sullivan Cnty
Cheryl Babcock, Fiscal Manager

Independent living center that serves Orange & Sullivan counties. Provides programs and services to individuals who have disabilities and to their families. These services include peer
counseling, individual & systems advocacy, independent living,
skills training, information and referral, benefits advisement,
recreation and a drop in center. We are designed to enable people
with disabilities to achieve independence, inclusion and
participation in their communities.

4342 Action Toward Independence: Monticello
309 E Broadway
Suite A
Monticello, NY 12701-8810   845-794-4228
                                    FAX: 845-794-4475
                                    TTY:845-794-4228
                                    szecchini@atitoday.org
                                    www.atitoday.org
Steve McLaughlin, Executive Director
Joann Hargabus, Director of Services

A not-for-profit, non residential, peer run, referral and advocacy
agency for persons with disaiblities in Orange and Sullivan counties. Our services are aimed at promoting accessibility, community integration, and equal opportunity in all aspects of society
for persons with all types of disabilities.

4343 Bronx Independent Living Services
4419 Thrid Avenue
Suite 2C
Bronx, NY 10457   718-515-2800
                                    FAX: 718-515-2844
                                    TTY:718-515-2803
                                    webmaster@bils.org
                                    www.bils.org

Barbara Linn, President
Anita Richichi, Vice President
Sheldon Mann, Treasurer
Brett L. Eisenberg, Executive Director

BILS is a not-for-profit community agency serving people with
all kinds of disabilities. The mission is to empower people with
disabilities toward living independent lives. BILS assists individuals by providing advocacy, peer counseling, housing information, and independent living training/counseling.

4344 Brooklyn Center for Independence of the Disabled
27 Smith Street
Suite #200
Brooklyn, NY 11201   718-998-3000
                                    FAX: 718-998-3743
                                    TTY:718-998-7406
                                    advocate@bcid.org
                                    www.bcid.org

Joan Peters, Executive Director
Sandrina Kingston, Program Director
Princess Davis, Office Manager
Stanley Stephen, Office Assistant

Operated by a majority of people with disabilities, BCID is dedicated to guaranteeing the civil rights of people with disabilities.
BCID exists to improve the quality of life of brooklyn residents
with disabilities thgouh programs that empower them to gain
greater control of their lives and achieve full and equal
integration into society.

4345 Capital District Center for Independence
845 Central Ave
South 3
Albany, NY 12206-1342   518-459-6422
                                    FAX: 518-459-7847
                                    TTY:518-459-6422
                                    info@cdciweb.com
                                    www.cdciweb.com

Laurel Kelley, Executive Director
Dawn Werner, Deputy Director
Judy Zuchero, Program Director
G. W. Barr, Advocate

One of 37 Independent Living Centers in New York State, the
Center is a non-residential, community based organization,
which primarily serves Albany and Schenetady Counties. The
Center's mission is to assist people with disabilities to acquire
self-advocacy skills and by teaching through example, consumers achieve greater control over the direction of their lives.

4346 Catskill Center for Independence
6104 State Highway 23
Oneonta, NY 13820   607-432-8000
                                    FAX: 607-432-6907
                                    TTY:607-432-8000
                                    ccfi@ccfi.us
                                    www.ccfi.us

Chris Zachmeyer, Executive Director
Christine Worden, Assistant Director

One of 37 community-based independent living centers located
throughout the state of New York. As an advocacy agency, we
provide a variety of services to people with disabilities, their
friends and family members. In addition, we provide advocacy,
training, and technical assistance to our community members, organizations, businesses and state and local governments in a variety of disability related areas. Serves Otsego, Delaware and
Schoharie counties.

4347 Center for Community Alternatives
115 E Jefferson St
Suite #300
Syracuse, NY 13202-2018   315-422-5638
                                    FAX: 315-471-4924
                                    cca@communityalternatives.org
                                    www.communityalternatives.org

Kwame Johnson, President
Susan R. Horn, Esq., Vice-President
Carole A. Eady, Secretary
Marsha Weissman, Executive Director

Promotes reintegrative justice and a reduced reliance on incarcer-
ation through advocacy, services and public policy development
in pursuit of civil and human rights.

4348   Center for Independence of the Disabled of New York
80-02 Kkew Garden Rd.
Suite 107
Kew Gardens, NY 11415   646-442-1520
FAX: 347-561-4883
TTY:718-886-0427
info@cidny.org
www.cidny.org

Martin Eichel, President
Anne M. Davis, Vice President
John O'Neill, Vice President
Susan Dooha, Executive Director
To ensure full integration, independence and equal opportunity
for all people with disabilities by removing barriers to the social,
economic, cultural and civic life of the community.

4349   Center for Independence of the Disabled of New York
841 Broadway
Suite #301
New York, NY 10003-4708   212-674-2300
FAX: 212-254-5953
TTY:212-674-5619
info@cidny.org
www.cidny.org

Martin Eichel, President
Anne M. Davis, Vice President
John O'Neill, Vice President
Susan Dooha, Executive Director
To ensure full integration, independence and equal opportunity
for all people with disabilities by removing barriers to the social,
economic, cultural and civic life of the community.

4350   DD Center/St Lukes: Roosevelt Hospital Center
St Lukes Roosevelt
1000 10th Ave
New York, NY 10019-1192   212-473-2045
FAX: 212-473-0501

Charles Raimondo, VP
Farooq Chaudry, MD
Independent living center that advocates for people with disabilities by assisting with the application process of housing, benefits,
etc.

4351   Finger Lakes Independence Center
215 5th St
Ithaca, NY 14850-3403   607-272-2433
FAX: 607-272-0902
TTY:607-272-2433
flic@clarityconnect.com
www.fliconline.org

Lenore Schwager, Executive Director
FLIC assists all people with disabilities, their families and
friends to promote independence and make informed decisions in
pursuit of their goals. The servides provided are free of charge,
and services are primarily served to residents of Tompkins,
Schyler counties.

4352   Harlem Independent Living Center
289 St. Nicholas Avenue
Suite #21
New York, NY 10027- 4805   212-222-7122
800-673-2371
FAX: 212-222-7199
harlemilc@aol.com
www.hilc.org

Christina Curry, Executive Director
Edward Randolph, Resource Specialist
Dr. Herbert Thornhill, Emeritus
Vanessa J. Young, Chair
A non-profit agency that advocates for people with disabilities by
assisting with the application process of housing, benefits, etc.
Our services are free of charge.
Monthly

4353   Independent Living
5 Washington Terrace
Newburgh, NY 12550-5383   845-565-1162
FAX: 845-565-0567
TTY:845-565-0337
info@myindependentliving.org
www.myindependentliving.org

Matthew Migliaccio, President
Charles Walwyn, III, Vice President
Douglas J. Hovey, Executive Director
Anne Miller, Director of Development
A consumer directed, cross-disability advocacy organization
dedicated to enhancing quality of life for persons with
disabilities.

4354   Long Island Center for Independent Living
3601 Hempstead Tpke
Suites 208 & 500
Levittown, NY 11756-1331   516-796-0144
FAX: 516-520-1247
TTY:516-794-0135
licil@aol.com
www.licil.net

Joan Lynch, Executive Director
LICIL is committed to the empowerment of consumers with disabilities. LICIL staff functions as ambassadors to the belief that
individuals with disabilities have a responsibility to take an active role in their own lives and self determined view of their
futures.

4355   Massena Independent Living Center
156 Center St
Massena, NY 13662-1495   315-764-9442
877-397-9613
FAX: 315-764-9464
TTY: 315-764-9442
mindepli@twcny.rr.com
www.milcinc.org

Jeff Reifensnyder, Executive Director
Courtnie Toms, Deputy Director
Provides a variety of non-residential direct services as well as ed-
ucating the public through community awareness campaigns.
Also seeks to address the current appropriate unmet needs of per-
sons experiencing a disability - primarily in St Lawrence and
Franklin Counties.

4356   NYS Independent Living Council
111 Washington Ave
Suite #101
Albany, NY 12210-2280   518-427-1060
877-397-4126
FAX: 518-427-1139
bradw@nysilc.org
www.nysilc.org

Brad Williams, Executive Director
Patty Black, Administrative Assistant
Provides support and technical assistance to 37 independent living centers-community-based organizations directed by and for
people with disabilities.

4357   Nassau County Office for the Physically Challenged
60 Charles Lindberg Blvd
Uniondale, NY 11553-4812   516-227-7399
www.nassaucountyny.gov

Edward P. Mangano, County Executive
This agency serves as the ADA compliance coordinating office
for all Nassau County governmental facilities, programs and services. It also serves in an advisory capacity to local, regional and
national policy-making organizations, planning committees and
legislative bodies and conducts advocacy as well as direct programs and services to enhance inclusion by people with disabilities to employment, consumerism and transportation.

4358 North Country Center for Independent Living
80 Sharron Avenue
Plattsburgh, NY 12901-3827
518-563-9058
FAX: 518-563-0292
TTY: 518-563-9058
andrew@ncci-online.com
www.ncci-online.com

Ted Graser, President
Kathy Latinville, Vice President
Robert Poulin, Executive Director
Deb Piper, Program Director
To empower people with disabilities to live more independent and productive lives, and to promote beneficial policies and community understanding of disability issues.

4359 Northern Regional Center for Independent Living: Watertown
210 Court St
Suite #107
Watertown, NY 13601-4546
315-785-8703
800-585-8703
FAX: 315-785-8612
TTY: 315-785-8704
nrcil@nrcil.net
www.nrcil.net

Ronald Griffin, Chair
Michael Simmons, Vice Chair
Melanie Adkins, Secretary
Aileen Martin, Executive Director
A disability rights and resource center that promotes community efforts to end discrimination, segregation, and prejudice against people with disabilities.

4360 Northern Regional Center for Independent Living: Lowville
7632 N State St
Lowville, NY 13367-1318
315-376-8696
FAX: 315-376-3404
TTY: 315-376-8696
karenb@nrcil.net
www.nrcil.net

Ronald Griffin, Chair
Michael Simmons, Vice Chair
Melanie Adkins, Secretary
Aileen Martin, Executive Director
A disability rights and resource center that promotes community efforts to end discrimination, segregation, and prejudice against people with disabilities.

4361 Options for Independence: Auburn
75 Genesee St
Auburn, NY 13021-3667
315-255-3447
FAX: 315-255-0836
gguy@optionsforindependence.org
www.ariseinc.org

Tania Anderson, President
Sue Judge, Vice President
Michael Cook, Treasurer
Tom McKeown, Executive Director
Options for Independence is an Independent Living Center which assists people with disabilities to gain opportunities, make their own decisions, pursue activities and become part of comunity life. Options provides a variety of services to all people with disabilities, their families, friends, and service providers in Cayuga and Seneca Counties.

4362 Putnam Independent Living Services
1961 Route 6
2nd Floor
Carmel, NY 10512-2324
845-228-7457
FAX: 845-228-7460
TTY: 866-933-5390
info@wilc.org
www.putnamils.org

Joe Bravo, Executive Director
Mildred Caballero-Ho, Deputy Executive Director
Margaret Valenzuela, Program Director, IL Services
Jessica Baumann, Program Director, Educational Ad

A non-profit, community-based advocacy and resource center that serves people with all types of disabilities.

4363 Regional Center for Independent Living
497 State St
Rochester, NY 14608-1642
585-442-6470
FAX: 585-271-8558
TTY: 585-442-6470
bdarling@rcil.org
www.rcil.org

Shelly Perrin, Chairperson
Bobbi Wallach, Vice Chairperson
Bruce E Darling, Executive Director
Jennifer Smouse, Director of Finance
To empower people with disabilities to self-advocate, to live independently and to enhance the quality of community life.

4364 Resource Center for Accessible Living
727 Ulster Ave
Kingston, NY 12401-1709
845-331-0541
FAX: 845-331-2076
TTY: 845-331-4527
office@rcal.org
www.rcal.org

Paul Scarpati, President
Paula Kindos-Carberry, Co-Vice President
Bernadette Mueller, Co-Vice President
Susan Hoger, RCAL Executive Director
RCAL is a non-profit, community based service and advocacy run by and for people with any type of disability. RCAL is dedicated to assisting and empowering individuals, of all ages, to live independently and participate in all aspects of community life.

4365 Resource Center for Independent Living
347 W Main St
Amsterdam, NY 12010-2225
518-842-3561
FAX: 518-842-0905
TTY: 518-842-3593
bdanovitz@rcil.com
www.rcil.ocom

Shelly Perrin, Chairperson
Bobbi Wallach, Vice Chairperson
Bruce E Darling, Executive Director
Jennifer Smouse, Director of Finance
Peer counseling, advocacy, independent living skills training, information and referral services, self-advocacy training, ADA consultation, home and community based services, community education, benefits advisement and more. All programs and services are available in English and Spanish.

4366 Rockland Independent Living Center
873 Route 45
Suite 108
New City, NY 10956-2712
845-624-1366
FAX: 845-624-1369
TTY: 845-624-0848
info@rilc.org
www.rilc.org

Audrey Rosenfield, President
Myrna Wulfson, Vice President / Secretary
David Aron, CPA, Treasurer
George Hoehmann M.A., Executive Director
RILC serves all individuals with disabilities. We promote philosophy consumer empowerment and control. The services we provide include benefit and advisement information and referral and consumer directed personal assistants.

4367 Southern Adirondack Independent Living
418 Geyser Rd
Country Club Plaza
Ballston Spa, NY 12020-6002
518-584-8202
FAX: 518-584-1195
sail@sail-center.org
www.sail-center.org

Karen Thayer, Executive Director
Anna Livingston, Assistant Director
Barbara Potvin, Executive Assistant
Michele Nicholson, Administrative Assistant

To assist individuals with disabilities to become independent empowered self-advocates.

4368   Southern Adirondack Independent Living Center
71 Glenwood Ave
Queensbury, NY 12804-1728

518-792-3537
FAX: 518-792-0979
TTY:518-792-0505
sail@sail-center.org
www.sail-center.org

Karen Thayer, Executive Director
Anna Livingston, Assistant Director
Shirley Dumont, Director of Advocacy
Barbara Potvin, Executive Assistant

To assist individuals with disabilities to become independent empowered self-advocates.

4369   Southern Tier Independence Center
135 E Frederick St
Binghamton, NY 13904-1224

607-724-2111
FAX: 607-772-3600
TTY:607-724-2111
stic@stic-cil.org
www.stic-cil.org

Maria Dibble, Executive Director
Frank Pennisi, Accessibility Services

STIC provides assistance and services to all people with disabilities of all ages to increase their independence in all aspects of integrated community life. STIC also serves their families and friends, and businesses, agencies, and goverments to enable them to better meet the needs of people with disabilities, and finally STIC educates and influences the community in pursuit of full inclusion of people with disabilities.

4370   Southwestern Independent Living Center
843 N Main St
Jamestown, NY 14701-3546

716-661-3010
FAX: 716-661-3011
TTY:716-661-3012
info@ilc-jamestown-ny.org
ilc-jamestown-ny.org

Marie T Carrubba, Executive Director
Linda Rumbaugh, Independent Living Specialist
Christine Ahlstrom, Independent Living Specialist
Helen Kern, Independent Living Specialist

A non-residential, private, nonprofit agency established to provide services throughout Chautauqua County that will assist individuals with disabilities in reaching maximum independence and an enriched quality of life.

4371   Staten Island Center for Independent Living, Inc.
470 Castleton Ave
Staten Island, NY 10301

718-720-9016
FAX: 718-720-9664
TTY:718-720-9870
ldesantis@siciliving.org
www.siciliving.org

Lorraine DeSantis, Executive Director
Claudia J. Stanton, Office Manager
Michelle Sabatino, Independent Living Specialist
John Mastellone, Community Consultant / Benefits

Mission is to provide all individuals with disabilities the information, life skills training, and facilitative assistance which contributes to independence, individuality, and integration in the community and provides the skills and knowledge necessary to function in the least restrictive, personally fulfilling, most self reliant and productive manner.

4372   Suffolk Independent Living Organization(SILO)
2111 Lakeland Ave.
Suite A
Ronkonkoma, NY 11779

631-880-7929
FAX: 631-946-6377
TTY:631-946-6585
www.siloinc.org/?

Edward Ahern, Manager
Glenn Campbell, Co-Executive Director

A not-for-profit organization that helps the disabled become more independent and more involved in the community by providing them with information on referrals on Housing, Education, Employment and Benefits.

4373   Taconic Resources for Independence
82 Washington St
Suite #214
Poughkeepsie, NY 12601-2305

845-452-3913
866-948-1094
FAX: 845-485-3196
tri@taconicresources.org
www.taconicresources.org

Cynthia L. Fiore, Executive Director
Patrick Muller, Program Director
Diane Barkstrom, Program Director/Staff Interpret
Jeanine Byrnes, Coordinator of Deaf & Hard of He

A center for independent living, benefits advisement information, and referral, advocacy, independent living skills, peer counseling, parent advocacy, sign language interpreters.

4374   Westchester Disabled on the Move
984 N. Broadway
Suite LL-10
Yonkers, NY 10701-1320

914-968-4717
FAX: 914-968-6137
info@wdom.org
www.wdom.org

Gail Cartenuto Cohn, President
Mattie Trupia, Vice President
Sandra Dolman, Secretary
Chandra Sookdeo, Assistant Recording Secretary

WDOM empowers people with disabilities to control their own lives; advocates for civil rights and a barrier free society; encourages people with disabilities to participate in the political process; educates government, business, other entities, and a society as a whole to understand, accept, and accommodate people with disabilities; creates an environment that inspires self-respect

4375   Westchester Independent Living Center
200 Hamilton Avenue
2nd Floor
White Plains, NY 10601- 1809

914-682-3926
FAX: 914-682-8518
TTY:866-933-5390
Contact@wilc.org
www.wilc.org

Joseph Bravo, Executive Director

A not-for-profit, community-based advocacy and resource center that serves people with all types of disabilities.

North Carolina

4376   Disability Awareness Network
609 Country Club Dr.
Suite C
Greenville, NC 27834-6210

252-353-5522
FAX: 252-353-5160
DAWNpittco@aol.com
consolidatedmachines.com

Jackie Hansley, Owner

Information and referral for diabled persons; peer counseling for diabled persons; advocacy on ADA issues; independent living skills and training.

4377   Disability Rights & Resources
5801 Executive Center Dr.
Suite #101
Charlotte, NC 28212-8870
704-537-0550
800-755-5749
FAX: 704-566-0507
TTY: 704-537-0550
mailto@disability-rights.org
www.disability-rights.org

Maura Chavez, President
Marta Fales, Vice President
Holly Howell, Secretary
Rick Griffiths, Treasurer
To guard the civil rights of people wtih disabilities by empowering ourselves and others to live as we choose.

4378   Joy: A Shabazz Center for Independent Living
235 N Greene St
Greensboro, NC 27401-2410
336-272-0501
FAX: 336-272-0575
TTY: 336-272-0501
aaron.shabazz@shabazzcenter.org
www.wangshuai.net

Aaron Shabazz, Executive Director
James Wells, President
Stephen Simpson, Vice-President
B. J. Gerald Covington, Secretary/Treasurer
A non-profit, consumer oriented, Center for Independent Living (CIL) providing advocacy, peer counseling and peer support, independent living skills, training, information and referrals, with other related services for persons with disabilites.

4379   Live Independently Networking Center
P.O.Box 1135
Newton, NC 28658-1135
828-464-0331
FAX: 828-464-7375
TTY: 828-464-2838
linc@twave.net
www.linconline.org

Donavon Kirby, Deputy Director
Private, nonprofit, federally funded center for independent living located in Western North Carolina.

4380   Live Independently Networking Center: Hickory
2830 16th St NE
Apt. 17
Hickory, NC 28601-8606
828-464-0331
FAX: 828-464-7375

4381   Pathways for the Future Center for Independent Living
525 Mineral Springs Dr
Sylva, NC 28779-9077
828-631-1167
FAX: 828-631-1169
TTY: 828-631-1167
bdavis@pathwayscil.org
www.pathwayscil.org

Barbara Davis, Executive Director
Dedicated to increasing independence, changing attitudes, promoting equal access and building a peer support network in western North Carolina through the use of community education, independent living services and advocacy.

4382   Western Alliance Center for Independent Living
30b London Rd
Asheville, NC 28803-2706
828-274-0444
FAX: 828-274-4461
wacil@main.nc.us
westernalliance.org

Katy Hollingsworth, Manager
Jerry Brewton, Independent Living Specialist
.

4383   Western Alliance for Independent Living
108 New Leicester Highway
Asheville, NC 28806
828-298-1977
FAX: 828-298-0875
khollingsworth@disabilitypartners.org
www.disabilitypartners.org

Kathy Hollingsworth, Associate Director
Rosemary Weaver, Independent Living Specialist
Mechelle Holt, Volunteer/Program Coordinator
Eva Reynolds, Emploment Network Coordinator

North Dakota

4384   Dakota Center for Independent Living: Dickinson
26-1st street East
Suite 103
Dickinson, ND 58601-5103
701- 48- 436
800-489-5013
FAX: 701- 48- 436
TTY: 800489501363
dcil@ndsupernet.com
www.dakotacil.org

Robin Were, President
Claudia Ziegler, Vice president
Carol Mihulka, Secretary/Treasurer
Royce Schultze, Executive Director
Believes in self-determination for people with disabilities and creates the environment in which it is achieved.

4385   Dakota Center for Independent Living: Bismarck
3111 E Broadway Ave
Bismarck, ND 58501-5085
701-222-3636
800-489-5013
FAX: 701-222-0511
TTY: 701-222-3636
maryr@dakotacil.org
www.dakotacil.org

Robin Were, President
Cladia Ziegler, Vice president
Carol Mihulka, Secretary/Treasurer
Royce Schultze, Executive Director
Believes in self-determination for people with disabilities and creates the environment in which it is achieved.

4386   Fraser
2902 University Drive South
Fargo, ND 58103-6053
701-232-3301
FAX: 701-237-5775
fraser@fraserltd.org
fraserltd.org

Sandra Leyland, Executive Director
Mark Brodshaug, President
Michael Kirk, Vice President
David A. Laske, Treasurer
Private non-profit, federally funded center for independent living

4387   Freedom Resource Center for Independent Living: Fargo
2701 9th Ave S
Suite H
Fargo, ND 58103-8712
701-478-0459
800-450-0459
FAX: 701-478-0510
TTY: 701-478-0459
freedom@freedomrc.org
www.freedomrc.org

Nate Aalgaard, Executive Director
Angie Bosch, Office Coordinator
Mark Mark Bourdon Bourdon, Program Director
Andrea Nelson, Independent Living Advocate
To work toward equality and inclusion for people with disabilities through programs of empowerment, community education, and systems change.

4388 Resource Center for Independent Living: Minot
300 3rd Ave SW
Suite F
Minot, ND 58701-4346   701-839-4724
                                    800-377-5114
                                    FAX: 701-838-1677
                                    TTY: 701-839-4724
                      independencecil@independencecil.org
                                www.independencecil.org/?

Susan Ogurek, Chair
Scott Burlingame, Executive Director
Dee Tischer, Senior Independent Living Specia
Jamie Hardt, Youth Transition Specialist
A resource center for independent living. Mission is to advocate for the freedom of choice for individuals with disabilities to live independently through the removal of all barriers.

Ohio

4389 Ability Center of Greater Toledo
5605 Monroe St
Sylvania, OH 43560-2702   419-885-5733
                                    866-885-5733
                                    FAX: 419-882-4813
                                    TTY: 419-885-5733
                                    www.abilitycenter.org

Tim Harrington, Executive Director
Lisa Justice, Executive Assistant
Dale Abell, Director of Programme Developmen
Debbie Keller, Tomorrow Planning Specialist
To assist people with disabilities to live, work and socialize within a fully accessible community.

4390 Ability Center of Greater Toledo: Defiance
5605 Monroe St
Sylvania, OH 43560-2702   419-885-5733
                                    866-885-5733
                                    FAX: 419-882-4813
                                    TTY: 419-885-5733
                                    www.abilitycenter.org

Tim Harrington, Executive Director
Lisa Justice, Executive Assistant
Dale Abell, Director of Programme Developmen
Debbie Keller, Tomorrow Planning Specialist
To assist people with disabilities to live, work and socialize within a fully accessible community.

4391 Ability Center of Greater Toledo: Port Clinton
1848 East Perry Street
Suite #110
Port Clinton, OH 43452-1802   419-734-0330
                                    877-734-0330
                                    FAX: 419-732-6864
                                    TTY: 419-734-0330
                                    www.abilitycenter.org

Tim Harrington, Executive Director
Lisa Justice, Executive Assistant
Dale Abell, Director of Programme Developmen
Debbie Keller, Tomorrow Planning Specialist
To assist people with disabilities to live, work and socialize within a fully accessible community.

4392 Access Center for Independent Living
901 S Ludlow St
Dayton, OH 45402-2614   937-341-5202
                                    FAX: 937-341-5217
                                    TTY: 937-341-5218
                                    info@acils.com
                                    www.acils.com/?

Darrell Price, IL Team Co-Leader
Tonya Banther, IL Team Co-Leader
Melody Burba, Information & Referral Specialis
John Dixon, Information & Referral Specialis
Offers peer counseling, disability education and other services to the community.

4393 Center for Independent Living Options
2031 Auburn Avenue
Cincinnati, OH 45219-2436   513-241-2600
                                    FAX: 513-241-1707
                                    TTY: 513-241-7170
                                    cilo@cilo.net.
                                    cilo.net

Lin Laing, Executive Director
Justin Bifro, President
Brian Frazier, Vice-President
Ed Klene, Treasurer
The oldest center for independent living in Ohio serving individuals with disabilities in the Greater Cincinnati/Northern Kentucky region.

4394 Fairfield Center for Disabilities and Cerebral Palsy
681 E 6th Ave
Lancaster, OH 43130-2602   740-653-5501
                                    FAX: 740-653-6046
                                    fcdcp@sbcglobal.net
                                    www.fcdcp.org

David Macioci, President
David Welsh, Vice-President
Mary Snider, Treasurer
Edwin R. Payne, Secretary
Adult Day Program and Transportation. The mission of the Fairfield Center for disabilities and Cerebral Palsy, Inc, is to create a better future for people with a disability by increasing and enhancing their lifestyle opportunities.

4395 Linking Employment, Abilities and Potential
2545 Lorain Ave.
Cleveland, OH 44113-3102   216-696-2716
                                    FAX: 216-687-1453
                                    www.leapinfo.org

Charles Heindrichs, President
Brian Roof, Vice President
Vincent Shemo, Treasurer
Betsey Kamm, Secretary
Consumer-directed to ensure a society of equal opportunity for all persons, regardless of disability.

4396 Mid-Ohio Board for an Independent Living Environment (MOBILE)
690 S High St
Columbus, OH 43206-1016   614-443-5936
                                    FAX: 614-443-5954
                                    TTY: 614-443-5957
                                    info@mobileonline.org
                                    www.mobileonline.org

Darry Moore, President
Thomas Shapaka, Vice-President
Mark Morton, Treasurer
Warren King, Secretary
A non-profit Center for Independent Living directed by persons with disabilities. MOBILE was founded on principles that affirm the right of persons with disabilities to live their lives with a full measure of liberty and human dignity.

4397 Ohio Statewide Independent Living Council
670 Morrison Road
Suite 200
Gahanna, OH 43230-5324   614-892-0390
                                    800-566-7788
                                    FAX: 614-861-0392
                                    www.ohiosilc.org

Kay Grier, Executive Director
Eugene Iacovetta, Special Projects Coordinator
Mary Butler, Systems Change Coordinator
Janae Miller, Office Manager
Committed to promoting a philosophy of consumer control, peer support, self-help, self-determination, equal acess, and individual and systems advocacy, in order to maximize leadership, empowerment, independence, productivity and to support full inclusion and integration of individuals with disabilities into the mainstream of American society.

4398 Rehabilitation Service of North Central Ohio
270 Sterkel Blvd
Mansfield, OH 44907-1508 419-756-1133
800-589-1133
FAX: 419-756-6544
info@therehabcenter.org
www.therehabcenter.org

Veronica L. Groff, President/CEO
Susan Baker, Chairman
Dan Wiegand, Vice-Chairman
Scott Donnenwirth, Secretary
Private nonprofit organization providing coordinated, team-oriented comprehensive outpatient rehabilitation services to children and adults of all ages. Serves 8 counties in N/C Ohio. Four umbrella areas of service include medical rehabilitation services, vocational rehabilitation services, behavioral health service and drug and alcohol addiction services. Medical rehabilitation services include physical therapy, occupational therapy, speech therapy and audiology.

4399 Samuel W Bell Home for Sightless
3775 Muddy Creek Rd
Cincinnati, OH 45238-2055 513-241-0720
FAX: 513-241-1481
swbellhome@fuse.net
www.samuelbell.org

Timothy Lighthal, President
Kevin Kappa, Vice-President
Miles L.Hoff, Treasurer
James Witte, Secretary
Offers a residential, independent living environment for blind and legally blind adults.

4400 Services for Independent Living
25100 Euclid Ave
Suite #105
Cleveland, OH 44117-2663 216-731-1529
FAX: 216-731-3083
TTY:216-731-1529
sil@sil-oh.org
www.sil-oh.org

Lynn Hildebrand, Executive Director
Offers support ADA, consultation and education, advocacy, transitional education services, independent living skills training, information and referrals.

4401 Society for Equal Access: Independent Living Center
1458 5th St NW
New Philadelphia, OH 44663-1224 330-343-9292
888-213-4452
FAX: 330-602-7425
TTY:330-602-2557
ilc@tusco.net
www.seailc.org

Scott Huston, President
Edna Fillinger, Vice-President
Victoria Eichel, Secretary
Twyla Mccartney, Treasurer
The Society works with individuals to become more independent. Our agency assists with peer support, advocacy, information and referral, independent living skills and transportation. Our goal is to move those with challenges in the direction ofn independence.

Oklahoma

4402 Ability Resources
823 S Detroit Ave
Suite #110
Tulsa, OK 74120-4223 918-592-1235
800-722-0886
FAX: 918-592-5651
webadmin@ability-resources.org
www.ability-resources.org
Carla Lawson, Executive Director
To assist people with disabilities in attaining and maintaining their personal independence.

4403 Green County Independent Living Resource Center
4100 S.E. Adams Rd
Suite C-106
Bartlesville, OK 74006- 8409 918-335-1314
800-559-0567
FAX: 918-333-1814
TTY: 918-335-1314

Vicki Haws, Executive Director
Independent living skills training, information and referrals, advocacy, a loan library of adaptive equipment and books. Services available to all individuals with disabilities and their family members who reside in Northeastern Oklahoma.

4404 Oklahomans for Independent Living
601 East Carl Albert Parkway
McAlester, OK 74501-5410 918-426-6220
800-568-6821
FAX: 918-426-3245
TTY: 918-426-6263
info@oilok.org
www.oilok.org

Pam Pulchny, Executive Director/ADAspecialist
Terry Yates, Administrative Assistant/Bookke
Leanna Amos, Service Management Specialist
Stephen Strickland, Living Choice Coordinator
OIL encourages individuals of all ages, with all types of disabilities to increase: personal dependence; empowerment and self determiniation; and ful integration and participation in their work, community, school and home activities.

4405 Progressive Independence
121 N Porter Avenue
Norman, OK 73071-5834 405-321-3203
800-801-3203
FAX: 405-321-7601
TTY: 405-321-2942
heathera@progind.org
www.progind.org

Scott Spray, Chairperson
Teresa Tisdell, Vice Chair
Mark Newman, Treasurer
Mary Dulan, Secretary
Preovides four cores services of Information & Referral, Individaul& Systems Advocacy, Peer Counseling, and Skills Training; in addition, offers accessible computer lab, short term DME loans, ande benefits counseling for SSI/SSDI.

Oregon

4406 Abilitree
2680 NE Twin Knolls Dr.
Suite 3
Bend, OR 97701 541-388-8103
FAX: 541-389-2337
TTY:541-388-8103
coril@coril.org
www.abilitree.org

Tim Johnson, Executive Director
Greg Sublett, Director of Operations
April O'Meara, Marketing Director
Jen Michelson, Access Manager
CORIL empowers people with disabilities to maximize their independence, productivity and inclusio in community life. CORIL envisions a society where all people have the opportunity to develop their full capabilities with independence, productivity and more meaningful involvment in local community events and activities.

4407 Eastern Oregon Center for Independent Living
1021 SW 5th Ave
Ontario, OR 97914-3301 541-889-3119
866-248-8369
FAX: 541-889-4647
eocil@eocil.org
www.eocil.org

Kirt Toombs, Executive Director

EOCIL is a nonprofit community based resource and advocacy center that promotes independent living and equal access for all persons with disabilities. EOCIL serves consumers in the counties of: Baker, Gilliam, Grant, harney, Malheur, Morrow, Umatilla, Union, Wallowa and Wheeler.

4408   HASL Independent Abilities Center
305 NE 'E' Street
Grants Pass, OR 97526

541-479-4275
800-758-4275
FAX: 541-479-7261
TTY: 541-479-3588
haslstaff@yahoo.com
www.haslonline.org

Randy Samuelson, Executive Director
To promote public awareness of the special needs and legal rights of individuals with cross-disabilities; to facilitate their integration into society and provide support through advocacy, peer counseling, skills training and information and referral to encourage independence.

4409   Independent Living Resources
1839 NE Couch Street
Portland, OR 97232-5308

503-232-7411
FAX: 503-232-7480
TTY: 503-232-8404
info@ilr.org
www.ilr.org/?

Barry Fox-Quamme, Executive Director
May Altman, LCSW, Associate Director
Barbara Norris, Office Manager, Executive Assist
Amy Camp, Independent Living Specialist, R
ILR looks to promote the philosophy of Independent Living by creating opportunities, encouraging choices, advancing equal access, and furthering the level of independence for all people with disabilities

4410   Laurel Hill Center
2145 Centennial Plaza
Eugene, OR 97401-2474

541-485-6340
FAX: 541-984-3124
TTY: 541-684-6822
info@laurel.org
www.laurel.org

Tom Fauria, President
DAVE Burtner, Vice-President
EDUARDO Sifuentez, Secretary
Lt. Jennifer Bills, Special operations
Provides natoinall-recognized, recovery-focused rehabilitation services in Lane County, Oregon, for people with severe and persistent mental illnesses

4411   Progressive Options
611 S.W. Hurbert Street
Suite A
Newport, OR 97365-9678

541-265-4674
FAX: 541-574-4313
TTY: 541-574-1927
progop541@yahoo.com
www.progressive-options.org

Rhonda Walker, Executive Director
Progressive Options seeks to provide free services and support to people with disabilities of all kinds to help them achieve and maintain maximum independence and self-sufficiency in Lincoln County and surrounding areas in Oregon.

4412   SPOKES Unlimited
1006 Main St
Klamath Falls, OR 97601-6029

541-883-7547
FAX: 541-885-2469
TTY: 541-883-7547
info@spokesunlimited.org
www.spokesunlimited.org

Wendy Howard, Executive Director
Mission is to enhance the ability of people with disabilities to live more independently.

4413   Umpqua Valley Disabilities Network
736 SE Jackson Street
Roseburg, OR 97470-110

541-672-6336
FAX: 541-672-8606
TTY: 541-440-2882
uvdn@uvdn.org
www.uvdn.org

David Fricke, Executive Director
Heather Vialpando, Executive Assistant
UVDN's mission is to promote independent living and community inclusion for people with disabilities.

Pennsylvania

4414   Abilities in Motion
210 N 5th St
Reading, PA 19601-3304

610-376-0010
888-376-0120
FAX: 610-376-0021
TTY: 610-228-2301
staff@abilitiesinmotion.org
www.abilitiesinmotion.org

Terry Graul, Board President
David Lerch, Vice-President
Bonnie Milke, Treasurer
Ralph Trainer, Executive Director
Dedicated to advancing the rights of persons with disabilities in orer to promote a full life in the community through the prevention and elimination of physical, psychological, social and attitudinal barriers which serve to deny them the rights and privileges common to the general public.

4415   Anthracite Region Center for Independent Living
Pennsylvania Council on Independent Living
8 West Broad St
Suite 228
Hazleton, PA 18201-6418

570-455-9800
800-777-9906
FAX: 570-455-1731
TTY: 570-455-9800
dcorcoran@anthracitecil.org
www.anthracitecil.org

Irene Mordosky, President
Margo Madden, Vice-President
Rand Martin, Treasurer
Tracy Clark, Secretary
Enables individuals with disabilities to attain their highest possible level of independence.

4416   Brian's House
757 Springdale Dr.
Exton, PA 19341-8531

610-399-1175
ekihara@brianshouse.org
brianshouse.org

Diana L. Ramsay, MPP, OTR, FAOT, Resident and Chief Executive Off
Peter M. Shubiak, MA, Executive Vice President and Chi
Lori Plunkettt, Executive Director
A non-profit organization that provides residential, vocational and recreational/respite programs for children and adults with intellectual and developmental disabilities.

4417   Community Resources for Independence
3410 W 12th St
Erie, PA 16505-3649

814-838-7222
800-530-5541
FAX: 814-838-8491
TTY: 814-838-8115
www.crinet.org

Timothy Finegan, Executive Director
William Essigmann, Administrative Program Manager
Carl Berry, Human Resources Director
Marty Pushchak, Controller
A community based, nonprofit, nonresidential organization that offers services and assistance to enable people with disabilities to

expand their options, pursue their goals, and achieve and maintain self-sufficient and producitve lives in the community.

4418 Community Resources for Independence, Inc., Bradford
3410 West 12th Street
Erie, PA 16505

814-838-7222
800-530-5541
FAX: 814-838-8491
TTY: 814-838-8115
crinet.org

Timothy J. Finegan, Executive Director
William Essigmann, Administrative Program Manager
Carl Berry, Human Resources Director
Marty Pushchak, Controller
Community Resources for Independence, Inc is committed to preserve, enhance and enrich the quality of life for all people with disabilities.

4419 Community Resources for Independence: Lewistown
33 East Hale Street
Suite L
Lewistown, PA 17044-2160

717-248-8011
800-309-0989
FAX: 717-248-8029
www.crinet.org

Timothy Finegan, Executive Director
William Essigmann, Administrative Program Manager
Carl Berry, Human Resources Director
Marty Pushchak, Controller
A community based, nonprofit, nonresidential organization that offers services and assistance to enable people with disabilities to expand their options, pursue their goals, and achieve and maintain self-sufficient and producitve lives in the community.

4420 Community Resources for Independence: Altoona
1331 Twelth Ave
Suite #103
Altoona, PA 16601

814-994-2645
866-944-2645
FAX: 814-944-2683
www.crinet.org

Timothy Finegan, Executive Director
William Essigmann, Administrative Program Manager
Carl Berry, Human Resources Director
Marty Pushchak, Controller
A community based, nonprofit, nonresidential organization that offers services and assistance to enable people with disabilities to expand their options, pursue their goals, and achieve and maintain self-sufficient and producitve lives in the community.

4421 Community Resources for Independence: Clarion
1200 Eastwood Drive
Suite #1
Clarion, PA 16214-8824

814-297-7141
800-372-0140
FAX: 814-297-7161
www.crinet.org

Timothy J. Finegan, Executive Director
William Essigmann, Administrative Program Manager
Carl Berry, Human Resources Director
Marty Pushchak, Controller
A community based, nonprofit, nonresidential organization that offers services and assistance to enable people with disabilities to expand their options, pursue their goals, and achieve and maintain self-sufficient and producitve lives in the community.

4422 Community Resources for Independence: Clearfield
209 E Locust St
Clearfield, PA 16830-2422

814-765-6405
866-619-6405
FAX: 814-765-1269
www.crinet.org

Timothy Finegan, Executive Director
William Essigmann, Administrative Program Manager
Carl Berry, Human Resources Director
Marty Pushchak, Controller
A community based, nonprofit, nonresidential organization that offers services and assistance to enable people with disabilities to

expand their options, pursue their goals, and achieve and maintain self-sufficient and producitve lives in the community.

4423 Community Resources for Independence: Hermitage
3875 East State St
Suite B
Hermitage, PA 16148-3415

724-347-4121
FAX: 724-347-5966
www.crinet.org

Timothy J. Finegan, Executive Director
William Essigmann, Administrative Program Manager
Carl Berry, Human Resources Director
Marty Pushchak, Controller
A community based, nonprofit, nonresidential organization that offers services and assistance to enable people with disabilities to expand their options, pursue their goals, and achieve and maintain self-sufficient and producitve lives in the community.

4424 Community Resources for Independence: Lewisburg
11 Reitz Blvd
Suite #105
Lewisburg, PA 17837-1493

570-524-4314
800-332-4135
FAX: 570-524-9236
www.crinet.org

Timothy J. Finegan, Executive Director
William Essigmann, Administrative Program Manager
Carl Berry, Human Resources Director
Marty Pushchak, Controller
A community based, nonprofit, nonresidential organization that offers services and assistance to enable people with disabilities to expand their options, pursue their goals, and achieve and maintain self-sufficient and producitve lives in the community.

4425 Community Resources for Independence: Oil City
250 Elm St
Oil City, PA 16301-1413

814-677-4655
866-209-3882
FAX: 814-677-4915
www.crinet.org

Tim Finegan, Executive Director
William Essigmann, Administrative Program Manager
Carl Berry, Human Resources Director
Marty Pushchak, Controller
A community based, nonprofit, nonresidential organization that offers services and assistance to enable people with disabilities to expand their options, pursue their goals, and achieve and maintain self-sufficient and producitve lives in the community.

4426 Community Resources for Independence: Warren
1003 Pennsylvania Ave W
Warren, PA 16365-1837

814-726-3404
866-579-3404
FAX: 814-726-3428
www.crinet.org

Timothy Finegan, Executive Director
William Essigmann, Administrative Program Manager
Carl Berry, Human Resources Director
Marty Pushchak, Controller
A community based, nonprofit, nonresidential organization that offers services and assistance to enable people with disabilities to expand their options, pursue their goals, and achieve and maintain self-sufficient and producitve lives in the community.

4427 Community Resources for Independence: Wellsboro
38 Plaza Ln
Wellsboro, PA 16901-1766

570-724-5852
866-401-7911
FAX: 570-724-3945
www.crinet.org

Timothy Finegan, Executive Director
William Essigmann, Administrative Program Manager
Carl Berry, Human Resources Director
Marty Pushchak, Controller
A community based, nonprofit, nonresidential organization that offers services and assistance to enable people with disabilities to expand their options, pursue their goals, and achieve and maintain self-sufficient and producitve lives in the community.

4428 Freedom Valley Disability Center
3607 Chapel Road
Suite B
Newtown Square, PA 19073-3602   610-353-6640
                                        800-427-4754
                                   FAX: 610-353-6753
                                   TTY: 610-353-8900
                                              fvdc.info

Ann Cope, Executive Director
Assists persons with disabilities in the achievement of independent living goals. Also promotes individual and community options to maximize independence for persons with disabilities. Serves people with disabilities in Chester, Delaware, and Montgomery Counties.

4429 Institute on Disabilities At Temple Univ.
Temple University
1755 N. 13th St
Student Center, Rm. 4115
Philadelphia, PA 19122-6099   215-204-1356
                                 FAX: 215-204-6336
                                   iod@temple.edu
                             www.disabilities.temple.edu

James Earl Davis, Phd, Interim Executive Director
Celia Feinstein, Co-Executive- Director
Amy Goldman, Co-Executive- Director
Ann Marie White, Deputy- Director
Leads by example, creating connections and promoting networks within and among communitites so that people with disabilities are recognized as integral to the fabric of community life.

4430 Lehigh Valley Center for Independent Living
713 North 13th Street
Allentown, PA 18102-9121   610-770-9781
                                   800-495-8245
                              FAX: 610-770-9801
                              TTY: 610-770-9789
                                   info@lvcil.org
                                   www.lvcil.org

Scott Berman, President
Michelle Mitchell, Vice President
Amy Beck, Executive Director
Cara Steidel, Fiscal Coordinator
Serves persons in Lehigh and Northampton Counties with any type of disability and/or his/her family.

4431 Liberty Resources
714 Market St
Suite #100
Philadelphia, PA 19106-2337   215-634-2000
                                      888-634-2155
                                 FAX: 215-634-6628
                                 TTY: 215-634-6630
                              lrinc@libertyresources.org
                              www.libertyresources.org

Edwin Bomba, Chairman
Mary Ellen Caffrey, Chairman
Estelle B. Richman, Vice-Chairman
Thomas J. Earle, CEO
A non-profit, consumer driven organization that advocates and promotes Independent Living for persons with disabilities.

4432 Life and Independence for Today
503 E Arch St
Saint Marys, PA 15857-1779   814-781-3050
                                      800-341-5438
                                 FAX: 814-781-1917
                                 TTY: 814-781-3050
                                   lift@liftcil.org
                                   www.liftcil.org

Stephen DePrater, President
Linda McKinstry, Vice-President
Larry Caggeso, Treasurer
Hope Weichman, Deputy Director
Offers services to enable people with disabilities to achieve new goals and broaden their horizons. It enables them to achieve and maintain self-sufficient and productive lives.

4433 Northeastern Pennsylvania Center for Independent Living
1142 Sanderson Ave
Suite #1
Scranton, PA 18509   570-344-7211
                             800-344-7211
                        FAX: 570-344-7218
                        TTY: 570-344-5275
                        nepacilinfo@nepacil.org
                             www.nepacil.org

Robert Treptow, President
Michael Sporer, Secretary
Chris Armone,Esq, Treasurer
Established to assist in removing barriers and expanding independent living options available to people with disabilities.

4434 South Central Pennsylvania Center for Independence Living
1019 Logan Blvd
Altoona, PA 16602-2434   814-949-1905
                                 800-237-9009
                            FAX: 814-949-1909
                            TTY: 814-949-1912
                            cilscpa@cilscpa.org
                                 www.cilscpa.org

Susan Estep, Executive Director
The missio of the Center for Independent Living of South Central PA is to empower people with disabilities to lead independent lives in their commnuitites. The Center covers Bedford, Blair, cambria, Fulton, Huntingdon, Indiana and Somerset counties.

4435 Three Rivers Center for Independent Living: New Castle
900 Rebecca Ave
Pittsburgh, PA 15221-9383   412-371-7700
                                    800-633-4588
                               FAX: 412-371-9430
                               TTY: 412-371-6230
                                   lgray@trcil.org
                            www.trcil.myfastsite.net/

Kourtney T. Diaz, Chairperson
Shanicka Kennedy, Esq, Vice-Chairperson
Stanley A Holbrook, President
Rachel Rogan, Chief Executive Officer
To empower people with disabilities to enjoy self-directed, personally meaningful lives by providing outstanding consumer controlled services and by advocating for effective community college.

4436 Three Rivers Center for Independent Livi ng: Washington
900 Rebecca Ave
Pittsburgh, PA 15221-4425   412-371-7700
                                    800-633-4588
                               FAX: 412-371-9430
                               TTY: 412-371-6230
                                   lgray@trcil.org
                            www.trcil.myfastsite.net/

Stanley A Holbrook, President
Kourtney T. Diaz, Chairperson
Shanicka Kennedy, Esq, Vice-Chairperson
Roxanne Huss, Director of Waiver Services
To empower people with disabilities to enjoy self-directed, personally meaningful lives by providing outstanding consumer controlled services and by advocating for effective community college.

4437 Three Rivers Center for Independent Living
900 Rebecca Ave
Pittsburgh, PA 15221-2938   412-371-7700
                                    800-633-4588
                               FAX: 412-371-9430
                               TTY: 412-371-6230
                                   lgray@trcil.org
                            www.trcil.myfastsite.net/

Stanley A Holbrook, President
Kourtney T. Diaz, Chairperson
Shanicka Kennedy, Esq, Vice-Chairperson
Roxanne Huss, Director of Waiver Services
To empower people with disabilities to enjoy self-directed, personally meaningful lives by providing outstanding consumer

451

controlled services and by advocating for effective community college.

4438 Tri-County Patriots for Independent Living
69 East Beau St
Washington, PA 15301-4711

724-223-5115
877-889-0965
FAX: 724-223-5119
TTY: 724-228-4028
www.tripil.com

Kathleen Kleinmann, Chief Executive Officer
Maxine Berton, Administrative Assistant
Jeffry D. Woods, Chief Information Officer
Jan Crockett, Chief Financial Officer
Brings together individuals who share common problems in equal access, education, housing, employment, attendant care, transportation, and access to technology.

4439 Voices for Independence
1107 Payne Ave
Erie, PA 16503-1741

814-874-0064
866-407-0064
FAX: 814-874-3497
TTY: 814-874-0064
web@vficil.org
www.vficil.org

Shona Eakin, Executive Director
Edna Anabui, Executive Administrative Assista
Doug McClintock, Director of Finances
Colleen Porath, Accountant
To empower people with disabilities and promote independent living.

Rhode Island

4440 Arc of Blackstone
500 Prospect St.
Wing B, Suite 203
Pawtucket, RI 2860- 4396

401-727-0150
800-257-6092
FAX: 401-727-1545
contact@bvcriarc.org
www.bvcriarc.org

Kathleen O'Neill, President
Thomas E. Hodge, Vice-President
Joseph F. McEnness, Treasurer
A. Melanie Cherry, Secretary

Committed to supporting people with developmental disabilities secure the opportunity to choose and realize their goals of where and how they live, learn, work and play

4441 Franklin Court Assisted Living
180 Franklin St
Bristol, RI 2809-3352

401-253-3679
FAX: 401-253-5855
mgargano@ebcdc.org
www.ebcdc.org

Michelle Belmore Cabana, Chief Financial Officer
Brenda Marshall, Administrator
Lynn A. Marshall, Property Manager
Jennifer Morra, Administrative Assistant
Offers local seniors an affordable assisted living option with first-rate services and gracious accommodations.

4442 IN-SIGHT Independent Living
43 Jefferson Blvd
Warwick, RI 2888-1078

401-941-3322
FAX: 401-941-3356
cbutler@in-sight.org
www.in-sight.org

Jean Saylor, Chairman
Robert Tyler, Vice-Chairman
James Hahn, Treasurer
Karl Sherry, Secretary
Creating opportunities and choices for people who are blind and visually impaired

4443 Ocean State Center for Independent Living
1944 Warwick Avenue
Warwick, RI 2889-2448

401-738-1013
866-857-1161
FAX: 401-738-1083
TTY: 401-738-1015
info@oscil.org
www.oscil.org

Lorna Ricci, Executive Director
OSCIL is a consumer controlled, community based, nonprofit organization established to provide a range of independent living services to enhance, through self direction, the quality of life of Rhode Islander with significant disability and to promote integration into the community.

4444 Office of Rehabilitation Services
40 Fountain St
Suite #4B
Providence, RI 2903-1898

401-421-7005
FAX: 401-421-7016
www.ors.ri.gov

Ronald Racine, Associate Director
Kathleen Brown, Acting Administrator ORD
Ron Racine, Deputy Administrator Blind
John Microulis, Deputy Administrator Disability
Their goal is to help individuals with physical and mental disabilities prepare for and obtain appropriate employment.

4445 PARI Independent Living Center
500 Prospect St
Pawtucket, RI 2860-6259

401-725-1966
FAX: 401-725-2104
TTY:401-725-1966
info@pari-ilc.org
www.pari-ilc.org

Leo Canuel, Executive Director
Sue Bilodau, Program Director
Offers information and referral services, personal care attendant services, home modifications, advocacy services and peer counseling, independent living skills training, and recycled equipment.

South Carolina

4446 Columbia Disability Action Center
136 Stonemark Lane
Suite #100
Columbia, SC 29210

800-681-6805
FAX: 803-779-5114
TTY:803-779-0949
www.able-sc.org/

David Dawson, President
Rochelle Gadson, Vice President
Joe Butler, Treasurer
Angela Jacildone, Secretary
A non-profit consumer governed Center for Independent Living. Programs and services support persons with disaibities in taking full advantage of community resources, enhancing personal opportunities, and determining the direction of their lives.

4447 Disability Action Center
330B Pelham Rd
Suite 100 A
Greenville, SC 29615-3116

864-235-1421
800-681-7715
FAX: 864-235-2056
TTY: 864-235-8798
amayne@dacsc.org
www.able-sc.org/

David Dawson, President
Rochelle Gadson, Vice President
Joe Butler, Treasurer
Angela Jacildone, Secretary
Empowering people with disabilities to reach their highest level of independence.

4448 **Graham Street Community Resources**
306 Graham St
Florence, SC 29501-4735 843-665-6674
FAX: 843-665-6674

Faye Thompson, Manager
Promotes independent living and empowers people with disabilities to reach their highest level of independence.

4449 **South Carolina Independent Living Council**
136 Stonemark Lane
Suite #100
Columbia, SC 29210-7318 803-217-3209
800-994-4322
FAX: 803-731-1439
TTY: 803-217-3209
scilc@scilconline.org
www.scsilc.com

Mike Le Fever, President
Committed to equal opportunity, equal access, self determination, independence, and choice for all people with disabilities and pursues these goals by the means available.

4450 **Walton Options for Independent Living: North Augusta**
325 Georgia Ave
North Augusta, SC 29841-3848 803-279-9611
FAX: 803-279-9135
tjohnston@waltonoptions.org
www.waltonoptions.org

Cynthia Anzek, Executive Director
Empowers persons of all ages with all types of disabilities to reach their highest level of independence, community inclusion and employment.

South Dakota

4451 **Adjustment Training Center**
607 N 4th St
Aberdeen, SD 57401-2733 605-229-0263
FAX: 605-225-3455
www.aspiresd.org

Jennifer Gray, Executive Director
Arlette Keller, Director of Service Coordination
Angela Huffman, Director of Nursing
Paul Schumacher, Director of Vocational Services
Offers peer counseling, attendant care registry and referrals.

4452 **Black Hills Workshop & Training Center**
Black Hills Workshop
3650 Range Road
PO Box 2104
Rapid City, SD 57709-2104 605-343-4550
FAX: 605-343-0879
TTY:800-877-1113
drosby@bhws.com
www.blackhillsworks.org

Brad Saathoff, Chief Executive Officer
Janet Niehaus, VP of Finance
Michelle Aman, VP of Residential Services
Helen Usera, VP of Development
Offers job placement, housing options, case coordination, supported employment and supported living for all disability groups, as well as specialized services for brian injury victims.

4453 **Communication Service for the Deaf: Rapid City**
200 W Cesar Chavez St
Suite 650
Austin, TX 78701-694 844-222-0002
800-642-6410
FAX: 605-394-6609
TTY: 866-273-3323
csd@csd.org
www.c-s-d.org

Dr. Benjamin Soukup, Founder, Chairman & CEO
Christopher Soukup, President
Brad Hermes, Chief Financial Officer
Christina Kokenge, Vice President, Human Resources

A private, nonprofit organization dedicated to providing broad-based services, ensuring public accessibility and increasing public awareness of issues affecting deaf and hard of hearing inividuals.

4454 **Native American Advocacy Program for Persons with Disabilities**
P.O.Box 527
Winner, SD 57580-527 605-842-3977
800-303-3975
FAX: 605-842-3983
TTY: 605-842-3977
officemgr@nativeamericanadvocacy.org
www.nativeamericanadvocacy.org

Marla Bull Bear, Executive Director
Charles Bull Bear, Specialist
Betty Farr, Il Specialist
Megan L. Garcia, Prevention Specialist
The mission is to encourage a healthy organization that assists Native Americans with disabilities, by providing prevention, education and training, advocacy, support, independent living skills and referrals.

4455 **Prairie Freedom Center for Independent Living: Sioux Falls**
4107 S Carnegie Cr
Suite #9
Sioux Falls, SD 57106-3100 605-362-3550
FAX: 605-367-5639
i-l-c@ilcchoices.org
www.ilcchoices.org

Steve Tripp, President
Cheri Raymond, Vice President
Matt Cain, Executive Director
Laura Staebner, Treasurer
Established to provide basic skills so many of us take for granted: to take care of our own needs and to make our own decisions to be independent.

4456 **Prairie Freedom Center for Independent Li ving: Madison**
4107 S Carnegie Cr
411 SE 10th St
Sioux Falls, SD 57106-3570 605-362-3550
FAX: 605-256-5071
i-l-c@ilcchoices.org
www.ilcchoices.org

Steve Tripp, President
Cheri Raymond, Vice President
Matt Cain, Executive Director
Laura Staebner, Treasurer
Established to provide basic skills so many of us take for granted: to take care of our own needs and to make our own decisions to be independent.

4457 **Prairie Freedom Center for Independent Living: Yankton**
4107 S Carnegie Cr
Suite #107
Sioux Falls, SD 57106-2800 605-362-3550
FAX: 605-668-3060
TTY:605-668-3060
i-l-c@ilcchoices.org
www.ilcchoices.org

Steve Tripp, President
Cheri Raymond, Vice President
Matt Cain, Executive Director
Laura Staebner, Treasurer
Established to provide basic skills so many of us take for granted: to take care of our own needs and to make our own decisions to be independent.

4458 South Dakota Assistive Technology Project: DakotaLink
1161 Deadwood Ave N
Suite #5
Rapid City, SD 57702-382

605-394-6742
800-645-0673
FAX: 605-394-6744
TTY: 605-394-6742
atinfo@dakotalink.net
dakotalink.tie.net

Pat Czerny, Manager
Patrick Czerny, Technical Services Coordinator
David Scherer, Program Coordinator
DakotaLink, the South Dakota Assistive Technology Program, provides resources and supports to individuals of all ages to ensure greater access to and acquisition of assistive technology devices and services.

4459 Western Resources for dis-ABLED Independence
405 East Omaha St
Suite D
Rapid City, SD 57701-2974

605-718-1930
888-434-4943
FAX: 605-718-1933
TTY: 605-718-1930
chad@wril.org
www.wril.org

Jeff Wangen, President
Dennis Coull, Vice-President
Linda Lockner, Secretary
Mike Pendo, Treasurer
WRDI advocates for the rights of equal inclusion of people with disabilities in all aspects of community life. WRDI also strives to identify and promote access to existing resources and to advocate for the development of new resources, which may enable people with disabilities to live more independently.

Tennessee

4460 Center for Independent Living of Middle Tennessee
955 Woodland St
Nashville, TN 37206-3753

615-292-5803
866-992-4568
FAX: 615-383-1176
TTY: 615-292-7790
cilmt@tndisability.org
www.cil-mt.org

Tom Hopton, Executive Director
Tria Bridgeman, Benefits Analyst-Jackson
Dylan Brown, Benefits Analyst-Nashville
Pattrick Gallaher, Employment Assistant-Nashville

CILMT provides persons with disabilities opportunities to be self advocates and make their own decisions regarding living arrangements, means of transportation, employment, social and recreational activities, as well as other aspects of everyday life. Serves Davidson, Cheatham, Wilson, Robertson, Rutherford, Sumner and Williamson Counties.

4461 DisAbility Resource Center: Knoxville
900 E Hill Ave
Suite 205
Knoxville, TN 37915-2567

865-637-3666
FAX: 865-637-5616
TTY: 865-637-6976
drc@drctn.org
www.drctn.org

Lillian Burch, Executive Director
Nicole Craig, Programme Director
Katherine Moore, Independent Living Specialist
Basil Farris, Employment Coach
DRCTN mission is to empower people with disabilities to fully integrate and participate in the community. DRC is a community-based non-residential program of services designed to assist people with disabilities to gain independence and to assist the community in eliminating barriers of independence.

4462 Jackson Center for Independent Living
1981 Hollywood Drive
Jackson, TN 38305-4388

731-668-2211
FAX: 731-668-0406
TTY: 731-664-3970
information@jcil.tn.org
www.j-cil.com

Glen Barr, Executive Director
JCIL works with people with significant disabilities and the Deaf Community in achieving their Independent Living Goals while assisting the community in eliminating barriers to Independent Living.

4463 Memphis Center for Independent Living
1633 Madison Ave
Memphis, TN 38104-2506

901-726-6404
800-848-0298
FAX: 901-726-6521
TTY: 901-726-6404
info@mcil.org
www.mcil.org

Kevin Lofton, Chairman
Marvin Glenn Bailey, Vice-Chairman
Charles M. Weirich, Jr., Board Counsel
MCIL is a community based non-profit organization whose primary mission is to facilitate the full integration of persons with disabilities into all aspects of community life.

4464 Tennessee Technology Access Program (TTAP)
400 Deaderick St
14th Fl
Nashville, TN 37243-1403

615-313-5183
800-732-5059
FAX: 615-532-4685
TTY: 615-313-5695
tn.ttap@state.tn.us
www.state.tn.us/humanserv/rehab/ttap.html

Kevin Wright, Director
TTAP's mission is to maintain a statewide program of technology-rated assistance that is timely, comprehensive and consumer driven to ensure that all Tennesseans with disabilities have the information, services and deices that they need to make choices about where and how they spend their time as independently as possible. .

4465 Tri-State Resource and Advocacy Corporation
6925 Shallowford Rd
#300
Chattanooga, TN 37421

423-892-4774
800-868-8724
FAX: 423-892-9866
TTY: 423-892-4774
4trac@bellsouth.net
www.1trac.org

Mark Woofall, Executive Director
Pam Jackson, Independent Living Facilitator
TRAC is dedicated to improving opportunities for individuals wuth disabilities.

Texas

4466 ABLE Center for Independent Living
1931 E 37th
St # 1
Odessa, TX 79762-6906

432-580-3439
info@ablecenterpb.org
www.ablecenterpb.org

Marilyn Hancock, Executive Director
Kathleen Story MA, Independent Living Specialist
Britni Veretto, HR Manager
To promote independent living for people with disabilities.

4467 Austin Resource Center for Independent Living
825 E. Rundberg Ln
Suite E6
Austin, TX 78753-4813

512-832-6349
800-414-6327
FAX: 512-832-1869
arcil@arcil.com
www.arcil.com

Ross Davis, Chair
Linda Loach, Vice-Chair
Sylvia Davis, Secretary/Treasurer
Vonnye Gardner, Member
Serving people with disabilities, their families and communities throughout Travis and surrounding counties.

4468 Austin Resource Center: Round Rock
525 Round Rock West
Suite A120
Round Rock, TX 78681-5020

512-828-4624
FAX: 512-828-4625
sally@arcil.com
www.arcil.com

Ross Davis, Chair
Linda Loach, Vice-Chair
Sylvia Davis, Secretary/Treasurer
Vonnye Gardner, Member
Serving peole with disabilities, their families and communities throughout Travis and surrounding counties.

4469 Austin Resource Center: San Marcos
618 South Guadalupe St
Suite #103
San Marcos, TX 78666- 6977

512-396-5790
800-572-2973
FAX: 512-396-5794
sanmarcos@arcil.com
www.arcil.com

Ross Davis, Chair
Linda Loach, Vice-Chair
Sylvia Davis, Secretary/Treasurer
Vonnye Gardner, Member
Serving people with disabilities, their families and communities throughout Travis and surounding counties.

4470 Brazoria County Center For Independent Living
1104D East Mullberry Street
Suite D
Angleton, TX 77515- 3952

979-849-7060
888-872-7957
FAX: 979-849-8465
TTY: 979-849-7060
bccil@neosoft.com
www.hcil.cc

Chamane Barrow, Manager
To promote the full inclusion, equal opportunity and participation of persons with disabilities in every aspect of community life. We believe that people with disabilities have the right to make choices affecting their lives, a right to take risks, a right to fail, and a right to succeed.

4471 Centre, The
3550 West Dallas Rd
Houston, TX 77019

713-525-8400
FAX: 713-525-8444
thecenterhouston.org

Bill Coorsh, President
Richard Rosenberg, Vice-President
Lisa F. Schott, Secretary
Glen Shepherd, Treasurer
Provides services for more than 600 children and adults with mental retardation and other developmental disabilities. The Center also offers a wide array of programs including education, vocational training and job placement services, three different residential options representing both urban and rural living environments, special programs designed to meet the needs of older adults, and a variety of therapeutic support services.

4472 Crockett Resource Center for Independent Living
1020 Loop 304 East
Crockett, TX 75835-1806

936-544-2811
FAX: 936-544-7315
TTY:936-544-2811
crcil@windstream.net
www.crockettresourcecenter.org

Sara Minton, Executive Director
Mary Killough, Chief Financial Officer
Cathy Newsome, Information/Outreach Coordinator
Debbie Oliver, Information and Outreach Coor.
Provides independent living services to cross-disability groups to increase their personal self-determination and minimize dependence on others. Maintain comprehensive information on availability of resources and provides referrals to such resources. Provides instruction to assist people with disabilities to gain skills that would empower them to live independently. Peer counseling, advocacy - both individual and community by assisting to obtain support services to make changes in society.

4473 Houston Center for Independent Living
6201 Bonhomme Rd
Ste 150
South Houston, TX 77036

713-974-4621
FAX: 713-974-6927
TTY:713-974-2703
hcil@neosoft.com
www.hcil.cc

Sandra Bookman, Executive Director
Advocacy organization created by and for people with disabilities (PWD) to empower and protect their rights. Services include but not limited to: peer support, individual and systems advocacy, independent living skills training, information and referral, disability cultural awareness, ASL classes, ADA technical assistance, computer technology training, work incentive counseling, equipment loan program.

4474 Independent Life Styles
215 North Benton Drive
Sauk Rapids, MN 56379-1874

320-529-9000
888-529-0743
FAX: 320-529-0747
ilicil@independentlifestyles.org
www.independentlifestyles.org

Karen Ahles, Chair
Jay Keller, Educator
Cara Ruff, Executive Director
Chad Hansen, Community Member
Offers peer counseling, advocacy and other services to the community.

4475 Independent Living Research Utilization Project
Institute For Rehabilitation & Research
1333 Moursund
Houston, TX 77030

713-520-0232
FAX: 713-520-5785
TTY:713-520-0232
ilru@ilru.org
www.ilru.org

Lex Frieden, Director
Linda CoVan, Grant Coordinator
Maria Del Bosque, Project Associate
Diego Demaya, Legal Specialist
ILRU is a national center for information, training, research and technical assistance in independent living. Its goal is to expand the body of knowledge in independent living and to improve utilization of results of research programs and demonstration projects in this field. ILRU is a program of The Institute for Rehabilitation and Research, a nationally recognized medical rehabilitation facility for persons with disabilities. TTY phone number: (713) 520-5136.

4476 LIFE/ Run Centers for Independent Living
8240 Boston Avenue
Lubbock, TX 79423-2342 806-795-5433
FAX: 806-795-5607
TTY:806-795-5433
wilmacrain@yahoo.com
www.liferun.org

Michelle Crain, Executive Director
Committed to providing individuals with disabilities the information and skills necessary to become independent and to achieve full inclusion in every aspect of their life.

4477 Office for Students with Disabilities, University of Texas at Arlington
701 South Nedderman Drive
Arlington, TX 76019-1 817-272-3364
800-735-2989
FAX: 817-272-1447
TTY: 800-735-2989
helpdesk@uta.edu
www.uta.edu/disability

Penny Acrey, Director
Demarice Ferguson, MS, CRC, Associate Director
Scott Holmes, Assistant Director for Testing
Gilda Williams, BSW, Office Manager
Offers disability counseling and academic accomodation to UT Arlington community.

4478 Palestine Resource Center for Independent Living
421 Avenue a St
Palestine, TX 75801-2903 903-729-7505
888-326-5166
FAX: 903-729-7540
TTY:903-729-7505
prcil@embarqmail.com
www.palestineresourcecenter.org/?

Sara Minton, Executive Director
Mary Killough, Chief Financial Officer
Cathy Newsome, Information/Outreach Coordinator
Debbie Oliver, Information and Outreach Coor.
Provides independent living services to cross-disability groups to increase their personal self-determination and minimize dependence on others. Maintain comprehensive information on availability of resources and provides referrals to such resources. Provides instruction to assist people with disabilities to gain skills that would empower them to live independently. Peer counseling, advocacy - both individual and community by assisting to obtain support services to make changes in society.

4479 Panhandle Action Center for Independent Living Skills
417 W. 10th Avenue
Amarillo, TX 79101-4316 806-374-1400
FAX: 806-374-4550
TTY:806-374-2774
info@panhandleilc.org
www.panhandleilc.org

Joe Rogers, Executive Director
Alma Benavides, Employment Director
Chris White, Development Director
Cynthia Hammett, Consumer Coordinator & Youth Tra
PILC is a non profit organization dedicated to the advancement of full participation in all aspects of life. PILC services are developed, directed, delivered, and governed primarily by individuals with disabilities.

4480 REACH of Dallas Resource Center on Independent Living
8625 King George Drive
Suite 210
Dallas, TX 75235-2286 214-630-4796
FAX: 214-630-6390
TTY:214-630-5995
reachdallas@reachcils.org
www.reachcils.org

Charlotte A. Stewart, Executive Director
Kevan Johnson, Employment Consultant
Janie Peachee, Information & Referral Specialis
Kiowanda Jasso, Information & Referral Specialis

Information and referral, peer support/peer counseling, independent living skills training and advocacy assistance.

4481 REACH of Denton Resource Center on Independent Living
405 S. Elm St
Suite 202
Denton, TX 76201-6068 940-383-1062
FAX: 940-383-2742
reachden@reachcils.org
www.reachcils.org

Charlotte A. Stewart, Executive Director
Missy Dickenson, Assistant Director
Murphy Hardinger, IL Skills Training & ADA Special
Becky Teal, Office Manager
To provide for people with disabilities so that they are enabled to lead self-directed lives and to educate the general public about disability-related topics in order to promote a barrier free community.

4482 REACH of Fort Worth Resource Center on Independent Living
1000 Macon Street
Suite 200
Fort Worth, TX 76102-4527 817-870-9082
FAX: 817-877-1622
TTY:817-870-9086
reachftw@reachcils.org
www.reachcils.org

Charlotte A. Stewart, Executive Director
Missy Dickenson, Assistant Director
Murphy Hardinger, IL Skills Training & ADA Special
Becky Teal, Office Manager
To provide services for people with disabilities so that they are enabled to lead self-directed lives and to educate the general public about disability-related topics in order to promote a barrier free community.

4483 RISE-Resource: Information, Support and Empowerment
755 11th Street
Suite 101
Beaumont, TX 77701-3723 409-832-2599
FAX: 409-838-4499
TTY:409-832-2599
www.risecil.org

Jim Brocato, Executive Director
Amanda Powe, Relocation Services Specialist
Cheryl Bass, Program Director
Gracie Jackson, Independent Living Specialist
A non-profit center for independent living.

4484 SAILS
1028 S Alamo St
San Antonio, TX 78210-1170 210-281-1878
800-474-0295
FAX: 210-281-1759
TTY: 210-281-1878
kbrietzke@sailstx.org
www.sailstx.org

Patricia Byrd, Chair
Dennis Wolf, Vice Chair
Jerry D. King, Treasurer
Donna McBee, Member
SAILS advocates for the rights and empowerment of people with disabilities in San Antonio; as well as surrounding areas. Services are provided to people with disabilities in the following counties: Atacosa, Bandera, Bexar, Calhoun, Comal, DeWitt, Dimmit, Edwards, Frio, Gillespie, Goliad, Gonzalez, Guadalupe, Jackson, Karnes, La Salle, Kendall, Kerr, Kinney, Lavaca, Maverick, Medina, Real, Uvalde, Val Verde, Victoria, Wilson and Zavala.

4485 Texas Department of Assistive and Rehabilitative Services
4800 N. Lamar Blvd
Austin, TX 78756

512-472-4138
800-628-5115
FAX: 512-472-0603
TTY: 866-581-9328
dars.inquiries@dars.state.tx.us
www.dars.state.tx.us

Bill West, Manager
Daniel Bravo, Chief Operating Officer
Rebecca Trevino, Chief Financial Officer
Glenn Neal, Deputy Commissioner

Provides technical assistance and other support services to the state's Independent Living Council, Independent Living Centers and Independent Living Counseling programs.

4486 VOLAR Center for Independent Living
1220 Golden Key Circle
El Paso, TX 79925-5825

915-591-0800
800-591-0800
FAX: 915-591-3506
TTY: 915-591-0800
volar@volarcil.org
www.volarcil.org

Luis Chew, Executive Director
Danny Monroe, Chief Financial Officer
Nena Garcia, Records Manager/Bookkeeper
Thelma Hernandez, Office Manager

VOLAR is committed to providing independent living ervices and information and referral, and to developing community options for persons with cross disabilities to empower them to live the kind of lives they choose. VOLAR is an organization of and for people with disabilities, advocating human and civil rights, community options and empowering people to live the lives they choose. Newsletter available.

4487 Valley Association for Independent Living (VAIL)
3012 N McColl Road
McAllen, TX 78501

956-668-8245
866-400-8245
FAX: 956-878-1601
info@vailrgv.org
vailrgv.org

Woodie Johnston, Executive Director

Offers information and referral, peer couseling, MS supprt group, independent living skills training, and advocacy, work incentives planning and assistance, transitioning people with disabilities from the nursing home into the community.

4488 Valley Association for Independent Living: Harlingen
1824 W. Jefferson Ave
Suite B
Harlingen, TX 78550-5247

956-428-1126
866-400-8245
FAX: 956-428-4339
smyers@valleyassociation.org
www.valleyassociation.org

Soledad Myers, Manager

Provides information and referral, peer counseling, support groups, independent living skills training, community rehab program and advocacy

Utah

4489 Active Re-Entry
10 S Fairgrounds Rd
Price, UT 84501

435-637-4950
FAX: 435-637-4952
TTY: 435-637-4950
active@arecil.org
www.arecil.org

Nancy Bentley, Executive Director

Active Re-Entry is a community based program which assists individuals with disabilities to acheive or maintain self-sufficient and productive live in their own communities. Active Re-Entry is committed to promoting the rights, dignity, and quality of life for all persons with disabilities.

4490 Active Re-Entry: Vernal
10 S Fairgrounds Rd
Price, UT 84501-9727

435-637-4950
FAX: 435-789-6090
TTY: 435-789-4021
active@arecil.org
www.arecil.org

Heather Moore, President

Active Re-Entry is a community based program which assists individuals with disabilities to achieve or maintain self-sufficient and productive lives in their own communities. We are committed to promoting the rights, dignity, and quality of life for all persons with disabilities.

4491 Central Utah Independent Living Center
3445 S Main St
Salt Lake City, UT 84115-2824

801-466-5565
877-421-4500
FAX: 801-466-2363
TTY: 801-373-5044
uilc@uilc.org
www.uilc.org

Debra Mair, Executive Director
Kim Meichle, Assistant Director
Patty Trent, Fiscal Manager
Shauna Brock, Independent Living Specialist

Empowers people with disabilities to reach their full potential in community settings through peer support, advocacy, and education.

4492 OPTIONS for Independence
Northern Utah Center for Independent Living
106 East 1120 N
Logan, UT 84341-2215

435-753-5353
FAX: 435-753-5390
TTY: 435-753-5353
jbiggs@optionind.org
www.optionsind.org

Cheryl Atwood, Executive Director

OPTIONS for Independence, the Northern Utah Center for Independent Living serves people of all ages with all types of disabilities. OPTIONS is a nonresidential Center that provides services to individuals with disabilities to facilitate their full participation in the community and raise the understanding of disability issues and access to the community. The Independent Living philosophy is strictly adhered to: consumer control and choice being the focus.

4493 OPTIONS for Independence: Brigham Satellite
106 East 1120 N
Logan, UT 84341-3379

435-753-5353
FAX: 435-753-5390
TTY: 435-723-2171
dcrockett@qwestoffice.net
www.optionsind.org

Cheryl Atwood, Executive Director
Deanna Crockett, Manager

OPTIONS is a nonresidential Independent Living Center where people with disabilities can learn skills to gain more control and independence over their lives. OPTIONS raises the vision and capability of the community at large to the point where people of all abilities will have equal access.

4494 Red Rock Center for Independence
515 W 300 N
Suite A
Saint George, UT 84770-4578

435-673-7501
800-649-2340
FAX: 435-673-8808
rrci@rrci.org
www.rrci.org

Barbara Lefler, Executive Director
Jerry Salkowe, President
Celeste Sorensen, Secretary
Joseph Gordon, Treasurer

Red Rock Center for Independence assists people with disabilities to live and participate independently.

4495 Tri-County Independent Living Center
P.O.Box 428
Ogden, UT 84402-428
801-612-3215
866-734-5678
FAX: 801-612-3732
TTY: 801-612-3215
www.uilc.org

Richard Fox, Chairperson
Kim Price, Vice-Chairperson
Greg Killpack, Secretary/Treasurer
Debra Mair, Executive Director
The mission of the Tri-County ILC is to enhance independence for all people with disabilities. Serves Davis, Weber and Morgan Counties.

4496 Utah Assistive Technology Program (UTAP) Utah State University
6855 Old Main Hill
Logan, UT 84322-6855
435-797-3811
800-524-5152
FAX: 435-797-2355
www.uatpat.org

Sachin Pavithran, UATP Program Director
Marilyn Hammond, Utah Assistive Technology Founda
Lois Summers, UATP Staff Assistant/UATF Busine
Alma Burgess, Data Collection Coordinator
Provides expertise, resources, and a structure to enhance and expand AT services provided by private and public agencies in Utah. Occcurs through monitoring, coordination, information dissemination, empowering individuals, the identification and removal of barriers, and expanding state resources.

4497 Utah Independent Living Center
3445 S Main St
Salt Lake City, UT 84115-4453
801-466-5565
800-355-2195
FAX: 801-466-2363
TTY: 801-466-5565
uilc@uilc.org
www.uilc.org

Debra Mair, Executive Director
Kim Meichle, Assistant Director
Julie Beckstead, Program Coordinator
Patty Trent, Fiscal Manager
Offers information and referral services. To assist persons with disabilities achieve independence by providing services and activities which enhance independent living skillspromote the public's understanding, accomodation, and acceptance of their rights, needs and abilities.

4498 Utah Independent Living Center: Minersville
P.O.Box 168
Minersville, UT 84752-168
435-691-7724
rrci@rrci.org
www.rrci.org

Barbara Lefler, Executive Director
Jerry Salkowe, President
Celeste Sorensen, Secretary
Joseph Gordon, Treasurer
To enhance independence for all people with disabilities.

4499 Utah Independent Living Center: Tooele
42 S Main St
Tooele, UT 84074-2132
435-843-7353
FAX: 435-843-7359
TTY:435-843-7353
angies@uilc.org
www.uilc.org

Debra Mair, Executive Director
Kim Meichle, Assistant Director
Julie Beckstead, Program Coordinator
Patty Trent, Fiscal Manager
Mission is to assist persons with disabilities achieve greater independence by providing services and activities which enhance independent living skills and promote the public's understanding, accomodation, and acceptance of their rights, needs and abilities.

Vermont

4500 Vermont Assistive Technology Program
Department of Aging and Independent Living
100 State Street
Montpelier, VT 05602-2305
802-871-3353
800-750-6355
FAX: 802-871-3048
TTY: 802-241-1464
dail.atinfo@state.vt.us
www.atp.vermont.gov/tryout-centers

Julie Tucker, Program Director
David Punia ATP, Information/Education Specialist
Encompasses a state coordinating council for assistive technology issues, regional centers for demonstration, trial and technical support with computer and augmentative communication equipment and regional seating and positioning centers.

4501 Vermont Center for Independent Living: Bennington
601 Main St
Bennington, VT 5201-2875
802-447-0574
800-639-1522
info@vcil.org
www.vcil.org

Colleen Arcodia, Peer Advocate Counselor
Michelle Grubb, Finance & Operations Officer
Sarah Launderville, Executive Director
Sue Booth, Business Office Coordinator
Believes that individuals with disabilities have the right to live with dignity and with appropriate support in their own homes, fully participate in their communities, and to control and make decisions about their lives.

4502 Vermont Center for Independent Living: Chittenden
11 East State Street
Montpelier, VT 05602
802-229-0501
800-639-1522
FAX: 802-229-0503
TTY: 802-229-0501
info@vcil.org
www.vcil.org

Colleen Arcodia, Peer Advocate Counselor
Nathan Besio, Peer Advocate Counselor
Chanda Beun, Receptionist/Admin Specialist
Sue Booth, Business Office Coordinator
Believes that individuals with disabilities have the right to live with dignity and with appropriate support in their own homes, fully participate in their communities, and to control and make decisions about their lives.

4503 Vermont Center for Independent Living: Montpelier
11 E State St
Montpelier, VT 05602-3008
802-229-0501
800-639-1522
FAX: 802-229-0503
info@vcil.org
vcil.org

Colleen Arcodia, Peer Advocate Counselor
Denise Bailey, Direct Services Coordinator
Dhiresha Blose, Development Officer
Sue Booth, Business Office Coordinator
Believes that individuals with disabilities have the right to live with dignity and with appropriate support in their own homes, fully participate in their communities, and to control and make decisions about their lives.

Virginia

4504 **Access Independence**
324 Hope Dr
Winchester, VA 22601-6800
540-662-4452
FAX: 540-662-4474
TTY:540-662-5556
askai@accessindependence.org
www.accessindependence.org

Donald Price, Executive Director
Brenda Ernst, Independent Living Specialist
Joan Davis, Manager Operations/Rep Payee
Michaela Zaraszczak, Executive Administrative Assis.

Offers support services to persons with disabilities to assist in maintaining or increasing their independence and self-determination. Includes housing assistance, independent living skills training, information, referral services, assistance and representative payee and advocacy.

4505 **Appalachian Independence Center**
230 Charwood Dr
Abingdon, VA 24210-2566
276-628-2979
FAX: 276-628-4931
TTY:276-676-0920
aicadmin@ntelos.net
aicadvocates.org

Greg Morrell, Executive Director
Donna Buckland, Development Director
Scarlett Cox, Operations Director

Mission is to advocate for and with people with disabilities to promote full participation in society

4506 **Blue Ridge Independent Living Center**
Ste B
1502 Williamson Rd NE
Roanoke, VA 24012-5100
540-342-1231
FAX: 540-342-9505
TTY:540-342-1231
brilc@brilc.org
brilc.org

Karen Michalski-Karn, Executive Director
Dana Jackson, Program Services Director
Lottie Diomedi, Independent Living Coordinator
Sallee Ebbett, Finance Manager

BRILC assists people with disabilities to live independently. The Center also serves the community at large by helping to create and environment that is accessible to all. BRILC offers a variety of services ranging from referrals to community resources, support services, and direct services. These include peer counseling, support groups, training and seminars, advocacy, education, support services, awareness, aid in obtaining specialized equipment, and much more.

4507 **Blue Ridge Independent Living Center: Christianburg**
210 Pepper Street S
Christiansburg, VA 24073-3571
540-381-8829
FAX: 540-381-8833
TTY:540-381-9149
brilc@brilc.org
brilc.org

Karen Michalski-Karney, Executive Director
Dana Jackson, Program Services Director
Lottie Diomedi, Independent Living Coordinator
Sallee Ebbett, Finance Manager

Assists people with disabilities to live independently. The center also serves the community at large by helping to create an environment that is accessible to all.

4508 **Blue Ridge Independent Living Center: Low Moor**
P.O.Box 7
Low Moor, VA 24457-7
540-862-0252
FAX: 540-862-0252
TTY:540-862-0252
brilc.org

Karen Michalski-Karney, Executive Director
Dana Jackson, Program Services Director
Lottie Diomedi, Independent Living Coordinator
Sallee Ebbett, Finance Manager

Assists to help people with disabilities to live independently. The center also serves the community at large by helping to create an environment that is accessible to all.

4509 **Clinch Independent Living Services**
1139C Plaza Drive
Grundy, VA 24614-6780
276-935-6088
800-597-2322
FAX: 276-935-6342
TTY: 276-935-6088
cils@clinchindependent.org
cils-online.org

Betty Bevins, Executive Director

Nonprofit organization providing information and referral, peer counseling, advocacy and independent living skills training to persons with disabilities.

4510 **Disability Resource Center**
409 Progress St
Fredericksburg, VA 22401-3337
540-373-2559
800-648-6324
FAX: 540-373-8126
TTY: 540-373-5890
drc@cildrc.org
www.cildrc.org

Debe Fults, Executive Director
Eric Barnes, Equipment Connection Assistant
Grace Marshall, Community Integration Coor.
Janet Lutkewitte, Accounting/IT

Mission is to assist people with disabilities, those who support them, and the community, through information, education and resources, to achieve the highest potential and benefit of independent living.

4511 **ENDependence Center of Northern Virginia**
2300 Claredon Blvd.
Suite 3305
Arlington, VA 22201-3367
703-525-3268
866-849-3852
FAX: 703-525-3585
TTY: 703-525-3553
info@ecnv.org
www.ecnv.org

Cynthia Evans, Director of Community Services
Layo Oyewole, Director of Medicaid Programs
Doris Ray, Director of Advocacy and Outreac
Brewster Thackeray, Executive Director

ECNV is a community-based resource and advocacy enter which is managed by and for people with disabilities. ENCV promotes independent living philosophy and equal access for all persons with disabilities and, like the nearly 400 centers for independent living across the country, ECNV grew from local disability rights and self-help movements.

4512 **Equal Access Center for Independence**
4031 University Drive
Suite #301
Fairfax, VA 22030-3409
703-934-2020
TTY:703-277-7730
drc@patriot.net

David Sharp, Executive Director

Provides information and referral, peer counseling, advocacy and independent living skills training to persons with disabilities.

4513 **Independence Empowerment Center**
8409 Dorsey Circle
Suite 101
Manassas, VA 20110-4414
703-257-5400
FAX: 703-257-5043
TTY:703-257-5400
info@ieccil.org
www.ieccil.org

Mary D Lopez, Executive Director
Roberta McEachern, Program Director
Sheree Thomas, Grants Coordinator
Alan Smiley, Service Facilitator
A non-profit Center for Independent Living. One of over 500 centers in the United States with roots in civil rights models of the 1960's.

4514 **Independence Resource Center**
815 Cherry Ave
Charlottesville, VA 22903-3448
434-971-9629
FAX: 434-971-8242
TTY:434-971-9629
tvandever@ntelos.net
www.charlottesvilleirc.org

Tom Vandever, Executive Director
Brenda Gianniny, Administrator
Carolyn Berry, Participant Services Coordinator
Nate Brown, Senior Peer Advocate
Information and referral services.

4515 **Independent Living Center Network: Department of the Visually Handicapped**
Ste 300
1809 Staples Mill Rd
Richmond, VA 23230-3515
FAX: 804-355-9297

Robert W Partin, Director
Robert Kastenbaum, Partner
Information and referral services.

4516 **Junction Center for Independent Living**
P.O.Box 1210
Norton, VA 24273-913
276-679-5988
FAX: 276-679-6569
TTY:276-679-5988
jcil1@junctioncenter.org
junctioncenter.org

Dennis Horton, Executive Director
Cindy Mefford, Assistant to the Executive Direc
Joe Brady, Deaf and Hard of Hearing Coordin
Brenda Cowden, Housing Specialist
To assist those who have significant disabilities so that they migh live independently in the least restrictive and most integrated environment possible.

4517 **Junction Center for Independent Living: Duffield**
P.O.Box 408
Duffield, VA 24244-408
276-431-1195
FAX: 276-431-1196
TTY:276-431-1195
jcil1@junctioncenter.org
junctioncenter.org

Dennis Horton, Executive Director
Cindy Mefford, Assistant to the Executive Direc
Joe Brady, Deaf and Hard of Hearing Coordin
Brenda Cowden, Housing Specialist
To assist those who have significant disabilities so that they might live independently in the least restrictive and most integrated environment possbile.

4518 **Lynchburg Area Center for Independent Living**
500 Alleghany Ave
Suite #520
Lynchburg, VA 24501-2610
434-528-4971
FAX: 434-528-4976
TTY:434-528-4972
lacil@lacil.org
www.lacil.org

Phil Theisen, Executive Director

LACIL is a private non-profit, non-residential consumer driven organization that promotes the efforts of persons with disabilities to live independently in the community and supports the efforts of the community to be open and accessible to all citizens.

4519 **Peidmont Independent Living Center**
Piedmont Living Center
601 S. Belvidere Street
Richmond, VA 23220
804-782-1986
800-828-1140
FAX: 877-VHD- 123
www.vhda.com

Kit Hale, Chairman
Timothy M. Chapman, Vice Chairman
Susan Dewey, Executive Director
Tammy Neale, Chief Learning Officer
Empowering indivials with disabilities to become self-sufficient and independent within their communities.

4520 **Peninsula Center for Independent Living**
2021-A Cunningham Drive
Suite #2
Hampton, VA 23666-3320
757-827-0275
FAX: 757-827-0655
TTY:757-827-8800
iepcil@hvacil.org
www.hvacil.org

Ralph Shelman, Executive Director
IEPCIL is a private non-profit non-residential Agency established to provide services to people with disabilities. The Centers Philosophy is that people with a disability should play a major role in deciding their future. The center provides services to people with disabilities in the cities of Hampton, Newport News, Poquoson, Williamsburg, and counties of James City, York, and Gloucester.

4521 **Piedmont Independent Living Center**
1045 Main Street
Suite #2
Danville, VA 24541-1800
434-797-2530
FAX: 434-797-2568
TTY:434-797-2530

Clarence Dickerson, Executive Director
Jeanette King, ILS Coordinator/BPAD
Lori Penn, Office Manager
Empowering indivials with disabilities to become self-sufficient and independent within their communities.

4522 **Resources for Independent Living**
4009 Fitzhugh Ave
Richmond, VA 23230-3953
804-353-6503
FAX: 804-358-5606
TTY:804-353-6583
info@ril-va.org
www.ril-va.org

Gerald O'Neill, Executive Director
Marcia Guardino, Program Manager
Kelly Hickok, Community Services Manager
Tom Allen, Chair
Assisting persons who are severly disabled to live independently in the community and to encourage necessary change within the community so independent living is a possibility.

4523 **Valley Associates for Independent Living (VAIL)**
Shenandoah Valley Workforce Investment Board
3210 Peoples Drive
Suite 220
Harrisonburg, VA 22801-869
540-433-6513
888-242-8245
FAX: 540-433-6313
vail@govail.org
www.govail.org

Marcia Du Bois, Executive Director
Bob Satterwhite, Executive Director
VAIL is a not-for-profit, private Center for Independent Living providing advocacy, information and referral, independent living skills training, supported employment, and peer counseling to individuals with disabilities in our planning district.

4524 Valley Associates for Independent Living: Lexington
205-B South Liberty St
Harrisonburg, VA 22801-3638
540-433-6513
888-242-8245
FAX: 540-433-6313
TTY: 540-438-9265
vail@govail.org
www.govail.org

Marcia Du Bois, Executive Director
Promoting self-direction among people with disabilities and removing barriers to independence in the community.

4525 Woodrow Wilson Rehabilitation Center Training Program
243 Woodrow Wilson Avenue
Fishersville, VA 22939-1500
540-332-7000
800-345-9972
FAX: 540-332-7132
TTY: 800-811-7893
WWRCInfo@wwrc.virginia.gov
www.wwrc.net

Rick Sizemore, Executive Director
Information & referral services. Six week Virginia residential programs and evaluation services.

Washington

4526 Alliance for People with Disabilities: Seattle
1120 E. Terrace St
Suite 100
Seattle, WA 98122
206-545-7055
866-545-7055
FAX: 206-545-7059
TTY: 206-632-3456
info@disabilitypride.org
www.disabilitypride.org

Kimberly Heymann, Executive Director
Elizabeth Kennedy, Executive Assistant
Bhelle Ollero, IL Specialist
Hope Drumond, Program Manager
The Alliance promotes equality and choice for people with disabilities. They provide advocacy, peer support, idependent living skills training, information and referral, transition assistance for youth, civil rights legal aid, assistive technology, training and nursing home transition back into the community.

4527 Alliance of People with Disabilities: Redmond
East King County Office
1150 140th Ave NE
Suite 101
Bellevue, WA 98005-3537
425-558-0993
800-216-3335
FAX: 425-558-4773
TTY: 425-861-4773
info@disabilitypride.org
www.disabilitypride.org

Kimberly Heymann, Executive Director
Elizabeth Kennedy, Executive Assistant
Bhelle Ollero, IL Specialist
Hope Drumond, Program Manager
Services include: information and referral, independent living skills training, peer groups, disAbility law project (DLP), access reviews, health insurance advising, and systems advocacy.

4528 Coalition of Responsible Disabled
612 N Maple St
Spokane, WA 99201-1801
509-326-6355
877-606-2680
FAX: 509-327-2420
TTY: 509-326-6355
info@scilwa.org
www.cordwa.info

Charley Lane, Transition Manager
MaryAnn S., Supervisor
Holly M., BS, Representative Payee
Judy M., MBA, Representative Payee

To improve the self-determination and self-reliance of people with disabilities through systems and individual advocacy, education and independent living services.

4529 Community Services for the Blind and Partially Sighted Store: Sight Connection
9709 Third Ave NE
Suite #100
Seattle, WA 98115-2027
206-525-5556
800-458-4888
FAX: 206-525-0422
info@sightconnection.org
www.sightconnection.org

Mary Lewis, Secretary
Shannon Grady Martsolf, President/CEO
Miles Otoupal, Chair
Jonathan Avedovech, Vice Chair
Over 300 practical products for living with vision loss selected by certified vision rehabilitation specialists from Community Services for the Blind and Partially Sighted. Easy-to-use online store features large print, large photos, secure transactions, and links to other vision-related resources.

4530 disAbility Resource Connection: Everett
607 SE Everett Mall Way
Suite 6C
Everett, WA 98208-3210
425-347-5768
800-315-3583
FAX: 425-710-0767
TTY: 425-347-5768
drcservices@drconline.net
www.drconline.net

Charley Lane, Executive Director
disAbility Resource Connection is all about living your life as you choose. The staff is committed to assisting every individual to connect to resources, connect to skills, connect to life.

4531 Kitsap Community Resources
845 8th St
Bremerton, WA 98337-1517
360-478-2301
FAX: 360-415-2706
info@kcr.org
www.kcr.org

Larry Eyer, Executive Director
Irmgard Davis, Fiscal Officer
Rudy Taylor, Board President
Kurt Wiest, Board Vice President
Kitsap Community Resources is a local, non-profit organization dedicated to helping people in need. KCR creates hope and opportunity for low-income Kitsap County Residents by providing resources that promote self-sufficiency.

4532 Tacoma Area Coalition of Individuals with Disabilities
6315 S 19th St
Tacoma, WA 98466-6217
253-565-9000
877-538-2243
FAX: 253-565-5578
TTY: 253-565-3486
tacid@tacid.org
www.tacid.org

Ken Gibson, Executive Director
Steve Pierce, CFO
Jo Ann Maxwell, Deputy Executive Director - Phil
Marsha Doman-Masters, Executive Assistant - Administra
Promotes the independence of individuals with disabilities.

West Virginia

4533 Appalachian Center for Independent Living
4710 Chimney Drive
Suite # C
Charleston, WV 25302-4841   304-965-0376
800-642-3003
FAX: 304-965-0377
TTY: 800-642-3003
acil@yahoo.com
www.mtstcil.org

Ann Weeks, President and CEO
Adam Elmer, Chief Financial Officer
Georgetta Stevens, VP, Corporate Operations
Debbie Conley, Board Chair
A resource center for persons with disabilities and their communities. Serves Kanawha, Clay, Boone and Putnam counties.

4534 Appalachian Center for Independent Living: Spencer
811 Madison Avenue
Suite #106
Spencer, WV 25276-1900   304-927-4080
FAX: 304-927-4330
TTY:800-642-3003
susanacil@yahoo.com
www.mtstcil.org

Ann Weeks, President and CEO
Adam Elmer, Chief Financial Officer
Georgetta Stevens, VP, Corporate Operations
Debbie Conley, Board Chair
A resource center for persons with disabilities and their communities. Serves Jackson, Roane, and Calhoun counties.

4535 Mountain State Center for Independent Living
329 Prince St
Beckley, WV 25801-4515   304-255-0122
FAX: 304-255-0157
TTY:304-255-0122
aoweeks@mtstcil.org
www.mtstcil.org

Ann Weeks, President and CEO
Adam Elmer, Chief Financial Officer
Georgetta Stevens, VP, Corporate Operations
Debbie Conley, Board Chair
This office provides individual and systems advocacy, independent living skills development, information and referral, peer support, personal assistance services, housing referral and training, transportation. Serves Raleigh counties.

4536 Mountain State Center for Independent Living
821 Fourth Avenue
Huntington, WV 25701-1406   304-525-3324
866-687-8245
FAX: 304-525-3360
TTY: 304-525-3324
aoweeks@mtstcil.org
www.mtstcil.org

Ann Weeks, President and CEO
Adam Elmer, Chief Financial Officer
Georgetta Stevens, VP, Corporate Operations
Debbie Conley, Board Chair
Services provided are: individual and systems advocacy, independent living skills development, information and referral, peer support, personal assistance services, supported employment, community integration program, housing referral and training, transportation. Serves Cabell and Wayne counties.

4537 Northern West Virginia Center for Independent Living
601-603 East Brockway
Suite A & B
Morgantown, WV 26501   304-296-6091
800-834-6408
FAX: 304-296-5217
TTY: 304-296-6091
nwvcil@nwvcil.org
www.mtstcil.org

Ann Weeks, President and CEO
Adam Elmer, Chief Financial Officer
Georgetta Stevens, VP, Corporate Operations
Debbie Conley, Board Chair
NWVCIL is committed to the philosophy that all persons have equal access and unconditional value, that all individuals shall be respected for their uniqueness and shall have the right to live within the community of their choice, having equal access to participate in and contribute to that community.

Wisconsin

4538 Center for Independent Living of Western Wisconsin
2920 Schneider Avenue East
Menomonie, WI 54751-2331   715-233-1070
800-228-3287
FAX: 715-233-1083
TTY: 800-228-3287

cilww@cilww.com
www.cilww.com

Tim Sheehan, Executive Director
Kay Sommerfeld, Assistant Director
Tammy Grage, Fiscal & HR Manager
Noelle Johnson, Resource Counselor Camp Quest
Advocates for the full participation in society of all persons with disabilities. Our goal is empwoering individuals to exercise choices to maintain or increase their indpendence. Our strategy is providing consumer-driven services at no cost to persons with disiabilities in Western Wisconsin

4539 Independence First
540 South 1st Street
Milwaukee, WI 53204-1516   414-291-7520
FAX: 414-291-7525
TTY:414-297-7520
lschulz@independencefirst.org
www.independencefirst.org

Lee Schulz, President and CEO
John Schmid, Chair
Judy Murphy, Vice Chair
Judi Wisla, Secretary
A non-profit agency directed by, and for the benefit of, persons with disabilities, primarily serving the four county metropolitan Milwaukee area.

4540 Independence First: West Bend
735 S Main St
West Bend, WI 53095-3965   262-306-6717
lschulz@independencefirst.org
www.independencefirst.org

Lee Schulz, President and CEO
John Schmid, Chair
Judy Murphy, Vice Chair
Judi Wisla, Secretary
A non-profit agency directed by, and for the benefit of, persons with disabilities, primarily serving the four county Metropolitan Milwaukee area.

4541   Inspiration Ministries
N2270 State Road 67
Walworth, WI 53184-948
262-275-6131
FAX: 262-275-3355
IMinfo@InspirationMinistries.org
inspirationministries.org

Robin Knoll, President
Richard Hall, Executive Vice President
Craig Pape, VP Ministry Services
Michael Scholl, VP Development
Formerly known as Christian League for the Handicapped, Inspiration Ministries is a vibrant community of adults with disabilities engaged in living, working, leisure and faith activities designed to provide a complete living experience. The campus consists of a modern residential facility offering a range of living accomodations; a work center and resale shop; and Inspiration Center, a retreat/camping center designed to be 100% wheelchair accessible.

4542   Mid-State Independent Living Consultants: Wausau
3262 Church Street
Suite #1
Stevens Point, WI 54481-5321
715-344-4210
800-382-8484
FAX: 715-344-4414
TTY: 800-382-8484
milc@milc-inc.org
www.milc-inc.org

Tom Vandehey, President
Becky Paulson, Independent Living Consultant
Working for persons with disabilities towards empowerment to make informed choices.

4543   Mid-state Independent Living Consultants: Stevens Point
3262 Church Street
Suite #1
Stevens Point, WI 54481-5321
715-344-4210
800-382-8484
FAX: 715-344-4414
TTY: 800-382-8484
milc@milc-inc.org
www.milc-inc.org

Jenny Fasula, Executive Director
Karalyn Peterson, Resource Director
Committed to enhancing personal and community relationships, providing opportunities for growth, and helping people with varying abilities achieve their personal goals.

4544   North Country Independent Living
69 N 28th St.
Suite 28
Superior, WI 54880-5138
715-392-9118
800-924-1220
FAX: 715-392-4636
john@northcountryil.org
northcountryil.com

John Nousaine, Executive Director
Gloria Hakkila-Johnson, Assistant Director
Jim Glaeser, Accountant
Russ Stover, Office Assistant
Empowers people with disabilities.

4545   North Country Independent Living: Ashland
422 3rd St. W.
Suite #114
Ashland, WI 54806-1553
715-682-5676
800-499-5676
FAX: 715-682-3144
TTY: 715-682-5676
ncilstew@superior-nfp.org
northcountryil.com

John Nousaine, Director
Empowers people with disabilities.

4546   Options for Independent Living
555 Country Club Road
Green Bay, WI 54307-1967
920-490-0500
888-465-1515
FAX: 920-490-0700
TTY:920-490-0600
info@optionsil.com
www.optionsil.com

Thomas Diedrick, Executive Director
Kathryn C. Barry, Assistant Director
Sandra L. Popp, Independent Living Coordinator
Vicky Lasch, Independent Living Coordinator
A non-profit organization committed to empowering people with disabilities to lead independent and productive lives in their community through advocacy, the provision of information, education, technology and related services.

4547   Options for Independent Living: Fox Valley
820 West College Ave
Suite #5
Appleton, WI 54914
920-997-9999
888-465-1515
FAX: 920-997-9381
TTY:920-490-0600
info@optionsil.com
www.optionsil.com

Thomas Diedrick, Executive Director
Kathryn C. Barry, Assistant Director
Sandra L. Popp, Independent Living Coordinator
Vicky Lasch, Independent Living Coordinator
A non-profit organization committed to empowering people with disabilities to lead independent and productive lives in their community through advocacy, the provision of information, education, technology and related services.

4548   Society's Assets: Elkhorn
615 E Geneva St
Elkhorn, WI 53121-2301
262-723-8181
800-261-8181
FAX: 262-723-8184
TTY: 866-840-9763
info@societysassets.org
www.societysassets.org

Bruce Nelson, Director
Jill Vigueres, Manager
To ensure the rights of all persons with disabilities to live and function as independently as possible in the community of their choice, through supporting individual's efforts to achieve control over their lives and become integrated into community life.

4549   Society's Assets: Kenosha
5455 Sheridan Road
Suite 101
Kenosha, WI 53140-4103
262-657-3999
800-317-3999
FAX: 262-657-1672
TTY: 866-840-9762
info@societysassets.org
www.societysassets.org

Sue Liu, Manager
Bruce Nelsen, Executive Director
To ensure the rights of all persons with disabilities to live and function as independently as possible in the community of their choice, through supporting individuals efforts to achieve controll over their lives and become integrated into community life. Offers home care and independent living services.

4550   **Society's Assets: Racine**
5200 Washinton Ave
Suite #225
Racine, WI 53406-4238

262-637-9128
800-378-9128
FAX: 262-637-8646
TTY: 886-840-9761
info@societysassets.org
www.societysassets.org

Deb Pitsch, Administrator
Karen Olufs, Director Independent Living
Jean Rumachik, Director Home Care Services
Society's Assets assists people with disabilities to live as independently as possible. A non-profit human services agency, Society's Assets provides information and referal, independent living skills training, peer support, advocacy, and supportive home care. Home health care is provided by SAI Home Health Care. The agency serves 5 counties in southeastern Wisconsin and also provides information about interpreters, employment, benefits, home modifications, assistive equipment and accessibility.
Fees vary

Wyoming

4551   **RENEW: Gillette**
35 Fairgrounds Road
Newcastle, WY 82701

307-746-4733
888-253-4653
FAX: 307-746-9701
www.renew-wyo.com

Donna Bombeck, Chairwoman
Carolyn Holso, Vice Chairwoman
Renee Nack, Secretary
Bryan Bergstreser, Treasurer
Empowering persons with disabilities to enrich their lives.

4552   **RENEW: Rehabilitation Enterprises of North Eastern Wyoming**
1969 S Sheridan Ave
Sheridan, WY 82801-6108

307-672-7481
888-309-2020
FAX: 307-674-5117
pr@renew-wyo.com
www.renew-wyo.com

Donna Bombeck, Chairwoman
Carolyn Holso, Vice Chairwoman
Renee Nack, Secretary
Bryan Bergstreser, Treasurer
Multi-disciplinary organization dedicated to the highest possible economic and social independence for persons with disabilities. Extensive referral service, specialized employment placement, occupational therapy, psychological services, evaluation services, and coordination of external services as needed to meet client plans and objectives.

4553   **Rehabilitation Enterprises of North Eastern Wyoming: Newcastle**
35 Fairgrounds Rd
Newcastle, WY 82701-2625

307-746-4733
888-693-9245
FAX: 307-746-9701
pr@renew-wyo.com
www.renew-wyo.com

Donna Bombeck, Chairwoman
Carolyn Holso, Vice Chairwoman
Renee Nack, Secretary
Bryan Bergstreser, Treasurer
Empowering persons with disabilities to enrich their lives.

4554   **Wyoming Services for Independent Living**
1156 South 2nd
Lander, WY 82520-3905

307-332-4889
800-266-3061
FAX: 307-332-2491
TTY: 307-332-7582
sjuergens@wyoming.com
www.wysil.org

Susan Hoesel, Business Manager
Donna Langelier, Program Manager
Marcia Henthorn, Program Manager
Valentina Knutson, Independent Living Specialist
Committed to enhancing personal and community relationships, providing opportunities for growth, and helping people with varying abilities achieve thier personal goals.

Law

Associations & Referral Agencies

4555   AIDS Legal Council of Chicago
180 N Michigan Ave
Ste 2110
Chicago, IL 60601   312-427-8990
866-506-3038
FAX: 312-427-8419
info@aidslegal.com
aidslegal.com

Tom Yates, Executive Director
D. Matthew Feldhaus, Esq., President
Mike Sullivan, Esq., Vice-President
Andrew Skiba, CRSP, Treasurer
Legal assistance for people with HIV/AIDS related issues.
Greater Chicago area.

4556   AIDSLAW of Louisiana
3801 Canal Street
New Orleans, LA 70119   504-568-1631
800-375-5035
info@aidslaw.org
www.aidslaw.org

Don Paul Landry, Executive Director
Stacy Morris, Deputy Executive Director
Joshua Holmes, Full-time Staff Attorney
Louise Bienvenu, Supervising Attorney
The mission of AIDSLaw is to provide excellent, specialized legal services for people living with HIV/AIDS in Louisiana, to improve their quality of life and access to health care, related to their HIV/AIDS status.
1989

4557   Center for Disability and Elder Law, Inc.
79 West Monroe Street
Suite 919
Chicago, IL 60603-4908   312-376-1880
866-519-2413
FAX: 312-376-1885
info@cdelaw.org
www.cdelaw.org

Michael Roth, Executive Director
M. Catherine Taylor, Associate Director
Thomas Wendt, Chief Legal Officer
A not-for-profit, 501(c)(3) legal services organization which provides legal services to low income persons residing in Chicago and Cook County, Il., who are either elderly and/or persons with disabilities. CDEL provides legal services by matching qualified candidates with volunteer attorneys who represent them, pro bono, in a wide range of civil legal matters;and (2) through special initiatives including the Senior Center Initiative (SCI) and the Senior Tax Opportunity program (STOP).

4558   Chicago Lawyers' Committee for Civil Rights Under Law
100 N Lasalle Street
Suite 600
Chicago, IL 60602-2403   312-630-9744
FAX: 312-630-1127
opportunities@clccrul.org
www.clccrul.org

Jay Readey, Executive Director
Promotes and protects civil rights, particularly the civil rights of poor, minority, and disadvantaged people in the social, economic, and political systems of the nation.

4559   DNA People's Legal Services
PO Box 306
Window Rock, AZ 86515   928-871-4151
800-789-7287
FAX: 928-871-5036
www.dnalegalservices.org

Kathy Gallagher, Development Director
Tom Parker, Development Assistant

A nonprofit legal aid organization working to protect civil rights, promote tribal sovereignty and alleviate civil legal problems for people who live in poverty in the Southwestern United States.
1967

4560   Disability Rights Education and Defense Fund
3075 Adeline Street
#210
Berkeley, CA 94703-2219   510-644-2555
800-348-4232
FAX: 510-841-8645
info@dredf.org
dredf.org

Sue Henderson, Executive Director
Nonprofit organization dedicated to advancing the civil rights of individuals with disabilities through legislation, litigation, informal and formal advocacy and education and training of lawyers, advocates and clients with respect to disability issues. DREDF also provides training, advocacy, technical assistance and referrals for parents of disabled children.

4561   Disability Rights Texas
2222 West Braker Lane
Austin, TX 78758-1024   512-454-4816
FAX: 512-302-4936
www.disabilityrightstx.org

Mary Faithfull, Executive Director
The federally designated legal protection and advocacy agency (P&A) for people with disabilities in Texas. Helps people with disabilities understand and exercise their rights under the law, ensuring their full and equal participation in society.

4562   Equal Employment Advisory Council
1501 M Street NW
Suite 400
Washington, DC 20005   202-629-5650
FAX: 202-629-5651
info@eeac.org
www.eeac.org

Jeffrey A Norris, President
Nicole McDuffie, Administrator
Nonprofit employer association founded in 1976 to provide guidance to its member companies on understanding and complying with their EEO and affirmative action obligations.

4563   Guardianship Services Associates
41A South Blvd
Oak Park, IL 60302-2777   708-386-5398
FAX: 708-386-5970
GSAoakpark@sbcglobal.net

Robert R. Wohlgemuth, Owner
Information and counseling on guardianship and its alternatives. Can provide direct assistance in obtaining guardianship for disabled adults in Cook County. Also provides information and direct assistance on durable powers of attorney. Can assume appointment as guardian in selected cases.

4564   Independence Council for Economic Development
201 N Forest Avenue
Suite 120
Independence, MO 64050- 2753   816-252-5777
FAX: 816-254-1641
tlesnak@inedc.biz
www.iced.org

Tom Lesnak, President
A non-profit, public/private partnership established for the purpose of supporting and enhancing the economic growth of independence.

4565   Judge David L Bazelon Center for Mental Health Law
1101 15th Street NW
Suite 1212
Washington, DC 20005   202-467-5730
                                   FAX: 202-223-0409
                                   TTY:202-467-4232
                            communications@bazelon.org
                                      www.bazelon.org

Robert Berstein, Executive Director

A nonprofit organization devoted to improving the lives of people with mental illnesses through changes in policy and law.

4566   Legal Action Center
236 Massachusetts Avenue NE
Suite 505
Washington, DC 20002-4980   202-544-5478
                                   FAX: 202-544-5712
                                      lacdc@lac.org
                                        www.lac.org

Paul N Samuels, Director/President

The only non-profit law and policy organization in the United States whose sole mission is to fight discrimination against people with histories of addiction, HIV/AIDS, or criminal records, and to advocate for sound public policies in these areas.

4567   Legal Center for People with Disabilities& Older People
455 Sherman Street
Suite 130
Denver, CO 80203   303-722-0300
                                   FAX: 303-722-0720
                              tlcmail@thelegalcenter.org
                                www.thelegalcenter.org

Peter Lindquist, Esq., President

Protects and promotes the rights of people with disabilities and older people in Colorado through direct legal representation, advocacy, education and legislative analysis.

4568   Legislative Handbook for Parents
NAPVI
1 North Lexington Avenue
8th Floor
White Plains, NY 10601   617-972-7441
                                        800-562-6265
                                   FAX: 617-972-7444
                                napvi@guildhealth.org
                                       www.napvi.org

Susan LaVenture, Executive Director
Julie Urban, President
Venetia Hayden, Vice President
Randi Sher, Secretary

A helpful publication for parents who make direct contact with public officials on behalf of their children. Sample letters, do's-and-dont's, and a glossary of legislative terms are some of the useful topics that are contained in this manual. *$5.50*

24 pages Paperback

4569   NHeLP
3701 Wilshire Blvd
Suite 750
Los Angeles, CA 90010   310-204-6010
                                   FAX: 213-368-0774
                                 nhelp@healthlaw.org
                                    www.healthlaw.org

Abbi Coursolle, Staff Attorney
Kimberly Lewis, Managing Attorney

A national public interest law firm that seeks to improve health care for America's working and unemployed poor, minorities, the elderly and people with disabilities. NHeLP serves legal services programs, community-based organizations, the private bar, providers and individuals who work to preserve a health care safety net for the millions of uninsured or underinsured low-income people.
1970

4570   National Right to Work Legal Defense and Education Foundation
8001 Braddock Rd, Ste 600
Springfield, VA 22160-1   703-321-8510
                                        800-336-3600
                                   FAX: 703-321-9319
                                     legal@nrtw.org
                                         nrtw.org

Raymond LaJeunesse, Director

Provides free legal aid to employees whose human and civil rights are being violated by compulsory unionism abuses.

4571   Pocket Guide to the ADA: Accessibility Guidelines for Buildings and Facilities
Wiley Publishing
111 River St
Hoboken, NJ 07030-5774   201-748-6000
                                   FAX: 201-748-6088
                                    info@wiley.com
                                      www.wiley.com

Evan Terry, Editor

Helps readers understand the facilities requirements of the Americans with Disabilities Act Accessibility Guidelines. Presents the technical requirements for accessible elements and spaces in new construction, alterations and additions. *$30.00*

198 pages Paperback
ISBN 0-470108-70-3

4572   Public Law 101-336
US Department of Justice
950 Pennsylvania Ave NW
Washington, DC 20530-9   202-307-0663
                                        800-514-0301
                                   FAX: 202-307-1197
                                   TTY: 800-514-0383
                                        www.ada.gov

Rebecca B. Bond, Chief
Zita Johnson Betts, Deputy Chief
Sally Conway, Deputy Chief
James Bostrom, Deputy Chief

Text of the Americans with Disabilities Act, as enacted on July 26, 1990.

4573   Questions and Answers: The ADA and Hiring Police Officers
US Department of Justice
950 Pennsylvania Ave NW
Washington, DC 20530   202-307-0663
                                        800-574-0301
                                   FAX: 202-307-1197
                                        www.ada.gov

Rebecca B. Bond, Chief
Zita Johnson Betts, Deputy Chiefs
James Bostrom, Deputy Chiefs
Sally Conway, Deputy Chiefs

Provides information on ADA requirements for interviewing and hiring police officers.

5 pages

4574   REACH/Resource Centers on Independent Living
1000 Macon Street
Suite 200
Fort Worth, TX 76102-4527   817-870-9082
                                   FAX: 817-877-1622
                                   TTY:817-870-9086
                                reachfwt@reachcils.org
                                    www.reachcils.org

Charlotte A Stewart, Executive Director
Missy Dickenson, Assistant Director
Murphy Hardinger, IL Skills Training & ADA Specialist
Becky Teal, Office Manager

Providing services for people with disabilities so that they are empowered to lead self-directed lives and educating the general public on disability-related topics in order to promote a barrier-free community.

4575 **Strengthening the Roles of Independent Living Centers Through Implementing Legal Service**
Independent Living Research Utilization ILRU
1333 Moursund
Houston, TX 77030-7031
713-520-0232
FAX: 713-520-5785
TTY:713-520-0232
ilru@ilru.org
ilru.org

Lex Frieden, Director
Jacquie Brennan, Legal Specialist
Linda CoVan, Grant Coordinator
Maria Del Bosque, Project Associate
Featuring the Disability Law Clinic at Community Resources for Independence (CRI) in Northern California.
10 pages

4576 **Summaries of Legal Precedents & Law Review**
Through the Looking Glass
3075 Adeline Street
Suite 120
Berkeley, CA 94703
510-848-1005
800-644-2666
FAX: 510-848-4445
TLG@lookingglass.org
www.lookingglass.org

Stephanie Miyashiro, Board President
Thomas Spalding, Board Treasurer
Alice Nemon, Board Secretary
Christina Jopes, Board Member
Summarized legal precedents and law review articles relevant to marital custody and child protection situations of parents with diverse disabilities. *$25.00*
24 pages

4577 **TASH Connections**
1001 Connecticut Avenue NW
Suite 325
Washington, DC 20036
202-540-9020
FAX: 202-540-9019
info@tash.org
www.tash.org

Barbara Trader, Executive Director
Jonathan Riethmaier, Advocacy Communications Manager
Haley Kimmet, Program Manager
Patrick Allen, Program Assistant
Received as a member benefit that keeps readers informed on best practices, family concerns, advocacy events and policy changes.
Quarterly

Resources for the Disabled

4578 **ABDA/ABMPP Annual Conference**
American Board of Disability Analysts
4525 Harding Road
2nd Floor
Nashville, TN 37205
615-327-2984
FAX: 615-327-9235
americanbd@aol.com
www.americandisability.org

Alexander E. Horowitz, Executive Officer Emeritus
Kenneth N. Anchor, Administrative Officer/Editor
Gabriel Sella, Education Coordinator
Lela Boggs, Business Manager
February workshop. Workshop leader: Dr. William Tsushima.

4579 **Americans with Disabilities Act Manual**
US Department of Justice
950 Pennsylvania Ave NW
Washington, DC 20530-9
202-307-0663
800-514-0301
FAX: 202-307-1197
TTY: 800-514-0383
www.ada.gov

Rebecca B. Bond, Chief
Zita Johnson Betts, Deputy Chief
Sally Conway, Deputy Chief
James Bostrom, Deputy Chief
An in-depth analysis of the legal and practical implications of the ADA using non-technical language. *$20.00*

4580 **Americans with Disabilities Act: Selected Resources for Deaf**
Gallaudet University Bookstore
800 Florida Avenue NE
Washington, DC 20002-3695
202-651-5000
800-621-2736
FAX: 202-651-5508
clerc.center@gallaudet.edu
www.gallaudet.edu

Priscilla O'Donnell, Bookstore Manager
Iva Williams, Bookstore Secretary
Elaine Vance, Human Resources Director
Marteal Pitts, Circulation Coordinator
This resource identifies programs and publications specific to the ADA and deafness and also lists ADA materials and programs for people with any disability.

4581 **Approaching Equality**
T J Publishers
Ste 108
2544 Tarpley Rd
Carrollton, TX 75006-2288
972-416-0800
800-999-1168
FAX: 301-585-5930
TJPubinc@aol.com

Frank Bowe, Author
Public education laws guarantee special education for all deaf children, but may find the special education system confusing, or are unsure of their rights under current laws. For anyone with an interest in education, advocacy and the deaf community, this book reviews dramatic developments in education of deaf children, youth and adults since COED's 1988 report, Toward Equality.. *$12.95*
112 pages
ISBN 0-93266 -39-6

4582 **Assessment of the Feasibility of Contracting with a Nominee Agency**
Mississippi State University
PO Drawer 6189
Mississippi State, MS 39762
662-325-2001
FAX: 662-325-8989
rrtc@colled.msstate.edu
www.blind.msstate.edu

Michelle Capella McDonnall, Interim Director
Stephanie Hall, Business Manager
Douglas Bedsaul, Research and Training Coordinator
Jacqui Bybee, Research Associate II
Only five State Licensing Agencies currently utilize nominee agreements. This study compared the Pennsylvania BE program with four states that utilize nominee agencies and four states that do not. *$20.00*
152 pages Paperback

4583 **Bluebook: Explanation of the Contents of the ADA**
Disability Rights Education and Defense Fn
3075 Adeline Street
Suite 210
Berkeley, CA 94703
510-644-2555
800-348-4232
FAX: 510-841-8645
TTY: 510-841-8645
info@dredf.org
dredf.org

Claudia Center, President and Chair
Ann Cupolo Freeman, Secretary and Treasurer
Susan Henderson, Executive Director
Arlene B. Mayerson, Directing Attorney
Written in narrative form for both professionals and lay people,
DREDF's bluebook offers detailed, thorough analysis of all of
the law's provisions, encompassing ADA legislative history, the
statute and regulations. Available in alternative formats. *$100.00*
214 pages

4584 **Can America Afford to Grow Old?**
Brookings Institution
1775 Massachusetts Ave NW
Washington, DC 20036-2103
202-797-6000
FAX: 202-797-6004
bibooks@brookings.edu
www.brookings.edu

William Antholis, Managing Director
Steven Bennett, Vice President and Chief Operating Officer
Kimberly Churches, Vice President for Development
Kemal Dervis, Vice President and Director, Global Economy and
Development
Social security laws and regulations. *$8.95*
144 pages Paperback
ISBN 0-815700-43-1

4585 **Childcare and the ADA**
Eastern Washington University
Rm 223
705 W 1st Ave
Spokane, WA 99201-3909
509-623-4200
FAX: 509-623-4230
susan.vanmeter@mail.ewu.edu

Nancy Ashworth, Director Child Development
Allen Barrom, Manager
Provides information on how childcare providers must comply
with the ADA. Eight videotapes plus an instructional manual
with examples of situations and problems.. *$85.00*
Set

4586 **Common ADA Errors and Omissions in New Construction
and Alterations**
US Department of Justice
950 Pennsylvania Ave NW
Washington, DC 20530
202-307-0663
800-574-0301
FAX: 202-307-1197
www.ada.gov

Rebecca B. Bond, Chief
Zita Johnson Betts, Deputy Chiefs
James Bostrom, Deputy Chiefs
Sally Conway, Deputy Chiefs
Lists a sampling of common accessibility errors or omissions that
have been identified through the Department of Justice's ongoing
enforcement efforts.
13 pages

4587 **Commonly Asked Questions About Child Care Centers and
the Americans with Disabilities Act**
US Department of Justice
950 Pennsylvania Ave NW
Washington, DC 20530
202-307-0663
800-574-0301
FAX: 202-307-1197
www.ada.gov

Rebecca B. Bond, Chief
Zita Johnson Betts, Deputy Chiefs
James Bostrom, Deputy Chiefs
Sally Conway, Deputy Chiefs
Explains how the requirements of the ADA apply to Child Care
Centers. Also describes some of the Department of justice's on-
going enformcement efforts in the child care area and it provides
a resource list on sources of information on the ADA.
13 pages

4588 **Commonly Asked Questions About Title III of the ADA**
US Department of Justice
950 Pennsylvania Ave NW
Washington, DC 20530-9
202-307-0663
800-574-0301
FAX: 202-307-1197
TTY: 800-514-0383
www.ada.gov

Rebecca B. Bond, Chief
Zita Johnson Betts, Deputy Chief
Sally Conway, Deputy Chief
James Bostrom, Deputy Chief
A 6-page publication providing information for state and local
governments about ADA requirements for ensuring that people
with disabilities receive the same services and benefits as
provided to others.
on-line

4589 **Commonly Asked Questions About the ADA and Law
Enforcement**
US Department of Justice
950 Pennsylvania Ave NW
Washington, DC 20530-9
202-307-0663
800-574-0301
FAX: 202-307-1197
TTY: 800-514-0383
www.ada.gov

Rebecca B. Bond, Chief
Zita Johnson Betts, Deputy Chief
Sally Conway, Deputy Chief
James Bostrom, Deputy Chief
A publication explaining ADA requirements for ensuring that
people with disabilities receive the same law enforcement ser-
vices and protections as provided to others.
13 pages on-line

4590 **Complying with the Americans with Disabilis Act**
Greenwood Publishing Group
130 Cremona Drive
Santa Barbara, CA 93117
805-968-1911
800-368-6868
FAX: 866-270-3856
CustomerService@abc-clio.com
www.greenwood.com

Don Fresh, Author
Peter W Thomas, Co-Author
John Gosden, Library Resource Consultants
Lina Gosden, Library Resource Consultants
A guidebook for management and people with disabilities. This
unique guidebook presents a comprehensive analysis of the new
Americans with Disabilities Act (ADA), the most significant federal civil rights law in almost 30 years, and its impact on over four
million American businesses, state and local governments, non-
profit associations, 87 percent of American's private sector jobs,
and 22.7 million working-age people with disabilities. *$117.95*
280 pages Hardcover
ISBN 0-899307-14-0

4591 Court-Related Needs of the Elderly and Persons with Disabilities
Mental Health Commission
2700 Martin Luther King Jr Ave SE
Washington, DC 20032- 2601
202-282-0027
FAX: 202-373-7982
276 pages

4592 Criminal Law Handbook on Psychiatric & Psychological Evidence & Testimony
New York City Bar
42 West 44th Street
New York, NY 10036-6604
212-382-6600
FAX: 212-768-8116
phynes@nycbar.org
www.nycbar.org

Bret Parker, Executive Director
Debra Raskin, President
Alan Rothstein, General Counsel
Maria Cilenti, Director Legislative Affairs
The Criminal Law Handbook provides lawyers, judges and forensic experts with comprehensive, in-depth treatment of admissibility (and limitations on admissibility) of psychiatric and psychological evidence and testimony pertaining to key criminal mental health law standards. *$47.00*

4593 Department of Justice ADA Mediation Program
US Department of Justice
950 Pennsylvania Ave NW
Washington, DC 20530
202-307-0663
800-574-0301
FAX: 202-307-1197
TTY: 800-514-0383
www.ada.gov

Rebecca B. Bond, Chief
Zita Johnson Betts, Deputy Chiefs
James Bostrom, Deputy Chiefs
Sally Conway, Deputy Chiefs
Provides an overview of the Department's Mediation Program and examples of successfully mediated cases.
6 pages

4594 Dimensions of State Mental Health Policy
Greenwood Publishing Group
130 Cremona Drive
Santa Barbara, CA 93117
805-968-1911
800-368-6868
FAX: 866-270-3856
CustomerService@abc-clio.com
www.greenwood.com

Christopher Hudson, Author
Arthur J Cox, Co-Author
John Gosden, Library Resource Consultants
Lina Gosden, Library Resource Consultants
Introduces students to the emerging field of state mental health policy, its history, current policies, organizational models and required programming knowledge. *$86.95*
320 pages Hardcover
ISBN 0-275932-52-7

4595 Disability Compliance for Higher Education
LRP Publications
360 Hiatt Dr
Palm Beach Gardens, FL 33418
561-622-6520
800-341-7874
FAX: 561-622-0757
lrpitvp@lrp.com
www.lrp.com

Kenneth Kahn, CEO
Gives guidance on the most difficult issues faced, such as supporting students with psychological disabilities, ensuring accessibility, understanding OCR rulings, and more. *$57.29*
300 pages

4596 Disability Discrimination Law, Evidence and Testimony
ABA Commission on Mental & Physical Disability Law
1050 Connecticut Ave. N.W.
Suite 400
Washington, DC 20036
202-662-1000
800-285-2221
FAX: 202-442-3439
cmpdl@americanbar.org
www.americanbar.org

John W Parry JD, Author
Explains and analyzes key aspects of disability discriminiation law from several different perspectives to guide you through the myriad federal and state statutes, court cases, and regulations.
$105.00
694 pages Paperback
ISBN 1-604420-12-8

4597 Disability Law in the United States
William Hein & Company
2350 North Forest Rd.
Getzville, NY 14068-1296
716-882-2600
800-828-7571
FAX: 716-883-8100
mail@wshein.com
www.wshein.com

Dr Bernard D Reams Jr, Author
Peter J McGovern, Co-Author
Jon S Schultz, Co-Author
Offers thousands of pages of information on the laws and legislation affecting the disabled in the United States. Its purpose is to provide a clear and comprehensive mandate to end discrimination against individuals with disabilities and to bring disabled persons into the economic and social midstream of American Life.
$675.00
5750 pages
ISBN 0-899417-97-3

4598 Disability Rights Now
Disability Rights Education and Defense Fund
3075 Adeline Street
Suite 210
Berkeley, CA 94703
510-644-2555
800-348-4232
FAX: 510-841-8645
TTY: 510-841-8645
info@dredf.org
dredf.org

Claudia Center, President and Chair
Ann Cupolo Freeman, Secretary and Treasurer
Susan Henderson, Executive Director
Arlene B. Mayerson, Directing Attorney
Free quarterly publication describing the activities of the Disability Rights Education and Defense Fund, available in alternative formats.
Quarterly

4599 Disability Under the Fair Employment & Housing Act: What You Should Know About the Law
California Department of Fair Employment & Housing
2218 Kausen Drive
Suite 100
Elk Grove, CA 95758
916-478-7251
800-884-1684
FAX: 916-227-2870
contact.center@dfeh.ca.gov
www.dfeh.ca.gov

Phyllis W Cheng, Director
Intended to highlight and summarize workplace disability laws enforced by the California Department of Fair Employment and Housing. It will familiarize people with the content of these laws, including recent changes and amendments to state statutes and attendent accommodation responsibilities.

4600 Discrimination is Against the Law
California Department of Fair Employment & Housing
2218 Kausen Drive
Suite 100
Elk Grove, CA 95758 916-478-7251
800-884-1684
FAX: 916-227-2870
contact.center@dfeh.ca.gov
www.dfeh.ca.gov

Phyllis Cheng, Director
Enforces California state laws that prohibit harassment and discrimination in employment, housing, and public accomodations and that provide for pregnancy leave and family and personal leave.

4601 Education of the Handicapped: Laws, Legislative Histories and Administrative Document
William S Hein & Co Inc
2350 North Forest Rd.
Getzville, NY 14068-1296 716-882-2600
800-828-7571
FAX: 716-883-8100
mail@wshein.com
www.wshein.com

Bernard D Reams Jr, Editor
Focuses upon Elementary and Secondary Education Act of 1965 and its amendment, Education For All Handicapped Children Act of 1975 and its amendments and acts providing services for the blind, deaf, mentally retarded, etc. *$2950.00*
55 volumes
ISBN 0-899411-57-6

4602 ElderLawAnswers.com
150 Chestnut Street
4th Floor, Box 15
Providence, RI 02903 617-267-9700
866-267-0947
support@elderlawanswers.com
www.elderlawanswers.com

Harry S Margolis, Founder/President
Mark Miller, Director of Product and Business Development
Ken Coughlin, Managing Editor
Supports seniors, their families and their attorneys in achieving their goals by providing

4603 Employment Discrimination Based on Disability
California Department of Fair Employment & Housing
2218 Kausen Drive
Suite 100
Elk Grove, CA 95758 916-478-7251
800-884-1684
FAX: 916-227-2870
contact.center@dfeh.ca.gov
www.dfeh.ca.gov

Phyllis W Cheng, Director
Prohibits employment discrimination and harassment based on a person's disability or perceived disability. Also requires employers to reasonably accommodate individuals with mental or physical disabilities unless the employer can show that to do so would cause an undue hardship.

4604 Employment Standards Administration Department of Labor (ESA)
200 Constitution Ave NW
Washington, DC 20210-1 800-321-6742
TTY:877-889-5627
osha.gov

David Michaels, Assistant Secretary
Jordan Barab, Deputy Assistant Secretary
Richard Fairfax, Deputy Assistant Secretary
Deborah Berkowitz, Chief of Staff
Monitors compliance with sub-minimum wage requirements for handicapped workers in sheltered workshops, competitive industry and hospitals and institutions under Section 14 of the Fair Labor Standards Act of 1938.

4605 Enforcing the ADA: A Status Report from the Department of Justice
US Department of Justice
950 Pennsylvania Ave NW
Washington, DC 20530 202-307-0663
800-514-0301
FAX: 203-307-1197
www.ada.gov

Rebecca B. Bond, Chief
Zita Johnson Betts, Deputy Chiefs
James Bostrom, Deputy Chiefs
Sally Conway, Deputy Chiefs
A brief report issued by the Justice Department each quarter providing timely information about ADA cases and settlements, building codes that meet ADA accessibility standards, and ADA technical assistance activities.

4606 Federal Laws of the Mentally Handicapped: Laws, Legislative Histories and Admin. Documents
William Hein & Company
2350 North Forest Rd.
Getzville, NY 14068-1296 716-882-2600
800-828-7571
FAX: 716-883-8100
mail@wshein.com
www.wshein.com

Bernard D Reams Jr, Editor
Chronological compilation of all relevant federal laws dealing with the mentally handicapped along with supporting documentation necessary to create a complete legislative history. *$3500.00*
42 Volume/Set
ISBN 0-899411-06-1

4607 Formed Families: Adoption of Children with Handicaps
Haworth Press
711 Third Avenue
New York, NY 10017 212-216-7800
800-354-1420
FAX: 212-244-1563
subscriptions@tandf.co.uk.
www.haworthpress.com

William Cohen, Owner
Provides broad coverage of the issues relating to the adoption of children with handicaps. Concerned professionals can find here all the answers about clinical programs, legal issues, estimates of frequency, and important factors related to positive and negative outcomes of these adoptions. *$74.95*
242 pages Hardcover
ISBN 0-866569-14-6

4608 Free Appropriate Public Education: The Law and Children with Disabilities
Love Publishing Company
9101 E Kenyon Avenue
Suite 2200
Denver, CO 80237 303-221-7333
FAX: 303-221-7444
lpc@lovepublishing.com
www.lovepublishing.com

H Rutherford Turnbull III, Author
Matthew J Stowe, Co-Author
Nancy E Huerta, Co-Author
Includes the 2004 IDEA reauthorization and the proposed regulations. This up-to-the-minute resource brings you the most recent developments in legislation, case law techniques, due process, parent participation and much, much more. *$78.00*
448 pages Hardcover
ISBN 0-891083-25-2

4609 **Health Care Quality Improvement Act of 1986**
William Hein & Company
2350 North Forest Rd.
Getzville, NY 14068-1296

716-882-2600
800-828-7571
FAX: 716-883-8100
mail@wshein.com
www.wshein.com

Bernard D Reams Jr, Editor
In order to encourage more stringent peer review by doctors and hospitals, and to protect reporting physicians and institutions from retaliatory lawsuits, Congress enacted The Health Care Quality Improvement Act. The Act was also intended to address the increasing incidence of medical malpractice and to prevent the ease with which incompetent practitioners moved from state to state. Hardcover. *$125.00*
721 pages
ISBN 0-899416-93-4

4610 **Housing and Transportation of the Handicapped**
William Hein & Company
2350 North Forest Rd.
Getzville, NY 14068-1296

716-882-2600
800-828-7571
FAX: 716-883-8100
mail@wshein.com
www.wshein.com

Bernard D Reams Jr, Editor
National laws, recognizing the problems encountered by the handicapped in the areas of Housing and Transportation and providing assistance in an effort to surmount those problems, span more than half a century. *$1552.50*
30000 pages 250 documents
ISBN 0-899412-47-5

4611 **Human Resource Management and the Americans with Disabilities Act**
Greenwood Publishing Group
130 Cremona Drive
Santa Barbara, CA 93117

805-968-1911
800-368-6868
FAX: 866-270-3856
CustomerService@abc-clio.com
www.greenwood.com

John G Veres, Author
Ronald R Sims, Co-Author
John Gosden, Library Resource Consultants
Lina Gosden, Library Resource Consultants
Concrete advice for human resource professionals on how to cope with the vague, often obscure provisions of the Americans with Disabilities Act. *$107.95*
232 pages Hardcover
ISBN 0-899308-57-9

4612 **International Handbook on Mental Health Policy**
Greenwood Publishing Group
130 Cremona Drive
Santa Barbara, CA 93117

805-968-1911
800-368-6868
FAX: 866-270-3856
CustomerService@abc-clio.com
www.greenwood.com

John Gosden, Library Resource Consultants
Lina Gosden, Library Resource Consultants
Steve Pearson, Library Resource Consultants
Lou Pingitore, Library Resource Consultants
The first major reference book for academics and practitioners that provides a systematic survey and analysis of mental health policies in twenty representative countries. *$179.95*
512 pages Hardcover
ISBN 0-313275-67-8

4613 **Knowing Your Rights**
A AR P Fulfillment
601 E St NW
Washington, DC 20049-1

202-434-3525
800-687-2277
FAX: 202-434-3443
TTY: 877-434-7598
member@aarp.org
www.aarp.org

William D. Novelli, CEO
Lynn Smith, Director of Human Resources
Describes how changes in Medicare's reimbursement policies are designed to reduce health care costs and suggests steps that Medicare beneficiaries, their families and friends can take to assure that they continue to receive quality care under the Prospective Payment System.
19 pages

4614 **Law Center Newsletter**
Public Interest Law Center of Philadelphia
1709 Benjamin Franklin Parkway
United Way Building
Philadelphia, PA 19103

215-627-7100
FAX: 215-627-3183
general@pilcop.org
www.pilcop.org

Eric J Rothschild, Chair
Brian T Feeney, Vice Chair
Jennifer R. Clarke, Executive Director
Ellen S Friedell, Treasurer
Information on mental health, foster care and public education. Provides all updates concerning the law in these areas.

4615 **Legal Center for People with Disabilities& Older People**
455 Sherman St
Suite 130
Denver, CO 80203

303-722-0300
800-288-1376
FAX: 303-722-0720
TTY: 303-722-3619
tlcmail@thelegalcenter.org
www.thelegalcenter.org

Mary Anne Harvey, Executive Director
John R. Posthumus, President
Stephen P. Rickles, Vice President
John Paul Anderson, Treasurer
Uses the legal system to protect and promote the rights of people with disabilities and older people in Colorado through direct legal representation, advocacy, education and legislative analysis. The Legal Center is Colorado's Protection and Advocacy System. We are also the State Ombudsman for nursing homes and assisted living facilities. Call for a free publications and products list.

4616 **Legal Right: The Guide for Deaf and Hard of Hearing People**
National Association of the Deaf
8630 Fenton Street
Suite 820
Silver Spring, MD 20910- 3819

301-587-1789
FAX: 301-587-1791
TTY:301-587-1789
www.nad.org

Christopher Wagner, Board Chair
Howard A. Rosenblum, Chief Executive Officer
Marc P. Charmatz, Staff Attorney
Lizzie Sorkin, Director of Communications
This revised fifth edition is in easy-to-understand language, offering the latest state and federal statues and administrative procedures that prohibit discrimination against the deaf, hard of hearing and other physically challenged people. *$32.50*
264 pages Paperback
ISBN 1-563680-00-9

4617 **Legal Rights of Persons with Disabilities**
LRP Publications
360 Hiatt Dr
Palm Beach Gardens, FL 33418-7106

561-622-6520
800-341-7874
FAX: 561-622-0757
lrpitvp@lrp.com
www.lrp.com

Kenneth Kahn, CEO
Shows what is required, permitted and guaranteed by federal disability laws-including the ADA, Section 504 of the Rehabilitation Act and the IDEA. Explores the boundaries of accceptable behavior under disability laws and provides guidelines to help clients fulfill their legal obligations. *$365.00*
2722 pages

4618 **Legislative Network for Nurses**
Business Publishers
2222 Sedwick Drive
Durham, NC 27713

800-223-8720
FAX: 800-508-2592
custserv@bpinews.com
www.bpinews.com

8 pages Newsl./BiMonthly

4619 **Loving Justice**
Exceptional Parent Library
P.O.Box 1807
Englewood Cliffs, NJ 7632-1207

201-947-6000
800-535-1910
FAX: 201-947-9376
eplibrary@aol.com
www.eplibrary.com

4620 **Making News: How to Get News Coverage of Disability Rights Issues**
Advocado Press
PO Box 406781
Louisville, KY 40204

888-739-1920
FAX: 502-899-9562
contact145@avocadopress.org
www.advocadopress.org

Tari Susan Hartman, Author
Mary Johnson, Co-Author
This book gives examples and tips on how to fight back and get on the front pages, lead the newscasts and influence public debate. *$10.95*
165 pages Paperback
ISBN 0-962706-43-4

4621 **Medicare and Medicaid Patient and Program Protection Act of 1987**
William Hein & Company
2350 North Forest Rd.
Getzville, NY 14068-1296

716-882-2600
800-828-7571
FAX: 716-883-8100
mail@wshein.com
www.wshein.com

Bernard D Reams Jr, Editor
Enables the HHS to protect patients and federal health care programs from censured practitioners. The Act broadens the authority of HHS to exclude practitioners from Medicare and Medicaid programs; strengthens the monetary penalities HHS may impose on violators; provides for criminal penalties in certain cases; and requires states to inform HHS regarding sanctions against health care providers. *$195.00*
3 Volumes
ISBN 0-899416-95-0

4622 **Mental & Physical Disability Law Reporter**
American Bar Association
1050 Connecticut Ave. N.W.
Suite 400
Washington, DC 20036-1019

202-662-1570
800-285-2221
FAX: 202-442-3439
cmpdl@abanet.org
www.abanet.org

Robert M Carlson, Chair
James R Silkenat, President
Jack L Rives, Executive Director
G. Nicholas Casey, Treasurer
Contains over 2,000 summaries per year of federal and state court decisions and legislation that affect persons with mental and physical disabilities. Includes bylined articles by experts in the field regarding disability law developments and trends. *$384.00*
350+ pages BiMonthly

4623 **Mental Disabilities and the Americans with Disabilities Act**
Greenwood Publishing Group
130 Cremona Drive
Santa Barbara, CA 93117

805-968-1911
800-368-6868
FAX: 866-270-3856
CustomerService@abc-clio.com
www.greenwood.com

John Gosden, Library Resource Consultants
Lina Gosden, Library Resource Consultants
Steve Pearson, Library Resource Consultants
Lou Pingitore, Library Resource Consultants
A clear, practical compliance guide, written by a psychologist, to help organizations conform to provisions on mental disabilities in the Americans with Disabilities Act. Hardcover. *$91.95*
216 pages Hardcover
ISBN 0-899308-26-5

4624 **Mental Disability Law, Evidence and Testimony**
ABA Commission on Mental & Physical Disability Law
1050 Connecticut Ave. N.W.
Suite 400
Washington, DC 20036-1019

202-662-1000
800-285-2221
www.abanet.org

Robert M Carlson, Chair
James R Silkenat, President
Jack L Rives, Executive Director
G. Nicholas Casey, Treasurer
Provides a comprehensive analysis of federal and state statues and case law with a disability discrimination focus. *$95.00*
491 pages Paperback
ISBN 1-590318-32-3

4625 **Mental Health Law Reporter**
Business Publishers
2222 Sedwick Drive
Durham, NC 27713

240-514-0600
800-223-8720
FAX: 800-508-2592
custserv@bpinews.com
www.bpinews.com

Leonard A Eiserer, Publisher
Jeremy Bond, Editor MHLR
Bob Grupe, Editor MHLR
Adam Goldstein, President
MHLR brings you the most timely, focused and thorough information on the legal issues that concern mental health practitioners in mental health litigation. Topics include: malpractice litigation, patient-therapist confidentiality, sexual victimization of patients, the insanity defense, social security administrative case law and much more.. *$286.00*
8 pages Monthly

4626   Mental and Physical Disability Law Reporter
American Bar Association
1050 Connecticut Ave. N.W.
Suite 400
Washington, DC 20036-1019   202-662-1000
                                             800-285-2221
                                    service@americanbar.org
                                        www.americanbar.org
Wm T Robinson III, President
The only periodical that comprehensively covers civil and criminal mental disability law and disability discrimination law. *$324.00*
150+ pages Bimonthly

4627   Mentally Disabled and the Law
William S Hein & Company
2350 North Forest Rd.
Getzville, NY 14068-1296   716-882-2600
                                              800-828-7571
                                     FAX: 716-883-8100
                                         mail@wshein.com
                                           www.wshein.com
Samuel Brakel, Author
John Parry, Co-Author
Barbara A Weiner, Co-Author
Chapters retained from 1961 and 1971 editions have been substantially rewritten. Two subjects-sterilization and sexual psychopathy-have been integrated into chapters on family law. Three new chapters on treatment rights, provider-patient relationship and rights of mentally disabled persons in the community. Sixteen new tables supplement the existing revised 41. *$92.00*
845 pages
ISBN 0-910059-05-5

4628   Myths and Facts
US Department of Justice
950 Pennsylvania Ave NW
Washington, DC 20530-9   202-307-0663
                                              800-514-0301
                                     FAX: 202-307-1197
                                     TTY: 800-514-0383
                                              www.ada.gov
Rebecca B. Bond, Chief
Zita Johnson Betts, Deputy Chief
Sally Conway, Deputy Chief
James Bostrom, Deputy Chief
A 3-page publication dispelling some common misconceptions about the ADA's requirements and implementation.

4629   NAD Broadcaster
National Association of the Deaf
8630 Fenton Street
Suite 820
Silver Spring, MD 20910- 3819   301-587-1789
                                     FAX: 301-587-1791
                                     TTY:301-587-1789
                                         nad.info@nad.org
                                              www.nad.org
Christopher Wagner, Board Chair
Howard A. Rosenblum, Chief Executive Officer
Marc P. Charmatz, Staff Attorney
Lizzie Sorkin, Director of Communications
National newspaper published 11 times a year by the nation's largest organization safeguarding the accessbility and civil rights of 28 million deaf and hard of hearing Americans in education, employment, health care, and telecommunications. Membership: individual $30 per year. *$7.00*

4630   No Longer Disabled: the Federal Courts & the Politics of Social Security Disability
Greenwood Publishing Group
130 Cremona Drive
Santa Barbara, CA 93117   805-968-1911
                                              800-368-6868
                                     FAX: 866-270-3856
                                CustomerService@abc-clio.com
                                        www.greenwood.com
John Gosden, Library Resource Consultants
Lina Gosden, Library Resource Consultants
Steve Pearson, Library Resource Consultants
Lou Pingitore, Library Resource Consultants
This book is a case study of judicial policy making. It focuses on the role of adjudication in the making and refining of federal policy. *$107.95*
208 pages Hardcover
ISBN 0-313254-24-9

4631   Nolo's Guide to Social Security Disability Getting and Keeping Your Benefits
NOLO
950 Parker St
Berkeley, CA 94710-2524   800-955-4775
                                     FAX: 800-645-0895
                                              www.nolo.com
David Morton, Author
This guide demystifies the program and tells you everything you need to know about qualifying and applying for benefits, maintaining your benefits, and appealing the denial of a claim. *$25.49*
512 pages paperback
ISBN 1-413311-04-4

4632   Opening the Courthouse Door: An ADA Access Guide for State Courts
American Bar Association
1050 Connecticut Ave. N.W.
Suite 400
Washington, DC 20036-1019   202-662-1000
                                              800-285-2221
                                    service@americanbar.org
                                        www.americanbar.org
Wm T Robinson III, President
Practical step-by-step guide walks the reader through the courthouse and court process, presenting a menu of straightforawrd access ideas to enhance communications in court, make the facility more accessbile, and nodify rules and procedures. *$12.00*
78 pages

4633   PAL News
Parent Professional Advocacy League
45 Bromfield Street
10th Floor
Boston, MA 02108-4106   866-815-8122
                                     FAX: 617-542-7832
                                              info@ppal.net
                                              www.ppal.net
Earl N. Stuck, Chair
Lisa Lambert, Executive Director
Deborah A. Fauntleroy, Associate Director
Anne Metzger, Treasurer
Parent/Professional Advocacy Leage (PPAL) is an organization that promotes a strong voice for families of children and adolescents with mental health needs. PAL advocates for supports, treatment and policies that enable families to live in their communities in an environment of stability and respect.
Quarterly

4634   Power of Attorney for Health Care
Center for Public Representation
P.O.Box 260049
Madison, WI 53726-49   608-251-4008
                                            800-369-0388
                                       FAX: 606-251-1263

132 pages
ISBN 0-93262 -38-0

4635   Title II & III Regulation Amendment Regarding Detectable Warnings
U S Department of Justice
950 Pennsylvania Ave NW
Washington, DC 20530-9   202-307-0663
                                            800-514-0301
                                       FAX: 202-307-1197
                                       TTY: 800-514-0383
                                            www.ada.gov

Rebecca B. Bond, Chief
Zita Johnson Betts, Deputy Chief
Sally Conway, Deputy Chief
James Bostrom, Deputy Chief
This document suspends the requirements for detectable warnings at curb ramps, hazardous vehicular areas, and reflecting pools.

4636   Title II Complaint Form
US Department of Justice
950 Pennsylvania Ave NW
Washington, DC 20530   202-307-0663
                                            800-514-0301
                                       FAX: 202-307-1197
                                            www.ada.gov

Rebecca B. Bond, Chief
Zita Johnson Betts, Deputy Chiefs
James Bostrom, Deputy Chiefs
Sally Conway, Deputy Chiefs
Standard form for filing a complaint under title II of the ADA or section 504 of the Rehabilitation Act of 1973, which prohibit discrimination on the basis of disability by State and local governments and by recipients of federal financial assistance.

4637   Title II Highlights
US Department of Justice
950 Pennsylvania Ave NW
Washington, DC 20530   202-307-0663
                                            800-514-0383
                                       FAX: 202-307-1197
                                            www.ada.gov

Rebecca B. Bond, Chief
Zita Johnson Betts, Deputy Chiefs
James Bostrom, Deputy Chiefs
Sally Conway, Deputy Chiefs
Outline of the key requirements of the ADA for State and local governments. Provides detailed information in bullet format for quick reference.
8 pages

4638   Title III Technical Assistance Manual and Supplement
U S Department of Justice
950 Pennsylvania Ave NW
Washington, DC 20530   202-307-0663
                                            800-574-0301
                                       FAX: 202-307-1197
                                            www.ada.gov

Rebecca B. Bond, Chief
Zita Johnson Betts, Deputy Chiefs
James Bostrom, Deputy Chiefs
Sally Conway, Deputy Chiefs
Explains in lay terms what businesses and non-profit agencies must do to ensure access to their goods, services, and facilities.
83 pages

4639   Toward Independence
National Council on Disability
81 E. Main Street
Xenia, OH 45385   937-376-3996
                                       FAX: 937-376-2046
                                            info@ti-inc.org
                                            www.ti-inc.org
Mary Rose Zink, Chair
Paul Osterfeld, Vice Chair
Mark Schlater, Executive Director
Bob Groskopf, Treasurer
A 1986 report to the U.S. Congress on the federal laws and programs serving people with disabilities, and recommendations for legislation.

4640   UCP Washington Wire
United Cerebral Palsy
1825 K Street NW
Suite 600
Washington, DC 20006-1601   202-776-0406
                                            800-872-5827
                                       FAX: 202-776-0414
                                            info@ucp.org
                                            www.ucp.org
Stephen Bennett, President/CEO
Publication that provides a comprehensive source of information on federal legislation, agency regulations, court decisions and other issues of interest to the disability community.
weekly

4641   US Department of Health and Human Services Office for Civil Rights
200 Independence Ave SW
Room 509F, HHH Building
Washington, DC 20201   202-619-0403
                                            800-368-1019
                                       TTY:800-537-7697
                                            ocrmail@hhs.gov
                                            www.hhs.gov
Georgina Verdugo, Director
The Department's civil rights and health privacy law enforcement agency, OCR investigates complaints, enforces rights, and promulgates regulations, develops policy and provides technical assistance and public education to ensure understanding of and compliance with non-discrimination and health information privacy laws.

4642   US Department of Labor
200 Constitution Ave NW
Washington, DC 20210
                                            866-487-2365
                                            talktosolis@dol.gov
                                            www.dol.gov
Hilda L Solis, Secretary of Labor
Seth D Harris, Deputy Secretary
To foster, promote, and develop the welfare of the wage earners, job seekers, and retirees of the United States; improve working conditions, advance opportunities for profitable employment; and assure work-related benefits and rights.

4643   US Department of Labor Office of Federal Contract Compliance Programs
200 Constitution Ave NW
Washington, DC 20210   312-596-7010
                                            866-487-2365
                                       FAX: 312-596-7044
                                            OFCCP-MW-PreAward@dol.gov
                                            www.dol.gov
Melissa L Speer, Interim Regional Director
To enforce, for the benefit of job seekers and wage earners, the contractual promise of affirmative action and equal employment opportunity required of those who do business with the Federal government.

4644 **University Legal Services AT Program**
Ste 130
220 i St NE
Washington, DC 20002-4364

202-547-4747
877-221-4638
FAX: 202-547-2083
TTY: 202-547-2657
atpdc@uls-dc.org
dcpanda.org

Jane Brown, Executive Director
Designed to empower individuals with disabilities; to promote consumer involvement and advocacy, and provide information, referral and training as they relate to accessing assistive technology services and devices; and to identify and improve access to funding resources..

4645 **William S Hein & Company**
2350 North Forest Rd.
Getzville, NY 14068-1296

716-882-2600
800-828-7571
FAX: 716-883-8100
mail@wshein.com
www.wshein.com

Kevin Marmion, President
Offers a catalog of periodicals, publications and reprints, microforms and government publications on medical, handicapped and health law.

Libraries & Research Centers

Alabama

4646 Alabama Institute for Deaf and Blind Library and Resource Center
205 E South Street
P.O. Box 698
Talladega, AL 35160
256-761-3206
FAX: 256-761-3352
aidb.org

Dr. John Mascia, President
Teresa Lacy, Director, Library & Resource Center
Book collection includes discs, cassettes, braille and large print. Also closed-circuit TV and magnifiers. Offers braille production and binding.

4647 Alabama Radio Reading Service Network(ARRS)
Public Radio WBHM 90.3 FM
650 11th St S
Birmingham, AL 35233-1
205-934-2606
800-444-9246
FAX: 205-934-5075
wbhm.org

Audrey Atkins, Marketing Manager
Scott E Hanley, General Manager
Theresa Kidd, Office Manager
Michael Krall, Program Director
Services and readings are broadcast over a subcarrier service of public radio WBHM. This is a statewide service devoted to Alabama's blind and handicapped community.

4648 Alabama Regional Library for the Blind and Physically Handicapped
Alabama Public Library Service
6030 Monticello Dr
Montgomery, AL 36130-1
334-213-3906
800-392-5671
FAX: 334-213-3993
revans@apls.state.al.us
webmini.apls.state.al.us

Mike Coleman, Blind & Physically Handicapped Division
Tim Emmons, Blind & Physically Handicapped Division
Nancy Pack, Director
Kelyn Ralya, Assistant Director
Recreational reading in special format for persons unable to use standard print. Reference materials offered include materials on blindness and other handicaps, films, local subjects and authors.

4649 Dothan Houston County Library System
Formerly Houston-Love Memorial Library
445 N Oates St
Dothan, AL 36303
334-793-9767
dhcls@dhcls.org
www.dhcls.org

Jason DeLuc, Library Director
Charlotte Mitchell, Main Library Manager
Offers magnifiers, summer reading programs and more for the blind and physically handicapped. Scanner, software, jaws for Windows.

4650 Huntsville Subregional Library for the Blind & Physically Handicapped
Huntsville-Madison County Public Library
915 Monroe St SW
Huntsville, AL 35804-0000
256-532-5980
FAX: 256-532-5994
bphdept@hmcpl.org
www.hmcpl.org

Laurel Best, Executive Director
Talking books for people who are blind or disabled offering reference materials on the blind and other disabilities, large-print photocopier, thermaform duplicator and more.

4651 Public Library Of Anniston-Calhoun County
108 E 10th St
Anniston, AL 36201
256-237-8501
library@publiclibrary.cc
publiclibrary.cc

4652 Technology Assistance for Special Consumers
UCP Huntsville
1856 Keats Drive
Huntsville, AL 35810
256-859-8300
FAX: 256-859-4332
tasc@ucphuntsville.org
ucphuntsville.org

Cheryl Smith, Chief Executive Officer
Provide individuals with disabilities, their families and/or advocates, and associated professionals access to assistive technology devices and services to increase independence at home, school, and work.

Alaska

4653 Alaska State Library Talking Book Center
State of Alaska
344 W 3rd Ave
Ste 125
Anchorage, AK 99501-2338
907-465-1304
888-820-4525
FAX: 907-269-6580
tbc@alaska.gov
talkingbooks.alaska.gov

Patience Frederiksen, Director, Division of Libraries, Archives & Museums
Freya Anderson, Requisitions Librarian
Ginny Jacobs, Library Assistant
The Alaska State Library Talking Book Center is a cooperative effort between the Library of Congress National Library Service for the Blind and Physically Handicapped and the Alaska State Library to provide print handicapped Alaskans with talking book and Braille service. The Talking Book Center has 55,000 audiobooks that can be checked out to eligible Alaskans whose visual or physical handicap prevents them from reading standard print materials.

Arizona

4654 Arizona Braille and Talking Book LibraryArizona State Library
1030 N 32nd St
Phoenix, AZ 85008-5108
602-255-5578
800-255-5578
FAX: 602-286-0444
btbl@lib.az.us
www.azlibrary.gov

Linda Montgomery, Director
Audio and braille books and magazines, summer reading program, volunteer-produced audio books, audo described, films and more.

4655 Books for the Blind of Arizona
Unit A107
6120 E 5th St
Tucson, AZ 85711-2536
602-792-9153
FAX: 520-886-9839

Betty Evans, Chairperson
Offers large print photocopier, textbooks, recreational, career, vocational, braille books, talking books, cassettes, large print books and more for the visually impaired K-12, college students and adults..

4656 Children's Center for Neurodevelopmental Studies
5430 W Glenn Dr
Glendale, AZ 85301-2628   623-915-0345
                                          FAX: 623-937-5425
                                          admin@ccnsaz.org
                                          www.thechildrenscenteraz.org
Kent Rideout, Executive Director
Dawna Sterner, Preschool & Education Informatio
Catherine Orsak, Therapy Information
Alicia Bolan, Teaching Staff
The Center is a non-profit school and therapy center for children
with autism and other developmental delays specializing in the
use of sensory integration.

4657 Flagstaff City-Coconino County Public Library
300 W Aspen Ave
Flagstaff, AZ 86001-5304   928-779-7670
                                          TTY:928-214-2417
                                          www.flagstaffpubliclibrary.org

4658 Fountain Hills Lioness Braille Service
P.O.Box 18332
Fountain Hills, AZ 85269-8332   480-837-3961

Jean Hauck, Chairperson
Braille and large print books on the subjects of recreation, career
and vocations, religion, novels and cookbooks for the visually
impaired..

4659 Prescott Public Library
215 E Goodwin St
Prescott, AZ 86303-3911   928-777-1500
                                          FAX: 928-771-5829
                                          prescottlibrary.info
Roger Saft, Director
Martha Baden, Public Services Manager
Teresa Vonk, Support Services Manager
Lisa Zierke, Technical Services
Large print, braille and audio books; magnifiers; text to voice
scanner; talking book machine application; toy library for chil-
dren with special needs; special needs product catalogs; home
book delivery; descriptive videos; 43 point PC monitor..

4660 Special Needs Center/Phoenix Public Library
1221 N Central Ave
Phoenix, AZ 85004-1867   602-262-4636
                                          TTY:602-254-8205
                                          www.phoenixpubliclibrary.org

4661 World Research Foundation
P.O. Box 20828
Sedona, AZ 86341-8804   928-284-3300
                                          FAX: 928-284-3530
                                          info@wrf.org
                                          wrf.org
Steven A Ross, President
LaVerne Boeckmann, Co-Founder
Large research library of alternative medicine; offers a computer
search and printout of specific health issues for a nominal fee.

Arkansas

**4662 Arkansas Regional Library for the Blind and Physically
Handicapped**
900 West Capitol Avenue
Suite 100
Little Rock, AR 72201-3108   501-682-2053
                                          www.library.arkansas.gov
J D Hall, Manager of BPH Services
Dwain Gordon, Deputy Director
Danny Koonce, Public Information Specialist
Ruth Hyatt, Manager of Extension Services
Public library books in recorded or braille format. Popular fiction
and nonfiction books for all ages, books and players are on free
loan, sent to patrons by mail and may be returned postage free.

Anyone who cannot see well enough to read regular print with
glasses on or who has a disability that makes it difficult to hold a
book or turn the pages is eligible.

4663 Arkansas School for the Blind
P.O.Box 668
Little Rock, AR 72203-668   501-296-1810
                                          800-362-4451
                                          FAX: 501-296-1831
                                          www.arkansasschoolfortheblind.org
Khayyam Eddings, Chairperson
Jennifer Benedetti, Elementary Principal
Teresa Doan, Special Education Supervisor
William Harrison, Technology Director
Students at the ASB receive a quality education from specially
trained instructors of the Visually Impaired in all academic areas.
ASB features a comprehensive Music and Art program, as well as
extensive extra-curricular activities. ASB is a proud member of
the Arkansas Activities Association and The North Central
Association of Schools for the Blind.

4664 Educational Services for the Visually Impaired
2402 Wildwood Avenue
Suite 112
Sherwood, AR 72120-5085   501-835-5448
                                          FAX: 501-835-6840
                                          Angyln.Young@arkansas.gov
                                          www.esvi.org
Angyln Young, State Coordinator
Cindy Lester, Data Management Specialist
Cynthia Kelly, ESVI Office Manager
Offers textbooks, braille books and more to the visually impaired
grades K-12 in the Arizona area.

**4665 Library for the Blind and Physically Handicapped SW
Region of Arkansas**
P.O.Box 668
2057 North Jackson St
Magnolia, AR 71754-668   870-234-1991
                                          FAX: 870-234-5077
                                          library@cocolib.org
                                          www2.youseemore.com/Columbia
Rhonda Rolen, Director
Dana Thornton, Assistant Director
Becky Verschage, Processing Clerk
Lisa Lewis, Bookkeeping
A free library service that serves adults and children who meet the
eligiblity requirements, offers free loan of cassette machine and
recorded books, which meet the reading preferences of a highly
diverse clientele.

**4666 Northwest Ozarks Regional Library for the Blind and
Handicapped**
Fayetteville, AR 72701   479-575-2000
                                          www.uark.edu

California

4667 Braille Institute Library
741 N Vermont Ave
Los Angeles, CA 90029-3594   323-663-1111
                                          800-808-2555
                                          FAX: 323-663-0867
                                          la@brailleinstitute.org
                                          brailleinstitute.org
Leslie E. Stocker, President
Sally H. Jameson, Vice President of Programs and S
Peter A. Mindnich, Executive Vice President
Reza Rahman, Vice President of Finance/Chief
Braille Institute provides an environment of hope and encourage-
ment for people who are blind and visually impaired through inte-
grated educational, social and recreational programs and
services.

4668 Braille Institute Santa Barbara Center
2031 De La Vina St
Santa Barbara, CA 93105-3895 805-682-6222
805-272-4553
FAX: 805-687-6141
sb@brailleinstitute.org
brailleinstitute.org

Leslie E. Stocker, President
Sally H. Jameson, Vice President of Programs and S
Peter A. Mindnich, Executive Vice President
Reza Rahman, Vice President of Finance/Chief
Offers programs, services and information for persons with visual impairments.

4669 Braille Institute Sight Center
741 N Vermont Ave
Los Angeles, CA 90029-3594 323-663-1111
800-808-2555
FAX: 323-663-0867
la@brailleinstitute.org
brailleinstitute.org

Sally H. Jameson, Vice President of Programs and S
Leslie E Stocker, President
Peter A. Mindnich, Executive Vice President
Reza Rahman, Vice President of Finance/Chief
Offers help, programs, services and information to the blind and visually impaired children and adults.

4670 Braille and Talking Book Library: California
P.O. Box 942837
Sacramento, CA 94237-0001 916-654-0640
800-952-5666
www.library.ca.gov/services/btbl.html
Stacey A. Aldrich, State Librarian
Debbie Newton, Bureau Chief, Administrative Ser
Phyllis Smith, Manager, Human Resources and Bus
Sharleen Finn, Budget Officer, Fiscal Services
Free service for eligible Northern California residents.

4671 California State Library Braille and Talking Book Library
P.O. Box 942837
Sacramento, CA 94237-0001 916-654-0640
800-952-5666
www.library.ca.gov/services/btbl.html
Stacey A. Aldrich, State Librarian
Debbie Newton, Bureau Chief, Administrative Ser
Phyllis Smith, Manager, Human Resources and Bus
Sharleen Finn, Budget Officer, Fiscal Services
Provides library services to people in Northern California who are unable to read standard print books because of visual or physical disabilities. Braille and talking books, magazines, machines, catalogs and postage are provided free to qualified appicants. The service is conducted by mail.

4672 Clearinghouse for Specialized Media and Translations
1430 N St
Ste 3207
Sacramento, CA 95814-5901 916-319-0800
FAX: 916-323-9732
EHughes@cde.ca.gov.
www.cde.ca.gov/re/pn/sm
Jonn Paris-Salb, Manager
Provides materials in accessible formats; aural media, braille, large print, digital talking books and electronic media access technology.

4673 Dental Amalgam Syndrome (DAMS) Newsletter
725-9 Tramway Ln NE
Albuquerque, NM 87122-1672 505-291-8239
FAX: 505-294-3339

4674 Fresno County Free Library Blind and Handicapped Services
2420 Mariposa Street
Fresno, CA 93721-3640 559-600-7323
800-742-1011
wendy.eisenberg@fresnolibrary.org
www.fresnolibrary.org/tblb
Wendy Eisenberg, Manager
Laurel Prysiazny, County Librarian
Magnifiers, home visits, volunteer-produced cassette books, discs and cassettes.

4675 Glaucoma Research Foundation
251 Post St
Ste 600
San Francisco, CA 94108-5017 415-986-3162
800-826-6693
FAX: 415-986-3763
question@glaucoma.org
glaucoma.org
Tom Brunner, President and CEO
Nancy Graydon, Executive Director of Development
Andrew L. Jackson, Director of Communications
Catalina San Agustin, Director of Operations
Clinical and laboratory studies of glaucoma. We work to prevent vision loss from glaucoma by investing in innovative research, education and support with the ultimate goal of finding a cure..

4676 Herrick Health Sciences Library
Alta Bates Medical Center
2001 Dwight Way
Berkeley, CA 94704-2608 510-869-6777
FAX: 510-204-4091
www.altabatessummit.org
Laurie Bagley, Librarian
Carol Hirsch-Butler, Administrator
Carolyn Kemp, Regional Manager of Public Relations
Information on rehabilitation, psychiatry and psychoanalysis.

4677 Kuzell Institute for Arthritis and Infectious Diseases
Medical Research Institute Of San Francisco
2200 Webster St
San Francisco, CA 94115-1821 415-923-3262
FAX: 415-441-8548
Lowell S Young, Director
Edward Byrd, Owner
One of seven units comprising the Medical Research Institute of San Francisco that offers basic and applied research in arthritis and related diseases.

4678 New Beginnings: The Blind Children's Center
4120 Marathon St
Los Angeles, CA 90029-3584 323-664-2153
800-222-3566
FAX: 323-665-3828
blindchildrenscenter.org
Lena French, Executive Director
Kimberlee Jones, Director of Development
Ross Vergara, Director of Finance
Manuel Ayala, Director of Facilities
The purpose of the Center is to turn initial fears into hope. Helps children and their families become independent by creating a climate of safety and trust. Children learn to develop self confidence and to master a wide range of skills. Services include an infant stimulation program, educational preschool, interdisciplinary assessment services, family services, correspondence program, toll free national hotline and a publication and research service.

4679 Research & Training Center on Mental Health for Hard of Hearing Persons
California School of Professional Psychology
Ste 140
6215 Ferris Sq
San Diego, CA 92121-3279
619-282-4443
800-HEA-R619
FAX: 800-642-0266

Raymond J Trybus, Director
Thomas J Goulder, Associate Director
Funded by the National Institute on Disability and Rehabilitation Research, this training center aims to address issues of psychological relevance to persons who are hard of hearing or late deafened (as distinct from prelingually, culturally deaf persons). Also serves as information clearinghouse on this topic.

4680 Rosalind Russell Medical Research Center for Arthritis
Suite 600
350 Parnassus Ave
San Francisco, CA 94117
415-476-1141
FAX: 415-476-3526
rrac@medicine.ucsf.edu
www.rosalindrussellcenter.ucsf.edu

Ephraim P Engleman, MD, Center Director
David Wofsy, MD, Associate Director
Paula R. Gambs, Chair
Christine Abele, Volunteer
Arthritis research and its probable causes.

4681 San Francisco Public Library for the Blind and Print Handicapped
100 Larkin St
San Francisco, CA 94102-4705
415-557-4400
FAX: 415-557-4252
TTY:415-557-4433
webmail@sfpl.org
www.sfpl.org

Toni Cordova, Chief of Communications, Program
Toni Bernardi, Special Projects Manager
Laura Lent, Chief of Collections & Technical
Edward Melton, Chief of Branches
Foreign-language books on cassette, children's books on cassettes and more.

4682 San Jose State University Library
150 E San Fernando St
San Jose, CA 95112-3580
408-808-2000
FAX: 408-924-1118
office@wahoo.sjsu.edu
www.sjlibrary.org

Don W Kassing, President
Jane Light, Library/Executive Director
Jeff Barber, Security Officer
Luann Budd, Administrative Officer
Information on physical disabilities, accessibility and learning disabilities.

Colorado

4683 AMC Cancer Research Center
3401 Quebec Street
Suite 3200
Denver, CO 80207
303-233-6501
800-321-1557
FAX: 303-239-3400
contactus@amc.org
amc.org

Gary Kortz, Chairman
Steven D. Toltz, Treasurer
Cheryl Kisling, Secretary
Karen Padgett, President and CEO
Provides trained counselors who provide understanding and support for cancer patients; information and referral services; and screening programs.

4684 Boulder Public Library
1001 Arapahoe Ave
Boulder, CO 80302-6015
303-441-3100
www.boulderlibrary.org

Melinda Mattling, Manager
Priscilla Hudson, Manager
Offers braille books, cassettes, talking books, large print photocopier, large print books and more for the visually impaired.

4685 Colorado Talking Book Library
180 Sheridan Blvd
Denver, CO 80226-8101
303-727-9277
800-685-2136
FAX: 303-727-9281
ctbl.info@cde.state.co.us
www.cde.state.co.us/ctbl/index.htm

Debbie Macleod, Executive Director
Provides free library service to Coloradans of all ages who are unable to read standard print due to visual, physical or learning disabilities whether permanent or temporary. Provides audio, braille and large-print books and magazines.

4686 National Jewish Medical & Research Center
1400 Jackson St
Denver, CO 80206-2762
303-388-4461
877-225-5654
www.nationaljewish.org

Michael Salem, MD, President and CEO
Richard A. Schierburg, Chair
Robin Chotin, Vice Chair
Robin Chotin, Secretary
The only medical center in the country whose research and patient care resources are dedicated to respiratory and immunologic diseases.

Connecticut

4687 Connecticut Braille Association
107 Vanderbilt Ave
West Hartford, CT 6110-1514
860-953-4445
FAX: 860-378-0205

Nick Martino, Owner
Offers textbooks, cassettes, large print books, braille books and more.

4688 Connecticut Library for the Blind and Physically Handicapped
231 Capitol Avenue
Hartford, CT 06106-1569
860-757-6500
860-866-4478
FAX: 860-721-2056
ctaylor@cslib.org
www.cslib.org

Kendall Wiggin, State Librarian
Ursula Hunt, Administrative Assistant
Shelley Delisle, IT Manager
Jane Beaudoin, Administrative Assistant
Network library of the National Library Service for the Blind and Physically Handicapped, Library of Congress. Lends books and magazines in Braille or recorded formats along with the necessary playback equipment, free, for any Connecticut adult or child who is unable to read regular print due to a visual or physical disability. All materials are mailed to and from library patrons by postage-free mail

4689 Connecticut State Library
Connecticut State Government
231 Capitol Ave
Hartford, CT 06106-1569

860-757-6500
866-866-4478
FAX: 860-721-2056
isref@cslib.org
www.cslib.org

Kendall Wiggin, State Librarian
Ursula Hunt, Administrative Assistant
Shelley Delisle, IT Manager
Jane Beaudoin, Administrative Assistant
Discs, cassettes, braille, reference materials on blindness and other handicaps, closed-circuit TV and large-print photocopier.

4690 Connecticut Tech Act Project: Connecticut Department of Social Services
Bureau of Rehabilitations Services
25 Sigourney St
11th Floor
Hartford, CT 06106-5041

860-424-4881
800-537-2549
FAX: 860-424-4850
TTY: 860-424-4839
arlene.lugo@ct.gov
www.cttechact.com

Arlene Lugo, Program Director
Single point of entry, advocacy, information and referral, peer counseling, and access to objective expert advice and consultation for people with disabilities.

4691 Prevent Blindness Connecticut
101 Whitney Avenue
New Haven, CT 06510

203-722-4653
800-850-2020
FAX: 203-722-4691
info@preventblindnesstristate.org
tristate.preventblindness.org

Kathryn Garre-Ayars, President and CEO
Tahesha Bryan, Administrative Assistant
Naomi Hayner, Connecticut Program Manager
Maria Giarratana, Grants Manager
The mission of Prevent Blindness Connecticut is to save sight and prevent blindness through eye screenings, education, safety activities and research.

4692 Yale University: Vision Research Center
310 Cedar St, LH 108
PO Box 208023
New Haven, CT 06520- 8023

203-785-2759
800-395-7949
FAX: 203-785-7303
pamela.berkheiser@yale.edu
medicine.yale.edu/pathology

George Shafranov, Chairman
Pam Burkheiser, Manager
Robert J. Alpern, Dean
Vision including studies on growth and development.

Delaware

4693 Delaware Assistive Technology Initiative (DATI)
Alfred I. duPont Hospital for Children
461 Wyoming Road
Newark, DE 19716-0269

302-831-0354
800-870-3284
FAX: 302-831-4690
TTY: 302-651-6794
dati@asel.udel.edu
www.dati.org

Beth Mineo Mollica, Director
Sonja Rathel, Project Coordinator
The Delaware Assistive Technology Initiative (DATI) connects Delawareans who have disabilities with the tools they need in order to learn, work, play and participate in community life safely and independently. DATI services include: Equipment demonstration centers in eah county; no-cost, short-term equipment loans that let you try before you buy; Equipment Exchange Program; AT workshops and other training sessions; advocacy for improved AT access policies and funding and several more.

4694 Delaware Library for the Blind and Physically Handicapped
Government
121 Duke of York Street
Dover, DE 19901-7430

302-739-4748
800-282-8676
FAX: 302-739-6787
debph@lib.de.us
libraries.delaware.gov/default.shtml

Dr. Annie E. Norman, Director
Sonja Brown, Administrative Specialist
Beth-Ann Ryan, Deputy Director
Diann Colose, Administrative Librarian
Books on cassette and playback equipment are provided to patrons who are unable to read regular printed books.

4695 Elwyn Delaware
111 Elwyn Road
Elwyn, PA 19063-3499

610-891-2000
FAX: 302-654-5815
info@elwyn.org
www.elwyn.org

Vicki Haschak, Contact
Kendra Johnson, Contact
Provides work training, job placement and supported employment, and elder care services.

District of Columbia

4696 District of Columbia Public Library: Services for the Deaf Community
District of Columbia Public Library
901 G St NW, Room 215
Washington, DC 20001-4531

202-727-0321
FAX: 202-727-0321
TTY:202-559-5368
library_deaf_dc@yahoo.com
dclibrary.org

Venetia Demson, Chief Adaptive Services
Janice Roseu, Library for the Deaf Community
Offers reference services through videophone, signers for library programs, sign language classes, information about deafness, print and non-print materials for persons who have hearing disabilities. Book talks on deaf culture and American Sign Language story hours for kids, and Saturday sessions on employment-related skills are offered. Videophones for public use are available at the MLK Library.

4697 District of Columbia Regional Library for the Blind and Physically Handicapped
901 G St NW
Washington, DC 20001-4531

202-727-0321
FAX: 202-727-1129
TTY:202-727-2145
lbphb_2000@yahoo.com
www.dclibrary.org

Richard Reyes-Gavilan, Executive Director
Jonathan Butler, Director of Business Services
Barbara Kirven, Director of Human Resources
Joi Mecks, Director of Communications
Regional library/RPH is network library in the Library of Congress, National Library Services for the Blind and Physically Handicapped.

4698 Georgetown University Center for Child and Human Development
P.O.Box 571485
Washington, DC 20057-1485   202-687-5000
                                     FAX: 202-687-8899
                                     TTY:202-687-5000
                                  gucdc@georgetown.edu
                                  gucchd.georgetown.edu

Phyllis R Magrab, Phd, Director
John J DeGioia, President
Established over four decades ago to improve the quality of life for all children and youth, especially those with, or at risk for, special needs and their families. Located in the nation's capital, this center both directly serves vulnerable children and their families, as well as influences local, state, national and international programs and policy.

4699 National Institute on Disability and Rehabilitation Research
U S Department of Education
400 Maryland Ave SW
Washington, DC 20202-1   202-401-2000
                                        800-872-5327
                                   FAX: 202-401-0689
                                   TTY: 800-437-0833
                                customerservice@inet.ed.gov
                                            ed.gov

Arne Duncan, Secretary of Education
Jim Shelton, Deputy Secretary
Ted Mitchell, Secretary
A national leader in sponsoring research. Mission is to generate, disseminate and promote new knowledge to improve the options available to disabled persons.

Florida

4700 Brevard County Talking Books Library
Brevard County Libraries
2725 Judge Fran Jamieson Way
Viera, FL 32940   321-633-2000
                                   FAX: 321-633-1964
                                   TTY:321-633-1838
                                      kbriley@brev.org
                          www.brevardcounty.us/PublicLibraries

Camille Johnson, Manager
Catherine J Schweinsburg, Library Services Director
Subregional library for the blind and physically handicapped, assistive reading devices collection, reference materials on blindness and other handicaps, descriptive videos, CCTV, phonic ear, reading edge and LOUD-R assistive listening devices available.

4701 Broward County Talking Book Library
100 S Andrews Ave
Fort Lauderdale, FL 33301-1830   954-357-7444
                                   FAX: 954-357-5548
                                      www.broward.org

Robert E. Cannon, Director
Carolyn Kayne, Manager
Reference materials on blindness and other handicaps, films, closed-circuit TV, discs, cassettes and a book discussion group is offered.

4702 Dade County Talking Book Library
Miami Dade Public Library System
101 West Flagler Street
Miami, FL 33130   305-375-2665
                                        800-451-9544
                                   FAX: 305-757-8401
                                  talkingbooks@mdpls.org
                                        www.mdpls.org

Raymond Sanpiago, Executive Director
Lainey Brooks, Development Officer
Sylvia Mora Oria, Assistant Director
Ian D. Rosenior, Operations Administrator
A free Outreach Service of the Miami-Dade Public Library System. A network library, or subregional, of the National Library

Service for the Blind and Physically Handicapped, Library of Congress, and of the Florida Bureau of Braille and Talking Books Library Service.

4703 Florida Division of Blind Services
Regional Library
325 West Gaines Street
Turlington Building, Suite 1114
Tallahassee, FL 32399-0400   850-245-0300
                                        800-342-1828
                                   FAX: 850-245-0363
                               mike-gunde@dbs.doe.state.fl.us
                                     dbs.myflorida.com

Mike Gunde, Manager
Susan Roberts, Bureau Chief
Robert Doyle, Director
Edward Hudson, Bureau Chief
Discs, cassettes, closed-circuit TV, large-print photocopier, films, children's books on cassettes and more.

4704 Florida Instructional Materials Center forthe Visually Impaired (FIMC-VI)
4210 W Bay Villa Ave
Tampa, FL 33611-1206   813-837-7826
                                        800-282-9193
                                   FAX: 813-837-7979
                             FloridaBrailleChallenge@gmail.com
                                       www.fimcvi.org

Mary Stoltz, Database Manager
Jeffrey Fitterman, Technology Specialist
Teresa Gutierrez, Administrative Secretary
Kay Ratzlaff, Coordinator
Operates a clearinghouse depository and production center for braille, large print and digital texts. Provides assistance in assessment of materials and specialized apparatus, organizes and trains volunteers for material production for the visually impaired, and provides professional development for teachers of the visually impaired. Provides electronic texts to NIMAS-eligible students in Florida.

4705 Hillsborough County Talking Book Library
Tampa-Hillsborough County Public Library
900 N Ashley Dr
Tampa, FL 33602-3704   813-273-3652
                                   FAX: 813-273-3707
                                   TTY:813-273-3610
                                       www.hcplc.org

Joe Stines, Director of Libraries
Marcee Challener, Assitant Director
David Wullschleger, Chief of Operations
Linda Gillon, Manager of Staff & Administrativ
Serves as the reference hub and resource center for all citzens of Hillsborough County and as the flagship library of the Tampa-Hillsborough County Public Library System.

4706 Jacksonville Public Library: Talking Books/Special Needs
303 N Laura St
Jacksonville, FL 32202-3505   904-630-2665
                                   FAX: 904-630-0604
                                       jerryr@coj.net
                            www.jpl.coj.net/lib/talkingbooks.html

Barbara Gubbin, Executive Director
Offers cassettes and digital books, reference materials on blindness and ADA issues, newsline, descriptive videos, and some assistive devices.

4707 Lee County Library System: Talking Books Library
2001 N. Tamiami Trail N.E.
North Fort Myers, FL 33903-4855   239-533-4320
                                        800-854-8195
                                   FAX: 239-485-1146
                                   TTY: 239-995-2665
                                  talkingbooks@leegov.com
                                  www.lee-county.com/library

Cynthia N Cobb, Director
Terri Crawford, Deputy Director
Debbie Parrott, Manager
Karen McLeish-Delgado, Librarian

Provides free books and magazines to Lee County residents of all ages who have any disability that prevents them from reading printed material. Books are played on special players provided free by the National Library Service. Circulates low tech assistive aids and devices for temporary loan to Lee County Library card holders. Directs people to assistive technology and disability related resources.

4708 Louis de la Parte Florida Mental Health Institute Research Library
University of South Florida
4202 E. Fowler Ave. LIB122
Tampa, FL 33620
813-974-2729
FAX: 813-974-7242
library@fmhi.usf.edu
lib.usf.edu/fmhi

William A. Garrison, Dean
Florence Jandreau, CAP, Senior Assistant to the Dean
Claudia Dold, Assistant University Librarian
Tomaro Taylor, Associate University Librarian / Certified Archivist
Information offered on mental illness, autism and pervasive development disabilities mental health research and archives management.

4709 Orange County Library System: Audio-Visual Department
101 E Central Blvd
Orlando, FL 32801-2429
407-835-7323
FAX: 407-835-7649
TTY:407-835-7641
comments@ocls.info
www.ocls.info

Ted Maines, President
Lisa Franchina, Vice President
Bob Tessier, Comptroller
Craig Wilkins, Public Service Administrator
Serves the residents of the Orange County Library District, with headquarters in downtown Orlando.

4710 Pearlman Biomedical Research Institute
Mt Sinai Medical Center
1600 NW 10th Ave
Miami Beach, FL 33140
305-674-2121
FAX: 305-674-2198
william-abraham@msmc.com

William Abraham, Director
A 32,000 square feet facility located on the main campus of Mount Sinai. The institute consists of laboratory space, research and administrative offices. The studies conducted within the facility are primarily pre-clinical research.

4711 Pinellas Talking Book Library for the Blind and Physically Handicapped
1330 Cleveland St
Clearwater, FL 33755-5103
727-441-8408
FAX: 727-441-8398
TTY:727-441-3168
contactus@pplc.us
www.pplc.us

William Horne, Chair
Cheryl Morales, Executive Director
David Saari, Facilities Manager
Rosa Rodriguez, Deaf Literacy Coordinator at Saf
The Pinellas Public Library Cooperative serves Pinellas County residents in member cities and the unincorporated county. The Cooperative Office provides cooridination of activities and funding as well as marketing services for the the member counties. The Talking Book Library servces Pinellas, Manatee, and Sarasota counties.

4712 Talking Book Service: Mantatee County Central Library
1112 Manatee Avenue West
Bradenton, FL 34206-1000
941-748-4501
FAX: 941-751-7098
www.mymanatee.org

Patricia Schubert, Manager
Offers children's books on disc and cassette and more reference materials for the blind and physically handicapped.

4713 Talking Books Library for the Blind and Physically Handicapped
Palm Beach County Library
3650 Summit Blvd
West Palm Beach, FL 33406-4114
561-233-2600
888-780-4962
FAX: 561-233-2627
webmaster@pbclibrary.org
www.pbclibrary.org

John Callahan, Executive Director
Bill Rautenberg, Chair
Harriet Helfman, Vice Chair
John Callahan III, Library Director
Established in 1967, today the County Library system serves Palm Beach County through the Main Library, 2 Regional Libraries, 11 Branch Libraries, a Bookmobile and a library annex. It continues to expand through our involvement with library networks, the Internet, and the World Wide Web.

4714 Talking Books/Homebound Services
Brevard County Library System
2725 Judge Fran Jamieson Way
Viera, FL 32940
321-633-2000
FAX: 321-633-1838
kbriley@brev.org
www.brevardcounty.us/PublicLibraries

Kay Briley, Librarian
Camille Johnson, Executive Director
Offers reference materials on blindness and other handicaps. Subregional library for the blind and physically handicapped, assistive reading devices collection, reference materials on blindness and other handicaps; CCTV, phonic ear, reading edge and LOUD-R assistive listening devices available.

4715 University of Miami: Bascom Palmer Eye Institute
Department Of Ophthalmalogy
900 NW 17th St
Miami, FL 33136-1119
305-243-2020
888-845-0002
FAX: 305-326-7000
www.bascompalmer.org

Michael Gittelman, CEO
Teresa Spaulding, Manager
Eduardo C. Alfonso, M.D., Professor and Chairman
Jennifer Cohen, Executive Director
Clinical and basic research into blindness and visual impairments.

4716 University of Miami: Mailman Center for Child Development
1601 NW 12th Ave
Miami, FL 33136-1005
305-243-6395
FAX: 305-326-7594
pedsinformation@med.miami.edu
pediatrics.med.miami.edu

William Donelan, Vice President for Medical Admin
William W. O'Neill, M.D., Executive Dean, Chief Medical Of
Pascal J. Goldschmidt, M.D., SVP, Dean, CEO
Steven Falcone, M.D., Executive Dean
Focuses on birth defects and children's illnesses.

4717 West Florida Regional Library
200 W Gregory St
Pensacola, FL 32502-4822
850-436-5060
FAX: 850-436-5039
TTY:850-436-5063
hhudson@ci.pensacola.fl.us
wfrl.lib.fl.us

Eugene Fischer, Executive Director
Helen Hudson, Outreach Librarian
Offers children's print/braille books.

Georgia

4718 Athens Talking Book Center-Athens-Clarke County Regional Library
2025 Baxter St
Athens, GA 30606-6331
706-613-3655
800-531-2063
FAX: 706-613-3660
www.clarke.public.lib.ga.us/talkingbooks/inde
Stacey Chandler, Manager
Discs, cassettes, large print books, reference materials on blindness, descriptive videos, films, closed-circuit TV, magnifiers, braille writer, summer reading programs, cassette books and magazines and more.

4719 Augusta Talking Book Center
823 Telfair Street
Augusta, GA 30901-2232
706-821-2600
FAX: 706-724-6762
TTY: 706-722-1639
priced@ecgrl.org
www.ecgrl.org
Lillie Hamilton, Board Of Trustee
Audrey Bell, Manager
Loran Gray, Board Of Trustee
Brenda Morton, Board Of Trustee
Discs, cassettes, braille writer, films, large print books, summer reading program, magnifiers and reference materials on blindness and other handicaps.

4720 Bainbridge Subregional Library for the Blind & Physically Handicapped
S W Georgia Regional Library
301 S Monroe St
Bainbridge, GA 39819-4029
229-248-2665
800-795-2680
FAX: 229-248-2670
lbph@swgrl.org
www.swgrl.org
Susans Wittle, Manager
Kathy Hutchins, Supervisor
The library houses a large collection of recorded materials as well as reference materials. For recorded and Braille materials that are provided by the National Library Service (NLS) but not currently in stock at the Bainbridge Library, the Regional Library in Atlanta can be contacted to Interlibrary Loan the requested materials.

4721 Columbus Subregional Library For The Blind And Physically Handicapped
1120 Bradley Dr
Columbus, GA 31906-2813
706-649-0780
800-652-0782
FAX: 706-649-1914
TTY: 706-649-0974
Dorothy Bowen, Librarian
Braille writer, magnifiers, closed-circuit TV, large-print photocopier, cassette books and magazines, children's books on cassette, home visits and other reference materials on blindness and other handicaps.

4722 Emory Autism Resource Center
Emory University
1551 Shoup Ct
Decatur, GA 30033
404-727-8350
FAX: 404-727-3969
tohannon@emory.edu
www.emory.edu/HOUSING/CLAIRMONT/autism.html
James W. Wagner, President
Larry Hagan, IT Manager
Paul B. Pruett, MD, Director of Residency Education
Terri Trotter, Coordinator of Residency Educati
Offers on-line bulletin boards which are relevant to autism.

4723 Emory University Laboratory for Ophthalmic Research
1365b Clifton Rd NE
Atlanta, GA 30322-1013
404-778-4530
FAX: 404-778-4002
pbennet@emory.edu
www.eyecenter.emory.edu/education/resi
James W. Wagner, President
Larry Hagan, IT Manager
Paul B. Pruett, MD, Director of Residency Education
Terri Trotter, Coordinator of Residency Educati
Various studies into the aspects of blindness.

4724 Georgia Library for the Blind and Physically Handicapped
Georgia Public Library
1800 Century Place
Suite 150
Atlanta, GA 30345-4304
404-235-7200
800-248-6701
FAX: 404-756-4618
dscott@georgialibraries.org
georgialibraries.org
Stella Cone, Director
Deborah Scott, Business Manager
Dr. Lamar Veatch, Librarian
Julie Walker, State Librarian
Discs, cassettes, braille, films, closed-circuit TV, braille writer, large-print photocopier, cassette books and magazines.

4725 Hall County Library: East Hall Branch and Special Needs Library
127 Main St NW
Gainesville, GA 30501-3614
770-532-3311
FAX: 770-532-4305
TTY: 770-531-2520
info@hallcountylibrary.org
www.hallcountylibrary.org
Adrian Mixson, Manager
Summer reading programs, braille writer, magnifiers, scanners and readers, audio described videos, closed captioned videos, closed-circuit TV, large-print photocopier, cassette books and magazines, large print books, children's books on cassette, home visits and other reference materials on blindness and other handicaps.

4726 Macon Library for the Blind and Physically Handicapped
Washington Memorial Library
1180 Washington Ave
Macon, GA 31201-1762
478-744-0800
FAX: 478-742-3161
jonest@bibblib.org
www.co.bibb.ga.us/library
Thomas Jones, Director
Leila Brittain, Finance Officer
Hannah Warren, Office Manager
Viveca Jackson, Librarian, West Bibb Branch
Summer reading programs, braille writer, magnifiers, closed-circuit TV, large-print photocopier, cassette books and magazines, children's books on cassette, home visits and other reference materials on blindness and other handicaps.

4727 National Center on Birth Defects and Developmental Disabilities
Centers for Disease Control and Prevention
1600 Clifton Rd NE
MS E-87
Atlanta, GA 30333
404-639-3311
800-232-4636
FAX: 404-498-3070
TTY: 888-232-6348
cdcinfo@cdc.gov
www.cdc.gov/ncbddd/
Coleen A. Boyle, PhD, MSHyg, Director
Stephanie Dulin, MBA, Deputy Director
Vicki Kipreos, PMP, Management Officer
Lisa Richardson, MD, Director, Division of Blood Diso
Promotes child development, prevents birth defects and developmental disabilities.

4728 North Georgia Talking Book Center
LaFayette-Walker Public Library
305 S Duke St
La Fayette, GA 30728-2936

706-638-8312
888-506-0509
888-506-0509
FAX: 706-638-4028
cstubblefield@chrl.org
www.chrl.org

Tim York, Manager
June DeLong, Library Assistant
Martha McKeehan, Library Assistant
Kaylee Smith, Library Assistant

We offer books on cassette for the visual and physically disabled induvidual, books in braille, magazines on cassette, zoom text screen magnifier, computer voice program, large-print photocopier, summer reading program, home visits na dother reference materials on blindness and other disabilities.

4729 Oconee Regional Library
801 Bellevue Ave
Dublin, GA 31021-4847

478-272-5710
FAX: 478-275-5381
georgialibraries.org

Stella Cone, Director
Deborah Scott, Business Manager
Dr. Lamar Veatch, Librarian
Leard Daughety, Director

Summer reading programs, braille writer, magnifiers, closed-circuit TV, large-print photocopier, cassette books and magazines, children's books on cassette, home visits and other reference materials on blindness and other handicaps.

4730 Rome Subregional Library for the Blind and Physically Handicapped
205 Riverside Pkwy
Rome, GA 30161-2922

706-236-4611
888-263-0769
FAX: 706-236-4631
TTY: 706-236-4618
www.floyd.public.lib.ga.us

Diana Mills, Librarian
Delana Hickman, Manager

The regional library system serves Floyd and Polk counties. System headquarters are located in Rome, Georgia, within the Rome/Floyd County Library Branch.

4731 South Georgia Regional Library-Valdosta Talking Book Center
300 Woodrow Wilson Dr
Valdosta, GA 31602-2532

229-333-0086
FAX: 229-333-0364
commissioner@lowndescounty.com
sgrl.org

Chuck Gibson, Manager

Summer reading programs, Braille writer, magnifiers, closed-circuit TV, large print photocopier, cassette books and magazines, children's books on cassette, home visits and other reference materials on blindness and other handicaps.

4732 Talking Book Center Brunswick-Glynn County Regional Library
208 Gloucester St
Brunswick, GA 31520-7007

912-267-1212
FAX: 912-267-9597
bransom@trll.org
www.trrl.org/tbc

Betty Ransom, Librarian
Joe Shinnick, Executive Director

The Three Rivers Regional Library system is named for 3 rivers that flow through all 7 counties of the library system. The Three Rivers Regional Library system serves patrons in Brantley, Camden, Charlton, Glynn, Long, McIntosh, and Wayne counties in southeast Georgia.

Hawaii

4733 Assistive Technology Resource Centers of Hawaii (ATRC)
200 North Vineyard Boulevard
Suite 430
Honolulu, HI 96817-5362

808-532-7110
800-645-3007
FAX: 808-532-7120
TTY: 808-532-7110
atrc-info@atrc.org
www.atrc.org

Barbara Fischlowitz-Leong, Executive Director
Jeff Ah Sam, Technical Assisstant
Jodi Asato, Deputy Director
Edna Kaahaaina, Office Manager

Provides information and training on assistive technology devices, services, and funding resources. Conducts presentations and demonstrations in the community to increase AT awareness and promote self-advocacy among people with disabilities.

4734 Hawaii State Library for the Blind and Physically Handicapped
874 Dillingham Blvd
Honolulu, HI 96817-4505

808-845-9221
800-559-4096
FAX: 808-733-8449
honcclib@hawaii.edu
www2.honolulu.hawaii.edu/library

Fusako Miyashiro, Manager

Supported by the Hawaii State Public Library System and the National Library Service for the Blind and Physically Handicapped, Library of Congress. Staff with knowledge of sign language; Special interest periodicals; Books on deafness and sign language; captioned media; Special Services: Radio Reading Service, Talking Books Reader's Club, educational and cultural programs, machine lending agency. Braille, cassette and large type. Regional and National service, quarterly newsletter.

Idaho

4735 Idaho Assistive Technology Project
University of Idaho
121 West Sweet Ave
Moscow, ID 83843-2268

208-885-3557
800-432-8324
FAX: 208-885-6145
idahoat@uidaho.edu
www.idahoat.org

Janice Carson, Project Director
Irene Lunsford, Loan Program Manager
Julie Magelky, Loan Program Coordinator
Dan Dyer, Training Coordinator

A federally funded program managed by the Center on Disbailities and Human Development at the University of Idaho. The goal of the IATP is to increase the availability of assistive technology devices and services for Idahoans with disabilities. The IATP offers free trainings and technical assistance, a low-interest loan program, assistive technology assessments for children and agriculture workers, and free informational materials.

4736 Idaho Commission for Libraries: Talking Book Service
325 W State St
Boise, ID 83702-6055

208-334-2150
800-458-3271
FAX: 208-334-4016
talkingbooks@libraries.idaho.gov
www.libraries.idaho.gov/tbs

Ann Joslin, Manager
Irene Lunsford, Library Consultant
David Harrell, IT & Telecommunications Resources Manager
Erica Compton, Project Coordinator

Offers audio and braille books and magazines, equipment, and accessories. All materials are mailed free to users' homes. Service is available free to all Idaho residents with a disability which limits their ability to use print materials.

Illinois

4737 Chicago Public Library Talking Book Center
400 S State St
Chicago, IL 60605-1216

312-747-4300
800-757-4654
FAX: 312-747-4962
dtaylor@chipublib.org
www.chipublib.org

Linda Johnson Rice, President
Christopher Valenti, Vice President
Cristina Benitez, Secretary
Joselyn Bell, Director, Finance

Summer reading programs, braille writer, closed-circuit TV, large print photocopier, cassette books and magazines, children's books on cassette, home visits and other reference materials on blindness and other handicaps. Three assistive technology centers designed and equipped for the blind and visually impaired, funded by the National Library Service for the Blind and Handicapped, a division of the Library of Congress. All services FREE!

4738 Department of Ophthalmology and Visual Science
1855 W Taylor St
Chicago, IL 60612-7242

312-996-7000
800-625-2013
FAX: 312-996-7770
TTY: 312-413-0123
adriadel@uic.edu
www.uic.edu

Paula Allen-Meares, Chancellor
Lon S. Kaufman, Vice Chancellor for Academic Aff
Mitra Dutta, Vice Chancellor for Research
Barbara Henley, Vice Chancellor for Student Affa
Offers help, support, information and research for persons with vision problems, including Retinitis Pigmentosa.

4739 Guild for the Blind
65 E. Wacker Place
Suite 1010
Chicago, IL 60601-7463

312-236-8569
FAX: 312-236-8128
info@guildfortheblind.org
www.second-sense.org

Brett Christenson, President
Laura Rounce, Vice President
Michael P. Wagner, Treasurer
Toria Emas, Secretary
provides worship on vision rehabilitation, training on computers and other adaptive technology, career counseling, and professional development workshops and offers assistive devices for sale.

4740 Horizons for the Blind
125 Erick Street
A103
Crystal Lake, IL 60014-4404

815-444-8800
800-318-2000
FAX: 815-444-8830
TTY: 815-444-8800
mail@horizons-blind.org
www.horizons-blind.org

Camille Caffarelli, Executive Director
Jeff T. Thorsen, First Vice President/Treasurer
Keith Myers, Second Vice President
Maryann Bartkowski, Secretary
HORIZONS for the BLIND is a nonprofit organization dedicated to providing products and services to people who are blind or visually impaired. In addition, Horizons is a leading provider of Braille transcription services to the business community; specialing in partnering with companies and nonprofits to provide billing and financial statements, newsletters, and documents in Braille, large print, and audio formats.

4741 Illinois Early Childhood Intervention Clearinghouse
51 Gerty Drive
Champaign, IL 61820-7469

217-333-1386
877-275-3227
FAX: 217-244-7732
Illinois-eic@illinois.edu
www.eiclearinghouse.org

Charlton Brandt, Manager
Patricia Traylor, Project Associate
Free lending library of materials related to early childhood and disability. Books, audiovisuals and articles available. Computerized database with more than 31,000 items available to Illinois residents.

4742 Illinois Machine Sub-Lending Agency
607 S Greenbriar Rd
Carterville, IL 62918-1602

618-985-8375
800-455-2665
FAX: 618-985-4211
imsastaff@imsa.lib.il.us
www.imsa.lib.il.us

Loretta Broomfield, Director
The Illinois Machine Sublending Agency (IMSA) is a division of the Illinois Network of Talking Book and Braille Libraries. The primary responsibility of IMSA is to maintain Talking Book equipment and accessories and to issue Talking Book equipment and accessories to Illinois residents who are registered for the service. IMSA is also the support center for patrons in need of assistance with the Braille and Audio Reading Download (BARD) service.

4743 Illinois Regional Library for the Blind and Physically Handicapped
1055 W Roosevelt Rd
Chicago, IL 60608-1559

312-746-9210
800-331-2351
FAX: 312-746-9192

Shawn Thomas, Reference Librarian
Barbara Perkins, Acting Director
Summer reading programs, braille writer, magnifiers, closed-circuit TV, large-print photocopier, cassette books and magazines, descriptive videos, children's books on cassette, home visits and other reference materials on blindness and other handicaps.

4744 Mid-Illinois Talking Book Center
600 High Point Ln
East Peoria, IL 61611-9396

309-694-9200
800-426-0709
info@mitbc.org
mitbc.org

Rose Chenoweth, Director
Michelle Moran, Assistant
Rebecca Rollings, Assistant
Jane Furrh, Assistant
Providing a free library service to anyone unable to read regular print because of a visual or physical disability. There are books and magazines on tape and playback equipment; and also in Braille. Books and magazines are mailed free to and from library patrons, wherever they reside.

4745 National Eye Research Foundation (NERF)
Ste 207a
910 Skokie Blvd
Northbrook, IL 60062-4033

847-564-4652
800-621-2258
FAX: 847-564-0807
info@nerf.org
www.nerf.org

Joel Tenner, Manager
Dedicated to improving eye care for the public and meeting the professional nees of eye care practitioners; sponsors eye research projects on contact lens applications and eye care problems. Special study sections in such fields as orthokertology, primary eyecare, pediatrics, and through continuing education programs. Provides eye care information for the public and professionals. Educational materials including pamphlets. Program activities include education and referrals.

4746 National Lekotek Center
2001 N. Clybourn
Chicago, IL 60614

773-528-5766
800-366-7529
FAX: 773-537-2992
lekotek@lekotek.org
www.lekotek.org

Elaine D. Cottey, Chair
Joanna Horsnail, Chair Elect
Eric Gastevich, Treasurer
Carol Neiger, Secretary
Toy library and play-centered programs for children with special needs and their families with branches in 17 states. Sliding fee scale. Lekotek also has a Toy Resource Helpline that provides individualized assistances in the selection of toys and play materials and general resources for families with children with disabilities.

4747 Northwestern University Multipurpose Arthritis & Musculoskeletal Center
420 East Superior Street
Chicago, IL 60611-4296

312-503-8194
FAX: 312-503-1204
med-webteam@northwestern.edu
www.feinberg.northwestern.edu

Cynthia Barnard, MBA, Director, Quality Strategies
John Vozenilek, MD, Assistant Professor
Eric G. Neilson, MD, Vice President for Medical Affairs
Sherri L. LaVela, PhD, MPH, MBA, Assistant Professor
Conducts biomedical, educational and health services research into musculoskeletal diseases.

4748 Skokie Accessible Library Services
Skokie Public Library
5215 Oakton St
Skokie, IL 60077-3680

847-673-7774
FAX: 847-673-7797
TTY:847-673-8926
tellus@skokielibrary .info
www.skokie.lib.il.us

Carolyn A. Anthony, Director
John J. Graham, President
Diana Hunter, Vice President/President Emerita
Karen Parrilli, Secretary
Library services for people with disabilities, including electronic aids, materials in special formats, programs and special services.

4749 University of Illinois at Chicago: Lions of Illinois Eye Research Institute
University of Illinois at Chicago
1855 West Taylor Street, m/c 648
Room 3.138
Chicago, IL 60612

312-996-6591
FAX: 312-996-7770
eyeweb@uic.edu
www.uic.edu

Rolanda Geddis, Manager
Paula Alen Meares, Chancellor
Jerry Bauman, Vice President for Health Affairs
James Schmidt, Director of Athletics
Visual impairments and blindness research, including glaucoma studies.

4750 Voices of Vision Talking Book Center at DuPage Library System
125 Tower Drive
Burr Ridge, IL 60527-2771

630-734-5055
800-426-0709
FAX: 630-208-0399
info@illinoistalkingbooks.org
www.illinoistalkingbooks.org

Karen L. Odean, Director
Provides library service to persons who are unable to use standard printed material because of visual or physical disabilities. Part of the Illinois network of Talking Book Libraries. The service is free to those who are eligable. Provides books and magazines on audio-cassettes. Special playback equipment needed to use the books is also loaned. Braille books and magazines are also avail-

able. The collection includes popular books, classics and children's literature.

Indiana

4751 Allen County Public Library
900 Library Plaza
Fort Wayne, IN 46802-3699

260-421-1200
FAX: 260-421-1386
TTY:260-421-1302
Genealogy@ACPL.Info
www.acpl.lib.in.us

Jeffrey R. Krull, Director
Martin E. Seifert, President
Alan McMahan, Vice President
Paul G. Moss, Secretary
Summer reading programs, braille writer, magnifiers, closed-circuit TV, large-print photocopier, cassette books and magazines, children's books on cassette, home visits and other reference materials on blindness and other handicaps.

4752 Bartholomew County Public Library
536 5th St
Columbus, IN 47201-6225

812-379-1255
FAX: 812-379-1275
library@barth.lib.in.us
barth.lib.in.us

Beth Poor, Executive Director
Summer reading programs, braille writer, magnifiers, closed-circuit TV, large-print photocopier, cassette books and magazines, children's books on cassette, home visits and other reference materials on blindness and other handicaps.

4753 Elkhart Public Library for the Blind and Physiclly Handicapped
300 S 2nd St
Elkhart, IN 46516-3109

574-522-2223
800-622-4970
FAX: 574-522-2174
webmaster@myepl.org
www.myepl.org/epl

Connie Jo Ozinga, Executive Director
Barbara G. Anderson, President
Janice E. Dean, Vice-President
Krystal Anderson, Secretary
Summer reading programs, braille writer, magnifiers, closed-circuit TV, large-print photocopier, cassette books and magazines, children's books on cassette, home visits and other reference materials on blindness and other handicaps.

4754 Indiana Resource Center for Autism
2853 E 10th St
Bloomington, IN 47408-2696

812-855-6508
800-825-4733
FAX: 812-855-9630
TTY: 812-855-9396
iidc@indiana.edu
www.iidc.indiana.edu/irca

Dr Cathy Pratt Ph.D., BCBA, Director
Donna Beasley, Administrative Program Secretary
Pamela Anderson, Outreach/Resource Specialist
Marci Wheeler, M.S.W., Social Work Specialist
The Indiana Resource Center for Autism staff conduct outreach training and consultations, engage in research and develop and disseminate information focused on building the capicity of local communities, organizations, agencies and families to support children and adults across the autism spectrum in typical work, school, home and community settings. Please check our website for a complete list of publications.

4755 Indiana University: Multipurpose Arthritis Center
School Of Medicine, Rheumatology Division
509 E. 3rd Street
Bloomington, IN 47401-3654　　　　812-855-0516
　　　　　　　　　　　　　　FAX: 812-855-9943
　　　　　　　　　　　　　　dbrandt@iupui.edu
　　　　　　　　　　　　　　research.iu.edu

Dr. Kenneth Brandt MD, Director
Carmichael Center, Vice President for Research
Steven A Martin, Associate Vice President for Research
Marisa Pratt, Executve Financial & Operations Officer
The mission of the center is to pursue major biomedical research interests relevant to the rheumatic diseases. Current areas of emphasis include; articular cartilage biology, pathogenesis of articular cartilage breakdown in osteoarthritis, causes of pain and disability in QA, the pathogenesis and treatment of various forms of amyloidosis, the pathogenesis of dermatomyositis, and immunologic and biochemical markers of cartilage breakdown and repair.

4756 Lake County Public Library Talking Books Service
1919 W 81st Ave
Merrillville, IN 46410-5488　　　　219-769-3541
　　　　　　　　　　　　　　FAX: 219-769-0690
　　　　　　　　　　　　webmaster@lakeco.lib.in.us
　　　　　　　　　　　　　　www.lcplin.org
Larry Acheff, Manager
Large-print books, descriptive videos, braille writer, magnifiers, closed-circuit TV, large-print photocopier, cassette books and magazines, children's books on cassette, and other reference materials on blindness and other handicaps.

4757 Special Services Division: Indiana State Library
140 N Senate Ave
Indianapolis, IN 46204-2207　　　　317-232-3675
　　　　　　　　　　　　　　800-622-4970
　　　　　　　　　　　　　　FAX: 317-253-3209
　　　　　　　　　　　　　　TTY: 317-232-7763
　　　　　　　　　　　delivery@statelib.lib.in.us
　　　　　　　　　　　　www.in.gov/isloutage

Roberta Brooker, Manager
Barbara Maxwell, State Librarian
C Ewick, Manager
Circulates a collection of braille, recorded, and large print books and magazines and the special equipment needed to play the recorded materials to anyone in Indiana who cannot read regular print due to a visual or physical disability.

4758 St. Joseph Hospital Rehabilitation Center
700 Broadway
Fort Wayne, IN 46802-1402　　　　260-425-3000
　　　　　　　　　　　　　　FAX: 260-425-3741
　　　　　　　　　　　　　www.stjoehospital.com

Kirk Ray, CEO
Bob Hailes, Vice President
Information offered on rehabilitation.

4759 Talking Books Service Evansville Vanderburgh County Public Library
200 SE Martin Luther King Jr Blvd
Evansville, IN 47713- 1802　　　　812-428-8200
　　　　　　　　　　　　　　866-645-2536
　　　　　　　　　　　　　　FAX: 812-428-8397
　　　　　　　　　　　　　　tbs@evpl.org
　　　　　　　　　　　　　　www.evpl.org

Marcia Learned Au, COO
Connie Davis, Vice President
Marcia Au, Executive Director
Barbara Shanks, Talking Book Manager
The Talking Book Service of the Evansville Vanderburgh Public Library is part of a nationwide network of cooperating libraries headed by the National Library Service & a division of the Library of Congress. This free program provides library services and materials in alternative formats to person who are unable to use standard print material due to a visual or physical handicap.

4760 Iowa Department for the Blind Library
State Of Iowa
524 4th Street
Des Moines, IA 50309-2364　　　　515-281-1333
　　　　　　　　　　　　　　800-362-2587
　　　　　　　　　　　　　　FAX: 515-281-1263
　　　　　　　　　　　　　　TTY: 515-281-1355
　　　　　　　　　　　contact@blind.state.ia.us
　　　　　　　　　　　　www.IDBonline.org
Richard Sorey, Director
Mike Hoenig, Chair
Steve Hagemoser, Commision Board Member
Peggy Elliott, Commision Board Member
Summer reading programs, large print, disc, Braille and cassette books and magazines, descriptive videos and reference materials on blindness and other handicaps.

4761 Iowa Registry for Congenital and Inherited Disorders
University of Iowa
Department of Epidemiology, Univers
100 BVC, Room W260
Iowa City, IA 52242-5000　　　　319-335-4107
　　　　　　　　　　　　　　866-274-4237
　　　　　　　　　　　　　　FAX: 319-335-4030
　　　　　　　　　　　　　ircid@uiowa.edu
　　　　　　　　www.public-health.uiowa.edu/ircid/
Paul Romitti, Ph.D, Director
Kim Keppler-Noreuil, M.D, Clinical Director for Birth Defects
Katherine. Mathews, M.D, Clinical Director for Neuromuscular Disorders
James Torner, Ph.D., Chair
The mission of the Iowa Registry for Congenital and Inherited Disorders is; maintain statewide surveillance for collecting information on selected congenital and inherited disorders in Iowa, monitor annual trends in occurrence and mortality of these disorders, provide data for research studies and educational activities for the prevention and treatment of these disorders.

4762 Library Commission for the Blind
State Of Iowa
524 4th Street
Des Moines, IA 50309-2364　　　　515-281-1333
　　　　　　　　　　　　　　800-362-2587
　　　　　　　　　　　　　　FAX: 515-281-1263
　　　　　　　　　　　　　　TTY: 515-281-1355
　　　　　　　　　　　contact@blind.state.ia.us
　　　　　　　　　　　　www.blind.state.ia.us
Karen A Keninger, Director
Aldini Jodi, Library Support Staff
Barber Kim, Independent Living Supervisor
Bauer Marcia, Rehabilitation Teacher
Summer reading programs, Braille writer, magnifiers, closed-circuit TV, large print photocopier, cassette books and magazines, children's books on cassette and other reference materials on blindness and other handicaps.

4763 Center for the Improvement of Human Functioning
3100 N Hillside St
Wichita, KS 67219-3904　　　　316-682-3100
　　　　　　　　　　　　　　FAX: 316-682-5054
　　　　　　　　　　　information@riordanclinic.org
　　　　　　　　　　　　www.riordanclinic.org

Hugh D Riordan, President
Ron Hunninghake MD, Chief Medical Officer
Brian Riordan, Chief Executive Officer
Danae , Certified Medical Assistant
Medical, research, and educational facility specializing in the treatment of chronic illness.

4764   Central Kansas Library Systems Headquarters (CSLS)
1409 Williams St
Great Bend, KS 67530-4020
620-792-4865
800-362-2642
FAX: 620-793-7270
cbobbitt@ckls.org
www.ckls.org

Harry Williams, Administrator
Vickie Herl, Adminstrative Manager
Marquita Boehnke, Department Head
Connie Bobbitt, Assistant
Summer reading programs, braille writer, magnifiers, closed-circuit TV, large-print photocopier, cassette books and magazines, children's books on cassette, home visits and other reference materials on blindness and other handicaps. Assistive technology available. Serving 17 counties in Central Kansas.

4765   Kansas State Library
Esu Memorial Union
300 SW 10th Avenue
Room 312-N
Topeka, KS 66612-1593
785-296-3296
800-432-3919
FAX: 620-343-7124
infodesk@library.ks.gov
kslib.info

Christie Brandau, Manager
Jo Kord, Manager
Budler Jo, State Librarian
Turner Barbara, Administrative Officer
Summer reading programs, braille writer, magnifiers, closed-circuit TV, large-print photocopier, cassette books and magazines, children's books on cassette, home visits and other reference materials on blindness and other handicaps.

4766   Kansas Talking Books Regional Library
300 SW 10th Avenue
Room 312-N
Topeka, KS 66612-4401
785-296-3296
800-432-3919
FAX: 620-343-7124
talkingbooks@kslib.info
kslib.info

Toni Harrell, Director
Christie Brandau, Manager
Jo Kord, Manager
Budler Jo, State Librarian
Summer reading programs, Braille writer, closed-circuit TV, large-print photocopier, cassette books and magazines, children's books on cassette, home visits and other reference materials on blindness and other handicaps.

4767   Manhattan Public Library
629 Poyntz Ave
Manhattan, KS 66502-6131
785-776-4741
800-432-2796
FAX: 785-776-1545
refstaff@mhklibrary.org
manhattan.lib.ks.us

Linda Knupp, Director
John Pecoraro, Assistant Director
Brice Hobrock, President
Thomas Giller, Vice President
Summer reading programs, Braille writer, magnifiers, closed-circuit TV, large-print photocopier, cassette books and magazines, children's books on cassette, home visits and other reference materials on blindness and other disabilities.

4768   Northwest Kansas Library System Talking Books
2 Washington Square
Norton, KS 67654-1615
785-877-5148
800-432-2858
FAX: 785-877-5697
tbook@ruraltel.net
www.nwkls.org

George Seamon, Director
Alice Evans, Business Manager & Acquisitions
David Fischer, Technology Consultant
Marry Boller, Children's and Talking Book Consultant
Offers books on disc and cassette. Library of Congress talking book and program for qualified individuals. Also offers descriptive videos to eligible persons.

4769   South Central Kansas Library System
321 North Main Street
South Hutchinson, KS 67505-1145
620-663-3211
800-234-0529
FAX: 620-663-9797
sckls.info

Paul Hawkins, Director
Sharon Barnes, Technology Consultant
Larry Papenfuss, Director of Information Technology
Jill Stern, Continuing Education Specialist
Serving public, school, academic and special libraries in 12 counties since 1968, the South Central Kansas Library System (SCKLS) is the "go to" resource for innovative services, quality member awareness and assistance.

4770   Topeka & Shawnee County Public Library Talking Books Service
1515 SW 10th Ave
Topeka, KS 66604-1374
785-580-4400
800-432-2925
FAX: 785-580-4496
TTY: 785-580-4544
tbooks@tscpl.lib.ks.us
www.tscpl.org

Stephanie Hall, Manager
Gina Millsap, Chief Executive Officer
Robert Banks, Chief Operating Officer
Sheryl Weller, Chief Financial Officer
Talking books is a free service that provides cassette and digital books and equipment to people who are unable to read or use standard print materials because of a visual or physical impairment. There are no fees. To apply for Talking Books you must fill out and submit an application, have it certified by the appropriate authority and return it to the library. You can find an application on our website or have one mailed out to you by contacting our office.

4771   Wichita Public Library/Talking Book Service
Wichita Public Library
223 S Main St
Wichita, KS 67202-3795
316-261-8500
FAX: 316-262-4540
TTY:316-262-3972
admin@wichita.lib.ks.us
www.wichita.lib.ks.us

Cynthia Berner-Harris, Executive Director
Eric J. Larson, Member of the Board
Furnish recorded reading material (books and magazines) for visually and physically challenged citizens.

4772   Wichita Public Library/Talking Book Service
223 S Main St
Wichita, KS 67202-3795
316-261-8500
FAX: 316-262-4540
TTY:316-262-3972
admin@wichita.lib.ks.us
www.wichita.lib.ks.us

Cynthia Berner-Harris, Executive Director
Eric J. Larson, Member of the Board
Furnish recorded reading material (books and magazines) for visually and physically challenged citizens.

Kentucky

4773   EnTech: Enabling Technologies of Kentuckiana
Spaulding University
851 South 3rd Street
Louisville, KY 40203-2115
                                    502-585-9911
                                    800-896-8941
                              FAX: 502-585-7103
                              admissions@spalding.edu
                                    www.spalding.edu

Laura Strickland, Manager
Mary Kaye Steinmietz, Outreach Coordinator
Tori Murden McClure, President
Assistive technology resource and demonstration center, serving persons of all ages and disabilities in Kentucky and Southern Indiana. Services include: assistive technology information, demonstration, evaluation, training, technical support and short-term loan of equipment.

4774   Kentucky Talking Book LibraryKentucky Dept. for Libraries and Archives
300 Coffee Tree Road
PO Box 537
Frankfort, KY 40602-0537
                                    502-564-8300
                                    800-372-2968
                              FAX: 502-564-5773
                              ktbl.mail@ky.gov
                                    www.kdla.ky.gov

Barbara Penegor, Regional Librarian
Lauren Abner, Field Services
Katherine K. Adelberg, E-Rate Coordinator
Jackie Arnold, Local Records Regional Administrator
Provides library service to those who are physically unable to read print. Audio and braille books and magazines are available via mail or download.

4775   Louisville Free Public Library
301 York Street
Louisville, KY 40203-2257
                                    502-574-1611
                              FAX: 502-574-1666
                              webteam@lfpl.org
                                    lfpl.org

Craig Buthod, Manager
Summer reading programs, braille writer, magnifiers, closed-circuit TV, large-print photocopier, cassette books and magazines, children's books on cassette, home visits and other reference materials on blindness and other handicaps.

Louisiana

4776   Central Louisiana State Hospital Medical and Professional Library
P.O.Box 5031
Pineville, LA 71361-5031
                                    318-484-6200
                              FAX: 318-484-6501
                              http://wwwprd.doa.louisiana.gov/laservices/pu

Patrick Kelly, CEO
Carol Gee, Manager
Information offered on psychiatry, psychology and mental health.

4777   Louisiana State Library
701 North 4th St
Baton Rouge, LA 70802-5345
                                    225-342-4913
                                    800-543-4702
                              FAX: 225-219-4804
                              admin@state.lib.la.us
                                    www.state.lib.la.us

Rebecca Hamilton, Assistant Secretary, State Libra
Diane Brown, Deputy State Librarian
Beverly Dugas, Business Manager
Meg Placke, Associate State Librarian
Summer reading programs, braille writer, magnifiers, closed-circuit TV, large-print photocopier, cassette books and magazines,

children's books on cassette. Descriptive videoss and other reference materials on blindness and other handicaps.

4778   Louisiana State University Genetics Section of Pediatrics
533 Bolivar St
New Orleans, LA 70112-1349
                                    504-568-6151
                              FAX: 504-568-8500
                              postmaster@lsuhsc.edu
                                    www.medschool.lsuhsc.edu

Steve Nelson, MD, Dean
Janis Letourneau, MD, Associate Dean for Faculty & Ins
Cathi Fontenot, MD, Associate Dean for Alumni Affair
Charles Hilton, MD, Associate Dean for Academic Affa
Our goal is to continue building a strong department in which all of the faculty are successful in attracting funding, and committed to establishing productive programs that bring credit to the Department and to the Health Sciences Center as a whole.

4779   State Library of Louisiana: Services for the Blind and Physically Handicapped
701 North 4th St
Baton Rouge, LA 70802-5345
                                    225-342-4913
                                    800-543-4702
                              FAX: 225-219-4804
                              sbph@state.lib.la.us
                                    www.state.lib.la.us

Rebecca Hamilton, Assistant Secretary, State Libra
Diane Brown, Deputy State Librarian
Beverly Dugas, Business Manager
Meg Placke, Associate State Librarian
Summer reading programs, braille publications, cassette books and magazines, children's books on cassette and other reference materials on blindness and other handicaps. Louisiana Hotlines - quarterly newsletter. Affiliated with National Library Service for the Blind and Physically Handicapped, Washington, DC. Louisiana Voices recording program uses volunteers to record books for the blind.

Maine

4780   Bangor Public Library
145 Harlow St
Bangor, ME 04401-4900
                                    207-947-8336
                              FAX: 207-945-6694
                              bpill@bpl.lib.me.us
                                    www.bpl.lib.me.us

Barbara Mc Dade, Executive Director
Norman Minsky, President
Franklin E. Bragg II, MD, Vice President
Lee Chick, Treasurer
Summer reading programs, braille writer, magnifiers, closed-circuit TV, large-print photocopier, cassette books and magazines, children's books on cassette, home visits and other reference materials on blindness and other handicaps.

4781   Cary Library
107 Main Street
Houlton, ME 04730-2196
                                    207-532-1302
                              FAX: 207-532-4350
                              faucher!@carey.lib.me.us
                                    www.cary.lib.me.us

Iva Sussman, Chair
Forrest Barnes, Treasurer
Gary Hagan, Secretary
Linda Faucher, Library Director
Summer reading programs, braille writer, magnifiers, closed-circuit TV, large-print photocopier, cassette books and magazines, children's books on cassette, home visits and other reference materials on blindness and other handicaps.

4782 Lewiston Public Library
200 Lisbon St
Lewiston, ME 04240-7234

207-513-3004
FAX: 207-784-3011
TTY:207-200-1511
LPLReference@LewistonMaine.gov
lplonline.org

Rick Speer, Library Director
Marcela Peres, Adult Services Librarian
David Moorhead, Children's Librarian
Beth Martel, Circulation Services Supervisor
Summer reading programs, braille writer, magnifiers, closed-circuit T.V., large-print photocopier, cassette books and magazines, children's books on cassette, home visits and other reference materials on blindness and other handicaps.

4783 Maine State Library
Maine State
64 State House Sta
Augusta, ME 04333-64

207-287-5650
800-762-7106
FAX: 207-287-5624
TTY: 888-577-6690
benitad@ursus3.ursus.maine.edu
maine.gov

Chris Boynton, Manager
J Gary Nichols, State Librarian
Melora Norman, Manager
Summer reading programs, cassette books and magazines, children's books on cassette, home visits and other reference materials on blindness and other handicaps.
Newsl./BiAnnual

4784 New England Regional Genetics Group
P.O.Box 920288
Needham, MA 02492-4

781-444-0126
FAX: 781-444-0127
mfgnergg@verizon.net
www.nergg.org

Marinell Newtown, President
Jennifer Walsh, Secretary
Merrill Henderson, Treasurer
Mary Frances Garber, MS, CGC, Executive Director
New Englands primary network for collaborative exchange of genetic health information and education.

4785 Portland Public Library
5 Monument Sq
Portland, ME 04101-4072

207-871-1700
FAX: 207-871-1703
reference@portland.lib.me.us
portlandlibrary.com

Stephen J. Podgajny, Executive Director
Clare E. Hannan, Head of Finance and Operations
Linda Albert, Head of Human Resources
Linda Putnam, Head of Reference and Informatio
Summer reading programs, magnifiers, closed-circuit T.V., large-print photocopier, cassette books and magazines, children's books on cassette, home visits and other reference materials on blindness and other handicaps.

4786 Waterville Public Library
73 Elm Street
Waterville, ME 04901-6078

207-872-5433
FAX: 207-873-4779
wplhelpdesk@waterville.lib.me.us
www.watervillelibrary.org

Sarah Sugden, Executive Director
Marnie Terhune, President
William Grant, Treasurer
Cindy Jacobs, Secretary
Summer reading programs, braille writer, magnifiers, closed-circuit T.V., large-print photocopier, cassette books and magazines, children's books on cassette, home visits and other reference materials on blindness and other handicaps.

Maryland

4787 Johns Hopkins University Dana Center for Preventive Ophthalmology
Wilmer Ophthalmology Institute
600 N Wolfe St
Wilmer Suite 122
Baltimore, MD 21287-9019

410-955-2777
FAX: 410-955-2542
boland@jhu.edu
www.hopkinsmedicine.org/wilmer/danacenter

Harry Quigley, Director
Emily W. . Gower, Ph.D, Director
Joanne . Katz, Sc.D, Director/Professor and Associate Chair
Oliver D. Schein, M.D., MPH, MBA, Director
Established in 1979, the Dana Center for Preventive Ophthalmology is dedicated to improving knowlege of risk factors for ocular disease and public health approaches to the prevention of these diseases and their ensuing visual impairment and blindness worldwide.

4788 Johns Hopkins University: Asthma and Allergy Center
5501 Hopkins Bayview Cir
Baltimore, MD 21224-6821

410-550-0545
FAX: 410-550-1733
jhuallergy@jhmi.edu
hopkins-arthritis.org

Lawrence Lichtenstein, Director
Studies of allergic diseases and individuals with allergic disease, pulmonary diseases and diseases involving inflammation and immunological processes.

4789 Maryland State Library for the Blind and Physically Handicapped
Maryland State Department of Education
415 Park Avenue
Baltimore, MD 21201-3603

410-230-2424
800-964-9209
FAX: 410-333-2095
TTY: 800-934-2541
referenc@lbph.lib.md.us
www.lbph.lib.md.us

Jill Lewis, Manager
Diana Jarvis, Administrative Specialist
LaTarsha Wilson, Secretary
Provide comprehensive library services to the eligible blind and physically handicapped residents of the State of Maryland. The vision is to provide innovative and quality services to meet the needs and expectations of the patrons of Maryland.

4790 Montgomery County Department of Public Libraries/Special Needs Library
6400 Democracy Blvd
Bethesda, MD 20817-1638

240-777-0922
TTY:301-897-2203
http://www6.montgomerycountymd.gov/apps/libra

Susan F Cohen, Assistant Head Librarian
James Montgomery, Owner
Joseph Eagan, Branch Manager
Serves the library information and reading needs of people with disabilities, family members, students and service providers. Some of its services include books, periodicals, and videos on disability issues, adaptive technology, community information; the National Library for the Blind and Physically Handicapped Talking Book program; large print books; and computer room with adaptive technology.

4791   National Epilepsy Library (NEL)
Epilepsy Foundation
8301 Professional Pl
Landover, MD 20785-7223

866-330-2718
800-332-1000
FAX: 877-687-4878
ContactUs@efa.org
www.epilepsyfoundation.org

Marl A Finucane, Executive Vice President
Patty Dukes, Vice President Operations/Human
Mimi Browne, Director, HRSA programs
Chad Hartman, Director of Major Gifts
Contains information about epilepsy and seizure disorders and serves physicians and other health professionals. Provides in-house bibliographic database (ESDI), searches and documents delivery and interlibrary loans. Maintains the Albert and Ellen Grass Archives.

4792   National Federation of the Blind JerniganInstitute
200 E. Wells St.
at Jernigan Place
Baltimore, MD 21230

410-659-9314
FAX: 410-685-5653
nfb@nfb.org
nfb.org/jernigan-institute

Anil Lewis, Executive Director, NFB Jernigan Institute
Patricia Maurer, Director of Reference, Jacobus tenBroek Library
Cutting-edge research and training is conducted through the NFB Jernigan Institute to address the real problems of blindness, such as model education and rehabilitation methods to empower the blind or improved instruction in Braille.

4793   National Rehabilitation Information Center(NARIC)
8400 Corporate Drive
Suite 500
Landover, MD 20785-2245

301-459-5984
800-346-2742
FAX: 301-459-4263
TTY: 301-459-5984
naricinfo@heitechservices.com
www.naric.com

Heidi W Gerding, CEO
Mark X. Odum, Project Director
Jessica H. Chaiken, Media and Information Services Manager
Birgitta Chaiken, Research Associate
NARIC is a federally-funded library and information center that focuses on disability and rehabilitation information.

4794   Red Notebook
Friends of Libraries for Deaf Action
2930 Craiglawn Rd
Silver Spring, MD 20904-1816

301-572-5168
FAX: 301-572-5168
TTY:301-572-5168
folda86@aol.com
www.folda.net

Alice L Hagemeyer, MLS, Founder/President
Merrie A. Davidson, Associate
Ricardo Lopez, MS, Associate
Joan Naturale, M.Ed, MLIS, Associate
A binder containing fact sheets, library reprints, announcements and other printed informational materials that are related to both deaf and library issues. It is designed to help build communication among individuals and groups within the deaf community. The focus is on assisting libraries in providing cost-effective and efficient library and information services to these consumers in a unbiased fashion.

4795   Social Security Library
U S Social Security Administration
6401 Security Blvd
Baltimore, MD 21235-6401

800-772-1213
TTY:800-325-0778
www.socialsecurity.gov

Bill Vitek, Manager
Jo B Barnhart, Chief Executive Officer
Information on social security and disability insurance.

4796   Warren Grant Magnuson Clinical Center
National Institue Health
9000 Rockville Pike
Bethesda, MD 20892-1

301-496-2563
800-411-1222
FAX: 301-480-2984
TTY: 866-411-1010
prpl@mail.cc.nih.gov
www.cc.nih.gov

John I Gallin, MD, Clinical Center Director
Clare Hastings, PhD, RN, FAA, Chief Nurse Officer
Maureen E. Gormley, MPH, MA, RN, Chief Operating Officer
Maria D. Joyce, MBA, CPA, Chief Financial Officer
Established in 1953 as the research hospital of the National Institutes of Health. Designed so that patient care facilities are close to research laboratories so new findings of basic and clinical scientists can be quickly applied to the treatment of patients. Upon referral by physicians, patients are admitted to NIH clinical studies.

Massachusetts

4797   Boston University Arthritis Center
Boston University
715 Albany St
Boston, MA 02118-2526

617-638-4640
FAX: 617-638-5226
www.bumc.bu.edu

Karen Antman, Dean & Provost, Medical School
Meg Aranow, Director
Barbara A. Cole, Associate VP for Research Admin
Christopher Dorney, Director
The Arthritis Center focuses its educational, research and patient care efforts on the diagnosis and treatment of rheumatic diseases. These include the many forms of arthritis; the auto-immune diseases such as Scleroderma, Systemic Lupus, Erythematosus, Rheumatoid Arthritis; localized pain syndromes such as tendonitis, bursitis, and carpal tunnel syndrome; and metabolic bone disorders such as osteoporosis.

4798   Boston University Center for Human Genetics
840 Memorial Drive
Suite 101
Cambridge, MA 02139

617-638-7083
FAX: 617-638-7092
amilunsk@bu.edu
www.chginc.org

Aubrey Milunsky, Co-Director
Jeff Milunsky, M.D., F.A.C., Director of Clinical Genetics
Research and molecular diagnosis.

4799   Boston University Robert Dawson Evans Memorial Dept. of Clinical Research
75 East Newton St
Boston, MA 02118-2657

617-247-5019
FAX: 617-638-8728

Norman G Levinsky, Director
Jack Ansel, MD
Integral unit of the University Hospital specializing in arthritis and connective tissue studies.

4800   Braille and Talking Book Library, Perkins School for the Blind
175 North Beacon Street
Watertown, MA 02472-2751

617-972-3434
800-852-3133
FAX: 617-926-2027
Info@Perkins.org
www.perkins.org

Frederic M. Clifford, Chairman
Philip L. Ladd, Vice Chairman
Dave Power, CEO & President
Michael Schnitman, Secretary
The Braille and Talking Book Library loans braille and recorded reading materials and the playback equipment necessary to use them. You are eligible for services if you are unable to read print due to a disability.

4801 Brigham and Women's Hospital: Asthma and Allergic Disease Research Center
75 Francis St
Boston, MA 02115-6110
617-732-5500
855-278-8010
FAX: 617-730-2858
arc@partners.org
www.brighamandwomens.or

Matthew H Liang, Director
Elizabeth G Nabel, President
Arthur Mombourquette, Vice President of Support Servic
Joel T. Katz, M.D., Director
Integral unit of the hospital focusing research attention on asthma and allergy related disorders.

4802 Brigham and Women's Hospital: Robert B Brigham Multipurpose Arthritis Center
Brigham and Women s Hospital
75 Francis St
Boston, MA 02115-6110
617-732-5500
855-278-8010
FAX: 617-432-0979
www.brighamandwomens.org

Matthew H Liang, Director
Elizabeth G Nabel, President
Arthur Mombourquette, Vice President of Support Servic
Joel T. Katz, M.D., Director
Research studies into arthritis and rheumatic diseases.

4803 Caption Center
One Guest Street
Boston, MA 02135
617-300-3600
FAX: 617-300-1020
access@wgbh.org
www.wgbh.org/caption

Pat McDonald, Director
Lauren Madden, Business Manager
Ian McDonald, Business Manager
Ira Miller, Production Manager
Has been pioneering and delivering accessible media to disabled adults, students and their families, teachers and friends for over 30 years. Each year, the Center captions more than 10,000 hours worth of broadcast and cable programs, feature films, large-format and IMAX films, home videos, music videos, DVDs, teleconferences and CD-Roms.

4804 Center for Interdisciplinary Research on Immunologic Diseases
Childrens Hospital Medical Center
300 Longwood Avenue
Boston, MA 02115-5724
617-355-6000
800-355-7944
FAX: 617-355-0443
TTY: 617-730-0152
webteam@tch.harvard.edu
www.childrenshospital.org

Sandra L. Fenwick, President and Chief Executive Officer
Kevin Churchwell, MD, Executive Vice President
Dick Argys, Senior Vice President and Chief Administrative Officer
Jean Mixer, Vice President, Strategy
Organizational research unit of the Children's Hospital that focuses on the causes, prevention and treatments of asthma, infections and allergies.

4805 Harvard University Howe Laboratory of Ophthalmology
Massachusetts Eye & Ear Infirmary
243 Charles Street
Boston, MA 02114-3002
617-523-7900
FAX: 617-573-4380
TTY: 617-573-5498
richard.godfrey@schepens.harvard.edu
www.masseyeandear.org/

Wycliffe Grousbeck, Chairman
John Fernandez, President and CEO
Jonathan Uhrig, Treasurer
Lily H. Bentas, Secretary
Development ophthalmology and eye research.

4806 Laboure College Library
303 Adams Street
Dorchester Center, MA 02124-5698
617-296-8300
FAX: 617-296-7947
admissions@laboure.edu
laboure.edu

Andrew Callo, Manager
Maureen A. Smith, President
Offers information on physical disabilities, independent living, peer counseling and advocacy.

4807 Massachusetts Rehabilitation Commission
600 Washington Street
Boston, MA 02111
617-204-3603
800-245-6543
FAX: 617-727-1354
TTY: 800-245-6543
www.mass.gov/mrc

Elmer C Bartels, Commissioner
Deval L. Patrick, Governor
Timothy P. Murray, Lieutenant Governor
John Polanowicz, Secretary
Vacational Rehabilitation and Independent Living for people with disabilities.

4808 Schepens Eye Research Institute
20 Staniford Street
Boston, MA 02114-2508
617-912-0100
FAX: 617-912-0118
geninfo@vision.eri.harvard.edu
www.theschepens.org

John Fernandez, President and CEO
Debra Rogers, Vice President for Ophthalmology
Alan A Ryan, Director Research Finance
Frances Ng, M.B.A., Director of Human Resources
Prominent center for research on eye, vision, and blinding diseases; dedicated to research that improves the understanding, management, and prevention of eye diseases and visual deficiencies; fosters collaboration among its faculty members; trains young scientists and clinicians from around the world; promotes communication with scientists in allied fields; leader in the worldwide dispersion of basic scientific knowledge of vision.

4809 Talking Book Library at Worcester Public Library
3 Salem Sq
Worcester, MA 01608-2015
508-799-1730
800-762-0085
FAX: 508-799-1676
talkbook@cwmars.org
www.worcpublib.org/talkingbook

James Izatt, Dept Head
Braille embosser, magnifiers, closed-circuit TV, adapted computers, cassette books and magazines, children's books on cassette, reference materials on blindness and other disabilities.

Michigan

4810 Artificial Language Laboratory
Michigan State University
220 Trowbridge Rd
East Lansing, MI 48824-1042
517-353-5940
FAX: 517-353-4766
finaid@msu.edu
www.msu.edu

Dr. John B Eulenberg, Phd, Director
Stephen R. Blosser, BSME, Technical Director
Shawn A. Miller, Laboratory Manager
Rebecca Ann Baird, Editor, Communication Outlook
Multidisciplinary research center in the Audiology & Speech Science department, Michigan State University. Its basic research program includes speech analysis and synthesis. Applied research is carried out on computer-based systems for persons who are blind and for persons with cerebral palsy and head injury. The laboratory develops physical, cognitive and linguistic assessment technology.

4811 Burger School for the Autistic
31735 Maplewood St.
Garden City, MI 48135-1993
734-793-1830
FAX: 734-762-8533
garden-city.lib.mi.us

James B Lenze, Library Director
Dan Lodge, Adult Librarian
Lindsay Fricke, Youth Librarian
Marti Boyn Tamaroglio, Library Aide
Burger school for students with autism is the largest public school in the United States that specializes in the education of students with autism.

4812 Chi Medical Library
Ingham Regional Medical Center
401 West Greenlawn
Lansing, MI 48910-2819
517-975-6000
irmc.org

Judy Barnes, Manager
Consumer health and patient education collection in books, videotapes, pamphlets. Open to the public.

4813 Glaucoma Laser Trial
Sinai Hospital of Detroit: Dept. of Opthalmology
31 Center Drive
Bethesda, MI 20892-2510
301-496-5248
kcl@nei.nih.gov
www.nei.nih.gov/neitrials

Paul A. Sieving, M.D., Ph.D., Director
The purpose of the trial is to compare the safety and long-term efficacy of argon laser treatment of the trabecular meshwork with standard medical treatment for primary open-angle glaucoma.

4814 Grand Traverse Area Library for the Blind and Physically Handicapped
610 Woodmere Ave
Traverse City, MI 49686-3103
231-932-8500
877-931-8558
FAX: 231-932-8578
webmaster@tadl.tcnet.org
www.tadl.org

Metta Lansdale, Library Director
Thomas Kachadurian, President
Jason Gillman, Vice President
Jerry Beasley, Secretary
The LBPH was established as a sub-regional library in 1972 and currently provides services for 783 registered individuals in 16 counties, 171 of these registrants are Grand Traverse County residents. Anyone unable to read regular printed materials because of visual or physical limitations may be eligible.

4815 Kent District Library for the Blind and Physically Handicapped
814 West River Center Dr. NE
Comstock Park, MI 49321-3420
616-784-2007
877-243-2466
FAX: 616-336-3256
WyomingYouthStaff@kdl.org
www.kdl.org

Charles R Myers, Chair
Vickie Hoekstra, Vice Chair
Carol Simpson, Secretary
Lance Werner, Director
Summer reading programs, braille writer, magnifiers, large-print photocopier, cassette books and magazines, children's books on cassette, and other reference materials on blindness and other handicaps.

4816 Library of Michigan Service for the Blind
P.O.Box 30007
702 W. Kalamazoo St
Lansing, MI 48909-7507
517-373-5614
877-932-6424
FAX: 517-373-4480
sbph@michigan.gov
www.michigan.gov

Sue Chinault, Manager

Braille writer, magnifiers, closed-circuit T.V., large-print photocopier, cassette books and magazines, children's books on cassette, and other reference materials on blindness and other handicaps.

4817 Macomb Library for the Blind & Physically Handicapped
40900 Romeo Plank
Clinton Township, MI 48038-1132
586-226-5020
800-203-5274
FAX: 586-286-0634
mlbph@cmpl.org
www.cmpl.org

Larry Neal, Library Director
Fred L. Gibson, Jr., President
Peter M. Ruggirello,, Vice Chairman
Barbara S. Brown, Treasurer
Braille writer, closed-circuit T.V., large-print books, cassette books and magazines, children's books on cassette, other reference materials on blindness and other handicaps, descriptive videos and bifokal kits. Assistive technology including JAWS, Zoomtext, OpenBook, and Duxbury.

4818 Michigan's Assistive Technology Resource
Physically Impaired Association of Michigan
1023 S Us Highway 27
Saint Johns, MI 48879-2423
989-224-0333
800-274-7426
FAX: 989-224-0330
matr@edzone.net
www.cenmi.org/mits

Jeff Diedrich, Manager
Maryann Jones, Coordinator
Barbara Warren, Information Specialist
Provides information services, support materials, technical assistance, and training to local and intermediate school districts in michigan to increase their capacity to address the needs of students with disabilities for assistive technology.

4819 Mideastern Michigan Library Co-op
503 S Saginaw St
Suite 711
Flint, MI 48502-1807
810-232-7119
800-641-6639
FAX: 810-232-6639
dhooks@mmlc.info
www.mmlc.info

Denise Hooks, Director
Irene Bancroft, Admin. Assistant
Ruth Helwig, Board Member
Robert Cierzniewski, Board Member
Summer reading programs, braille writer, magnifiers, closed-circuit T.V., large-print photocopier, cassette books and magazines, children's books on cassette, home visits and other reference materials on blindness and other handicaps.

4820 Muskegon Area District Library for the Blind and Physically Handicapped
4845 Airline Rd
Unit 5
Muskegon, MI 49444-4503
231-737-6248
877-569-4801
FAX: 231-737-6307
TTY: 231-722-4103
mclsm@llcoop.org
madl.org

Stephen Dix, Director
Richard Schneider, Assistant Director
Brenda Hall, Business Manager
Michele Wittkopp, Youth Services Coordinator
Braille typewriter, magnifiers, closed-circuit TV, large-print photocopier, cassette books and magazines, children's books on cassette, home visits and other reference materials on blindness and other handicaps, The Reading Edge, and large print books.

4821 Northland Library Cooperative
Library Cooperative/ Library for the blind
220 W. Clinton St.
Charlevoix, MI 49720
231-855-2206
webmaster@nlc.lib.mi.us
www.nlc.lib.mi.us

Jennifer Dean, Director
Christine Johnston, Executive Director
Roger Mendel, Director
Summer reading programs, Braille writer, magnifiers, closed-circuit TV, large-print photocopier, cassette books and magazines, children's books on cassette and other reference materials on blindness and other handicaps.

4822 Oakland County Library for the Visually & Physically Impaired
1200 N Telegraph Rd
Pontiac, MI 48341-1032
248-858-5050
800-774-4542
FAX: 248-858-1153
TTY: 248-452-2247
lvpi@.oakgov.com
www.oakgov.com/lvpi

Dave Conklin, Manager
The Oakland County Library for the Visually and Physically Impaired was established in 1974 to provide access to free library service for County residents who are unable to read standard printed material because of a visual impairment or physical limitation.

4823 St. Clair County Library Special Technologies Alternative Resources (S.T.A.R.)
210 McMorran Blvd
Port Huron, MI 48060-4014
810-982-3600
800-272-8570
FAX: 810-982-3600
TTY: 810-455-0200
lbph@sccl.lib.mi.u
www.sccl.lib.mi.us/LBPH.aspx

Arnold H. Larson, Chairperson
Arlene M. Marcetti, Trustee
Kathleen J. Wheelihan, Trustee
Laurie Crisenbery, Trustee
Offers library services to the blind, deaf and blind, visually disabled, phsyically disabled, and reading disabled.

4824 University of Michigan: Orthopaedic Research Laboratories
1500 E. Medical Center Drive
Ann Arbor, MI 48109
734-936-6641
800-211-8181
FAX: 734-647-0003
patient-customer-service@umich.edu
www.med.umich.edu

Steve Goldstein, Lab Director
Paul Castillo, C.P.A., Chief Financial Officer
Michael ME Johns, M.D., Interim Executive Vice President for Medical Affairs
Quinta Vreede, Chief Administrative Officer,
Develops and studies the causes and treatments for arthritis including new devices and assistive aids.

4825 Upper Peninsula Library for the Blind
1615 Presque Isle Ave
Marquette, MI 49855-2811
906-228-7697
800-562-8985
FAX: 906-228-5627
TTY: 906-228-7697
webmaster@uproc.lib.mi.us
www.uplibraries.org

Suzanne Dees, Executive Director
Summer reading programs, braille writer, magnifiers, closed-circuit T.V., large-print photocopier, cassette books and magazines, children's books on cassette, home visits and other reference materials on blindness and other handicaps.

4826 Washtenaw County Library for the Blind & Physically Handicapped
P.O.Box 8645
Ann Arbor, MI 48107-8645
734-222-6860
FAX: 734-222-6803
lbpd@ewashtenaw.org
ewashtenaw.org

Mary Udoji, Manager
Michigan Subregional Library, Library of Congress National Library Service network. General library service for persons unable to use standard print materials for various physical reasons. Lends audio books and listening equipment, large type books, descriptive videos. Provides reference information and programs. Kurzweil scanner with components which convert standard print to Braille, large type or audio and closed circuit TV magnifier on site.

4827 Wayne County Regional Library for the Blind
30555 Michigan Ave
Westland, MI 48186-5310
734-727-7300
888-968-2737
FAX: 734-727-7333
TTY: 734-727-7330
wcrlbph@wayneregional.lib.mi.us
www.wayneregional.lib.mi.us

Vanessa Morris, Regional Librarian
Sue Steiger, Librarian
Rebecca Farmer, Student Intern
Mariya Webb, Student Intern
Summer reading programs, braille writer, magnifiers, closed-circuit T.V., large-print photocopier, cassette books and magazines, children's books on cassette, and other reference materials on blindness and other handicaps.

4828 Wayne State University: CS Mott Center for Human Genetics and Development
42. W. Warren Avenue
Detroit, MI 48202-1405
313-577-1485
FAX: 313-577-8554
rsokol@med.wayne.edu
www.media.wayne.edu

Robert Sokol, Director
Matthew Lockwood, Director of Communications
Tom Reynolds, Associate Director of Public Relations
Mike Brinich, Associate Director of Communicaitons
Human growth and development disorders.

Minnesota

4829 Century College
3300 Century Ave North
White Bear Lake, MN 55110-1252
651-779-3300
800-228-1978
FAX: 651-779-3417
TTY: 651-773-1715
century.edu

Dr. Ron Anderson, President
Steven Ritt, Vice President
Harold M. Johnson, Treasurer
Ralph Olsen, Jr., Secretary
Programs of study - Orthotic Practitioner, Orthotic Technician, Prosethetic Practitioner, Prosthetic Technician. In addition, Century College offers more than 50 other programs in liberal arts, career and occupational programs.

4830 Communication Center/Minnesota State Services for the Blind
Services for the Blind
332 Minnesota Street
Suite 200
Saint Paul, MN 55101-1351
651-642-0500
800-652-9000
FAX: 651-649-5927
DEED.CustomerService@state.mn.us
www.mnssb.org

Katie Clark Sieben, Commissioner
Brian Allie, Chief Information Officer
Kim Babine, Director

Government Affairs
Richard Strong, Executive Director

Special library service for the blind and physically handicapped providing tape and Braille transcription of textbooks and vocational materials; Minnesota Radio Talking Book providing current newspaper, magazines and best selling books; Dial-in-News, a touch tone phone accessed newspaper service; Library of Congress cassette and phonograph talking book equipment; repair services for special audio reading equipment, with most services free to Minnesota Residents.

4831 Duluth Public Library
520 W Superior St
Duluth, MN 55802-1578
218-730-4200
FAX: 218-723-3822
webmail@duluth.lib.mn.us
www.duluth.lib.mn.us

Carla Powers, Library Manager
Renee Zurn, Digital & Outreach Manager
Davis Ouse, Public Services Manager
Dave Lull, Technical Services Manager

Main library computer lab contains one Sorenson Relay and accessibility computer with zoom text JAWS software.

4832 Minnesota Library for the Blind and Physically Handicapped
Department of Education
1500 Highway 36 West
Roseville, MN 55113
651-582-8200
800-722-0550
FAX: 507-333-4832
charlene.briner@state.mn.us
education.state.mn.us

Catherine A. Durivage, Manager
Rene Perrance, Librarian
Charlene Briner, Chief of Staff
Dr. Brenda Cassellius, Commissioner

Provides books and magazines in Braille, large print, records, and cassettes to qualified residents of Minnesota who have a visual or physical impairment, including reading disabilities due to an organic cause certified by a medical doctor, that prevents residents from reading standard print or physically handling a book. Equipment for in-house use include magnifiers, braillers, listening equipment, and CCTV. Reference collection for in-house use only on visual impairment topics.

4833 Special U
University of Minnesota
P.O.Box 721-Umhc
Minneapolis, MN 55455
612-625-3846
800-276-8642
FAX: 612-624-0997
kdwb-var@umn.edu

Mississippi

4834 Blind and Physically Handicapped Library Services
Mississippi Library Commission
3881 Eastwood Dr
Jackson, MS 39211-6473
601-432-4492
877-594-5733
FAX: 601-432-4478
mlcref@mlc.lib.ms.us
www.mlc.lib.ms.us

Shellie Zeigler, BPHLS Director
Christy Williams, Director of Administrative Services Bureau
Gloria Washington, Public Relations Director
Jennifer Walker, Director of Development Services Bureau

BPHLS serves as the MS Regional Library for the Library of Congress, NLS for the Blind and Physically Handicapped. Book collections include audio cassette, CDs, digital books, Braille, large print, children's 18-20 point large print, and standard print reference collection. Descriptive videos, magazines in Braille or on cassette are available, as well as equipment: adaptive workstation, Braille embosser, closed-circuit TV, magnifier, speech input/output, and more. Check for eligibility.

4835 Mississippi Library Commission
3881 Eastwood Dr
Jackson, MS 39211-6473
601-432-4111
800-647-7542
FAX: 601-354-4181
TTY: 601-354-6411
mslib@mlc.lib.ms.us
www.mlc.lib.ms.us/index.html

Susan Cassagne, Executive Director
Katherine Buntin, Senior Library Consultant
Tracy Carr, Library Services Bureau Director
David Collins, Grant Program Director

Summer reading programs, braille writer, magnifiers, closed-circuit T.V., large-print photocopier, cassette books and magazines, children's books on cassette, home visits and other reference materials on blindness and other handicaps.

4836 Mississippi Library Commission\Talking Book and Braille Services
3881 Eastwood Dr
Jackson, MS 39211-6473
601-432-4111
800-446-0892
FAX: 601-354-4181
mslib@mlc.lib.ms.us
www.mlc.lib.ms.us/index.html

Susan Cassagne, Executive Director
Katherine Buntin, Senior Library Consultant
Tracy Carr, Library Services Bureau Director
David Collins, Grant Program Director

Library service for the print handicapped braille, cassette and disc materials (books & periodicals) for children and adults. Large print RG production (copier & printer), braille embosser and other handicaps.

Missouri

4837 Assemblies of God Center for the Blind
1445 N Boonville Ave
Springfield, MO 65802-1894
417-862-2781
855-642-2011
FAX: 417-863-6614
blind@ag.org
myhealthychurch.com

Thomas Trask, Manager
Caryl Weingartner, Administrative Assistant

Offers braille and cassette lending library, braille and cassette Sunday School materials for all ages, braille and cassette periodicals, resource assistance, and resources for blind children and children of blind parents. CHildren's braille books with tactile graphics for purchase or loan. Books in digital media for adaptive reading services.

4838 Church of the Nazarene
Nazarene Publishing House
P.O. Box 843116
Kansas City, MO 64184-3116

816-333-7000
800-877-0700
FAX: 800-849-9827
it@nazarene.org
www.nazarene.org

Dr.Eugenio R Duarte, Board of General Superintendents
Dr.Jerry D. Porter, Board of General Superintendents
Dr. David A Busic, Board of General Superintendents
Dr. David W. Graves, Board of General Superintendents
Offers braille and large print books. Also offers a lending library and cassettes for the blind.

4839 Judevine Center for Autism
1333 W Lockwood Avenue
Saint Louis, MO 63132-3252

314-432-6200
800-780-6545
FAX: 888-507-4453
judevine@judevine.org
www.judevine.org

Becky Blackwell, President
Evaluations and assessments, parent and professional training programs, consultations, workshops, seminars, family support, clinical therapies, adult programs and support, residential services.

4840 Lutheran Blind Mission
7550 Watson Rd
Saint Louis, MO 63119-4409

314-918-0415
888-215-2455
FAX: 314-963-0738
blind.mission@blindmission.org
www.blindmission.org

Sherry Lambing, Manager
Dave Andrus, Executive Director
Nancy Crawford, Manager
Offers Christian books in braille and large print books and cassettes for the blind and visually impaired, on loan, as well as Christian periodicals in braille, large print and cassette tape.

4841 University of Missouri: Columbia Arthritis Center
University of Missouri
1 Hospital Dr
Columbia, MO 65212-1

573-882-4141
FAX: 573-884-3996
webeditor@missouri.edu
www.muhealth.org

James Ross, Chief Executive Officer
Mitch Wasden, Chief Operating Officer
Anita Larsen, Chief Nurse Executive
Jeri Doty, Chief Planning Officer
Research into arthritis and rheumatic diseases. One of the most comprehensive health-care networks in Missouri, our 5 hospitals and numerous clinics, all staffed by University Physicians, offer the finest primary, secondary, and tertiary health-care services. We also provide education for future health-care providers and participate in important research.

4842 Wolfner Talking Book & Braille Library
Secretary State Office
600 West Main Street
PO Box 387
Jefferson City, MO 65101-387

573-751-4936
800-392-2614
FAX: 573-526-2985
TTY: 800-347-1379
wolfner@sos.mo.gov
www.sos.mo.gov/wolfner/

Richard J Smith, Division Director
Paul Mathews, Reader Advisor, A-CO
Brandon Kempf, Reader Advisor, CP-G & Wi-Z
Virginia Ryan, Reader Advisor, H-L
Wolfner Library provides reading material for Missouri State residents unable to read standard print due to a visual or physical disability. Book formats are recorded books on digital cartridge and cassette, braille and some childrens books in large print. Wolfner

Library also lends out descriptive videos, playback equipment for the cartridges and cassettes are also on loan.

Montana

4843 MonTECH, Montana's Statewide Assistive Technology Program
700 SW Higgins Ave
Suite 250
Missoula, MT 59803

406-243-5751
877-243-5511
montech@ruralinstitute.umt.edu
montech.ruralinstitute.umt.edu

Kathy Laurin PhD, Project Director
Chris Clasby MSW MATP, Project Coordinator
James Poelstra MA, Info Technology Specialist
Specializing in Assistive Technology and oversee a variety of AT related grants and contracts. The overall goal is to develop a comprehensive, statewide system of assistive technology related assistance. Striving to ensure that all people in Montana with disabilities have equitable access to assistive technology devices and services in order to enhance their independence, productivity, and quality of life.

4844 Montana State Library-Talking Book Library
1515 East 6th Ave
P.O. Box 201800
Helena, MT 59620-1800

406-444-2064
800-332-5087
FAX: 406-444-0266
TTY: 406-444-4799
mtbl@mt.gov
msl.mt.gov/talking_book_library

Christie Briggs, Regional Librarian/Supervisor
Erin Harris, Director Recording and Volunteer Programs
Carolyn Meier, Library Clerk/Circulation
Martin Landry, Readers' Advisor
The Library offers FREE alternative audio and Braille reading materials for Montana citizens who cannot read standard print materials because of a visual, physical or reading handicap. Over 50,000 titles on 4-track cassette, WebBraille, Web0pac, WebBlud, summer reading programs, braille writer, magnifiers, closed-circuit T.V., large-print photocopier, cassette books and magazines, children's books on cassette, home visits and other reference materials on blindness and other handicaps.

Nebraska

4845 Nebraska Assistive Technology Partnership Nebraska Department of Education
Ste C
5143 S 48th St
Lincoln, NE 68516-2261

402-471-0734
888-806-6287
888-806-6287
FAX: 402-471-6052
TTY:402-471-0734
atp@atp.state.ne.us
nlc.nebraska.gov/tbbs/

Steve Miller, Manager
Lilly Blase, Program Coordinator
Provides statewide assistive technology and home modification services for Nebraskans of all ages and disabilities.

4846   Nebraska Library Commission: Talking Book and Braille Service
Talking Book and Braille Service
Ste 120
1200 N St
Lincoln, NE 68508-2020   402-471-4016
                                             800-307-2665
                               FAX: 402-471-6244
                               TTY: 402-471-4083
                          talkingbook@nlc.state.ne.us
                                  nlc.nebraska.gov

David Oertli, Executive Director
Kay Goehring, Reader Services Coordinator
Bill Ainsley, Audio Production Studio Manager
Scott Scholz, Circulation & Audio Prod. Coor.
Summer reading programs, braille writer, magnifiers, closed-circuit T.V., large-print photocopier, audio books and magazines, children's audio books, and in braille and reference materials on blindness and other disabilities.

Nevada

4847   Las Vegas-Clark County Library District
7060 W. Windmill Lane
Las Vegas, NV 89113   702-734-7323
                               FAX: 702-507-6187
                          administration@lvccld.org.
                                  www.lvccld.org

Keiba Crear, Chair
Michael Saunders, Vice Chair
Randy Ence, Secretary
Ydoleena Yturralde, Treasurer
Summer reading programs, braille writer, magnifiers, closed-circuit T.V., large-print photocopier, cassette books and magazines, children's books on cassette, home visits and other reference materials on blindness and other handicaps.

4848   Nevada State Library and Archives
100 North Stewart Street
Carson City, NV 89701-4285   775-684-3313
                                             800-922-2880
                               FAX: 775-684-3330
                          ddeleon@nevadaculture.org
                               nsla.nevadaculture.org

Michael Fischer, Director
Ann Brinkmeyer, Head of Government Publications
Kathy Edwards, Government Publications Libraria
Sherry Glick, Library Assistant
Summer reading programs, braille writer, magnifiers, closed-circuit T.V., large-print photocopier, cassette books and magazines, children's books on cassette, home visits and other reference materials on blindness and other handicaps.

New Hampshire

4849   New Hampshire State Library: Talking Book Services
117 Pleasant St
Concord, NH 03301-3852   603-271-3429
                                             800-491-4200
                               FAX: 603-271-8370
                               TTY: 800-735-2964
                          michael.york@dcr.nh.gov
                          www.nh.gov/nhsl/talking_books

Michael York, State Librarian
Janet Eklund, Administrator of Library Operations
Donna Gilbreth, Supervisor
Marilyn Stevenson, Supervisor
Regional Library for National Library Service for the Blind & Physically Handicapped offers digital and cassette books, magazines on cassette, children's books on digital and on cassette, descriptive videos, playaways, and downloadable digital audio books, and Braille services.

New Jersey

4850   Children's Specialized Hospital Medical Library - Parent Resource Center
150 New Providence Rd
Mountainside, NJ 07092-2590   908-518-5806
                                             888-244-5373
                               FAX: 908-233-4176
                          jbrooks@childrens-specialized.org
                               www.childrens-specialized.org

Amy B Mansue, President and CEO
Robin A. Walton, Chairwoman
Victoria Wicks, Treasurer
Sueanne D. Korn, Secretary
Contains some 3,000 books, and journals specializing in nursing, pediatrics, child neurology, and rehabilitation. Also provides a Parent Resource Center, a special collection of books, videos and pamphlets designed to meet the information needs of parents and families, as well as the local community.

4851   Christopher & Dana Reeve Foundation Resource Center
636 Morris Turnpike
Suite 3A
Short Hills, NJ 07078-2608   973-379-2690
                                             800-539-7309
                               FAX: 973-912-9433
                          infospecialist@christopherreeve.org
                               www.christopherreeve.org

John M. Hughes, Chairman
John E. McConnell, Vice Chairman
Peter T. Wilderotter, President and CEO
Robert L. Guyett, Treasurer
A national clearinghouse for information, referral and educational materials on paralysis. Offers a free book 'Paralysis Resource Guide' in English or Spanish. Free lending library.

4852   Eye Institute of New Jersey
New Jersey Medical School
Suite 6100
PO Box 1709
Newark, NJ 07101-1709   973-972-2065
                               FAX: 973-972-2068
                          bhagatne@umdnj.edu
                               www.umdnj.edu/eyeweb

Jacinta Ogbonna, Administrative director
Department A
Tatiana Forofonova, Program Coordinator
Ophthamology, including research into cornea, retina and neuro-ophthamalogy.

4853   Mycoclonus Research Foundation
Apt 17d
200 Old Palisade Rd
Fort Lee, NJ 7024-7060   201-585-0770
                               FAX: 201-585-0770
                          research@myoclonus.com
                          http://www.pspinformation.com/index.html

Mark Seiden, VP
Supports clinical and basic research into the cause and treatment of myoclonus; four international workshops facilitated the sharing of information by physicians, scientists, and investigators active in the field, resulted in three publications; supports promising research projects, clinical neurological fellows, with special emphasis on posthypoxic myoclonus and encourages all who are interested in futhering the understanding, treatment, and cure of myoclonus.

4854 **New Jersey Center for Outreach and Services for the Autism Community (COSAC)**
500 Horizon drive
Suite 530
Robbinsville, NJ 8691-2951 609-588-8200
800-4AU-TISM
FAX: 609-588-8858
information@autismnj.org
www.autismnj.org

Suzanne Buchanan, Executive Director
Genare A. Valiant, President
Kathleen Moore, Vice President
James Grasselino, Treasurer

Purpose is to assist families, individuals and agencies concerned with the welfare and education of children and adults with autism and other pervasive development disorders.

4855 **New Jersey Library for the Blind and Handicapped**
2300 Stuyvesant Ave
Trenton, NJ 8618-3226 609-530-4000
800-792-8322
FAX: 609-406-7181
TTY: 609-530-4000
tbbc@njstatelib.org
njlbh.org

Adam Szczepaniak, Director
Maria Baratta, Assistant Director
Information Technology

Summer reading programs, braille writer, magnifiers, closed-circuit T.V., large-print, cassette, braille books and magazines, children's books on cassette, and other reference materials on blindness and other handicaps. Provides reading material on audio, cassette, large print and braille to eligible NJ residents.

New Mexico

4856 **New Mexico State Library for the Blind and Physically Handicapped**
1209 Camino Carlos Rey
Santa Fe, NM 87507-4400 505-476-9700
1-0-6 5
FAX: 505-476-9776
TTY: 800-659-4915
lbph@state.nm.us
www.nmstatelibrary.org

David L. Caffey, Chairperson
Norice Lee, Vice Chairperson
Eugene Gant, Public Education Department Appointee
Dean Smith, Professional Member

Summer reading programs, braille writer, magnifiers, closed-circuit T.V., large-print photocopier, cassette books and magazines, children's books on cassette, home visits and other reference materials on blindness and other handicaps.

New York

4857 **Andrew Heiskell Braille and Talking Book Library**
New York Public Library
40 W 20th St
New York, NY 10011-4211 212-206-5400
FAX: 212-206-5418
TTY:212-206-5458
ahlbph@nypl.org
www.nypl.org/locations/heiskell

Tony Marx, President and CEO
Mary Lee Kennedy, Chief Library Officer
Anne L. Coriston, Vice President for Public Service
Jeff Roth, Vice President for Finance and Strategy

The library provides talking books and talking book players to the five boroughs of New York City, and braille books to New York City and Long Island. These items may be circulated in person or through the mail without charge to the borrower. Deposit collections may be arranged with agencies that provide service to people with visual impairments. The library also circulates large print books and materials in other formats.

4858 **Center on Human Policy: School of Education**
Syracuse University
805 S Crouse Ave
Syracuse, NY 13244-2280 315-443-3851
800-894-0826
FAX: 315-443-4338
thechp@syr.edu
www.thechp.syr.edu

Steven Taylor, Executive Director
Rachael Zubal-Ruggieri, Information Coordinator

The Center on Human Policy is a disability policy organization concerned with ensuring the rights of people with disabilities.

4859 **DREAMMS for Kids**
190 Whispering Oaks Dr
Longs, SC 29568-6973 607-539-3027
FAX: 607-539-9930
janet@dreamms.org
www.dreamms.org

Janet Hosmer, Executive Director

DREAMMS is committed to increasing the use of computers, high quality instructional technology, and assistive technologies for students with special needs in schools, homes and the workplace.

4860 **Ehrman Medical Library**
New York University Medical Center
577 First Avenue
Room 117
New York, NY 10016-6402 212-263-5394
FAX: 212-263-6534
HSL_admin@nyumc.org
hsl.med.nyu.edu

N. Rambo, Chair/Director
D. Peters, Executive Assistant
N. Romanosky, Department

Administrator
J. Williams, Associate Director

Our mission of the Fredrick L. Ehrman Library is to enhance learning, research and patient care and New York University Medical Center by effectively managing knowledge-based resources, providing client-centered information services and education, and extending access through new initiatives in information technology.

4861 **Finger Lakes Developmental Disabilities Service Office**
44 Holland Avenue
Albany, NY 12229-0001 518-474-3625
866-946-9733
FAX: 585-461-8764
folwelbe@nysomr.emi.com
www.opwdd.ny.gov/opwdd_contacts/local_

Mike Feeney, Director
Carolyn Bassett, Manager
Andrew M Cuomo, Governor

Information on mental retardation and developmental disabilities.

4862 **Helen Keller International**
Fl 12
352 Park Ave S
New York, NY 10010-1723 212-532-0544
877-535-5374
FAX: 212-532-6014
info@hki.org
hki.org

Henry C. Barkhorn III, Chairman
Desmond G. FitzGerald, Vice Chairman
Mary Crawford, Secretary

Nonprofit international organization whose mission is to combat the causes and consequences of blindness and malnutrition.

4863   Helen Keller National Center for Deaf - Blind Youths And Adults
141 Middle Neck Rd
Sands Point, NY 11050-1218   516-944-8900
                                      FAX: 516-944-7302
                                      TTY:516-944-8637
                                      hkncinfo@hknc.org
                                      www.hknc.org

Joseph McNulty, Executive Director
HKNC is the only national vocational and rehabilitation program providing services exclusively to youth and adults who are deaf-blind.

4864   Institute for Basic Research in Developmental Disabilities
1050 Forest Hill Rd
Staten Island, NY 10314-6399   718-494-0600
                                      FAX: 718-698-3803
                                      ibr@opwdd.ny.gov
                                      www.opwdd.ny.gov

W. Ted Brown, MD, PhD, Director
Joseph Maturi, MS, Deputy Director
Ann Marie Pannell, Director of Human Resources
Theresa Troiano, Head of Grants Management Office
More than 40 years after IBR opened its doors, its mission has grown from solely conducting research in the developmental disabilities to also providing services and offering educational programs: in 1980, IBR's George A. Jervis Diagnostic and Research Clinic opened, and since 1987, IBR has been providing educational, training and mentoring opportunities, and access to resources for neuroscience research and scholarship to over 125 graduate-level students through the Programs in Developmental Ne

4865   Institute for Visual Sciences
221 E 71st St
New York, NY 10021-4139   212-517-0400
                                      FAX: 212-472-0295
                                      www.mmm.edu/

Judson R. Shaver, Ph.D., President
Paul Ciraulo, Executive Vice President for Administration and Finance
Carol L Jackson, Vice President for Student Affairs and Dean of Students
David Podell, Vice President for Academic Affairs & Dean of the Faculty
Ophthalmology with emphasis on the development of care for the eye.

4866   JGB Cassette Library International
15 W 65th St
New York, NY 10023-6601   212-769-6200
                                      800-284-4422
                                      FAX: 212-769-6266
                                      info@guildhealth.org
                                      www.guildhealth.org

Jerry Bechhofer, President
Summer reading programs, braille writer, magnifiers, closed-circuit T.V., large-print photocopier, cassette books and magazines, children's books on cassette, home visits and other reference materials on blindness and other handicaps.

4867   Nassau Library System
900 Jerusalem Ave
Uniondale, NY 11553-3097   516-292-8920
                                      FAX: 516-565-0950
                                      outreach@nassaulibrary.org
                                      nassaulibrary.org

Ken Ulric, President
Barbara Behrens, Vice President
Kathy Seyfried, Treasurer
Joe Carroll, Secretary
Information about public library services in Nassau County, including services for people with disabilities and the Senior Connections volunteer project (information and referral for seniors and their families).

4868   National Braille Association
95 Allens Creek Road
95 Allens creek road
Suite 202
Rochester, NY 14618   585-427-8260
                                      FAX: 585-427-0263
                                      nbaoffice@nationalbraille.org
                                      www.nationalbraille.org

David Shaffer, Executive Director
Jan Carroll, President
Cindi Laurent, Vice President
Heidi Lehmann, Secretary
Only national organization dedicated to the professional development of individuals who prepare and produce braille materials.

4869   New York State Talking Book & Braille Library
New York State Library and Education
Cultural Education Center
222 Madison Avenue
Albany, NY 12230-1   518-474-5930
                                      800-342-3688
                                      FAX: 518-474-5786
                                      tbbl@mail.nysed.gov
                                      nysl.nysed.gov/tbbl

Loretta Ebert, Research library director
Lends audio and braille books and specialized playback equipment to eligible borrowers with print disabilities. Service is completely free. Serves 55 counties of upstate NY (Westchester and above). Also provides service to schools, nursing homes, and other facilities.

4870   Postgraduate Center for Mental Health
124 E 28th St
New York, NY 10016-8402   212-576-4150
                                      FAX: 212-696-1679
                                      www.dvguide.com/newyork/postgrad.html

Marge Slobetz, Assistant Director
Marie Serrano, Manager
Evaluations and psychotherapy by social workers psychologists for children, adolescents, families and couples. Neuropsychological testing and remedation for learning disabilities.

4871   Rehabilitation Research Library
Human Resources Center
Albertson, NY 11507   516-741-2010
                                      FAX: 516-746-3298

Amnon Tishler, Research Librarian
Susan Feifer, Manager
Information on rehabilitation and occupational rehabilitation.

4872   State University of New York Health Sciences Center
450 Clarkson Avenue
Brooklyn, NY 11203-2098   718-270-1000
                                      FAX: 718-778-5397
                                      www.downstate.edu

Meg O'Sullivan, Assistant Vice President
Jennifer Hayes, Staff Assistant
Child psychiatry research programs.

4873   Suffolk Cooperative Library System: Long Island Talking Book Library
Long Island Talking Book Library System
2 Penn Plaza
Suite 1102
New York, NY 10121   212-502-7600
                                      888-545-8331
                                      FAX: 631-286-1647
                                      TTY: 631-286-4546
                                      communications@afb.net
                                      www.afb.org

Carl R Augusto, President & CEO
Kelly Bleach, Chief Administrative Officer
Rick Bozeman, Chief Financial Officer
Robin Vogel, Vice President Resource Development
Offers a variety of support services to its 55 member libraries and other patrons including, an extensive talking book program,

assistive technology and other services for people with disabilities.

4874 United Spinal Association
75-20 Astoria Blvd
Suite 100
East Elmhurst, NY 11370- 1177 718-803-3782
800-404-2898
FAX: 718-803-0414
info@unitedspinal.org
www.unitedspinal.org

Lex Frieden, Chairman of the Board
Denise A. Mc Quade, Vice Chairman of the Board
Michael B. Kinne, Secretary
Paul J. Tobin, President
United Spinal Association's mission is to improve the quality of life of all people living with spinal cord injuries and disorders (SCI/D).

4875 Wallace Memorial Library
Rochester Institute Of Technology
90 Lomb Memorial Dr
Rochester, NY 14623-5603 585-475-2551
FAX: 585-475-7220
TTY:585-475-2760
twc@rit.edu
wallacecenter.rit.edu

Lynn Wild, Associate Provost for Faculty Development
Shirley Bower, Director RIT Libraries
Julia Lisuzzo, Director of TWC Administration
Steven Wunrow, Director of RIT Production Services
Information on physical disabilities and deafness.

4876 Xavier Society for the Blind
Two Penn Plaza,
Suite 1102
New York, NY 10121-4595 212-473-7800
800-637-9193
FAX: 212-473-7801
info@xaviersocietyfortheblind.org
www.xaviersocietyfortheblind.org

Fr. John Sheehan, SJ, Chairman of the Board / CEO
Fr. Claudio Burgaleta, SJ, Vice-President
Mr. Victor Gainor, Secretary
Ms. Margaret O'Brien, Operations Manager
Provides spiritual and inspirational reading material to visually impaired persons in suitable format: braille, large print and cassette, throughout U.S. and Canada. Services are provided both by way of regular periodical publications sent through the mail and non-returnable; and by means of a lending library where books are returned. All services are provided free.

North Carolina

4877 Genova Diagnostics
63 Zillicoa St
Asheville, NC 28801-1038 828-253-0621
800-522-4762
FAX: 828-252-9303
gdx.net

Ted Hull, President and Chief Executive Officer
Darrly Landis, Vice President and Chief Medical Officer
Ceco Ivanov, Chief Information Officer
Jennifer Gillen, Director of Marketing
Laboratory serves over 8000 primary/specialty physicians and healthcare providers, offering over 125 specialized diagnostic assessments. These innovative tests cover a wide range of physiological areas, including digestive, immune, nutritional, endocrine, and metabolic function. To date, the lab has performed over 2 million individual diagnostic tests.

4878 North Carolina Library for the Blind and Physically Handicapped
109 East Jones Street
Raleigh, NC 27635-1 919-807-7450
888-388-2460
FAX: 919-733-6910
TTY: 919-733-1462
nclbph@ncdcr.gov
statelibrary.dcr.state.nc.us

Francine Martin, Manager
Carl Ginger Rush, Secretary
James Benton, President
Dennis Thurman, Vice president
Free loan of large print, braille, and cassette tape books and magazines and specialized playback equipment to registered eligible North Carolinians. Call for an application form. Collection contains general fiction and nonfiction titles. Registered borrowers may subscribe to receive descriptive videos for a one time fee.

4879 Pediatric Rheumatology Clinic
Duke Medical Center
P.O.Box 3212
Durham, NC 27708-3212 919-684-8111
FAX: 919-684-6616
rabin001@mc.duke.edu
www.duke.edu

Rebecca H. Buckley, Medical Director
Michael Duke, Owner
Clinical and laboratory pediatric rheumatoid studies.

4880 University of North Carolina at Chapel Hill: Neuroscience Research Building
115 Mason Farm Road
Chapel Hill, NC 27599-7250 919-843-8536
FAX: 919-966-9605
www.med.unc.edu/ophth/

Ricky D. Bass, MBA, MHA, Associate Chair for Administration
Sandy Scarlett, Development Director
Cassandra J. Barnhart, MPH, Manager of Research Administration
An interdepartmental research center on the campus of the UNC-Chapel Hill School of Medicine. Mission is to promote neuroscience research with specific emphasis on developmental , cellular, and disease-related processes.

North Dakota

4881 North Dakota State Library Talking Book Services
604 E Boulevard Ave
Bismarck, ND 58505-0800 701-328-4622
800-472-2104
FAX: 701-328-2040
TTY: 800-892-8622
statelib@snd.gov
ndsl.lib.state.nd.us

Doris Ott, Manager
Hullen E. Bivins, State Lbirarian
Susan Hammer-Schneider, Head Disability Serves
The Talking Books Program provides patrons with free access to cassette books and magazines. The Talking Books Program is administered by the National Library Service for the Blind and Physically Handicapped.

Ohio

4882 Case Western Reserve University
10900 Euclid Ave
Cleveland, OH 44106-4901 216-368-2000
president@case.edu
www.case.edu

Barbara R. Snyder, President
Stanton L. Gerson, MD
W.A. Bud Baeslack, Provost and Executive Vice President
Steven M. Altschuler, M, Chief Executive Officer

Programs which encompass the arts and sciences, engineering, health sciences, law, management, and social work.

4883 Case Western Reserve University Northeast Ohio Multipurpose Arthritis Center
11100 Euclid Ave
Cleveland, OH 44106-1716

216-844-3969
888-844-8447
www.uhhs.com

Fred Rothstein, Executive Director
Basic and clinical research into the causes, diagnosis and treatment of arthritis.

4884 Cincinnati Children's Hospital Medical Center
University Of Cincinnati Uap
3333 Burnet Ave
Cincinnati, OH 45229-3026

513-636-4200
800-344-2462
FAX: 513-636-2837
TTY: 513-636-4900
oopes0@chmcc.org
www.cincinnatichildrens.org

James Anderson, CEO
James M Anderson, Chief Executive Officer
David Schonfeld, Executive Director
Richard G Azizkhan, Member of the Board
Dedicated to providing the highest level of pediatric care. As Greater Cincinnati's only pediatric hospital, Cincinnati Children's is committed to bringing the very best medical care to children in our community.

4885 Cleveland FES Center
11000 Cedar Ave
Suite 230
Cleveland, OH 44106-3056

216-231-3257
FAX: 216-231-3258
TTY: 216-231-3257
info@fesc.org
fescenter.case.edu

Robert Kirsch, Executive Director
Peckham P Hunter, Director
Research and development center on functional electrical stimulation. Houses the FES Information Center, a resource center with a library. Publications, newsletters and videotapes for persons with disabilities and others interested in electrical stimulation are offered.

4886 Cleveland Public Library
325 Superior Ave E
Cleveland, OH 44114-1271

216-623-2800
FAX: 216-623-2800
info@library.cpl.org
cpl.org

Felton Thomas, Executive Director
Thomas D. Corrigan, President
Maritza Rodriguez, Vice President
Alan Seifullah, Secretary
Summer reading programs, braille writer, magnifiers, closed-circuit T.V., large-print photocopier, cassette books and magazines, children's books on cassette, and other reference materials on blindness and other handicaps.

4887 Ohio Regional Library for the Blind and Physically Handicapped
National Library Office
800 Vine St
Cincinnati, OH 45202-2009

513-369-6900
800-582-0335
FAX: 513-369-3111
TTY: 516-665-3384
info@cincinnatilibrary.org
www.cincinnatilibrary.org

Kimber L. Fender, Director
Ross A Wright, President
Paul G Sittenfeld, Vice President
Elizabeth H LaMachhia, Secretary
Summer reading programs, braille writer, magnifiers, closed-circuit T.V., large-print photocopier, cassette books and magazines,

children's books on cassette, and other reference materials on blindness and other handicaps.

4888 State Library of Ohio: Talking Book Program
National Library Service in Washington
Ste 100
274 E 1st Ave
Columbus, OH 43201-3692

614-644-7061
800-686-1531
FAX: 614-466-3584
jbudler@sloma.state.oh.us
library.ohio.gov

Jo Budler, Manager
Jim Buchman, Dir Patron & Catalog Services
Peter Bates, Deputy Director
A machine-lending agency for the visually impaired. Provides free recorded books, and magazines to approximately 26,000 eligible blind, visually impaired, physically handicapped, and reading disabled Ohio residents.

Oklahoma

4889 Oklahoma Library for the Blind & Physically Handicapped
300 NE 18th St
Oklahoma City, OK 73105-3296

405-521-3514
800-523-0288
FAX: 405-521-4582
TTY: 405-521-4672
library@drs.state.ok.us
www.library.state.ok.us

Paul Adams, Library Director
Vicky Golightly, Public Information Officer
Braille writer, magnifiers, closed-circuit T.V., large-print photocopier, cassette books and magazines, children's books on cassette, home visits and other reference materials on blindness and other handicaps.

4890 Oklahoma Medical Research Foundation
825 NE 13th St
Oklahoma City, OK 73104-5097

405-271-6673
800-522-0211
FAX: 405-271-7510
contact@omrf.org
www.omrf.org

Dr. Stephen Prescott, President
Mike D. 'Chip' Morgan, Executive VP and COO
Adam Cohen, Senior VP and General Counsel
Lisa Day, VP of Business and Government Affairs
Focuses on arthritis and muscoloskeletal disease research.

4891 Tulsa City-County Library System: Outreach Services
Tulsa City: County Library System
400 Civic Centre
Tulsa, OK 74103-3857

918-549-7323
FAX: 918-596-2841
os@tulsalibrary.org
www.ohsu.edu

Susan Babbitt, Manager
Linda Saferite, Director
Homebound delivery of library services for the physically disabled.

Oregon

4892 Oregon Health Sciences University, Elks' Children's Eye Clinic
Casey Eye Institute
3181 S.W. Sam Jackson Park Rd.
Portland, OR 97239-3098

503-494-3000
888-222-8311
FAX: 503-494-4286
Roystere@ohsu.edu
www.ohsucasey.com

Earl A Palmer, Director
Eleen Reyster, Clinic Manager
James Rosenbaum, Manager
The elks children's eye clinic is the major charitable project of the Oregon State Elks association. The clinic would not be possible without the organization's dedication and commitment to providing eye care for babies and children.

4893 Oregon Talking Book & Braille Services
250 Winter St NE
Salem, OR 97301-3950

503-378-5389
800-452-0292
FAX: 503-585-8059
TTY: 503-378-4334
tbabs.info@state.or.us
www.oregon.gov/OSL/TBABS/Pages/index.aspx

Mary Kay Dahlgreen, Interim State Librarian
Robin Speer, Fund Development Officer
Susan Westin, Program Manager
Joel Henderson, Admin Program Coordinator
We serve the blind and physically disabled. Cassette books and magazines, Braille books-magazines, for children and adults. Descriptive videos. Audiocassette machines are provided free of charge. Call us for an application.

4894 Talking Book & Braille Services Oregon State Library
250 Winter St NE
Salem, OR 97301-3950

503-378-5389
800-452-0292
FAX: 503-585-8059
TTY: 503-378-4334
tbabs.info@state.or.us
www.oregon.gov/OSL/TBABS/Pages/index.aspx

Mary Kay Dahlgreen, Interim State Librarian
Robin Speer, Fund Development Officer
Susan Westin, Program Manager
Joel Henderson, Admin Program Coordinator
Braille writer, magnifiers, large-print photocopier, cassette books and magazines, children's books on cassette and braille books.

Pennsylvania

4895 Associated Services For The Blind & Visually Impaired
919 Walnut St
Philadelphia, PA 19107-5237

215-627-0600
FAX: 215-922-0692
asbinfo@asb.org
asb.org

Patricia C. Johnson, President and CEO
Dolores Ferrara-Godzieba, Director
John Corrigan, Director
Derby Ewing, Director HumanService
A service of Associated Services for the Blind. 26 magazines are available on cassette through this subscription service. A magazine list can be sent, in both large print and on audio cassette.
$18.00

4896 Carnegie Library of Pittsburgh Library for the Blind & Physically Handicapped
4400 Forbes Ave
Pittsburgh, PA 15213-4007

412-622-3114
800-242-0586
FAX: 412-687-2442
info@carnegielibrary.org
carnegielibrary.org

Cathy Chaparro, Manager
Sue Murdock, Manager
Jane Dayton, Assistant Director
Jacqueline Flanagan, Executive Director
Loans recorded books/magazines and playback equipment, large print books and described videos to western PA residents unable to use standard printed materials due to a visual, physical, or physically-based reading disability.

4897 Free Library of Philadelphia: Library for the Blind and Physically Handicapped
1901 Vine Street
Philadelphia, PA 19103

215-686-5322
reardons@freelibrary.org
www.library.phila.gov

Tobey Gordon Dichter, Chair
Richard A. Greenawalt, First Vice Chair
Miriam Spector, Vice Chair
Siobhan A. Reardon, President and Director
Summer reading programs for children and teens. Closed-circuit T.V.for enlarging print for low vision; computers with screen readers and large print; cassette books and magazines; braille books and magazines; and descriptive videos for the blind and visually impaired. Unique and acclaimed adult education program for all disabilities. State of the art book recording facilities.

4898 Pennsylvania College of Optometry Eye Institute
8360 Old York Rd
Elkins Park, PA 19027-1598

215-780-1400
FAX: 215-780-1336
www.pco.edu

4899 Reading Rehabilitation Hospital
Box 250
Rr 1
Reading, PA 19607

610-796-6297
FAX: 610-796-6353
rehab.fsnhospitals.com/USA/PA/Pottstow

Richard Kruczek, CEO
Doug Mehrkam, Owner
Information on physical disabilities, stroke, head injuries, aging and spinal cord injuries.

Rhode Island

4900 Office Of Library & Information Services for the Blind and Physically Handicapped
1 Capitol Hill
4th Floor
Providence, RI 02908-5803

401-574-9300
FAX: 401-574-9320
olis.webmaster@olis.ri.gov
www.olis.ri.gov

Howard Boksenbaum, Chief Library Officer
Chaichin Chen, Library Program Specialist: LORI
Debbie Cullerton, Information Services Technician:
Jeremy Cutler, Information Services Technician
Offers information and services for the visually impaired including reference materials, braille printers, braille writers, large-print books and more.

4901 **Talking Books Plus**
Library for the Blind & Physically Handicapped
1 Capitol Hill
4th Floor
Providence, RI 02908-5803   401-574-9300
                                    FAX: 401-574-9320
                            olis.webmaster@olis.ri.gov
                                        www.olis.ri.gov

Howard Boksenbaum, Chief Library Officer
Chaichin Chen, Library Program Specialist: LORI
Debbie Cullerton, Information Services Technician:
Jeremy Cutler, Information Services Technician
Offers talking book services for the blind and physically handicapped. Collection includes reference materials, braille printer, braille writer, large-print books, adaptive computer workstations and referrals to appropriate agencies/programs for other services.

South Carolina

4902 **Medical University of South Carolina Arthritis Clinical/Research Center**
171 Ashley Avenue
Charleston, SC 29425-100   843-792-1414
                                            800-424-MUSC
                                        FAX: 843-792-7121
                        academicdepartments.musc.edu/musc/

Jennie Ariail, Director
Tom Gasque Smith, Associate Director
Dr. David Cole, President
Mark S Sothmann, Ph.D., Vice President for Academic Affairs and Provost
Offers patient care services and basic and clinical research on various types of arthritis and connective tissue diseases.

4903 **South Carolina State Library**
1500 Senate Street
P.O.Box 11469
Columbia, SC 29211-1469   803-734-8026
                                        FAX: 803-734-4757
                            reference@statelibrary.sc.gov
                                        statelibrary.sc.gov

Debbie Anderson,, Administrative Coordinator
Flora A. DuBose, Administrative Specialist
Leesa Benggio, Acting Director
Paula James, Director of Finance and Administration
Summer reading programs, braille writer, magnifiers, closed-circuit T.V., large-print photocopier, cassette books and magazines, children's books on cassette, home visits and other reference materials on blindness and other handicaps.

South Dakota

4904 **South Dakota State Library**
800 Governors Dr
Pierre, SD 57501-2294   605-773-3131
                                            800-423-6665
                                        FAX: 605-773-6962
                                        TTY: 605-773-4950
                                    library@state.sd.us
                                            library.sd.gov

Dr. Lesta V. Turchen, President
Monte Loos, Vice President
Sarah Easter, Secretary
Daria Bossman, State Librarian
Summer reading programs, braille writer, magnifiers, closed-circuit T.V., large-print photocopier, cassette books and magazines, children's books on cassette, home visits and other reference materials on blindness and other handicaps.

Tennessee

4905 **Tennessee Library for the Blind and Physically Handicapped**
Tennessee State Library Archives
403 7th Ave N
Nashville, TN 37243-1409   615-741-3915
                                            800-342-3308
                                        FAX: 615-532-8856
                                        tlbph.tsla@tn.gov
                            www.tennessee.gov/tsla/lbph/

Ruth Hemphill, Director
Ed Byrne, Assistant Director
Blake Fontenay, Communications Director
Provides free public library service to residents of Tennessee who are unable to read standard print due to a physical disability. Cooperating library with national network of libraries serving people with print disabilities, operating under the auspices

Texas

4906 **Baylor College of Medicine Birth Defects Center**
One Baylor Plaza
Houston, TX 77030-2348   713-798-4951
                                        FAX: 832-825-3141
                                    www.bcm.edu/obgyn/tcfs

Frank Greenberg, Director
Dr. Paul Klotman, President
One of the few centers in the world that performs fetal surgery. Provides integrated, multidisciplinary care for mothers, carrying babies with genetic or anatomic birth defects requiring therapy before or immediately after birth. This collaboration enable.

4907 **Baylor College of Medicine: Cullen Eye Institute**
Baylor College of Medicine
One Baylor Plaza
Houston, TX 77030-2743   713-798-4951
                                            888-562-3937
                                        FAX: 713-798-1521
                    http://www.bcm.edu/eye/index.cfm?pmid=0

Dan B. Jones, Professor and Chair
Al Vaughan, Manager
Michael Cassidy, Plant Manager
Dr. Paul Klotman, President
Research activities focus on restoring vision and preventing blindness through a better understanding of the disease.

4908 **Brown-Heatly Library**
4800 N Lamar Blvd
P O Box 149198
Austin, TX 78756-2316   800-252-5204
                                            800-628-5115
                            DARS.Inquiries@dars.state.tx.us
                                        www.dars.state.tx.us

Veronda L. Durden, Commissioner
Glenn Neal, Deputy Commissioner
Daniel Bravo, Chief Operating Officer
Rebecca Trevino, Chief Financial Officer
Houses a collection of books, audio and video tapes and periodicals focusing on rehabilitation, disabilities, employment skills and practices and management for the Texas Rehabilitation Commission. Houses materials on developmental and other disabilities.

4909 **Center for Research on Women with Disabilities**
Baylor College of Medicine
One Baylor Plaza
Houston, TX 77030-3411   713-798-5782
                                       800-443-7693
                                  FAX: 713-798-4688
                                  crowd@bcm.tmc.edu
                                  www.bcm.edu/crowd

Kathy Fire, Administrator
Margaret A. Nosek, Executive Director
Martha Mendez, Secretary
Susan Robin Whelen, Investigator
Research organization dedicated to conducting research and promoting, developeing, and disseminating information to expand
the life choices of women with disabilities. Conducts research
and training activities on issues related to the health,
independence

4910 **Christian Education for the Blind**
Suite 702
4200 S Freeway Dr
Fort Worth, TX 76115   817-920-0044
                                  FAX: 817-920-0777
                                       bceb@evl.net

Rodger Dyer, Executive Director
Offers braille and large print books and cassettes for the visually
impaired.

4911 **Houston Public Library: Access Center**
500 McKinney St
Houston, TX 77002-5000   832-393-1313
                                  FAX: 832-393-1474
                                  TTY:832-393-1539
                                  website@hpl.lib.tx.us
                                  houstonlibrary.org
Rhea Brown Lawson, Director
Roosevelt Weeks, Deputy Director
Greg Simpson, Assistant Director
Offers full library services to the visually and hearing impaired in
Houston, TX at no charge. Houses unique and critical services for
its users including online access to the Internet in a private and
secure area.

4912 **Talking Book Program/Texas State Library**
Talking Book Program
1201 Brazos St.
PO Box 12927
Austin, TX 78711-2927   512-463-5458
                                       800-252-9605
                                  FAX: 512-936-0685
                                  tbp.services@tsl.state.tx.us
                                  www.texastalkingbooks.org
Ava M Smith, Director
Providing free library service to Texans of all ages who are unable
to read standard print material due to visual, physical, or reading
disabilities-whether permanent or temporary. The program offers
more than 80,000 titles in fiction and nonfiction, plus 80 national
magazines for adults and children.

4913 **University of Texas Southwestern Medical Center/Allergy &
Immunology**
5323 Harry Hines Blvd
Dallas, TX 75390-7208   214-648-3111
                                  philip.schoch@utsouthwestern.edu
                                  www.utsouthwestern.edu
Diane Jeffries, Director
Priscilla Alderman, Executive Assistant
Daniel K Podolsky, President
Mission is to improve the health care in our community, Texas,
our nation, and the world through innovation and education. To
educate the next generation of leaders in patient care, biomedical
science and disease prevention. To conduct high-impact, intern

4914 **University of Texas at Austin Library**
101 E 21st St
Austin, TX 78712-900   512-495-4350
                                  FAX: 512-495-4347
                                  webform@lib.utexas.edu
                                  www.lib.utexas.edu
Douglas Dempster, Manager
Sheldon Ekland-Olson, Chief Executive Officer
Dr. Fred Heath, Vice Provost and Director
Provides access to information for all users, including those with
disabilities, in accordance with the overall mission of the General
Libraries of the University of Texas at Austin.

Utah

4915 **Utah State Library Division: Program for the Blind and
Disabled**
250 North 1950 West
Suite A
Salt Lake City, UT 84116- 7901   801-715-6789
                                       800-662-5540
                                  FAX: 801-715-6767
                                  TTY: 801-715-6721
                                       blind@utah.gov
                                  www.blindlibrary.utah.gov
Donna Morris, Director
Lisa Nelson, Program Manager
Michael Sweeney, Readers Advisor Librarian
Scott Brooks, Multistate Manager
The Program for the Blind and Disabled provides the kinds of materials found in public libraries in formats accessible to the blind
and disabled. Books and magazines are available in braille, in
large print, on audio cassettes, and on audio digital books. Services are provided by the Utah State Library Division in cooperation with the Library of Congress, National Library Service for
the Blind and Physically Handicapped. Services are provided
free of charge to eligible readers.

Vermont

4916 **Vermont Department of Libraries - Special Services Unit**
578 Paine Tpke N
Berlin, VT 05602   802-828-3273
                                       800-479-1711
                                  FAX: 802-828-3109
                                  lib.ssu@state.vt.us
                                  www.libraries.vermont.gov/ssu
Teresa Faust, Special Services Librarian
Sara Blow, Library Assistant
Jennifer Hart, Librarian
Aidan Sammis, Library Assistant
Regional network library pf the National Library Service for the
Blind & Physically Handicapped. The SSU makes available read-
ing material in large print and NLS talking book formats, includ-
ing these special collections: children's print braille books, audio
described videos and DVDs.

4917 **Vermont Department of Libraries -Special Services Unit**
578 Paine Tpke N
Berlin, VT 05602-9139   802-828-3273
                                       800-479-1711
                                  FAX: 802-828-3109
                                  lib.ssu@state.vt.us
                                  www.libraries.vermont.gov/ssu
Teresa Faust, Special Services Librarian
Sara Blow, Library Assistant
Jennifer Hart, Librarian
Aidan Sammis, Library Assistant

Virginia

4918   Access Services
Fairfax County Public Library
12000 Government Center Pkwy
Suite 123
Fairfax, VA 22035-1   703-324-7329
                                    FAX: 703-222-3193
                                    TTY:703-324-8365
                              access@fairfaxcounty.gov
                                       fairfaxcounty.gov

Janice Kuch, Branch Manager
Beena Pandey, Volunteer Coordinator
Ken Plummer, Outreach Manager
Offers talking books, TDD access, assistive devices such as de-coders for three-week loans, support groups for people who are visually impaired, adapted computer work station with braille printer and assistive listening devices.

4919   Alexandria Library Talking Book Service
5005 Duke St
Alexandria, VA 22304-2903   703-746-1702
                                    FAX: 703-519-5917
                                    TTY:703-519-5911
                          emccaffrey@alexandria.lib.va.us
                                  www.alexandria.lib.va.us

Rose T. Dawson, Director
Renee DiPilato, Deputy Director
Linda Wesson, Communications Officer
Kym Robertson, Talking Book Service
Summer reading programs, braille writer, magnifiers, closed-cir-cuit T.V., large-print photocopier, cassette books and magazines, children's books on cassette, home visits and other reference ma-terials on blindness and other handicaps.

4920   Arlington County Department of Libraries
Arlington County Library
1015 N Quincy St
Arlington, VA 22201-4603   703-228-5990
                                    FAX: 703-228-7720
                                    TTY:703-228-6320
                               libraries@arlingtonva.us
                                       arlingtonva.us

Diane Kresh, Director
Margaret Brown, Chief
Anne Gable, Administrative Services/Technology Division Chief
Peter Golkin, Public Information Officer
Summer reading programs, braille writer, magnifiers, closed-cir-cuit T.V., large-print photocopier, cassette books and magazines, children's books on cassette, home visits and other reference ma-terials on blindness and other handicaps.

4921   Braille Circulating Library for the Blind
2700 Stuart Ave
Richmond, VA 23220-3305   804-359-3743
                                    FAX: 804-359-4777
                                       bclministries.org

Rev. Brian J Barton, Sr., Executive Director
Offers library materials for the blind and visually impaired on a free-loan basis. Serves the entire USA and 41 foreign countries with cassette tapes, reel to reel tapes, braille books, large print books along with talking book records.

4922   Central Rappahannock Regional Library
1201 Caroline St
Fredericksburg, VA 22401-3701   540-372-1144
                                    FAX: 540-899-9867
                                    TTY:540-371-9165
                                    webmaster@crrl.org
                                    www.librarypoint.org

Donna Cote, Executive Director
Alison Heartwell, Librarian
Offers reference materials on blindness and other disabilities.

4923   Council for Exceptional Children
2900 Crystal Drive
Suite 1000
Arlington, VA 22202-3557   888-232-7733
                                    FAX: 703-264-9494
                                  service@cec.sped.org
                                       www.cec.sped.org

Robin D. Brewer, President
James P. Heiden, President Elect
Christy A. Chambers, Immediate Past President
Members are teachers, college faculty members, administrators, supervisors and others concerned with the education and welfare of visually handicapped and blind children and youth. This is a di-vision of the Council For Exceptional Children.

4924   James Branch Cabell Library
Virginia Commonwealth University
901 Park Avenue
PO Box 842033
Richmond, VA 23284-2033   804-828-1110
                                         866-828-2665
                                         866-828-2665
                                    FAX: 804-828-0151
                                       library@vcu.edu
                                       www.library.vcu.edu

John Birch, Media Specialist II
Wesley Chenault, Head
Yuki Hibben, Assistant Head
Ray Bonis, Coordinator
Provides individualized orientations and assistance with library research and equipment.

4925   Newport News Public Library System
2400 Washington Ave
3rd Floor
Newport News, VA 23607- 4301   757-926-8000
                                    FAX: 757-926-1365
                          icieszyn@ci.newport-news.va.us
                                       newportnewsva.com

Thomas P. Herbert, P.E., Chair
Wendy C. Drucker, Vice Chair
Sam Workman, Assistant Director of Development
Matt Johnson, Business Retention Coordinator
Summer reading programs, braille writer, magnifiers, closed-cir-cuit T.V., large-print photocopier, cassette books and magazines, children's books on cassette, home visits and other reference ma-terials on blindness and other handicaps.

**4926   Northern Virginia Resource Center for Deafand Hard of
Hearing Persons**
3951 Pender Dr
Suite 130
Fairfax, VA 22030-6035   703-352-9056
                                    FAX: 703-352-9058
                                    TTY:703-352-9056
                                       info@nvrc.org
                                       nvrc.org

William Boyd, Chair
Jim Faughnan, Vice Chair
Steve Williams, Treasurer
Donna Grossman, Secretary
Empowering deaf and hard of hearing individuals and their fami-lies through education, advocacy and community involvement.

4927   Roanoke City Public Library System
706 S Jefferson St
Roanoke, VA 24016-5191   540-853-2473
                                    FAX: 540-853-1781
                              main.library@roanokeva.gov
                                  www.roanokegov.com/library

Michael L. Ramsey, President
Barbara Lemon, Vice President
Summer reading programs, braille writer, magnifiers, closed-cir-cuit T.V., large-print photocopier, cassette books and magazines, children's books on cassette, home visits and other reference ma-terials on blindness and other handicaps.

4928 Staunton Public Library Talking Book Center
1 Churchville Ave
Staunton, VA 24401-3229
540-885-6215
800-995-6215
FAX: 540-332-3906
talking books@ci.staunton.va.us
www.talkingbookcenter.org

Lisa Eye, Reader Advisor
Lynn Harris, President
Daniel Swift, Treasurer
Betsy Little, Secretary

Offers free library service by circulating recorded books, magazines, and playback equipment to individuals unable to use standard print materials because of visual or physical impairment.

4929 University of Virginia Health System General Clinical Research Group
P.O.Box 800787
Charlottesville, VA 22908-0787
434-924-2394
FAX: 434-924-9960
gcrc@virginia.edu
gcrc.med.virginia.edu

Pamela Sprouse, Administrator
Eugene J. Barrett, Program Director
Mary Lee Vance, Associate Director

Provides investigators with the specialized resources necessary to conduct advanced clinical research. The facility includes ten inpatient beds, skilled research nurses, a core assay laboratory, a metabolic kitchen, outpatient facilities, computing and st

4930 Virginia Autism Resource Center
4100 Price Club Blvd
PO Box 842020
Richmond, Virginia, VA 23284-2020
804-674-8888
877-667-7771
877- -
FAX: 804-276-3970
info@varc.org
www.varc.org

Carol Schall, Ph.D., Director
Florence McLeod, Administrative Assistant
Dawn Hendricks, Ph.D., Faculty/instructor

VARC promotes and facilitates best practices for those diagnosed within the autism spectrum. Information, resources, and education and training help parents, educators, service providers and medical professionals provide effective support from early childhood through adulthood.

4931 Virginia Beach Public Library Special Services Library
936 Independence Blvd
Virginia Beach, VA 23455-6006
757-385-2680
FAX: 757-464-6741
spaddock@vbgov.com
www.vbgov.com/dept/library

Marcy Sims, Library Director
David Palmer, Public Services Manager
Susan Paddock, Library Manager

A public library for people with visual and physical disabilities, braille writer, magnifiers, closed-circuit T.V., large-print photocopier, cassette books and magazines, children's books on cassette, and other reference materials on blindness and other d

4932 Virginia Chapter of the Arthtitis Foundation
2201 W. Broad St
Suite 100
Richmond, VA 23220-3937
800-365-3811
800-456-4687
FAX: 804-359-4900
cmogel@arthritis.org
www.arthritis.org/virginia

Gail Norman, Interim President/CEO
Terri Harris, Chief Financial Officer
Nick Turvas, Senior VP of Health/Wellness
Cecil Wallace, Senior VP Policy and Communication

Provides free information, services and counseling to the public. Services include assistance in locating and accessing government and other health care programs for persons with arthritis, referral to doctors specializing in the treatment of arthritis,

4933 Virginia State Library for the Visually and Physically Handicapped
395 Azalea Ave
Richmond, VA 23227-3623
804-266-2477
800-552-7015
FAX: 804-266-2478
barbara.mccarthy@dbvi.virginia.gov
virginiavoice.org

Paula I. Otto, President
Susan C. Rucker, Secretary/Treasurer
Nicholas B Morgan, Executive Director
Rebecca Emmett, Office Manager

Summer reading programs, braille writer, magnifiers, closed-circuit T.V., large-print photocopier, cassette books and magazines, children's books on cassette, home visits and other reference materials on blindness and other handicaps.

Washington

4934 Meridian Valley Clinical Laboratory
801 SW 16th St
Suite 126
Renton, WA 98057-2632
425-271-8689
855-405-8378
FAX: 425-271-8674
meridian@meridianvalleylab.com
www.meridianvalleylab.com

Dr. Jonathan Wright, Medical Director

A clinical test facility dedicated to providing the most accurate and informative data for patient diagnosis and therapeutic monitoring. With our current research and up-to-date information and various aspects of clinical nutritional medicine, our methodo

4935 Ophthalmic Research Laboratory Eye Institute/First Hill Campus
747 Broadway
Seattle, WA 98122-4307
206-386-6000
800-833-8879
TTY:206-386-2022
www.swedish.org

Bryan Mueller, CEO
Dan Harris, CFO
Heidi Aylsworth, Chief Strategy Officer
Naren Balasubramaniam, Chief Human Resources Officer

Color vision physiology, vision disorders and blindness research.

4936 Washington Talking Book and Braille Library
2021 9th Ave
Seattle, WA 98121-2783
206-615-0400
800-542-0866
FAX: 206-615-0437
TTY: 206-615-0418
wtbbl@sos.wa.gov
wtbbl.org

Danielle Miller, Director and Regional Librarian
Amy Ravenholt, Assistant Program Manager
Mandy Gonnsen, Youth Services Librarian
David Gonnsen, Volunteer and Outreach Services

Summer reading programs, braille writer, magnifiers, closed-circuit T.V., large-print photocopier, cassette books and magazines, children's books, and other reference materials on blindness and other handicaps, online catalog, reference station with assis

West Virginia

4937 Cabell County Public Library/Talking Book Department/Subregional Library for the Blind
455 9th St
Huntington, WV 25701-1417
304-528-5700
FAX: 304-528-5739
cabelllibrary@cabell.lib.wv.us
cabell.lib.wv.us

Judy K. Rule, Director
Angela Straight, Assistant Director
Mary Lou Pratt, Adult Services Coordinator
Breana Brown, Youth Service Manager
Summer reading programs, Braille writer, magnifiers, closed-circuit TV, cassette books and magazines, children's books on cassette reference materials on blindness and other handicaps, enlargers and Arkenstone Reader.

4938 Division of Rehabilitation Services: Staff Library
107 Capitol St
Charleston, WV 25301-2609
304-356-2060
800-642-8207
FAX: 304-766-4913
carolc@mail.drs.state.wv.us
wvdrs.org

Carol Johnson, Manager
Specialized library with information on disabilities and the rehabilitation there of special collections: deaf and hard of hearing, visually impaired/blind, wellness center, literacy and career. The library has assistive devices such as CCTV, scanner and

4939 Kanawha County Public Library
123 Capitol St
Charleston, WV 25301-2686
304-343-4646
FAX: 304-348-6530
webmaster@kanawha.lib.wv.us
kanawha.lib.wv.us

Cheryl Morgan, President
Jennifer Pauer, First Vice President
Elizabeth O. Lord, Second Vice President
Michael Albert, Board Member
Summer reading programs, large print PC option, magnifiers, large type books, cassette books, and magazines, children's books on cassette, home visits and other reference materials on blindness and other handicaps

4940 Ohio County Public Library Services for the Blind and Physically Handicapped
52 16th St
Wheeling, WV 26003-3671
304-232-0244
FAX: 304-232-6848
ocplweb@weirton.lib.wv.us
wheeling.weirton.lib.wv.us

Jimmie McCamic, Chairman
Michael Baker, Secretary-Treasurer
Greg Marquart, Trustee
Anthony Werner, Trustee
The Ohio Public Library exists to provide books and related materials that will assist the residents of the community in the pursuit of knowledge, information, education, research, and recreation in order to promote an enlightned citizenry and to enrich t

4941 Talking Book Department, Parkersburg and Wood County Public Library
3100 Emerson Ave
Parkersburg, WV 26104-2414
304-420-4587
FAX: 304-420-4589
bhdept@park.lib.wv.us

Lindsay Place, Talking Books Dept. Coordinator
Brian Raitz, Director
Free program loaning recorded books and magazines, braille books and magazines to people who are unable to read or use standard print due to a visual or physical impairment.

4942 West Virginia Autism Training Center
Marshall University College Of Educational & Human
Old Main 316
1 John Marshall Drive
Huntington, WV 25755-1
304-696-2332
800-344-5115
FAX: 304-696-2846
www.marshall.edu/atc/

Amanda Plumley, Executive Office Manager
Ginny Painter, Communications Director
Joe Ciccarello, Associate Executive Director
J. T. Schneider, Grants Officer
Provides education, training, and treatment programs for W Virginians who have autism, pervasive devolopmental disorders or Asperger's disease and have formally been registered with the center.

4943 West Virginia Library Commission
1900 Kanawha Blvd E
Charleston, WV 25305-9
304-558-2041
800-642-9021
FAX: 304-558-2044
web_one@wvlc.lib.wv.us
www.librarycommission.wv.gov

Karen Goff, Secretary
Deborah McNeal, Personnel Officer
Steve Tyler, Supervisor
Denise Seabolt, Library Administrative Services Director
Summer reading programs, braille writer, magnifiers, closed-circuit T.V., large-print photocopier, cassette books and magazines, children's books on cassette, home visits and other reference materials on blindness and other handicaps.

4944 West Virginia School for the Blind Library
301 E Main St
Romney, WV 26757-1828
304-822-4840
FAX: 304-822-3370
cjohn@access.mountain.net
wvde.state.wv.us

Patsy Shank, Administrator
Cynthia Johnson, Librarian
Summer reading programs, braille writer, magnifiers, closed-circuit T.V., large-print photocopier, cassette books and magazines, children's books on cassette, home visits and other reference materials on blindness and other handicaps.

Wisconsin

4945 Brown County Library
Central Library Downtown
515 Pine Street
Green Bay, WI 54301-3743
920-448-4400
FAX: 920-448-4376
TTY:920-448-4400
bc_library@co.brown.wi.us
www.co.brown.wi.us/library

Terry Watermelon, President
Kathy Pletcher, Vice President
Carla Buboltz, Secretary
John Hickey, Financial Secretary
Summer reading programs, braille writer, magnifiers, closed-circuit TV, large-print photocopier, cassette books and magazines, children's books on cassette, home visits and other reference materials on blindness and other handicaps.

4946 Eye Institute of the Medical College of Wisconsin and Froedtert Clinic
925 N 87th St
Milwaukee, WI 53226-4812
414-456-2020
FAX: 414-456-6300
eyecare@mcw.edu
doctor.mcw.edu

Jane D Kivlin, Director
Richard Schultz, MD, Director
A national leader as a full-service academic opthalmology program. Dedicated to the highest quality patient care, education,

and vision research, the faculty and staff strive to provide state-of-the-art clinical and surgical patient care in a compassionat

4947 Trace Research and Development Center
2107 Ecb
Madison, WI 53706

608-262-6966
FAX: 608-262-8848
info@trace.wisc.edu
trace.wisc.edu

Kate Vanderheiden, Program Manager
Research focused on how standard information and communication technology products may be designed so that more people with disabilities can use them.

4948 Wisconsin Regional Library for the Blind& Physically Handicapped
813 W Wells St
Milwaukee, WI 53233-1436

414-286-3045
800-242-8822
FAX: 414-286-3102
TTY: 414-286-3548
lbph@mpl.org
talkingbooks.dpi.wi.gov

Marsha J Valance, Manager
Meredith Wittmann, Regional Librarian
Circulates recorded materials, playback equipment and braille materials to print-handicapped Wisconsin residents.

Wyoming

4949 Wyoming Services for the Visually Impaired
Wyoming Department of Education
2300 Capitol Ave
Cheyenne, WY 82002-0050

307-777-7690
FAX: 307-777-6234
jackie.miller@wyo.gov
edu.wyoming.gov/in-the-classroom/special-prog

Ron Micheli, Chairman
Scotty Ratliff, Vice-Chair
Pete Ratliff, Treasurer
Cindy Hill, Superintendent
Services for the Visually Impaired assists people of all ages who have low vision or are blind. The goal is to provide information, education, and support to individuals with low vision in order that they may lead enjoyable and productive lives with maxim

4950 Wyoming's New Options in Technology(WYNOT) - University of Wyoming
1000 E University Ave
Laramie, WY 82071-2000

307-766-2761
888-989-9463
FAX: 307-766-2763
TTY: 800-908-7011
wind.uw@uwyo.edu
wind.uwyo.edu/wynot

William MacLean Jr., Ph.D., Executive Director
Designed to develop and implement a consumer oriented statewide system of technology-related assistance for people with disabilities of all ages.

Media, Print

Children & Young Adults

4951 **Assistive Technology for Infants and Toddlers with Disabilities Handbook**
Idaho Assistive Technology Project
University of Idaho
1187 Alturas Dr.
Moscow, ID 83843- 2268

800-432-8324
FAX: 208-885-6102
idahoat@uidaho.edu
www.idahoat.org

LaRae Rhoads, Author
Ron Seiler, Author
This handbook is designed as a guide for parents and families in Idaho who have infants and toddlers with developmental delays or disabilities.

4952 **Assistive Technology for School-Age Children with Disabilities - Handbook**
Idaho Assistive Technology Project
University of Idaho
1187 Alturas Dr.
Moscow, ID 83843- 2268

208-885-3557
800-432-8324
FAX: 208-885-6102
idahoat@uidaho.edu
www.idahoat.org

LaRae Rhoads, Author
Ron Seiler, Author
Michelle Doty, Author
A handbook designed to provide guidance and information for parentswho have school-aged children with disabilities, focusing on resources for assistive technologies available for their children.

4953 **Children's Understanding of Disability**
Routledge (Taylor & Francis Group)
711 Third Ave.
New York, NY 10017

212-216-7800
800-634-7064
FAX: 202-564-7854
enquiries@taylorandfrancis.com
www.routledge.com

Ann Lewis, Author
Children's Understanding of Disability is a valuable addition to the debate surrounding the integration of children with special needs into ordinary schools. Taking the viewpoint of the children themselves, it explores how pupils with severe learning difficulties and their non-disabled classmates interact.Ann Lewis examines what happens when non-disabled children and pupils with severe learning difficulties work together regularly over the course of a year.
Hardcover

4954 **Complete IEP Guide: How to Advocate for Your Special Ed Child (8th Edition)**
NOLO (Internet Brands)
909 N. Sepulveda Blvd
11th Fl.
El Segundo, CA 90245

310-280-4000
www.nolo.com

Lawrence Siegel, Attorney/Author
This all-in-one guide will help you understand special education law, identify your child's needs, prepare for meetings, develop the IEP and resolve disputes.
384 pages

4955 **Don't Call Me Special: A First Look at Disability**
Barron's Educational Series
250 Wireless Blvd
Hauppauge, NY 11788

800-645-3476
FAX: 631-494-3723
barrons@barronseduc.com
www.barronseduc.com

Pat Thomas, Author
This picture book explores questions and concerns about physical disabilities in a simple and reassuring way. Youger children can find out about individual disabilities, special equipment that is available to help the disabled, and how people of all ages can deal with disabilities and live happy and full lives.
Paperback

4956 **Everything Parent's Guide to Special Education**
Adams Media
4868 Innovation Dr
Bldg 2
Fort Collins, CO 80525

855-278-0402
www.adamsmediastore.com

Amanda Morin, Author
This handbook offers parents assistance, advice, and aid on navigating special education for their child, with information on assessment, evaluation, specific needs for specific disabilities, current law, and dealing with parent-school conflict. It includes worksheets, forms, and sample documents to help parents be effective advocates for their child's learning.

4957 **It isn't Fair!: Siblings of Children with Disabilities**
Praeger - ABC-CLIO
130 Cremona Dr
Santa Barbara, CA 93117

805-968-1911
800-368-6868
FAX: 866-270-3856
CustomerService@abc-clio.com
www.abc-clio.com/praeger

Stanley D. Klein, Editor
Maxwell J. Schleifer, Editor
This book presents a wide range of perspectives on the relationship of siblings to children with disabilities. These perspectives are written in the first person by parents, young adult siblings, younger siblings, and professionals.
200 pages

4958 **Life Beyond the Classroom: Transition Strategies for Young People with Disabilities**
Brookes Publishing
P.O.Box 10624
Baltimore, MD 21285-0624

410-337-9580
800-638-3775
FAX: 410-337-8539
custserv@brookespublishing.com
www.brookespublishing.com

Paul Wehman, Author
This textbook is an essential guide to planning, designing, and implementing successful transition programs for students with disabilities.
616 pages

4959 **Mayor of the West Side**
Fanlight Productions
32 Court St
21st Fl.
Brooklyn, NY 11201

718-488-8900
800-876-1710
FAX: 718-488-8642
info@fanlight.com
www.fanlight.com

Judd Ehrlich, Director
What happens when love gets in the way of letting go? As a teenager with multiple disabilities prepares for his Bar Mitzvah, his family and community consider what Mark's life will be like when they are no longer able to protect him.

4960   New Horizons Independent Living Center
8085 E Manley Dr
Prescott Valley, AZ 86314-6154   928-772-1266
                                        800-406-2377
                                        FAX: 928-772-3808
                                        TTY: 928-772-1266
                                        www.nhilc.org

Gale Dean, Executive Director
Alan Loosley, President
Sharon Geddes, Vice President
Mary Russell, Secretary
The mission of New Horizons Independent Living Center is to provide programs and services in Northern Arizona which encourage and empower people with disabilities to self-determine the goals and activities of their lives.

4961   Rolling Along with Goldilocks and the Three Bears
Woodbine House
6510 Bells Mill Rd
Bethesda, MD 20817
                                        800-843-7323
                                        info@woodbinehouse.com
                                        www.woodbinehouse.com

Cindy Meyers, Author
Carol Morgan, Illustrator
The familiar fairytale with a special needs twist. Ages 3-7.
28 pages

4962   Shriner's Hospitals for Children Newsletter
3101 SW Sam Jackson Park Rd
Portland, OR 97201   503-241-5090
                                        FAX: 503-221-3498
                                        mthoreson@shrinenet.org
                                        www.shrinershospitalforchildren.org

4963   Sibling Forum: A FRA Newsletter
Family Resource Associates
35 Haddon Ave
Shrewsbury, NJ 07702-4007   732-747-5310
                                        FAX: 732-747-1896
                                        info@frainc.org
                                        www.frainc.org

Quarterly

4964   Sibshops: Workshops for Siblings of Children with Special Needs
Sibling Supporting Project
322-6512 23rd Ave NW
Seattle, WA 98117
                                        206-297-6368
                                        info@siblingsupport.org
                                        www.siblingsupport.org

Don Meyer, Author
Patricia Vadasy, Author
Sibshops is a program that brings together 8-to 13-year-old brothers and sisters of children with special needs. The siblings receive support and information in a recreational setting, so they have fun while they learn.
264 pages

4965   Special Education Report
LRP Publications
360 Hiatt Dr
Dept. 150F
Palm Beach Gardens, FL 33418
                                        800-341-7874
                                        FAX: 561-622-2423
                                        custserv@lrp.com
                                        www.lrp.com

Monthly Newsletter

4966   Special Format Books for Children and Youth Ages 3-19
New York State Talking Book and Braille Library
Cultural Education Center
222 Madison Ave
Albany, NY 12230-0001   518-474-5935
                                        800-342-3688
                                        FAX: 518-474-7041
                                        tbbl@nysed.gov
                                        www.nysl.nysed.gov/tbbl/index.html

4967   The Sibling Slam Book: What It's Really Like To Have a Brother or Sister with Special Needs
Sibling Support Project
6512 23rd Ave NW
Ste 322
Seattle, WA 98117   206-297-6368
                                        info@siblingsupport.org
                                        www.siblingsupport.org

Don Meyer, Author
A brutally honest, non-PC look at the lives, experiences, and opinions of siblings without disabilities who have siblings with disabilities. Formatted like the slam books passed around in many junior high and high schools, this one poses a series of 50 personal questions, with responses drawn from the author's interviews with over 80 teens from across the United States. It reflects experiences that range from positive to negative.

4968   The Sibling Survival Guide
Sibling Support Project
6512 23rd Ave. NW
Ste 322
Seattle, WA 98117   206-297-6368
                                        info@siblingsupport.org
                                        www.siblingsupport.org

Don Meyer, Author
Emily Holl, Author
Edited by experts in the field of disabilities and sibling relationships, The Sibling Survival Guide focuses on the topmost concerns identified in a survey of hundreds of siblings.

4969   Views from Our Shoes
Sibling Support Project
6512 23rd Ave NW
Ste 322
Seattle, WA 98117   206-297-6368
                                        info@siblingsupport.com
                                        www.siblingsupport.org

Don Meyer, Author
Siblings share what it is like to have a brother or sister with a disability. Age 9 and up.
106 pages Paperback

4970   What About Me? Growing Up with a Developmentally Disabled Sibling
Da Capo Press/ Perseus Books Group
Order Department
210 American Dr
Jackson, TN 38301
                                        800-343-4499
                                        FAX: 800-351-5073
                                        dacapo.info@perseusbooks.com
                                        www.perseusbooksgroup.com

Bryna Siegel, Author
Stuart Silverstein, Author
A compassionate and accessible guide on living with and caring for a developmentally disabled sibling.
316 pages Paperback

4971   What It's Like to be Me
Friendship Press
P.O.Box 37844
Cincinnati, OH 45222-844   513-948-8733
                                        FAX: 513-761-3722

Community

4972 'Cultural Life,' Disability, Inclusion, and Citizenship: Moving Beyond Leisure in Isolation
Routledge (Taylor & Francis Group)
711 Third Ave
New York, NY 10017   212-216-7800
800-634-7064
FAX: 202-564-7854
enquiries@taylorandfrancis.com
www.routledge.com
Simon Darcy, Editor
Jerome Singleton, Editor
This book concentrates on disability citizenship in leisure.
90 pages Hardback

4973 Active Citizenship and Disability: Implementing the Personalization of Support
Cambridge University Press
Shaftesbury Rd
Cambridge, UK CB2-8BS
information@cambridge.org
www.cambridge.org
Andrew Power, Author
Janet E. Lord, Author
Allison S. DeFranco, Author
This book provides an international comparative study of the implementation of disability rights law and policy focused on the emerging principles of self-determination and personalisation. The case studies examine how different jurisdictions have reformed disability law and policy and reconfigured how support is administered and funded to ensure maximum choice and independence is accorded to people with disabilities.
518 pages Paperback; Hardcover

4974 California Community Care News
Community Residential Care Association of CA
1924 Alhambra Blvd
P.O. Box 163270
Sacramento, CA 95816-9270   916-455-0723
FAX: 916-455-7201
information@crcac.com
www.crcac.com
Charles W Skoien Jr, Director/Lobbyist
Denise Johnson, Consultant
Forum for the exchange of ideas, information and opinions among clients, families and service providers. Information regarding services and assisted living programs for the elderly, mentally ill and disabled.
Monthly

4975 Community Disability Services: An Evidence-Based Approach to Practice
Purdue University Press
Stewart Center 190
504 W State St
West Lafayette, IN 47907-2058   265-494-2038
pupress@purdue.edu
www.thepress.purdue.edu
Ian Dempsey, Editor
Karen Nankervis, Editor
Articles by an array of international experts provide as an excellent resource for professionals and students involved in the area of disability studies. The book is divided into three parts: (1) disability and modern society; (2) working with people who are challenged; and (3) working within a disability-services environment. This approach mirrors the contemporary debate within a practice framework reflecting how individuals, organizations, and communities deal with the problem and solutions.
304 pages Paperback

4976 Comprehensive Care Coordination for Chronically Ill Adults
Wiley-Blackwell
111 River St
Hoboken, NJ 07030-5774   201-748-6000
877-762-2974
FAX: 201-748-6088
info@wiley.com
www.wiley.com
Cheryl Schraeder, Editor
Paul S. Shelton, Editor
A combination of theory and case studies, this book presents the growing demographic of chronically ill adults in the U.S., offering models for change and improvement in quality of care; recommendations on relevant and current literature; and descriptions of successful care outcomes.
440 pages Paperback

4977 Hallmarks and Features of High-Quality Community-Based Services
Independent Living Research Utilization (ILRU)
1333 Moursund
Houston, TX 77030   713-520-0232
FAX: 713-520-5785
ilru@ilru.org
ilru.org

4978 Human Exceptionality: School, Community, and Family (12th Edition)
Cengage Learning
20 Channel Center St
Boston, MA 02210   617-289-7700
FAX: 617-289-7844
www.cengage.com/us
Michael L. Hardman, Author
M. Winston Egan, Author
Clifford J. Drew, Author
An evidence-based testament to the critical role of cross-professional collaboration in enhancing the lives of exceptional individuals and their families. This text's unique lifespan approach combines powerful research, evidence-based practices, and inspiring stories, engendering passion and empathy and enhancing the lives of individuals with exceptionalities.
544 pages Hardcover

4979 Inclusive Leisure Services (3rd Edition)
Venture Publishing Inc.
1999 Cato Ave
State College, PA 16801   814-234-4561
FAX: 814-234-1651
www.venturepublish.com
John Dattilo, Author
This text will educate future and current leisure services professionals about attitude development and actions that promote positive attitudes about people who have experienced discrimination and segregation. It provides strategies that will facilitate meaningful leisure participation by all participants, while respecting their rights.
560 pages Hardcover

4980 Independent Living for Persons with Disabilities and Elderly People
IOS Press
6751 Tepper Dr
Clifton, VA 20124   703-830-6300
FAX: 703-830-2300
sales@iospress.com
www.iospress.nl
Mounir Mokhtari, Editor
Discusses the need for assistive technology in making homes more accessible for the elderly and people with disabilities. Goes on to suggest the application of these technologies in other areas of the community, such as hospitals and schools, which allow those with disabilities and the elderly to live their lives with some independence and autonomy.
216 pages Softcover

4981 Independent Living for Physically Disabled People
People With Disabilities Press (iUniverse)
1663 Liberty Dr
Bloomington, IN 47403

812-330-2909
800-288-4677
FAX: 812-355-4085
media@iuniverse.com
www.iuniverse.com

Nancy M. Crewe, Author
Irving Kenneth Zola, Author
This book describes the philosophy of independent living, from legislative strides to community centres, as well as future trends.
436 pages

4982 Pathways To Inclusion (2nd Edition)
Captus Press
1600 Steeles Ave W
Concord, ON, Canada L4K-4M2

416-736-5537
FAX: 416-736-5793
info@captus.com
www.captus.com

John Lord, Author
Peggy Hutchison, Author
Pathways to Inclusion 2nd edition addresses the organizational strategies that have been used in the past and highlights areas for change. Human service organizations are examined, pinpointing common characteristics that have led to improved quality of life for people with disabilities and other vulnerable citizens.
328 pages Paperback

Employment

4983 A Supported Employment Workbook: Individual Profiling and Job Matching
Jessica Kingsley Publishers
73 Collier St
London, UK N19BE

hello@jkp.com
www.jkp.com

Steve Leach, Author
Created with the goal of helping job developers, this guide offers practical tools and strategies to help job development professionals assist their clients. The workbook includes vocational forms, job analysis forms, and support review charts, and offers aid to professionals in assisting disabled persons to find and secure stable jobs in their communities.
224 pages Paperback

4984 Career Success for Disabled High-Flyers
Jessica Kingsley Publishers
73 Collier St
London, UK N19BE

hello@jkp.com
www.jkp.com

Sonali Shah, Author
Drawing on case studies of 31 disabled adults, this book suggests that individual traits and patterns of behaviour are key factors in career success, and shows that it is often society rather than impairment that hinders professional progression. It will provide role models and valuable insights for young career-minded disabled people.
208 pages Paperback

4985 Job Success for Persons with Developmental Disabilities
Jessica Kingsley Publishers
73 Collier St
London, UK N19BE

hello@jkp.com
www.jkp.com

David B. Wiegan, Author
This book provides a comprehensive approach to developing a successful jobs program for persons with developmental disabilities, drawn from the author's extensive experience and real success.
160 pages Paperback

4986 Making News: How to Get News Coverage of Disability Rights Issues
The Advocado Press

contact145@advocadopress.org
www.advocadopress.org

165 pages

4987 Making Self-Employment Work for People with Disabilities
Brookes Publishing
P.O.Box 10624
Baltimore, MD 21285-0624

410-337-9580
800-638-3775
FAX: 410-337-8539
custserv@brookespublishing.com
www.brookespublishing.com

Cary Griffin, Author
David Hammis, Author
Beth Keeton, Author
Molly Sullivan, Author
Practical support for individuals with significant disabilities in starting and maintaining a small business. Covers building a business plan; pinpointing interests, strengths, and goals; and finding helpful information and support
288 pages

4988 Road Ahead: Transition to Adult Life for Persons with Disabilities (3rd Edition)
IOS Press
6751 Tepper Dr
Clifton, VA 20124

703-830-6300
FAX: 703-830-2300
sales@iospress.com
www.iospress.nl

Keith Storey, Editor
Dawn Hunter, Editor
Explores transition planning, assessment, instructional strategies, career development and support, social life, quality of life, supported living, and post-secondary education for people with disabilities.
318 pages

4989 The Job Developer's Handbook: Practical Tactics for Customized Employment
Brookes Publishing
P.O. Box 10624
Baltimore, MD 21285-0624

410-337-9580
800-638-3775
FAX: 410-337-8539
custserv@brookespublishing.com
www.brookespublishing.com

Cary Griffin, Author
David Hammis, Author
Tammara Geary, Author
Michael Callahan, Author
One of the most practical employment books available, this forward-thinking guide walks employment specialists step by step through customized job development for people with disabilities, revealing the best ways to build a satisfying, meaningful job around a person's preferences, skills, and goals.
264 pages

General Disabilities

4990 A Guide to Disability Rights Laws
U.S. Department of Justice
950 Pennsylvania Ave NW
Washington, DC 20530-0001

202-514-2000
www.ada.gov

Available in Large Print & Braille

4991   A Practical Guide to Art Therapy Groups
Routledge (Taylor & Francis Group)
711 Third Ave
New York, NY 10017   212-216-7800
                                        800-634-7064
                                   FAX: 202-564-7854
                   enquiries@taylorandfrancis.com
                              www.routledge.com

Diane Fausek, Author
Unique approaches, materials, and device will inspire you to tap
into your own well of creativity to design your own treatment
plans. It lays out the ingredients and the skills to get the results
you want. Includes strategies that have been used for people with
Alzheimer's, geri-psychiatric conditions and developmental
disabilities.
124 pages Hardcover; Paperback

4992   A World Awaits You
Mobility International USA
132 E. Broadway
Ste 343
Eugene, OR 97401   541-343-1284
                                   FAX: 541-343-6812
                                        info@miusa.org
                                        www.miusa.org
Yearly

4993   ADA Guide for Small Businesses
U.S. Department of Justice, Civil Rights Division
950 Pennsylvania Ave NW
Washington, DC 20530-0001   202-514-4609
                                   FAX: 202-307-1197
                                   TTY:202-514-0716
                                        www.ada.gov

4994   ADA Information Services
U.S. Department of Justice, Civil Rights Division
950 Pennsylvania Ave NW
Washington, DC 20530-0001   202-514-4609
                                        800-514-0301
                                   FAX: 202-307-1197
                                   TTY: 800-514-0383
                                        www.ada.gov

4995   ADA Pipeline
DRTAC: Southeast ADA Center
1419 Mayson Street NE
Atlanta, GA 30324   404-385-0636
                                        800-949-4232
                                   FAX: 404-385-0641
                   sedbtacproject@law.sgr.edu
                              www.sedbtac.org

Cyndi Smith, B.S., Office Assistant
Mary Morder, Information Technology Support
Sally Z. Weiss, B.A., Director
*Rebecca Williams, B.A., M.S., Information Specialist / Technical
Assistance*

16 pages Quarterly

4996   ADA Questions and Answers
U.S. Department of Justice, Civil Rights Division
950 Pennsylvania Ave NW
Washington, DC 20530-0001   202-514-4609
                                        800-514-0301
                                   FAX: 202-307-1197
                                   TTY: 800-514-0383
                                        www.ada.gov

4997   ADA Tax Incentive Packet for Business
US Department of Justice
950 Pennsylvania Ave NW
Washington, DC 20530-9   202-586-5000
                                        800-574-0301
                                   FAX: 202-307-1197
                                   TTY: 800-514-0383
                                        www.ada.gov

James Bostrom, Deputy Chiefs
Zita Johnson Betts, Deputy Chiefs
Sally Conway, Deputy Chiefs
Jana Erickson, Deputy Chiefs
A 13-page packet of information to help businesses understand
and take advantage of the tax credit and deduction available for
complying with the ADA.

4998   ADA and City Governments: Common Problems
US Department of Justice
950 Pennsylvania Ave NW
Washington, DC 20530-9   202-586-5000
                                        800-574-0301
                                   FAX: 202-307-1197
                                   TTY: 800-514-0383
                                        www.ada.gov

James Bostrom, Deputy Chiefs
Zita Johnson Betts, Deputy Chiefs
Sally Conway, Deputy Chiefs
Jana Erickson, Deputy Chiefs
A 9-page document that contains a sampling of common prob-
lems shared by city governments of all sizes, provides examples
of common deficiencies and explains how these problems affect
persons with disabilities.

**4999   ADA-TA: A Technical Assistance Update from the
Department of Justice**
US Department of Justice
950 Pennsylvania Ave NW
Washington, DC 20530-9   202-586-5000
                                        800-574-0301
                                   FAX: 202-307-1197
                                   TTY: 800-514-0383
                                        www.ada.gov

James Bostrom, Deputy Chiefs
Zita Johnson Betts, Deputy Chiefs
Sally Conway, Deputy Chiefs
Jana Erickson, Deputy Chiefs
A serial publication that answers Common Questions about ADA
requirements and provides Design Details illustrating particular
design requirements. The first edition addresses Readily Achiev-
able Barrier Removal and Van Accessible Packing Spaces.

5000   AEPS Family Report: For Children Ages Birth to Three
Brookes Publishing
P.O.Box 10624
Baltimore, MD 21285-0624   410-337-9580
                                        800-638-3775
                                   FAX: 410-337-8539
                   custserv@brookespublishing.com
                              www.brookespublishing.com

Diane Bricker, Author
Betty Capt, Author
JoAnn Johnson, Author
Kristine Slentz, Author
This is a 64-item questionnaire that asks parents to rank their
child's abilities on specific skills. In packages of 10.
28 pages Saddle-stiched

5001   ARC's Government Report
Arc of the District of Columbia
817 Varnum St NE
Washington, DC 20017-2144   202-636-2950
                                   FAX: 202-636-2996
                                        arcdc@arcdc.net
                                        www.arcdc.net

Mary Lou Meccariello, Executive Director
Ed Cabatic, Director of Finance
Randy Shingler, Chief Operating Officer
Denize Stanton-Williams, Director of Supports & Services

Reports on government activities related to individuals with disabilities with a focus on persons with mental retardation. *$50.00*

5002 ARCA Newsletter
ARCA - Dakota County Technical College
1300 145th St E
Rosemount, MN 55068-2932   651-423-8301
                                 877-937-3282
                            FAX: 651-423-7028
                                      dctc.edu
Ron Thomas, President
Offers information on support groups, conventions, books, manuscripts and programs for the rehabilitation professional and the disabled.
Monthly

5003 Accent on Living Magazine
Cheever Publishing
P.O.Box 700
Bloomington, IL 61702-700   309-378-2961
                                 800-787-8444
                            FAX: 309-378-4420
Julie Cheever, Marketing Manager
A magazine published for forty four years, serves physically disabled people, with general interest, travel, and home modification features. *$12.00*
112 pages Quarterly

5004 Access Design Services: CILs as Experts
Independent Living Research Utilization ILRU
1333 Moursund
Houston, TX 77030   713-520-0232
                            FAX: 713-520-5785
                                  ilru@ilru.org
                                       ilru.org
Lex Frieden, Director, ILRU
Richard Petty, Consultant
Rose Shepard, Office Manager
Featuring the Access Design Services of Alpha One in Maine, this month's Readings is another of the winners of the recent competition for innovative CIL programs.
10 pages

5005 Access To Independence Inc.
Access to Independence
3810 Milwaukee Street
Madison, WI 53714   608-242-8484
                                 800-362-9877
                            FAX: 608-242-0383
                            TTY: 608-242-8485
                            info@accesstoind.org
                            www.accesstoind.org
Dee Truhn, Executive Director
Jason Belaungy, Assistant Director
Geri , Finances/HR
Janie , Administrative Assistant
Independent Living Center serving people of any age and all types of disabilities in south-central Wisconsin. Empower people with disabilities, through advocacy, education, and support.
24 pages Semi-Annual

5006 Access for 911 and Telephone Emergency Services
US Department of Justice
950 Pennsylvania Ave NW
Washington, DC 20530-9   202-586-5000
                                 800-574-0301
                            FAX: 202-307-1197
                            TTY: 800-514-0383
                                   www.ada.gov
James Bostrom, Deputy Chiefs
Zita Johnson Betts, Deputy Chiefs
Sally Conway, Deputy Chiefs
Jana Erickson, Deputy Chiefs
A 10-page publication explaining the requirements for direct, equal access to 911 for persons who use teletypewritters (TTYs).

5007 Achieving Diversity and Independence
Independent Living Research Utilization ILRU
1333 Moursund
Houston, TX 77030   713-520-0232
                            FAX: 713-520-5785
                                  ilru@ilru.org
                                       ilru.org
Lex Frieden, Director, ILRU
Richard Petty, Consultant
Rose Shepard, Office Manager

10 pages

5008 Activity-Based Intervention: 2nd Edition
Brookes Publishing
P.O.Box 10624
Baltimore, MD 21285-0624   410-337-9580
                                 800-638-3775
                            FAX: 410-337-8539
                    custserv@brookespublishing.com
                                 readplaylearn.com
Paul H. Brooks, Chairman
Jeffrey D. Brookes, President
Melissa A. Behm, Executive Vice President
This 14 minute video illustrates how activity-based intervention can be used to turn everyday events and natural interactions into opportunities to promote learning in young children who are considered at risk for developmental delays or who have mild to significant disabilities. *$39.00*

ISBN 1-55766 -86-3

5009 Ad Lib Drop-In Center: Consumer Management, Ownership and Empowerment
Independent Living Research Utilization ILRU
1333 Moursund
Houston, TX 77030   713-520-0232
                            FAX: 713-520-5785
                                  ilru@ilru.org
                                       ilru.org
Lex Frieden, Director, ILRU
Richard Petty, Consultant
Rose Shepard, Office Manager
Joe describes how Ad Lib ensured consumer control in their Drop-In Center: the DIC came about because of consumer input, and consumers are involved in planning the program; members can choose to become volunteers or paid staff members. All of the staff at the DIC are consumers; and active consumer advisory board helps develop policies and programs and provides input to the Ad Lib board.
10 pages

5010 Adobe News
Santa Barbara Foundation
15 E Carrillo St
Santa Barbara, CA 93101-2706   805-963-1873
                                 805-966-2345
                            FAX: 805-966-2345
Ron Gallo, CEO

8 pages Bi-Annually

5011 Advocate
Arc Massachusetts
217 South St
Waltham, MA 02453-2710   781-891-6270
                            FAX: 781-891-6271
                            arcmass@arcmass.org
                            www.arcmass.org
Leo V. Sarkissian, Executive Director
Judy Zacek, Associate Editor
Beth Rutledge, Production Coordinator/Ad
Brenda Asis, Director of Development
Advocate is The Arc of Massachusetts' quarterly newsletter. This is one of the ways in which we inform and educate people about current topics in the field of developmental disabilities. *$20.00*
8-12 pages Quarterly

5012 **American Herb Association Newsletter**
P.O.Box 353
Nevada City, CA 95959-353
530-265-9552
FAX: 530-274-3140
www.ahaherb.com

5013 **Americans with Disabilities Act Checklist for New Lodging Facilities**
US Department of Justice
950 Pennsylvania Ave NW
Washington, DC 20530-9
202-586-5000
800-574-0301
FAX: 202-307-1197
TTY: 800-514-0383
www.ada.gov

James Bostrom, Deputy Chiefs
Zita Johnson Betts, Deputy Chiefs
Sally Conway, Deputy Chiefs
Jana Erickson, Deputy Chiefs
This 34-page checklist is a self-help survey that owners, franchisors, and managers of lodging facilities can use to identify ADA mistakes at their facilities.

5014 **Americans with Disabilities Act Handbook**
Aspen Publishers
76 9th Ave
7th Floor
New York, NY 10011-4962
212-790-2000
FAX: 212-771-0885
customerservice@aspenpublishers.com
www.aspenpublishers.com

Henry H Perritt Jr Esq, Author
Bob Lemmond, President and CEO
Gustavo Dobles, Vice President & Chief Content Officer
Susan Pikitch, Vice President & CFO
The Americans With Disabilities Act (ADA) Handbook provides comprehensive coverage of the ADA's employment, commercial facilities, and public accommodations provisions as well as coverage of the transportation, communication, and federal, local, and state government requirements. *$599.00*
1671 pages 2X per year
ISBN 0-735531-48-X

5015 **An Interdisciplinary Journal for the Social Study of Health, Illness and Medicine**
Sage Publications
2455 Teller Rd
Thousand Oaks, CA 91320-2218
805-499-0721
800-818-7243
FAX: 805-499-0871
hea.sagepub.com

Alan Radley, Editor
Blaise Simqu, Chief Executive Officer

Quarterly

5016 **Annual Report Sarkeys Foundation**
530 E Main St
Norman, OK 73071-5823
405-364-3703
FAX: 405-364-8191
susan@sarkeys.org
sarkeys.org

Kim Henry, Executive Director
Lorri Sutton, Executive Assistant
Susan C. Frantz, Senior Program Officer
Linda English Weeks, Senior Program Officer

Yearly

5017 **Applied Kinesiology: Muscle Response in Diagnosis, Therapy and Preventive Medicine**
Inner Traditions
P.O.Box 388
Rochester, VT 05767-388
802-767-3174
800-246-8648
FAX: 802-767-3726
orders@innertraditions.com
www.InnerTraditions.com

Jessica Arsenault, Sales Associate
Rob Meadows, VP Sales & Marketing
$12.95
144 pages
ISBN 0-892813-28-8

5018 **Arc Connection Newsletter**
Arc of Tennessee
151 Athens Way
Suite 100
Nashville, TN 37228-1367
615-248-5878
800-835-7077
FAX: 615-248-5879
pcooper@thearctn.org
thearctn.org

Carrie Hobbs Guiden, Executive Director
Peggy Cooper, Membership, Chapter and Communications Manager
Nicole Davidson, Business Manager
Lori Israel, Office Manager
The Arc of Tennessee is a nonprofit organization that offers advocacy, information, referral and support to people with intellectual or developmental disabilities and their families. This is their publication. It is free to members. *$10.00*
12 pages Quarterly

5019 **Aromatherapy Book: Applications and Inhalations**
North Atlantic Books
1435a 4th St
Berkeley, CA 94710
510-559-8277
FAX: 510-559-8279
info@northatlanticbooks.com
www.northatlanticbooks.com

Alla Spector, Director of Finance & Office Operations
Doug Reil, Executive Director
Ed Angel, Director of Office Administration
Janet Levin, Senior Director of Sales & Distribution
Considered a bible for those interested in aromatherapy. *$18.95*

ISBN 1-556430-73-6

5020 **Aromatherapy for Common Ailments**
Simon & Schuster
100 Front St
Delran, NJ 8075-1181
856-461-6500
800-323-7445
FAX: 856-824-2402
www.simonsays.com

David Schaeffer, VP
Explains aromatherapy with emphasis on medicinal uses.
96 pages
ISBN 0-671731-34-3

5021 **As I Am**
Fanlight Productions
32 Court Street
21st Floor
Brooklyn, NY 11201
718-488-8900
800-876-1710
FAX: 718-488-8642
info@fanlight.com
www.fanlight.com

Ben Achtenberg, Owner
Anthony Sweeney, Marketing Director

Three young people with developmental disabilities speak for themselves about their lives, the problems they face and their hopes and expectations for the future. *$99.00*

ISBN 1-572950-58-7

5022 Attitudes Toward Persons with Disabilities
Springer Publishing Company
11 West 42nd Street
15th Floor
New York, NY 10036
212-431-4370
877-687-7476
FAX: 212-941-7842
marketing@springerpub.com
www.springerpub.com

James C. Costello, Vice President, Journal Publishing
Diana Osborne, Production Manager
Megan Larkin, Managing Editor, Journals
Theodore C. Nardin, Chief Executive Officer and Publisher
This volume examines what is known of people's complex and multifaceted attitudes toward persons with disabilities. Divided into five areas of concern: theory, origin of attitudes, attitude measurement, attitudes of specific groups and attitude change. *$38.95*
352 pages Hardcover
ISBN 0-82616-90-1

5023 Authoritative Guide to Self- Help Resourcein Mental Health
Guilford Press
72 Spring St
New York, NY 10012-4019
212-431-9800
800-365-7006
FAX: 212-966-6708
info@guilford.com
www.guilford.com

Linda F Campbell PhD, Author
Thomas P Smith PsyD, Author
Robert Sommer PhD, Author
Bob Matloff, President
Reviews and rates 600+ self-help books, autobiographies, and popular films, and evaluates hundreds of Internet sites. Addresses 28 of the most prevalent clinical disorders and life challenges- from ADHD, Alzheimer's, and anxiety disorders, to marital problems, mood disorders and weight management. Also in cloth at $45.00 (ISBN# 1-57230-506-1) *$25.00*
377 pages Paperback
ISBN 1-572305-80-0

5024 AwareNews
Services for Independent Living
26250 Euclid Ave
Suite 801
Euclid, OH 44132
216-731-1529
FAX: 216-731-3083
sil@stratos.net
www.sil-oh.org

Molly Foos, Executive Director
Katherine Foley, Director of Advocacy
Lisa Marn, Assistant Director
Laura A. Gold, Director

12 pages Quarterly

5025 Bach Flower Therapy: Theory and Practice
Inner Traditions
1 Park St
Rochester, VT 05767
802-767-3174
FAX: 802-767-3726
customerservice@InnerTraditions.com
www.innertraditions.com

Ehud Sperling, Owner
Contemporary study of Bach's techniques, intended for practitioners and lay readers alike. Includes lists of symptoms to facilitate diagnosis, ans aims to provide an understanding of psychosomatic elements in relation to physical complaints.

ISBN 0-892812-39-7

5026 Barrier Free Travel: A Nuts and Bolts Guide for Wheelers and Slow Walkers (3rd Edition)
Demos Health Publishing
11 W 42nd St
15th Fl
New York, NY 10036
212-683-0072
barrierfreetravel.net

Candy Harrington, Author
Billed as the definitive guide to accessible travel, this indispensable resource contains detailed information about the logistics of planning accessible travel by plane, train, bus and ship. *$19.95*
200 pages Paperback
ISBN 1-932603-83-2

5027 Beliefs, Values, and Principles of Self Advocacy
Brookline Books
34 University Rd
Brookline, MA 02445-4533
800-666-2665
FAX: 617-734-3952
brbooks@yahoo.com
www.brooklinebooks.com

48 pages Paperback
ISBN 0-57129 -22-2

5028 Beliefs: Pathways to Health and Well Being
Metamorphous Press
P.O.Box 10616
Portland, OR 97296-616
503-228-4972
FAX: 503-223-9117
www.metamodels.com/meta/bks/hea1.htm

David Balding, Publisher
Explores behavioral technologies and belief change strategies that can alter beliefs that support unhealthy habbits such as smoking, overeating, and drug use. Also covers the changing of thinking processes that create phobias and unreasonable fears, retraining the immune system to eliminate allergies and to deal optinally with cancer, AIDS, and other diseases. Includes strategies to transform unhealthy beliefs into lifelong constructs of wellness.

5029 Bench Marks
Govennor's Council on Developmental Disabilities
1717 W Jefferson St
Phoenix, AZ 85007-3202
602-542-4049
800-889-5893
FAX: 602-542-5320
mward@mail.dc.state.us

Micheal Ward, Executive Director
Susan Madison, Manager

Quarterly

5030 Bodie, Dolina, Smith & Hobbs, P.C.
21 W Susquehanna Ave
Suite 110
Towson, MD 21204-5218
410-823-1250
877-739-1013
FAX: 443-901-0802
chobbs@bodie-law.com
www.bodie-law.com

Chester Hobbs, Esquire
Thomas G. Bodie, Lawyer
Wallace Dann, Lawyer
Thomas J. Dolina, Lawyer
Law firm; provides estates, trusts and guardianship administration, estate planning, elder law, tax issues, bankruptcy, foreclosures, and real estate issues. *$25.00*
Quarterly

5031 Body Reflexology: Healing at Your Fingertips
Parker Publishing Company
Ste 2605
1501 Broadway
New York, NY 10036-5600
212-869-6350

Hy Dubin, President

Features step-by-step instructions of how to send healing flows of energy through the body to relieve back pain, headaches, arthritis, and other afflictions. Illustrated.
343 pages Hardcover
ISBN 0-132997-36-3

5032   Body Silent: The Different World of the Disabled
WW Norton & Company
324 State St
Santa Barbara, CA 93101-2362
800-333-6867
FAX: 805-962-5087
www.specialneeds.com/store/

256 pages
ISBN 0-393320-42-1

5033   Body of Knowledge/Hellerwork
406 Berry St
Mount Shasta, CA 96067-2548
530-926-2500
thehellher@aol.com
www.josephheller.com

Joseph Heller, Owner
Information, referral directory, training and certification.

5034   Bridge Newsletter
Arizona Bridge to Independent Living
1229 E Washington St
Phoenix, AZ 85034-1101
602-256-2245
800-280-2245
FAX: 602-254-6407
azbridge@abil.org
abil.org

Phil Pangrazio, President & CEO
Regina Mitzel, V. P. & Chief Administrative Officer
Amina Kruck, V.P. of Advocacy
Ann Pasco, V.P. of Operations

12 pages Monthly

5035   Bridging the Gap: A National Directory of Services for Women & Girls with Disabilities
Educational Equity Concepts
71 Fifth Avenue
New York, NY 10016-5506
212-725-1803
FAX: 212-725-0947
TTY:212-725-1803
infomration@edequity.org
www.edequity.org

Ellen Rubin, Coordinator Disability Programs
Merle Froschl, Editor
Contains a resource section of publications and videos geared specifically to women and girls with disabilities. Available in print, on cassette, and also in braille. *$24.95*

ISBN 0-931629-16-0

5036   Bulletin of the Association on the Handicapped
Assoc. on Handicapped Student Service Program
P.O.Box 21192
Columbus, OH 43221-0192
614-365-5216
FAX: 614-365-6718

5037   CDR Reports
Council for Disability Rights
Ste 1540
20 N Wacker Dr
Chicago, IL 60606-2903
312-201-4800
FAX: 312-444-1977
cdrights@interaccess.com
www.disabilityrights.org

Jo Holzer, Executive Director/Editor
Bruce Moore, Employment Specialist
$15.00
8 pages Monthly

5038   California Financial Power of Attorney
NOLO
950 Parker St
Berkeley, CA 94710-2524
510-549-1976
800-955-4775
FAX: 510-548-5902
www.nolo.com

Maira Dizgalvis, Trade Customer Service Manager
Susan McConnell, Director Sales
Natasha Kaluza, Sales Assistant
David Rothenberg, CEO
A plain-English book packed with forms and instructions to give a trusted person the legal authority to handle your financial affairs.
Paperback

5039   Caring for America's Heroes
Oklahoma City VA Medical Center
921 NE 13th St
Oklahoma City, OK 73104-5007
405-270-0501
FAX: 405-270-1560
www.oklahoma.va.gov

Steven Gentlin, Director
Kathleen Fogarty, Associate Director
D Robert McCaffree MD, Chief of Staff
Tom Duchene, Plant Manager

5040   Center for Health Research: Eastern Washington University
Showalter 209a
Cheney, WA 99004
509-359-2279
800-221-9369
FAX: 509-359-2778
sharon.wilson@mail.ewu.edu
iceberg.ewu.edu

5041   Center for Libraries and Educational Improvement
400 Maryland Ave SW
Washington, DC 20202-1
202-260-2226
800-872-5327
FAX: 202-401-0689
TTY: 800-437-0833
www.ed.gov

5042   Centering Corporation Grief Resources
7230 Maple Street
Omaha, NE 68134
402-553-1200
866-218-0101
FAX: 402-533-0507
j1200@aol.com
www.centering.org

Joy Johnson, Founder
Dr. Marvin Johnson, Founder
Janet Roberts, Executive Director
Kelsey Novacek, Director of Marketing
A full catalog of all our available bereavement resources. We are a small, non-profit organization providing help to families in crisis situations.
32 pages BiAnnually

5043   Centers for Disease Control and Prevention
US Department of Health and Human Services
1600 Clifton Rd NE
Atlanta, GA 30329-4018
404-639-3311
800-232-4636
FAX: 404-498-1177
inquiry@cdc.gov
www.cdc.gov

Robert Delaney, Plant Manager
Publishes an annually updated list of infectious and communicable diseases transmitted through the handling of food in accordance with Section 103 of Title I.

5044 **Child With Special Needs: Encouraging Intellectual and Emotional Growth**
Addison-Wesley Publishing Company
Ste 300
75 Arlington St
Boston, MA 02116-3988
617-848-7500
800-238-9682
FAX: 617-944-7273
www.awprofessional.com

Bill Barke, CEO
Covering all kinds of disabilities — including cerebral palsy, autism, retardation, ADD, and language problems — this guide offers parents specific ways of helping all special needs chidren reach their full intellectual and emotional potential. *$32.00*
496 pages
ISBN 0-201407-26-4

5045 **Chinese Herbal Medicine**
Shambhala Publications
300 Massachusetts Avenue
Boston, MA 02115
617-424-0030
FAX: 617-236-1563
editors@shambhala.com
shambhala.com

Richard Reoch, President
Gives an in-depth look into herbal medicine.
176 pages
ISBN 0-877733-98-8

5046 **Christian Approach to Overcoming Disability: A Doctor's Story**
Haworth Press
10 Alice St
Binghamton, NY 13904-1503
607-722-5857
800-429-6784
FAX: 607-722-6362
orders@haworthpress.com
www.haworthpress.com

William Cohen, Owner
$29.95
128 pages
ISBN 0-789022-57-5

5047 **Closing the Gap**
526 Main Street
P.O.Box 68
Henderson, MN 56044-68
507-248-3294
FAX: 507-248-3810
info@closingthegap.com
www.closingthegap.com

Dolores Hagen, Founder
Delores Hagen, Founder
Connie Kneip, Vice President
Megan Turek, Managing Editor
Explores use of microcomputers as personal and educational tools for persons with disabilities.
36+ pages BiMonthly

5048 **Constellations**
Minnesota STAR Program
Ste 309
50 Sherburne Ave
Saint Paul, MN 55155-1402
651-296-2771
800-657-3862
FAX: 651-282-6671
star.program@state.mn.us
www.admin.state.mn.us/assistivetechnology

Chuck Rassbach, Executive Director
Free quarterly publication from the Minnesota STAR Program.
8 pages Quarterly

5049 **Consumer Buyer's Guide for Independent Living**
American Occupational Therapy Association (AOTA)
4720 Montgomery Ln
Bethesda, MD 20814-5320
301-652-2682
800-SAY-AOTA
FAX: 301-652-7711
TTY: 800-377-8555
www.aota.org

Florence Clark, President
A buyer's directory of products and publications for the general public listing suppliers' names, addresses and telephone numbers. This directory lists AOTA publications on numerous topics (back pain, Alzheimers, Carpal Tunnel Syndrome, etc.) and suppliers of equipment to assist in activities of daily living for individuals with disabilities.
60 pages Annual

5050 **Coping+Plus: Dimensions of Disability**
Greenwood Publishing Group
130 Cremona Drive
Santa Barbara, CA 93117
805-968-1911
800-368-6868
FAX: 866-270-3856
CustomerService@abc-clio.com
www.abc-clio.com

Matt Laddin, Vice President of Marketing
Mike Saltzman, Director-Eastern Territories & National Accounts
James Lingle, International Sales & Marketing
Everyone can learn new or more effective coping skills and strategies to deal with times of loss, crisis and disability. $55-$59.95
280 pages Hardcover
ISBN 0-275945-44-8

5051 **Council News**
Northern Nevada Center for Independent Living
999 Pyramid Way
Sparks, NV 89431-4471
775-353-3599
FAX: 775-353-3588
nncil@sbcglobal.net
www.nncil.org

Lisa Bonie, Executive Director
Hilda Velasco, Operations Manager
Joni Inglis, Independent Living Advocate
Patti Rodriguez, Life Skills Coordinator
NNCIL was founded in 1982 by a small group of people with disabilities, who believe that each person, regardless of the severity of his or her disability, has the potential to grow, develop and share fully the joys and responsibilities of our society.
12 pages Quarterly

5052 **Counseling in Terminal Care & Bereavement**
Brookes Publishing
P.O.Box 10624
Baltimore, MD 21285-0624
410-337-9580
800-638-3775
FAX: 410-337-8539
custserv@brookespublishing.com
readplaylearn.com

Paul H. Brooks, Chairman
Jeffrey D. Brookes, President
Melissa A. Behm, Executive Vice President
Provides practical suggestions for addressing the needs of patients and family members who are anticipating or currently dealing with grief and bereavement, such as hospice care, hospitals, or at home care. *$34.00*
210 pages Paperback
ISBN 1-85433-78-7

5053 **Creating Wholeness: Self-Healing Workbook Using**
Dynamic Relaxation, Images and Thoughts
Plenum Publishing Corporation
233 Spring St
7th Floor
New York, NY 10013-1522   212-620-8000
                                 800-644-4831
                                 FAX: 212-460-1575
                                 ainy@aveda.com
                                 www.aveda.edu

232 pages
ISBN 0-306441-72-1

5054 **DRS Connection**
Disabled Resource Services
Ste 101
424 Pine St
Fort Collins, CO 80524-2421   970-482-2700
                                     FAX: 970-407-7072
                                     drs@frii.com

Nancy Jackson, Executive Director

4 pages Quaterly

5055 **Demand Response Transportation Through a Rural ILC**
Independent Living Research Utilization ILRU
1333 Moursund
Houston, TX 77030   713-520-0232
                           FAX: 713-520-5785
                           ilru@ilru.org
                           ilru.org

Lex Frieden, Director, ILRU
Richard Petty, Consultant
Rose Shepard, Office Manager
Oklahomans for Independent Living's transportation program
was selected as exemplary becuase they marketed it by emphasizing people with disabilities as economic constituency.
10 pages

5056 **Developing Organized Coalitions and Strategic Plans**
Independent Living Research Utilization ILRU
1333 Moursund
Houston, TX 77030   713-520-0232
                           FAX: 713-520-5785
                           ilru@ilru.org
                           ilru.org

Lex Frieden, Director, ILRU
Richard Petty, Consultant
Rose Shepard, Office Manager

10 pages

5057 **Dictionary of Congenital Malformations& Disorders**
Informa Healthcare
Fl 16
52 Vanderbilt Ave
New York, NY 10017-3846   212-520-2777
                                 FAX: 212-661-5052
                                 orders@crcpress.com
                                 www.tandfonline.com

193 pages
ISBN 0-850705-77-1

5058 **Dictionary of Developmental Disabilities Terminology**
Brookes Publishing
P.O.Box 10624
Baltimore, MD 21285-0624   410-337-9580
                                  800-638-3775
                                  FAX: 410-337-8539
                                  custserv@brookesopublishing.com
                                  www.brookespublishing.com

Paul H. Brooks, Chairman
Jeffrey D. Brookes, President
Melissa A. Behm, Executive Vice President
George S. Stamathis, Vice President & Publisher

With more than 3,000 easy-to-understand entries, this dictionary
provides thorough explanations of terms associated with developmental disabilities and disorders. *$55.95*
368 pages Hardcover
ISBN 1-557662-45-2

5059 **Directory of Members**
American Network of Community Options & Resources
1101 King St
Suite 380
Alexandria, VA 22314-2962   703-535-7850
                                   FAX: 703-535-7860
                                   ancor@ancor.org
                                   ancor.org

Dave Toeniskoetter, President
Chris Sparks, Vice President
Julie Manworren, Secretary/Treasurer
Wendy Swager, Past president
The Directory lists over 600 agencies that provide residential services and supports in 48 states and the District of Columbia. The
listings include the name of the Executive Directors, the name,
address, and phone number of the agency, describe the types of
services that are provided and how many individuals receive services from that agency. *$25.00*
189 pages

5060 **Disability Awareness Guide**
Central Iowa Center for Independent Living
655 Walnut St
Suite 131
Des Moines, IA 50309-3930   515-243-1742
                                   FAX: 515-243-5385
                                   cicil@raccoon.com
                                   centraliowacil.com

Bob Jeppesen, Executive Director
Frank Strong, Assistant Director Programs
Bob Jepson, Manager
The Disability Awareness Guide contains information about our
center; who we are and what we do. It also contains the telephone
numbers of local and national agencies and resources available
for people with disabilities.

5061 **Disability Rights Movement**
Children's Press
Sherman Tpke
Danbury, CT 6813   800-621-1115
                          FAX: 800-374-4329

Elena Rockman, Marketing Manager
Author Deborah Kent illuminates both the history of the National
Disability Rights Movement and the inspiring personal stories of
individuals with various disabilities. *$18.00*
32 pages Hardcover
ISBN 0-53106 -32-3

5062 **Disabled People's International Fifth World Assembly as**
Reported by Two US Participants
Independent Living Research Utilization ILRU
1333 Moursund
Houston, TX 77030   713-520-0232
                           FAX: 713-520-5785
                           ilru@ilru.org
                           ilru.org

Lex Frieden, Director, ILRU
Richard Petty, Consultant
Rose Shepard, Office Manager
This report describes the international conference on independent living held in Mexico City in December 1998 as experienced
by staff members from two U.S. centers. Kaye Beneke interviewed Luis Chew and Marco Antonio Coronado for this edition
of Readings in Independent Living.
10 pages

5063   Disabled We Stand
Brookline Books
34 University Rd
Brookline, MA 02445-4533

800-666-2665
FAX: 617-734-3952
brbooks@yahoo.com
www.brooklinebooks.com

Paperback
ISBN 0-25331-80-0

5064   Disabled, the Media, and the Information Age
Greenwood Publishing Group
130 Cremona Drive
Santa Barbara, CA 93117

805-968-1911
800-368-6868
FAX: 866-270-3856
CustomerService@abc-clio.com
www.abc-clio.com

Matt Laddin, Vice President of Marketing
Mike Saltzman, Director-Eastern Territories & National Accounts
James Lingle, International Sales & Marketing
A short and easy-to-read overview of how disabled Americans have been portrayed by the media and how images and the role of the handicapped are changing. *$55.00*
264 pages Hardcover
ISBN 0-313284-72-5

5065   Discovery Newsletter
North Dakota State Library Talking Book Services
Dept 250
604 E Boulevard Ave
Bismarck, ND 58505-605

701-328-2000
800-843-9948
FAX: 701-328-2040
sbschneider@nd.gov
ndsl.lib.state.nd.us/DisabilityServices.html

Doris Ott, Manager
The North Dakota State Library Disability Services produces the Doscovery Newsletter containing information on services, books, catalogs and of interest to the patron.
6 pages Bi-Annually

5066   EP Resource Guide
Exceptional Parent Library
P.O.Box 1807
Englewood Cliffs, NJ 7632-1207

201-947-6000
800-535-1910
FAX: 201-947-9376
eplibrary@aol.com
www.eplibrary.com

5067   ESCIL Update Newsletter
Eastern Shore Center for Independent Living
9 Sunburst Ctr
Cambridge, MD 21613-2057

410-221-7701
800-705-7944
FAX: 410-221-7714
escil@comcast.net
www.escil.org

Shirley Tarbox, Executive Director
Jean Reed, Administrative Assistant
Lisa Morgan, Director IL Services

6 pages Quarterly

5068   Easy Things to Make Things Simple: Do It Yourself Modifications for Disabled Persons
Brookline Books
34 University Rd
Brookline, MA 02445-4533

800-666-2665
FAX: 617-734-3952
brbooks@yahoo.com
www.brooklinebooks.com

160 pages Paperback
ISBN 1-571290-24-9

5069   Enabling Romance: A Guide to Love, Sex & Relationships for the Disabled

Ken Kroll, Author
Erica Levy Klein, Author
An uncensored, illustrated guide to intimacy and sexual expression for persons with physical disabilities.

5070   Encyclopedia of Disability
Sage Publications
2455 Teller Rd
Thousand Oaks, CA 91320-2218

805-499-0721
info@sagepub.com
www.sagepub.com

Gary L Albrecht, Editor
Blaise Simqu, Chief Executive Officer
A five volume set that covers disabilities A-Z *$850.00*
2500 pages
ISBN 0-761925-65-1

5071   EveryBody's Different: Understanding and Changing Our Reactions to Disabilities
Brookes Publishing
P.O.Box 10624
Baltimore, MD 21285-0624

410-337-9580
800-638-3775
FAX: 410-337-8539
custserv@brookespublishing.com
readplaylearn.com

Paul H. Brooks, Chairman
Jeffrey D. Brookes, President
Melissa A. Behm, Executive Vice President
This book discusses the emotions, questions, fears, and stereotypes that people without disabilities sometimes experience when they interact with people who do have disabilities. The author teaches readers to become more at ease with the concept of disability and to communicate more effectively with each other. Features activities and exercises that encourage self-examination, helping people to create more enriching personal relationships and work toward a fully inclusive society.
Paperback
ISBN 1-55766-59-9

5072   Everybody's Guide to Homeopathic Medicines
Jeremy P Tarcher
375 Hudson St
New York, NY 10014-3658

212-366-2000
academic@penguin.com
www.us.penguingroup.com

John Makinson, Chairman and CEO
Coram Williams, CFO
Covers alternative treatments in homeopathic medicines.
375 pages
ISBN 0-874778-43-3

5073   Everyday Social Interaction: A Program for People with Disabilities
Brookes Publishing
P.O.Box 10624
Baltimore, MD 21285-0624

410-337-9580
800-638-3775
FAX: 410-337-8539
custserv@brookespublishing.com
readplaylearn.com

Paul H. Brooks, Chairman
Jeffrey D. Brookes, President
Melissa A. Behm, Executive Vice President
This source guides teachers and human services professionals in helping people with disabilities acquire social interaction skills and develop satisfying relationships. Included is a checklist and task analyses that shows how complex skills can be broken down into major components for easy performance monitoring accompanied by tips on social courtesies, rewards, praise, and criticism.
$41.95
342 pages Paperback
ISBN 1-55766-58-4

5074 Family Challenges: Parenting with a Disability
Aquarius Health Care Videos
P.O.Box 1159
Sherborn, MA 01770-7159
508-650-1616
888-440-2963
FAX: 508-650-4216
aqvideos@tiac.net
www.aquariusproductions.com

Lesile Kussmann, Owner
When a parent has a disability, everyone in the family is affected. For children, these experiences may profoundly influence their lives and views of the world. In this sensitive film, you will hear about different roles that all the family members take on at varying times. *$195.00*

5075 Force A Miracle
Writer's Showcase Press

244 pages
ISBN 0-595226-88-4

5076 Forum
Coalition for the Education of Disabled Children
165 W Center St
Marion, OH 43302-3742
740-382-7362
800-374-2806
FAX: 740-382-3428
oceed@gte.net
www.oceed.org

Tracie Wilson, Manager
Leeann Derugen, Manager
Forum is a newsletter reporting on legislative and other developments affecting persons with disabilities.
Quarterly

5077 Foundation Fundamentals for Nonprofit Organizations
Foundation Center
Department Ze
79 5th Ave
New York, NY 10003-3034
212-620-4230
800-424-9836
FAX: 212-807-3677
order@foundationcenter.org
www.fdncenter.org

Bradford K. Smith, President
Lisa Philip, Vice President for Strategic Philanthropy
Lawrence T. McGill, Vice President for Research
Lisa Brooks, Director of Knowledge Management Systems
This video is designed to give fundraisers a general overview of the foundation funding process and to introduce them to the many resources available through our libraries and cooperating collections. The video gives clear, step-by-step instructions on how to build a fundraising program. *$24.00*
Video

5078 Four-Ingredient Cookbook
Laurel Designs
Apt A
1805 Mar West St
Belvedere Tiburon, CA 94920-1962
FAX: 415-435-1451
laureld@ncal.verio.com

Janet Sawyer, Owner
Lynn Montoya, Owner
Simple, easy to follow recipes, each containing four ingredients. Particularly suited to persons with limited physical ability. Includes 400 recipes, appetizers to desserts. *$9.00*

5079 Frequently Asked Questions About Multiple Chemical Sensitivity
Independent Living Research Utilization ILRU
1333 Moursund
Houston, TX 77030
713-520-0232
FAX: 713-520-5785
ilru@ilru.org
ilru.org

Lex Frieden, Director, ILRU
Richard Petty, Consultant
Rose Shepard, Office Manager
This FAQ covers important information about multiple chemical sensitivity and environmental illness. The FAQ describes the conditions, recommends strategies for improving access, and lists resources for CILs and other organizations. As the fact sheet states, centers must set an example in assuring that all people can enter their offices.
10 pages

5080 Genetic Disorders Sourcebook
Omnigraphics
155 W. Congress
Suite 200
Detroit, MI 48226-3900
313-961-1340
800-234-1340
FAX: 800-875-1340
contact@omnigraphics.com
www.omnigraphics.com

Paul Rogers, Publicity Associate
Georgiann Fratoni, Customer Service Manager
Provides information on hereditary diseases and disorders. *$7800.00*
650 pages
ISBN 0-789892-41-1

5081 Genetic Nutritioneering
McGraw-Hill Company
2460 Kerper Blvd
Dubuque, IA 52001-2224
563-588-1451
800-338-3987
FAX: 614-755-5654
www.mhhe.com/hper/physed

Kurt Strand, VP
Describes how to modify the expression of genetic traits, potentially preventing heart disease, cancer, arthritis, and hormone-related problems. Features how to slow biological aging and reduce the risk of age-related diseases. *$16.95*
288 pages
ISBN 0-879839-21-X

5082 Going to School with Facilitated Communication
Syracuse University, School of Education
230 Huntington Hall
Syracuse, NY 13244-1
315-443-4752
FAX: 315-443-2258
jhrusso@syr.edu
www.soe.syr.edu

Shirley Adamczyk, Administrative Assistant
Rachael Gazdick, Executive Director
Isabelle M. Glod, Administrative Assistant
Angela Flanagan, Development Assistant
A video in which students with autism and/or severe disabilities illustrate the use of facilitated communication focusing on basic principles fostering facilitated communication.
Video

5083 Grief: What it is and What You Can Do
Centering Corporation
7230 Maple Street
Omaha, NE 68134

402-553-1200
866-218-0101
FAX: 402-533-0507
j1200@aol.com
www.centering.org

Joy Johnson, Founder
Dr. Marvin Johnson, Founder
Janet Roberts, Executive Director
Kelsey Novacek, Director of Marketing
General grief information for all grief issues. *$3.50*
32 pages Paperback

5084 Guidelines on Disability
US Department of Housing & Urban Development
451 7th St SW
Washington, DC 20410-1

202-708-1112
TTY:202-708-1455
portal.hud.gov/hudportal/HUD

Shaun Donovan, Secretary
Helen R. Kanovsky, Acting Deputy Secretary
Jennifer Ho, Senior Advisor to the Secretary
Mike Anderson, Chief Human Capital Officer
Contains information on housing and accessibility for persons
with disabilities.

5085 Handbook of Services for the Handicapped
Greenwood Publishing Group
130 Cremona Drive
Santa Barbara, CA 93117

805-968-1911
800-368-6868
FAX: 866-270-3856
CustomerService@abc-clio.com
www.abc-clio.com

Matt Laddin, Vice President of Marketing
Mike Saltzman, Director-Eastern Territories & National Accounts
James Lingle, International Sales & Marketing
A handy reference book offering information and services for dis-
abled individuals. $59.95-$65.00.
291 pages Hardcover
ISBN 0-313213-85-2

5086 Healing Herbs
Rodale Press
33 E Minor St
Emmaus, PA 18098-1

610-967-5171
FAX: 610-967-8963
www.rodale.com

Maria Rodale, Chairman/Chief Executive Officer
Scott D. Schulman, President
*Heather Rodale, Board Member/Vice President/ Leadership Devel-
opment*
Thomas A. Pogash, EVP/Chief Financial Officer
Covers everything from growing the herbs to home remedies.

**5087 Helen Keller National Center for Deaf- Blind Youths And
Adults**
141 Middle Neck Rd
Sands Point, NY 11050-1218

516-944-8900
FAX: 516-944-7302
hkncinfo@hknc.org
www.hknc.org

Joseph McNulty, Executive Director
HKNC is the only national vacational and rehabilitation program
providing services exclusively to youth and adults who are
deaf-blind.

5088 Hospice Alternative
Harper Collins Publishers/Basic Books
10 E 53rd St
New York, NY 10022-5244

212-207-7000
800-242-7737
FAX: 212-207-7203

Jane Friedman, CEO

An account of the hospice experience. An innovative and humane
way of caring for the terminally ill. *$8.95*
256 pages
ISBN 0-46503 -61-0

5089 How to File a Title III Complaint
US Department of Justice
950 Pennsylvania Ave NW
Washington, DC 20530-9

202-307-0663
800-574-0301
FAX: 202-307-1197
TTY: 800-514-0383
www.ada.gov

Rebecca B. Bond, Chief
Zita Johnson Betts, Deputy Chiefs
Sally Conway, Deputy Chiefs
James Bostrom, Deputy Chiefs
This publication details the procedure for filing a complaint un-
der Title III of the ADA.

5090 How to Live Longer with a Disability
Accent Books & Products
PO Box 700
Bloomington, IL 61702-700

309-378-2961
800-787-8444
FAX: 309-378-4420
acmtlvng@aol.com

Raymond C Cheever, Publisher
Betty Garee, Editor
Eleven chapters to help you enjoy every aspect of your life, and
live easier and happier. Includes sexuality and disability, getting
more from the medical community and benefit programs.
Co-authored by Robert Mauro, sociologist and Elle Becker,
counselor and psychologist, both disabled. *$11.50*
266 pages Paperback
ISBN 0-19570 -38-8

5091 Ideas for Kids on the Go
Accent Books & Products
PO Box 700
Bloomington, IL 61702-700

309-378-2961
800-787-8444
FAX: 309-378-4420
acmtlvng@aol.com

Raymond C Cheever, Publisher
Betty Garee, Editor
This guide shows kids with physical disabilities how to go for it!
Lists products and where to get them, and includes tips from oth-
ers for having fun and getting ahead. Ages 1-18. *$6.95*
69 pages Paperback
ISBN 0-91570 -17-5

5092 If I Only Knew What to Say or Do
AARP Fulfillment
601 E St NW
Washington, DC 20049-1

202-434-2277
800-424-3410
FAX: 202-434-3443
TTY: 877-434-7598
member@aarp.org
www.aarp.org

Carol Raphael, Chair
Ronald E. Daly, Sr., Board Vice Chair
Jeannine English, President
A. Barry Rand, Chief Executive Officer
Provides a concise discussion of how to help a friend in crisis.
Learn what to say and what not to say.

5093 If it Weren't for the Honor: I'd Rather Have Walked
Accent Books & Products
PO Box 700
Bloomington, IL 61702-700

309-378-2961
800-787-8444
FAX: 309-378-4420
acmtlvng@aol.com

Raymond C Cheever, Publisher
Betty Garee, Editor

Revealing, often humorous, highly interesting and important reading. This book offers an account told by the author who was on the scene and actually saw and participated in many events that paved the way for progress for all those with disabilities. *$14.50*
262 pages Paperback
ISBN 0-91570 -41-8

5094   Imagery in Healing Shamanism and Modern Medicine
Shambhala Publications
300 Massachusetts Avenue
Horticultural Hall
Boston, MA 02115   617-424-0030
                                    888-424-2329
                                FAX: 617-236-1563
                                editors@shambhala.com
                                www.shambhala.com

Richard Reoch, President
Patients use self imagery to fight sickness and pain throughout their lives. *$15.95*
272 pages
ISBN 1-570629-34-x

5095   Independence
Easter Seals
1219 Dunn Ave
Daytona Beach, FL 32114-2405   386-255-4568
                                    877-255-4568
                                FAX: 386-258-7677
                                info@eseals-vf.org
                                www.easterseals-volusiaflagler.org

Jeff Blass, Chairman
Austin Brownlee, Chair-Elect
Becky Rutland, Vice Chair
Lynn Sinnott, President/ CEO

4-6 pages Quarterly

5096   Independent Living Centers and Managed Care: Results of an ILRU Study on Involvement
Independent Living Research Utilization ILRU
1333 Moursund
TIRR Memorial Hermann Research Cent
Houston, TX 77030-7031   713-520-0232
                                FAX: 713-520-5785
                                ilru@ilru.org
                                www.ilru.org

Lex Frieden, Director, ILRU
Richard Petty, Program Director
Vinh Nguyen, Program Director
Roxy Funchess, Administrative Secretary
This month's Readings presents findings from an ILRU study of roles centers are taking vis-a-vis managed care. Initiated in spring 1998, we asked Drew Batavia to take the lead in conducting this study for us. We were interested in collecting data on frequency with which centers are contacted by consumers with managed care problems. This is a study that will need to be repeated periodically as our experiences with managed care evolves. Meanwhile, here are the initial findings.
10 pages

5097   Independent Living Challenges the Blues
Independent Living Research Utilization ILRU
1333 Moursund
TIRR Memorial Hermann Research Cent
Houston, TX 77030-7031   713-520-0232
                                FAX: 713-520-5785
                                ilru@ilru.org
                                www.ilru.org

Lex Frieden, Director, ILRU
Richard Petty, Program Director
Vinh Nguyen, Program Director
Roxy Funchess, Administrative Secretary
Patricia's article highlights the Georgia SILC's health care advocacy efforts: the Georgia legislature passed a bill enabling Georgia Bleu to convert to for-profit status without a distribution of assets to similar nonprofit corporations; the Georgia SILC joined other health care advocates in filing a class action law suit to chal-

lenge the legality of the conversion; the Georgia SILC continues advocacy efforts to involve people with disabilities in developing and monitoring health care policy.
10 pages

5098   Independent Living Office
Department of Housing & Urban Development (HUD)
451 7th St SW
Washington, DC 20410-1   202-863-2800
                                www.portal.hud.gov

Ted Tozer, President
Rafael Diaz, Chief Information Officer/Chief Information Officer
Mike Anderson, Chief Human Capital Officer
Shaun Donovan, Secretary
This office within HUD is charged with encouraging the construction of housing that is accessible to handicapped persons. The Office of Independent Living encourages modifications of apartments and other dwellings so that handicapped persons can enter without assistance.

5099   Independent Newsletter
Easter Seals Nebraska
12565 West Center Road
Suite 100
Omaha, NE 68144-8144   402-345-2200
                                    800-650-9880
                                FAX: 402-345-2500
                                kginder@ne.easterseals.com
                                www.easterseals.com/ne/

James C. Summerfelt, President/Chief Executive Officer
Angela Howell, Vice President
Lily Sughroue, Director of Camp
Terrific fun for campers and a much needed respite for families and care givers from the daily challenges of caring for special needs indviduals
4 pages Quarterly

5100   Information Services for People with Developmental Disabilities
Greenwood Publishing Group
130 Cremona Drive
Santa Barbara, CA 93117   805-968-1911
                                    800-368-6868
                                FAX: 866-270-3856
                                CustomerService@abc-clio.com
                                www.abc-clio.com

Matt Laddin, Vice President of Marketing
Mike Saltzman, Director - Eastern Territories
James Lingle, International Sales & Marketing
Overviews the information needs of people with developmental disabilities and tells librarians how to meet them. $65.oo-$75.00.
368 pages Hardcover
ISBN 0-313287-80-5

5101   Innovative Programs: An Example of How CILs Can Put Their Work in Context
Culture
1333 Moursund
TIRR Memorial Hermann Research Cent
Houston, TX 77030-7031   713-520-0232
                                FAX: 713-520-5785
                                ilru@ilru.org
                                www.ilru.org

Lex Frieden, Director, ILRU
Richard Petty, Program Director
Vinh Nguyen, Program Director
Roxy Funchess, Administrative Secretary
Another winner in the innovative CIL competition- Steve Brown describes the Talking Books Program of Southeast Alaska Independent Living, discussing their efforts to record the oral history and life experiences of people with disabilities in the larger context of disability culture.
10 pages

5102 Insurance Solutions: Plan Well, Live Better
Demos Medical Publishing
11 West 42nd Street
15th Floor
New York, NY 10036   212-683-0072
                                   800-532-8663
                              FAX: 212-683-0118
                       support@demosmedical.com
                            www.demosmedpub.com

Paul Choi, Vice-President of Finance and Operations
Matt Conmy, Sr. Director of Sales
Thomas Hastings, Marketing Manager
Beth Kaufman Barry, Publisher
Learn how to look at various insurance options from a new perspective — including life, disability, health, and long-term care. Concrete information for dealing with potential problems in your coverage, to secure your financial future. *$24.95*
192 pages 2002
ISBN 1-888799-55-2

5103 International Directory of Libraries for the Disabled
KG Saur/Division of RR Bowker
121 Chanlon Rd
New Providence, NJ 7974-1541   908-286-1090
                                   800-521-8110

Michael Cairns, CEO
An essential resource for improving the quality and quantity of materials available to the print-handicapped audience. Featuring talking books, braille books, large print books as well as production centers for these materials. *$46.00*
257 pages
ISBN 3-59821 -81-1

5104 Issues in Independent Living
Independent Living Research Utilization
1333 Moursund
TIRR Memorial Hermann Research Cent
Houston, TX 77030-7031   713-520-0232
                              FAX: 713-520-5785
                                   ilru@ilru.org
                                   www.ilru.org

Laurie Redd, Executive Director
Lex Frieden, Manager
Vinh Nguyen, Program Director
Roxy Funchess, Administrative Secretary
This booklet is a report of the National Study Group on the Implications of Health Care Reform for Americans with Disabilities and Chronic Health Conditions.
30 pages

5105 JAMA: The Journal of the American Medical Association
American Medical Association
PO Box 10946
Chicago, IL 60654-4820   312-670-7827
                                   800-262-2350
                              FAX: 312-464-5909
                    subscriptions@jamanetwork.com
                        www.jama.jamanetwork.com
Howard Bauchner, MD, Editor-in-Chief
Articles cover all aspects of medical research and clinical medicine. *$66.00*

5106 JCIL Advocate Times
Jackson Center for Independent Living
409 Linden Ave
Jackson, MI 49203-4065   517-782-6054
                              FAX: 517-782-3118
Lesia Pikaart, Executive Director
JoAnn Lucas, Associate Director

Quarterly

5107 Jason & Nordic Publishers, Inc.
PO Box 441
Hollidaysburg, PA 16648-441   814-696-2929
                              FAX: 814-696-4250
                      turtlbks@jasonandnordic.com
                          www.jasonandnordic.com

Norma Mc Phee, Owner/CEO
Norma Phee
Turtle Books for children with disabilities present heroes who look like them, have problems like theirs, have similar doubts and feelings in non-threatening, fun stories. They are motivational, bridge the gap and promote understanding among peers and siblings. 22 children's books (grades preK-3) plus Sensitivity and Awareness Guide containing lesson plans, activities, background information keyed to the series. Disabilities include: Down syndrome, cerebral palsy, blindness, deafness and more.

5108 Journal of Social Work in Disabilty & Rehabilitation
Haworth Press
10 Alice St
Binghamton, NY 13904-1503   607-722-5857
                                   800-429-6784
                              FAX: 607-722-6362
                        orders@haworthpress.com
                           www.haworthpress.com

William Cohen, Owner
John T Oardeck PhD, Editor
S Harrington-Miller, Advertising
Presents and explores issues related to disabilities and social policy, practice, research, and theory. Reflecting the broad scope of social work in disabilty practice, this interdisciplinary journal examines vital issues aspects of the field — from innovative practice methods, legal issues, and literature reviews to program descriptions and cuttinf-edge practice research.
Quarterly

5109 Just Like Everyone Else
World Institute on Disability
3075 Adeline Street
Suite 155
Oakland, CA 94703-1520   510-225-6400
                              FAX: 510-225-0477
                              TTY:510-225-0478
                                   wid@wid.org
                                   www.wid.org

Paul W. Schroeder, Chair
Linda M. Dardarian, Vice Chair
Mary Brooner, Treasurer
Cassandra Malry, Secretary
The oversize-format publication, intended for general audiences, provides perspective, inspiration and information about the Independent Living Movement and the Americans with Disabilities Act. *$5.00*
16 pages

5110 Keep the Promise: Managed Care and People with Disabilities
American Network of Community Options & Resource
1101 King St
Ste 380
Alexandria, VA 22314-2962   703-535-7850
                              FAX: 703-535-7860
                                   ancor@ancor.org
                                   www.ancor.org

Dave Toeniskoetter, President
Chris Sparks, Vice President
Julie Manworren, Secretary/Treasurer
Renee L. Pietrangelo, PhD, Chief Executive Officer
This publication presents a detailed review of the process and the lessons learned. Details a way for all stake holders to work together for a state or local system.
119 pages $18 - $22

5111 **Keeping Our Families Together**
Through the Looking Glass
3075 Adeline St.
Ste. 120
Berkeley, CA 94703-2212 510-848-1112
800-644-2666
FAX: 510-848-4445
TTY: 510-848-1005
tlg@lookingglass.org
www.lookingglass.org

Maureen Block, J.D., Board President
Thomas Spalding, Board Treasurer
Alice Nemon, D.S.W.,, Board Secretary
Report of the National Task Force on parents with disabilities and
their families. Available in braille, large print or cassette. *$2.00*
12 pages

5112 **Learn About the ADA in Your Local Library**
US Department of Justice
950 Pennsylvania Ave NW
Washington, DC 20530-9 202-307-0663
800-574-0301
FAX: 202-307-1197
TTY: 800-514-0383
www.ada.gov

Rebecca B. Bond, Chief
Zita Johnson Betts, Deputy Chiefs
Sally Conway, Deputy Chiefs
A 10-page annotated list of 95 ADA publications and one video-
tape that are available in 15,000 public libraries throughout the
country.

5113 **LifeLines**
Disabled & Alone/Life Services for the Handicapped
1440 Broadway
23rd Floor
New York, NY 10018-2326 212-532-6740
800-995-0066
FAX: 212-532-3588
info@disabledandalone.org
www.disabledandalone.org

Leslie D. Park, Chairman
Rex L. Davidson, Vice President
William G. Shannon, J.D., Treasurer
Lee Alan Ackerman, B.A., Executive Director
Newsletter providing current and valuable information about
lifetime care and planning for persons with disabilities and their
families and the organizations serving them. Free upon request.
4-10 pages BiAnnual

5114 **Lifelong Leisure Skills and Lifestyles for Persons with
Developmental Disabilities**
Brookes Publishing
PO Box 10624
Baltimore, MD 21285-0624 410-337-9580
800-638-3775
FAX: 410-337-8539
custserv@brookespublishing.com
www.readplaylearn.com

Paul H. Brooks, Chairman
Jeffrey D. Brookes, President
Melissa A. Behm, Executive Vice President
This instructional manual offers ideas and detailed examples that
describe how to guide individuals of all ages through popular activities using adaptations that foster skill acquisition and inclusion. Some of the concepts explored are home-school-community
collaboration, choice making and the dignity of risk, and leisure
skill acquisition for the life span. *$35.00*
352 pages Paperback
ISBN 1-55766 -47-2

5115 **Livin'**
Lehigh Valley Center for Independent Living
435 Allentown Dr
Allentown, PA 18109-9121 610-770-9781
FAX: 610-770-9801
info@lvcil.org
www.lvcil.org

Amy Beck, Executive Director
Cara Steidel, Director of Finance
Greg Bott, Director of Development
Jessica DeMaio, Administrative Services Coordinator

4 pages Quarterly

5116 **Living in a State of Stuck**
Brookline Books
8 Trumbull Rd
Suite B-001
Northampton, MA 01060 413-584-0184
800-666-2665
FAX: 413-584-6184
brbooks@yahoo.com
www.brooklinebooks.com

3rd ed., paper
ISBN 1-571290-27-3

5117 **Living in the Community**
Independent Living Research Utilization ILRU
1333 Moursund
TIRR Memorial Hermann Research Cent
Houston, TX 77030-7031 713-520-0232
FAX: 713-520-5785
ilru@ilru.org
www.ilru.org

Lex Frieden, Director, ILRU
Richard Petty, Program Director
Vinh Nguyen, Program Director
Roxy Funchess, Administrative Secretary
James, Lori, and Jamey describe the elements of their successful
program to move people out of nursing homes and into the community: providing funding for deposits, first month's rent and
other neccessities, including assistive technology; providing
training and the other core services before and after consumers
leave the nursing home; developing relationships with housing
and other service providers.
10 pages

5118 **Loud, Proud and Passionate**
Mobility International USA
132 E. Broadway, Suite 343
PO Box 10767
Eugene, OR 97401 541-343-1284
FAX: 541-343-6812
info@miusa.org
www.miusa.org

Susan Sygall, CEO
Cerise Roth-Vinson, COO
Cindy Lewis, Director of Programs
Stephanie Gray, Program Managers
A resource book for international development and women's or-
ganization about including women with disabilities in projects in
the community. Informs women sith disabilities about the efforts
and successes of their peers worldwide. *$30.00*

5119 **Love: Where to Find It, How to Keep It**
Accent Books & Products
PO Box 700
Bloomington, IL 61702-700 309-378-2961
800-787-8444
FAX: 309-378-4420
acmtlvng@aol.com

Raymond C Cheever, Publisher
Betty Garee, Editor

Offers ideas such as how to meet other single people, avoid the wrong type; communications skills and much more for the disabled person wanting to date. *$6.95*
104 pages Paperback
ISBN 0-91570-31-0

5120 MOOSE: A Very Special Person
Brookline Books
8 Trumbull Rd
Suite B-001
Northampton, MA 01060

413-584-0184
800-666-2665
FAX: 413-584-6184
brbooks@yahoo.com
www.brooklinebooks.com

Paperback
ISBN 0-91479-73-5

5121 Mainstream Magazine
2973 Beech St
San Diego, CA 92102-1529

619-232-2727
FAX: 619-234-3155
editor@mainstream.mag.com
www.mainstream-mag.com

Cyndi Jones, Executive Director
The authoritative, national voice of people with disabilities, publishes in-depth reports on employment, education, new products and technology, legislation and disability rights advocacy, recreation and travel, disability arts and culture, plus personality profiles and challenging commentary. *$24.00*
Monthly

5122 Making Changes: Family Voices on Living Disabilities
Brookline Books
8 Trumbull Rd
Suite B-001
Northampton, MA 01060

413-584-0184
800-666-2665
FAX: 413-584-6184
brbooks@yahoo.com
www.brooklinebooks.com

216 pages Paperback
ISBN 0-91479-93-

5123 Making Informed Medical Decisions: Where to Look and How to Use What You Find
Patient-Centered Guides
1005 Gravenstein Highway North
Sebastopol, CA 95472-3836

707-827-7019
800-889-8969
FAX: 707-824-8268
orders@oreilly.com
www.patientcenters.com

Tim O'Reilly, CEO
Making Informed Medical Decisions acts like a friendly reference librarian, explaining: tips for researching for someone else; medical journal articles; statistics and risk; standard treatment options; clinical trial; making an ally of your doctor; and determining your own best course. Authors Oster, Thomas, and Joseff-a patient advocate, medical librarian, and medical doctor-also share examples and stories. *$17.95*
280 pages Paperback
ISBN 1-565924-59-2

5124 Making Wise Decisions for Long-Term Care
AARP Fulfillment
601 E St NW
Washington, DC 20049-1

202-434-2277
800-424-3410
FAX: 202-434-3443
TTY: 877-434-7598
member@aarp.org
www.aarp.org

Carol Raphael, Chair
Ronald E. Daly, Sr., Board Vice Chair
Jeannine English, President
A. Barry Rand, Chief Executive Officer

Here's a comprehensive consumer education effort in the area of long-term care.
28 pages

5125 Making a Difference
Georgia Council On Developmental Disabilities
2 Peachtree St N.W.
Suite 26-246
Atlanta, GA 30303-3141

404-657-2126
888-275-4233
FAX: 404-657-2132
TTY: 404-657-2133
eejacobson@dhr.state.ga.us
www.gcdd.org

Eric E Jacobson, Executive Director
Pat Nobbie, Deputy Director
Dottie Adams, Family/Individual Support Dir.
Valerie Meadows Suber, Public Information Director
The Georgia Council on Developmental Disabilities collaborates with Georgia's citizens, public and private advocacy organizations and policymakers to positively influence public policies that enhance the quality of life for people with disabilities and their families. GCDD provides this through education and advocacy activities, program implementation, funding and public policy analysis and research.

5126 Making a Difference: A Wise Approach
Easter Seals
233 South Wacker Drive
Suite 2400
Chicago, IL 60606-4703

312-726-0653
800-221-6827
FAX: 312-726-1494
www.easterseals.com

Richard W. Davidson, Chairman
Sandra L. Bouwman, 1st Vice Chairman
Joseph G. Kern, 2nd Vice Chairman
Ralph F. Boyd, Jr., Treasurer
The town of Wise, Virginia, and its leading citizen, Virgil Craft, personify what Making a Difference is all about when a community supports implementing the provisions of the Americans with Disabilities Act. Craft, a person with a disability, has spent his life giving back to the community. The community, in turn, has supported Craft's efforts to improve the environment, education, healthcare and access for disabled persons. A must buy for companies of all sizes, clubs and organizations. *$50.00*

5127 Managing Your Activities
Arthritis Foundation
PO Box 78423
Atlanta, GA 30357-0669

404-237-8771
800-933-7023
FAX: 404-872-0457
help@arthritis.org
www.arthritis.org

John H Klippel, CEO/ President

5128 Managing Your Health Care
Arthritis Foundation
PO Box 78423
Atlanta, GA 30357-0669

404-237-8771
800-933-7023
FAX: 404-872-0457
help@arthritis.org
www.arthritis.org

John H Klippel, CEO/ President

5129 Medical Aspects of Disability: A Handbook For The Rehabilitation Professional
Springer Publishing Company
11 West 42nd Street
15th Floor
New York, NY 10036 212-431-4370
877-687-7476
FAX: 212-941-7842
cs@springerpub.com
www.springerpub.com

Ursula Springer, President
Theodore C. Nardin, CEO/Publisher
Jason Roth, VP/Marketing Director
James C. Costello, Vice President, Journal Publishing
$62.92
744 pages
ISBN 0-826179-71-1

5130 Meeting the Needs of Employees with Disabilities
Resources for Rehabilitation
22 Bonad Road
Ste 19a
Winchester, MA 01890-4330 781-368-9080
FAX: 781-368-9096
orders@rfr.org
www.rfr.org

Susan Greenblatt, Editor
Provides information to help people with disabilities retain or obtain employment. Information on government programs and laws, supported employment, training programs, environmental adaptations and the transition from school to work are included. Chapters on mobility impairment, vision impairment and hearing and speech impairments. *$ 47.95*
167 pages Biennial
ISBN 0-92971 -13-5

5131 NCD Bulletin
National Council on Disability
1331 F Street Northwest
Suite 850
Washington, DC 20004- 1138 202-272-2004
FAX: 202-272-2022
ncd@ncd.gov
www.ncd.gov

Jeff Rosen, Chairperson
Kamilah Oni Martin-Proctor, Co-Vice Chair
Lynnae Ruttledge, Co-Vice Chair
Rebecca Cokley, Executive Director
Reports on the latest issues and news affecting people with disabilities.
2 pages Monthly

5132 NCDE Survival Strategies for Oversease Living for People with Disabilities
National Clearinghouse on Disability and Exchange
132 E. Broadway, Suite 343
PO Box 10767
Eugene, OR 97401 541-343-1284
FAX: 541-343-6812
info@miusa.org
www.miusa.org

Susan Sygall, CEO
Cerise Roth-Vinson, COO
Cindy Lewis, Director of Programs
Stephanie Gray, Program Managers
This book will provide individuals with disablilities information, resources and guidance on pursuing international exchange opportunities. It addresses disability-related aspects of the international exchange process such as choosing a program, applying, preparing for the trip, adjusting to a new country and returning home.

5133 NOD E-Newsletter
National Organization on Disability
77 Water Street
Suite 204
New York, NY 10005 646-505-1191
FAX: 646-505-1184
zchizar@a-g.com
www.nod.org

George H W Bush, President
Thomas J. Ridge, Chairman
Charles F. Dey, Vice Chairman
Carol Glazer, President
Monthly E-Newsletter from the National Organization on Disability. Free.
3 pages Monthly

5134 National Hookup
ISC
16 Liberty St
Larkspur, CA 94939-1520 415-924-3549
FAX: 415-927-9556
russbo@microweb.com

Russ Bohlke, Manager
Newsletter published by ISC, a national organization of people with physical disabilities. *$6.00*
12-16 pages Quarterly

5135 New Horizons in Sexuality
Accent Books & Products
PO Box 700
Bloomington, IL 61702-700 309-378-2961
800-787-8444
FAX: 309-378-4420
acmtlvng@aol.com

Raymond C Cheever, Publisher
Betty Garee, Editor
This manual helps both males and females progress toward a satisfying post-injury relationship. *$7.95*
50 pages Paperback
ISBN 0-91570 -42-6

5136 New Voices: Self Advocacy By People with Disabilities
Brookline Books
8 Trumbull Rd
Suite B-001
Northampton, MA 01060 413-584-0184
800-666-2665
FAX: 413-584-6184
brbooks@yahoo.com
www.brooklinebooks.com

274 pages Paperback
ISBN 1-57129 -04-4

5137 North Star Community Services
3420 University Ave
Waterloo, IA 50701-2050 319-236-0901
888-879-1365
FAX: 319-236-3701
jmuller@northstarcs.org
www.northstarcs.org

Mark Witmer, Executive Director
Matt Hinders, Director of Operations & Safety
Bridget Hartmann, Director of Human Resources
Terri Davis, Director of Financial Services
North Star Community Services is a rehabilitative services organization with home office in Waterloo, IA and several branch offices in Northeast, Northern and Central Iowa. North Star helps indiviuals with disabilities live and work in their communities. Services include: adult day services, supported community living services, employment services, and case management/service coordination.

5138 **Nothing is Impossible: Reflections on a New Life**
Ballantine Books
1745 Broadway
10th Floor
New York, NY 10019
212-782-9000
rhkidspublicity@randomhouse.com
www.atrandom.com
Edward Warren, Owner
Reeve offers a uniquely powerful message of hope on topics ranging from the controversial stem cell debate to the mind-body connection he credits with his recent physical improvements. *$6.99*
224 pages
ISBN 0-345470-73-7

5139 **Nutritional Desk Reference**
Keats Publishing
P.O.Box 876
New Canaan, CT 06840
203-966-8721
800-323-4900

5140 **Nutritional Influences on Illness:**
Third Line Press
4751 Viviana Dr
Tarzana, CA 91356-5038
818-996-0076
third-line.com
Melvyn R Werbach, Owner
A comprehensive summary of the world's knowledge concerning the relationship between dietary and nutrtional factors and illness. This book does not try to promote any particular school of thought. Instead of the author telling readers his opinion as to what research says, he makes it easy for them to see data for themselves and then form their own opinions.
504 pages
ISBN 0-879835-31-1

5141 **Oregon Perspectives**
Oregon Council on Developmental Disabilities
540 24th Pl NE
Salem, OR 97301-4517
503-945-9941
800-292-4154
FAX: 503-945-9947
ocdd@ocdd.org
www.ocdd.org
Laura Bronson, Office Manager
Beth Kessler, Planning & Communications Coordi
A quarterly publication from the Oregon Council on Developmental Disabilities.

5142 **Organ Transplants: Making the Most of Your Gift of Life**
Patient-Centered Guides
1005 Gravenstein Highway North
Sebastopol, CA 95472-3836
707-827-7000
800-998-9938
FAX: 707-824-8268
orders@oreilly.com
www.patientcenters.com
Linda Lamb, Series Editor
Shawnde Paull, Marketing
Tim O'Reilly, CEO
Over 64,000 people in the US are awaiting an organ transplant. Although transplant surgeries are now fairly routine and can give their recipients the gift of new life, the road to getting a transplant can be long and harrowing. Living with immunosuppressive drugs and strong emotional responses can also be more challenging than families imagine. Medical journalist Robert Finn answers the concerns of these families, with the latest facts about transplantation - as well as the stories behind them. *$19.95*
326 pages Paperback
ISBN 1-565926-34-X

5143 **PEAK Parent Center**
611 N Weber St
Suite 200
Colorado Springs, CO 80903-1072
719-531-9400
800-284-0251
FAX: 719-531-9452
info@peakparent.org
www.peakparent.org
Barbara Buswell, Executive Director
PEAK Parent Center is a federally-designated Parent Training and Information Center (PTI). As a PTI, PEAK supports and empowers parents, providing them with information and strategies to use when advocating for their children with disabilities. PEAK works one-on-one with families and educators helping them realize new possibilities for children with disabilities by expanding knowledge of special education and offering new strategies for success.

5144 **Parallels in Time**
MN Governor's Council on Development Disabilities
658 Cedar St
Saint Paul, MN 55155-1603
651-296-4018
877-348-0505
FAX: 651-297-7200
admin.dd@state.mn.us
www.mncdd.org
Colleen Wieck PhD, Executive Director
Parallels in Time traces present attitudes and the treatment of people with disabilities, and supplements the first weekend seesion of Partners in Policymaking. This CD-ROM includes the History of the Parent Movement and the History of the Independent Living Movement, as well as personal stories of self advocates, leaders in the self advocacy movement.

5145 **Part of the Team**
Easter Seals
Ste 1800
230 W Monroe St
Chicago, IL 60606-4851
312-726-6800
FAX: 312-726-1494
Janet D Jamieson, Communications Manager
James Williams Jr, Chief Executive Officer
Designed for employers of all sizes, rehabilitation organizations and all others concerned with the employment of people with disabilities. It addresses managers' concerns and questions about supervising persons with disabilities and can be used as a discussion/team-building tool for employees with and without disabilities. The video recognizes people with disabilities as strong contenders for almost any job. *$15.00*

5146 **Partnering with Public Health: Funding& Advocacy Opportunities for CILs and SILCs**
Independent Living Research Utilization ILRU
1333 Moursund
Houston, TX 77030-7031
713-520-0232
FAX: 713-520-5785
ilru@ilru.org
ilru.org
Lex Frieden, Director, ILRU
Richard Petty, Program Director
Roxy Funchess, Administrative Secretary
George Powers, Legal Specialist
Laura Rauscher discusses how CILs and SCILs can use funding from the Centers for Disease Control and partnerships with public health agencies to provide innovative programs promoting the health of people with disabilities.
10 pages

5147 Peer Counseling: Roles, Functions, Boundaries
Independent Living Research Utilization ILRU
1333 Moursund
Houston, TX 77030-7031 713-520-0232
FAX: 713-520-5785
ilru@ilru.org
ilru.org

Lex Frieden, Director, ILRU
Richard Petty, Program Director
Roxy Funchess, Administrative Secretary
George Powers, Legal Specialist
In this article, the following points were discussed: describing peer support as counseling suggests safeguards and expectations which cannot be provided by nonprofessionals; the purpose of peer counseling is to promote the independent living philosophy and encourage consumers to embrace it; peer counseling cannot and is not intended to help individuals deal with intense emotional stress, whether it is related to their disability or to something else.
10 pages

5148 Peer Mentor Volunteers: Empowering People for Change
Independent Living Research Utilization ILRU
1333 Moursund
Houston, TX 77030-7031 713-520-0232
FAX: 713-520-5785
ilru@ilru.org
ilru.org

Lex Frieden, Director, ILRU
Richard Petty, Program Director
Roxy Funchess, Administrative Secretary
George Powers, Legal Specialist
Arizona Bridge to Independent Living (ABIL) in Phoenix, featured in this issue, is another winner in the innovative CIL program competition.
10 pages

5149 People and Families
New Jersey Council on Developmental Disabilities
20 West State Street, 6th Floor
P.O.Box 700
Trenton, NJ 08625-0700 609-292-3745
800-792-8858
FAX: 609-292-7114
TTY: 609-777-3238
njcdd@njcdd.org
www.njcdd.org

Elaine Buchsbaum, Chairman
Christopher Miller, Vice Chair
Alison M. Lozano, Ph.D, Executive Director
Shirla Rufo Simpson, M.A., DRCC, Deputy Director
A free magazine for people with disabilities, their families and the public about disability topics such as personal assistance, deinstitutionalization, health care and community living. Published by the New Jersey council on Developmental Disabilities, a federally funded advocacy and policy advisory body. The council has 25 members - 15 consumer/product volunteers and 10 professionals.
48 pages Quarterly

5150 People with Disabilities & Abuse: Implications for Center for Independent Living
Independent Living Research Utilization ILRU
1333 Moursund
P.O.Box 700
Houston, TX 77030-7031 713-520-0232
FAX: 713-520-5785
ilru@ilru.org
ilru.org

Lex Frieden, Director, ILRU
Richard Petty, Program Director
Roxy Funchess, Administrative Secretary
George Powers, Legal Specialist

10 pages

5151 People with Disabilities Who Challenge the System
Brookes Publishing
P.O.Box 10624
Baltimore, MD 21285-0624 410-337-9580
800-638-3775
FAX: 410-337-8539
custserv@brookespublishing.com
readplaylearn.com

Paul H. Brooks, Chairman
Jeffrey D. Brookes, President
Melissa A. Behm, Executive Vice President
Jeffrey D. Brookes, President
Helpful forms, tables, and case studies plus an emphasis on self-determination point the way to the development of supports so that people who are deaf-blind, have severe to profound physical and cognitive disabilities, or have serious behavior problems can be fully included in the classroom, workplace, and community. *$34.00*
464 pages Paperback
ISBN 1-55766-29-0

5152 People's Voice
Independence CIL
300 3rd Ave SW
Suite F
Minot, ND 58701-4346 701-839-4724
800-377-5114
FAX: 701-838-1677
independencecil@independencecil.org
independencecil.org

Susan Ogurek, Chair
Heather Wittliff, Vice Chair
Scott Burlingame, Executive Director
Emily Rodacker, Secretary/Treasurer

8 pages Quarterly

5153 Personal Perspectives on Personal Assistance Services
World Institute on Disability
3075 Adeline Street
Suite 155
Berkeley, CA 94703 510-225-6400
FAX: 510-225-0477
TTY:510-225-0478
wid@wid.org
www.wid.org

Anita Shafer Aaron, Executive Director
Thomas Foley, Deputy Director
Bruce Curtis, International Program Director
Marsha Saxton, Director of Research and Training.
This collection of personal essays explores a wide range of perspectives on Personal Assistance Services. Family issues and PAS concerns for people with various different disabilities, of different ages and as members of minority groups are addressed. *$5.00*
80 pages Paperback

5154 Perspectives
National Assoc of State Directors of DD Services
113 Oronoco St
Alexandria, VA 22314-2015 703-683-4202
FAX: 703-684-1395
dberland@nasddds.org
Nancy Thaler, Executive Director
Nancy Thaler, Executive Director
Provides a concise summary of national policy developments and initiatives affecting persons with devlopmental disabilities and the programs that serve them. From bills pending before Congress, to the growth in Medicaid-funded services, to changes in federal-state Medicaid policies and the shift of responsibility from Washington to the states, keeps readers in tune with the latest national issues shaping publically funded disability services. *$95.00*
Monthly

5155 Place to Live
Accent Books & Products
P.O.Box 700
Bloomington, IL 61702-700   309-378-2961
                                    800-787-8444
                              FAX: 309-378-4420
                              acmtlvng@aol.com

Raymond C Cheever, Publisher
Betty Garee, Editor
Raymond C Cheever, Publisher
Many disabled people have found that group housing or accessible apartments are the best alternative to living in a nursing home. These articles tell about some of the alternatives people have found so they can live independently. Just one idea might be the answer for better living for you. $4.95
64 pages Paperback
ISBN 0-91570 -30-2

5156 Proceedings
AHEAD
107 Commerce Center Drive
Suite 204
Huntersville, NC 28078   704-947-7779
                          FAX: 704-948-7779
                          information@ahead.org
                          www.ahead.org

Stephan Haml Smith, Director
Bea Awoniyi, President
Michael Johnson, Treasurer
Terra Beethe, Secretary
National conferences, innovative programs, research, evaluation services, auxiliary aids, career information and other vital information.

5157 Psychological & Social Impact of Disability
Springer Publishing Company
11 West 42nd Street
15th Floor
New York, NY 10036   212-431-4370
                            877-687-7476
                      FAX: 212-941-7842
                      cs@springerpub.com
                      www.springerpub.com

James C. Costello, Vice President, Journal Publishing
Diana Osborne, Production Manager
Megan Larkin, Managing Editor, Journals
$49.95
488 pages
ISBN 0-826122-13-2

5158 Psychology and Health
Springer Publishing Company
11 West 42nd Street
15th Floor
New York, NY 10036   212-431-4370
                            877-687-7476
                      FAX: 212-941-7842
                      cs@springerpub.com
                      www.springerpub.com

James C. Costello, Vice President, Journal Publishing
Diana Osborne, Production Manager
Megan Larkin, Managing Editor, Journals
Content of this book spans a wide range of clinical conditions, including somatization disorders, chronic pain, migraine, anxiety and cancer. $29.95
256 pages

5159 Psychology of Disability
Springer Publishing Company
11 West 42nd Street,
15th Floor
New York, NY 10036-3915   212-431-4370
                                  877-687-7476
                            FAX: 212-941-7842
                            cs@springerpub.com
                            www.springerpub.com

James C. Costello, Vice President, Journal Publishing
Diana Osborne, Production Manager
Megan Larkin, Managing Editor, Journals
Theodore C Nardin, Chief Executive Officer
Reactions to the disabled. $27.95
288 pages
ISBN 0-82613 -40-1

5160 Quality of Life for Persons with Disabilities
Brookline Books
8 Trumbull Road
Suite B-001
Northampton, MA 01060   413-584-0184
                                800-666-2665
                          FAX: 413-584-6184
                          brbooks@yahoo.com
                          www.brooklinebooks.com

James C. Costello, Vice President, Journal Publishing
Quality of life generally refers to a person's subjective experience of his or her life and focuses attention on how the individual with a disabling condition experiences the world. This book presents a comprehensive and international view of this concept as applied to a broad range of settings in which persons with disabilities live, work and play. $35.00
Paperback
ISBN 0-91479 -92-1

5161 REACHing Out Newsletter
REACH of Dallas Resource on Independent Living
8625 King George Drive
Suite 210
Dallas, TX 75235-2286   214-630-4796
                          FAX: 214-630-6390
                          TTY:214-630-5995
                          reachdallas@reachcils.org
                          reachcils.org

Charlotte A. Stewart, Executive Director
Kiowanda Jasso, Information & Referral Specialist
Kevan Johnson, Employment Consultant
Janie Peachee, Administrative Assistant
Quarterly newsletter from REACH of Dallas Resource Center on Independent Living.
16 pages Quarterly

5162 RTC Connection
Research and Training Center
University of Wisconsin Stou
Menomonie, WI 54751   715-232-2236
                          FAX: 715-232-2251
                          menz@uwstout.edu
                          www.rtc.uwstout.edu

Julie Larson, Program Assistant
Bi-annual reports on disability and rehabilitation research and policy topics.
Newsletter

5163 Rehabilitation Gazette
Gazette International Networking Institute
4207 Lindell Blvd
Suite 110
Saint Louis, MO 63108-2930   314-534-0475
                          FAX: 314-534-5070
                          info@post-polio.org
                          www.post-polio.org

Joan L Headley, Executive Director
William G. Stothers, President/Chairperson
Saul J. Morse, Vice President
Marny K. Eulberg, Secretary

International journal of independent living for people with disabilities. *$12.00*
8 pages Bi-Annually

5164   Relaxation: A Comprehensive Manual for Adults and Children with Special Needs
Research Press
2612 N. Mattis Ave.
P.O.Box 7886
Champaign, IL 61822- 9177   217-352-3273
                                             800-519-2707
                                        FAX: 217-352-1221
                                   orders@researchpress.com
                                    www.researchpress.com

Paperback
ISBN 0-878221-86-8

5165   Resources for People with Disabilities and Chronic Conditions
Resources for Rehabilitation
Ste 19a
33 Bedford St
Lexington, MA 02420-4330   781-890-6371
                                        FAX: 781-861-7517
Susan Greenblatt
A comprehensive resource directory that helps people with disabilities and chronic conditions achieve their maximum level of independence. Chapters on spinal cord injuries, low back pain, diabetes, hearing and speech impairments, epilepsy, multiple sclerosis. Describes organizations, products and publications. *$49.95*
215 pages Biennial
ISBN 0-92971 -12-7

5166   Role Portrayal and Stereotyping on Television
Greenwood Publishing Group
130 Cremona Drive
P O Box 1911
Santa Barbara,, CA 93117-4208   203-226-3571
                                           800-368-6868
                                           805-968-1911
                                      FAX: 866-270-3856
                              customerservice@abc-clio.com
                                        www.abc-clio.com

214 pages $55 - $59.95
ISBN 0-313248-55-9

5167   Screening in Chronic Disease
Oxford University Press
2001 Evans Rd
Cary, NC 27513-2009   800-445-9714
                                            877-773-4325
                                       FAX: 919-677-1303
                                    custserv.us@oup.com
                                         global.oup.com

Thomas Carty, Senior Vice President
Early detection, or screening, is a common strategy for controlling chronic disease, but little information has been available to help determine which screening procedures are worthwhile, until this textbook. *$42.50*
256 pages

5168   Sexual Adjustment
Accent Books & Products
P.O.Box 700
Bloomington, IL 61702-700   309-378-2961
                                            800-787-8444
                                       FAX: 309-378-4420
                                       acmtlvng@aol.com

Raymond C Cheever, Publisher
Betty Garee, Editor
Essential information concerning sexual adjustment for the paraplegic male. *$4.95*
73 pages Paperback
ISBN 0-19570 -00-0

5169   Sexuality and Disabilities: A Guide for Human Service Practitioners
Haworth Press
2&4 Park Square
Abingdon, FL 33487-1503   561-994-0555
                                       FAX: 561-241-7856
                              orders@taylorandfrancis.com
                                 taylorandfrancisgroup.com

159 pages Hardcover
ISBN 1-560243-75-9

5170   Sickened: The Memoir of a Muchausen by Proxy Childhood
Bantam Books
1745 Broadway
10th Floor
New York, NY 10019-4039   212-782-9000
                                       FAX: 212-572-6066
                              crownpublicity@randomhouse.com
                                   www.randomhouse.com

256 pages Hardcover
ISBN 0-553803-07-7

5171   Socialization Games for Persons with Disabilities
Charles C. Thomas
2600 S First St
Springfield, IL 62704-4730   217-789-8980
                                            800-258-8980
                                       FAX: 217-789-9130
                                     books@ccthomas.com
                                       www.ccthomas.com

Michael P. Thomas, President
This text will assist those who want to teach severely multiple disabled students by providing information on: general principles of intervention and classroom organization; managing the behavior of students; physically managing students and using adaptive equipment; teaching eating skills; teaching toileting, dressing, and hygiene skills; teaching cognition, communication, and socialization skills; teaching independent living skills; and teaching infants and preschool students. *$38.95*
176 pages Paperback
ISBN 0-398067-46-5

5172   Sometimes You Just Want to Feel Like a Human Being
Brookes Publishing
P.O.Box 10624
Baltimore, MD 21285-0624   410-337-9580
                                            800-638-3775
                                       FAX: 410-337-8539
                              custserv@brookespublishing.com
                                       readplaylearn.com

Paul Brooks, Owner
Case studies of empowering psychotherapy with people with disabilities. This text reveals how counseling can be beneficial to individuals with disabilities of all kinds, including autism, mental retardation, sensory impairment, cerebral palsy, or HIV infection. *$ 26.95*
272 pages Paperback
ISBN 1-55766 -96-0

5173   South Carolina Assistive Technology Program
8301 Farrow Road
University Center for Excellence
Columbia, SC 29203-2920   803-935-5263
                                            800-915-4522
                                       FAX: 803-935-5342
                              carol.page@uscmed.sc.edu
                                       www.sc.edu/scatp/

Carol Page, Ph.D, Program Director
Mary r Alice Bechtle, Program Coordinator
Janet Jendron, Program Coordinator
Lydia Durham, Administrative Assistant
The South Carolina Assistive Technology Program (SCATP) is a federally funded program concerned with getting technology into the hands of people with disabilities so that they might live, work, learn and be a more independent part of the community. We provide an equipment loan and demonstration program, an on-line equipment exchange program, training, technical assistance,

publications, an interactive CDROM (SC Curriculum Access through AT), an information listserv and work with various state com
7-8 pages Bi-annually

5174 Space Coast CIL News
Space Coast Center for Independent Living
571 Haverty Court,
Suite W
Rockledge, FL 32955-2566

321-633-6011
FAX: 321-633-6472
TTY:321-784-9008
agrau@bellsouth.net
www.sccil.net

Michael Lavoie, President
Howard Fetes, Vice-President
Non-profit organization that provides services which enable people with disabilities to live as independently as possible.
12 pages Quarterly

5175 Special Needs Trust Handbook
Aspen Publishers
7th Fl
76 9th Ave
New York, NY 10011-4962

301-644-3599
800-638-8437
customerservice@aspenpublishers.com
www.aspenpublishers.com

Bob Lemmond, President and CEO
Gustavo Dobles, Vice President and Chief Content Officer
Susan Pikitch, Vice President and Chief Financial Officer
Alan Scott, Vice President & Chief Marketing Office
The Special Needs Trusts Handbook is the single-volume, comprehensive resource that provides information on how to handle the complex requirements of drafting and administering trusts for clients who are mentally or physically disabled, or who wish to provide for others with disabilities. *$245.00*
900 pages
ISBN 0-735572-88-7

5176 Special Siblings: Growing Up With Someone with A Disability
Brookes Publishing
P.O.Box 10624
Baltimore, MD 21285-0624

410-337-9580
800-638-3775
FAX: 410-337-8539
custserv@brookespublishing.com
readplaylearn.com

Paul Brooks, Owner
The author reveals what she experienced as the sister of a man with cerebral palsy and mental retardation — and shares what others have learned about being and having a special sibling. Weaving a lifetime of memories and reflections with relevant research and interviews with more than 100 other siblings and experts, McHugh explores a spectrum of feelings — from anger and guilt to love and pride — and helps readers understand the issues siblings may encounter. *$21.95*
256 pages Paperback
ISBN 1-557666-07-5

5177 TERI
251 Airport Rd
Oceanside, CA 92058-1321

760-721-1706
teriinc.org

Cheryl Kilmer, CEO & Founder
William E. Mara, Chief Operating Officer
Krysti DeZonia, Ed.D, Director of Education & Research
Joe Michalowski, Chief Financial Officer
A private, nonprofit corporation which has been developing and operating programs for individuals with developmental disabilities since 1980. Offers staff training videos, staff training tools and technique manuals.

5178 That All May Worship: An Interfaith Welcome to People with Disabilities
American Association of People with Disabilities
2013 H St NW
5th Fl
Washington, DC 20006-1207

202-521-4316
800-840-8844
communications@aapd.com
www.aapd.com/publications

5179 The Ultimate Guide to Sex and Disability
Read How You Want Large Print Books

800-797-9277
support@readhowyouwant.com
www.readhowyouwant.com

Miriam Kaufman, Author
For everyone, men and women of all ages and sexual identities, The Ultimate Guide to Sex and Disability covers the span of disabilities - from chronic fatigue and back pain to spinal cord injury, multiple sclerosis, cystic fibrosis, cerebral palsy, and many others.

5180 To Live with Grace and Dignity
World Institute on Disability
3075 Adeline Street
Suite 155
Berkeley, CA 94703-1520

510-225-6400
FAX: 510-225-0477
TTY:510-225-0478
wid@wid.org
www.wid.org

Anita Shafer Aaron, Executive Director
Thomas Foley, Deputy Director
Bruce Curtis, International Program Director
Marsha Saxton, Director of Research and Training.
This unique book combines photographs and essays to allow the reader to enter some of the real day to day relationships that develop between individuals with disabilities and their personal assistants. Looking at and listening to what these relationships are all about is what motivated and inspired this book, says author Lydia Gans. The individuals included in this book represent a wide range of ages, disabilities and cultural backgrounds. *$26.00*
72 pages Paperback

5181 Touch/Ability Connects People with Disabilities & Alternative Health Care Pract.
Independent Living Research Utilization ILRU
1333 Moursund
Houston, TX 77030-7031

713-520-0232
FAX: 713-520-5785
ilru@ilru.org
ilru.org

Lex Frieden, Director, ILRU
Richard Petty, Program Director
Roxy Funchess, Administrative Secretary
George Powers, Legal Specialist
The people at DIRECT center for Independence and Touch/Ability in Tuscon, Arizona, have collaborated to develop a wellness program that makes alternative health care choices available to people with disabilities. The Touch/Ability Wellness program was selected as one of last year's winners in the Innovative CILs competition because of this outcome of increased options open to people with disabilities.
10 pages

5182 US Role in International Disability Activities: A History
World Institute on Disability
3075 Adeline Street
Suite 155
Berkeley, CA 94703-1520   510-225-6400
                                      FAX: 510-225-0477
                                      TTY:510-225-0478
                                           wid@wid.org
                                           www.wid.org

Anita Shafer Aaron, Executive Director
Thomas Foley, Deputy Director
Bruce Curtis, International Program Director
Marsha Saxton, Director of Research and Training.
This study was undertaken to present an initial introduction to US involvement in the field of international rehabilitation and disability. *$12.00*
169 pages Paperback

5183 Understanding and Accommodating Physical Disabilities: Desk Reference
Greenwood Publishing Group
130 Cremona Drive
P O Box 1911
Santa Barbara,, CA 93117-4208   203-226-3571
                                           800-368-6868
                                           805-968-1911
                                      FAX: 866-270-3856
                              customerservice@abc-clio.com
                                           www.abc-clio.com

200 pages $52.95 - $55
ISBN 0-899308-14-7

5184 Vestibular Disorders Association
Vestibular Disorders Association
5018 NE 15th Ave
PO Box 13305
Portland, OR 97211-305   503-229-7705
                                           800-837-8428
                                      FAX: 503-229-8064
                                        info@vestibular.org
                                           www.vestibular.org

Cynthia Ryan MBA, Executive Director
Tony Staser, Development Director
Kerrie Denner, Outreach Coordinator
Karen Ilari, Administrative Support Coordinator
The mission of the Vestibular Disorders Association is to serve people with vestibular disorders by providing access to information, offering a support network, and elevating awareness of the challenges associated with these disorders. *$15.00*

ISBN 0-963261-15-0

5185 Visions & Values
Idaho Council on Developmental Disabilities
650 W. State St., Room 100
P. O. Box 83720
Boise, ID 83720-5840   208-332-1824
                                           800-544-2433
                                      FAX: 208-334-2307
                                           www.state.id.us/icdd

C. L. Butch Otter, Governor
A quarterly publication from the Idaho Council on Developmental Disabilities.

5186 Weiner's Herbal
Quantum Books
355 Middlesex Avenue
Wilmington, MA 01887-1406   978-988-2470
                                      FAX: 617-577-7282
                                        orders@quantumbk.com
                                           www.quantumbooks.com

William Szabo, Owner
A-Z index covering all aspects of herbs.
Paperback
ISBN 0-812825-86-1

5187 When the Brain Goes Wrong
Fanlight Productions
32 Court Street,
21st Floor
Brooklyn, NY 11201-1731   718-488-8900
                                           800-876-1710
                                      FAX: 718-488-8642
                                        info@fanlight.com
                                           www.fanlight.com

Ben Achtenberg, Owner
Nicole Johnson, Publicity Coordinator
Anthony Sweeney, Marketing Director
An extraordinary and provocative series of seven short films which profile individuals with a range of brian dysfunctions. The seven brief segments focus on schizophrenia, manic depression, epilepsy, head injury, headaches and addiction. In addition to the personal stories, the segments include interviews with physicians who speak briefly about what is known about the disorders and treatment. #131 *$245.00*

ISBN 1-572951-31-1

5188 Women with Physical Disabilities: Achieving & Maintaining Health & Well-Being
Spina Bifida Association of America
1600 Wilson Blvd.
Suite 800
Arlington, VA 22209-4226   202-944-3285
                                           800-621-3141
                                      FAX: 202-944-3295
                                        sbaa@sbaa.org
                              www.spinabifidaassociation.org

Ana Ximenes, Chair
Sara Struwe, President & CEO
Cindy Brownstein, CEO
George Sturm, Treasurer
Introduces the critical concept of womens health in the context of physical disabilities. *$42.00*

5189 Work in the Context of Disability Culture
Independent Living Research Utilization ILRU
1333 Moursund
Houston, TX 77030-7031   713-520-0232
                                      FAX: 713-520-5785
                                           ilru@ilru.org
                                           ilru.org

Lex Frieden, Director, ILRU
Richard Petty, Program Director
Roxy Funchess, Administrative Secretary
George Powers, Legal Specialist
Another winner in the innovative CIL competition-Steve Brown describes the Talking Books Program of Southeast Alaska Independent Living, discussing their efforts to record the oral history and life experiences of people with disabilities in the larger context of the disability culture.
10 pages

Parenting: General

5190 AEPS Family Report: Birth to Three Years
Brookes Publishing
P.O. Box 10624
Baltimore, MD 21285-0624   410-337-9580
                                           800-638-3775
                                      FAX: 410-337-8539
                              custserv@brookespublishing.com
                                           www.brookespublishing.com

Diane Bricker, Author
Betty Capt, Author
JoAnn Johnson, Author
Misti Waddell, Author
This Family Report was developed for use in conjunction with the AEPSr for children birth to 3 years to obtain information from parents and other caregivers about their children's skills and abil-

ities across major areas of development. Available in packages of 10.

28 pages Saddle-stitched

5191 AEPS Family Report: For Children Ages Three to Six
Brookes Publishing
P.O.Box 10624
Baltimore, MD 21285-0624
410-337-9580
800-638-3775
FAX: 410-337-8539
custserv@brookespublishing.com
www.brookespublishing.com

Diane Bricker, Author
Betty Capt, Author
JoAnn Johnson, Author
Elizabeth Straka, Author
This is a 64-item questionnaire that asks parents to rank their child's abilities on specific skills. In packages of 10 paperback.
28 pages Saddle-stiched

5192 Adapted Physical Activity
Human Kinetics
1607 N Market St
P.O.Box 5076
Champaign, IL 61820-5076
800-747-4457
FAX: 217-351-1549
info@hkusa.com
www.humankinetics.com

5193 Assistive Technology for Parents with Disabilities Handbook
Idaho Assistive Technology Project
University of Idaho
1187 Alturas Dr.
Moscow, ID 83843- 2268
208-885-3557
800-432-8324
FAX: 208-885-6102
idahoat@uidaho.edu
www.idahoat.org

5194 Babyface: A Story of Heart and Bones
Penguin Books USA
375 Hudson St
New York, NY 10014
212-366-2000
consumerservices@penguinrandomhouse.com
www.penguin.com

Jeanne McDermott, Author
A must read for families that seek insight into coping with a chronic condition. Many useful resources provided.
288 pages Paperback

5195 Backyards and Butterflies: Ways to Include Children with Disabilities in Outdoor Activities
Brookline Books
8 Trumbull Rd
Ste B-001
Northampton, MA 01060
413-584-0184
800-666-2665
FAX: 413-584-6184
brbooks@yahoo.com
www.brooklinebks.com

Doreen Greenstein, Author
Suzanne Bloom, Author
An illustrated book with dozens of imaginative ways parents can include children with physical disabilities in outdoor activities. Offers clear concise, how-to directions for constructing home-made toys, utensils, and other items that can be enjoyed outside safely and comfortably.
72 pages Paperback

5196 Beyond Tears: Living After Losing a Child
St. Martin's Griffin (Macmillan Publishers)
75 Varick St
New York, NY 10013
212-226-7521
press.inquiries@macmillan.com
us.macmillan.com/smp

Ellen Mitchell, Author

Meant to comfort and give direction to bereaved parents, Beyond Tears is written by nine mothers who have each lost a child. This revised edition includes a new chapter written from the perspective of surviving siblings. The death of a child is that unimaginable loss no parent ever expects to face. In this book, nine mothers share their individual stories of how to survive in the darkest hour.

5197 Broken Dolls: Gathering the Pieces: Caringfor Chronically Ill Children
St. Paul Press

Jennifer Travis Cox, Author
Told from the point of view of the author, this book tracks the challenges faced by parents and caregivers of chronically ill-children - both in terms of medical care and emotional impact. It offers advice based on the author's own experiences caring for her child, as well as insights from other families who have gone through the same experience.
164 pages Paperback

5198 Building the Healing Partnership: Parents, Professionals and Children
Brookline Books
8 Trumbull Road
Suite B-001
Northampton, MA 01060
413-584-0184
800-666-2665
FAX: 413-584-6184
brbooks@yahoo.com
www.brooklinebooks.com

Paperback
ISBN 0-91479 -63-8

5199 Children with Disabilities
Brookes Publishing
P.O.Box 10624
Baltimore, MD 21285-0624
410-337-9580
800-638-3775
FAX: 410-337-8539
custserv@brookespublishing.com
www.brookespublishing.com

Mark L Batshaw MD, Editor
Paul Brooks, Owner
Lauren Rohe, Regional Sales Consultant
Cary Gold, Educational Sales Representative
Extensive coverage of genetics, heredity, pre- and postnatal development, specific disabilities, family roles, and intervention. Features chapters on substance abuse, HIV and AIDS, Down syndrome, fragile X syndrome, behavior management, transitions to adulthood, and health care in the 21st century. Also reveals the causes of many conditions that can lead to developmental disabilities. $69.95
912 pages Hardcover
ISBN 1-557665-81-8

5200 Conditional Love: Parents' Attitudes Toward Handicapped Children
Greenwood Publishing Group
130 Cremona Drive
P O Box 1911
Santa Barbara,, CA 93117-4208
203-226-3571
800-368-6868
805-968-1911
FAX: 866-270-3856
customerservice@abc-clio.com
www.abc-clio.com

312 pages
ISBN 0-89789 -24-7

5201 **Coordinacion De Servicios Centrado En La Familia**
Brookline Books
8 Trumbull Road
Suite B-001
Northampton, MA 01060
413-584-0184
800-666-2665
FAX: 413-584-6184
brbooks@yahoo.com
www.brooklinebooks.com

34 pages Paperback
ISBN 0-91479 -90-5

5202 **Developing Personal Safety Skills in Children with Disabilities**
Brookes Publishing
P.O.Box 10624
Baltimore, MD 21285-0624
410-337-9580
800-638-3775
FAX: 410-337-8539
custserv@brookespublishing.com
readplaylearn.com

Paul Brooks, Owner
A guide for teachers, parents, and caregivers, this volume explores the issue of personal safety for children with disabilities and offers strategies for empowering and protecting them at home and in school. Recognizing that children with disabilities are vulnerable to abuse, this work explores why children with disabilities need personal safety skills, offers, curriculum ideas and exercises, and advocates the development of self-esteem and assertiveness so that children can protect themselves. *$34.00*
220 pages Paperback
ISBN 1-557661-84-7

5203 **Developmental Disabilities in Infancy and Childhood**
Brookes Publishing
P.O.Box 10624
Baltimore, MD 21285-0624
410-767-6100
800-638-3775
FAX: 410-767-5850
custserv@brookespublishing.com
readplaylearn.com

Paul Brooks, Owner
This two volume set explores advances in assessment and treatment, retains a clinical focus, and incorporates recent developments in research and theory. Can be purchased individually or as a set (Vol. 1: Neurodevelopmental Diagnosis and Treatment Vol. 2: The Spectrum of Developmental Disabilities). *$210.00*
Hardcover
ISBN 1-55766O-CA-P

5204 **Dictionary of Developmental Disabilities Terminology**
Brookes Publishing
P.O.Box 10624
Baltimore, MD 21285-0624
410-337-9580
800-638-3775
FAX: 410-337-8539
custserv@brookespublishing.com
readplaylearn.com

Paul Brooks, Owner
Answers thousands of questions for medical or human services professionals, parents or advocates of children with disabilities, or students preparing for their careers. Provides thorough explanations of the most common terms associated with disabilities. *$ 55.95*
368 pages Hardcover
ISBN 1-557662-45-2

5205 **Encyclopedia of Genetic Disorders & Birth Defects**
Facts on File
132 W 31st St
17th Floor
New York, NY 10001-3406
800-322-8755
FAX: 800-678-3633
custserv@factsonfile.com
www.infobasepublishing.com/

Mark Donnell, President
Layperson-accessible entries on genetic terminology and genetically-influenced conditions. *$71.50*
474 pages
ISBN 0-816038-09-0

5206 **Exceptional Parent Magazine**
Psy-Ed Corporation
416 Main Street
Johnstown, PA 15901-2032
814-361-3860
877-372-7368
FAX: 814-361-3861
cmellott@eparent.com
www.eparent.com

Vanessa B Ira, Contributing Writer / Editor
Joseph M. Valenzano, Jr., President, CEO & Publisher
Rick Rader, MD, Editor-in-Chief
Lois Keegan, Human Resources Manager
Magazine that provides information, support, ideas, encouragement, and outreach for parents and families of children with disabilities and the professionals who work with them. *$39.95*
85 pages Monthly

5207 **Face of Inclusion**
Special Needs Project
Ste H
324 State St
Santa Barbara, CA 93101-2364
805-962-8087
800-333-6867
FAX: 805-962-5087
eplibrary@aol.com
www.eplibrary.com

Hod Gray, Owner
A unique and moving parents' perspective of inclusion for administrators, teachers, and parents of children with disabilities. *$99.00*

5208 **Families Magazine**
New Jersey Developmental Disabilities Council
20 West State Street, 6th Floor
P.O.Box 700
Trenton, NJ 08625-0700
609-292-3745
800-792-8858
FAX: 609-292-7114
TTY: 609-777-3238
njcdd@njcdd.org
www.njddc.org

Elaine Buchsbaum, Chairman
Christopher Miller, Vice Chair
Alison M. Lozano, Ph.D, Executive Director
Shirla Rufo Simpson, M.A., DRCC, Deputy Director
Quarterly magazine for people with disabilities, their families and the public, features family profiles, news, columns and the New Jersey Family support councils newsletter.
Quarterly

5209 **Families, Illness & Disability**
Through the Looking Glass
3075 Adeline St
Ste. 120
Berkeley, CA 94703-2212
510-848-1112
800-644-2666
FAX: 510-848-4445
TTY: 510-848-1005
tlg@lookingglass.org
www.lookingglass.org

Maureen Block, J.D., Co-Founder
Karen Fessel, Ph.D., Executive Director
$35.00
320 pages

5210 Family Interventions Throughout Disability
Springer Publishing Company
11 West 42nd Street,
15th Floor
New York, NY 10036-3915   212-431-4370
                                              877-687-7476
                                         FAX: 212-941-7842
                                         cs@springerpub.com
                                         www.springerpub.com

Theodore C Nardin, Chief Executive Officer
James C. Costello, Vice President, Journal Publishing
Diana Osborne, Production Manager
Megan Larkin, Managing Editor, Journals
Family attitudes throughout chronic illness and disability. *$31.95*
320 pages
ISBN 0-82615-80-4

5211 Family-Centered Service Coordination: A Manual for Parents
Brookline Books
8 Trumbull Road
Suite B-001
Northampton, MA 01060   413-584-0184
                                              800-666-2665
                                         FAX: 413-584-6184
                                         brbooks@yahoo.com
                                         www.brooklinebooks.com

34 pages Paperback
ISBN 0-91479-90-5

5212 Handbook About Care in the Home
AARP Fulfillment
601 E St NW
Washington, DC 20049-1   202-434-2277
                                              888-687-2277
                                         TTY:877-434-7598
                                         member@aarp.org
                                         www.aarp.org

24 pages

5213 LifeLines
Disabled & Alone/Life Services for the Handicapped
1440 Broadway,
23rd Floor
New York, NY 10006-2734   212-532-6740
                                              800-995-0066
                                         FAX: 212-532-6740
                                         info@disabledandalone.org
                                         www.disabledandalone.org

Leslie D. Park, Chairman
Rex L Davidson, Vice President
Disabled and Alone is a national, nonprofit organization whose sole purpose is to assure the well being of disabled individuals, particularly those whose families have died and have engaged Disabled and Alone to provide advocacy and oversight for the lifetime of their disabled children. This newsletter provides information about 'future planning' for a person with a disability.
8-16 pages Bi-annual

5214 Living with a Brother or Sister with Special Needs: A Book for Sibs
Sibling Support Project
6512 23rd Ave NW
Ste 322
Seattle, WA 98117   206-297-6368
                                         info@siblingsupport.org
                                         www.siblingsupport.org

Don Meyer, Author
Patricia Vadasy, Author
Living with a Brother or Sister with Special Needs focuses on the intensity of emotions that brothers and sisters experience when they have a sibling with special needs, and the hard questions they ask. It talks about the good and not-so-good parts of having a brother or sister who has special needs, and offers suggestions for how to make life easier for everyone in the family.
144 pages Paperback

5215 Loving & Letting Go
Centering Corporation
7230 Maple Street
Omaha, NE 68134-5064   402-553-1200
                                              866-218-0101
                                         FAX: 402-533-0507
                                         j1200@aol.com
                                         www.centering.org

Joy Johnson, Founder
Dr. Marvin Johnson, co-Founder
For parents who decide to turn away from aggressive medical intervention for their critically ill newborn. *$5.95*
48 pages Paperback

5216 Mobility Training for People with Disabilities
Charles C. Thomas
2600 S First St
Springfield, IL 62704-4730   217-789-8980
                                              800-258-8980
                                         FAX: 217-789-9130
                                         books@ccthomas.com
                                         www.ccthomas.com

Michael P. Thomas, President

5217 Mother to Be
Through the Looking Glass
3075 Adeline St
Ste. 120
Berkeley, CA 94703-2212   510-848-1112
                                              800-644-2666
                                         FAX: 510-848-4445
                                         TTY: 510-848-1005
                                         tlg@lookingglass.org
                                         www.lookingglass.org

Maureen Block, J.D., Co-Founder
Karen Fessel, Ph.D., Executive Director
Guide to pregnancy and birth for women with disabilities. *$34.00*
410 pages

5218 New Language of Toys: Teaching Communication Skills to Children with Special Needs
Spina Bifida Association of America
1600 Wilson Blvd.
Suite 800
Arlington, VA 22209-4226   202-944-3285
                                              800-621-3141
                                         FAX: 202-944-3295
                                         sbaa@sbaa.org
                                         www.spinabifidaassociation.org

Ana Ximenes, Chair
Sara Struwe, President & CEO
Cindy Brownstein, CEO
George Sturm, Treasurer
A guide for parents and teachers and a reader-friendly resource guide that provides a wealth of information on how play activities affect a child's language development and where to get the toys and materials to use in these activities. *$19.00*

5219 NewsLine
Federation for Children with Special Needs
45 Bromfield Street
10th Floor
Boston, MA 02108   866-815-8122
                                         FAX: 617-542-7832
                                         info@ppal.net
                                         www.ppal.net

Lisa Lambert, Executive Director
Deborah A. Fauntleroy, MSW, Associate Director
Offers information for parents and families on resources, medical updates, activities, fund-raising events and association news for their disabled children.
Quarterly

5220 **On the Road to Autonomy: Promoting Self- Competence in Children & Youth with Disabilities**
Brookes Publishing
P.O.Box 10624
Baltimore, MD 21285-0624
410-337-9580
800-638-3775
FAX: 410-337-8539
custserv@brookespublishing.com
readplaylearn.com

Paul Brooks, Owner
This book provides detailed conceptual, practical, and personal information regarding the promotion of self-esteem, self-determination, and coping skills among children and youth with and without disabilities. *$48.00*
432 pages Paperback
ISBN 1-55766 -35-5

5221 **Pain Erasure**
M Evans and Company
2'16 E 49th St
New York, NY 10017-1546
212-979-0880
FAX: 212-486-4544

Mary Evans, Owner
This book explains Bonnie Prudden's method for pain relief using myotherapy, a method hailed by doctors and patients.

ISBN 0-345331-02-8

5222 **Parent Centers and Independent Living Centers: Collectively We're Stronger**
Independent Living Research Utilization ILRU
1333 Moursund
Houston, TX 77030-7031
713-520-0232
FAX: 713-520-5785
ilru@ilru.org
ilru.org

Lex Frieden, Director, ILRU
Richard Petty, Program Director
Roxy Funchess, Administrative Secretary
George Powers, Legal Specialist
This article describes several examples of effective working relationships of PTIs and CILs. The examples highlight how parent and consumer organizations have identified complimentary strengths and formed partnerships to better support children with disabilities and their families. These partnerships can also be a very important way of involving youth in the disability movement so they may become leaders of tomorrow.
10 pages

5223 **Parent-Child Interaction and Developmental Disabilities**
Greenwood Publishing Group
130 Cremona Drive
P O Box 1911
Santa Barbara,, CA 93117
800-368-6868
805-968-1911
FAX: 866-270-3856
customerservice@abc-clio.com
www.abc-clio.com

395 pages Hardcover
ISBN 0-275928-35-7

5224 **Parenting**
Accent Books & Products
P.O.Box 700
Bloomington, IL 61702-700
309-378-2961
800-787-8444
FAX: 309-378-4420
acmtlvng@aol.com

Raymond C Cheever, Publisher
Betty Garee, Editor
Experienced parents (who are disabled) discuss: raising children from infant to teens, balancing career and motherhood, discipline methods and more when both parents are disabled. *$7.95*
83 pages
ISBN 0-91570 -26-4

5225 **Parenting with a Disability**
Through the Looking Glass
3075 Adeline St
Ste. 120
Berkeley, CA 94703-2212
510-848-1112
800-644-2666
FAX: 510-848-4445
TTY: 510-848-1005
tlg@lookingglass.org
www.lookingglass.org

Maureen Block, J.D., Board President
Rusty Hendlin, M.A., LMFT, Director of Medi-Cal Services
Thomas Spalding, Board Treasurer
Alice Nemon, D.S.W., Board Secretary
International newsletter. Available in braille, large print or cassette.
3 per year

5226 **Perspectives on a Parent Movement**
Brookline Books
8 Trumbull Rd
Suite B-001
Northampton, MA 1060-4533
413-584-0184
800-666-2665
FAX: 413-584-6184
brbooks@yahoo.com
www.brooklinebooks.com

Paperback
ISBN 0-91479 -74-3

5227 **Sexuality and the Developmentally Handicapped**
Edwin Mellen Press
P.O.Box 450
Lewiston, NY 14092-450
716-754-2266
FAX: 716-754-4056
jrupnow@mellenpress.com
mellenpress.com

Herbert Richardson, Owner
Presents the knowledge, attitudes, and skills pertinent to responding to the sexual problems of developmentally handicapped persons, their families and communities. Details fully documented cases, issues concerning the law, and resource materials available. *$89.95*
245 pages Hardcover
ISBN 0-88946 -32-5

5228 **Shattered Dreams-Lonely Choices: Birth Parents of Babies with Disabilities**
Greenwood Publishing Group
130 Cremona Drive
Santa Barbara, CA 93117-4208
203-226-3571
800-368-6868
805-968-1911
FAX: 866-270-3856
customerservice@abc-clio.com
www.abc-clio.com

208 pages Hardcover
ISBN 0-897892-86-0

5229 **Since Owen, A Parent-to-Parent Guide for Care of the Disabled Child**
Special Needs Project
Ste H
324 State St
Santa Barbara, CA 93101-2364
818-718-9900
800-333-6867
FAX: 818-349-2027
editor@specialneeds.com
www.specialneeds.com

Hod Gray, Owner
Against the background of his experience as the parent of a severely disabled young man, Callahan writes conscientiously to other parents. *$16.95*
486 pages

5230   **Sleep Better! A Guide to Improving Sleep for Children with Special Needs**
Brookes Publishing
P.O.Box 10624
Baltimore, MD 21285-624

410-337-9580
800-638-3775
FAX: 410-337-8539
custserv@brookespublishing.com
readplaylearn.com

Paul Brooks, Owner
This book offers step-by-step, how to instructions for helping children with disabilities get the rest they need. For problems ranging from bedtime tantrums to night waking, parents and care-givers will find a variety of widely tested and easy-to-implement techniques that have already helped hundreds of children with special needs. *$21.95*
288 pages Paperback
ISBN 1-55766-15-7

5231   **Something's Wrong with My Child!**
Charles C. Thomas
2600 S First St
Springfield, IL 62704-4730

217-789-8980
800-258-8980
FAX: 217-789-9130
books@ccthomas.com
www.ccthomas.com

Michael P. Thomas, President
This text provides professionals and parents with the opportunity to gain insights into a family that has benefited positively and constructively from the presence of a member with a disability. The author presents a compilation of easy-to-read material that's based on real-life experiences. *$39.95*
234 pages Paperback 1998
ISBN 0-398068-99-8

5232   **Sometimes I Get All Scribbly**
Exceptional Parent Library
P.O.Box 1807
Englewood Cliffs, NJ 7632-1207

201-947-6000
800-535-1910
FAX: 201-947-9376
eplibrary@aol.com
www.eplibrary.com

5233   **Son-Rise: The Miracle Continues**
2080 South Undermountain Road
Sheffield, MA 01257-9643

413-229-2100
877-766-7473
FAX: 413-229-3202
sonrise@option.org
www.son-rise.org

Barry Neil Kaufman, Co-Founder/ Co-Originator/Senior Teacher/Trainer
Samahria Lyte Kaufman, Co-Founder/ Co-Originator/Senior Teacher/Trainer
Bryn Hogan, ATCA Senior Staff
William Hogan, ATCA Senior Staff
Documents Raun Kaufman's astonishing development from a lifeless, autistic, retarded child into a highly verbal, lovable youngster with no traces of his former condition. Details Raun's extraordinary progress from the age of four into young adulthood, also shares moving accounts of five families that successfully used the Son-Rise Program to reach their own special children.
372 pages
ISBN 0-915811-53-7

5234   **Special Kids Need Special Parents: A Resource for Parents of Children With Special Needs**
Berkley Publishing Group
375 Hudson Street
New York, NY 10014-3657

212-366-2372
FAX: 212-366-2933
ecommerce@us.penguingroup.com
www.us.penguingroup.com

319 pages Paperback
ISBN 0-425176-62-2

5235   **Special Parent, Special Child**
Exceptional Parent Library
P.O.Box 1807
Englewood Cliffs, NJ 7632-1207

201-947-6000
800-535-1910
FAX: 201-947-9376
eplibrary@aol.com
www.eplibrary.com

Hardcover

5236   **Strategies for Working with Families of Young Children with Disabilities**
Brookes Publishing
P.O.Box 10624
Baltimore, MD 21285-624

410-337-9580
800-638-3775
FAX: 410-337-8539
custserv@brookespublishing.com
readplaylearn.com

Paul Brooks, Owner
This text offers useful techniques for collaborating with and supporting families whose youngest members either have a disability or are at risk for developing a disability. The authors address specific issues such as cultural diversity, transitions to new programs, and disagreements between families and professionals. *$33.00*
272 pages Paperback
ISBN 1-55766-57-6

5237   **That's My Child**
Exceptional Parent Library
P.O.Box 1807
Englewood Cliffs, NJ 7632-1207

201-947-6000
800-535-1910
FAX: 201-947-9376
eplibrary@aol.com
www.eplibrary.com

5238   **The Complete Guide to Creating a SpecialNeeds Life Plan**
Jessica Kingsley Publishers
73 Collier St
London, UK N19BE

hello@jkp.com
www.jkp.com

Hal Wright, Author
The purpose of special needs planning is to create the best possible life for an adult with a disability. This book provides comprehensive guidance on creating a life plan to transition a special needs child to independence or to ensure they are well cared for in the future.
360 pages

5239   **They Don't Come with Manuals**
Fanlight Productions
32 Court Street, 21st Floor
Brooklyn, NY 11201-1731

718-488-8900
800-876-1710
FAX: 718-488-8642
orders@fanlight.com
www.fanlight.com

Ben Achtenberg, Owner
Anthony Sweeney, Marketing Director
Nicole Johnson, Publicity Coordinator
The parents and adoptive parents in this video speak candidly of their day to day experiences caring for children with physical and mental disabilities. *$145.00*

5240   They're Just Kids
Aquarius Health Care Videos
30 Forest Road
P.O. Box 249
Millis, MA 02054-7159
                                            508-376-1244
                                       FAX: 508-376-1245
                                       aqvideos@tiac.net
                                   www.aquariusproductions.com

Lesile Kussmann, President
Joyce Farmer, Assistant Director
The importance and value of inclusion, excellent for anyone
working with kids with disabilities. The documentary explores
the advantages of the inclusion of disabled children in the classroom, cub scouts and other extracurricular activities. *$99.00*
Video

5241   To a Different Drumbeat
Alliance for Parental Involvement in Education
P.O. Box 59
East Chatham, NY 12060-59
                                            518-392-6900
                                       FAX: 518-392-6900

5242   Uncommon Fathers
Woodbine House
6510 Bells Mill Rd
Bethesda, MD 20817-1636
                                            301-897-3570
                                            800-843-7323
                                     info@woodbinehouse.com
                                       woodbinehouse.com

Irv Shapell, Owner
Nineteen fathers talk about the life-altering experience of having
a child with special needs and offer a welcome, seldom-heard perspective on raising kids with disabilities, including autism, cerebral palsy, and Down syndrome. Uncommon Fathers is the first
book for fathers by fathers, but it is also helpful to partners, family, friends, and service providers. *$14.95*
206 pages Paperback
ISBN 0-933149-68-9

**5243   We Can Speak for Ourselves: Self Advocacy by Mentally
Handicapped People**
Brookline Books
8 Trumbull Rd
Suite B-001
Northampton, MA 1060-4533
                                            413-584-0184
                                            800-666-2665
                                       FAX: 413-584-6184
                                      brbooks@yahoo.com
                                    www.brooklinebooks.com

246 pages Paperback
ISBN 0-25336 -65-9

5244   You May Be Able to Adopt
Through the Looking Glass
3075 Adeline St
Ste. 120
Berkeley, CA 94703-2212
                                            510-848-1112
                                            800-644-2666
                                       FAX: 510-848-4445
                                       TTY: 510-848-1005
                                       tlg@lookingglass.org
                                     www.lookingglass.org

Maureen Block, J.D., Board President
Rusty Hendlin, M.A., LMFT, Director of Medi-Cal Services
Thomas Spalding, Board Treasurer
Alice Nemon, D.S.W., Board Secretary
A guide to the adoption process for prospective mothers with dis-
abilities and their partners. Available in braille, large print or cas-
sette. *$10.00*
112 pages

5245   You Will Dream New Dreams
Kensington Publishing
119 West 40th Street
New York, NY 10018
                                            800-221-2647
                                   www.kensingtonbooks.com

Steven Zacharius, Chairman, President & CEO
A parent's support group in print. The shared narratives come
from those with newly diagnosed children, adult disabled children, and everything in between. *$13.00*
278 pages Paperback
ISBN 1-575665-60-3

**5246   Your Child Has a Disability: A Complete Sourcebook of
Daily and Medical Care**
Brookes Publishing
P.O. Box 10624
Baltimore, MD 21285-624
                                            410-337-9580
                                            800-638-3775
                                       FAX: 410-337-8539
                                custserv@brookesopublishing.com
                                       readplaylearn.com

Paul Brooks, Owner
Offers expert advice on a wide range of issues-from finding the
right doctor and investigating the medical aspects of a child's
condition to learning care techniques and fulfilling education requirements. *$24.95*
368 pages Paperback
ISBN 1-557663-74-2

Parenting: Specific Disabilities

**5247   Cancer Clinical Trials: A CommonsenseGuide to
Experimental Cancer Therapies and Trials**
DiaMedica Inc.
2 Carlson Pkwy N
Ste 165
Minneapolis, MN 55447
                                            763-270-0603
                                       FAX: 763-710-4456
                                      info@diamedica.com
                                       www.diamedica.com

Tomasz M. Beer, Author
Larry W. Axmaker, Author
Cancer Clinical Trials is a comprehensive, no-nonsense, and
readable guide for anyone who is considering therapeutic options
in addition to standard cancer therapy. The book seeks to share
knowledge about cancer clinical trials with people living with
cancer, their families and loved ones. It will help readers decide if
a clinical trial is a good option for them, to choose an appropriate
trial, and to navigate through the clinical trial process.
192 pages

**5248   Different Dream Parenting: A PracticalGuide to Raising a
Child with Special Needs**
Discovery House Publishers
3000 Kraft Ave SE
P.O. Box 3566
Grand Rapids, MI 49512
                                            800-653-8333
                                       support@dhp.org
                                            dhp.org

Jolene Philo, Author
In Different Dream Parenting, author Jolene Philo offers guidance and encouragement through biblical insights and her own
personal experiences. Find spiritual wisdom, practical resources,
and tools that can help you become an extraordinary advocate for
your child. Discover how you can move beyond the challenges
and experience the joy of being your childs biggest and best
supporter.
336 pages

5249 Essential First Steps for Parents of Children with Autism
Woodbine House
6510 Bells Mill Rd
Bethesda, MD 20817
301-897-3570
800-843-7323
info@woodbinehouse.com
www.woodbinehouse.com

Lara Delmolino, Author
Sandra L. Harris, Author

When autism is diagnosed or suspected in young children, over-whelmed parents wonder where to turn and how to begin helping their child. Drs. Delmolino and Harris, experienced clinicians and ABA therapists, eliminate the confusion and guesswork by outlining the pivotal steps parents can take now to optimize learning and functioning for children ages 5 and younger.
154 pages Paperback

5250 Final Report: Challenges and Strategies of Disabled Parents: Findings from a Survey (1997)
Through the Looking Glass
3075 Adeline St
Ste. 120
Berkeley, CA 94703-2212
510-848-1112
800-644-2666
FAX: 510-848-4445
TTY: 510-848-1005
tlg@lookingglass.org
www.lookingglass.org

Linda Toms Barker, Author
Vida Maralani, Author

This milestone TLG-directed report presents findings from the first national survey of parents with disabilities. The report includes a description of parents with disabilities, barriers to parenting among adults with disabilities, transportation issues, personal assistance, adaptive parenting equipment, housing, as well as recommendations for legal and service system changes.

5251 Pervasive Developmental Disorders: Finding a Diagnosis and Getting Help
Patient-Centered Guides/O'Reilly Media
1005 Gravenstein Hwy N
Sebastopol, CA 95472
707-827-7019
800-889-8969
FAX: 707-824-8268
orders@oreilly.com
shop.oreilly.com

Mitzi Waltz, Author

This unique book encompasess both the practical aspects as well as ther personal stories and emotional facets of living with PDD-NOS, the most common pervasive developmental disorder. Parents of an undiagnosed child may suspect many things, from autism to servere allergies. Pervasive Developmental Disorders is for parents (or newly diagnosed adults) who struggle with this neurological condition that profoundly impacts the life of child and family.
580 pages Paperback 1999

5252 Teaching Children with Down Syndrome about Their Bodies, Boundaries, and Sexuality
Woodbine House
6510 Bell Mills Rd
Bethesda, MD 20817
800-843-7323
info@woodbinehouse.com
www.woodbinehouse.com

Terri Couwenhoven, Author

Drawing on her unique background as both a sexual educator and mother of a child with Down syndrome, the author blends factual information and practical ideas for teaching children with Down syndrome about their bodies, puberty, and sexuality. This book gives parents the confidence to speak comfortably about these sometimes difficult subjects.
332 pages Paperback

5253 Thinking Differently: An Inspiring Guide for Parents of Children with Learning Disabilities
William Morrow Paperbacks (HarperCollins)
195 Broadway
New York, NY 10007
212-207-7000
orders@harpercollins.com
www.harpercollins.com

David Flink, Author

An innovative, comprehensive guide—the first of its kind—to help parents understand and accept learning disabilities in their children, offering tips and strategies for successfully advocating on their behalf and helping them become their own best advocates.

5254 Your Child in the Hospital: A Practical Guide for Parents (3rd Edition)
Childhood Cancer Guides/O'Reilly Media
1005 Gravenstein Hwy N
Sebastopol, CA 95472
707-827-7019
800-889-8969
FAX: 707-824-8268
orders@oreilly.com
shop.oreilly.com/category/publishers/ccg.do

Nancy Keene, Author

This book offers advice from dozens of veteran parents on how to cope with a child's hospitalization, relieving anxious parents so they can help dispel their child's fears and concerns. Parents will find easy-to-read tips on preparing their child, handling procedures without trauma, and preventing insurance snafus. The second edition features a journal to help open communication and give the child a measure of control over the experience.
176 pages Paperback

Parenting: School

5255 Allergy & Asthma Today
Allergy & Asthma Network
8229 Boone Blvd
Ste 260
Vienna, VA 22182
800-878-4403
FAX: 703-288-5271
canderson@allergyasthmanetwork.org
www.allergyasthmanetwork.org

Tonya Winders, President
Charmayne Anderson, Director, Advocacy
Gary Fitzgerald, Managing Editor
Laurie Ross, Associate Editor

Practical, medical,information for school patients, physicians, caregivers and families.

5256 Carolina Curriculum for Infants and Toddlers with Special Needs (3rd Edition)
Brookes Publishing
P.O.Box 10624
Baltimore, MD 21285-0624
410-337-9580
800-638-3775
FAX: 410-337-8539
custserv@brookespublishing.com
www.brookespublishing.com

Nancy M. Johnson-Martin, Author
Susan M. Attermeier, Author
Bonnie J. Hacker, Author

This book includes detailed assessment and intervention sequences, daily routine integration strategies, sensorimotor adaptations, and a sample 24-page Assessment Log that shows readers how to chart a child's individual progress.
504 pages Spiral-bound

5257 Choosing Outcomes and Accommodations for Children (COACH) (2nd Edition)
Brookes Publishing
P.O.Box 10624
Baltimore, MD 21285-0624
410-337-9580
800-638-3775
FAX: 410-337-8539
custserv@brookespublishing.com
www.brookespublishing.com

Michael F. Giangreco, Author
Chigee J. Cloninger, Author
Virginia Salce Iverson, Author
A guide to educational planning for students with disabilities, second edition. Focuses on life outcomes such as social relationships and participation in typical home, school, and community activities.
232 pages Spiral bound

5258 Complete IEP Guide: How to Advocate for Your Special Ed Child (8th Edition)
NOLO (Internet Brands)
909 N. Sepulveda Blvd
11th Fl.
El Segundo, CA 90245
310-280-4000
www.nolo.com

Lawrence Siegel, Author/Attorney
This all-in-one guide will help you understand special education law, identify your child's needs, prepare for meetings, develop the IEP and resolve disputes.
384 pages

5259 Exceptional Student in the Regular Classroom (6th Edition)
Pearson
330 Hudson St
New York, NY 10013
212-641-2400
www.pearsoned.com

Bill R. Gearheart, Author
Mel W. Weishan, Author
Carol J. Gearheart, Author
Offers good, solid information through a practical understandable presentation unencumbered by specialized jargon. Covers topics associated with special learners.
517 pages

5260 Study Power Workbook: Exercises in StudySkills to Improve Your Learning and Your Grades
Brookline Books
8 Trumbull Rd
Ste B-001
Northampton, MA 1060-4533
413-584-0184
800-666-2665
FAX: 413-584-6184
brbooks@yahoo.com
www.brooklinebks.com

Sara Beth Huntley, Author
William Luckie, Author
Wood Smethurst, Author
The techniques in the easy-to-use, self-teaching manual have yielded remarkable success for students from elementary to medical school, at all levels of intelligence and achievement. Key skills covered include: listening, note taking, concentration, summarizing, reading comprehension, memorization, test taking, preparing papers and reports, time management, and more. These abilities are vital to success throughout every stage of learning; the benefits will last a lifetime.

Parenting: Spiritual

5261 A Good and Perfect Gift: Faith, Expectations, and a Little Girl Named Penny
Bethany House Publishers (Baker Publishing Group)
6030 E Fulton Rd
Ada, MI 49301
616-676-9185
800-877-2665
FAX: 616-676-9573
bakerpublishinggroup.com

Amy Julia Becker, Author
When her first baby, Penny, is given a frightening diagnosis, Amy Julia's world comes crashing down. Could she continue to trust God's goodness through what felt like personal tragedy? But challenging surprises often lead to unforeseen joy, and disappointments can turn into blessings. This wise and beautiful book is more than a courageous story of raising a child against the odds—it is a journey through the unexpected ups and downs of life and the discoveries that come along the way.
240 pages

5262 Before and After Zachariah
Chicago Review Press
814 N Franklin St
Chicago, IL 60610
312-337-0747
800-888-4741
FAX: 312-337-5110
www.chicagoreviewpress.com

Fern Kupfer, Author
This intimate chronicle of one family's life with a severely brain damaged child is recently back in print.
247 pages 1982

5263 Bethy and the Mouse: A Father Remembers His Children with Disabilities
Brookline Books
8 Trumbull Rd
Ste B-001
Northampton, MA 1060-4533
413-584-0184
800-666-2665
FAX: 413-584-6184
brbooks@yahoo.com
www.brooklinebks.com

Donald C. Bakely, Author
A moving collection of poetry, photographs, and prose following a father's experiences with two disabled children—one with Down Syndrome and one with an underdeveloped brain.
184 pages Paperback 1999

5264 Disabled God: Toward a Liberatory Theologyof Disability
Abingdon Press
2222 Rosa L. Parks Blvd
Nashville, TN 37288
615-749-6615
800-251-3320
orders@abingdonpress.com
www.abingdonpress.com

Nancy L. Eisland, Author
Draws on themes of the disability rights movement to identify people with disabilities as members of a socially disadvantaged minority group rather than as individuals who need to adjust. Highlights the history of people with disabilities in the church and society.
139 pages Paperback 1994

5265 Farewell, My Forever Child
CreateSpace, an Amazon Company
4900 Lacross Rd
North Charleston, SC 29406
843-760-8000
www.createspace.com

Kalila Smith, Author
Based on her own experiences following the loss of her 29-year-old daughter, Kalila Smith discusses the complex grief felt by parents who have lost a developmentally disabled child, and offers strategies to help families achieve peace and deal with the loss.
134 pages

5266 In Time and with Love: Caring for the Special Needs Infant and Toddler

William Morrow Paperbacks (HarperCollins)
195 Broadway
New York, NY 10007
212-207-7000
orders@harpercollins.com
www.harpercollins.com

Marilyn Segal, Author
Roni Leiderman, Author
Wendy S. Masi, Author
For families and caregivers of preteen and handicapped children in their first three years - more than one hundred tips for adjusting and coping. Part of the Your Child At Play series.
240 pages

5267 Journal of Disability & Religion

Routledge (Taylor & Francis Group)
711 Third Ave
New York, NY 10017
212-216-7800
800-354-1420
FAX: 202-564-7854
orders@taylorandfrancis.com
www.tandfonline.com

Quarterly

5268 Spiritually Able: A Parents Guide to Teaching Faith To Children with Special Needs

Loyola Press
3441 N Ashland Ave
Chicago, IL 60657
800-621-1008
FAX: 773-281-0555
customerservice@loyolapress.com
www.loyolapress.com

David Rizzo, Author
Both memoir and manual, Spiritually Able: A Parent's Guide to Teaching the Faith to Children with Special Needs is a life-preserver to parents who are seeking ways to grow and nourish a deeper relationship to God and their faith for their child with special needs. Full of tips, advice, and personal accounts, Spiritually Able helps bridge the gap and invites all into the welcoming embrace of the Church.
140 pages

5269 The Spiritual Art of Raising Children withDisabilities

Judson Press
P.O. Box 851
Valley Forge, PA 19482
800-458-3766
www.judsonpress.com

Kathleen Deyer Bolduc, Author
In The Spiritual Art of Raising Children with Disabilities, Bolduc uses the metaphor of the mosaic to life as parents of children with disabilities. Readers are walked through the process using the spiritual disciplines to help you recognize God's presence in your life and regain the balance we all need. this book offers readers the unique perspective of a parent raising a child with disabilities and dealing with it through faith and spiritual direction.
192 pages Paperback

5270 Worst Loss: How Families Heal from the Death of a Child

Holt Paperbacks (Macmillan Publishers)
75 Varick St
New York, NY 10013
212-226-7521
press.inquiries@macmillan.com
us.macmillan.com/henryholt

Barbara D. Rosof, Author
Combines anecdotal case histories and the latest research to help bereaved parents cope with the loss of a child, offering practical and comforting advice on how to overcome the disabling symptoms of grief.
304 pages 1995

Professional

5271 American Journal of Physical Medicine &Rehabilitation

Lippincott, Williams & Wilkins
2001 Market St
Ste 5
Philadelphia, PA 19103-1551
215-521-8300
800-638-3030
FAX: 215-521-8902
orders@lww.com
www.lww.com

Walter R. Frontera, MD, PHD, Editor-in-Chief
Journal of the Association of Academic Psychiatrists. Articles covering research and clinical studies and applications of new equipment, procedures and therapeutic advances.
Monthly

5272 American Journal of Psychiatry

American Psychiatric Association
1000 Wilson Blvd
Ste 1825
Arlington, VA 22209-3924
703-907-7322
800-368-5777
FAX: 703-907-1091
ajp@psych.org
ajp.psychiatryonline.org

Robert Freedman, Editor
Peer-reviewed articles focus on developments in biological psychiatry as well as on treatment innovations and forensic, ethical, economic, and social topics.
Monthly

5273 American Journal of Public Health

American Public Health Association
800 I St NW
Washington, DC 20001
202-777-2471
888-320-2742
FAX: 202-777-2534
TTY: 202-777-2500
comments@msmail.apha.org
www.apha.org

Alfredo Morabia, Editor-in-Chief
Association journal containing professional articles and sections such as Notes from the Field and Association News.
Monthly

5274 Art Therapy

American Art Therapy Association
4875 Eisenhower Ave
Ste 240
Alexandria, VA 22304-3302
703-548-5860
888-290-0878
FAX: 703-783-8468
info@arttherapy.org
www.arttherapy.org

Quarterly

5275 CAREERS & the disABLED Magazine

Equal Opportunity Publications
445 Broad Hollow Rd
Ste 425
Melville, NY 11747-3615
631-421-9421
FAX: 631-421-1352
info@eop.com
www.eop.com

Barbara Capella Loehr, Editor
A career magazine for professional career seekers who have disabilities. Profiles disabled people who have achieved successful careers. Features a career section in Braille, career guide.

5276   Clinician's Practical Guide to Attention-Deficit/Hyperactivity Disorder
Brookes Publishing
P.O.Box 10624
Baltimore, MD 21285-0624

410-337-9580
800-638-3775
FAX: 410-337-8539
custserv@brookespublishing.com
www.brookespublishing.com

Marianne Mercugliano, Author
Quick reference volume with comprehensive data on psychoeducational and neuropsychological assessment, related symptoms, drug and counseling therapies and critical issues.
368 pages

5277   Counseling Parents of Children with Chronic Illness or Disability
Wiley
111 River St
Hoboken, NJ 07030-5774

201-748-6000
877-762-2974
FAX: 201-748-6088
info@wiley.com
www.wiley.com

Hilton Davis, Author
This book aims to help medical staff and carers relate to parents in ways that facilitate their adaptation to their child's illness. The key to this is in effective communication.
148 pages Paperback

5278   Creating Options for Family Recovery: A Provider's Guide to Promoting Parental Mental Health
Employment Options Inc.
82 Brigham St
Marlboro, MA 01752-3137

508-485-5051
FAX: 508-485-8807
options@employmentoptions.org
www.employmentoptions.com

Joanne Nicholson, Author
Toni Wolf, Author
Chip Wilder, Author
Kathleen Biebel, Author
This book seeks to advise professionals and providers on strategies to use when working with families who are dealing with mental illness, assisting them with the promotion of a healthy recovery. The resources in this guide are drawn from over 20 years of research and practice, and the lived experiences of parents, children and family members.
120 pages Paperback

5279   Cystic Fibrosis: Medical Care
Lippincott, Williams & Wilkins
16522 Hunters Green Pkwy
Hagerstown, MD 21740

301-223-2300
800-638-3030
FAX: 301-223-2400
orders@lww.com
www.lww.com

David M. Orenstein, Author
Beryl J. Rosenstein, Author
Robert C. Stern, Author
A guide to the medical community to the principles and practices of cystic fibrosis care. After chapters on the molecular and cellular bases of CF and its diagnosis, they cover the major organ systems affected by CF and deal with surgery for CF patients, transplantation (lung and liver), hospitalization, and terminal care. Also included are chapters on special populations, exercise, and laboratory testing.
365 pages

5280   Disability & Rehabilitation Journal
Taylor & Francis Online
6000 Broken Sound Pkwy NW
Ste 300
Boca Raton, FL 33487

212-216-7800
800-634-7064
FAX: 212-564-7854
enquiries@taylorandfrancis.com
www.taylorandfrancis.com

Dave Muller, Editor-in-Chief
Peer-reviewed journal offering the latest news, research, and insights on disability and rehabilitation medicine.
Bi-weekly

5281   Disability Analysis Handbook: Tools forIndependent Practice
American Board of Disability Analysts
4525 Harding Rd
2nd Fl
Nashville, TN 37205-1520

615-327-2978
FAX: 615-327-9235
americanbd@aol.com
www.americandisability.org

Kenneth N. Anchor, Editor
Official newsletter of the American Board of Disability Analysts; features Healthnews Headlines, Meeting Calendar, Application Packet and much more. Free to members; $20 per year for non-members.
396 pages

5282   Enhancing Everyday Communication for Children with Disabilities
Brookes Publishing
P.O.Box 10624
Baltimore, MD 21285-0624

410-337-9580
800-638-3775
FAX: 410-337-8539
custserv@brookespublishing.com
www.brookespublishing.com

Jeff Sigafoos, Author & Editor
Michael Arthur-Kelly, Author
Nancy Butterfield, Author
Practical and concise, this introductory guide is filled with real-world tips and strategies for anyone working to improve the communication of children with moderate, severe, and multiple disabilities. Emphasizing the link between behavior and communication, three respected researchers transform up-to-date research and proven best practices into instructional procedures and interventions ready for use at home or in school.
176 pages Paperback

5283   Ethical Issues In Home Health Care (2ndEdition)
Charles C. Thomas
2600 S First St
Springfield, IL 62704-4730

217-789-8980
800-258-8980
FAX: 217-789-9130
books@ccthomas.com
www.ccthomas.com

Sheri Smith, Author
Rosalind Ekman Ladd, Author
Lynn Pasquerella, Author
This book will help to answer some of the growing number of ethical questions and more complex issues that home health care nurses face. The cases presented in each chapter of the book are fictionalized situations based on interviews conducted with home health care nurses in both hospital-sponsored and private agencies, in hospices, and in urban and rural settings. Each chapter of the book is devoted to one of the main areas of concern for home health care nurses.
258 pages

5284   Journal of Public Health
Oxford Journals, Oxford University Press
2001 Evans Rd
Cary, NC 27513
919-677-0977
800-852-7323
FAX: 919-677-1714
www.oxfordjournals.org

Eugene Milne, Editor
Ted Schrecker, Editor
Scholarly articles on issues that relate to public health and the
healthcare system.

5285   National Rehabilitation Association AnnualReport
National Rehabilitation Association (NRA)
633 S Washington St
P.O. Box 150235
Alexandria, VA 22315-4109
703-836-0850
888-258-4295
FAX: 703-836-0848
TTY: 703-836-0849
info@nationalrehab.org
www.nationalrehab.org

Fredric Schroeder, Executive Director
Sandra Mulliner, Administrative Assistant
Association newsletter containing news, programs and informa-
tion of interest to the Association and its members.
Annual

5286   PM&R Journal
American Academy of Physical Medicine & Rehab
9700 W Bryn Mawr Ave
Ste 200
Rosemont, IL 60018-5701
847-737-6000
877-227-6799
FAX: 847-737-6001
TTY: 800-437-0833
info@aapmr.org
www.pmrjournal.org

Stuart M. Weinstein, Editor-in-Chief
Cathy Mendelsohn, Managing Editor
Covers medical, social and employment aspects of vocational rehabilitation. The content of PM&R includes articles that are contemporary and important to both research and clinical practice.
The various sections of the journal include original research such
as clinical trials, outcomes studies, and clinically relevant
translational science; reviews (narrative and analytical); case
presentations; point/counterpoint debates; ethical/legal topics;
practice management updates; and statistical themes.
Monthly

5287   Provider Magazine
American Health Care Association
1201 L St NW
Washington, DC 20005-4024
202-842-4444
888-656-6669
FAX: 202-842-3860
sales@ahca.org
www.providermagazine.org

Joanne Erickson, Editor-in-Chief
Amy Mendoza, Managing Editor
Magazine for long-term healthcare professionals.
Monthly

5288   Public Health Reports
Association of Schools & Programs of Public Health
1900 M St NW
Ste 710
Washington, DC 20036
202-296-1099
FAX: 202-296-1252
support@publichealthreports.org
www.publichealthreports.org

Frederic E. Shaw, Editorn-in-Chief
Sasha M. Ruiz, Acting Managing Editor
PHR is a peer-reviewed journal published on a bi-monthly basis.
Each issue offers recurring guest columns such as Local Acts,
Global Health Matters, ASPPH From the Schools and Programs
of Public Health, Law and the Public's Health, Public Health

Chronicles, NCHS Dataline, and the Surgeon General's
Perspectives.
Bi-monthly

5289   Sociopolitical Aspects of Disabilities(2nd Edition)
Charles C. Thomas
2600 S First St
Springfield, IL 62704-4730
217-789-8980
800-258-8980
FAX: 217-789-9130
books@ccthomas.com
www.ccthomas.com

Willie V. Bryan, Author
Provides understanding of the social and political histories of
people with disabilities in the United States. This understanding
is pivotal in working with persons with disabilities, to provide
background and perspective on current policies and attitudes.
284 pages

5290   Starting and Sustaining Genetic Support Groups
Johns Hopkins University Press
2715 N Charles St
Baltimore, MD 21218-4363
410-516-6900
FAX: 410-516-6968
webmaster@jhupress.jhu.edu
www.press.jhu.edu

Joan O. Weiss, Author
Jayne S. Mackta, Author
Guide to the establishment and maintenance of genetic support
groups for individuals with genetic disorders and their families.
For therapists and group leaders. Discusses practical matters including finding a leader, fund-raising, organizing peer support
training programs.
152 pages

5291   The Essential Brain Injury Guide (5th Edition)
Brain Injury Association of America
1608 Spring Hill Rd
Ste 110
Vienna, VA 22182
703-761-0750
FAX: 703-761-0755
customerservice2@biausa.org
shop.biausa.org

5292   What Psychotherapists Should Know about Disabilty
Guilford Press
370 Seventh Ave
Ste 1200
New York, NY 10001-1020
800-365-7006
FAX: 212-966-6708
info@guilford.com
www.guilford.com

Rhoda Olkin, Author
This comprehensive volume provides the knowledge and skills
that mental health professionals need for more effective, informed work with clients with disabilities. Topics addressed include etiquette with clients with disabilities; special concerns in
assessment, evaluation, and diagnosis. Filled with clinical examples and observations, the volume also discusses strategies for
enhancing teaching, training, and research.
368 pages

**5293   Women with Visible & Invisible Disabilitiees: Multiple
Intersections, Issues, Therapies**
Routledge (Taylor & Francis Group)
711 Third Ave
New York, NY 10017
212-216-7800
800-634-7064
FAX: 202-564-7854
enquiries@taylorandfrancis.com
www.routledge.com

Martha E. Banks, Editor
Ellyn Kaschak, Editor
Addresses the issues faced by women with disabilities, examines
the social construction of disability, and makes suggestions for

the development and modification of culturally relevant therapy to meet the needs of disabled women.
414 pages Hardcover; Paperback

Specific Disabilities

5294 **inMotion Magazine**
Amputee Coalition
9303 Center St
Ste 100
Manassas, VA 20110
865-524-8772
888-267-5669
www.amputee-coalition.org
Bi-monthly

Vocations

5295 **Ability Magazine**
P.O. Box 10878
Costa Mesa, CA 92627
www.abilitymagazine.com
Bi-monthly

5296 **Demystifying Job Development: Field-Based Approaches to Job Development for the Disabled**
Training Resource Network
266 Roaring Dr.
St. Augustine, FL 32084
FAX: 904-823-3554
www.trn-store.com

David Hoff, Author
Cecilia Gandolfo, Author
Marty Gold, Author
Melanie Jordan, Author
A guide to successful placement of individuals with severe disabilities in quality jobs in the community.
105 pages

5297 **Hiring Idahoans with Disabilities**
Idaho Assistive Technology Project
University of Idaho
1187 Alturas Dr.
Moscow, ID 83843- 8331
208-885-3557
800-432-8324
FAX: 208-885-6102
idahoat@uidaho.edu
www.idahoat.orh

Jane Frederickson, Author
Kristen Hagen, Author
The purpose of this handbook is to inform employers in Idaho business and industry about the promise of hiring Idahoans with disabilities.

5298 **Life Beyond the Classroom: Transition Strategies for Young People with Disabilities**
Brookes Publishing
P.O.Box 10624
Baltimore, MD 21285-0624
410-337-9580
800-638-3775
FAX: 410-337-8539
custserv@brokespublishing.com
www.brookespublishing.com

Paul Wehman, Author
Specialists in a variety of disciplines use creative and practical techniques to ensure careful transition planning, to build young people's confidence and competence in work skills, and to foster support from businesses and community organizations for training and employment programs.
616 pages

5299 **More Than a Job: Securing Satisfying Careers for People with Disabilities**
Brookes Publishing
P.O. Box 10624
Baltimore, MD 21285-0624
800-638-3775
FAX: 410-337-8539
custserv@brookespublishing.com
www.brookespublishing.com

Paul Wehman, Editor
John Kregel, Editor
This book transforms job placement into career counseling for people with physical and developmental disabilities. It presents step-by-step guidelines for helping people with disabilities to identify their own interests.
384 pages 1998

5300 **OT Practice Magazine**
American Occupational Therapy Association
4720 Montgomery Ln
Bethesda, MD 20814-3449
301-652-6611
800-729-2682
FAX: 301-652-7711
TTY: 800-377-8555
otpractice@aota.org
www.aota.org/publications-news.aspx

5301 **Occupational Therapy and Vocational Rehabilitation**
Wiley
111 River St
Hoboken, NJ 07030-5774
201-748-6000
877-762-2974
FAX: 201-748-6088
info@wiley.com
www.wiley.com

Joanne Ross
This book introduces the occupational therapist to the practice of vocational rehabilitation. As rehabilitation specialists, Occupational Therapists work in a range of diverse settings with clients who have a variety of physical, emotional and psychological conditions. This book highlights the contribution, which can be made by occupational therapists in assisting disabled, ill or injured workers to access, remain in and return to work.
280 pages Paperback

5302 **Teaching Chemistry to Students with Disabilities: A Manual**
American Chemical Society
1155 16th St NW
Washington, DC 20036-4839
202-872-4600
800-227-5558
FAX: 202-872-4574
TTY: 202-872-6355
cwd@acs.org
www.acs.org

Todd Pagano, Author
Annemarie Ross, Author
Promotes the full involvement of individuals with physical and learning disabilities in educational and career opportunities in the chemical and allied sciences. CWD members lead the American Chemical Society's efforts to help: individuals with disabilities who seek education or employment in chemical and allied sciences; employers and educators of persons with disabilities; other committees, offices and members of ACS who are interested in the full involvement of persons with disabilities.

5303 **Work and Disability: Contexts, Issues & Strategies for Enhancing Employment Outcomes**
PRO-ED Inc.
8700 Shoal Creek Blvd
Austin, TX 78757-6897
512-451-3246
800-897-3202
FAX: 800-397-7633
general@proedinc.com
www.proedinc.com

Edna Mora Szymanski, Editor
Randall M. Parker, Editor

492 pages

Media, Electronic

Audio/Visual

5304 A Place for MeEducational Productions
Educational Productions
9000 SW Gemini Dr
Beaverton, OR 97008-7151   503-644-7000
                                         800-950-4949
                                         FAX: 503-350-7000
                                         custserve@edpro.com
                                         www.teachingstrategies.com
Diane Trister Dodge, Founder/President/Lead Author
Arnitra Duckett, VP, Sales & Strategic Marketing
In this video, parents discuss the issues they face in planning for
their child's future. This program is designed to stimulate discussion of these issues and help increase awareness of the options
available in your local community.

5305 Able to LaughFanlight Productions/Icarus Films
Fanlight Productions
32 Court St.
21st Floor
Brooklyn, NY 11201-4421   718-488-8900
                                         800-876-1710
                                         FAX: 718-488-8642
                                         info@fanlight.com
                                         www.fanlight.com
Jonathan Miller, President
Patricio Guzman, Director
Meredith Miller, Sales Manager
Anthony Sweeney, Acquisitions
An exploration of the world of disability as interpreted by six pro-
fessional comedians who happen to be disabled. It is also about
the awkward ways disabled and able-bodied people relate to one
another. *$199.00*

ISBN 1-572951-05-2

5306 Acting BlindFanlight Productions/Icarus Films
Fanlight Productions
32 Court St.
21st Floor
Brooklyn, NY 11201-4421   718-488-8900
                                         800-876-1710
                                         FAX: 718-488-8642
                                         info@fanlight.com
                                         www.fanlight.com
Jonathan Miller, President
Patricio Guzman, Director
Meredith Miller, Sales Manager
Anthony Sweeney, Acquisitions
Takes audiences behind the scenes as a company of non-profes-
sional actors rehearse a play about life without sight. The per-
formers have no problem imagining themselves in these roles:
they are blind themselves. *$229.00*

5307 Adaptive Baby Care
Through the Looking Glass
3075 Adeline St
Suite 120
Berkeley, CA 94703-2577   510-848-1112
                                         800-644-2666
                                         FAX: 510-848-4445
                                         TTY: 510-848-1005
                                         tlg@lookingglass.org
                                         www.lookingglass.org
Megan Kirshbaum, Executive Director
Paul Preston, Assoc. Dir
This publication is presented as a catalyst for problem-solving regarding the development of adaptive baby care equipment. This
newest publication is designed for parents, family members and
professionals. It includes: guidelines for problem-solving baby
care barriers; photographs and descriptions of prototypes and resources for adaptive baby care equipment; adaptive baby care
techniques; adaptive baby care equipment checklist; commercial
product safety commission guidelines; and local and natio
$250.00

**5308 Adaptive Baby Care Equipment Video and Book Through
the Looking Glass**
Through the Looking Glass
3075 Adeline St
Suite 120
Berkeley, CA 94703-2577   510-848-1112
                                         800-644-2666
                                         FAX: 510-848-4445
                                         TTY: 510-848-1005
                                         tlg@lookingglass.org
                                         www.lookingglass.org
Stephanie Miyashiro, Board President
Thomas Spalding, Board Treasurer
Alice Nemon, D.S.W., Board Secretary
Christina Jopes, Board Members
Includes Adaptive Baby care Equipment: Guide Lines; Proto-
types and Resources, plus a twelve minute video. Available in
braille, large print or cassette. *$79.00*

5309 All About Attention Deficit Disorders, Revised
Parent Magic
800 Roosevelt Rd
B-309
Glen Ellyn, IL 60137-5839   630-208-0031
                                         800-442-4453
                                         FAX: 630-208-7366
                                         ordercenter@parentmagic.com
                                         www.parentmagic.com
Nancy Roe, Administrator/Exec Admin
Thomas Phelan, Owner/President/CEO
A psychologist and expert on ADD outlines the symptoms, diag-
nosis and treatment of this neurological disorder. Video ($49.95 -
2 parts) and audio cassette ($24.95). Also in DVD format (1
disk-$39.93).

5310 AutismAquarius Health Care Media
Aquarius Health Care Media
30 Forest Rd
PO Box 249
Millis, MA 2054-1511   508-376-1244
                                         FAX: 508-376-1245
                                         lann@aquariusproductions.com
                             www.nmm.net/storage/guide-2011/Aquarius_Hea lt
Lesile Kussmann, Owner/President/Producer
Kathy Newkirk, Director
Jane Hutchinson, Assoc. Director
This video takes you into the lives of autistic people and their
families to understand more about autism. What defines autism
and how can we help those living with the disability? Children,
teens, and adults are also profiled and we begin to see the varying
levels of development and new technology to help these people
communicate. Preview Available. *$149.00*
Video

**5311 Basic Course in American Sign Language(B100) Harris
Communications, Inc.**
Harris Communications
15155 Technology Dr
Eden Prairie, MN 55344-2273   952-906-1180
                                         800-825-6758
                                         FAX: 952-906-1099
                                         TTY: 800-825-9187
                                         info@harriscomm.com
                                         www.harriscomm.com
Robert Harris, Owner/President
Kevin Horsky, Business Director
Randall Moore, Manager
This series of four one-hour tapes is designed to illustrate the var-
ious exercises and dialogues in the text. *$39.95*
Video

5312   **Beginning ASL Video CourseHarris Communications, Inc.**
Harris Communications
15155 Technology Dr
Eden Prairie, MN 55344-2273   952-906-1180
                                               800-825-6758
                                        FAX: 952-906-1099
                                        TTY: 800-825-9187
                                        info@harriscomm.com
                                        www.harriscomm.com

Robert Harris, Owner/President
Kevin Horsky, Business Director
Randall Moore, Manager
You'll watch a family teach you to learn American Sign Language during funny and touching family situations. A total of 15 tapes in the course. *$599.40*
Video

5313   **BlindnessLandmark Media, Inc.**
Landmark Media
3450 Slade Run Dr
Falls Church, VA 22042-3940   703-241-2030
                                               800-342-4336
                                        FAX: 703-536-9540
                                        info@landmarkmedia.com
                                        www.landmarkmedia.com

Michael Hartogs, President/Owner
Joan Hartogs, Owner/Vice President
Peter Hartogs, Vice President
Richard Hartogs, Vice President
Landmark Media is an independent family-owned company currently celebrating our 28th anniversary. We have been fortunate to be able to offer the finest quality educational DVDs available. *$250.00*
Video

5314   **Boy Inside, TheFanlight Productions/Icarus Films**
Fanlight Productions
32 Court St.
21st Floor
Brooklyn, NY 11201-4421   718-488-8900
                                               800-876-1710
                                        FAX: 718-488-8642
                                        info@fanlight.com
                                        www.fanlight.com

Jonathan Miller, President
Patricio Guzman, Director
Meredith Miller, Sales Manager
Anthony Sweeney, Acquisitions
Filmmaker Marianne Kaplan tells the personal and often distressing story of her son Adam, a 12-year-old with Asperger Syndrome, during a tumultuous year in the life of their family.

5315   **Braille Documents**
Metrolina Association for the Blind
704 Louise Ave
Charlotte, NC 28204-2128   704-887-5118
                                               800-926-5466
                                        FAX: 704-372-3872
                                        bschmiel@mabnc.org
                                        www.mabnc.org

Robert Scheffel, President
Richard Hartness, Vice President, Product Design & Development
Barbara Schmiel, Vice President, Accessible Braille Services
Chris Wilkins, Vice President, Information Technology
This production shop creates Braille and large-print documents. We work with our clients to find the most cost effective solutions for their needs. Unlike other modified statement service providers, we accept your existing style of statement or allow you to design your own statement.Documents may be received in electronic data files as encrypted data sent over public networks, data sent to a file transfer protocol drop box, or data sent over a dedicated data line. ABS also accepts paper hardcopi

5316   **Bringing Out the Best**
PO Box 9177
Dept. 11W
Champaign, IL 61826-9177   217-352-3273
                                               800-519-2707
                                        FAX: 217-352-1221
                                        orders@researchpress.com
                                        www.researchpress.com

David Parkinson, Chairman
Russell Pence, President
Gail Salyards, Dir. Of Marketing/President

5317   **Business as UsualFanlight Productions/Icarus Films**
Fanlight Productions
32 Court St.
21st Floor
Brooklyn, NY 11201-4421   718-488-8900
                                               800-876-1710
                                        FAX: 718-488-8642
                                        info@fanlight.com
                                        www.fanlight.com

Jonathan Miller, President
Patricio Guzman, Director
Meredith Miller, Sales Manager
Anthony Sweeney, Acquisitions
An enlightening documentary, brings a unique international perspective to this struggle. This film examines five innovative programs which create opportunities for people with mental and physical disabilities to own and operate their own businesses. *$145.00*

5318   **Buying Time: The Media Role in Health CareFanlight Productions/Icarus Films**
Fanlight Productions
32 Court St.
21st Floor
Brooklyn, NY 11201-4421   718-488-8900
                                               800-876-1710
                                        FAX: 718-488-8642
                                        info@fanlight.com
                                        www.fanlight.com

Jonathan Miller, President
Patricio Guzman, Director
Meredith Miller, Sales Manager
Anthony Sweeney, Acquisitions
This video program is a thoughtful and disturbing examination in the role of the media in determining the allocation of health care resources. This program is a powerful tool on ethics, policy, journalism, sociology, medicine and nursing as well as for professional workshops, and continuing education programs. *$99.00*

5319   **Caring for Persons with Developmental Disabilities**
PO Box 9177
Dept. 11W
Champaign, IL 61826-9177   217-352-3273
                                               800-519-2707
                                        FAX: 217-352-1221
                                        www.researchpress.com

David Parkinson, Chairman
Russell Pence, President
Gail Salyards, Dir. Of Marketing/President

5320   **Clockworks**
Learning Corporation of America
6493 Kaiser Dr
Fremont, CA 94555-3610   510-490-7311

Oonchia Chia, Owner
Scotty, who has Down Syndrome, is fascinated by clocks. This film follows him on his adventures of employment in the clock shop.
Film

5321 Close Encounters of the Disabling Kind
Mainstream
6930 Carroll Ave
Suite 204
Takoma Park, MD 20912-4468   301-891-8777
FAX: 301-891-8778
info@mainstreaminc.org
www.mainstreaminc.org

Lillie Harrison, Information Programs Clerk
Fritz Rumpel, Editor
A training video that provides a hiring manager with information on how to learn the basics of disability etiquette and, by the end of the video, seems much better prepared and willing to interview qualified individuals with disabilities. Includes trainer and trainee guides. *$99.95*
Video

5322 Deaf Children Signers
Harris Communications
15155 Technology Dr
Eden Prairie, MN 55344-2273   952-906-1180
800-825-6758
FAX: 952-906-1099
TTY: 800-825-9187
info@harriscomm.com
www.harriscomm.com

Robert Harris, Owner
Kevin Horsky, Business Director
Randall Moore, Manager
Graduate to voicing for Deaf children ages 5-11. Adding new meaning to the phrase, Out of the mouths (hands?) of babes..., this unique tape lets eleven young children demonstrate their abilities by signing about what is important to them. *$39.95*
Video

5323 Deaf Culture Series
Harris Communicatin
15155 Technology Dr
Eden Prairie, MN 55344-2273   952-906-1180
800-825-6758
FAX: 952-906-1099
TTY: 800-825-9187
info@harriscomm.com
www.harriscomm.com

Robert Harris, Owner
Kevin Horsky, Business Director
Randall Moore, Manager
Each video in this five-part series features a topic dealing with the unique culture of deaf people. It is an excellent resource for deaf studies programs, Interpreter Preparation programs and Sign Language programs. *$49.95*
Video

5324 Deaf Mosaic
Harris Communications
15155 Technology Dr
Eden Prairie, MN 55344-2273   952-906-1180
800-825-6758
FAX: 952-906-1099
TTY: 800-825-9187
info@harriscomm.com
www.harriscomm.com

Robert Harris, Owner
Kevin Horsky, Business Director
Randall Moore, Manager
Deaf Mosaic: Deaf President Now documents the most extraordinary week in deaf history, including interviews with student leaders; exclusive footage of the demonstrations; and an interview with Gallaudet president, Dr. I. King Jordan. *$29.95*
Video

5325 Do You Hear That?
Alexander Graham Bell Association
3417 Volta Pl NW
Washington, DC 20007-2737   202-337-5220
FAX: 202-337-8314
info@agbell.org
www.agbell.org

Todd Houston, Executive Director
This video shows auditory-verbal therapy sessions of a therapist working individually with 11 children who range in age from 7 months to 7 years old and have hearing aids or cochlear implants.
Video

5326 Doing Things Together
Britannica Film Company
345 4th St
San Francisco, CA 94107-1206   415-928-8466
FAX: 415-928-5027

Dave Bekowich, Owner
Steve went with his parents to an amusement park. He met another boy named Martin who at first was shocked by Steve's prosthetic hand.
Film

5327 Emerging Leaders
Mobility International USA
132 E. Broadway
Suite 343
Eugene, OR 97401-2767   541-343-1284
FAX: 541-343-6812
info@miusa.org
www.miusa.org

Susan Sygall, CEO/Founder
Susan Dunn, Exec. Asst./Project Specialist
Cindy Lewis, Director of Programs
Estelle Coreris-Moore, Financial Manager
Pioneering short-term international disability leadership programs in the U.S. and abroad with 2,000 youth, young adults and professionals from over 100 countries. *$49.00*
Video

5328 Face FirstFanlight Productions/Icarus Films
Fanlight Productions
32 Court St.
21st Floor
Brooklyn, NY 11201-4421   718-488-8900
800-876-1710
FAX: 718-488-8642
info@fanlight.com
www.fanlight.com

Jonathan Miller, President
Patricio Guzman, Director
Meredith Miller, Sales Manager
Anthony Sweeney, Acquisitions
In this documentary, the stories told reflect the reality faced by all those who are seen as different. Despite their difficult experiences, the survival of the profiled individuals affords comic relief &, by adulthood, they possess unusual strengths that shape their careers in pediatrics, disability care, public speaking, and journalism. *$ 195.00*

5329 Family-Guided Activity-Based Intervention for Toddlers & Infants
Brookes Publishing
PO Box 10624
Baltimore, MD 21285-0624   410-337-9580
800-638-3775
FAX: 410-337-8539
custserv@brookespublishing.com
www.readplaylearn.com

Paul Brooks, Owner
This 20-minute video was created to assist early childhood professionals to incorporate therapeutic intervention into daily living. It includes a discussion and demonstration of how intervention professionals actively may involve caregivers in the

planning and implementation of activities aimed at encouraging development of a child's target skills *$37.00*
20 Minutes
ISBN 1-55766 -19-3

5330   Filmakers Library
124 E 40th St
Suite 901
New York, NY 10016-1798   212-808-4980
                                          FAX: 212-808-4983
                                          info@filmakers.com
                                          www.filmakers.com

Sue Oscar, Co-President
Linda Gottesman, Co-President
Andrea Traubner, Dir., Broadcast Sales
Filmakers Library has been a leading source of outstanding films for the education, library, and non-theatrical markets. Now, as an imprint of award-winning online publisher Alexander Street Press, Filmakers Library is able to offer online streaming access to most of our titles, ensuring that our films receive the greatest possible exposure and accessibility through the most flexible delivery platforms. We market and promote our films throughout the world by direct mail, print advertising, exhib

5331   Filmakers Library: An Imprint Of AlexanderStreet Press
124 E 40th St
Suite 901
New York, NY 10016-1798   212-808-4980
                                          FAX: 212-808-4983
                                          info@filmakers.com
                                          www.filmakers.com

Sue Oscar, Co-President
Linda Gottesman, Co-President
Andrea Traubner, Dir., Broadcast Sales
Filmakers Library has been a leading source of outstanding films for the education, library, and non-theatrical markets. Now, as an imprint of award-winning online publisher Alexander Street Press, Filmakers Library is able to offer online streaming access to most of our titles, ensuring that our films receive the greatest possible exposure and accessibility through the most flexible delivery platforms. We market and promote our films throughout the world by direct mail, print advertising, exhib
$100 - $300

5332   Films & Videos on Aging and Sensory Change
Lighthouse International
111 E 59th St
New York, NY 10022-1202   212-821-9200
                                          800-829-0500
                                          FAX: 212-821-9706
                                          info@lighthouse.org

Joanna Mellor, VP Information Services
Tara Cortes, President
Ah annotated list of over 80 films and videos dealing with age-related sensory change, divided into sections on vision impairment, hearing impairment, and multiple sensory impairments. *$5.00*

5333   Heart to HeartBlind Childrens Center, Inc
Blind Children's Center
4120 Marathon St
Los Angeles, CA 90029-3584   323-664-2153
                                          800-222-3567
                                          FAX: 323-665-3828
                                          info@blindchildrenscenter.org
                                          www.blindchildrenscenter.org

Lena French, Executive Director
Fernanda Armenta-Schmitt, PhD, Director of Education & Family Services/Assistant Executive
Muriel Scharf, Director of Development
Ross Vergara, Director of Finance
Parents of blind and partially sighted children talk about their feelings. *$35.00*
Video

5334   Helping HandsFanlight Productions/Icarus Films
Fanlight Productions
32 Court St.
21st Floor
Brooklyn, NY 11201-4421   718-488-8900
                                          800-876-1710
                                          FAX: 718-488-8642
                                          info@fanlight.com
                                          www.fanlight.com

Jonathan Miller, President
Patricio Guzman, Director
Meredith Miller, Sales Manager
Anthony Sweeney, Acquisitions
The ADA mandates equal access and opportunity for the 43 million people with disabilities in the United States. These individuals may have limited speech, sight or mobility; a developmental disability; or a medical condition which limits some life activities. Many, however, are ready, willing and very able to join the workforce. This video demonstrates that many modifications or adaptations can be made simply by using ingenuity or common sense — such as keeping the aisles clear, etc. *$145.00*
37 Minutes

5335   Home is in the Heart: Accommodating Peoplewith Disabilities in the Homestay Experience
Mobility International USA
132 E. Broadway
Suite 343
Eugene, OR 97401-2767   541-343-1284
                                          FAX: 541-343-6812
                                          info@miusa.org
                                          www.miusa.org

Susan Sygall, CEO/Founder
Susan Dunn, Exec. Asst./Project Specialist
Cindy Lewis, Director of Programs
Estelle Coreris-Moore, Financial Manager
Provides information and ideas for exchange organizations. Discusses how to recruit homestay families, meet accessibility needs and accommodate international participants with disabilities. *$49.00*
Video

5336   How Difficult Can This Be ? (Fat City)Rick Lavoie
CACLD
PO Box 210
Barnstable, MA 02630-210   508-362-1052
                                          scheduling@ricklavoie.com
                                          www.ricklavoie.com

Rick Lavoie, Film Maker
This unique program allows viewers to experience the same frustration, anxiety and tension that children with learning disabilities face in their daily lives. Teachers, social workers, psychologists, parents and friends who have participated in Richard Lavoie's workshop reflect upon their experience and the way it changed their approach to L.D. children. 1989.

5337   How We PlayFanlight Productions/Icarus Films
Fanlight Productions
32 Court St.
21st Floor
Brooklyn, NY 11201-4421   718-488-8900
                                          800-876-1710
                                          FAX: 718-488-8642
                                          info@fanlight.com
                                          www.fanlight.com

Jonathan Miller, President
Patricio Guzman, Director
Meredith Miller, Sales Manager
Anthony Sweeney, Acquisitions
Though most of the people in this new, short documentary are in wheelchairs, and one is blind, they are anything but handicapped. Playing tennis, snorkeling, whitewater canoeing, practicing karate - they are living proof that a disability can be a challenge, not an obstacle. *$99.00*

5338 I'm Not DisabledLandmark Media, Inc.
Landmark Media
3450 Slade Run Dr
Falls Church, VA 22042-3940
703-241-2030
800-342-4336
FAX: 703-536-9540
info@landmarkmedia.com
www.landmarkmedia.com

Michael Hartogs, President
Joan Hartogs, Vice President
Peter Hartogs, Vice President
Richard Hartogs, Vice President
Young people talk about their disabilities and the importance of sports in their lives. The afflictions range from blindness and missing limbs to paralysis. Through physical education and therapy they enjoy freedom of movement and participate in sports such as tennis, basketball, kayaking, skiing, and swimming. *$195.00*
Video

5339 Imagery Procedures for People with Special Needs
Research Press
PO Box 9177
Dept. 11W
Champaign, IL 61826-9177
217-352-3273
800-519-2707
FAX: 217-352-1221
rp@researchpress.com
www.researchpress.com

David Parkinson, Chairman
Russell Pence, President
Gail Salyards, Dir. Of Marketing/President
This video was developed at the Groden Center and illustrates imagery based procedures including the use of positive reinforcement, covert modeling, and a self-control triad to assists individuals to self-regulate their behaviors in stressful situations or under conditions that may evoke extreme fear. Recommended for professionals and family members interested in teaching self-control strategies that individuals with autism spectrum disorders can use in community settings. *$195.00*
32 Minutes

5340 Include Us
Exceptional Parent Library
PO Box 1807
Englewood Cliffs, NJ 7632-1207
201-947-6000
800-535-1910
FAX: 201-947-9376
eplibrary@aol.com
www.eplibrary.com

5341 Intensive Early Intervention and Beyond
PO Box 9177
Dept. 11W
Champaign, IL 61826-9177
217-352-3273
800-519-2707
FAX: 217-352-1221
www.researchpress.com

David Parkinson, Chairman
Russell Pence, President
Gail Salyards, Dir. Of Marketing/President

5342 Invisible Children
Learning Corporation of America
6493 Kaiser Dr
Fremont, CA 94555-3610
510-490-7311

Oonchia Chia, Owner
Renaldo was blind, Mandy was deaf, and Mark had Cerebral Palsy and used a wheelchair. These child-size puppet characters interacted with non-handicapped puppets.
Film

5343 Look Who's LaughingAquarius Health Care Media
Aquarius Health Care Videos
30 Forest Rd
PO Box 249
Millis, MA 2054-1511
508-376-1244
FAX: 508-376-1245
aqvideos@tiac.net
www.aquariusproductions.com

Lesile Kussmann, Owner/President/Producer
Kathy Newkirk, Director
Jane Hutchinson, Assoc. Director
This video is packed with laugh-out-loud comedic moments, but is also full of intelligent and inspiring messages. Look Who's Laughing introduces viewers to some of today's funniest comedians - who just happen to be physically disabled. We hear them talk openly and honestly about their limitations as well as their abilities and talents. Helpful for those who work with the disabled and motivational to both the disabled and able-bodied. Preview option available. *$95.00*
Video

5344 My Body is Not Who I AmAquarius Health Care Media
Aquarius Health Care Videos
30 Forest Rd
PO Box 249
Millis, MA 2054-1511
508-376-1244
FAX: 508-376-1245
aqvideos@tiac.net
www.aquariusproductions.com

Lesile Kussmann, Owner/President/Producer
Kathy Newkirk, Director
Jane Hutchinson, Assoc. Director
This thought-provoking video introduces viewers to people who openly discuss the struggles and triumphs they have experienced living in a body that is physically disabled. They talk honestly about the social stigma of their disability and the problems they face in terms of mobility, health care and family relationships, as well as the challenges of emotional and sexual intimacy. Preview option available. *$195.00*
Video

5345 My CountryAquarius Health Care Media
Aquarius Health Care Videos
30 Forest Rd
PO Box 249
Millis, MA 2054-1511
508-376-1244
FAX: 508-376-1245
aqvideos@tiac.net
www.aquariusproductions.com

Lesile Kussmann, Owner/President/Producer
Kathy Newkirk, Director
Jane Hutchinson, Assoc. Director
By telling the stories of three people with disabilities and their struggle for equal rights under the law, this film draws a powerful parallel between the efforts of disability rights activists and the civil rights struggle of the 1960s. Great for disability awareness programs, and for discussions of disability rights issues. Should be part of every college curriculum on disabilities. Awarded Best of Show Superfest 98. Preview option available. *$195.00*
Video

5346 No BarriersAquarius Health Care Media
Aquarius Health Care Videos
30 Forest Rd
PO Box 249
Millis, MA 2054-1511
508-376-1244
FAX: 508-376-1245
aqvideos@tiac.net
www.aquariusproductions.com

Lesile Kussmann, Owner/President/Producer
Kathy Newkirk, Director
Jane Hutchinson, Assoc. Director
Everyone faces the world with different abilities and disabilities. But everyone has at least one goal in common...to break through their own barriers says Mark Wellman. Mark, a paraplegic, knows this well. No Barriers takes us into Mark's world where he defies the odds for most able bodied individuals by climbing Yosemite's Half Dome and El Capitan. This video is more than inspiring and

fun to watch...it helps one make that paradigm shift from can't do to can do! Preview option available *$90.00*
Video

5347   **On The SpectrumFanlight Productions/Icarus Films**
Fanlight Productions
32 Court St.
21st Floor
Brooklyn, NY 11201-4421
718-488-8900
800-876-1710
FAX: 718-488-8642
info@fanlight.com
www.fanlight.com

Jonathan Miller, President
Patricio Guzman, Director
Meredith Miller, Sales Manager
Anthony Sweeney, Acquisitions
Adults living with Asperger syndrome describe the ways AS has affected their lives, their work and their relationships. They discuss learning to cope with the disorder and the comfort and reinforcement of participating with others 'like them' in an Asperger's support group. 53 min. *$199.00*

5348   **Open for Business**
Disability Rights Education and Defense Fund
3075 Adeline Street
Suite 210
Berkeley, CA 94703-2219
510-644-2555
800-841-8645
FAX: 510-841-8645
info@dredf.org
www.dredf.org

Sue Henderson, Executive Director
Jenny . Kern, Esq, President/Chair
Claudia Center, Esq, Treasurer
Vikki Davis, Secretary
Documentary video captures the drama and emotions of the historic civil rights demonstration of people with disabilities in 1977, resulting in the signing of the 504 Regulations, the first Federal Civil Rights Law protecting people with disabilities. Includes contemporary news footage and news interviews with participants and demonstration leaders. *$179.00*

5349   **Open to the PublicAquarius Health Care Media**
Aquarius Health Care Videos
30 Forest Rd
PO Box 249
Millis, MA 2054-1511
508-376-1244
FAX: 508-376-1245
aqvideos@tiac.net
www.aquariusproductions.com

Lesile Kussmann, Owner/President/Producer
Kathy Newkirk, Director
Jane Hutchinson, Assoc. Director
Provides an overview of the Americans with Disabilities Act as it applies to state and local governments. The ADA doesn't provide recommendations for solving common problems, but this film could provide enough information for governments to solve some common problems without turning to high-priced consultants. Preview option available. *$125.00*
Video

5350   **Our Own RoadAquarius Health Care Media**
Aquarius Health Care Videos
30 Forest Rd
PO Box 249
Millis, MA 2054-1511
508-376-1244
FAX: 508-376-1245
aqvideos@tiac.net
www.aquariusproductions.com

Lesile Kussmann, Owner/President/Producer
Kathy Newkirk, Director
Jane Hutchinson, Assoc. Director
This video shows the disabled helping other people who are disabled and portrays the sense of pride they get from helping others. This multicultural program features many different healing techniques, and teaches the importance of helping those who are disabled become independent and productive. *$99.00*

5351   **Outsider: The Life and Art of Judith ScottFanlight Productions/Icarus Films**
Fanlight Productions
32 Court St.
21st Floor
Brooklyn, NY 11201-4421
718-488-8900
800-876-1710
FAX: 718-488-8642
info@fanlight.com
www.fanlight.com

Jonathan Miller, President
Patricio Guzman, Director
Meredith Miller, Sales Manager
Anthony Sweeney, Acquisitions
Judith Scoot has Down Syndrome, is deaf, and does not speak. Yet after 35 years of institutionalization, with the help of a sister who never gave up on her, she emerged to create a series of sculptures that have fascinated and mystified art experts and collectors around the world. 26 minutes. *$199.00*

5352   **Passion for Justice**
Fanlight Productions
32 Court St.
21st Floor
Brooklyn, NY 11201-4421
718-488-8900
800-876-1710
FAX: 718-488-8642
info@fanlight.com
www.fanlight.com

Jonathan Miller, President
Patricio Guzman, Director
Meredith Miller, Sales Manager
Anthony Sweeney, Acquisitions
An unusually penetrating examination of the question of inclusion, this is an engaging portrait of Bob Perske, the author of Unequal Justice, and a crusader for the legal rights of people with developmental disabilities. A Passion for Justice asks challenging questions about society's responsibility to this population, and about ways to protect everyone's rights to equality and justice. *$99.00*
29 Minutes

5353   **Phoenix DanceFanlight Productions/Icarus Films**
Fanlight Productions
32 Court St.
21st Floor
Brooklyn, NY 11201-4421
718-488-8900
800-876-1710
FAX: 718-488-8642
info@fanlight.com
www.fanlight.com

Jonathan Miller, President
Patricio Guzman, Director
Meredith Miller, Sales Manager
Anthony Sweeney, Acquisitions
A heroic journey of transformation and healing, Phoenix Dance challenges our expectations of what it means to be disabled. In March, 2001, renowned dancer Homer Avila discovered that the pain in his hip was cancer. A month later, his right leg and most of his hip were amputated. *$199.00*

5354   **Pool Exercise ProgramArthritis Water Exercise / Arthritis Foundation**
Arthritis Foundation Distribution Center
PO Box 932915
Atlanta, GA 31193-2915
440-872-7100
800-283-7800
FAX: 404-872-0457
aforders@arthritis.org
www.arthritis.org

John Klippel, President/CEO
This video features water exercises that will help you increase and maintain joint flexibility, strengthen and tone muscles, and increase endurance. All exercises are performed in water at chest level. No swimming skills are necessary. *$19.50*

5355 Potty Learning for Children who Experience Delay
Exceptional Parent Library
PO Box 1807
Englewood Cliffs, NJ 7632-1207

201-947-6000
800-535-1910
FAX: 201-947-9376
eplibrary@aol.com
www.eplibrary.com

5356 Pushin' ForwardFanlight Productions/Icarus Films
Fanlight Productions
32 Court St.
21st Floor
Brooklyn, NY 11201-4421

718-488-8900
800-876-1710
FAX: 718-488-8642
info@fanlight.com
www.fanlight.com

Jonathan Miller, President
Patricio Guzman, Director
Meredith Miller, Sales Manager
Anthony Sweeney, Acquisitions

Growing up poor and Latino, James Lilly was a gang member and drug dealer until, at fifteen, he was shot in the back and paralyzed. Today, he shares his story with inner city kids, and tells them about one thing that helped him move on; wheelchair racing. In Pushin' Forward he takes on the world's longest wheelchair race, from Fairbanks to Anchorage, Alaska, in six days! 39 minutes. *$229.00*

5357 Recognizing Children with Special Needs
Films Media Group
132 W. 31st St
16th Fl.
New York, NY 10001

800-322-8755
FAX: 800-678-3633
custserv@films.com
www.films.com

DVD/Video

5358 Relaxation Techniques for People with Special Needs
Research Press
PO Box 9177
Dept. 11W
Champaign, IL 61826-9177

217-352-3273
800-519-2707
FAX: 217-352-1221
rp@researchpress.com
www.researchpress.com

David Parkinson, Chairman
Russell Pence, President
Gail Salyards, Dir. Of Marketing/President

The developers discuss and demonstrate how to use special relaxation procedures with children and adolescents who have developmental disabilities. They emphasize the need for students to learn relaxation as a means of coping with stress and developing self-control. During the scenes of Dr June Groden conducting relaxation training, viewers will see how to correctly use the training procedures, how to use reinforcement during training and how to use guided imagery. 23 minutes. Includes book. *$195.00*
Video

5359 Right at HomeAquarius Health Care Media
Aquarius Health Care Videos
30 Forest Rd
PO Box 249
Millis, MA 2054

508-376-1244
FAX: 508-376-1245
aqvideos@tiac.net
www.aquariusproductions.com

Lesile Kussmann, Owner/President/Producer
Kathy Newkirk, Director
Jane Hutchinson, Assoc. Director

Shows simple solutions for complying with the Fair Hoiusing Act amendments. Emphasizes low-cost, practical solutions, and working with people with disabilities to find the best applicable solution. Ideal for people with disabilities and their families, as well as housing providers, university courses, and disability awareness organizations. Preview option is available. *$99.00*
Video

5360 Seat-A-Robics
PO Box 630064
Little Neck, NY 11363-64

718-631-4007

Daria Alinovi, President

Offers a variety of safe, affordable and medically approved video exercise programs that are listed in our video chapter. In addition the company offers two resources. The first Healthy Eating & Facts For Kids is geared specifically to health professionals and educators that work with disabled children ($39.95). The second is a recreational resource guide that stimulates children to be creative and get involved. It keeps them actively engaged while having fun and getting fit ($29.95).

5361 Shining Bright: Head Start Inclusion
Brookes Publishing
PO Box 10624
Baltimore, MD 21285-624

410-337-9580
800-638-3775
FAX: 410-337-8539
custserv@brookespublishing.com
www.readplaylearn.com

Paul Brooks, Owner

This documentary depicts the collaborative efforts of a Head Start and a local education agency to include children with severe disabilities in a Head Start program. This video addresses issues such as support for children with severe health impairments, benefits of participating in Head Start, ability of teachers with a general education background to serve children with severe disabilities, and staff relations. Includes a 28-page saddle-stitched booklet. *$45.00*
23 Minutes
ISBN 1-55766 -95-9

5362 Small DifferencesAquarius Health Care Media
Aquarius Health Care Videos
30 Forest Rd
PO Box 249
Millis, MA 2054-1511

508-376-1244
FAX: 508-376-1245
aqvideos@tiac.net
www.aquariusproductions.com

Lesile Kussmann, Owner/President/Producer
Kathy Newkirk, Director
Jane Hutchinson, Assoc. Director

What happens when you give children with and without disabilities a camera and ask them to produce a video about disabilities? The result is an uplifting, award-winning disability video that both children and adults can relate to. The kids interviewed adults and children with physical and sensory disabilities. A top-quality production that increases understanding and awareness. Winner, Columbus International Film & Video Festival. Winner, National Education Media Network. Preview option availabe *$110.00*
Video

5363 Someday's ChildEducational Productions
Educational Productions
9000 SW Gemini Dr
Beaverton, OR 97008-7151

503-644-7000
800-950-4949
FAX: 503-350-7000
custserv@edpro.com
www.edpro.com

Diane Trister Dodge, Founder/President/Lead Author
Arnitra Duckett, VP, Sales & Strategic Marketing

This video focuses on three families' search for help and information for their children with disabilities.

5364 Sound & FuryAquarius Health Care Media
Aquarius Health Care Videos
30 Forest Rd
PO Box 249
Millis, MA 2054-1511

508-376-1244
FAX: 508-376-1245
aqvideos@tiac.net
www.aquariusproductions.com

Lesile Kussmann, Owner/President/Producer
Kathy Newkirk, Director
Jane Hutchinson, Assoc. Director
This film takes viewers inside the seldom seen world of the deaf to witness a painful family struggle over a controversial medical technology called the cochlear implant. Some of the family members celebrate the implant as a long overdue cure for deafness while others fear it will destroy their language and way of life. This documentary explores this seemingly irreconcilable conflict as it illuminates the ongoing struggle for identity among deaf people today. *$195.00*
Video

5365 Special Children/Special Solutions
Option Indigo Press
2080 S Undermountain Rd
Sheffield, MA 1257-9643

413-229-8727
800-714-2779
FAX: 413-229-8727
indigo@option.org
www.optionindigo.com

Barry Kaufmans, Owner/Founder/Author
Samahria Kaufmans, Owner/Founder
This four-tape audio series presents concrete, down-to-earth, no-nonsense alternatives which are full of love and acceptance for the special child while being wholly supportive of parents, professionals and helpers who want to reach out. The accepting (nonjudgmental) attitude presented is the basis of all Samahria's work and is the foundation for the nurturing teaching process that has encouraged and helped parents, children and others to accomplish more than most would have believed. *$55.00*
Audio

5366 Technology for the DisabledLandmark Media, Inc.
Landmark Media
3450 Slade Run Dr
Falls Church, VA 22042-3940

703-241-2030
800-342-4336
FAX: 703-536-9540
info@landmarkmedia.com
landmarkmedia.com

Michael Hartogs, President
Joan Hartogs, Vice President
Peter Hartogs, Vice President
Richard Hartogs, Vice President
Physically disabled people cope with the frustrations of a body they cannot control. The computer age has made many disabled more self-reliant; armless feed themselves, the blind read newspapers and the voiceless speak through marvelous technological breakthroughs. *$195.00*
Video

5367 Three R's for Special Education: Rights, Resources, Results
Brookes Publishing
PO Box 10624
Baltimore
MD, 21 0624-624

410-337-9580
800-638-3775
FAX: 410-337-8539
custserv@brookespublishing.com
www.readplaylearn.com

Paul Brooks, Owner
This is a guide for parents, and a tool for educators. Through this video parents learn how to work through the steps of the special education system and work toward securing the best education and services for their children. Reviews the laws to protect children with disabilities in easy to understand language. Also pro-

vides a list of national organizations that can offer resources, information and advice to parents. *$49.95*
50 Minutes
ISBN 0-96461 -80-7

5368 Tools for StudentsAquarius Health Care Media
Aquarius Health Care Videos
30 Forest Rd
PO Box 249
Millis, MA 2054-1511

508-376-1244
FAX: 508-376-1245
aqvideos@tiac.net
www.aquariusproductions.com

Lesile Kussmann, Owner/President/Producer
Kathy Newkirk, Director
Jane Hutchinson, Assoc. Director
Provides a series of 26 fun occupational therapy sensory processing activities. Designed as an in-home, in-workshop, and in-class exercise leader with students. Activities include: Strenghten the muscles necessary for normal activities, provide the muscles necessary to enhance alertness and concentration, increase the ability to use good posture, help social skills and fitting in and increase coordination; concludes with emphasis on team collaboration between the student, teacher, and parents. *$99.00*
Video

5369 Video Guide to Disability AwarenessAquarius Health Care Media
Aquarius Health Care Videos
30 Forest Rd
PO Box 249
Millis, MA 2054-1511

508-376-1244
FAX: 508-376-1245
aqvideos@tiac.net
www.aquariusproductions.com

Lesile Kussmann, Owner/President/Producer
Kathy Newkirk, Director
Jane Hutchinson, Assoc. Director
President Clinton opens and concludes this informative video about disability awareness. A series of candid interviews with people who have a wide range of disabilities provide personal insights into the issues surrounding visual, hearing, physical and mental disabilities. Video comes with written reference guide and is also available with open or closed captioning. Preview option available. *$195.00*
Video

5370 Video Intensive Parenting
Systems Unlimited/LIFE Skills
1556 S 1st Ave
Iowa City, IA 52240-6007

319-356-5412

Geoffrey Lauer, Program Director
Bill Gorman, President
Ginny Kirschling, Public Information Specialist
Parents who have children with special needs share their reactions to their child's diagnosis and how they have learned to cope with their feelings. *$69.95*

5371 Vital Signs: Crip Culture Talks BackFanlight Productions/Icarus Films
Fanlight Productions
32 Court St.
21st Floor
Brooklyn, NY 11201-4421

718-488-8900
800-876-1710
FAX: 718-488-8642
info@fanlight.com
www.fanlight.com

Jonathan Miller, President
Patricio Guzman, Director
Meredith Miller, Sales Manager
Anthony Sweeney, Acquisitions
This edgy, raw video documentary explores the politics of disability through the performances, debates and late-night conversations of artists at a recent national conference of disabilities

and the art's. Vital Signs conveys the intensity, variety and vitality of disability culture today. *$225.00*
Video

5372 What About Me?Educational Productions
Educational Productions
9000 SW Gemini Dr
Beaverton, OR 97008-7151   503-644-7000
      800-950-4949
      FAX: 503-350-7000
      custserve@edpro.com
      www.teachingstrategies.com
Diane Trister Dodge, Founder/President/Lead Author
Arnitra Duckett, VP, Sales & Strategic Marketing
This video focuses on two siblings of children with disabilities. The siblings (Brian and Julie) share their perspectives, their worries, concerns and victories about living with a sibling with a disability.

5373 When Billy Broke His Head...and OtherFanlight Productions/Icarus Films
Fanlight Productions
32 Court St.
21st Floor
Brooklyn, NY 11201-4421   718-488-8900
      800-876-1710
      FAX: 718-488-8642
      info@fanlight.com
      www.fanlight.com
Jonathan Miller, President
Patricio Guzman, Director
Meredith Miller, Sales Manager
Anthony Sweeney, Acquisitions
When Billy Golfus, an award-winning journalist, became brain damaged as the result of a motor scooter accident, he joined the ranks of the 43 million Americans with disabilities, this country's largest and most invisible minority. He helped create this video, which blends humor with politics and individual experience with a chorus of voices, to explain what it is really like to live with a disability in America. #136 *$195.00*

ISBN 1-57295 -36-2

5374 When I Grow Up
Britannica Film Company
345 4th St
San Francisco, CA 94107-1206   415-928-8466
      FAX: 415-928-5027
Dave Bekowich, Owner
At a costume party each child was to come as what they wanted to be when they grew up. Some of the children had handicaps, and they talked about why their handicaps would not prevent them from fulfilling their desires.
Film

5375 When Parents Can't Fix ItFanlight Productions/Icarus Films
Fanlight Productions
32 Court St.
21st Floor
Brooklyn, NY 11201-4421   718-488-8900
      800-876-1710
      FAX: 718-488-8642
      info@fanlight.com
      www.fanlight.com
Jonathan Miller, President
Patricio Guzman, Director
Meredith Miller, Sales Manager
Anthony Sweeney, Acquisitions
This documentary looks at the lives of five families who are raising children with disabilities - the problems they face, how they have learned to cope, and the rewards and stresses of adapting to their child's condition. It explores the medical complexities and financial pressures families encounter, the emotional and physical toll on parents and siblings, and the dangers of child abuse in

this population. It offers a very realistic look at different family strengths and coping styles.
58 Min. DVD/VHS
ISBN 1-572958-76-6

5376 White Cane and WheelsFanlight Productions/Icarus Films
Fanlight Productions
32 Court St.
21st Floor
Brooklyn, NY 11201-4421   718-488-8900
      800-876-1710
      FAX: 718-488-8642
      info@fanlight.com
      www.fanlight.com
Jonathan Miller, President
Patricio Guzman, Director
Meredith Miller, Sales Manager
Anthony Sweeney, Acquisitions
Carmen and Steve once dreamed of lives on stage and screen, but their plans were cut short by her blindness and his muscular dystrophy. This program is a funny and touching exploration of a relationship filled with frustration, but held together with patience, stubborness, forgiveness, and love. 26 minutes. *$169.00*

5377 Why My Child
976 Lake Baldwin Lane
Suite 104
Orlando, FL 32814   407-895-0802
      800-313-ABDC
      staff@birthdefects.org
      www.birthdefects.org

Web Sites

5378 ADA Questions and Answers
U.S. Department of Justice, Civil Rights Division
950 Pennsylvania Ave NW
Washington, DC 20530-0001   202-514-4609
      FAX: 202-307-1197
      TTY:202-514-0716
      www.ada.gov

5379 Ability Jobs
Ability Magazine
P.O. Box 10878
Costa Mesa, CA 92627
      www.abilityjobs.com

5380 AbleApparelAffordable Adaptive Clothing and Accessories
2121 Hillside Ave
New Hyde Park, NY 11040-2712   516-873-6552
      FAX: 516-248-7308
      sales@abledata.com
      www.ableapparel.com
Mary Ann Tenaglia, Partner
Marie Harmon, Partner
Donna Lo Monica, Partner/Designer
AbleApparel is always designing and creating new products that will make Matty's life and others with disabilities a little easier. Most of the people spoken to regardless of age want to be able to wear clothes that are functional, affordable and, above all, fashionable.

5381 Abledata
8630 Fenton Street
Suite 930
Silver Spring, MD 20910- 3820   301-608-8998
      800-227-0216
      FAX: 301-608-8958
      TTY: 301-608-8912
      abledata@macrointernational.com
      www.abledata.com
Katherine Belknap, Project Director
Steve Lowe, Associate Project Manager/Webmaster
David Johnson, Publications Director
Juanita Hardy, Information Specialist

AbleData provides objective information on assistive technology and rehabilitation equipment available from domestic and international sources to consumers, organizations, professionals, and caregivers within the United States. We serve the nation's disability, rehabilitation, and senior communities.

5382   Access Unlimited
570 Hance Rd
Binghamton, NY 13903-5700   607-669-4822
                                    800-849-2143
                            FAX: 607-669-4595
                            www.accessunlimited.com

Thomas Egan, President/Owner
Tom 'TC' Cole, National Sales Manager
Adaptive transportation and mobility equipment for people with disabilities. ccess Unlimited products empower people with disabilities to regain control of their mobility.

5383   Ai Squared
130 Taconic Business Park
Manchester Center, VT 05255-9752   802-362-3612
                                          800-859-0270
                                 FAX: 802-362-1670
                                 sales@aisquared.com
                                 www.aisquared.com

David Wu, CEO
Jost Eckhardt, VP of Engineering
Doug Hacker, VP of Business Development
Scott Moore, VP of Marketing
Ai Squared has been a leader in the assistive technology field for over 20 years. Our flagship product, ZoomText, is the world's best magnification and reading software for the vision impaired. We pride ourselves on delivering the highest quality software products and superior technical support.

5384   Alternatives in Education for the Hearing Impaired (AEHI)
9300 Capitol Drive
Wheeling, IL 60090-7207   847-850-5490
                        FAX: 847-850-5493
                        info@agbms.org
                        www.agbms.org

Sandra L. Mosetick, Board President Emeritus
Bridget Chevez, Board President
Daniel Konopacki, Treasurer
Debra Trude-Suter, Ph.D., CEO/Executive Director
AEHI is a program of the Alexander Graham Bell Montessori School in Mt. Prospect, IL, that fosters literacy and empowers people with hearing impairments to achieve their full potential through unique educational options. AEHI provides Cued Speech workshops, individualized parental training and support, educational consulting, professional development opportunities, and access to a wide variety of information on Cued Speech and its benefits.

5385   American Academy of Audiology
11480 Commerce Park Drive
Suite 220
Reston, VA 20190- 4748
                                    800-222-2336
                            FAX: 703-476-5157
                            infoaud@audiology.org
                            www.audiology.org

Cheryl Kreider Carey, Executive Director
Edward Sullivan, Deputy Executive Director
Deborah Carlson, PhD, President
Shilpi Banerjee, PhD, Board Member
The American Academy of Audiology is the world's largest professional organization of, by, and for audiologists. The active membership of more than 11,000 is dedicated to providing quality hearing care services through professional development, education, research, and increased public awareness of hearing and balance disorders.

5386   American Association of People with Disabilities
2013 H Street, NW
5th Floor
Washington, DC 20006-1675   202-457-0046
                                    800-840-8844
                            FAX: 866-536-4461
                            www.aapd.com

Mark Perriello, President/CEO
Henry Claypool, Executive Vice President
Ginny Thornburgh, Director of Interfaith Initiative
TaKeisha Walker, Director of Workplace & Leadership Initiatives
The American Association of People with Disabilities is the nation's largest disability rights organization. We promote equal opportunity, economic power, independent living, and political participation for people with disabilities. Our members, including people with disabilities and our family, friends, and supporters, represent a powerful force for change.

5387   American Botanical Council
6200 Manor Rd
PO Box 144345
Austin, TX 78723-4345   512-926-4900
                                800-373-7105
                        FAX: 512-926-2345
                        abc@herbalgram.org
                        www.abc.herbalgram.org

Mark Blumenthal, Founder/Executive Director
Gayle Engels, Special Projects Director
Matthew Magruder, Art Director
Denise Meikel, Development Director
Provide education using science-based and traditional information to promote responsible use of herbal medicine - serving the public, researchers, educators, healthcare professionals, industry and media.

5388   American College of Rheumatology, Researchand Education Foundation
2200 Lake Boulevard NE
Atlanta, GA 30319-5310   404-633-3777
                        FAX: 404-633-1870
                        acr@rheumatology.org
                        www.rheumatology.org

Audrey B. Uknis, MD, President
David I. Daikh, MD, PhD, Foundation President
Jan K. Richardson, PT, PhD, O, ARHP President
E. William St.Clair, MD, Treasurer
The American College of Rheumatology's mission is advancing rheumatology. The organization represents over 8,500 rheumatologists and rheumatology health professionals around the world. The ACR offers its members the support they need to ensure that they are able to continue their innovative work by providing programs of education, research, advocacy , and practice support.

5389   American Liver Foundation
39 Broadway
Suite 2700
New York, NY 10006-3054   212-668-1000
                        FAX: 212-483-8179
                        www.liverfoundation.org

Ryan Reczek, National Director, Field Development
Rolf Taylor, National Director, Corporate Relations
Pritha Kuchaculla, National Director, Programs
David Ticker, Chief Financial Officer
Is the only national voluntary health organization dedicated to preventing, treating, and curing hepatitis and other liver and gall bladder diseases through research and education.

5390   American Mobility: Personal Mobility Solutions
60 Island St
Lawrence, MA 1840-1835   978-794-3030
                        www.americanmobility.com

David Lacroix, President
Source of Pride Scooters, Jazzy Power Chairs, personal mobility vehicles, and lift and recline chairs.

5391 American Speech-Language and Hearing Association
2200 Research Blvd
Rockville, MD 20850-3289   301-296-5700
800-638-8255
FAX: 301-296-8580
TTY: 301-296-5650
actioncenter@asha.org
www.asha.org
*Wayne A. Foster, PhD, CCC-SLP/A, Chair, Audiology Advisory
Council*
Patricia A. Prelock, PhD, CCC-SLP, President
Carolyn W. Higdon, EdD, CCC-SLP, Vice President for Finance
*Howard Goldstein, PhD, CCC-SL, Vice President for Science and
Research*
Exhibits by companies specializing in alternative and
augmentative communications products, publishers, software
and hardware compinies, and hearing aid testing equipment
manufacturers.

5392 Americans with Disabilities Act: ADA Home Page
800-514-0301
TTY:800-514-0383
webmaster@usdoj.gov
www.ada.gov

5393 Appliance 411
www.appliance411.com

5394 Arc of the United States
1825 K Street, NW
Suite 1200
Washington, DC 20006-5689   202-534-3700
800-433-5255
FAX: 202-534-3731
info@thearc.org
www.thearc.org
Gary Bass, Director
Carol Wheeler, Director
Nancy Webster, President
Ronald Brown, Vice President
We are the largest national community-based organization advocating for and serving people with intellectual and developmental
disabilities and their families. We encompass all ages and all
spectrums from autism, Down syndrome, Fragile X and various
other developmental disabilities.

**5395 Association for the Cure of Cancer of the Prostate (CaP
CURE)-Prostate Cancer Foundation**
1250 Fourth St
Suite 360
Santa Monica, CA 90401-1444   310-570-4700
800-757-2873
FAX: 310-570-4701
info@pcf.org
www.pcf.org
Mike Milken, Founder/Chairman
Jonathon Simons, MD, President/CEO
Ralph Finerman, Chief Financial Officer/Treasurer/Secretary
*Howard R. Soule, PhD, Executive Vice President /Chief Science
Officer*
CURE is a nonprofit public charity that is dedicated to supporting
prostate cancer research and hastening the conversion of research
into cures or controls.

5396 Asthma and Allergy Foundation of America
8201 Corporate Drive
Suite 1000
Landover, MD 20785-2266
800-727-8462
info@aafa.org
www.aafa.org
Lynn Hanessian, Chair
Michele Abu Carrick, LICSW, Co-Chair, Governance
Judi McAuliffe, RN, Co-Chair, Programs & Services
Calvin Anderson, Chair/Finance/Treasurer

AAFA is dedicated to improving the quality of life for people with
asthma and allergic diseases through education, advocacy and
research.

5397 Auditory-Verbal InternationalAG Bell
3417 Volta Place, NW
Washington, DC 20007-2737   202-204-4700
FAX: 202-337-8314
academy@agbell.org
www.agbell.org
Anita Bernstein, Director
Kathleen Treni, President of the Association
Cheryl Dickson, President
Focus on education, guidance, advocacy, family support and the
rigorous application of techniques to promote optimal acquision
of spoken language

5398 BDRC Newsletter
Birth Defect Research for Children
976 Lake Baldwin Ln
Ste. 104
Orlando, FL 32814   407-895-0802
FAX: 407-895-0824
staff@birthdefects.org
www.birthdefects.org
Betty Mekdeci, Executive Director
A monthly electronic newsletter offering the latest news, re-
search, and updates on birth defects.
Monthly

**5399 Cancer Immunology Research Foundation(CIRF) Cancer
Research Institute National Headquar**
Concern Foundation
One Exchang Plaza, 55 Broadway
Suite 1802
New York, NY 10006-3724   212-688-7515
800-992-2623
FAX: 212-832-9376
bbrewer@cancerresearch.org
www.cancerresearch.org
Brian M. Brewer, Director of Marketing and Communications
*Lynne Harmer, Director of Grants Administration and Special
Events*
*Alfred R. Massidas, Chief Financial Officer and Director of Human
Resources*
Alexandra S. Mulvey, Associate Director of Communications
Immunology research will discover why the immune system fails
and cancer develops. Herein lies the cure for cancer, AIDS, and
other autoimmune diseases.

5400 Cancer Immunotherapy and Gene Therapy
www.skcc.org

5401 Cancer Research Institute
One Exchang Plaza, 55 Broadway
Suite 1802
New York, NY 10006-3724   212-688-7515
800-992-2623
FAX: 212-832-9376
bbrewer@cancerresearch.org
www.cancerresearch.org
Brian M. Brewer, Director of Marketing and Communications
*Lynne Harmer, Director of Grants Administration and Special
Events*
*Alfred R. Massidas, Chief Financial Officer and Director of Human
Resources*
Alexandra S. Mulvey, Associate Director of Communications
Immunology research will discover why the immune system fails
and cancer develops. Herein lies the cure for cancer, AIDS, and
other autoimmune diseases.

5402 **Center on the Social & Emotional Foundations for Early Learning (CSEFEL)**
Vanderbilt University 110 Magnolia
Box 328 GPC
Nashville, TN 37203   615-322-8150
                                                        FAX: 615-343-1570
                                              ml.hemmeter@vanderbilt.edu
                                                www.csefel.vanderbilt.edu

Mary-Louise Hemmeter, Principal Investigator
Rob Corso, Project Coordinator
Tweety Yates, Project Coordinator
Glen Dunlap, Key Center Personnel

The center will: focus on promoting the social and emotional developmental of children as a means of preventing challenging behaviors; collaborate with existing T/TA providers for the purpose of ensuring the implementation and sustainability of practices at the local level; provide ongoing identification of training needs and preferred delivery formats of local programs and T/TA providers; disseminate evidence-based practices.

5403 **Damon Runyon Cancer Research Foundation**
Walter Winchell Foundation
One Exchange Plaza, 55 Broadway
Suite 302
New York, NY 10006-3720   212-455-0500
                                                            877-722-6237
                                                    info@damonrunyon.org
                                                     www.damonrunyon.org

Lorraine Egan, President/Chief Executive Officer
Elizabeth Portland, Director of Development
Marialice C. Pagnotta, Director of the Damon Runyon Broadway Tickets Service
Kimberly Kubert, Director of Special Events

The Damon Runyon Cancer Research Foundation funds early career cancer researchers who have the energy, drive and creativity to become leading innovators in their fields. We identify the best young scientists in the nation and support them through four award programs: our Fellowship, Pediatric Cancer Fellowship, Clinical Investigator and Innovation Awards.

5404 **DisAbility Information and Resources**
                                                      jlubin@eskimo.com
                                                         www.makoa.org

Jim Lubin, Creator/Owner

Offers dozens of links to sites with information, services and products for the disabled.

5405 **Disability Net**
                                              www.bargione.co.uk/disabled.htm

5406 **Disability Rights Activist**
                                                         www.disrights.org

5407 **Disability and Medical Resources Mall**
                                          www.icdri.org/Medical/disabilitymall.hmt

5408 **DisabilityResources.org**
Four Glatter Lane
Dept. IN
Centereach, NY 11720-1032   631-585-0290
                                                        FAX: 631-585-0290
                                               info@disabilityresources.org
                                                www.disabilityresources.org

Julie Klauber, Co-founder/Managing Editor
Avery Klauber, Co-Founder/Executive Director
Sally Rosenthal, Contributing Editor
Ruth Porfert, Editorial Assistant

Disability Resources, inc. is a nonprofit 501(c)(3) organization established to promote and improve awareness, availability and accessibility of information that can help people with disabilities live, learn, love, work and play independently.

5409 **Discover Technology**
Houston, TX   713-885-1519
                                                     dtinc8888@hotmail.com
                                                  www.discovertechnology.com

Amantha Cole, Founder

The primary mission of Discover Technology, Inc.is to create and administer computer labs for persons with disabilities, to encourage communication between persons with and without disabilities and to educate the general population about the disabled population.

5410 **Dynamic Living**
125 Old Iron Ore Road
Bloomfield, CT 06002-1315   860-683-4442
                                                            888-940-0605
                                                        FAX: 860-243-1910
                                                    info@dynamic-living.com
                                                     www.dynamic-living.com

Andrea Tannenbaum, Owner

Kitchen products, bathroom helpers, and unique daily living products that provide a convenient, comfortable, and safe environment for people with disabilities.

5411 **ElderLawAnswers.com**
150 Chesnut St
4th Floor, Box #15
Providence, RI 02903
                                                            866-267-0947
                                               support@elderlawanswers.com
                                                 www.elderlawanswers.com

Harry S. Margolis, Founder/President
Ken Coughlin, Editor
Mark Miller, Director of Product and Business Development
Wendy Miki Glaus, Attorney

Provides information about legal issues facing senior citizens and a searchable directory of attorneys.

5412 **Exploring Autism: A Look at the Genetics of Autism**
Box 3445 DUMC
Durham, NC 27710
                                                      FAX: 919-684-0952
                                                  info@exploringautism.org
                                                    www.exploringautism.org

Chantelle Wolpert, Project Director

Dedicated to helping families who are living with the challenges of autism stay informed about the exciting breakthroughs involving the genetics of autism. Report and explain new genetic research findings. Explain genetic principles as they relate to autism, provide the latest research news, and seek your imput.

5413 **FHI 360**
1825 Connecticut Ave., NW
Suite 800
Washington, DC 20009-5721   202-884-8000
                                                        FAX: 202-884-8400
                                              CareerCenterSupport@fhi360.org
                                                          www.fhi360.org

Willard Cates Jr, MD, MPH, President Emeritus
Albert J. Siemens, PhD, Chief Executive Officer
Patrick C. Fine, MS, Chief Operating Officer
Robert S. Murphy, MBA, Chief Financial Officer

FHI 360 is a nonprofit human development organization dedicated to improving lives in lasting ways by advancing integrated, locally driven solutions.

5414 Foundation Fighting Blindness
7168 Columbia Gateway Dr.
Ste 100
Columbia, MD 21046   410-423-0600
800-683-5555
FAX: 410-363-2393
TTY: 800-683-5551
info@fightblindness.org
www.blindness.org

William T. Schmidt, Chief Executive Officer
Valerie Navy-Daniels, Chief Development Officer
Stephen M. Rose, Chief Research Officer
Rhea K. Farberman, Senior Director, Communications &
Marketing
The urgent mission of the Foundation Fighting Blindness, Inc. is to drive the research that will provide preventions, treatments and ures for people affected by retinitis pigmentosa (RP), macular degeneration, Usher syndrome, and the entire spectrum of retinal degenerative diseases.

5415 Freedom Scientific
11830 31st Court North
St. Petersburg, FL 33716-1805   727-803-8000
800-444-4443
FAX: 727-803-8001
info@freedomscientific.com
www.freedomscientific.com

Lee Hamilton, President/CEO/Chairman
Mike Self, Sales Representative
Joseph McDaniel, Sales Representative
Bobby Lakey, Sales Representative
Assistive technology for blind and visually impaired computer users.

5416 Gallaudet University Press
800 Florida Ave, NE
Washington, DC 20002-3695   202-651-5488
FAX: 202-651-5489
gupress@gallaudet.edu
www.gupress.gallaudet.edu

5417 Glaucoma Research Foundation
251 Post Street
Suite 600
San Francisco, CA 94108-5017   415-986-3162
800-826-6693
question@glaucoma.org
www.glaucoma.org

Andrew Iwach, MD, Board Chair/Executive Director
Thomas r M. Brunne, President/CEO
H. Allen Bouch, Vice Chair
Fred H. Brinkmann, Treasurer
Our mission is to prevent vision loss from glaucoma by investing in innovative research, education, and support with the ultimate goal of finding a cure.

5418 Helen Beebe Speech and Hearing Center
www.helenbeebe.org

5419 Herb Research Foundation
5589 Arapahoe Ave
Suite 205
Boulder, CO 80303-8115   303-449-2265
www.herbs.org

Rob McCaleb, President
John Lowe, Director of Research
Research and public education on the health benefits of medicinal plants. Dedicated to world health through the informed use of herbs.

5420 Hypokalemic Periodic Paralysis Resource Page
155 West 68th St
Suite 1732
New York, NY 10023-5830   407-339-9499
lfeld@cfl.rr.com
www.periodicparalysis.org

Jacob Levitt, President/Medical Director
Linda Feld, Vice President
Provides understandable information on HKPP, dynamia linkage to several additional sources of helpful information on the Internet, and offers several online networking opportunities.

5421 INCLUDEnyc
Formerly Resources for Children with Special Needs
116 E. 16th St.
5th Fl.
New York, NY 10003   212-677-4650
FAX: 202-254-4070
info@includenyc.org
www.includenyc.org

Barbara Glassman, Executive Director
Todd Dorman, Senior Director of Communications and Outreach
Mariko Sakita, Director of Parent & Family Services
Lori Podvesker, Senior Manager of Disability and Education Policy
Provides free services and resources for youth and families with disabilities in all five state boroughs. Organizational services include: Parenting & Advocacy; School and Community Activities; Parent counseling and Training for students with Autism; Medicaid Waiver services; Transition and Adult Services; and Social skills and building relationships.

5422 Innovation Management Group
179 Niblick Road
Suite 454
Paso Robles, CA 93446-4845   818-701-1579
800-889-0987
FAX: 818-936-0200
sales@imgpresents.com
www.imgpresents.com

5423 Interstitial Cystitis Association
1760 Old Meadow Road
Suite 500
McLean, VA 22102-2651   703-442-2070
800-435-7422
FAX: 703-506-3266
icamail@ichelp.org
www.ichelp.org

Barbara Gordon, Co-Chair/Executive Director
Eric Zarnikow, MBA, Co-Chair
Marilynn Schreibstein, CFO
F. Neal Thompson, Treasurer
The Interstitial Cystitis Association (ICA) advocates for interstitial cystitis (IC) research dedicated to discovery of a cure and better treatments, raises awareness, and serves as a central hub for the healthcare providers, researchers and millions of patients who suffer with constant urinary urgency and frequency and extreme bladder pain called IC. (IC is also referred to as painful bladder syndrome, bladder pain syndrome, and chronic pelvic pain.)

5424 LD OnLineWETA Public Television
2775 S. Quincy Street
Arlington, VA 22206-2269   703-998-2060
FAX: 703-998-2060
ldonline@weta.org
www.ldonline.org

Noel Gunther, Executive Director
Christian Lindstrom, Director
Tina Chovanec, Director
Shalini Anand, Senior Mangager
LD OnLine seeks to help children and adults reach their full potential by providing accurate and up-to-date information and advice about learning disabilities and ADHD. The site features hundreds of helpful articles, multimedia, monthly columns by noted experts, first person essays, children's writing and artwork, a comprehensive resource guide, very active forums, and a Yel-

low Pages referral directory of professionals, schools, and products.

5425   Lyme Disease Foundation
PO Box 332
Tolland, CT 6084-332
860-870-0070
FAX: 860-870-0080
info@lyme.org
www.lyme.org

Karen Forschuer, Chairman
Thomas Forschuer, Executive Director
Provides critical information about tick-borne disease prevention, improves healthcare and funds research for solutions. 500,000 children, adults, and professionals assisted 25 countries.

5426   Mainstream Living
333 SW 9th St
Des Moines, IA 50309
515-243-8115
FAX: 515-243-5017
www.mainstreamliving.org

5427   Mainstream Online Magazine of the Able-Disabled

www.mainstream-mag.com
Cyndi Jones, Publisher
William G. Stothers, Editor
The leading news, advocacy and lifestyle magazine for people with disabilities.

5428   Microsoft Accessibility Technology for Everyone
One Microsoft Way
Redmond, WA 98052-6399
425-882-8080
800-642-7676
FAX: 425-936-7329
TTY: 800-892-5234
www.microsoft.com/enable

William Gates III, Chairman
Steven Ballmer, CEO/Director
Information about accessibility features and options included in Microsoft products.

5429   MossRehab ResourceNet
1200 West Tabor Road
Philadelphia, PA 19141-3099
215-456-9900
800-225-5567
NOSPAMkennedyd@einstein.edu
www.mossresourcenet.org
John Whyte, Owner
Ruth Lefton, COO
Anthony Allonardo, Director of Technology
MossRehab, a modern, 147-bed facility, offers comprehensive care to people with a broad range of conditions—including stroke, brain injury, orthopaedic and musculoskeletal disabilities, spinal cord dysfunction, pulmonary disorders, amputations, and other forms of disability.

5430   Multiple Sclerosis National Research Institute
11350 SW Village Parkway
Port St. Lucie, FL 34987-2352
858-597-3872
866-676-7400
FAX: 858-597-3804
info@ms-research.org
www.ms-research.org

Robin Offord, Chairman
Richard Houghten, President/CEO
Donald B. Cooper, C.F.O
Karen Douthitt, VP & Corporate Secretary
Multiple Sclerosis National Research Institute is a division of Torrey Pines Institute for Molecular Studies, a not-for-profit basic research center dedicated to the discovery and development of innovative research methods that lead to treatments for major medical conditions, including multiple sclerosis, AIDS, Alzheimer's disease, pain, heart disease, many types of cancer, and more.

5431   National Alliance of the Disabled(NAOTD)

turtle@dnaco.net
www.naotd.wheelboat.com
Walton Dutcher, Executive Director/Operations
Fred Temple, Director
Spike Spikberg, Director
Donna Eustice, Director
The National Alliance OF The DisAbled is an online informational and advocacy organization dedicated to working towards gaining equal rights for the disAbled in all areas of life.

5432   National Association for Visually Handicapped Lighthouse International
111 E 59th St
New York, NY 10022-1202
212-821-9497
800-829-0500
FAX: 212-821-9707
TTY: 212-821-9713
kcampbell@lighthouse.org
www.lighthouse.org/navh

Karen Campbell, Director of Social Services
Mark Ackermann, President/CEO
Jonathan Wainwright, VP & Secretary
Since 1905, Lighthouse International has led the charge in the fight against vision loss through prevention, treatment and empowerment.

5433   National Brain Tumor FoundationNational Brain Tumor Society
55 Chapel Street
Suite 200
Newton, MA 02458-2599
617-924-9997
800-770-8287
FAX: 617-928-9998
info@braintumor.org
www.braintumor.org

Jeffrey Kolodin, Chair
Michael Nathanson, Vice Chair
N. Paul TonThat, Executive Director
Michele Rhee, Director of Program Initiatives
An organization serving people whose lives are affected by brain tumors. The organization is dedicated to promoting a cure for brain tumors, improving the quality of life and giving hope to the brain tumor community by funding meaningful research and providing patient resources, timely information and education.

5434   National Business & Disability Council
201 I.U. Willets Road
Albertson, NY 11507-1516
516-465-1516
lfrancis@viscardicenter.org
www.business-disability.com
Michael C. Pascucci, Executive Leadership Team Chairman
Laura Francis, Executive Director
John D. Kemp, President
The NBDC is the leading resource for employers seeking to integrate people with disabilities into the workplace and companies seeking to reach them in the consumer marketplace.

5435   National Organization on Disability
77 Water Street
Suite 204
New York, NY 10005-538
646-505-1191
FAX: 646-505-1184
info@nod.org
www.nod.org
Kate Brady, Director of Research and Public Funding
Erika Byrnes, Director of Development
Dwayne D. Beason, Sr, Deputy Director, Wounded Warrior Careers Program
Howard Green, Deputy Director, Corporate Programs
Promotes full and equal participation of America's 54 million men, women, and children with disabilities in all aspects of life. Today, NOD focuses on increasing employment opportunities for the 79 percent of working-age Americans with disabilities who are not employed.

559

5436   National Rehabilitation Information Center
8400 Corporate Drive
Suite 500
Landover, MD 20785-2266   301-459-5900
                                           800-346-2742
                                      FAX: 301-459-4263
                                      TTY: 301-459-5984
                           naricinfo@heitechservice.com
                                           www.naric.com

Mark X. Odum, Director
Jessica H. Chaiken, Media and Information Services Manager
Natalie J. Collier, Library and Acquisitions Manager
Tamara J. Pyle, Library and Information Services Coordinator
Serves both professionals and the general public intersted in disability and rehabilitation.

5437   National Women's Health Resource Center
157 Broad Street
Suite 200
Red Bank, NJ 07701-2029
                                           877-986-9472
                                      FAX: 732-530-3347
                                  info@healthywomen.org
                                     www.healthywomen.org

Eve Dryer, Chair
Kathleen Dyer, Board Member
Erin Graves, Director of Communications and New Media
Elizabeth Battaglino Cahill, Chief Executive Officer
Provides information for women with disabilities, health professionals, researchers, and caretakers.

5438   NeuroControl Corporation
8333 Rockside Rd
Valley View, OH 44125-6134   216-912-0101
                                           800-378-6955
                                      FAX: 216-912-0129
                                skrebs@neurocontrol.com
                                     www.neurocontrol.com

5439   Newsletter of PA's AT Lending Library
Temple University Institute on Disabilities
1755 N 13th Street
Student Center, Room 411S
Philadelphia, PA 19122-6024   215-204-1356
                                           800-204-PIAT
                                      FAX: 215-204-6336
                                      TTY: 215-204-1805
                                        iod@temple.edu
                        www.disabilities.temple.edu/atlend

Celia Feinstein, Co-Executive Director of the Institute on Disabilities
Amy Goldman, Co-Executive Director of the Institute on Disabilities
Ann Marie, Deputy Director
Kristin Ahrens, PA Consumer & Family Training Project Assistant Director
Newsletter from the Assistive Technology Lending Library in Pennsylvania. It is produced quarterly, is free of charge, and is available online only.
4-8 pages Quarterly

5440   Office of Juvenile Justice and Delinquency Prevention
810 Seventh St NW
Washington, DC 20531-3718   202-307-5911
                                           800-851-3420
                                      FAX: 301-519-5600
                           Robert.L.Listenbee@usdoj.gov
                                          www.ojjdp.gov

Kathi Grasso, Director, Concentration of Federal Efforts Program
Robert Listenbee, Jr., Administrator
Melodee Hanes, Principal Deputy Administrator
Nancy Ayers, Deputy Administrator for Operations
The Office of Juvenile Justice and Delinquency Prevention (OJJDP) provides national leadership, coordination, and resources to prevent and respond to juvenile delinquency and victimization. OJJDP supports states and communities in their efforts to develop and implement effective and coordinated prevention and intervention programs and to improve the juvenile justice system so that it protects public safety, holds offenders ac-

countable, and provides treatment and rehabilitative services tailored

5441   Osteogenesis Imperfecta Foundation
804 W. Diamond Ave.
Suite 210
Gaithersburg, MD 20878- 1414   301-947-0083
                                          800-981-2663
                                     FAX: 301-947-0456
                                       bonelink@oif.org
                                           www.oif.org

Mary Beth Huber, Director of Program Services
Tom Costanzo, Director of Finance & Administration
Erika r Ruebensaal Carte, Director of Communications & Development
Tracy Smith Hart, Chief Executive Officer
Strives to improve the quality of life for indivduals with this brittle bone disorder through research, education, awareness, and mutual support.

5442   Quantum Technologies
25242 Arctic Ocean Drive
Lake Forest, CA 92630-6217   949-930-3400
                                     FAX: 949-399-4600
                                       info@qtww.com
                                          www.qtww.com

Dale Rasmussen, Chairman
Alan Niedzwieck, President/Director
W. Brian Olson, Chief Executive Officer
Bradley J. Timon, Chief Financial Officer
Provides access to information and tools for independence to serve the visually impaired and those with a learning disability.

5443   Regional Resource Centers Program
1 Quality Street
Suite 721
Lexington, KY 40507   859-257-4921
                                     FAX: 859-257-4353
                                     TTY: 859-257-2903
                                   mike.abell@uky.edu
                                     www.rrcprogram.org

Shauna Crane, RRCP Coordinator
Perry Williams, OSEP, Team Member
Mike Abell, Team Member
Betty Beale, Team Member
The Regional Resource Centers Program provides service to all states as well as the Pacific jurisdictions, the Virgin Islands, and Puerto Rico. The six regional program centers are funded by the federal Office of Special Education Programs (OSEP) to assist state education agencies in the systemic improvement of education programs, practices, and policies that affect children and youth with disabilities.

5444   Research!America
1101 King Street
Suite 520
Alexandria, VA 22314-2960   703-739-2577
                                         800-366-2873
                                    FAX: 703-739-2372
                             info@researchamerica.org
                                 www.researchamerica.org

Hon. John Edward Porter, Chair
Hon. Michael Castle, Vice Chair
Mary Woolley, President/CEO
Barbara Love, Executive Assitant to the President
Builds active public support for more government and private-industry research to find treatments and cures for both physical and mental disorders.

5445 Social Security Online
5 Park Centre Court
Suite 100
Owings Mills, MD 21117-1

800-772-1213
TTY:800-325-0778
www.ssa.gov

Carolyn W. Colvin, Commissioner
James A. Kissko, Chief of Staff
Katherine A. Thornton, Deputy Chief of Staff
Karena L. Kilgore, Executive Secretary,Office of Executive Operations
Official website of the Social Security Administration.

5446 Special Clothes for Children
PO Box 333
E. Harwich, MA 02645-333

508-430-2410
FAX: 508-430-2410
TTY:508-430-2410
lou@lnrmusic.com
www.special-clothes.com

A catalog of adaptive clothing for children with disabilities - helping boys and girls with special needs meet the world with pride and confidence since 1987.

5447 V Foundation for Cancer Research
106 Towerview Court
Cary, NC 27513-3595

919-380-9505
800-454-6698
info@jimmyv.org
www.jimmyv.org

Sherrie Mazur, Director of Marketing & Communication
Danielle Smith, Director of Corporate and Market Development
Mark Steudel, Associate Director of Development for Prospect Research
Nick Valvano, President Emeritus
Named after basketball coach and broadcaster, Jim Valvano. The V Foundation funds critical stage research conducted by young researchers at NCI approved cancer research facilities.

5448 ValueOptions
240 Corporate Blvd.
Norfolk, VA 23502-4900

757-459-5100
FAX: 501-707-0940
TTY:877-334-0077
www.valueoptions.com

Heyward R. Donigan, President/CEO
Scott Tabakin, Chief Financial Officer
Kyle A. Raffaniello, Executive Vice President and Chief Strategy Officer
Paul Rosenberg, Executive Vice President and General Counsel
Serves over 22 million people in behavioral healthcare through publicaly funded, federal, and commercial contracts.

5449 Wardrobe Wagon: The Special Needs Clothing Store
258B Route 46 E
Fairfield, NJ 7004-2324

973-244-2414
800-992-2737
wardrobew@aol.com
www.wardrobewagon.com

E Oppenberg, President
Bonnie Oppenberg
Jerome Oppenberg, Owner
Wearing apparel for individuals with special clothing needs.

5450 We Magazine
130 William St
New York, NY 10038

646-769-2722
FAX: 212-375-6266
TTY:212-375-6235
sales@wemedia.com
www.icdri.org/NEWS/WEMedia.htm

5451 We Media
1801 Reston Parkway
Suite 300
Reston, VA 20190-4303

703-880-2659
help@wemedia.com
www.wemedia.com

Andrew Nachison, Founder
Dale Peskin, Founder
Online network for people with disabilities.

5452 WebABLE

www.hisoftware.com/press/webable.html

5453 WheelchairNet
6425 Penn Ave
Suite 401 BAKSQ, Department of Reha
Philadelphia, PA 15206

412-624-6279
ruffing@pitt.edu
www.wheelchairnet.org

Joseph Ruffing, Communications Specialist
A virtual community of people who care about wheelchairs.

5454 World Association of Persons with Disabilities
2441 N Sterling Ave
302W
Oklahoma, OK 73127-2009

405-672-4440
execvp@wapd.org
www.wapd.org

Byron R. Kerford, Founder/Leader
Thomas J. Mecke, Executive Director
Sierra Hebron, Director of Human Resources
Ashley Wardle, Director of Internet Marketing
Dedicated to improving the quality of life for those with disabilities.

Support Groups & Hotlines

General

5455 MedicAlert Foundation International
5226 Pirrone Crt
Salida, CA 95368
800-432-5378
customer_service@medicalert.org
www.medicalert.org

Barton G. Tretheway, CAE, Chairt
David Leslie, President & CEO
Melody Howard, Vice President Of Call Center Operations

A trusted emergency support network dedicated to educating
emergency responders and medical personnel for facing everyday emergency situations, as well as providing emergency care
services for members.

Toys & Games

General

5456 Age Appropriate Puzzles
7756 Winding Way
Fair Oaks, CA 95628-5735
916-961-3507
FAX: 916-961-0765
miltcher@spcglobal.net

Cheryl Meyers, President

These unique puzzles teach numerous concepts: picture, name, color and shape recognition. Each of the two themes (holidays, and clothing) comes with self-adhesive stickers that name each picture in English, Hmong, Russian, Spanish and Vietnamese. A notch at each puzzle piece makes grasping and lifting the pieces easy to use., They are designed for children from 18 months and up. Special needs children, preschool through high school would also benefit. *$9.95*

5457 All-Turn-It Spinner
AbleNet, Inc.
2625 Patton Road
Roseville, MN 55113-1308
651-294-2200
800-322-0956
FAX: 651-294-2222
customerservice@ablenetinc.com
www.ablenetinc.com

Jennifer Thalhuber, President/CEO
Cheryl Volkman, Co-founder
Bill Sproull, Chairman of the Board
William Mills, Board of Directors

The All-Turn-It Spinner is a random spinner that comes with a dice overlay allowing user's to participate in any commercially-available game that require dice. Activate the spinner with its built-in switch or connect an external switch. Overlays are interchangeable with AbleNet designed spinner games or create your own overlay. A great inclusion tool!. *$89.00*

5458 Anthony Brothers Manufacturing
Convert-O-Bike
9 Capper Drive
Dailey Industrial Park,
Pacific, MO 63069-5196
636-257-0533
800-346-6313
FAX: 636-257-5473
www.angelesstore.com

Tim Lynch, Director of Sales
David Curry, General Manager
Michelle Vondera, Customer Service Manager
Sally Perrin, National Account Manager

Manufacture wheeled toys and goods for disabled children.

5459 Automatic Card Shuffler
Maxi Aids
42 Executive Blvd
Farmingdale, NY 11735-4710
631-752-0521
800-522-6294
FAX: 631-752-0689
TTY: 631-752-0738
sales@maxiaids.com
www.maxiaids.com

5460 Backgammon Set: Deluxe
Maxi Aids
42 Executive Blvd
Farmingdale, NY 11735-4710
631-752-0521
800-522-6294
FAX: 631-752-0689
TTY: 631-752-0738
sales@maxiaids.com
www.maxiaids.com

5461 Board Games: Snakes and Ladders
Maxi Aids
42 Executive Blvd
Farmingdale, NY 11735-4710
631-752-0521
800-522-6294
FAX: 631-752-0689
TTY: 631-752-0738
sales@maxiaids.com
www.maxiaids.com

5462 Board Games: Solitaire
Maxi Aids
42 Executive Blvd
Farmingdale, NY 11735-4710
631-752-0521
800-522-6294
FAX: 631-752-0689
TTY: 631-752-0738
sales@maxiaids.com
www.maxiaids.com

5463 Braille Playing Cards: Plastic
Maxi Aids
42 Executive Blvd
Farmingdale, NY 11735-4710
631-752-0521
800-522-6294
FAX: 631-752-0689
TTY: 631-752-0738
sales@maxiaids.com
www.maxiaids.com

5464 Braille: Bingo Cards, Boards and Call Numbers
Maxi Aids
42 Executive Blvd
Farmingdale, NY 11735-4710
631-752-0521
800-522-6294
FAX: 631-752-0689
TTY: 631-752-0738
sales@maxiaids.com
www.maxiaids.com

5465 Braille: Rook Cards
Maxi Aids
42 Executive Blvd
Farmingdale, NY 11735-4710
631-752-0521
800-522-6294
FAX: 631-752-0689
TTY: 631-752-0738
sales@maxiaids.com
www.maxiaids.com

5466 Card Holder Deluxe
Maxi Aids
42 Executive Blvd
Farmingdale, NY 11735-4710
631-752-0521
800-522-6294
FAX: 631-752-0689
TTY: 631-752-0738
sales@maxiaids.com
www.maxiaids.com

5467 Cards: Musical
Sense-Sations
919 Walnut St
Philadelphia, PA 19107-5237
215-627-0600
FAX: 215-922-0692
asbinfo@asb.org
www.asb.org

Richard Forsythe, Director
Patricia Johnson, CEO
Robert Bivenour, IT Manager
Brian Rusk, Public Relations Officer

These cards, for all occasions, play music when they are opened, for the visually impaired and blind persons. *$2.50*

5468 Cards: UNO
Maxi Aids
42 Executive Blvd
Farmingdale, NY 11735-4710
631-752-0521
800-522-6294
FAX: 631-752-0689
TTY: 631-752-0738
sales@maxiaids.com
www.maxiaids.com

5469 Checker Set: Deluxe
Maxi Aids
42 Executive Blvd
Farmingdale, NY 11735-4710
631-752-0521
800-522-6294
FAX: 631-752-0689
TTY: 631-752-0738
sales@maxiaids.com
www.maxiaids.com

5470 Chess Set: Deluxe
Maxi Aids
42 Executive Blvd
Farmingdale, NY 11735-4710
631-752-0521
800-522-6294
FAX: 631-752-0689
TTY: 631-752-0738
sales@maxiaids.com
www.maxiaids.com

5471 Dice: Jumbo Size
New Vision Store
919 Walnut St
Philadelphia, PA 19107-5237
215-629-2990
www.asb.org

Richard Forsythe, Director
Patricia Johnson, CEO
Robert Bivenour, IT Manager
Brian Rusk, Public Relations Officer
The large white and black dice are over-sized and have grooved dots to indicate the numbers, for easy reading for the visually handicapped. *$4.95*

5472 Early Learning 1
MarbleSoft
12301 Central Ave NE
Suite 205
Blaine, MN 55434-4902
763-755-1402
888-755-1402
FAX: 763-862-2920
sales@marblesoft.com
www.marblesoft.com

Vicki Larson, Manager
Early learning 2.1 includes four activities that teach prereading skills. Single and dual-switch scanning are built in and special prompts allow blind students to use all levels of difficulty. Includes Matching Colors, Learning Shapes, Counting Numbers and Letter Match. Runs on Windows 98 or later and MAC OS 9 or OSX (classic not required). *$70.00*

5473 Enabling Devices
50 Broadway
Hawthorne, NY 10532-2837
914-747-3070
800-832-8697
FAX: 914-747-3480
info@enablingdevices.com
www.enablingdevices.com

Steven Kanor, Owner
Karen O'Connor, Vice President Operations
Elizabeth Bell, Marketing Manager
Enabling Devices is a company dedicated to developing affordable learning and assistive devices to help people of all ages with disabling conditions. Founded by Steven E. Kanor, Ph.D. and orginally known as Toys for Special Children, the company has been creating innovative communicators, adapted toys and switches for the physically challenged for more than 35 years.

5474 Hands-Free Controller
Nintendo
PO Box 957
Redmond, WA 98073-957
800-255-3700
www.nintendo.com

Yoshio Tsuboike, Editor-in-Chief
Nintendo controller for the physically disabled.

5475 Let's Count Braille and Tactile Numbers Poster
Maxi Aids
42 Executive Blvd
Farmingdale, NY 11735-4710
631-752-0521
800-522-6294
FAX: 631-752-0689
TTY: 631-752-0738
sales@maxiaids.com
www.maxiaids.com

5476 National Lekotek Center
2001 N. Clybourn Av.
1st Floor
Chicago, IL 60614-3716
773-528-5766
800-366-PLAY
FAX: 773-537-2992
TTY: 773-973-2180
lekotek@lekotek.org
www.lekotek.org

Elaine D. Cottey, Chair
Joanna Horsnail, Chair
Eric Gastevich, Treasurer
Carol Neiger, Secretary
Maximizes the development of children with special needs through play. Supports families through nationwide family play centers, toy lending libraries and computer play programs. Publishes six-page newsletter three times per year.

5477 New Language of Toys: Teaching Communication Skills to Children with Special Needs
Spina Bifida Association of America
4590 MacArthur Blvd,NW,
Suite 250
Washington, DC 20007- 4226
202-944-3285
800-621-314
FAX: 202-944-3295
sbaa@sbaa.org
www.spinabifidaassociation.org

Lisa Raman, Director-National Resource Center
Mary Nethercutt, National Walk Director
Christopher Vance, Director of Development
Cindy Brownstein, President /CEO
A guide for parents and teachers and a reader-friendly resource guide that provides a wealth of information on how play activities affect a child's language development and where to get the toys and materials to use in these activities. *$19.00*

5478 Puzzle Games: Cooking, Eating, Community and Grooming
PCI
PO Box 34270
San Antonio, TX 78265-4270
210-670-3866
800-594-4263
FAX: 218-210-3771
www.pci.edu.com

Janie Haugen, Program Director
Jeff McLane, President/CEO
Rebecca Phillips, Executive Director
Each game has 63 pieces which are 2 inches in size. The completed full color puzzle is 19 inch x 15 inch. Step 1 - Work the puzzle. Step 2 - Match picture or word cards to the correct space on the puzzle. These puzzles teach basic life skills. *$19.95*

5479 Single Switch Games
MarbleSoft
12301 Central Ave NE
Suite 205
Blaine, MN 55434-4902

763-755-1402
888-755-1402
888-755-1402
FAX: 763-862-2920
sales@marblesoft.com
www.marblesoft.com

Vicki Larson, Manager
Mark Larson

Theres alot of educational software for single switch users, but how about something that's just fun? We've taken some games similar to the ones you enjoyed as a kid and made them work just right for single switch users. Includes Single Switch Maze, A Frog's Life, Switching Lanes, Switch Invaders, Slingshot Gallery and Scurry. Runs on Windows 98 or later and MAC OS9 or OSX (classic not required) *$60.00*

5480 Single Switch Latch and Timer
AbleNet
2625 Patton Road
Roseville, MN 55113-1308

651-294-2200
800-322-0956
FAX: 651- 29- 225
customerservice@ablenetinc.com
www.ablenetinc.com

Bill Sproull, Chairman of the Board
William Mills, Board of Directors, Chair
Jennifer Thalhuber, President/CEO
Paul Sugden, Vice President of Finance, IT & CFO, Trustee

A Single Switch Latch and Timer allows a user to activate a battery-operated toy or appliance in the latch, timed seconds and timed minutes modes of control. Choose for one user and one device at a time. *$63.00*

5481 Socialization Games for Persons with Disabilities
Charles C. Thomas
2600 S First St
Springfield, IL 62704-4730

217-789-8980
800-258-8980
FAX: 217-789-9130
books@ccthomas.com
www.ccthomas.com

Michael P. Thomas, President
Nevalyn Nevil, Author
Marna Beatty, Author
David Moxley, Author

This text will assist those who want to teach severely multiple disabled students by providing information on: general principles of intervention and classroom organization; managing the behavior of students; physically managing students and using adaptive equipment; teaching eating skills; teaching toileting, dressing, and hygiene skills; teaching cognition, communication, and socialization skills; teaching independent living skills; and teaching infants and preschool students. *$38.95*

176 pages Paperback
ISBN 0-398067-46-5

5482 Take a Chance
Speech Bin
1965 25th Ave
Vero Beach, FL 32960-3062

772-770-0007
800-477-3324
FAX: 772-770-0006
info@speechbin.com
www.store.schoolspecialty.com

Jan J Binney, Senior Editor
Card game for practice of commonly misarticulated speech sounds. *$18.75*

16 pages Book & Cards
ISBN 0-93785 -46-7

5483 Tic Tac Toe
Maxi Aids
42 Executive Blvd
Farmingdale, NY 11735-4710

631-752-0521
800-522-6294
FAX: 631-752-0689
TTY: 631-752-0738
sales@maxiaids.com
www.maxiaids.com

5484 Turnabout Game
Maxi Aids
42 Executive Blvd
Farmingdale, NY 11735-4710

631-752-0521
800-522-6294
FAX: 631-752-0689
TTY: 631-752-0738
sales@maxiaids.com
www.maxiaids.com

Travel & Transportation

Newsletters & Books

5485 A Guide for the Wheelchair Traveler
Access for Disabled Americans
3240 Burnt Mill Drive
Orinda, CA 94563-2317
925-254-1499
FAX: 925-254-6167
psmither@aol.com
www.accessfordisabled.com

Neal Smither, President
Patricia Smither, Editor/Secretary
All you need to know when traveling in a wheelchair. *$30.00*
165 pages Paperback
ISBN 1-928616-00-3

5486 A World Awaits You
Mobility International USA
132 E. Broadway
Suite 343
Eugene, OR 97401-2767
541-343-1284
FAX: 541-343-6812
info@miusa.org
www.miusa.org

Susan Sygall, CEO/Founder
Susan Dunn, Exec. Asst./Project Specialist
Cindy Lewis, Director of Programs
Estelle Coreris-Moore, Financial Manager
A journal of success stories and tips of people with disabilities participating in international exchange programs.
40 pages Yearly

5487 Access Travel: Airports
Consumer Information Center
Department 575a
Pueblo, CO 81009-1
719-948-3334
catalog.pueblo@gsa.gov

Michael Clark, Public Affairs
Alfred Pino, Manager
Tips and suggestions for easier travel for persons with disabilities and the elderly. Lists designs, facilities, and services at 553 airport terminals worldwide.

5488 Architectural Barriers Action League
PO Box 57088
Tucson, AZ 85732-7088
520-628-8118

Martin Floerchinger, Owner
Offers guides to accessible hotels and motels across the country.

5489 Directory of Travel Agencies for the Disabled
Twin Peaks Press
PO Box 129
Vancouver, WA 98666-129
206-694-2462
800-637-2256
twinpeak@pacifier.com

David Lynch, Director
Directory lists more than 360 travel agents specializing in arrangements for people with disabilities. Handbook provides information about accessibility. *$19.95*
40 pages Paperback
ISBN 0-93326 -04-8

5490 Elderly Guide to Budget Travel/Europe
Pilot Books
PO Box 2102
Greenport, NY 11944-893
631-477-1094
FAX: 631-661-4379

5491 Ideas for Easy Travel
Accent Books & Products
PO Box 700
Bloomington, IL 61702-700
309-378-2961
800-787-8444
FAX: 309-378-4420
acmtlvng@aol.com

Raymond C Cheever, Publisher
Betty Garee, Editor
Ideal for helping the new traveler get started having fun. Points out favorite accessible high-spots as reported by two travel experts (one is disabled), and offers basic ideas to help wherever you go. *$3.25*
55 pages Paperback
ISBN 0-91570 -36-1

5492 Sports n' Spokes Magazine
Paralyzed Veterans of America
801 18th St NW
Washington, DC 20006-3517
202-872-1300
800-424-8200
888-888-2201
FAX: 202-785-4432
TTY:800-795-4327
info@pva.org
www.pva.org

Homer S. Townsend, Jr., Executive Director
Larry Dodson, National Secretary
Bill Lawson, National President
Al Kovach, Jr, Natonal Senior Vice President
Publication of the PVA, a congressionally chartered veterans service organization, with unique expertise on a wide variety of issues involving the special needs of our members— veterans of the armed forces who have experienced spinal cord injury or dysfunction.

5493 Survival Strategies for Going Abroad, A Guide for People with Disabilites
132 E. Broadway
Suite 343
Eugene, OR 97401-2767
541-343-1284
FAX: 541-343-6812
info@miusa.org
www.miusa.org

Susan Sygall, Executive Director
Melissa Mitchell, Public Relations
$16.95
225 pages

5494 Travel Information Service/Moss Rehab Hospital
Moss Rehabilitation Hospital
1200 W Tabor Rd
Philadelphia, PA 19141-3099
215-456-9900
800-225-5667
staff@mossresourcenet.org
www.mossresourcenet.org

John Whyte, Owner
Ruth Lefton, COO
Anthony Allonardo, Director of Technology
Alberto Esquenazi, Plant Manager
Offers information and resources, to telephone callers only, for persons with special traveling/accessibility needs.

5495 United States Department of the Interior National Park Service
Superintendent of Documents
1849 C St NW
Washington, DC 20240-1
202-208-3100
FAX: 202-619-7302
feedback@ios.doi.gov
www.doi.gov

Mainella, Director
Gale Norton, Chief Executive Officer
Offers an informational packet containing books, guides and tours for the disabled and elderly.

5496 **Wheelin Around**
Wheelers Handicapped Accessible Van Rentals
6614 W Sweetwater Ave
Glendale, AZ 85304-1040

602-776-8830
800-456-1371
FAX: 623-412-9920
info@wheelersvanrentals.com
www.wheelersvanrentals.com

Tammy Smith, President
Ron Smith, Corporate Treasurer
Wheelers has been breaking travel barriers through innovative service and products since 1989. Our mission is to have Wheelers rental affiliates available in every city in the United States, Canada and all around the globe. Wheelers' objective is to connect you to the best possible solution for your transportation challenges and continue to find new and innovative ways in making the world a more accessible place.

5497 **Where to Stay USA**
Council On International Educational Exchange
633 3rd Ave
New York, NY 10017-6706

212-822-2600
888-COU-NCIL
FAX: 212-822-2649

Priscilla Tovey, Information Services
A guide to low-cost lodging throughout the United States including information on whether the establishment is accessible. $15.95
250 pages
ISBN 0-67179-49-5

Associations & Programs

5498 **Access America**
Northern Cartographic
4050 Williston Rd
South Burlington, VT 5403-6062

802-860-2886
FAX: 802-865-4912

Cynthia Belliveau, President
Offers information on 36 national parks, providing detailed information on accessibility.

5499 **Access Yosemite National Park**
Special Needs Project
324 State Street
Santa Barbara, CA 93101-2364

805-962-8087
800-333-6867
books@specialneeds.com
www.specialneeds.com

Hod Gray, Owner
Represents unprecedented combinations of intensive information survey data with high quality cartography. $7.95
31 pages

5500 **American Hotel and Lodging Foundation**
1201 New York Ave NW
Suite 600
Washington, DC 20005-3931

202-289-3100
FAX: 202-289-3199
membership@ahla.com
www.ahla.com

Barbara DiRocco, Director, Conventions & Events
Katherine Lugar, President/CEO
Pam Inman, IOM, CAE, CMHS, Executive Vice President/COO
Joori Jeon, CPA, CAE, Executive Vice President/CFO, President of AH&LEF
Will disseminate information, develop and conduct a series of seminars for the hotel and motel industry at state-level association conferences, and develop and distribute an ADA Compliance handbook for use by the lodging industry.

5501 **Amtrak**
50 Massachusetts Ave NE
Washington, DC 20002-4214

202-000-1111
800-872-7245
FAX: 202-906-4564
TTY: 800-523-6590
access@w0.amtrak.com
www.amtrak.com

Joseph H. Boardman, President/CEO
Eleanor D. Acheson, Vice President, General Counsel and Corporate Secretary
Stephen J. Gardner, Vice President, NEC Infrastructure and Investment Developmen
DJ Stadtler, Vice President, Operations
Amtrak is committed to making travel for passengers with disabilities more accessible. Anyone interested should contact Amtrak's Special Services Desk at 1-800-USA-RAIL at least 24 hours in advance to arrange for special assistance. The type of equipment and accessibility vary from train to train and station to station.

5502 **Easter Seals Project ACTION**
1425 K St NW
Suite 200
Washington, DC 20005-3508

202-347-3066
800-659-6428
FAX: 202-737-7914
TTY: 202-347-7385
project_action@easterseals.com
www.projectaction.org

Judy Shanley,Ph. D, Director
Donna Smith, Director of Training
C. Marie Maus, Assistant Director
Mary Leary, Vice President
A national technical assistance program designed to improve access to transportation services for people with disabilities and assist transit providers in implementing the Americans with Disabilities Act. Publishes quarterly newsletter.

5503 **General Motors Mobility Program for Persons with Disabilities**
GM Mobility Program
PO Box 5053
Troy, MI 48007

800-323-9935
TTY:800-833-9935
www.gmmobility.com

Frederick A Henderson, CEO
GM Mobility Program provides up to $1000 reimbursement toward mobility adaptations for drivers or passengers and/or vehicle alerting devices for drivers who are deaf or hard of hearing. Provided on eligible new Chevrolet, Pontiac, Oldsmobile, Buick, Cadillac, and GMC vehicles. Complete GMC financing available. GM Mobility also offers free resource information, including list of area adaptive equipment installers, plus free resource video.

5504 **Kenny Foundation**
21700 Northwestern Hwy
Suite 730
Southfield, MI 48075-4930

810-552-0202
800-237-3422
comnet@uwcs.org

Susan Burstein, Executive Director
Provides education, advocacy & direct services to people with mobility impairments throughout Michigan. Services include Equipment Connection, a database, available online, that connects buyers & sellers of used adaptive equipment; Attitudes is a disability awareness program for 1st & 2nd graders; Information & Referral services; and Accessbility, a program that uses volunteer labor and donated materials to buid ramps for people who can't afford them.

5505

MedEscort International
PO Box 8766
Allentown, PA 18105-8766
610-791-3111
800-255-7182
FAX: 610-791-9189
serice@medescort.com
www.medescort.com

Craig Poliner, President
MedEscort International was founded over a decade ago with these basic principles and philosophies as its foundation. MedEscort has served the health care community, throughout the world, and has strived to perfect the techniques of moving patients from one place to another. Our medical staff includes registered nurses, respiratory therapists, paramedics, and physicians. MedEscort has developed comprehensive, individual aeromedical services to meet each patient's needs with a personal touch.

5506

Nantahala Outdoor Center
13077 Highway 19 W
Bryson City, NC 28713-9165
828-488-2176
888-905-7238
FAX: 828-488-2498
TTY:800-877-8339
rafting@noc.com
www.noc.com

Sutton Bacon, CEO
Nantahala Outdoor Center, the leader in outdoor recreation and education for more than 30 years, strongly encourages and supports participants with disabilities. We offer whitewater rafting adventures on six rivers in the Southeast for all skill and thrill levels for groups, also kayak and canoe adaptive instruction. NOC will tailor a whitewater program to your skill and ability level, modify the gear, and pace instruction for you. We also offer a Ropes Challenge Course and team building program

5507

Paralysis Society of America
Paralyzed Veterans of America
801 18th St NW
Washington, DC 20006-3517
202-872-1300
800-424-8200
FAX: 202-785-4432
TTY: 800-795-4327
info@pva.org
www.pva.org

Homer S. Townsend, Jr., Executive Director
Larry Dodson, National Secretary
Bill Lawson, National President
Al Kovach, Jr, Natonal Senior Vice President
A national organization whose members are people with spinal cord injury or disease, their family members and caregivers, health-care professionals, and others with an interest in the disciplines of spinal cord medicine and paralsis. One year membership includes NewsWheels, a quarterly newsletter.

5508

Shilo Inns & Resorts
11707 NE Airport Way
Portland, OR 97220-5995
503-252-7500
800-222-2244
FAX: 503-254-0794
franchiseinfo@shiloinns.com
www.shiloinns.com

Mark S. Hemstreet, Founder/Owner
Ivan Mc Affee, VP
Shilo Inns offers affordable excellence with special assist rooms at many of our locations throughout the western United States. These rooms include larger sized bathrooms equipped with assistance railings and wheelchair access. Special assist dogs are welcome free of charge ar most Shilo Inns. Call 1-800-222-2244 for details or make reservations or check out www.shiloinns.com

5509

Travelers Aid International
1612 K St. NW
Suite 206
Washington, DC 20006-2849
202-546-0599
FAX: 202-546-9112
info@travelersaid.org
www.travelersaid.org

Joan Lowden, Chair
Brian Rogers, Vice Chair
Edward Powers, Vice Chair
Jessica M. Rooney, Treasurer
Provides crisis intervention and casework services, limited financial assistance, protective travel assistance and information and referrals for travelers, transients and newcomers.

5510

US Airways/America West Airlines
4000 E Sky Harbor Blvd
Phoenix, AZ 85034-3802
480-693-0800
800-327-7810
FAX: 480-693-3702
TTY: 800-245-2966
www.usairways.org

Douglas Parker, CEO
This airline trains employees to make sure that passengers with disabilities enjoy convenient, safe and comfortable travel.

5511

US Servas
1125 16th Street
Suite 201
Arcata, CA 95521-5585
707-825-1714
FAX: 707-825-1762
info@usservas.org
www.usservas.org

Judy Sears, Administrator
International network that links travelers with hosts in 130+ countries with the hope of building world peace through understanding and friendship.
Quarterly

5512

Westin Hotels and Resorts
270 West 43rd Street
New York, NY 10036
212-201-2700
FAX: 212-201-2701
info@westinny.com
www.starwoodhotels.com

Sue A Brush, Senior VP
Westin Hotels & Resortsr indulge our guests in elements of well-being. Our refreshing ambience, innovative programs and thoughtful amenities help provide a stay that leaves you feeling better than when you arrived.

5513

Wheelers Handicapped Accessible Van Rentals
6614 W Sweetwater Ave
Glendale, AZ 85304-1040
602-418-5076
800-456-1371
FAX: 623-412-9920
info@wheelersvanrentals.com
www.wheelersvanrentals.com

Tammy Smith, President
Rental wheelchairs and scooter accessible vans. Technically advanced engineering features bring a world of independence to the user. Locations throughout the U.S. call 800-456-1371 to make reservations at any of our locations nationwide.

5514

Wilderness Inquiry
808 14th Ave SE
Minneapolis, MN 55414-1516
612-676-9400
800-728-0179
FAX: 612-676-9401
TTY: 612-676-9475
info@wildernessinquiry.org
www.wildernessinquiry.org

Greg Lais, Executive Director
Lee Friedman, Business and Outreach Director
Megan O'Hara, Youth Outdoor Employment Director
Beth Dooley, Communications Director

Allows people of all ages and abilities to share the adventure of wilderness travel. This nonprofit organization was formed in 1978 and conducts tours to some of the most beautiful and remote parts of the world.

Tours

5515   Able Trek Tours
P.O. Box 384
Reedsburg, WI 53959   608-524-3021
                                             800-205-6713
                                        FAX: 608-524-8302
                                    info@abletrektours.com
                                         abletrektours.com

5516   AccessToThePlanet
Accessible Journeys
35 W Sellers Ave
Ridley Park, PA 19078-2113   610-521-0339
                                             800-846-4537
                                        FAX: 610-521-6959
                              sales@disabilitytravel.com
                            www.accessiblejourneys.com

Howard Mc Coy, Owner
Kathy Pagliei, Director
Howard J. McCoy, President/CEO
Contains new product announcements, organizing land groups and world travel news.
Monthly

5517   Accessible Journeys
35 West Sellers Ave
Ridley Park, PA 19078-2113   610-521-0339
                                             800-846-4537
                                        FAX: 610-521-6959
                           sales@accessiblejourneys.com
                            www.accessiblejourneys.com

Howard Mc Coy, Owner
Kathy Pagliei, Director
Howard J. McCoy, President/CEO
Accessible Journeys is a vacation planner and tour operator exclusively for wheelchair travelers, their families and friends.

5518   American The Beautiful; National Parks & Federal Recreation Lands
National Parks Service
1849 C St NW
Washington, DC 20240-1   202-208-6843
                                             888-275-8747
                                        FAX: 202-219-0910
                                       webteam@ios.doi.gov
                                             www.nps.gov

Mary A Bomar, CEO
A free lifetime passport to federally operated parks, monuments, historic sites, recreation areas and wildlife refuges for persons who are blind or permanently disabled.

5519   Anglo California Travel Service
4250 Williams Rd
San Jose, CA 95129-3344   408-257-2257
                                        FAX: 408-257-2664
                                       www.acts4travel.com

Audrey Cooper, President
Plans for one and two week accessible tours.

5520   Cunard Line
24305 Town Center Drive
Suite 200
Valencia, CA 91355- 2079   305-463-3000
                                             800-528-6273
                                        FAX: 305-463-3010
                                           www.cunard.com

Pamela C Conover, CEO
Cunard Line, one of the world's most recognized brand names with a classic British heritage, operated by Cunard Line Limited,

has provided the ultimate in deluxe ocean travel experience for the past 158 years. The fleet consists of famed liner Queen Elizabeth 2 and the Caronia, a classic ship formerly identified as Vistafjord. The Cunard Line brand, the epitome of British essence, focuses on recalling the golden age of sea travel for those who missed the first.

5521   Dell Rapids Sportsmens Club
PO Box 126
Dell Rapids, SD 57022-126   605-428-3522
                                        FAX: 605-428-5502
                                   billybuckww@sio.midco.net
                                   www.sdshootingsports.org

Wayne Coffaa, President
Pat Weinacht, Vice President
Bill Weber, Secretary/Treasurer
Robin Anderson, Board Member
Offers leage shooting for trap, as well as shooting on individual basis for archery, trap and pistol.

5522   Diabetic Cruise Desk
Hartford Holidays
500 Old Country Rd
Suite 110
Garden City, NY 11530-536   516-746-6670
                                             800-828-4813
                                        FAX: 516-746-6690
                                     info@hartfordholidays.com
                                     www.hartfordholidays.com

Scott M. Kertes, President
Les Kertes, Chief Executive Officer
Stacey Ganca, Chief Financial Officer
Sally Kertes, Business Development Manager / Senior Travel Counselor
Offers a seven-day cruise to Alaska for people with diabetes. Includes seminars on diabetes, self management, planning, special guidance for exercise classes and individual dietary advice.

5523   Dialysis at Sea Cruises
2504 Merchant Ave
Odessa, FL 33556-3468   813-775-4040
                                             800-544-7604
                                             001-813-775
                                        FAX: 727-372-7396
                                       info@dialysisatsea.com
                                         www.dialysisatsea.com

Steve Debroux, Owner
Been in the business of providing travel opportunities for persons on hemodialysis and CAPD since 1977. Handle all aspects of their travel and medical requirements. Not Sold Through Travel Agents! Make all reservations and coordinates the total set-up and operation of an onboard ship mobile dialysis clinic. Cruises run from seven days to three weeks and have departures from cities around the world on a variety of cruise lines.

5524   Directions Unlimited Acccessible Tours
Empress Travel
720 N. Bedford Rd
Bedford Hills, NY 10507-1508   914-241-1700
                                             800-533-5343
                                        FAX: 914-241-0243

Lois Bonanni, Director
Charles Digiacomo, Manager
Arrange vacations throughout the world for all disabilities including accessible cruises, African safari, rafting and scuba diving, European and Caribbean vacations.

5525   Dvorak Expeditions
17921 Us Highway 285
Nathrop, CO 81236-9701   719-539-6851
                                             800-824-3795
                                        FAX: 719-539-3378
                                    info@dvorakexpeditions.com
                                    www.dvorakexpeditions.com

Bill Dvorak, Owner
Jaci Dvorak, Co-Owner

This organization does river trips for people who are deaf, visually impaired, physically or mentally disabled. Rafting trips with groups and families and whitewater instruction.

5526 Environmental Traveling Companions
Fort Mason Center, 2 Marina Blvd.
Bldg. C
San Francisco, CA 94123
415-474-7662
FAX: 415-474-3919
info@etctrips.org
www.etctrips.org

Diane Poslosky, Executive Director
Maureen O'Hagan, Associate Director
Jessica Heyman, Development Manager
Davido Crow, River Program Manager
Aids travelers regardless of physical or financial limitations to experience the beauty and challenge of the wilderness.

5527 Flying Wheels Travel
143 W. Bridge St.
PO Box 382
Owatonna, MN 55060-382
507-451-5005
877-451-5006
FAX: 507-451-1685
barbaraj@flyingwheelstravel.com
www.flyingwheelstravel.com

Barbara Jacobson, Owner
Timothy Holtz
Arranges worldwide custom independent travel and cruises for the physically challenged.

5528 Guide Service of Washington
734 15th St NW
Suite 701
Washington, DC 20005-1023
202-628-2842
FAX: 202-638-2812
sales@dctourguides.com
www.dctourguides.com

Neil Amrine, President
A guide service offering tours of Washington DC and vicinity.

5529 Guided Tour for Persons 17 & Over with Developmental and Physical Challenges
7900 Old York Rd
Suite 111-B
Elkins Park, PA 19027-2310
215-782-1370
800-783-5841
FAX: 215-635-2637
gtour400@aol.com
www.guidedtour.com

Irv Segal, DCSW, LSW, Owner/Director
Jon Fash, Administration
Lynsey Trohoske, Office/Program Co-ordinator
The Guided Tour is a very special program that offers opportunities for personal growth, recreation and socialization through travel.

5530 Hostelling North America
Hostelling International
8401 Colesville Road
Suite 600
Silver Spring, MD 20910- 6339
301-495-1240
FAX: 240-650-2094
netanya.trimboli@hiusa.org
www.hiusa.org

Russ Hedge, CEO
Demetria Trent, Manager
Netanya Trimboli, Communications & PR Manager
Hostels are very inexpensive accommodations for travelers of all ages. They provide dorm-style sleeping rooms with separate quarters for males and females, fully equipped self-service kitchens, dining areas and common rooms for relaxing and socializing. HI-AYH has hostels in major cities, in national and state parks, near beaches and in the mountains. Send for a copy of Hostelling North America, a directory of hostels in U.S. and Canada, which lists hostels that are handicap accessible. *$ 3.00*
400 pages Yearly

5531 New Courier Travel
532 Duane St
Glen Ellyn, IL 60137-4695
630-469-0511
888-777-4453
FAX: 630-469-7390
www.travelcourierinc.com

Fred Mueller, Owner
Offers specialized assistance for independent travel or tours for persons with disabilities including cruises and travel in the USA and abroad. Fee charged for out-of-state clients, long-distance calls and clients who have free air.

5532 New Directions For People With Disabilities, Inc.
5276 Hollister Avenue
Suite 207
Santa Barbara, CA 93111-3068
805-967-2841
888-967-2841
FAX: 805-964-7344
hello@newdirectionstravel.org
www.newdirectionstravel.org

Dee Duncan, Executive Director
Jeanne Mohle, Director of Operations
Danna Mead, Program Director
Colette Piacentini, Business Manager
A non-profit organization providing high quality local, national, and international travel vacations and holiday programs for people with mild to moderate developmental disabilities.

5533 Norwegian Cruise Line
7665 Corporate Center Drive
Miami, FL 33126-1201
866-234-0292
800-327-7030
FAX: 305-436-4117
www.ncl.com

Tan Sri Lim Kok Thay, Director
David Chua Ming Huat, Director
Marc J. Rowan, Director
Steve Martinez, Director
Has accessible cabins but urges mobility impaired passengers to travel in the same cabin with a person who is not mobility impaired. Cruise fares vary.

5534 ROW Adventures
202 Sherman Ave
PO Box 579
Coeur D Alene, ID 83816
208-765-0841
800-451-6034
FAX: 208-667-6506
info@rowadventures.com
www.rowadventures.com

Brad Moss, Adventure Administration - Director - Marketing & Sales
Betsy Bowen, Adventure Administration - Founder
Morag Prosser, Adventure Administration - International Sales Manager
Candy Bening, Adventure Administration - Domestic Sales Manager
Offers one to six day rafting trips to physically disadvantaged people. Designs custom itineraries, or trips with a special focus for small groups. For those with special dietary needs, they prepare special meals. So come ride the rapids and enjoy life. They also offer canoe trips aboard 34' voyager canoes along the trail of Lewis and Clark on Montana's upper Missouri River. Free brochure upon request.

5535 Sundial Special Vacations
750 Marine Dr.
Suite 100
Astoria, OR 97103
503-325-4536
800-547-9198
FAX: 503-325-4536
thomas@sundial-travel.com
www.sundialtour.com

Terry Conner, VP
Provides special vacations for developmentally disabled persons. Provides quality vacations for persons with developmental disabilities. Ratio is 1 for 7 or 1 for 5 depending on tour. Only two people to a room. Exciting destinations. 3 to 4 star properties. Great fun.

5536 Trips Inc.
P.O. Box 10885
Eugene, OR 97440

541-686-1013
800-686-1013
FAX: 541-465-9355
trips@tripsinc.com
www.tripsinc.com

Jim Peterson, President & Founder
Leslie Peterson, Executive Director
Trips Inc. Special Adventures provides travel outings to adults of various abilities in a safe, respectful and fun atmosphere. Our trips are designed for people with developmental disabilities and special needs who require staff assistance for a safe and enjoyable vacation.

5537 Ventures Travel
3600 Holly Lane N.
Suite 95
Plymouth, MN 55447-1619

952-852-0107
866-692-7400
FAX: 952-852-0123
vt@venturestravel.org
www.venturestravel.org

Nikki Adegun, Director
Lisa Moore, Director
Maggie Venell
A limited liability company is a service of Friendship Ventures-a nonprofit organization that has been enriching the lives of people with mental retardation and related developmental disabilities since 1985. Contact us to learn about our other programs, employment information, volunteer openings or donor opportunities.

5538 Wheelchair Getaways
PO Box 1098
Mukilteo, WA 98275-1098

425-353-8213
800-536-5518
FAX: 425-355-6159
info@wheelchairgetaways.com
www.wheelchairgetaways.com

Edward Van Artsdalen, Director
Wheelchair Getaways, the largest wheelchair/scooter accessible van rental company in the US, has 50 franchise locations serving major cities and airports throughout the continental US and Hawaii. Rentals by the day, week, month or longer. Delivery/pickup available.

5539 Wilderness Inquiry
808 14th Ave SE
Minneapolis, MN 55414

612-676-9400
FAX: 612-676-9401
info@wildernessinquiry.org
www.wildernessinquiry.org

Greg Lais, Executive Director
Jenny Lavine, Associate Director
Nell Holden, Programs Director
Jonathan Houlihan, Business Operations Director
Wilderness Inquiry is a non-profit adventure travel organization on a mission to connect everyone to great places through activities such as sea kayaking, canoeing, rafting, hiking, safaris and dogsledding. Adventures provide high-quality experiences featuring carefully crafted itineraries, excellent food, top-notch gear and, highly-skilled trail guides who aim to provide the very best experience possible.

Vehicle Rentals

5540 ABC Union, ACE, ANLV, Vegas Western Cab
5010 S Valley View Blvd
Las Vegas, NV 89118-1705

702-798-3498
FAX: 702-736-8813
www.lvcabs.com

Phyllis Frias, President
Charles Frias, President
Taxi service in Las Vegas that uses vans with wheelchair lifts at regular taxi rates.

5541 Accessible Vans Of America

866-224-1750
www.accessiblevans.com

5542 Avis Rent A Car
379 Parsippany Road
Parsippany, NJ 07054-5111

973-428-3900
TTY:800-331-2323
access@avis.com
www.avis.com

F Robert Salerno, President
Avis Access is a program of Avis Rent A Car that provides a full range of complementary products and services to drivers and passengers with physical disabilities. Renters can simply call the designated Avis Access Reservation line (888-TRY-HARDER) at 24 hours in advance. Products or services include transfer boards, hand controls, swivel seats, and more.

5543 Consulting & Engineering for the Handicapped (CEH)
4457 63rd Cir
Pinellas Park, FL 33781-5981

727-522-0364
866-244-1150
FAX: 727-522-9024
ceh@liftsandramps.com
www.liftsandramps.com

Al Crisp, Owner
Brenda Crisp, Owner
New vans, used vans, specializing in quad conversions, all types of handicap equipment. Celebrating 33 years in business. Hand controls, lifts & ramps, porch lifts, hand-crank bikes.

5544 Mobile Care
6201 Riverdale Rd
Suite 101
Riverdale, MD 20737-2174

301-277-7371
FAX: 301-699-1865
jaklimo@aol.com

Maurice Naccache, Manager
Specializing in non-emergency wheelchair service for the elderly and physically challenged.

5545 National Car Rental System
600 Terminal Drive
Suite 202
Fort Lauderdale, FL 33315- 3618

954-359-3020
877-222-9058
888-826-6890
FAX: 954-359-8313
www.nationalcar.com

William Decker, Manager
Accommodates special requests subject to availability. Offers hand controls, bench seats, extra mirrors and vans with lifts at many major locations.

5546 Northwest Limousine Service
9950 Lawrence Ave
Suite 314
Schiller Park, IL 60176-1216

847-698-0000
800-376-5466
chiohare@aol.com
www.oharelimousine.com

Sam Malas, Manager
Offers wheelchair accessible mini vans, sedans, stretch and super stretch limousines for hourly or daily rental.

5547 Over the Rainbow Disabled Travel Services& Wheelers Accessible Van Rentals
186 Mehani Cir
Kihei, HI 96753-8072

808-879-5521
800-303-3750
FAX: 808-871-7533

David McKown, VP
Offers the disabled traveler Hawaii airport arrangements and ticketing accessible accommodations, hotels and condos including roll-in showers, Wheelers' Accessible Van Rentals on Maui and Honolulu or cars with hand controls, personal care attendants, medical or recreational equipment rentals and activities

such as: helicopter rides, luau's, whalewatching, boating and more. Airfare varies from departure points and time of the year.

5548 Public Technology
US Department of Transportation
1301 Pennsylvania Ave NW
Washington, DC 20004
202-626-2400
FAX: 202-626-2498

J Rutter, CEO
One of a series of reports concerned with improving transportation for elderly and disabled persons.
28 pages

5549 Rehabilitation Engineering Center for Personal Licensed Transportation
University Of Virginia School Of Engineering
PO Box 400246
Charlottesville, VA 22904-4246
434-924-3072

Tom Connors, VP
Mitch Rosen, Director

5550 Wheelchair Getaways Wheelchair/Scooter Accessible Van Rentals
4443 Dixie Highway
PO Box 1098
Mukilteo, WA 98275-2864
425-353-8213
800-536-5518
FAX: 425-355-6159
info@wheelchairgetaways.com
www.wheelchairgetaways.com

Jennifer Richardson, Owner
Dale Richardson, Owner
Rebecca Heim, Manager
Moon Ko, Owner
Rents wheelchair/scooter accessible vans by the day, week, month or longer and offers delivery to major airports and other convenient locations in more than 200 cities in 42 states and Puerto Rico. Also offers full size and mini vans with automatic lifts and ramps. Some vans are equipped with hand controls, six-way power seats and remote controls for powered door operation and lifts.

5551 WheelersMarauatha Baptist Church
9120 N 95th Avenue
Peoria, AZ 85345-2501
623-937-7866
800-456-1371
FAX: 623-934-3971

Greg Iehl, Religious Leader, Pastor
Gene Noel, Assn't Pastor
Offers delivery to airports in 29 states and Washington, D.C. In about 40 cities, Wheelers works directly with Avis Rent-a-Car. Wheelers offers a variety of van configurations with capacity for up to three wheelchairs, automatic ramps or lifts and nylon tie-downs, hand controls or other modifications.

5552 Wheelers Handicapped Accessible Van Rentals
6614 W Sweetwater Ave
Glendale, AZ 85304-1040
602-418-5076
800-456-1371
FAX: 623-412-9920
info@wheelersvanrentals.com
www.wheelersvanrentals.com

Tammy Smith, President
Ron Smith, Corporate Treasurer
Wheelers has been breaking travel barriers through innovative service and products since 1989. Our mission is to have Wheelers rental affiliates available in every city in the United States, Canada and all around the globe. Wheelers' objective is to connect you to the best possible solution for your transportation challenges and continue to find new and innovative ways in making the world a more accessible place.

Veteran Services

National Administrations

5553 DAV National Service Headquarters
807 Maine Ave SW
Washington, DC 20024-2410
                                         202-554-3501
                                   FAX: 202-554-3581
                              feedback@davmail.org
                                         www.dav.org

Donald L. Samuels, Chairman
Joseph W. Johnston, Vice-Chairman
Marc Burgess, Secretary
Joseph R. Lenhart, Treasurer

Serves America's disabled veterans and their families. Direct services include legislative advocacy; professional counseling about compensation, pension, educational and job training programs and VA health care; and assistance in applying for those entitlements.

5554 Department of Medicine and Surgery Veterans Administration
810 Vermont Ave NW
Washington, DC 20420
                                         202-273-8504
                                   FAX: 202-273-9108
                                   TTY:800-273-8255
                                         www.va.gov

Eric K. Shinseki, Secretary
Stephen W. Warren, Principal Deputy Assistant Secretary
W. Todd Grams, Chief Financial Officer
Glenn D. Haggstrom, Principal Executive Director

Provides hospital and outpatient treatment as well as nursing home care for eligible veterans in Veterans Administration facilities. Services elsewhere provided on a contract basis in the United States and its territories. Provides non-vocational inpatient residential rehabilitation services to eligible legally blinded veterans of the armed forces of the United States.

5555 Department of Veterans Affairs Regional Office - Vocational Rehab Division
380 Westminster St
Providence, RI 02903-3246
                                         401-222-2488
                                         800-827-1000
                                   FAX: 401-254-1340
                              dhs.state.ri.us/dhs/dvetsff.htm
                                         www.va.gov

Eric K. Shinseki, Secretary
Stephen W. Warren, Principal Deputy Assistant Secretary
W. Todd Grams, Chief Financial Officer
Glenn D. Haggstrom, Principal Executive Director

Vocational rehabilitation is a program of services administered by the Department of Veterans Affairs for service members and veterans with service-connected physical or mental disabilities. If persons are compensibly disabled and are found in need of rehabilitation services because they have an employment handicap, this program can prepare them for a suitable job; get and keep that job; assist persons to become fully productive and independent.

5556 Department of Veterans Benefits
810 Vermont Ave NW
Suite 727
Washington, DC 20420
                                         202-461-6913
                                         800-827-1000
                                   FAX: 202-275-3689
                              vacoOAO@va.gov
                                         www.va.gov

Eric K. Shinseki, Secretary
Stephen W. Warren, Principal Deputy Assistant Secretary
W. Todd Grams, Chief Financial Officer
Glenn D. Haggstrom, Principal Executive Director

Furnishes compensation and pensions for disability and death to veterans and their dependents. Provides vocational rehabilitation services, including counseling, training, assistance and more towards employment, to blinded veterans disabled as a result of service in the armed forces during World War II, Korea and the Vietnam era; also provides rehabilitation services to certain peace-time veterans.

5557 Disabled American Veterans
PO Box 14301
Cincinnati, OH 45250-0301
                                         859-441-7300
                                         877-426-2838
                                         877-426-2838
                                   FAX: 859-441-1416
                                         www.dav.org

Donald L. Samuels, Chairman
Joseph W. Johnston, Vice-Chairman
Marc Burgess, Secretary
Joseph R. Lenhart, Treasurer

Advises veterans of their rights and employers of their obligations, under the Rehabilitation Act, the Americans with Disabilities Act, and legislation governing the employment and training of Vietnam era veterans with disabilities.

5558 Federal Benefits for Veterans and Dependents
Government Printing Office
810 Vermont Ave NW
Washington, DC 20420
                                         202-273-6763
                                         800-827-1000
                                   FAX: 202-275-3689
                                         www.benefits.va.gov

Eric K. Shinseki, Secretary
Stephen W. Warren, Principal Deputy Assistant Secretary
W. Todd Grams, Chief Financial Officer
Glenn D. Haggstrom, Principal Executive Director

Offers information on benefits for veterans and their families.
93 pages
ISBN 0-16048 -58-

5559 Hospitalized Veterans Writing Project
5920 Nall Ave
Room 101
Mission, KS 66202-3456
                                         913-432-1214
                                   FAX: 913-432-1214
                              veteransvoices@sbcglobal.net
                                         www.veteransvoices.org

Margaret (Th Clark, Veterans' Voices Editor in Chief/President HVWP/ VAVS Deputy
Jerry D. Brown, Vice President HVWP
Eileen Wirtz, Recording Secretary HVWP
Tess (John) Raydo, Treasurer HWVP

Individuals and organizations united to encourage VA veterans to write for pleasure and rehabilitation. Maintains speakers' bureau and audio tape version for the blind in Cooperation with Ku Audio. Bestows numerous monetary awards including article; book review; cartoon and drawing; light verse; poetry and short story.
$15.00
64 pages Magazine
ISSN 0504-07 9

5560 US Department of Veterans Affairs National Headquarters
1120 Vermont Ave NW
Washington, DC 20420-2
                                         202-273-5400
                                         800-827-1000
                              washingtondc.query@vba.va.gov
                                         www.va.gov

Eric K. Shinseki, Secretary
Stephen W. Warren, Principal Deputy Assistant Secretary
W. Todd Grams, Chief Financial Officer
Glenn D. Haggstrom, Principal Executive Director

Administers the laws providing benefits and other services to veterans, their dependents, and their beneficiaries. Acts as their principal advocate in ensuring that they recieve medical care, benefits, social support, and lasting memorials promoting the health, welfare, and dignity of all veterans in recognition of their service to this nation. As the DVA heads into the 21st century, they will strive to meet the needs of the Nation's veterans today and tomorrow. Publishes a monthly magazine.
80 pages

5561   US Veteran's Affairs
810 Vermont Ave NW
Washington, DC 20420-2   202-273-5400
                                      800-827-1000
                         veteransvoices@sbcglobal.net
                                      www.va.gov

Eric K. Shinseki, Secretary
Stephen W. Warren, Principal Deputy Assistant Secretary
W. Todd Grams, Chief Financial Officer
Glenn D. Haggstrom, Principal Executive Director
Provides a wide range of services for those who have been in the
military and their dependents, as well as offering information on
driver assessment and education programs.

Alabama

5562   Alabama VA Benefits Regional Office -Montgomery
U.S. Department of Veteran Affairs
345 Perry Hill Rd
Montgomery, AL 36109
                                      800-827-1000
                              FAX: 334-213-3565
                     montgomery.query@vba.va.gov
                                      www.va.gov

Cory A. Hawthorne, Director
Erica P. Worthington, Assistant Director
Jamie Bozeman, Vocational Rehabilitation & Employment Officer
Lolita McClung-Shepherd, Veterans Service Center Manager
The Veterans Benefits Administration (VBA) provides a variety
of benefits and services to Servicemembers, Veterans, and their
families.

5563   Alabama VA Medical Center - Birmingham
Veterans Health Administration U.S. Dept. of VA
700 S. 19th St
Birmingham, AL 35233   205-933-8101
                                 www.birmingham.va.gov

Thomas Smith, Director
Veterans medical clinic offering disabled veterans medical treatments.

5564   Central Alabama Veterans Healthcare System
Veterans Health Administration, U.S. Dept. of VA
215 Perry Hill Rd
Montgomery, AL 36109-3798   334-272-4670
                                      800-214-8387
                              www.centralalabama.va.gov

Paul Bockelman, Interim Director
Thomas Huettemann, Associate Director for Resources
Linda Townsend-Green, Acting Associate Director, Operations
Vic Malabonga, Chief of Staff
CAVHCS exists to provide excellent services to veterans across
the continuum of healthcare. We take pride in providing delivery
of timely quality care by staff who demonstrate outstanding customer service, the advancement of health care through research,
and the education of tomorrow's health care providers.

5565   Tuscaloosa VA Medical Center
Veterans Health Administration, U S Dept. of V A
3701 Loop Rd E
Tuscaloosa, AL 35404-5015   205-554-2000
                                      888-269-3045
                              FAX: 205-554-2845
                                 www.tuscaloosa.va.gov

John F. Merkle, Medical Center Director
*David L. Carden, Associate Director, Nursing & Patient Care Ser-
vices*
Carlos Berry, Chief of Staff
To serve America's Heroes by improving their health and
well-being through Veteran and Family Centered Care.

Alaska

5566   Alaska VA Healthcare System - Anchorage
1201 North Muldoon Road
Ste 115
Anchorage, AK 99504-5914   907-257-4700
                                      888-353-7574
                              FAX: 907-561-7183
                                      www.alaska.va.gov

Linda L. Boyle, Interim Director
Shawn Bransky, Associate Director
Veterans medical clinic offering disabled veterans medical treat-
ments.

5567   DAV Department of Alaska
2925 Debarr Rd
Room 3101
Anchorage, AK 99508-2983   907-257-4803
                              FAX: 907-258-9828
                         www.davmembersportal.org

Pamela F. Beale, Alaska Commander
Robert W. Bingham, Membership Chairman

5568   Veteran Benefits AdministrationAnchorage Regional Office
U.S. Department of Veteran Affairs
1201 Muldoon Rd
Anchorage, AK 99504   907-257-4803
                                      800-827-1000
                     anchorage.query@vba.va.gov
                         www.benefits.va.gov/anchorage

Robert A. McDonald, Secretary of Veterans
Robert D. Snyder, Chief of Staff
The Anchorage Regional Office is remotely managed by the Salt
Lake City Regional Office. The VBA operation includes a
one-stop Veterans Service Center made up of the merged Adjudi-
cation and Veterans Service Divisions. There is also a one person
Loan Guaranty Division and a Vocational Rehabilitation and
Employment Division.

Arizona

5569   Carl T Hayden VA Medical Center
Veterans Health Administration, U S Dept. of V A
650 E Indian School Rd
Phoenix, AZ 85012-1839   602-277-5551
                                      800-554-7174
                              FAX: 602-222-6472
                              g.vhacss@forum.va.gov
                                      www.phoenix.va.gov

D Gregg Gordon, President
Marva Greene, Vice President
John Fears, CEO
Linda Herrly MSW, LCSW, Caregiver Support Coordinator

5570   Northern Arizona VA Health Care System
Veterans Health Administration, US Dept. of VA
500 Hwy 89N
Prescott, AZ 86313-5001   928-445-4860
                                      800-949-1005
                              FAX: 928-768-6076
                              g.vhacss@forum.va.gov
                                      www.prescott.va.gov

Deborah Thompson, Manager

5571   Southern Arizona VA Healthcare System
Veterans Health Administration, U S Dept. of V A
3601 S 6th Ave
Tucson, AZ 85723   520-792-1450
                                               800-470-8262
                                          FAX: 520-629-1818
                                     g.vhacss@forum.va.gov
                                         www.tucson.va.gov

Jonathan H. Gardner, MPA, FACHE, Director
Jennifer S Gutowski, MHA, FACHE, Associate Director
Katie A. Landwehr, MBA, Assistant Director
Fabia Kwiecinski, MD, FACP, Chief of Staff
The Southern Arizona VA Health Care System (SAVAHCS) located in Tucson AZ serves over 170,000 Veterans located in eight counties in Southern Arizona and one county in Western New Mexico.

Arkansas

5572   Eugene J Towbin Healthcare Center
Veterans Health Administration, U S Dept. of V A
2200 Fort Roots Dr
North Little Rock, AR 72114-1706   501-257-1000
                                               800-827-1000
                                          FAX: 501-257-1779
                                     g.vhacss@forum.va.gov
                                      www.littlerock.va.gov

Michael R. Winn, Director
Toby T. Mathew, MHA/MBA, Deputy Director
Cyril O. Ekeh, MHA, Associate Director
Julie A. Brandt, MSN, RN, CNA-B, Associate Director for Patient Care Service/Nurse Executive
CAVHS is reaching out to veterans through its community-based outpatient clinics in Mountain Home, El Dorado, Hot Springs, Mena, Pine Bluff, Searcy, Conway, Russellville, its Home Health Care Service Center in Hot Springs, and a VA Drop-In Day Treatment Center for homeless veterans in downtown Little Rock.

5573   Fayetteville VA Medical Center
Veterans Health Administration, US Dept. of VA
1100 N College Ave
Fayetteville, AR 72703-1944   479-443-4301
                                               800-691-8387
                                     g.vhacss@forum.va.gov
                                     www.fayettevillear.va.gov

W. Todd Grams, Chief Financial Officer
Glenn D. Haggstrom, Principal Executive Director
Stephen W. Warren, Principal Deputy Assistant Secretary
Honor America's Veterans by providing exceptional health care that improves their health and well-being.

5574   John L McClellan Memorial Hospital
Veterans Health Administration, US Dept. of VA
4300 W 7th St
Little Rock, AR 72205-5446   501-257-1000
                                               800-827-1000
                                     g.vhacss@forum.va.gov
                                      www.littlerock.va.gov

Michael R. Winn, Director
Toby T. Mathew, MHA/MBA, Deputy Director
Cyril O. Ekeh, MHA, Associate Director
Julie A. Brandt, MSN, RN, CNA-B, Associate Director for Patient Care Service/Nurse Executive
CAVHS is reaching out to veterans through its community-based outpatient clinics in Mountain Home, El Dorado, Hot Springs, Mena, Pine Bluff, Searcy, Conway, Russellville, its Home Health Care Service Center in Hot Springs, and a VA Drop-In Day Treatment Center for homeless veterans in downtown Little Rock. Throughout its rich 90 year history, CAVHS has been widely recognized for excellence in education, research, and emergency preparedness, and -first and foremost -for a tradition of quality an

5575   North Little Rock Regional Office
Veterans Benefits Administration, U S Dept. of V A
2200 Fort Roots Drive
Building 65
N Little Rock, AR 72114-1756   501-370-3820
                                               800-827-1000
                                          FAX: 501-370-3829
                                   littlerock.query@vba.va.gov
                                             www.va.gov

Eric K. Shinseki, Secretary
Stephen W. Warren, Principal Deputy Assistant Secretary
W. Todd Grams, Chief Financial Officer
Glenn D. Haggstrom, Principal Executive Director
The Little Rock VA Regional Office offers services to veterans in the State of Arkansas and the city of Texarkana in Bowie County, Texas. Based on 2004 information provided by the Office of Policy, Planning, and Preparedness, the veteran population of Arkansas is 268,000 and the city of Texarkana, Texas, has a veteran population of 3,545. With a staff of approximately 124 employees, the Regional Office determines entitlement to disability compensation and pension, survivors' benefits, vocational

California

5576   Jerry L Pettis Memorial VA Medical Center
Veterans Health Administration, U S Dept. of V A
11201 Benton St
Loma Linda, CA 92357-1000   909-825-7084
                                               800-741-8387
                                     g.vhacss@forum.va.gov
                                       www.lomalinda.va.gov

Barbara Fallen, RD, MPA, FACHE, Acting Director
Prachi V. Asher, FACHE, Assistant Director
Dwight C. Evans, M.D., Chief of Staff
Shane M. Elliott, MBA, AD for Administration
Since 1977, VA Loma Linda Healthcare System has been improving the health of the men and women who have so proudly served our nation. We consider it our privilege to serve your health care needs in any way we can.

5577   Long Beach VA Medical Center
Veterans Health Administration, U S Dept. of V A
5901 E 7th St
Long Beach, CA 90822-5201   562-826-8000
                                               800-827-1000
                                               888-769-8387
                                     g.vhacss@forum.va.gov
                                       www.longbeach.va.gov

Isabel Duff, Medical Center Director
John M. Tryboski, MSN, Associate Director
Anthony DeFrancesco, FACHE, Associate Director
Sherrie Schuldheis, Ph.D., RN, Assistant Director, Systems Redesign

5578   Los Angeles Regional Office
Veterans Benefits Administration, U S Dept. of V A
11000 Wilshire Blvd
Los Angeles, CA 90024-3602
                                               800-827-1000
                                   losangeles.query@vba.va.gov
                                             www.va.gov

Eric K. Shinseki, Secretary
Stephen W. Warren, Principal Deputy Assistant Secretary
W. Todd Grams, Chief Financial Officer
Glenn D. Haggstrom, Principal Executive Director
The Los Angeles Regional Office (RO) provides benefits and services to approximately 706,000 veterans residing in the Southern California counties of Los Angeles, San Bernardino, Riverside, Ventura, Santa Barbara, San Luis Obispo, and Kern. VA benefits expenditures for veterans residing within the jurisdiction of the RO exceed $800 million annually. All Loan Guaranty activities for the six counties are under jurisdiction of the Phoenix Regional Office.

5579 Martinez Outpatient Clinic
Veterans Health Administration, U S Dept. of V A
150 Muir Rd
Martinez, CA 94553-4668
925-372-2000
800-382-8387
g.vhacss@forum.va.gov
www.va.gov

John H Simms, Director
Brian E. Schuman, Chief of Police
The Martinez Outpatient Clinic offers a full range of medical, surgical, mental health, and diagnostic outpatient services, including nuclear medicine, ultrasound, CT and MRI. The Center for Rehabilitation and Extended Care is located adjacent to the outpatient clinic.

5580 Oakland VA Regional Office
Veterans Benefits Administration U S Dept. of V A
1301 Clay Street
12th Floor
Oakland, CA 94612-5217
800-827-1000
oakland.query@vba.va.gov
www.benefits.va.gov/oakland

Geri Spearman, Director
The jurisdiction includes all Northern California, except for Modoc, Lassen, Alpine and Mono counties, which are assigned to the Reno Regional Office. All Loan Guaranty activities are under the jurisdiction of the Phoenix Regional Office. Seven service organizations are collocated on the eleventh floor of the Federal Office building occupied by the regional office.

5581 Rehabilitation Research and Development Center
Department of Veteran s Affairs
810 Vermont Avenue, NW
Washington, DC 94304-1207
202-443-0575
FAX: 202-495-6153
tiffany.asqueri@va.gov
www.rehab.research.va.gov
Patricia A. Dorn, Ph.D., Acting Director, Rehab R&D Service
Ricardo Gonzalez, Administrative Officer
Gloria Winford, Staff Assistant
Sarah Armstrong, Budget Technician
The VA Center of Excellence on Mobility in Palo Alto, CA is dedicated to developing innovative clinical treatments and assistive devices for veterans with physical disabilities to increase their independence and improve their quality of life. The clinical emphasis of the center is to improve mobility, either ambulation or manipulation, in individuals with neurologic impairments or orthopaedic impairments. We do not publish any printed books, journals or periodicals.

5582 Sacramento Medical Center
Veterans Health Administration U S Department of V
10535 Hospital Way
Mather, CA 95655-4200
916-843-7000
800-382-8387
g.vhacss@forum.va.gov
www.northerncalifornia.va.gov
David G. Mastalski, Interim Director
Donna Iatarola, RN, MSN, Associate Director
William T. Cahill, MD, Chief of Staff
It is an integrated health care delivery system, offering a comprehensive array of medical, surgical, rehabilitative, mental health and extended care to veterans in Northern California. The health system is comprised of a medical center in Sacramento; a rehabilitation and extended care facility in Martinez, and seven outpatient clinics.

5583 San Diego VA Regional Office
Veterans Benefits Administration, U S Dept. of V A
8810 Rio San Diego Dr
San Diego, CA 92108-1698
858-552-8585
800-827-1000
FAX: 858-552-7436
oakland.query@vba.va.gov
www.benefits.va.gov/sandiego
Janet M Peyton, Administrative Officer

The San Diego VA Regional Office provides benefit services for over 600,000 Veterans and their dependents in the Southern California Counties of Imperial, Orange, Riverside and San Diego. Since the Regional Office shares occupancy of the building with a VA Outpatient Clinic and the Employment Development Department of the State of California, it truly offers a one stop Service Center.

5584 VA Central California Health Care System
Veterans Health Administration, U S Dept. of V A
2615 E Clinton Ave
Fresno, CA 93703-2223
559-225-6100
888-826-2838
FAX: 559-268-6911
g.vhacss@forum.va.gov
www.fresno.va.gov

Joanne Krumberger, Director
Susan Shyshka, Associate Director
Patricia Richardson Ed.D, RN, N, Nursing Executive
Wessel Meyer MB ChB, FCP (SA), Chief of Staff
VA Central California Health Care System (VACCHCS) has been improving the health of the men and women who have so proudly served our nation. We consider it our privilege to serve your health care needs in any way we can.

5585 VA Greater Los Angeles Healthcare System
Veterans Health Administration U S Deptartment of
11301 Wilshire Blvd
Los Angeles, CA 90073-1003
310-478-3711
800-827-1000
FAX: 310-268-4848
g.vhacss@forum.va.gov
www.losangeles.va.gov

Donna M. Beiter, RN, MSN, Director
Christopher Sandles, Assistant Director
Marlene Brewster, RN, MSN, Acting Associate Director, Nursing and Patient Care Services
Carrie J Dekorte, Associate Director for Administration / Operations
The VA Greater Los Angeles Healthcare System is the largest, most complex healthcare system within the Department of Veterans Affairs.GLA consists of three ambulatory care centers, a tertiary care facility and 10 community based outpatient clinics. GLA serves veterans residing throughout five counties: Los Angeles, Ventura, Kern, Santa Barbara, and San Luis Obispo. There are 1.4 million veterans in the GLA service area. GLA is affiliated with both UCLA School of Medicine and USC School of Medici

5586 VA Northern California Healthcare System
Veterans Health Administration, U S Dept. of V A
150 Muir Rd
Martinez, CA 94553-4668
925-372-2000
800-382-8387
g.vhacss@forum.va.gov
www.northerncalifornia.va.gov

David G. Mastalski, Interim Director
Donna Iatarola, RN, MSN, Associate Director
William T. Cahill, MD, Chief of Staff
VA Northern California Health Care System (VANCHCS) is an integrated health care delivery system, offering a comprehensive array of medical, surgical, rehabilitative, mental health and extended care to veterans in Northern California. The health system is comprised of a medical center in Sacramento; a rehabilitation and extended care facility in Martinez, and seven outpatient clinics.

5587 VA San Diego Healthcare System
Veterans Health Administration, U S Dept. of V A
3350 La Jolla Village Dr
San Diego, CA 92161
858-552-8585
800-331-8387
g.vhacss@forum.va.gov
www.sandiego.va.gov

Jeffrey T. Gering, FACHE, Director
Cynthia Abair, MHA, Associate Director
Robert M. Smith, MD, Chief of Staff/Medical Director
Sandra Solem, PhD, RN, Associate Director, Patient Care Services/Nurse Executive

We provide medical, surgical, mental health, geriatric, spinal cord injury, and advanced rehabilitation services. VASDHS has 296 authorized beds, including skilled nursing beds and operates several regional referral programs including cardiovascular surgery and spinal cord injury. The facility also supports three Vet Centers at the following locations: Chula Vista, San Diego, and San Marcos.

Colorado

5588   Boulder Vet Center
4999 Pearl East Circle
Suite 106
Boulder, CO 80301   303-440-7306
                                            877-927-8387
                                       FAX: 303-449-3907
                                             www.va.gov

Gail N Bennett, Office Manager
Michael J Pantaleo, Team Leader
Annette Matlock, Counselor
Collette M Archibald, Counselor
Offers trauma and readjustment from military and civilian life counseling and assistance with disability claims, military benefits and employment are provided.

5589   Colorado/Wyoming VA Medical Center
Veterans Benefits Administration U S Dept. of V A
155 Van Gordon St
Suite 395
Lakewood, CO 80225   303-914-2680
                                            800-827-1000
                                   denver.query@vba.va.gov
                                          www.denver.va.gov

Forest Farley Jr, Medical Center Director
Thomas E Bowen, Chief of Staff

5590   Denver VA Medical Center
Veterans Health Administration, U S Dept. of V A
1055 Clermont St
Suite 6A138
Denver, CO 80220-3808   303-393-2869
                                            888-336-8262
                                          judi.guy@va.gov
                                          www.denver.va.gov

Lynnette Roth, Executive Director
Peggy Kearns MS, RD, FACHE, Associate Director
Judith Burke RN, MS, NEA-BC, Associate Director, Patient Care Services
Rebecca Keough MPA, VHA-CM, Assistant Director
Construction of our 1.1m sq foot, $800m replacement facility is well under way! Concrete is being poured, steel is being put in, and we're working hard to open in 2015.

5591   Grand Junction VA Medical Center
Veterans Health Administration
2121 North Ave
Grand Junction, CO 81501-6428   970-242-0731
                                            866-206-6415
                                       FAX: 970-244-1300
                                   g.vhacss@forum.va.gov
                                      www.grandjunction.va.gov

Patricia A. Hitt, MS, Acting Director
Michael Murphy, Manager
Randal France, M.D., Chief Psychiatry Service/ Int. Chf. of Staff
Angela T Brothers, AD/ Patient Care Svcs
The VAMC operates 53 beds comprised of 23 acute care and 30 Transitional Care Unit beds. The VAMC provides primary and secondary care including acute medical, surgical, and psychiatric inpatient services, as well as a full range of outpatient services.

Connecticut

5592   Hartford Regional Office
Veterans Benefits Administration U S Department of
555 Willard Ave
Building 2E
Newington, CT 6111-2631   860-666-6951
                                            800-827-1000
                                   hartford.query@vba.va.gov
                                      www.vba.va.gov/ro/hartford

Jeanette A Chirico Post, Network Director
The Hartford Regional Office now provides one-stop service to veterans and their families seeking assistance in compensation, pension, and vocational rehabilitation and employment in an accessible campus environment.

5593   Hartford Vet Center
25 Elm St
Suite A
Rocky Hill, CT 06067-2305   860-563-8800
                                            877-927-8387
                                       FAX: 860-563-8805
                                   donna.hryb@med.va.gov
                                             www.va.gov

Donna Hryb LCSW, Team Leader
Pedro Ortiz, Counselor
Amy Otzel, Counselor
Laura Hall, Military Sexual Trauma Counselor
A U.S. Department of Veterans Affairs counseling center offering counseling to Vietnam era and combat veterans. Sexual trauma/harassment counseling, medical screening and benefit referral is available to all veterans.

5594   VA Connecticut Healthcare System: Newington Division
Veterans Health Administration U S Department. of
555 Willard Ave
Newington, CT 6111-2631   860-666-6951
                                            800-827-1000
                                       FAX: 860-667-6764
                                   g.vhacss@forum.va.gov
                                      www.connecticut.va.gov

Janice M. Boss, MS, Director
Margaret Veazey, RN, MSN, Associate Director for Patient Care Services
John Callahan, Associate Director
Al Montoya, Assistant Director
The mission of VA Connecticut Healthcare Systems is to fulfill a nation's commitment to its veterans by providing quality healthcare, promoting health through prevention and maintaining excellence in teaching and research. Provides primary, secondary and tertiary care in medicine, geriatrics, neurology, psychiatry and surgery with an operating capacity of 211 hospital beds.

5595   VA Connecticut Healthcare System: West Haven
Veterans Health Administration, U S Dept. of V A
950 Campbell Ave
West Haven, CT 06516-2770   203-932-5711
                                            800-827-1000
                                       FAX: 203-937-3868
                                   g.vhacss@forum.va.gov
                                      www.connecticut.va.gov

Janice M. Boss, MS, Director
Margaret Veazey, RN, MSN, Associate Director for Patient Care Services
John Callahan, Associate Director
Al Montoya, Assistant Director
The mission of VA Connecticut Healthcare Systems is to fulfill a nation's commitment to its veterans by providing quality healthcare, promoting health through prevention and maintaining excellence in teaching and research. Provides primary, secondary and tertiary care in medicine, geriatrics, neurology, psychiatry and surgery with an operating capacity of 211 hospital beds.

Delaware

5596 **Delaware VA Regional Office**
Veterans Benefits Administration U S Dept. of V A
1601 Kirkwood Hwy
Wilmington, DE 19805-4917   302-994-2511
                                  800-461-8262
                             FAX: 302-633-5516
                             wilmington.query@vba.va.gov
                             www.wilmington.va.gov
Daniel D. Hendee, FACHE, MHA, Director
Mary Alice Johnson, MS, RN, Associate Director for Patient Care
Services
William E. England, Associate Director for Finance and Operations
Enrique Guttin, MD, MMM, CPE,, Chief of Staff
We offer comprehensive services ranging from preventive
screenings to long-term care. Wilmington VAMC proudly serves
Veterans in multiple locations for convenient access to the ser-
vices we provide.

5597 **Wilmington VA Medical Center**
Veterans Health Administration, US Dept. of VA
1601 Kirkwood Hwy
Wilmington, DE 19805-4917   302-994-2511
                                  800-461-8262
                             FAX: 302-633-5516
                             g.vhacss@forum.va.gov
                             www.wilmington.va.gov
Daniel D. Hendee, FACHE, MHA, Director
Mary Alice Johnson, MS, RN, Associate Director for Patient Care
Services
William E. England, Associate Director for Finance and Operations
Enrique Guttin, MD, MMM, CPE,, Chief of Staff
We offer comprehensive services ranging from preventive
screenings to long-term care. Wilmington VAMC proudly serves
Veterans in multiple locations for convenient access to the ser-
vices we provide.

5598 **Wilmington Vet Center**
2710 Centerville Road
Suite 103
Wilmington, DE 19808- 4917   302-994-1660
                                    877-927-8387
                               FAX: 302-994-8361
                               www.va.gov
Joan Spencer, Team Leader
Patricia Elwood, Office Manager
Valerie Feeley, Counselor
Barbara F Blevins, Counselor
Veterans counseling program offering individual counseling ser-
vices, advocacy services and group counseling. The focus is the
counseling of all veterans coping with the aftermath of war, sexual abuse/harassment in the military and all veterans of the Vietnam era. The center also has an active outreach program to seek
veterans needing services. Hours of operation are between 8:00
AM - 4:30 PM, Monday - Friday and other times by appointment
only. Services are free.

District of Columbia

5599 **Disabled American Veterans, National Service & Legislative**
Headquarters
807 Maine Ave SW
Washington, DC 20024-2410   202-554-3501
                             FAX: 202-554-3581
                             www.dav.org
Donald L. Samuels, Chairman
Joseph W. Johnston, Vice-Chairman
Marc Burgess, Secretary
Joseph R. Lenhart, Treasurer
Our mission simply is one of service and advocacy on behalf of
the men and women who put their lives on the line to ensure our
safety, to protect our freedoms and cherished way of life.

5600 **PVA Sports and Recreation Program**
Paralyzed Veterans of America
801 18th St NW
Washington, DC 20006-3517   202-872-1300
                                   800-424-8200
                                   888-888-2201
                             FAX: 202-785-4432
                             TTY:800-795-4327
                             info@pva.org
                             www.pva.org
Randy Pleva, President
Homer S. Townsend, Jr., Executive Director
Larry Dodson, National Secretary
Bill Lawson, National President
Today, the work continues to create an America where all veter-
ans and people with disabilities, and their families, have every-
thing they need to live full and productive lives.

5601 **VA Medical Center, Washington DC**
50 Irving St NW
Washington, DC 20422-1   202-745-8000
                                800-827-1000
                                877-328-2621
                             g.vhacss@forum.va.gov
                             www.washingtondc.va.gov
Brian A. Hawkins, MHA, Medical Center Director
Bryan C. Matthews, MBA, Associate Medical Center Director
Natalie Merckens, Assistant Medical Center Director
Ross D. Fletcher, MD, Chief of Staff
Acute general and specialized services in medicine, surgery, neu-
rology, and psychiatry.

5602 **Washington DC VA Medical Center**
Veterans Health Administration, U S Dept. of V A
50 Irving St NW
Washington, DC 20422-1   202-745-8000
                                800-827-1000
                                877-328-2621
                             FAX: 202-754-8530
                             g.vhacss@forum.va.gov
                             www.washingtondc.va.gov
Brian A. Hawkins, MHA, Medical Center Director
Bryan C. Matthews, MBA, Associate Medical Center Director
Natalie Merckens, Assistant Medical Center Director
Ross D. Fletcher, MD, Chief of Staff
Acute general and specialized services in medicine, surgery, neu-
rology, and psychiatry.

Florida

5603 **Bay Pines VA Medical Center**
Veterans Health Administration, U S Dept. of V A
10000 Bay Pines Blvd
PO Box 5005
Bay Pines, FL 33744   727-398-6661
                             800-827-1000
                             888-820-0230
                             g.vhacss@forum.va.gov
                             www.baypines.va.gov
Suzanne M. Klinker, Medical Center Director
Kristine Brown, MPH, Associate Director
Teresa Kumar, RN, MSN, CPHQ,, Associate Director for Patient /
Nursing Services
Keith Neeley, FACHE, Assistant Director
Since 1933, Bay Pines VA Healthcare System has been improving
the health of the men and women who have so proudly served our
nation. We consider it our privilege to serve your health care
needs in any way we can. Our services are available to Veterans
living in a ten county catchment area in west central Florida.

5604 **Gainesville Division, North Florida/South Georgia Veterans Healthcare System**
Veterans Health Administration, U S Dept. of V A
1601 SW Archer Rd
Gainesville, FL 32608-1611
352-376-1611
800-324-8387
FAX: 352-379-7445
g.vhacss@forum.va.gov
www.northflorida.va.gov/northflorida

Thomas Wisnieski, MPA, FACHE, Director
Nancy Reissener, Deputy Director
Maureen Wilkes, Associate Director
LeAnne Whitlow, RN, MSHSA, MB, Associate Director, Nursing Service

In addition to our medical centers in Gainesville and Lake City, we offer services in three satellite outpatient clinics and several community-based outpatient clinics across North Florida and South Georgia.

5605 **James A Haley VA Medical Center**
Veterans Health Administration, U S Dept. of V A
13000 Bruce B Downs Blvd
Suite T72
Tampa, FL 33612-4745
813-972-2000
800-827-1000
888-811-0107
g.vhacss@forum.va.gov
www.tampa.va.gov

Kathleen R. Fogarty, Director
Roy L. Hawkins Jr., Deputy Director
David J. VanMeter, Associate Director
Suzanne Tate, Assistant Director

Comprehensive health care is provided through primary care, tertiary care, and long-term care in areas of medicine, surgery, psychiatry, physical medicine and rehabilitation, spinal cord injury, neurology, oncology, dentistry, geriatrics, and extended care.

5606 **Miami VA Medical Center**
Veterans Health Administration, U S Dept. of V A
1201 NW 16th St
Suite B822
Miami, FL 33125-1693
305-575-7000
800-827-1000
888-276-1785
FAX: 305-575-3266
g.vhacss@forum.va.gov
www.miami.va.gov

Paul M. Russo, Director
Mark E. Morgan, Associate Director
Marcia Lysaght, Associate Director, Patient Care Services
P. Gwendolyn Findley, Ph.D., Assistant Director

The Miami VA is an accredited comprehensive medical provider, providing general medical, surgical, inpatient and outpatient mental health services, the Miami VA Healthcare System includes an AIDS/HIV center, a prosthetic treatment center, spinal cord injury rehabilitative center, and Geriatric Research, Education, and Clinical Center (GRECC).

5607 **St. Petersburg Regional Office**
Veterans Benefits Administration, U S Dept. of V A
9500 Bay Pines Blvd
St Petersburg, FL 33708
727-319-7492
800-827-1000
stpete.query@vba.va.gov
www.va.gov

Warren McPherson, Executive Director

5608 **West Palm Beach VA Medical Center**
Veterans Health Administration, U S Dept. of V A
7305 N Military Trl
West Palm Beach, FL 33410-7417
561-422-8262
800-972-8262
FAX: 561-882-6707
g.vhacss@forum.va.gov
www.westpalmbeach.va.gov

Charleen R. Szabo, FACHE, Medical Center Director
Cristy McKillop, FACHE, MHA, Medical Center Associate Director
Gloria A. Bays, MSN, ARNP, NE-BC, Associate Director for Patient Care Services
Deepak Mandi, MD, Chief of Staff

The medical center is a general medical, psychiatric and surgical facility. It is a teaching hospital, providing a full range of patient care services, with state-of-the-art technology as well as education and limited research. Comprehensive healthcare is provided through primary care and long-term care in the areas of dentistry, extended care, medicine, neurology, oncology, pharmacy, physical medicine, psychiatry, rehabilitation and surgery. The West Palm Beach VA Medical Center operates a Blin

Georgia

5609 **Atlanta Regional Office**
Veterans Benefits Administration, U S Dept. of V A
1700 Clairmont Road
Decatur, GA 30033-1210
404-463-3100
800-827-1000
FAX: 404-929-5819
atlanta.query@vba.va.gov
www.va.gov

Chick Krautler, Executive Director

The Atlanta VA Regional Office is responsible for delivering non-medical VA benefits and services to Georgia Veterans and their dependent family members. This is accomplished through the administration of comprehensive and diverse benefit programs established by Congress. Our goal is to deliver these benefits and services in a timely, accurate, and compassionate manner.

5610 **Atlanta VA Medical Center**
Veterans Health Administration, U S Dept. of V A
1670 Clairmont Rd
Decatur, GA 30033-4004
404-321-6111
800-827-1000
FAX: 404-728-7734
g.vhacss@forum.va.gov
www.atlanta.va.gov

Leslie B. Wiggins, Director
Tom Grace, MBA/MHA, Associate Director
Sheila Meuse, PhD, Assistant Director
Sandy Leake, MSN, RN, Associate Director for Nursing/Patient Services

The Atlanta VA Medical Center (VAMC), located on 26 acres in Decatur, is one of eight medical centers in the VA Southeast Network. It is a teaching hospital, providing a full range of patient care services complete with state-of-the-art technology, education, and research.

5611 **Augusta VA Medical Center**
Veterans Health Administration, U S Dept. of V A
950 15th Street Downtown/1 Freedom
Augusta, GA 30904-6258
706-733-0188
800-827-1000
FAX: 706-731-7227
g.vhacss@forum.va.gov
www.agusta.va.gov

Robert U. Hamilton, MHA, FACHE, Medical Center Director
Richard Rose, Associate Director
Michelle Cox-Henley, MS, RN, Associate Director for Nursing/Patient Services
Luke M. (Mik Stapleton, MD, Chief of Staff

The Charlie Norwood VA Medical Center is a two-division Medical Center that provides tertiary care in medicine, surgery, neurology, psychiatry, rehabilitation medicine, and spinal cord injury. The Downtown Division is authorized 155 beds (58 medicine, 37 surgery, and 60 spinal cord injury). The Uptown Division, located approximately three miles away, is authorized 315 beds (68 psychiatry, 15 blind rehabilitation and 40 medical rehabilitation. In addition, a 132-bed Restorative/Nursing Home C

5612 Carl Vinson VA Medical Center
Veterans Health Administration, U S Dept. of V A
1826 Veterans Blvd
Dublin, GA 31021-3699
478-272-1210
FAX: 478-277-2717
dana.doles@med.va.gov
www.dublin.va.gov

John S. Goldman, Director
Gerald M. DeWorth, Associate Director
Sue Preston, RN, Associate Director for Patient and Nursing Services
Nomie Finn, M.D, Chief of Staff
Since 1948, Carl Vinson VA Medical Center has been improving the health of the men and women who have so proudly served our nation. We consider it our privilege to serve your health care needs in any way we can. Services are available to veterans living in the Middle Georgia area.

5613 Southeastern Paralyzed Veterans of America(PVA)
4010 Deans Bridge Rd
U.S. Highway 1
Hephzibah, GA 30815-5616
706-796-6301
800-292-9335
FAX: 706-796-0363
homercpva@gmail.com
www.southeasternpva.org
Dr. Chuck Turek, National Director
Linda Hutchinson, Advocacy & Legislative Director for North and South Carolina
Homer Cole, Chapter President
Larry Dodson, Chapter Vice President
Works to maximize the quality of life for its members and all people with SCI/D as a leading adovocate for healthcare, SCI/D research and education, veteran's benefits, and rights, accessibility and the removal of architectural barriers, sports programs, and disability rights.

Hawaii

5614 Hilo Vet Center
70 Lanihuli St
Suite 102
Hilo, HI 96720-2067
808-969-3833
877-927-8387
FAX: 808-969-2025
www.va.gov

Felipe Sales, Team Leader
Samuelito Labasan, Office Manager
Peter Ehlich, Counselor
Nancy G Waller, Counselor
Veterans medical clinic offering disabled veterans medical treatments, readjustment and PTSD counseling to combat veterans

5615 Honolulu VBA Regional Office
Veterans Benefits Administration, U S Dept. of V A
459 Patterson Road, E-Wing
Honolulu, HI 96819-1522
808-566-1412
800-827-1000
FAX: 808-433-0478
honolulu.query@vba.va.gov
www.vba.va.gov/ro/honolulu
Claude M Kicklighter, Chief of Staff
Alan Furuno, Manager
Alvin Kalawe, Elderly Program Coordinator
Karin Frazier, Women Veteran's Program Coordinator
The Honolulu Regional Office is responsible for administering VA's benefit programs under the leadership and direction of the Under Secretary for Benefits for the Veterans Benefits Administration. Formerly part of the Honolulu VA Medical & Regional Office Center (VAMROC), the Honolulu Regional Office (RO) was renamed as a stand alone RO on June 2, 2003. The office is co-located with the Spark M. Matsunaga Pacific Islands Health Care System medical center, on the grounds of the Tripler Army Medic

5616 Pacific Islands Health Care System
Veterans Health Administration, US Dept. of VA
459 Patterson Rd
Honolulu, HI 96819-1522
808-433-0600
800-214-1306
FAX: 808-433-0390
g.vhacss@forum.va.gov
www.hawaii.va.gov
William F. Dubbs, M.D., Acting Director
Brandon K. Yamamoto, Acting Associate Director
Jane Wellman, APRN, Associate Director of Patient Care Services
David M. Bernstein, M.D, Acting Chief of Staff
The VA Pacific Islands Health Care System (VAPIHCS) Honolulu provides a broad range of medical care services, serving an estimated 127,600 veterans throughout Hawaii and the Pacific Islands. The VAPIHCS provides outpatient medical and mental health care through a main Ambulatory Care Clinic on Oahu (Honolulu) and through five Community Based Outpatient Clinics (CBOCs) on the neighboring islands including: Hawaii (Hilo and Kona), Maui, Kauai, and Guam. Traveling clinicians also provide episodi

Idaho

5617 Boise Regional Office
Veterans Benefits Administration, U S Dept. of V A
444 W. Fort Street
Boise, ID 83702-4531
800-827-1000
boise.query@vba.va.gov
www.va.gov
Jim Vance, Director
Pat Teague, Service Officer
Tom Ressler, Manager
The Boise Regional Office administers monetary benefits to 17,283 veterans in Idaho, Utah, and Oregon. The Regional Office issued monthly disability and death benefit payments of over $15 million in January 2007. VBA's annual compensation and pension benefits for veterans residing within the RO's jurisdiction now exceed $185 million

5618 Boise VA Medical Center
Veterans Health Administration, U S Dept. of V A
500 W Fort St
Boise, ID 83702-4531
208-422-1000
800-827-1000
FAX: 208-422-1326
g.vhacss@forum.va.gov
www.boise.va.gov
Jennifer T Shalz, Chief of Staff
We truly hope to improve your health and well-being and will make your visit or stay as pleasant as possible. We are committed to veterans and the nation and strive to continually enhance the care we provide. We also train future healthcare professionals, conduct research and support our nation in times of emergency. In all of these activities, our employees will respect and support your rights as a patient.

Illinois

5619 Edward Hines Jr Hospital
Veterans Health Administration, U S Dept. of V A
5000 South 5th Avenue
Hines, IL 60141 708-202-8387
800-827-1000
FAX: 708-202-2684
g.vhacss@forum.va.gov
www.hines.va.gov

Joan Ricard, FACHE, Hospital Director
Dr. Daniel Zomchek, Associate Director
Carol A. Gouty, RN, MSN, PhD, Associate Director of Patient Care
Karandeep Sraon, Assistant Director
Specialized clinical programs include Blind Rehabilitation, Spinal Cord Injury, Neurosurgery, Radiation Therapy and Cardiovascular Surgery. The hospital also serves as the VISN 12 southern tier hub for pathology, radiology, radiation therapy, human resource management and fiscal services. Hines VAH currently operates 471 beds and six community based outpatient clinics in Elgin, Kankakee, Oak Lawn, Aurora, LaSalle, and Joliet.

5620 Marion VA Medical Center
Veterans Health Administration U S Department of V
2401 W Main St
Marion, IL 62959-1188 618-997-5311
800-827-1000
kimberly.travelstead@va.gov
www.marion.va.gov

Paul Bockelman, Medical Center Director
Frank Kehus, Associate Director
The VA Medical Center in Marion, Illinois, is a general medical and surgical facility that operates 55 acute care beds and a 60 bed Community Living Center. Ten Outpatient Clinics that provide primary care and behavioral medicine services are located in Harrisburg; Carbondale; Effingham; and Mt. Vernon, IL; Paducah; Hanson; Owensboro; and Mayfield, Kentucky; Vincennes and Evansville, IN.

5621 North Chicago VA Medical Center
Veterans Health Administration, U S Dept. of V A
3001 North Green Bay Rd
North Chicago, IL 60064-3048 847-688-1900
800-393-0865
g.vhacss@forum.va.gov
www.lovell.fhcc.va.gov

Patrick L. Sullivan, Director
Captain Jos, A. Acosta, MC, US, Commanding Officer/Deputy Director
Captain Jami Kersten, Associate Director
Dr. Sarah Fouse, Associate Director of Patient Services/Nurse Executive
The arrangement incorporates facilities, services and resources from the North Chicago VA Medical Center (VAMC) and the Naval Health Clinic Great Lakes (NHCGL). A combined mission of the health care center means active duty military, their family members, military retirees and veterans are all cared for at the facility.

5622 VA Illiana Health Care System
Veterans Health Administration, U S Dept. of V A
1900 E Main St
Danville, IL 61832-5198 217-554-3000
800-320-8387
FAX: 217-554-4552
g.vhacss@forum.va.gov
www.danville.va.gov

Emma Metcalf, MSN, RN,, Director
Diana Carranza, Associate Director
Alesia Coe, MSN, RN,, Associate Director for Patient Care Services
Nirmala Rozario, M.D., Ph.D, Chief of Staff
Since 1898, our buildings, facilities, patients, and missions have changed, but remaining constant is VA Illiana Health Care System's endeavor in improving the health of the men and women who have so proudly served our nation. Being the 8th oldest VA facility, we consider it our privilege to serve your health care needs in any way we can.

Indiana

5623 Indianapolis Regional Office
Veterans Benefits Administration U S Department of
575 N Pennsylvania St
Indianapolis, IN 46204-1563 317-226-7860
800-827-1000
TTY:800-829-4833
indianapolis.query@vba.va.gov
www.benefits.va.gov/indianapolis

5624 Richard L Roudebush VA Medical Center
Veterans Health Administration, U S Dept. of V A
1481 W 10th St
Indianapolis, IN 46202-2803 317-554-0000
800-827-1000
FAX: 317-554-0127
g.vhacss@forum.va.gov
www.indianapolis.va.gov

Thomas Mattice, Director
Jeff Nechanicky, Associate Director
Kimberly Radant, Associate Director for Patient Care Services
Cathy Lee, Assistant Director
Since 1932, Richard L. Roudebush VA Medical Center has been improving the health of the men and women who have so proudly served our nation. We consider it our privilege to serve your health care needs in any way we can. Services are available to more than 196,000 veterans living in a 45-county area of Indiana and Illinois.

5625 VA North Indiana Health Care System: Fort Wayne Campus
Veterans Health Administration, U S Dept. of V A
2121 Lake Ave
Fort Wayne, IN 46805-5100 260-426-5431
800-360-8387
g.vhacss@forum.va.gov
www.northernindiana.va.gov

Denise M. Deitzen, Medical Center Director
Audrey L. Frison, MHA, RN, Associate Director
Helen Rhodes MPA, RN, Associate Director for Operations
Ajay Dhawan MD FACHE, Chief of Staff
The Fort Wayne Campus offers primary and secondary medical and surgical services. Primary care clinics are available at both medical center campuses and at Community Based Outpatient Clinics (CBOCs) located in South Bend, Goshen, Peru and Muncie Indiana. Recently completed renovations and construction, and continuous maintenance, ensure an attractive, state-of-the-art healthcare environment.

5626 VA Northern Indiana Health Care System: Marion Campus
Veterans Health Administration, U S Dept. of V A
1700 E 38th St
Marion, IN 46953-4568 765-674-3321
800-360-8387
g.vhacss@forum.va.gov
www.northernindiana.va.gov

Denise M. Deitzen, Medical Center Director
Audrey L. Frison, MHA, RN, Associate Director
Helen Rhodes MPA, RN, Associate Director for Operations
Ajay Dhawan MD FACHE, Chief of Staff
The Marion Campus offers a full range of mental health, nursing home care, and extended care services. Primary care clinics are available at both medical center campuses and at Community Based Outpatient Clinics (CBOCs) located in South Bend, Goshen, Peru and Muncie Indiana.

Iowa

5627 Des Moines VA Medical Center
Veterans Health Administration, U S Dept. of V A
3600 30th St
Des Moines, IA 50310-5753
515-699-5999
800-294-8387
FAX: 515-699-5862
g.vhacss@forum.va.gov
www.centraliowa.va.gov

Donald Cooper, Director
Susan Martin, Associate Director for Resources and Operations
Tammy Neff, RN, MBA, MSN, M, Acting Associate Director for Patient Services/Nurse Executi
Fredrick Bahls, MD, Chief of Staff
The VA Central Iowa Health Care System (VACIHCS) operates a Veterans Health Administration (VHA) medical facility in Des Moines, with Community Based Outpatient Clinics (CBOCs) in Mason City, Fort Dodge, Knoxville, Marshalltown and Carroll. The medical center provides acute and specialized medical and surgical services, residential outpatient treatment programs in substance abuse and post-traumatic stress and a full range of mental health and long-term care services, as well as sub-acute and r

5628 Des Moines VA Regional Office
Veterans Benefits Administration, U S Dept. of V A
210 Walnut Street
Des Moines, IA 50309-2115
515-323-7580
800-827-1000
FAX: 515-323-7580
leander@vba.va.gov
www.va.gov

Rich Anderson, Service Director
The Des Moines VA Regional Office provides Compensation, Pension and Vocational Rehabilitation and Counseling services for all military veterans in the State of Iowa. The Des Moines VA Regional Office currently provides approximately $260 million in benefits to the approximately 270,000 veterans in Iowa.

5629 Iowa City VA Medical Center
Veterans Health Administration, U S Dept. of V A
601 Highway 6 West
Iowa City, IA 52240-2202
319-338-0581
800-637-0128
866-687-7382
FAX: 319-339-7171
g.vhacss@forum.va.gov
www.iowacity.va.gov

Barry Sharp, Director
Timothy McMurry, Associate Director for Operations
Dawn Oxley, RN, Associate Director Patient Care Services/Nurse Executive
Stanley Parker, MD, Acting Chief of Staff
Tertiary care facility, affiliated teaching hospital, and research center seving an aging veteran populatiaon in eastern Iowa and western Illinois. Satellite clinics are located in Bettendord, Dubuque, and Waterloo, Iowa and in Quincy and Galesburg, Illinois.

5630 Knoxville VA Medical Center
Veterans Health Administration, U S Dept. of V A
1515 W Pleasant St
Knoxville, IA 50138-3399
641-842-3101
800-816-8878
FAX: 641-828-5124
g.vhacss@forum.va.gov
www.centraliowa.va.gov

Claudia M Kicklighter

5631 VA Central Iowa Health Care System
3600 30th St
Des Moines, IA 50310-5753
515-699-5999
800-294-8387
FAX: 515-699-5862
www.centraliowa.va.gov

Donald Cooper, Director
Susan Martin, Associate Director for Resources and Operations
Tammy Neff, RN, MBA, MSN, M, Acting Associate Director for Patient Services/Nurse Executi
Fredrick Bahls, MD, Chief of Staff
The VA Central Iowa Health Care System (VACIHCS) operates a Veterans Health Administration (VHA) medical facility in Des Moines, with Community Based Outpatient Clinics (CBOCs) in Mason City, Fort Dodge, Knoxville, Marshalltown and Carroll. The medical center provides acute and specialized medical and surgical services, residential outpatient treatment programs in substance abuse and post-traumatic stress and a full range of mental health and long-term care services, as well as sub-acute and r

Kansas

5632 Colmery-O'Neil VA Medical Center
Veterans Health Administration, U S Dept. of V A
2200 SW Gage Blvd
Topeka, KS 66622
785-350-3111
800-574-8387
g.vhacss@forum.va.gov
www.topeka.va.gov

A. Rudy Klopfer, FACHE, Director
John Moon, Associate Director
Nelson L. Dean, RN, BSN, MA, Associate Director for Patient Care Services
Christine M Kleckner, MBA, RD, Assistant Director
Since 1946, the staff of the Colmery-O'Neil VA Medical Center has been serving veterans. Today, we proudly serve our nation's veterans with excellent health care as part of the VA Eastern Kansas Health Care System (VAEKHCS). We consider it our privilege to serve your health care needs in any way we can.

5633 Dwight D Eisenhower VA Medical Center
Veterans Health Administration, U S Dept. of V A
4101 4th Street Trafficway
Leavenworth, KS 66048-5014
913-682-2000
800-952-8387
g.vhacss@forum.va.gov
www.leavenworth.va.gov

A. Rudy Klopfer, FACHE, Director
John Moon, Associate Director
Nelson L. Dean, RN, BSN, MA, Associate Director for Patient Care Services
Christine M Kleckner, MBA, RD, Assistant Director
Since 1886, the staff of the Dwight D. Eisenhower VA Medical Center has been serving veterans. Today, we proudly serve our nation's veterans with excellent health care as part of the VA Eastern Kansas Health Care System (VAEKHCS). We consider it our privilege to serve your health care needs in any way we can.

5634 Kansas VA Regional Office
Veterans Benefits Administration, U S Dept. of V A
5500 E Kellogg Dr
Wichita, KS 67218-1607
800-827-1000
wichita.query@vba.va.gov
www.benefits.va.gov/wichita

Edgar L Tucker, Medical Center Director

5635 Robert J Dole VA Medical Center
Veterans Health Administration, U S Dept. of V A
5500 E Kellogg Dr
Wichita, KS 67218-1607   316-685-2221
                                               800-827-1000
                                               888-827-6881
                                          FAX: 316-651-3666
                                          g.vhacss@forum.va.gov
                                          www.wichita.va.gov

Kevin Inkley, MA, Director
Vicki Bondie, MBA, Associate Director
Carol A. Kaster, MA, RN, Associate Director of Patient Care/Nurse Executive
M. Ganga Hematillake, MD, Chief of Staff
For over 70 years, the Dole VA Medical and Regional office center has been honored to serve Kansas area veterans. The center provides a full range of primary and specialty acute and extended care services to veterans in 59 counties of Kansas. Special emphasis programs include substance abuse, post traumatic stress disorder (PTSD), women's health, spinal cord injury, visual impairment, prosthetic and sensory aids, and homeless services.

Kentucky

5636 Lexington VA Medical Center
Veterans Health Administration, U S Dept. of V A
1101 Veterans Dr
Lexington, KY 40502-2235   859-281-4900
                                               800-352-4000
                                          g.vhacss@forum.va.gov
                                          www.lexington.va.gov

Martin J. Traxler, Acting Medical Center Director
Patricia Breeden, MD, Acting Chief of Staff
Laura Faulkner, Acting Associate Medical Center Director
Agnes Therady, RN, NEA-BC, F, Acting Associate Director Patient Care Services
The Lexington Veterans Affairs Medical Center is a fully accredited, two-division, tertiary care medical center with an operating bed complement of 199 hospital beds. Acute medical, neurological, surgical and psychiatric inpatient services are provided at the Cooper Division, located adjacent to the University of Kentucky Medical Center. Other available services include: emergency care, medical-surgical units, acute psychiatry, ICU, progressive care unit, (includes Cardiac Cath Lab) ambulatory s

5637 Louisville VA Medical Center
Veterans Health Administration, U S Dept. of V A
800 Zorn Ave
Louisville, KY 40206-1433   502-287-4000
                                               800-376-8387
                                          g.vhacss@forum.va.gov
                                          www.louisville.va.gov

Wayne L. Pfeffer, MHSA, FACHE, Medical Center Director
Douglas V Paxton, Sr, Associate Director / Operations
Pamala Thompson, RN, MSA, MSN, Associate Director for Patient Care Services
Marylee Rothschild, M.D., Chief of Staff
Since 1952, Robley Rex VAMC has been improving the health of the men and women who have so proudly served our nation. We consider it our privilege to serve your health care needs in any way we can. Services are available to more than 166,000 veterans living in a 35-county area of the Kentuckiana area.

5638 Louisville VA Regional Office
Veterans Benefits Administration, U S Dept. of V A
800 Zorn Avenue
Louisville, KY 40206-1433   502-287-4000
                                               800-376-8387
                                          louisville.query@vba.va.gov
                                          www.louisville.va.gov

Wayne L. Pfeffer, MHSA, FACHE, Medical Center Director
Douglas V Paxton, Sr, Associate Director / Operations
Pamala Thompson, RN, MSA, MSN, Associate Director for Patient Care Services
Marylee Rothschild, M.D., Chief of Staff

Since 1952, Robley Rex VAMC has been improving the health of the men and women who have so proudly served our nation. We consider it our privilege to serve your health care needs in any way we can. Services are available to more than 166,000 veterans living in a 35-county area of the Kentuckiana area.

Louisiana

5639 Alexandria VA Medical Center
Department of Veterans Affairs
2495 Shreveport Highway
Pineville, LA 71360-9004   318-466-4000
                                                800-375-8387
                                           FAX: 318-483-5029
                                           richard.wright2@va.gov
                                           www.alexandria.va.gov

Martin J. Traxler, Medical Center Director
Yolanda Sanders-Jackson, Associate Director
Jose N Rivera, MD, Acting Chief of Staff
Amy Lesniewski, RN MS, Nurse Executive
The VAMC Alexandria is categorized as a primary and secondary care facility. It is a teaching hospital, providing a full range of primary care services with state-of-the-art technology and education. Comprehensive acute and extended health care is provided on a primary and secondary basis in areas of medicine, surgery, psychiatry, physical medicine and rehabilitation, neurology, oncology, dentistry, geriatrics, and extended care. The Medical Center serves a potential veteran population of over 1

5640 New Orleans VA Medical Center
Veterans Health Administration, U S Dept. of V A
1601 Perdido St
New Orleans, LA 70112-1262   504-412-3700
                                                800-935-8387
                                           FAX: 504-589-5210
                                           Stacie.Rivera@med.va.gov
                                           www.neworleans.va.gov

John D Church Jr, Medical Director/President
Fernando Rivera, Association Medical Center Direc
Sam Lucero, Special Assistant to Director
Stacie M Rivera, Public Affairs Officer
A teaching hospital, providing a full range of patient care services, with state-of-the-art technology as well as education and research. Comprehensive health care is provided through primary care, tetiary care, and long-term care in areas of medicine, surgery, psychiatry, physical medicine and rehabilitation, neurology, oncology, dentistry, geriatrics, and extended care.

5641 Shreveport VA Medical Center
Veterans Health Administration, U S Dept. of V A
510 E Stoner Ave
Shreveport, LA 71101-4295   318-221-8411
                                                800-827-1000
                                           www.shreveport.va.gov

Shirley M. Bealer, Medical Center Director
Todd M. Moore, Assistant Medical Center Director
Erik J. Glover, Associate Medical Center Director
Ruth Davis, DNS, Associate Director for Patient Care Services

Maine

5642 Maine VA Regional Office
Veterans Benefits Administration, U S Dept. of V A
1 VA Center
Augusta, ME 4330-6719   207-623-8411
                                                877-421-8263
                                           togus.query@vba.va.gov
                                           www.va.gov

Dale Demers, Director
Scott Karczewski, Manager

5643 Togus VA Medical Center
Veterans Health Administration, U S Dept. of V A
1 VA Center
Augusta, ME 04330-6795

207-623-8411
877-421-8263
FAX: 207-623-5792
g.vhacss@forum.va.gov
www.togus.va.gov

Scott Karczewski, Regional Office Director
Denise Benson, Veterans Sevice Center Manager
Gregg Morin, Assistant Veterans Service Center Manager
Tracy Sinclair, Support Services Chief

Maryland

5644 Baltimore Regional Office
Veterans Benefits Administration, U S Dept. of V A
31 Hopkins Plz
Baltimore, MD 21201-2825

800-827-1000
baltimore.query@vba.va.gov
www.va.gov

Jerry L Calhoun
The Baltimore Regional Office serves 484,013 veterans living in the State of Maryland, 2% of the national veteran population. The Regional Office's jurisdiction includes all counties in the State of Maryland. The Baltimore Regional Office has an assigned staffing of 218. We provide services at the VA Medical Center in Baltimore and Transition Assistance throughout the State. We actively participate in a homeless veterans outreach program based at the Maryland Center for the Veterans Educatio

5645 Baltimore VA Medical Center
Veterans Health Administration, U S Dept. of V A
10 N Greene St
Baltimore, MD 21201-1524

410-605-7000
800-463-6295
FAX: 410-605-7901
g.vhacss@forum.va.gov
www.maryland.va.gov

Dennis H. Smith, Director
Nancy Quailey-Giannopoulis, Associate Director for Operations
Frederick P. Soetje, Associate Director for Finance
David O. Barrett, Acting Chief of Staff
The Baltimore Medical Center is nationally recognized for its outstanding patient safety and state-of-the-art technology, the VA Maryland Health Care System is proud of its reputation as a leader in veterans' health care, research and education.

5646 Fort Howard VA Medical Center
Veterans Health Administration, U S Dept. of V A
9600 N Point Rd
Fort Howard, MD 21052-3050

410-477-1800
800-351-8387
FAX: 410-477-7177
md.veterans@erols.com
www.mdva.state.md.us

Thomas Hutchins, Secretary

5647 Maryland Veterans Centers
10 N Greene St
Baltimore, MD 21201-1524

410-605-7000
800-463-6295
FAX: 410-605-7901
www.maryland.va.gov

J Y Jacks, Manager
Dennis H Smith, Executive Director
Veterans medical clinic offering disabled veterans medical treatments.

5648 Perry Point VA Medical Center
Veterans Health Administration, U S Dept. of V A
Circle Drive
Perry Point, MD 21902

410-642-2411
800-949-1003
FAX: 410-642-1165
g.vhacss@forum.va.gov
www.maryland.va.gov

Dennis H. Smith, Director
Nancy Quailey-Giannopoulis, Associate Director for Operations
Frederick P. Soetje, Associate Director for Finance
David O. Barrett, Acting Chief of Staff
It is nationally recognized for its outstanding patient safety and state-of-the-art technology, the VA Maryland Health Care System is proud of its reputation as a leader in veterans' health care, research and education.

5649 VA Maryland Health Care System
10 N Greene St
Baltimore, MD 21201-1524

410-605-7000
800-463-6295
FAX: 410-605-7900
www.maryland.va.gov

Dennis H. Smith, Director
Nancy Quailey-Giannopoulis, Associate Director for Operations
Frederick P. Soetje, Associate Director for Finance
David O. Barrett, Acting Chief of Staff
A dynamic and exciting health care organization that is dedicated to providing quality, compassionate and accessible care and service to Maryland's veterans. As a part of one of the largest health care systems in the United States, the VAMHCS has a reputation as a leader in veterans' health care, reserch and education. Provides comprehensive service to veterans including medical, surgical, rehabilitative, nurological and mental health care on both an inpatient and outpatient basis.

Massachusetts

5650 Boston VA Regional Office
Veterans Benefits Administration, U S Dept. of V A
15 New Sudbury Street
JFK Bldg
Boston, MA 2203-9928

617-232-9500
800-827-1000
boston.query@vba.va.gov
www.boston.va.gov

Liza Catucci, Administrative Officer
Michael Lawson, President

5651 Edith Nourse Rogers Memorial Veterans Hospital
Veterans Health Administration U S Deptartment of
200 Springs Rd Bldg #23
Bedford, MA 1730-1114

781-687-2000
800-827-1000
FAX: 781-687-3536
g.vhacss@forum.va.gov
www.bedford.va.gov

Michael Mayo-Smith, Manager

5652 Northampton VA Medical Center
Veterans Health Administration, U S Dept. of V A
421 N Main St
Leeds, MA 1062

413-584-4040
800-827-1000
g.vhacss@forum.va.gov
www.northhampton.va.gov

Richard Woloss, Manager

5653 VA Boston Healthcare System: Brockton Division
Veterans Health Administration, U S Dept. of V A
940 Belmont St
Brockton, MA 02301-5596   508-583-4500
                                 800-865-3384
                                 FAX: 617-323-7700
                                 g.vhacss@forum.va.gov
                                 www.boston.va.gov

Vincent Ng, Acting Director
Susan A. MacKenzie, PhD, Associate Director
Cecilia McVey, BSN, MHA, CAN, Associate Director Nursing & Patient Care Services
VA Boston Healthcare System's consolidated facility consists of the Jamaica Plain campus, located in the heart of Boston's Longwood Medical Community; the West Roxbury campus, located on the Dedham line; and the Brockton campus, located 20 miles south of Boston in the City of Brockton.

5654 VA Boston Healthcare System: Jamaica Plain Campus
Veterans Health Administration, U S Dept. of V A
150 S Huntington Ave
Boston, MA 2130-4817   617-232-9500
                                 800-865-3384
                                 FAX: 617-278-4549
                                 g.vhacss@forum.va.gov
                                 www.boston.va.gov

Vincent Ng, Acting Director
Susan A. MacKenzie, PhD, Associate Director
Cecilia McVey, BSN, MHA, CAN, Associate Director Nursing & Patient Care Services
VA Boston Healthcare System's consolidated facility consists of the Jamaica Plain campus, located in the heart of Boston's Longwood Medical Community; the West Roxbury campus, located on the Dedham line; and the Brockton campus, located 20 miles south of Boston in the City of Brockton.

5655 VA Boston Healthcare System: West Roxbury Division
Veterans Health Administration, U S Dept. of V A
1400 VFW Pkwy
West Roxbury, MA 2132-4927   617-323-7700
                                 800-865-3384
                                 g.vhacss@forum.va.gov
                                 www.boston.va.gov

Susan A Mac Kenzie, Associate Director
VA Boston Healthcare System's consolidated facility consists of the Jamaica Plain campus, located in the heart of Boston's Longwood Medical Community; the West Roxbury campus, located on the Dedham line; and the Brockton campus, located 20 miles south of Boston in the City of Brockton.

Michigan

5656 Aleda E Lutz VA Medical Center
Veterans Health Administration, U S Dept. of V A
1500 Weiss St
Saginaw, MI 48602-5251   989-497-2500
                                 800-827-1000
                                 FAX: 989-791-2428
                                 g.vhacss@forum.va.gov
                                 www.saginaw.va.gov

Jeff Nechanicky, Acting Medical Center Director
Stephanie Young, Associate Director
Penny Holland, R.N., MSN, Associate Director for Patient Care Svcs
Robert W. Dorr, D.O., JD, CHCQM,, Chief of Staff
Since 1950, the Aleda E. Lutz VA Medical Center has been improving the health of the men and women who have so proudly served our nation. We consider it our privilege to serve your health care needs in any way we can. Services are available to more than 31,000 veterans living in the Central and Northern 35 counties of Michigan's Lower Peninsula.

5657 Battle Creek VA Medical Center
Veterans Health Administration, U S Dept. of V A
5500 Armstrong Rd
Battle Creek, MI 49037-7314   269-966-5600
                                 888-214-1247
                                 888-214-1247
                                 FAX: 269-966-5483
                                 g.vhacss@forum.va.gov
                                 www.battlecreek.va.gov

Mary Beth Skupien, Director
Edward Dornoff, Associate Director
Kay Bower, Associate Director for Patient Care Services
Dr. Shah, Acting Chief of Staff
Since 1924, the Battle Creek, Michigan VA Medical Center has been improving the health of the men and women who have so proudly served our nation. The Battle Creek VA Medical Center consists of 104 medical and psychiatric beds, 32 residential rehabilitation beds, and 103 nursing home care unit beds. In addition, specialized services offered include a Palliative Care Unit, a Substance Abuse Clinic, a Post Traumatic Stress Disorder Program and a Domicilliary.

5658 Iron Mountain VA Medical Center
Veterans Health Administration, U S Dept. of V A
325 East H Street
Iron Mountain, MI 49801-4760   906-774-3300
                                 800-827-1000
                                 FAX: 906-779-3114
                                 g.vhacss@forum.va.gov
                                 www.ironmountain.va.gov

James W. Rice, Medical Center Director
William Caron, FACHE, Associate Medical Center Director
Andrea Collins, RN, MSN, Associate Director for Nursing and Patient Care Service
Grace L. Stringfellow, M.D., Chief of Staff
OGJVAMC is a primary and secondary level care facility with 17 acute care beds, 13 in the medical/surgical ward and 4 in the intensive care unit (ICU). The main facility provides limited emergency and acute inpatient care, and collaborates with larger VA Medical Centers in Milwaukee and Madison, WI, to provide higher-level emergency and specialty care services. OGJVAMC also provides rehabilitation and extended care, including palliative and hospice care, in its 40-bed Community Living Center.

5659 John D Dingell VA Medical Center
Veterans Health Administration, U S Dept. of V A
4646 John R St
Detroit, MI 48201-1916   313-576-1000
                                 800-827-1000
                                 FAX: 313-576-1112
                                 g.vhacss@forum.va.gov
                                 www.detroit.va.gov

Pamela J. Reeves, M.D., Director
Annette Walker, M.S.H.A., B.S., Associate Director
Ann M. Herm, R.N., B.S.N., M., Associate Director, Patient Care Services
Scott A. Gruber, M.D., Ph.D.,, Chief of Staff
Our mission is to provide timely, compassionate and high quality care to those we serve by encouraging teamwork, education, research, innovation, and continuous improvement.

5660 Michigan VA Regional Office
Veterans Benefits Administration, U S Dept. of V A
477 Michigan Ave
Patrick V McNamara Federal Building
Detroit, MI 48226-1217
                                 800-827-1000
                                 detroit.query@vba.va.gov
                                 www.benefits.va.gov/detroit

David Leonard, Director
Dennis W Paradowski, Assistant Director
The Regional Office Staff are dedicated to providing responsive and timely service to the veterans of Michigan and their families. Their duties include processing and making decisions on claims for disability compensation, and assisting with applications for a wide range of VA benefits.

5661 VA Ann Arbor Healthcare System
Veterans Health Administration, U S Dept. of V A
2215 Fuller Rd
Ann Arbor, MI 48105-2303

734-769-7100
800-361-8387
FAX: 734-761-7870
g.vhacss@forum.va.gov
www.annarbor.va.gov

Robert P. McDivitt, FACHE, Director
Randall E. Ritter, Associate Director
Stacey Breedveld, R.N., Associate Director Patient Care
Ginny Creasman, Assistant Director
Since 1953, the VA Ann Arbor Healthcare System (VAAAHS) has provided state-of-the-art healthcare services to the men and women who have so proudly served our nation. We consider it our privilege to serve your healthcare needs in any way we can.

5662 Vet Center Readjustment Counseling Service
1940 Eastern Ave SE
Grand Rapids, MI 49507-2771

616-285-5795
800-905-4675
FAX: 616-285-5898
www.va.gov

William Busby, Executive Director
Branden K Lyon, Counselor
Lynn Hall, Clinical Coordinator
Providing a broad range of counseling outreach and referral services to eligible veterans in order to help make readjustments to cilvilian life.

Minnesota

5663 Minneapolis VA Medical Center
Veterans Health Administration, U S Dept. of V A
1 Veterans Dr
Minneapolis, MN 55417-2399

612-725-2000
866-414-5058
FAX: 612-725-2049
g.vhacss@forum.va.gov
www.minneapolis.va.gov

Judy Johnson-Mekota, Director
Erik J. Stalhandske, Associate Director
Kent Crossley, Chief of Staff
Helen Pearlman, Nurse Executive
Minneapolis VA Health Care System (VAHCS) is a teaching hospital providing a full range of patient care services with state-of-the-art technology, as well as education and research. Comprehensive health care is provided through primary care, tertiary care and long-term care in areas of medicine, surgery, psychiatry, physical medicine and rehabilitation, neurology, oncology, dentistry, geriatrics and extended care.

5664 St. Cloud VA Medical Center
Veterans Health Administration, U S Dept. of V A
4801 Veterans Dr
Saint Cloud, MN 56303-2015

320-252-1670
800-247-1739
FAX: 320-255-6472
g.vhacss@forum.va.gov
www.stcloud.va.gov

Barry I. Bahl, Director
Cheryl Thieschafer, Associate Director
Meri Hauge, BSN, MSN Nurse, Executive/Associate Director for Patient Care Services
Susan Markstrom, MD, Chief of Staff
Specialty care services include audiology, cardiology, dentistry, hematology, oncology, optometry, orthopedics, podiatry, pulmonology, urology and rheumatology. A new Ambulatory Surgery (same-day) Center opened in the fall of 2011 and will provide access to additional outpatient surgical procedures. The medical center offers extensive mental health programming, including acute psychiatric care, Residential Rehabilitation Treatment programs and an outpatient mental health clinic. The programs u

5665 St. Paul Regional Office
Veterans Benefits Administration, U S Dept. of V A
1 Federal Dr
Fort Snelling, MN 55111-4080

800-827-1000
stpaul.query@vba.va.gov
www.benefits.va.gov/stpaul

Vincent Crawford, Director

5666 Vet Center
405 E Superior St
Ste 160
Duluth, MN 55802-2240

218-722-8654
877-927-8387
FAX: 218-723-8212
www.vetcenter.va.gov

Cynthia Macaulay MEd, Counselor
Rob Evanson, Counselor
Debbie Burt, Office Manager
Counseling, social services and benefits assistance for combat veterans and those sexually traumatized in the military.

Mississippi

5667 Biloxi/Gulfport VA Medical Center
Veterans Health Administration, U S Dept. of V A
400 Veterans Ave
Biloxi, MS 39531-2410

228-523-5000
800-296-8872
FAX: 228-563-2898
g.vhacss@forum.va.gov
www.biloxi.va.gov

Anthony L. Dawson, Director
Nancy Weaver, Associate Director
Kenneth Shimon, Chief of Staff
Margaret G Givens, Assciate Director

5668 Jackson Regional Office
Veterans Benefits Administration, U S Dept. of V A
1600 E Woodrow Wilson Ave
Jackson, MS 39216-5100

601-364-7000
800-827-1000
FAX: 601-364-7007
jackson.query@vba.va.gov
www.benefits.va.gov/jackson

Neil Anthony Mcphie, Chairman
Barbara Sapin, Vice Chairman

Missouri

5669 Harry S Truman Memorial Veterans' Hospital
Veterans Health Administration, U S Dept. of V A
800 Hospital Dr
Columbia, MO 65201-5275

573-814-6000
800-827-1000
FAX: 573-814-6551
g.vhacss@forum.va.gov
www.columbiamo.va.gov

Sallie Houser-Hanfelder, Director
Robert Ritter, Associate Director
Lana Zerrer, Chief of Staff

5670 John J Pershing VA Medical Center
Veterans Health Administration, U S Dept. of V A
1500 N Westwood Blvd
Poplar Bluff, MO 63901-3318
573-686-4151
888-557-8262
FAX: 573-778-4156
g.vhacss@forum.va.gov
www.poplarbluff.va.gov

Merk Hedstrom, Medical Center Director
Linda Haga, Research Contact

5671 Kansas City VA Medical Center
Veterans Health Administration, U S Dept. of V A
4801 E Linwood Blvd
Kansas City, MO 64128-2226
816-861-4700
800-827-1000
g.vhacss@forum.va.gov
www.kansascity.va.gov

Kenneth Grasing, Research/Development
Ram Sharma, Administrative Officer
Kent Hill, Executive Director
The Kansas City VA Medical Center is a modern, well-equipped teriary care inpatient and outpatient center. As the third largest teaching hospital in the metropolitan area, it maintains educational affiliations with the University of Kansas School of Medicine.

5672 St. Louis Regional Office
Veterans Benefits Administration, U S Dept. of V A
400 S 18th St
Saint Louis, MO 63103-2265
800-827-1000
stlouis.query@vba.va.gov
www.stlouis.va.gov

5673 St. Louis VA Medical Center
Veterans Health Administration, U S Dept. of V A
915 N Grand Blvd
Saint Louis, MO 63106-1621
314-652-4100
800-228-5459
FAX: 314-289-7009
g.vhacss@forum.va.gov
www.stlouis.va.gov

Dolores Minor, Administrative Officer

Montana

5674 Montana VA Regional Office
3633 Veterans Drive
Fort Harrison, MT 59636-188
406-442-7310
800-827-1000
www.va.gov

5675 V A Montana Healthcare System
U S Dept. of V A
3687 Veterans Drive
PO Box 1500
Fort Harrison, MT 59636-1500
406-442-6410
877-468-8387
FAX: 406-447-7916
ftharrison.query@vba.va.gov
www.montana.va.gov

Christine Gregory, Director
Vicki Thennis, Interim Associate Director
Trena Bonde, Chief of Staff
Norlynn Nelson, Associate Director for Patient Care
This is a complete, medically reliable dictionary of congenital malformations and disorders. As the authors explain, 'Down syndrome is the only common congenital disorder, the other defects and disorders are rare or very rare, some having been reported fewer than 20 times worlwide.' This dictionary covers them all. Examples: Aagenaes syndrome, Acrocallosal syndrome, and Acrodysostosis

5676 VA Montana Healthcare System
Veterans Health Administration, U S Dept. of V A
1892 William St
Fort Harrison, MT 59636
406-447-7945
800-827-1000
FAX: 406-447-7965
g.vhacss@forum.va.gov
www.montana.va.gov

Joseph Underkofel, Executive Director
Gregory Johnson, MD

5677 Vet Center
Readjusment Counciling Service Western Mountain Re
2795 Enterprise Ave.
Suite 1
Billings, MT 59102-3238
406-657-6071
FAX: 406-657-6603
www.va.gov

Bob Phillips, Manager
Luanne Anderson, Office Manager
Barry Osgard MS, Counselor
Readjustment counseling service for counseling veterans who are having difficulty adjusting from military service especially those diagnosed with PTSD.

Nebraska

5678 Grand Island VA Medical System
Veterans Health Administration, U S Dept. of V A
2201 N Broadwell Ave
Grand Island, NE 68803-2153
308-382-3660
866-580-1810
g.vhacss@forum.va.gov
www.nebraska.va.gov/visitors/grand_island.asp
John Hilbert, Executive Director
Daniel L Parker, Deputy Director

5679 Lincoln Regional Office
Veterans Benefits Administration, U S Dept. of V A
3800 Village Dr.
Lincoln, NE 68501-4103
402-471-4444
800-827-1000
FAX: 402-479-5124
lincoln.query@vba.va.gov
www.veteranprograms.com

Bill Gibson, CEO
Daniel Parker, Deputy Director

5680 Lincoln VA Medical Center
Veterans Health Administration, U S Dept. of V A
600 S 70th St
Lincoln, NE 68510-2451
402-489-3802
800-827-1000
FAX: 402-486-7860
g.vhacss@forum.va.gov
www.nebraska.va.gov/visitors/lincoln.asp
Ryon L Adams, Research/Development Coordinator

5681 VA Nebraska-Western Iowa Health Care System
Veterans Health Administration, U S Dept. of V A
4101 Woolworth Ave
Omaha, NE 68105-1850
402-449-0610
800-451-5796
FAX: 402-449-0684
www.nebraska.va.gov

Marci Mylan, Director
Rowen Zetterman, Chief of Staff

Nevada

5682 **Las Vegas Veterans Center**
1919 S. Jones, Suite A
Las Vegas, NV 89146-905
702-251-7873
FAX: 702-388-6664
www.lasvegas.va.gov

Daryl Harding, Resident Counselor LCSW
Matt Watson, Team Leader MSW
Veterans clinical counseling center for veterans and their dependent individual and group counseling, marital and family counseling, alcohol and drug assessment referral or treatment. Community education and consultation, employment counseling.

5683 **Reno Regional Office**
Veterans Benefits Administration U S Deptartment o
1000 Locust St
Reno, NV 89502-2597
775-328-1486
800-827-1000
FAX: 775-328-1447
reno.query@vba.va.gov
www.reno.va.gov

Joseph E Dardillo, Administrative Officer

5684 **VA Sierra Nevada Healthcare System**
Veterans Health Administration, U S Dept. of V A
957 Kirman Ave
Reno, NV 89502-2597
775-786-7200
888-838-6256
FAX: 775-328-1816
https://iris.custhelp.com
www.reno.va.gov

Kurt W. Schlegelmich, Director
Michael C. Tadych, Associate Director
Rachel Crossley, Associate Director
Steve E. Brilliant, Chief of Staff

5685 **VA Southern Nevada Healthcare System**
Veterans Health Administration, U S Dept. of V A
6900 North Pecos Rd
Las Vegas, NV 89086
702-791-9000
800-827-1000
FAX: 707-636-3027
g.vhacss@forum.va.gov
www.lasvegas.va.gov

Isabel M. Duff, Acting Director
Ramu Komanduri, Chief of Staff
Sandra L. Solem, Acting Nurse Executive
John L. Stelsel, Assistant Director

New Hampshire

5686 **Manchester Regional Office**
Veterans Benefits Administration, U S Dept. of V A
275 Chestnut St
Manchester, NH 3101-2411
800-827-1000
manchester.query@vba.va.gov
www.va.gov

Jerry Beale, Director

5687 **Manchester VA Medical Center**
Veterans Health Administration, U S Dept. of V A
718 Smyth Rd
Manchester, NH 03104-7007
603-624-4366
800-892-8384
g.vhacss@forum.va.gov
www.manchester.va.gov

Susan MacKenzie, Acting Med Center Director
Tammy A. Krueger, Associate Director
Andrew J. Breuder, Chief of Staff
Carol Williams, Associate Director for Patients

5688 **New Hampshire Veterans Centers**
103 Liberty St
Manchester, NH 3104-3118
603-668-7060
800-562-3127
FAX: 603-666-7404
www.va.gov

Caryl Ahern, Manager
Paulette Landry, Office Manager
Veterans clinic offering combat veterans outpatient counseling

New Jersey

5689 **Disabled American Veterans: Ocean County**
P.O.Box 1806
Toms River, NJ 8754-1806
732-929-0907
bvenga@thecore.com
community.nj.com/cc/dav24

Mary Bencivenga, Contact

5690 **East Orange Campus of the VA New Jersey Healthcare System**
385 Tremont Ave
East Orange, NJ 07018-1023
973-676-1000
FAX: 973-676-4226
www.newjersey.va.gov

Kenneth Mizrach, Director
Glen Giaquinto, Associate Director
John A. Griffith, Associate Director
Patrick J. Troy, Nurse Executive

5691 **Lyons Campus of the VA New Jersey Healthcare System**
Veterans Health Administration, U S Dept. of V A
151 Knollcroft Rd
Lyons, NJ 7939-5001
908-647-0180
800-827-1000
FAX: 908-647-3452
g.vhacss@forum.va.gov
www.newjersey.va.gov

James J Farsetta, Director
Donna Henderson, Coordinator

5692 **Newark Regional Office**
Veterans Benefits Administration, U S Dept. of V A
20 Washington Pl
Newark, NJ 07102-3174
973-645-1441
800-827-1000
newark.query@vba.va.gov
www.newjersey.va.gov

Stephen G Abel, Deputy Commissioner for Veterans

New Mexico

5693 New Mexico State Veterans' Home
992 South Broadway
Truth or Consequences, NM 87901-927   575-894-4200
800-964-3976
FAX: 575-894-4270
www.nmveteranshome.org/index/shtml
Lori S Montgomery, Administrator
Carol B Wilson, Admission Coordinator
Veterans medical clinic offering disabled veterans medical treatments.

5694 New Mexico VA Healthcare System
Veterans Health Administration, US Dept. of VA
1501 San Pedro Dr SE
Albuquerque, NM 87108-5154   505-265-1711
800-465-8262
FAX: 505-256-2855
g.vhacss@forum.va.gov
www.albuquerque.va.gov
George Marnell, Executive Director
Pamela Crowell, Acting Associate Director
Peter Woodbridge, Chief of Staff
Jennifer DeWinne, Acting Assistant Director

New York

5695 Albany VA Medical Center: Samuel S Stratton
Veterans Health Administration, U S Dept. of V A
113 Holland Ave
Albany, NY 12208-3410   518-626-5000
800-233-4810
888-838-7890
FAX: 518-626-5500
g.vhacss@forum.va.gov
www.albany.va.gov
Donald W Stuart, Associate Director (Interim)
Linda W Weiss, Director
Laurdes Irzarry, Chief of Staff
Deborah Spath, Associate Director for Patient/N

5696 Albany Vet Center
Ste 2
17 Computer Dr W
Albany, NY 12205-1618   518-458-7998
FAX: 518-458-8613
Lloyd Mc Omber, Owner
Melodie Krahula, Team Leader
Provides readjustment counseling for combat veterans and also provides benefits and job counseling for all veterans.

5697 Bath VA Medical Center
Veterans Health Administration U S Deptartment of
76 Veterans Avenue
Bath, NY 14810   607-664-4000
877-845-3247
888-823-9659
FAX: 607-664-4000
g.vhacss@forum.va.gov
www.bath.va.gov
Michael Swartz, Medical Center Director
David B. Krueger, Associate Director
Felipe Diaz, Chief of Staff
Shirley A. Pikula, Associate Director for Patient Services

5698 Bronx VA Medical Center
Veterans Health Administration, U S Dept. of V A
130 W Kingsbridge Rd
Bronx, NY 10468-9938   718-584-9000
800-877-6976
FAX: 718-733-1223
g.vhacss@forum.va.gov
www.bronx.va.gov
Eric Langhoff, Director
Vincent F Immiti, Associate Director
Kathleen M. Capitulo, Chief of Staff
Kathleen M Capitulo, Associate Director for Patient C

5699 Brooklyn Campus of the VA NY Harbor Healthcare System
Veterans Health Administration, U S Dept. of V A
800 Poly Place
Brooklyn, NY 11209-7104   718-836-6600
800-827-1000
g.vhacss@forum.va.gov
www.nyharbor.va.gov
Martina A Parauda, Director
Veronica J Foy, Associate Director, Facilities &
Michael S Simberkoff, Executive Chief of Staff
Elizabeth H Weinshel, Deputy Chief of Staff

5700 Buffalo Regional OfficeDepartment of Veterans Affairs
Veterans Benefits Administration
130 South Elmwood Avenue
Buffalo, NY 14202-2465   716-852-3028
800-827-1000
www.va.gov

5701 Canandiagua VA Medical Center
Veterans Health Administration, U S Dept. of V A
400 Fort Hill Ave
Canandaigua, NY 14424-1159   585-394-2000
800-204-9917
g.vhacss@forum.va.gov
www.canandaigua.va.gov
Craig S Howard, Medical Center Director
Margaret Owens, Associate Director
Dr. Robert B Babcock, Chief of Staff
Patricia Hryzak Lind, Associate Director for Patient/N

5702 Castle Point Campus of the VA Hudson Valley Healthcare System
Veterans Health Administration, U S Dept. of V A
Route 9D
Castle Point, NY 12511   845-831-2000
800-827-1000
FAX: 845-838-5193
g.vhacss@forum.va.gov
www.hudsonvalley.va.gov
Gerald F Culliton, Director
John M. Gary, Associate Director
Patricia A. Burke, Associate Director
Joanne J. Malina, Chief of Staff

5703 New York City Campus of the VA NY Harbor Healthcare System
Veterans Health Administration, U S Dept. of V A
423 E 23rd St
New York, NY 10010-5011   212-686-7500
800-827-1000
FAX: 718-567-4082
g.vhacss@forum.va.gov
www.nyharbor.va.gov
Camille R Varacchi, Administrative Officer

5704 New York Regional Office
Veterans Benefits Administration, U S Dept. of V A
245 W Houston St
New York, NY 10014-4805
212-714-0699
800-827-1000
FAX: 212-807-4042
newyork.query@vba.va.gov
www.va.gov

Ronna Brown, President

5705 Northport VA Medical Center
Veterans Health Administration, U S Dept. of V A
79 Middleville Rd
Northport, NY 11768-2296
631-261-4400
800-827-1000
FAX: 631-266-6710
g.vhacss@forum.va.gov
www.northport.va.gov

Philip C Moschitta, Medical Center Director
Rosie A Chatman, Associate Director for Patient &
Maria Favale, Associate Director
Edward Mack, Chief of Staff

5706 Syracuse VA Medical Center
Veterans Health Administration, U S Dept. of V A
800 Irving Ave
Syracuse, NY 13210-2716
315-425-4400
800-792-4334
888-838-7890
g.vhacss@forum.va.gov
www.syracuse.va.gov

James Cody, VA Medical Center Director
Judy Hayman, Associate Medical Center Director
William H Marx, Chief of Staff
Nancy Schmid, Associate Director for Patient/N

5707 Torah Alliance of Families of Kids with Disabilities
T AF KI D
1433 Coney Island Ave
Brooklyn, NY 11230-4119
718-252-2236
FAX: 718-252-2216
tafkid@worldnet.att.net
www.tafkid.org

Juby Shapiro, Manager
Serves over 1k families whose children have a variety of disabilities and special needs. Many of these families are large families in the low socioeconomic level. Offers monthly meetings, guest lectures, parent matching, information of new developments in software, technology and techniques, sibling support groups, pen pal lists, audio and video library, alternative medicine and nutrition information and education on legal awareness and rights of disabled citizens.

5708 VA Hudson Valley Health Care System
Veterans Health Administration, U S Department of
2094 Albany Post Road
Montrose, NY 10548-1454
914-737-4400
FAX: 845-788-4244
www.hudsonvalley.va.gov

James J Farsette, Network Director
Michael Sabo, Executive Director

5709 VA Western NY Healthcare System, Batavia
Veterans Health Administration, U S Dept. of V A
222 Richmond Ave
Batavia, NY 14020-1227
585-297-1000
800-827-1000
FAX: 585-786-1258
g.vhacss@forum.va.gov
www.va.gov

William F Feeley, Medical Center Director
Miguel Rainstein, Chief of Staff
Jason C Petti, Associate Medical Center Directo
Royce Calhoun, Assistant Director

5710 VA Western NY Healthcare System, Buffalo
Veterans Health Administration, U S Dept. of V A
3495 Bailey Ave
Buffalo, NY 14215-1129
716-834-9200
800-532-8387
www.buffalo.va.gov

Brian Stiller, Medical Center Director
Jason C. Petti, Chief of Staff
Royce Calhoun, Associate Medical Center Directo
Miguel Rainstein, Chief of Staff

North Carolina

5711 Asheville VA Medical CenterCharles George
Veterans Health Administration, U S Dept. of V A
1100 Tunnel Rd
Asheville, NC 28805-2043
828-298-7911
800-932-6408
FAX: 828-299-2502
g.vhacss@forum.va.gov
www.asheville.va.gov

Cynthia Beyfogle, Executive Director
David A. Pattillo, Assistant Medical Director
James Wells, Chief of Staff
Dennis J. Mehring, Public Affairs Officer

5712 Charlotte Vet Center
2114 Ben Craig Drive
Charlotte, NC 28262-2350
704-549-8025
FAX: 704-549-8261
www.va.gov

Loretta Deaton, Team Leader
Cynthia Algra, Office Manager
Billy Moore, Counselor
Melissa L Saunders, Counsilor
Preadjustment Counseling for Combat Veterans with Post Traumatic Stress Disorder (PTSD).

5713 Durham VA Medical Center
Veterans Health Administration, U S Dept. of V A
508 Fulton St
Durham, NC 27705-3875
919-286-0411
800-827-1000
888-878-6890
FAX: 919-286-5944
leola.jenkins@med.va.gov
www.durham.va.gov

Deanne M Seekins, Director
Rudy A Klopfer, Associate Director
John D Shelburne, Chief of Staff
Kathryn Ward-Presson, Associate Director for Nursing P
Since 1953, Durham Veterans Affairs Medical Cetner has been improving the health of the men and women who have so proudly served our nation. We consider it our privilege to serve your health care needs in any way we can. Services are available to more than 200,000 veterans living in a 26-county area of central and eastern North Carolina.

5714 Fayetteville VA Medical Center
Veterans Health Administration, U S Dept. of V A
2300 Ramsey St
Fayetteville, NC 28301-3856
910-488-2120
800-771-6106
FAX: 910-822-7926
g.vhacss@forum.va.gov
www.va.gov

Elizabeth Goolsby, Director
James Galkowski, Associate Director, Operations
Jesse Howard III, Acting Chief of Staff
Joyce Alexander-Hines, Associate Director, Patient Care
Since 1940,the Fayetteville VA Medical Center (VAMC) hasimproved the health of the men and women who have so

proudly served our nation. We consider it our privilege to serve your health care needs in any way we can. Medical, mental health, women's health careand specialty servicesare available to more than 157,000 veterans living in a 21-county area of North Carolina and South Carolina.

5715 WG Hefner VA Medical CenterSalisbury
Vet Health Administration U S Department of VA
1601 Brenner Ave
Salisbury, NC 28144-2515   704-638-9000
                                           800-469-8252
                                           FAX: 704-638-3395
                                           g.vhacss@forum.va.gov
                                           www.salisbury.va.gov

Kaye Green, Director
Linette Barker, Associate Medical Center Directo
Subbarao Pemmaraju, Chief of Staff (Interim)
Michele Hill, Associate Director for Patient C

Since 1953, Hefner VAMC has been improving the health of the men and women who have so proudly served our nation. We consider it our privilege to serve your health care needs in any way we can. Primary and secondary inpatient health care are available to more than 287,000 veterans living in a 24-county area of the Central Piedmont Region of North Carolina. This includes the Charlotte area with over 100,000 veterans, and the Winston-Salem area with 65,000 veterans.

5716 Winston-Salem Regional Office
Veterans Benefits Administration, U S Dept. of V A
251 N Main St
Winston-Salem, NC 27155-2   336-768-5560
                                           800-827-1000
                                           FAX: 336-768-7295
                                           TTY: 800-829-4833
                                           winsalem.query@vba.va.gov
                                           www.va.gov

Glenn Cobb, Executive VP

North Dakota

5717 Fargo VA Medical Center
Veterans Health Administration, U S Dept. of V A
2101 North Elm
Fargo, ND 58102-2417   701-232-3241
                                           800-410-9723
                                           FAX: 701-239-7166
                                           g.vhacss@forum.va.gov
                                           www.va.gov

Michael J Murphy, Healthcare Center Director
Dale DeKrey, Associate Director for Operation
J Brian Hancock, Chief of Staff
Julie Bruhn, Associate Director for Patient C

5718 North Dakota VA Regional OfficeFargo Regional Office
Veterans Benefits Administration, U S Dept. of V A
2101 Elm St N
Fargo, ND 58102-2417   701-451-4690
                                           800-410-9723
                                           FAX: 701-451-4690
                                           fargo.query@vba.va.gov
                                           www.fargo.va.gov

Thomas Santoro, Director Research Department

Ohio

5719 Chillicothe VA Medical Center
Veterans Health Administration, U S Dept. of V A
17273 State Route 104
Chillicothe, OH 45601-9718   740-773-1141
                                           800-358-8262
                                           888-838-6446
                                           FAX: 740-772-7023
                                           g.vhacss@forum.va.gov
                                           www.chillicothe.va.gov

Wendy J. Hepker, Medical Center Director
Keith Sullivan, Associate Medical Center Directo
Deborah M Meesig, Chief of Staff
Ruth Yerardi, Associate Director for Patient C

The Chillicothe VA Medical Center provides acute and chronic mental health services, primary and secondary medical services, a wide range of nursing home care services, specialty medical services as well as specialized women Veterans health clinics. The facility is an active ambulatory care setting and serves as a chronic mental health referral center for VA Medical Center in southern Ohio and parts of West Virginia and Kentucky

5720 Cincinnati VA Medical Center
Veterans Health Administration, U S Dept. of V A
3200 Vine St
Cincinnati, OH 45220-2213   513-861-3100
                                           800-827-1000
                                           888-267-7873
                                           FAX: 513-475-6500
                                           g.vhacss@forum.va.gov
                                           www.cincinnati.va.gov

Linda Smith, Director
David Ninneman, Associate Director
Robert Falcone, Chief of Staff
Katheryn Cook, Nurse Executive

5721 Cleveland Regional Office
Veterans Benefits Administration, U S Dept. of V A
1240 E 9th St
Cleveland, OH 44199-2068   800-827-1000
                                           FAX: 216-522-8262
                                           cleveland.query@vba.va.gov
                                           www.va.gov

P Hunter Peckham, Director
Robert Ruff, Assistant Director
William Bunkley, Minority Veterans Program Coordi

5722 Dayton VA Medical Center
Veterans Health Administration U S Department of V
4100 W 3rd St
Dayton, OH 45428-9000   937-268-6511
                                           800-368-8262
                                           888-838-6446
                                           FAX: 937-262-2170
                                           g.vhacss@forum.va.gov
                                           www.dayton.va.gov

Glenn Costie, Acting Director
Mark Murdock, Associate Director
James T. Hardy, Chief of Staff
Anna Jones, Associate Director, Patient Care

The Dayton VAMC is a state of the art teaching facility that has been serving Veterans for 146 years, having accepted its first patient in 1867. The Dayton VA Medical Center provides a full range of health care through medical, surgical, mental health (inpatient and outpatient), home and community health programs, geriatric (nursing home), physical medicine and therapy services, neurology, oncology, dentistry, and hospice.

5723 Louis Stokes VA Medical CenterWade Park Campus
Veterans Health Administration, U S Dept. of V A
10701 East Blvd
Cleveland, OH 44106-1702   216-791-3800
                                        877-838-8262
                                        888-838-6446
                                        FAX: 440-838-6017
                                        g.vhacss@forum.va.gov
                                        www.cleveland.va.gov

Susan M Fuehrer, Medical Center Director
Darwin Goodspeed, Associate Medical Center Director
Murray D. Altose, Chief of Staff
Inette Sarduy, Associate Director Patient

Oklahoma

5724 Jack C. Montgomery VA Medical Center
Veterans Benefits Administration, U S Dept. of V A
1011 Honor Heights Dr
Muskogee, OK 74401-1318   918-577-3000
                                        800-827-1000
                                        muskogee.query@vba.va.gov
                                        www.muskogee.va.gov

Alef Nancy Graham, Manager

5725 Jack C. Montomery VA Medical Center
1011 Honor Heights Dr
Muskogee, OK 74401-1318   918-577-3000
                                        800-827-1000
                                        muskogee.query@vba.va.gov
                                        www.muskogee.va.gov

James R. Floyd, Medical Director
Inez Reitz, Acting Associate Director
Thomas D. Schneider, Chief of Staff
Bonnie R Pierce, Associate Director for Patient C

5726 Oklahoma City VA Medical Center
Veterans Health Administration, U S Dept. of V A
921 NE 13th St
Oklahoma City, OK 73104-5007   405-456-1000
                                        800-827-1000
                                        FAX: 405-270-1560
                                        www.oklahoma.va.gov

Jimmy A. Murphy, Director
Debra A. Colombe, Associate Director
Mark Huycke, Chief of Staff
Donna DeLise, Associate Director for Patient C

5727 Oklahoma Veterans Centers Vet Center
3033 N Walnut Ave
Ste W101
Oklahoma City, OK 73105-2833   405-270-5184
                                        FAX: 405-270-5125

Peter Sharp, Manager
Steve Kenzie, Owner
PTSP counseling for all combat Veterans and victims of sexual
trauma/sexual harassment.

Oregon

5728 Oregon Health Sciences University
3181 SW Sam Jackson Park Rd
Portland, OR 97239-3098   503-494-8311
                                        ohsu.edu

Joe Robertson, President
James Morgan, Executive Director
Offers services for the totally blind, legally blind, visually impaired, mentally retarded blind and more with health, counseling,
educational, recreational, rehabilitation, computer training and
professional training services.

5729 Portland Regional Office
Veterans Benefits Administration, U S Dept. of V A
100 SW Main St, Floor 2
Portland, OR 97204-2802   503-373-2388
                                        800-827-1000
                                        portland.query@vba.va.gov
                                        www.va.gov

5730 Portland VA Medical Center
Veterans Health Administration, U S Dept. of V A
3710 SW U.S. Veterans Hospital Rd.
Portland, OR 97239-2964   503-220-8262
                                        800-949-1004
                                        FAX: 503-273-5319
                                        g.vhacss@forum.va.gov
                                        www.portland.va.gov

John E Patrick, Director
David Stockwell, Deputy Director of Administratio
Tom Anderson, Chief of Staff
Kathleen M Chapman, Deputy Director for Patient Care
The Portland VA Medical Center (PVAMC) is a 303-bed consolidated facility with two main divisions. The medical center serves
as the quaternary referral center for Oregon, Southern Washington, and parts of Idaho for the U.S. Department of Veterans Affairs. The Portland VAMC is located atop Marquam Hill on 28.5
acres overlooking the city of Portland. In addition to comprehensive medical and mental health services, the Portland VAMC supports ongoing research and medical education, including nati

5731 Roseburg VA Medical Center
Veterans Health Administration, U S Dept. of V A
913 NW Garden Valley Blvd
Roseburg, OR 97471-6523   541-440-1000
                                        800-549-8387
                                        FAX: 541-440-1225
                                        g.vhacss@forum.va.gov
                                        www.roseburg.va.gov

Jim Willis, Director
Mark Traines, MD

5732 Southern Oregon Rehabilitation Center & Clinics
Veterans Health Administration, U S Dept. of V A
8495 Crater Lake Hwy
White City, OR 97503   541-826-2111
                                        800-809-8725
                                        FAX: 541-830-3500
                                        g.vhacss@forum.va.gov
                                        www.southernoregon.va.gov

George Andries, Executive Director

Pennsylvania

5733 Butler VA Medical Center
Veterans Health Administration, U S Dept. of V A
325 New Castle Rd
Butler, PA 16001-2418   724-282-7171
                                        800-362-8262
                                        FAX: 724-282-7640
                                        g.vhacss@forum.va.gov
                                        www.butler.va.gov

John Gennaro, Director
Rebecca Hubscher, Associate Director
Sharon Parson, Nurse Executive
Timothy Burke, Chief of Staff
VA Butler Healthcare is located in the heart of Butler County, on
the bus line, and convenient to community support services for
Western Pennsylvania and Eastern Ohio-area Veterans. We have
been attending to Veterans' total care since 1947 and are the
health care choice for over 18,000 Veterans - providing comprehensive Veteran care including primary, specialty, and mental
health care - as well as health maintenance plans, management of
chronic conditions and preventative medicine needs.

5734 **Coatesville VA Medical Center**
Veterans Health Administration, U S Dept. of V A
1400 Blackhorse Hill Rd
Coatesville, PA 19320-2040
610-384-7711
800-290-6172
888-558-3812
g.vhacss@forum.va.gov
www.coatesville.va.gov

Gary Devansky, Director
Sheila Chelleppa, Chief of Staff
Nancy Schmid, Associate Director Patient Care
Jonathan Eckman, Associate Director

5735 **Erie VA Medical Center**
Veterans Health Administration, U S Dept. of V A
135 E 38th Street Blvd
Erie, PA 16504-1559
814-868-8661
800-274-8387
888-860-2124
FAX: 814-860-2425
g.vhacss@forum.va.gov
www.erie.va.gov

Michael Adelman, Medical Center Director
Melissa Sundin, Associate Medical Center Directo
Dr. Anthony Behm, Chief of Staff
Dorene Sommers, Associate Director for Patient C

5736 **James E Van Zandt VA Medical Center**
Veterans Health Administration, U S Dept. of V A
2907 Pleasant Valley Blvd
Altoona, PA 16602-4377
814-943-8164
800-827-1000
FAX: 814-940-7898
g.vhacss@forum.va.gov
www.va.gov

Cecil B Hengeveld, Director
Gerald Williams, Executive Director

5737 **Lebanon VA Medical Center**
Veterans Health Administration, U S Dept. of V A
1700 S Lincoln Ave
Lebanon, PA 17042-7597
717-272-6621
800-409-8771
FAX: 717-228-5907
g.vhacss@forum.va.gov
www.lebanon.va.gov

Robert (Bob) Callahan Jr., Director
Robin C. Aube-Warren, Associate Director
Kanan Chatterjee, Chief of Staff
Margaret G Wilson, Associate Director for Patient C

5738 **Pennsylvania Veterans Centers**
Veterans Health Administration, U S Department of
135 E 38th St
Erie, PA 16504
814-868-8661
800-274-8387
FAX: 717-861-8589
www.erie.va.gov

Michael Aldeman, medical Center Director
Melissa Sundin, Associate Director
Anthony Behm, Chief of Staff
Veterans medical clinic offering disabled veterans medical treatments.

5739 **Philadelphia Regional Office and Insurance Center**
Veterans Benefits Administration, U S Dept. of V A
5000 Wissahickon Ave
Philadelphia, PA 19144-4867
215-336-3003
800-827-1000
FAX: 215-336-5542
phillyro.query@vba.va.gov
www.va.gov

Sonny Dicrecchio, Executive Director

5740 **Philadelphia VA Medical Center**
Veterans Health Administration, U S Dept. of V A
3900 Woodland Avenue
Philadelphia, PA 19104
215-823-5800
800-949-1001
g.vhacss@forum.va.gov
www.philadelphia.va.gov

Joseph M Dalpiaz, Director
Ralph Schapira, Chief of Staff
Margaret O'Shea Caplan, Associate Director for Finance
Patricia O'Kane, Acting Associate Director for Cl

5741 **Pittsburgh Regional Office**
Veterans Benefits Administration U S Deparment of
1000 Liberty Avenue
Pittsburgh, PA 15222
412-688-6100
800-827-1000
FAX: 412-688-6121
pittsburgh.query@vba.va.gov
www.pittsburgh.va.gov

Micahel E Moreland

5742 **VA Pittsburgh Healthcare System, University Drive Division**
Veterans Health Administration, U S Dept. of V A
University Dr
Pittsburgh, PA 15240-2400
412-688-6000
866-482-7488
FAX: 412-688-6901
g.vhacss@forum.va.gov
www.pittsburgh.va.gov

Timothy Mar Carlos, CEO

5743 **VA Pittsburgh Healthcare System, Highland Drive Division**
Veterans Health Administration, U S Dept. of V A
7180 Highland Dr
Pittsburgh, PA 15206-1206
412-688-6000
800-827-1000
FAX: 412-365-4213
g.vhacss@forum.va.gov
www.pittsburgh.va.gov

Kristin Best, Deputy Adjutant General
Roger Sutton, MD

5744 **Wilkes-Barre VA Medical Center**
Veterans Health Administration, U S Dept. of V A
1111 E End Blvd
Wilkes Barre, PA 18711-30
570-824-3521
877-928-2621
FAX: 570-821-7278
g.vhacss@forum.va.gov
www.wilkes-barre.va.gov

William H Mills, Director (Interim)
Douglas V Paxton Sr., Associate Director
Mirza Z Ali, Chief of Staff
Linda Stout, Associate Director for Nursing S

Rhode Island

5745 **Providence Regional Office**
Veterans Benefits Administration, U S Dept. of V A
380 Westminster St
Providence, RI 2903-3246
401-462-0324
800-827-1000
FAX: 401-254-2320
providence.query@vba.va.gov
www.va.gov

Daniel Evangelista, Acting Associate Director

5746 **Providence VA Medical Center**
Veterans Health Administration, U S Dept. of V A
830 Chalkstone Ave
Providence, RI 02908-4799   401-273-7100
                                             866-363-4486
                                             FAX: 401-457-3360
                                             g.vhacss@forum.va.gov
                                             www.providence.va.gov

Vincent W Ng, Medical Center Director
William J Burney, Medical Center Associate Directo
Gregory M Gillette, Medical Center Chief of Staff
Deborah A Clickner, Medical Center Associate Directo

To fulfill President Lincoln's promise To care for him who shall have borne the battle, and for his widow, and his orphan by serving and honoring the men and women who are America's veterans.

South Carolina

5747 **Columbia Regional Office**
Veterans Benefits Administration, U S Dept. of V A
6437 Garners Ferry Rd
Columbia, SC 29209-2401   803-401-1094
                                             800-827-1000
                                             columbia.query@vba.va.gov
                                             www.va.gov

Jimmie Ruff, Executive Director

5748 **Ralph H Johnson VA Medical Center**
Veterans Health Administration, U S Dept. of V A
109 Bee St
Charleston, SC 29401-5703   843-577-5011
                                             800-827-1000
                                             888-878-6884
                                             FAX: 843-876-5384
                                             g.vhacss@forum.va.gov
                                             www.charleston.va.gov

Carolyn L Adams, Director
Scott Isaacks, Associate Director
Florence N Hutchinson, Chief of Staff
Mary C Fraggos, Associate Director for Patient/N

5749 **William Jennings Bryan Dorn VA Medical Center**
Veterans Health Administration U S Department of V
6439 Garners Ferry Rd
Columbia, SC 29209-1638   803-776-4000
                                             800-293-8262
                                             FAX: 803-695-6739
                                             Carolyn.Adams@va.gov
                                             www.columbiasc.va.gov

Carolyn L Adams, Director
Barbara Temeck, Chief of Staff
David L. Omura, Chief of Staff
Ruth Mustard, Director for Patient Care/Nursin

South Dakota

5750 **Royal C Johnson Veterans Memorial Medical Center**
Veterans Health Administration, U S Dept. of VA
2501 W. 22nd St
Sioux Falls, SD 57105-5046   605-336-3230
                                             800-316-8387
                                             FAX: 605-333-6878
                                             g.vhacss@forum.va.gov
                                             www.siouxfalls.va.gov

Patrick J Kelly, Director
Sara Ackert, Associate Director
Victor Waters, Chief of Staff
Barbara Teal, Associate Director, Patient Care

5751 **Sioux Falls Regional Office**
Veterans Benefits Administration, U S Dept. of V A
2501 W. 22nd St
Sioux Falls, SD 57105-5046   605-336-3230
                                             800-827-1000
                                             FAX: 605-333-5316
                                             siouxfalls.query@vba.va.gov
                                             www.siouxfalls.va.gov

Tennessee

5752 **Alvin C York VA Medical Center**
Veterans Health Administration, U S Dept. of V A
3400 Lebanon Pike
Murfreesboro, TN 37129-1237   615-867-6000
                                             800-876-7093
                                             FAX: 615-867-5768
                                             g.vhacss@forum.va.gov
                                             www.tennesseevalley.va.gov

Juan Morales, Medical System Director
Janice Cobb, Associate Director, Nursing Serv
Emma Metcalf, Chief Operating Officer

5753 **Memphis VA Medical Center**
Veterans Health Administration, U S Dept. of V A
1030 Jefferson Ave
Memphis, TN 38104-2127   901-523-8990
                                             800-636-8262
                                             g.vhacss@forum.va.gov
                                             www.memphis.va.gov

Jay Robinson III, Associate Medical Center Directo
Douglas D Southall, Assistant Medical Center Directo
Margarethe Hagemann, Chief of Staff
Marilyn Kerkhoff, Interim Associate Medical Center

5754 **Mountain Home VA Medical CenterJames H Quillen VA Medical Center**
Veterans Health Administration, US Dept. of VA
Corner of Lamont & Veterans Way
Mountain Home, TN 37684   423-926-1171
                                             877-573-3529
                                             g.vhacss@forum.va.gov
                                             www.mountainhome.va.gov

Charlene S Ehret, Medical Center Director
Jimmy H McGlawn, Associate Director
David R Reagan, Chief of Staff
Linda M McConnell, Associate Director, Patient/Nurs

5755 **Nasheville Regional Office**
Veterans Benefits Administration, U S Dept. of V A
110 9th Ave S
Nashville, TN 37203-3817
                                             800-827-1000
                                             nashville.query@vba.va.gov
                                             www.va.gov

Michael R Walsh, Administrative Officer
Donald H Rubin, Research/Development Coordinator

5756 **Nashville VA Medical Center**
Veterans Health Administration, US Dept. of VA
1310 24th Ave S
Nashville, TN 37212-2637   615-327-4751
                                             800-228-4973
                                             FAX: 615-321-6350
                                             g.vhacss@forum.va.gov
                                             www.tennesseevalley.va.gov

Juan Morales, Medical System Director
Michael A Doukas, Chief of Staff
Gary D Trende, Associate Director, Nursing Serv
Gary D Trende, Chief Operating Officer

Texas

5757   Amarillo VA Healthcare System
Veterans Health Administration, U S Dept. of V A
6010 Amarillo Blvd West
Amarillo, TX 79106-1991   806-355-9703
                                 800-687-8262
                            FAX: 806-354-7869
                         g.vhacss@forum.va.gov
                            www.amarillo.va.gov

David Welch, Director
Lance Robinson, Associate Director
Grace Stringfelow, Chief of Staff
Louise Anderson, Executive/Chief, Nursing Service

5758   Amarillo Vet Center
Department of Veterans Affairs
3414 Olsen Blvd
Suite E
Amarillo, TX 79109-3072   806-351-1104
                            FAX: 806-351-1104
                                 www.va.gov

Pedro Garcia Jr., Team Leader
Simon Camarillo, Counsilor
William C Santer, Family Therapist
Cathy L Williams, Office Manager
Provides individual, group and family counseling to veterans
who served in combat theaters of World War II and Korea, veterans
of the Vietnam Era, and veterans of conflicts zones in Lebanon,
Grenada, Panama, the Persian Guld and Somalia.

5759   El Paso VA Healthcare Center
Veterans Health Administration, U S Dept. of V A
5001 N Piedras
El Paso, TX 79930-4210   915-564-6100
                                 800-672-3782
                            FAX: 915-564-7920
                         g.vhacss@forum.va.gov
                             www.elpaso.va.gov

John A. Mendoza, Director
Elizabeth Lowery, Associate Director
Homer LeMar, Interim Chief of Staff
Timothy McMurry, Associate Director, Patient Care

5760   Houston Regional Office
Veterans Benefits Administration, U S Dept. of V A
6900 Almeda Rd
Houston, TX 77030-4200   713-791-1414
                                 800-827-1000
                      houston.query@vba.va.gov
                                 www.va.gov

Cecil Aultman, Executive Director
Edgar Tucker, Chief Executive Officer

5761   Michael E. Debakey VA Medical Center
Veterans Health Administration, U S Dept. of V A
2002 Holcombe Blvd
Houston, TX 77030-4211   713-791-1414
                                 800-553-2278
                         g.vhacss@forum.va.gov
                            www.houston.va.gov

Adam C Walmus, Director
J Kalavar, Chief of Staff
Francisco Vazquez, Associate Director
Thelma Grey-Becknell, Associate Director for Patient C

5762   South Texas Veterans Healthcare System
Veterans Health Administration, U S Dept. of V A
7400 Merton Minter
San Antonio, TX 78229-4404   210-617-5300
                                 877-469-5300
                                 888-686-6350
                         g.vhacss@forum.va.gov
                           www.southtexas.va.gov

Marie L. Wedon, Director
Wade Vlosich, Associate Director
Joe A. Perez, Assistant Director
Julianne Flynne, Chief of Staff

**5763   VA North Texas Health Veterans Affairs Care System:
Dallas VA Medical Center**
Veterans Health Administration, U S Dept. of V A
4500 S Lancaster Rd
Dallas, TX 75216-7167   214-742-8387
                                 800-849-3597
                            FAX: 214-857-1171
                   www.northtexas.va.gov/index.asp

Jeffrey Milligan, Director
Peter Dancy, Associate Director
Clark R. Gregg, Chief of Staff
Alan Bernstein, Assistant Director
Health care system which serves veterans with medical care and
rehabilitation services including spinal cord injury center. For
VA benefit inquiries contact 1-800-827-1000. This system has locations
in Bonham, Dallas, and Fort Worth.

5764   Waco Regional Office
Veterans Benefits Administration, U S Dept. of V A
4800 Memorial Dr
Waco, TX 76711-1   254-752-6581
                                 800-423-1111
                            TTY:800-829-4833
                        waco.query@vba.va.gov
                          www.centraltexas.va.gov

William F. Harper, Chief of Staff
Russell E. Lloyd, Associate Director of Resources
Karen Spada, Associate Director for Patients
Andrew Garcia, Assistant Director for Operations
Mission is to honor America's Veterans by providing exceptional
health care that improves their health and well being.

5765   West Texas VA Healthcare System
Veterans Health Administration, U S Dept. of V A
300 Veterans Blvd
Big Spring, TX 79720-5566   432-263-7361
                                 800-472-1365
                            FAX: 915-264-4834
                         g.vhacss@forum.va.gov
                           www.bigspring.va.gov

Andrew M. Welch, Interim Director
Kenneth Allensworth, Associate Director
Raul Zambrano, Chief of Staff
Charles V. Silveri, Associate Director
The West Texas VA Health Care System (WTVAHCS) proudly
serves Veterans in 33 counties across 53,000 square miles of rural
geography in West Texas and Eastern New Mexico. The George
H. O'Brien, Jr. VA Medical Center is located in Big Spring, Texas
and the six Community Based Outpatient Clinics (CBOC's) that
comprise the remainder of the health care system are located in
Abilene, TX, Stamford, TX, San Angelo, TX, Odessa, TX, Fort
Stockton, TX, and Hobbs, NM.

Utah

5766 Utah Division of Veterans Affairs
Utah Division of Veterans Affairs
550 Foothill Blvd
Ste 202
Salt Lake City, UT 84113-1106   801-582-1565
                                        800-894-9497
                                        FAX: 801-326-2369
                                        tandrews@utah.gov
                                        www.saltlakecity.va.gov

David J Peifer, Director
Todd Andrews, Assistant to the Director
Karen H. Gribbin, Manager
Our mission is to serve the veteran who served us. The VA Salt Lake City Health Care System is committed to providing our patients with the highest Quality of Care in an environment that is safe. We do this by focusing on Continuous Process Improvement and by supporting a Culture of Safety

5767 VA Salt Lake City Healthcare System
Veterans Health Administration, U S Dept. of V A
500 Foothill Drive
Salt Lake City, UT 84148-1   801-582-1565
                                     800-613-4012
                                     FAX: 801-584-1289
                                     www.saltlakecity.va.gov

Steven W Young, Director
Warren E Hill, Associate Director
Karen H. Gribbin, Chief of Staff
Shella Stovall, Associate Director, Patient Care
Our mission is to serve the veteran who served us. The VA Salt Lake City Health Care System is committed to providing our patients with the highest Quality of Care in an environment that is safe. We do this by focusing on Continuous Process Improvement and by supporting a Culture of Safety

Vermont

5768 Vermont VA Regional Office Center
Veterans Benefits Administration U S Department V
215 N Main St
White River Junction, VT 05009-1   802-295-9363
                                           866-687-8387
                                           FAX: 802-290-6354
                                           whiteriver.query@vba.va.gov
                                           www.whiteriver.va.gov

Deborah Amdur, Executive Director
Danielle S. Ocker, Associate Director
Melanie Thompson, Acting Chief of Staff
Laura F. Miraldi, Associate Director for Nursing
The White River Junction VA Medical Center (WRJ VAMC) is responsible for the delivery of health care services to eligible Veterans in Vermont and the 4 contiguous counties of New Hampshire. These services are delivered at the Medical Center's main campus located in White River Junction, Vermont, and at its seven Outpatient Clinics (Bennington, Brattleboro, Colchester, Newport, and Rutland, Vermont; Keene and Littleton, New Hampshire). The White River Junction VA is closely affiliated with the Ge

5769 Vermont Veterans Centers
359 Dorset St
South Burlington, VT 05403-6210   802-862-1806
                                          877-927-8387
                                          FAX: 802-865-3319
                                          www.va.gov

Fred Forehand, Team Leader
William Newkirk, Counsilor
George Troutman, Counsilor
Tamara R Thompson, Family Therapist
Veterans medical clinic offering disabled veterans medical treatments.

Virginia

5770 Hampton VA Medical Center
Veterans Health Administration, U S Dept. of V A
100 Emancipation Dr
Hampton, VA 23667-1   757-722-9961
                              800-827-1000
                              FAX: 757-728-3135
                              mike.eisenberg@med.va.gov
                              www.hampton.va.gov

Deanne M Seekins, Medical Center Director
Benita K Stoddard, Associate Director for Operation
G. Arul, Chief of Staff
Shedale Tindall, Associate Director for Patient C

5771 Hunter Holmes McGuire VA Medical Center
Veterans Health Administration, U S Dept. of V A
1201 Broad Rock Blvd
Richmond, VA 23249-1   804-675-5000
                               800-784-8381
                               FAX: 804-675-5236
                               g.vhacss@forum.va.gov
                               www.richmond.va.gov

Charles E Sepich, Director
David P Budinger, Associate Director
Julie Beales, Interim Chief of Staff
Rita A Duval, Associate Director for Patient C

5772 Roanoke Regional Office
Veterans Benefits Administration, U S Dept. of V A
116 North Jefferson St
Roanoke, VA 24016-1906   540-362-1999
                                 800-827-1000
                                 FAX: 540-563-4838
                                 anne.atkins@vdvs.virginia.gov
                                 www.va.gov

Roger Bohm, Executive
Bert Boyd, COO/Executive Director

5773 Salem VA Medical Center
Veterans Health Administration, U S Dept. of V A
1970 Roanoke Blvd
Salem, VA 24153-6478   540-982-2463
                               800-827-1000
                               888-982-2463
                               FAX: 540-983-1096
                               g.vhacss@forum.va.gov
                               www.salem.va.gov

Miguel H LaPuz, Director
Carol S Bogedain, Associate Director
Maureen McCarthy, Chief of Staff
Pearl Washington, Nurse Executive

5774 Virginia Department of Veterans Services
270 Franklin Rd SW
Roanoke, VA 24011-2204   540-857-7102
                                 FAX: 540-857-6437
                                 pmigrand131@worldnet.att.net
                                 dvs.virginia.gov

Colbert Boyd, Manager

Washington

5775 Jonathan M Wainwright Memorial VA Medical Center
Veterans Health Administration, U S Dept. of V A
77 Wainwright Dr
Walla Walla, WA 99362-3975
509-525-5200
888-687-8863
FAX: 509-946-3062
www.va.gov

Michael W Parnicky, R and D Coordinator

5776 Seattle Regional Office
Veterans Benefits Administration U S Department of
915 2nd Ave
Seattle, WA 98174-1060
206-762-1010
800-827-1000
seattle.query@vba.va.gov
www.va.gov

Va Ad Harabanim, Executive Director
Timothy Williams, Chief Executive Officer

5777 Spokane VA Medical Center
Veterans Health Administration, U S Dept. of V A
4815 N Assembly St
Spokane, WA 99205-6185
509-434-7000
800-325-7940
FAX: 509-434-7119
g.vhacss@forum.va.gov
www.spokane.va.gov

Alan Prentiss, Chief of Staff
Dirk Minatre, Coordinator
Joseph Manley, Executive Director

5778 VA Puget Sound Health Care System
Veterans Health Administration, U S Dept. of V A
1660 S Columbian Way
Seattle, WA 98108-1532
206-762-1010
800-329-8387
g.vhacss@forum.va.gov
www.pugetsound.va.gov

Michael Fisher, Director
Michael Tadych, Deputy Director
Walt Dannenberg, Assistant Director
William Campbell, Chief of Staff

West Virginia

5779 Huntington Regional Office
Veterans Benefits Administration, U S Dept. of V A
640 4th Ave
Huntington, WV 25701-1340
304-525-5131
800-827-1000
FAX: 304-399-9344
huntington.query@vba.va.gov
www.va.gov

Mark Bugher, President

5780 Huntington VA Medical Center
Veterans Health Administration, U S Dept. of V A
1540 Spring Valley Dr
Huntington, WV 25704-9300
304-429-6741
800-827-8244
FAX: 304-429-6713
www.huntington.va.gov

Edward H Seiler, Director
Suzanne Jene, Associate Director
Jeffery B Breaux, Chief of Staff
Catherine J Locher, Associate Director for Nursing S

5781 Louis A Johnson VA Medical Center
Veterans Health Administration, U S Dept. of V A
1 Medical Center Drive
Clarksburg, WV 26301-4155
304-623-3461
800-733-0512
FAX: 304-626-7048
g.vhacss@forum.va.gov
www.clarksburg.va.gov

William E Cox, Director
Jeffrey A Beiler II, Associate Director
Glenn R Snider, Chief of Staff
Theresa J White, Nurse Executive

5782 Martinsburg VA Medical Center
Veterans Health Administration, U S Dept. of V A
510 Butler Avenue
Martinsburg, WV 25405-9990
304-263-0811
800-817-3807
FAX: 304-262-7433
g.vhacss@forum.va.gov
www.martinsburg.va.gov

Ann R Brown, Director
Timothy J Cooke, Associate Medical Center Directo
Jonathan E Fierer, Chief of Staff
Susan George, Nursing Programs and Education

5783 US Department Veterans Affairs Beckley Vet Center
200 Veterans Ave
Beckley, WV 25801-4301
304-255-2121
877-902-5142
FAX: 304-254-8711
www.beckley.va.gov

Karin L. McGraw, Director
Vet Center services includes individual and group readjustment counseling, referral for benefits assistance, liason with community agencies, marital and family counseling, substance abuse counseling, job counseling and referral, sexual trauma counseling, and community education.

Wisconsin

5784 Clement J Zablocki VA Medical Center
Veterans Health Administration U S Department of V
5000 W National Ave
Milwaukee, WI 53295-1
414-384-2000
888-827-1000
888-469-6614
FAX: 414-382-5319
www.milwaukee.va.gov

Robert H Beller, Director
Michael D Erdmann, Chief of Staff
Judith A Murphy, Associate Director for Patient/N
In an effort to improve access to veterans in Milwaukee County, the VAMC has deployed a mobile clinic that provides primary care four days a week to veterans. The Medical Center also assists the Vet Center located in the City of Milwaukee. In addition, this Medical Center participates in a four-way partnership with the WDVA, the Center for Veterans Issues, Ltd., and the Social Development Commission, to operate Vets Place Central, a 72-bed transitional housing program.

5785 Tomah VA Medical Center
Veterans Health Administration, U S Dept. of V A
500 E Veterans St
Tomah, WI 54660-3105
608-372-3971
800-872-8662
FAX: 608-372-1224
g.vhacss@forum.va.gov
www.tomah.va.gov

Mario V. DeSanctis, Medical Center Director
David Huffman, Associate Director
David J. Houlihan, Chief of Staff
Judith E. Broad, Associate Director

VAMCTomah has been improving the health of the men and women who have so proudly served our nation. We consider it our privelege to serve your health care needs in any way we can. Services are available to veterans living in a Western/Central area of Wisconsin.

5786 William S Middleton Memorial VA Hospital Center
Veterans Health Administration, U S Dept. of V A
2500 Overlook Ter
Madison, WI 53705-2254

608-256-1901
888-478-8321
888-256-1901
FAX: 608-280-7244
g.vhacss@forum.va.gov
www.madison.va.gov

Judy McKee, Director
John Rohrer, Associate Director
Alan J. Bridges, Chief of Staff
Rebecca Kordahl, Associate Director

5787 Wisconsin VA Regional Office
Veterans Benefits Administration, U S Dept. of V A
5000 W National Ave
Milwaukee, WI 53295-1

414-384-2000
800-827-1000
FAX: 414-382-5374
milwaukee.query@vba.va.gov
www.milwaukee.va.gov

Philip L Cook, Executive Director
Neil S Mandel, Research/Development Coordinator
Glen Grippen, CEO
In an effort to improve access to veterans in Milwaukee County, the VAMC has deployed a mobile clinic that provides primary care four days a week to veterans. The Medical Center also assists the Vet Center located in the City of Milwaukee. In addition, this Medical Center participates in a four-way partnership with the WDVA, the Center for Veterans Issues, Ltd., and the Social Development Commission, to operate Vets Place Central, a 72-bed transitional housing program.

Wyoming

5788 Casper Vet Center
1030 N. Poplar Suite B
Casper, WY 82601-2665

307-261-5355
FAX: 307-261-5439
www.vetcenter.va.gov

James Whipps, Office Manager
Vet Center offering re-adjustment counseling for combat veterans.

5789 Cheyenne VA Medical Center
Veterans Health Administration, U S Dept. of V A
2360 E Pershing Blvd
Cheyenne, WY 82001-5356

307-778-7370
877-927-8387
888-483-9127
FAX: 307-638-8923
g.vhacss@forum.va.gov
www.va.gov

Cynthia McCormack, Medical Center Director
Elizabeth Lowery, Associate Director
Jerry Zang, Chief of Staff
Polly Baird, Associate Director

5790 Sheridan VA Medical Center
Veterans Health Administration, U S Dept. of V A
1898 Fort Rd
Sheridan, WY 82801-8320

307-672-3473
800-827-1000
866-822-6714
FAX: 307-672-1639
g.vhacss@forum.va.gov
www.sheridan.va.gov/index.asp

Debra L Hirschman, Director
Michele Beach, Director
Wendell Robison, Chief of Staff
Jane Votaw, Nurse Executive

5791 Wyoming/Colorado VA Regional Office
Veterans Benefits Administration, U S Dept. of V A
155 Van Gordon St
Lakewood, CO 80228-1709

303-894-7474
800-827-1000
FAX: 303-894-7442
denver.query@vba.va.gov
www.va.gov

E William Belz, Director

Vocational & Employment Programs

Alabama

5792 ADRS Lakeshore
Alabama Department Of Rehabilitation Services
3830 Ridgeway Dr
Birmingham, AL 35259-9127   205-870-5999
                                    800-441-7609
                              FAX: 205-879-2685
                              www.rehab.alabama.gov

Stephen G. Kayes, District 1, Mobile
Jimmy Varnado, District 2, Montgomery
Eddie C. Williams, District 5, Huntsville
Roger McCullough, District 6, Birmingham
Rehabilitation offering employment services to severely disabled persons. Programs include Adaptive Driving Training, Assistive Technology; Employability Development, and Vocational Evaluation.

5793 Alabama Goodwill Industries
2350 Green Springs Highway S
Birmingham, AL 35205-6834   205-323-6331
                              FAX: 205-324-9059
                        caroline.goodwill@yahoo.com
                              www.alabamagoodwill.org

Don Smith, President & CEO
Paul Beasley, Chairman
Herbert L. Boring, Vice Chairman
Roger Cartwright, Treasurer
The mission of Goodwill is to provide rehabilitation services, training, employment, and opportunities for personal growth to the disabled/disadvantaged.

5794 Arc of Jefferson County
6001 Crestwood Blvd
Birmingham, AL 35212   205-323-6383
                              FAX: 205-323-0085
                              www.arcofjeff.org

Chris B. Stewart, President & CEO
Scarlet Thompson, Vice President, Development
Clarissa McKinney, Director, Day Programs - Jefferson County
Mary Frances Colley, Assistant Director, Development
The ARC has four primary components. The HOPE Program provides early intervention therapy services to developmentally delayed infants and toddlers up to the age of three years. The ARC also provides services to adults ages 21 and over with intellectual disabilities. Adult services provides education, pre-vocational screening, and socialization skills training. Employment services provides vocational training, a sheltered workshop, off-site job skills training, job coach services and more.

5795 Coffee County Training Center
801 Aviation Blvd
P.O.Box 311343
Enterprise, AL 36330   334-393-1732
                              FAX: 334-347-0252
                              vflorence@enter.twcbc.com

Vickie Florence, Manager
Clients 21 years and up receive training in Independent Living Skills, Self-Care, Language Skills, Learning, Self-Direction and Economic Self-Sufficiency. Transportation is also provided to clients of the center.

5796 Easter Seals: Achievement Center
Easter Seals of Alabama
510 W Thomason Circle
Opelika, AL 36801-5499   334-745-3501
                                866-239-2237
                          FAX: 334-749-5808
                      info@achievement-center.org
                      www.achievement-center.org

Furrel Bailey, Executive Director
Rick Dudley, Vocational Instructor
Star Wray, Director Of Industrial & Vocational Services
George Dunn, Employment Specialist
Provides vocational development and extended employment programs for physically, mentally, and developmentally disabled individuals and to non-disabled persons who are culturally, socially, or economically disadvantaged.

5797 Easter Seals: Opportunity Center
6300 McClellan Blvd
Anniston, AL 36206   256-820-9960
                        FAX: 256-820-9592
                        www.opportunity-center.com

Steven D. Miles, Administrator
Marty Gwin, Assistant Administrator Director of Rehabilitation
Lisa Fincher, Employment Specialist
Debra Wood, Vocational Instructor
A nationally accredited non-profit organization providing vocational evaluation/assessment, paid work training, and employment services for people with disabilities in Calhoun, Cleburne, Clay, Talladega, Coosa and Randolph counties.

5798 Montgomery Career Center: Alabama Employment Services Division
Alabama Department of Labor
649 Monroe St
Montgomery, AL 36131   334-286-1746
                          FAX: 334-288-7286
                    montgomery@alcc.alabama.gov
                          joblink.alabama.gov

5799 Vocational Rehabilitation Service - Opelika
Alabama Department of Rehabilitation Services
520 W Thomason Circle
Opelika, AL 36801   334-749-1259
                            800-671-6835
                      FAX: 334-749-8753
                      TTY: 800-499-1816
                          www.rehab.state.al.us

5800 Vocational Rehabilitation Service - Dothan
Alabama Department of Rehabilitation Services
795 Ross Clark Circle NE
Ste 2
Dothan, AL 36303   334-699-8600
                            800-275-0132
                      FAX: 334-792-1783
                          www.rehab.state.al.us

5801 Vocational Rehabilitation Service - Homewood
Alabama Department Of Rehabilitation Services
236 Goodwin Crest Dr
Birmingham, AL 35209   205-290-4400
                                800-671-6837
                          FAX: 205-290-0486
                          www.rehab.state.al.us

Roger McCullough, Manager
Availiable through any of the 21 VRS offices statewide, services can include educational services, vocational assesment, evaluation and counseling, job training, assistive technology, orientation and mobility training, and job placement.

5802 **Vocational Rehabilitation Service - Huntsville**
3000 Johnson Rd SW
Huntsville, AL 35805-5847 256-650-1700
800-671-6840
FAX: 256-650-1795
www.rehab.state.al.us

Eddie C. Williams, Manager
Available through any of the 21 VRS offices statewide, services
can include educational services, vocational assesment, evaluation and counseling, job training, assistive technology, orientation and mobility training, and job placement.

5803 **Vocational Rehabilitation Service - Jackson**
1401 Forest Ave
P.O.Box 1005
Jackson, AL 36545 251-246-5708
800-671-6836
FAX: 251-246-5224
www.rehab.state.al.us

5804 **Vocational Rehabilitation Service - Jasper**
Alabama Department of Rehabilitation Services
4505 Hwy 78 E
Ste 300
Jasper, AL 35501 205-221-7840
800-671-6841
FAX: 205-221-1062
www.rehab.state.al.us

5805 **Vocational Rehabilitation Service - Mobile**
Alabama Department of Rehabilitation Services
2419 Gordon Smith Dr
Mobile, AL 36617 251-479-8611
800-671-6842
FAX: 251-478-2197
www.rehab.state.al.us

Stephen G. Kayes, Manger
Available through any of the 21 VRS offices statewide, services
can include educational services, vocational assesment, evaluation and counseling, job training, assistive technology, orientation and mobility training, and job placement.

5806 **Vocational Rehabilitation Service - Muscle Shoals**
Alabama Department of Rehabilitation Services
1450 E Avalon Ave
Muscle Shoals, AL 35661 256-381-1110
800-275-0166
FAX: 256-389-3149
www.rehab.state.al.us

5807 **Vocational Rehabilitation Service - Selma**
Alabama Department of Rehabilitation Services
722 Alabama Ave
Selma, AL 36701 334-877-2927
888-761-5995
FAX: 334-877-3796
www.rehab.state.al.us

5808 **Vocational Rehabilitation Service - Talladega**
Alabama Department of Rehabilitation Services
31 Arnold St
Talladega, AL 35160 256-362-1300
800-441-7592
FAX: 256-362-6387
www.rehab.state.al.us

5809 **Vocational Rehabilitation Service - Troy**
Alabama Department of Rehabilitation Services
1109 Troy Plaza St
Troy, AL 36081 334-566-2491
800-441-7608
FAX: 334-566-9415
www.rehab.state.al.us

5810 **Vocational Rehabilitation Service - Tuscaloosa**
Alabama Department of Rehabilitation Services
1305 James I Harrison Jr Parkway E
Tuscaloosa, AL 35405 205-554-1300
800-331-5562
FAX: 205-554-1369
www.rehab.state.al.us

William Strickland, Manager
Available through any of the 21 VRS offices statewide, services
can include educational services, vocational assessment, evaluation and counseling, job training, assistive technology, orientation and mobility training, and job placement.

5811 **Vocational Rehabilitation Service- Gadsden**
Alabama Department of Rehabilitation Services
1100 George Wallace Dr
Gadsden, AL 35903-6501 256-547-6974
800-671-6839
FAX: 256-543-1784
www.rehab.state.al.us

5812 **Vocational Rehabilitation Service: Scottsboro**
Alabama Department of Rehabilitation Services
203 S Market St
P.O. Box 296
Scottsboro, AL 35768-0296 256-574-5813
800-418-8823
FAX: 256-574-6033
www.rehab.alabama.gov

5813 **Vocational Rehabilitation Services - Andalusia**
Alabama Department of Rehabilitation Services
1082 Village Square Dr
Ste 1
Andalusia, AL 36420 334-222-4114
800-671-6833
FAX: 334-427-1216
www.rehab.state.al.us

5814 **Vocational Rehabilitation Services - Anniston**
Alabama Department of Rehabilitation Services
1910 Coleman Rd
Anniston, AL 36207 256-240-8800
800-671-6834
FAX: 256-240-6580
www.rehab.state.al.us

5815 **Vocational and Rehabilitation Service - Decatur**
Alabama Department of Rehabilitation Services
621 Cherry St NE
Decatur, AL 35602 256-353-2754
800-671-6838
FAX: 256-351-2476
www.rehab.state.al.us

5816 **Vocational and Rehabilitation Services - Montgomery**
Alabama Department of Rehabilitation Services
602 S Lawrence St
Montgomery, AL 36104 334-293-7500
800-441-7578
FAX: 334-293-7372
www.rehab.state.al.us

Jimmy Varnado, Manager
Available through any of the 21 VRS offices statewide, services
can include educational services, vocational assessment, evaluation and counseling, job training, assistive technology, orientation and mobility training and job placement.

5817 Wiregrass Rehabilitation Center, Inc.
795 Ross Clark Circle
Dothan, AL 36303
334-792-0022
800-395-7044
FAX: 334-712-7632
cgreen@wcrjobs.com
www.wrcjobs.com

Ben Slingluff, Chairman
Jeff Coleman, Vice-Chairman
Cynthia Green, Director, Development
Trains individuals to become employable and assists them in finding jobs withing their communities. Also assists individuals who have difficulty maintaining employment, those who are on forms of public assistance such as welfare and those who are employable and underemployed.

5818 Workshops, Inc.
4244 3rd Ave S
Birmingham, AL 35222-2008
205-592-9683
888-805-9683
FAX: 205-592-9687
TTY:205-592-8006
email@workshopsinc.org
www.workshopsinc.org

Susan Crow, Executive Director
Dana Chang, Director, Programs
Kathy Dunn, Director, Operations
Mary Hendley, Director, Development & Marketing
Provides vocational training, sheltered employment and other support services to people with disabilities in central Alabama.

Alaska

5819 Alaska Division of Vocational Rehabilitation
Department of Labor & Workforce Development
1111 W. 8th St
Ste 210
Juneau, AK 99801-1894
907-465-2814
800-478-2815
FAX: 907-465-2856
TTY: 800-478-2815
dol.dvr.info@alaska.gov
www.labor.state.ak.us/dvr

John Cannon, Director
Assist individuals with disabilities to obtain and maintain employment.

5820 Alaska Fair Employment Practice Agency
Alaska State Commission for Human Rights
800 A St
Ste 204
Anchorage, AK 99501-3669
907-276-7474
800-478-4692
FAX: 907-278-8588
TTY: 907-276-3177
www.humanrights.alaska.gov

5821 Alaska Job Center Network
Alaska Department of Labor & Workforce Development
P.O. Box 115509
Juneau, AK 99811-5509
907-465-2712
FAX: 907-465-4537
www.jobs.alaska.gov

Arizona

5822 Downtown Neighborhood Learning Center
1001 W Jefferson St
Phoenix, AZ 85007-2913
602-254-6524
800-869-8521
FAX: 602-256-2524
dnlc@swlink.net
www.swlink.net

Scott Ritchey, Manager
Mattie Johnson, Receptionist
Peg Osinski, El Mirage Learning Lab
Adult education agency providing basic skills, GED, ESOL, life skills, computer skills, resume assistance and career testing.

5823 Fair Employment Practice Agency: Arizona
Arizona Civil Rights Division
1275 W Washington St
Phoenix, AZ 85007-2926
602-542-5025
800-352-8431
FAX: 602-542-4085
www.azag.gov

Virginia Gonzales, Director
Bruna Pedrini, Manager
Provides legal advice to most state agencies. The office also investigates and prosecutes consumer fraud, white collar crime, organized crime, public corruption, and civil rights.

5824 JOBS Administration Job Opportunities & Basic Skills
1717 W Jefferson St
Phoenix, AZ 85007-3202
602-542-9596
FAX: 602-542-5171

Gretchen Evans, Program Administrator
Assist applicants and recipients of temporary assistance to needy families to obtain job training and employment that will lead to economic independence.

5825 TETRA Services
Beacon Group SW Inc
2222 N 24th Street
Phoenix, AZ 85008
602-685-9703
FAX: 602-244-2435
info@tetraservices.org
www.tetraservices.org

5826 Vocational and Rehabilitation Agency Rehabilitation Services Administrations
Division of Employment & Rehabilitation Services
1789 W Jefferson St
Phoenix, AZ 85007-3202
602-604-8835
800-563-1221
800-563-1221
FAX: 602-604-8901
TTY:602-542-6049
tazrsa@azdes.gov
azdes.gov/rsa

Michelle Nitschke, Manager
Katharine Levandowsky, Administrator
Moises Gallegos, Manager
This program serves individuals with disabilities seeking jobs and job training.

5827 Yavapai Regional Medical Center-West
1003 Willow Creek Rd
Prescott, AZ 86301-1668
928-445-2700
877-843-9762
FAX: 928-445-0994
yrmc.org

Tim Barnett, CEO
Widely recognized for the quality and success of the physical, occupational, and speech therapy programs it offers. Provides a wide range of programs and services that enable our patients to reach their maximum level of function and independence- and enjoy the highest possible quality of life.

Arkansas

5828 Arkansas Employment Service Agency and Job Training Program
Arkansas Employment Security Department
Capitol Mall
Ste 2
Little Rock, AR 72201-2981   501-682-2033
                                    FAX: 501-682-2273
                                    www.arkansas.gov/esd

Artee Williams, Manager
Wide range of services including employment services, unemployment insurance, and labor market information.

5829 Easter Seal Work Center
3920 Woodland Heights Rd
Little Rock, AR 72212-2406   501-227-3600
                                    FAX: 501-227-7180
                                    mail@ar.easterseals.com
                                    www.ar.easterseals.com

Lauren Zilk, Administrator
Mission is to provide exceptional services to ensure that all people with disabilities or special needs have equal opportunities to live, learn work and play in their communities.

5830 VCT/A Job Retention Skill Training Program
Arkasas Rehab Services
P.O.Box 1358
Hot Springs, AR 71902-1358   501-624-4411
                                    FAX: 501-624-0019

Barbara Lewis, Administrator
Mae Robinson, Assistant Administrator
A training program designed for use in rehabilitation and educational settings. Using a social skill training strategy, VCT helps participants learn how to solve on-the-job problems and cope with common supervisory demands.

5831 Vocational and Rehabilitation Agency Division of Services for the Blind
700 Main St
Little Rock, AR 72201-4608   501-686-9433
                                    800-960-9270
                                    FAX: 501-686-9418
                                    TTY: 501-682-0093
                                    jim.hudson@mail.state.ar.us
                                    www.state.ar.us

Lyndel Lybarger, Field Adminstrator
James Hudson, Executive Director

5832 Vocational and Rehabilitation Agency for Persons Who Are Visually Impaired
Arkansas Department of Human Services
P.O.Box 3237
Little Rock, AR 72203-3237   501-686-9433
                                    800-960-9270
                                    FAX: 501-686-9418
                                    TTY: 501-324-9271
                                    arkblind@edu.gte.net

James C Hudson, Executive Director
Furnishes a wide variety of services to help people with disabilities return to work.

California

5833 ABLE Industries
8127 Avenue 304
Visalia, CA 93291   559-651-8150
                                    888-813-2253
                                    FAX: 559-651-0357
                                    www.ableindustries.org

Wende-Leigh Ayers, Executive Director
Committed to improving the lives of people with disabilities by creating opportunities to maximize their independence.

5834 ARC-Adult Vocational Program
1500 Howard St
San Francisco, CA 94103-2525   415-255-7200
                                    FAX: 415-255-9488
                                    info@thearcsanfrancisco.org
                                    www.thearcsanfrancisco.org

Timothy Hornbecker, Executive Director
Job placement programs, remunerative work services and work adjustment training programs.

5835 AbilityFirst
1300 E Green Street
Pasadena, CA 91106   626-396-1010
                                    877-768-4600
                                    FAX: 626-396-1021
                                    info@abilityfirst.org
                                    www.abilityfirst.org

Lori E Gangemi, President
Steve S. Schultz, CFO
Keri Castaneda, Chief Program Officer
Syed Kazmi, Controller
Provides programs and services to help children and adults with physical and developmental disabilities reach their full potential throughout their lives. Offers a broad range of employment, recreational and socialization programs and operate 12 accessible residential housing complexes.

5836 Achievement House & NCI Affiliates
496 Linne Road
Paso Robles, CA 93446   805-238-6630
                                    FAX: 805-239-9073
                                    conact@nciaffiliates.org
                                    www.achievementhouse.org

5837 Bakersfield ARC
2240 S Union Ave
Bakersfield, CA 93307-4158   661-834-2272
                                    800-834-3160
                                    FAX: 661-834-1694
                                    lplank@barc-inc.org
                                    www.barc-inc.org

Jim Baldwin, President/CEO
William Froning, Senior VP/CFO
Dave Kyle, Senior VP/Chief Compliance Officer
Mike Grover, Senior VP/Chief Programmes Officer
A non-profit organization that has been providing essential job training, employment and support services for the developmentally disabled and their families.
1949

5838 California Department of Fair Employment& Housing
2218 Kauden Drive
Suite 100
Elk Grove, CA 95758   916-478-7251
                                    800-884-1684
                                    contact.center@dfeh.ca.gov
                                    www.dfeh.ca.gov

Phyllis W Cheng, Director
Annmarie Billotti Esq, Chief Deputy Director
To protect Californians from employment, housing and public accomodation discrimination, and hate violence.

5839 Career Connection Transition Program
Whittier Union High School District
9401 Painter Ave
Whittier, CA 90605-2729   562-698-8121
                                    FAX: 562-693-4414
                                    Richard.Rosenberg@wuhsd.k12.ca.us
                                    www.wuhsd.k12.ca.us

Richard L Rosenberg PhD, Vocational Coordinator
Bonnie Bolton, Transition Department Head
Job placement programs, remunerative work services and work adjustment training programs. Transition services.

5840 Career Development Program (CDP)
260 W Grand Ave
Escondido, CA 92025-2604   760-738-0277
                                 FAX: 760-741-9452

Richard Brady MD
Wendy Hope, Supported Employment
Jill Hennessy, Independent Living
Work hardening and disciplinary programs.

5841 Colton-Redlands-Yucaipa Regional Occupational Programs
1214 Indiana Ct
PO Box 8640
Redlands, CA 92374-2896   909-793-3115
                                 FAX: 909-793-6901
                                 www.cryrop.org

Stephanie Houston, Superintendent
Sandra Moritensen, Manager Student Services
Provides quality hands-on training programs in over 40 high demand career fields to assist high school students and adults in acquiring marketable job skills. Works in cooperation with local
high schools, adult education colleges, and employers providing
a collaborative team of academic and ROP occupational teachers
who integrate academic and vocational competencies to provide
sequenced paths within career majors. Support services, career
guidance and services are provided to disabled people.

5842 Community Outpatient Rehabilitation Center
2823 Fresno Street
Fresno, CA 93721   559-459-6000
                                 FAX: 559-459-1004
                                 complaint@jointcommission.org
                                 www.communitymedical.org

Tim A. Joslin, Chief Executive Officer
Thomas Utecht, M.D., Senior Vice President
Craig S. Castro, Senior Vice President
Vicki Anderson, Vice President, Managed Care
Physical, occupational and speech therapy, neuropsychology ser-
vices available for orthopedic and neurological diagnosis.
Lymphedema program.

5843 Desert Haven Enterprises
43437 Copeland Circle
PO Box 2110
Lancaster, CA 93535   661-948-8402
                                 FAX: 661-948-1080
                                 kmiller@desrthaven.org
                                 www.deserthaven.org

Jenni Moran, Executive Director
Kathleen Miller, Program Services Director
Lisa Enos, Director Contract Services
Kathy Burcina, Job Developer
A private, nonprofit organization dedicated to developing, en-
hancing, and promotingthe capabilities of persons with mental
retardation and other developmental disabilities.

5844 ESS Work Center
858 Stanton Rd
Burlingame, CA 94010-1404   650-697-2642
                                 FAX: 650-697-2405

Ed Mentzer, Owner
Work adjustment and remunerative work programs.

5845 Employment Service: California
Employment Development Department
800 Capitol Mall
P.O. Box 826880
Sacramento, CA 95814- 0001   916-653-0707
                                 www.edd.ca.gov

5846 Feather River Industries
1811 Kusel Rd
Oroville, CA 95966-9528   530-534-1112
                                 FAX: 530-534-3137
                                 www.featherriverindustries.com

Randy Guild, Rehabilitation Counselor
Ed Turner, Production Coordinator
Judy Smith, President
Steve Wattenberg, Vice President
Vocational training for persons with developmental disabilities
provided through wood products fabrication and assembly tasks.
Instructor to trainer rating ranging from 1 to 12, 1 to 8, 1 to 6, and
1 to 4 depending on individual needs and complexity of tasks.

5847 Fit to Work
Ste 401
3581 Palmer Dr
Cameron Park, CA 95682-8238   530-676-7485
                                 FAX: 530-676-9114
                                 www.trueyellow.com

Helen Cheng
Provides remunerative work.

5848 Fresno City College: Disabled Students Programs and Services
Fresno City College
1101 E University Ave
Fresno, CA 93741-1   559-442-4600
                                 FAX: 559-489-2281
                                 janice.emerzian@fresnocitycollege.edu
                                 fresnocitycollege.edu

Dr Janice Emerzian Ed D, District Director
Tony Cantu, President
Ginna Bearden, Director of TRIO Programs
Cris Monahan Bremer, Director of Marketing and Commun
This program offers programs and services to students with physical, learning and/or psychological disabilities beyond those provided by conventional Fresno City College Programs and enables
students to successfully pursue their individual educational, vocational and personal goals.

5849 Heartland Opportunity Center
323 N E Street
Madera, CA 93638   559-674-8828
                                 FAX: 559-674-8857
                                 kanderson@heartlandopportunity.com
                                 www.heartlandopportunity.com

Kristy Anderson, CEO
Maria Alvarado, CFO
Provides employment, job placement, vocational and life skills
training to adults with mental, physical and/or emotional disabilities in order to help them reach their personal and vocational
goals.

5850 Hollister Workshop
Hope Rehabilitation Services
185 Berry Street
Suite 4000
San Francisco, CA 94107-2536   415-243-4200
                                 888-567-7442
                                 415-764-1622
                                 FAX: 831-637-8726
                                 salesteam@loopnet.com
                                 www.loopnet.com

Fred Saint, President
Wayne Warthen, CTO & SVP, Information Technology
Curtis Kroeker, President, LoopNet Marketplace Verticals
Leah McMurtry, Vice President, Member Services
Work adjustment and remunerative work programs.

5851 **Job Training Program Liaison: California**
Employment Development Department
800 Capitol Mall
Sacramento, CA 95814-4807

916-654-8210
800-300-5616
FAX: 916-657-5294
edd.ca.gov

Patrick Henning, Manager
Provides information on filing an Unemployment Insurance or Disability Insurance claim, on-line job and resume bank which boasts thousands of job openings.

5852 **King's Rehabilitation Center**
494 E Hanford-Armona Road
Hanford, CA 93232

559-583-5051
FAX: 559-582-1182
www.kingsrehab.com

Robert Knudseon, President
Steve Mendoza, Executive Director
Pat Vestal, VP
Renee Castro, Treasurer
To enhance the lives of adults with disabilities by providing day program services, vocational training and employment opportunities to assist such persons to attain their full potential.

5853 **Morongo Basin Work Activity Center**
74325 Joe Davis Dr
Twentynine Palms, CA 92277

760-366-8474
www.guidestar.org

Sheree Fraser
Job placement programs, remunerative work services and work adjustment training programs.

5854 **Mother Lode Rehabilitation Enterprises**
399 Placerville Dr
Placerville, CA 95667

530-622-4848
FAX: 530-622-0204
www.morerehab.org

Susan Peters, Chair
Henry Jeter, VP Finance
Christa K. Campbell, Secretary
A private, non-profit organization dedicated to supporting persons with disabilities. MORE was established by a group of parents, educators, rehabilitation professionals and concerned citizens and first began serving adults with disabilities in 1973.

5855 **Napa Valley PSI Inc.**
P.O.Box 600
Napa, CA 94559-600

707-255-0177
FAX: 707-255-0802
admin@napavalleypsi.org
http://www.napavalleypsi.org

Kimberly Alexander-Yarbor, President
Carol Gonsalves , Vice President
Eleanor Cullum, Secretary
Worthy Brooks, Directors
Work adjustment, work training and educational services for developmentally disabled adults. Emphasis is on manufacture of quality wood products, primarily wooden office furniture.

5856 **Oakland Work Activity Area**
6315 San Leandro St
Oakland, CA 94621-3727

510-639-9350
oaklandlocal.com

Greg Whalley
Dennis Scharssenberg, Manager
Susan Mernit, Editor/Publisher
Abraham Hyatt, Editor
Job placement programs, remunerative work services and work adjustment training programs.

5857 **Opportunities for the Handicapped**
P.O.Box 322
New York, NY 10040-0322

419-855-2742
www.giveindia.org

Kathy Dodd
Pradeep Jayaraman, President
Harendra Guturu, Secretary
Uttara Diwan, Treasurer
Work adjustment and remunerative work programs.

5858 **Orange County ARC**
225 W Carl Karcher Way
Anaheim, CA 92801

714-744-5301
FAX: 714-744-5312
jhearn2001@yahoo.com
ocarc.net

Joyce Hearn, CEO
Richard Farmer, VP Finance
Michael Galliano, VP Operations
Patrick Faraday, VP Sales
To provide quality care, training and services to our intellectually/developmentally disabled clients.

5859 **PRIDE Industries**
10030 Foothills Boulevard
Roseville, CA 95747-7102

916-788-2100
800-550-6005
FAX: 800-888-0447
info@prideindustries.com
http://www.prideindustries.com

Michael Ziegler, CEO
Tim Yamauchi, Executive Vice President and Chi
John Vaughan, Senior Vice President, Manufactu
Pete Berghuis, Senior Vice President, Integrate
Vocational rehabilitation and employment services creating jobs for people with disabilites; services include career counseling, vocational assessment, work adjustment, work services, job seeking skills, job development, job placement, on-the-job support (coaching), mentoring, independent living skills, transition services and case management.

5860 **Parents and Friends, Inc**
350 Cypress St
PO Box 656
Fort Bragg, CA 95437

707-964-4940
FAX: 707-964-8536
rmoon@parentsandfriends.org
www.parentsandfriends.org

Rick Moon, Executive Director
Serves people with developmental disabilities.

5861 **PathPoint**
315 W Haley Street
Ste 102
Santa Barbara, CA 93101

805-966-3310
info@pathpoint.org
www.pathpoint.org

Barbara Stevenson, Chair
Christopher Jones, Vice Chair/Treasurer
Mary E. Tiffany, Secretary
Jeffery Dodds, Director
To provide comprehensive training and support serviceds that empower people with disabilities of disadvantages to live and work as valued members of the community.

5862 **People Services, Inc**
4195 Lakeshore Blvd
Lakeport, CA 95453

707-263-3810
FAX: 707-263-0552
idumont@nctac.com
www.peopleservices.org

Ilene Dumont, Executive Director
To serve as the local community agency, providing the delivery of quality services for people with disabilities.

5863 **Pomona Valley Workshop**
4650 Brooks St
Montclair, CA 91763
909-624-3555
FAX: 909-624-5675
karen@pvwonline.org
www.pvwonline.org

Karen Jones, Executive Director
Mitch Gariador, Director of Administration
Kitty Dubois, Director of Human Resources
Terri Perkins, Director of Work Services
To assist adults with disabilities reach their potential in vocationsl and socialization skills in order tthat they may achieve their highest level of employment and community integration.

5864 **Porterville Sheltered Workshop**
194 West Poplar Avenue
Porterville, CA 93257-3449
559-784-1399
FAX: 559-781-5651
info@pswrehab.com
http://www.portervillesshelteredworkshop.com/
Steve Tree, Executive Director
Work adjustment and remunerative work programs. Mission is to assist disabled individuals achieve a more independent and productive life.

5865 **Project Independence**
3505 Cadillac Ave
Suite O-103
Costa Mesa, CA 92626
714-549-3464
877-444-0144
FAX: 714-549-3559
info@proindependence.org
www.proindependence.org

Debra Marsteller, Executive Director
Promote civil rights for people with developmental disabilities through services which expand independence and choice.

5866 **Sacramento Vocational Services**
6950 21st Ave
Sacramento, CA 95820
916-381-1300
FAX: 916-381-9026
info@inallianceinc.com
inallianceinc.com

5867 **San Francisco Vocational Services**
Ste 600
490 Golf Club Road
Pleasant Hill, CA 94523-1553
925-682-6343
FAX: 925-682-6375
sfvs@sfvocational.org
rsnc-centers.org

Gina Chenoweth, Executive Director
Jeffrey Faircloth, Manager Case Management
Rita Hays, Chair/President
William Wilson, Vice Chair
Comprehensive vocational rehabilitation center offering vocational evaluation, rehabilitative counseling, business office training, work experience, and job placement.

5868 **Shasta County Opportunity Center**
1265 Redwood Blvd
Redding, CA 96003-1965
530-225-5781
FAX: 530-225-5751
oppcenter_info@co.shasta.ca.us
www.co.shasta.ca.us

Del Lockwood, Manager
Leonard Moty, 2012 Chairman
David A. Kehoe, Board of Supervisor
Glenn Hawes, Board of Supervisor
An employment training program for people with disabilities in Shasta County. These individuals perform paid work in a number of different work environments and at the same time learn the skills necessary to obtain competetive employment in the local community.

5869 **Social Vocational Services**
Ste A104
350 Crenshaw Blvd
Torrance, CA 90503-1725
310-783-0633
FAX: 310-783-0636
nto@svsinc.org
socvoc.org

Sabrina Silva, Manager
Dan Strohm, Manager
The leading provider of services for people with developmental disabilities in the state of California

5870 **South Bay Vocational Center**
1526 W 240th St
Harbor City, CA 90710
310-784-2032
FAX: 310-539-6342
corey@sbvc1.com
www.sbvc1.com

Corey Sylve, President/CEO
Clare Grey, Vice President/COO
Santiago Lindo, Operations Specialist
Celia Bennett, CFO
A not-for-profit organization that has been providing excellent vocational programs and services for individuals with disabilities.

5871 **Tri-County Independent Living Center**
2822 Harris Street
Eureka, CA 95503
707-445-8404
877-576-5000
FAX: 707-445-9751
aa@tilinet.org
http://www.tilinet.org

Chris Jones, Executive Director
Allan Daniel, Information & Referral / Indepen
Mary Bullwinkel, Outreach & Resource Development
Cindy Calderon, Systems Change Advocate
To provide programs, services and information for people with disabilities living in Humboldt, Del Norte and Trinity Counties in northern California in an effort to allow choices for individuals to optimize their independence.

5872 **Unyeway**
Suite E
2330 Main Street
Ramona, CA 92065-2595
760-789-5960
FAX: 760-789-8156
http://www.unyeway.com

Kim Metli, Executive Director
Lisa Oertling, President
Dr. Richard Ferguson, Vice President/Audit Committee C
Pearl Aiello, Director
Job placement programs, remunerative work services and work adjustment training programs.

5873 **V-Bar Enterprises**
720 Gordon Cir
Suisun City, CA 94585
707-864-1334
government-contractors.findthebest.com

Lu Brunet
Job placement programs, remunerative work services and work adjustment training programs.

5874 **Valley Light Industries**
5360 Irwindale Avenue
Irwindale, CA 91706
626-332-6200
info@valleylightindustries.org
valleylightind.org

5875 **Visalia Workshop**
2031 S. Mooney Blvd.
Visalia, CA 93277-6711
559-622-9650
FAX: 866-575-6627
www.buildabear.com

Hortensia Venegas
Work hardening and disciplinary programs.

5876 Westside Opportunity Workshop
9503 Jefferson Blvd
Culver City, CA 90232-2917
310-836-4262
FAX: 310-825-0676
ayokota@mednet.ucla.edu
http://www.semel.ucla.edu

Peter Whybrow, Director
Fawzy Fawzy, Associate Director
Mark Wheeler, Media Relations
Alan Han, Director of Development
Job placement programs, remunerative work services and work adjustment training programs.

5877 Work Training Center
2255 Fair Street
Chico, CA 95928
530-343-7994
FAX: 530-343-4619
carlo@ewtc.org
www.wtcinc.org

Carl Ochsner, Executive Director
Brett Barker, Vocational Services Director
Deb Royat, Rehabilitation Services Director
A nonprofit organization providing services to people with disabilities.

Colorado

5878 Blue Peaks Developmental Services
703 Fourth Street
Alamosa, CO 81101-2638
719-589-5135
FAX: 719-589-0680
info@bluepeaks.org
http://www.bluepeaks.org

John Kreiner, Director
Randall P. Johnson, Human Resources/Staff Developmen
Brooke Hayden, Residential Director
George Garcia, Operations Director
Provides remunerative work.

5879 Cheyenne Village
6275 Lehman Drive
Colorado Springs, CO 80918
719-592-0200
FAX: 719-548-9947
TTY:719-592-0224
info@cheyennevillage.org
www.cheyennevillage.org

Ann M Turner, Executive Director
B. Jeanne Solze, Business Director
Serves adults with developmental disabilities such as Autism, Down syndrome, Cerebral Palsy, and Mental Retardation in El Paso, Teller and Park Counties.

5880 Colorado Civil Rights Divsion
1560 Broadway
Ste 110
Denver, CO 80202
303-894-7855
800-866-7675
FAX: 303-894-7885
www.dora.state.co.us

Barbara J. Kelly, Executive Director
Fred J. Joseph, Banking Division
Steven Chavez, Civil Rights Division
Chris Mykelbust, Division of Financial Services
Embraces the Department's mission of consumer protection and works to protect individuals from discrimination in employment, housing and at places of public accommodation through enforcement and outreach consistent with the Colorado Civil Rights Laws.

5881 Colorado Employment Service
Department of Labor and Employment
Suite 400
1800 Grant Street
Denver, CO 80203-3528
303-860-4200
855-216-7740
FAX: 303-860-4299
employeeservices@cu.edu
www.cu.edu/employee-services

Clara Capano, Manager
Job placement programs, remunerative work services and work adjustment training programs.

5882 Developmental Training Services
4600 North Fairfax Drive
Suite 402
Arlington, VA 22203
703-465-9388
FAX: 703-465-9344
www.onlinedts.com

Roger Jensen, CEO
Linda Davis, Administrator
Indira Kaur Ahluwalia,, Founder and President
Viresh Desai, Vice President
Residential and employment programs for adults with developmental disabilities.

5883 Dynamic Dimensions
701 Cypress Street
Sulphur, LA 70663
337-527-7034
FAX: 719-346-6010
https://www.wcch.com

Cheryl Reese, Executive Director
Vocational, evaluation and assessment, training and placement for most disabilities. Group homes and day programs for the developmentally disabled.

5884 Gray Street Workcenter
11177 West 8th Avenue
Lakewood, CO 80215-2821
303-233-3363
FAX: 303-467-2793
http://services.ddrcco.com

Tammy Drumright, Manager
C. David Pemberton, II, President
Neal Berlin, Vice President
Joanne Elliott, M.A., Secretary
Residental and employment programs for adults with developmental disabilities.

5885 Hope Center
3400 Elizabeth St
Denver, CO 80205-4801
303-388-4801
FAX: 303-388-0249
gghope@comcast.net
www.hopecenterinc.org

Charlse T. Smith, Chairperson
Sid Davidson, Vice Chairperson
John Hanson, Treasurer
Barbara Batey, Secretary
Provides educational and vocational opportunities for special-needs and at-risk children and adults from 2 1/2 to adulthood.

5886 Imagine: Innovative Resources for Cognitive & Physical Challenges
1400 Dixon St
Lafayette, CO 80026-2790
303-665-7789
FAX: 303-665-2648
caroline@imaginecolorado.org
www.imaginecolorado.org

Mark Emery, Executive Director
Judy James-Anderson, Behavioral Health Services Dir
Provides support services to more than 2,600 people of all ages with developmental delays and cognitive disabilities including autism, cerebral palsy and Down syndrome.

5887 Las Animas County Rehabilitation Center
P.O.Box 781
Trinidad, CO 81082-781
719-846-3388
FAX: 719-846-4543
www.scdds.com

Duane Roy, Executive Director
Bernice Whalen, Human Resources Manager
Jeannette Vialobos, SPCC Director
Leslie Lark, Finance Director
Job placement programs, remunerative work services and work adjustment training programs.

5888 NORESCO Workshop
903 E Burlington Ave
Fort Morgan, CO 80701-3637
970-867-5702
fort-morgan.gopickle.com

Ramona Proctor, Executive Director
Nancy Study, Manager
Provides remunerative work.

5889 Regional Assessment and Training Center
1145 Gayley Avenue
Suite 304
Los Angeles, CA 90024-3108
303-866-7253
www.srphtc.ucla.edu

Russell Porter, Executive Director
Work adjustment and renumerative work programs.

5890 Sedgwick County Workshop
7001 W. 21 st St.
North Wichita, KN 67205-1759
316-660-0100
FAX: 316-722-1432
sedgwickinfo@k-state.edu
www.sedgwick.ksu.edu

Maria Contreras, Manager
Provides remunerative work.

5891 Vocational and Rehabilitation Agency
Unit B
2 Peachtree Street, NW
Atlanta, GA 30303-3855
404-232-1998
866-489-0001
FAX: 404-232-1800
TTY: 303-866-3980
GVRAcustomer-service@gvra.ga.gov
https://gvra.georgia.gov

Diana Huerta, Director
James N. Defoor, Chair
Louise Hill, Vice Chair
Purpose is to assist eligible individuals with disabilities to become productive members of the Colorado workforce and to live independently.

5892 Yuma County Workshop
710 E 2nd Ave
Yuma, CO 80759
970-848-2874
www.yellowpages.com/yuma-co

Robert Stephens
Andrea Anderson, Manager
Provides remunerative work.

Connecticut

5893 Abilities Without Boundaries
615 W Johnson Avenue
Cheshire, CT 06410
203-272-5607
FAX: 203-272-4284
cconway@abilitieswithoutboundaries.org
www.abilitieswithoutboundaries.or g

Charlie Conway, Executive Director
Christopher Fanelli, Business Manager
Nancy Knapp, Office Manager
Richard Ambro Jr., Employment Specialist
Formerly known as Cheshire Occupational & Career Opportunities (COCO), provides opportunities in the community through employment and social experiences for people with developmental disabilities.

5894 Allied Community Services
Six Craftsman Road
East Windsor, CT 06088
860-741-3701
FAX: 860-741-6870
TTY:860-741-3701
www.alliedgroup.org

Dean M Wern, President/CEO
Provides individuals with disabilities or other challenges the opportunity to live and enjoy a productive, independent, and fulfilling life

5895 Area Cooperative Educational Services(ACES)
350 State St
North Haven, CT 06473
203-498-6800
acesinfo@aces.org
www.aces.org

Craig W Edmondson EdD, Executive Director
Claudette J. Beamon, Human Resources Director
Carolyn McNally, Program Development Director
Exists to improve public education through high quality, cost effective programs and services.

5896 CW Resources
200 Myrtle Street
New Britain, CT 06053
860-229-7700
FAX: 860-229-6847
info@cwresources.org
www.cwresources.org

Ronald H Buccilli, President
CW Resources is dedicated to serving the needs of persons with disabilities through the creation of integrated vocational training and employment opportunities for those individuals who are physically, developmentally, emotionally and/or socio-economically challenged.

5897 Central Connecticut Association For Retarted Citizens
950 Slater Rd
New Britain, CT 06053-1658
860-229-6665
FAX: 860-826-6883
ccarc@ccarc.com
www.ccarc.com

Anne Ruwet, CEO
Julie Erickson, Senior Vice President
William allyn, Vice President of Residential Services
Anna Cardona, Vice President
Empowerment through Employment

5898 Community Enterprises
441 Pleasant Street
Northampton, MA 01060
413-584-1460
info@communityenterprises.com
www.communityenterprises.com

Dick Venne, President/CEO
William Donohue, Chairman
Donald Milner, Vice Chairman
Joanne Carlisle, Clerk
Support self-determination for individuals with disabilities and/or other challenges to actively live, learn, and work in the community.

5899 Connecticut Governor's Committee on Employment of People With Disabilities
200 Folly Brook Boulevard
Wethersfield, CT 06109-1153
860-263-6000
FAX: 860-263-6039
dol.webhelp@ct.gov
http://www.ctdol.state.ct.us

Dennis Murphy, Acting Commissioner
Dannel P. Malloy, Governor
Work adjustment and remunerative work programs.

5900 Fotheringhay Farms
84 Waterhole Rd
Colchester, CT 06415-2323
860-267-4463
FAX: 860-267-7628
http://caringcommunityct.org

Wesley Martins, Executive Director
Job placement programs, remunerative work services and work adjustment training programs.

5901 George Hegyi Industrial Training Center
5 Coon Hollow Rd
Derby, CT 06418-1149
203-735-8727
FAX: 203-735-2204
bob.wood@snet.net
http://www.varcainc.com

Joan Bucci, Executive Director
Robert Wood, President
Cecelia Staiano-Hayes, Program Manager
Work adjustment and remunerative work programs.

5902 Kennedy Center
2440 Reservoir Ave
Trumbull, CT 06611-4757
203-365-8522
FAX: 203-365-8533
info@kennedyctr.org
www.thekennedycenterinc.org

Martin D. Schwartz, President & CEO
Stuart Gordon, Vice President of Finance
Lynn Pellegrino, Vice President of HR
Marie Farina, HR Generalist
Provides vocational rehabilitation, job training and job placement services to 1,000 adults with disabilities including mental retardation, traumatic brain injury, psychiatric disabilities and more. Residential services, well integrated within the community, serve 97 individuals on a daily basis. Children's programs provide support to 85 children age birth to three, in addition to after hours and recreation programs to appromxately 100 school age children. Staff size is presently 450 employees.

5903 Quaezar
285 Riverside Avenue
Suite 300
Westport, CT 06880-4806
203-226-8711
FAX: 203-454-5780
sterlinglp.com

William J Sedarweck, President
Agency for adult mentally retarded/autistic people providing residential care in a group home or apartment setting. Also provides placement in community employment.

5904 Valley Memorial Health Center
435 E Main St
Ansonia, CT 06401-1964
203-736-2601
FAX: 203-736-2641
info@bghealth.org
www.bghealth.org

Marilyn Cormack, CEO
Provides innovative, exceptional behavioral health care through quality services and programs that focus on, and respect the consumer.

5905 Vocational and Rehabilitation Agency
2 Peachtree Street, NW
Atlanta, GA 30303-4536
404-232-1998
866-489-0001
FAX: 404-232-1800
TTY: 860-602-4221
GVRAcustomer-service@gvra.ga.gov
https://gvra.georgia.gov

Keith Maynard, Deputy Director
Brian Sigman, Executive Director
Alan Sylvestre, Chairman
Mission is to provide quality educational and rehabilitative services to all people who are legally blind or deaf/blind and children who are visually impaired at no cost to our clients or their families.

5906 Vocational and Rehabilitation Agency: State Department of Social Services
Department of Social Services
25 Sigourney St
11th Floor
Hartford, CT 06106-5041
860-424-4844
800-537-2549
FAX: 860-424-4850
TTY: 860-424-4839
brs.dss@po.state.ct.us
www.ct.gov/brs

Amy L Porter, Director
Roderick L Bremby, Commissioner
Provides a broad range of services to the elderly, disabled, families, and individuals who need assistance in maintaining or achieving their full potential for self-direction, self-reliance and independent living.

Delaware

5907 Delaware Division of Vocational Rehabilitation
Delaware Department of Labor
4425 N Market Street
Wilmington, DE 19802
302-761-8085
www.delawareworks.com

John McMahon, Secretary of Labor
The state's public program that helps people with physical and mental disabilities obtain or retain employment. Also, and Independent Living Program helps people with disabilities function in the community. DVR's commitment is to help people with disabilities increase independence through employment.

5908 Delaware Fair Employment Practice Agency
Delaware Department of Labor
Ste 6
820 North French Street
Wilmington, DE 19801-3509
302-577-8278
FAX: 302-577-6561
delarts@state.de.us
artsdel.org

Karen Gimbutas, VP
Paul Weagraff, Director
Susan Salkin, Deputy Director
Dana Wise, Administrative Specialist
Provides opportunities and resources to eligible individuals with disabilities leading to success in employment and independent living.

5909 Delaware Job Training Program Liaison
Division of Employment & Training
P.O.Box 9828
820 N. French Street
Wilmington, DE 19801- 828
302-577-8977
FAX: 302-577-3996
www.jobaps.com

Harold Stafford, Manager
Work adjustment and remunerative work programs. Also offers career guidance, supported employment, work readiness and job placement.

5910 Service Source
3030 Bowers St
Wilmington, DE 19802
302-762-0300
800-738-1733
FAX: 302-762-8797
www.servicesource.org

Michelle Lee, President/CEO
Rhonda VanLowe, Legal Counsel
Joseph J. Sorota, President
Marilynn Bersoff, BTG
ServiceSource is a leading nonprofit disability resource organization with regional offices and programs located in eight states and the District of Columbia. We serve more than 14,000 individuals with disabilities annually through a range of innovative and valued employment, training, habilitation, housing and other support services. ServiceSource directly employs more than

1,500 individuals on government and commercial affirmative employment contracts.

District of Columbia

5911 **District of Columbia Department of Employment Services**
4058 Minnesota Avenue NE
Washington, DC 20019
202-724-7000
FAX: 202-673-6993
does@dc.gov
does.dc.gov

5912 **District of Columbia Dept. of Employment Services: Office of Workforce Development**
4058 Minnesota Avenue, NE
Washington, DC 20019
202-671-1633
877-319-7346
FAX: 202-673-6993
TTY: 202-673-6994
does@dc.gov
www.does.dc.gov

Diana C Johnson, Public Information Officer
Marianna Lourenco, Specialist/ADA Coordinator
To foster economic development and growth in the District of Columbia by providing workforce training, bringing together job seekers and employers, compensating unemployed and injured workers and promoting safe and healthy workplaces.

5913 **District of Columbia Fair Employment Practice Agencies**
D C Office of Human Rights
Ste 570n
441 4th Street NW
Washington, DC 20001-2714
202-727-3400
FAX: 202-347-8922
TTY:202-727-3400
oag@dc.gov
http://oag.dc.gov

Elizabeth Noel, Executive Director
Irvin B. Nathan, Attorney General
Ariel B. Levinson-Waldman, Senior Counsel to the Attorney G
Victor Bonett, Legislative Director FOIA Office
Investigations and discrimination complaints.

5914 **Goodwill of Greater Washington**
2200 South Dakota Ave NE
Washington, DC 20018-1622
202-636-4225
888-817-4323
FAX: 202-526-3994
info@dcgoodwill.org
dcgoodwill.org

Catherine Meloy, CEO
Brendan Hurley, Vice President Marketing & Commu
Judy Sklar, Regional Director Retail Operati
Colleen Paletta, Vice President Workforce Develop
Offers vocational training, job training, sheltered employment and work experience.

5915 **Green Door**
1221 Taylor Street, NW
Washington, DC 20011-3063
202-464-9200
FAX: 202-464-5730
info@greendoor.org
www.greendoor.org

Judith Johnson, Executive Director
Brenda Randall, Assistant Director
Richard R. Bebout, Ph.D., President and CEO
Linda Wheeler Banton, Chair
Green Door is a community program which prepares people with a severe and persistent mental illness to live and work independently. Since 1976, Green Door has provided comprehensive services to mentally ill people, including housing, job training, job placement, education, homeless outreach, case management, support for people with substance abuse problems, family support,and specialized help for people who have had repeated hospitalizations.

5916 **Operation Job Match**
National Multiple Sclerosis Society
Suite 750 South
1800 M St NW
Washington, DC 20036-5802
202-887-0136
FAX: 202-296-3425
OJM@nmss.org
operationjobmatch.org

Steven Nissen, Manager
Jeanne Angulo, Executive Director
Job readiness program for individuals with adult-onset physical disabilities.

5917 **Rehabilitation Services Administration**
10th Floor
810 First Street NE
Washington, DC 20002-4227
202-442-8663
FAX: 202-442-8742
dds@dc.gov
rsa.dhs.dc.gov

Elizabeth Parker, Administrator
Mark D. Back, FOIA Officer
Laura L. Nuss, Director, Department on Disabili
State Rehabilitation Agency providing services to eligible persons with disabilities.

5918 **WAVE Work, Achievement, Value, & Education**
Suite 500
525 School St SW
Washington, DC 20024-2762
202-484-0103
800-274-2005
FAX: 202-488-7595
wave4kids@aol.com
www.waveinc.org

Dr. Steven W Edwards, President & CEO
Arthur Griffin, Senior Vice President
Dr. Beth P. Reynolds, Executive Director
Dr. Sandy Addis, Associate Director
Job placement programs, remunerative work services and work adjustment training programs for 18 and 21 years of age in many cities across the country including Drop-Out Recovery Programs and Drop-Out Prevention Programs. Programs also available for youth ages 12-18. Youth Professionals Development and Training and key aspects of WAVE services, as well.

Florida

5919 **Abilities of Florida: An Affiliate of Service Source**
2735 Whitney Road
Clearwater, FL 33760-1610
727-538-7370
FAX: 727-538-7387
abilities@ourpeoplework.org
servicesource.org

Janet Samuelson, President & CEO
Mark Hall, Executive Vice President, Corpor
David Hodge, Executive Vice President & Chief
Bruce Patterson, Executive Vice President & Chief
Provides a full range of employment services including work evaluation, training, job coaching, job placement, advocacy and education. Also provides housing assistance and specialized to adults with cystic fibrosis.

5920 **Able Trust, The**
3320 Thomasville Road
Suite 200
Tallahassee, FL 32308
850-224-4493
888-838-2253
888-838-2253
FAX: 850-224-4496
TTY:850-224-4493
info@abletrust.org
www.abletrust.org

Susanne Homant, President & CEO
Guenevere Crum, Senior Vice President
Ray Ford, Assistant Director of Communicat
Jessica Taylor, Assistant to the President & CEO

Provides grant funds for employment-related programs for non-profit agencies in Florida. Assists families, individuals and agencies through educational conferences, and youth training programs. Provides businesses free resources for hiring people with disabilities.

5921 Career Assessment & Planning Services
Goodwill Industries - Suncoast Incorporated
10596 Gandy Blvd
St Petersburg, FL 33702-1422   727-523-1512
                                  888-279-1988
                                  FAX: 727-563-9300
                                  TTY: 727-579-1068
                                  gw.marketing@goodwillhisuncoast.com
                                  www.goodwill-suncoast.org

Oscar J. Horton, Chair
Martin W. Gladysz, Sr. Vice Chair
Heather Ceresoli, Vice Chair
Deborah A. Passerini, President
Career assessment and planning services help determine how prepared an individual is for employment, training, or future education. It is a comprehensive assessment that can predict current and future employment and potential adjustment factors for physically, emotionally or developmentally disabled persons who may be unemployed or underemployed.

5922 Choices to Work Program
Goodwill Industries-Suncoast
10596 Gandy Blvd
St Petersburg, FL 33702-1422   727-523-1512
                                  888-279-1988
                                  FAX: 727-563-9300
                                  TTY: 727-579-1068
                                  gw.marketing@goodwill-suncoast.com
                                  goodwill-suncoast.org

Oscar J. Horton, Chair
Martin W. Gladysz, Sr. Vice Chair
Heather Ceresoli, Vice Chair
Deborah A. Passerini, President
Assisting individuals currently eligible for Workman's Compensation, this program allows those recovering from injury on the job to prepare to return to independent employment, either through increasing ability and confidence in using adaptive behaviors and/or equipment to return to related employment, or adjusting to a more compatible employment environment.

5923 Florida Division of Vocational Rehabilitation
Bldg A
4070 Esplanade Way
Tallahassee, FL 32399-7016   800-451-4327
                                  800-451-4327
                                  FAX: 850-245-3316
                                  TTY: 866-515-3692
                                  ombudsman@vr.fldoe.org
                                  rehabworks.org

Bill Palmer, Manager
Debra Thompson, Florida Rehabilitation Council C
Roy Cosgrove, Administrator
Andrea Schwendinger, Government Analyst
Rehabilitation services are important when a physical or mental handicap interferes with your ability to work. Our purpose is to help prepare for, and return to, gainful employment.

5924 Florida Fair Employment Practice Agency
Florida Commission on Human Relations
Suite 100
2009 Apalachee Parkway
Tallahassee, FL 32301- 4830   850-488-7082
                                  800-342-8170
                                  FAX: 850-488-5291
                                  TTY: 800-955-1339
                                  fchrinfo@fchr.myflorida.com
                                  http://fchr.state.fl.us

Michelle Wilson, Executive Director
Gilbert Singer, Chairman
Mario Valle, Vice Chairman
Gayle Cannon, Commissioner

The Commission is the state agency charged with enforcing the state's civil rights laws and serves as a resource on human relations for the people of Florida.

5925 Goodwill Industries-Suncoast Adult Day Training
10596 Gandy Blvd N
St Petersburg, FL 33702-1422   727-523-1512
                                  888-279-1988
                                  FAX: 727-563-9300
                                  gw.marketing@goodwill-suncoast.com
                                  goodwill-suncoast.org

Lee Waits, President
Goodwill's adult day training programs enable people with developmental disabilities to set and achieve personal goals within a work-like setting. Participants work at various jobs throughout Goodwill and engage in a variety of activities that will allow them to become more self-sufficients.

5926 Goodwill Industries-Suncoast Inc. Adult Day Training
10596 Gandy Blvd.
St. Petersburg, FL 33702-3305   727-523-1512
                                  888-279-1988
                                  FAX: 727-563-9300
                                  TTY: 727-579-1068
                                  gw.marketing@goodwill-suncoast.com
                                  www.goodwill-suncoast.org

Oscar J. Horton, Chair
Martin W. Gladysz, Sr. Vice Chair
Heather Ceresoli, Vice Chair
Deborah A. Passerini, President
Goodwill's adult day training programs enable people with developmental disabilities to set and achieve personal goals within a work-like setting. Participants work at various jobs throughout Goodwill and engage in a variety of activities that will allow them to become more self-sufficients.

5927 Goodwill Industries-Suncoast Inc. Adult Day Training
10596 Gandy Blvd.
St. Petersburg, FL 33702-3704   727-523-1512
                                  888-279-1988
                                  FAX: 727-563-9300
                                  TTY: 727-579-1068
                                  gw.marketing@goodwill-suncoast.com
                                  www.goodwill-suncoast.org

Oscar J. Horton, Chair
Martin W. Gladysz, Sr. Vice Chair
Heather Ceresoli, Vice Chair
Deborah A. Passerini, President
Goodwill's adult day training programs enable people with developmental disabilities to set and achieve personal goals within a work-like setting. Participants work at various jobs throughout Goodwill and engage in a variety of activities that will allow them to become more self-sufficients.

5928 Goodwill Industries-Suncoast Non-Residential Supports And Services Program
10596 Gandy Blvd N
St Petersburg, FL 33702-1422   727-523-1512
                                  888-279-1988
                                  FAX: 727-563-9300
                                  TTY: 727-579-1068
                                  gw.marketing@goodwill-suncoast.com
                                  goodwill-suncoast.org

Lee Waits, President
Jean-Marie Moore, Director Of Operations
Goodwill's adult day training programs enable people with developmental disabilities to set and achieve personal goals within a work-like setting. Participants earn paychecks working at various jobs throughout Goodwill and engage in a variety of activities that will allow them to become more self-sufficients.

5929   Goodwill Industries-Suncoast Supported Living
10596 Gandy Blvd
St Petersburg, FL 33702-1422   727-523-1512
                                      888-279-1988
                                 FAX: 727-563-9300
                                 TTY: 727-579-1068
                        gw.marketing@goodwill-suncoast.com
                                 goodwill-suncoast.org

Oscar J. Horton, Chair
Martin W. Gladysz, Sr. Vice Chair
Heather Ceresoli, Vice Chair
Deborah A. Passerini, President
Goodwill's supported living program helps people with developmental disabilities expand their skills so they can lead increasingly independentlives. Individuals receive training and assistance with daily living activities while living in the community. Additional support includes assistance with legal issues, adocacy, community resources, banking, safety procedures, self-medication, household management, meal preparation, interpersonal relationships and parenting training.

5930   Goodwill Industries-Suncoast,Adult Day Training
10596 Gandy Blvd
St Petersburg, FL 33702-5654   727-523-1512
                                      888-279-1988
                                 FAX: 727-563-9300
                                 TTY: 727-579-1068
                        gw.marketing@goodwill-suncoast.com
                                 goodwill-suncoast.org

Oscar J. Horton, Chair
Martin W. Gladysz, Sr. Vice Chair
Heather Ceresoli, Vice Chair
Deborah A. Passerini, President
Goodwill's adult day training programs enable people with developmental disabilities to set and achieve personal goals within a work-like setting. Participants work at various jobs throughout Goodwill and engage in a variety of activities that will allow them to become more self-sufficients.

5931   Goodwill Temporary Staffing
Goodwill Industries- Suncoast
10596 Gandy Blvd
St Petersburg, FL 33702-1422   727-523-1512
                                      888-279-1988
                                 FAX: 727-576-1314
                                 TTY: 727-579-1068
                        gw.marketing@goodwill-suncoast.com
                                 goodwill-suncoast.org

Oscar J. Horton, Chair
Martin W. Gladysz, Sr. Vice Chair
Heather Ceresoli, Vice Chair
Deborah A. Passerini, President
Provides employment links from potential employees, both disabled and non-disabled alike to employers with immediate employment opportunities seeking qualified candidates. Pre-screening on all applicants include: Employment history, personal references, law enforcement background checks and substance screening.

5932   Impact: Ocala Vocational Services
Goodwill Industries- Suncoast
10596 Gandy Blvd
St Petersburg, FL 33702-1422   727-523-1512
                                      888-279-1988
                                 FAX: 727-563-9300
                                 TTY: 727-579-1068
                        gw.marketing@goodwill-suncoast.com
                                 goodwill-suncoast.org

Oscar J. Horton, Chair
Martin W. Gladysz, Sr. Vice Chair
Heather Ceresoli, Vice Chair
Deborah A. Passerini, President
Designed to enable individuals with disabilities to work in integrated settings in the community, receiving wages and benefits matching those of non-handicapped workers.

5933   JobWorks NISH Food Service
Goodwill Industries- Suncoast
10596 Gandy Blvd
St Petersburg, FL 33702-1422   727-523-1512
                                      888-279-1988
                                 FAX: 727-563-9300
                                 TTY: 727-579-1068
                        gw.marketing@goodwill-suncoast.com
                                 goodwill-suncoast.org

Oscar J. Horton, Chair
Martin W. Gladysz, Sr. Vice Chair
Heather Ceresoli, Vice Chair
Deborah A. Passerini, President
An enclave style (or group) supported employment program designed to give consumers additional supports that allow and encourage increasingly independent employment opportunities within a food services environment.

5934   JobWorks NISH Postal Service
Goodwill Industries - Suncoast
10596 Gandy Blvd
St Petersburg, FL 33702-1422   727-523-1512
                                      888-279-1988
                                 FAX: 727-563-9300
                                 TTY: 727-579-1068
                        gw.marketing@goodwill-suncoast.com
                                 goodwill-suncoast.org

Oscar J. Horton, Chair
Martin W. Gladysz, Sr. Vice Chair
Heather Ceresoli, Vice Chair
Deborah A. Passerini, President
An enclave style (or group) supported employment program designed to give consumers additional supports that allow and encourage increasingly independent employment opportunities within a mailroom environment.

5935   Lighthouse Central Florida
215 East New Hampshire Street
Orlando, FL 32804-6403   407-898-2483
                                     888-898-2483
                                FAX: 407-898-0236
                              lvaneepoel@lcf-fl.org
                           lighthousecentralflorida.com

Lee Nasehi, Executive Director
Lee Van Eepoel, Program Service Director
Donna Esbensen, Vice President, Chief Financial
Kimberly Pawling, Director of Education & Rehabili
Lighthouse Central Florida (LCF) is the only non-profit organization offering comprehensive, professional, vision rehabilitation services to Central Floridians of all ages with low vision or blindness.

5936   MAClown Vocational Rehabilitation Workshop
6390 NE 2nd Ave
Miami, FL 33138-6036   305-759-0212

Sabrina Shelton, Manager
Provides remunerative work.

5937   One-Stop Service
Goodwill Industries- Suncoast
10596 Gandy Blvd.
St Petersburg, FL 33702-1422   727-523-1512
                                      888-279-1988
                                 FAX: 727-563-9300
                                 TTY: 727-579-1068
                        gw.marketing@goodwill-suncoast.com
                                 goodwill-suncoast.org

R. Lee Waits, President and CEO
Deborah A. Passerini, Executive Vice President and Chi
Gary Hebert, Corporate Treasurer and Chief Fi
Lee C. Zeh, Corporate Secretary and Vice Pre
Provides universal job search and placement related services are available to any person entering the service center. Each One-Stop Services Center provides on-site representation from a variety of employment-related service providers. All One-Stops host and/or facilitate local employment fairs and provides access to computerized job-postings.

5938 Palm Beach Habilitation Center
4522 South Congress Avenue
Lake Worth, FL 33461-4797   561-965-8500
                                        FAX: 561-433-8816
                                        postman@pbhab.com
                                              pbhab.com

Jeffrey Chapman, Chief Financial Officer
David Lin, Vice President of Programs & Services
Roxanne Jacobs, Director of Developmen
Tina Philips, President/CEO
Providing work evaluation, work adjustment, job placement, employment, residential and retirement services for mentally, emotionally and physically disabled adults.

5939 Primrose Supported Employment Programs
2733 South Ferncreek Ave
Orlando, FL 32806-5538   407-898-7201
                                        FAX: 407-898-2120
                                        www.primrosecenter.org

Mary Vanburen, Executive Director
Leslie North, Chairman
Helen Galloway, Board Director
Faye Scott-Evans, Board Director
Mission is to transform the lives of people with developmental disabilities by providing opportunities to achieve their fullest potential.

5940 Quest
500 E. Colonial Drive
Orlando, FL 32803-4504   407-218-4300
                                             888-807-8378
                                        FAX: 407-218-4301
                                        contact@questinc.org
                                              questinc.org

John Gill, President / CEO
Todd Thrasher, Chief Financial Officer
Eb Blakely, Vice President, Behavioral Services
Karenne Levy, Chief Operating Officer
Quest has built communities where people with disabilities have achieved their goals for nearly 50 years. Through a variety of residential and employment options, behavioral therapy, therapeutic day programs, charter schools and even a recreational summer camp, Quest serves more than 1000 individuals each day in the Orlando and Tampa areas.

5941 Quest - Tampa Area
1404 Tech Blvd
Tampa, FL 33619   813-423-7700
                                             888-807-8378
                                        FAX: 813-423-7701
                                        contact@questinc.org
                                             www.questinc.org

John Gill, President / CEO
Todd Thrasher, Chief Financial Officer
Eb Blakely, Vice President, Behavioral Services
Karenne Levy, Chief Operating Officer
Quest has built communities where people with disabilities have achieved their goals for nearly 50 years. Through a variety of residential and employment options, behavioral therapy, therapeutic day programs, charter schools and even a recreational summer camp, Quest serves more than 1000 individuals each day in the Orlando and Tampa areas.

5942 SCARC, Inc Evaluation, Training + Emploment Center
213 West McCollum Avenue
Bushnell, FL 33513-5916   352-793-5156
                                        FAX: 352-793-6545
                                        marshaperkins@embargmail.com
                                        http://scarcinc.com

Marsha Perkins, Administrator
Training and employment program for adults with disabilities. SCARC offers vocational evaluation, training, work services, transportation, supported independent living and community based training.

5943 Seagull Industries for the Disabled
3879 Byron Drive
West Palm Beach, FL 33404-3311   561-842-5814
                                        FAX: 561-881-3554
                                        main@seagull.org
                                             www.seagull.org

Fred Eisinger, Executive Director
Linda Moore, Assistant Executive Director, Se
Joyce Hambrick, Director of Program Services
Ellen Hoffacker, Director of Finance
Dedicated to improving the quality of life of mentally, physically and emotionally challenged adults in Palm Beach County, Florida through advocacy and the provision of a variety of social service, vocational training and residential programs designed to encourage self reliance and independence.

5944 Supported Employment Program
Goodwill Industries - Suncoast
10596 Gandy Blvd.
St Petersburg, FL 33702-1422   727-523-1512
                                             888-279-1988
                                        FAX: 727-563-9300
                                        TTY: 727-579-1068
                                        gw.marketing@goodwill-suncoast.com
                                             www.goodwill-suncoast.org

R. Lee Waits, President and CEO
Deborah A. Passerini, Executive Vice President and Chi
Gary Hebert, Corporate Treasurer and Chief Fi
Lee C. Zeh, Corporate Secretary and Vice Pre
Goodwill's supported employment program enables people with developmental disabilities to work in the community, earning wages and benefits marching those of non-disabled workers. Participants receive intensive on-the-job training at job sites that have been carefully chosen for their suitability. A support facilitator provides follow-up job coaching to ensure success. Serving people in Pinellas, Hillsborough and Pasco counties.

5945 Vocational and Rehabilitation Agency Department of Education
Bldg A
4070 Esplanade Way
Tallahassee, FL 32399-7016   850-245-3399
                                             800-451-4327
                                        FAX: 850-245-3316
                                        TTY: 850-488-0867
                                        speaker@vr.fldoe.org
                                             rehabworks.org

Bill Palmer, Manager
Aleisa McKinlay, Director
Work adjustment and remunerative work programs.

5946 Vocational and Rehabilitation Agency: Division of Blind Services
401 Platt Street
Daytona Beach, FL 32114-2803   386-254-3856
                                             800-522-5078
                                        FAX: 386-252-3800
                                        craig_kiser@dbe.doe.state.fl.us
                                             www.state.fl.us/dbs

Bill Palmer, Manager
Carl Augusto, President and CEO
Kelly Bleach, Chief Administrative Officer
Rick Bozeman, Chief Financial Officer
Mission is to ensure blind and visually impaired Floridians have the tools, support, and opportunity to achieve success.

5947 Work Exploration Center
3000 N West 83rd Street i 40
Gainesville, FL 32606   352-395-5265
                                        FAX: 352-395-5271
                                        admin.sfcc.edu

Karla Wooten, Coordinator
The Work Exploration Center embraces a holistic approach to Comprehensive Vocational Evaluation and Community Employment services, encouraging individual understanding, hope and growth for a productive and fulfilling future.

Georgia

5948 Employment and Training Division, Region B
Goodwill Industries of North Georgia
1123 Progress Rd
Ellijay, GA 30540-5504

706-276-4722
888-514-8112
FAX: 706-276-4732
vti@ellijay.com

Linda Rau, Director Programs/Services
Employment training, assessment and job placement for people who have disabilities and/or are disadvantaged. Serving 15 counties in Northern Georgia.

5949 Fair Housing and Equal Employment
Georgia Commission on Equal Opportunity
7 Martin Luther King, Jr. Drive, S.
3rd Floor
Atlanta, GA 30334-9000

404-656-1736
800-473-6736
FAX: 404-656-4399
gceo@gceo.state.ga.us
www.gceo.state.ga.us

Teresa Chappell, Fair Housing Division Director
Stephanie Randolph, Intake Coordinator/Housing
Abdul Wali Khadeem, Equal Employment Division Director
Melvin J. Everson, Executive Director/Administrator
To investigate housing and employment discrimination in the state of Georgia.

5950 Griffin Area Resource Center Griffin Community Workshop Division
931 Hamilton Boulevard
Post Office Box 83
Griffin, GA 30224

770-229-4212
FAX: 770-229-4212
united_way@bellsouth.net
http://www.gscunitedway.org

Cary Grubbs, Executive Director
Charles Cary Grubbs, Garc Executive Director
Rodney Shurman, President
Dr. Curtis Jones, Vice-President
A CARF (The Rehabilitation Accreditation Commission) accredited Employment and Community Support organization providing daily services to participants with disabilities from 16 years of age and up in a 5 county area.

5951 IBM National Support Center
Special Needs Systems
P.O.Box 2150
Atlanta, GA 30301-2150

404-577-7995
800-426-2133
FAX: 561-982-6059
TTY: 800-284-9482
www.skepticfiles.org/md001/mobility.htm

5952 Kelley Diversified
P.O.Box 967
Athens, GA 30603-967

706-549-4398
FAX: 706-549-4479
ibizprofile.com/biz/kelley-diversified-inc-30

Mary Patton, Executive Director
Sherry Burns, Rehabilitation Services Director
Jenny Taylor, Business Operations Manager
Patricia Horne, Bookkeeper
Work adjustment and remunerative work programs.

5953 New Ventures
306 Fort Dr
Lagrange, GA 30240-5900

706-882-7723
FAX: 706-882-5401
customersvc@newventures.org
newventures.org

Dave Miller, CEO
Kelly Anderson, Quality Director
Jeff Chamberlain, Director of Business Services
Mike Wilson, Director of Industrial Marketing

A rehabilitation and work training facility for individuals with barriers to employability. The program utilizes community based industrial work of varying levels of difficulty. A return to work conditioning program for the industrially injured is offered which features: first-day contact, workers compensation rehabilitation team management, and light-duty work conditioning. A training stipend is paid to defray costs associated with training.

Hawaii

5954 Assets School
One Ohana Nui Way
Honolulu, HI 96818-4497

808-423-1356
FAX: 808-422-1920
info@assets-school.net
assets-school.net

John F. Morton, Chairman
Kristi L. Maynard, Vice Chairman
Robert W. Wo, Secretary
Russell J. Lau, Treasurer
ASSETS is an independent school for gifted and or dyslexic children that provides an individualized, integrated learning enviroment. ASSETS' enviroment empowers these children to maximize their potential and to find their place as lifelong learners in school and society.

5955 Hawaii Fair Employment Practice Agency
Room 411
830 Punchbowl St
Honolulu, HI 96813-5080

808-586-8636
800-586-8800
FAX: 808-586-8655
TTY: 808-586-8692
DLIR.HCRC.INFOR@hawaii.gov
http://hawaii.gov/labor/hcrc

Michael O Yamamoto
William Hoshijo, Executive Director
HCRC enforces state laws prohibiting discrimination in employment.

5956 Hawaii Vocational Rehabilitation Division
1901 Bachelot St.
Honolulu, HI 96817

808-586-9744
FAX: 808-586-9755
TTY: 808-586-9744
info@hawaiivr.org
hawaiivr.org

Jonathan Chun, Chair
Albert Perez, Administrator
Susan Foard, Assistant Administrator
Katie Keim, Staff Specialist
Mission is our committed staff strive, day-in day-out, to provide timely efficient and effective programs, services and benefits, for the purpose of achieving the outcome of empowering those who are the most vulnerable in our state to expand thier capacity for self sufficiency , self-determination, independence, healthy choices, quality of life and personal dignity.

5957 Lanakila Rehabilitation Center
1809 Bachelot St
Honolulu, HI 96817-2430

808-531-0555
FAX: 808-533-7264
TTY: 808-531-0555
info@lanakilahawaii.org
www.lanakilahawaii.org

Marian Tsuji, President
Wayne Fujishige, Vice President
Dwayne MASUTANI, Director Budget & Finance
Rachael Young, Director Human Resources
Lanakila is a private nonprofit organization whose mission is to provide services and supports that assist individuals with physical, mental, or age-related challenges to live as independently as possible within our community. A broad range of services are offered which include meal/senior services, community based adult day programming for individuals with disabilities, work training

opportunities, and extended/supported employment for individuals with special needs.

5958 Vocational and Rehabilitation Agency
P.O.Box 339
601 Kamokila Boulevard, Room 515
Kapolei, HI 96707-339

808-692-7719
FAX: 808-692-7727
TTY:808-692-7715
sfoard@dhs.hawaii.gov
http://www.hawaiivr.org/

Albert Perez, Manager
Work adjustment and remunerative work programs.

5959 Wahiawa Family
302 California Ave
#204
Wahiawa, HI 96786-1883

808-621-7407
wpf-dentalcare.com/

Leslie Chinna
Work adjustment and remunerative work programs.

Idaho

5960 Idaho Employment Service and Job Training Program Liaison
Idaho Department of Employment
317 W Main St
Boise, ID 83735-1

208-332-3578
FAX: 208-327-7470
idahocis@labor.idaho.gov
http://labor.idaho.gov

Roger Madsen, Manager
C.L Butch Otter, Governor
Roger B. Madson, Director
Renee Cox, Program Manager
Work adjustment and remunerative work programs.

5961 Idaho Fair Employment Practice Agency
Idaho Human Rights Commission
P.O.Box 83720
450 West State Street
Boise, ID 83720-3

208-334-2873
FAX: 208-334-2664
www2.state.id.us/ihrc/ihrchome.htm

David Rogers, Administrator
Mission is to admininster state and federal anti-discrimination laws in Idaho in a manner that is fair, accurate, and timely; and to work towards ensuring that all people withink the state are treated with dignity and respect in their places of employment, housing, education, and public accomodations.

5962 Idaho Governor's Committee on Employment of People with Disabilities
317 W Main St
Boise, ID 83735-1

208-332-3750
FAX: 208-327-7331
www.dol.gov

5963 Idaho Vocational Rehabilitation Agency
Room 150
650 W. State St.
Boise, ID 83704-8780

208-334-3390
FAX: 208-327-7417
TTY:208-327-7040
department.info@vr.idaho.gov
vr.idaho.gov

Darrell Quist, Manager
Janet Thaldorf, Supervisor
Vocational Rehabilitation assists many individuals with disabilities to go to work. With VR assistance, these individuals have overcome numerous obstacles and disability related barriers to achieve employment.

5964 Vocational and Rehabilitation Agency
Idaho Commission for the Blind & Visually Impaired
341 W Washington St
PO Box 83720
Boise, ID 83720-0012

208-334-3220
800-542-8688
FAX: 208-334-2963
aroan@icbvi.state.id.us
icbvi.state.id.us

Angela Roan, Manager
Raelene Thomas, Management Assistant
Bruce Christopherson, Rehabilitation Services Chief
Dana Ard, Vocational Rehabilitation Counse
Vocational rehabilitation, independent living training, medical intervention, adaptive technology and devices and employer advocacy.

Illinois

5965 Ada S McKinley Vocational Services
1359 W Washington Blvd
Chicago, IL 60607-4577

312-554-0600
FAX: 312-554-0292
TTY:312-697-9794
info@adasmckinley.org
adasmckinley.org

George Jones, Jr., Executive Director
Marion G. Sleet, Chief Operating Officer
Hans J. Schuster, Chief Financial Officer
Kathleen D. Chappell, Chief Development Officer
Mission is to serve those who, because of disabilities or other limiting conditions, need help in finding and pursuing paths leading to healthy, productive, and fulfilling lives.

5966 Anixter Center
2001 N. Clybourn Ave.
3rd Floor
Chicago, IL 60614

773-973-7900
FAX: 773-973-5268
TTY:773-973-2180
AskAnixter@anixter.org
anixter.org

Kevin Limbeck, President and CEO
Stacy Brown, Executive Vice President
Lauren K. Hill, Managing Director
Dan Sabol, Vice President and Business Deve
A Chicago-based human services agency that assists people with disabilities to live and work successfully in the community. Anixter Center provides vocational training, employment services, residences, special education, prevention programs, community services and health care. In addition, Anixter Center offers Illinois' only substance abuse treatment programs specifically for people with disabilities including Addiction Recovery of the Deaf.

5967 C-4 Work Center
4740 North Clark St.
Chicago, IL 60640

773-769-0205
infoc4@c4chicago.org
www.c4chicago.org

Eileen Durkin, President and CEO
Bruce Seitzer, LCPC, Senior Vice President
John Troy, MBA, CPA, Vice President of Finance
Danielle Byron, MS, Vice President of Information Systems
Aftercare, case finding, information and referrals, vocational training and work activities offered to mentally ill persons.

5968 Clearbrook
1835 W Central Rd
Arlington Heights, IL 60005-2410

847-870-7711
FAX: 847-870-7741
TTY: 847-870-2239
info@clearbrook.org
www.clearbrook.org

Carl M La Mell, President
Tracy Martin, Admissions Director
Bernie Andersen, Assistant to the President
Rosa Baez-Lopez, Vice President of Human Resource
Offers educational, employment and residential services to the developmentally disabled children and adults.

5969 Cornerstone Services
777 Joyce Rd
Joliet, IL 60436-1876

815-741-7600
FAX: 815-723-1177
jhogan@cornerstoneservices.org
cornerstoneservices.org

James A Hogan, CEO
Susan Murphy, Coordinator Public Relations
Ben Stortz, President/Chief Executive Officer
Don Hespell, Vice-President/Chief Operating Officer
Cornerstone Services provides progressive, comprehensive services for people with disabilities, promoting choice, dignity and the opportunity to live and work in the community. Established in 1969, the agency provides developmental, vocational, employment, residential and behavioral health services at various community-based locations. The nonprofit social service agency helps approximately 750 people each day.

5970 Fulton County Rehab Center
500 N Main St
Canton, IL 61520-1844

309-647-6510
FAX: 309-647-7965
www.fultoncountyrehabilitationcenter.com

Rex L. Lewis, Executive Director
John C. Harmon, Public Relations / Marketing
Rhonda S. Dawson, Production Director
Residential rehab center with health care incidental; manufactures wood pallets and skids; job training and vocational rehabilitation services.

5971 Glenkirk
3504 Commercial Ave
Northbrook, IL 60062-1863

847-272-5111
FAX: 847-272-7350
info@glenkirk.org
glenkirk.org

Allan G. Spector, CEO
Helps infants, children and adults with developmental disabilities reach higher levels of independence. A non-profit organization serving people in north and northwest Chicago suburbs. Glenkirk's residential, vocational, educational and support programs include services which provide individual evaluation, therapeutic treatment and training.

5972 Illinois Employment Service
Department of Employment Security
Fl 4
401 S State St
Chicago, IL 60605-1293

312-793-4880
800-247-4984
www.state.il.us/agency/

5973 Jewish Vocational Services
216 West Jackson Blvd.
Suite 700
Chicago, IL 60606-4602

312-673-3400
FAX: 312-553-5544
jvschgo@jvschicago.org
http://jvschicago.org/

H. Debra Levin, President
Alan S. Crane, Vice President
Marc Jacobs, Vice President
Benn Feltheimer, Secretary

Occupational training and job placement for handicapped persons of all religions.

5974 JoDavies Workshop
P.O.Box 6087
706 West Street
Galena, IL 61036-6087

815-777-2211
FAX: 815-777-3386
theworkshopgalena@theworkshopgalena.org
www.jdwi.org

Jean Muchow, Treasurer
Peg Tonne, Chairperson
Dale Gereau, Plant Manager
Lynn Berning, Vice Chairperson
Intake and referral, early intervention for children only, vocational evaluation and work adjustment training services offered.

5975 Kennedy Job Training Center
18350 Crossing Drive
Tinley Park, IL 60487-6122

708-342-5246
FAX: 708-594-7156
Information@stcolettail.org
http://www.stcolettail.org

Robin Mertes, Placement Manager
Kandy Stamer, QMRP/Intake Coordinator
Bob Loquercio, Board of Director
Wayne A. Kottmeyer, Executive Director
Offers vocational evaluation, vocational training work adjustment training, and job placement services for developmentally disabled and hearing impaired persons.

5976 Knox County Council for Developmental Disabilities
2015 Windish Dr
Galesburg, IL 61401-9774

309-344-2600
FAX: 309-344-1754
mcrittenden@kccdd.com
kccdd.com

Mary Crittenden, Executive Director
Pam Green, Director of Operations
Jeff Gomer, Director of Finance
Lynndel Messmore, Director of Rehabilitation
Developmental training, vocational evaluation, work adjustment training, extended training, placement, supported employment.

5977 Kreider Services
500 Anchor Road
Dixon, IL 61021-366

815-288-6691
FAX: 815-288-1636
TTY: 815-288-5931
info@kreiderservices.org?subject=Kreider%20Se
kreiderservices.org

Dr. Richard Piller, President
Dr. Vernon Brickley, Vice President
Cheryl Ebens, Director
Mike Hickey, Director
Offers day service programs, vocational training programs, job placement, supported employment, respite care, residential and family support for ages birth to three years.

5978 Lambs Farm
14245 W Rockland Rd
Libertyville, IL 60048-9745

847-362-4636
FAX: 847-362-9688
info@lambsfarm.org
lambsfarm.org

Dianne Yaconetti, President & CEO
Kathy Buresch, Director, Operations, Marketing
Nikki Bonamarte, Director, Development
Jose Martinez, Director, Quality Assurance
Person-centered, comprehensive program of residential, vocational and social support service for adults with developmental disabilities.

5979 **Land of Lincoln Goodwill Industries**
1220 Outer Park Drive
Springfield, IL 62704
217-789-0400
FAX: 217-789-0540
info@llgi.org
www.llgi.org

Sharon Durbin, CEO and President
Valerie Ausmus, VP of Finance
Deborah Clark, VP of Retail Operations
Kim Wonnell, VP of Human Resources
Empowers people with special needs to become self-sufficient through the power od work.

5980 **Orchard Village**
7660 Gross Point Road
Skokie, IL 60077-2628
847-967-1800
FAX: 847-967-9543
info@orchardvillage.org
www.orchardvillage.org

Joy Decker, President & CEO
Sally Ruecking, Vice President, Development
Allison Stark, Vice President, Programs
Jennifer Burgess, Director, Residential Services
Vocational program and counseling, respite services and community living group homes for the disabled and cognitively impaired. Orchard village also operates a private hope school especially devoted to teaching young adults independent living and skills necessary to flourish in the community.

5981 **President's Committee on Employment of Employment of the Disabled**
1331 F Street, NW,
Suite 300
Washington, DC 20004-1614
202-376-6200
800-ASK-DORI
FAX: 202-376-6219
TTY: 202-376-6205
info@pcepd.gov
www.usccr.gov/pubs/crd/federal/pcepd.htm
Carol Adams, President
John Lancaster, Executive Director
Work adjustment and remunerative work programs.

5982 **Sertoma Centre**
4343 W 123rd St
Alsip, IL 60803-1807
708-371-9700
FAX: 708-371-9747
info@sertomacentre.org
sertomacentre.org

Gus Vanden Brink, Executive Director
Paula Phillips, Assistant Director
A nationally accredited, not-for-profit agency that provides services to students and adults with developmental disabilities and mental illness. MIssion is to provide opportunities that empower individuals with disabilities to achieve success.

5983 **Shore Training Center**
Shore Community Services
4232 Dempster Street
Skokie, IL 60076
847-982-2030
FAX: 847-982-2039
TTY:847-581-0076
info@shoreservices.org
shoreinc.org

Debora K. Braun, Executive Director
Kirsten Luna, Director of Residential Services
Debbie Shulruf, Director of SHORE Lois Lloyd Cen
Lisa Wright, Director, SHORE Joseph Koenig, S
Mission is to improve the quality of life for citizens with developmental disabilities through community based services providing education/training.

5984 **Skills Inc.**
44 Morris Street
Webster, MA 01570-1233
508-943-0700
FAX: 508-949-6129
life-skills@life-skillsinc.org
skills-inc.org

Robert Miller, President
Pamela Guanci, Vice President
Raymond Bembenek, Treasurer
Janice Smith, Secretary
Accredited through the Commission on Accreditation of Rehabilitation Facilities; offers job training partnership act and vocational evaluation services offered.

5985 **Thresholds AMISS**
12145 Western Ave
Blue Island, IL 60406-1387
708-597-7997
FAX: 708-597-8073

Julia Rupp, Executive Director
Camille Rucks, Team Leader
Services offered include psychosocial, vocational and residential programs for ages 18 or older with a primary diagnosis of mental illness. Facility is wheelchair accessible.

5986 **Vocational and Rehabilitation Agency**
207 Staehouse
Springfield, IL 62706-1
217-782-0244
800-843-6154
FAX: 217-524-6262
TTY: 888-261-3336
ITTF.Web@illinois.gov
www.state.il.us
Pat Quinn, Governor
Provides work adjustment and remunerative skills.

5987 **Washington County Vocational Workshop**
781 E Holzhauer Dr
Nashville, IL 62263-2055
618-327-4461
FAX: 618-327-4477
www.mapquest.com

Keith Curran, Executive Director
Provides job training and related services and vocational rehabilitation services.

5988 **Westside Parents Work Activity Center**
3395 Mottman Road SW
Olympia, WA 98512
360-339-7297
blackhillsgym.com/family-activity-center
Theresa McKenzieSullivan, General Manager
Offers developmental training programs providing basic skills in self care for multiply and physically handicapped persons.

Indiana

5989 **ADEC Resources for Independence**
19670 State Road 120
Bristol, IN 46507-9162
574-848-7451
877-342-8954
FAX: 574-848-5917
shivelyp@adecinc.com
adecinc.com

Donna Belusar, President & CEO
Mitch Walorski, CFO
Sally Russell, Vice President
Joe Blocher, Vice President of Human Relation
Serves Elkhart County and surrounding area.

5990   ARC of Allen County
4919 Coldwater Rd
Fort Wayne, IN 46825-5532
260-456-4534
800-234-7811
FAX: 260-745-5200
delbrecht@esarc.org
www.easterseals.com

Bill Martin, Chairperson
Larry Graham, Senior Vice Chairperson
Donna K. Elbrecht, President/CEO
Susan Klug, Chief Operating Officer
Primary list of services includes: community living services, production and work training services, residential services, 24 hour medicaid waiver services, employment services, child care center, adult day services, and recreation.

5991   Arc Bridges
2650 W 35th Ave
Gary, IN 46408-1416
219-985-6562
FAX: 219-980-7315
mailbox@thearcnwindiana.com
www.thearcnwindiana.com

Brian Davis, Contact
Kris Prohl, Executive Director
Mission is to improve the welfare of people with intellectual and development disabilities and their families.

5992   BI-County Services
425 East Harrison Rd
Bluffton, IN 46714-9013
260-824-1253
FAX: 260-824-1892
info@adifferentlight.com
www.bi-countyservices.com

John Whicker, President
Serves Wells and Adam Counties. Infant services, Medicaid waivers, music therapy, ICF, MR, group homes, sheltered employment, pay program and supported employment services available.

5993   Balance Centers of America
3831 Hughes Ave.
Ste 504B
Culver, CA 90232-2630
310-625-5657
americanbalancecenters.com/

Jane Labar, Contact
Offers developmental training programs providing basic skills in self care for physically handicapped persons.

5994   Bridge Pointe Services & Goodwill of Southern Indiana, Inc
Goodwill International
1329 Applegate Lane
P.O. Box 2488
Clarksville, IN 47131-2488
812-283-7908
800-660-3355
FAX: 812-283-6248
comments@goodwillsi.org
http://www.goodwillsi.org/

Candice C. Barksdale, Chief Executive Director
Joel Henderson, PHR, Vice President of Human Resource
Bonnie Davis, Vice President of Donated Goods
Michelle Dayvault, Vice President of Development an
Career assesment, job readiness and placement, office skills training. Pediatric family support services. Childrens Academy, a developmental preschool.

5995   Carey Services
2724 S Carey St
Marion, IN 46953-3515
765-668-8961
FAX: 765-664-6747
www.careyservices.com

Bonnie Smith, Human Resources Manager
James Allbaugh, Chief Executive Officer
Gary Hendricks, Corporate Compliance
David Sprowl, Intake Coordinator
The mission of Carey Services is to create pathways towards self-sufficiency with personal satisfaction.

5996   Evansville Association for the Blind
500 North 2nd Avenue
Evansville, IN 47710-2355
812-422-1181
FAX: 812-424-3154
eabcdc@evansville.net
http://www.evansvilleblind.org/

Karla Horrell, Executive Director
Daniel Dana, President
Larry Arp, Vice President
Pam Doerter, Vice President
An community rehabilitation facility untilizing individual goals to assist persons with disabilities achieve or maintain potenial

5997   Four Rivers Resource Services
P.O.Box 249
Hwy. 59 South
Linton, IN 47441-249
812-847-2231
FAX: 812-847-8836
fourrivers@frrs.org
frrs.org

Kenton Barnes, President
Mary Lou Chapman, Vice-President
Ray Hart, Treasurer
Kathy Pennington, Secretary
Employment, community living, connections, follow-along, early intervention, preschool, healthy families, child care resource and referral and child care voucher program, impact, and transpotation services.

5998   Gateway Services/JCARC
P.O.Box 216
3500 North Morton Street
Franklin, IN 46131-216
317-738-5500
888-494-8069
FAX: 317-738-5522
www.gatewayarc.com

Karen Luehmann, Executive Director
Utilizes individual goals to assist persons with disabilities achieve or maintain potential.

5999   Goodwill Industries of Central Indiana
1635 West Michigan St
Indianapolis, IN 46222-3852
317-524-4313
FAX: 317-524-4336
TTY:317-524-4309
goodwill@goodwillindy.org
goodwillindy.org

James M. Mc Clelland, President & CEO
Nicki Washburn, Disability Services Coordinator
Kent A. Kramer, Senior Vice President and Chief Operating Officer
Daniel J. Riley, Senior Vice President, Administration and Chief Financial Of
Goodwill is in the business of helping people find jobs and provides programs and services for people who want to work. Goodwill is a community resource committed to deploying our assets and leveraging our resources with those of others in the community to create more opportunities for people who need assistance to improve their ability to earn a living.

6000   Indiana Civil Rights Commission
100 North Senate Avenue
Suite N103
Indianapolis, IN 46204-2208
317-232-2600
800-628-2909
FAX: 317-232-6580
TTY: 800-743-3333
info@icrc.in.gov
www.in.gov/icrc

Jamal Smith, Executive Director
Works to develop public policies that ensure equal opportunity in education to all.

6001 Indiana Employment Services and Job Training Program Liaison
10 North Senate Avenue
Indianapolis, IN 46204-2201
317-232-6702
FAX: 317-233-5499
www.in.gov/dwd/

6002 Michigan Resources
4315 East Michigan Blvd
Michigan City, IN 46360-3151
219-874-4288
FAX: 219-874-2689
TTY:219-873-2245
michiana@michianaresources.org
michianaresources.org

Nancy J Matela, Board Member
Matt Hollander, Chair
Gretchen Kalk, Treasurer
Andie Wolfinsohn, Secretary

Vocational training center for persons 16 and older with disabilities.

6003 New Hope Services
725 Wall Street
Jeffersonville, IN 47130-3616
812-288-8248
800-237-6604
FAX: 812-288-1206
info@newhopeservices.org
newhopeservices.org

James A. Bosley, President and CEO
John Broady, Senior Vice President and CFO
Bonnie Long, Senior Vice President, CAO
Jody Kitch, Chief Operating Officer

Mission is to provide hope through services which are responsive to individual needs.

6004 New Horizons Rehabilitation
P.O.Box 98
237 Six Pine Ranch Road
Batesville, IN 47006-98
812-934-4528
FAX: 812-934-2522
mdausch@nhrinc.org
www.nhrehab.org

Marie Dausch, Executive Director

Serves Ripley, Franklin, Ohio, Switzerland Dearborn, and Decatur. Provides training and services to adults with mental/physical disabilities and infants birth to age 3 with developmental delays or conditions of risk which could result in a developmental delay.

6005 Noble Of Indiana
Noble, Inc.
7701 East 21st Street
Indianapolis, IN 46219-2406
317-375-2700
FAX: 317-375-2719
rita.davis@nobleofindiana.org
www.nobleofindiana.org

Julia Huffman, President & CEO
Rita Davis, Director, Community Relations
Julie Brown, Director of Human Resources
Jeanine Coleman, Director of Community Living

Since 1953, Noble of Indiana has been dedicated to its mission: to create opportunities for people with developmental disabilities to live meaningful lives.

6006 Office of State Coordinator of Vocational Education for Students with Disability
Rm 212
10 N Senate Ave
Indianapolis, IN 46204-2201
317-232-1829
800-891-6499
tfields@dwd.state.in.us
www.state.in.us/dwd/techd

Scott B. Sanders, Commissioner
Randy Gillespie, Chief Financial Officer
Jeff Gill, General Counsel
Michelle Marshel, Deputy Commissioner of Communica

Manages and impliments innovative employment programs, unemployment insurance systems, and facilitates regional economic growth initiatives for Indiana.

6007 Putnam County Comprehensive Services
630 Tennessee St
Greencastle, IN 46135-2102
765-653-9763
877-653-9763
FAX: 765-653-3646
cns_pccs@yahoo.com
www.pccsinc.org

Chuck Schroeder, CEO
Charles Schroeder, Executive Director
Teresa Human, Community Living Services Director
Josi Blunton, Residential Director

A not-for-profit organization serving individuals with disabilities and similar characteristics in Indiana. Their mission is to provide services to individuals with disabilities in order for them to reach their optimum potential in attitudes, habits, and skills through training and integration, making them contributing members of their community, and to promote community awareness and acceptance of people with different abilities.

6008 Southern Indiana Resource Solutions
1579 S Folsomville Rd
Boonville, IN 47601-9465
812-897-4840
FAX: 812-897-0123
kelly@sirs.org
www.sirs.org

Kelly Mitchell, CEO/President
Don Critchlow, Chairperson
Larry Oathout, Vice-Chairperson
Jeff Hagedorn, Board Member

Adult services including jobs, community connections, and residential, childrens services, including service coordination and all therapies.

6009 Sycamore Rehabilitation Services
1001 Sycamore Lane
Danville, IN 46122-1474
317-745-4715
888-573-0817
FAX: 317-745-8271
info@sycamoreservices.com
sycamoreservices.com

Ralph Dunkin, President
Terry Kessinger, Vice President
Steve Patterson, Treasurer
Peg Murphy, Secretary

Provides individuals training and services for persons with disabilities that enhance independence in all areas of life.

6010 Vocational and Rehabilitation Agency
P.O.Box 7083
2 Peachtree Street, NW
Atlanta, GA 30303- 7083
404-232-1998
800-545-7763
FAX: 404-232-1800
GVRAcustomer-service@gvra.ga.gov
gvra.georgia.gov

Mike Hedden, Executive Director
James N. Defoor, Chair
Louise Hill, Vice Chair

Vocational training center for persons with disabilities.

6011 Wabash/Employability Center
201 I.U. Willets Road
S C6395 Earl Ave
Albertson, NY 11507
516-465-1400
FAX: 765-447-6456
info@viscardicenter.org
http://www.nbdc.com

Bill Carmichael, Contact
John D. Kemp, Esq., President & CEO
Kenneth J. Kunken, Esq., County Court Deputy Bureau Chief
Constantina Petallides-Markou, Human Resources Manager

Serves Tippecanoe County.

Iowa

6012   ACT Assessment Test Preparation Reference Manual
American College Testing Program
P.O.Box 168
500 ACT Drive
Iowa City, IA 52243-168   319-337-1000
                                       FAX: 319-339-3021
                                                act.org

Jon Whitmore, Chief Executive Officer
Janet E. Godwin, Chief of Staff and Accountability Officer
Jon L. Erickson, President, Education and Career Solutions
Martin L. Scaglione, President, Workforce Development
This reference manual was developed as a resource for high school teachers and counselors in assisting students with test preparation.

6013   Franklin County Work Activity Center
20 5th St NW
Hampton, IA 50441-1908   641-456-2532
                                       FAX: 641-456-4682
                                 www.accessincorportated.org

Harry Jacoby, Executive Director
Jim Koenen, Owner
Nonprofit organization providing residential and vocational services in Franklin and Hardin counties in the state of Iowa. Residential Services include RCF/MR services, Supported Community Living Services and Community Supervised Apartment Living Arrangement Services. Vocational Services include Work Services and Supported Employment Services. Accredited by the Commission on Accreditation of rehabilitation Facilities since 1984, and serves individuals with a wide range of needs.

6014   Innovative Industries
405 E Madison St
Box 41205
Cleveland, OH 44141-2402   330- 46- 260
                                         800-THE-M IR
                                       FAX: 330- 46- 260
                               info@innovativeindustries.com
                               www.innovativeindustries.com

Duane Nelson, Program Manager

6015   Iowa Civil Rights Commission
400 E 14th Street
Des Moines, IA 50319-201   515-281-4121
                                         800-457-4416
                                       FAX: 515-242-5840
                                   don.grove@iowa.gov
                             www.state.ia.us/government/crc

Ralph Rosenberg, Executive Director
Ron Pothast, Acting Executive Director
Corlis Moody, Executive Director
Beth Townsend, Executive Director
A neutral, fact-finding administrative agency that enforces the 'Iowa Civi Rights Act of 1965,' Iowa's anti-discrimination law. The commission doesn not provide legal representation. The commission's vision is a state free of discrimination.

6016   Iowa Employment Service
1000 East Grand Ave
Suite 140
Des Moines, IA 50309   515-282-5823
                                       FAX: 515-288-2184
                              fering@iowacareerconnection.com
                               www.iowacareerconnection.com

L.M. (Al) Fering, SPHR, FLMI, President
Miles Morrow, CPC
Specializes in accounting and human resources talent aquisition in the Upper-Midwest.

6017   Iowa Job Training Program Liaison
Iowa Department of Economic Development
200 East Grand Ave
Des Moines, IA 50309-1856   515-725-3000
                                       FAX: 515-725-3010
                                     info@iowa.gov
                                   iowalifechanging.com

David Lyons, President
Debi Durham, Director
Kathy Anderson, Director, Communications Team
Jody Benz, Director, Iowa Commission on Vol
To engender and promote economic development policies and practices which stimulate and sustain Iowa's economic growth and climate and that integrate efforts across public and private sectors.

6018   Iowa Valley Community College
3700 S. Center St.
Marshalltown, IA 50158-4783   641-752-7106
                                         866-622-4748
                                       FAX: 641-752-5909
                                   mccinfo@iavalley.edu.
                                   http://www.iavalley.edu/

Dr. Chris Wynes, Chancellor
Robin Anctil, Director of Marketing
Dr. Lisa Breja, Institutional Researcher/AQIP Li
Nate Chua, MCC Director of Retention & Lear
Offers two levels of specialized vocational preparatory programming for adults with disabilities. The Career Development Center serves dependent adults. The goal of the program is to maintain or improve skills to enable persons served to enter sheltered or supported employment. The IRP/CBVT programs are non-credit specialized vocational programs for independent adults served by Vocational Rehabilitation and our programs. The goals are for competitive placements in jobs. CARF accredited.

6019   Iowa Vocational Rehabilitation Services
510 East 12th Street
Jessie Parker Building
Des Moines, IA 50319-0240   515-281-4211
                                       FAX: 515-281-7645
                                       TTY:515-281-4211
                             Victoria.Carrington@iowa.gov
                                     www.ivrs.iowa.gov

David Mitchell, Administrator
Matthew Coulter, Chief Financial Officer
Kenda Jochimsen, Bureau Chief
Charlie Levine, Assistant Bureau Chief
The mission is to work for and with individuals who have disabilities to achieve their employment, independence and economic goals.

6020   New Focus
102 W Washington St
Centerville, IA 52544-1550   641-437-1722
                                       FAX: 641-437-1028

Peggy Oden, Executive Director
Provides vocational services for adults with disabilities. Includes work activity, supported employment and supported community living.

6021   Second Time Around
560 Harrison Ave
Suite 501
Boston, MA 02118-1709   641-437-7355
                                press@secondtimearound.net
                                 www.secondtimearound.net/

Monica Blizeck, Manager
Debbie Steen, Store Supervisor
Deana Edwards, Manager
Work training site for adults with disabilities.

Kansas

6022 Clay Center Adult Training Center
40 Beech Street
Port Chester, NY 10573-2903
914-937-2047
FAX: 914-935-1205
mail@clayartcenter.org
www.clayartcenter.org

Michael Spielman, Manager
Robert Rattet, President
Bruce Fern, Vice President
Reena Kashyap, Treasurer
Work training site for adults with disabilities.

6023 Kansas Fair Employment Practice Agency
Suite 568-South
900 SW Jackson St
Topeka, KS 66612-2818
785-296-3206
FAX: 785-296-0589
khrc@ink.org
www.state.ks.us/public/khrc

Mostafa Kamal, Manager
William V. Minner, Executive Director
Melvin Neufeld, Chair
Terry Crowder, Vice Chair

6024 Kansas Vocational Rehabilitation Agency
915 SW Harrison
8th Floor West
Topeka, KS 66612-1995
785-368-7471
866-213-9079
FAX: 785-368-7467
TTY: 785-368-7478
jac@srkspo.wpo.state.ks.us
www.srskansas.org/rehab

Michael Donnelly, Director
Helps people with disabilities achieve employment and self-sufficiency. Also links employers with qualified and productive individuals to meet thier work force needs.

Kentucky

6025 Kentucky Committee on Employment of Peoplewith Disabilities
2nd Floor
275 East Main St
Frankfort, KY 40601-2321
502-564-7456
800-648-6057
FAX: 502-564-7459
VivianL.Bettis@ky.gov
www.oet.ky.gov

Greg Higgins, Manager
Tom Bowell, Manager
Shane Smith, Manager
Terri Bradshaw, Communications Director
Provides qualified people for jobs, quality jobs for people, temporary financial support for the unemployed, comprehensive labor market information, and preserve the integrity and viability of the Unemployment Insurance Trust Fund.

6026 Kentucky Department for Employment Serviceand Job Training Program Liaison
275 E Main Street 2-W
Frankfort, KY 40621-1
502-564-5331
FAX: 502-564-7452
VivianL.Bettis@ky.gov
http://www.oet.ky.gov

Gina Oney, Assistant Director
Linda Prewitt, Acting Division Director/ Assist
Linda Pierce, Compliance Support Branch Manage
Gregory Higgins, Acting Unemployment Insurance Di
Provides qualified people for jobs, quality jobs for people, temporary financial support for the unemployed.

6027 Kentucky Department for the Blind
275 East Main Street
Frankfort, KY 40621
502-564-7456
800-321-6668
FAX: 502-564-2951
TTY: 502-564-2929
JenniferN.Wright@ky.gov
www.blind.ky.gov

Christopher Smith, Executive Director
Michelle McElmurray, Executive Assistant
Allison Jessee, Director of Consumer Services
Cora McNabb, VR Administrator, Training and H
Provides career services and assistance to adults with severe visual handicaps who want to become productive in the home or work force. Also provides the Client Assistance Program established to provide advice, assistance and information available from rehabilitation programs to persons with handicaps.

6028 Kentucky Office for the Blind
275 East Main Street
Frankfort, KY 40621
502-564-7456
800-321-6668
FAX: 502-564-2951
TTY: 502-564-2929
JenniferN.Wright@ky.gov
blind.ky.gov

Christopher Smith, Executive Director
Michelle McElmurray, Executive Assistant
Allison Jessee, Director of Consumer Services
Cora McNabb, VR Administrator, Training and H
Our mission is to provide opportunities for employment and independence to individuals with visual impairments.

6029 Kentucky Vocational Rehabilitation Agency
275 East Main Street
Frankfort, KY 40621
502-564-4440
800-372-7172
FAX: 502-564-6745
WFD.VOCREHAB@ky.gov
http://ovr.ky.gov

Dr. David Beach, Executive Director
Holly Hendricks, Assistant Director of Program Se
Jason Jones, Director of Community Relations
Mindy Yates, Administrative Services Branch M
Assists eligible individuals with disabilities achieve their employment goals.

6030 Pioneer Vocational/Industrial Services
150 Corporate Drive
P.O Box 1396
Danville, KY 40422-1396
859-236-8413
800-527-4198
FAX: 859-238-7115
TTY: 859-236-1251
pioneer@pioneerservices.org
pioneerservices.org

Mike Pittman, Chief Executive Officer / Executive Director
Danny Rigney, Director of Marketing and Operations
Dot Carman, Office Administration Director / Safety / Compliance Officer
Mike Fayne, Director of Services Assistant
Mission is to provide vocational development and extended employment programs to people who are disabled and or disadvantaged to assist them in obtaining employment and maximizing independent living skills.

6031 Work Enhancement Center of Western Kentucky
1906 College Heights Blvd.
Bowling Green, KY 42101-3576
270-745-0111
FAX: 502-767-3600
wku@wku.edu
www.wku.edu

Steve Passmore, Director
John O'Shaughnessy, Chief Executive Officer
J. David Porter, Chair
Frederick A. Higdon, Vice Chair
The center has been established in order to service industry in the three state area surrounding Kentucky. This service includes

job/skill evaluation, job design consultation, pre-employment employee evaluations and economic evaluation.

Louisiana

6032   Community Opportunities of East Ascension
1121 E Ascension Complex Blvd
Gonzales, LA 70737   225-621-2000
                                       FAX: 225-621-2022
                                       http://coea.homestead.com

Mark Thomas, Director
Committed to affording individuals the opportunities that reflect and support choices, dignity, individuality, self-determination, community, coherency and commen sense. Programs incloude Respite, Personal Care Attendant, Support Living, Support Environment, Adult Day Training, and Elderly/Adult Waiver Services.

6033   Louisiana Employment Service and Job Training Program Liaison
1001 North 23rd Street
Post Office Box 94094
Baton Rouge, LA 70804-9094   225-342-3111
                                       800-259-5154
                                       FAX: 225-342-7960
                                       owd@lwc.la.gov
                                       http://www.laworks.net

Curt Eysink, Executive Directo
Carey Foy, Deputy Executive Director
Jay Augustine, Executive Counsel
Renee Ellender Roberie, Chief Financial Officer
Provides services for job seekers and job training programs.

6034   Louisiana Vocational Rehabilitation Agency
950 N 22nd St
Baton Rouge, LA 70802-6109   225-219-2225
                                       800-737-2958
                                       FAX: 225-219-4993
                                       www.dss.state.la.us/departments/lrs

James Gaston, Manager
Ed Barras, Manager
Mark Martin, Director
Offers individuals with disabilities a wide range of services designed to provide them with skills, resources, attitudes, and expectations needed to compete in the interview process, get the job, keep the job, and develop a lifetime career.

6035   St. James Association for Retarded Citizens
29150 Health Unit St
Vacherie, LA 70090-4221   225-265-2181
                                       FAX: 225-265-7427
                                       info@brightscope.com
                                       www.brightscope.com

Judy Bastian, Manager
Bruce Hansen, Chairman
John Sarkisian, Board of Directors
A private sheltered work program for mentally retarded and developmentally disabled adults.

6036   Westbank Sheltered Workshop
606 OPELOUSAS AVE
New Orleans, LA 70114-4344   504-362-1311
                                       www.taxexemptworld.com

Maine

6037   Addison Point Specialized Services
P.O.Box 207
Addison, ME 04606-207   207-483-6500
                                       FAX: 207-483-2817
                                       www.faqs.org

Paula Chartrand, Owner
Provides services to individuals who are deaf/blind, mentally retarded, autistic, behaviorally challenged and/or dual diagnosed.

Training services to place these individuals in community employment.

6038   Bangor Veteran Center: Veterans Outreach Center
Veteran's Administration
368 Harlow St
Bangor, ME 04491   207-947-3391
                                       FAX: 207-941-8195
                                       Patricia.Albert-Dehetre@va.gov
                                       http://www.maine.va.gov

Joseph A Degrasse, Team Leader
Robert L Daisey LCSW, Clinical Coordinator
Eric K. Shinseki, Secretary
W. Scott Gould, Deputy Secretary
Readjustment counseling services for veterans of Vietnam, Vietnam Era, Persian Gulf, Panama, Grenada, Lebanon, Somalia, WWII and Korean conflicts, as well as Iraq, Afganistan, and military sexual trauma.

6039   Creative Work Systems
619 Brighton Ave
Portland, ME 04102   207-879-1140
                                       FAX: 207-879-1146
                                       kraye@creativeworks.com
                                       creativeworksystems.com

Susan Percy, Executive Director
Edward McGeachey, President
Jim Houle, Vice President
Provides residential, day habilitation and supported emploment in Central and Southern Maine.

6040   Maine Department Of Labor
45 Commerce Drive
Augusta, ME 04330   207-623-7900
                                       FAX: 207-287-3042
                                       mdol@maine.gov
                                       www.state.me.us/labor

Patrick Fleming, Executive
Jeanne Shorey Paquette, Commissioner
Provides a wide range of services such as employment, labor market information, rehabilitation/disability and others.

6041   Maine Governor's Committee on Employment of the Disabled
45 Commerce Drive
Augusta, ME 04330-7880   207-621-5087
                                       800-794-1110
                                       FAX: 207-624-5302
                                       www.maine.gov

6042   Maine Human Rights Commission
Maine Human Rights Commission
51 State House Station
Augusta, ME 04333-51   207-624-6290
                                       FAX: 207-624-8729
                                       Amy.Sneirson@maine.gov
                                       www.maine.gov/mhrc

Amy Sneirson, Executive Director
Barbara Archer Hirsch, Commission Counsel
Victoria Ternig, Chief Investigator
Jill Duson, Compliance Manager
State agency with the responsibility of enforcing Maine's anti-discrimination laws. The commission investigates complaints of unlawful discrimination in employment, housing, education, access to public accommodations, extension of credit and offensive names.

6043   Northeast Occupational Exchange
29 Franklin Street
Bangor, ME 04401-3857   207-942-3685
                                       800-857-0500
                                       FAX: 207-561-4725
                                       TTY: 207-992-2298
                                       www.noemaine.org

Charles O Tingley, Executive Director
A fully licensed, comprehensive mental health and substance abuse treatment and rehabilitation facility.

6044 Vocational and Rehabilitation Agency
Division for the Blind and Visually Impaired
55 State House Station
Augusta, ME 04333-55
                                           207-623-7981
                                           888-457-8883
                                           FAX: 207-624-5980
                                           TTY: 800-794-1110
                                    jobbank.careercenter@maine.gov
                                           www.mainecareercenter.com

Jill Busond, Bureau Director

The Maine CareerCenter provides a variety of employment and training services at no charge for Maine workers and businesses. Whether you are looking to improve your job qualifications, explore a different profession, find a new career or hire an employee, the CareerCenter can help.

Maryland

6045 Ardmore Developmental Center
3000 Lottsford Vista Road
Bowie, MD 20721-4001
                                           301-577-2575
                                           FAX: 301-306-9799
                                    grow@ArdmoreEnterprises.org
                                    www.ardmoreenterprises.org

Patrick L. Carter, President
Eileen Baker, Vice-President
Marilynn W. Riley, Secretary
Daphne Pallozzi, Chief Executive Officer

Offers supported employment programs and vocational education for persons who are mentally retarded as well as residential services and Emergency Respite Care.

6046 Job Opportunities for the Blind
National Federation of the Blind
200 East Wells Street at Jernigan P
Baltimore, MD 21230- 4914
                                           410-659-9315
                                           FAX: 410-685-5653
                                           nfb@nfb.org
                                           www.nfb.org

Marc Mauer, President
John Berggren, Executive Director for Operation
John G. Paré Jr., Executive Director for Strategic
Mark Riccobono, Executive Director, NFB Jernigan

This free service allows individuals touch-tone telephone access to the thousands of jobs listed in America's Job Bank, and internet service run by the Department of Labor. Any person registered with either a state rehabilitation agency or a state employment service can search across the country for jobs by either type of work or location.

6047 Mainstream
9800 Mt. Pyramid Ct.
Suite 360
Englewood, CO 80112-6301
                                           303-268-1920
                                           FAX: 303-268-1926
                                           mainstrm@aol.com
                                           investigativerisk.com

Patricia M Jackson, Executive Director
Charles Moster

Nonprofit organization dedicated to improving competitive employment opportunities for persons with disabilities. Provides specialized services and acts as a bridge that links service providers, employers and persons with disabilties. Provides training, educational publications, and videos on disabiltyemployment issues. Educationa materials include a magazine, brochures, and audio-visual aids.

6048 Maryland Employment Services and Job Training Program Liaison
500 North Calvert Street
#401
Baltimore, MD 21202-2201
                                           410-230-6001
                                           det@dllr.state.md.us
                                           http://www.dllr.state.md.us

Maria Simms
Maureen O'Connor, Communications and Media Relatio
Jill Porter, Director of Legislative Services
Kathleen Spencer, Human Resources

Provides job development and placement and services

6049 Maryland Fair Employment Practice Agency
9th Fl
6 Saint Paul St
Baltimore, MD 21202-6806
                                           410-767-8600
                                           800-637-6247
                                           FAX: 410-333-1841
                                           TTY: 410-333-1737
                                    nbell@mccr.state.md.us
                                    www.mchr.state.md.us

Adrienne Jones, Executive Director
James Neil Bell, Deputy Director
Glendora Hughes, General Counsel
Benny F. Short, Assistant Director

Mission is to ensure equal opportunity to all through the enforcement of Maryland's laws against discrimination in employment, housing, and public accomodations; to provide educational and outreach services related to the provisions of this law: and to promote and improve human relations in Maryland.

6050 Maryland State Department of Education
Division of Rehabilitation Services (DI RS)
200 West Baltimore Street
Baltimore, MD 21218-1628
                                           410-767-0100
                                           888-246-0016
                                           FAX: 410-554-9412
                                           TTY: 410-333-6442
                                    http://www.marylandpublicschools.org

Robert Burns, Manager

The Vocational Rehabilitation Program delivers to eligible individuals with physical and/or mental disabilities to enable them to become employed. The Independent Living Program's goal is to assist people in remaining in their homes and communities. The Division operates the Maryland Rehabilitation Center, a comprehensive evaluation and training center that has dormitory space. There are field offices located statewide with counselors to advise and manage the provision of services offered.

6051 Melwood
5606 Dower House Road
Upper Marlboro, MD 20772-3432
                                           301-599-8000
                                           FAX: 301-599-0180
                                           services@melwood.org
                                           www.melwood.org

Donald A. Donahue, DHEd, MBA, FA, Chair
Richard Mahan, CPA, Vice Chair
George Watkins, CPA, Treasurer
Shelly Gardeniers, Secretary

Melwood is a dynamic nonprofit that creates jobs and opportunities to improve the lives of people with disabilities. Melwood serves more than 1900 people with disabilities in the greater Washington DC area.

6052 PWI Profile
Projects W Industry Goodwill Industries of America
16120 W Bernardo Dr
San Diego, CA 92127
                                           858-673-6050
                                           FAX: 858-673-0085
                                    kicthermal.com/process-window-index-pwi

6053 Project LINK
Mainstream
Suite 700
3 Bethesda Metro Ctr
Bethesda, MD 20814-6301   301-215-9100
                                        800-247-1380
                                    FAX: 301-891-8778
                                info@cosmoscorp.com
                                        cosmoscorp.com

Charles Moster
Provides job development and placement in services to dislocated workers with disabilities in the Washington, DC and Dallas, TX areas.

6054 Treatment and Learning Centers (TLC)
14901 Dufief Mill Road
Suite 100
North Potomac, MD 20878   301-738-6424
                                    FAX: 301-340-6082
                                    TTY:301-424-5203
                                        www.ttlc.org

Dr Patricia Ritter, Executive Director
Suellyn Sherwood, Operations Director
Rhona Schwartz, High School Program Director
Janet Graves-Wright, Outpatient Services Director
A non-profit organization that specializes in educational, therapeutic and vocational services for invididuals with special needs. Programs include speech-language and occupational therapy, psycho-educational testing, tutoring, audiology, employment opportunities and the Katherine Thomas School for students with moderate to severe language and learning disabilities and/or high-functioning autism.
Preschool-12

Massachusetts

6055 Department Of Workforce Development
State of Massachusetts
Rm 2112
1 Ashburton Pl
Boston, MA 02108-1518   617-626-7100
                                        800-439-0183
                                    TTY:800-439-2370
                                    Dhurley@detma.org
                                www.massworkforce.org

Suzanne M. Bump, Secretary
Deval L. Patrick, Governor
Timothy P. Murray, Lt. Governor
Serves as the Governor's principal advisory board on workforce development.

6056 Gateway Arts Center: Studio, Craft Store& Gallery
Vinsen Corporation
60-62 Harvard St
Brookline, MA 02445-7993   617-734-1577
                                    FAX: 617-734-3199
                                    gateway@vinfen.org
                                    www.gatewayarts.org

Rae Edelson, Director
Stephanie Schmidt, Program Director
Mona Thaler, Marketing Director
Stephen De Fronzo, Artistic Director
Award winning, nationally recoginzed Arts based rehabilitation service with over 100 talented adults with disabilities.

6057 Massachusetts Fair Employment Practice Agency
Rm 601
1 Ashburton Pl
Boston, MA 02108-1524   617-994-6000
                                    FAX: 617-720-6053
                                    TTY:617-994-6196
                        Barbara.Green@massmail.state.ma.us
                                www.state.ma.us/mcad

Julian T. Tynes, Chairman
Sunila Thomas George, Commissioner
Jamie R. Williamson, Commissioner
Joel Berner, Esq., Chief of Enforcement
The commission works to eliminate discrimination on a variety of bases and areas, and strives to advance the civil rights of the people of commonwealth through law enforcement, outreach and training.

6058 Massachusetts Governor's Commission on Employment of Disabled Persons
11th Floor
One Ashburton Place
Boston, MA 02108-2502   617-573-1600
                                appointments.state.ma.us

Theodore Schipani, Owner
John Polanowicz, Secretary
Kathleen Betts, Assistant Secretary
Claudia Henderson, Chief of Staff
State vocational rehabilitation agency.

6059 Vocational Rehabilitation Agency
2 Peachtree Street, NW
Atlanta, GA 30303-1616   404-232-1998
                                        866-489-0001
                                    FAX: 404-232-1800
                                    TTY: 800-764-0200
                        elmer.bartels@mrc.state.ma.us
                                disabilitycompendium.org

Charles Carr, Commissioner of Rehabilitation
Kasper M. Goshgarian, Deputy Commissioner
Debra Kamen, Assistant Commissioner, Communit
Barbara Kinney, Assistant Commissioner, Disabili
Provides residential, day habilitation and supported employment

6060 Vocational and Rehabilitation Agency Massachusetts Commission for the Blind
600 Washington Street
Boston, MA 02111-4718   617-727-5550
                                        800-392-6450
                                    FAX: 617-626-7685
                                    TTY: 800-392-6556
                    Ronald.Gallagher@MassMail.State.MA.US
                    www.mass.gov/eohhs/gov/departments/mcb/

Charles Carr, Commissioner of Rehabilitation
Kasper M. Goshgarian, Deputy Commissioner
Debra Kamen, Assistant Commissioner, Communit
Barbara Kinney, Assistant Commissioner, Disabili
Provides residentail, habilitation, and supported employment

6061 Work Inc.
25 Beach Street
Dorchester, MA 02122-2734   617-691-1500
                                    FAX: 617-691-1595
                                        workinc.org

James Cassetta, CEO
James R. Flanagan, Chairman
Philip Dould, Vice Chairman
David Anderson, Treasurer (CFO)
Mission is all individuals have the ability to grow, the right to make choices and to participate in community life. It is the mission of WORK inc. to join with others in creating the conditions under which all persons with disablilities will experience.

Michigan

6062 Department Of Human Services
P.O.Box 30037
235 S. Grand Ave.
Lansing, MI 48909-8152
517-887-9400
800-292-4200
FAX: 517-335-5140
TTY: 5173734025
kreinerc@state.mi.us
www.michigan.gov.dhs

Maura D. Corrigan, Director
Duane Berger, Chief Deputy Director/Chief Oper
Terrence Beurer, Director, Field Operations
Susan Kangas, Deputy Director, Financial Servi
The DHS is Michigan's public assistance, child and family welfare agency. DHS directs the operations of public assistance and service programs through a network of over 100 county department of human service offices around the state.

6063 Lamplighter's Work Center
1320 W State St
Cheboygan, MI 49721-1402
231-627-4319
www.usa.com/frs/lamplighters-work-center.html
Robert Spinella, Executive Director
Offers small business counseling and training to individuals with disabilities

6064 Michigan Department of Civil Rights
3054 W Grand Blvd
Ste 3-600
Detroit, MI 48202-6054
313-456-3700
800-482-3604
FAX: 313-456-3791
TTY: 877-878-8464
MDCR-INFO@michigan.gov
www.michigan.gov/mdcr
Daniel H. Krichbaum, Director
Investigates and resolves discrimination complaints and works to prevent discrimination through educational programs that promote voluntary compliance with civil rights laws

6065 Michigan Employment Service
201 N. Washington Square
Lansing, MI 48913-3165
517-335-5858
888-605-6722
FAX: 517-241-8217
TTY: 888-605-6722
www.michigan.gov/mdcd
Christine Quinn, Director, Michigan Rehabilitatio
Job development and placement in services to dislocated workers with disabilities

6066 Michigan Rehabilitation Services: Dept ofLabor & Regulatory Affairs
235 S Grand Ave
PO Box 30037
Lansing, MI 48909-7510
517-373-3390
800-605-6722
FAX: 517-335-7277
TTY: 888-605-6722
porterj3@michigan.gov
www.michigan.gov/mrs
Jaye N Porter, Director
Laurie Eggers, Administrative Assistant
State vocational rehabilitation agency.

6067 Small Business Development Center
Ann Arbor Center for Independent Living
409 3rd St, SW
Washington, DC 20416-6832
800-827-5722
FAX: 313-971-0826
answerdesk@sba.gov
www.sba.gov

Sarah Bard, Director
Phil Zepeda, Manager
Maria Contreras-Sweet, SBA Administrator
Fred Baldassaro, Assistant Administrator
Offers small business counseling and training to individuals with disabilities in the state of Michigan.

Minnesota

6068 Jewish Vocational Service of Jewish Familyand Children's Services
401 N 3rd St
Suite 605
Minneapolis, MN 55401-1388
612-692-8920
FAX: 612-692-8921
jfcs@jfcsmpls.org
http://www.jfcsmpls.org
Nancy Rhein, Vice President of Board Development
Howard Zack, President
Sherri Feuer, Vice President of Fund Development
Eileen Kohn, Vice President of Marketing
The mission of JVS is to be a recognized leader in delivering employment, training, and career development services that positively impact individuals of all backgrounds, business and society.

6069 Minnesota Department of Employment and Economic Development - Vocational Rehab Services
332 Minnesota St
1st National Bank Bldg #E-200
Saint Paul, MN 55101-1314
651-259-7114
800-657-3858
FAX: 651-296-3900
TTY: 800657397373
DEED.CustomerService@state.mn.us
www.positivelyminnesota.com
Kim Peck, Director
Service for people with disabilities who need skills to prepare for work, or to find and keep a job.

6070 Minnesota Employment Practice Agency
Minnesota Dept. Of Human Rights
Freeman Building
625 Robert Street North
Saint Paul, MN 55155
651-539-1100
800-657-3704
FAX: 651-296-9042
TTY: 651-296-1283
Info.MDHR@state.mn.us
humanrights.state.mn.us
Kevin Lindsey, Commissioner
Denise Romero-Zasada, Executive Assistant to the Commi
Ytmar Santiago, Deputy Commisioner
Gregory Torrence, Assistant Commisioner
Mission and vision is to make Minnesota discrimination free.

6071 PWI Forum
Multi Resource Centers
1900 Chicago Ave
Minneapolis, MN 55404-1903
612-752-8138
pwi-forum.perfectworld.com/

6072 **Vocational and Rehabilitation Agency**
332 Minnesota Street
Suite E200
Saint Paul, MN 55101- 1351
651-259-7114
800-657-3858
FAX: 651-649-5927
TTY: 612-642-0506
info@ngwmail.des.state.mn.us
www.mnssb.org

Richard Strong, Executive Director
People seeking work, businesses seeking employees, students, and those looking for a first job or returning to the workforce, will find services to meet their needs.

Mississippi

6073 **Allied Enterprises of Tupelo**
Ability Works Incorporated
1281 Highway 51
Madison, MS 39110
800-443-1000
FAX: 662-287-1463
mdrs.state.ms.us

Michael Byrd, Manager
Jack Virden, Chairman
Jean Massey, Associate State Superintendent of Education
Carey Wright, Superintendent of Education
Vocational evaluation, work adjustment and job placement of disabled persons in a rehabilitation workshop.

6074 **Mississippi Department of Rehabilitation Services**
1281 Highway 51
Madison, MS 39110-1698
601-853-5100
800-443-1000
FAX: 601-359-1695
TTY: 800-443-1000
bmcmillan@mdrs.state.ms.us
http://www.mdrs.state.ms.us/

Ed LeGrand, Executive Director
Shelia Browning, Deputy Director
Chris Howard, Deputy Director
Richard Sorey, Director
Offers low vision aids and appliances, counseling, social work, educational and professional training, residential services, recreational services, computer training and employment opportunities for the handicapped.

6075 **Mississippi Employment Secutity Commission**
P.O.Box 1699
1235 Echelon Parkway
Jackson, MS 39215-1699
601-321-6000
FAX: 601-961-7405
comments@mdes.ms.gov.
www.mdes.ms.gov

Mark Henry, Executive Director
Phil Bryant, Governor
A federally funded state agency. The programs of MDES, under direction of the governor of Mississippi, report to the federal government.

6076 **Worksight**
Mississippi State University
PO Drawer 6189
108 Herbert - South, Room 150
Mississippi State, MS 39762-6189
662-325-2001
800-675-7782
FAX: 662-325-8989
TTY: 662-325-2694
nrtc@colled.msstate.edu
www.blind.msstate.edu

Michele Capella McDonnall, Research Professor and Interim D
Jacqui Bybee, Research Associate II
Jessica Thornton, Business Manager
Angela Shelton, Coordinator of Instructional Mat
Discusses news, activities, research projects and training programs of the Center.

Missouri

6077 **Missouri Commission on Human Rights**
421 EastDunklinSt.
P.O. Box 59
Jefferson City, MO 65102-0059
573-751-3215
800-320-2519
FAX: 573-751-4945
mchr@labor.mo.gov
http://www.labor.mo.gov

Alisa Warren, Executive Director
Tracey Allan, Intake Officer
Nia Ray, Director
The Missouri Commission on Human Rights enforces the state's anti-discrimination law that prohibits discrimination in housing, employment and places of public accommodations. It prohibits discrimination due to race, color, religion, national origin, ancestry, sex, disability, age and familial status. Complaints must be filed within 180 days of the alleged discrimination. If discrimination is found after investigation, the Commission can hold hearings to enforce the law.

6078 **Missouri Governor's Council on Disability**
P.O. Box 687
1706 East Elm
Jefferson City, MO 65102-1668
573-751-8676
800-877-8249
FAX: 573-526-4109
TTY: 573-751-2600
gcd@oa.mo.gov
www.gcd.oa.mo.gov

Douglas E. Nelson, Acting Commissioner
James Trout, Acting Chair and Council Members
Linda Baker, Executive Director Governor's Co
Dawn Evans, Disability Program Specialist
Advocate training, civil rights, community education services, community resource referral, conferences, consumer education, disability awareness program, educational information and resources, information and education services, information and referral, newsletter, policy issues and services, publications, resource directory, seminars, technical assistance, training and seminars.

6079 **Missouri Job Training Program Liaison**
221 Metro Dr
Jefferson City, MO 65109-4412
573-634-2321

Joe Jerkins, Manager
Services for individuals with disabilities who want to become employed.

6080 **Missouri Vocational Rehabilitation Agency**
205 Jefferson St.
Jefferson Cty, MO 65101-6188
573-751-4212
877-222-8963
FAX: 573-751-1441
TTY: 573-751-0881
info@vr.dese.mo.gov
www.vr.dese.mo.gov

Jeanne Loyd, Assistant Commissioner
Michelle Scherer, Administrator
A team of decicated individuals working for the continuous improvement of education and services for all citizens.

6081 **WX: Work Capacities**
Suite 103
17331 E 40th Hwy
Independence, MO 64055
816-478-2333
FAX: 816-478-2335

Chris Walters, Manager
Mike Heinz, Manager
Services for individuals with disabilities who want to become employed.

Montana

6082 **Montana Fair Employment Practice Agency**
1805 Prospect Avenue
PO Box 1728
Helena, MT 59624-1728
406-444-2840
800-542-0807
FAX: 406-444-2978
TTY: 406-444-9696
erdquestions@mt.gov
www.erd.dli.mt.gov

Marieke Chief, Bureau Chief
Kathleen Hel , Case Manager
Advocate training, civil rights, community education services, community resource referral and conferences

6083 **Montana Governor's Committee on Employment of Disabled People**
PO Box 200801
Helena, MT 59620-127
406-444-4405
800-243-4091
FAX: 406-444-4151
Boards@mt.gov
svc.mt.gov/gov/boards/

Nebraska

6084 **Nebraska Employment Services**
Department of Labor
140 S 27th St Ste C
Lincoln, NE 68510-2601
402-474-9675
www.yellowpages.com

6085 **Nebraska Fair Employment Practice Agency**
301 Centennial Mall South, 5th Floo
PO Box 94934
Lincoln, NE 68509-4394
402-471-2024
800-642-6112
FAX: 402-471-4059
www.nol.org/home/neoc

Royce Jeffries, Chairperson
Kristin Yates, Vice-Chairman
Ms.Barbara Albers, Executive Director
he Nebraska Equal Opportunity Commission is a neutral administrative agency created by statute in 1965 to enforce the public policy of the state against discrimination. The principal function of the NEOC is to receive, investigate and pass upon charges of unlawful discrimination occurring anywhere within the State of Nebraska in the areas of Employment, Housing, and Public Accommodations.

6086 **Nebraska Vocational Rehabilitation Agency**
3901 N 27th St, Ste 6
Lincoln, NE 68521-2529
402-471-3231
800-472-3382
FAX: 402-471-0788
vr_stateoffice@vocrehab.state.ne.us
vocrehab.state.ne.us

Cheryl Ferree, Manager
Rod Armstrong, Vice President of Strategic Part
Mitch Arnolds, President
Amanda Jedlicka, Executive Director
Services for individuals with disabilities who want to become employed. Services are free to those who qualify.

Nevada

6087 **Nevada Equal Rights CommissionDepartment Of Employment,Training & Rehabilitation**
1820 E Sahara Ave
Ste 314
Las Vegas, NV 89104-6512
702-486-7161
800-326-6868
FAX: 702-486-7054
http://detr.state.nv.us/nerc

6088 **Nevada Governor's Committee on Employment of Persons with Disabilities**
Suite#202
896 W. Nye Lane
Carson City, NV 89703-5062
775-684-8619
FAX: 775-684-8626
www.nevadaddcouncil.org

Sherry Manning, Executive Director
Kari Horn, Projects Manager
Diana Peachay, Executive Assistant
Services for individuals with disabilities who want to become employed.

6089 **Vocational and Rehabilitation Agency**
State of Nevada
Ste 502
1933 N. Carson Street
Carson City, NV 89701-3705
775-684-0400
FAX: 775-684-4186
TTY:775-684-0360
mryasmer@nvdetr.org
detr.state.nv.us

Frank Woodbeck, Director
Dennis Perea, Deputy Director
Renee Olson, Administrator for the Employment
William Anderson, Chief Economist for the Research

New Hampshire

6090 **Fit for Work at Exeter Hospital**
5 Alumni Drive
Exeter, NH 03833-2160
603-778-7311
FAX: 603-580-6592
http://www.exeterhospital.com

Kevin Calahan, President
Staffed by a team of allied health professionals, our outpatient rehabilitation program offers functional restoration, work therapy, diagnostic testing and physical therapy.

6091 **New Hampshire Employment Security**
32 S Main St
Concord, NH 03301-4857
603-224-3311
800-852-3400
FAX: 603-228-4010
TTY: 800-735-2964
webmaster@nhes.state.nh.us
www.nh.gov/nhes

George Copadis, Commissioner
Darrell Gates, Deputy Commissioner
Zandy L. Dezonie, Administrative Assistant
Operates a free public employment service and provides assisted and self directed employment and career related services and labor market information for employers and the general public.

6092 New Hampshire Fair Employment Practice Agency
2 Chenell Dr Unit 2
Concord, NH 03301-8501
603-271-2767
FAX: 603-271-6339
humanrights@nhsa.state.nh.us
www.nh.gov/hrc

Joni N. Esperian, Esquire, Executive Director
Roxanne Juliano, Assistant Director
Deborah M Evans, Administrative Secretary
Nancy Rodgers, Secretary
Established for the purpose of eliminating discrimination in employment, public accomodations and the sale or rental of housing or commercial property.

6093 New Hampshire Job Training Program Liaison
26 College Drive
Concord, NH 03301-7317
603-230-3500
FAX: 603-271-2725
info@ccsnh.edu
www.ccsnh.edu/

Dr. Ross Gittell, Chancellor
Ron Rioux, Vice Chancellor
Michael Marr, Director of Financial Operations
Sara Sawyer, Director of Human Resources
Services for individuals with disabilities who want to become employed.

6094 Vocational and Rehabilitation Agency
Department of Education
101 Pleasant Street
Concord, NH 03301-3860
603-271-3494
FAX: 603-271-1953
TTY:603-271-3471
Lori.Temple@doe.nh.gov
www.ed.state.nh.us

Paul K Leather, Manager
Virginia Barry, Commissioner
Trisha Allen, Administrative Assistant
Steven Aylward, Rehabilitation Counselor
Offers services for the totally blind, legally blind, visually impaired, mentally retarded blind and more with health, counseling, educational, recreational, rehabilitation, computer training and professional training services.

New Jersey

6095 ARC of Gloucester County
1555 Gateway Blvd
West Deptford, NJ 08096-1018
856-629-9061
FAX: 856-848-7753
webmaster@thearcgloucester.org
www.thearcgloucester.org

Robert.H Weir, President
Charles Funk, VP
Ethel Lucas, Board Member
Ralph Sundy, Board Member
Non-profit organization serving people with intellectual and related developmental disabilities and their families through education, advocacy and direct services.

6096 ARC of Hunterdon County, The
1465 Route 31 South
Suite 23
Annandale, NJ 08801-3127
908-730-7827
FAX: 908-730-7726
jeff@archunterdon.org
www.archunterdon.org

Jeffrey Mattison, Executive Director
Colleen Dennis, Deputy Executive Director
Gail Stepka, Executive Assistant
Our mission is to support, training and opportunities to individuals with intellectual & developmental disabilities to achieve the greatest degree of independence and productivity to become contributing, responsible, and proud members of society.

6097 ARC of Mercer County
180 Ewingville Road
Ewing, NJ 08638-2425
609-406-0181
FAX: 609-406-9258
arc@arcmercer.org
www.arcmercer.org

Geoffrey Morris, President
Rick Koreyva, 1st Vice President
Ethel Lucas, Board Member
Ralph Sundy, Board Member
Committed to securing for all people with disabilities mental retardation and developmental disabilities the opportunity to choose and realize their goals.

6098 ARC of Monmouth
1158 Wayside Road
Tinton Falls, NJ 7712-3148
732-493-1919
FAX: 732-493-3604
info@arcofmonmouth.org
www.arcofmonmouth.org

Joyce Quarles, President
Roger Trendowski, Immediate Past President
Rachel Weiss, First Vice-President
Bill Mirkin, Treasurer
A non-profit organization providing services and supports for individuals who have cognitive and developmental disabilities and for their families.

6099 Abilities Center of New Jersey
1208 Delsea Drive
Westville, NJ 08093-2227
856-848-1025
FAX: 856-848-8429
info@abilities4work.com
abilities4work.com

Susan Spies Perron, President/CEO
Sharon Kneubuehl, VP
Karen Weitzman, Director of Finance and Adminidt
Bill Urie, Director of Operations
A non-profit organization dedicated to developing employment opportunities for people with disabilities or other disadvantages through education, training and job placement.

6100 Abilities of Northwest New Jersey
264 Rt 31 North
Washington, NJ 07882
908-689-1118
info@abilitiesnw.com
abilities-nw.com

a.B Wildermuth, CEO
Private not-for-profit community rehabilitation program providing vocational training and employment services since 1974 to the disabled and disadvantaged population.

6101 Alliance for Disabled in Action New Jersey
629 Amboy Ave
Edison, NJ 08837-3579
732-738-4388
FAX: 732-738-4416
TTY:732-738-9644
ctonks@adacil.org
www.adacil.org

Carole Tonks, Executive Director
Luke Koppisch, Deputy Director
Salma Harris, Office Manager
Iris Hernandez, Bookkeeper
A private not-for-profit center for independence living. A dynamic membership organization run by people with disabilities for people with disabilities.

6102 Alternatives for Growth: New Jersey
137 W. Hanover St.
Trenton, NJ 08618
609-393-0008
FAX: 609-393-1189
experts@afg-lca.com
www.njfuture.org

Donna Flannery, Contact
Peter Kasabach, Executive Director
Elaine Clisham, Director of Communications and Development
Nicholas Dickerson, Planning and Policy Analyst

Serves all New Jersey.

6103 Arc of Bergen and Passaic Counties
223 Moore Street
Hackensack, NJ 7601-7402   201-343-0322
FAX: 201-343-0401
arc@arcbp.com
arcbergenpassaic.org

Kathy Walsh, President/CEO
Alice Siegel, Senior VP
Olga Podolsky, Director of Family Support Servi
Anne Gallucci, Vocational Services Director
Serving persons with disabilities and their families in Bergen and Passaic Counties, NJ.

6104 Career Opportunity Development of New Jersey
901 Atlantic Avenue
Egg Harbor City, NJ 08215-1810   609-965-6871
FAX: 609-965-3099
njcodi.org

Linda L. Carney, President & CEO
Ellen Loughney, Vice Chairperson
Joe Silipena, Board Chairperson
Joe Cella, Secretary
Serves Bergen and Passaic Counties. Provides services to individuals with varying forms of physical, mental and economic disabilities and disadvantages. Provides services to more than 1,000 unduplicated consumers annually.

6105 Center for Educational Advancement New Jersey
11 Minneakoning Road
Flemington, NJ 08822-5726   908-782-1480
FAX: 908-782-5370
jkunz@ceaemployment.com
ceaemployment.com

Michael Skoczek, President & CEO
John Reardon, Secretary
Michael Collins, Treasurer
Nancy Vargas, Employee Relations
Serves Somerset and Hunterdon Counties. Skills training in office technology and food service. Job placement and job coaching services are available. Employer Network for Ticket to Work.

6106 Cerebral Palsy Association of Middlesex County
10 Oak Drive
Edison, NJ 08837-2313   732-549-6187
800-852-7897
FAX: 732-549-0629
Info@cpamc.org
cpamc.org

Dominic M. Ursino, President
Robert Ferrara, Executive Director
Rob Gross, MBA, Controller
Debra Gilbert, M.S.I.L.R, Director of Human Resources
Dedicated to the provision of comprehensive, superior, multi-faceted programs of service to individuals with developmental and related disabilities

6107 Easter Seal Society of New Jersey Highlands Workshop
Easter Seals
133 Main St
Franklin, NJ 7416-1542   973-827-9066
FAX: 973-827-3828
pskipp@nj.easterseals.com
www.nj.easterseals.com

Peggy Skipp, Manager
Enabling individuals with special needs or disabilities and their families to learn, live, work and play in their communities with equality, dignity and independence.

6108 Easter Seal of Ocean County
25 Kennedy Blvd.
Suite 600
East Brunswick, NJ 08816   732-257-6662
FAX: 732-257-7373
http://nj.easterseals.com

Brian.J Fitzgerald, President/CEO

Helping people and families with disabilities and special needs live, work, and play in their communities with equality, dignity and independence.

6109 Easter Seals New Jersey
25 Kennedy Blvd
Ste 600
E Brunswick, NJ 08816-2035   732-257-6662
FAX: 732-257-7373
TTY:732-545-1317
www.eastersealsnj.org

Brian Fitzgerald, CEO
Cheryl Young, CFO
Helen Drobnis, VP Corporate Affairs
To enable individuals with disabilities or special needs and their families to live, work and play in their communities with equality, dignity, and independence.

6110 Eden Acres Administrative Services
2 Merwick Road
Princeton, NJ 08540-5711   609-987-0099
FAX: 609-734-0069
www.nj.com/mercer/index.ssf/

Peter H. Bell, President & CEO
Jennifer Bizub, Chief Operating Officer
Carol Markowitz, M.A., M.Ed, Chief Program Officer
Melinda Gorny McAleer, Chief Development Officer
Provides services for the disabilitated.

6111 Edison Sheltered Workshop
328 Plainfield Avenue
Edison, NJ 08817-3117   732-985-8834
FAX: 732-985-2216
info@eswnj.org
http://www.eswnj.org

Veronica Valez, Executive Director
Robert.A Ellymer, President
John J. Hogan, First Vice President
Pat Colletto, Treasurer
Serves Middlesex County. Vocational training and job placement services.

6112 First Occupational Center of New Jersey
861 Asbury Avenue
Ocean City, NJ 08226-2809   609-399-6111
800-894-6265
FAX: 973-672-0065
ocnj@idt.net
www.ocnj.org

Rocco Meola, CEO
Tanya M. Edghill, VP Of Program Services
A private, nonprofit multi-service community rehabilitation program. Services are offered to all people, such as developmentally disabled, visually impaired, hearing impaired and welfare recipients. Services include vocational evaluation and training, respite care, basic and remedial education and job placement and community support services.

6113 Goodwill Industries of Southern New Jersey
2835 Route 73
Maple Shade, NJ 08052-1620   856-439-0200
FAX: 856-439-0843
esmith@goodwillnj.org
goodwillnj.org

Mark B Boyd, President and CEO
Michael Shaw, Chief Operating Officer
Stephen Castro, Chief Financial Officer
Deb Eckenhoff, Vice President of Goodwill Home Medical Equipment
A non profit, community-based organization governed by a volunteer bard of trustees.

6114 Hausmann Industries
130 Union Street
Northvale, NJ 7647-2290
201-767-0255
888-428-7626
FAX: 201-767-1369
info@hausmann.com
hausmann.com

David Hausmann, CEO
George Batchelor, Director Sales & Marketing
Michelle Riley, Mail order Sales
Julie Skoda, Sales and Marketing Adminitrator
Wheelchair acessible exam tables, treatment tables and mat platforms.

6115 Jersey Cape Diagnostic Training & Opportunity Center
152 Crest Haven Road
Cape May Court House, NJ 08210-1651
609-465-4117
FAX: 609-465-3899
paulann@capeworkshop.com
www.sjworks.org/

George J Plewa, Executive Director
George Plewa, Executive Director
Serves Cape May County. Employment training services. A vocational rehabilitation center that serves individuals with disabilities, the disabled, and the handicapped or others having barriers to work.

6116 New Jersey Commission for the Blind and Visually Impaired
Department of Human Services
153 Halsey St
6th Floor, PO Box 47017
Newark, NJ 07101- 8004
973-648-3333
877-685-8878
FAX: 973-648-3388
Vito.DeSantis@cbvi.nj.us
www.state.nj.us/humanservices/cbvi/home/index

Vito J Desantis, Executive Director
Bernice Davis, Executive Assistant
Marcus Stabile Esq., Manager Human Resources
Frank Scheik, Fiscal Operations
The Commission for the Blind and Visually Impaired (CBVI) promotes and provides services in the areas of education, employment, independence and eye health for persons who are blind or visually impaired, their families and the community. It seeks to provide or ensure access to services that will enable consumers to obtain their fullest measure of self-reliance and quality of life and fully integrated into their community.

6117 New Jersey Employment Service and Job Training Program Services
Department of Labor
John Fitch Plaza
Trenton, NJ 08625
609-292-1040
wd.dol.state.nj.us/

Roland Machold, Manager
Harold J. Wirths, Commissioner
Aaron R. Fichtner, Ph.D., Deputy Commissioner
Frederick J. Zavaglia, Chief of Staff
Services for individuals with disabilities who want to become employed.

6118 Occupational Center of Hudson County
68-70 Tuers Avenue
Jersey City, NJ 07306
201-434-3303
FAX: 201-434-3660
info@hudsoncommunity.org
http://www.hudsoncommunity.org

Christine Remler, Executive Director
Services for individuals with disabilities who want to become employed.

6119 Occupational Center of Union County
301 Cox St
Roselle, NJ 07203-1797
908-241-7200
FAX: 908-241-2025
ocuc@OCUCNJ.com
www.occupationalcenter.org

Michele Ford, VP
The Occupational Center is the only agency in the State of New Jersey which offers a unique combination of individualized training leading to long term employment for people with disabilities in the competitive job market or in our on-site industrial work center. This comprehensive package helps ensure on-the-job success and a productive, dignified life for those with disabilities.

6120 Occupational Training Center of Burlington County
2 Manhattan Drive
Burlington, NJ 08016-4408
609-267-6677
otcbc.org

Joseph S Bender, CEO
Mission is to assist individuals with disabilities in reaching their maximum potential.

6121 Occuptational Training Center of Camden County, New Jersey
520 Market Street
Suite 306
Camden, NJ 08102-1300
866-226-3362
FAX: 856-767-1378
camcofreeholders@gmail.com
www.camdencounty.com

Matt Treihart, President
Serves Camden County.

6122 Pathways to Independence, Inc.
60 Kingsland Ave
Kearny, NJ 07032-3305
201-997-6155
FAX: 201-997-7070
PTI450@aol.com
www.pathwaysnj.org

Alvin Cox, Executive Director
Tessa Farrell, Program Director
Marie Yakabofski, Financial Director
Lisa M. Johnson, Qualilty Assurance Director
Pre-vocational and vocational programming for people with disabilities. Specializing in Developmental Disabilities, Learning Disabilities and Mental Health issues. Serving over 100 people in Hudson, South Bergen, Passaic and East Essex counties. CARF accredited.

6123 Somerset Training and Employment Program
900 Hamilton Street
Somerset, NJ 08873-3206
732-846-8888
FAX: 732-246-7257
www.somersetcap.org/

Laurie Falka, Executive Director
Courtney Throckmorton, Owner
Services for individuals with disabilities who want to become employed.

6124 St. John of God Community Services Vocational Rehabilitation
1145 Delsea Dr
Westville, NJ 8093-2252
856-848-4700
FAX: 856-848-3965
devctr@stjohnofgod.org
www.stjohnofgod.org

Dr. Jerome Knast, Manager
Serves Gloucester and Camden Counties providing exemplary special education, vocational and habilitative services to residents of southern New Jersey since 1967.

6125 United Cerebral Palsy Associations of New Jersey
Suite 1
1005 Whitehead Road Ext
Ewing, NJ 08638-2424   609-882-4182
     888-322-1918
     FAX: 609-882-4054
     TTY: 609-882-0620
     cpofnj.org

Warren Kelemen, President
Jim Bartolomei, CPA, Vice President
Elizabeth R. Faircloth, Secretary
Michael Yarrow, Treasurer
Dedicated to changing lives and bringing independence to people
with all types of disabilities.

6126 Vocational and Rehabilitation Agency
P.O.Box 398
Trenton, NJ 08625   609-659-3045
     FAX: 609-292-8347
     TTY:609-292-2919
     tjennings@dol.state.nj.us
     http://lwd.dol.state.nj.us

Brian Fitzgibbons, Manager
Frederick J. Zavaglia, Chief of Staff
Harold J. Wirths, Commissioner
Programs and services for people with disabilities.

6127 West Essex Rehab Center
83 Walnut St
C
Montclair, NJ 07042-4088   973-744-7733
     FAX: 973-744-3744
     businessfinder.nj.com

Eugene Sefanelli, Executive Director
Shannon Williams, Contact
Eugene Stefanelli, Executive Director
Services and programs for individuals with disabilities who want
to become employed.

New Mexico

6128 Adelante Development Center
3900 Osuna Rd Ne
Albuquerque, NM 87109   505-341-2000
     FAX: 505-341-2001
     info@GoAdelante.org
     www.goadelante.org

Mike Kivitz, President
Pamela Sullivan, Board Chair
Mike Lowrimore, Borad Treasurer
Richard Cronin, Physician
Serves Albuquerque and Belen.

6129 Goodwill Industries of New Mexico
5000 San Mateo Blvd NE
Albuquerque, NM 87109-2499   505-881-6401
     866-376-0182
     FAX: 505-884-3157
     goodwillnm.org

Mary Best, President/CEO
Michael P. Keoghan, Chief Operating Officer
Roberta Valesquez, Finance Director
Ricky Sanchez, Facilities Logistics Director
Serves Albuquerque, Santa Fe and Rio Rancho.

6130 New Mexico Employment Services and Job Training Liaison
P.O.Box 1928
Albuquerque, NM 87103-1928   505-898-3599
     FAX: 505-827-6812
     djones2@state.nm.us
     http://www.dws.state.nm.us

Reese Suliten, Director
Celina Bussey, Secretary
Provides employment to improve economic progress.

6131 RCI
1111 Menaul Blvd NE
Albuquerque, NM 87107-1614   505-255-5501
     FAX: 505-255-9971
     info@LifeROOTSnm.org
     http://www.liferootsnm.org

Kathleen Cates, President/CEO
Gwendolyn Kiwanuka, Director of Adult Services
Trudy Eberhardt, Director of Finance
David Griffis, Director of Contracts
Serves Bernalillo County. Mission is to improve the abilities, in-
terests, and choices of children and adults with physical, develop-
mental or behavioral challenges toward achieving their highest
levels of self-sufficiency.

6132 Tohatchi Area of Opportunity & Services
100 Manuelita Drive, P.O.Box 49
Tohatchi, NM 87325   505-733-2027
     FAX: 505-733-2161
     patkeptner@yahoo.com
     http://taos-inc.org

Patrick Keptner, CEO
Carol Charles, Administrative Assistant
Judith Woodie, Accounting Clerk
Melinda Golden, Program Manager
Serves McKinley County, San Jose County and the Havanjo Na-
tion.

6133 Vocational Rehabilitation Agency
Ste D
435 Saint Michaels Dr
Santa Fe, NM 87505-7679   505-954-8500
     800-224-7005
     FAX: 505-954-8562
     TTY: 877-954-8583
     dvris@state.nm.us
     www.dvrgetsjobs.com

Gary Beene, Manager
Purpose is to help people with disabilities achieve a suitable employment outcome.

6134 Vocational and Rehabilitation Agency
Bldg 4
2905 Rodeo Park Dr E
Santa Fe, NM 87505-6342   505-827-4479
     888-513-7968
     greg.trapp@state.nm.us
     www.state.nm.us/cftb

Greg Trapp, Executive Director
James Salas, Deputy Director
Adelmo Vigil, Deputy Director-IL/OB
Catherine Cross-Maple, Manager
The Commission for the Blind provides vocational rehabilitation
and independent living services designed to enable persons who
are blind to become more participating and contributing members
of society. Blind people lead normal lives, have families, raise
children, participate in community activities, and work in a wide
range of jobs. They are secretaries, lawyers, teachers, engineers,
machinists, scientists, supervisors and business owners.

New York

6135 JOBS VI and SAGE
P ES CO International
21 Paulding St
Pleasantville, NY 10570-3108   914-769-4266
     800-431-2016
     FAX: 914-769-2970
     pesco@pesco.org
     www.pesco.org

Joseph Kass, President
A computerized matching system matching people to occupations, training, local jobs, local employers and giving job out-
looks for the year 2005. Computerized Sage is online
computerized testing with the ability for system to read all questions, and job descriptions. Manual Sage is a hands on-computer

scored test battery with various adaptation. Braille, large print, bi-lingual and special devices.

6136 Just One Break (JOBS)
6th Floor
570 Seventh Aveune
New York, NY 10018-1653

212-785-7300
FAX: 212-785-4513
TTY:212-785-4515
jobs@justonebreak.com
www.justonebreak.com

Orin Lehman, Founder
John D Kemp, President
Angela Burgess, Board of Director
C.Jeffrey Knittel, Board of Director
A not-for-profit organization that is dedicated to supporting and increasing the employment of people with disabilities.

6137 New York State Department of Labor
Building 12
State Office Campus
Albany, NY 12240

518-457-9000
888-469-7365
TTY:800-662-1220
nysdol@labor.state.ny.us
www.labor.state.ny.us

James J Mcgowan, Commissioner
Fredda Peritz, Employment Service Division Dire
Thomas Malone, Unemployment Insur Div Dir
The missin of the New York State Department of Labor is to help New York work by preparing individuals for the jobs of today and tomorrow. Provides direct job search and counseling services to job seekers, and can refer people who have disabilities for training opportunities. Provides unemployment insurance for those out of work through no fault of their own.

6138 Rational Effectiveness Training Systems
IRET Corporate Services Division
45 E 65th St
New York, NY 10021-6508

212-535-0822
FAX: 212-249-3582
www.yelp.com

Michael Broder, Owner
Offers advanced training for employee assistance professionals, full service outpatient counseling, consulting services and on-site workshops for the disabled.

6139 Special Education and Vocational Rehabilitation Agency: New York
Room 580 EBA
89 Washington Ave.
Albany, NY 12234

518-474-2925
800-222-5627
accesadm@mail.nysed.gov
www.vesid.nysed.gov

Richard Mills, Manager
Mission is to promote educational equity and excellence for students with disabilitites while ensuring that they receive the rights and protection to which they are entitled.

North Carolina

6140 Division Of Workforce Development
NC Department of Commerce
313 Chapanoke Road
Suite 120
Raleigh, NC 27603

919-814-0400
800-562-6333
FAX: 919-662-4770
http://www.nccommerce.com

Sherry Allen, Accountant
Delores Amogida, Program Assistant V
Barbara Barner, Business & Technology Applicatio
Robbin Broome, Training Manager
Offers vocational assessment and training, adult developmental activities.

6141 Iredell Vocational Workshop
200 Clanton Rd
Charlotte, NC 28217-1446

704-944-5100
www.lifespanservices.org

John Cervantes, Secretary
Davan Cloninger, President & CEO
Robert L. Mendenhall, Vice Chairperson
Jeff Hay, Chairperson
Mission of lifespan is to transform the lives of children and adults with developmental disabilities by providing education, employment, and enrichment programs that promote inclusion, choice, family supports, and other best practices.

6142 North Carolina Division of Services for the Blind
Department of Health and Human Services
2601 Mail Service Center
Raleigh, NC 27699-2601

919-733-9822
800-222-1546
FAX: 919-715-8711
TTY: 919-733-9700
VRStatePlan2015@dhhs.nc.gov
www.dhhs.state.nc.us/dsb

Eddie Weaver, Director
Carla Parker, Executive Assistant
Mary Flanagan, Assistant Director
Marvin Gilmore, LAN Administrator
Since 1935, the mission of the North Carolina Division of Services for the Blind has been to enable people who are blind or visually impaired to reach their goals of independence and employment.

6143 Rowan County Vocational Workshop
2728 Old Concord Rd
Salisbury, NC 28146-1338

704-637-9592
FAX: 704-633-6224
salisbury.marketplaceminer.com

Carl Rapsher, Executive Director
Offers vocational assessment and training, adult developmental activities.

6144 Rutherford Vocational Workshop
230 Fairground Rd
Spindale, NC 28160

828-286-4352
FAX: 828-287-3295
rutherfordlifeservices.com

Amanda Freeman, Program Supervisor
Christy Beddinfield, Staff
Larry Brown, Executive Director
John Jarrett, Human Resource Director
Offers vocational assessment and training, adult developmental activities.

6145 Transylvania Vocational Services
11 Mountain Industrial Drive
P.O. Drawer 1115
Brevard, NC 28712-6723

828-884-3195
info@tvsinc.org
tvsinc.org

Nancy Stricker, Executive Director
A private non-profit corporation with the mission to provide skills development, career opportunities and related services in a supportive environment for people with barriers to employment.

6146 Vocational and Rehabilitation Agency
2001 Mail Service Center
Raleigh, NC 27699-2001

919-855-4800
800-689-9090
FAX: 919-733-7968
TTY: 919-733-9700
dvr.WebInfoRequest@dhhs.nc.gov
http://www.ncdhhs.gov

Albert Delia, Acting Secretary
Beth Melcher, PhD, Chief Deputy Secretary for Healt
Maria. F Spaulding, Deputy Secretary for Long-Term C
Steven Cline, DDS, Assistant Secretary for Health I

Mission statement is to promote employment and independence for people with disabilities through customer partnership and community leadership.

6147 Vocational and Rehabilitation Agency: Department of Health and Human Services
2001 Mail Service Center
Raleigh, NC 27699-2001
919-855-4800
800-689-9090
FAX: 919-733-7968
TTY: 919-733-5924
dvr.WebInfoRequest@dhhs.nc.gov
dvr.dhhs.state.nc.us

Albert Delia, Acting Secretary
Beth Melcher, PhD, Chief Deputy Secretary for Healt
Maria. F Spaulding, Deputy Secretary for Long-Term C
Steven Cline, DDS, Assistant Secretary for Health I
Mission statement is to promote employment and independence for people with disabilities through customer partnership and community leadership.

6148 Webster Enterprises Inc.
140 Little Savannah Rd
Sylvia, NC 28779-220
828-586-8981
800-978-2681
FAX: 828-586-8125
grobinson@websterenterprises.org
www.websterenterprises.org

Gene Robinson, Executive Director
Wendy Cagle, Vice-Chair
Bob Cochran, Secretary/Treasurer
Tom Stovall, Chair
A community based employment and training program for people with disabilities. A full service program which includes a youth transitional program for life beyond high school, job coaching, vocational assessment and job placement.

6149 Western Regional Vocational Rehabilitation Facility Clifford File, Jr.
P.O.Box 1443
200 Enola Rd.
Morganton, NC 28655
828-433-2423
dvr.dhhs.state.nc.us

Connie Barnette, Facility Director
Elizabeth Watson, Executive Director
Frances Battle, Director of Training
Karen Romito, Program Assistant
Vocational Evaluation, Work Adjustment, Job Placement, On-site Work Services Program. Serves most disability groups including CMI, DD, Deaf and Physically impaired.

North Dakota

6150 North Dakota Department of Labor, Human Rights Division
Dept 406
600 East Boulevard Avenue
Bismarck, ND 58505- 0340
701-328-2660
800-582-8032
800-366-6888
FAX: 701-328-2031
humanrights@nd.gov
www.nd.gov

Mark Nelson, Manager
Kathy Kulesa, Human Rights Director
Robin Bosch, Business Manager
Peg Haug, Compliance Investigator
Through a work-sharing agreement with the Equal Employment Opportunity Commission (EEOC), the North Dakota Department of Labor's Human Rights Division enforces the Americans with Disabilities Act (ADA) as related to employment discrimination.

6151 North Dakota Employment Service and Job Training Program Liaison
Job Service North Dakota
1601 E. Century Avenue
PO Box 5507
Bismarck, ND 58506- 5507
701-328-2825
FAX: 701-328-4000
TTY:800-366-6888
www.jobsnd.com/

Leslie Weiss, Manager
Offers vocational assessment and training, adult developmental activities.

6152 North Dakota Vocational Rehabilitation Agency
Suite 1b
Prairie Hills Plaza 1237 W D
Bismarck, ND 58501-1208
701-328-8950
800-756-2745
FAX: 701-328-8969
dhsvr@nd.gov
www.nd.gov/dhs/dvr/

Russ Cusack, State Director
Cheryl Wescott, Chief of Field Services
Harley Engelman, Business Relations/Marketing Dir
Robin Throlson, Planning and Evaluation Administ
Offers services for the totally blind, legally blind, visually impaired, mentally retarded blind and more with health, counseling, educational, recreational, rehabilitation, computer training and professional training services.

Ohio

6153 Cornucopia
18120 Sloane Ave
Lakewood, OH 44107-3108
216-521-4600
FAX: 216-521-9460
Ronda.mohammad@cornucopia-inc.org
www.cornucopia-inc.org

Wm. Scott Duennes, Executive Director
Anthony Rospert, President
Judy DeFrancesco, 1st Vice President
David Westerfield, Treasurer
Provides work adjustment training for people with and developmental disabilities in a unique community based setting; Nature's Bin, a natural fresh foods market. Consumers learn through participation in retail operations in produce, grocery, bakery, deli, maintenance and customer service areas. Retail revenues help offset the cost of the program. Job search skills training and placement assistance available to program graduates.

6154 Great Oaks Joint Vocational School
3254 E Kemper Rd
Cincinnati, OH 45241-1581
513-771-8881
800-441-6257
FAX: 513-771-4932
http://www.greatoaks.com/

Harold Carr, Medical Director
Deb Graw, Manager
Jim Perdue, Chair
Sue Steele, Vice Chair
Offers vocational assessment and training, adult developmental activities.

6155 Hearth Day Treatment and Vocational Services
8301 Detroit Ave
Cleveland, OH 44102-1805
216-281-2660

Don Cook, Manager
Hearth offers time-limited, paid work adjustment experiences to consumers with mental illness. The goal of Hearth Programs is to prepare the consumer for success in the competitive workforce.

6156   Highland Unlimited Business Enterprises of CRI
1501 Madison Road
Cincinnati, OH 45206-2223   513-354-5200
                                         FAX: 513-354-7115
                                         ddutton@cricincy.com
                                         gcbhs.com

Tony Datillo, CEO
Debbie Dutton Lambert, Director Employment Programs
Tony Carter, Chairman of GCB Board
Adrienne Russ, Secretary
Offers vocational assessment and training, adult developmental
activities.

6157   Ohio Civil Rights Commission
Rhodes State Office Tower
30 East Broad Street, 5th Floor
Columbus, OH 43215-3414   614-466-5928
                                         TTY:614-753-2391
                                         http://crc.ohio.gov

Leonard Hubert, Chairman
Eddie Harrell, Jr, Commissioner
Rashmi Yajnik, Commissioner
Stephanie Mercado, Commissioner
Primary function is to enforce state laws against discrimination.

6158   Ohio Commission On Minority Health
77 S High Street
18th Floor
Columbus, OH 43215-6108   614-466-4000
                                         FAX: 614-752-9049
                                         minhealth@mih.ohio.gov
                                         www.mih.ohio.gov

Angela C Dawson, Executive Director
Sheronda Whitner, Executive Assistant
Reina M. Sims, MSA, Program Manager
Venita O'Bannon, Fiscal Specialist
Offers vocational assessment and training, adult developmental
activities.

6159   Vocational and Rehabilitation Agency
400 East Campus View Boulevard
Columbus, OH 43235-4604   614-438-1210
                                              800-282-4536
                                         FAX: 614-438-1257
                                         TTY: 614-438-1334
                                         john.connellyu@rsc.state.oh.us
                                         www.state.oh.us

John M Connelly, Administrator
Rose Reed, Manager
State agency that provides vocational rehabilitation services to
help people with disabilities become employed and independent.

Oklahoma

6160   Oklahoma Department of Rehabilitation Services
Ste 500
3535 NW 58th St
Oklahoma City, OK 73112-4824   405-424-4932
                                              800-845-8476
                                         FAX: 405-951-3529
                                         jharlan@okdrs.gov
                                         www.okrehab.org

Michael O'Brien, Director
Jody Harlan, Public Information Administrator
The Oklahoma Department of Rehabilitation Services (DRS)
provides assistance to Oklahomans with disabilities through vocational rehabilitation, employment, independent living, residential and outreach programs, and the determination of medical
eligibility for disability benefits.

**6161   Oklahoma Employment Services and Job Training Program
Liaison**
2401 North Lincoln Boulevard
Oklahoma City, OK 73105-4409   405-557-7100
                                         FAX: 405-557-5368
                                         TTY:800-722-0353
                                         http://www.ok.gov

Richard McPherson, Executive Director
Teresa Keller, Deputy Director
Mike Evans, Chief Information Technology Officer
*Lisa Graven, Reemployment Services/Customer Service Division
Director*
As the primary agency dedicated to disability services in
Oklahoma, we offer a wide range of programs for many individu-
als each year.

**6162   Oklahoma Governor's Committee on Employment of People
with Disabilities**
Ste 90
2401 NW 23rd
Oklahoma City, OK 73107-2423   405-521-3756
                                              800-522-8224
                                         FAX: 405-522-6695
                                         www.odc.ok.gov

Steve Stokes, Executive Director
Doug MacMillan, Director
William Ginn, Disability Program Specialist
Dalene Barton, Office Manager
Mission is to promote the employment of people with disabilities.
The vision of the committee is to facilitate partnerships with com-
mitment to full, high quality employment of people with
disabilities.

Oregon

6163   Bend Work Activity Center
P.O. Box 430 835 E Hwy 126
Redmond, OR 97756   541-548-2611
                                         FAX: 541-548-9573
                                         info@ofco.org
                                         www.ofco.org

James Booth, Chairperson
Bill Schertzinger, Vice Chairperson
Cam Chambers, Manager
Seth Johnson, Executive Director
Offers vocational assessment and training, adult developmental
activities and programs.

6164   Oregon Fair Employment Practice Agency
Oregon Bureau of Labor & Industry
Suite 1045
800 NE Oregon St
Portland, OR 97232-2180   971-673-0761
                                         FAX: 971-673-0762
                                         mailb@boli.state.or.us
                                         www.boli.state.or.us/civil

6165   State of Oregon Office of Vocational Rehabilitation Service
Ste 500
3165 10th St
Baker City, OR 97814-1480   541-524-1800
                                              800-578-9990
                                         FAX: 541-523-5667
                                         wendy.m.wall@state.or.us
                                         www.oregon.gov/dhs/vr

Wendy Wall, Voc Rehab Counselor
Allan McCandless, Voc Rehab Counselor
Offers vocational assessments and training, adult developmental
activities, and helps remove disability related barriers to
employment.

6166 Vocational and Rehabilitation Agency
500 Summer St NE E-87
Salem, OR 97301-1063
503-945-5880
877-277-0513
FAX: 503-947-5010
vr.info@state.or.us
www.oregon.gov/dhs/vr/index.shtml

Stephanie Taylor, Administrator
Offers vocational assessments and training, adult developmental activities and programs.

6167 Vocational and Rehabilitation Agency: Oregon Commission for the Blind
535 SE 12th Avenue
Portland, OR 97214-2408
971-673-1588
888-202-5463
FAX: 503-234-7468
TTY: 971-673-1577
ocb.mail@state.or.us
www.oregon.gov/Blind

Linda Mock, Administrator
Frank Armstrong, Representative
Pat MacDonell, Director
Jodi.C Roth, Chair
A resource for visually impaired Oregonians, as well as their families, friends, and employers. Nationally recognized programs and staff that make a difference in people's lives every day.

Pennsylvania

6168 ACLD/An Association for Children and Adults with Learning Disabilities: Greater Pittsburgh
4900 Girard Rd
Pittsburgh, PA 15227-1440
412-881-2253
info@acldonline.org
acldonline.org

Thomas Fogarty, Administrator
Kathleen Donahoe, Director ACLD Tillotson School
Jackie Lulich, Director Business Services
Dedicated to helping children, adolescents, and adults with Specific Learning Disabilities and related disorders succeed in school, employment and life.

6169 Office of Vocational Rehabilitation
7th and Forester St
Harrisburg, PA 17120-1
717-787-4746
FAX: 717-783-5221
www.dli.state.pa.us

Barry Brandt, Rehabilitation Specialist
Information in vocational counseling and the governor's committee on Employment of People with Disabilities. Also serves persons with disabilities that present a substantial handicap to employment and independence. Services are provided when there is a reasonable expectation that employment is possible as a result of those services.

6170 Pennsylvania Employment Services and Job Training
P A Department of Labor and Industry
Room 1700
7th and Forster St
Harrisburg, PA 17120-1
717-787-2500
FAX: 717-772-8284
www.dli.state.pa.us

Edward G Rendell, Manager
Stephen Schmerin, Manager
Administers benefits to unemployed individuals, oversees the administration of worker's compensation benefits to individuals with job related injuries, and provides vocational rehabilitation to individuals with disabilities.

6171 Pennsylvania Governor's Committee on Employment of Disabled Persons
121 N Sixth Street
Harrisburg, PA 17120-1
717-772-6382
FAX: 717-783-5221
www.dli.state.pa.us/landi/cwp

6172 Pennsylvania Human Relations Commission Agency
8th Floor
333 Market St.
Harrisburg, PA 17101-2210
717-787-4410
FAX: 717-772-4340
TTY: 717-787-7279
phrc@pa.gov
phrc.state.pa.us

JoAnn. L Edwards, Executive Director
Gerald.S Robinson, Chairman
Tom Corbett, Governor
Dr. Raquel O Yiengst, Vice Chairperson
Mission is to administer and enforce the PHRAct and the PFEOA of the Commonwealth of Pennsylvania for the identification and elimination of discrimination and the providing of equal opportunity for all persons.

6173 US Healthworks
25124 Springfield Court
Suite 200
Valencia, CA 91355- 3333
661-678-2600
800-720-2432
FAX: 610-926-6225
www.ushealthworks.com

Beverly Shaeff, Manager
Stephanie Makovsky, Sales Consultant
Daniel D. Crowley, President & Chief Executive Officer
Joseph T. Mallas, Chief Operating Officer
Offers employers comprehensive occupational health services and state-of-the-art physical and occupational therapy. Staff works as a team to produce the best possible patient care while delivering cost savings through workers compensation disability management programs.

6174 Vocational and Rehabilitation Agency
1521 North Sixth Street
Harrisburg, PA 17102-1100
717-787-5244
800-442-6351
FAX: 717-783-5221
TTY: 717-787-4885
ovr@dli.state.pa.us
dli.state.pa.us

William Gannon, Manager
Thomas Washic, Manager
Mission is to assist with disabilities, to secure and maintain employment and independence.

6175 Vocational and Rehabilitation Agency: Department of Labor and Industry
909 Green St
Harrisburg, PA 17102-2913
717-236-6211
800-622-2842
FAX: 717-236-3390
TTY: 717-787-6176
cboone@state.pa.us

Thomas Carlock, CEO
Mission is to assist people with disabilities, to serve and maintain employment and independence.

Rhode Island

6176 Goodwill Industries of RI
100 Houghton Street
Providence, RI 02904-1013
401-861-2080
FAX: 401-454-0889
TTY: 401-331-2830
www.goodwillri.org

Jeffrey D. Machado, President/CEO
Justine Beatini, Transitional Resource Specialist
Shirl Berger, Employee Development & Program
Daniel Burgess, Finance Director
The mission of Goodwill Industries of Rhode Island is to provide training, education and other services which result in employment and expanded opportunities for people with disabilities and other barriers to employment in order to enhance their capacity for independent living, increased quality of life and work.

6177 Groden Center
86 Mount Hope Avenue
Providence, RI 02906-1648   401-274-6310
grodencenter.org

Helen Morcos, Chief Executive Officer
Jane I Carlson, Ph.D., BCBA, Vice President Day & Residential
Programs
Cooper Woodard, Ph.D., Vice President Clinical Services
Peggy H. Stocker, Admissions Coordinator
The Groden Center is a school and residential treatment center in
Rhode Island enhancing the lives of children and youth with au-
tism, behavioral disorders, and developmental disabilities by
providing early autism intervention services, an early childhood
education program as well as providing functional and social de-
velopment instruction to school-age children with learning
disabilities.

6178 Newport County Chapter of Retarded Citizens
P.O.Box 4390
906 Aquidneck Avenue
Middletown, RI 02842   401-846-0340
FAX: 401-847-9459
danam@mahercenter.org
mahercenter.org

John Maher, Executive Director
Daniel J Oakley, VP
Barbara Burns, Secretary
Walter Jachna, Chairman
Vocational training and job placement services.

6179 Office of Rehabilitation Services
40 Fountain Street
Providence, RI 02903-1898   401-421-7005
FAX: 401-222-3574
TTY:401-421-7016
garyw@ors.ri.gov
ors.ri.gov

Ron Racine, Deputy Administrator
Steve Brunero, Acting Deputy Administrator-ORS
John Microulis, Deputy Administrator-Disability
Walter Jachna, Chairman Board of Directors
Their goal is to help individuals with physical and mental disabil-
ities prepare for and obtain appropriate employment.

**6180 Vocational and Rehabilitation Agency: Department of
Human Services**
RI Services for the Blind and Visually Impaired
40 Fountain St
Providence, RI 02903-1830   401-421-7005
FAX: 401-222-3574
TTY:401-421-7016
garyw@ors.ri.gov
ors.ri.gov

Ron Racine, Deputy Administrator
Steve Brunero, Acting Deputy Administrator-ORS
John Microulis, Deputy Administrator-Disability
Walter Jachna, Chairman Board of Directors
Their goal is to help individuals with physical and mental disabil-
ities prepare for and obtain appropriate employment.

South Carolina

**6181 South Carolina Employment Security Commission South
Carolina Center**
P.O.Box 567
Columbia, SC 29201   803-777-2400
800-436-8190
jobs@sces.org
www.sces.org

Camille Fallow, Disability Program Navigator
Regina Ratterros, Program Coordinator/State Office
Public agency taht offers job search assistance. Unemployment
Benefits and WIA program. Also offered is Disability Program
Navigator who helps persons with disabilities to find needed
resources

**6182 South Carolina Governor's Committee on Employment of
the Handicapped**
1410 Boston Avenue
P.O.Box 15
West Columbia, SC 29171-15   803-896-6500
800-832-7526
FAX: 803-896-1224
TTY: 806-896-6553
http://www.scvrd.net/

Barbara G. Hollis, Executive Director
Derle A. Lowder Sr., Agency Board Chairman
Dr. Roxzanne Breland, Vice Chair
Joseph A. Thomas, Vice Chair
Goal is to help individuals with physical and mental disabilities
prepare for and obtain appropriate employment.

6183 South Carolina Vocational Rehabilitation Department
P.O.Box 15
1410 Boston Avenue
West Columbia, SC 29171-15   803-896-6500
800-832-7526
TTY:806-896-6553
info@scvrd.state.sc.us
www.scvrd.net

Larry C Bryant, Commissioner
Barbara G Hollis, Executive Director
Dr. Roxzanne Breland, Vice Chair
Derle A Lowder Sr., Agency Board Chairman
The SCVRD's mission is to enable eligible South Carolinians
with disabilities to prepare for, achieve and maintain competitive
employment.

**6184 Vocational and Rehabilitation Agency: Commission for the
Blind**
Vocational and Rehabilitation Agency
P.O.Box 79
1430 Confederate Avenue
Columbia, SC 29201-79   803-898-8764
800-922-2222
FAX: 803- 89- 879
publicinfo@sccb.sc.gov
http://www.sccb.state.sc.us/

Zertie Johnson, Manager
James Kirby, Commissioner
Don Bradley, Director Consumer Affairs
Rhonda Thompson, Director, Prevention & Older Blind
Goal is to help individuals with physical and mental disabilities
prepare for and obtain appropriate employment.

South Dakota

**6185 South Dakota Governor's Advisory Committeeon
Employment of the Disabled**
700 Governors Drive
Pierre, SD 57501-2291   605-773-3101
FAX: 605-773-6184
http://dlr.sd.gov

Patrick Keating, Manager
Marcia Hultman, Secretary of Labor and Regulation
Lyle Harter, Director of Administrative Services
Bret Afdahl, Director of the Division of Banking
Goal is to help individuals with physical and mental disabilities
prepare for and obtain appropriate employment.

6186 South Dakota State Vocational Rehabilitation
Department of Human Services
3800 E Highway 34 Hillview Plz
Pierre, SD 57501   605-773-3195
FAX: 605-773-5483
eric.weiss@state.sd.us
www.state.sd.us

Jeff Pierce, Manager
Bernie Grimme, Assistant Director, DRS
Eric Weiss, Director
South Dakota State Vocational Rehabilitation consists of two
agencies; Rehab Services and service to the Blind and Visually

Impaired. There mission is the same to provide individualized rehabilitation services that result in optimal employment and independent living outcomes for individuals with disabilities.

6187 South Dakota Workforce Investment Act Training Programs
700 Governors Dr
Pierre, SD 57501-2291

605-773-3101
800-952-3216
FAX: 605-773-6184
www.sdjobs.org

Michael Ryan, Administrator
Patrick Keating, Manager
Marcia Hultman, Secretary of Labor and Regulation
Lyle Harter, Director of Administrative Services
Mission is to enhance the South Dakota workforce by providing business with employment-related solutions and helping people with job placement and career transition services

6188 Vocational and Rehabilitation Agency: Division of Services to the Blind/Visually Impaired
3800 E Highway 34 Hillview Plz
Pierre, SD 57501

605-773-3195
FAX: 605-773-5483
gaye.mattke@state.sd.us
www.state.sd.us

Dawn Backer, Manager, Rehabilitation Center for the Blind
Eric Weiss, Director
Gaye Mattke, Division Director, Service to the Blind and Visually Impaire
Nancy Hoyme, Program Specialist
To provide individualized rehabilitation services that result in optimal employment and independent living outcomes for people with disabilities.

Tennessee

6189 Division of Rehabilitative Services
Tennessee Department Human Services
400 Deaderick Street
15th Floor
Nashville, TN 37243-1403

615-313-4700
FAX: 615-741-4165
mandy.johnson@tn.gov
www.state.tn.us/humanserv/rehabilitation.htm

Raquel Hatter, Commisioner

6190 Tennessee Department of Labor: Job Training Program Liaison
220 French Landing Drive
Nashville, TN 37243-1712

615-741-6642
FAX: 615-741-5078
www.tn.gov

Ruth S Letson, Manager
Burns Phillips, Commissioner
Dustin Swayne, Deputy Commissioner
Stephanie Mitchell, Mitchell
Goal is to help individuals with physical and mental disabilities prepare for and obtain appropriate employment.

6191 Tennessee Fair Employment Practice Agency
Human Rights Commission
23rd floor
312 Rosa L Parks Ave
Nashville, TN 37243-1

615-741-5825
800-251-3589
FAX: 615-253-1886
www.state.tn.us/humanrights

Tricia Crawford, Manager
Beverly L. Watts, Executive Director
Sabrina Hooper, Deputy Director
Shalini Rose, General Counsel
An independent state agency charged with preventing and eradicating discrimination in employment, public accomodations, and housing.

Texas

6192 C-CAD Center of United Cerebral Palsy of Metropolitan Dallas
8802 Harry Hines Blvd.
Dallas, TX 75235

800-999-1898
info@ucpdallas.org
www.ucpdallas.org

Mark Denzin, President/Chief Operating Officer
Frank Pickens, CPA, Chief Financial Officer
April Allen, Chief Program Officer
Shea Needham, Regional Director
Offers a wide range of technology opportunities for persons with all types of disabilities, their families and the professionals who serve them. Services include assements, traiing, technology access showroom, and workshops for rehabilitation and educational personnel.

6193 Handbook of Career Planning for Students with Special Needs
Pro- Ed Publications
8700 Shoal Creek Boulevard
Austin, TX 78757-6897

512-451-3246
800-897-3202
FAX: 512-451-8542
general@proedinc.com
www.proedinc.com

Donald D Hammill, Owner
Courtney King, Marketing Coordinator
Thomas F. Harrington, Editor
The practitioner's guide will show you how to help special needs adolescents and young adults overcome barriers to employment by identifying goals and problems, assessing interests and aptitudes, involving client families and developing communication skills. *$42.00*
358 pages

6194 Texas Employment Services and Job Training Program Liaison
Texas Workforce Commission
101 E 15th St
Rm 665
Austin, TX 78778-0001

512-463-2236
866-938-4444
TTY:700-735-2989
ombudsman@twc.state.tx.us
http://www.twc.state.tx.us

Larry Temple, Executive Director
Lasha Lenzy, Division Director
Reagan Miller, Division Director
Tom McCarty, Division Director
State government agency charged with overseeing and providing workforce development services to employers and job seekers of Texas. Offers career development information, job search resources, training programs, and, as appropriate, unemployment benefits.

6195 Vocational and Rehabilitation Agency: State Rehabilitation Commission
Vocational and Rehabilitation Agency
4800 N Lamar Blvd
Austin, TX 78756-3106

512-383-7000
800-628-5115
FAX: 512-424-4730
TTY: 800-628-5115
DARS.Inquiries@dars.state.tx.us
www.dars.state.tx.us

Marilyn Hancock, Executive Director
Michelle Crain, Executive Director
Veronda L. Durden, Commissioner
Glenn Neal, Deputy Commissioner
Helps people with disabilities prepare for, find and keep jobs. Work related services are individualized and may include counseling, training, medical treatment, assistive devices, jon placement assistance and other services.

Utah

6196 **Utah Employment Services**
P.O. Box 45249
2292 South Redwood Road
West Valley, UT 84119-0249 801-978-0378
FAX: 801-978-0374
info@utahemploy.com
www.utahemploy.com

Kristen Cox, Executive Director
To help individuals prepare and obtain appropriate employment.

6197 **Utah Governor's Committee on Employment of the Handicapped**
195 North 1950 West
Salt Lake City, UT 84116-5238 801-538-4200
800-837-6811
FAX: 801-538-4279
dspd@utah.gov
dspd.utah.gov

George Kelner, Executive Director
Promotes opportunities and provide support for persons with disabilities to lead self-determined lives.

6198 **Utah Veterans Centers**
Ste 105
200 South Central Campus Drive
Salt Lake City, UT 84112-1686 801-587-7722
800-246-1197
FAX: 801-377-0227
www.military.com/benefits/veteran-benefits

Dennis Stevens, Executive Director
Brent Price, Manager
Roger Perkins, Director of Veterans Support
Sylvia O'Hara, Executive Assistant
Readjustment counseling services to veterans.

6199 **Utah Vocational Rehabilitation Agency**
Utah State Office of Rehabilitation
P.O. Box 144200
1501 M Street, NW Seventh Floor
Washington, DC 20005-4200 202-466-6550
800-473-7530
FAX: 202-785-1756
duchida@utah.gov
www.ppsv.com/

Donald Uchida, Executive Director
Heidi Kubbe, Executive Assistant
Jennifer Smart, Training Coordinator
Coy Jackson, Program Specialist
Vocational Rehabilitation Services for individuals with disabilities. To assist individuals with disabilities to prepare for and obtain employment and increase their independence.

6200 **Vocational and Rehabilitation Agency: Division of Services for the Blind/Visually Imp.**
1st Floor
160 E 300 S
Salt Lake City, UT 84111-7902 801-530-4849
877-526-3994
FAX: 801-530-6438
wgibson@utah.gov
utah.gov

Willam G Gibson, Executive Director
Cheryl Ritchie, Administrative Secretary
LuWana Martin, Network Specialist
Sharon Pipkin, Office Specialist
Mission is to assist individuals who are blind or visually impaired to obtain employment or increase their independence.

Vermont

6201 **State of Vermont Department of Disabilities, Aging and Independent Living**
Agency of Human Services
103 South Main Street
Weeks IC
Waterbury, VT 05671-2304 802-241-2210
888-405-5005
FAX: 802-241-2128
Info@ahs.state.vt.us
www.ahs.state.vt.us/dbvi

Fred Jones, Director
Stacy Rollins, Executive Administrative Assistant
Carl Augusto, President and CEO
Rick Bozeman, Chief Financial Officer
Mission is to support the efforts of Vermonters who ar blind and visually impaired to achieve or sustain their economic independence, self reliance, and social integration to a level consistent with thier interests, abilities and informed choices.

6202 **Vermont Employment Services and Job Training**
5 Green Mountain Drive P.O.Box 488
Montpelier, VT 05601- 488 802-828-4000
FAX: 802-828-4022
TTY:802-828-4203
tdouse@labor.state.vt.us
www.labor.vermont.gov

Annie Noonan, Commissioner
Deborah Bruce, Human Resource Administrator
Richard Gray, State Director
Tracy Phillips, Director, Unemployment Insurance & Wages
The primary focus is to help support the efforts to make Vermont a more competitive place to do business and create good jobs.

6203 **Vermont Governor's Committee on Employment of People with Disabilities**
103 South Main Steet
Weeks 1A
Waterbury, VT 05671-2303 802-241-6757
866-879-6757
FAX: 802-241-3359
melita@gcepd.org.
www.vocrehabvermont.org

Diane Dalmasse, Manager
Melita DeBeliss, Staff
Committed to facilitating successful, long-term relationships between employers and people with disabilities in Vermont.

Virginia

6204 **Alexandria Community Y Head Start**
418 S Washington St
Alexandria, VA 22314-3673 703-549-0111
FAX: 703-549-2097
www.campagnacenter.org/

Tammy.L Mann, Ph.D, President and CEO
Raj Kapur, Chief Financial Officer
Karla Kelley, Senior Director of Out-of-School
Chrystal Starr Brown, Senior Director, Early Childhood
Offers social services, on-the-job-training for parents, play therapy, physical therapy, speech therapy and any other specialized services.

6205 **Department Of Rehabilitative Services**
8004 Franklin Farms Drive
Henrico, VA 23229-5019 804-662-7000
FAX: 804-662-9532
dars@dars.virginia.gov
vadrs.org

Jay Windsor, Contact Pers
Jim Rothrock, Commissioner
Helps people with disabilities get ready for, find, and keep a job.

6206 Didlake
8641 Breeden Ave
Manassas, VA 20110-8431
703-361-4195
866-361-4195
FAX: 703-369-7141
www.didlake.com

Rex Parr, CEO
John S Craig, VP Rehabilitation Services
Tammara L. Hoover, Treasurer
Patty Tracy, Secretary
Offers situational assessments, work training, employment and job placement services to people with disabilities.

6207 Learning Services: Shenandoah
204 Howe Hall
1460 University Drive
Winchester, VA 22601-5829
540-665-4928
FAX: 540-665-3470
www.su.edu/academic

Peter Patrick, Administrator
Michelle Shenk, Director of Learning Resources and Services
Jeremai Santiago, M.S., Assistant Director & Learning Enrichment Coach
Erin Beaupre, Learning Services Specialist
Postacute rehabilitation program.

6208 NISH
8401 Old Courthouse Road
Vienna, VA 22182-3820
571-226-4660
FAX: 703-849-8916
nish.org

E. Robert Chamberlin, President and CEO
Dennis.A Fields, Chief Operating Officer
Elizabeth W. Goodman, Chief Financial Officer
Paul W. Plattner, Vice President of Operations
A nonprofit agency desigated by the Committee for Purchase from People Who Are Blind or Severely Disabled to provide technical assistance to rehabilitation programs interested in obtaining federal contracts under Public Law 92-28, the Javits-Wagner-O'Day Act. NISH's primary objective is to assist community rehabilitation programs in providing jobs for people with severe disabilities.

6209 Richmond Research Training Center
P.O.Box 842011
1314 West Main Street
Richmond, VA 23284-2011
804-828-1851
FAX: 804-828-2193
TTY:804-828-2494
RRTC@vcu.edu
http://www.worksupport.com

Paul Wehman Ph.D., Professor and Director
Dolores Taylor, Executive Director
John Kregel, Ed.D, Associate Director
Vicki Brooke, M. Ed., Director of Training and Knowledge Translation
Research and training center report on the supported employment of persons with developmental and other disabilities.

6210 ServiceSource
Suite 175
6295 Edsall Rd
Alexandria, VA 22312-2670
703-461-6000
800-244-0817
FAX: 703-461-3906
www.ourpeoplework.org

Janet Samuelson, President & CEO
Edie Castner, Assistant Director
Mark Hall, Executive Vice President, Corporate Development
David Hodge, Executive Vice President & Chief Financial Officer
Provides training, job placement and employment services in private sector and government contract employment.

6211 Sheltered Occupational Center of Virginia
750 23rd St
Arlington, VA 22202-2452
703-521-4441
FAX: 703-521-3443
socent.org

Perla Ni, CEO
Hayley Gefell, Chief Business Development Offic
Marshall Henson, Chief Operating Officer
Donnell Karimah, Chief Administrative Officer
Assists, empowers and supports people with disabilities to achieve employment, independence and integration in the workplace and community. Our services include: printing, copying, hand work, mail shop, fulfillment and distribution.

6212 Vocational and Rehabilitation Agency: Department for the Blind/Visually Impaired
397 Azalea Avenue
Richmond, VA 23227-3623
804-371-3140
800-622-2155
FAX: 804-371-3154
Kimberley.Jennings@dbvi.virginia.gov
www.vdbvi.org

Raymond E. Hopkins, Commissioner
James A Taylor, Chief Deputy
Kimberley Jennings, Contact Person
Dr. Rick L. Mitchell, Deputy Commissioner, Services Delivery
DBVI envisions a world in which blind, vision impaired and deafblind people can access all that society has to offer and can, in turn, contribute to the greater community. We believe this is achievable.

Washington

6213 Career Connections
P.O.Box 141806
431 East Colfax Ave.
South Bend, IN 46617-1806
574-232-5400
866-404-5867
FAX: 574-245-5822
carconn@mindspring.com
www.peoplelinking.com

Susan Warwick, Executive Director
Teresa Antosyn, Program Coordinator
Dan Moody, CFO
Sadie Takila, Production Manager
Offers structured work sites at several locations. Production work at various skill levels, with training as needed.

6214 Department of Services for the Blind National Business & Disability Council
Department of Services for the Blind
P.O.Box 40933
4565 7th Avenue SE
Olympia, WA 98504-933
360-725-3830
FAX: 360-407-0679
info@dsb.wa.gov
www.dsb.wa.gov

Louana Durand, Executive Director
A state rehabilitation agency that offers assistance to persons who are blind or visually impaired. Also provides various services for employers interested in accomodating or hiring workers with vision loss.

6215 Division of Developmental Disabilities: Department of Social & Health Services
P.O.Box 45310
Olympia, WA 98504-5310
360-725-3413
800-737-0617
FAX: 360-407-0955
dddcoreception@dshs.wa.gov
www1.dshs.wa.gov/ddd/index.shtml

Robin Arnold-Williams, Secretary
Colleen Cawston, Senior Director
Steve Lowe, Senior Director
Tracy Guerin, Chief of Staff

The Division of Developmental Disabilities offers persons with developmental disabilities quality supports and services that are individual/family driven, stable and flexible, satisfying to the person and their family, and able to meet individual needs.

6216 SL Start and Associates
901 N Monroe St.
Suite 200
Spokane, WA 99201-4800
509-328-2740
888-355-7155
FAX: 509-326-9207
info@slstart.com
slstart.com

Stephen L Start, Owner
A diversified and innovative human and health services company focused on a wide range of social, employment and long-term services.

6217 School of Piano Technology for the Blind
2510 E Evergreen Blvd
Vancouver, WA 98661-4323
360-693-1511
FAX: 360-693-6891
info@pianotuningschool.org
pianotuningschool.org

Len Leger, Executive Director
Jeff Lane, Executive Director
Donald L. Mitchell, Director of Instructional Operat
Les Fitzpatrick, Technician/Instructor
Teaches piano tuning and repair to blind and visually impaired menand women, leading to employment and/or self-employment in the piano service industry. Licensed by Washington State and accredited by the Accrediting Commission of Career Schools and Colleges of Technology (ACCSCT). 20-month course.

6218 Vocational and Rehabilitation Agency: Division of Vocational Rehabilitation
Department of Social and Health
P.O.Box 45340
Olympia, WA 98504-5340
360-704-3560
800-637-5627
FAX: 360-570-6941
TTY: 360-438-8000
krulik@dshs.wa.gov
www1.dshs.wa.gov/dvr

Patrick Raines, Manager
Andres , Director
Mission is to empower individuals with disabilities to achieve a greater quality of life by obtaining and maintaining employment.

West Virginia

6219 West Virginia Division of Rehabilitation Services
P.O.Box 50890
107 Capitol Street
Charleston, WV 25301- 2609
304-356-2060
800-642-8207
FAX: 304-766-4905
TTY: 304-766-4809
www.wvdrs.org

Deborah Lovely, Director
Donna Ashworth, Assistant Director
DRS specializes in helping people with disabilities who want to find a job or maintain current employment. Rehabilitation counselors at more than 30 field offices help with applications. Once eligibility is determined, counselors & clients work as a team to develop a plan to meet the individuals employment goal. Services may include work-related counseling/guidance, evaluation/assessment, job development & placement assistance, vocational training, college assistance & assistive technology.

6220 West Virginia Employment Services and Job Training Programs Liaison
112 California Ave
Charleston, WV 25305-12
304-558-2660
FAX: 304-558-1343
workforcelmi@wv.gov
http://workforcewv.org

Valerie Comer, Director
Allan Galloway, Manager
Workforce West Virginia, a division of the Department of Commerce, effectively coordinates all avaiilable state and federal resources by orchestrating the efforts of state agencies and local organizations.

6221 West Virginia Vocational Rehabilitation
P.O.Box 1004
107 Capitol Street
Charleston, WV 25301- 2609
304-356-2060
800-642-8207
www.wvdrs.org

Earl Wolfe, Director
Offers services for the totally blind, legally blind, visually impaired, mentally retarded blind and more with health, counseling, educational, recreational, rehabilitation, computer training and professional training services.

Wisconsin

6222 Vocational and Rehabilitation: State of Wisconsin
201 E Washington Ave
Madison, WI 53702-1
608-266-0050
800-442-3477
FAX: 608-266-3131
TTY: 888-877-5939
dvr@dwd.wisconsin.gov
www.dwd.state.wi.us/dvr

Tamara Monsees, Office Manager/Admin. Support
Offers vocational rehabilitation services for the totally blind, legally blind, visually impaired, mentally retarded blind and more with health, counseling, educational, rehabilitation, computer training and professional training services, and displaced worker.

Wyoming

6223 Division of Vocational Rehabilitation of Wyoming
Wyoming Department of Workforce Services
1100 Herschler Buiding
Cheyenne, WY 82002-1
307-777-7364
wyomingworkforce.org/how/vr.aspx

Jim Mcintosh, Administrator
Kathy Emmones, Director Workforce Services
Provides only those services which are necessary for eligible individuals to reach the employment goal agreed to in the Individualized Plan for Employment.

6224 Vocational Rehabilitation, Division of Department of Workforce Services
Suite 1e
1510 East Pershing Blvd.
Cheyenne, WY 82002-1
307-777-7364
866-804-3678
FAX: 307-777-3759
TTY: 307-777-7386
jmcint@state.wy.us
www.wyomingworkforce.org

Jim McIntosh, Administrator
Joan K. Evans, Director
Lisa M. Osvold, Deputy Director
Provides only those services which are necessary for eligible individuals to reach the employment goal agreed to in the individualized plan for employment.

6225 Wyoming Department of Employment Unemployment Insurance
P.O.Box 2760
100 West Midwest
Casper, WY 82602-2760

307-235-3264
FAX: 307-235-3277
doe.state.wy.us

Randy Hopper, Manager
A combined state/federally funded agency of the state of Wyoming, headed by a Department Director who is appointed by the Governor.

6226 Wyoming Governor's Committee on Employment of the Handicapped
Room 1126
1510 East Pershing Blvd.
Cheyenne, WY 82002-1

307-777-3700
FAX: 307-777-5870
workforceservices@state.wy.us
doe.state.wy.us/Inetclaims

Brenda Oswald, Manager
Joan K. Evans, Director
Lisa M. Osvold, Deputy Director
Assists, empowers and supports people with disabilities to achieve employment, independence and intergration in the workplace and community.

Rehabilitation Facilities, Acute

Alabama

6227 **HealthSouth Lakeshore Rehabilitation Hospital**
3800 Ridgeway Dr
Birmingham, AL 35209-5599
205-868-2000
FAX: 205-868-2029
www.healthsouthlakeshorerehab.com
Vickie Demers, Chief Executive Officer
April Cobb, Chief Nursing Officer
Al Rayburn, Director, Therapy Operations
A 100 bed facility whos key services is physical rehabilitation. Also specialized services (inpatient) infection isolation room. In addition, also has outpatient physical rehabilitation and sports medicine. Patient family support services include patient representative, transportation for elderly/handicapped and patient support groups. Imaging services(diagnostic & theraputic) include ct scanner, diagnostic diagnostic radioisotope facility, MRI, and ultrasound.

6228 **HealthSouth Rehabilitation Hospital of North Alabama**
107 Governors Dr
Huntsville, AL 35801
256-535-2300
FAX: 256-428-2608
www.healthsouthhuntsville.com
Douglas H. Beverly, Chief Executive Officer
Susan Creekmore, Director, Therapy Operations
Risha Hoover, Director, Marketing Operations
Joy McMinn, Director, Nursing
A comprehensive 50 bed rehabilitation hospital serving the need of patients in the North Alabama area. Guides patients with physically disabling conditions along an individualized treatment pathway so they can reach their highest level of physical, social and emotional well-being. A wide range of medical and theraputic services are delivered by qualified and experienced professionals.

6229 **J.L. Bedsole/Rotary Rehabilitation Hospital**
Infirmary Health
5 Mobile Infirmary Circle
Mobile, AL 36607-3513
251-435-3417
www.infirmaryhealth.org
D. Mark Nix, President & CEO
Kenneth C. Brewington, Chief Medical Office, Mobile Infirmary
Jennifer Eslinger, President, Mobile Infirmary
Provides rehabilitation for patients affected by stroke, spinal cord injury, brain injury or other neurological illnesses.

6230 **More Than Just a Job**
Institute On Disability/UCED
60 5th Avenue
Suite 101
New York, NY 10011
212-366-8900
FAX: 603-862-0555
www.forbes.com

6231 **Rocky Mountain Resource & Training Institute**
3630 Sinton Road
Suite 103
Colorado Springs, CO 80907- 5072
719-444-0268
800-949-4262
FAX: 719-444-0269
TTY: 800-949-4232
www.adainformation.org
Jana Copeland, Principal Investigator
Patrick Going, Senior Advisor
Serves people with disabilities and provides training to the agencies that assist them. Facilitates disabled individuals' transition from school to adult life; provides information and resources concerning assistive technology, devices, and services; promotes and ensures compliance with the federal Americans with Disabilities Act (ADA) and other legislation promoting the rights and inclusion of people with disabilities; promotes supported employment, strategic planning and development.

Arkansas

6232 **Central Arkansas Rehab Hospital**
2201 Wildwood Ave
Sherwood, AR 72120-5074
501-834-1800
FAX: 501-834-2227
www.stvincentrehabhospital.com
Lee Frazier, MPH, Dr, CEO
Dr. Sean Foley, Medical Director
Debbie Taylor, Director of Marketing Operations
Stacy Sawyer, Director Of Therapy Operations
A nonprofit hospital licensed for 69 acute care beds with all private rooms. Opened in 1999the hospital offers a full range of outpatient diagnostic services, including MRI,CT,PET along with surgical procedures, cardiology, neurology, neurosurgery, othopedic, rehab and a 24 hour emergency department staffed with board certified emergency room physicians. Includes an outpatient surgery center, rehabilitation hospital, senior health program, diabetic program and physician offices.

6233 **HealthSouth Rehabilitation Hospital**
1401 South J St
Fort Smith, AR 72901-5158
479-785-3300
FAX: 479-785-8599
www.healthsouth.com
Juli Stec, CEO
Provides physical rehabilitation as its key services. Also provides other services such as end-of-life services, pain management and an infection isolation room.

6234 **Northwest Arkansas Rehabilitation Hospital**
153 E Monte Painter Dr
Fayetteville, AR 72703-4002
479-444-2233
FAX: 479-444-2390
www.healthsouthfayetteville.com
Marty Hurlbut, Medical Director
Denise Wilson, Director Of Clinical Services
A 60-bed acute medical rehabilitation hospital that offers comprehensive inpatient and outpatient rehabilitation services.

6235 **Rebsamen Rehabilitation Center**
P.O.Box 159
Jacksonville, AR 72078-159
501-985-7000
FAX: 501-985-7384
www.rebsamenmedicalcenter.com
Mack McAlister, Chairperson
Murice Green, Vice Chairman
Tommy Swaim, Secretary
Mission is to provide personal healthcare for your family. Vision is to develop a family of caregivers to become your community hospital. A 113 bed acute care facility operated by a volunteer Board of Directors made up of community leaders. Rebsamen Medical Center is accredited by the Joint Commission on Accreditation of Healthcare Organizations as well as the Arkansas Department of Health. Through JCAHO we voluntary sumbit to evaluations of our compliance with nationwide hospital standards.

Arizona

6236 **Barrow Neurological Institute Rehab Center**
350 W Thomas Rd
Phoenix, AZ 85013-4409
602-406-3000
FAX: 602-406-4104
www.stjosephs-phx.org
Jackie Aragon, VP Care Management
Linda Hunt, President
Dedicated resources to delivering compassionate, high-quality, affordable health services; serving and advocating for our sisters and brothers who are poor and disenfranchised; and partnering with others in the community to improve the quality of life. Our vision:a growing and diversified health care ministry distinguished by excellent quality and committed to expanding access to those in need.

6237 **HealthSouth Sports Medicine Center**
5111 N Scottsdale Rd
Ste 100
Scottsdale, AZ 85250-7076   480-990-1379
                                 FAX: 480-423-8458
                        chamine@wiley@healthsouth.com
                                 www.healthsouth.com

Troy Meiners, Manager
An out patient facility specialising in sports medicine and treatment of sports injuries.

6238 **Healthsouth Rehab Institute of Tucson**
2650 N Wyatt Dr
Tucson, AZ 85712-6108   520-325-1300
                                 800-333-8628
                             FAX: 520-327-4045
                        www.rehabinstituteoftucson.com

Lee Sanford, Plant Manager
Jon Larson, Medical Director
An accredited member of the Joint Commission On Accreditation of Health Care Organizaions (JCAHO) An 80 bed facility specializing in rehabilitation

6239 **Scottsdale Healthcare**
9630 E Shea Blvd
Scottsdale, AZ 85260-6285   480-551-5400
                                 FAX: 480-551-5401
                                     preiley@shc.org
                                     www.shc.org

Thomas Sadvary, CEO
Pegg Reiley, Chief Nursing Officer
Kathy Zarubi, Associate VP of Nursing Practice
Lisa Sandoval, Director fo Marketing
A 343 bed full-service hospital providing medical/surgical, critical care, obstetrics, pediatrics, surgery, cardiovascular, and oncology services, as well as the Sleep Disorder Center. All patient rooms are private. Emergency department is a level II Trauma Center. The Radiology Department offers state-of-the-art diagnostic equipment, including MRI, PET/CT scanning, nuclear medicine and ultrasound. Also located are the Piper Surgery Center, Cancer Center, and several medical office plazas.

6240 **St. Joseph Hospital and Medical Center**
350 W Thomas Rd
Phoenix, AZ 85013-4496   602-406-3000
                                 FAX: 602-406-4190
                    http://hospitals.dignityhealth.org/stjosephs/
Linda Hunt, President
Rehabilitation programs offered by the clinic assists clients with rehabilitation health needs in the comfort of their own home. The home care rehabilitation team of professionals focuses on correcting deficiencies in self-care, mobility skills and communication. Services offered include physical therapy, occupational therapy, speech pathology, rehabilitative nursing and restorative nursing assistants.

California

6241 **Bakersfield Regional Rehabilitation Hospital**
5001 Commerce Dr
Bakersfield, CA 93309-648   661-323-5500
                                 800-288-9829
                             FAX: 661-633-5254
                        www.healthsouthbakersfield.com

Chris Yoon, Medical Director
Sandra Hegland, Chief Executive Officer
A specialty hospital that treats an array of physical disabilities. It has 60 beds and offers physical rehabilitation services including support groups and education classes on illnesses such as arthritis, asthma and strokes. No surgery facilities on site.

6242 **Brotman Medical Center: RehabCare Unit**
3828 Delmas Ter
Culver City, CA 90232-6806   310-836-7001
                                 FAX: 310-202-4141
                                 info@brotmanmed.com
                             www.brotmanmedicalcenter.com

Howard Levine, CEO
The mission of Brotman Medical Center is to deliver innovative, quality health care to our patients and their families in an environment of compassion, respect, patient saftey, education, and fiscal responsibility.

6243 **Casa Colinas Centers for Rehabilitation**
255 E Bonita Ave
Pomona, CA 91767-1923   909-596-7733
                                 866-724-4127
                             FAX: 909-593-0153
                             TTY: 909-596-3646
                                 rehab@casacolina.org
                                 www.casacolina.org

Felice Loverso, CEO/President
Steve Norin, Chairman
Stephen W. Graeber, Vice Chairman
Mary Lou Jensen, Secretary
Casa Colina will provide individuals the opportunity to maximize their medical recovery and rehabilitation potential efficiently in an environment that recognizes their uniqueness, dignity and self esteem. The vision is to strategically reposition themselves at the forefront of the post-acute continuum by becoming the center of excellence in the provision of services to persons who can benefit from rehabilitation care.

6244 **Community Hospital of Los Gatos Rehabilitation Services**
815 Pollard Rd
Los Gatos, CA 95032-1400   408-378-6131
                                 FAX: 408-866-4003
                        communityhospitallosgatos.com
Ned Borgstrom, CEO
Rehabilitation Services provide individualized treatment programs for inpatient/outpatient care. The team is supervised by a Physiatrist and may include Nurses, Physical Therapists, Occupational Therapists, Speech/Language Therapists, Psychologists, Case Managers, Dietitians, Respiratory Therapists, Recreation Therapists and/or Prosthetists/Orthotists.

6245 **Garfield Medical Center**
525 N Garfield Ave
Monterey Park, CA 91754-1205   626-573-2222
                                 FAX: 626-571-8972
                             www.garfieldmedicalcenter.com

Philip Cohen, CEO
Provides quality care to all citizens of all ages. We are foreward looking to meet the changing health care needs of Forsyth and the surrounding area. At the same time, we are a stable organization that is financially sound. We involve all of our medical staff through good communication. We support them by trying to meet their professional needs in training, equipment and services. We emphasize good communication with all county citizens who support us financially and through the use of services

6246 **Grossmont Hospital Rehabilitation Center**
5555 Grossmont Center
La Mesa, CA 91942   619-740-6000
                                 800-827-4277
                             FAX: 619-644-4159
                                 www.sharp.com

Michael Murphy, President/CEO
Daniel Gross, EVP
It is our mission to improve the health of those we serve with a commitment to excellence in all that we do. Our goal is to offer quality care and programs that set community standards, exceed patients' expectations and are provided in a caring, convenient, cost-effective and accessible manner.

6247 **Health South Tustin Rehabilitation Hospita**
14851 Yorba St
Tustin, CA 92780-2925   714-832-9200
                             FAX: 714-508-4550
                             www.healthsouth.com

Sandra Yule, CEO

6248 **Holy Cross Comprehensive Rehabilitation Center**
15031 Rinaldi St
Mission Hills, CA 91345-1207   818-365-8051
                                 888-432-5464
                             FAX: 818-898-4472
                             www.providence.org

Larry Bowe, CEO
Derek Berz, COO
Known for providing exceptional treatment through its Cancer Centers, Heart Center, Orthopedics, Neurosciences and Rehabilitation Services, as well as Woman's and Children's Services. As a 254-bed, not-for-profit facility, Providence offers a full continuum of health services, from outpatient to inpatient to home health care. Providence operates one of the only round-the-clock trauma centers in the San Fernando Valley and surrounding communities.

6249 **Job Hunting Tips for the So-Called Handicapped**
Special Needs Project
324 State St
Ste H
Santa Barbara, CA 93101-2364   805-962-8087
                                 800-333-6867
                             FAX: 805-962-5087
                             editor@specialneeds.com
                             www.specialneeds.com

Hod Gray, Owner
This nifty booklet from the guru of job hunting himself is sincere, useful and brief. *$4.95*

6250 **Kentfield Rehabilitation Hospital & Outpatient Center**
1125 Sir Francis Drake Blvd
Kentfield, CA 94904-1418   415-456-9680
                             FAX: 415-485-3563
                             info@kentfieldrehab.com
                             www.kentfieldrehab.com

Deborah Doherty, MD
Provides specialized inpatient and outpatient programs. We provide quality services that are patient centered and family-oriented. Under the medical direction of board-certified hospitalists and other physician specialists, our dedicated interdisciplinary teams provide a coordinated, comprehensive treatment approach to a wide range of neurological, orthopedic, pulmonary and complex medical problems.

6251 **Laurel Grove Hospital: Rehab Care Unit**
20103 Lake Chabot Rd
Castro Valley, CA 94546-4093   510-537-1234
                             FAX: 510-727-2778
                             nissims@sutterhealth.org
                             www.edenmedcenter.org

George Bischalaney, CEO & President
Kent Myers, Treasurer
Jeffrey Randall, Secretary
David Davini, CPA Chairman
The mission of Eden Medical Center is carried out by our Board of Directors, employees, physicians and volunteers who are committed to providing our patients and their families with the highest quality medical care and customer service. Creating standards of excellence to ensure quality and value for our patients. Maintaining a financially sound organization through effective clinical and administrative support. Encouraging a culture that supports employees and physicians in development.

6252 **Lodi Memorial Hospital West**
Lodi Memorial Hospital
975 S Fairmont Ave
Lodi, CA 95240   209-334-3411
                                 800-323-3360
                             FAX: 209-333-7131
                             lmh@lodihealth.org
                             www.lodihealth.org

Joseph Harrington, President
Ron Kreutner, Vice President And CFO
Judy Begley RN, MSN, Chief Nursing Officer
Our vision is to provide a system of health-care services which is clinically effective, quality driven and community focused in an environment that supports and encourages excellence. In partnership with our medical staff, we will assume accountability for the health of our community, be responsible for illness and injury prevention and provide care for the ill and injured. We will measure our success on quality outcomes and customer satisfaction.

6253 **Long Beach Memorial Medical Center Memorial Rehabilitation Hospital**
2801 Atlantic Ave
Long Beach, CA 90806-1701   562-933-2000
                             FAX: 562-933-9018
                             www.memorialcare.org

Nissar Syed, Administrator
Barry Arbuckle, President
The hospital offers rehabilitation after catastrophic injury of disabling disease to give patients the opportunity for maximum recovery. The Hospital offers many of the area's finest rehabilitation specialists and most advanced technology, making it one of Southern California's most respected rehabilitation centers.

6254 **North Coast Rehabilitation Center**
1165 Montgomery Drive
Santa Rosa, CA 95405-4869   707-546-3210
                             FAX: 707-525-8413
                             www.santarosamemorial.org

Joyce Cavagnaro, Admissions
Combines state-of-the-art medicine, compassionate care, and the widest array of resources to enhance your health and promote healthy communities. Dedicated to continually introducing new programs and services that help you live life to the fullest.

6255 **Northridge Hospital Medical Center**
18300 Roscoe Blvd
Northridge, CA 91328   818-885-8500
                             FAX: 818-885-5435
                             www.northridgehospital.org

Mike Wall, CEO
dedicating resources to delivering compassionate, high-quality, affordable health services; serving and advocating for our sisters and brothers who are poor and disinfranchised; and partnering with others in the community to improve the quality of life.

6256 **PEERS Program**
8912 W Olympic Blvd
Beverly Hills, CA 90211-3514   310-553-4833
                             FAX: 310-553-4833

Paul Berns, Medical Director
Offers a new approach for wheelchair users. PEERS uses a combination of modern physical therapy, the DOUGLAS Reciprocating Gait System and when necessary, functional electrical stimulation to assist selected individuals to walk with recently patented specially made lightweight braces.

6257 PIRS Hotsheet
Placer Independent Resource Services
11768 Atwood Rd
Ste 29
Auburn, CA 95603
530-885-6100
800-833-8453
FAX: 530-885-3032
TTY: 530-885-0326
lbrewer@pirs.org
pirs.org

Susan Miller, Executive Director
Harry Powell, President
Paul Opper, Vice President
Dawn Davidson, Secretary
Monthly newletter to customers and other constituents.
6 pages Monthly

6258 Providence Holy Cross Medical Center
Providence Health System
15031 Rinaldi St
Mission Hills, CA 91345-1285
818-365-8051
818-898-4603
FAX: 818-365-4472
www.providence.org

Kerry Carmody, CEO
Physicains and nurses are among the best and are recoginzed nationally for clinical excellence. We are committed to improving your health and wellness as you journey through life. Our services span beyond the latest advancements in medical procedures, equipment and medication to also include education and wellness services-all provided with compassion and respect. We help our patients understand and use some of the healthiest tools at their disposal, including nutrition & excercise.

6259 Queen of Angels/Hollywood Presbyterian Medical Center
1300 N Vermont Ave
Los Angeles, CA 90027-6005
213-413-3000
FAX: 213-413-3500
info@hollywoodpresbyterian.com
www.hollywoodpresbyterian.com

Kathy Wong, Manager
A 434 bed acute-care facility that has been caring for the Hollywood community and surrounding areas since 1924. The hospital is committed to serving local multicultural communities with quality medical and nursing care. With more then 500 physicians representing virtually every speciality. Ready to serve your medical needs and those of your loved ones and strive to distinguish itself as a leading healthcare provider, recognized for providing quality, innovative care in a compassionate manner.

6260 Queen of the Valley Hospital
1000 Trancas St
Napa, CA 94558-2941
707-252-4411
FAX: 707-257-4032
www.thequeen.org

Walt Mickens, President
Vincent Morgese, Vice President
For more then 40 years, Queen of the Valley Hospital has been the premiere medical facility in the Napa Valley. Our long history of providing high quality and caring service is founded on 4 core values:Dignity, Service, Excellence and Justice. These central principals inspire us to reach out to those in need and to help heal the whole person-mind, body and spirit.They are the driving force behind our mission to improve the health and quality of life of people in the community we serve.

6261 Rancho Los Amigos National Rehabilitation Center
7601 E Imperial Hwy
Downey, CA 90242-3496
562-401-7111
877-726-2461
888-RAN-CHO1
FAX: 562-401-6690
TTY:562-401-8450
inquiry@rancho.org
www.rancho.org

Jorge Orozco, CEO
Mindy Lipson Aisen, Chief Medical Officer
Michelle Sterling, Interim Chief Nursing Officer
Robin Bayus, CFO
Internationally renowned in the field of medical rehabilitation, consistently ranked in the top Rehabilitation Hospitals in the United States by U.S. News and World Report. It is one of the largest comprehensive rehabilitaion centers in the United States. Licensed for 395 beds, providing service through over 20 centers of excellence.

6262 San Joaquin Valley Rehabilitation Hospital
7173 N Sharon Ave
Fresno, CA 93720-3329
559-436-3600
FAX: 559-436-3606
jpage@svjrehab.com
sjvrehab.com

Edward Palacios, CEO
Complete comprehensive rehabilitation services from acute rehab, outpatient and community fitness services.

6263 Santa Clara Valley Medical Center
County of Santa Clara
751 S Bascom Ave
San Jose, CA 95128-2699
408-885-5000
www.scvmed.org

Paul E. Lorenz, CEO
Jeffrey Arnold, Medical Officer
Trudy Johnson, Director of Patient Care Services & Nursing
Carolyn Brown, Director of Quality & Patient Safety
The mission of the medical center is to provide high-quality, cost-effective medical care to all residence of Santa Clara County regardless of their ability to pay. Make availiable a wide range of inpatient, outpatient, emergency services within resource constraints. Maintain an environment within which the needs of our patients are paramount and where patients, their families and all our visitors are treated in a compassionate, supportive, friendly, and dignified manner.

6264 Scripps Memorial Hospital at La Jolla
9888 Genesee Ave
La Jolla, CA 92037-1205
858-626-4123
800-727-4777
FAX: 858-626-6122
www.scripps.org

Sean A Deitch, President/CEO
Gary Fybel, Executive Director/Administrator
One of the county's 6 designated trauma centers, offers a wide range of clinical and surgical services including 24-hour emergency services; intensive care; interventional cardiology and radiology; radiation oncology; cardiothoracic and orthopedic services; neurology; ophthalmology; and mental health and psychology services.

6265 South Coast Medical Center
12 Mason
Ste A
Irvine, CA 92618-2733
714-669-4446
FAX: 714-669-4448
info@southcoastmedcenter.com
www.southcoastmedcenter.com

Leigh Erin Connealy, Manager
Bruce Christian, President
A 208 bed acute care hospital. Services include maternity, surgical, subacute care, psychiatric program, eating disorder treatment, chemical dependency treatment, radiology, ICU/CCU, comprehensive rehabilitation services, bariatric surgery and movement disorders program..

6266   St. Joseph Rehabilitation Center
St. Joseph Health System
2200 Harrison Ave
Eureka, CA 95501-3215

707-441-4414
FAX: 707-441-4429
www.stjosepheureka.org

6267   St. Jude Brain Injury Network
St. Jude Hospital
130 W Bastanchury Rd
Fullerton, CA 92835-1058

714-446-5626
866-785-8332
FAX: 714-446-5979
ocrcuser@stjoe.org
www.tbioc.org

Jana Gable, Program Coordinator
David Bogdan, Service Coordinator
Lina Marroquin, Servicer Coordinator
Provides comprehensive planning, program referral, assists with funding possibilities, and interagency coordination of services. Areas of emphasis include day treatment, vocational and housing options, and the requirements are adults who have suffered a brain injury from an external force.

6268   St. Jude Medical Center
101 E Valencia Mesa Dr
Fullerton, CA 92835-3809

714-871-3280
800-627-8106
FAX: 714-992-3029
stjudemedicalcenter.org

Robert Fraschetti, President
We are one of Southern California's most respected and technologically advanced hospitals, and our four core values: dignity, excellence, service and justice are the guiding principles for everything we do. St. Jude is synonymous with exceptional care that extends beyond good medicine to a commitment to caring for you - mind, body and spirit.

6269   St. Mary Medical Center
1050 Linden Ave
Long Beach, CA 90813-3393

562-491-9000
FAX: 562-491-9053
www.stmarymedicalcenter.org

Chris Desicco, CEO

6270   Sunnyside Nursing Center
22617 S Vermont Ave
Torrance, CA 90502-2595

310-320-4130
FAX: 310-212-3232
businessdevelopment@sunnysidenursing.com
www.sunnysidenursing.com

Shane Dahl, Administrator
Manny Cordero, Director of Nursing
El Sayad, Medical Director
Skilled nursing care facility; residential care facility; intermediate care facility; specialty hospital.

6271   UCLA Medical Center: Department of Anesthesiology, Acute Pain Services
U CL A Medical Center
1245 16th Street Medical Plz
Ste 225
Santa Monica, CA 90404

310-794-1841
FAX: 310-794-1511
access@mednet.ucla.edu
www.medcnt.ucla.edu

Michael Ferrante, Clinical Director
A 337-bed acute-care medical center, has been serving the healthcare needs of West Los Angeles and Santa Monica since 1926. Highly regarded for its primary and specialty care, the medical center features many outstanding clinical programs, including its women's and children's services, emergency services, and family medicine programs.

Colorado

6272   Children's Hospital Rehabilitation Center
University of Colorado Health Sciences Center
1056 E 19th Ave
Denver, CO 80218-1007

303-861-8888
800-624-6553
webmaster@tchden.org
chipteam.org

Lou Blankenship, CEO
Michael J Farrell, Chief Operating Officer
Helen Martinez, Manager
Private not-for-profit pediatric healthcare network, the hospital is 100 percent dedicated to caring for kids of all ages and stages of growth. That dedication is evident in more then 1000 pediatric specialists and more then 2400 employees. It is also our continual dedication that has placed us at the forefront of research in childhood disease with several nationally and internationally recognized medical programs.

6273   Craig Hospital
3425 S Clarkson St
Englewood, CO 80113-2899

303-789-8000
FAX: 303-789-8214
khosack@craighospital.org
www.craighospital.org

Michael Fordyce, President
Thomas Balazy, Medical Director
Julie Keegan, VP of Finance
Dona Polonsky, VP of Clinical Services
A 93-bed, private, not-for-profit, free-standing, acute care and rehabilitation hospital that provides a comprehensive system of inpatient and outpatient medical care, rehabilitation, neurosurgical rehabilitative care, an equipment company, and long-term follow up services.

6274   HealthSouth Rehabilitation Hospital of Colorado Springs
HealthSouth Corporation
325 S Parkside Dr
Colorado Springs, CO 80910-3134

719-630-8000
FAX: 719-520-0387
www.healthsouthcoloradosprings.com

Steve Schaefer, CEO
A 56 bed rehabilitation hospital, its key services are: cardiology department, physical rehabilitation, and orthopedics department. Accredidted to the Joint Commission on Accreditation of Health Care Organizations (JCAHO)

6275   Mapleton Center
North Broadway & Balsam
Boulder, CO 80301-9130

303-440-2273
FAX: 303-441-0536
pr@bch.org
www.bch.org

David Gehant, President/CEO
Comprehensive inpatient and outpatient rehabilitation services for all age groups. Treatment provided by interdisciplinary teams and staff physicians. CARF accredited in brain injury rehabilitation, pediatric rehabilitation, pain management, work hardening and inpatient rehabilitation.

6276   Mediplex Rehab: Denver
Vibra Health Care
8451 Pearl St
Thornton, CO 80229-4804

303-288-3000
FAX: 303-496-1120
info@vhdenver.com
www.northvalleyrehab.com

Walter Sacckett, CEO
Encompasses the broadest mix of professional talent, the finest technology and a total commitment by our people to deliver the highest quality care today, and well into the future. The services can be divided into 4 main categories: long term Acute Care and rehab. Skilled nursing facility and residential ventilator program. Outpatient services and pain management. Adult and Geriatric inpatient psychiatric services.

Connecticut

6277 Mariner Health Care: Connecticut
23 Liberty Way
Niantic, CT 06357   860-739-4007
                                     FAX: 860-701-2202

District of Columbia

6278 National Rehabilitation Hospital
102 Irving St NW
Washington, DC 20010-2949   202-877-1760
                                     FAX: 202-829-2789
                                     www.nrhrehab.org

Edward Healton, Medical Director
Robert Bunning, Associate Medical Director
A private facility dedicated solely to medical rehabilitation. The hospital offers intensive inpatient programs and full-service outpatient programs.

Florida

6279 Florida Hospital Rehabilitation Center
601 E Rollins St
Orlando, FL 32803-1248   407-303-1527
                                     855-303-3627
                                     FAX: 407-303-7566
                                     fh.web@flhosp.org
                                     www.flhosp.org

Rex Alleyne, President
Florida Hospital Orlando uses the latest technology to treat over 32,000 inpatients and 53,600 outpatients annually. This 881-bed, acute-carecommunity hospital also serves as a major tertiary facility for much of the Southeast, the Caribbean and South America

6280 HealthSouth Regional Rehab Center/Florida
20601 Old Cutler Rd
Miami, FL 33189-2441   305-251-3800
                                     FAX: 305-259-0498
                                     www.healthsouth.com

Murray Rolnick, Medical Director
Elizabeth Izquierdo, Chief Executive Officer
HealthSouth Rehabilitation Hospital of Miami is a member of the HealthSouth Corporation, the nation's largest healthcare services provider, The hospital is accredited by the Joint Commission on Accreditation of Healthcare Organizations (JCAHO) and Commission on Accreditaion of Rehabilitation Facilities (CARF). Services offered include dietary services, occupational therapy, and respitory care.

6281 HealthSouth Rehab Hospital: Largo
901 Clearwater Largo Rd N
Largo, FL 33770-4121   727-586-2999
                                     FAX: 727-588-3404
                                     www.healthsouthlargo.com

Elaine Ebaugh, CEO
Linda Russo, Director, Therapies
A specialty hospital devoted to providing comprehensive medical rehabilitation services. The hospital is licensed as a Comprehensive Medical Rehabilitation Hospital by the state of Florida, and accredited by the Joint Commission on Accreditation of Healthcare Organizations (JCAHO). HealthSouth of Largo is the only free standing Rehabilitation Hospital in the Tampa Bay region, and serves patients of all ages. Provides inpatient medical rehabilitation services as well as outpatient programs.

6282 HealthSouth Sports Medicine & Rehabilitation Center
3280 Ponce De Leon Blvd
Coral Gables, FL 33134-7252   305-444-0909
                                     FAX: 305-444-5760
                                     www.healthsouth.com

Jay Greeney, President
Ray Jaffet, Administrator
Provides specialized medical and therapeutic services designated to help physically disabled individuals reach their optimum level of independence and function by providing inpatient and outpatient comprehensive medical rehabilitation services.

6283 HealthSouth Sports Medicine and Rehabilitation Center
2141 South Highway A1A Alt
Jupiter, FL 33477   561-743-8890
                                     FAX: 561-743-8795

Diane Reiley, Manager
Outpatient orthopedic and sports medicine/physical therapy.

6284 HealthSouth Treasure Coast Rehabilitation Hospital
Health South Corporation of Alabama
1600 37th St
Vero Beach, FL 32960-4863   772-778-2100
                                     FAX: 772-567-7041
                                     www.healthsouthtreasurecoast.com

Jimmy Lockhart, Medical Director
HealthSouth Treasure Coast Rehabilitation Hospital is a 90-bed inpatient comprehensive rehabilitation hospital serving Indian River, St. Lucie, Martin and Okeechobee counties. Outpatient services are available at the hospital and at four other clinics. Therapies include physical, occupational, speech and psychology services.

6285 Manatee Springs Care & Rehabilitation Center
5627 9th St E
Bradenton, FL 34203-6105   941-753-8941
                                     FAX: 941-739-4409
                                     info@manateespringsrehab.com
                                     www.manateespringsrehab.com

Donna Steiermann, Administrator
Skilled rehabilitation facility specializing in PT, OT, speech therapy, aquatic therapy and an indoor pool. Piped oxygen bed for specialized respiratory care. Compassionate end of life care. Some Medicare, private insurance, and Medicaid.

6286 Perry Health Facility
207 Marshall Dr
Perry, FL 32347-1897   850-584-6334
                                     FAX: 850-838-1801

Rebkah Hatch, Administrator
Full rehabilitation team available, Physiatrist, DOR, Psychiatrist, Psychologist, RD, Geriatric Nursing, PT/OT/ST/RT, Orthotiet/Prosthetist. Provider for PPO's & HMO's as well as medicare, private insurance and medicare/medicaid.

6287 Pinecrest Rehabilitation Hospital and Outpatient Centers
Tenet South Florida
5352 Linton Blvd
Delray Beach, FL 33484-6514   561-498-4440
                                     800-283-8326
                                     FAX: 561-495-3103
                                     www.pinecrestrehab.com

Mark Bryan, CEO
Pinecrest Rehabilitation Hospital is a 90 bed, accredited hospital and is comprised of a Specialty Unit, a Neuro Trauma Unit and Joint Replacement Unit. Additional services at Pincrest include six outpatient rehab centers throughout Palm Beach County. The Outpatient Centers each focus on various specialties such as orthopedic and neurological rehab, pain management, cardiac and pulmonary rehab, occupational medicine, Hearing Institute, dizziness and balance and wellness.

6288 Rehabilitation Institute of Sarasota
3251 Proctor Rd
Sarasota, FL 34231-8538   941-921-8796
                                     FAX: 941-922-6228

Stacy Shepherd, Director Clinical Services

a 75-bed hospital that offers individualized medical and theraputic services tailored to patients and clinics for those affected with stroke, multiple sclerosis, Parkinson's, muscular dystrophy and Lou Gehrig's disease (ALS)

6289   Sea Pines Rehabilitation Hospital
101 E Florida Ave
Melbourne, FL 32901-8398   321-984-4600
                                             FAX: 321-727-7440
                                   ellen.lyons-olski@healthsouth.com
                                   www.healthsouthseapines.com

Stuart Miller, Medical Director
Donna Bohdal, Director of Therapy Operations
Denise McGrath, Administrator
A 90-bed facility specializing in rehabilitation of brain and spinal injuries.

6290   Shriners Hospitals for Children: Tampa
12502 USF Pine Dr
Tampa, FL 33612-9411   813-972-2250
                                                 813-281-0300
                                             FAX: 813-975-7125
                                     aargiz-lyons@shrinenet.org
                                 www.shrinershq.org/hospitals/tampa

David Ferrell, FACHE
Maureen Maciel, Chief of Staff
Alicia Argis-Lyons, Develpoment Officer
Recognizing that the family plays a vital role in a child's ability to overcome an illness or injury, Shriners Hospitals helps the family provide the support the child needs by involving the family in all aspects of the child's care and recovery. The purpose of all Shriners Hospitals for Children is to provide care to children with orthopedic problems and burn injuries to help them lead fuller, more productive lives.

6291   South Miami Hospital
6200 SW 73rd St
South Miami, FL 33143-4679   786-662-4000
                                             FAX: 786-662-5302
                                             www.baptisthealth.net

Brian E. Keely, CEO
The mission is to improve the health and well-being of individuals, and to promote the sanctity and preservation of life, in the communities we serve. We are committed to maintaining the highest standards of clinical and service excellence, rooted in utmost integrity and moral practice.

6292   St. Anne's Nursing Center
11855 Quail Roost Dr
Miami, FL 33177-3956   305-252-4000
                                             FAX: 305-969-6752
                                   www.catholichealthservices.org

Tony Farinella, Executive Director
Francisco Cruz, Medical Director
Julia Shillingford, Director of Nursing
Provides spacious, comfortable accommodations with ample recreational areas in a beautifully landscaped setting.

6293   St. Anthony's Hospital
1200 7th Ave N
St Petersburg, FL 33705-1388   727-825-1100
                                             www.stanthonys.com

William Ulbricht, President
James McClint, VP
Ron Colaguori, VP Operations
Mary McNally, VP Mission
A not-for-profit, 395-bed hospital established in 1931. St. Anthony's is dedicated to improving the health of the community through community-owned health care that sets the standard for high-quality, compassionate care.

6294   St. Anthony's Rehabilitation Hospital
3487 NW 35th Ave
Lauderdale Lakes, FL 33311-1107   954-485-4023
                                                 954-739-6233
                                   www.catholichealthservices.org

Linda Motte, Hospital Administrator
Kathy Torbertsonn, Dir. Rehab.
Provides spacious, comfortable accommodations with ample recreational areas in a beautifully landscaped setting.

6295   St. Catherine's Rehabilitation Hospital and Villa Maria Nursing Center
1050 NE 125th St
North Miami, FL 33161-5805   305-357-1735
                                                 305-891-3361
                                   www.catholichealthservices.org

Virginia Irving, Hospital Administrator
Jim Reiss, Executive Director
Greg Hartley, Director Rehab
St. Catherine's Rehabilitation Hospital is a CARF accredited, 60 bed facility offering inpatient and outpatient rehabilitation and medical clinics; including physical, occupational, and speech therapy, neurology, neurodiagnostics, wound care, and hyperbaric medicine. Villa Maria Nursing center is a JCAHO accredited, 212 bed skilled nursing center providing short term nursing and rehabilitation , as well as long term care.

6296   St. John's Nursing Center
3075 NW 35th Ave
Lauderdale Lakes, FL 33311-1107   954-739-6233
                                             FAX: 954-733-9579
                                   www.catholichealthservices.org

Ralph E. Lawson, Chairman
Elizabeth Worley, Vice Chairman
Thomas Marin, Assistant Secretary
Provides spacious, comfortable accommodations with ample recreational areas in a beautifully landscaped setting.

6297   Successful Job Accommodation Strategies
LRP Publications
36- Hiatt Dr
Palm Beach Gardens, FL 33418   561-622-6520
                                                 800-341-7874
                                             FAX: 561-622-0757
                                             webmaster@lrp.com
                                             www.lrp.com

Honora McDowell, Product Group Manager
Kenneth Kahn, Chief Executive Officer
This monthly newsletter provides you with quick tips, new accommodation ideas and innovative workplace solutions. You learn the outcomes of the latest cases involving workplace accommodations. *$ 140.00*
12 pages Monthly

6298   Tampa General Rehabilitation Center
1 Tampa General Circle
Tampa, FL 33601-1289   813-844-7000
                                             FAX: 813-844-1477
                                             jstone@tgh.org
                                             tgh.org

Ron Hytoff, President/CEO
Devanand Mangar MD, Vice Chief of Staff
Thomas L. Bernasek MD, Chief of Staff
Offers a full range of inpatient and outpatient programs all aimed at helping patients achieve their full potentials. JCAHO and CARF accredited and V.R. designated center. A wide range of inpatient and outpatient programs are available such as Brain and Spinal Cord Injury Programs, Comprehensive Medical Rehabilitation, Pain Management, Cardiac Rehab, Pediatric Therapy Service, Sleep Disorders, Epilepsy, and Wheelchair Seating.Hosts the Florida Alliance for Assistive Services and Technolgy.

6299 **University of Miami: Jackson Memorial Rehabilitation Center**
University of Miami
1611 NW 12th Ave
Miami, FL 33136-1005
305-585-6970
FAX: 305-585-6092
info@jhsmiami.org
www.jhsmiami.org

Michael Butler, Chief Medical Officer
An accredited, non-profit, tertiary care hospital and the major teaching facility for the University of Miami School of Medicine. With more then 1,550 beds, Jackson Memorial is a referral center, a magnet for medical research, and home to the Ryder Trauma Center- the only adult and pediatric level 1 trauma center in Miami-Dade County.

6300 **Winter Park Memorial Hospital**
Florida Hospital
200 N Lakemont Ave
Winter Park, FL 32792-3273
407-646-7000
FAX: 407-646-7639
healthcare@winterparkhospital.com
www.winterparkhospital.com

Ken Bradley, CEO
Offers Acute Rehabilitation.

Georgia

6301 **Candler General Hospital: Rehabilitation Unit**
5353 Reynolds St
Savannah, GA 31405-6015
912-819-6000
FAX: 912-819-8829
www.sjchs.org/body.cfm?id=383

Paul Hinchey, President/CEO
Special Physical Therapy Services at Candler Outpatient Center: Aquatic therapy, pediatric services, outpaitient neurological rehabilitation program, woman's health therapy, orthotics, and spine specialty

6302 **Children's Healthcare of Atlanta at Egleston**
1405 Clifton Rd NE
Atlanta, GA 30322-1060
404-785-6000
FAX: 404-315-2158
www.choa.org

Donna Hyland, President/CEO
Ruth Fowler, CFO
Patrick Friars, Chief Children's Physician
Ron Frieson, Chief Public Policy Officer
Rehabilitation Center at Egleston accepts children from birth to age 18 with acute or chronic problems. The length of rehab stay varies for each child according to the determined program of care. The center offers inpatient, outpatient & day rehab programs for comprehensive evaluation & treatment. The program emphasizes the development of the child's abilities & concentrates on helping the family & child compensate for any long-term disabilities. Short term stays require one or two weeks.

6303 **Cobb Hospital and Medical Center: Rehab Care Center**
3950 Austell Rd
Austell, GA 30106-1121
770-732-5126
generalinfo@wellstar.org
www.wellstar.org

David Anderson, Executive VP
Michael Andrews, Chief Cancer Network Officer
Avril Beckford, Chief Pediatrics Officer
To deliver world class healthcare we equip our healthcare facilities and employees with the best technology, resources and education availiable. To deliver world class healthcare we keep seeking ways to improve the way we deliver care knowing each day holds more miracles, more life, more chances, more compassion, and more opportunities.

6304 **HealthSouth Central Georgia Rehabilitation Hospital**
3351 Northside Dr
Macon, GA 31210-2587
478-201-6500
FAX: 478-471-6536
www.centralgarehab.com

6305 **Specialty Hospital**
Floyd Healthcare Resources
304 Turner McCall Blvd SW
Rome, GA 30165-5621
706-509-5000
FAX: 706-802-4175
contactus@floyd.org
www.floyd.org

Kurt Stuenkel, CEO
Dee Russell, Chief Medical Officer
Our mission is to be responsive to the communities we serve with a comprehensive and technologically advanced heal care system commited to the delivery of care that is characterized by continually improving quality, accessability, affordability and personal dignity.

Hawaii

6306 **Shriners Hospital for Children: Honolulu**
1310 Punahou St
Honolulu, HI 96826-1099
808-941-4466
888-888-6314
FAX: 808-942-8573
jburda@shrinenet.org
www.shrinershospitalsforchildren.org

Kenneth Guidera, Chief Medical Officer
Eugene D'Amore, Vice President
Kathy A. Dean, Vice President Human Resources
Sharon Russell, VP Finance & Accounting
One of 22 hospitals across North America that provide excellent, no-cost medical care to children with orthopedic problems and burn industries.

Idaho

6307 **Pocatello Regional Medical Center**
777 Hospital Way
Pocatello, ID 83201-2797
208-234-6154
FAX: 208-239-3719
robbieo@portmed.org
www.portmed.org

Mark Bukalew, Chairman
John Abreu, VP Finance
Stephen Weeg, Vice-Chairman
David Swindell, Treasurer
Pocatello Regional Medical Center offers 24-hour emergency care, specialized heart services, a dialysis center, a full service rehabilitation unit including transition care, and the Woman's Center For Health including obstetrics.

Illinois

6308 **Builders of Skills**
515 Busse Hwy
Park Ridge, IL 60068-3154
847-318-0870
FAX: 847-292-0873
avenues@avenuesonline.org
www.avenuestoindependence.org

Jacqueline Kinmel, Chair
Peg O'herron, Vice Chair
Eric Johnson, Treasurer
Bob Healy, Secretary
Residential setting for hearing-impaired, developmentally disabled adults who are assisted with daily living skills.

6309 Center for Learning
National-Louis University
2840 Sheridan Rd
Evanston, IL 60201-1730
847-256-5150
FAX: 845-256-1057
kadamle@nl.edu

Jerry Dachs, Manager
Psycho-educational evaluations for children, adolescents, and adults. Individualized remedial academic programs, individual counseling

6310 DBTAC-Great Lakes ADA Center
1640 W Roosevelt Road
Room 405
Chicago, IL 60608-1316
312-413-1407
800-949-4232
FAX: 312-413-1856
gldbtac@uic.edu
www.adagreatlakes.org

Robin Jones, Project Director
Glenn Fujiura, PhD, Director of Research and Co-Inve
Claudia Diaz, Associate Project Director
Peter Berg, Project Coordinator for Technica
Provides training, technical assistance and consultation on the rights and resposibilities of indiviualsand entities covered by the ADA. Toll free number for technical assistance and materials provided electronically or via mail at no cost.

6311 Institute of Physical Medicine and Rehabilitation
6501 N Sheridan Rd
Peoria, IL 61614-2932
309-692-8110
800-957-4767
FAX: 309-692-8673
foundation@ipmr.org
ipmr.org

Lisa Snyder, Medical Director
Comprehensive CARF accredited programs in outpatient medical rehabilitation services. Eight outpatient locations, specialty programs include adult day services, driving evaluations, balance and visual rehabilitation board certified physiatrists.

6312 LaRabida Children's Hospital and Research Center
E 65th At Lake Michigan
Chicago, IL 60649
773-363-6700
FAX: 773-363-9554
pr@larabida.org
www.larabida.org

Brenda Wolf, President/CEO
Dedicated to excellence in caring for children with chronic illness, disabiliesm or who have been abused, allowing them to achieve their fullest potential through expertise and innovation within the health care and academic communities.

6313 Marianjoy Rehabilitation Hospital and Clinics
26W171 Roosevelt Rd
Wheaton, IL 60187-6078
630-909-8000
800-462-2366
FAX: 630-909-8001
dlebloch@marianjoy.org
www.marianjoy.org

Maureen Beal, Chairperson
John Oliverio, Vice Chairman
Kathleen Dvorakk, Treasurer
Thomas A. Keiser, Secretary
Goal at Marianjoy Rehabilitation Hospital is to help you and your family return to the lifestyle you enjoyed before your illness or injury. To meet this goal, we provide you with a dedicated team of experienced professionals to assist you every step of the way.

6314 Rush Copley Medical Center-Rehab Neuro Physical Unit
2040 Ogden Ave
Ste 303
Aurora, IL 60504-7222
630-898-3700
866-426-7539
FAX: 630-898-3681
clord@rsh.net
www.rushcopley.com

Barry Finn, CEO
Mary Shilkaitis, VP, Patient Care Services
The mission of the medical center and the medical staff is to work together to serve your healthcare needs through excellence in education, technology and a caring touch. Rush-Copley Medical Center will be the leading healthcare provider of the greater Fox Valley area. At Rush-Copley we pride ourselves on providing everyone with extrodinary service.

Indiana

6315 ATTAIN
U S Department of Education/ NI DR R
32 E Washington St
Ste 1400
Indianapolis, IN 46204-3552
317-534-0236
800-528-8246

Gary Hand, Executive Director
The mission of Attain is to create solutions that enable people with functional limitations to live, learn, work and play in the community of their choice. All will have access to assistive devices. We will do this in partnership with people with functional limitations, families and members of the community through training, system change, services and support, research, dissemination and consumer advocacy.

6316 About Special Kids
7172 Graham Rd
Suite 100
Indianapolis, IN 46250-2879
317-257-8683
800-964-4746
FAX: 317-251-7488
FamilyNetw@aboutspecialkids.org
www.aboutspecialkids.org

Joe Brubaker, Executive Director
Jane Scott, Director Of Information
Nancy Stone, Project Director
A Parent to Parent organization that works throughout the state of Indiana to answer questions and provide support, information and resources. We are parents and family members of children with special needs and we help other families and professionals understand the various systems that are encountered related to special needs. Our central office is where parents from the entire state can access information, resources and support.

6317 Clark Memorial Hospital: RehabCare Unit
1220 Missouri Ave
Jeffersonville, IN 47130-3743
812-282-6631
FAX: 812-283-2656
humanresources@clarkmemorial.org
clarkmemorial.org

Martin Padgett, CEO
The mission of Clark Memorial Hospital is to provide superior health services to the people and communities we serve. The vision of Clark Memorial Hospital is to be the best community healh care provider in the United States. We value each individual and work together to explore new ways to improve the quality of life of all. We persue excellence in all we do. We treat all individuals with the same compassion, dignity, and privacy that we want in ourselves.

6318 Developmental Disabilities Planning Council
402 W Washington St
Indianapolis, IN 46204-2855 317-232-7770
FAX: 317-233-3712
gpcpd@gpcpd.org
www.state.in.us/gpcpd

Suellen Jackson-Boner, Executive Director
Christine Dahlberg, Associate Director
Jim Geswein, CFO
Betty Jones, Secretary
The mission of the Indiana Governor's Council is to promote public policy which leads to the independence, productivity and inclusion of people with disabilities in all aspects of society. This mission is accomplished through planning, evaluation, collaboration, education, research and advocacy. The Council is consumer-driven and is charged with determining how the service delivery system in both the public and private sectors can be most responsible to the people with disabilities.

6319 Easter Seals Wayne/Union Counties
P.O.Box 86
Centerville, IN 47330-86 765-855-2482
FAX: 756-855-2482
eastersealswu@comcast.net
eastersealswu.tripod.com

Kathy Stephen, Treasurer
Vickey Allen, President
Leslie Mayl Whitney, Secretary
Helps people discover nature and much more at camps equipped to offer physcial, social and emotional support and fun for campers with physical and/or developmental disabilities.

6320 IN-SOURCE
Indiana Resource Center for Families with Special
1703 S Ironwood Dr
South Bend, IN 46613-3414 574-234-7101
800-332-4433
FAX: 574-234-7279
insource@insource.org
insource.org

Richard Burden, Executive Director
Scott Carson, Assistant Director
Dory Lawrence, Project Director
Sally Hamburg, Project Director
The mission of IN*SOURCE is to provide parents, families and service providers in Indiana the information and training necessary to assure effective educational programs and appropriate services for children and young adults with disabilities.

6321 Indiana Congress of Parent and Teachers
2525 N Shadeland Ave
Ste D4
Indianapolis, IN 46219-1770 317-357-5881
FAX: 317-357-3751
info@indianapta.org
www.indianapta.org

Sharon Wise, President
Theresa Distelrath, VP
Job Wise, Secretary
Julie Klingenberger, Treasurer
The mission of the Indiana PTA is three-fold: to support and speak on behalf of children and youth in the schools, community and before governmental agencies and other organizations that make decisions affecting children; to assist parents in developing the skills they need to raise and protect their children; and, to encorage parent and community involvement in the public schools of this state and nation.

6322 Indiana Protection and Advocacy Services Commission
4701 N Keystone Ave
Ste 222
Indianapolis, IN 46205-1561 317-722-5555
800-838-1131
FAX: 317-722-5564
dward@ipas.IN.gov
www.in.gov/ipas

Karen Pedevilla, Education and Training Director

IPAS was created in 1977 by state law to protect and advocate the rights of people with disabilities and its Indiana's federally designated Protection (P&A) system and client assist program. It is an independent state agency, with receives no state funding and is independent from all service providers, as required by federal and state law.

6323 Kokomo Rehabilitation Hospital
829 N Dixon Rd
Kokomo, IN 46901-7709 765-452-6700
FAX: 765-452-7470

Brenda Harry, Admissions Director
a 60 bed facility specializing in rehabilitation services to the people of Indiana.

6324 Memorial Regional Rehabilitation Center
615 N Michigan St
South Bend, IN 46601-1033 574-647-1000
www.qualityoflife.org

6325 Methodist Hospital Rehabilitation Institute
8701 Broadway
Merrillville, IN 46410-7035 219-738-5500
FAX: 219-755-0448
methodisthospitals.org

Ian McFadden, President/CEO
Matthew Doyle, VP & CFO
Wright Alcorn, VP Operations
Michael Davenport, Vp Medical Affairs
Methodist Hospitals, of all the hospitals in Northwest Indiana, attracts the most complex cases across a range of specialties, including stroke, brain tumor, cancer, trauma and high-risk pregnancy. This is the result of our commitment to providing the expertise and technology needed to offer the most advanced clinical care.

6326 NAMI Indiana
P.O.Box 22697
Indianapolis, IN 46222-697 317-925-9399
800-677-6442
FAX: 317-925-9398
info@namiindiana.org
www.namiindiana.org

Marilynn Walker, President
Joshua Sprunger, Executive Director
Linda Williams, Program Coooridnator
Leslie Gay, Office Manager
NAMI Indiana is a non-profit grassroots organization dedicated to improving the lives of people afflicted by serious and persistant mental illness. We are dedicated to helping families through a network of support, education, advocacy, and promotion of research. NAMI's goal is to help establish a system of care that provides community based services for persons with serious mental illness, as well as support for them and their families.

6327 Parkview Regional Rehabilitation Center
2200 Randallia Dr
Fort Wayne, IN 46805-4638 260-373-4000
888-480-5151
FAX: 260-373-4288
www.parkview.com

Mike Packnett, President & CEO
Mike Browning, CFO
Rick Henvey, Chief Administrative Officer
Sue Ehinger, President (Parkview & Affiliates)
Provides a full range of inpatient, theraputic services and programs for patients as young as 3 years of age to the very elderly. Our acute care rehabilitation center, is well equipped to care for patients with neurological and orthopedic injuries and diseases.

6328 Programs for Children with Disabilities: Ages 3 through 5
Indiana Department of Education
151 W Ohio St
Indianapolis, IN 46204-1905
317-232-0570
877-851-4106
FAX: 317-232-0589
specialed@doe.in.gov
www.doe.in.gov/exceptional

Heather Neal, Chief of Staff

The division provides leadership and state-level support for public school gifted and talented (grades K-12) programs and for students with disabilities from ages 3-21. The division ensures that Indiana, in its compliance with the federal Individuals With Disabilities Education Act, through monitoring of special education programs, oversight of community and residential programs, provision of mediation and due process rights, and sound fiscal management.

6329 Programs for Children with Special Health Care Needs
Indiana State Department of Health
2 N Meridian St
Indianapolis, IN 46204-3021
317-233-1325
wgettelf@isdh.state.in.us
www.in.gov/isdh/

Sean Keefer, Chief of Staff

The Children's Special Health Care Services (CSHCS) program provides financial assistance for needed medical treatment to children with serious and chronic medical conditions to reduce complications and promote maximum quality of life.

6330 Programs for Infants and Toddlers with Disabilities: Ages Birth through 2
402 W Washington St
Indianapolis, IN 46204-2773
317-232-1144
800-441-7837
firststepsweb@fssa.state.in.us

6331 Riley Child Development Center
705 Riley Hospital Drive
Rm 5837
Indianapolis, IN 46202-5128
317-274-7819
FAX: 317-944-9760
info@child-dev.com
child-dev.com

Cristy James, Communication Coordinator

Riley Hospital for Children is Indiana's only comprehensive children's hospital, with pediatric specialists in evry field of medicine and surgery. Riley is committed to providing the highest quality health care to children in a compassionate, family-centered environment. Riley is a national leader in cutting edge research and medical education, ensuring health care excellence for children for generations to come. Riley provides medical care to all children, regardless of family's ability to pay.

6332 St. Anthony Memorial Hospital: Rehab Unit
301 W Homer St
Michigan City, IN 46360-4358
219-879-8511
FAX: 219-877-1409
www.saintanthonymemorial.org

Joseph Allegreti, Board of Directors
Calvin Bellamy, Board of Directors

Saint Anthony Memorial is an acute care hospital located in Michigan City, primary serving La Porte and Porter Counties in Indiana as well as Berrien County Michigan.

6333 State Division of Vocational Rehabilitation
402 W Washington St
P O Box 7083
Indianapolis, IN 46207-7083
317-233-4475
800-545-7763
FAX: 317-232-6478
vrcommission@fssa.in.gov
www.state.in.us/fssa

Megan Ornellas, Chief of Staff
Susie Howard, Deputy Chief of Staff

6334 VSA Indiana
Harrison Center for the Arts
1505 N Delaware St
Indianapolis, IN 46202-4466
317-974-4123
FAX: 317-974-4124
info@vsai.org
www.vsai.org

Gayle Holtman, President
Linda Wisler, Vice President
Ron Lenz, Chairman of the Board
Bruce Westpahl, Vice Chairman

For over 25 years VSA arts of Indiana has led the movement to make the arts accessable to people with disabilitites. VSA arts of Indiana offers a variety of opportunities for people with disabilities of all ages to engage the power of the arts as a means of education, creative self-expression, and personal and professional growth. As a result, VSA promotes change in public perceptions and raises public awareness, and advocates for increased accessability in providing art experiences for all.

Iowa

6335 Younker Rehabilitation Center of Iowa Methodist Medical Center
1776 W Lakes Pkwy
Des Moines, IA 50266
515-241-6161
888-584-6311
FAX: 515-241-5137
www.ihs.org

Bill Leaver, President
Kevin Vermeer, EVP
Danny Drake, VP
Kara Dunham, VP Finance

Iowa Health System is the state's first and largest integrated healthcare system. We are physicians, hospitals, civic leaders and local volunteers committed to providing the highest possible quality and the lowest possible cost. We serve over 70 communities in Iowa, Western Illinois, and Eastern Nebraska.

Kansas

6336 Kansas Rehabilitation Hospital
1504 SW 8th Ave
Topeka, KS 66606-2714
785-235-6600
FAX: 785-232-8545
www.kansasrehabhospital.com

Mark LeNeave, CEO
Mindy Mitchell, Chief Nursing Officer

A free standing physical rehabilitation hospital located in Topeka Kansas. Designated to provide a barrier-free access to all treatment and patient service areas. This 79-bed facility offers a total rehabilitation environment in a warm, caring setting that encourages patient, family and staff interaction.

6337 Mid-America Rehabilitation Hospital HealthSouth
Health South Corporation
5701 W 110th St
Overland Park, KS 66211-2503
913-491-2400
FAX: 913-491-1097
tiffany.kiehl@healthsouth.com
www.midamericarehabhospital.com

Kristen De Hart, CEO
Tiffany Kiehl, Director Marketing/Operations
Paul Matlack, Director Therapy Operations
Damon Parker, Chief Nursing Officer

97 bed Acute Rehab hospital offering full continuum from in-patient, day treatment and outpatient services for individuals with physical limitations due to CVA, TBI, SCI, other traumas, joint replacement, etc.

Kentucky	Louisiana

6338   Cardinal Hill Rehabilitation Hospital
2050 Versailles Rd
Lexington, KY 40504-1499   859-254-5701
                                  800-233-3260
                              FAX: 859-231-1365
                       webmaster@cardinalhill.org
                            www.cardinalhill.org

Kerry Gillihan, CEO
William J. Lester, Medical Director
Russell Travis, Assistant Medical Director
CARF-accredited rehab center provides comprehensive inpatient and outpatient services in two locations to people with physical and cognitive disabilities. We provide diagnosis-specific programs to 100 inpatients, outpatient clinics, outpatient therapies, pain management and therapeutic pool services. The Pediatric Center serves children from birth to age 18 years of age.

6339   HealthSouth Rehabilitation of Louisville
1227 Goss Ave
Louisville, KY 40217-1287   270-769-3100
                              FAX: 502-636-0351
                            www.healthsouth.com

Tim Nichol, Manager
Regina Durbin, Administrator
HealthSouth Rehabilitation Hospitals lead the way, consistently outperforming peers with a unique, intensive approach to rehabilitative care, partnering with every patient to find a treatment plan that works for them. We offer a wide range of comprehensive rehabilitation programs for a wide variety of diagnoses. At HealthSouth, we provide access to independent private practice physicians, specializing in physical medicine and rehabilitation, who work in conjunction with HealthSouth's highly qual

6340   Lakeview Rehabilitation Hospital
134 Heartland Dr
Elizabethtown, KY 42701-2778   270-769-3100
                                  FAX: 270-769-6870
                            www.healthsouthlakeview.com

Lori Jarboes, CEO
Chris Koford, Medical Director
HealthSouth Rehabilitation Hospitals lead the way, consistently outperforming peers with a unique, intensive approach to rehabilitative care, partnering with every patient to find a treatment plan that works for them. We offer a wide range of comprehensive rehabilitation programs for a wide variety of diagnoses. At HealthSouth, we provide access to independent private practice physicians, specializing in physical medicine and rehabilitation, who work in conjunction with HealthSouth's highly qual

6341   Shriners Hospitals for Children, Lexington
1900 Richmond Rd
Lexington, KY 40502-1204   859-266-2101
                                  800-444-8314
                              FAX: 859-268-5636
                       Dwallenius@shrinenet.org
                  www.shrinershq.org/hospitals/lexington

Warren E. Hopkins, Chairman
Kirk E. Carter, Vice Chairman
Ken R. Dougherty, Treasurer
David E. Hager, Secretary
Shriners Hospitals for Childrenr - Lexington, is a 50-bed pediatric orthopaedic hospital. Our family-centered approach to care is designed to support the whole family during the acute and reconstructive phases of a child's injury. Located in Lexington, Ky., our hospital treats children from all over the country and around the world, and has unique relationships with some of the top hospitals and universities in the world.

6342   HealthSouth Specialty Hospital Of North Louisiana
1401 Ezelle St
Ruston, LA 71270-7218   318-251-3126
                                  800-548-9157
                              FAX: 318-251-1594
                       mark.rice@lifecare-hospitals.com
                            www.healthsouth.com

Mark Rice, CEO
A 90-bed specialty hospital offering both inpatient and outpatient services. Acute long term care.

6343   Our Lady of Lourdes Rehabilitation Center
4801 Ambassador Caffery Pkwy
Lafayette, LA 70508   337-470-2000
                              FAX: 318-289-2681
                       info@lourdesrmc.com
                            www.lourdesrmc.com

William Barrow, CEO
Gerald R. Boudreaux, Chairman of the Board
D. Wayne Elmore, Secretary
Our Lady of Lourdes outpatient physical medicine and rehabilitation department is compprised of a multi-disciplinary team of physical therapists, oppcuptational therapists and speech languare pathologists.

6344   Rehabilitation Center of Lake Charles Memorial Hospital
1701 Oak Park Boulevard
Lake Charles, LA 70601-8911   337-494-3000
                                  FAX: 337-494-2656
                       webmaster@lcmh.com
                            www.lcmh.com

Dale Shearer, Director
Larry Graham, President/CEO
Ben F. Thompson, MD, Medical Staff President
Ronald Lewis, Jr., Medical Staff President - Elect
Rehabilitation center offering intensive physical, occupational, speech, neuropsychology, recreational therapies along with rehabilitation nursing.

6345   Shriners Hospital for Children-Shreveport
3100 Samford Ave
Shreveport, LA 71103-4239   318-222-5704
                              FAX: 318-424-7610
                       jburda@shrinenet.org
                  www.shrinershospitalsforchildren.org

Richard McCall, Chief of Staff
Phillip Gates, Assistant Chief
An interdisciplinary approach is used in patient care programs to ensure comprehensive care for each patient. The staff includes orthopaedists, pediatricians, nurses, therapists, social workers, child life specialists, and more. The Shreveport Hospital is equipped and staffed to provide care for virtually all pediatric orthopaedic problems, with the exception of acute trauma.

6346   South Louisiana Rehabilitation Hospital
715 W Worthy Rd
Gonzales, LA 70737-3844   225-647-8277
                              FAX: 225-647-2446
                       sober@powerhouseprograms.com
                            www.powerhouseprograms.com

Cody Gautreux, Executive Director
Tonja Randolph, President
Power House Programs is a male only facility for the treatment of Chemical Dependency/Dual Diagnosis, located in Gonzales, Louisiana. Applicants must have participated in a primary treatment program for substance abuse prior to acceptance. Our program is divided into 3 phases and is staffed by Board Certified Social Workers and Board Certified Substance Abuse Counselors. We provide individual, group and family therapy; plus 12 step meetings in a community setting.

6347 **St. Frances Cabrini Hospital: Rehab Unit**
St Frances Cabrini Hospital
3330 Masonic Dr
Alexandria, LA 71301-3899   318-487-1122
                                          FAX: 318-448-6822
                              www.christusstfrancescabrini.org

Curman Gaines, Chairperson
Dallas Hixson, Vice Chairperson
CHRISTUS St. Frances Cabrini Hospital is a 265-bed facility located in Alexandria, Louisiana. Employing approximately 1,400 Associates and with a staff of neary 320 physicians, CHRISTUS St. Frances Cabrini Hospital offers a comprehensive array of services providing the highest quality patient care in a compassionate setting.

6348 **St. Patrick Hospital: Rehab Unit**
524 Doctor Michael Debakey Dr
Lake Charles, LA 70601-5725   337-491-7577
                                          888-722-9355
                                          FAX: 337-430-4284
                              www.christusstpatrick.org

Ellen Jones, CEO
Committed to providing care and service of the highest quality for children and adults, and to ensuring that the basic human rights of expression, decision making and personal dignity are preseved. We are also committed to treating our patients with respect, understanding and Christian love. We realize that this committment involves much more then attending to your medical needs.

6349 **Thibodaux Regional Medical Center**
602 N Acadia Rd
PO Box 1118
Thibodaux, LA 70301-4847   985-447-5500
                                          800-822-8442
                                          FAX: 985-449-4600
                                          info@thibodaux.com
                              www.thibodaux.com

Greg Stock, CEO
Jacob Giardina, Chairman
Andrew Hoffman, Chief of Staff
Mission is to provide the highest quality, most cost effective health care services possible to the people of Thibodaux and surrounding areas. The vision is to be the regional medical center of choice for health care services in the southeast Louisiana by recognizing the value of physicians and employees, committing to quality improvement, partnering with other health care providers, and remaining financially viable in a competitive environment.

Maine

6350 **Brewer Rehab and Living Center**
74 Parkway S
Brewer, ME 04412-1628   207-989-7300
                                          800-359-7412
                                          FAX: 207-989-4240
                              www.brewerrehab.com

Janet Hope, Executive Director
Brewer Rehab and Living Center accomodates 106 residents. We are located in Brewer, Maine. We have a 24-hour nursing staff and experienced dedicated on-site physical therapists, occupational therapists and speech language pathologists. We have a specialized inpatient program for individuals with brain injury resulting from a traumatic injury or neurological event such as a stroke. We also have a specialized care unit for individuals with Alzheimer's disease and other dementias.

6351 **New England Rehabilitation Hospital of Portland**
335 Brighton Ave
Portland, ME 04102-2363   207-662-8000
                                          FAX: 207-879-8168
                                          jaye.sewall@healthsouth.com
                              www.nerhp.org

Elissa Charbonneau, Medical Director
Amy Morse, CEO

Mission is to provide individuals with guidance, education, support, and motivation while helping them achieve maximum independence and function. Our professionals work with the patient and family through a team approach, to establish and implement an individualized rehabilitation plan designed to meet specific patient goals.

Maryland

6352 **Mt. Washington Pediatric Hospital**
1708 W Rogers Ave
Baltimore, MD 21209-4596   410-578-8600
                                          FAX: 410-466-1715
                              www.mwph.org

Sheldon Stein, President
Richard Katz, VP, Medical Affairs
Provides inpatient, outpatient and day programs for infants and children with rehabilitation and/or complex medical needs. We are dedicated to maximizing the rehabilitation and development of our patients through the delivery of interdisciplinary services and programs and providing every resource availiable to enable our patients to attain the highest quality of life within their families and their communities.

Massachusetts

6353 **New Bedford Rehabilitation Hospital**
4499 Acushnet Ave
New Bedford, MA 02745-4707   508-995-6900
                                          FAX: 508-998-8131
                              www.newbedfordrehab.com

6354 **New England Rehabilitation Hospital: Massachusetts**
2 Rehabilitation Way
Woburn, MA 01801-6098   781-939-5050
                                          FAX: 781-933-9257
                              www.newenglandrehab.com

Deniz Ozel, Medical Director
A 168-bed comprehensive inpatient rehabilitation hospital, which includes 2 off-campus satellite units. Offers an array of area outpatient rehabilitation centers. New England Rehabilitation Hospital remains committed to a personal caring approach. The vision is to provide the communities with a complete continuum of acute rehabilitative programs and services.

6355 **Shriners Burns Hospital: Boston**
51 Blossom St
Boston, MA 02114-2623   617-722-3000
                                          800-255-1916
                                          FAX: 617-523-1684
                                          sberkowitz@shrinenet.org
                   www.shrinershospitalsforchildren.org/Hospital

Thomas D'Esmond, Administrator
Matthias Donelan, Chief of Staff
Provides treatment for children to their 18th birthday with acute, fresh burns, plastic reconstructive surgery for patients with healed burns, severe scarring and facial deformity. Some non-burn conditions such as Scalded Skin Syndrome, Cleft Lip, Cleft Palate and purpura fulminians are also treated. Call the Hospital for information. All medical treatment is without cost to the patient, parents, or any third party.

6356 **Shriners Hospital Springfield Unit Springfield Unit for Crippled Children**
516 Carew St
Springfield, MA 01104-2330   413-787-2000
                                          800-237-5055
                                          FAX: 413-787-2009
                   www.shrinershospitalsforchildren.org

Kenneth Guidera, Chief Medical Officer
Eugene D'Amore, Vice President
Kathy A. Dean, Vice President Human Resources
Sharon Russell, VP Finance & Accounting

Shriners Hospital for Children is fully equipped and staffed to provide care for pediatric orthopaedic conditions and disorders.

Michigan

6357 Covenant Healthcare Rehabilitation Program
1447 N Harrison
Saginaw, MI 48602-4316

989-583-2930
FAX: 989-583-0000
www.covenanthealthcare.com

Spence Maidlow, President
Juli Martin, Program Director
Offers a broad spectrum of programs and services ranging from obstetrics, neonatal and pediatric care, to acute care including cardiology, oncology, surgery and many other services on the leading edge of medicine. All our programs and services exemplify our commitment to providing quality, compassionate care. As a medical facility with more then 700 beds, and a complete range of medical services, Covenant stands ready to meet the healthcare needs of the 15 counties in Michigan we serve.

6358 Farmington Health Care Center
34225 Grand River Ave
Farmington, MI 48335-3440

248-477-7373
FAX: 248-477-2888
www.farmingtonhealthcarecenter.com

Brian Garavaglia, Administrator
Skilled nursing facility specializing in ventilator dependent residents.

6359 Flint Osteopathic Hospital: RehabCare Unit
3921 Beecher Rd
Flint, MI 48532-3602

810-606-5000
FAX: 810-762-2153
TTY:888-633-2368
www.genesys.org

Susan Malone, Program Manager
Joy Finkenbiner, Executive Director
Genesys Health System takes great pride in the fact that we strive to deliver the highest quality health care, in a model healing environment, for the entire continuum of care needed throughout one's life. From birth to the twilight years, and everywhere in between, Genesys is there to get you back to the things you love to do.

6360 Integrated Health Services of Michigan at Clarkston
4800 Clintonville Rd
Clarkston, MI 48346-4297

248-674-0903
FAX: 248-674-3359
donna.cook@fundltc.com
www.clarkstonspecialtyhealthcare.com

Carol Doll, Admissions Director
Margaret Canny, Administrator
At Clarkston Specialty Healthcare Center, our mission is to deliver personalized care to the members of our community at a time when our support is most needed. We strive to maximize and enhance the quality of life in a compassionate and professional environment.

6361 St. John Hospital: North Shore
Ascension Health
26755 Ballard St
Harrison Township, MI 48045-2419

586-465-5501
866-501-3627
FAX: 586-466-5352
webcenter@stjohn.org
www.stjohnprovidence.org

David Sessions, CEO
A 96-bed specialty hospital that provides comprehensive physical medicine and rehabilitation, along with a wide range of medical and surgical services. St. John North Shores Hospital also provides emergency and urgent care, extensive outpatient rehabilitation services, and most ancillary diagnostic services.

Minnesota

6362 Alinna Health
800 E 28th St
Minneapolis, MN 55407-3798

612-863-4200
866-880-3550
FAX: 612-863-5698
sisterkenny@allina.com
www.allinahealth.org/ahs/ski.nsf/

Helen Kettner, Nurse-Liaison
Courage Kenny Rehabilitation Institute provides a continuum of rehabilitation services for people with short- and long-term conditions and disabilities in communities throughout Minnesota and western Wisconsin. Our goal is to improve health outcomes, make it easier for clients and families to get the right services for their needs, and reduce costs by preventing complications.

Missouri

6363 Columbia Regional Hospital: RehabCare Unit
404 N Keene St
Columbia, MO 65201-6698

573-882-2501
FAX: 573-449-7588
www.muhealth.org

James Ross, CEO
Anita Larsen, COO
A medical and physical rehabilitation program serving patients throughout Mid-Missouri with functional deficits due to neurologic, orthopaedic or other medical conditions.

6364 Jewish Hospital of St. Louis: Department of Rehabilitation
1 Barnes Jewish Hospital Plz
Saint Louis, MO 63110-1003

314-747-3000
855-925-0631
FAX: 314-454-5277
www.barnesjewish.org

Richard Liedweg, President
Mark Krieger, VP/CFO
John Lynch, Chief Medical Officer
Craig D. Schnuck, Chairman
We take exceptional care of people by providing world-class healthcare, delivering care in a compassionate, respectful and responsive way. By advancing medical knowledge and continously improving our practices. By educating current and future generations of healthcare professionals.

6365 St. Mary's Regional Rehabilitation Center
201 NW R D Mize Rd
Blue Springs, MO 64014-2513

816-228-5900
FAX: 816-655-5348
www.stmaryskc.com

Fleury Yelvington, President/CEO
Amy McKay, Executive Director of Nursing
A 143-bed inpatient physical rehabilitation unit offering PT, OT, ST, recreational therapy, psychiatry and all other ancillary services of a full-service hospital. Specialize in orthopedic and neurologic disabilities.

6366 Three Rivers Health Care
2620 N Westwood Blvd
Poplar Bluff, MO 63901-3396

573-785-7721
800-582-9533
FAX: 573-686-5388
info@pbrmc.hma-corp.com
www.poplarbluffregional.com

Charles Stewart, Market CEO
Gerald Faircloth, Administrator
Melissa Samuelson, Chief Nursing Officer
Kevin Fowler, CFO
Poplar Bluff Regional Medical Center is a regional medical center with 2 hospital campuses and more then 100 active physicians. The 423-bed facility is the largest medical center in Southeast Missouri and is located in ButlerCounty. With outreach clinics in Bloomfield, Dexter, Malden, Piedmont, and Puxico, Poplar Bluff

Regional Medical Center is committed to serving its 6 county region.

Montana

6367   St. Vincent Hospital and Health Center
1233 N 30th St
Billings, MT 59101-165
　　　　　　　　　　　　　　　　406-657-7000
　　　　　　　　　　　　　　FAX: 406-657-8817
　　　　　　　　　　　　　　　　www.svhhc.org

Jason Barker, CEO
Steve Loveless, COO
Joan Thullberry, Chief Nursing Officer
Ron Oldfield, VP Finance

Vision is to be recognized for our vitality, best in class performance and providing easy access to compassionate and trust-worthy healthcare. The healthcare we offer is based on community need. We strive to improve the health status of the community, with a special concern for the poor and those who have limited access to healthcare.

Nebraska

6368   Madonna Rehabilitation Hospital
5401 South St
Lincoln, NE 68506-2150
　　　　　　　　　　　　　　　　402-489-7102
　　　　　　　　　　　　　　　　800-676-5448
　　　　　　　　　　　　　　FAX: 402-483-9406
　　　　　　　　　　　　　　info@madonna.org
　　　　　　　　　　　　　　www.madonna.org

Marsha Lommel, CEO

Provides a complete range of inpatient and outpatient rehabilitation for patients of all ages and abilities. Through highly specialized programs and services, Madona offers individualized treatment and support to help every patient.

Nevada

6369   University Medical Center
1800 W Charleston Blvd
Las Vegas, NV 89102-2386
　　　　　　　　　　　　　　　　702-383-2000
　　　　　　　　　　　　　　FAX: 702-383-2536
　　　　　　　　　　　　　　feedback@umcsn.com
　　　　　　　　　　　　　　　　www.umcsn.com

Brian Brannman, CEO
Lawrence Barnard, Chief Operating Officer
Joan Brookhyser, Chief Medical Officer
Stephanie Merril, Chief Financial Officer

University Medical Center is dedicated to providing the highest level of health care possible by maintaining its ongoing commitment to personal, individualized care for each patient.Through the latest treatment techniques, comfortable surroundings and a dedicated staff, that commitment is expressed every day, in every area of the hospital.

New Hampshire

6370   Head Injury Treatment Program at Dover
307 Plaza Dr
Dover, NH 03820-2455
　　　　　　　　　　　　　　　　603-742-2676
　　　　　　　　　　　　　　FAX: 603-749-5375
　　　　　　　　　　　　　　　　www.doverrehab.com

Sue Mills, Program Rep
Jill Bosa, Administrator

A provider of postacute services in the greater New Hampshire Seacost area. We accomodate 112 residents and are licensed by the state of New Hampshire. We employ nearly 150 licensed nurses, therapists, and other healthcare professionals, who strive to provide quality care. The goal of our patient service model is to bridge the gap between hospitalization and home so that recovery

and physical functioning are maximized and hospital re-admission is minimized.

6371   Lakeview NeuroRehabilitation Center
244 Highwatch Road
Effingham, NH 03882
　　　　　　　　　　　　　　　　603-539-7451
　　　　　　　　　　　　　　　　800-473-4221
　　　　　　　　　　　　　　FAX: 603-539-8815
　　　　　　　　　　　　　　www.lakeviewsystem.com

Anton Merka, Chairman
Carolyn McDermott, President
Christopher Slover,, Chief Executive Officer
Tina M. Trudel, PhD,, Chief Operating Officer

Residential treatment center serving individuals with neurologic/behavioral disorders. Lakeview serves both children and adults in functionally based program environment. Transistional programs in various group homes also available to clients as they progress in their treatment.

6372   Northeast Rehabilitation Hospital
70 Butler St
Salem, NH 03079-3974
　　　　　　　　　　　　　　　　603-893-2900
　　　　　　　　　　　　　　　　800-825-7292
　　　　　　　　　　　　　　FAX: 603-893-1638
　　　　　　　　　　　　　　TTY: 800-439-2370
　　　　　　　　　　　　　webmaster@northeastrehab.com
　　　　　　　　　　　　　　www.northeastrehab.com

John Prochilo, CEO

NRHN is an organization characterized by the positive and proactive commitment to the delivery of customer centered care. Our employees exemplify our organizational commitment to providing quality rehabilitation services throughout the continuum. NRHN will be prudent with all resources and will take individual and collective responsibility for fiscal health. NRHN will remain a model by which other rehabilitation and post acute networks seek to emulate.

6373   St. Joseph Hospital Rehabilitation
172 Kinsley St
Nashua, NH 03060-3688
　　　　　　　　　　　　　　　　603-595-3076
　　　　　　　　　　　　　　　　800-210-9000
　　　　　　　　　　　　　　FAX: 603-595-3635
　　　　　　　　　　　　　　www.stjosephhospital.com

Judy Grilli, Medical Staff Officer

A comprehensive healthcare system that serves the Greater Nashua area, western New Hampshire and Northern Massachusetts. Our hospital is licensed for 208 beds and includes a Level 2 Trauma Center. In addition to the hospital, St. Joseph Healthcare system also includes a satellite emergency center in Milford, 5 family medical centers, a large network of primary care and specialty physician practices.

New Jersey

6374   Betty Bacharach Rehabilitation Hospital
61 W Jimmie Leeds Rd
Pomona, NJ 08240-9102
　　　　　　　　　　　　　　　　609-652-7000
　　　　　　　　　　　　　　FAX: 609-652-7487
　　　　　　　　　　　　　　chrism@bacharach.org
　　　　　　　　　　　　　　www.bacharach.org

Philip J. Perskie, Esq., Chairman
Roy Goldberg, Vice Chairman
Craig Anmuth, Medical Director
Ross Berlin, Medical Director

Therapists, nurses and other specialists, led by physiatrists - doctors specially trained in the medical practice of physical medicine and rehabilitation.

6375 Children's Specialized Hospital
150 New Providence Rd
Mountainside, NJ 07092-2590
908-259-3330
888-344-5373
FAX: 908-233-4176
jbrooks@childrens-specialized.org
www.childrens-specialized.org

Robin A. Walton, Chairwoman
Margaret M. Pego, First Vice Chairwoman
Steven M. Rosenberg, Esq, Second Vice Chairman
Victoria Wicks, Treasurer
New Jersey's largest comprehensive pediatric rehabilitation hospital, treats children and adolescents from birth through 21 years of age. Programs include spinal dysfunction, brain injury, respiratory, burn, Day Hospital, early intervention, preschool, and cognitive rehabilitation. Locations in Fairwood, Roselle Park, Newark, Toms River and Hamilton

6376 HealthSouth Rehabilitation Hospital
14 Hospital Dr
Toms River, NJ 08755-6402
732-244-3100
FAX: 732-244-7790
www.rehabnj.com/tomsriver/

Patty Ostaszewski, CEO
Joseph Stillo, Medical Director
A comprehensive 131-bed medical rehabilitation hospital dedicated to treating individuals with a variety of physical disabilities resulting from injury and illness. We serve all of New Jersey, Manhattan, and Philiadelphia. Accredited by the Joint Commission on Accreditation of Healthcare Organizations (JCAHO). The mission of the hospital is to get people back to work, to play, to living.

6377 JFK Johnson Rehab Institute
65 James St
Edison, NJ 08820-3947
732-321-7070
FAX: 732-321-0994
jfkjri@solarishs.org
www.njrehab.org

Krishna Urs, Physician
David Brown, Physician
JRI has developed programs in such specialties as stroke rehabilitation, orthopedic programs, fitness, cardiac rehabilitation, women's health, pediatrics and brain injury rehabilitation. We also offer the most sophisticated diagnostic services available.

6378 Kessler Institute for Rehabilitation, Welkind Facility
201 Pleasant Hill Rd
Chester, NJ 07930-2141
973-252-6300
FAX: 973-252-6343
jkment@kessler-rehab.com
kessler-rehab.com

Sue Kida, CEO
Sam Bayoumy, Director of Rehabilitation
Bruce Pomeranz, MD, Medical Director
Norma Glennon, Associate Director of Outpatient Rehabilitation
Set in the rolling hills of Morris County, this 72 bed facility provides specialized services to brain injury patients, including our unique Cognitive Redmediation Program, as well as a full range of stroke, amputee and orthopedic services. Kessler's team of dedicated rehabilitation professionals, including physicians, nurses and therapists, work with each patient to build physical strength, optimize movement, maximize independence, increase cognitive skills and address any other issues.

6379 Mediplex Rehab: Camden
1 Cooper Plz
Camden, NJ 08103-1461
856-342-2300
FAX: 856-342-7979
www.cooperhealth.org/content/locationsCamden

John P. Sheridan, Jr. President/CEO
Adrienne Kirby, Phd, President/CEO
Raymond L. Baraldi, Interim Chief Medical Officer
Celeste Johnson, Administrator
Cooper University Hospital is the leading provider of comprehensive health services, medical education and clinical research in Southern New Jersey and the Delaware Valley. With over 550 physicians in over 75 specialties, Cooper is uniquely equipped to provide an almost unlimited number of medical services. The hospital is committed to excellence in medical education, patient care, and research. Offers training programs to medical students, residents, and nurses in a variety of specialties.

6380 Universal Institute Rehabilitation & Fitness Center
15 Microlab Rd
Ste 101
Livingston, NJ 07039
973-992-8181
800-468-5440
FAX: 973-992-7178
www.uirehab.com

Adam Steinberg, President
Lisa Lasso, Vice President, Chief Financial Officer
Universal institute is a 15,000 square foot, state of the art rehabilitation facility that specializes in neurological disorders such as brain injuries, spinal cord injury, strokes, etc. Services include PT, OT, speech patholgy, cognitive remediation, aqua therapy and EMG biofeedback.

New Mexico

6381 HealthSouth Rehabilitation Center: New Mexico
7000 Jefferson St NE
Albuquerque, NM 87109-4357
505-344-9478
800-293-7226
FAX: 505-345-6722
www.healthsouthnewmexico.com

Sylvia Kelly, CEO
Rocky BigCrane, Director of Plant Operations
Lisa Brower, Director of Therapy Operations
Angela Eaton-Walker, M.D, Medical Director
Our hospital offers highly specialized inpatient rehabilitation services. From hip fractures to joint replacements and stroke to Parkinson's disease - our hospital has the experts, technology and experience to meet your rehabilitation needs.

6382 St. Joseph Rehabilitation Hospital and Outpatient Center
Ardence
505 Elm St NE
Albuquerque, NM 87102-2500
505-727-4700
FAX: 505-727-4793
www.sjhs.org

Janelle Raborn, Administrator/CEO
Sherrie Peterson, Director
A member of the four hospital, St. Joseph healthcare system, this facility provides inpatient and outpatient care for those requiring physical medicine and rehabilitation. Specialty programs include brain injury, stroke, spinal cord, orthopedics, occupational and physical therapies, clinical psychology, speech/language pathology, hand clinic and functional capacity evaluations. The only facility in New Mexico accredited in four areas by the commission on accreditation of rehab facilities.

New York

6383 Burke Rehabilitation Hospital
785 Mamaroneck Ave
White Plains, NY 10605-2523
914-597-2500
888-99 -URKE
FAX: 914-946-0866
web@burke.org
www.burke.org

John Ryan, Executive Director
Mary Beth Walsh, M.D., Executive Medical Director/CEO
Brett Langley, Physician .
We provide inpatient and outpatient care for a broad range of neurological, musculoskeletal, cardiac, and pulmonary disabilities caused by disease or injury. Burke treats patients who have suffered a stroke, spinal cord injury, brain injury, amputation, joint replacement, complicated fracture, arthritis, cardiac and pulmonary disease, and neurological disorders. Patients are most frequently transferred to Burke from acute care hospitals once their condition is stable and they are able to partici

6384 **Occupational Therapy Strategies and Adaptations for Independent Daily Living**
Haworth Press
10 Alice St
Binghamton, NY 13904-1503
607-722-5857
800-429-6784
FAX: 607-722-6362
orders@haworthpress.com
www.tandf.co.uk

186 pages Softcover
ISBN 0-866563-50-4

6385 **Rusk Institute of Rehabilitation Medicine**
301 East 17th Street
Second Avenue (in the Hospital for
New York, NY 10016-4901
212-263-6034
FAX: 212-263-8510
DevelopmentOffice@nyumc.org
www.med.nyu.edu/rusk

Steven Flanagan, Chairman
Operates under the auspices of the Dept. Of Rehabilitation Medicine of New York University School of Medicine, one of the nations foremost medical schools. The relationship between Rusk and other clinical and research units within the medical center contributes to an environment which provides the optimal rehabilitation setting for patients. Rusk provides patients with access to treatment across a continuum of care depending on their individual medical needs.

6386 **Silvercrest Center for Nursing & Rehabilitation**
144-45 87th Ave
Briarwood, NY 11435-3109
718-480-4000
800-645-9806
FAX: 718-658-2367
admissions@silvercrest.org
www.silvercrest.org

Andrea Gibbon, Clinical Care Coordinator
Penny Blakely, Unit Manager
The Silvercrest Center for Nursing and Rehabilitation has earned a wide-spread reputatiopn for combing the best in clinical care with the best in nursing care and for making available to its communities the broadest menu of services to ease a patients' path to recovery from hospital to home. The Center is for the treatment of medically complex patients beginning their recovery, for the rehabilitation of patients who need restorative therapy before going home and much more.

6387 **Vocational Rehabilitation and Employment**
Books on Special Children
PO Box 305
Congers, NY 10920-305
845-638-1236
FAX: 845-638-0847
www.vba.va.gov/bln/vre/

372 pages Hardcover

North Carolina

6388 **Horizon Rehabilitation Center**
Trans Health Incorporated
3100 Erwin Rd
Durham, NC 27705-4505
919-383-1546
800-541-7750
FAX: 919-383-0862

6389 **Integrated Health Services of Durham**
Duke University Medical Center
3100 Erwin Rd
Durham, NC 27705-4505
919-383-1546
FAX: 919-383-0862

Aaron Lony, Administrator

6390 **Learning Services Corporation**
Corporate Office
10 Speen St
Ste 4
Framingham, MA 01701-4661
508-626-3671
888-419-9955
FAX: 866-491-7396
www.learningservices.com

Susan Snow, Director of Admissions
Deb. Braunling-McMorrow, Ph, President and CEO
A licensed postacute rehabilitation program for adults who have an acquired brain injury. Individuals who are enrolled in the program participate in active, intensive rehabilitation carried out by a team of neuropsychology, speech/language therapy, physical therapy, occupational therapy, vocational services, family services and life skills training. Services include residential rehabilitation, home based treatment, day treatment, subacute rehabilitation and supported living.

Ohio

6391 **Columbus Rehab & Subacute**
44 S Souder Ave
Columbus, OH 43222-1539
614-228-5900
FAX: 614-228-3989
columbusrehab@extendicare.com
www.columbusrehabskillednursing.com

Kelly Fligor, Administrator
Columbus Rehabilitation and Subacute Institute is a leading provider of long-term skilled nursing care and short-term rehabilitation solutions. Our 120 bed facility offers a full continuum of services and care focused around each individual in today's ever-changing healthcare environment.

6392 **Great Lakes Regional Rehabilitation Center**
3700 Kolbe Rd
Lorain, OH 44053-1611
440-960-3470
FAX: 440-960-4636

Julie Jones, Manager
Provides excellent, innovative and comprehensive rehabilitation programs to people in our community. Committed to a better quality of life for all individuals, the Rehabilitation Center has grown to become a regional resource for individuals needing all types of rehabilitation services.

6393 **HCR Health Care Services**
1 Seagate
Toledo, OH 43604-1541
419-321-5470
800-736-4427
FAX: 419-252-5543
www.harborfund.net

6394 **Heather Hill Rehabilitation Hospital**
Heather Hill
12340 Bass Lake Rd
Chardon, OH 44024-8327
440-285-4040
800-423-2972
FAX: 440-285-0946
info@heatherhill.org

Ed Davis, Operations
Donald Goddard, Chief Medical Officer
Individualized treatment programs for adults and adolescents can participate in and benefit from three-plus hours a day of active therapy.

6395 **Parma Community General Hospital Acute Rehabilitation Center**
7007 Powers Blvd
Parma, OH 44129-5437
440-743-3000
FAX: 440-843-4387
www.parmahospital.org

David Nedrich, Chairman
Thomas P. O'Donnell, First Vice Chairman
Nancy E. Hatgas, Second Assistant Treasurer
Alex I. Koler, First Assistant Treasurer

Parma Hospital offers acute and subacute inpatient care including specialty centers for heart, cancer, robotic surgery, orthopedics, pain management, acute rehabilitation and bariatric care.

6396 Rehabilitation Institute of Ohio at Miami Valley Hospital
1 Wyoming St
Dayton, OH 45409-2793   937-208-8000
                               TTY:937-208-2006
                               www.miamivalleyhospital.com

Vanessa Sandarusi, Executive Director
Anita Marie Greer, Program Manager, Acute Therapy Services
Jessica Hallum, Nurse Manager of the Inpatient Rehabilitation Unit
Phillip Boarman, Clinical Coordinator for Acute Care Occupational Therapy and

The Miami Valley Hospital Rehabilitation Institute of Ohio (RIO) is one of the largest and most comprehensive rehabilitation services providers in the United States. RIO offers a full spectrum of specialized rehabilitation programs delivered by the region's most experienced rehabilitation experts.

6397 Shriners Burn Institute: Cincinnati Unit
Shriners Hospitals for Children Cincinnati
3229 Burnet Ave
Cincinnati, OH 45229-3095   513-872-6000
                                   800-875-8580
                              FAX: 513-872-6999
                              vmosley@shrinenet.org
                   www.shrinershospitalsforchildren.org

Richard Kagan, Chief of Staff
Petra Warner, Assistant Chief of Staff
Tony Lewgood, Interim Administrator
Vanessa Mosley, Development Officer

All the attention and resources are focused on just one kind of patient-the burn-injured child. Shriners combine excellent clinical skill, compassionate care, and innovative research, providing comprehensive pediatric burn care and reconstructive rehabilitation to achieve the best possible outcome for a child that has suffered a burn injury. There is never a charge to the patient or family for any of the medical care or services provided by the Shriners Hospitals throughout North America.

6398 St. Francis Health Care Centre
401 N Broadway St
Green Springs, OH 44836-9653   419-639-2626
                                      800-248-2552
                                 FAX: 419-639-6225
                                 hr@sfhcc.org
                                 www.sfhcc.org

Kim Eicher, CEO
Jane Holmer, Admissions Coordinator

Provides compassionate care for the elderly and physically challenged. We are a healthcare ministry under the sponsorship of the Franciscan Sisters of Our Lady of Perpetual Help. As a Catholic facility. we respectfully offer those we serve, care hope and dignity in a joyful and compassionate manner.

6399 St. Rita's Medical Center Rehabilitation Services
730 W Market St
Lima, OH 45801-4602   419-227-3361
                             800-232-7762
                        FAX: 419-226-9750
                        www.ehealthconnection.com

James Reber, CEO

The St. Rita's Inpatient Acute Care Rehabilitation service provides individualized service to you or your family member 7 days a week, wherever you might stay in the hospital. Acute rehabilitation care includes physical, occupational, and speech therapy services. Our goal is to make you as independent as possible before your discarge to home or, when necessary to extended services in other parts of the hospital.

6400 University of Cincinnati Hospital
Health Alliance
234 Goodman St
Cincinnati, OH 45219-2316   513-584-1000
                              FAX: 513-584-7712
                   www.universityhospital.uchealth.com

James Kingsbury, President/CEO

University Hospital has an international reputation, bringing thousands of people, from the region and around the world to Cincinnati to receive care from world renowned physicians in state-of-the-art medical facilities.

6401 Upper Valley Medical/Rehab Services
3130 N County Road
25-A
Troy, OH 45373-1309   937-440-4000
                        FAX: 937-440-7337
                        info@uvmc.com
                        www.uvmc.com

Rafay Atiq, Director Rehab Services

A not-for-profit health care system serving the health care needs of Miami County and the surrounding area. The health care system features a state-of-the-art acute care hospital which opened in 1998. Comprehensive inpatient and outpatient services are provided with a full compliment of diagnostic and treatment services and behavioral health care programs.

Oklahoma

6402 Hilcrest Medical Center: Kaiser Rehab Center
1125 S Trenton Ave
Tulsa, OK 74120-5498   918-579-7100
                         FAX: 918-579-7110
                         www.hillcrest.com/kaiser

Perri Craven, Medical Director

Kaiser Rehabilitation Center offers a wide range of services to help people regain functionality and independence after a debilitating injury or illness. Our approach to rehabilitation is a team approach, bringing the expertise of physicians, therapists, nurses and other health professionals together with patient family to achieve the best possible outcome. Each patient is given an individualized treatment plan that stimulates and challenges them to achieve their maximum potential.

6403 Jane Phillips Medical Center
Jane Phillips Medical Center
3500 E Frank Phillips Blvd
Bartlesville, OK 74006-2464   918-333-7200
                                 FAX: 918-331-1360
                                 webmaster@jpmc.org
                                 www.jpmc.org

David Stire, CEO
Mike Moore, CFO

Jane Phillips Health System is sponsored by St. John Health System. This partnership helps our patients by ensuing access to the most sophisticated levels of care availiable in this area. It offers a wide range of services, including general medicine, surgery, cardiopulmonary care, maternal and infant care, cancer treatment, geriatric care, orthopedics, and physical medicine.

6404 Jim Thorpe Rehabilitation Center at Southwest Medical Center
Southwest Medical Center
4100 S. Douglas Ave.
Oklahoma City, OK 73109   405-644-5445
                                 800-677-1238
                            FAX: 405-644-5384
                            www.integris-health.com

Al Moorad, Medical Director

Provides inpatient rehabilitation for people with head injuries, spinal cord injuries, orthopedic conditions, pain management, neurological diseases, strokes and a variety of diagnoses that stop individuals from being able to take care of themselves independently. Services available include medical direction, physical therapy, social work, occupational therapy, speech therapy, recreational therapy, and aftercare follow-up.

6405 Mercy Memorial Health Center-Rehab Center
1011 14th Ave NW
Ardmore, OK 73401-1828   580-223-5400
                                          800-572-1182
                                    FAX: 580-220-6463
                                          www.mercy.net

Jan Shores, Manager
Lynn Britton Britton, President/CEO
Randy Combs, Executive Vice President Strategic Growth
Michael McCurry, Executive Vice President/Chief Operating Officer
A full service tertiary hospital with 176 licensed beds, 913 co-workers and 100 physicians. Four primary care clinics

6406 St. Anthony Hospital: Rehabilitation Unit
St. Anthony Hospital
1000 N Lee Ave
Oklahoma City, OK 73102-1036   405-272-7000
                                          800-851-0888
                                    FAX: 405-272-7075
                                    st_anthony@ssmhc.com
                                          www.saintsok.com

S Beaver, President
18 spacious private rooms, each with bathroom, and furnishings designed with patient safety in mind. Horticulture room where patients can work with plants and flowers as part of their rehabilitation. And a residential-style training apartment with fully equipped kitchen, bathroom, and bedroom to make the patient feel more at home.

6407 Valir Health
700 NW 7th St
Oklahoma City, OK 73102-1212   405-609-3600
                                         888-898-2080
                                   FAX: 405-605-8638
                                         info@valir.com
                                         www.valir.com

Dirk O'Hara, Principal
Tonya Purvine, Corporate Compliance Officer
Inpatient Rehab Facility including all therapy services serving people who have been injured and had an illness resulting in a decreased level of independence.

Oregon

6408 Shriners Hospitals for Children: Portland
3101 SW Sam Jackson Park Rd
Portland, OR 97239-3095   503-241-5090
                                          800-237-5055
                                    FAX: 503-221-3701
                                    mthoreson@shrinenet.org
                            www.shrinershospitalsforchildren.org

Michael Aiona, Chief of Staff
Craig Patchin, Administrator
Mark Thoreson, Development Officer
Joslyn Davidson, M.D, Anesthesiology
Pediatric orthopedic and plastic surgery; inpatient and outpatient services. No charge for any services provided at the Hospital. Diagnosis, rehabilitation, surgery, sports and recreation for ages 0-18 for people with physical disabilities involving bones, muscles or joints or in need of plastic surgery for burn scars or cleft lip/palate.

Pennsylvania

6409 Allied Services John Heinz Institute of Rehabilitation Medicine
150 Mundy St
MAC III Building, 1st Floor
Wilkes Barre, PA 18702-6830   570-826-3900
                                    FAX: 570-830-2027
                                    tpugh@allied-services.org
                                          www.allied-services.org

Gerald Franceski, Chairman
Thomas Speicher, Vice-Chairman
William Conaboy, CEO
Gregory Basting, VP Medical Affairs
John Heinz Rehab is one of the foremost providers of rehabilitation in the country. Under the supervision of board-certified psychiatrists, a team of highly qualified professionals provides a broad range of specialized services and therapies for inpatients, with speacialized programs in the areas of brain injury, injured worker recovery and pediatrics. John Heinz Rehab is the only CARF accredited program in northeastern Pennsylvania for treatment of brain injury rehabilitation.

6410 Allied Services Rehabilitation Hospital
475 Morgan Hwy
Scranton, PA 18508-2656   570-348-1359
                                    FAX: 570-341-4548
                                          www.allied-services.org

Gerald Franceski, Chairman
Thomas Speicher, Vice-Chairman
William Conaboy, CEO
Gregory Basting, VP Medical Affairs
We are committed to the people of our community, to help them overcome challenges and reach their greatest potential by providing quality care, people-oriented services and comfort. Our approach is a hands-on, people-oriented style which places the physical and emotional needs of those in our care at the center of all we do. Whether in our rehabilitation hospitals, our skilled nursing facilities, or mental health/mental retardation program, we strive to help people reach their potential.

6411 Brighten Place
131 North Main St
Chalfont, PA 18914-245   215-997-7746
                                    FAX: 215-997-2517
                                    brightenplace@enter.net
                                          www.brightenplace.org
William Koffros, CEO
A residential brain injury program with the mission to encourage growth and foster independence on an individual level for each resident. We are CARF accredited and provide additional services which include a day program and respite care.

6412 Chestnut Hill Rehabilitation Hospital
8601 Stenton Ave
Wyndmoor, PA 19038-8312   215-233-6200
                                    FAX: 215-233-6879
                                          www.extendedcare.com

Cammi Lubking, Administrator
Chestnut Hill Rehab Hospital is dedicated to meeting patients' physical, emotional, social, and vocational goals. Through innovative programs, sophisticated equipment, and support by specially trained staff members committed to the progress of every patient, Chestnut Hill achieves results.

6413 Doylestown Hospital Rehabilitation Center
595 W State St
Doylestown, PA 18901-2597   215-345-2200
                                    FAX: 215-345-2512
                                          www.dh.org

James Brexler, President and Chief Executive Officer
Eleanor Wilson, RN, MSN, MHA, Vice President, Patient Services/Chief Operating Officer
Dan Upton, Vice President, Chief Financial Officer
Scott S. Levy, MD, Vice President, Chief Medical Officer
The mission of Doylestown Hospital is to provide a responsive healing environment for patients and their families, and to im-

prove the quality of life for all members of our community. We combine the creative energies of Medical Staff, Board, Associates and Volunteers to make Doylestown Hospital a place where each patient and family feels healed and whole, even when disease cannot be cured.

6414   **Health Care Solutions**
500 Abbott Dr
Ste B
Broomall, PA 19008-4301   610-544-6023
                                       800-451-1671
                                  FAX: 610-544-6035
                                   www.lincare.com

John Byrnes, CEO
Shawn Schabel, President/COO
Develops unique containment programs, offers equipment set-up, patient instruction, patient assessment and equipment usage. Offers clinical services that include oxygen systems, ventilators, aerosol therapy, suction equipment, T.E.N.S. programs, compression pumps, custom orthotics, enteral feeding.

6415   **HealthSouth Harmarville Rehabilitation Hospital**
P.O. Box 11460
320 Guys Run Road
Pittsburgh, PA 15238-460   412-828-1300
                                        877-937-7342
                                  FAX: 412-828-7705
                          www.healthsouthharmarville.com
Ken Anthony, Chief Executive Officer
Thomas Franz, M.D., Medical Director
Catherine M. Birk, M.D., Staff Physiatrist
Brian Cicuto, D.O., Staff Physiatrist
A 202-bed facility providing inpatient and outpatient physical medicine and rehabilitation to adults and adolescents in Pennsylvania, West Virginia, Ohio and Maryland.

6416   **HealthSouth Nittany Valley Rehabilitation Hospital**
Health South of Nittany Valley
550 W College Ave
Pleasant Gap, PA 16823-7401   814-359-3421
                                        800-842-6026
                                  FAX: 814-359-5898
                           www.nittanyvalleyrehab.com
Richard Allatt, Medical Director
Susan Hartman, CEO
Sara Godwin, CNO
Ann Foster, Therapy Operations Director
Comprehensive inpatient and outpatient facilities. Treatment for symptoms relating to: stroke, head injury, pulmonary disease, orthopedic conditions, neurological disorders, cardiac illnesses and spinal cord injuries. Healthsouth Nittany Valley Rehabilitation Hospital is a part of Healthsouth's national network of more than 2,000 facilities in 50 states.

6417   **HealthSouth Rehab Hospital Of Erie**
143 E 2nd St
Erie, PA 16507-1501   814-878-1200
                                        800-234-4574
                                  FAX: 814-878-1399
                              www.healthsoutherie.com
Douglas Grisier, Medical Director
Shelly Mayes, Director of Therapy Operations
An acute inpatient rehabilitation hospital that was founded in 1986. HealthSouth Erie is one of the only rehabilitation hospitals in the country to hold a triple-certification by the Joint Commission in the areas of Brain Injury, Stroke and Parkinson's disease Rehabilitation.

6418   **HealthSouth Rehabilitation Hospital of Altoona**
2005 Valley View Blvd
Altoona, PA 16602-4548   814-944-3535
                                        800-873-4220
                                  FAX: 814-944-6160
                            www.healthsouthaltoona.com
Scott Filler, Chief Executive Officer
Paul Sutton, Director Of Clinical Services
Rakesh (Rock Patel, D.O., Medical Director
Mary Gen Boyles, Director of Nursing Services

Inpatient and outpatient physical rehabilitation programs and services.

6419   **Healthsouth Rehabilitation Hospital of Greater Pittsburgh**
2380 McGinley Rd
Monroeville, PA 15146-4400   412-856-2400
                                  FAX: 412-856-9320
                           www.lifecare-hospitals.com
Mary Lee Dadey, Administrator
Rehabilitation and long-term acute care hospital that treats brain injury, stroke, multiple sclerosis, Parkinson's disease, back and spinal cord injuries, cancer, pulmonary disease, cardiac disease, traumatic and work injuries.

6420   **Healthsouth Rehabilitation Hospital of Mechanicsburg**
175 Lancaster Blvd
Mechanicsburg, PA 17055-3562   717-691-3700
                                        800-933-3831
                                  FAX: 717-697-6524
                         annette.bates@healthsouth.com
                              www.healthsouthpa.com
Mark Freeburn, CEO
Annette Bates, Director of Marketing Operations
Jeff Brandenburg, MPT, Director of Therapy Operations
Michael F. Lupinacci, M.D., Medical Director
HealthSouth provides comprehensive rehabilitation and recovery services to patients with stroke, brain injury, hip fracture, medically complex, pulmonary, wound, spinal cord injury, amputation, and other neuro-muscular, and orthopedic impairments. Our primary goal is to provide individualized treatment programs to people requiring physical rehabilitation and medical recovery in order to help patients get back to work, to play, to living.

6421   **Healthsouth Rehabilitation Hospital of York**
1850 Normandie Dr
York, PA 17408-1552   717-767-6941
                                  FAX: 717-767-8776
                              www.healthsouthyork.com
Sally Arthur, Director of Human Resources
Bruce Sicilia, Medical Director
Elaine Charest, Director of Therapy Operations
Daniel C. DeFalcis, M.D., Associate Medical Director
A 120-bed rehabilitation hospital dedicated to providing advanced, comprehensive services to patients who have suffered head injury, spinal cord injury, stroke, burns, amputation, chronic pain and other neurological and musculoskeletal disorders. HRH of York provides outpatient services in seven locations. Healthsouth is located in York, Pennsylvania, approximately 50 miles north of Baltimore and 25 miles south of Harrisburg.

6422   **Magee Rehabilitation Hospital**
1513 Race St
Philadelphia, PA 19102-1177   215-587-3000
                                        800-966-2433
                                  FAX: 215-568-3736
                           hskoczen@mageerehab.org
                               www.mageerehab.org
Jack Carroll, CEO
A not-for-profit health organization which is the home to the nation's first brain injury rehabilitation program to be accredited by the Commission on the Accreditation of Rehabilitation Facilities (CARF) and is one of 14 federally designated Regional Spinal Cord Injury Centers. Our staff and management are committed to restoring the highest level of independence possible to individuals with disabilities.

6423   **Moss Rehabilitation Hospital**
1200 W Tabor Rd
Philadelphia, PA 19141-3099   215-456-9800
                                  FAX: 215-456-9381
                               www.mossrehab.com
Alberto Esquenazi, Plant Manager
Alberto Esquenazi, MD, Director
Carmen Angles, MD, Director
Cynthia Farrell, DO, Director
The Philadelphia region's major resource for medical rehabilitation since 1959. This 152 bed facility offers comprehensive care

to people with broad ranges of conditions, diagnostic laboratories and a multidisciplinary team of rehabilitation professionals.

6424   Shriners Hospitals for Children, Philadelphia
Shrinners Hospitals for Children
3551 N Broad St
Philadelphia, PA 19140-4131   215-430-4000
                                             800-281-4051
                                        FAX: 215-430-4126
                                         www.shrinershq.org
Alan W. Madsen, Chairman of the Board
John A. Cinotto, 1st Vice President
Dale W. Stauss, 2nd Vice President
Ernest Perilli, Administrator
At Shriners Hospitals for Childrenr - Philadelphia, we provide state-of-the-art medical care for children with spinal cord injuries, as well as a host of orthopaedic and neuromusculoskeletal disorders and diseases

6425   Shriners Hospitals for Children, Erie
1645 W 8th St
Erie, PA 16505-5007   814-875-8700
                                        FAX: 814-875-8756
                                         www.shrinershq.org
John Lubahn, Chief of Staff
Charles Walczak, Administrator
The Shriners Hospitals for Children, Erie, is a 30-bed pediatric orthopaedic hospital providing comprehensive orthopaedic care to children at no charge. The hospital is one of 22 Shriners Hospitals throughout North America. The Erie Hospital accepts and treats children with routine and complex orthopaedic and neuromuscular problems, utilizing the latest treatments and technology available in pediatric orthopaedics, resulting in early ambulation and reduced length of stay.

6426   Shriners Hospitals, Philadelphia Unit, for Crippled Children
3551 N Broad St
Philadelphia, PA 19140-4105   215-430-4000
                                        FAX: 215-430-4079
                                www.shrinershq.org/hospitals/philadelphia
Randal Betz, Chief of Staff
Ernest Perilli, Administrator
Provides comprehensive medical, surgical and rehabilitative care for children with orthopaedic conditions and spinal cord injuries. All services are provided at no charge. The hospital is one of 22 located throughout North America. In addition to treating children with routine and complex orthopaedic problems, the Philadelphia hospital provides a comprehensive and individualized rehabilitation program for children and adolescents who have sustained a traumatic injury to their spine.

South Carolina

6427   Colleton Regional Hospital: RehabCare Unit
501 Robertson Blvd
Walterboro, SC 29488-5714   843-782-2000
                                        FAX: 843-549-7562
                                       www.colletonmedical.com
Mitchell Mongel, CEO
Colleton Medical Center's 8-bed physical and mental rehabilitation department is the oldest in the Lowcountry and has been serving the community for nearly 20 years. Strives to provide patient-centered care in a family atmosphere. The team includes nurses, physical therapists, occupational therapists, speech therapists, and nutritionists. The typical patient requires rehabilitation following a stroke, spinal injury, close head injury, and orthopedic rehabilitation.

6428   HealthSouth Rehab Hospital: South Carolina
2935 Colonial Dr
Columbia, SC 29203-6811   803-254-7777
                                        FAX: 803-414-1414
                                    www.healthsouthcolumbia.com
W. Anthony Jackson, CEO
Lydia Carpenter, Director of Therapy Operations
Devin Troyer, M.D., Medical Director
Luanne Burton, Director of Human Resources
Offers a wide range of specialized medical and therapeutic services designed to help physically disabled individuals reach their optimum level of function and independence.

6429   Shriners Hospitals for Children, Greenville
950 W Faris Rd
Greenville, SC 29605-4255   864-271-3444
                                             866-459-0013
                                        FAX: 864-271-4471
                                      tmcreynolds@shrinenet.org
                              www.shrinershq.org/hospitals/greenville
Randall Romberger, Administrator
Peter Stasikelis, Chief of Staff
Tracy McReynolds,, Development Officer
A 50-bed pediatric orthopaedic hospital providing comprehensive orthopaedic care to children at no charge to their families. The hospital is one of 22 Shriners Hospitals throughout North America. The hospital accepts and treats children with routine and complex orthopaedic problems, utilizing the latest tretments and technology availiable in pediatric orthopaedics, resulting in early ambulatory and reduced length of stay.

Tennessee

6430   Health South Cane Creek Rehabilitation Center
Health South Corporation
180 Mount Pelia Rd
Martin, TN 38237-3812   731-587-4231
                                        FAX: 731-588-1454
                                   dayle.unger@healthsouth.com
                                    www.healthsouthcanecreek.com
Eric Garrard, CEO
William Eason, Medical Director
Lindsey Box-Rotger, BSN, RN, C, Director of Quality and Risk Management
Cindy Cooper, RN, Director of Case Management
Offers a wide variety of programs and services for patients in need of acute rehabilitation. Programs and services are availiable through inpatient and outpaitent. Thereapy services availiable are physical, occupational, speech, and respiratory.

6431   HealthSouth Chattanooga Rehabilitation Hospital
2412 McCallie Ave
Chattanooga, TN 37404-3398   423-697-9129
                                             800-763-5189
                                        FAX: 423-697-9124
                                  www.healthsouthchattanooga.com
Scott Rowe, CEO
Amjad Munir, Medical Director
Karen Jonakin, Director Clinical Services
Offers orthopaedic rehabilitation, stroke rehabilitation, amputee rehabilitation, brain injury program, pain management, ventilator weaning, carpal tunnel screening, low intensity program, oncology program, aquatic therapy, day treatment, burn program and outpatient services.

6432   HealthSouth Rehabilitation Cntr/Tennessee
1282 Union Ave
Memphis, TN 38104-3414   901-722-2000
                                        FAX: 901-729-5171
                                      healthsouthmemphis.com
Tracy Willis, CEO
Toni Wackerfuss, Director of Therapy Operation
An 80-bed acute medical rehabilitation hospital that offers comprehensive inpatient and outpatient rehabilitation services.

6433   James H And Cecile C Quillen Rehabilitation Hospital
2511 Wesley St
Johnson City, TN 37601-1723   423-952-1700
                                            800-235-1994
                                     FAX: 423-283-0906
                                            www.msha.com

Tammy Bishop, Manager
A 60-bed, freestanding comprehensive medical rehabilitation hospital. Full range of outpatient and day treatment, 14-bed traumatic brain injury unit, in ground therapeutic pool, transitional living apartment, outdoor ambulation course. All inpatient and outpatient programs utilize an interdisciplinary team approach designed to improve a patient's physical and cognitive functioning.

6434   Nashville Rehabilitation Hospital
610 Gallatin Ave
Nashville, TN 37206-3225   615-650-2600
                                            800-227-3108
                                     FAX: 615-650-2562
                                            www.nrhcares.com

Alan Miller, CEO
Marc Miller, President
A free-standing physical rehabilitation facility offering services to patients on an inpatient and outpatient basis. Programs include CVA, orthopedic, neuromuscular, traumatic brain injury, spinal cord injury, general rehabilitation and Bridges - geriatric psychiatric unit. Intra-disciplinary team approach is utilized to assist patients in obtaining their maximum fuctional level.

6435   Patricia Neal Rehab Center : Ft. Sanders Regional Medical Center
Covenant Health
1901 W Clinch Ave
Knoxville, TN 37916-2307   865-541-1111
                                            800-728-6325
                                     FAX: 865-541-2247
                                            www.patneal.org

J.E. Henry, Co-Chair
David Kugley, Co-Chair
Mary Dillon, M.D., Medical Director, Patricia Neal Rehabilitation Center
Sharon E. Glass, M.D., Stroke Program Director, Patricia Neal Rehabilitation Center
A CARF accredited 73-bed facility, it offers a comprehensive team approach to care. Physical, occupational, recreational, behavioral medicine and speech language therapists work with physiatrists to develop individual plans of care designed to return patients to a normal lifestyle as quickly as possible. In addition, rehabilitation nurses collaborate with specialists to teach self-care techniques and provide education to help patients reach optimal functionality.

6436   Rehabilitation Center Baptist Hospital
137 E Blount Ave
Suite 6-B
Knoxville, TN 37920-1643   865-632-5520

6437   Rehabilitation Center at McFarland Hospital
University Medical Center
500 Park Ave
Lebanon, TN 37087-3721   615-449-0500
                                     FAX: 615-453-7405
                                     www.universitymedicalcenter.com
Saad Ehtisham, CEO
Matt Caldwell, Chief Executive Officer
Michael Cherry, Chief Financial Officer
Greg Carda, Chief Operating Officer
An Acute Inpatient Rehab, located on the hospital's second floor. The center has 26 patient rooms, three therapy treatment rooms, a patient dining area, and an 'activities of daily living' area which includes a kitchen/laundry area and a patient apartment, for those individuals who will be returning home.

6438   St. Mary's Medical Center: RehabCare Center
900 E Oak Hill Ave
Knoxville, TN 37917-4505   865-545-7962
                                     FAX: 865-545-8133
                                            www.tennova.com

Jeffrey Ashin, President
Committed to providing individualized and flexable treatment programs designed for individuals who have been disabled by an injury or illness. The primary mission of the RehabCare Center is to help patients achieve basic skills that may allow independent living and working.

6439   Sumner Regional Medical Center
555 Hartsville Pike
Gallatin, TN 37066-2400   615-328-8888
                                     FAX: 615-328-3903
                                     www.mysumnermedical.com

Susan Peach, BSN, MBA, CEO
Kevin Rinks, Chief Financial Officer
Michael S. Herman, Chief Operating Officer
Anne Melton, RN, MSN, Chief Nursing Officer
SRMC operates as a 155-bed healthcare facility and provides quality Gallatin hospital and medical care services in numerous areas, including cancer treatment, cardiac care, same- day surgery, orthopaedics, diagnostics, women's health and rehabilitation services. As the community grows, SRMC strives to continually improve its services and programs to meet the changing needs of its service area.

Texas

6440   Bayshore Medical Center: Rehab
4000 Spencer Hwy
Pasadena, TX 77504-1202   713-359-2000
                                     FAX: 713-359-1283
                                     www.bayshoremedical.com

Dr. Charles Bessire, Board
Jeanna Barnard, FACHE,, CEO
Alice Hopkins Adams, Board
Wilfred J. Broussard, Board
A 345-bed facility, providing the award-winning care for which we have been nationally recoginzed. Members are here to care for the physical and emotional well-being of those who arrive at Bayshore Medical Center often frightned, in pain and perhaps even alone. We offer patients solace and security through constant communication and compassionate listening in the midst of their medical emergencies and surgical or diagnostic procedures. Kindness, empathy & quality are triats that patients trust.

6441   Cecil R Bomhr Rehabilitation Center of Nacogdoches Memorial Hospital
1204 N Mound St
Nacogdoches, TX 75961-4027   936-564-4611
                                     FAX: 936-564-4616
                                            info@nacmem.org
                                            www.nacmem.org

Jerry Whitaker, Chairperson
Larry Walker, M.D., Vice-Chairperson
Lisa King, Secretary
Walter Scott, Board Member
The goal of Nacogdoches Memorial Hospital's rehabilitation services is to assist patients in attaining their highest potential activity level for independent daily living, thereby reducing the number of necessary hospitalizations. Keeping folks healthy and in their homes lowers healthcare costs for all of us.

6442   Covenant Health Systems Owens White Outpatient Rehab Center
9812 Slide Rd
Lubbock, TX 79424-1116   806-725-5627
                                     FAX: 806-723-6009
                                     www.covenanthealth.org

Walt Cathey, Manager
A comprehensive rehabilitation program designed to help patients attain their maximum level of independence following a debilitating stroke, illness or injury. Our fully accredited program

features outpatient physical, occupational and speech language therapies, as well as certified athletic trainers and a certified strength and conditioning specialist.

6443 Gonzales Warm Springs Rehabilitation Hospital
200 Memorial Dr
Luling, TX 78648-3213
830-875-8400
FAX: 830-875-5029
www.warmsprings.org

Anthony Misitano, President/CEO
Vonnie Cromwell, Operations Manager

Statewide not-for-profit system of inpatient and outpatient rehabilitation speciality centers. Throughout the communities we serve, the Warm Springs Rehabilitation System offers hope and acts as a catalyst for achieving an optimal quality of life by providing comprehensive physical and/or cogenitve care. Investing resources in educational and recreational programs. Supporting research efforts.

6444 Harris Methodist Fort Worth Hospital Mabee Rehabilitation Center
1301 Pennsylvania Ave
Fort Worth, TX 76104-2122
817-250-2760
866-847-7342
FAX: 814-250-6846
www.texashealth.org

Lillie Biggins, B.S.N., M.S.N, CEO/President
Elaine Nelson, R.N., M.S.N., Chief Nursing Officer
Joseph Prosser, M.D., M.B.A., Chief Medical Officer

Professionals at the Harris Methodist Fort Worth Hospital's Mabee Rehabilitation Center work closely with each patient to develop a specialzed treatment plan for personal achievement. The center offers highly trained clinical staff members and spacious facilities An incredibly wide range of treatment programs and educational services are provided for both inpatient and outpatient needs.

6445 HealthSouth Plano Rehabilitation Hospital
6701 Oakmont Blvd.
Fort Worth, TX 76132-7526
817-370-4700
FAX: 972-423-4293
www.healthsouth.com

Jon F. Hanson, Chairman
John W. Chidsey, Board of director
Donald L. Correll, Board of director
Yvonne M. Curl, Board of director

A 62-bed medical reahabilitation facility serving inpatient and out patient needs in the Northern Dallas area. The team coordinate all aspects of the patient's rehabilitation to maximize results. The overall effort is directed by board-certified physical medicine and rehabilitation physicians who specialize in medical rehabilitation. Whatever the cause of the disability, our services can benefit patients who have functional limitations in such areas as mobility, communication and self care.

6446 HealthSouth Rehab Hospital Of Arlington
3200 Matlock Rd
Arlington, TX 76015-2911
817-468-4000
FAX: 817-468-3055
www.healthsouth.com

Jon F. Hanson, Chairman
John W. Chidsey, Board of director
Donald L. Correll, Board of director
Yvonne M. Curl, Board of director

A modern 65-bed hospital dedicated to providng inpatient programs in a general rehabilitation setting for persons recovering for a disabling injury or illness. As part of our continuum of care, we also offer outpatient therapy, a day program, and individual therapy services. Our goal is to help our patients resume a productive and more meaningful life through appropriate rehabilitative care and restorative nursing in a wellness-oriented environment that promotes healing and functional recovery.

6447 HealthSouth Rehab Hospital Of Austin
1215 Red River St
Austin, TX 78701-1921
512-474-5700
FAX: 512-479-3765
www.healthsouthaustin.com

Duke Saldiver, CEO
Corey Helm Swartz, Director of Therapy Operations
Maria Arizmendez, M.D., Medical Director
Debbie Belcher, Human Resource Director

A comprehensive 83 bed medical rehabilitation hospital serving the needs of patients in the Central Texas area. The mission is to promote recovery for persons with disabling conditions by providing individualized treatment so they can reach the highest level of physical, social and emotional well-being.

6448 HealthSouth Rehabilitation Center of Humble Texas
19002 McKay Blvd
Humble, TX 77338
281-446-6148
FAX: 281-446-5616
www.healthsouthhumble.com

Angie Simmons, CEO
Mikael Simpson, Director of Therapy Operations
Emile Mathurin, Jr., M.D., Medical Director
Christy Dixon, Human Resources Director

Offers comprehensive rehabilitation services for patients with diverse diagnoses. Rehabilitation can be defined as multidisciplinary therapy designed to increase patient's overall functioning to a level that meets or exceeds where the patient was prior to illness or injury or to maximize current level of ability. The benefits of these services to patients and their families is invaluable.

6449 HealthSouth Rehabilitation Hospital
6701 Oakmont Blvd
Fort Worth, TX 76132-2957
817-370-4700
FAX: 817-370-4977
www.healthsouthcityview.com

Deborah Hopps, CEO
Mark Bussell, Medical Director
Mark Bussell, M.D., Medical Director
Kenneth Akwar, PharmD, Director of Pharmacy

A 62-bed acute medical rehabilitation hospital that offers comprehensive inpatient and outpatient rehabilitation services.

6450 HealthSouth Rehabilitation Hospital of Beaumont
3340 Plaza 10 Dr
Beaumont, TX 77707-2551
409-835-0835
FAX: 409-835-0898
www.healthsouthbeaumont.com

Sam Coco, Director of Therapy Operations
HJ Gaspard, CEO
Linda Smith, M.D., Medical Director
Sam Coco, PT, Director of Therapy Operations

A state of the art freestanding 61-bed comprehensive physical rehabilitation hospital. The hospital is specifically designed to meet the needs of individuals and their families who have experienced a disabling injury or illness or are recovering from a surgery. An experienced team of physicians, nurses, therapists, treat conditions and other disorders.

6451 HealthSouth Rehabilitation Institute Of San Antonio (RIOSA)
9119 Cinnamon Hill
San Antonio, TX 78240-5401
210-691-0737
FAX: 210-558-1297
www.hsriosa.com

Scott Butcher, CEO
Richard Senelick, Medical Director
Christine Chesnut, OTR, MPH, Director of Therapy Operations
Linda Hart, LVN, Director of Marketing

HealthSouth Rehabilitation Institute of San Antonio is the largest free-standing physical rehabilitation hospital in San Antonio and is proud to enter our 11th year of delivering quality, comprehensive medical rehabilitation in a pristine environment. HealthSouth annually serves over 1,500 inpatients and more then 20,000 outpatient visits from throughout San Antonio and Mexico. 108-bed hospital has more then 300 personell on staff providing extensive experience.

6452   Hillcrest Baptist Medical Center: Rehab Care Unit
100 Hillcrest Medical Blvd
Waco, TX 76712-3239   254-202-2000
                                   FAX: 254-202-8975
                           marketing@hillcrest.net
                                   www.hillcrest.net

Fred Walters, President
Jon Ellis, Secretary
A fully accredited 393-bed acute care facility in Waco including a
Level II Trauma Center, Hillcrest Family Health Center, a network of family medicine clinics; and many key services. Hillcrest
is a ministry of Texas Baptists and is one of 7 health care institutions affiliated with the Baptist General Convention of Texas.

6453   Institute for Rehabilitation & Research
1333 Moursund St
Houston, TX 77030-3405   713-942-6159
                                        800-447-3422
                                   FAX: 713-942-5289
                       tirr.referrals@memorialhermann.org
                           www.memorialhermann.org

Jeffrey Berliner, Physician
Michelle Pu, Physician
A national center for information, training, research, and technical assistance in independent living. The goal is to extend the
body of knowledge in independent living and to improve the utilization of results of research programs and demonstration projects
in this field. It has developed a variety of strategies for collecting,
synthesizing, and disseminating information related to the field
of independent living.

6454   Midland Memorial Hospital & Medical Center
400 Rosalind Redfern Grover Parkway
Midland, TX 79701-9980   432-685-1111
                                        800-833-2916
                       russell.meyers@midland-memorial.com
                           www.midland-memorial.com

J.T. Lent Jr., President
Russell Meyers, CEO
Greg Wright, Board of Directors
Pete Hulder, Board of Directors
The Occupational and Physical Therapy Center is a specialzed
outpatient clinic. The clinic provides a wide variety of rehabilitation services designed to adequately assist you in returning back
to your normal duties. Our highly trained professionals are here
to help you with all your rehabilitation needs.

6455   Navarro Regional Hospital: RehabCare Unit
Navarro Hospital
3201 W State Highway 22
Corsicana, TX 75110-2469   903-654-6800
                                   FAX: 903-654-6955
                                   www.navarrohospital.com

Xavier Villarreal, CEO
Glenda Teri, Chief Nursing Officer
The rehab unit is located on the 4th floor and is designed for individuals who require intense rehab for an injury or disease process
where the goal would be to return home. Our team is committed to
helping individuals return to the highest level of functioning. Our
team consists of physicians, nurses, physical therapist, occupational therapist, speech therapist, social workers, dieticians and
other professionals as needed.

6456   Rebound: Northeast Methodist Hospital
12412 Judson Rd
Live Oak, TX 78233-3255   210-757-7000
                                   FAX: 210-757-5072
                                   www.nemh.sahealth.com

Joe Hernandez, Manager
Methodist Healthcare provides quality, comprehensive rehabilitation services for children and adults. Working as a team, rehabilitation professionals help patients define and achieve
individual goals in restoring function and productivity.

6457   Rio Vista Rehabilitation Hospital
1740 Curie Dr
El Paso, TX 79902-2900   915-544-8336
                                        800-999-8392
                                   FAX: 915-544-4838

Gene Miller, Administrator

6458   San Antonio Warm Springs Rehabilitation Hospital
5101 Medical Dr
San Antonio, TX 78229-4801   210-595-2380
                                   FAX: 210-614-0649
                                   www.warmsprings.org

Kurt Meyer, SVP Operations
Rick Marek, VP Post Acute Medical
A statewide not-for-profit system of inpatient and outpatient rehabilitation specialty centers. Warm Springs Rehabilitation System offers hope and acts as a catalyst for achieving an optimal
quality of life by providing comprehensive physical and/or cognitive rehabilitative care. Invensting resources in educational
and recreational programs. Supporting research efforts.

6459   Shannon Medical Center: RehabCare Unit
120 E Harris Ave
San Angelo, TX 76903-5904   325-653-6741
                                   FAX: 325-657-5706
                                   www.shannonhealth.com

Bryan Horner, CEO
Irv Zeitler, VP Medical Affairs
Shane Plymell, Chief financial officer
Gary Gibian, Executive director
Committed to improving the health of our community, using the
latest technologies available in the spirit of caring and integrity.
Strives to create an environment committed to the values of accountability, service, pride, integrity, respect and excellence. We
foster growth toward the highest quality care and customer service and strive for excellent financial performance. We hire and
develop the best people to accomplish these tasks.

6460   Shriners Burn Institute: Galveston Unit
815 Market St
Galveston, TX 77550-2725   409-770-6600
                                   FAX: 409-770-6919
                                   www.totalburncare.com

David Herndon, Chief Of Staff
David Ferrell, F.A.C.H.E., Administrator
Providing expert, orthopaedic and burn care to children under 18
regardless of ability to pay.

6461   Shriners Hospitals for Children, Houston
6977 Main St
Houston, TX 77030-3701   713-797-1616
                                        800-853-1240
                                   FAX: 713-797-1029
                                   www.shrinershq.org

David Ferrell, Administrator
Douglas Barnes, Chief of Staff
Melanie Lux, M.D.,, Director
Gloria Gogola, M.D., Doctor
Shriners Hospitals provides at no charge quality pediatric orthopedic serivces to children ages newborn to 18 years old. These
services include both outpatient and inpatient needs. Specialties
include cerebrel palsy, spina bifida, scoliosis, hand, hip and feet
problems. An application is required and may be completed by
phone.

6462   South Arlington Medical Center: Rehab Care Unit
3301 Matlock Rd
Arlington, TX 76015-2908   817-472-4849
                                   FAX: 817-472-4946
                                   mca@hcahealthcare.com
                           www.medicalcenterarlington.com

Patrice Oliver, Manaager
Above all else, we are committed to the care and improvement of
human life. In recognition of this committment, we strive to deliver high-quality, cost-effective healthcare in the communities
we serve.

6463   South Texas Rehabilitation Hospital
Ernest Health
425 E Alton Gloor Blvd
Brownsville, TX 78526-3361   956-554-6000
                                         FAX: 956-350-6150
                                    askus@earnesthealth.com
                                      www.strh.ernesthealth.com

Christopher Wilson, Medical Director
Jessie Eason, CEO
Mary Valdez, Director of Marketing
STRH was designed for the provision of specialized rehabilitative care, in the only freestanding acute rehabilitation hospital
serving Brownsville and the Rio Grande Valley. The hospital provides rehabilitative services for patients with functional deficits
as a result of debilitating illnesses or injuries.

6464   St. David's Rehabilitation Center
St. David s Medical Center
621 Radam Lane
Suite 200
Austin, TX 78745-4237   512-447-1083
                                         FAX: 512-447-1338
                                              www.stdavids.com

Anisa Godinez, Medical Director
Everett Heinze, MD Neurology, Medical Director
Tom Hill, MD, Medical Director
Albert Horn, MD, Medical Director
Mission is to provide exceptional care to every patient every day
with a spirit of warmth, friendliness and personal pride. Values
are integrity, compassion, accountability, respect and excellence.

6465   Texas NeuroRehab Center
1106 W Dittmar Rd
Austin, TX 78745-6328   512-444-4835
                                              800-252-5151
                                         FAX: 512-462-6749
                                          www.texasneurorehab.com

Alison Crawford Sinsky, Inpatient and Outpatient Manager
Ed Varando, Occupational Therapy Manager
Internationally recognized provider in brain in-
jury/neurobehavioral treatment for children, adolescents, and
adults with complex medical, physical and/or behavioral issues.
Medical rehabilitation, neurobehavioral, and neuropsychiatric
programs combine traditional therapies with education, vocational, substance abuse, and sensory integration services.

6466   Texas Specialty Hospital at Dallas
7955 Harry Hines Blvd
Dallas, TX 75235-3305   214-637-0000

Robin Burns, CEO
66 beds offering active/acute rehabilitation, brain injury day
treatment, cognitive rehabilitation, complex care, extended rehabilitation and short term evaluation.

6467   Touchstone Neurorecovery Center
Nexus Health Systems
9297 Wahrenberger Rd
Conroe, TX 77304-2441   936-788-7770
                                              800-414-4824
                                         FAX: 936-788-7785
                                       tncinfo@nhsltd.com
                                       www.touchstoneneuro.com

John W. Cassidy, MD, Executive Medical Director
Jude Theriot, MD, Medical Director
Ron Tintner, MD, Associate Clinical Director
Nelson Valena, MD, Director of Physical Medicine and
Rehabilitation
Touchstone provides treatment and rehabilitation in a residential
environment on a tranquil, wooded 26-acre site just north of
Houston in Conroe, TX. Touchstone offers customized treatment
programs designed to help individuals with known or suspected
brain injury or neurological deficits progress to their highest
functional level possible. Touchstone offers both on-campus and
off-campus housing in home-like settings for residents based on
their needs.

6468   Valley Regional Medical Center: RehabCare Unit
100A E Alton Gloor Blvd
Brownsville, TX 78526-3328   956-350-7000
                                         FAX: 956-350-7111
                                  www.valleyregionalmedicalcenter.com

Billy Bradford Jr.,, Chair
Francisco Javier Del Castillo, M, Vice Chair
Subramaniam Anandasivam, MD, Board
Christopher Olson, MD, Board
Our mission is to treat our community as family by providing
quality compassionate care.

Utah

6469   HealthSouth Rehab Hospital Of Utah
8074 S 1300 E
Sandy, UT 84094-743   801-561-3400
                                              801-565-6666
                                         FAX: 801-565-6576
                                          www.healthsouthutah.com

Phil Eaton, CEO
William McNutt, Director of Therapy Operations
Mark Rada, M.D., Interim Medical Director
Richard Ashby, Western Regional Director of Plant Opera-
tions/Safety Officer
A full spectrum of services, including inpatient, outpatient, day
hospital and home health. Holistic patient care, education and
community assimilation are the hallmarks of our programs, and
evidence of our leadership in the field of rehabilitation. Working
together as a team, we are able to tailor the needs of our patients
and provide the highest quality services. We believe that education and involvement of family and friends, will assist them in
maintaining independence after discharge.

6470   LDS Hospital Rehabilitation Center
8th Ave & C Street
Salt Lake City, UT 84143-0001   801-408-1100
                                              800-527-1118
                                         FAX: 801-408-5610
                                   contactus@intermountainmail.org
                                      www.intermountainhealthcare.org

Lizz Daley, Administrator
Jim Sheets, Administrator
Located within a Trauma I Center, this facility provides comprehensive inpatient and outpatient rehabilitation to people with
physical disabilities. CARF/JCAHO accredited. Low cost family
housing is available and Medicaid/Medicare is accepted.

6471   Primary Children's Medical Center
100 Mario Capecchi Dr
Salt Lake City, UT 84113-1100   801-662-1000
                                         FAX: 801-588-2318
                                      www.intermountainhealthcare.org

Scott Parker, President
Kevin Jones, Manager
Ore-Ofe O. Adesina, MD, Ophthalmology
Zeinab A. Afify, MD, Pediatric Hematology Oncology
Primary Children's Medical Center is the pediatric center serving
5 states in the Intermountain West Utah, Idaho, Wyoming, Nevada and Montana. The 289-bed facility is equipped and staffed
to treat children with complex illness and injury. PCMC is owned
by Intermountain Healthcare, a non-profit health care system. In
addition, it is affiliated with the Dept. of Pediatrics, University of
Utah, integrating pediatric programs. The hospital is designed to
meet the needs of children & their families.

6472   Shriners Hospitals for Children: Intermountain
Fairfax Road at Virginia St
Salt Lake City, UT 84103   801-536-3500
                                              800-313-3745
                                         FAX: 801-536-3782
                                              www.shrinershq.org

Kevin Martin, Administrator
Jacques D'Astous, Chief of Staff
One of nineteen hospitals in North America specializing in pedi-
atric orthopedics (plus four hospitals providing pediatric burn

treatment). This hospital serves the Intermountain region. All services provided in the hospital are at no cost to family, insurance company, nor state/federal agency regardless of ability to pay.

6473   Stewart Rehabilitation Center: McKay Dee Hospital
4401 Harrison Blvd
Ogden, UT 84403-3195   801-387-2080
                                  FAX: 801-387-7720
                        contactus@intermountainmail.org
                        www.intermountainhealthcare.org

Corey Anden, Nurse Coordinator
Judy Grover, Manager

With 10 affiliated clinics, McKay-Dee serves northern Utah, and portions of southeast Idaho and western Wyoming. A part of Intermountain Healthcare's system of 21 hospitals, McKay-Dee Hospital Center offers nationally ranked programs such as the Heart & Vascular Institute, the Newborn ICU and a new Cancer Treatment Center.

6474   University Healthcare-Rehabilitation Center
50 N Medical Dr
Salt Lake City, UT 84132-1   801-587-3422
                                     801-58 -EHAB
                                  FAX: 801-581-2111
                        www.healthcare.utah.edu/rehab/

David Entwistle, Administrator
Trish Jensen, Program Coordinator

Provides quality, comprehensive, rehabilitation services to persons with complex rehabilitation needs, including spinal cord injuries, head trauma, stroke, and other disabling conditions. Rehabilitation Services has been serving physicians, their patients, and the community since 1965. Rehabilitation Services has been an established leader in comprehensive inpatient, outpatient and home/community rehabilitation programs. Accredited by CARF and JCAHO.

Vermont

6475   Vermont Achievement Center
88 Park St
Rutland, VT 05701-4715   802-775-2395
                                  FAX: 802-773-9656
                        kmcshane@vac-rutland.com
                        www.vac-rutland.com

Kiki Mc Shane, CEO
Rebecca Wisell, Administrator

Vermont Achievement Center is recognized as a catalyst in building a community where all people are capable of change. Individuals flourish because they are nutured, valued and treated with respect. Education is empowering. The family is the primary influence in a person's life. Children belong in a family. Families are enhanced by support of the community. Children and family services are flexible and responsive to changing needs.

Virginia

6476   Inova Mount Vernon Hospital Rehabilitation Program
Inova Rehabilitation Center
2501 Parkers Ln
Alexandria, VA 22306-3209   703-664-7000
                                     800-554-7342
                                  FAX: 703-664-7423
                                  www.inova.com

Barbara Doyle, CEO

Inova Mount Vernon Hospital is a 237-bed hospital offering patients convenience and state-of-the-art care in a community environment. Our hospital sits on 26 acres of beautifully landscaped open space, where patients can find moments of serenity in our specially designed gardens..

6477   Kluge Children's Rehabilitation Center
University of Virginia
2270 Ivy Rd
Charlottesville, VA 22903-4977   434-924-5161
                                     800-627-8596
                                  FAX: 434-924-5559
                        www.healthsystem.virginia.edu

Janet Allaire, Administrator
Richard Stevenson, Research Director

The Kluge Childrens's Rehabilitation Center (KCRC) is a place dedicated to serving children with special needs. Children between the ages of birth and 21 come to the KCRC from all over Virginia, the United States, and even overseas for many reasons. Some need specific therapy or rehabilitation after injuries, accidents, or surgery. Others have chronic illness such as diabetes, and cystic fibrosis. Many families come to find out why their child is experiencing behavior problems.

Washington

6478   Good Samaritan Healthcare Physical Medicine and Rehabilitation
Good Samaritan Hospital
407 14th Ave SE
Puyallup, WA 98372-3770   253-697-4000
                                  FAX: 253-697-5157
                        info@goodsamhealth.org
                        www.multicare.org

Glenn Kassman, President
Vince Schmitz, CFO

Good Samaritan is part of the Multi-Care Health System, a non-for-profit medical system serving the growing populations of Pierce and King Counties in the greater Puget Sound region of Washington. Our medical staff includes 1,600 of the regions most respected primary care physicians and specialists.

6479   Northwest Hospital Center for Medical Rehabilitation
1550 N 115th St
Seattle, WA 98133-9733   206-364-0500
                                  FAX: 206-364-0500
                                  TTY:877-694-4677
                                  www.nwhospital.org

Peter Evans, Chairman
Scott L. Hardman, Vice Chairman
James K. Anderson, Board
C W Schneider, CEO

Provides complete medical and surgical services in both inpatient and outpatient settings. Services across multiple specialties include: 24hr emergency services, critical care, cardiac care, stroke program, cancer care, childbirth center, rehabilitation center, diagnostic imaging and education and wellness services. Mission is to raise the long-term health status of our community by providing personalized, quality care with compassion dignity, and respect.

6480   Providence Medical Center
500 17th Ave
Seattle, WA 98122-5711   206-000-1111
                                  FAX: 206-320-3387
                                  www.providence.org

6481   Providence Rehabilitation Services
Providence Rehabilitation Services
1321 Colby Ave
Everett, WA 98201-1665   425-261-3825
                                  FAX: 425-261-3823
                                  www.providence.org

Jim Phillips, Manager
Leslie Baumgarten, Manager

Continuum of care available: Acute Care, Inpatient Rehabilitation Unit, Transitional Care, Outpatient therapies, and In-home services.

6482 **Shriners Hospitals for Children: Spokane**
Shriners Hospitals
911 W 5th Ave
Spokane, WA 99204-2901   509-455-7844
                              FAX: 509-744-1223
                  www.shrinershq.org/hospitals/spokane
Kristin Monasmith, Public Relations Director
Craig Patchin, Administrator
Paul M. Caskey, M.D., Chief of Staff
Provides pediatric orthopedic services plus burn scar revision to
children birth to 18. All services at no charge to the family.

West Virginia

6483 **HealthSouth Mountain View Regional Rehab Hospital**
1160 Van Voorhis Rd
Morgantown, WV 26505-3437   304-598-1100
                                   800-388-2451
                              FAX: 304-598-1103
                       healthsouthmountainview.com
                       www.healthsouthmountainview.com/
Vicki Demers, Chief Executive Officer
Govind Patel, M.D., Medical Director
Robbin Butler, OTR/L, Director of Therapy Operations
Ginger Dearth, RN, Director of Marketing Operations
A 96-bed inpatient accute rehabilitation hospital. Outpatient ser-
vices, physical, occupational and speech therapy, and interior
therapy pool. Programs include neuro/stroke, brain injury, spinal
cord injury and pediatric.

6484 **HealthSouth Western Hills Regional Rehab Hospital**
3 Western Hills Dr
Parkersburg, WV 26105-8122   304-420-1392
                              FAX: 304-420-1374
                       www.healthsouthwesternhills.com
Kalapala Rao, Medical Director
Candace Ross, Director of Human Resources
Greg Holland, Director of Marketing Operations
Michelle Lowers, MS, LSW, Director of Care Management
A 40-bed medical rehabilitation hospital serving inpatient and
outpatient needs in the western West Virginia area. Our hospital is
accredited by the Joint Commission on Accreditation of
Healthcare Organizations (JCAHO) Our mission is to guide patients whtih physically disabling conditions along an individualized treatment pathway so they can reach the highest level of
physical, social and emotional well-being. We strive to provide
the highest quality care for you and your family.

Wisconsin

6485 **Extendicare Health Services, Inc.**
3540 South 43rd Street
Milwaukee, WI 53220-2903   414-541-1000
                                   800-395-5000
                              FAX: 414-541-1942
                       www.extendicare.com
Timothy Lukenda, CEO
Douglas Harris, SVP
David Pearce, Vice President, General Counsel
Sunrise Care Center is a leading provider of long-term skilled
nursing care and short-term rehabilitation solutions. Our 99 bed
facility offers a full continuum of services and care focused
around each individual in today's ever-changing healthcare environment. Our facility is Medicare and Medicaid certified.

6486 **St. Catherine's Hospital**
9555 76th St
Pleasant Prairie, WI 53158   262-577-8000
                              FAX: 262-653-5795
                       www.uhsi.org
Vicki Lewis, Manager
Committed to living out the healing ministries of the
Judeo-Christian faiths by providing exceptional and compas-
sionate healthcare service that promotes the dignity and
well-being of the people we serve.

6487 **St. Joseph Hospital**
611 Saint Joseph Ave
Marshfield, WI 54449-1898   715-387-1713
                              FAX: 715-389-3939
                       sjhweb@stjosephs-marshfield.org
                       www.ministryhealth.org
Michael Schmidt, CEO
Catherine Olson, Director
A values-driven healthcare delivery network of aligned hospitals, clinics, long-term care facilities, home care agencies, dialysis centers and many other programs and services in Wisconsin
and Minnesota.

Wyoming

6488 **Spalding Rehabilitation Hospital at Memorial Hospital of
Laramie**
2301 House Ave
Suite 300
Cheyenne, WY 82001-3748   307-635-4141
                                   800-374-7687
                              FAX: 307-638-2656
                       www.imgwy.com
Mitchell Schwarzbach, Executive Director
Tanya Boerkircher, Wyoming Endoscopy Center Manager
Andrea Bailey, Charge Entry Supervisor
Michelle Flanagan, Front Office Supervisor
We are a professional corporation of physicians trained in various
medical specialties and subspecialties including Internal Medi-
cine, Gastroenterology and Chest Diseases.It is our mission to
provide the highest quality, cost-effective primary and
subspecialty medical care, and education to the people of southern Wyoming, western Nebraska, and northern Colorado.

Rehabilitation Facilities, Post-Acute

Alabama

6489   Alabama Department of Rehabilitation Services
602 S Lawrence St
Montgomery, AL 36104-4787   334-293-7500
                                   800-441-7607
                              FAX: 334-293-7383
                              www.rehab.alabama.gov

Cary F. Boswell, Commissioner
Anna Taylor
State agency which provides services and assistance to Alabama's children and adults with disabilities.

6490   Briarcliff Nursing Home & Rehab Facility
3201 North Ware Road
McAllen, TX 78501   956-631-5542
                              FAX: 956-631-5777
                    http://www.briarcliffnursingcenter.com

6491   Butler Adult Training Center
South Central Alabama Mental Health
680 Hardscramble Rd
Greenville, AL 36037   334-382-2353
                              FAX: 334-382-9518
                                   www.scamhc.org

6492   Centers for The Developmentally DisabledNorth Central Alabama
1602 Church St SE
P.O. Box 2091
Decatur, AL 35602   256-350-1458
                              FAX: 256-350-1485
                                   info@cddnca.org
                                   www.cddnca.org

Earl Brightwell, Executive Director
CDD NCA provides services and programs for individuals who are mentally and/or physically challenged, or developmentally delayed. These services range from early intervention services for infants and toddlers to residential and employment programs for adults. All services are typically provided at no cost to the individual or their family, regardless of income. Funding sources for the CDD NCA include DMH, United Way, and ADRS.

6493   Cheaha Regional Mental Health Center
351 W 3rd St
Sylacauga, AL 35150   256-245-1340
                              FAX: 256-245-1343
                                   crmhc.org

Cynthia L. Atkinson, Executive Director
Dr. Shakil Khan, Medical Director
Karen McKinney, Clinical Director, Mental Health Services
Ann Cunningham, Director, Intellectual Disabilities Services
CRMHC provides a continuum of services for persons with intellectual disabilities, serious mental illness and substance abuse in a four county area in east Alabama, which includes Clay, Coosa, Randolph, and Talladega Counties.

6494   Children's Rehabilitation Service -District Office, Montgomery
Alabama Department of Rehabilitation Services
602 S. Lawrence St.
Montgomery, AL 36104   334-293-7500
                                   800-568-9034
                              FAX: 334-293-7374
                              www.rehab.alabama.gov

6495   Chilton-Shelby Mental Health Center
110 Medical Center Dr
Calera, AL 35045   205-755-8800
                              FAX: 205-668-4957
                                   chiltonshelby.org

Melodie D. Crawford, Chief Executive Officer
Vicki M. Potts, Chief Financial Officer
Kathryn T. Crouthers, Chief Operations Officer
Dena Smitherman, Intellectual Disabilities Division Director
Mental health rehabilitation services and more for the recovery of mentally disabled adults. Serves Chilton and Shelby counties.
Business Office Location

6496   Darden Rehabilitation Center
1001 E Broad Street
Ste C
Gadsden, AL 35903-2400   256-547-5751
                              FAX: 256-547-5761
                              darden@dardenrehab.org
                                   dardenrehab.org

Lynn Curry, Executive Director
Derek Coburn, Operations Manager
Dana Johnson, Program Coordinator
Lisa Wilson, Executive Assistant
Work adjustment and job placement programs. Serves the counties of Etawah, Marshall, Dekalb, Clair and Cherokee.

6497   Easter Seals Central Alabama
2125 E. South Blvd
Montgomery, AL 36116-2409   334-288-0240
                              FAX: 334-288-7171
                              info@eastersealsca.org
                                   www.eastersealsca.or

Debbie Lynn, Executive Director
Ed Collier, Director, Programs
Sharis LeMay, CNA Instructor
Frankie Thomas, Senior Employment Program
A private, nonprofit organization offering services audiology, physical, occupational, lymphedemia and speech therapy, psychological counseling, vocational evaluation and assessment, person, social and work adjustment training, GED preparation, computer service training, job placement and follow-up, and special learning disabilities service and supported employment service.

6498   Easter Seals Northwest Alabama
1450 Avalon Ave
Muscle Shoals, AL 35660-3110   256-391-1110
                              FAX: 256-314-5105
                                   www.eastersealsnwal.org

Danny Prince, Administrator
John Ives, Chairman
Tommy Hester, Treasurer
Susie White, Secretary
Easter Seals has been helping individuals with disabilities and special needs, and their families live better lives for more then 80 years. From child development centers to physical rehabilitation and job training for people with disabilities, Easter Seals offers a variety of services to help people with disabilities address life's challenges and achieve personal goals.

6499   Easter Seals West Alabama
1110 Dr. Edward Hillard Drive
Tuscaloosa, AL 35401-7446   205-759-1211
                                   800-726-1216
                              FAX: 205-349-1162
                              eswa@eswaweb.org
                                   eswaweb.org

Ronny Johnston, Executive Director
Dusty Beam, Administrative Coordinator
Holly Hillard, Director, Development
Leading organization in helping children and adults with disabilities to live with equality, dignity and independence. Rehabilitation services are provided in two divisions: outpatient rehabilitation division (physical therapy, occupational therapy, speech therapy, hearing evaluation, sell and service hearind aids) and vocational division (vocational evaluation and vocational

development). Services are rendered regardless of age, race, sex, color, creed, national origin, veteran's status.

6500 **Easter Seals West Central Alabama Rehabilitation Center**
2906 Citizens Pkwy
P.O. Box 750
Selma, AL 36702-0750
334-872-8421
800-801-4776
FAX: 334-872-3907
wcarcdw@tomnet.com
www.eswcarc.us

6501 **Geer Adult Training Center**
P.O.Box 419
83 South Canaan Road
Canaan, CT 06018-419
860-824-7067
FAX: 205-367-8032
geercares.org/content/about-geer

Yvonne Williams, Program Coordinator

6502 **Goodwill Easter Seals of the Gulf Coast**
2440 Gordon Smith Dr.
Mobile, AL 36617-2319
251-471-1581
info@al.easterseals.com
www.gesgc.org

Peter D'Olive, Chairman
Frank Harkins, President & CEO
Bill Dillman, Vice President, Marketing & Development
Vocational, medical, pre-school education, day care, recreation and other support services.

6503 **HealthSouth Corporation**
3660 Grandview Parkway
Ste 200
Birmingham, AL 35243-3332
205-967-7116
800-765-4772
FAX: 225-928-0317
healthsouth.com

Jacque Shadle, CEO
Derrick Landreneau, Director of Nursing services
Dedicated to one field of medicine - physical rehabilitation medicine - and are committed to one goal, helping patients achieve the highest level of functioning possible after a debilitating injury or illness.

6504 **Indian Rivers Mental Health Center - Bibb**
2439 Main St
Brent, AL 35034
205-926-4681
FAX: 205-296-6016
www.irmhc.org

6505 **Indian Rivers Mental Health Center - Pickens**
890 Reform St.
Carrollton, AL 35447
205-367-8032
FAX: 205-367-9291
www.irmhc.org

6506 **Indian Rivers Mental Health Center - Tuscaloosa**
2209 - 9th St
Tuscaloosa, AL 35401
205-391-3131
FAX: 205-391-3135
http://www.irmhc.org

Barbara Friedman, President
Elizabeth Rice, First Vice President
Services are available to adults who have serious mental illness resulting in personal, family or work-related problems. Counseling may take place in either individual or group settings, identification, evaluation and treatment services are available to persons who experience problems related to alcohol and drug abuse and counseling services are available for children and adolescents who have a severe emotional disturbance causing discipline problems at home and school.

6507 **Mobile ARC**
2424 Gordon Smith Dr
Mobile, AL 36617-2397
251-479-7409
FAX: 251-473-7649
jzoghby@mobilearc.org
mobilearc.org

Jeff Zoghby, Executive Director
Amy Odom, Public Relations and Development Director
Mobile Arc, Inc. (MARC) offers a wide range of services for persons with intellectual and developmental disabilities.

6508 **Southeastern Blind Rehabilitation Center**
U.S. Department of Veteran Affairs
700 S 19th St
Birmingham, AL 35233-1927
205-558-4706
FAX: 205-933-4484
george.sands@med.va.gov
www.rehab.va.gov/blindrehab/

6509 **UAB Eye Care**
University Of Alabama at Birmingham
1716 University Blvd
Birmingham, AL 35233
205-975-2020
FAX: 205-934-6755
www.uab.edu/optometry/home/eyecare

Rodney W. Nowakowski, Dean
Dr. Marsha Snow, Chief, Low Vision Patient Care
Brittney Bolen, Optometric Technician
Joseph Fleming, D.D., Chief Of Staff
Complete eye services, including low vision services and materials.

6510 **Vaughn-Blumberg Services**
2715 Flynn Rd
P.O. Box 8646
Dothan, AL 36304
334-793-3102
FAX: 334-793-7740
www.vaughnblumbergservices.com

Ed Dorsey, Executive Director
Linda Cunningham, Director of Human Resources
Billy McCarthy, Director of Finance
Karen Amos, Director of Nursing
Provides comprehensive services for people with intellectual disabilities that reside in Houston County as well as assist in facilitating their participation in society to the fullest extent of their individual capabilities. Offers early intervention services for the mentally handicapped adult including diagnosis and evaluation and physical, speech, and occupational therapies. They also offer counseling, day training,employment assistance and residential homes.

Alaska

6511 **Alaska Center for the Blind and Visually Impaired**
3903 Taft Drive
Anchorage, AK 99517-3069
907-248-7770
800-770-7517
FAX: 907-248-7517
info@alaskabvi.org
www.alaskabvi.org

Regan Mattingly, Executive Director
Robert Tasso, Program Manager
Caren Ailleo, Development & Communications Director
Bonnie Lucas, Visually Impaired Senior Coordinator
Services to help the adult residential or community-based student become independent and self-sufficient by offering independent travel, Braille reading and writing, use of assiative technology such as talking computers, manual skills and personal, as well as home management. There is a special program for those 55 years of age and older who are experiencing a vision loss and another program for rural Alaska Native youth who are visually impaired.

Arizona

6512 Arizona Center for the Blind and Visually Impaired
3100 E Roosevelt St
Phoenix, AZ 85008-5036   602-273-7411
                                  FAX: 602-273-7410
                                  jlamay@acbvi.org
                                  acbvi.org

James La May, CEO
Frank Vance, Director
Christine Boisen, Chair
Alexia Matek, Secretary
A private, nonprofit organization that provides comprehensive rehabilitation services and more for the blind and visually handicapped. The staff includes 20 instructional and adminstrative professionals.

6513 Arizona Industries for the Blind
Suite 130
515 N 51st Avenue
Phoenix, AZ 85043-2711   602-771-9100
                                  FAX: 602-353-5701
                                  DanielMartinez@azdes.gov
                                  www.azdes.gov/aib

Richard Monaco, General Manager
Daniel Martinez, Community Services Liaison
Offers rehabilitation services, vocational/pre-vocational evaluation and training, work adjustment, job development and employment and training opportunties for individuals who are blind.

6514 Banner Good Samaritan Medical Center
1111 E McDowell Road
Phoenix, AZ 85006-2666   602-839-2000
                                  FAX: 602-239-5868
                                  www.bannerhealth.com

Steve Narang, MD, Chief Executive Officer
Lorraine Hudspeth, Controller
Letty Cerpa, Senior Accountant
Larry Mann, IT Manager
Nearly 1,700 physicians representing more than 50 specialties work with Banner Good Samaritan staff to care for more then 36,000 inpatients a year. Houses more then 650 licensed patient care beds. A teaching hospital that trains more then 220 physicians annually and a premier medical center in Arizona and the Southwest. Provides a comprehensive foundation of major programs and an equally impressive offering of highly specialized programs not availiable in most hospitals.

6515 Beacon Foundation for the Mentally Retarded
308 W. Glenn St.
Tucson, AZ 85703   520-622-4874
                                  FAX: 520-620-6620
                                  sking@beacongroup.org
                                  http://beacongroup.org

Steven R King, President
Chuck Tiller, Vice President Rehabilitation Se
Greg Natvig, Vice President of Business Opera
Michelle Kroeger, CFO
Committed to effectively assisting adults with disabilities to maximize their personal, social, vocational and educational skills in order to attain a successful and meaningful independence within the Tucson community.

6516 Carondelet Brain Injury Programs and Services (Bridges Now)
2202 N. Forbes Blvd.
Tucson, AZ 85745-2602   520-872-7324
                                  FAX: 520-873-3743
                                  comments@carondelet.org
                                  carondelet.org

Daisy M Jenkins, Executive VP, Chief HR/Administr
James K Beckmann, President/Chief Executive Officer
Alan Strauss, Executive VP, Finance and Chief Financial Officer
Christen Castellano, MBA, Executive VP and Chief Strategy Officer
Comprehensive outpatient rehabilitation post program. PT, OT, ST, Psychology and Rehab Counseling Services.

6517 Desert Life Rehabilitation & Care Center
1919 W Medical St
Tucson, AZ 85704-1133   520-369-9620
                                  FAX: 520-867-6612
                                  www.desertlifercc.com

Amad Nazifi, Executive Director
Accomodates 240 residents. Provides skilled and intermediate nursing with occupational, physical, speech and respiratory therapy services. Offers special programs including an Alzheimer's Unit and a Young Adult program

6518 Devereux Advanced Behavioral HealthArizona - Scottsdale
Administrative Office
11000 N. Scottsdale Rd.
Ste 260
Scottsdale, AZ 85254   480-998-2920
                                  www.devereux.org

Lane Barker, Executive Director
Services include evidenced based approaches in: Early Intervention for birth to five, Parent Training, ABA Strategies for Autism Spectrum Disorder Population, Day School, Facility Based Respite, Group Homes, Foster Care, Outpatient Counseling and Psychiatric Support, Crisis Stabilization, and Residential Treatment with a wellness focus incorporating Cognitive Behavioral therapy approaches, Positive Behavior Intervention and Supports, Recreation Therapy, and Substance Abuse treatment.

6519 Devereux Advanced Behavioral Health Arizona - Tucson
Administrative Office
6141 E. Grant Rd.
Tucson, AZ 85712   520-296-5551
                                  FAX: 520-296-8244
                                  www.devereux.org

6520 Freestone Rehabilitation Center
10617 E Oasis Drive
Mesa, AZ 85208   480-986-1531
                                  FAX: 480-986-1538
                                  Marccenter.com
                                  www.manta.com

Randy Gray, Executive Director
Cherie Vance, Manager

6521 HealthSouth Valley Of The Sun Rehabilitation Hospital
13460 N 67th Ave
Glendale, AZ 85304-1000   623-878-8800
                                  FAX: 623-878-5254
                                  healthsouth.com

Beth Bacher, Manager
A 60-bed free-standing hospital that offers acute physical rehabilitation, outpatient therapy services and day hospital treatment. Works in cooperation with local, regional and national managed care organizations and other sources to maximise patient recovery while conserving financial resources.

6522 Institute for Human Development
Northern Arizona University
912 Riordan Rd. P.O.Box 5630
Flagstaff, AZ 86011-5630   928-523-4791
                                  FAX: 928-523-9127
                                  TTY:928-523-1695
                                  ihd@nau.edu
                                  www.nau.edu/ihd

Levi Esguerra, Director
Lisa Andrew, Advisory Commitee
Lynn Black, Advisory Commitee
Maria Bravo, Advisory Commitee
The Institute values and supports the independence, productivity and inclusion of Arizona's citizens with disabilities. Based on the values and beliefs, the Institute conducts training, research and services that further these goals.

6523 John C Lincoln Hospital North Mountain
250 E Dunlap Ave
Phoenix, AZ 85020-2871
602-943-2381
FAX: 602-944-8062
webmaster@jcl.com
www.jcl.com/content/northmountain/default.htm
Rhonda Forsyth, President
Bruce Pearson, FACHE, Senior Vice President
Maggi Griffin, RN, MS, Vice President & Chief Executive Officer
Jessica Rivas, RN, MSN, Vice President and Chief Nursing Officer
Mission is to assist each person entrusted to our care to enjoy the fullest gift of health possible, and work with others to build a community where a helping hand is available for our most vulnerable members.

6524 La Frontera Center
504 W 29th St
Tucson, AZ 85713-3394
520-884-9920
FAX: 520-792-0654
www.lafronteraaz.org
Kevin Heath, Board Chair
Frank Valenzuela, Vice Chair
Celestino Fernandez, Treasurer
Susan Agrillo, Recording Secretary
A nonprofit community-based behavioral health agency that has been helping southern Arizona children, adults, and families since 1968.

6525 Manor Care Nursing and Rehab Center: Tucson
3705 N Swan Rd
Tucson, AZ 85718-6939
520-299-7088
FAX: 520-529-0038
www.hcr-manorcare.com
Clifton J. Porter II, Vice President - Government Rela
Martin Allen, Vice President
A leading provider of short-term post-acute medical care and rehabilitation and long-term skilled nursing care. High quality medical care is provided through registered (RN) and licensed practical (LPN) nurses and certified nursing assistants (CNA) in concert with physical , occupational and speech rehabilitation therapists. Our more then 275 skilled nursing centers are Medicare-and Medicaid-certified.

6526 Nova Care
Second Floor
680 American Avenue
King of Prussia, PA 19406-2607
800-331-8840
FAX: 602-256-7292
novacare.com
Scott Lusted, General Manager
Brian Beal, Market Manager
NovaCare Rehabilitation's highly respected clinical team provides preventative and rehabilitative services that maximize functionality and promote well-being. NovaCare Rehabilitation also provides physical therapy and athletic training services to more then 20 professional sports teams and 300 universities, colleges, and highschools thoughout the nation.

6527 Perry Rehabilitation Center
3146 E Windsor Avenue
Phoenix, AZ 85008-1199
602-956-0400
FAX: 602-957-7610
perrycenter@qwest.net
www.azafh.com
Diana Casillas, Human Resources Director
Jim Musick, President
Provides services for people with disabilities, cognitive disabilities including residential services, day treatment, job training and job placement.

6528 Phoenix Veterans Center
Ste 100
1544 W. Grant St.
Phoenix, AZ 85004-1554
602-358-8494
FAX: 602-379-4130
www.azcremationcenter.com/?
Ken Benckwitz, Manager

Veterans medical clinic offering disabled veterans medical treatments.

6529 Progress Valley: Phoenix
10505 North 69th Street
Suite 1100
Paradise Valley, AZ 85253-6106
480-922-9427
FAX: 602-274-5473
mailto:recovery@progressvalley.org
alcoholism.about.com
Susanne Lambert, Executive Director
Jennifer White, Director of Programs
Cathie Scott, Sober Housing Manager
Kristine Peltier, Finance Director
Residential aftercare for alcoholism and chemical dependency. Certified chemical dependency counselors provide individual treatment.

6530 Rehabilitation Services Administration
Suite 102
3425 East Van Buren
Phoenix, AZ 85008-3202
602-771-9100
800-563-1221
FAX: 602-250-8584
TTY: 855-475-8194
azrsa@azdes.gov
azdes.gov/rsa
Katharine Levandowsky, Administrator
Provides a variety of specialized services to assist in removing barriers to employment and/or independent living for individuals with physical or mental disabilities. RSA offers 3 major service programs and several specialized programs/services.

6531 Southern Arizona Association For The Visually Impaired
3767 East Grant Rd
Tucson, AZ 85716-2935
520-795-1331
FAX: 520-795-1336
reception@saavi.us
www.saavi.us
Michael Gordon, Executive Director
Amy Murillo, Associate Director
Carol Lopez, Finance Director
Lenetta Lefko, Tucson Services Manager
Offers health services, counseling, social work, home and personal management, computer training, low vision aids and more for the visually handicapped 18 years or older.

6532 Toyei Industries
Hc 58 Box 55
Ganado, AZ 86505-55
928-736-2417
888-45T-OYEI
FAX: 928-736-2495
www.yelp.com/biz/toyei-industries-inc-ganado-
Anthony Lincoln, CEO
Serves the needs of developmentally disabled and the severely mentally impaired adult citizens of the Navajo Nation and other Indian Nations. Staff of 60+ serves the needs of all the Navajo adults. Services include day treatment programs, and residential and group home services.

6533 Yuma Center for the Visually Impaired
328 W. Spears Street
Yuma, AZ 85365-6580
928-247-8890
FAX: 928-344-1863
https://www.azdes.gov
Calvin Roberts, Executive Director
Kathy Lucero, Store Manager
Dana Clayton, Human Resources Specialist
Lorraine Hudspeth, Controller
A private nonprofit agency offering services for totally blind and legally blind children and adults in the Arizona area.

Arkansas

6534 Arkansas Lighthouse for the Blind
P.O.Box 192666
6818 Murray St.
Little Rock, AR 72209- 2666   501-562-2222
                              FAX: 501-568-5275
                         info@arkansaslighthouse.org
                              arkansaslighthouse.org

Bill Johnson, Chief Executive Officer
Danny Novielli, COO
John McAtee, Chief Financial Officer
Ronnie Cates, Director of Communications & Procurement
Manufacturer of textiles, apparel and paper products and employs blind and legally blind individuals.

6535 Beverly Enterprises Network
1 Thousand Beverly
Fort Smith, AR 72901-2629   479-201-2000
                              800-666-9996
                         FAX: 479-452-5131
               www.yelp.com/biz/beverly-enterprises-inc-fort
Randy Churchey, CEO
Offers a progressive approach to subacute care. The goal of this organization is to assist injured and disabled individuals regain the level of independence to which they have been accustomed. Provides support and training programs, patient and family services and specialty programs for patients.

6536 Easter Seals: Arkansas
3920 Woodland Heights Rd
Little Rock, AR 72212-2495   501-227-3600
                              877-533-3700
                         FAX: 501-227-4021
                         TTY: 501-227-3686
                    lrogers@ar.easterseals.com
                         www.eastersealsar.com
Sharon Moone-Jochums, President/ CEO
Linda Rogers, VP Programs
Michael E. Stock, Treasurer
Cindy Nash, Secretary
Their mission is to provide exceptional services to ensure that all people with disabilities or special needs have equal opportunities to live, learn, work and play in their communitites.

6537 HealthSouth Rehabilitation Hospital Of Fort Smith
1401 South J. Street
Fort Smith, AR 72901-5158   479-785-3300
                              FAX: 479-785-8599
                              healthsouth.com
Ryan Cassedy, CEO
Cygnet Schroeder, M.D., Medical Director
Donna Beallis, D.O., Director of Medical Management
Brandi Denham, Director of Human Resources
A free-standing 80-bed comprehensive physical medicine and rehabilitation hospital offering inpatient and outpatient services. Provides specialized medical and therapy services, designed to assist physically challenged persons to reach their highest level of independent function.

6538 Lions World Services for the Blind
2811 Fair Park Blvd
Little Rock, AR 72204-5044   501-664-7100
                              800-248-0734
                         FAX: 501-664-2743
                         training@lwsb.org
                         www.wsblind.org/
Larry Dickerson, President/ CEO
Tony Woodell, President & Chief Executive Officer
Bill Smith, Director of Development
Melanie Jones, Marketing & Communications Director
Offers services in the areas of health education, recreation, rehabilitation, counseling, employment, computer training and more for all legally blind residents of the U.S. The staff includes 56 full time employees.

6539 Little Rock Vet Center #0713
Department of Veterans Affairs of Washington DC
Suite A
201 W Broadway St
North Little Rock, AR 72114- 5505   501-324-6395
                              877-927-8387
                         FAX: 501-324-6928
               www.hud.gov/offices/cpd/about/hudvet/state/ar
Elizabeth N Ruggiero, Team Leader
Ida L Fogle, Counselor
Van A Hall, Counselor
Darryl A Lasker, Office Manager
Vet Center provides PTSD counseling to veterans of a combat zone. No medical care provided.

6540 Timber Ridge Ranch NeuroRestorative Services
4500 W Commerce Dr
North Little Rock, AR 72116   501-758-8799
                              800-743-6802
                         FAX: 501-758-8778
                    neuroinfo@thementornetwork.com
                         www.neurorestorative.com
Bill Duffy, Chief Operating Officer
Michael E. Hofmeister, MS, MBA, Vice President of Operations
Sean Byrne, MBA, Chief Financial Officer
Roger P. Carrillo, M.Ed, Vice President of Business Development
Comprehensive, individualized services from a transdisciplinary team of licensed professionals assist clients along a course to greater independence. A separate team is dedicated to the needs of children, adolescents, and their families. A clinical team may include professionals from the disciplines of: behavior analysis, neuropsychology, physiatry, psychology, speech-language pathology, occupational therapy, physical therapy, social work, couseling, education, nursing, and case management.

California

6541 ARC Fresno-Kelso Activity Center
4567 N Marty Ave
Fresno, CA 93722-7810   559-226-6268
                              FAX: 559-226-6269
                         arcfresno@arcfresno.org
                              arcfresno.org
Lori Ramirez, Executive Director
Catherine Wooliever, Director of Human Resources
Jamie Marrash, Director of Program Services
Pamela Wirth, Director of Finance
The Arc Fresno is a private, non-profit 501(c)(3) organization who was founded in 1953. They provide services and supports for over 550 individuals with developmental disabilities throughout Fresno County. They currently offer eight (8) programs, and do so with the help of 145 employees.

6542 ARC Of San Diego-ARROW Center, The
3030 Market Street
San Diego, CA 92102-3297   619-685-1175
                              FAX: 619-234-3759
                              arc-sd.com
Dwight Stratton, Chair
Jerry Wechsler, 1st Vice Chairman
David W. Schneider, President & CEO
Anthony J. DeSalis, Executive Vice President & COO
The ARC of San Diego will be the premier provider of services to persons with disabilities. Arc-SD will be an advocate for diversity of opportunities, enhancing individual life choices as a member of the community. Our values: Everyone will be be treated equally, without prejudice and with respect. Will provide Quality Services and Supports with a well trained and caring staff. State of the art equipment and methods. A willingness to innovate and collaborate.

6543 ARC Of San Diego-East County Training Center, The
1374 E Lexington Ave
El Cajon, CA 92019-2312   619-444-9417
                                      FAX: 619-234-3759
                                           arc-sd.com

Dwight Stratton, Chair
Jerry Wechsler, 1st Vice Chairman
David W. Schneider, President & CEO
Anthony J. DeSalis, Executive Vice President & COO
Work adjustment and remunerative work programs.

6544 ARC Of San Diego-Rex Industries, The
9575 Aero Dr
San Diego, CA 92123-1803   858-571-4369
                                           800-748-5575
                                      FAX: 858-715-3788
                                           arc-sd.com

Dwight Stratton, Chair
Jerry Wechsler, 1st Vice Chairman
David W. Schneider, President & CEO
Anthony J. DeSalis, Executive Vice President & COO
Offers many different programs including: North County Parent/Infant Program which is an educational program for children, birth to three years who are showing delays in development or who are at risk for developmental delays. The Adult Development Center is a program for adults, eighteen and over, with a developmental disability in the severe to profound range. The program focuses on self-help, communication, daily living and pre-vocational skills. Other programs are available..

6545 ARC Of San-Diego-South Bay
1280 Nolan Avenue
Chula Vista, CA 91911-3738   619-427-7524
                                      FAX: 619-427-4657
                                        info@arc-sd.com
                                    www.arc-sd.com/locations

Becky Thaller, Director
Steve Hojsan, Arc Enterprises Director
Michael Bruce, Workshop Manager
David W. Schneider, President & CEO
Provides remunerative work.

6546 ARC Of Southeast Los Angeles-Southeast Industries
9501 Washburn Rd
Downey, CA 90242-2913   562-803-1556
                                      FAX: 562-803-4080
                                       sales@arcselac.org
                                        www.arcselac.org/

6547 ARC: VC Community Connections West
5103 Walker Street
Ventura, CA 93003-7358   805-650-8611
                                      FAX: 805-644-7308
                                           www.arcvc.org

Robert Hogan, President
Gene West, First Vice President
Eve Liebman, Recording Secretary
Kathy Raffaelli, Treasurer
Caring and experienced staff is dedicated to serving participants with a variety of physical, mental and social disabilities who require a higher level of support and supervision. Using a person-centered planning approach, Arc Ventura County promotes self-directed services for all clients and families served. Adult development centers serve individuals with physical and mental disabilities, as well as people with challenging behaviors, who require assistance with basic skills such as self care.

6548 ARC: VC Ventura
5103 Walker Street
Ventura, CA 93003-7358   806-650-8611
                                      FAX: 806-644-7308
                                           www.arcvc.org

Robert Hogan, President
Gene West, First Vice President
Eve Liebman, Recording Secretary
Kathy Raffaelli, Treasurer

Arc Ventura County is a private, nonprofit organization that provides educational, vocational and residential services for people with developmental disabilities. Informed decisions, positive changes, and integration in the community are fundamental principals in all programs. As evidence of our programming excellence, Arc Ventura County has been accredited by CARF (The Rehabilitation Accreditation Commission.

6549 AbilityFirst
1300 E Green Street
Pasadena, CA 91106-2606   626-396-1010
                                           877-768-4600
                                      FAX: 626-396-1021
                                        info@abilityfirst.org
                                         www.abilityfirst.org

Lori E. Gangemi, President
Steve S. Schultz, Chief Financial Officer
Keri Castaneda, Chief Program Officer
Syed Kazmi, Controller
AbilityFirst serves children and adults with special needs through 24 locations in Southern California.

6550 Accentcare
17855 North Dallas Pkwy
Dallas, TX 75287-2468   972-201-3800
                                           800-834-3059
                                        info@accentcare.com
                                           accentcare.com

Mark Pacala, Chairman of the Board and CEO (i
Vincent E. Cook, EVP and Chief Financial Officer
Melvin Warriner, SVP and Chief Culture Officer
Mel Deutsch, General Counsel
Postacute rehabilitation program: home care aides follow through with rehabilitation instructions given by physical, occupational and speech therapists. Other home care services are available, serving special needs for Alzheimer's, blind, brain injury, MS, ostomies, parkinsonism, spinal injury and stroke.

6551 Anaheim Veterans Center
859, South Harbor Blvd
Anaheim, CA 92805-4680   714-776-0161
                                           800-225-8387
                                      FAX: 714-776-8904
                                 anaheimvetcenter@yahoo.com
                           www.longbeach.va.gov/visitors/vet_center.asp

6552 Association for Retarded Citizens: Alameda County
1101 Walpert St
Hayward, CA 94541-3721   510-582-8151
                                      FAX: 510-639-4684
                                           www.sbn.com

Ram Sirck, Director
Offers the Right Track program in which selected workers are grouped together on a contract basis to maximize work productivity. Provides a full benefit package, as well as a permanent supervisor. A worker is matched to a job of at least 20 hours per week and then trained by the staff of The Right Track.

6553 Azure Acres Recovery Center
5777 Madison Avenue
Suite 1210
Sacramento, CA 95841-9034   877-977-3755
                                           877-762-3735
                                      FAX: 707-823-8972
                                        info@azureacres.com
                                          azureacres.com

Joe Tinervin, MSW, Executive Director
Michael Roeske, Psy.D., Clinical Director
Christie Splitstone, MA, Counselor/Case Manager
James Canter, CATC, Counselor/Case Manager
Offers rehabilitation services and residential care for the person with an alcohol or drug abuse related problems.

6554 Back in the Saddle
2 BITS Trail
P.O. Box 3336
Chelmsford, MA 01824-0936   800-865-2478
                                   877-756-5068
                      FAX: 800-866-3235
                      help@BackInTheSaddle.com
                      www.thesaddle.com

Richard Smith PhD, Owner
Erika Reed, Co-Director
A long term community residential facility for head injured
adults. House parents live on-site; and oversee a variety of programs which are individually designed and might include classes
in community college, placement in a workshop or on a workstation, volunteer positions and home skills assignments. Recreational outing range from horseback riding to weekend camping.
Apartment programs available as set-up. Price: $2800-$3000 per
month.

6555 Ballard Rehabilitation Hospital
1760 W 16th St
San Bernardino, CA 92411-1150   909-473-1200
                                       800-761-1226
                          FAX: 909-473-1276
                          www.ballardrehab.com

Edward C. Palacios, RN,MPH, Administrator
Mary Hunt, Chief Operating Officer
Patty Meinhardt, Director Marketing/Admissions
Ballard Rehab Hospital is a free standing specialty hospital and
provides the complete continuum of acute rehabilitation and outpatient rehabilitation, dedicated to providing rehab care to adults
and children. The following inpatient and outpatient programs
are available: CNA (Stroke) Rehab; Spinal Cord Injury Rehab;
Brain Injury Rehab; Pain Management Rehab; Bariatric program,
pulmonary program, injured Worker Programs; and Post
Amputation Rehab.

6556 Bayview Nursing and Rehabilitation
516 Willow Street
Alameda, CA 94501-6132   510-521-5600
                     FAX: 510-865-6441
                     TTY:800-735-2922
                     kleger.org@comcast.net.
                     http://www.bayviewnursing.com/
Richard S Espinoza, Administrator
Offers a full range of medical services to meet the individual
needs of our residents, including short-term rehabilitative services and long termed skilled care. Working with the resident's
physician, our staff-including medical specialists, nurses, nutritionists, dietitians, and social workers-establishes a comprehensive treatment plan intended to restore you or your loved one to
the highest practicable potential.

6557 Belden Center
606 Humboldt St
Santa Rosa, CA 95404-4219   707-579-2735
                          FAX: 707-579-4145
Casey Harding, Owner
Pamela Fadden, Owner
Postacute rehabilitation program.

6558 Blind Babies Foundation
Suite 300
1814 Franklin St
Oakland, CA 94612-3487   510-446-2229
                      FAX: 510-446-2262
                      bbfinfo@blindbabies.org
                      blindbabies.org

Dottie Bridge, President
Aben Hill, 1st Vice President
Clare Friedman, PhD, 2nd Vice President
Beverly Libaire, Treasurer
Mission: when an infant or pre school child is identified as blind
or visually impaired, provides family-centered services to sup-
port the child's optimal development and access to the world.

6559 Brotman Medical Center: RehabCare Unit
Brotman Medical Center
3828 Delmas Terrace
Culver City, CA 90232-2713   310-836-7000
                                    800-677-1238
                        FAX: 310-202-4105
                        info@brotmanmed.com
                        phvc.com

Jennifer Cortez, Program Manager
Kevin O'Connor, CEO
Scott Leonard, CTO
Ben Taylor, Senior Editor
Culver City is centrally located within the city of Los Angeles.
These are two programs offering inpatient rehabilitation. The
acute rehab program is designed for patients who need physical
rehabilitation due to injury or medical disability. This program
requires patients to participate in 3 hours therapy per day. The
sub-acute program is designed especially for patients who need
rehab but cannot tolerate the intensity of the acute rehab
program..

6560 Build Rehabilitation Industries
12432 Foothill Blvd
Sylmar, CA 91342   818-898-0020
                     FAX: 818-898-1949
                     buildindustries.com

6561 California Elwyn
18325 Mt. Baldy Circle
Fountain Valley, CA 92708-6115   714-557-6313
                               FAX: 714-963-2961
                               info@elwyn.org
                               elwyn.org
Sandra S. Cornelius, President of Elwyn
*Daniel M. Reardon, Senior Vice President and Chief Operating Of-
ficer*
Stan H. Retif, Vice President for Development a
Richard T. Smith, Vice President for Information Technology
Provides opportunities for people challenged by physical and
mental disabilities who are 18 or older. California Elwyn develops an Individual Rehabilitation Plan for all consumers. Contract
work, shrinkwrap, janitorial are just some of the types of jobs
done. Supported Employment Services are available and over
100 consumers currently are employed. Funded by the State Department of Rehabilitation and Vocational Rehabilitation.

6562 California Eye Institute
1360 E Herndon Ave
Fresno, CA 93720-3326   559-449-5000
                          www.samc.com
Nancy Hollingsworth, President and CEO
Michael W. Martinez, EVP/Chief Operating and Financial Officer
Stephen Soldo, Chief Medical Officer
Christine Sarrico, Chief Financial Officer
A private, nonprofit agency offering services such as health, edu-
cational, recreational, rehabilitation and employment counseling
to the totally blind, legally blind and visually impaired. The staff
includes two full time workers.

6563 Camp Recovery Center
3192 Glen Canyon Rd
Scotts Valley, CA 95066-4916   877-557-6237
                             FAX: 831-438-2789
                             camprecovery.com
Michael Johnson, Ph.D, Executive Director
Tim Sinnott, Clinical Director
Zoe R., Case Manager
Jeff Geiger, Clinical Tech Director
A free-standing social model recovery center for chemical dependency located on 25 wooded acres in the Santa Cruz Mountains. The services include: medical detoxification, complete
medical evaluation, psychiatric evaluation and counseling, psychological testing, individual counseling and more. Helps the recovery from chemical dependency in a easier, warm and caring
environment.

6564   Campobello Chemical Dependency Recovery Center
2448 Guerneville Road
Suite 400
Santa Rosa, CA 95402- 4030   707-546-1547
                                              800-805-1833
                                              FAX: 707-579-1603
                                              campobello.org

6565   Casa Colina Centers for Rehabilitation
P.O.Box 6001
255 East Bonita Avenue
Pomona, CA 91767- 6001   909-596-7733
                                               866-724-4127
                                               FAX: 909-593-0153
                                               TTY: 909-596-3646
                                               casacolina.org

Steve Norin, Chairman
Felice L Loverso, President
Chandrahas Agarwal, Medical Director
Elmer B. Pineda, M.D., Chief Of Medical Staff
Casa Colina, has pioneered effective programs to create opportunity for health, productivity and self-esteem for persons with disability since 1936. Through medical rehabilitation, transitional living, residential, community, and prevention and wellness programs. Casa Colina serves more than 7,000 persons annually. Casa Colina, a non-profit organization, offers a unique spectrum of opportunities, achievement and results to patients and their families.

6566   Casa Colina Padua Village
P.O.Box 6001
255 East Bonita Avenue
Pomona, CA 91767- 6001   909-596-7733
                                               866-724-4127
                                               FAX: 909-593-0153
                                               TTY: 909-596-3646
                                               casacolina.org
Steve Norin, Chairman
Chandrahas Agarwal, Medical Director
Felice L Loverso, President
Elmer B. Pineda, M.D., Chief Of Medical Staff
Long term residential services for adults with developmental disability. Residences include Malmquist House, Woodbend House, and Hillsdale House, all located in Claremont, California.

6567   Casa Colina Residential Services: Rancho Pino Verde
Casa Colina Center for Rehabilitation
P.O.Box 6001
255 East Bonita Avenue
Pomona, CA 91767- 7517   909-596-7733
                                               866-724-4127
                                               FAX: 909-593-0153
                                               TTY: 909-596-3646
                                               www.casacolina.org
Steve Norin, Chairman
Randy Blackman, Vice Chairman
Felice L. Loverso, President
Elmer B. Pineda, M.D., Chief Of Medical Staff
Long term residential services in rural environment for adults with brain injury.

6568   Casa Colina Transitional Living Center
255 East Bonita Avenue
P.O.Box 6001
Pomona, CA 91767- 1923   909-596-7733
                                               866-724-4127
                                               FAX: 909-593-0153
                                               TTY: 909-596-3646
                                               casacolina.org
Steve Norin, Chairman
Felice L Loverso, President
Chandrahas Agarwal, Medical Director
Elmer B. Pineda, M.D., Chief Of Medical Staff
Postacute rehabilitation program.

6569   Casa Colina Transitional Living Center: Pomona
P.O.Box 6001
255 East Bonita Avenue
Pomona, CA 91767- 6001   909-596-7733
                                               866-724-4127
                                               FAX: 909-593-0153
                                               TTY: 909-596-3646
                                               casacolina.org

Steve Norin, Chairman
Felice L Loverso, President
Chandrahas Agarwal, Medical Director
Elmer B. Pineda, M.D., Chief Of Medical Staff
Post acute short term residential program for persons with brain injury. In a home-like setting, therapy promotes successful re-entry to home and community living.

6570   Cedars of Marin
PO Box 947
Ross, CA 94957-947   415-454-5310
                                               FAX: 415-454-0573
                                     lauren@thecedarsofmarin.org
                                               thecedarsofmarin.org

Jefferson Rice, Board Chair
James Brentano, Board Vice President
Andrew Hinkelman, Board Treasurer
Chuck Greene, Executive Director
The Cedars of Marin has provided residential and day programs for adults with developmental disabilities for over 91 years. Our award-winning programs help our clients to live creative, productive, joyous lives.

6571   Center for Neuro Skills
5215 Ashe Rd.
Bakersfield, CA 93313-2988   661-872-3408
                                               800-922-4994
                                               FAX: 661-872-5150
                                     skatomski@neuroskills.com
                                               neuroskills.com
Mark J Ashley, President/CEO and Co-Founder
A comprehensive, post-acute, community based head-injury rehabilitation program serving over 100 clients per year. Since 1980, CNS has effectively treated the entire spectrum of head-injured clients, including those with severe behavioral disorders, cognitive/perceptual impairments, speech/language problems, physical disabilities and post-concussion syndrome.

6572   Center for the Partially Sighted
Suite 150
6101 W. Centinela Ave.
Culver City, CA 90230   310-988-1970
                                               FAX: 310-988-1980
                                               info@low-vision.org
                                               low-vision.org
La Donna S. Ringering, Ph.D, President/CEO
Pam Thompson, Director of Psychological Servic
Phyllis Amaral, Clinical Director
Laura Valencia, Psychosocial Services Coordinato
Services for partially sighted and legally blind people include low vision evaluations, the design and prescription of low vision devices and adaptive technology, as well as counseling and rehabilitation training (independent living skills and orientation/mobility training). Special programs include children's program, diabetes and vision loss program, Technology demonstrations. Store carries low vision aids. Catalog available.

6573   Central Coast Neurobehavioral Center OPTIONS
P.O.Box 877
800 Quintana Road Suite 2C
Morro Bay, CA 93442-877   805-772-6066
                                               FAX: 805-772-6067
                                               info@optionsccnbc.org
                                               www.optionsccnbc.org
Michael Mamot, CEO
Ole von Frausing-Borch, COO
Serves adults with developmental disabilities, traumatic head injuries, or other neurological impairments. OPTIONS operates two transitional living centers, eight licensed residential facilities, two licensed community integration day programs and a li-

censed short term stabilization center. Services offered include: supported and independent living services, group and individual vocational services, neuropsychological assessment, occupational therapy, cognitive therapy, speech therapy and more.

6574 Cerebral Palsy: North County Center
#209
8525 Gibbs Drive
San Diego, CA 92123-1758   858-571-7803
                                 FAX: 858-571-0919
                                 info@ucpsd.org
                                 www.ucpsd.org

David Carucci, Executive Director
Mary Krieger, Associate Executive Director
Bruce Neufeld, Chief Financial Officer
Sophia Williams, Director of Human Resources
The mission of UCP San Diego County is to advance the independence, productivity and full citizenship of people affected by cerebral palsy and other disabilities. By making solid steps, UCP can build a better community for all in the process.

6575 Children's Hospital Central California Rehabilitation Center
9300 Valley Childrens Place
Madera, CA 93636-8762   559-353-3000
                                 www.valleychildrens.org
Todd Suntrapak, President & Chief Executive Officer
David Christensen, MD, SVP Medical Affairs & Chief Medical Officer
Beverly Hayden-Pugh, Vice President & Chief Nursing Officer
Kirk Larson, Vice President & Chief Informati
A 297-bed pediatric medical center on a 50-acre campus. We now have more then 500 doctors practicing in over 40 pediatric subspecialties with clinics and services throughout the state.

6576 Children's Hospital Los Angeles Rehabilitation Program
4650 W Sunset Blvd
Los Angeles, CA 90027-6062   323-361-4155
                                 888-631-2452
                                 FAX: 323-361-8101
                                 webmaster@chla.usc.edu
                                 www.childrenshospitalla.org
Richard D. Cordova, President & CEO
Rodney B. Hanners, Senior Vice President and Chief
Henri R. Ford, M.D.
Lawrence L. Foust, J.D.,, Secretary
Designated as a Level I Pediatric Trauma Canter by the Los Angeles County EMS Agency, the hospital treats more then 1,500 pediatric trauma patients per year. Performs more then 13,900 pediatric surgeries a year, including more complex surgical procedures then any other hospital in Southern California

6577 Children's Therapy Center
Ste 120
770 Paseo Camarillo
Camarillo, CA 93010-6092   805-383-1501
                                 FAX: 805-383-1504
                                 ctcinc@isle.net
Beth Maulhardt, Owner
Provides individual occupational therapy, speech/language therapy, family/child consulting, education services and physical therapy consultation for children. Evaluations and treatment are on an individual basis and special emphasis is placed on a multidisciplinary approach with information sharing, and often team treatment.

6578 Clausen House
88 Vernon Street
Oakland, CA 94610-4217   510-839-0050
                                 info@clausenhouse.org
                                 clausenhouse.org
Deborah Levy, Interim Executive Director
Michael A. Scott, Director of Development
Stan Nicholson, Director of Human Resources
Jaynette Underhill, Director of Program Services
Residential, supported employment, independent and supported living, adult education, and social recreation activities. Serving the developmentally disabled since 1967.

6579 Community Gatepath
1764 Marco Polo Way
Burlingame, CA 94010-4503   650-259-8544
                                 helpmychild@gatepath.com
                                 communitygatepath.com
Sheryl Young, Chief Executive Officer
John Marvuglio, Chief Financial Officer
Gabrielle Karampelas, Vice President of Strategic Initiatives & Collaborations
Anne Jarchow, Director of Internal Communications and Culture
Popular center and Peninsula Care merged into a new organization named Community Gatepath. Driving forces behind the merger were to be able to provide expanded and/or better services to indidviduals throughout San Mateo County, using the best practices of both organizations.

6580 Community Hospital and Rehabilitation Center of Los Gatos-Saratoga
815 Pollard Rd
Los Gatos, CA 95032-1438   408-378-6131
                                 FAX: 408-866-4003
                                 communityhospitallosgatos.com
Gary Honts, CEO
Offers rehabilitation services, inpatient and outpatient care, physical therapy, occupational therapy and more for the physically challenged adult. We have a commitment to health care excellence. It is in this commitment that we have dedicated ourselves to provide personal and professional service to our patients. Our goal is to work closely with staff, physicians and the community to attain shared goals and positive changes, now and in the future..

6581 Contra Costa ARC
1340 Arnold Drive
Suite 127
Martinez, CA 94553-4189   925-370-1818
                                 FAX: 925-370-2048
                                 feedback@arcofcc.org
                                 www.ContraCostaARC.com
Barbara Maizie, Executive Director
Diana Jorgensen, Program Coordinator
Andrey George, Administrative Coordinator
A private nonprofit membership-based organization dedicated to enhancing the quality of life of individuals with mental retardation and other developmental disabilities.

6582 Corona Regional Medical Center- Rehabiltation Center
800 S. Main St.
Corona, CA 92882-3117   951-737-4343
                                 FAX: 951-736-7276
                                 www.coronaregional.com
Diane Mc Donald, Manager
Mark Uffer, Chief Executive Officer
Doreen Dann, Chief Nursing Officer
Douglas Crouse, Chairman of the Board
Offers inpatient and outpatient rehabilitation services. The Center consists of an acute rehab unit, a subacute rehab unit containing modules for long-term ventilator care, respiratory rehab, coma intervention and orthopedics. In addition to inpatient therapies, the Center's outpatient programs include sports and industrial medicine.

6583 Critical Air Medicine
Montgomery Field
8775 Aero Drive
Suite 235
San Diego, CA 92123-1705   858-300-0224
                                 800-247-8326
                                 FAX: 858-300-0228
                                 criticalair.ops@criticalair.com
                                 www.aircharterguide.com
Frank Craven, Publisher of the Air Charter Guide
Offers emergency medical care by air medical transport carriers. These carriers are fully equipped with medical equipment and supplies for cardiovascular emergencies, respiratory supplies, orthopedic supplies and medications..

6584   Crutcher's Serenity House
P.O.Box D
50 Hillcrest Drive
Deer Park, CA 94576-504   707-963-3192
                                   FAX: 707-963-2309
                                   crutcherssh@earthlink.net
                                   www.crutcherssh.com

Robert Crutcher, Owner/CEO
Lu Crutcher, Executive Director
A privately owned and operated facility that introduces to residents a new lifestyle free of all chemicals, and a new awareness of their total being. The length of the program is four weeks and is within five minutes of an acute care hospital. The Center is licensed for 19 beds, male and female located in a home-like setting with an emphasis on maintaining a family atmosphere.

6585   Daniel Freeman Rehabilitation Centers
333 N Prairie Ave
PO Box 28990
Santa Ana, CA 92799-4501   714-230-3150
                                   FAX: 714-850-0153
                                   advertising@acupuncturetoday.com
                                   www.acupuncturetoday.com

H Arndt, Associate Administrator
Gabrielle Lindsley, Business Development Manager
Evelyn Petersen, Human Resources / Payroll Manager
Andrea Weeks, Accountant
Comprehensive rehabilitation services which address needs and issues of the physically diabled and their families. We offer acute input rehabilitation, outpatient and short term skilled nursing rehabilitaion. Specialty areas include: brain injury, stroke, spinal chord injury, chronic pain, arthritis..

6586   Delano Regional Medical Center
1401 Garces Highway
Delano, CA 93215-3690   661-725-4800
                                   info@drmc.com
                                   drmc.com

Bahram Ghaffari, President
Jeremy Klemm, HealthStream Regional Director
Robert A. Frist, HealthStream CEO
Delano Regional Medical Center (DRMC) is proud to be known throughout California & beyond as an innovative regional hospital, deeply rooted in the local communities and committed to providing an exceptional patient experience. A non-profit acute-care facility serving a region of 10 rural central Californiatowns. With over 100 physicians on our active medical staff and additional courtesy or consulting physicians, patients are assured of receiving high-quality care in multiple specialties.

6587   Desert Regional Medical Center
1150 N Indian Canyon Dr
Palm Springs, CA 92262   760-323-6511
                                       800-491-4990
                                   www.desertmedctr.com

Carolyn Caldwell, Chief Executive Officer
Tracey Cowles, Physician Relations Manager
Jeanne Stanton, RN, Chair
Lee Bledsoe, Physician Relations Manager
Our dedicated physicians and caregivers provide a broad array of quality programs and services, including comprehensive cancer care, women's health services, heart care, surgical weight loss reduction and orthopedics.

6588   Devereux Advanced Behavioral HealthCalifornia
P.O.Box 6784
Santa Barbara, CA 93160-6784   805-968-2525
                                   FAX: 805-968-3247
                                   www.devereuxca.org

Amy Evans, Executive Director
Rebecca Popke, Marketing & Admissions Manager
Cassi Noel, Manager of External Affairs
Sherry Davis, Clinical Case Manager
Serves adults age 18 through life span who have intellectual and developmental disabilities, emotional disturbances, neurological impairments, brain injuries, schizophrenia, autism, and dual diagnosis. Devereux California currently provides a continuum of services, including on-campus residential, day programs, behavior management, and supported living services in the community.

6589   Division of Physical Medicine and Rehabilitation
San Joaquin General Hospital
500 W Hospital Rd
French Camp, CA 95231-9693   209-468-6000
                                   FAX: 209-468-6501
                                   pmradministration@sjgh.hs.co.san-joaquin.ca.u
                                   www.sjphysicalmedicine.com

6590   Dr. Karen H Chao Developmental Optometry Karen H. Chao. O.D.
Suite A
121 S Del Mar Ave
San Gabriel, CA 91776-1345   626-287-0401
                                   FAX: 626-287-1457
                                   drkhchao@yahoo.com
                                   www.healthgrades.com

Karen Chao, Owner
Karen Chao OD, Owner
Roger C. Holstein, Chief Executive Officer
Jeff Surges, President
Developmental optometrist specializing in the testing and treatment of vision problems and the enhancement of visual performance. Performs visual perceptual testing and training for children and adults. Undetected vision problems interfere with the ability to achieve and are highly correlated with learning difficulties and developmental problems. Provides the opportunity to overcome vision and visual-perceptual dysfunctions..

6591   Early Childhood Services
Desert Area Resources and Training
201 E Ridgecrest Blvd
Ridgecrest, CA 93555-3919   760-375-9787
                                   FAX: 760-375-1288
                                   dart@dartontarget.org
                                   www.dartontarget.org/

Peter V. Berns, Chief Executive Officer
Cris Bridges, Chief of Client Services
Bob Beecroft, Chief Operations Officer
Jeannie Luke, Human Resources Director/Risk Ma
Provides early intervention services to children who have disabilities or are experiencing delays in development. Provides developmental activities to promote the attainment of developmental milestones so that each child may reach his/her maximum potential. The program also provides therapeutic and educational intervention and offers support and guidance to families.

6592   East Los Angeles Doctors Hospital
4060 Whittier Boulevard
Los Angeles, CA 90023-2526   323-268-5514
                                   www.elalax.com

Hector Hernandez, Chief Executive Officer
Kamlesh Dhawan, Chief Of Staff
Michael Austerlitz, Vice-Chief Of Staff
Horacio Fleischman, Secretary Treasurer
Postacute rehabilitation program.

6593   Easter Seals Disability Svcs: Bay Area
Suite 250
391 Taylor Boulevard
Pleasant Hill, CA 94523- 4851   925-849-8999
                                       800-221-6827
                                   FAX: 312-726-1494
                                   info@easterseals.com
                                   www.bayarea.easterseals.com

6594 Easter Seals Superior California
Sacramento Center & Regional Offices
2617 A & B Alta Arden Expy.
Sacramento, CA 95825-1306
916-679-3113
888-877-3257
FAX: 916-485-2653
www.superiorca.easterseals.com
Harry Johns, President and CEO
Kathie Wright, Program Director
Terry Colborn, VP Programs/Government Affairs
Joanne Budge, Chief Financial Officer
Provides outpatient rehabilitation services including day training programs for adults with disabilities and traumatic brain injuries, warm water therapy, non-public agency services to children including pediatric OT and PT services, work training/employment services, medical equipment loans, early intervention services for infants and toddlers. Serving the counties of Alpine, Calaveras, El Dorado, Sacramento, San Joaquin, Sutter, Tuolumne, Yolo, Yuba, Amador, Stanislaus, Nevada and Placer, CA.

6595 Exceed: A Division of Valley Resource Center
P.O.Box 1773
1285 N. Santa Fe
Hemet, CA 92543-1773
951-766-8659
800-423-1227
FAX: 951-929-9758
vrctwohip@aol.com
www.exceed-solutions.org
Pattie Robert, Business Development Specialist
Mary Morse, Marketing Director
Kathy Cooke, Manager
Our vision is an environment where each client is valued as an individual and is provided the opportunity to reach his/her maximum potential. Our mission is to provide service and advocacy, which creates choices and opportunities, for adults with disabilities to reach their maximum potential..

6596 Eye Medical Center of Fresno
Eye Medical Center
1360 E. Herndon Avenue
Suite 301 & 210
Fresno, CA 93720-1498
559-486-5000
emcfresno.com

6597 Fontana Rehabilitation Workshop
Industrial Support Systems
8333 Almeria Ave
Fontana, CA 92335-3283
909-428-3883
800-755-4755
FAX: 909-428-3835
ceo@industrialsupport.org
www.industrial-support.org
Silvia Anderson, Executive Director
U. Jones, CFO
C.Steven Bowen Plant, Operations manager
Bonnie Edwards, Operations Manager
The Fontana Rehabilitation Workshop, Inc., through its business divisions is committed to maintaining a stable environment wherein people with disabilities are provided with those services and supports that enable them to overcome barriers to employment and empower them to maximize their employment potential.

6598 Foothill Vocational Opportunities
789 North Fair Oaks Avenue
Pasadena, CA 91103-3045
626-449-0218
FAX: 626-449-0218
info@foothillvoc.org
foothillvoc.org

6599 Fred Finch Youth Center
3800 Coolidge Ave
Oakland, CA 94602-3399
510-482-2244
FAX: 510-488-1960
receptionist@fredfinch.org
fredfinch.org
Vonza Thompson, President/CEO
Kathie Jacobson, COO
Ed Hsu, CFO
Sue Guy, Chief Human Resource Officer
Seeks to provide a continum of high quality programs for the care and treatment of children, youth, young adults and their families, whose changing needs can best be met by a variety of mental health and social services. The goal is for clients to be professionally served in the least restricitive environment appropriate to their needs so that they may function at their highest potential.

6600 Gateway Center of Monterey County
850 Congress Ave
Pacific Grove, CA 93950-4898
831-372-8002
FAX: 831-372-2411
info@gatewaycenter.org
gatewaycenter.org
Stephanie Lyon, Executive Director
Mike Price, Chief Financial Officer
Desiree Boller, Accounting Assistant
Heidy Welch, Human Resources
Our mission is to be a caring and stimulating environment for the Developmentally Disabled where all people can achieve their individual goals safely and with dignity. Our goal is to continue our programs and to find new and innovative ways of assisting the developmentally disabled to live in our community in surroundings compatable with their ability to live and work at the highest level possible.

6601 Gateway Industries: Castroville
7055 Veterans Blvd
Unit A
Burr Ridge, IL 60527
630-321-1333
888-473-3744
FAX: 630-321-1321
growth@redshft.com
www.redshift.com

6602 Gilroy Workshop
7471 Monterey Street
Gilroy, CA 95020-3629
408-430-2810
FAX: 408-842-6770
info@leadershipgilroy.org
www.leadershipgilroy.org/
Kristi Alarid, Manager
Sally French, Manager
Denise Martin, Executive Director
Andrea Gamble, Administrative Director
Work adjustment and remunerative work programs..

6603 Glendale Adventist Medical Center
1509 Wilson Ter
Glendale, CA 91206-4098
818-409-8000
FAX: 818-546-5609
www.glendaleadventist.com/services/rehab
Kevin Roberts, President/CEO
Warren Tetz, Sr. Vice President and COO
Kelly Turner, Sr. Vice President and CFO
Judy Blair, Sr. Vice President and CNO
Rehabilitative team is made up of physician specialists, as well as professional and certified staff nurses, thereapists and others who meet regularly to ensure tht each patients progress is carefully planned and closely monitored.

6604 Glendale Memorial Hospital and Health Center Rehabilitation Unit
Glendale Memorial Hospital and Health Center
1420 South Central Ave
Glendale, CA 91204-2508
818-502-1900
FAX: 818-409-7688
www.glendalememorialhospital.org
Catherine M. Pelley, President

Offers rehabilitation services, occupational therapy, physical therapy, residential services and more for the disabled.

6605 Goleta Valley Cottage Hospital
Cottage Health System
351 S Patterson Ave
Santa Barbara, CA 93111-2496   805-967-3411
FAX: 805-681-6437
cverkiak@cottagehealthsystem.org
www.sbch.org

Ronald C. Wreft, President & CEO
Rosemary Bray, Clinical Manager
Diana Gray Miller, Administrator
Betty Jane Petrich, Manager

A 122-bed acute care hospital was founded in 1966 to serve the growing community of Goleta Valley. Today, we admit more then 2,000 patients a year, see more then 17,000 emergency visits, and welcome nearly 400 newborns to our designated 'Baby Friendly' Birth Center each year. We are also recognized for our Level IV trauma designation. We take great pride in fulfilling our goal of providing each patient with comfortable, personalized care.

6606 HealthSouth Tustin Rehabilitation Hospital
Health South Corporation
14851 Yorba St
Tustin, CA 92780-2925   714-832-9200
www.tustinrehab.com/

Diana Hanyak, Chief Executive Officer
Rodric Bell, Medical Director
Lindsey Barrett, Director of Case Management
Maryam Jouharzadeh, Pharm.D., Director, Pharmacy

HealthSouth Tustin Rehabilitation Hospital is part of the HealthSouth Corportation, the nation's largest provider of rehabilitative healthcare services, we are the only facility of its kind in Orange County. Fully accredited by the Joint Commission on Accreditation of Healthcare Organizations (JACHO) we provide inpatient and outpatient care designed to meed individual needs of patients and their families.

6607 Hi-Desert Medical Center
6601 White Feather Road
Joshua Tree, CA 92252-760   760-366-3711
hdmc.org

Lionel Chadwick, Chief Executive Officer
Tom Duda, Chief Financial Officer
Judy Austin, Chief Operating Officer & Chief
Barbara Staresinic, Director, Human Resources

Postacute rehabilitation program.

6608 Home of the Guiding Hands
Suite 200
1825 Gillespie Way
El Cajon, CA 92020-0501   619-938-2850
FAX: 619-938-3055
info@guidinghands.org
guidinghands.org

Mary Miller, President
Debby McNeil, Vice President
Michael Harris, Treasurer
Mark Klaus, Executive Director

The mission of Home og the Guiding Hands is to provide quality services, training and advocacy for people with developmental disabilities, their families, and others who will benefit.

6609 Hospital of the Good Samaritan Acute Rehabilitation Unit
1225 Wilshire Blvd
Los Angeles, CA 90017-1901   213-977-2121
800-366-8338
FAX: 213-482-2770
info@goodsam.org
goodsam.org

Andrew B Leeka, President and CEO
Charles T. Munger, Chairman

Physicians, researchers and staff are united by a common mission: to foster growth into one of the most comprehensive medical centers in the West. Services offered include: cardiology and cardiovascular services, neurosciences, movement disorders and Parkinsons disorder, wound care center and transfusion-medicine and surgery center.

6610 Innovative Rehabilitation Services
Hacienda La Puente Unified School District
15959 E. Gale Ave
City Of Industry, CA 91745   626-933-1000
FAX: 626-934-2900
info@hlpusd.k12.ca.us
www.hlpusd.k12.ca.us

Matthew Smith, Site Administrator
George Stransky, Counselor
Crystal Ontiveros, Counselor

Provides innovative student-centered learning opportunities and support services to a diverse population that enable individuals to achieve thier goals as lifelong learners, productive workers and effective communicators.

6611 Janus of Santa Cruz
Suite 150
200 7th Ave
Santa Cruz, CA 95062-4669   831-462-1060
866-526-8772
janussc.org

Rod Libbey, Executive Director
Bill Morris, Medical Director
Margie Storms, Clinical Director
Chris Storms, Intake Manager

A private not-for-profit corporation, licensed by the state of California. The Janus Clinic has a 3 year accreditation by the Council on Accreditation for Health Care Facilities.

6612 John Muir Medical Center Rehabilitation Services, Therapy Center
1601 Ygnacio Valley Rd
Walnut Creek, CA 94598-3122   925-939-3000
FAX: 925-308-8944
www.johnmuirhealth.com

Calvin Knight, President and CEO
Helen Doughty, Librarian

A 324-bed acute care facility that is designated as the only trauma center for Contra Costa County and portions of Solano County. Recognized as one of the region's premier healthcare providers, areas of specialty include high-and low-risk obstetrics, orthopedics, neurosciences, cardiac care and cancer care. The campus is accredited by the Joint Commission on Accreditation of Healthcare Organizations (JCAHO), a national surveyor of quality patient care.

6613 Kindred Hospital-La Mirada
14900 E. Imperial Hwy
La Mirada, CA 90638-2172   562-944-1900
FAX: 562-906-3455
TTY:800-735-2922
www.kindredlamirada.com

April Myers, Administrator
Adam Darvish, Executive Director

Committed to the delivery of high quality care in a cost-effective manner to enable us to become 'a model of excellence' in Long-Term Acute Care. Committed to treat our patients and families with dignity and respect, in the same manner we would want to be treated.

6614 King's View Work Experience Center- Atwater
559 East Bardsley Avenue
P. O. Box 688
Tulare, CA 93275-0688   559-688-7531
FAX: 559-688-3509
info@kingsview.org
www.kingsview.org

Leon Hoover, Chief Executive Officer
Vida Jalali, Chief Financial Officer Interim
Sue Essman, Director of Human Resources
Jeff Gorski, Director of Business Development

The primary mission of the Kings View Work Experience Center (KVWEC) is to serve people who have developmental disabilities. We believe in the dignity and worth of each person and in their right to rehabilitation, education and community integration. It is Kings View's aim to provide quality services to people who need assistance in the development of social, vocational and independent living skills.

6615 LaPalma Intercommunity Hospital
7901 Walker St
La Palma, CA 90623-1764   714-670-7400
LPIHInfo@primehealthcare.com
www.lapalmaintercommunityhospital.com
Virg Narbutas, Regional CEO
Sami Shoukair, Chief Medical Officer
Linda Gonzaba, Medical Staff Office Director
Hilda Manzo-Luna, Chief Nursing Officer
Lapalma Intercommunity Hospital endeavors to provide comprehensive, quality healthcare in a convenient, compassionate and cost effective manner. Lapalma is consistenty at the forefront of evolving national healthcare reform. Our organization provides an innovative and integrated healthcare delivery system. We remain ever cognizant of our patient's needs and desires for high quality affordable healthcare.

6616 Learning Services of Northern California
131 Langley Drive
Suite B
Lawrenceville, GA 30046-9315   408-848-4379
                                          888-419-9955
                                     FAX: 866-491-7396
www.learningservices.com
Dr. Debra Braunling-McMorrow, President and CEO
Jeanne Mack, Chief Financial Officer and Vice President of Operations
Michael Weaver, Chief Development Officer
Susan Snow, Director of Admissions
Located on 10 acres of ranchland in rural Santa Clara Valley, our Gilroy Program offers treatment, structure, and support in a spacious, campus-based living environment. Sharing living residences are complimented by a treatment and recreation facility for individuals who require intensive support.

6617 Learning Services: Morgan Hill
131 Langley Drive
Suite B
Lawrenceville, GA 30046-9315   408-848-4379
                                          888-419-9955
                                     FAX: 866-491-7396
www.learningservices.com
Dr. Debra Braunling-McMorrow, President and CEO
Jeanne Mack, Chief Financial Officer and Vice President of Operations
Michael Weaver, Chief Development Officer
Susan Snow, Director of Admissions
Located in the quaint rural town within walking distance from the old main street of Morgan Hill. Our Morgan Hill program offers the convenience and amenities of small-town living within the supportive community of Morgan Hill.

6618 Learning Services: Supported Living Programs
131 Langley Drive
Suite B
Lawrenceville, GA 30046-9315   408-848-4379
                                          888-419-9955
                                     FAX: 866-491-7396
www.learningservices.com
Dr. Debra Braunling-McMorrow, President and CEO
Jeanne Mack, Chief Financial Officer and Vice President of Operations
Michael Weaver, Chief Development Officer
Susan Snow, Director of Admissions
We offer a variety of diverse and stimulating environments for people with different needs, capabilities and personal goals. Within comfortable, homelike, age-appropriate settings we provide the structure and support necessary to ensure the richest possible quality of life. Program offered in both Northern and Southern facilities of California

6619 Leon S Peters Rehabilitation Center
2823 Fresno St
Fresno, CA 93721-1324   559-459-6000
www.communitymedical.org
Florence Dunn, Chairwoman
John McGregor, Esquire, Secretary
Tim A. Joslin, President, Chief Executive Officer
Patrick Rafferty, Executive Vice President, Chief Operating Officer
Community's flagship hospital that offers world class specialized critical care with the area's only stroke unit with 24-hour vascular neurology and neurosurgery coverage and a team of specially trained stroke nurses. The world's first G4 CyberKnife. The table Mountain Rancheraia Level 1 Trauma Center. The Leon S. Peters burn center. The region's only perinatology program for high rish pregnancies and deliveries. The Da-Vinci robotic surgical system, and 3 helicopeter landing pads.

6620 Lion's Blind Center of Diablo Valley, Inc. Lions Center For The Visually Impaired
175 Alvarado Ave
Pittsburg, CA 94565-4862   925-432-3013
                                          800-750-3937
                                     FAX: 925-432-7014
edward.329@comcast.net
www.seniorvision.org
Edward Schroth, Executive Director
Barbara Cronin, President
Charles Dunham, First Vice President
Phillis Neitling, Secretary
A private, nonprofit agency offering services such as health, educational, recreational, rehabilitation, employment and counseling to the totally blind, legally blind and visually impaired. The staff includes two full time workers..

6621 Lion's Blind Center of Oakland
2115 Broadway
Oakland, CA 94612-2698   510-450-1580
                                     FAX: 510-654-3603
info@lbcenter.org
lbcenter.org
Michelle Taylor Lagunas, Executive Director/ CEO
Christina Easiley, Administrative Manager
Scott Blanks, Director of Rehabilitation Servi
Danette Davis, Orientation & Mobility Instructor
A private nonprofit organization offering services for the totally blind, legally blind, deaf-blind and multihandicapped blind. Services include: professional training, rehabilitation, education, counseling, social work, self help and more. The staff includes 12 full time and 1 part time worker.

6622 Living Skills Center for the Visually Impaired
2430 Road 20
#B112
San Pablo, CA 94806-5005   510-234-4984
                                     FAX: 510-234-4986
info@hcblind.org
www.hcblind.org
Patricia Williams, Executive Director
Patricia Maffei, Program Director
Ronald Hideshima, Adaptive Technology Instructor
Lee Staub, Orientation and Mobility Instruc
A private, nonprofit agency offering services such as independent living skills training, recreational, employment and accessible technology training to the totally blind, legally blind and visually impaired. The staff includes six full time teachers.

6623 Loma Linda University Orthopedic and Rehabilitation Institute
25333 Barton Rd
Loma Linda, CA 92354-3123   909-558-1000
                                     FAX: 909-558-0308
www.llu.edu
Richard H. Hart, MD, DrPH, President & Chief Executive Officer
Ronald L. Carter, PhD, Senior Vice President, Educational Affairs
Cari Dominguez, DHS, Senior Vice President, Human Resources
Mark L. Hubbard, Senior Vice President, Risk Management
Offers a full range of clinical programs for both inpatients and outpatient. The specific diagnosis leading to patient admission

includes stroke, spinal cord injury, traumatic or anoxic brain damage, amputation, post neurosurgery, chronic neurological disease, Guillain-Barre syndrome, arthritis, multiple trauma or other complex orthopedic problems. The facilities and professional services are comprehensive and ensure that the best care is provided to pediatric and adult patients..

6624   Manor Care Health Services- Citrus Heights
7807 Uplands Way
Citrus Heights, CA 95610-7500   916-967-2929
                                  FAX: 916-965-8439
                                  hcr-manorcare.com

Steven M. Cavanaugh, Chief Financial Officer
Paul A. Ormond, Chairman, President and Chief Ex
The nations leader in skilled nursing and rehabilitation care. Our facility has been serving the Sacramento area for more then 12 years. We are known for our beautiful decor, outstanding rehabilitation staff and loving nursing care. We offer short term rehabilitation, long term skilled nursing care, respite care and post hospital surgical care.

6625   Manor Care Health Services- Palm Desert
74-350 Country Club Dr
Palm Desert, CA 92260-1608   760-341-0261
                                  FAX: 760-779-1563
                                  hcr-manorcare.com

Steven M. Cavanaugh, Chief Financial Officer
Paul A. Ormond, Chairman, President and Chief Ex
Centrally located in the Coachella Valley, specializing in skilled nursing whith an emphasis on rehabilitation, post surgery recovery, hospice, alzheimer's care and long term care. In addition, we offer 2 unique service options for the discriminating consumer. Our Arcadia unit offers a specialized Alzheimer's care program in a dedicated secure wing. ManorCare offers rehabilitation services including physical, occupational and speech therapies for those recovering from illness injury or surgery.

6626   Manor Care Health Services-Fountain Valley
11680 Warner Ave
Fountain Valley, CA 92708-2513   714-241-9800
                                  FAX: 714-966-1654
                                  hcr-manorcare.com

Steven M. Cavanaugh, Chief Financial Officer
Paul A. Ormond, Chairman, President and Chief Ex
Provides 24-hour skilled nursing, rehabilitative therapies and specialized Alzheimer's care. Our in-house therapists provide physical, occupational and speech therapies in our rehabilitation area. Our team is goal oriented and focuses on producing positive outcomes for those recovering from illness, injury or surgery. Our respite care program provides a full range of services for a few days, a week or even a season.

6627   Manor Care Health Services-Hemet
1717 W Stetson Ave
Hemet, CA 92545-6882   951-925-9171
                                  FAX: 951-925-8186
                                  hcr-manorcare.com

Steven M. Cavanaugh, Chief Financial Officer
Paul A. Ormond, Chairman, President and Chief Ex
Provides skilled nursing, Rehabilitation services, and specialized Alzheimer's care. In addition we offer short term respite stays for family caregivers that simply need a break from the stress of daily care. Our Arcadia unit staff is specially trained in the care of residents with Alzheimer's disease. The secured unit is designed to provide a soothing and homelike environment while enhancing each resident's remaining abilities.

6628   Manor Care Health Services-Sunnyvale
1150 Tilton Dr
Sunnyvale, CA 94087-2440   408-735-7200
                                  FAX: 408-736-8629
                                  hcr-manorcare.com

Steven M. Cavanaugh, Chief Financial Officer
Paul A. Ormond, Chairman, President and Chief Ex
Our in-house therapists provide physical, occupational and speech therapies in our rehabilitation area. Our team is goal oriented and focuses on producing positive outcomes for those recovering from illness, injury or surgery. Our skilled nursing staff

works with our therapy department and dietary department to provide positive wound care programs for patients requiring skin management care.

6629   Manor Care Health Services-Walnut Creek
1226 Rossmoor Pkwy
Walnut Creek, CA 94595-2538   925-975-5000
                                  FAX: 925-937-1132
                                  hcr-manorcare.com

Steven M. Cavanaugh, Chief Financial Officer
Paul A. Ormond, Chairman, President and Chief Ex
Provides luxurious long term care and rehabilitation services. In house therapists provide, physical, occupational and speech therapies in our rehabilitation area. Our team is goal oriented and focuses on producing positive outcomes for those recovering from illness, injury or surgery. Our years of combined management experience add value to our resident's quality of life.

6630   Maynord's Chemical Dependency Recovery Centers
19325 Cherokee Road
Tuolumne, CA 95379-1657   209-928-3737
                                       800-228-8208
                                  FAX: 209-928-1152
                                  maynords.com

James Berry, Director
Maynord's Recovery Centers has always been dedicated to the recovery of good people whose lives are being destroyed by alcohol and drugs. Since 1978, Maynord's residential program has helped thousands of people put their lives back together after addiction has taken its toll. Today, Maynord's offers a treatment system over much of the San Joaquin Valley and the San Francisco Bay Area.

6631   Maynord's Ranch for Men
19325 Cherokee Road
Tuolumne, CA 95379-1657   209-928-3737
                                       800-228-8208
                                  FAX: 209-928-1152
                                  maynords.com

James Berry, Director
Provides treatment for chemical dependency problems to men. The treatment addresses their recovery through a comprehensive plan created for their individual needs. Also offers a program for women called the Meadows.

6632   Meadowbrook Manor
431 West Remington Boulevard
Bolingbrook, IL 60440   630-759-1112
                                  FAX: 630-759-6925
                                  jmolen@meadowbrookmanor.com
                                  www.meadowbrookmanor.com

6633   Meadowview Manor
41 Crestview Terrace
Bridgeport, WV 26330   304-842-7101
                                  FAX: 304-842-7104
                                  info@meadowviewmanor.com
                                  www.meadowviewmanor.com

6634   Memorial Hospital of Gardenia
1145 West Redondo Beach Blvd
Gardena, CA 90247-3528   310-532-4200
                                       800-782-2288
                                  www.avantihospitals.com/memorial-hospital-of-
Edward Mirzabegian, Corporate Chief Executive Officer
Postacute rehabilitation program..

6635   Mercy Medical Group
Mercy Hospital
3000 Q Street
Sacramento, CA 95816   916-733-3333
                                  www.mymercymedicalgroup.org

6636 Napa County Mental Health Department
2344 Old Sonoma Road
Bldg. D
Napa, CA 94559-3708 707-259-8151
800-648-8650
www.countyofnapa.org/MentalHealth/

6637 Napa Valley Support Systems
1700 Second Street Suite 212
Napa, CA 94559-1344 707-253-7490
FAX: 707-253-0115
napavalleysupportservices.org

Beth Kahiga, Executive Director
Heather Jump, Administrative Manager
Katy Vanzant, Program Director
Emmy Lesko, Program Supervisor
Work hardening and disciplinary programs.

6638 North Valley Services
1040 Washington
Red Bluff, CA 96080-4509 530-527-0407
FAX: 530-527-7091
www.northvalleyservices.org

Joe Brown, President
Larry Donnelley, Vice President
Lynn DeFreece, CEO
Delbert Brownfield, COO
Provides vocational rehabilitation services, such as job counseling, job training, and work experience, to unemployed and underemployed persons, persons with disabilities.

6639 Northridge Hospital Medical Center Rehabiltation Medicine
18300 Roscoe Blvd
Northridge, CA 91328-4167 818-885-8500
FAX: 818-701-7367
www.northridgehospital.org/index.htm

Mike L. Wall, President
Thomas L. Hedge, Medical Director
Joel S. Rosen, Associate Medical Director
Alex L. Lin, Managing Director
A full service, comprehensive rehabilitation program suited to treat patients of all ages who have suffered catastrophic or debiltating injury or illness. The goal of the program is to deliver exceptional patient care to maximise each individual's skills and independence.

6640 Northridge Hospital Medical Center: Centerfor Rehabilitation Medicine
18300 Roscoe Blvd
Northridge, CA 91328-4167 818-885-8500
FAX: 818-701-7367
www.northridgehospital.com

Mike L. Wall, President
Thomas L. Hedge, Medical Director
Joel S. Rosen, Associate Medical Director
Alex L. Lin, Managing Director
Committed to serving the health needs of our communities with particular attention to the needs of the poor, the disadvantaged, and vulneralbe, and the comfort of the suffering and dying. Catholic Healthcare West has a commitment to quality-quality healthcare services and the promotion of optimal quality of life for all of life.

6641 Old Adobe Developmental Services
1301A Rand Street
Suite A
Petaluma, CA 94954-5697 707-763-9807
FAX: 707-763-7708
webmaster@oadsinc.org
www.oadsinc.org

Elizabeth Clary, Executive Director
Marie Padgett, Controller
The mission of Old Adobe to provide opportunities for individuals with developmental challenges to reach thier fullest potentials. Our job at OADS is to find ways for these individuals to find full expression in all parts of their lives. We have a partnership with the Adult Education Department of the Petaluma School District in providing services to persons with developmental challenges. We are funded by the Dept. of Rehabilitation and the Dept. Of Developmental services.

6642 Old Adobe Developmental Services-Rohnert Park Services (Behavioral)
5401 Snyder Ln.
Rohnert Park, CA 94928-3124 707-584-5859
FAX: 707-664-8057
www.oadsinc.org

Elizabeth Clary, Executive Director
Helen Gunderson, Administrative Assistant
The program services are designed to assist individuals who demonstrate basic work skills, to develop social skills and work habits necessary to succeed in supported or competitive employment. Most often individual program services involve working with the client to replace those behavioral excesses that have been a barrier to vocational placement.

6643 PRIDE Industries
10030 Foothills Blvd
Roseville, CA 95747-7102 916-788-2100
800-550-6005
FAX: 800-888-0447
info@prideindustries.com
prideindustries.com

Michael Ziegler, President & CEO
Bob Selvester, Vice Chair
Mike Snegg, Treasurer
Tim Yamauchi, Executive Vice President and Chi
To provide opportunities through employment, training, evaluation and placement maximizing community access, independence and quality of life for people with barriers to employment.

6644 Pacific Hospital Of Long Beach-Neuro Care Unit
2776 Pacific Ave
Long Beach, CA 90806-2613 562-997-2000
webmaster@phlb.org
www.phlb.org

Michael D. Drobot, CEO
Clark Todd, President
Teri Plemmons, Administrative Assistant
Our mission is to heal with compassion and to perform with distinction. Our vision: to improve the hospital's orthopedic and Spine Center of Excellence. Achieve exceptional financial performance to enhance hospital services. Improve the vertically integrated ancillary, outpatient and inpatient surgery system. Develop a professionally challenging work environment that reflects an agile, peak performance culture.

6645 Paradise Vally Hospital-South Bay Rehabilitation Center
2400 East 4th St
National City, CA 91950-2026 619-470-4321
paradisevalleyhospital.net

Prem Reddy, Chairman
Neerav Jadeja, Administrator
Luis Leon, President
Gemma Rama-Banaag, Chief Nursing Officer
South Bay Rehabilitation Center, offers a complete range of treatment for patients with physical disabilities. Our specialized inpatient and outpatient programs are designed to meet each person's individual needs or injuries, with the goal of restoring as much independence as possible and significantly improving their lives.

6646 Parents and Friends
350 South Main Street
Fort Bragg, CA 95437-5408 707-964-4940
moon@parentsandfriends.org
parentsandfriends.org

Rick Moon, Executive Director
Jessica Dickey, Administrative Assistant
Kristy Tanguay, Manager
Kathy Connell, Bookkeeper
Parents and Friends provides opportunities for persons with developmental challenges and similar needs to participate fully in our community.

6647   **People Services**
4195 Lakeshore Blvd
Lakeport, CA 95453-6411   707-263-3810
idumont@nctac.com
peopleservices.org

Ilene Dumont, Executive Director
Martin Diesman, Director
Vicki Cole, Director
Kathy Ryan, Director
Providing an array of services for adults with developmental disabilities and other people with disabilities. Services include supported employment, work services, supported living, personal, social and community training, transportation, specialized individual services and much more.

6648   **Petaluma Recycling Center**
Old Adobe Developmental Services
315 2nd St
Petaluma, CA 94952-4230   707-763-4761
FAX: 707-763-4921
davide@oadsinc.org
www.oadsinc.org/petarecycle

Elizabeth Clary, Executive Director
Began in 1974; has been one of the major employers of persons with developmental challenges for 26 years; is the primary recycling facility in the growing city of 52,000; accepts over 20 different kinds of recyclables; employs 20-25 persons a day.

6649   **Pomerado Rehabilitation Outpatient Service**
15615 Pomerado Rd
Poway, CA 92064-2405   858-485-6511
FAX: 858-613-4248

Bob Blake, Director Rehab Services
Jonathan Pee, Manager
A 107-bed acute care hospital. In addition to a round-the-clock Emergency Department, Pomerado offers the area's finest outpaitent surgery center and general medical/surgical services. Pomerado Hospital also is home to a world-class Birth Center and a Level II NICU. Fully JCAHO-accredidted, Pomerado is well-known for offering only private rooms, each with a scenic view of the North Countryside, which enhances the healing atmosphere..

6650   **Pride Industries: Grass Valley**
12451 Loma Rica Dr
Grass Valley, CA 95945-9059   530-477-1832
800-550-6005
FAX: 530-477-8038
info@prideindustries.com
www.prideindustries.com

Bob Olsen, Chairman
Bob Selvester, Vice Chairman
Walt Payne, President/CEO
Mike Snegg, Treasurer
Work adjustment and remunerative work programs. We offer an adult day program as well.

6651   **Rancho Adult Day Care Center**
Rancho Los Amigos Medical Center
7601 Imperial Hwy
Downey, CA 90242-3456   562-401-7111
FAX: 562-401-7991
TTY:562-401-8450
radscenter@aol.com
www,rancho.org/ser_adultday

Valerie Orange, CEO
Margaret L Campbell, Research Director
Provides personal care, social services and a therapeutic program to older adults in order to improve their quality of life. Offers a Clinical Gerontology Service, an Alzheimer's Disease Diagnostic and Treatment Center and a Geriatric Assessment and Rehabilitation Unit..

6652   **Regional Center for Rehabilitation**
2288 Auburn Blvd
Sacramento, CA 95821-1618   916-421-4167
FAX: 916-925-1586

6653   **Rehabilitation Institute of Santa Barbara**
2415 De La Vina St
Santa Barbara, CA 93105-3819   805-569-8999
FAX: 805-687-3707
risb.org

Ralph Pollock, President
Scott Silic MBA, Vice President Of Operations
Cheryl Ellis MD, MHA, VP Medical Services
A regional rehabilitation system with an acute care hospital at the center, the Institute provides specialized inpatient and outpatient programs for brain injury, spinal cord injury, stroke, work-related injury, chronic pain, orthopedic problems and more. Offers a 46-bed acute-care rehabilitation hospital, a free-standing outpatient center, the brain injury continuum, chronic pain program..

6654   **Rehabilitation Institute of Southern California**
1800 E La Veta Ave
Orange, CA 92866-2902   714-633-7400
FAX: 714-633-4586
adults@rio-rehab.com
riorehab.org

Praim S. Singh, Executive Director
Carol Reese, Executive Assistant
Grace Lee, Administrative Assistant
Dana Patton, Personnel Officer
Outpatient rehabilitation serving physically and disabled children and adults. Child development programs, adult day care for disabled seniors, child care for disabled and non-disabled children, outpatient therapy, aquatics, adult day healthcare, independent living, vocational services, social services, and housing.

6655   **Rubicon Programs**
2500 Bissell Avenue
Richmond, CA 94804-1815   510-235-1516
FAX: 510-235-2025
rubicon@rubiconpgms.org
www.rubiconprograms.org

Rob Hope, Chief Program Officer
Jane Fischberg, President and Executive Director
Roger Contreras, CFO
Kelly Dunn, General Counsel and Director of Legal Services
Rubicon Programs Inc. helps people and communities build assets to achieve greater independence. Since 1973, Rubicon has built and operated affordable housing and provided employment, job training, mental health, and other supportive services to individuals who have disabilities, are homeless, or are otherwise economically disadvantaged.

6656   **San Bernardino Valley Lighthouse for the Blind**
762 North Sierra Way
San Bernardino, CA 92410-4438   909-884-3121
FAX: 909-884-2964
lighthouse4blind@aol.com
www.afb.org

Robert Mc Bay, Executive Director
Sandra Wood, Administrative Assistant
Provides training in independent living skills - cooking, mobility and orientation, sewing, Braille and typing. Also, we have classes in macrame, ceramics and basket weaving. Weekly support group and Bible study..

6657   **Santa Clara Valley Blind Center, Inc.**
101 N Bascom Ave
San Jose, CA 95128-1805   408-295-4016
FAX: 408-295-1398
info@visionbeyondsight.org
visionbeyondsight.org

Arnold Chew, President
John Glass, Vice President
Arlene Holmes, Secretary
Sue Szucs, Treasurer
SCVBC's mission is to increase the confidence, independence, and quality of life of the blind and visually impaired through educational, recreational, and rehabilitative programs.

6658 Scripps Memorial Hospital: Pain Center
4275 Campus Point Ct.
San Diego, CA 92121-1205   858-626-4123
                                   800-727-4777
              clinicalresearch@scrippshealth.com
                                   www.scripps.org

Chris Van Gorder, President and CEO
Richard K Rothberger, Vice President, Chief Financial Officer
Robin B Brown, Chief Executive
Richard R Sheridan, Corporate Senior Vice President

Offers both inpatient and outpatient programs including: physical activity management, individual pain management, group therapy, medication adjustment, pain control classes, occupational therapy, biofeedback training, family counseling, vocational and leisure counseling and recreational therapy.

6659 Sharp Coronado Hospital
250 Prospect Place
Coronado, CA 92118-1999   619-522-3600
              erica.carlson@sharp.com
                                   sharp.com

Marcia Hall, CEO
Mark Tamsen, Chairman
Tom Smisek, Vice Chairman
Dan Gensler, Secretary

Providing medical and surgical care, intensive care, sub-acute and long-term care, rehabilitation therapies and emergency services in a peaceful setting is part of our live+heal+grow philosophy. We are one of the county's few community-owned hospitals and are proud of our history of providing convenient, award-winning heath care to Coronado and San Diego.

6660 Shriners Hospitals For Children-Northern California
2425 Stockton Blvd.
Sacramento, CA 95817   916-453-2000
              patientreferrals@shrinenet.org
              www.shrinershospitalsforchildren.org
John McCabe, Executive Vice President
Dale W Stauss, Chairman
Jerry G Gantt, 1st Vice President
Chris L Smith, 2nd Vice President

The only hospital in the Shriners system that houses facilities for treatment of all 3 Shriner specialties -spinal cord injuries, orthopaedic, and burns. The hospital features 80 patient beds, 9 parent apartments, 5 state-of-the-art operating rooms, a high-tech Motion Analysis lab, and an entire floor devoted to research.

6661 Shriners Hospitals for Children: Los Angeles
3160 Geneva Street
Los Angeles, CA 90020-1199   213-388-3151
              patientreferrals@shrinenet.org
              www.shrinershospitalsforchildren.org
John McCabe, Executive Vice President
Dale W Stauss, Chairman
Jerry G Gantt, 1st Vice President
Chris L Smith, 2nd Vice President

Shriners Hospitals for Children: Los Angeles, treats children under age 18 with burn scars, orthopedic conditions, cleft lip and palate and limb deficiencies at no cost to the patient or their families.

6662 Society for the Blind
1238 S St.
Sacramento, CA 95811-3256   916-452-8271
                                   FAX: 916-492-2483
              info@societyfortheblind.org
              societyfortheblind.org

Shari Roesler, Executive Director
Shane Snyder, Director of Programs

A private, local nonprofit organization providing blind and visually impaired people with the training supplies and support they need to live independent, productive and fulfilled lives with limited vision. Services include the Low Vision Clinic, Braille classes, computer training, support groups, living skills instruction, mobility training and the Products for Independence Store.

6663 Solutions at Santa Barbara: Transitional Living Center
1135 N Patterson Ave
Santa Barbara, CA 93111-1113   805-683-1995
                                   FAX: 805-683-4793
              sol1135@aol.com
              solutionsatsantabarbara.com

Sue Hannigan, Director

Postacute rehabilitation program. Short-term transitional living program for individuals with traumatic brain injury, stroke, aneurysm and other neurological disorders.

6664 St. John's Pleasant Valley Hospital Neuro Care Unit
2309 Antonio Ave
Camarillo, CA 93010-1414   805-389-5800
                                   shw.org

Jerry Conway, President
Maureen M. Malone, Administrator
Raye Burkhardt, Vice President and Chief Nursing

Houses 82 acute-care beds, a 99-bed extended care unit, and the only hyperbaric medicine unit in Ventura County. Employ's 1,800 people and count 250 active medical staff.

6665 St. John's Regional Medica Center- Industrial Therapy Center
1600 North Rose Ave
Oxnard, CA 93030-3723   805-988-2500
                                   www.stjohnshealth.org
Gudrun Moll, Vice President and Chief Nursing
Laurie Harting, President & CEO
Kim Wilson, Vice President
Chris Champlin, Senior Vice President

A non-profit health care facility offering multi-disciplinary programs for pain management and work hardening, as well as physical and occupational therapy.

6666 Sub-Acute Saratoga Hospital
13425 Sousa Lane
Saratoga, CA 95070-4663   408-378-8875
                                   FAX: 408-378-7419
              subacutesaratoga.com

Jack Stephens, President & CEO
Paul Quintana, Medical Director
Gary Vernon, NHA Administrator
Lindsay Zarcone, Marketing Manager

Dedicated to the fulfillment of human needs, desires, and wishes in illness and in health. The cohesiveness of caring in a family community of staff, patients, and their loved ones. The celebration of each unique life through their therapeutic journey, while preserving their individual spirit. The achievement of advanced medical expertise, knowledge, and skill given with the human touch of caring toward the ultimate goal: enhancing the healing process from acute illness to the joy of going home.

6667 Synergos Neurological Center: Hayward
27200 Calaroga Avenue
Hayward, CA 94545-4383   510-264-4000
                                   FAX: 510-264-4007
                                   strosehospital.org

Richard C. Hardwig, Chair
Alan McIntosh, Vice Chair
Lex Reddy, President and CEO
Roger Krissman, Chief Financial Officer
Postacute rehabilitation program.

6668 Synergos Neurological Center: Mission Hills
27200 Calaroga Avenue
Hayward, CA 94545-4383   510-264-4000
                                   FAX: 510-264-4007
                                   www.strosehospital.org
Richard C. Hardwig, Chair
Alan McIntosh, Vice Chair
Lex Reddy, President and CEO
Roger Krissman, Chief Financial Officer

For over 30 years, St. Rose Hospital Rehabilitation Services Department has helped thousands of patients recover from illness and injury through the help of our specially trained therapists.

These therapists have been trained in specific rehabilitative areas such as physical, occupational, and speech therapies.

6669 Temple Community Hospital
235 N Hoover St
Los Angeles, CA 90004-3672
213-382-7252
FAX: 213-382-1874
info@templecommunityhospital.com
templecommunityhospital.com

6670 Tunnell Center for Rehab
680 South Fourth Street
Louisville, CA 40202-4807
502-596-7300
FAX: 800-545-0749
web_administrator@kindred.com
kindredhealthcare.com

Mary R., Activities Assistant
Kristen W., Health and Rehabilitation Center
The Tunnell Center for Rehabilitation and Healthcare accomodates 178 residents. We are dedicated to short-term complex medical and rehabilitative care. Using a holistic care management approach we work with residents who have suffered debilitating injury or illness, and who need comprehensive nursing and rehabilitation services to achieve their highest practicable level of functional ability and independence.

6671 Ukiah Valley Association for Habilitation
Ukiah, CA 95482-689
707-468-8824
FAX: 707-468-9149
TTY:800-735-2929
www.uvah.org

Pamela Jensen, Executive Director
Kris Vipond, Business Manager
Sharrae Elston, Director
Suzanne Warner, Employment Training Specialist
Work adjustment and suppoted employment and social and community services.

6672 Valley Center for the Blind
2491 W Shaw Avenue
Suite 124
Fresno, CA 93711-3331
559-222-4088
FAX: 559-222-4844
info@valleycenterblind.org
www.valleycenterblind.org

Bud Breslin, Executive Director
Millie Marshall, Marriage Family Therapist
Saramarie Katich, Office Mngr/Program Director
Connie Parrick, Secretary
A private, nonprofit organization that offers educational, health, recreational and professional training services to the totally blind, legally blind or severely visually impaired.

6673 Villa Esperanza Services
2060 East Villa Street
Pasadena, CA 91107
626-449-2919
FAX: 626-449-2850
info@villaesperanzaservices.org
www.villaesperanzaservices.org

Candice Rogers, Chairman
Richard Hubinger, President
Vicky Castillo, CFO
Kelly White, Chief Executive Officer
Serving disabled infants to seniors in a school, adult day program, adult work program and residences and adult day health care program and care management program.

6674 Village Square Nursing And Rehabilitation Center
Kindred Healthcare, Inc.
1586 West San Marcos Blvd
San Marcos, CA 92078-4019
760-471-2986
www.villagesquarerehab.com

6675 Vista Center for the Blind & Visually Impaired
2470 El Camino Real,
Suite 107
Palo Alto, CA 94306-1715
650-858-0202
800-660-2009
FAX: 650-858-0214
info@vistacenter.org
www.vistacenter.org

Pam Brandin, Executive Director
Nacole Barth-Ellis, Co-Director of Development
Terry Kurfess, Co-Director of Development
Meg Faville, Administrative Services Manager
Private nonprofit agency that serves the visually impaired in the San Mateo, Santa Clara, San Benito and Santa Cruz Counties with offices in Palo Alto and Santa Cruz. Offers Low Vision Evaluations, mobility training, daily living skills training, social services, counseling, support groups, computer training, other rehabilitation services, and a store.

6676 Winways at Orange County
7732 E Santiago Canyon Rd
Orange, CA 92869-1829
714-771-5276
FAX: 714-771-1452
winwaysrehab.com

Pamela Kauss, Director
The program offers clients highly personalized, comprehensive programs to meet the needs of individuals with traumatic brain injury, stroke, tumors, aneurysm, post concussive syndrome or other neurological disorders. Winways also has a special program that provides services to Spanish speaking clients, called Contigo Adelante with materials in Spanish, and Spanish speaking interpreters to assist in the therapy process.

Colorado

6677 Capron Rehabilitation Center
Penrose Hospital/ St. Francis Healthcare System
2222 N Nevada Ave
Colorado Springs, CO 80907-6819
719-776-5000
penrosestfrancis.org

Margaret Sabin, President & CEO
Nate Olson, Chief Executive Officer
Jameson Smith, Senior VP & Chief Admnistrative Officer
Gil Porat, Chief Medical Officer
Southern Colorado's most complete inpatient and outpatient rehabilitation center.

6678 Cerebral Palsy of Colorado
801 Yosemite Street
Denver, CO 80230
303-691-9339
FAX: 303-691-0846
abilityconnectioncolorado.org

Judith I Ham, CEO
James Reuter, Chairman of the Board
Penfield Tate, Vice Chairman
Kathy Higgins, Treasurer
Provides services for children birth-5 years, employment services for adults, information and referral, donation pickup and cell phone/ink cartridge recycling services.

6679 Cherry Hills Health Care Center
Kindred
3575 S Washington St
Englewood, CO 80110-3807
303-789-2265
www.cherryhillshc.com

6680 Community Hospital Back and Conditioning Clinic
1060 Orchard Ave
Grand Junction, CO 81501-2997
970-243-3400
800-621-0926
FAX: 970-856-6510

Amy Hibberd, Executive Director
David Scherman, Manager
Post-accute rehabilitation program .

6681 Devereux Advanced Behavioral HealthColorado - Cleo Wallace Center
8405 Church Ranch Blvd.
Westminster, CO 80021
303-466-7391
800-456-2536
www.devereux.org

6682 Laradon Hall Society for Exceptional Children and Adults
5100 Lincoln St
Denver, CO 80216-2056
303-296-2400
866-381-2163
FAX: 303-296-4012
laradon.org
William Mitchell, Chair
Suzanne Bradeen, Vice Chair
Jason Adams, Treasurer
Nancy Hodges, Secretary
Laradon provides educational, vocational and residential services to children and adults with developmental disabilities and other special needs. Laradon was founded in 1948. It is among the largest and most comprehensive service providers in Colorado.

6683 Learning Services: Bear Creek
7201 W Hampden Ave
Lakewood, CO 80227-5305
303-989-6660
888-419-9955
FAX: 866-491-7396
lengland@learningservices.com
learningservices.com
Susan Snow, Director of Admissions
Dr. Debra Braunling-McMorrow, President and CEO
Jeanne Mack, Chief Financial Officer
Michael Weaver, Chief Development Officer
Supported living program for persons with acquired brain injury.

6684 MOSAIC In Colorado SpringsMOSAIC
888 W. Garden of the Gods Road
Ste 100
Colorado Springs, CO 80907-6251
719-380-0451
FAX: 719-380-7055
mosaic_cosprings@mosaicinfo.org
www.mosaicincoloradosprings.org
Tom Maltais, Executive Director
Mosaic in Colorado Springs provides a variety of services to assist adults and families in achieving positive goals. Services to persons with intellectual disabilities include community living options, vocational training and supported employment, spiritual growth and personal development options, and day programs habilitation and community participation.

6685 Manor Care Nursing and Rehabilitation Center: Boulder
Manor Care Ohio
2800 Palo Pkwy
Boulder, CO 80301-1540
303-440-9100
FAX: 303-440-9251
www.hcr-manorcare.com
Steven M. Cavanaugh, Chief Financial Officer
Paul A. Ormond, Chairman, President and Chief Ex
150 bed center offers a full spectrum of nursing care and rehabilitation. This includes our Arcadia Special Care Unit for Alzheimer's patients. Specialized unit for post acute skilled nursing care. Physical and massage therapies. And a 48 bed upscale Heritage unit offering additional amenities and furnishings.

6686 Manor Care Nursing: Denver
290 S Monaco Pkwy
Denver, CO 80224-1105
303-355-2525
FAX: 303-333-6960
www.hcr-manorcare.com
Steven M. Cavanaugh, Chief Financial Officer
Paul A. Ormond, Chairman, President and Chief Ex
Our center has delveloped a reputation for its luxurious environment, comprehensive rehabilitation service and focus on quality care. A wide range of individual and group activities and many gracious amenities create the finest combination of elegance and professional skilled nursing care. Arcadia, our special care unit for persons with Alzheimer's disease and related memory impairments, promotes independence and preserves dignity within a safe and secure environment.

6687 Mediplex of Colorado
8451 Pearl St
Thornton, CO 80229-4804
303-288-3000
FAX: 303-286-5136
info@vhdenver.com
www.northvalleyrehab.com
Jan Eyer, Chief Executive Officer
Our programs and services help each patient along the road to recovery toward our ultimate aim; the greatest possible restoration of the individual's self-esteem, ability to set goals, and self-sufficiency. Also offer specialized acute inpatient rehabilitative services, including special programs in Trauma Rehabilitation.

6688 Platte River Industries
490 Bryant St
Denver, CO 80204-4808
303-825-0041
FAX: 303-825-0564
pri01_lil@attglobal.net
Bob Smith, Executive Director
Postacute rehabilitation facility and program..

6689 Pueblo Diversified Industries
2828 Granada Blvd
Pueblo, CO 81005-3198
800-466-8393
FAX: 719-564-3407
info@pdipueblo.org
www.pdipueblo.net
Karen K Lillie, President & CEO
Robin Forbes, Director Human Services
Tom Drolshagen, Chief Operating Officer
Tom Denslow, Manager, Human Resources
A place where people can turn limitations into opportunities. People can experience the independence, pride and self worth of securing and maintaining a job.

6690 SHALOM Denver
2498 W 2nd Ave
Denver, CO 80223-1007
303-623-0251
FAX: 303-620-9584
akover@jewishfamilyservice.org
shalomdenver.com
Arnie Kover, Disability and Employment Servic
Sara Leeper, Coordinator of Client Services
Vicky Brittain, Mailing Business Manager
Bari Belinsky, Work Services Manager
SHALOM Denver provides employment, training, and job placement opportunities to people with disabilities, resettled immigrants, and people moving from welfare to work.

6691 SPIN Early Childhood Care & Education Cntr
1333 Elm Ave
Canon City, CO 81212-4431
719-275-0550
www.starpointco.com/spin
Diane Trujillo, Manager
SPIN center is a fully inclusive non-discriminating community early childhood program, offering a variety of schedule choices for families. The philosophy of the SPIN program is to promote each child's growth and development. Special attention is given to cognitive, physical, speech language and social-emotional growth. Staff is specifically trained to facilitate and prepare environments that promote exploration, key experiences, creativity and self-expression..

6692 Schaefer Enterprises
500 26th Street
P.O. Box 200009
Greeley, CO 80631-8427
970-353-0662
FAX: 970-353-2779
schaefenterprises@comcast.net
www.schaeferenterprises.com
Valorie Randall, Executive Director
Alex Witt, Executive Assistant
Veronica Griego, Production Director

Schaefer Enterprises, Inc., located in Greely, Colorado, is a vauluable community resource that has been fulfilling the outsourcing needs of businesses in Weld County and outlying areas since 1952.

6693 Spalding Rehab Hospital West Unit
150 Spring St
Morrison, CO 80465
303-697-4334
FAX: 303-697-0570

Connecticut

6694 ACES/ACCESS Inclusion Program
350 State Street
North Haven, CT 06473-3218
203-498-6800
FAX: 203-234-1369
acesinfo@aces.org
www.aces.org

Thomas M Danehy, Executive Director
Erika Forte, Assistant Executive Director
Evelyn Rossetti, Manager
Provides a person centered planning approach for integrated employment, volunteer community based opportunities for adults who have developmental disabilities..

6695 Apria Healthcare
26220 Enterprise Court
Lake Forest, CA 92630-1015
800-277-4288
contact_us@apria.com
www.apria.com

Lisa M. Getson, Executive Vice President, Govern
Nichola Denney, Executive Vice President, Revenue Management
Dan Stark, Chief Executive Officer
Debra L Morris, Chief Financial Officer
Provides a broad range of high quality and cost effective specialty infusion therapies and related services to patients in their homes throughout the Northeastern United States. Offer home infusion antibiotic therapy, quality pharmacy services, skilled nursing services and related support services.

6696 Arc Of Meriden-Wallingford, Inc.
200 Research Parkway
Meriden, CT 06450
203-237-9975
FAX: 203-639-0946
info@mwsinc.net
www.arcmw.org

Pamela Fields, Executive Director
Joseph Palfini, Board President
Becky Blazejowski, Financial Director
Maritza Dell, Director of Program Services
A membership agency that provides comprehensive, full-service, community-based opportunities for people with disabilities. Guided by over 120 community members and an active Board of Directors, the Arc always has its focus on improving the lives of people with disabilities. The Arc of Meriden-Wallingford offers advocacy and assistance to our members along with advocating for the rights and choices of people with disabilities in our community.

6697 Arc of the Farmington Valley
225 Commerce Drive
Canton, CT 06019-2478
860-693-6662
FAX: 860-693-8662
rcipolla@favarh.org
favarh.org

George Kral, President
Ernest E Mack, Vice President
Larry Pollock, Treasurer
Robin Dinicola, Secretary
Serving over 300 mentally retarded adults through a comprehensive program of residential and support services. These include three group homes, three apartments, competitive and supported employment options, a day program for mentally retarded seniors, community experience day services for severe and profoundly disabled adults, recreation and leisure services,

advocacy, transportation, case management, in-home respite and other support services.

6698 Connecticut Subacute Corporation
19 Tuttle Pl
Middletown, CT 06457-1881
860-347-6300
FAX: 860-347-2446
www.cpl-usa.com

Evan K Lyle, Managed Care Director
Cheri Kauset, Corporate Rep.
Specializes in subacute medical and rehabilitation programming. The strength of our system is in its' ability to service a broad range of clinical and psychosocial needs which enable each individual to attain his/her optimal potential. Programming includes neurological and orthopedic rehabilitation, post-surgical and wound care management, intravenous therapy, pulmonary rehabilitation including ventilator services, and long term care..

6699 Datahr Rehabilitation Institute
4 Berkshire Blvd
Bethel, CT 06801-1001
203-775-4700
888-8DA-TAHR
FAX: 203-775-4688
abilitybeyonddisability.com

Thomas Fanning, CEO
Providers of comprehensive rehabilitation services with a history of nearly 5 decades of service. This institute is recognized as a leading resource in meeting the needs of those disabled by illness, injury or developmental disorders in Connecticut and New York. A team of rehabilitation and health care professionals offering career development, residential services, supported employment, volunteer services, occupational therapy, day activities and more.

6700 Eastern Blind Rehabilitation Center
810 Vermont Avenue
Washington, DC 20420
202-461-7600
800-273-8255
www1.va.gov/blindrehab

Eric K. Shinseki, Secretary of Veterans Affairs
W. Scott Gould, Deputy Secretary of Veterans Aff
Jose D Riojas, Chief of Staff
Richard J Griffin, Acting Inspector General
Provides residential rehabilitation services to eligible legally blind veterans in the Northeast and Middle Atlantic portions of the country. Referral applications by Veterans Administration Medical Centers and Outpatient Clinics in the geographical area served by the Blind Rehabilitation Center.

6701 FAVRAH Senior Adult Enrichment Program
23 W Avon Rd
Avon, CT 06001
860-674-8839
FAX: 860-676-0275

Nancy Ralston, Manager
Provides remunerative work. Post acute rehabilitation programs and facility.

6702 Gaylord Hospital
Gaylord Farm Road
P.O.Box 400
Wallingford, CT 06492-7048
203-284-2800
866-429-5673
FAX: 203-284-2894
TTY: 203-284-2700
lcrispino@gaylord.org
www.gaylord.org

James Cullen, President
Works to restore ability and build courage. Offers rehabilitation care with one goal in mind: to help patients return to their homes, communities and jobs.

6703 Hockanum Greenhouse
Hockanum Industry
290 Middle Tpke
Storrs Mansfield, CT 06268-2908   860-429-6697
FAX: 860-429-7496
hockanumindustries.org

Christopher Campbell, Manager
Beth Chaty, Director
Betsy Treiber, Director
A non profit agency that strives to provide gainful employment, training, support and retirement services for developmentally disabled individuals through the dignity of work, community interaction and structured activities.

6704 Kuhn Employment Oppurtunities
1630 North Colony Road
P.O.Box 941
Meriden, CT 06450   203-235-2583
860-347-5843
www.kuhngroup.org

Paul O'Sullivan, Chairperson
Mark DuPuis, Vice Chairperson
John J. Ausanka III, Treasurer
James Anderson, Secretary
Kuhn is committed to developing quality skill enhancement programs which provide meaningful employment for persons with disabilities so that they will become independentm gain self-esteem, and be accepted by the community. Our vision is that all individuals have the ability to fully participate in the community through work. Kuhn believes that all participants have a right to integrated community employment.

6705 Norwalk Hospital Section Of Physical Medicine And Rehabilitation
34 Maple Street
Norwalk, CT 06856   203-852-2000
FAX: 800-789-4584
marketing@norwalkhealth.org
www.norwalkhosp.org

Diane M. Allison, Chair
Edward A. Kangas, Vice Chair
Andrew J. Whittingham, Treasurer
Barbara Butler, Secretary
A 25 bed inpatient Rehabilitation Unit. This CARF and JCAHO accredidted rehab unit is located on the 8th floor of Norwalk Hospital. The focus of the rehab unit is to restore lost function and assist patients in returning to the community. Who have recently experienced a life changing medical event. The progam is tailored to meet individual therapy needs and address activities of daily living. Family and caregiver participation in the program is welcomed and encouraged.

6706 Rehabilitation Associates, Inc.
1931 Black Rock Tpke
Fairfield, CT 06825-3506   203-384-8681
FAX: 203-384-0956
info@rehabassocinc.com
www.rehabilitationassociatesinc.com

Carol Landsman, Director
A comprehensive outpatient rehabilitation facility offering physical therapy, occupational therapy, speech-language pathology, clinical social work services and nutritional services to all age groups. Facility locations in Fairfield, Stratford, Milford, Shelton and Westport.

6707 Reliance House
40 Broadway
Norwich, CT 06360-5702   860-887-6536
FAX: 860-885-1970
reliancehouse.org

Jack Malone, President
Jackie Falman, Vice President
Sam Bliven, Secretary
Raul Walker, Treasurer
A residential vocational and recreational support network. An active and productive clubhouse where people with mental illness can gain skills, strength and self-esteem.

6708 Yale New Haven Health System-Bridgeport Hospital
789 Howard Avenue
New Haven, CT 06519   203-384-3000
www.yalenewhavenhealth.org

Marna P. Borgstrom, President and CEO
Richard D'Aquila, Executive Vice President
Peter N. Herbert, MD, Senior VP, Medical Affairs
Kevin Myatt, Senior VP of Human Resources
Medical services are provided by physicians who are specialists in physical medicine and rehabilitation. The physical therapy department provides a variety of services and utilizes sophisticated modalities to restore and reinforce physical abilities.

Delaware

6709 Alfred I DuPont Hospital for Children
Division of Rehabilitation
1600 Rockland Road,
PO Box 269
Wilmington, DE 19803-269   302-651-4000
888-533-3543
FAX: 302-651-4055
infodupont@nemours.org
www.nemours.org

William G. Mackenzie, MD, Chair
David J. Bailey, President and Chief Executive Officer
Robert D. Bridges, Executive Vice President, Enterprise Services/Chief Financia
Roy Proujansky, Executive Vice President, Health Operations and Chief Operat
The hospital is a division of Nemours, which operates one of the nations largest subspecialty group practices devoted to pediatric patient care, teaching, and research. A 180-bed hospital that offers all the specialties of pediatric medicine, surgery, and dentistry in a spacious, comfortable, and family focused facility.

6710 Community Systems Inc.
2 Penns Way
Suite 301
New Castle, DE 19720   302-325-1500
FAX: 302-325-1505
info@csi-del.org
communitysystems.org

David Paige, Executive Director
Amy Yento, Chair
A 4 state family of non-profit, tax exempt corporations whose mission is helping persons with disabilities to find happiness in their own homes, in their personal relationships, and as contributing members of their community.

6711 DDDS/Georgetown Center
5 Academy St
Georgetown, DE 19947-1915   302-856-5366
FAX: 302-856-5305
dhss.delaware.gov/dhss

6712 Delaware Association for the Blind
2915 Newport Gap Pike
Landis Lodge Building
Wilmington, DE 19808   302-998-5913
888-777-3925
FAX: 302-691-5810
contact@dabdel.org
dabdel.org

Janet L. Berry, Executive Director
Ken Rolph, President
Jennifer Smith, Secretary
Robert Mosch, Treasurer
A private, nonprofit organization that offers adjustment to blindness counseling, recreation activities, summer camps and financial assistance for the legally blind. The staff includes five full time, nine part time and twelve seasonal. Operates a store selling items for the blind.

6713   Delaware Veterans Center
810 Vermont Avenue
Washington, DC 20420
302-994-2511
800-273-8255
FAX: 302-633-5591
www1.va.gov/directory/guide

Slaon D Gibson, Acting Secretary of Veterans Affairs
Jose D Riojas, Chief of Staff
Richard J Griffin, Acting Inspector General
A 60-bed hospital and 60-bed NHCU, both accredited by the Joint Commission on Accreditation of Healthcare Organizations with a VBA Regional Office and 2 Vet Centers (one on campus) offering veterans the unique opportunity to obtain heathcare, benefits services, and Readjustment Counseling at one location. The center provides a wide spectrum of primary and tertiary acute and extended care inpatient and outpatient activities an an academic setting..

6714   Easter Seals Delaware & Maryland's Eastern Shore
233 South Wacker Drive
Suite 2400
Chicago, IL 60606
302-324-4444
800-221-6827
FAX: 302-324-4441
TTY: 302-324-4442
easterseals.com

Richard W. Davidson, Chairman
Sandy Tuttle, President
Ralph F. Boyd, Treasurer
Eileen Howard Boone, Secretary
Provides exceptional services to ensure that all people with disabilities or special needs and their families have equal opportunities to live, learn, work and play in their communities.

6715   Edgemoor Day Program
500 Duncan Rd
Wilmington, DE 19809-2369
302-762-9077
FAX: 302-762-1652
www.dhss.delaware.gov/dhss/main/maps/other/ed

Scott Borino, Executive Director
Carol Koyste, Manager, Finance & Administratio
Brandon Furrowh, Director, Recreation & Youth Pro
Avani Patel, Administrative Assistant
Our mission is providing affordable and accessible services which help improve the quality of life for community members of all ages through a broad range of educational, recreational, self-enrichment, and family support services. ECC is a not-for-profit, community-based, multi-service agency located just north of Wilmington. We provide a broad range of educational, recreational, self-enrichment, and family support services.

6716   Elwyn Delaware
321 E 11th St
Wilmington, DE 19801-3422
302-658-8860
FAX: 302-654-5815
info@elwyn.org
www.elwyn.org

Sandra S. Cornelius, President of Elwyn
Daniel M. Reardon, Senior Vice President and Chief
H. Scott Campbell, Vice President
Richard T. Smith, Vice President for Information T
A non-profit human services organization recognized nationally and internationally as experts in the education and care of individuals with special challenges and disadvantages. Today Elwyn is a leading provider of services for people with special needs of all ages.

6717   First State Senior Center
291a N Rehoboth Blvd
Milford, DE 19963-1303
302-422-1510
dhss.delaware.gov/dhss/main/maps/other/dddssr

6718   Woodside Day Program
941 Walnut Shade Rd
Dover, DE 19901-7765
302-739-4494
FAX: 302-697-4490

Connie Grace, Supervisor
Joyce Oliver, Manager

District of Columbia

6719   Barbara Chambers Children's Center
1470 Irving St NW
Washington, DC 20010-2804
202-387-6755
FAX: 202-319-9066
bcchildrencenter@erols.com
barbarachambers.org

Barbara Chambers, Founder
Mission is to provide comprehensive, quality child care services to the community at large, by offering a variety of opportunities for childrens's intellectual, emotional, social and physical development in a clean, safe, and nurturing environment. Our philosophy is to provide a supportive environment in which children can be children..allowing each child to learn at his/her pace and most of all allowing the child to learn through his/her daily play.

6720   District of Columbia General Hospital Physical Medicine & Rehab Services
Room 1358
19th and Mass Ave
Washington, DC 20003
202-727-6055
FAX: 202-675-7819

Dr. Maribel Bieberach, Chairperson PM&R
Dr. Raman Kapur, Staff Physiatrist
Offers comprehensive physical medicine and rehabilitation services including in and outpatient consultations and electrodiagnostic testing; in and outpatient physical and occupational therapy; inpatient recreational therapy, and a multidisciplinary prosthetic clinic which meets once a month..

6721   George Washington University Medical Center
George Washington University Medical Center
2150 Pennsylvania Ave NW
Washington, DC 20037-3201
202-741-3000
FAX: 202-741-3183
www.gwdocs.com

6722   HSC Pediatric Center, The
1731 Bunker Hill Rd NE
Washington, DC 20017-3026
202-832-4400
800-226-4444
FAX: 202-467-0978
efowler@cscn.org
www.hscpediatriccenter.org

Debbie Zients, CEO
Dr Murry M Pollack, VP, Medical Affairs
Eva Fowler, Media Contact
Provides the highest quality rehabilitative and transitional care for infants, children, adolescents, and young adults with special health care needs and their families in a supportive environment that respects their needs, strengths, vslues and priorities..

6723   Howard University Child Development Center
1911 5th St NW
Washington, DC 20001-2314
202-797-8134
FAX: 202-986-6580

Connie Siler, Manager
Offers children with developmental problems diagnosis, treatment, evaluation and follow along visits..

6724 Psychiatric Institute of Washington
4228 Wisconsin Ave NW
Washington, DC 20016-2138
202-885-5600
800-369-2273
FAX: 202-885-5614
ceo@piw-dc.com
psychinstitute.com

Ken Courage, Chairman
Carol Desjuns, Chief Operations Officer
Howard Hoffman, Executive Medical Director
Aarti Subramanian, VP/Chief Financial Off
Psychiatric intensive care, crisis intervention, adult day treatment, drug treatment and other services to children and adults who have psychiatric and chemical dependency problems.

6725 Spina Bifida Program of DC Children's Hospital
Department of Physical Medicine and Rehabilitation
111 Michigan Ave NW
Washington, DC 20010-2916
202-476-5000
FAX: 202-476-2270
childrensnational.org

Kurt Newman, President and Chief Executive Of
Elizabeth Flury, Chief Strategy Officer
Kathleen E. Chavanu Gorman, Chief Operating Officer
Mary Anne Hilliard, Chief Risk Counsel
Offers neurosurgery, orthopedics, physical medicine, social work, urology and nursing. Mission is to improve health outcomes for children regionally, nationally, and internationally. Be a leader in creating innovative solutions to pediatric healthcare problems. Excel in Care, Advocacy, Research, and Education to meet the unique needs of children, adolescents and their families.

Florida

6726 Bayfront Rehabilitation Center
Bayfront Medical Center
701 6th St S
St Petersburg, FL 33701-4814
727-823-1234
www.bayfrontstpete.com

Kathryn Gillette, President and CEO
Eric Smith, Chief Financial Officer
Lavah Lowe, Chief Operating Officer
Karen Long, Chief Nursing Executive
Bayfront Medical Center has an Inpatient Rehabilitation Hospital and two outpatient rehabilitation clinics that each provide progressive, comprehensive, individualized treatment. Specialized care in Physiatry (physical medicine), rehab nursing, occupational therapy, speech language pathology, recreational therapy, patient/family services and psychology is tailored to each patient from admission to community and/or school reintegration.

6727 Brain Injury Rehabilitation Center Dr. P. Phillips Hospital
Brain Injury Rehabilitation Center Dr. P. Phillips
9400 Turkey Lake Rd
Orlando, FL 32819-8001
407-351-8580
www.orlandohealth.com/drpphillipshospital/ind

Shannon Elswick, President
Linda Chapin, Chairman
Mark Swanson, Chief Quality Officer
John Hillenmeyer, CEO Emeritus, Orlando Health
Dedicated to restoring brain injured patients with rehabilitation potential to their highest level of functioning. This is accomplished through an interdisciplinary team demonstrating personal responsibility to the patient, their family and each other.

6728 Brooks Memorial Hospital Rehabilitation Center
3599 University Blvd. South
Jacksonville, FL 32207-6215
904-858-7600
FAX: 904-858-7619
louise.spierre@brookshealth.org
www.brookshealth.org

Douglas Baer, Chief Executive Officer/ Preside
Holly Morris, Director, Brooks Rehabilitation
Louise Spierre, Medical Director
Floris Singletary, Research Manager, Clinical Resea

An entire care facility featuring five day inpatient evaluation, pre-operative evaluation programs, five week pain management program, referral criteria and treatment goals, therapy services, psychological services and more to the physically challenged.

6729 Center for Pain Control and Rehabilitation
Ste 607
2780 Cleveland Ave
Fort Myers, FL 33901-5858
239-337-4332

Mary Bonnette, Owner

6730 Comprehensive Rehabilitation Center at Lee Memorial Hospital
2776 Cleveland Ave
Fort Myers, FL 33901-5864
239-343-2000
leememorial.org

James R. Nathan, Chief Executive Officer System P
Larry Antonucci, Chief Operating Officer
Jon Cecil, Chief Human Resources Officer
Mike German, Chief Financial Officer
Lee Memorial hospital has achieved national recognition as one of the top 100 hospitals for stroke, orthopedics, and Intensive Care Unit (ICU) It is a 367 bed hospital that provides 24-hour emergency and trauma care, inpatient rehabilitation, orthopedics, neuroscience, trauma, cancer, diabetes, digestive, general surgery, urology, endocrinology, gastroenterology, opthamology, and many others.

6731 Comprehensive Rehabilitation Center of Naples Community Hospital
350 7th Street North
Naples, FL 34102
239-436-5000
FAX: 239-436-5250
www.nchmd.org

Allen S. Weiss, CEO
Mariann MacDonald, Chairman
Thomas Gazdic, Chairman/Treasurer
John Lewis, Secretary
Offers rehabilitation services, inpatient and outpatient care at 5 locations in the county and more for the benefit of the disabled.

6732 Conklin Center for the Blind
405 White St
Daytona Beach, FL 32114-2999
386-258-3441
FAX: 386-258-1155
info@conklincenter.org
www.conklincenter.org

Robert T Kelly, Executive Director
The Conklin Center's mission is to empower children and adults who are blind and have one or more additional disabilities to develop their potential to be able to obtain competitive employment, live independently and fully participate in community life.

6733 Davis Center for Rehabilitation Baptist Hospital of Miami
8900 N Kendall Dr
Miami, FL 33176-2118
786-596-1960
corporatepr@baptisthealth.net
www.baptisthealth.net/bhs

Brian E. Keeley, President and Chief Executive Of
Calvin Babcock, Chairman
A full-service, nonprofit community hospital providing a full range of inpatient and outpatient rehabilitation services. The overall commitment to excellence has extended to this specialized field. Access to medical expertise and services ensures that the best in medical resources are available should an unforeseen medical problem arise.

6734 Devereux Advanced Behavioral HealthFlorida - Titusville Campus
1850 S. Deleon Ave.
Titusville, FL 32780
800-338-3738
www.devereux.org

6735 **Devereux Advanced Behavioral Health -Florida**
Corporate Office
5850 T.G. Lee Blvd.
Ste 400
Orlando, FL 32822

800-338-3738
www.devereux.org

Steven Murphy, Executive Director

6736 **Devereux Advanced Behavioral Health Florida - Orlando Campus**
6147 Christian Way
Orlando, FL 32808

800-338-3738

6737 **Devereux Advanced Behavioral Health Florida - Viera Campus**
8000 Devereux Dr.
Viera, FL 32940

800-338-3738

6738 **Devereux Threshold Center for Autism**
Devereux Advanced Behavioral Health Florida
3550 N. Goldenrod Rd.
Winter Park, FL 32792

800-338-3738
www.devereux.org

6739 **Division of Blind Services**
325 West Gaines Street
Suite 1114
Turlington Building, FL 32399-0400
850-245-0300
800-342-1828
FAX: 850-245-0386
ana.saint-ford@dbs.fldoe.org
dbs.myflorida.com

Aleisa McKinlay, Interim Director
Phyllis Vaughn, Bureau Chief, Administrative Services
William Findley, Bureau Chief, Business Enterprise Program
Edward Hudson, Bureau Chief of the Rehabilitation Center for the Blind and
Serves the totally blind, legally blind, visually impaired, deaf-blind, learning disabled, mentally retarded and other multiply handicapped by offering health, counseling, educational, recreational and computer training services.

6740 **Easter Seals Broward County**
1475 N.W. 14th Ave.
Miami, FL 33125
305-325-0470
FAX: 305-325-0578
www.easterseals.com/southflorida

Loreen Chant, President and Chief Executive Officer
ESBC provides direct services to children and adults with physical, neurological and communications disabilities and their families.

6741 **Easter Seals South Florida**
1475 NW 14th Avenue
Miami, FL 33125-1616
305-325-0470
FAX: 305-325-0578
info@southflorida.easterseals.com
www.southflorida.easterseals.com

Luanne Welch, President
The mission of Easter Seals South Florida is to provide exceptional services to ensure that all children and adults with disabilities or special needs and their families have equal opportunities to live, learn, work and play in their communities.

6742 **Easter Seals Southwest Flordia**
Sarasota, FL 34243-2001
941-355-7637
themeadowscup.com

6743 **Easter Seals: Volusia and Flagler Counties, FL**
Easter Seals National
233 South Wacker Drive
Suite 2400
Chicago, IL 60606-2405
800-221-6827
easterseals.com

Richard W. Davidson, Chairman
Ralph F. Boyd, Jr., Treasurer
Eileen Howard Boone, Secretary
James E. Williams, Jr., Assistant Secretary
Provides early intervention services: inclusive pre-school, aquatherapy and sensory processing therapy, OT, PT, ST and parenting programs, audiology services, equipment loan program, assistive technology information and referral. Residential summer camp and respite.

6744 **Florida CORF**
Columbia Medical Center: Peninsula

www.memorial-health.com

John Feore, Executive VP
Sandra Trovato, Executive Director
Offers Medicare authorized therapy programs for seniors, disabled and others who need rehabilitation. CORF can provide coordinated and extended services in the home after a hospital stay, or when physical status changes. Patients who are treated at CORF, include amputations, arthritis, chronic/acute pain, depression/anxiety, nerve injury, sports injury, stroke and swallowing problems.

6745 **Florida Community College at Jacksonville/ Services for Students with Disabilities**
501 State St W
Jacksonville, FL 32202-4086
904-646-2300
877-578-6801
equityofficer@fscj.edu
fscj.edu

Steven R. Wallace, President
James E. McCollum, Chairman
Patti Williams, Project Coordinator
Shirley Hendley, Administrative Assistant II
Florida Community College provides educational support services through the Auxiliary Aids Program within the Office of Services for Students With Disabilities.

6746 **Florida Institute Of Rehabilitation Education (FIRE)**
3071 Highland Oaks Terrace
Tallahassee, FL 32301-4876
850-942-3658
888-827-6033
FAX: 850-942-4518
info@lighthousebigbend.org
www.firesight.org

Barbara Ross, Executive Director
Evelyn Worley, Assistant Director
Wayne Warner, Vocational Program Director
Toni King, Independent Living Specialist
Provides independent living and vocational rehabilitation services to Florida residents who are legally blind. Services include instruction in orientation and mobility, accessible technology, daily living skills and employability skills. Information, referral and counseling services are also offered. All services are provided without charge.

6747 **Florida Institute for Neurologic Rehabilitation, Inc**
1962 Vandolah Road
P O Box 1348
Wauchula, FL 33873-1348
863-773-2857
800-697-5390
FAX: 863-773-0867
finr.net

John Richards, Administrator
Stephanie Ortiz, RN, Director of Nursing
Kevin E. O'Keefe, Program Director
Dana Lucas, Director of Nursing
A residential rehabilitation facility providing a therapeutic environment in which children, adolescents and adults who have sur-

vived head-injury can develop the independence and skills necessary to re-enter the community.

6748 Fort Lauderdale Veterans Medical Center
713 NE 3rd Ave
Fort Lauderdale, FL 33304-2619   954-356-7926
                                    FAX: 954-356-7609
                                    www.va.gov/directory/guide/

Robert White, Executive Director
Sloan D Gibson, Acting Secretary
Jose D Riojas, Chief of Staff
Richard J Griffin, Acting Inspector General
Veterans medical clinic offering disabled veterans medical treatments.

6749 Halifax Hospital Medical Center Eye Clinic Professional Center
308 Farmington Avenue
Farmington, CT 06032   860-658-4388
                          888-444-3598
                          webmaster@evariant.com
                          www.evariant.com

Bill Moschella, CEO
Rob Grant, Executive Vice President
Michael Clark, Chief Operating Officer
James Orsillo, Chief Financial Officer
Offers services for the totally blind, legally blind, visually impaired, mentally retarded blind and more with health, counseling, educational, recreational, rehabilitation, computer training and professional training services.

6750 HealthQuest Subacute and Rehabilitation Programs
Regenta Park
8700 a C Skinner Pkwy
Jacksonville, FL 32256-836
                          FAX: 904-641-7896

6751 HealthSouth Emeral Coast Sports & Rehabilitation Center
1847 Florida Avenue
Panama City, FL 32405-3730   850-784-4878
                                FAX: 850-769-7566
                                www.healthsouthpanamacity.com
Tony Bennett, CEO
Michelle Miller, Manager
Outpatient sports medicine and rehabilitation center providing physical therapy, occupational therapy, industrial rehab, work hardening/work simulation, worksite and ergonomic analysis, FCE's, work assessment and pre-employment goals of returning the clients back to work, and returning to all recreational, sports and functional activities safely..

6752 HealthSouth Rehabilitation Hospital of Tallahassee
Healthsouth Corporation
1675 Riggins Rd
Tallahassee, FL 32308-5315   850-656-4800
                                www.healthsouthtallahassee.com
Heath Phillips, Chief Executive Officer
Robert Robert Rowland, Medical Director
Tom Abbruscato, Controller
Deborah Baird, Director of Quality and Risk Man
North Florida's sole acute rehabilitation hospital between Jacksonville \, Panama City, and Gainesville. With 250 employees providing a full continuum of care form its 70 bed facility, the hospital is accredited by JCAHO, CARF and state designated and certified by Vocational Rehabilitation for traumatic brain injury, as well as a wide variety of other diagnoses. With the addition of our outpatients, the facility has served the greater community by touching the lives of over 50,000 patients.

6753 HealthSouth Rehabilitation Hospital Of Miami
20601 Old Cutler Rd
Miami, FL 33189-2441   305-251-3800
                          www.healthsouthmiami.com
Elizabeth Izquierdo, Chief Executive Officer
Angelo Appio, Director of Marketing Operations
Reyna M. Hernandez, Chief Financial Officer
Paige Keil, Director of Quality and Risk Man

A comprehensive source of medical rehabilitation services for Pinellas County, Florida area residents, their families and their physicians. Offers the people of Florida all the clinical, technical and professional resources of the nation's leading provider of comprehensive rehabilitation care.

6754 HealthSouth Rehabilitation Hospital of Sarasota
Health South Corporation in Burmingham Alabama
6400 Edgelake Drive
Sarasota, FL 34240-8813   941-921-8600
                             866-330-5822
                             www.healthsouthsarasota.com
Marcus Braz, Chief Executive Officer
Alexander DeJesus, Medical Director
Nancy Arnold, Director of Marketing Operations
Brenda Benner, Director of Human Resources
HealthSouth Rehabilitation Hospital of Sarasota is a 96-bed inpatient rehabilitation hospital that offers comprehensive inpatient rehabilitation services designed to return patients to leading active and independent lives.

6755 HealthSouth Sea Pines Rehabilitation Hospital
Sea Pines Rehabilitation Hospital
101 E Florida Ave
Melbourne, FL 32901-8398   321-984-4600
                              FAX: 321-952-6532
                              www.healthsouthseapines.com
Stuart Miller, Medical Director
Denise McGrath, Chief Executive Officer
Donna Anderson, Director of Human Resources
Jerry Bishop, Director of Quality and Risk Man
Designed to return patients to leading active, independent lives, HealthSouth Sea Pines Rehabilitation Hospital is a 90-bed rehabilitation hospital that provides a higher level of comprehensive rehabilitation services.

6756 Holy Cross Hospital
Catholic Southwest
4725 North Federal Hwy
Fort Lauderdale, FL 33308-4668   954-771-8000
                                    www.holy-cross.com
Patrick Taylor, President & Chief Executive Offi
Luisa Gutman, Senior Vice President & Chief Op
Linda Wilford, Senior Vice President & Chief Fi
Kenneth Homer, Chief Medical Officer & Medical
Holy Cross Hospital in Fort Lauderdale is a full-service, non-profit Catholic hospital, sponsored by the Sisters of Mercy. Holy Cross is a US News & World Report 'Best Hospital' and HealthGrades Distinguished Hospital for Clinical Excellence, 2004 and 2005

6757 Lee Memorial Hospital
2776 Cleveland Ave
Fort Myers, FL 33901-5855   239-343-2000
                               www.leememorial.org
Sanford Cohen, Chairman
Chris Hansen, Vice Chairman
David Collins, Treasurer
Diane Champion, Secretary
Offers a complete inpatient program of intensive rehabilitation designed to restore a patient to a more independent level of functioning. The comprehensive care includes medical rehabilitation and training for spinal cord injury, brain injury, stroke and neurological disorders.

6758 Lighthouse for the Blind of Palm Beach
1710 Tiffany Drive East
West Palm Beach, FL 33407-3224   561-586-5600
                                    FAX: 561- 84- 80
                                    lighthousepalmbeaches.org
Marvin A. Tanck, President and CEO
Dont, Mickens, Chair
John R. Banister, Vice Chairman
David B. Cano, MD
A private, non-profit rehabilitation and education agency in its 55th year of service. Offers programs to assist persons who areblind or visually impaired, an on-site Industrial Center, a technology training center, an Aids and appliances Store, special

equipment grant programs, outreach services for children and adults, Early Intervention and Preschool Services, and a variety of support groups. These programs provide services and education for blind children and their parents.

6759   Lighthouse for the Visually Impaired and Blind
8610 Galen Wilson Blvd
Port Richey, FL 34668-5974   727-815-0303
                                                           866-962-5254
                                                      FAX: 727-815-0203
                                                      lighthouse@lvib.org
                                                          www.lvib.org

Sylvia Stinson-Perez, Executive Director
Dr. John Mann, President
Melissa M. Suess, Orientation and Mobility Instruc
Peter James, Business Development Specialist
The Lighthouse offers services for visually impaired or blind adults and children ages 0-5 years old. Counseling, educational services, recreational services, rehabilitation, computer training and support groups.

6760   MacDonald Training Center
5420 W Cypress Street
Tampa, FL 33607-1706   813-870-1300
                                                          866-948-6184
                                                      FAX: 813-872-6010
                                                      TTY: 813-873-7631
                                               jfreyvogel@macdonaldcenter.org
                                                     macdonaldcenter.org

Jim Freyvogel, President/CEO
Judith DeStasio, CFO
Debi Hamilton, Director of Services
Joe Donato, COO
A private, non-profit, community-based human services organization serving adults with disabilities (since 1953). Persons are provided the opportunity to achieve their highest potential through the Center's various programs that include day training, employment, community living and various support services.

6761   Medicenter of Tampa
4411 North Habana Avenue
Tampa, FL 33614-7211   813-872-2771
                                                      FAX: 813-871-2831
                                       rehabilitationandhealthcarecenteroftampa.com

Dan Davis, President
Mariluz G, Social Services Director
Brenda Pace, Secretary
Hilda B, Medicaid Coordinator
Postacute rehabilitation program. A 174 bed non-profit facility with postacute reahbilitation programs..

6762   Miami Heart Institute Adams Building
4300 Alton Rd
Miami Beach, FL 33140-2997   305-674-2121
                                                          www.msmc.com

Steven D. Sonenreich, President/CEO
The mission is to provide high quality health care to our diverse community enhanced through teaching, research, charity care and financial responsibility.

6763   Miami Lighthouse for the Blind
601 SW 8th Ave
Miami, FL 33130-3200   305-856-2288
                                                      FAX: 305-285-6967
                                               info@miamilighthouse.com
                                                    miamilighthouse.org

Virginia A. Jacko, President & Chief Executive Officer
Sharon Caughill, Special Projects Manager
Jeannie Reinoso, Executive Assistant
Arnie Paniagua, Chief Financial Officer
Offers services for the legally blind and severely visually impaired (including those who are developmentally delayed) of all ages in the areas of counseling and educational, recreational, rehabilitation, computer and vocational training services.

6764   Mount Sinai Medical Center Rehabilitation Unit
4300 Alton Rd
Miami Beach, FL 33140-2997   305-674-2121
                                                          www.msmc.com

Steven D. Sonenreich, President/CEO
A comprehensive inpatient and outpatient rehabilitation programs have been helping patients recover for more then 20 years. Fully customized treatment plans based on the needs of each patient is 1 reason why our services are among the best in South Florida. Our team approach takes into account the medical, physical, psychological, social, spiritual, cultural and economic needs of patients and their families.

6765   Neurobehavioral Medicine Center
Ste 1
4821 Us Highway 19
New Port Richey, FL 34652-4259   727-849-2005
                                                      FAX: 727-849-2087

Otsenre Matos, Medical Director
Gerard Taylor PhD, Counseling/Stress Management
Donna Taylor RN, Manager
Joyce Park Matos ARNP, Clinical Specialist
A multidisciplinary outpatient program for the evaluation and treatment of chronic pain. Consultation services for hospitalized patients are also provided upon request. Comprehensive treatment of individuals with closed traumatic brain injuries..

6766   North Broward Rehab Unit
North Broward Medical Center
201 E Sample Rd
Deerfield Beach, FL 33064-3596   954-941-8300
                                                      www.browardhealth.org

Douglas Ford, Chiefs of Staff
Pauline Grant, Chief Executive Officer
CARF accredited, 30-bed inpatient rehabilitation unit treating adults with brain injuries, spinal cord injuries, stroke, orthopedic and neurologic injuries.

6767   Northwest Medical Center
Health Care Corporation of America
2801 North State Road 7
Margate, FL 33063-5727   954-974-0400
                                                          866-256-7720
                                                      northwestmed.com

Mark Rader, CEO
Above all else, we are committed to the care and improvement of human life. In recognition of this commitment, we strive to deliver high quality, cost effective healthcare in the communities we serve. We recognize and affirm the unique and intrinsic work of each individual. We treat all those we serve with compassion and kindness. We act with absolute honesty, integrity, and fairness in the way we conduct our business and the way we live our lives.

6768   Pain Institute of Tampa
4178 N Armenia Ave
Tampa, FL 33607-6429   813-875-5913
                                                      www.barsahealth.com

John E Barsa, Founder & MD
Offers a comprehensive and multidisciplinary approach to pain controll and management. Most services are provided on-site but other services may require you to be referred elsewhere. We will monitor and coordinate your care in a manner to provide optimal recovery potential.

6769   Pain Treatment Center, Baptist Hospital of Miami
8900 N Kendall Dr
Miami, FL 33176-2118   786-596-1960
                                               corporatepr@baptisthealth.net
                                                     www.baptisthealth.net

Calvin Babcock, Chairman
Brian E. Keeley, President and Chief Executive Of
Since 1960, Baptist Hospital of Miami has been one of the most respected medical centers in South Florida. The hospitals full range of medical and technological services is the natural choice for a growing number of people throughout the world.

6770 **Pine Castle**
4911 Spring Park Rd
Jacksonville, FL 32207-7496
904-733-2650
FAX: 904-733-2681
info@pinecastle.org
pinecastle.org

Jonathan May, Executive Director
Randall Duncan, Associate Executive Director
Leigh Griffin, Director of Finance
Cliff Evans, Director of Development
Provides remunerative work, training, community employment and community living options for adults with developmental disabilities.

6771 **Polk County Association for Handicapped Citizens**
1038 Sunshine Dr E
Lakeland, FL 33801-6338
863-858-2252
FAX: 863-665-2330
sbaloghweb@pcahc.org
www.pcahc.org

Kecia Howell, Owner
Anthony J. Senzamici Jr., 1st Vice Chairman
Carol N. Asbill, 2nd Vice Chairman
A private non-profit organization that provides an adult day training program to people with developmental disabilities and is under the direction of a volunteer board of directors. The primary goal for our services is to provide people with knowledge and practical experience to be independent adults so they can become contributing members of their community..

6772 **Quest**
500 E Colonial Drive
P O Box 531125
Orlando, FL 32853- 4504
407-218-4300
888-807-8378
FAX: 407-218-4301
questinc.org

David Canora, Chair
James Gallagher, Vice-Chair
Suzanne Bennett, Treasurer
Ruth Bresnick, Secretary
Quest has built communities where people with disabilities have achieved their goals for nearly 50 years. Through a variety of residential and employment options, behavioral therapy, therapeutic day programs, charter schools and even a recreational summer camp, Quest serves more than 1000 individuals each day in the Orlando and Tampa areas.

6773 **Quest - Tampa Area**
1404 Tech Blvd
Tampa, FL 33619
813-423-7700
888-807-8378
FAX: 813-423-7701
contact@questinc.org
www.questinc.org

David Canora, Chair
James Gallagher, Vice-Chair
Suzanne Bennett, Treasurer
Ruth Bresnick, Secretary
Quest has built communities where people with disabilities have achieved their goals for nearly 50 years. Through a variety of residential and employment options, behavioral therapy, therapeutic day programs, charter schools and even a recreational summer

6774 **Rehabilitation Center for Children and Adults**
300 Royal Palm Way
Palm Beach, FL 33480-4305
561-655-7266
FAX: 561-655-3269
info@rcca.org
rcca.org

John C. Whelton, Chairman
Jacob L. Lochner, Co-Chairman
Christopher Adams, MD
A private, nonprofit organization whose purpose is to improve physical function, independence and communication of people with physical disabilities. Any child or adult with a physical or speech disability is eligible for services.

6775 **Renaissance Center**
3599 University Blvd
Suite 604
Jacksonville, FL 32216- 9249
904-399-0905
FAX: 904-743-5109
www.obiplasticsurgery.com/index.php

Lewis Obi, MD

6776 **Rosomoff Comprehensive Pain Center, The**
5200 NE 2nd Avenue
Miami, FL 33137-2706
305-532-7246
FAX: 305-534-3974
painrelief@rosomoffpaincenter.com
www.rosomoffpaincenter.com

Elsayed Abdel-Moty, Director
Hubert Rossomoff, Owner
A state-of-the-art Center of Excellence offering inpatient, outpatient, outpatient rehabilitation services and seniors programs. The Center became an internationally renowned model for the evalutation and treatment of all persons seeking pain relief.

6777 **Sarasota Memorial Hospital/Comprehensive Rehabilitation Unit**
1700 S Tamiami Trail
Sarasota, FL 34239-3509
941-917-9000
FAX: 941-917-2211
www.smh.com

Marguerite G Malone, Chair
Gregory Carter, First Vice Chair
Alex Miller, Second Vice Chair
Joseph J. DeVirgilio, Jt. Treasurer
The goal of the 34-bed Comprehensive Rehabilitation Unit (CRU) is to increase patient functional independence, adjust to illness or disability and successfully return to the community. The unit is dedicated to patients who have experienced conditions such

6778 **Strive Physical Therapy Centers**
2620 SE Maricamp RD
Ocala, FL 34471-4517
352-732-8868
FAX: 352-732-8890
www.striverehab.com

R W Shutes, Owner
Johanna Solbato, Administrator
R.W. Shutes, President and CEO
Certified as an Outpatient Rehabilitation Agency, providing a comprehensive approach to patient evaluation and treatment. Our objective is to return our patients back to a productive life as quickly as possible and safely as possible.

6779 **Sunbridge Care and Rehabilitation**
101 East State Street,
Kennett Square, FL 19348-6105
610-444-6350
FAX: 610-925-4000
info@genesishcc.com
www.genesishcc.com

Dan Hirschfeld, President
George V Hager, Chief Executive Officer
Robert A Reitz, Executive Vice President & Chief Operating Officer
Michael Sherman, Senior VP
A comprehensive medical rehabilitation facility that is committed to helping individuals with disabilities improve their quality of life. This is a 120-bed facility offering a full range of acute and sub-acute inpatient programs as well as community-based

6780 **Tampa Bay Academy**
12012 Boyette Rd
Riverview, FL 33569-5631
813-677-6700
800-678-3838
FAX: 813-671-3145
tlamb@tampahope.org
www.tampahope.org

Renee Scott, Chair
Amy McClure, Vice-Chair
Titania Lamb, Executive Director

A psychiatric residential treatment center and partial hospitalization program for ages 7 to 17.

6781 Tampa General Rehabilitation Center
1 Tampa General Circle
P.O.Box 1289
Tampa, FL 33606-3571
813-844-7700
866-844-1411
FAX: 813-844-1477
jstone@tgh.org
tgh.org

James R. Burkhart, *President & CEO*
Bruce Zwiebel, *Chief Of Staff*
Deana L. Nelson, *Chief Operating Officer*
Steve Short, *Cheif Financial Officer*
Offers a full range of programs all aimed at helping patients achieve their full potentials. It is one of three centers in the state that provides Driver Training and Evaluation Programs for persons with disabilities, and also an Assisted Reproduction Pro

6782 Tampa Lighthouse for the Blind
1106 West Platt Street
Tampa, FL 33606-2142
813-251-2407
FAX: 813-254-4305
tlh@templelighthouse.org
tampalighthouse.org

Sheryl Brown, *Executive Director*
Offers services for the totally blind, legally blind, visually impaired, mentally retarded blind and more with health, counseling, educational, recreational, rehabilitation, computer training and professional training services.

6783 Upper Pinellas Association for Retarded Citizens
1501 N Belcher Rd
Suite 249
Clearwater, FL 33765-1300
727-799-3330
FAX: 727-799-4632
info@uparc.com
www.uparc.com

Karen Crown, *Executive Director*
Offers services to more than 500 persons with mental retardation and other developmental disabilities. Services include two early intervention pre-schools, physical, speech and occupational therapies, homebound education and family support for children, b

6784 Visually Impaired Persons of Southwest Florida
35 W Mariana Ave
North Fort Myers, FL 33903-5515
239-997-7797
FAX: 239-997-8462
mmcgrael@vipcenter.org
vipcenter.org

Doug Fowler, *Executive Director*
Margaret Ruhe Lincoln, *Director of operations*
Provides training in independent living skills, orientation and mobility, counseling, computer and other communication skills, family support groups, peer counseling, socialization and a low vision clinic. Second location in Charlotte County. Phone: 941-6

6785 West Florida Hospital: The Rehabilitation Institute
8383 North Davis Hwy
Pensacola, FL 32514-6039
850-494-4000
800-342-1123
FAX: 850-494-4881
www.westfloridahospital.com

Roman S Bautista, *President/CEO*
Carol Saxton, *Senior VP Patient Care Services*
A 58-bed comprehensive rehabilitation facility offering inpatient and outpatient services. JCAHO and CARF accredited and a State designed head and spinal cord injury center. CARF accredited programs include: comprehensive inpatient rehab, spinal cord inju

6786 West Gables Health Care Center
2525 SW 75th Ave
Miami, FL 33155-2800
305-262-6800
FAX: 888-453-1928
www.westgablesrehabhospital.com

Jose Vargas, *Medical Director*
Walter Concepcion, *Chief Executive Officer*
Cesar Sepulveda, *Materials Manager*
Zely Santos, *Admissions Director*
Services provide by West Gables Health Center: activities services are provided onsite to residents. Clinical laboratory services are provided, dental, dietary, housekeeping, mental health services, nursing services, occupational therapy, pharmacy, physic

6787 Willough at Naples
9001 Tamiami Trail East
Naples, FL 34113-3397
239-775-4500
800-722-0100
FAX: 239-793-0534
info@thewilloughatnaples.com
thewilloughatnaples.com

James O'Shea, *President*
A licensed psychiatric hospital in Southwest Florida which provides quality management and treatment for eating disorders and chemical dependency in adults.

Georgia

6788 Annandale Village
3500 Annandale Ln
Suwanee, GA 30024-2150
770-945-8381
FAX: 770-945-8693
administration@annandale.org
annandale.org

Adam Pomeranz, *Chief Executive Officer*
Melissa Burton, *Chief Financial Officer*
Keith Fenton, *Chief Development & Marketing Officer*
Nancy Trujillo, *Chief Operating Officer*
Private nonprofit residential facility for adults with developmental disabilities. Located on 124 acres just north of Atlanta. Annandale provides full program and 24 hour residential services, pay program services, respite care and skilled nursing services.

6789 Atlanta Institute of Medicine and Rehabilitation
Ste E
2911 Piedmont Rd NE
Atlanta, GA 30305-2782
404-365-0160
FAX: 404-365-0751
contact@atlantaimr.com
www.atlantaimr.com

Lawrence E Eppelbaum, *Founder*
Galina Vayner, *MD*
One of the most famous medical centers in the state of Georgia. The Institute employs more then 40 highly qualified medical professionals and fully equipped with the latest medical equipment. It has gathered recognition and respect from the people of Atla

6790 Bobby Dodd Institute (BDI)
2120 Marietta Blvd NW
Atlanta, GA 30318-2122
678-365-0071
FAX: 678-365-0098
TTY:678-365-0099
wmcmillan@bdi-atl.org
bobbydodd.org

Rodney Hall, *Chair*
Christopher Rosselli, *Vice Chair*
Wayne McMillan, *President & CEO*
John Ralls, *Treasurer*
BDI annually serves approximately 400 clients in Atlanta, GA. BDI works primarily with people with developmental disabilities such as autism, down syndrome or mental retardation, but includes clients with physical or acquired disabilities. Client age va

6791 **Cave Spring Rehabilitation Center**
Georgia Department of Labor
7 Georgia Ave
P.O.Box 303
Cave Spring, GA 30124-2718
706-777-2341
FAX: 706-777-2366
russell.fleming@dol.state.ga.us
gvra.georgia.gov/cave-spring-center-cont acts-
Russell Fleming, Director
Karen Hulsey, Administrative Operations Coordinator
Renee Lambert, Rehabilitation Assistant
Renaultha Houston, Residential Program Supervisor

6792 **Center for Assistive Technology and Environmental Access**
490 10th St
Atlanta, GA 30332-0156
404-894-4960
800-726-9119
FAX: 404-894-9320
catea@coa.gatech.edu
www.catea.org
Carrie Bruce, Research Scientist
Charlie Drummond, Administrative Assistant
Summer Ienuso, Wen Developer
Trin Intra, Financial Administrator
The Center for Assistive Technology and Environmental Access (CATEA) promotes maximum function, activity and access of persons with disabilities through the use of technology. The foci of the Center includes the development, evaluation and utilization of

6793 **Center for the Visually Impaired**
739 West Peachtree St NW
Atlanta, GA 30308-1137
404-875-9011
FAX: 404-607-0062
info@cviatlanta.org
cviga.org
Susan Hoy, Chair
Fontaine M. Huey, President
Doreen Zaksheske, Vice President of Finance & Operations
Anisio Correia, Vice President for Programs
Offers services to people of all ages who are blind or visually impaired with training in orientation and mobility, computer technology, activities of daily living, communication skills and employment readiness. Aso offers two children's programs, a comm

6794 **Devereux Advanced Behavioral Health Georgia**
1291 Stanley Rd.
Kennesaw, GA 30152-8688
770-427-0147
800-342-3357
FAX: 770-427-4030
cfrost@devereux.org
www.devereuxga.org
Gwen Skinner, Executive Director
Mary Esposito, Assistant Executive Director
Yolanda Graham, Medical Director
Facility serving those from birth to 21 years old. Services includePsychiatric Residential Treatment Facility (PRTF), Foster Care Program, Therapeutic Group Homes, and SACS-Accredited School. Facility also offers a wide range of psychiatric, behavioral and emotional disorders with expertise in dual diagnoses and academic remediation.

6795 **Easter Seals East Georgia**
1500 Wrightsboro Road
Augusta, GA 30904-2441
706-667-9695
866-667-9695
FAX: 706-667-8831
sthomas@esega.org
www.easterseals.com/eastgeorgia
Sheila H. Thomas, CEO
Patrick Clayton, Chairman
Easter Seals East Georgia assists people with disabilities and other special needs to maximize opportunities for employment, independence and full inclusion into society.

6796 **Georgia Industries for the Blind**
700 Faceville Highway
Bainbridge, GA 39819-218
229-248-2666
FAX: 229-248-2669
gvra.georgia.gov/gib/about-us
James Hughes, Executive Director
Offers services for the totally blind, legally blind, visually impaired, mentally retarded blind and more with health, counseling, educational, recreational, rehabilitation, computer training and professional training services.

6797 **Hillhaven Rehabilitation**
26 Tower Rd NE
Marietta, GA 30060-6947
770-422-8913
800-526-5782
FAX: 770-425-2085
Leslie Ann Marie Parrish, Case Manager
Valerie Hamilton, Administrator
Routine skilled and subacute medical and rehabilitation care including physical therapy, occupational therapy, speech pathology and therapeutic recreation. Programs include stroke and head injury rehab; orthopedic rehab; complex IV therapy; woundcare; can.

6798 **In-Home Medical Care**
Care Master Medical Services
240 Odell Rd
P.O.Box 278
Griffin, GA 30223-4787
770-227-1264
800-542-8889
FAX: 770-412-0014
caremaster@accesunited.com
caremastermedical.com
Nancy Frederick, VP
Eddie Grogan, Chief Executive Officer
Offers the devoted attention of a professional nurse, the use of I.V. therapies, pain management and provision of medical equipment and supplies right where the patient wants to be.

6799 **Learning Services: Harris House Program**
131 Langley Drive
Suite B
Lawrenceville, GA 30046-4446
404-298-0144
888-419-9955
FAX: 866-491-7396
learningservices.com
Dr. Debra Braunling-McMorrow, President and CEO
Susan Snow, Director of Admissions
Michael Weaver, Chief Development Officer
Jeanne Mack, Chief Financial Officer
Situated in the small, historic district of Stone Mountain, just outside of Atlanta, this 6 bed program is designed to encourage independence while providing appropriate support for each individuals needs. Community-based productive activities are customi

6800 **Pain Control & Rehabilitation Institute of Georgia**
Ste 120
2784 N Decatur Rd
Decatur, GA 30033-5993
404-297-1400
FAX: 404-297-1427
Shulim Spektor, CEO
Anna Britman, Office Manager
Provides pain management for chronic and acute pain resulted from injuries, diseases of muscles and nerve, Reflex Sympathetic Dystrophy, perform disabilities and impairment ratings.

6801 **Savannah Association for the Blind**
214 Drayton Street
Savannah, GA 31401-4021
912-236-4473
FAX: 912-234-9286
www.sabinc.org
Gregory Hodges, President
Robert Falligant, Vice-president
Gary Sadowski, Treasurer
Lula Baker, Secretary

Offers services for the totally blind, legally blind, visually impaired, mentally retarded blind and more with health, counseling, educational, recreational, rehabilitation, computer training and professional training services.

6802 Shepherd Center for Treatment of Spinal Injuries
2020 Peachtree Rd NW
Atlanta, GA 30309-1465
404-352-2020
FAX: 404-350-7479
admissions@shepherd.org
www.shepherd.org

Gary R. Ulicny, President & CEO
David F. Apple, Jr., M.D., Medical Director
Angela Beninga, D.O., Staff Physiatrist
ChiChi Berhane, M.D., MBA, Director, Reconstructive Surgery
Dedicated exclusively to the care of patients with spinal cord injuries and other paralyzing spinal disorders. It serves predominately residents of Georgia and neighboring states as one of the only 14 hospitals designated by the U.S. Department of Educati

6803 Transitional Hospitals Corporation
Ste 1000
7000 Central Pkwy NE
Atlanta, GA 30328-4592
770-821-5328
800-683-6868
FAX: 770-913-0015
staff@csins.com
csins.com

Dean Kozee, Owner
Carolyn Norton, Special Projects Consultant/Broker
Amaury Rentas, Event Insurance/Broker
A national network of intensive care hospitals providing care for patients who suffer from a chronic illness and/or catastrophic accident. The mission is founded on providing quality health care to patients who require highly skilled nursing care and acce.

6804 Walton Rehabilitation Health System
1355 Independence Dr
Augusta, GA 30901-1037
706-823-8584
866-492-5866
FAX: 706-724-5752
vickig@waltonfoundation.net
www.waltonfoundation.net

Robert Taylor, Chair
Dennis Skelley, President/CEO
David Dugan, Treasurer
Brent Smith, Secretary
A 58-bed comprehensive physical rehabilitation hospital offering inpatient and outpatient services. Services offered include: stroke recovery, orthopedic injury, pediatrics, head injury, pain management for chronic pain syndrome, TMJ/Craniofacial pain and

Hawaii

6805 Rehabilitation Hospital of the Pacific
226 N Kuakini St
Honolulu, HI 96817-2498
808-531-3511
FAX: 808-566-3411
rehabfoundation@rehabhospital.org
www.rehabhospital.org

John Komeiji, Chair
Glenn O. Sexton, Vice Chair
E. Lynne Madden, Secretary/Treasurer
Timothy J. Roe, President & Chief Executive Officer
The only acute care medical rehabilitation organization serving both Hawaii and the Pacific. For over 52 years, the hospital and its 7 outpatient clinics on Oahu, and Maui and Hawaii have been dedicated to providing comprehensive, cost effective rehabilit

Idaho

6806 Ashton Memorial Nursing Home and Chemical Dependency Center
700 N 2nd
Ashton, ID 83420
208-652-7461
FAX: 208-652-7595
ashmem@frtel.com
ashtonmemorial.com

Sheila Kellogg, Administrator

6807 Easter Seals-Goodwill Northern Rocky Mountains
Easter Seals National
1465 S Vinnell Way
Boise, ID 83709-1659
208-378-9924
800-374-1910
FAX: 208-378-9965
www.easterseals.org

Richard W. Davidson, Chairman
Ralph F. Boyd, Jr., Treasurer
Eileen Howard Boone, Secretary
James E. Williams, Jr., Assistant Secretary
Provides services for children and adults with disabilities and other special needs, and support to their families

6808 Idaho Elks Rehabilitation Hospital
600 N Robbins Rd
Boise, ID 83702
208-489-4444
FAX: 208-344-8883
info@elksrehab.org
www.elksrehab.org

Joseph P. Caroselli, CEO
Doug Lewis, Chief Financial Officer
Mellisa Honsinger, Chief Operating Officer
A nonprofit hospital serving Idaho and the Pacific Northwest. All inpatient and outpatient programs and services are supervised by the hospital's full-time medical directors whose specialty is physical rehabilitative medicine. Services include: occupation

6809 Portneuf Medical Center Rehabilitation
777 Hospital Way
Pocatello, ID 83201-4004
208-239-1000
charlesa@portmed.org
www.portmed.org

Mark Buckalew, Chairman
Michael Nosacka, MD
Dan Ordyna, CEO
John Abreu, Vice President
Provides compassionate, quality health care services needed by the people of eastern Idaho in collaboration with other providers and community resources.

Illinois

6810 Advocate Christ Hospital and Medical Center
4440 W 95th St
Oak Lawn, IL 60453-2600
708-684-8000
FAX: 708-684-4440
advocatehealth.com

Jim Skogsbergh, CEO
Bill Santulli, COO
Kate K, Director
A 665-bed, not-for-profit teaching, research and referral medical center in Oak Lawn, Illinois. It also is home to the Advocate Hope Childrens's Hospital, one of the most comprehensive providers of pediatric care in the state. The medical center is a lead

6811

Advocate Christ Medical Center & Advocate Hope Children's Hospital
4440 W 95th St
Oak Lawn, IL 60453-2600
708-684-8000
FAX: 708-684-4440
advocatehealth.com

Kenneth Lukhard, CEO
Darcie Brazel, Market Chief Nurse Executive
Jan McCrea, Rehab Services Director
William Adair MD, Medical Director/Rehab Services

The largest fully integrated not-for-profit health care delivery system in metropolitan Chicago and is recognized as one of the top 10 systems in the country. The mission of Advocate Health Care is to serve the health needs of individuals, families and co

6812

Advocate Illinois Masonic Medical Center
836 W Wellington Ave
Chicago, IL 60657-5147
773-975-1600
www.advocatehealth.com/immc

Jim Skogsbergh, CEO
Ajay V. Maker, MD

Consultation, education, family counseling, parent training in behavior modification techniques offered to developmentally disabled adults.

6813

Alexian Brothers Medical Center
800 Biesterfield Rd
Elk Grove Village, IL 60007-3396
847-437-5500
AlexianBrothersMedicalCenter @alexian.net
www.alexian.org

Mark Frey, President/CEO
Tracy Rogers, Senior Vice President and Chief Operating Officer
Paul Belter, Senior Vice President and Chief Financial Officer
Patricia Cassidy, Senior Vice President and Chief Strategy Officer

A threefold mission: Works toward maximizing physical function, enhance independent social skills and optimize communication skills consistent with an individual's ability. The Center helps those disabled by accident or illness achieve a new personal best

6814

Back in the Saddle Hippotherapy Program
Corcoran Physical Therapy
4200 W Peterson Ave
Chicago, IL 60646-6074
312-286-2266
847-604-4145
FAX: 847-673-8895
info@hippotherapychicago.com

Julie Naughton, Program Coordinator
Maureen Corcoran, Physical Therapist
Tom Corcoran, Owner

A direct medical treatment used by licensed physical therapists who have a strong treatment background in posture and movement, neuromotor function and sensory processing. The benefits of Hippotherapy are available to individuals with just about any disab

6815

Barbara Olson Center of Hope
3206 N Central Ave
Rockford, IL 61101-1797
815-964-9275
FAX: 815-964-9607
info@b-olsoncenterofhope.org
b-olsoncenterofhope.org

Carm Herman, Executive Director
Pam Sondell, Director of Programs and Services
Pam Carey, Director of Human Resources
Mike Marvell, Director of Business Development

We provide vocational employment, educational and social opportunities for adults with developmental disabilities.

6816

Bartolucci Center, The- ILC Enterprises
6415 Stanley Ave
Berwyn, IL 60402-3130
708-745-5277
FAX: 708-698-5090
www.pillarscommunity.org

Zada Clarke, Chairman
Ann Schreiner, President & CEO
Jennifer Hogberg, Vice Chair
Sheila Eswaran, Secretary

A nonprofit tax exempt private social service agency serving suburban Chicago offering day treatment and vocational counseling to individuals who encountered a pattern of job loss due to emotional problems.

6817

Baxter Healthcare Corporation
1 Baxter Pkwy
Deerfield, IL 60015-4625
224-948-2000
800-422-9837
224-948-1812
FAX: 800-568-5020
baxter.com

Phillip L. Batchelor, Corporate Vice President - Quality and Regulatory Affairs
Jean-Luc Butel, Corporate Vice President - President, International
Robert M. Davis, Corporate Vice President - President, Medical Products
Robert Parkinson Jr, Chairman of the Board and Chief Executive Officer

Baxter International Inc. is a global healthcare company that, through its subsidiaries assists healthcare professionals and their patients with treatment of complex medical conditions including hemophelia, immune disorders, kidney disease, cancer, trauma and other conditions. Baxter applies its expertise in medical devices, pharmaceuticals, and biotechnology to make a meaningful difference in patient's lives.

6818

Beacon Therapeutic Diagnostic and Treatment Center
10650 S Longwood Dr
Chicago, IL 60643-2617
773-881-1005
FAX: 773-881-1164
www.beacon-therapeutic.org

Susan Reyha-Guerrero, President & CEO
Cheryl Thompson, Deputy CEO
Paul Morley, Chief Operating Officer

Offers community day treatment, education, diagnostic services, family counseling, learning disabled, speech and hearing and psychiatric services.

6819

Blind Service Association
17 N State St
Ste 1050
Chicago, IL 60602-3510
312-236-0808
blindserviceassociation.org

Ann Lousin, President
Linda Schwartz, Executive Vice President
Arthur M. Shapiro, Secretary
John Powen, Treasurer

Offers services for the totally blind, legally blind and visually impaired with reading and recording low vision network, social services, referrals and support groups.

6820

Brandecker Rehabilitation Center
1939 West 13th Street
Suite 300
Chicago, IL 60643-6316
312-491-4110
FAX: 312-733-0247
www.easterseals.com/chicago

Richard W. Davidson, Chairman
Ralph F. Boyd, Jr., Treasurer
Eileen Howard Boone, Secretary
James E. Williams, Jr., Assistant Secretary

We offer early intervention services for infants and toddlers with developmental delays and disabilities. Our outpatient Medical Rehabilitation Program offers direct therapy services for children from age birth-16.

6821   Brentwood Subacute Healthcare Center
T HI Brentwood
5400 W 87th St
Burbank, IL 60459-2913
866-300-3257
www.savaseniorcare.com

Audrey Protrowski, Director Business Development
Jill Sattersield, Administrator
John Walton, CEO

Seeks to help patients and their families through what can be a very emotional decision-making process. We provide guidance and consultation on everything from how to properly choose the facility to providing resources that help you cope with the nature of the decision itself.

6822   Caremark Healthcare Services
2211 Sanders Rd
Northbrook, IL 60062-6128
847-559-4700
800-423-1411
FAX: 847-559-3905
phu@caremark.com
www.caremark.com

Larry J. Merlo, President & CEO
Mark Cosby, Executive Vice President

An 80-service-center network providing services anywhere in the U.S. Offers 24 hour access to nursing and pharmacy services, case management resource centers, HIV/AIDS services, women's health services, transplant care services, nutrition support services

6823   Centegra Northern Illinois Medical Center
4209 West Shamrock Lane
Suite B
McHenry, IL 60050-8499
815-759-8017
877-236-8347
FAX: 815-759-8062
www.centegra.org

Michael S. Eesley, CEO
Jason Sciarro, President
David L. Tomlinson, Executive Vice President
Kumar Nathan, MD

Providing rehabilitation services in Lake and McHenry Counties, the Rehabilitation Unit is a complete living environment for up to 15 patients after a debilitating illness of trauma. Various locations offering a multitude of services: PT, OT, speech, HT,

6824   Center for Comprehensive Services
Mentor Network
P.O.Box 2825
Carbondale, IL 62902-2825
618-457-4008
800-582-4227
FAX: 618-457-5372
dayna.foreman@thementornetwork.com
mentorabi.com

Bill Duffy, Chief Operating Officer
Michael E. Hofmeister, Vice President
Sean Byrne, Chief Financial Officer

Post-acute rehabilitation services for adults and adolescents with acquired brain injuries. Residential, day-treatment and out-patient services tailored to individual needs.

6825   Center for Rehabilitation at Rush Presbyterian: Johnston R Bowman Health Center
1653 W Congress Parkway
Chicago, IL 60612-3833
312-942-5000
FAX: 312-942-3601
TTY:312-942-2207
teri_sommerfeld@rush.edu
www.rush.edu

Larry J. Goodman, CEO

A 613-bed hospital serving adults and children, the John R. Bowman Health Center and Rush University is home to one of the first medical colleges in the Midwest and one of the nation's top-ranked nursing colleges, as well as graduate programs in allied he

6826   Center for Spine, Sports & Occupational Rehabilitation
345 E Superior St
Chicago, IL 60611-2654
312-238-7767
800-354-7342
FAX: 312-238-7709
webmaster@ric.org
www.rehabchicago.org

Joanne C. Smith, President & CEO
Edward B. Case, Executive Vice President
M. Jude Reyes, Chair

Offers evaluation and treatment of patients with acute and sub-acute musculoskeletal and sports injuries. RIC offers different levels of care, including inpatient, day rehabilitation, and outpatients services, according to the special needs of each patient

6827   Children's Home and Aid Society of Illinois
125 South Wacker Drive
14th Floor
Chicago, IL 60606-4448
312-424-0200
contact@chasi.org
www.childrenshomeandaid.org

Beverley Sibblies, Chairman
Chris Leahy, Vice-Chairman
Mark Tresnowski, Secretary
David Gookin, Treasurer

Private state-wide. Multi-service, racially integrated staff and client populations. Provides educational, placement and community services for children-at-risk and their families. Advocacy, consultation and follow-up services provided according to our ph

6828   Clinton County Rehabilitation Center
1665 North Fourth Street
P O Box 157
Breese, IL 62230- 1791
618-526-8800
FAX: 618-526-2021
info@commlink.org
commlink.org

Wesley A. Gozia, President
Judge Joseph L. Heimann, Vice President
John L. Lengerman, Treasurer
Jerry Albers, Secretary

Provides Adult Day Programs (developmental training, work training, job readiness and job placements); Residentail Programs (CILA Intermittent Care, CILA 24 hour care); Infant Programs (early interventions, early head start); Community Services (specializ

6829   Continucare, A Service of the Rehab Institute of Chicago
West Suburban Hospital Medical Center
3 Erie Ct
Oak Park, IL 60302-2519
708-383-6200
800-354-7342
FAX: 312-908-1369
www.westsuburbanmedicalcenter.research.org

Heidi Asbury MD

We respond to the needs of the whole person: body, mind and spirit. We foster a climate of care, hospitality and a spirit of community. We develop systems and structures that attend to the needs of those at risk of discrimination because of age, gender, lifestyle, ethnic background, religious beliefs or socioeconomic status.

6830   Delta Center
1400 Commercial Ave
Cairo, IL 62914-1978
618-734-2665
800-471-7213
FAX: 618-734-1999
delta1@midwest.net
deltacenter.org

Lisa Tolbert, Executive Director
Lisa Tholbert, Assistant Executive Director

The Delta Center is a non-profit mental health center, substance abuse counseling facility, and also provides various community services to Alexander and Pulaski County, Illinois. The purpose and mission is to promote, encourage, foster and engage exclusi

6831 Division of Rehabilitation-Education Services, University of Illinois
Beckwith Hall
201 E. John Street
Champaign, IL 61820- 6901 217-333-4603
FAX: 217-333-0248
disability@uiuc.edu
www.disability.ui.uc.edu

Ann Fredricksen, Disability Specialist
Jon Gunderson, Coordinator
Pat Malik, Director
Dennis Cable, Accountant
Offers services for the totally blind, legally blind, visually impaired, mentally retarded blind and more with health, counseling, educational, recreational, rehabilitation, computer training and professional training services.

6832 Easter Seals
Easter Seals Joliet Region
233 South Wacker Drive
Suite 2400
Chicago, IL 60606-5272 312-726-6200
800-221-6827
FAX: 312-726-1494
www.easterseals.com

Richard W. Davidson, Chairman
Sandra L. Bouwman, 1st Vice Chairman
Joseph G. Kern, 2nd Vice Chairman
Ralph F. Boyd, Treasurer
Services for children and adults with disabilities and their families. Pediatric outpatient medical rehabilitation, inclusive childcare, fostercare, residential homes, clinics.

6833 Easter Seals DuPage And The Fox Valley Region
830 S Addison Ave
Villa Park, IL 60181-2877 630-620-4433
FAX: 630-620-1148
info@eastersealsdfvr.org
www.eastersealsdfvr.org

Theresa Forthofer, President & CEO
Erik Johnson, Vice President of Development
Roger Hendrick, Vice President of Operations
Kathy Schrock, Vice President of Clinical Services
The mission of Easter Seals DuPage & the Fox Valley Region is to enable infants, children & adults with disabilities to achieve maximum independence and to provide support to the families who love and care for them. Key services include: physical, occupational, speech-language, nutrition and assistive technology therapies and audiology services for all ages.

6834 Easter Seals Gilchrist-Marchman Rehab Center
1939 West 13th Street
Suite 300
Chicago, IL 60608-1226 312-491-4110
FAX: 312-733-0247
Mcancel@eastersealschicago.org
www.easterseals.com/chicago

David A. Pearre, Chairman
Jeff Buchanan, Vice Chairman
Mark O'Toole, Secretary
John G. Anos, Treasurer
Provides comprehensive services for individuals with disabilities or other special needs and their families to improve quality of life and maximize independence.

6835 Easter Seals Jayne Shover Center
799 S McLean Blvd
Elgin, IL 60123-6704 847-742-3264
FAX: 847-742-9436
il-ja.easter-seals.org
dfvr.easterseals.com

Dr. Haydee Muse, Chair
Kelly N. Taira, Vice Chairman
Karen Janousek, Secretary
Roger McDougal, Treasurer
A free-standing, comprehensive outpatient rehabilitation center serving children and adults with physical and developmental disabilities.

6836 El Valor Corporation
Early Intervention Program
1850 W 21st St
Chicago, IL 60608-2799 312-666-4511
FAX: 312-666-6677
info@elvalor.net
www.elvalor.org

Paul Gaughan, Chairman
Philip K. Fuentes, Vice Chairman
Rey B. Gonzalez, President & CEO
Michael J. Cabrera, Secretary
Mission is to challenge people with disabilities. It is a center for people with disabilities and their families and serves Chicago and surrounding areas, providing services in English and Spanish to individuals whose lives would be drastically impoverish

6837 Elgin Training Center
Association For Individual Development Elgin Area
1135 Bowes Road
Elgin, IL 60123-1321 847-931-6200
FAX: 847-888-6079
www.the-association.org

Chuck Miles, Chairmen
Patrick Flaherty, Vice Chairmen
Walter Dwyer, Treasurer
Lynn O'Shea, Executive Director
Day training services to develop work habits and attitudes while providing training in small product assembly, sorting, packaging, collating, & material handling. Instruction also offered in job related knowledge & in personal, social and independent living skills. There is also an on-site specialized Autism Program. Additionally, residential programs (group homes & apartments) are also available for people with developmental disabilities.

6838 Family Counseling Center
PO Box 759
Golconda, IL 62938 618-683-2461
FAX: 618-683-2066
fccgolconda@shawneelink.com
fccinconline.org

Larry Mizell, Executive Director
Connie Duncan, Director
Nora Beth Hacker, Financial Director
Provides counseling, developmental training, evaluations, assisted living services, referrals, psychosocial rehabilitation, and a variety of work services.

6839 Family Matters
A RC Community Support Systems
1901 S. 4th St
Ste 209
Effingham, IL 62401-4123 217-347-5428
866-436-7842
FAX: 217-347-5119
deinhorn@arc-css.org
www.fmptic.org

Debbie Einhorn, Executive Director
Debbie Einhorn, Director Family Support
Nancy Mader, Project Coordinator
Barbara Utz, Vice President
Parent Training and Information Center and family support programs for families of children who have disabilities from the ages of birth through 21. Services include: Parent support and training, school advocacy, home visits, information and referral, pa

6840 Five Star Industries
1308 Wells Street Road
P O Box 60
Du Quoin, IL 62832-60 618-542-5421
FAX: 618-542-5556
fivestarinc@5starind.com
5starind.com

Susan Engelhardt, Executive Director
Incorporated as a private, non-profit corporation under the laws of the State of Illinois, is an equal opportunity employer and provides equal opportunity in compliance with the Civil Rights Act of 1964 and all other appropriate laws, rules and regulation

6841 HSI Austin Center For Development
1819 S Kedzie Ave
Chicago, IL 60623-2623
773-854-1676
FAX: 773-854-8300

6842 Hyde Park-Woodlawn
950 E 61st St
Chicago, IL 60637-2623
773-324-0280
FAX: 773-324-0285
jvshp@jvschicago.org

Clarissa Williams, Manager

6843 Illinois Center for Autism
548 South Ruby Lane
Fairview Heights, IL 62208-2614
618-398-7500
FAX: 618-394-9869
info@illinoiscenterforautism.org
illinoiscenterforautism.org

Hardy Ware, Chairperson
Thomas E. Berry, Vice Chairperson
Gary Guthrie, Secretary
Joy Rick, Treasurer
A community-based mental health/educational treatment center dedicated to serving autistic clients.

6844 Julius and Betty Levinson Center
1825 K Street NW
Suite 600
Washington, DC 60304-1557
202-776-0406
800-872-5827
FAX: 708-383-9025
info@ucp.net.org
www.ucp.org

Woody Connette, Chair
Ian Ridlon, Vice Chair
Mark Boles, Treasurer
Pamela Talkin, Secretary
Houses one of its three adult developmental training programs for substantially physically disabled men and women.

6845 Lake County Health Department
18 N. County Street
Waukegan, IL 60085
847-377-2000
FAX: 847-336-1517
www.lakecountyil.gov

Aaron Lawlor, Chairman
Stevenson Mountsier, Vice Chairman
Barry Burton, Administrator
Includes counseling, crisis intervention, emergency management, psychotherapy and chemotherapy management for individuals and families.

6846 Little Friends, Inc.
140 N Wright Street
Naperville, IL 60540-4799
630-355-6533
FAX: 630-355-3176
info@lilfriends.com
www.littlefriendsinc.com

Dan Casey, Chairman
Matt Johanson, Vice Chairman
Michele Calbi, Treasurer
Kathy West, Secretary
Little Friends has been serving children and adults with autism and other developmental disabilities for over 40 years. Based in Naperville, Little Friends operates three schools, vocational training programs, community-based residential services and the

6847 MAP Training Center
7th and Mc Kinley St
Karnak, IL 62956
618-634-9401
FAX: 618-634-9090

Larry Earnhart, President
Cindy Earnhart, Community Liaison
Training, employment, residential and support services, targeted for adults with developmental disabilities.

6848 Macon Resources
2121 Hubbard Ave.
P O Box 2760
Decatur, IL 62524-2760
217-875-1910
FAX: 217-875-8899
TTY:217-875-8898
jpatterson@maconresources.org
maconresources.org

Tom Hill, President
Michael Breheny, Vice President
Barb Nadler, Secretary
Chris Funk, Treasurer
The purpose is to provide a comprehensive array of habilitative/rehabilitative training programs and support services to assist individuals and/or family units of an individual with a developmental disability, mental illness, or other handicapping conditi

6849 Mary Bryant Home for the Blind
2960 Stanton
Springfield, IL 62703-4385
217-529-1611
888-529-1611
FAX: 217-529-6975
mbha@marybryanthome.org
marybryanthome.org

Jerry Curry, Executive Director
Robert E. Maxey, President
Allan J. Rupel, Vice President
Gary Rapaport, Secretary
Supportive living facility for blind or visually impaired adults over the age of 22. A supportive living facility remodeled to foster the move to increased independence for residents. The new apartment style housing combined with personal care and other a

6850 Northern Illinois Special Recreation Association (NISRA)
285 Memorial Drive
Crystal Lake, IL 60014-3650
815-459-0737
FAX: 815-459-0388
info@nisra.org
www.nisra.org

Brian Shahinian, Executive Director
Carol Amoroso, Manager of Finance and Personnel
Kerri Ruddy, Manager of Office Services
Sarah Holcombe, Manager of Communications & Marketing
Leisure and recreation services to those with disabilities who are unable to participate successfully in park district and city recreation programs.

6851 Oak Forest Hospital of Cook County
15900 Cicero Ave
Oak Forest, IL 60452
708-687-7200
FAX: 708-687-7979
TTY:708-687-4794
http://www.cchil.org

Robert Weinstein, Department Chair
Suja Mathew, Associate Chair
A 654 bed health care center devoted to the diagnosis, rehabilitation and long-term care of adults suffering from chronic illnesses, diseases and physical impairments.

6852 PARC
1913 W. Townline Road
P.O.Box 3418
Peoria, IL 61615-3418
309-691-3800
FAX: 309-689-3613
rricketts@arcpeoria.org
parcway.org

Pat Kawczynski, Chair
Heyl Royster, Vice Chair
Terry Waters, Treasurer
Alexis Duhon, Secretary
Serves all ages that are diagnosed with mental retardation and other developmental and physical disabilities. Programs include early intervention, family support, respite care, vocational training, supported employment, adult day programs and residential

6853 **Peoria Area Blind People's Center**
2905 W Garden St
Peoria, IL 61605-1316
309-637-3693
FAX: 309-637-3693
info@cicbvi.org
cicbvi.org

Carol Warren, President
Cora Quinn, Vice President
Prasad Parupalli, Treasurer
Offers services for the totally blind, legally blind, visually impaired, mentally retarded blind and more with health, counseling, educational, recreational, rehabilitation, computer training and professional training services.

6854 **Pioneer Center of McHenry County**
4001 W Dayton St
McHenry, IL 60050-8379
815-344-1230
FAX: 815-344-3815
TTY:815-344-6243
GetHelp@pioneercenter.org
www.pioneercenter.org

Michael T. Moushey, Chairman
Pam Allen, Secretary
Mark LeFevre, Treasurer
Rebecca Heisler, Board
Pioneer Center is the largest social service agency in McHenry County delivering direct services to more than 2,500 individuals annually. The organization also provides education and outreach to schools and community organizations reaching over 10,000 additional individuals. Pioneer Center delivers community-based services in the areas of:McHenery County PADS, Youth Service Bureau, Autism Services, Developmental Disabilities, Mental Illness, Traumatic Brain Injury and VOICE Sexual Assault.

6855 **Prosthetics and Orthotics Center in Blue Island**
2310 York St
Blue Island, IL 60406-2411
708-597-2611
800-354-7342
FAX: 800-908-1932
www.rehabchicago.org/about/blue_island.php

6856 **RB King Counseling Center**
2300 N Edward St
Decatur, IL 62526-4163
217-877-8121
FAX: 217-875-0966

Gordon Cross MD
Offers outpatient, individual, group, divorce and meditation, family and re-adjustment counseling.

6857 **REHAB Products and Services**
3715 N Vermilion St
Danville, IL 61832-1130
217-446-1146
FAX: 217-446-1191
rehab@soltec.net
workse.org

Frank L. Brunacci, President/CEO
Crystal Meece, Vice President Production
Todd Seabaugh, VP Programs
Scott Rudy, VP Operations
janitorial, lawn care, distribution services.

6858 **RIC Northshore**
Rehabilitation Institute of Chicago
345 E Superior St
Chicago, IL 60611-2654
312-238-1000
800-354-7342
webmaster@ric.org
www.rehabchicago.org

Joanne C. Smith, President/CEO
Edward B. Case, Vice President
Provides rehabilitation for sports-related injuries, musculoskeletal conditions, neurological conditions, stroke, arthritis, amputation, burns, and general deconditioning.

6859 **RIC Prosthetics and Orthotics Center**
Rehabilitation Institute of Chicago
345 E. Superior Street
Suite 101
Chicago, IL 60611-4615
312-238-1000
800-345-7342
FAX: 708-957-8353
webmaster@rehabchicago.org
ric.org

Martin Buckner, CPO, Inpatient Coordinator
Nicole T. Soltys, CP, Clinical Coordinator
Robert D. Lipschutz, CP, Director of Prosthetic and Orthotic Education
Walter Afable, CP, Clinical Operations Manager
Offers almost all the prosthetics and orthotics services provided at RIC's main hospital in downtown Chicago, including consultations, fittings and training.

6860 **RIC Windermere House**
5548 S Hyde Park Blvd
Chicago, IL 60637-1909
773-256-5050
800-354-7342
FAX: 773-256-5060
www.rehabchicago.org

Meghan Scalise, Manager
Evaluation, therapeutic services and patient education are offered in the areas of arthritis, multiple sclerosis, musculoskeletal conditions, orthopedics, stroke, spinal cord injury, brain injury and sports medicine.

6861 **Ray Graham Association for People with Disabilities**
901 Warrenville Road
Suite 500
Lisle, IL 60532-1038
630-620-2222
FAX: 630-628-2350
TTY:630-628-2352
cathyfickerterill@yahoo.com
ray-graham.org

Michael Komoll, Chairperson
Neville Bilimoria, Vice Chairperson
Kim zoeller, President & CEO
Jeff Park, Secretary/Treasurer
Provides developmental services at 15 sites to infants, children and adults with disabilities. Services range from 1 hr/wk respite to full-time residential.

6862 **Reach Rehabilitation Program: Americana Healthcare**
9401 S Kostner Ave
Oak Lawn, IL 60453-2697
708-423-1505
FAX: 708-423-3822

Jean M Roche, Owner
Postacute rehabilitation program.

6863 **Rehabilitation Achievement Center**
345 E Superior St
Chicago, IL 60611-4805
312-238-1000
800-354-7342
www.ric.org

M. Jude Reyes, Chair
Mike P. Krasny, Vice Chair
Joanne C. Smith, President & CEO
Ed Case, Treasurer
Rehabilitation Institute of Chicago (RIC) has aquired the assets of the Rehabilitation Achievement Center (RAC).

6864 **Rehabilitation Institute of Chicago: Alexian Brothers Medical Center**
800 Biesterfield Rd
Elk Grove Village, IL 60007-3361
847-437-5500
866-253-9426
FAX: 847-631-5663
TTY: 847-956-5116
www.alexianbrothershealth.org

Mark Frey, President and Chief Executive Officer
Tracy Rogers, Senior Vice President and Chief Operating Officer
Paul Belter, Senior Vice President and Chief Financial Officer
Janice Jastrowski, Manager

A 32-bed rehabilitation unit under the medical direction and supervision of the Rehabilitation Institute of Chicago.

6865   Riverside Medical Center
Mental Health Unit
350 N Wall St
Kankakee, IL 60901-2991   815-933-1671
                                            FAX: 815-935-8160
                                              rhuber@rsh.net
                                         riversidehealthcare.org

Phillip Kambic, CEO
Bill W. Douglas, Vice President
Offers recreation, parenting therapy, emergency services, psychological testing and inpatient treatment programs. Riverside is nationally recognized for its specialty programs in heart care, obstetrics, trauma, oncology, rehabilitation, geriatrics, occupa

**6866   Robert Young Mental Health Center Division of Trinity
         Regional Haelth System**
Trinity Health Foundation
2701 17th St
Rock Island, IL 61201-5351   309-779-2800
                                                 800-322-1431
                                            FAX: 309-779-2027
                                              www.unitypoint.org

Rick Seidler, President & CEO
Jim Hayes, CFO
Tamara Byram, VP, Legal/Compliance
Matt Behrens, Regional VP, UnityPoint Clinic
Services include comprehensive inpatient rehabilitation, chronic pain management programs, outpatient medical rehabilitation, work hardening programs, vocational evaluation, alcohol and other drug dependency rehabilitation programs, Burn Center, and menta

6867   Sampson-Katz Center
216 West Jackson Blvd
Suite 700
Chicago, IL 60606-2104   312-673-3400
                                            FAX: 312-553-5544
                                            TTY:773-761-6672
                                         jvsskc@jvschicago.org
                                          www.jvschicago.org

Andrew M. Glick, Chair
John L. Daniels, Vice Chair
H. Debra Levin, President
Benn Feltheimer, Secretary

6868   Shelby County Community Services
160 North Main Street
Memphis, TN 38103-650   901-222-2300
                                            FAX: 912-222-2090
                                         www.shelbycountytn.gov

Dottie Jones, Director
Primary focus is substance abuse treatment.

6869   Streator Unlimited
305 N Sterling St
P O Box 706
Streator, IL 61364-2369   815-673-5574
                                            FAX: 815-673-1714
                                      contact@streatorunlimited.org
                                        www.streatorunlimited.org

Jeffrey Dean, Executive Director
Lynn Fukar, Director of Day Services
Julie Caestens, Director Residential Services
Vocational and personal skills training, residential services, client and family support, supported and computerized employment. Serves adults with intellectual disabilities with the goal of enabling them to reach their fullest potential, live as independ

6870   Swedish Covenant Hospital Rehabilitation Services
5145 N California Ave
Chicago, IL 60625-3661   773-878-8200
                                            FAX: 773-561-0490
                                            ask_us@schosp.org
                                              www.schosp.org

Mark Newton, President & CEO
Provides acute rehabilitation services, subacute care and outpatient services for many types of disabling injuries and conditions, including amputation, arthritis, brain injury, general deconditioning, multiple sclerosis, musculoskeletal injuries, stroke,

6871   TCRC Sight Center
21310 Route 9
Tremont, IL 61568-2558   309-347-7148
                                            FAX: 309-925-4241
                                              info@tcrcorg.com
                                              www.tcrcorg.com

Jamie Durdel, President & CEO
Molly Anderson, Vice President
Offers services for persons who are totally blind, legally blind, partially sighted or visually impaired along with other disabilities. Have support group, rehabilitation classes, orientation and mobility services, counseling services, low vision clinic,

6872   Tazewell County Resource Center
Box 12
Rr 1
Tremont, IL 61568   309-347-7148
                                            FAX: 309-925-4241
                                              info@tcrcorg.com
                                         http://www.tcrcorg.com

Jamie Durdel, President & CEO
Molly Anderson, Vice President
A private, nonprofit agency providing programs for the special needs of infants, adults, children and their families residing in Tazewell County. Services offered include: birth-three infant/parent program, adult day care services, family support, residen

6873   Thresholds Bridge Deaf North Program
Thresholds Psychiatric Rehabilitation Centers
4101 N. Ravenswood Ave
Chicago, IL 60613   773-572-5500
                                            FAX: 773-989-1075
                                         thresholds@thresholds.org
                                            www.thresholds.org

Jana Barbe, President
Marianne Doan, Vice President
Harold E. D'Orazio, Treasurer
Kathy Graham, Secretary
A private, nonprofit psychosocial rehabilitation center that serves the deaf mental health consumers at the highest risk of hospitalization, those with serious and persistent mental illness. The program provides residential case management services focuse

6874   Thresholds South Suburbs
4101 N. Ravenswood Ave
Chicago, IL 60613   773-572-5500
                                            FAX: 708-597-8053
                                         thresholds@thresholds.org
                                            www.thresholds.org

Jana Barbe, President
Marianne Doan, Vice President
Harold E. D'Orazio, Treasurer
Kathy Graham, Secretary
Services offered include psychosocial, vocational and residential programs for ages 18 or older with a primary diagnosis of mental illness. Facility is wheelchair accessible.

6875   Trumbull Park
10530 S Oglesby Ave
Chicago, IL 60617-6140   773-375-7022
                                            FAX: 773-375-5528

Gregory Terry, Director
Diana Moore, Site Supervisor
Ada McKinley, Manager

Offers consultation, education, general counseling, recreation, self-help and social services for children and adults.

6876 University of Illinois Medical Center
1740 West Taylor Street
Chicago, IL 60612-7232
312-355-4000
866-600-2273
FAX: 312-996-7770
hospital.uillinois.edu

Rajiv Pai, Chief
Marilyn Plomann, Manager
Offers services for the totally blind, legally blind, visually impaired, mentally retarded blind and more with health, counseling, educational, recreational, rehabilitation, computer training and professional training services.

6877 VanMatre Rehabilitation Center
950 S Mulford Rd
Rockford, IL 61108-4274
815-381-8500
866-754-3347
FAX: 815-484-9953
webcontentcoordinator@rhsnet.org
www.vanmatrerehab.com

Gary E. Kaatz, President and Chief Executive Officer
Scott Craig, Medical Director
A CARF-accredited comprehensive rehabilitation center based within the Rockford Memorial Hospital providing inpatient and outpatient services for physically and cognitively challenged persons with debilitating illness and injuries.

6878 Warren Achievement Center
1220 E 2nd Ave
Monmouth, IL 61546-2404
309-734-3131
FAX: 309-734-7114
info@warrenachievement.com
warrenachievement.com

Rick Barnhill, President
Jim Kesse, Vice President
Sherry Waite, Chief Operations Officer
Linda Baker, Chief Financial Officer
For developmentally disabled children and adults. Parent-infant education programs are for parents of infants with disabilities or developmental delays; Children's Group Homes which serve children on a fulltime basis and can serve additional children on a

Indiana

6879 Ball Memorial Hospital
2401 W University Ave
Muncie, IN 47303-3499
765-747-3111
FAX: 765-747-3313
iuhealth.org/ball-memorial

Mike Haley, CEO
Offers rehabilitation services, occupational therapy, physical therapy and more for the physically challenged child or adult.

6880 Community Health Network
1500 N Ritter Ave
Indianapolis, IN 46219-3027
317-355-4275
800-775-7775
FAX: 317-351-7723
www.ecommunity.com

Keith Thompson, Manager
Anita Harden, President
A leading not-for-profit health system offering convenient access to expert physicians, advanced treatments and leading edge technology, all focused on getting patients well and back to their lives. With caring compassion, Community's 5 hospitals and 70 + sites of care continually strive to improve the health and well being of those individuals in central Indiana who entrust care to us.

6881 Crossroads Industrial Services
8302 E 33rd Street
Indianapolis, IN 46226
317-897-7320
FAX: 317-897-9763
info@crossroadsindustrialservices.com
www.crossroadsindustrialservices.c om

Anne Shupe, Finance Executive
Curtiss Quirin, CEO
Assisting customers with short-term, seasonal, and long-term outsourcing needs. Many consider Crossroads an extension of their company

6882 Department of Veterans Affairs Vet Center #418
302 W. Washington St
Room E120
Indianapolis, IN 46204- 2738
317-232-3910
800-490-4520
FAX: 317-232-7721
vcen418@evansville.net
www.in.gov/veteran/sso/fac

Charles T. Applegate, Director
Provides readjustment counseling to combat veterans. Onsite assistance for employment problems, vocational rehabilitation and sexual trauma counsel.

6883 Frasier Rehabilitation Center Division of Clark Memorial Hospital
2201 Greentree N
Clarksville, IN 47129-8957
812-218-6590
FAX: 812-218-6597
http://www.jhsmh.org/Frazier-Rehab-Institute-
Catherine Lucas Spalding, Administrator
Designed to help patients in their adjustment to a physically limiting condition, both psychologically and physically, by helping to maximize each patient's abilities so he or she can function as independently as possible. The program treats patients whos

6884 HealthSouth Deaconess Rehabilitation Hospital
4100 Covert Ave
Evansville, IN 47714-5559
812-476-9983
800-677-3422
FAX: 812-476-4270
www.healthsouthdeaconess.com

Barbara Butler, Chief Executive Officer
Ashok . Dhingra, M.D, Medical Director
Brett Hirt, Director, Therapy Operations
Doron Finn, M.D., Wound Care Program Director
AHealthSouth Deaconess Rehabilitation Hospital is a joint venture partner with Deaconess Health System. Our hospital is an 80-bed inpatient rehabilitation hospital that offers comprehensive inpatient and outpatient rehabilitation services designed to return patients to leading active and independent lives. - See more a t : http://www.healthsouthdeaconess.com/en/our-hospital#sthash.RCsNTk1u.dpuf

6885 Healthwin Specialized Care
20531 Darden Rd
South Bend, IN 46637-2999
574-272-0100
FAX: 574-277-3233
info@healthwin.org
healthwin.org

Connie McCahill, President
Lauren Davis, Vice President
John Cergnul, Treasurer
Stephen J. Gazdick, Chief Financial Officer
No other facility in the area has a homelike environment like ours. Its simply part of our culture. Rehabilitation therapy that includes physical, occupational, speech, respiratory and a full time in-house therapist. Other services include a wound special

6886 Memorial Regional Rehabilitation Center
615 N Michigan St
South Bend, IN 46601-1033
574-647-1000
877-282-0964
www.qualityoflife.org/rehab

Johan Kuitse, MSA, PT, Outpatient Clinical Manager
Anne Clifford, DPT, Physical Therapists
Shanti Shrestha Dalson, DPT, Physical Therapists
Brandi DeMont, DPT, Physical Therapists
20-bed CARF accredited inpatient rehabilitation, outpatient orthopedic clinic and work performance program, head injury clinic. Outpatient neuro rehab and a driver education and training program are provided.

6887 Saint Joseph Regional Medical Center- South Bend
5215 Holy Cross Parkway
Mishawaka, IN 46545-2814
574-335-5000
FAX: 574-237-7312
thefoundation@sjrmc.com
sjmed.com

Albert Gutierrez, President & CEO
Steven Gable, Vice President
Janice Dunn, CFO
Christopher Karam, Chief Operating Officer
Continuum of rehabilitation services offered. Included are: acute rehabilitation, a 26 bed CARF accredited comprehensive inpatient unit, a CARF certified inpatient brain injury program, a CARF outpatient day treatment brain injury program, comprehensive o

Iowa

6888 Crossroads of Western Iowa
1 Crossroads Pl
Missouri Valley, IA 51555-6069
712-642-4114
FAX: 712-642-4115
info@cwiowa.org
explorecrossroads.com

Brent Dillinger, CEO
Pat Kocour, President
Steven Van Riper, Vice President
Darci Tierney, Secretary
CWI provides services in Missouri Valley, Onawa and Council Bluffs, Iowa. An array of services for people with mental illness, mental retardation and brain injury are provided in each location.

6889 Des Moines Division-VA Central Iowa Health Care System
3600 30th St
Des Moines, IA 50310-5753
515-699-5999
800-294-8387
FAX: 515-699-5862
www.centraliowa.va.gov

Judith Johnson-Mekota, Director
Fredrick Bahls, Chief Of Staff
Susan A. Martin, Associate Director
Alton C. Alexander, Associate Director
VA Cental Iowa Health Care System is the result of the 1997 merger of the Des Moines and Knoxville, Iowa, VA Medical Centers. This integrated healthcare system brings 2 previously separate organizational structures, located 40 miles apart, into one cohesi

6890 Easter Seals Iowa
Easter Seals National
401 N.E. 66th Avenue
Des Moines, IA 50313-4002
515-289-1933
FAX: 515-289-1281
TTY:515-289-4069
infi@eastersealsia.org
ia.easterseals.com

Steve Niebuhr, Chair
Rochelle Burnett, Vice Chair
Sherri Nielsen, President & CEO
David Lester, Treasurer
Easter Seals is a leading nonprofit provider of services to Iowans with disabilities. Services include vocational and employment

training, camping recreation and respite services, craft training and sales, home and farm adaptations, transportation, schola

6891 Genesis Regional Rehabilitation Center
Genesis Health System
1227 E.Rusholme Street
Davenport, IA 52803-3396
563-421-1000
FAX: 563-421-3499
genesishealth.com

Doug Cropper, President & CEO
Kenneth Croken, Vice President
Joseph Lohmuller, Chief Medical Officer
Karen Bolton, Vice President
Serves persons of all ages experiencing a disability, whether acquired at birth or following a serious interdisciplinary service. Rehabilitation programs include acute rehabilitation; adult rehabilitation, pediatric rehabilitation, outpatient orthopaedics

6892 Homelink
Van G Miller & Associates
1101 W S Marnan Drive
Waterloo, IA 50701-2817
319-235-7173
866-575-8483
FAX: 319-235-7822
homelinkprivacyofficer@vgm.com
www.vgmhomelink.com

Dave Kazynski, President
Rick Hibben, Coordinator
A national network of home medical equipment, respiratory therapy, rehabilitation and infusion therapy service providers with over 2,500 locations serving all fifty states.

6893 Iowa Central Industries
127 Avenue M
Fort Dodge, IA 50501-5797
515-576-2126
FAX: 515-576-2251
bloglines@merchantcircle.com
www.bloglines.com/company/3495669/post

Tom Eckman, Executive Director
Services include evaluation and training in pre-vocational and vocational skills, personal behavior management, cognitive skills, communication skills, self-care skills and social skills. Services arranged include: independent living training, medical ser

6894 Life Skills Laundry Division
1510 Industrial Rd SW
Le Mars, IA 51031-3009
712-546-4785
FAX: 712-546-4985

Don Nore, Executive Director

6895 MIW
909 S 14th Ave
Marshalltown, IA 50158-3610
641-752-3697
FAX: 641-752-1614

Rich Byers, President/CEO
Vocational services for adults with disabilities. Includes organizational employment services, supported employment, job placement.

6896 Mercy Dubuque Physical Rehabilitation Unit
250 Mercy Drive
Dubuque, IA 52001-7320
563-589-8000
FAX: 563-589-8162
www.mercydubuque.com

Russel M. Knight, CEO
Provides services which open the door to improved communication, offering the opportunity to enrich the quality of life. Mercy offers many other branches of services including, rehabilitation services for children and a pulmonary rehabilitation program.

6897   Mercy Medical Center-Pain Services
1111 6th Ave
Des Moines, IA 50314-2611   515-247-3121
                                    FAX: 515-248-8867
                    webmaster@mercydesmoines.org
            www.mercydesmoines.org/services/painservice s

Dana L. Simon, MD
Dave Vellinga, President & CEO
Laurie Conner, Vice President
An outpatient program dedicated to helping people with chronic pain live more productive, satisfying lives. The program is not designed for conditions that are surgically curable, but rather approaches the problem using a comprehensive, holistic treatment.

6898   Nishna Productions-Shenandoah Work Center
902 Day Street
Shenandoah, IA 51601-70   712-246-1242
                                    FAX: 712-246-1243
                                      nci@nishna.org
                                        nishna.org

Mary Rolf, President
Sherri Clark, Executive Director
Melissa Mueller, Program Manager
Barb Hammer, Team Leader
Shelter, workshop and job training for the disabled. Some of the services we provide are Work Activity, Adult Day Activity Program, Personal & Social Adjustment, Residential Services, Home & Community Based Services & Employment Resources.

6899   Northstar Community Services
3420 University Avenue
Waterloo, IA 50701-2050   319-236-0901
                                        888-879-1365
                                    FAX: 319-236-3701
                                   info@northdstarcs.org
                                     www.northstarcs.org

Mark Witmar, Executive Director
Jeff Conrey, President
Kathy Folkerts, Vice President
Mary Wankowicz, Director of operations
Provides adult day services, employment services and supported community living so people with disabilities can live and work in the community.

6900   Options of Linn County
935 2nd street
SW
Cedar Rapids, IA 52404-3100   319-892-5000
                                    FAX: 319-892-5849
                                   optons@linncounty.org
                                        linncounty.org

Joel D. Miller, Auditor
Sharon Gonzalez, Treasurer
Options of Linn County works with community businesses in providing employment services to adults with disabilities. Options is a publicly operated service provider within the Linn County Community Services department.

6901   RISE
106 Rainbow Dr
Elkader, IA 52043-9075   563-245-1868
                                    FAX: 563-245-2859

Ed Josten, Manager

6902   Ragtime Industries
116 N 2nd St
Albia, IA 52531-1624   641-932-7813
                                    FAX: 641-932-7814
                                    ragtime@cknet.net
                                   www.ragtimeind.com

Lisa Glenn, Executive Director
A work-oriented rehabilitation organization which provides training for mentally and physically disabled adults in Monroe County. A variety of programs which help to develop each person's individual potential are offered.

6903   Sunshine Services
1106 East 9th St
Spencer, IA 51301-225   712-262-7805
                                    FAX: 712-262-8369
                                  info@sunshine-services.org
                                  www.sunshine-services.org

Ann Vandehar, Executive Director

6904   Tenco Industries
710 Gateway Dr
Ottumwa, IA 52501-2204   641-682-8114
                                    FAX: 641-684-4223
                                      clogan@tenco.org
                                        www.tenco.org

Ben Wright, Executive Director
Dixie Merritt, Vocational Director
Brenda Miller, Marketing and Development DirectoR
Joanie Lundy, Human Resources Director
To advocate and provide opportunities for people with disabilities, or conditions that limit their abilities, to develop and maintain the skills necessary for personal dignity and independence in all areas of life. Provide a wide array of services to individuals with disabilities. By looking at each person as individuals, we are able to work with them to maximize their skills. Residentials services, including HCBS and CSALA are also provided in all communities.

Kansas

6905   Arrowhead West
1100 E Wyatt Earp Blvd
Dodge City, KS 67801-5337   620-227-8803
                                    FAX: 620-227-8812
                                   web@arrowheadwest.org
                                   www.arrowheadwest.org

Kelly Mason, Chairperson
Michael Stein, Vice Chairperson
Lori Pendergast, President
Anita Allard, Treasurer
Services and programs offered include: developmental and therapy services for children birth to age 3; adult center-based work services and community integrated employment options; adult life skills and retirement programs; and adult residential services.

6906   Big Lakes Developmental Center
1416 Hayes Dr
Manhattan, KS 66502-5066   785-776-9201
                                    FAX: 785-776-9830
                                    biglakes@biglakes.org
                                        biglakes.org

Lori Feldkamp, President
Shawn Funk, Community Education Director
A private nonprofit Community Developmental Disability Organization (CDDO) serving individuals with developmental disabilities in Riley, Geary, Clay and Pottawatome counties in Kansas. Big lakes is supported by county mill levy and federal and state fundi

6907   Developmental Services of Northwest Kansas
2703 Hall St
Suite 10
Hays, KS 67601-1964   785-625-5678
                                        800-637-2229
                                    FAX: 785-625-8204
                                  comments@notes1.dsnwk.org
                                        dsnwk.org

Jerry Michaud, President
Ruth Lang, Administrative Assistant
A private nonprofit organization serving both children and adults with disabilities. Offers services to children ages birth to three years, youth and adults through a network of community-based and outreach programs and inter-agency agreements with other

6908 ENVISION
2301 S Water St
Wichita, KS 67213-4819 316-267-2244
FAX: 316-267-4312
Info@envisionus.com
www.envisionus.com

Sam Williams, Chair
Jon Rosell, PhD, Vice-Chair
Michael Monteferrante, President and CEO
Greg Unruh, Vice President, CFO
Provides jobs, job training and vision rehabilitation services to people who are blind or low vision. A private not-for-profit agency uniquely combining employment opportunitites with rehabilitation services and public education.

6909 Heartspring
8700 E 29th St N
Wichita, KS 67226-2169 316-634-8700
800-835-1043
FAX: 316-634-0555
kgrover@heartspring.org
www.heartspring.org

Gary W. Singleton, President and CEO
Paul Faber, Executive Vice President, Operations
Katie Grover, Director Of Marketing
David Dorf, CPA, Chief Financial Officer
Heartspring provides outpatient therapies, evaluations and consultations for children with special needs through Heartspring Pediatric Services. The Heartspring School is a residential and day school for children ages 5-21 with multiple disabilities. Children with autism and their families receive resources through the Heartspring CARE program. The Heartspring Hearing Center provides services to individuals of all ages.

6910 Indian Creek Nursing Center
6515 W 103rd St
Overland Park, KS 66212-1798 913-633-7000
FAX: 913-642-3982
www.savaseniorcare.com

Randy Sutterfield, Administrator
Postacute rehabilitation program. A 120-bed nursing home facility.

6911 Johnson County Developmental Supports
111 South Cherry Street
Olathe, KS 66061-1223 913-715-5000
FAX: 913-715-0800
info@jocogov.org
www.jocogov.org

Ed Eilert, Chairman
Michael Lally, Vice Chair
Scott Tschudy, Treasurer
Jessica Dain, Secretary
JCDS is the community Developmental Disability Organization for Johnson County, Kansas. Provides supports in the form of direct services to people on a daily basis. Through a person-centered process and within availiable resources services are shaped to f

6912 Ketch Industries
1006 E Waterman St
Wichita, KS 67211-1525 316-383-8700
800-766-3777
FAX: 316-383-8715
webmaster@ketch.org
ketch.org

Fred Badders, Chairman
Carla Bienhoff, Chairman
Loren Anthony, Secretary
Dan Crug, Treasurer
The mission of Ketch is to promote independence for persons with disabilities through innovative learning experiences that support individuals choices for working, living and playing in their community.

6913 Lakemary Center
100 Lakemary Dr
Paola, KS 66071-1855 913-557-4000
FAX: 913-557-4910
lakemaryctr.org

William Craig, President
Paul Sokoloff, Chair
Gayle Richardson, Vice Chair
Lydia Marien, Secretary
A private, not-for-profit day and residential training facility which provides for the assessment, education, training, therapy and social development of children and adults, moderate and severe mental retardation. The Center is based 28 miles southwest o

6914 Northview Developmental Services
700 E 14th St
Newton, KS 67117-5702 316-283-5170
FAX: 316-283-5196
nds@northviewdsi.com
http://northviewdev.mennonite.net/

Mary Holloway, CEO
The mission is to provide quality supportive and coordinating services to persons with developmental disabilities, assisting them to grow as they integrate into the community. Further, our mission is to improve the quality of their lives by providing acce

Kentucky

6915 Cardinal Hill Rehabilitation Hospital
Cadinal Hill Medical Center
2050 Versailles Rd
Lexington, KY 40504-1499 859-254-5701
800-233-3260
FAX: 859-231-1365
www.cardinalhill.org

Gary R. Payne, CEO
Provides occupational health services, therapy services and urgent medical treatment of injured workers.

6916 Frazier Rehab Institute
220 Abraham Flexner Way
Louisville, KY 40202-1887 502-582-7400
FAX: 502-582-7477
www.frazierrehab.org

Jamie Ochsner, Manager
Steve Ahr, VP Frazier Rehab/Neurscience
Frazier Rehab Institute is a regional healthcare system dedicated entirely to rehabilitation. Through an expansive network of inpatient and outpatient facilites in Kentucky and southern Indiana, Frazier offers a wide array of services based on one common

6917 HealthSouth Northern Kentucky Rehabilitation Hospital
201 Medical Village Dr
Edgewood, KY 41017-3407 859-341-2044
800-860-6004
FAX: 859-341-2813
www.healthsouthkentucky.com

Richard Evans, CEO
Mary Pfeffer, Director Therapy Operations
Neal Moser, M.D., Medical Director
Mary Beth Bauer, RD, CSG, LD, Director of Quality and Risk Management
Offers all types of inpatient and outpatient rehabilitation services such as occupational therapy, physical therapy, speech therapy. Respiratory therpay, Psychology, Aquatics, Case Managemenet/Social Work and Nutritional Services.

6918 King's Daughter's Medical Center's Rehab Unit/Work Hardening Program
2201 Lexington Ave
Ashland, KY 41101-2843 606-408-4000
888-377-5362
FAX: 606-327-7542
info@kdmc.net
www.kdmc.com

Kristie Whitlatch, President & CEO
Matt Ebaugh, VP / Chief Strategy and Information Officer
Philip Fioret, M.D., VP / Chief Medical Officer
Howard Harrison, Vice President, Facilities
Offers a 27-bed, inpatient rehabilitation services unit treating physical disabilities related to accident or illness. The program provides an interdisciplinary inpatient program designed to restore the individual to the highest level of independence. It

6919 LifeSkills Industries
380 Suwannee Trail St
Bowling Green, KY 42103-6499 270-901-5000
800-223-8913
FAX: 270-782-0058
sbell@lifeskills.com
lifeskills.com

Alice Simpson, CEO
LifeSkills will be the reliable advocate, dependable safety net and provider of choice, for high quality, accessable services and supports for the citizens of south-central Kentucky whos lives are affected by mental illness, developmental disabilities or

6920 Low Vision Services of Kentucky
120 N. Eagle Creek Drive
Suite 500
Lexington, KY 40509- 1827 859-263-3900
800-627-2020
FAX: 859-977-1136
jvanarsdall@retinaky.com
www.lowvisionky.com

Regina Callihan-May, O.D.
Jeanne Van Arsdall, Co-ordinator
Maryanne Inman, Practice Administrator
William J. Wood, MD, Physician
Offers educational, recreational and rehabilitational services and devices for the visually impaired, legally blind, totally blind.

6921 Muhlenberg County Opportunity Center
PO Box 511
Greenville, KY 42345-1416 270-754-5590
FAX: 270-338-5977
muhlon.com

Chuck Hammonds, Manager
Charles Hamonds, Director
Post-acute rehabilitation facility with programs including a workshop with hand packaging of manufactured goods.

6922 New Vision Enterprises
1900 Brownsboro Rd
Louisville, KY 40206-2102 502-893-0211
800-405-9135
FAX: 502-893-3885

Larry Sherman, Plant Manager
Offers employment training and services for the blind and legally blind.

6923 Park DuValle Community Health Center, Inc.
3015 Wilson Ave
Louisville, KY 40211-1969 502-774-4401
FAX: 502-775-6195
rjones@pdchc.org
www.pdchc.org

Richard K Jones, President
John Howard MD, Medical Director
Dave Gerwig, CFO
Ann Hagan, Administrator
Offers services for the totally blind, legally blind, visually impaired, mentally retarded blind and more with health, counseling,

educational, recreational, rehabilitation, computer training and professional training services.

Louisiana

6924 Alliance House
427 S Foster Drive
Baton Rouge, LA 70806-2723 225-987-0013
FAX: 225-346-0857

6925 Assumption Activity Center
4201 Highway 1
Napoleonville, LA 70390-8628 985-369-2907
FAX: 985-369-2657
arcoa.catbl.net

Warren Gonzales, Manager
A community work center providing prevocational training and extended employment for adults with disabilities. Services include: social services, work activities, specialized training and supported employment.

6926 Bancroft Rehabilitation Living Centers
425 Kings Highway East
P.O. Box 20
Haddonfield, NJ 08033-0018 504-482-3075
800-774-5516
FAX: 504-483-2135
lynn.tomaio@bancroft.org
www.bancroft.org

Dr. Robert Voogt, Owner
Toni Pergolin, President & CEO
Cynthia Boyer, Executive Director
Thomas J. Burke, MBA, Chief Financial Officer
Mission is to nurture abilities and independence of people with neurological challenges by providing a broad spectrum of advanced therapeutic and educational programs and by fostering the development of best practices in the field through research and pro

6927 Caddo-Bossier Association for Retarded Citizens
4103 Lakeshore Dr
Shreveport, LA 71109-1998 318-636-0258
FAX: 318-221-4262

Janet Parker, Director
A community operated workshop for male and female mentally retarded individuals. It provides work evaluation and transitional and extended employment.

6928 Deaf Action Center Of Greater New Orleans
Catholic Charities
1000 Howard Ave
Suite 200
New Orleans, LA 70113-1903 504-523-3755
866-891-2210
FAX: 504-523-2789
TTY: 504-615-4944
ccano@ccano.org
www.ccano.org

Tommie A. Vassel, Chairman
Sr.Marjorie Hebert, MSC, President & CEO
This community service and resource center serves deaf, deaf-blind, hard of hearing and speech-impaired persons in the greater New Orleans area regardless of age, religion, race or secondary disability. DAC provides interpreting services, equipment distri

6929 Donaldsville Association for Retarded Citizens
1030 Clay St
Donaldsonville, LA 70346-3518 225-473-4516
FAX: 225-473-4517
daarc@eatel.net

Marlene Domingue, Executive Director
A private, nonprofit sheltered work program working with the mentally retarded and developmentally disabled adults.

6930 East Jefferson General Hospital Rehab Center
4200 Houma Blvd
Metairie, LA 70006-2996   504-454-4000
                                           www.ejgh.org

Newell D. Normand, Chairman
Ashton J. Ryan, Jr., Vice Chairman
Mark J, Peters, President & CEO
*Judy Brown, CPA, MHA, FACHE, Executive Vice President / Chief
Operating Officer*
Provides the highest quality, compassionate healthcare to the
people we serve. East Jefferson General Hospital will be the re-
gion's healthcare leader providing the highest quality care
through innovation and collaboration with our team members,
medical st

6931 Family Service Society
2515 Canal Street
Suite 201
New Orleans, LA 70119-6489   504-822-0800
                                           FAX: 504-822-0831
                                           family@fsgno.org
                                           www.fsgno.org

L. Blake Jones, Chair
Jackie Sullivan, 1st Vice Chair
Kathleen Vogt, 2nd Vice Chair
Ronald P McClain JD, President & CEO
Offers services for the totally blind, legally blind, visually im-
paired, mentally retarded blind and more with health, counseling,
educational, recreational, rehabilitation, computer training and
professional training services.

6932 Foundation Industries
9995 Highway 64
Zachary, LA 70791   225-654-6288
                                           FAX: 225-654-3988

Jim Lambert-Oswald, President
Jim Oswald, General Manager
A private, nonprofit sheltered workshop providing extended employment and work activities for the mentally retarded and developmentally disabled clients. Objectives are to build work skills
through supervision, develop social interaction and manifest
basi.

6933 Handi-Works Productions
2700 Lee St
Alexandria, LA 71301-4358   318-442-3377
                                           FAX: 318-473-0858

6934 Iberville Association for Retarded Citizens
24615 J.Gerald Berret Blvd
Plaquemine, LA 70764-201   225-687-4062
                                           FAX: 225-687-3272
                                           arci@eatel.net

Paul Rhorer, Executive Director
A private sheltered work program operating out of one facility
and providing transitional, extended employment and work activities for mentally and developmentally ill adults.

6935 Lighthouse for the Blind in New Orleans
123 State St
New Orleans, LA 70118-5793   504-899-4501
                                           888-792-0163
                                           FAX: 504-895-4162
                                           lighthouselouisiana.org

Curtis Eustis, Chair
Paul Masinter, Chair Elect
Tabatha George, Secretary
Peyton Bush, Treasurer
Offers services for the totally blind, legally blind, visually im-
paired, mentally retarded blind and more with health, counseling,
educational, recreational, rehabilitation, computer training and
professional training services.

6936 Louisiana Center for the Blind
101 South Trenton Street
Ruston, LA 71270-4431   318-251-2891
                                           800-234-4166
                                           FAX: 318-251-0109
                                           pallen@lcb-ruston.com
                                           www.louisianacenter.org

Pam Allen, Executive Director
Neita Ghrigsby, Office Manager
Janette Woodard, Residential Manager
Jack Mendez, Director of Technology
A new kind of orientation and training center for blind persons.
The center is privately operated and provides quality instruction
in the skills of blindness. Offers employment assistance, com-
puter literacy training, summer training and employment project

6937 Louisiana State University Eye Center
Lousiana State University
433 Bolivar Street
New Orleans, LA 70112-2272   504-568-4808
                                           FAX: 504-412-1315
                                           www.lsuhsc.edu

Jayne S. Weiss, Director
Kelli McMichael, Manager
The LSU Eye Center is part of the LSU Medical Center complex
in downtown New Orleans. It is in the LSU-Lions Building at
2020 Gravier Street between South Bolivar and South Prieur
streets.

6938 New Orleans Speech and Hearing Center
1636 Toledano St
New Orleans, LA 70115-4598   504-897-2606
                                           FAX: 504-891-6048
                                           noshc.org

Mary Beth Green, President
Jessica Vinturella, Treasurer
Kindall James, Secretary
This non-residential facility serves male and female clients for
purposes of evaluating speech and hearing problems and providing speech therapy, hearing aids and other assistive technology
for speech and hearing.

6939 Port City Enterprises
836 North Seventh Street
Port Allen, LA 70767-113   225-344-1142
                                           877-344-1142
                                           FAX: 225-344-1192
                                           www.portcityenterprises.org

William Kleinpeter, President
Mark Graffeo, Vice President
L.J. Treuil Jr, Secretary
Philip Bourgoyne, Treasurer
Offers supported employment, sheltered work and supervised
programs for the mentally retarded, ages 22 and over.

6940 Rehabilitation Center at Thibodeaux Regional
Rehab Care
602 N Acadia Rd
Thibodaux, LA 70301-4847   985-493-4731
                                           800-822-8442
                                           FAX: 985-449-4600
                                           infoA@thibodaux.com
                                           www.thibodaux.com/rehabilitation.html

Jan Torres, Program Manager
Rose Pipes, Clinical Coordinator
Designed to help patients in their adjustment to a physically limiting condition, both physically and psychologically, by helping to
maximize each patients abilities so he or she can function as independently as possible.

6941 St. Patrick RehabCare Unit
RehabCare
524 Doctor Michael Debakey Dr
Lake Charles, LA 70601-5725   337-491-7590
                                     888-722-9355
                                FAX: 337-491-7157
          www.stpatrichospital.org/serv_rehab_main.htm
Larry A Hauskins, Manager
Ruth Thornton, Admissions
A comprehensive physical and cognitive rehabilitation program designed to help individuals who have experienced a disabling injury or illness.

6942 Touro Rehabilitation CenterLCMC (Louisiana Children's Medical Center)
1401 Foucher St
New Orleans, LA 70115-3515   504-897-8565
                                FAX: 504-897-8393
          GeneralRehabilitationProgram@touro.com
                          www.touro.com/rehab
Jeanette Ray, VP of Rehab and Post Acute Srv
Janet Clark, Director of Inpatient Rehabilitation Programs
Marylee Pontillas, Director of Outpatient Rehab Srv
Lynn Drake, Patient Care Manager
Located in New Orleans' Garden District, Touro Rehabilitation is a comprehensive rehabilitation facility dedicated to the restoration of function and independence for individuals with disabilities. The scope of rehabilitation services is broad, with 3 CARF accreditations for Brain Injury, Spinal Cord Injury and General Rehabilitation. TRC opened in 1984 and offers 69 rehab beds. TRC is part of Touro Infirmary which has a proud 150 year history as a nonprofit teaching hospital.

6943 Training, Resource & Assistive-Technology
2000 Lakeshore Drive
New Orleans, LA 70148-1   504-280-6000
                                888-514-4275
                            FAX: 504-280-5707
                            ggaglian@uno.edu
                                www.uno.edu
Ken Zangla, Director
Naomi Moore, Assistant Director
Connie Lanier, Coordinator
Peter J. Fos, President
Provides quality services to persons with disabilities, rehabilitation professionals, educators and employers. Built a solid reputation for its innovative training programs and community outreach efforts. The Center is recognized as a valuable resource st

Maine

6944 Charlotte White Center
572 Bangor Rd
Dover Foxcroft, ME 04426-3373   207-564-2426
                                       888-440-4158
                                  FAX: 207-564-2404
                              info@charlottewhite.org
                              charlottewhitecenter.com
Richard M. Brown, CEO
Charles G. Clemons, COO
Dale Shaw, CFO
Mary Louis McEwen, President
A nonprofit agency, devoted to assisting adults and children with mental retardation, mental health, physical handicaps, and elder age related issues. With headquarters in Dover-Foxcroft Maine, the agency provides multiple levels of social services, inclu

6945 Iris Network for the Blind
189 Park Avenue
Portland, ME 04102-2909   207-774-6273
                            FAX: 207-774-0679
                            ashah@theiris.org
                                  theiris.org
Leonard Cole, Chairman
Katharine Ray, 1st Vice Chairman
Bruce Roullard, 2nd Vice Chairman
James E. Phipps MBA/JD, Executive Director
A statewide resource and catalyst for people who are visually impaired or blind so they can attain their determined level of independence and integration into the community.

6946 Roger Randall Center
45 School St
Houlton, ME 04730-2010   207-532-4068
                            FAX: 207-532-7334
                          rlangworthy@cla-maine.org
                              www.cla-maine.org
Rob Moran, Executive Director
Tom Moakler, President
Vicki Moody, Vice President
Peter Crovo, Treasurer
The Roger Randall Cneter is one of five Day Habilitation Programs adminsitered by Community Living Association, a private, non-profit agency. These programs may provide a supportive environment that allows the individual to achieve their maximum growth po

6947 Sebasticook Farms-Great Bay Foundation
P.O.Box 65
Saint Albans, ME 04971   207-487-4399
                            FAX: 207-938-5670
                              tad@tdstelme.net
                          www.greatbayfoundation.org
Tom Davis, Executive Director
Pam Erskin, Program Coordinator
Provides residential, educational and vocational services to adults who are developmentally disabled in order to maximize independent living and to provide assistance in obtaining an earned income.

6948 Social Learning Center
10 Shelton McMurphey Blvd
Eugene, OR 97401-3363   541-485-2711
                              877-208-6134
                          FAX: 541-485-7087
                              www.oslc.org
Sam Vuchinich, Ph.D, Chair
Gordon Naga Hall, Ph.D., Vice President
Susan Miller, J.D., Secretary/Treasurer
Sally Guyer, Staff Representative
Post accute rehabilitation program.

Maryland

6949 Blind Industries and Services of Maryland
3345 Washington Blvd
Baltimore, MD 21227-1602   410-737-2600
                                  888-322-4567
                              FAX: 410-737-2665
                                  info@bism.org
                                      bism.org
Donald J. Morris, Chairperson
Walter A. Brown, Vice Chairperson
Fredrick J. Puente, President
James R. Berens, Treasurer
Offers a comprehensive residential rehabilitation training program for people who are blind. Areas of instruction: braille, cane travel, independent living, computer, adjustment and blindness seminars.

6950 Center for Neuro-Rehabilitation
2340238 N Cary St
Annapolis, MD 21223

410-263-1704
410-462-4711
cnrnhq@erols.com

Jeanne Fryer
Laurent Pierre-Philippe
Provide community-based inpatient and outpatient acute rehabilitation, vocational services and long-term care. Specializing in treating complex neurological conditions including spinal cord injuries, multiple sclerosis, strokes, and other brain injuries resulting from trauma, anoxia, tumors, genetic malformations and other related conditions. Locations in Annapolis, Bethesda, Frederick, Towson, MD and Fairfax, Va. CNR is licensed, a Medicare provider and CARF accredited.

6951 Child Find/Early Childhood Disabilities Unit Montgomery County Public Schools
Ste A4
10731 Saint Margarets Way
Kensington, MD 20895- 2831

301-929-2224
FAX: 301-929-2223

Julie Bader, Supervisor
Offers free developmental screening for children ages 3 years until eligible for kindergarten, evaluation and placement services.

6952 Greater Baltimore Medical Center
6701 N Charles St
Baltimore, MD 21204-6881

443-849-2000
800-597-9142
FAX: 443-849-2631
www.gbmc.org

John B. Chessare MD, President & CEO
Harold J. Tucker MD, Chief Of Staff
Eric L. Melchoir, Vice President & CFO
Keith Poisson, Executive VP & COO
Offers services for the visually impaired and blind with low vision exams. Rehabilitation teaching and orientation and mobility in the home or workplace. Also offers a bimonthly newsletter for $12/yr for Hoover patients and monthly share group.

6953 James Lawrence Kernan Hospital
2200 Kernan Drive
Baltimore, MD 21207-6697

410-285-6566
888-453-7626
FAX: 410-448-6854
www.umrehabortho.org

Michael Jablonover MD,MBA, President & CEO
John P. Straumanis MD, FAAP, Vice President
W. Walter x Augustin, III, CPA, Vice President of Financial Services
Cheryl D. Lee, RN, MSN, CRRN, Vice President, Patient Care Services
Kernan reigns as Maryland's origional orthopaedic hospital with a staff which consists of a support team of orthopaedic physician assistants and dedicated nurses in the Post Anesthesia Care Unit and on the Medical/Surgical Unit, guaranteeing the highest q

6954 Levindale Hebrew Geriatric Center
2401 W. Belvedere Ave.
Baltimore, MD 21215-5267

410-601-9000
FAX: 410-601-2700
www.lifebridgehealth.org

Jason A. Blavatt, Chair
David Uhlfelder, Vice Chair
Edward L. Morris, Treasurer
Sharon Caplan, Secretary
a 292-licensed bed facility, which includes 172-comprehensive care beds, 20 subacute beds, and a 26-bed dementia care unit. Levindale's 120-bed specialty hospital consists of 20 gerospsychiatric beds, 80 complex medical beds, some with ventilator capacity

6955 Meridan Medical Center For Subacute Care
770 York Rd
Towson, MD 21204

410-821-5500
FAX: 410-821-6735

Yvette Caldwell, Administrator
Patients receive around-the-clock professional nursing care; physical and occupational, speech and respiratory therapists also assist patients. Each patient's individualized plan of care is reviewed and updated as patient needs change. Careful discharge p.

6956 Rehabilitation Opportunities
5100 Philadelphia Way
Lanham, MD 20706-4412

301-731-4242
FAX: 301-731-4191
roiworks.org

Tom Purcell, President
Bruce Shapiro, Vice President
David Fierst, Secretary
Henry Neloms, Treasurer
Organization offering day programs, evaluation, work adjustments and sheltered workshops for persons who are mentally retarded or developmentally disabled.

6957 Rosewood Center

410-951-5000
888-300-7071
FAX: 410-581-6157
www.dhmh.state.md.us/dda/rosewood

Leslie Smith, Program Director
James Anzalone, Director
Rosewood Center is a State residential Center that supports adults with mental retardation from the central Maryland region. Rosewood will provide comprehensive supports to Maryland citizens with developmental disabilities and their families in a setting .

6958 TLC: Treatment and Learning Centers
2092 Gaither Road
Suite 100
Rockville, MD 20850-3316

301-424-5200
FAX: 301-424-8063
dpaton@ttlc.org
www.ttlc.org

Patricia Ritter Ph.D., CCC-SLP, Executive Director
Cathleen Burgess Ms Ed, CCC-SLP, Director
Bill McDonald, President
Michael Cogan, Vice President
Provides audiological evaluations, testing and hearing aids, physical and occupational therapy and evaluation; speech-language evaluation and therapy, psycho-educational testing and tutoring services for learning disabled students, head injury services an

6959 Workforce and Technology Center
Division of Rehabilitation Services
2301 Argonne Drive
Baltimore, MD 21218-1628

410-554-9442
888-554-0334
FAX: 410-554-9112
www.dors.state.md.us

Dan Frye, Chairperson
Josie Thomas, Vice Chairperson
Is one of nine state operated comprehensive rehabilitation facilities in the country providing a wide range of services to individuals with disabilities. The Maryland Division of Rehabilitation Services operates the Workforce and Technology Program. Avail

Massachusetts

6960 Baroco Corporation
136 West Street
Northampton, MA 01060-2711 413-534-9978
FAX: 413-585-9019
www.baroco.com

Rick Barnard, President/Owner
Suzanne Darby, Executive Administrator
Julia McLaughlin, Executive Administrator
Janet Lawlor, Executive Administrator
Provides training and therapeutic support for its recipients with developmental disabilities in order to aid them in securing and maintaining placement in a less-restrictive setting.

6961 Berkshire Meadows
160 Gould Street
Suite 300
Needham, MA 02494-2300 781-559-4900
FAX: 413-528-0293
lkelly@jri.org
berkshiremeadows.org

Andy Pond, President
Gregory Canfield, Vice President
Deborah Reuman, CFO
Stephen H. Webster, Executive Advisor
Private, non profit school for children, adolescents, young adults who are severely, developmentally disabled. Approved special education learning center, work site program and foster care. Physical therapy, speech and language development, behavioral pro *$8200.00*

6962 Blueberry Hill Healthcare
75 Brimbal Ave
Beverly, MA 01915-6009 978-927-2020
FAX: 978-922-5213
admissions@BlueberryHillRehab.com
www.blueberryhillrehab.com

Ralph Epstein, Medical Director
Accomodates 146 residents. We are centrally located close to Route 128 and Route 1A in Beverly Massachusetts. We offer short-term rehab care, long term care and Alzheimer's Special Care Programs. Our interdisciplinary team designs individual care plans fo

6963 Boston University Hospital Vision Rehabilitation Services
One Boston Medical Center Place
Boston, MA 02118-2371 617-638-8000
FAX: 617-638-7769
www.bmc.org/rehab.htm

Simona Manasian, Medical Director
Karen Mattie, Director
Jenn Blake, Clinical Outpatient Supervisor
Kara Schworm, Clinical In-patient Supervisor
Offers services for the totally blind, legally blind, visually impaired, mentally retarded blind and more with health, counseling, educational, recreational, rehabilitation, computer training and professional training services.

6964 Burbank Rehabilitation Center
275 Nichols Rd
Fitchburg, MA 01420-1919 978-343-5000
888-840-3627
FAX: 978-343-5342
www.umassmemorialhealthcare.org

David Bennett, Chair
Eric Dickson, President & CEO
The largest community hospital and regional referral center in the area. Offers the most extensive high quality, cost-effective healthcare services in the region. The hospital provides outstanding hospital-based services such as case management of high ri

6965 CPB/WGBH National Center for Access Media
W GB H Educational Foundation
One Guest Street
Boston, MA 02135 617-300-3400
FAX: 617-300-1035
TTY:617-300-2489
ncam@wgbh.org
www.wgbh.org/ncam

Larry Goldberg, Director
Marcia Brooks, Project Director
Geoff Freed, Director of Technology
Richard Caloggero, Technology Specialist
Dedicated to the issues of media and information technology for people with disabilities in their homes, schools, workplaces, and communities. NCAM's mission is to expand access to present and future media for people with disabilities; explore how existin

6966 Carroll Center for the Blind
770 Centre St
Newton, MA 02458-2597 617-969-6200
800-852-3131
FAX: 617-969-6204
joe.abely@carroll.org
www.carroll.org

Joseph Abely, President
Arthur O'Neill, Vice President
Brian Charlson, Director of Computer Training Services
Robert McGillivray, Director of Low Vision Services
Offers services for the totally blind, legally blind, visually impaired, mentally retarded blind and more with health, counseling, educational, in dependent living, tronell skills, computer traing, recreational, rehabilitation, computer training and professional training services.

6967 Center for Psychiatric Rehabilitation
Boston University
940 Commonwealth Ave
West
Boston, MA 02215-1203 617-353-3549
FAX: 617-353-7700
psyrehab@bu.edu
cpr.bu.edu

Kim T. Mueser, Executive Director
Deborah Dolan, Director of operations
Larry Kohn, Director of Development
E. Sally Rogers, Director of Research
The mission of the Center is to increase knowledge, to train treatment personnel, to develop effective rehabilitation programs and to assist in organizing both personnel and programs into efficient and coordinated service delivery systems for people with

6968 Clark House Nursing Center At Foxhill Village
Kindred Healthcare
30 Longwood Dr
Westwood, MA 02090-1132 781-326-5652
800-359-7412
FAX: 781-326-4034
www.clarkhousefhv.com

Chris Wasel, Administrator
Clark House At Fox Hill Village accomodates 70 residents. We are part of the Fox Hill Village Assisted Living and Retirement Center campus. Clark House Nursing center has been named a recipient of a 2005 step II quality Award from the American Health Care

6969 College Internship Program at the Berkshire Center
18 Park St
Lee, MA 01238-1702 413-243-2576
FAX: 413-243-3351
admissions@berkshirecenter.org
berkshirecenter.org

Lucy Gosselin, Program Director
Laina Hubbard, Admissions Coordinator
Charles D. Houff, Head Therapist
A highly individualized postsecondary program for learning disabled young adults 18-30. Provides job placement services and follow-ups; college support; money management and social

skills. Residential students share an apartment and have their own room. T

6970 Devereux Advanced Behavioral HealthMassachusetts & Rhode Island
60 Miles Rd.
P.O. Box 219
Rutland, MA 01543-0219 508-886-4746
www.devereux.org
Stephen Yerden, Executive Director
Serving ages 0 to 21. Services include residential treatment, community-based group homes, therapeutic foster care, special needs day school, substance abuse and autism spectrum programs, diagnostic services, in-home services and vocational training.

6971 Eagle Pond Rehabilitation and Living Center
1 Love Lane
P.O.Box 208
South Dennis, MA 02660-3445 508-385-6034
FAX: 508-385-7064
www.eaglepond.com
Paul Marchwat, Executive Director
Ellen Reil, Marketing Director
Eagle Pond accomodates 142 residents. Medicare and Medicaid certified as well as being accredited by the Joint Comission (formerly (JCAHO) which enables us to contract with many insurance companies.

6972 FOR Community Services
75 Litwin Ln
Chicopee, MA 01020-4817 413-592-6142
FAX: 413-598-0478
ggolash1@aol.com
Gina Golash, Executive Director
Providing a world of meaning for individuals with developmental disabilities throughout Western Massachusetts since 1967.

6973 Fairlawn Rehabilitation Hospital
189 May Street
Worcester, MA 01602-4399 508-791-6351
FAX: 508-831-1277
www.fairlawnrehab.org
Dave Richer, CEO
Peter Bagley MD, Medical Director
Matthew Akulonis, Director Of Support Operations
Judy Chuli, Chief Nursing Officer
Offers comprehensive rehabilitation on both an inpatient and outpatient basis. Specialty programs include: head injury, spinal cord injury, young/senior stroke, oncology, geriatrics and orthopedics.

6974 Greenery Extended Care Center: Worcester
59 Acton Street
Worcester, MA 01604-4899 508-791-3147
800-633-0887
FAX: 508-753-6267
worcester@wingatehealthcare.com
wingatehealthcare.com
Scott Schuster, Founder & President
Brian Callahan, CFO
Michael Benjamin, Vice President
Trent Guthrie, Senior Director
173 beds offering complex care, extended rehabilitation and neurobehavioral intervention. Offering life care homes and Nursing home services. Specialties include life events and physical care, long term and home health care, and nursing homes and nursing

6975 Greenery Rehabilitation & Skilled Nursing Center
P.O.Box 1330
Middleboro, MA 02346-4330 508-947-9295
FAX: 508-947-7974

6976 Harrington House Nursing And Rehabilitation Center
160 Main Street
Walpole, MA 02081-4037 508-660-3080
FAX: 508-660-1634
www.harringtonrehab.com
Joseph Haron, Medical Director
Accomodates 90 residents. Our state-of-the-art center offers post-accute services including rehabilitation and medical management. Our center also provides a long term care program including hospice services.

6977 HealthSouth Rehabilitation Hospital Of Western Massachusetts
222 State Street
Ludlow, MA 01056-3478 413-308-3300
FAX: 413-547-2738
www.healthsouthrehab.org
Victoria Healy, CEO
Adnan Dahdul, M.D., Medical Director
Deborah Cabanas, Chief Nursing Officer
AnnMaria Elder, M.D., Medical Staff President
A 53-bed acute Rehabilitation Hospital. The facility has been operating for 14 years and has provided rehabilitative care to patients and families in the greater Springfield area with an outstanding reputation for attention to detail and compassion. Becau

6978 Holiday Inn Boxborough Woods
242 Adams Pl
Boxborough, MA 01719-1735 978-263-8701
800-465-4329
FAX: 978-263-0518
box_sales@finc-hotels.com
www.ihg.com/holidayinn
Kevin Murray, Manager
Marcel Girard, Manager
Nancy Ellen Hurley, Chief Marketing Officer
Located on 35 acres of wooded countryside just off I-495 at exit #28. Minutes from the Mass Turnpike, Route 2, 290 and 9. Conference center located on main level with 30,000 square feet of meeting space. Guest rooms feature two-line telephones, voice mail
$129 - $159

6979 Lifeworks Employment Services
1400 Providence Highway
Suite 2300
Norwood, MA 02062- 4551 781-769-3298
FAX: 781-551-0045
able@lifeworksma.org
www.lifeworksma.org
Dan Burke, President & CEO
Chris Page, Vice President
Brenda Calder, CFO
Mary Hagen, Controller
Providing homes, jobs, education and supportive living for people with developmental disabilities.

6980 Massachusetts Eye and Ear Infirmary & Vision Rehabilitation Center
243 Charles Street
Boston, MA 02114-3002 617-523-7900
FAX: 617-573-4178
TTY:617-523-5498
www.masseyeandear.org
Wycliffe Grousbeck, Chairman
John Fernandaz, President & CEO
Lily H. Bentas, Secretary
Jonathan Uhrig, Treasurer
Visual rehabilitation encompasses a low vision rehabilitation evaluation, occupational therapy evaluation (with home visit if necessary), and social service evaluation.

6981 **New England Center for Children**
260 Tremont Street
Boston, MA 02116-2108
617-636-4600
FAX: 617-636-4866
cwelch@necc.org
necc.org

Lisel Macenka, Chair
James C. Burling, Vice Chair
L.Vincent Strully, President
Michael F. Downey, Treasurer
A comprehensive year-round program for students with autism
and PDD who require a highly specialized educational and behavior management program. Students are from all over the country
and receive intensive, positive, behavioral counseling and social
skil

6982 **New England Eye Center, Tufts Medical Center**
Vision Rehabilitation Service
260 Tremont Street
Boston, MA 02116-1533
617-636-4600
800-231-3316
FAX: 617-636-4866
eli@vision.eri.harvard.edu
www.necc.com

Harry P. Selker, Principal Investigator
Anastassios Pittas, Program Director
Tamsin A. Knox, Associate Director
June S. Wasser, Executive Director
Offers services for the legally blind, visually impaired, mentally
retarded blind and more with health, counseling, educational,
recreational, rehabilitation, computer training and professional
training services.

6983 **New Medico Rehabilitation and Skilled Nursing Center at
Lewis Bay**
89 Lewis Bay Rd
Hyannis, MA 02601-5207
508-775-7601
FAX: 508-790-4239

Edmund Steinle, Executive Director
Post acute rehabilitation services.

6984 **Protestant Guild Learning Center**
411 Waverley Oaks Rd
Suite 104
Waltham, MA 02452-8449
781-893-6000
FAX: 781-893-1171
admin@theguildschool.org
www.theguildschool.org

Eric H. Rosenberger, President
Thomas P. Corcoran, Vice President & Treasurer
Thomas Belski, Chief Executive Officer
Sandra L. Skinner, Clerk
Offers services for the diagnostically disabled children and ado-
lescents with ages 6-22 years with health, counseling, educa-
tional, recreational, rehabilitation, computer training and
professional training services.

6985 **Shaughnessy-Kaplan Rehabilitation Hospital**
1 Dove Ave
Salem, MA 01970
978-745-9000
FAX: 978-740-4730
skrhinfo@partners.org
spauldingrehab.org

Anthony Sciola, CEO
Maureen Banks, RN, MS, MBA, CN, President
Mary Beth DiFilippo, Vice President
Charles Pu, MD, Chief Medical Officer
A 160-bed private, non-profit hospital. We have been providing
care for residents of greater North Shore communities since 1975.
Shaughnessy has 120 long-term care hospital beds and a 40-bed
transitional care unit sometimes referred to as a skilled nursin

6986 **Son-Rise Program**
2080 South Undermountain Road
Sheffield, MA 01257-9643
413-229-2100
877-766-7473
FAX: 413-229-3202
correspondence@option.org
www.autismtreatmentcenter.org

Barry Neil Kaufman, Co Founder
Samahria Lyte Kaufman, Co Founder
THe Son-Rise Program is a powerful, effective and totally unique
treatment for children and adults challengedby Autism, Autuism
Spectrum Disorders, Pervasive Developmental Disorder (PDD),
Asperger's Syndrome and other developmental difficulties.

6987 **Southern Worcester County Rehabilitation Inc. D/B/A
Life-Skills, Inc.**
44 Morris St
Webster, MA 01570-1812
508-943-0700
FAX: 508-949-6129
life-skills@lifeskillsinc.org
www.life-skillsinc.org

J Thomas Amick, Executive Director
Kristin Nelson, Board President
Barbara Butrym, Board Vice President
Janice Smith, Board Secretary
Life-Skills, Inc. assists mentally and developmentally challenged adults with meeting their individual needs, and empowering them to take full advantage of meaningful opportunities in
their communities. We provide residential, employment, transportation, behavior, and theraputic day habilitation services to
350 adults in MA. We operate thrift & consignment stores, a small
cafe, an ice cream shop, mini golf & arcade center, vending and
greenhouse businesses, bank courier service, and others.

6988 **Vinfen Corporation**
950 Cambridge Street
Cambridge, MA 02141-1001
617-441-1800
877-284-6336
FAX: 617-441-1858
TTY: 617-225-2000
info@vinfen.org
www.vinfen.org

Philip A. Mason, Ph.D., Chairperson
Bruce L. Bird, Ph.D., CEO/ President
Elizabeth K. Glaser, Chief Operations Officer
Glen Mattera, Chief Financial Officer
A private, nonprofit company, Vinfen Corporation is the largest
human services provider in Massachusetts. Vinfen offers clinical, educational, residential and support services to individuals
of all ages with mental illness and or mental retardation, who also
may have another disability (e.g. substance abuse, homelessness,
AIDS). The company also trains professionals in the mental
health field and helps consumers to learn to live in community-based settings at the highest levels.

6989 **Visiting Nurse Association of North Shore**
5 Federal St
Danvers, MA 01923-3687
508-751-6926
800-728-1862
FAX: 978-777-0308
www.vnacarenetwork.org

Mary Ann O'Connor, CEO/ President
Stephanie Jackman-Havey, Chief Operating Officer/

Chief Financial Officer
David Rose, Vice President of Human Resources
Jane Woodbury, Vice President of Fund Development

Home health services including nurses, physical, occupational
and speech therapy, home health aides and more. Special programs include nutrition counseling, IV care, pediatric therapy,
HIV/AIDS services and wound management. Provides services 7

days a week, 365 days a year and we accept Medicare, Medicaid and most HMO's and health insurers.

6990   Weldon Center for Rehabilitation
233 Carew St
Springfield, MA 01104-2377

413-748-6800
FAX: 413-748-6806
mercycares.com

Barbara Haswell, Manager
One of the most vital, necessary health resources in the region by helping thousands of people toward restored health and independence. A comprehensive, integrated, non-profit facility offering inpatient, outpatient, day rehabilitation and pediatric services on one site.

6991   Youville Hospital & Rehab Center
1575 Cambridge St
Cambridge, MA 02138-4398

617-876-4344
FAX: 617-547-5501
www.youville.org

Michigan

6992   Botsford Center For Rehabilitation & Health Improvement-Redford
28050 Grand River Ave.
Farmington Hills, MI 48336-5919

248-471-8000
877-442-7900
FAX: 313-387-3838
info@botsfordsystem.org
www.botsford.org

John Darin, Manager
A 20 bed inpatient physical rehabilitation unit, servicing individuals who have experienced a stroke, amputation, orthopedic fracture, or other neurological impairment.

6993   Chelsea Community Hospital Rehabilitation Unit
775 South Main Street
Chelsea, MI 48118-1383

734-593-6000
800-231-2211
FAX: 734-475-4191
www.stjoeschelsea.org

Nancy K. Graebner, CEO/ President
Kathy Brubaker, RN, Vice President and Chief Nursing Officer
Randall Forsch, MD, Chief Medical Officer
Barbara Fielder, VP Finance
A private, non-profit, acute care facility that combines the best of small town values with national standards of healthcare excellence. The hospital has a 19-bed acute care inpatient rehabilitation unit with comprehensive outpatient programs, including a coordinated brain injury program.

6994   Clare Branch
790 Industrial Dr
Clare, MI 48617-9224

989-386-7707
888-773-7664
FAX: 989-386-2199
mail@mmionline.com
www.mmionline.org

Cris Zeigler, Executive Director
MMI will strive to be the premier provider of person-centered services to people with barriers to employment. We will connect individuals with community resources that provide mutual benefit to them and to the community. MMI will be known for excellence in service provision, ethical business practices, a quality work environment, and for providing services that enhance the dignity and value of the people we serve.

6995   Clarkston Spec Healthcare Center
4800 Clintonville Rd
Clarkston, MI 48346-4297

800-454-5909
fundltc.com

Margaret Canny, Administrator
120 beds offering active/acute rehabilitation, complex care, day treatment, extended rehabilitation, neurobehavioral intervention and short-term evaluation.

6996   DMC Health Care Center-Novi
42005 W 12 Mile Rd
Novi, MI 48377-3113

248-305-7575
FAX: 425-201-1450
novi@patch.com
novi.patch.com

Bud Rosenthal, CEO
Leigh Zareli Lewis, COO
Andreas Turanski, CTO
Melanie Pereira, VP of Finance
The Detroit Medical Center's record of service has provided medical excellence throughout the history of the Metropolitan Detroit area. From the founding of the Children's Hospital in 1886, to the creation of the first mechanical heart at Harpers Hospital 50 years ago, to our compassion for the underdeserved, our legacy of caring is unmatched.

6997   Eight CAP, Inc. Head Start
904 Oak Drive
Greenville, MI 48838-9277

616-754-9315
FAX: 616-754-9310
laurelm@8cap.org
www.8cap.org

Ralph Loeschner, Executive Director
Nancy Secor, Contact
Post accute rehabilitation programs.

6998   Greater Detroit Agency for the Blind and Visually Impaired
16625 Grand River Ave
Detroit, MI 48227-1419

313-272-3900
FAX: 313-272-6893
Information@gdabvi.org
gdabvi.org

Frederick J Simpson, Board Chairman
Charles L. Cone, Vice Chairman
Leonard W Robinson, Board Secretary
John W. Rhinesmith, CPA, Board Treasurer
Offers services for seniors 60 and over who are legally blind. Also provides eye health information, counseling, education and rehabilitation services.

6999   Hope Network Rehabilitation Services
Hope Network
1490 East Beltline Ave SE
Grand Rapids, MI 49506-4336

616-940-0040
800-695-7273
FAX: 616-940-8151
jbaker@hopenetwork.org
hopenetwork.org

Margaret Kroese, Vice President/Executive Directo
An office of Hope Network, one of the largest, private, nonprofit organizations of its kind in Michigan. The purpose is to assist people with brain injuries and/or physical disabilities in achieving an optimal level of self-determination, dignity, and independence as they develop and attain goals to overcome environmental barriers and mobilize adaptive skills.

7000   Lakeland Center
26900 Franklin Rd
Southfield, MI 48033-5312

248-350-8070
FAX: 248-350-8078
peggys@thelakelandcenter.net
thelakelandcenter.net

Irving Shapiro, CEO
Santhosh Madhavan, Director Physical Medicine
Gary Yashinsky, Associate Medical Director
Subacute rehabilitation program directed toward those with severe neurologic diagnoses, ie: TBI, cerebral aneurysm, anoxic encephalopathy, CVA and cerebral hemorrhage, orthopedic injuries, and spinal cord injury. Subacute rehabilitation is provided for those who recover slowly and require individualized treatment plans. Residential program available as well.

7001   Mary Free Bed Rehabilitation Hospital
235 Wealthy St SE
Grand Rapids, MI 49503-5247
616-493-9657
800-528-8989
FAX: 616-454-3939
info@maryfreebed.com
maryfreebed.com

Kent Riddle, CEO
John Butzer, MD, Medical Director
Randy DeNeff, Vice President of Finance
Founded more than 100 years ago, Mary Free Bed Rehabilitation Hospital is and 80-bed, not-for-profit, acute rehabilitation center. Its mission is to restore hope and freedom through rehabilitation to people with disabilities. Mary Free Bed offers comprehensive inpatient and outpatient rehabilitationfor children and adults using an interdisciplinary approach. Also available are numerous specialty programs designed to increase the quality of life and independence of people with disabilities.

7002   Michigan Career And Technical Institute
11611 Pine Lake Rd
Plainwell, MI 49080-9225
269-664-4461
877-901-7360
FAX: 269-664-5850

Dennis Hart, Executive Director
A residential vocational training center for adults with physical, mental or emotional disabilities.

7003   Michigan Commission for the Blind Training Center
1541 Oakland Dr
Kalamazoo, MI 49008
269-337-3848
800-292-4200
FAX: 269-337-3872
mossc@michigan.gov
www.mcb1.org

Christine Boone, Director
Bruce Schultz, Assistant Director
Residential facility that provides instruction to legally blind adults in braille, computer operation and assistive technology, handwriting, cane travel, cooking, personal management, industrial arts and also crafts. During training students will develop career plans which may include work experience, internships, volunteer opprtunities and even part-time paid employment.

7004   Mid-Michigan Industries
2426 Parkway Dr
Mt Pleasant, MI 48858-4723
989-773-6918
888-773-7664
888-773-7664
FAX: 989-773-1317
mail@mmionline.com
mmionline.com

Alan Schilling, President
Andrea Christopher, Director Admissions
Linda Wagner, Branch Director
Sheri Alexander, Director of Community Employment
Providing jobs and training for persons with barriers to employment. Services include vocational evaluation, job placement, supported employment, work services, prevocational training and case management

7005   New Medico Community Re-Entry Service
216 St Marys Lake Rd
Battle Creek, MI 49017-9710
FAX: 269-962-2241

James Rekshan, Executive Director

7006   Sanilac County Community Mental Health
171 Dawson St
Sandusky, MI 48471-1062
810-648-0330
888-225-4447
888-225-4447
FAX: 810-648-0319
deanr@sanilacmentalhealth.org
sanilacmentalhealth.org

Roger Dean, Executive Director

Post-acute rehabilitation facility and programs.

7007   Special Tree Rehabilitation System
600 Stephenson Highway
Troy, MI 48083-1110
248-616-0950
800-648-6885
FAX: 248-616-0957
info@specialtree.com
www.specialtree.com

Joseph Richart, CEO
Special Tree exists to provide hope, encouragement, and expertise for people who have experienced life-altering changes. Our team approach to rehabilitation, custom designed for each person's needs and goals, offers these individuals the best opportunity for healing and recovery.

7008   Thumb Industries
1263 Sand Beach Rd
Bad Axe, MI 48413-8817
989-269-9229
FAX: 989-269-2587
thumbindustries@hotmail.com
www.thumbindustries.com

Rhonda Wisenbaugh, Executive Director
Provides job training and employment for disabled persons. Vocational rehabilitation agency, manufactures household furnishings, direct mail advertising service.

7009   Visually Impaired Center
1422 W Court St
Flint, MI 48503-5008
810-767-4014
FAX: 810-767-0020
info@vicflint.org
www.vicflint.org

a pages

7010   Welcome Homes Retirement Community for the Visually Impaired
1953 Monroe Ave NW
Grand Rapids, MI 49505-6242
616-447-7837
888-939-9292
888-939-9292
FAX: 616-447-9891
info@welcomehomes.org

Beth Lucksted, Manager
Offers services for the totally blind, legally blind, visually impaired, mentally retarded blind and more with health, counseling, educational, recreational, rehabilitation, computer training and professional training services.

7011   William H Honor Rehabilitation Center Henry Ford Wyanclotte Hospital
Henry Ford Health System
2333 Biddle Ave
Wyandotte, MI 48192-4668
734-246-6000
FAX: 734-246-6926
www.henryfordwyandotte.com

Denise Dailing, Administration Leader/rehabilita
James Sexton, Chief Executive Officer
Henry Ford, Owner
Henry Ford Wyandotte Hospital offers an array of educational programs, health screenings, and support groups. The hospital is CARF accredited and has a CARF certified stroke specialty unit.

Minnesota

7012   Industries: Cambridge
601 Cleveland St S
Cambridge, MN 55008-1752
763-689-5434
FAX: 763-552-1281
jspicer@industriesinc.org
www.industriesinc.org

Daryl Peterson, Board Chair
Bruce Montgomery, Vice Chair
Marilyn Bachman, Secretary
Kevin Troupe, Treasurer

Nonprofit organization that does vocational assessment and training for people with disabilities.

7013 Industries: Mora
500 Walnut St S
Mora, MN 55051-1936 320-679-2354
FAX: 320-679-2355
jspicer@industriesinc.org
www.industriesinc.org

Daryl Peterson, Board Chair
Bruce Montgomery, Vice Chair
Marilyn Bachman, Secretary
Kevin Troupe, Treasurer
Nonprofit organization that does vocational assessment and training for people with disabilities.

7014 Shriners Hospitals for Children: Twin Cities
2025 E River Pkwy
Minneapolis, MN 55414-3696 612-596-6100
888-293-2832
888-293-2832
FAX: 612-339-5954
dengle@shrinenet.org
www.shrinershospitalsforchildren.org

Charles C. Lobeck, Administrator
Cary Mielke, M.D, Interim Chief of Staff
Don Engel, Development Officer
Shriners Hospital for Children-Twin Cities offers quality orthopedic medical care regardless of the patients' ability to pay. Shriners Hospitals provide inpatient and outpatient services, surgery, casts, braces, artificial limbs, x-rays and physical and occupational therapy to any child under the age of 18 who may benefit from treatment.

7015 Vision Loss Resources
1936 Lyndale Ave S
Minneapolis, MN 55403-3101 612-871-2222
FAX: 612-872-0189
TTY:612-382-8422
info@vlrw.org
www.visionlossresources.org

Barry Shear, Chair
Lisa David, Vice Chair
Mary McDougall, Secretary
Jackie Peichel, Treasurer
Offers services for the totally blind, legally blind, visually impaired, and more with health, counseling, educational, recreational, rehabilitation, computer training and professional training services.

Mississippi

7016 Addie McBryde Rehabilitation Center for the Blind
PO Box 5314
Jackson, MS 39296-5314 601-364-2700
800-443-1000
FAX: 601-364-2677
www.mdrs.ms.gov/VocationalRehabBlind/Pages/Ad
H. S. McMillan, Executive Director
Shelia Browning, Deputy Director Non-Vocational P
Offers services for the totally blind, legally blind, visually impaired, mentally retarded blind and more with health, counseling, educational, recreational, rehabilitation, computer training services and orientation and mobility.

7017 Mississippi Methodist Rehabilitation Center
1350 E Woodrow Wilson Ave
Jackson, MS 39216-5198 601-981-2611
800-223-6672
FAX: 601-364-3571
www.methodistonline.org

Mark A. Adams, President/ CEO
Matthew L. Holleman, III, Chair
Mike P. Sturdivant Jr, Vice Chairman
David L. McMillin, Secretary

Rebuild lives that have been broken by disabilities and impairments from serious illness or severe injury. The challenge is to help patients regain abilities, restore function and movement, and renew emotionally. It features personal rehabilitation treatment plans administered by specialized teams of health care professionals through a variety of outpatient programs, treatments and other services.

Missouri

7018 Alpine North Nursing and Rehabilitation Center
4700 NW Cliff View Dr
Kansas City, MO 64150-1237 816-741-5105
FAX: 816-746-1301

Mike Stacks, Executive Director
Bob Richard, Administrator
Postacute rehabilitation program.

7019 Christian Hospital Northeast
11133 Dunn Rd
Saint Louis, MO 63136-6119 314-653-5000
877-747-9355
FAX: 314-653-4130
christianhospital.org

Ron McMullen, President
Bryan Hartwick, Vice President Human Resources
Sebastian Rueckert, MD, Vice President and Chief Medical Officer
Jennifer Cordia, Vice President and Chief Nurse Executive
A non-profit organization, a 493 bed acute care facility on 28 acres. Christian Hospital has more then 600 physicians on staff and a diverse workforce of more then 2,5000 health-care professionals who are dedicated to providing the absolute best care with the latest technology and medical advances.

7020 Integrated Health Services of St. Louis at Gravois
10954 Kennerly Rd
Saint Louis, MO 63128-2018 314-843-4242
FAX: 314-843-4031

Lisa Niehaus, Administrator
Subacute, skilled and intermediate care; ventilator/tracheostomy management program; wound management program and complex rehabilitation program.

7021 Metropolitan Employment & Rehabilitation Service
M ER S Goodwill
1727 Locust St
Saint Louis, MO 63103-1703 314-241-3464
FAX: 314-241-9348
info@mersgoodwill.org
www.mersgoodwill.org

Lewis C. Chartock, Ph.D., President/ CEO
Dawayne Barnett, CFO
Mark Arens, Executive Vice President, Chief of Program Services
Mark Kahrs, Executive Vice President, Retail Services
Vocational rehabilitation, primarily with the disabled, skills training and placement services.

7022 Missouri Easter Seal Society: Southeast Region
233 South Wacker Drive
Suite 2400
Chicago, IL 60606 312-726-6200
800-221-6827
FAX: 312-726-1494
easterseals.com

Richard W. Davidson, Chairman
Sandra L. Bouwman, 1st Vice Chairman
Ralph F. Boyd, Jr., Treasurer
Eileen Howard Boone, Secretary
The mission of the Easter Seal Society is to work with individuals, their families and the community to enhance the independence and quality of life for persons with disabilities.

7023 Poplar Bluff RehabCare Program
Lucy Lee Hospital
2620 N Westwood Blvd
Poplar Bluff, MO 63901-3396
573-785-7721
FAX: 573-686-5987

Jim Martin, Program Manager
Chris Murray, Care Coordinator
Darlene Hill, Care Admissions Coordinator
Provides physical medicine and rehabilitation to individuals with a physically limiting condition. The program is designed to help individuals function as independently as possible by maximizing their strength and abilities.

7024 Shriners Hospitals for Children St. Louis
2001 S Lindbergh Blvd
Saint Louis, MO 63131-3597
314-432-3600
800-850-2960
FAX: 314-432-2930
www.shrinershq.org/hospitals/st.louis

John McCabe, Executive Vice President
Kenneth Guidera, M.D., Chief Medical Officer
Eugene R. D'Amore, Vice President, Hospital Operations
Kathy A. Dean, Vice President, Human Resources
Medical care is provided free of charge for children 18 and under with orthopaedic conditions.

7025 St. Louis Society for the Blind and Visually Impaired
8770 Manchester Rd
Saint Louis, MO 63144-2724
314-960-9000
FAX: 314-968-9003
socscrv@slsbvi.org
www.slsbvi.org

David Ekin, President
Chris Pickel, Chair
Ann Shapiro, Vice Chair
Sherine Apte, Secretary
Offers vision rehabilitation services for the totally blind, legally blind, visually impaired, including counseling, educational, recreational, rehabilitation, computer training and professional training services. Low vision aids and appliance available through low vision clinic by appointment.

7026 Truman Medical Center Low Vision Rehabilitation Program
Eye Foundation of Kansas City
2300 Holmes St.
Kansas City, MO 64108
816-404-1780
FAX: 816-404-1786
www.umkc-efkc.org

Nelson R. Sabates, M.D., Chairman
Monika Malecha, MD, Residency Program Director
Abraham Poulose, MD, Director of Clinics
Our program is designed to maximize daily tasks for a person with low vision. We are able to evaluate a person's home and provide recommendations as needed.

7027 Truman Neurological Center
12404 E. US 40 Highway
Independence, MO 64055-1354
816-373-5060
FAX: 816-373-5787
info@tnccommunity.com
tnccommunity.com

James Landrum, Executive Director
Ann Johnson, Finance Director
Terri Boyce, Office Assistant
Mary Beth Johnson, Compliance Director
A licensed habilitation center established for the purpose of assisting persons with developmental disabilities and/or mental retardation. The minimum age is 18. Residential care is provided in four group homes in the community licensed by the DMH and CARF accredited.

Montana

7028 Benefis Healthcare
1101 26th St S
Great Falls, MT 59405-5104
406-455-5000
FAX: 406-455-2110
benefis@benefis.org
www.benefis.org

John Goodnow, CEO
Laura Goldhahn-Konen, President
Forrest Ehlinger, Chief Financial & Treasury Officer
Paul Dolan, MD, Chief Medical Information Officer
Benefis Healthcare is a not-for-profit community asses governed by a 15-member local board of directors. Benefis is locally owned and controlled. Benefis is a Level II trauma center- one of only 4 in the state and 107 in the country.

7029 Disability Services Division of Montana
Department of Public Health
Helena, MT 59604
406-444-7734
FAX: 406-444-3465
dphhs@mt.gov
www.dphhs.state.mt.us/dsd

Keith Messmer, Manager
Sandi Gory, Administrative Assistant
Janice Frisch, Chief Management Operations
Responsible for coordinating, developing and implementing comprehensive programs to assist Montanans with disabilities with activities of daily living, community base services and coordinated programs of habilation, rehabilitation and independent living.

Nebraska

7030 Las Vegas Healthcare And Rehabilitation Center
680 South Fourth Street
Louisville, KY 40202
502-596-7300
TTY:800-545-0749
web_administrator@kindredhealthcare.com
kindredhealthcare.com

Paul J. Diaz, President/ CEO
Accomodates 79 residents. Serving the community for approximately 40 years. Located in close proximity to local hospitals and surrounded by medical complexes, out center offers both short-term rehabilitation and long term.care.

7031 Sierra Pain Institute
265 Golden Ln
Reno, NV 89502-1205
775-323-7092
FAX: 775-323-5259

Lyle Smith, Owner
The program consists of a medically supervised outpatient program managed by an interdisciplinary team with input from specialties of Pain Medicine, Physical Therapy and Occupational Science. The format insures that each patient receives the full range of behavioral techniques in a well-integrated, individually tailored therapeutic regimen.

New Hampshire

7032 Crotched Mountain Adult Brain Injury Center
Crotched Mountain Foundation
1 Verney Dr
Greenfield, NH 03047-5000
603-547-3311
800-966-2672
FAX: 603-547-3232
admissions@crotchedmountain.org
www.crotchedmountain.org

Donald Shumway, President, CEO
Michael Terrian, Vice President of Administration & Facilities
Tom Zubricki, Chief Financial Officer
Kathleen C. Brittan, Vice President of Development

Adult Brain Injury Center provides sub-acute rehabilitative services and individualized care to survivors of acquired (including traumatic) brain injury. Ambulatory and non-ambulatory adults are served. Ages range from 18-59, the staff to client ratio is 3:1 and services are provided by experienced interdisciplinary clinical and therapeutic teams. Crotched Mountain is a licensed Special Hospital providing 24 hour medical coverage and skilled nursing. Clients reside in semi-private rooms w/superv

7033 Department of Physical Medicine and Rehabilitation
Exeter Hospital
5 Alumni Dr
Exeter, NH 03833-2128   603-778-7311
                            FAX: 603-580-6592
                          www.exeterhospital.com

Kevin Calahan, President
Offers patient treatment, committed to enhancing the lives of individuals with short and long term physically disabling conditions.

7034 Farnum Rehabilitation Center
580 Court St
Keene, NH 03431-1718   603-354-6630
                            FAX: 603-355-2078

Susan Loughrey, Program Director
Judy Bell, Manager
Offers rehabilitation services, occupational therapy, physical therapy and more for the physically challenged individual.

7035 Hackett Hill Nursing Center and Integrated Care
191 Hackett Hill Rd
Manchester, NH 03102-8993   603-668-8161
                            FAX: 603-622-2584

Daniele Peckham, Administrator
Brett Lennerton, Administrator
A 68-bed certified nursing home.Postacute rehabilitation program.

7036 Mental Health Center: Riverside Courtyard, The
3 Twelfth St
Berlin, NH 03570-3860   603-752-7404
                            FAX: 603-752-5194

Eileen Theriault, Manager
A center to help people that have mental disabilities.

7037 New Hampshire Rehabilitation and Sports Medicine
Catholic Medical Center
Ste 201
769 S Main St
Manchester, NH 03102-5166   603-647-1899
                                    800-437-9666
                            FAX: 603-668-5348

Stuart Draper, Owner
Victor Carbone, Manager
A specialized facility for comprehensive rehabilitation for individuals who have been injured or have a disability.

7038 New Medico, Highwatch Rehabilitation Center
Highwatch Rd
Center Ossipee, NH 03814
                            FAX: 603-539-8888

William Burke, Executive Director
Post-acute rehabilitation service.

7039 Northern New Hampshire Mental Health and Developmental Services
87 Washington St
Conway, NH 03818-6044   603-447-3347
                            FAX: 603-447-8893
                              www.northernhs.org

Dennis Mackay, CEO
Provides mental health and developmental services to northern New Hampshire, including early intervention, elderly services, residential program, outpatient services, employee assistance programs, inpatient services, etc.

New Jersey

7040 All Garden State Physical Therapy
44 Ridge Road
North Arlington, NJ 07031   201-998-6300
                            FAX: 201-998-6344
                               gardenstatept.com

7041 Bancroft
425 Kings Highway East
PO Box 20
Haddonfield, NJ 08033- 1284   856-429-0010
                                    800-774-5516
                            FAX: 856-429-1613
                            TTY: 856-428-2697
                            inquiry@bancroft.org
                               www.bancroft.org

Cynthia Boyer, PhD, Executive Director, Brain Injury Services
Toni Pergolin, President and Chief Executive
Clair Rohrer, Med, Executive Director, Programs for Adults
Dennis . Morgan, M.Ed, Executive Director of Bancroft Special Education Programs
Private, not-for-profit organization serving people with disabilities since 1883. Based in Haddonfield, New Jersey, help more than 1000 children and adults with autism, developmental disabilities, brain injuries, and other neurological impairments. Operates more than 140 sites throughout the U.S. and abroad.

7042 Daughters of Miriam Center/The Gallen Institute
155 Hazel St
Clifton, NJ 07011-3423   973-772-3700
                            FAX: 973-253-5389
                   administration@daughtersofmiriamcenter.org
                    www.daughtersofmiriamcenter.o rg
Fred Feinstein, Executive Director
Dedicated to providing the highest quality care, the Center has far exceeded a stereotypical nursing home by offering a continuum of care environment, making us a leader in Jewish eldercare.

7043 Devereux Advanced Behavioral Health NewJersey
286 Mantua Grove Rd.
Bldg 4
West Deptford, NJ 08066   856-599-6400
                                    800-345-1292
                            FAX: 856-423-8916
                            ccirucci@devereux.org
                               www.devereux.org

Carole Cirucci, Interim Executive Director
Janine Dalton, Assistant Executive Director
Donnie Marie Renner, Developmental & External Affairs Department
Serves ages 3 to life. Individuals with emotional, behavioral, and developmental disabilities are served via a broad spectrum of treatment settings including community-based homes and apartments, vocational training programs, family care homes, and consulting services. DNJCCR also has a residential/educational center that serves individuals with autism spectrum disorders.

7044 Ladacain Network
Schroth School & Technical Education Center
1701 Kneeley Blvd
Wanamassa, NJ 07712-7622   732-493-5900
                            FAX: 732-493-5980
                                    ladacin.org

Patricia Carlesimo, Executive Director
Provides an array of services and programs specifically for children and adults with developmental and physical disabilities. Services include approved Department of Education school programs; adult education and training; vocational training, personal care assistance services, in-home and Saturday respite; child care programs, housing opportunities, and more.

7045 Lourdes Regional Rehabilitation Center
Our Lady of Lourdes Medical Center
1600 Haddon Ave
Camden, NJ 08103-3101   856-757-3864
                                           856-757-3500
                                      FAX: 856-968-2511
                                      info@lourdesnet.org
                                      www.lourdesnet.org

Alexander J. Hatala, President
Kimberly D. Barnes, Vice President, Planning and Development
Michael Hammond, Chief Financial Officer
Maureen Hetu, Chief Information Officer
The only comprehensive rehabilitation facility located within an acute care hospital in Southern New Jersey. Patients benefit from the proximity to the full range of state of the art medical and surgical services should the need arise.

7046 Mt. Carmel Guild
1160 Raymond Blvd
Newark, NJ 07102-4168   973-596-4100
                                      FAX: 973-639-6583

Anita Holland, Manager
Offers services for the totally blind, legally blind, visually impaired, mentally retarded blind and more with health, counseling, educational, recreational, rehabilitation, computer training and professional training services.

7047 Pediatric Rehabilitation Department, JFK Medical Center
65 James St
Edison, NJ 08818-3947   732-321-7362
                                           732-321-7000
                                      FAX: 732-548-7751
                                      www.jfkmc.org

Michael A. Kleiman, DMD, Chair
Douglas A. Nordstrom, Vice Chair
John L. Kolaya, PE, Secretary
Leonard Sendelsky, Treasurer
Comprehensive interdisciplinary, family focused outpatient pediatric rehabilitation services including evaluation and individual and group treatment programs for children birth-21.

7048 REACH Rehabilitation Program: Leader Nursing and Rehabilitation Center
550 Jessup Rd
West Deptford, NJ 08066-1921   856-848-9551

Karen Fattore, Case Manager
Anthony Stenson, Administrator
Postacute rehabilitation program.

7049 REACH Rehabilitation and Catastrophic Long-Term Care
1180 Us Highway 22
Mountainside, NJ 07092-2810   908-654-0020
                                      FAX: 908-654-8661

Allen Swanson, Manager
Archie Ordana, Manager
Postacute rehabilitation program.

7050 Rehabilitation Specialists
18-01 Pollitt Drive
Ste 1A
Fair Lawn, NJ 07410-2815   201-478-4200
                                           800-441-7488
                                      FAX: 201-478-4201
                                program@rehab-specialists.com
                                      www.rehab-specialists.com
Virgilio Caraballo, President/CEO
Dustin Gordon, Director of Neuropsychological and Clinical Services
Dr. Brian Greenwald, Medical Director
Cindy Dittfield, Director of Marketing & Public Relations
Rehabilitation Specialists, founded in 1983, is a quality, cost effective community re-entry center treating individuals with acquired brain injury. A non clinical environment based in the community is utilized that offers professional services enabling participants to learn skills they need to return to a productive life. Both our Day and Residential programming emphases focus on Functional Life Skills, Work Skills and Learning Skills. Each participant's program is tailored to meet their needs.

7051 Somerset Valley Rehabilitation and Nursing Center
Care-One
11300 Cornell Park Drive
Suite 360
Cincinnati, OH 45242   513-469-7222
                                      FAX: 513-469-7230
                                      info@healthbridge.org
                                      healthbridge.org

Trudi Matthews, Director of Policy and Public Re
Subacute rehabilitation program, long term care, respite care.

7052 Summit Ridge Center
101 East State Street
Kennett Square, PA 19348   973-736-2000
                                      FAX: 973-736-2764
                                      genesishcc.com

New Mexico

7053 SJR Rehabilitation Hospital
525 S Schwartz Ave
Farmington, NM 87401-5955   505-609-2625
                                      FAX: 505-327-6562
                                      eniemand@sjrmc.net
                                      www.sjrrh.com

Ena M Niemand, Executive Director
Sue Clay, Program Director
Jill Morgan, Nursing Director
Uses a team of professionals to provide a comprehensive rehabilitation program. Accomplishing the best possible physical and cognitive improvement is the aim of the following treatment members: nurses, physical therapists, physicians, speech and occupational therapists, therapeutic recreation specialist. Providing inpatient and out patient services.

7054 Southwest Communication Resource
P.O.Box 788
Bernalillo, NM 87004-788   505-867-3396
                                      FAX: 505-867-3398
                                      info@abrazosnm.org
                                      swcr.org

New York

7055 Aspire of Western New York
2356 N Forest Rd
Getzville, NY 14068-1224   716-838-0047
                                      FAX: 716-894-8257
                                      info@aspirewny.org
                                      aspirewny.org

Thomas A. Sy, Executive Director
Janet Hansen, Chief Operating Officer
Mary Anne Coombe, V.P. of Service Coordination & Fiscal Management Services
Helen Trowbridge Hanes, Vice President of Community Living
Provides comprehensive services to individuals with disabilities from infancy through adulthood. Also serves people with all types of developmental disabilities as well as providing clinical services to persons with other types of disabilities such as: spinal cord injury, head trauma and others. Aspire employs 1500 people.

7056 Bronx Continuing Treatment Day Program
1527 Southern Blvd
Bronx, NY 10460-5619   718-893-1414
                                      FAX: 718-893-0707

Mary Jane Purcell, Manager
Post-acute rehabilitation program.

7057 Brooklyn Bureau of Community Service
285 Schermerhorn St
Brooklyn, NY 11217-1098   718-310-5600
FAX: 718-855-1517
info@WeAreBCS.org
www.wearebcs.org

Marla Simpson, Executive Director
Anthony B. Edwards, MBA, CCF, MFM, CFO
Janelle Farris, Chief Operating Officer
Sonya Shields, Chief Officer for External Relations and Advancement
Offers independent living skills, counseling, work readiness, vocational trianing, job placement and job follow-up services to individuals with disabilities (to include individuals with psychiatric, physical, and developmental disabilities). Special programs to move disabled welfare recipients from welfare to work. Publishes a bi-annual newsletter.

7058 Buffalo Hearing and Speech Center
50 E North St
Buffalo, NY 14203-1002   716-885-8318
FAX: 716-885-4229
askbhsc.org

Frank J. Polino, Chairman
Dennis J. Szefel, First Vice Chairman
Kenneth J. Wilson, Treasurer
Gerald Chiari, Esq., Secretary
Assists individuals with speech, language and/or hearing impairments to achieve maximum communication potential.

7059 Cora Hoffman Center Day Program
2324 Forest Ave
Staten Island, NY 10303-1506   718-447-8205
FAX: 718-815-2182

Kevin Kenney, Manager
Post-acute rehabilitation program specializing in Cerebral Palsy. Part of the Cerebral Palsey Association of New York State.

7060 Devereux Advanced Behavioral Health New York
40 Devereux Way
Red Hook, NJ 12571   845-758-1899
FAX: 845-758-1817
www.devereux.org

John Lopez, Executive Director
Serving ages 8 to 21. Devereux Advanced Behavioral Health New York provides a wide range of educational, clinical, residential, and community-based programs and services to children, youth and adults with intellectual disabilities, Autism Spectrum Disorder, and dual diagnoses.

7061 Elmhurst Hospital Center
7901 Broadway
Elmhurst, NY 11373-1368   718-334-4000
www.nyc.gov/html/hhc/ehc/html/home/home.shtml
Chris D Constantino, Executive Director
Hospital is comprised of 525 beds and is a Level I Trauma Center, and Emergency Heart Care Stattion and a 911 recieving hospital. It is the premiere health care organization for key areas such as Surgery, Cardiology, Women's health, Pediatrics, Rehabilitation Medicine, Renal and Mental Health Services.

7062 Federation Employment And Guidance Service(F-E-G-S)
315 Hudson St
New York, NY 10013-1086   212-366-8400
FAX: 212-366-8441
info@fegs.org
www.fegs.org

Gail Magaliff, CEO
Ira Machowsky, Executive Vice President
Thomas M. Higgins, CFO
Kristin M. Woodlock, Chief Operating Officer
The largest and most diversified private, not-for-profit health related and human service organization in the United States. With operations in over 258 facilities, residences, and off-site locations, F-E-G-S has served more then 2 million people since its inception.

7063 Flushing Hospital
4500 Parsons Blvd
Flushing, NY 11355-2205   718-670-5000
FAX: 718-670-3082
flushinghospital.org

Robert V. Levine, Executive Vice President and COO
Bruce J. Flanz, President/ CEO
Mounir Doss, Executive Vice President/CFO
Offers services for the totally blind, legally blind, visually impaired, mentally retarded blind and more with health, counseling, educational, recreational, rehabilitation, computer training and professional training services.

7064 Gateway Community Industries Inc.,
1 Amy Kay Pkwy
Kingston, NY 12401-6444   845-331-1261
800-454-9395
FAX: 845-331-4920
info@gatewayindustries.org
gatewayindustries.org

Francoise C. Gunefsky, President/ CEO
Eva Graham, CFO
Ralph Smith, Chief Information Officer
Mary Ann Hildebrandt, Chief Quality and Compliance Officer
Gateway Community Industries, Inc., founded in 1957, is one of the leading independent not-for-profit vocational rehabilitation and training centers for people with mental and/or physical disabilities. The agency provides comprehensive services in vocational evaluation, job training, job placement, vocational work center employment, supported employment, psychiatric rehabilitation, continuing day treatment, and residential habilitation/rehabilitation.

7065 Henkind Eye Institute Division of Montefiore Hospital
111 East 210th Street
Bronx, NY 10467-2404   718-920-4321
www.montefiore.org
Philip O. Ozuah, MD, PhD, Executive Vice President/ COO
Steven M. Safyer, MD, President/ CEO
Joel A. Perlman, Executive Vice President, Chief Financial Officer
Alfredo Cabrera, Senior Vice President & Chief Human Resources Officer
Offers services for the totally blind, legally blind, visually impaired, mentally retarded blind and more with health, counseling, educational, recreational, rehabilitation, computer training and professional training services. Low vision services offered.

7066 Industries for the Blind of New York State
194 Washington Ave
Ste 300
Albany, NY 12210-6314   518-456-8671
800-421-9010
FAX: 518-456-3587
customercare@nyspsp.org
www.abilityone.com

Richard Healey, CEO
Offers services for the totally blind, legally blind, visually impaired, mentally retarded blind and more with health, counseling, educational, recreational, rehabilitation, computer training and professional training services.

7067 Inpatient Pain Rehabilitation Program
550 First Avenue
New York, NY 10016   212-263-7300
FAX: 212-598-6468
www.med.nyu.edu

William Pinter Phd, Administrative Director
The Inpatient Rehabilitation Program, established in 1983 specializes in the treatment of chronic pain. Our inpatient program is one of the oldest and well established pain programs in the country. It is the only interdisciplinary inpatient pain program in the tri-state area and one of only 20 pain programs in the entire US to have CARF accreditation. Upon completion of an extensive evaluation, patients are admitted for an 18-day inpatient stay.

7068 Koicheff Health Care Center
2324 Forest Ave
Staten Island, NY 10303-1506
718-447-0200
FAX: 718-981-1431

Paul Castello, Clinic Director
Post-accute rehabilitation programs.

7069 New York-Presbyterian Hospital
622 W 168th St
New York, NY 10032-3796
212-305-4600
FAX: 212-305-1017
www.nyp.org

Steven J. Corwin, MD, CEO
Robert E. Kelly, MD, President
New York Presbyterian Hospital is internationally recognized for its outstanding comprehensive services. Its medical, surgical, and emergency care services provide each patient with the highest possible level of care. In addition, as part of the Hospital's commitment to the total well-being of each patient, it offers a range of specialized services, as well as special healthcare programs for neighboring communities.

7070 Norman Marcus Pain Institute
30 E 40th St
Ste 1100
New York, NY 10016
212-532-7999
FAX: 212-532-5957
support@nmpi.com
backpainusa.com

Norman J Marcus, Medical Director
We focus on muscles as the cause of most common pains, i.e. back, neck, shoulders, and headaches. We make specific muscle diagnoses and have specific treatments that in many cases will eliminate the need for surgery or relieve the pain. Patients diagnosed with herniated disc, spinal stenosis, rotator cuff tear, impingement syndrome, sciatica, fibromyalgia and headache will generally find relief.

7071 Pain Alleviation Center
Comprehensive Pain Management Associates
125 S Service Rd
Jericho, NY 11753-1038
516-997-7246
FAX: 516-997-7281
www.paincenter.com

Alex Weingarten, Director
Phillip Fyman, Director
Marisa French, Manager
One of the first pain clinics to gain national accreditation from the Commission on Accreditation of Rehabilitation Facilities. This is due largely to a patient-centered program based on the latest research.

7072 Pathfinder Village
3 Chenango Rd
Edmeston, NY 13335-2314
607-965-8377
FAX: 607-965-8655
info@pathfindervillage.org
www.pathfindervillage.org

Paul Landers, CEO
Caprice S. Eckert, Chief Financial Officer
Kelly A. Meyers, Director of Admissions
Paula B. Schaeffer, Director of Enrichment Programs
Pathfinder Village is a warm, friendly community in the rolling hills of Central New York. Here children and adults with Down Syndrome gain independence, build lasting friendships, become partners in the world and take in all that life has to offer.

7073 Pilot Industries: Ellenville
845-331-4300
48 Canal St
Ellenville, NY 12428-1327
845-647-7711
FAX: 845-647-7711

Peter Pierri, Executive Director
Betty Marks, Plant Manager
Post-accute rehabilitation services.

7074 Skills Unlimited
405 Locust Ave
Oakdale, NY 11769-1695
631-567-3320
FAX: 631-567-3285
info@skillsunlimited.org
skillsunlimited.org

Richard Kassnove, Executive Director
Our basic goals is to offer persons with disabilities the opportunity to explore and develop their full vocational potential. Our programs are unique in that by offering comprehensive services, individuals are able to deal with many different issues that could potentially affect their vocational success. Any individual that has an impairment that interferes with their ability to work is entitles to the services that we offer.

North Carolina

7075 Center for Vision Rehabilitation
Academy Eye Associates
3115 Academy Rd
Durham, NC 27707-2652
919-493-7456
800-942-1499
FAX: 919-493-1718
henry.greene@academyeye.com
academyeye.com

Henry A Greene, Owner
Vision rehabilitation and low-vision care for the visually impaired, post-stroke, head trauma and for neuro-oncology vision complications.

7076 Diversified Opportunities
1010 Herring Ave E
Wilson, NC 27893-3311
252-291-0378
FAX: 252-291-1402
www.diversifiedopportunitiesinc.com

Cindy Dixon, Executive Director
Carlton Goff, Business Manager
Ericka Simmons, QP Program Manager
Ken Jones, Chairman
Vocational rehabilitation agency, better outcomes, lower cost, guaranteed performance standards.

7077 Forsyth Medical Center
3333 Silas Creek Pkwy
Winston Salem, NC 27103-3090
336-718-5000
FAX: 336-718-9250
www.novanthealth.org

Jeffrey T. Lindsay, President
Denise Mihal, Chief Operating Officer
Stephen J. Motew, MD, Senior Vice President
Bruce D. Walley, MD, Senior Vice President
Provides care that is state-of-the-art and second to none, both because of advanced treatments availiable through our clinical research and technology to the academic excellence-and caring nature-of our doctors and nurses.

7078 Industries of the Blind
914-920 W Lee St
Greensboro, NC 27403-2803
336-274-1591
800-909-7086
FAX: 336-544-3739
customerservice@iob-gso.com
industriesoftheblind.com

David Thompson, Chairperson
Scott Thornhill, 1st Vice Chairperson
Ashley S. James, Jr., 2nd Vice Chairperson
Chi Anyansi-Archibong, Secretary
Offers services for the totally blind, legally blind, visually impaired, mentally retarded blind and more with health, counseling, educational, recreational, rehabilitation, computer training and professional training services.

7079 Johnston County Industries
1100 East Preston Street
Selma, NC 27576-3162
919-743-8700
FAX: 919-965-8023
jcindustries.com

John Shallcross, Jr., President
Durwood Woodall, Vice President
Lina Sanders-Johnson, Secretary/Treasurer
JCI is an entrepreneurial not-for-profit corporation dedicated to empowering people with disabilities or disadvantages to succeed through training and employment

7080 Learning Services: Carolina
707 Morehead Ave
Durham, NC 27707-1319
919-688-4444
888-419-9955
FAX: 919-419-9966
learningservices.com

Debra Braunling-McMorrow, President and CEO
Jeanne Mack, Chief Financial Officer and Vice President of Operations
Michael Weaver, Chief Development Officer
Terri Dorman, V.P. of Customer Service and Care Management
Located in an historic neighborhood in the heart of Durham, this campus-style setting offers easy access to resources at 3 outstanding facilities: Duke University, The University of North Carolina at Chapel Hill, and Research Triangle Park. This program provides a range of services and activities that draw upon the many resources availiable in the community.

7081 LifeSpan
200 Clanton Road
Charlotte, NC 28217
704-944-5100
lifespanservices.org

Davan Cloninger, President & CEO
Ralph Adams, Treasurer & CFO
Christopher White, Vice President of Operations & Business Development
Lori Avery, Senior Development Director
Provide vocational and enrichment program for adults with developmental disabilities.

7082 Lions Club Industries for the Blind
4500 Emperor Blvd
Durham, NC 27703
919-596-8277
800-526-1562
FAX: 919-598-1179
inquire@buylci.com

Bill Hudson, President
Offers services for the totally blind, legally blind, visually impaired, mentally retarded blind and more with health, counseling, educational, recreational, rehabilitation, computer training and professional training services.

7083 Lions Services Inc.
5 Penn Plaza
New York, NY 10001
21 -62 -210
lsisale@aol.com

Jimmy R Cranford, President
Jimmy Cranford, President
Offers services for the totally blind, legally blind, visually impaired, mentally retarded blind and more with health, counseling, educational, recreational, rehabilitation, computer training and professional training services.

7084 Regional Rehabilitation Center Pitt County Memorial Hospital
2100 Stantonsburg Rd
Greenville, NC 27834-2818
252-847-4448
FAX: 252-816-7552
mdixon@pcmh.com
www.uhseast.com/rehab

Martha M Dixon, VP General Services
An accredited, comprehensive rehabilitation center-part of a statewide network- and we're the largest such facility in eastern North Carolina. Our service area covers 29 counties, and we offer a complete array of rehabilitation services for patients of all ages.

Because the Regional Rehabilitation Center is associated with both Pitt County Memorial Hospital And the Brody School of Medicine at East Carolina University, patients have access to a full range of state of the art medical services.

7085 Rehab Home Care
2660 Yonkers Rd
Raleigh, NC 27604-3384
800-447-8692
FAX: 919-831-2211

Alan Silver, CEO
Janis Hansen, Chief Operating Officer
A Medicare/Medicaid certified, state-licensed home health agency with emphasis on rehabilitation.

7086 Thoms Rehabilitation Hospital
Thoms Rehabilitation Hospital
68 Sweeten Creek Rd
Asheville, NC 28803-2318
828-277-4800
FAX: 828-277-4812
TTY:800-735-2962
www.carepartners.org

Tracy Buchanan, President & CEO
Gary Bowers, COO
Freestanding physical rehabilitation hospital, founded 1938 - 100 beds, including 90 acute and 10 transitional - JCAHO accredited.

7087 Winston-Salem Industries for the Blind
7730 N Point Blvd
Winston Salem, NC 27106-3310
336-759-0551
800-242-7726
FAX: 336-759-0990
info@wsifb.com
www.wsifb.com

Mike Faircloth, Chairman
Karen Carey, Vice Chairman, Secretary
W. Robert Newell, Treasurer
David Horton, Executive Director
Offers services for the totally blind, legally blind, visually impaired, mentally retarded blind and more with health, counseling, educational, recreational, rehabilitation, computer training and professional training services.

Ohio

7088 Bellefaire Jewish Children's Bureau
22001 Fairmount Blvd
Cleveland, OH 44118-4819
216-932-2800
800-879-2522
FAX: 216-932-6704
info@bellefairejcb.org
www.bellefairejcb.org

Adam Jacobs, CEO
Adam G. Jacobs PhD, Executive Vice President
Residential treatment for ages 12 to 17 1/2 at time of admission offering individualized psychotherapy, special education, and group living for severaly emotionally disturbed children and adolescents. Also offers a variety of other programs including specialized and therapuetic foster care, partial hospitilization, outpatient counseling, home-based intensive counseling and adoption services.

7089 Christ Hospital Rehabilitation Unit
2139 Auburn Ave
Cincinnati, OH 45219-2906
513-585-2737
FAX: 513-585-4353
www.thechristhospital.com

Mike Keating, President and CEO
Chris Bergman, Vice President and Chief Financial Officer
Berc Gawne, MD, Vice President and Chief Medical Officer
Peter Greis, Vice President and Chief Information Officer
Patients of this 555-bed, not-for-profit acute care facility receive personalized health care provided by trained specialists using the most sophisticated medical technology available, including state-of-the-art intensive care units, surgical facilities, cardiac

catheterization labs, three new electrophysiology labs, and the tristates first positron emission tomography (PET) scanning capabilities.

7090 Cleveland Society for the Blind
Cleveland Sight Center
P.O.Box 1988
1909 East 101st Street
Cleveland, OH 44106-8696

216-791-8118
FAX: 216-696-2582
jcarey@clevelandsightcenter.org
www.clevelandsightcenter.org

William L. Spring, Chair
Thomas J. Gibbons, Vice Chair
Gary W. Poth, Treasurer
Sheryl King Benford, Secretary

Social, rehabilitation, education and support services for blind and visually impaired children and adults, early intervention program for children birth to age 6, low vision clinic, aid and appliance shop, Braille and taping transcription, training for rehabilitation, orientation, mobility and computer access, employment services and job placement, recreation program, resident camping, talking books, radio reading services, food service training and snack bar employment. Free screening.

7091 Columbus Speech and Hearing Center
510 E North Broadway St
Columbus, OH 43214-4114

614-263-5151
FAX: 614-263-5365
columbusspeech.org

Dawn Gleason, Au.D., President/ CEO
Karen Deeter, Director of Operations

Serves persons who have speech-language and hearing challenges. Provides vocational rehabilitation services for individuals who are deaf, hard-of-hearing or deaf-blind.

7092 CommuniCare of Clifton Nursing and Rehabilitation Center
Communi Care Health Services
4700 Ashwood Drive
Cincinnati, OH 45241

513-489-7100
FAX: 513-281-2559
communicarehealth.com

Stephen L. Rosedale, Founder/ CEO

A long term care facility which specializes in rehabilitation. Offers a full range of rehabilitative services including physical therapy, occupational therapy and speech therapy.

7093 Doctors Hospital
5100 W Broad St
Columbus, OH 43228-1672

614-544-1000
800-837-7555
FAX: 614-544-1844
www.ohiohealth.com/homedoctors

David Blom, President/ CEO
Michael Bernstein, Senior Vice President and Chief

We believe our first responsibility is to the patients we serve. We respect the physical, emotional and spiritual needs of our patients and find that compassion is essential to fostering healing and wholeness.

7094 Dodd Hall at the Ohio State University Hospitals
410 W 10th Ave
Columbus, OH 43210-1240

614-293-3300
800-293-5123
OSUCareConnection@osumc.edu
www.medicalcenter.osu.edu

Steven G. Gabbe, MD, Senior Vice President / CEO
Larry Anstine, CEO
Gail Marsh, Chief Strategy Officer
Phyllis Teater, Chief Information Officer

Dodd Hall is a full service medical rehabilitation hospital offering comprehensive inpatient and outpatient rehabilitation.

7095 Easter Seal Society of Mahoning
National Easter Seals Chicago
299 Edwards Street
Youngstown, OH 44502-1599

330-743-1168
800-221-6827
FAX: 330-743-1616
www.easterseals.com/mtc

7096 Four Oaks Center
245 N. Valley Road
Xenia, OH 45385-2605

937-562-6500
FAX: 937-562-6520
www.greenedd.org

Todd McManus, President
Jill A. LaRock, Director
Dr. Vijay Gupta, Vice President
Melinda Mays, Recording Secretary

Starts children on the road to discovery by providing a learning environment rich in opportunities and encouragement. The program was designed to give children with delays or disabilities, or those at-risk the extra help needed to develop fully. Any child under the age of six who exhibits developmental delays, handicapping conditions, or is considered at risk may qualify to participate.

7097 Genesis Healthcare System
Rehabilitation Services
800 Forest Ave
Zanesville, OH 43701-2881

740-454-5000
800-322-4762
FAX: 740-455-7527
llynn@genesishcs.org
www.genesishcs.org

Matt Perry, President/ CEO
Paul Masterson, CFO
Richard Helsper, COO

A CARF and JACHO accredited 19-bed rehabilitation facility located within Genesis Healthcare System, a 732 bed, non-profit hospital system, located in Zanesville, Ohio. Freestanding outpatient services, including work hardening, pain management, vocational services, audiology, lymphedema, vestibular rehab, off-the-road driving evals, aquatic therpay, womens health and sports enhancement.

7098 George A Martin Center
3603 Washington Ave
Cincinnati, OH 45229-2009

513-221-1017
FAX: 513-221-3817

Karen Doggett, Executive Director

Offers services for the totally blind, legally blind, visually impaired, mentally retarded blind and more with health, counseling, educational, recreational, rehabilitation, computer training and professional training services.

7099 Grady Memorial Hospital
561 W Central Ave
Delaware, OH 43015-1489

740-615-1000
800-487-1115
FAX: 740-368-5114
ohiohealth.com

Bruce Hagen, Regional Executive and President

As a progressive healthcare leader, Grady Memorial Hospital is committed to excellence while providing the Deleware community with comprehensive quality service delivered with compassionate, personal care. Our membership in Ohio's largest healthcare system, Ohio Health, enables us to improve access to a broader range of healthcare services, enhance development of new programs and services, and provide a complete continuum of care for patients in the deleware area.

7100 Hamilton Adult Center
3400 Symmes Rd
Hamilton, OH 45015-1359

513-867-5970
FAX: 513-874-2977

Donald Musnuff, Executive Director

7101 Holzer Clinic
100 Jackson Pike
Gallipolis, OH 45631-1560
740-446-5000
FAX: 740-446-5532
info@holzer.org
www.holzer.org

T. Wayne Munro, MD, CEO
Brent A. Saunders, Chair
Christopher Meyer, Chief Medical Officer
John Cunningham, Chief Administrative Officer
Serves medical needs of patients in an 8 county area, including counties in Ohio and West Virginia.

7102 Holzer Clinic Sycamore
Holzer Medical Center
4th Avenue & Sycamore St
Gallipolis, OH 45631-1560
740-446-5244
FAX: 740-446-5448
info@holzer.org
www.holzer.org

T. Wayne Munro, MD, CEO
Brent A. Saunders, Chair
Christopher Meyer, Chief Medical Officer
John Cunningham, Chief Administrative Officer
Offers an individualized quality comprehensive rehabilitation program for people with disabilities by an interdisciplinary team including physical therapy, occupational, speech, nursing and social services to restore the patient to the highest degree of rehab outcomes attainable.

7103 IKRON Institute for Rehabilitative and Psychological Services
2347 Vine St
Cincinnati, OH 45213-1745
513-621-1117
FAX: 513-621-2350
ikron@ikron.org
ikron.org

Randy Strunk, MA, LPCC-S, Executive Director
Ken Carbonell, BBA, Fiscal Director
Melissa Harmeling, MA, PCC-S, Program Director
Jake Striker, President
An accredited mental health facility and a certified rehabilitation center. Through a variety of creative treatment and rehabilitation services, IKRON assists adults with mental health and/or substance abuse problems to attain greater independence, to lead lives of sobriety, to obtain competitive work and live more satisfying lives. IKRON places a strong emphasis on respect and support for persons with problems of adjustment. Special contracts to persons desiring job placement.

7104 Integrated Health Services at Waterford Commons
955 Garden Lake Pkwy
Toledo, OH 43614-2777
419-382-2200
FAX: 419-381-8508

Nicole Giesige, Executive Director
A subacute and rehabilitation program specializing in ventilator weaning and management, I.V. therapeutics and pain management, wound management and subacute rehabilitation.

7105 Lester H Higgins Adult Center
3041 Cleveland Ave SW
Canton, OH 44707-3625
330-484-4814
FAX: 330-484-9416
http://www.theworkshopsinc.com/

Margalie Belazaire, Manager
Ed Allar, Manager
Post-accute rehabilitation service

7106 Live Oaks Career Development Campus
5936 Buckwheat Rd
Milford, OH 45150
513-575-1906
FAX: 513-575-0805

Harold Carr MD, Superintendent
Robin White, President/CEO
Jim Dixon, Principal
Post-accute rehabilitation facility and services.

7107 Metro Health: St. Luke's Medical Center Pain Management Program
2500 Metrohealth Dr
Cleveland, OH 44109-1900
216-778-7800
www.metrohealth.org

Mark Moran, President
CARF accredited comprehensive multidisciplinary pain management program.

7108 MetroHealth Medical Center
2500 Metrohealth Dr
Cleveland, OH 44109-1900
216-778-7800
www.metrohealth.org

Mark Moran, President
Located on the near west side of Cleveland, is a leader in trauma, emergency, and critical care; women's and childrens's services, including high risk obstetrical care and neonatal intensive care; comprehensive medical and surgical subspecialties.

7109 Middletown Regional Hospital: Inpatient Rehabilitation Unit
105 McKnight Dr
Middletown, OH 45044-4838
513-422-1401
800-338-4057
FAX: 513-422-1520
www.middletownhospital.org

C N Reddy, Owner
Douglas McNeill, Chief Executive Officer
Our mission is to serve and help people, improving the status of their health and the quality of thier lives. Our vision is to be the premier integrated delivery system in Southwest Ohio. Our Values are quality, respect, service and teamwork

7110 Newark Healthcare Center
680 South Fourth Street
Louisville, KY 40202
502-596-7300
TTY:800-545-0749
web_administrator@kindred.com
kindredhealthcare.com

Paul J. Diaz, President/ CEO
Accomodates 300 residents. We are located in the heart of Newark, Ohio. Newark Healthcare is a 2004 recipient of the American Health Care Association's Quality Award.

7111 Parma Community General Hospital Acute Rehabilitation Center
7007 Powers Blvd
Parma, OH 44129-5495
440-743-3000
FAX: 440-843-4387
www.parmahospital.org

David Nedrich, Chairman
Thomas P. O'Donnell, First Vice Chairman
Alex I. Koler, First Assistant Treasurer
Sharon Martin, Assistant Secretary
The mission of this CARF accredited unit is to provide the most comprehensive, cost-effective, acute rehabilitation program possible in order for every patient and family to adjust to his/her disability and to achieve the maximum potential of independent functioning when returning to community living.

7112 Peter A Towne Physical Therapy Center
Ste 10
447 Nilles Rd
Fairfield, OH 45014-2626
513-829-7726
FAX: 513-829-7726
www.townept.com/fairfield

Debbie Wilkerson, Office Manager
Outpatient, private practice physical and occupational therapy. Three other offices in Hamilton, Monroe and West Chester.

7113   Philomatheon Society of the Blind
2701 Tuscarawas St W
Canton, OH 44708-4638
                                    330-453-9157
                                    www.philomatheon.com

David Miller, President
Denise Dessecker, Vice President
Angela Randall, Secretary
Paul Williams, Treasurer
Offers services for the totally blind, legally blind, visually impaired, mentally retarded blind and more with health, counseling, educational, recreational, rehabilitation, computer training and professional training services.

7114   Providence Hospital Work
2270 Banning Rd
Cincinnati, OH 45239-6621
                                    513-591-5600
                                    FAX: 513-591-5604

Kay Brogle, Executive Director
Post-acute rehabilitation services.

7115   Six County, Inc.
2845 Bell St
Zanesville, OH 43701-1794
                                    740-454-9766
                                    800-344-5818
                                    FAX: 740-588-6452
                                    info@sixcounty.org
                                    www.sixcounty.org

John A Creek, President
Tim Llewellyn, Senior VP/Community Intervention
Robert Santos, Ex Vp & Coo
Mary Denoble, Vp Qip
Six County, Inc., is a private, not-for-profit corporation under contract with the Mental Health and Recovery Services Board. Six County, Inc., provides comprehensive community mental health services to people of all ages in each of the six Southeastern Ohio counties served: Coshocton, Guernsey, Morgan, Muskingum, Noble, and Perry. SCI's counseling centers provide a full range of services including outpatient counseling; diagnostic assessment, referrals, and psychological testing.

7116   Society for Rehabilitation
9290 Lake Shore Blvd
Mentor, OH 44060-1664
                                    440-352-8993
                                    800-344-3159
                                    FAX: 440-352-6632
                                    info@societyhelps.org
                                    www.societyhelps.org

Richard Kessler, Executive Director
Vision is to provide individuals with comprehensive services to improve their quality of life. Our mission is to meet the needs of individuals and their families by delivering a wide range of affordable accessible and personalized services, providing treatment by a team of highly qualified, caring professionals. Collaborating with other agencies to meet community needs.

7117   Southeast Ohio Sight Center
425 E. Alvarado Street
Suite E
Fallbrook, CA 92028
                                    800-677-4180
                                    www.charityadvantage.com

7118   St. Francis Rehabilitation Hospital
401 N Broadway St
Green Springs, OH 44836-9638
                                    419-639-2626
                                    800-248-2552
                                    FAX: 419-639-6225
                                    www.sfhcc.org

Kim Eicher, CEO
Dan Schwanke, Chief Executive Officer
Program offers specialized treatment for patients who have suffered a head injury, spinal cord injury, or stroke, or who have an orthopedic injury. The Head Injury Program provides a continuum of care from coma stimulation through transitional living. Their physicians, nurses, counselors and therapists are dedicated to helping our patients develop the motivation, strength and skills needed to overcome or adapt to their disability.

7119   TAC Enterprises
2160 Old Selma Rd
Springfield, OH 45505-4600
                                    937-525-7400
                                    FAX: 937-525-7401
                                    info@tacind.com
                                    www.tacind.com

Clifford Meyer, CEO
TAC Enterprises provides employment opportunities for individuals to develop marketable skills by completing contract work in partnership with other industries. Work and self-help skills, social adjustment, and a variety of daily living experiences are offered to the workers by our specialized staff.

Oklahoma

7120   Dean A McGee Eye Institute
608 Stanton L Young Blvd
Oklahoma City, OK 73104-5065
                                    405-271-6060
                                    800-787-9012
                                    FAX: 405-271-4442
                                    www.mei.org

Gregory L. Skuta, M.D., President/CEO
Matthew D. Brown, Executive Vice President
Lana G. Ivy, Vice President of Development
Kimberly A. Howard, Chief Financial Officer and Vice President of Finance
Offers services for the totally blind, legally blind, visually impaired, mentally retarded blind and more with health, counseling, educational, recreational, rehabilitation, computer training and professional training services.

7121   Jane Phillips Medical Center
Rehab Care
3500 E Frank Phillips Blvd
Bartlesville, OK 74006-2464
                                    918-333-7200
                                    FAX: 918-333-7801
                                    webmaster@jpmc.org
                                    jpmc.org

David Stire, President/ COO
Mike Moore, Chief Financial Officer/Vice President Fiscal Services
Susan Herron, RN, Vice President Nursing Services
Paul W. McQuillen, MD, Chief Medical Officer
Comprehensive inpatient rehabilitation services are provided to patients with orthopedic, neurologic, and other medical conditions of recent onset or regression, who have experienced a loss of function in activities of daily living, mobility, cognition and communication.

7122   McAlester Regional Health Center RehabCare Unit
1 E Clark Bass Blvd
McAlester, OK 74501-4255
                                    918-426-1800
                                    FAX: 918-421-6832
                                    nbrinlee@mrhcok.com
                                    www.mrhcok.com

David Keith, President/ CEO
Cara Bland, Chairman
Evans McBride, Vice-Chairman
A 19-bed inpatient physical rehabilitation unit serving the Southeast Oklahoma area. Offers physical therapy, occupational therapy, social work, speech and psychological services in an interdisciplinary framework.

7123   Oklahoma League for the Blind
501 N Douglas Ave
Oklahoma City, OK 73106-5085
                                    405-232-4644
                                    888-522-4644
                                    FAX: 405-236-5438
                                    info@newviewoklahoma.org
                                    www.newviewoklahoma.org

Lauren White, President/ CEO
Carol Campbell, Executive Assistant
John Wilson, Chief Financial Officer
Randy Hearn, Chief Operations Officer
Offers services for the blind and visually impaired, counseling, educational, recreational, rehabilitation, computer training and professional training services.

7124 Valley View Regional Hospital-RehabCare Unit
430 N Monte Vista St
Ada, OK 74820-4657

580-332-2323
FAX: 580-421-1395
valleyview@wrh.com
www.valleyviewregional.org

W. Kent Rogers, President/ CEO
Comprehensive physical medicine and rehabilitation services designed to help patients in their adjustment to a physically limiting condition.

Oregon

7125 Garten Services
PO Box 13970
Salem, OR 97309

503-581-1984
FAX: 503-581-4497
garten@garten.org
garten.org

Tim Rocak, CEO
Pamela Best, CFO
Steve Babcock, Mail Services Manager
Stacie Braun, Custodial Services Manager
Garten's mission is to support people with disabilities in their effort to contribute to the community through employment, career, and retirement opportunities. Our actions increase society's awareness of human potential. Garten's vision is to be recognized as an organization positively demonstrating to the community that people with disabilities can be contributing and valued employees of a thriving business.

7126 Legacy Emanuel Rehabilitation Center
2801 N. Gantenbein
Portland, OR 97227-1542

503-413-2200
FAX: 503-413-1501
www.legacyhealth.org

Gary Guidetta, Executive Director
Gail Weisgerber, Manager
A non-profit tax-exempt corporation that includes 5 full-service hospitals and a children's hospital. The Legacy system provides an integrated network of healthcare services, including acute and critical care, inpatient and outpatient treatment, community health education and a variety of specialty services.

7127 Oakcrest Care Center
2933 Center St NE
Salem, OR 97301-4527

503-585-5850
FAX: 503-585-8781

7128 Oakhill-Senior Program
1190 Oakhill Ave SE
Salem, OR 97302-3496

503-364-9086
FAX: 503-365-2879
Jan Dillon, Senior Services Manager
Garten Senior Services provides an adult day service program to seniors with and without developmental disabilities. The program will provide community opportunities, college classes and a wide variety of leisure activities in group and individual settings.

7129 Pacific Spine and Pain Center
1801 Highway 99 N
Ashland, OR 97520-9152

541-488-2255
866-482-5515
FAX: 541-482-2433

Janel R Guyette, Manager

7130 Vision Northwest
9225 SW Hall Blvd
Portland, OR 97223-6794

503-684-8389
800-448-2232
FAX: 503-684-9359
marthaz@visionnw.com
visionnw.com

Evelyn Maizels, Executive Director

Offers services for the totally blind, legally blind, visually impaired, mentally retarded blind and more with health, counseling, educational, recreational, rehabilitation, computer training and professional training services.

7131 Willamette Valley Rehabilitation Center
1853 W Airway Rd
Lebanon, OR 97355-1233

541-258-8121
FAX: 541-451-1762
wvrc.org

Martin Baughman, Executive Director
Provides the best professional vocational services to those adults in the community who, by virtue of their physical or mental limitations, are negatively impacted by their ability to attain or maintain employment.

Pennsylvania

7132 Alpine Nursing and Rehabilitation Center of Hershey
Pennstate
405 Martin Ter
State College, PA 16803-3426

814-865-1710
FAX: 814-863-9423
geron@psu.edu
geron.psu.edu

Melissa A Hardy, Director
Anna Shuey, Administrative Assistant
Postacute rehabilitation program.

7133 Beechwood Rehabilitation Services A Community Integrated Brain Injury Program
469 E Maple Ave
Langhorne, PA 19047-1600

215-750-4299
800-782-3299
FAX: 215-750-4327
dcerra-tyl@wood.org
beechwoodrehab.com

Thomas Felicetti, President
Services include residential, day treatment and community based support services. Individuals with brain injury are served. The facility is Care Accredited.

7134 Blind & Vision Rehabilitation Services Of Pittsburgh
1800 West St
Homestead, PA 15120-2578

412-368-4400
800-706-5050
FAX: 412-368-4090
www.bvrspittsburgh.org

Erika M. Arbogast, President
Brian Glass, Director of Information Services and Facilities
Leslie Montgomery, Director of Development and Public Relations
Barbara Peterson, Director of Client Services
Offers services for the totally blind, legally blind, visually impaired, mentally retarded blind and more with health, counseling, educational, recreational, rehabilitation, computer training and professional training services.

7135 Bradford Regional Medical Center
116 Interstate Pkwy
Bradford, PA 16701-1036

814-368-4143
FAX: 814-368-4130
www.brmc.com

Marek Dzionara, Owner
Andrew Lehman, Executive Director
Timothy J. Finan, President and CEO
Offers rehabilitation services to individuals with an alcohol or drug related problem.

7136 Bryn Mawr Rehabilitation Hospital
414 Paoli Pike
Malvern, PA 19355-3311

610-251-5400
888-734-2241
888-734-2241
FAX: 610-647-3648
www.mainlinehealth.org

Donna M. Phillips, President

We are dedicated to serving individuals and their families whose lives can be enhanced through physical or cognitive rehabilitation. We continually strive for excellence by providing care and services which are valued by those we serve and by contributing to the community through education, research and prevention of disability.

7137 Devereux Advanced Behavioral Health -National Office
444 Devereux Dr
Villanova, PA 19085-1932 610-520-3000
800-345-1292
FAX: 610-542-3100
www.devereux.org
Carol Oliver, State Director
Devereux is a leading nonprofit behavioral health organization that supports many of the most underserved and vulnerable members of our communities.

7138 Devereux Pennsylvania
230 Highland Ave.
Devon, PA 19333 610-788-6565
800-345-1292
FAX: 610-430-0567
www.devereux.org
Carol Oliver, M.S., State Director
Melanie Beidler, M.S., Executive Director, Children's Intellectual/ Developmental D
Judy Lau, M.S., Executive Director, Adult Services
Mary Seeley LPN, Executive Director, Devereux Poconos
Devereux Pennsylvania has been an innovative leader in helping children and adults with intellectual, behavioral and emotional challenges accomplish their dreams by discovering their strengths and realizing personal fulfillment.

7139 Fox Subacute Center
2644 Bristol Rd
Warrington, PA 18976-1404 800-782-2288
WebAdmin@rehabcare.com
subacute.com
James Foulke, CEO
Vic Costenko, COO
Walter Dunsmore, CFO
Fox subacute recognizes the great need for alternative programs for today's medically compromised patients. Fox has developed Models of Care and offers subacute programs fore the management of ventilator-dependent patients. We recognize that the best road to recovery for these patients is an environment with special care in an alternative setting. We believe that setting should be outside the hospital, in facilities where the focus is on the management of individual patients.

7140 Fox Subacute at Clara Burke
251 Stenton Ave
Plymouth Meeting, PA 19462-1220 610-828-2272
800-424-7201
FAX: 610-828-7939
admissions@foxsubacute.com
www.foxsubacute.com
Terri Herd, Director of Marketing
Amy Swartley, RN,, Director of Admissions
Kathy Palladino, Director of Human Resources
Erik I. Soiferman, DO, FACOI, Chief Medical Officer
Fox Subacute at Clara Burke in Plymouth Meeting, PA offers attentive, nurturing management of ventilator dependent, medically compromised patients in the PA, NJ, DE, Tri-State area. This sixty-bed facility, with its picturesque setting on 16 acres in historic Plymouth Meeting, is ideal for the specialized services and programs offered by Fox. With a team of highly motivated professionals, we offer the discharge alternative to prolonged lengths of stay in more costly acute care settings.

7141 Good Samaritan Health System
4th & Walnut Sts
P.O.Box 1281
Lebanon, PA 17042-1281 717-270-7500
www.gshleb.org
Robin Weiler, Manager
Frederick Davis, VP Clinical Services

Offers services for the totally blind, legally blind, visually impaired, mentally retarded blind and more with health, counseling, educational, recreational, rehabilitation, computer training and professional training services.

7142 Good Samaritan Hospital-Health System Center
Good Samaritan Hospital
4th & Walnut Sts
P.O.Box 1281
Lebanon, PA 17042-1281 717-270-7500
www.gshleb.org
June Nafziger-Eberl, Manager
Stuart Hartman, Medical Director
Comprehensive inpatient rehab unit for adults regarding general physical rehabilitation. Specific programs include orthopedic, neurological, stroke, amputee, etc.

7143 Pediatric Center at Plymouth Meeting Integrated Health Services
491 Allendale Rd
King of Prussia, PA 19406-1426 610-265-9290
800-220-7337
Fran Currick, Manager
Subacute programs such as intensive respiratory care, stressing ventilator dependent children, pre and post transplant care, total parenteral nutrition, IV therapy, intensive/behavioral oral feeding programs. Provides extensive discharge planning including teaching or review for all the above programs with an emphasis on development and accessing community resources.

7144 Penn State Milton S. Hershey Medical Center College Of Medicine
500 University Dr
Hershey, PA 17033-2360 717-531-8521
800-243-1455
FAX: 717-531-4558
www.pennstatehershey.org
Harold L Paz, CEO
Alan L. Brechbill, Executive Director
Wayne Zolko, Associate Vice President for Finance and Business
Andrew S. Resnick, Chief Quality Officer
a non-sectarian, not-for-profit community hospital whose purpose is to provide high quality acute, rehabilitative and preventive health services for the entire community, regardless of creed, race, nationality, or ability to pay.

7145 Pennsylvania Pain Rehabilitation Center
Ste 2
252 W Swamp Rd
Doylestown, PA 18901-2465 215-230-9707
FAX: 215-348-5106
Kenneth Lefkowitz, Manager
Post acute rehabilitation facility and programs.

7146 Rehabilitation & Nursing Center at Greater Pittsburgh, The
890 Weatherwood Ln
Greensburg, PA 15601-5777 724-837-8076
FAX: 724-837-7456
www.healthbridgemanagement.com
Nancy Flenner, Administrator
Marsha Echard, Admissions Coordinator
Craig Stepien, Admissions Director
Subacute care, ventilator and pulmonary managment, comprehensive rehabilitation.

Rhode Island

7147   **In-Sight**
43 Jefferson Blvd
Warwick, RI 02888-6400   401-941-3322
FAX: 401-941-3356
cbutler@in-sight.org
in-sight.org

Chris Butler, Executive Director
Lucille Gaboriault, Director of Community Resources
Paul Hopkins, Director of First Impressions
Richard Andrade, Director of Vision Rehabilitation
Offers services for the totally blind, legally blind, visually impaired, mentally retarded blind and more with health, counseling, educational, recreational, rehabilitation, computer training and professional training services.

7148   **Vanderbilt Rehabilitation Center**
Newport Hospital
167 Point Street
Providence, RI 02903   401-444-3500
www.lifespan.org

Timothy J. Babineau, President/CEO
Kenneth E. Arnold, SVP, General Counsel
Carole M. Cotter, SVP, Chief Information Officer
Cathy Duquette, EVP, Nursing Affairs
The Vanderbilt Rehabilitation Center at Newport Hospital has been providing comprehensive rehabilitation sercices for more than 40 years and is known throughout the region for its unique programs and high-quality, patient focused care.

South Carolina

7149   **Association for the Blind**
One Carriage Lane
Building A
Charleston, SC 29407   843-723-6915
FAX: 843-577-4312
www.abvisc.org

J. Douglas Hazelton, President
Capers A. Grimball, Vice President
Lea B. Kerrison, Secretary
Mary Morrison, Executive Director
Offers services for people who are blind, or are visually impaired with health, counseling, educational, recreational, rehabilitation, computer training and professional training services.

7150   **Hitchcock Rehabilitation Center**
690 Medical Park Dr
Aiken, SC 29801-6348   803-648-8344
800-207-6924
FAX: 803-648-1631
mail@hitchcockhealthcare.org
www.hitchcockhealthcare.org

Karen Bowlen, Administrator
Dan Hillman, Case Manager
Carrie Morgan, Finance Director
Comprehensive outpatient rehabilitation for adults, children, geriatrics, pediatric therapy, special needs preschool, sports medicine, home health and hospice.

7151   **Mentor Network, The**
3600 Forest Drive
Suite 100
Columbia, SC 29204-1891   803-799-9025
800-297-8043
FAX: 803-931-8959
thementornetwork.com

Edward Murphy, Executive Chairman
Bruce Nardella, President and CEO
Denis Holler, Chief Financial Officer
Jeffrey Cohen, Chief Information Officer
Mentor provides a full network of individually tailored services for people with development disabilities and their families. Individuals may be served in their homes, shared living home, or in a host home.

Tennessee

7152   **Humana Hospital: Morristown RehabCare**
726 McFarland St
Morristown, TN 37814-3989   423-522-6000
www.lakewayregionalhospital.com

James Perry, Program Director
Designed to help patients in their adjustment to a physically limiting condition by helping to maximize each patient's abilities so he or she can function as independently as possible.

7153   **Opportunity East Rehabilitation Services for the Blind**
758 W Morris Blvd
Morristown, TN 37813-2136   423-586-3922
800-278-6274
FAX: 423-586-1479
bandit75@charter.net
volblind.org

Fred Overbay, CEO
Vic Mende, Director Rehabilitation Services
Offers services for the totally blind, legally blind, visually impaired, mentally retarded blind and more with health, counseling, educational, recreational, rehabilitation, computer training and professional training services.

7154   **Patrick Rehab Wellness Center**
Lincoln County Health System
106 Medical Center Blvd
Fayetteville, TN 37334-2684   931-433-0273
FAX: 931-433-0378
www.ichealthsystem.com

Gloria Meadows, Administrator
Jim Stewart, Principal
Provides rehabilitation services of physical, occupational, and speech therapy. Also, wellness memberships are available to the public.

7155   **PharmaThera**
1785 Nonconnah Blvd
Memphis, TN 38132-2104   901-348-8100
800-767-6714
FAX: 901-348-8270

7156   **Siskin Hospital For Physical Rehabilitation**
1 Siskin Plz
Chattanooga, TN 37403-1306   423-634-1200
info@siskinrehab.org
siskinrehab.org

Bob Main, CEO
Robert P. Main, President
Dedicated exclusively to physical rehabilitation and offers specialized treatment programs in brain injury, amputation, stroke, spinal cord injury, orthopedics, and major multiple trauma. The hospital also provides treatment for neurological disorders and loss of muscle strength and controll following illness or surgery.

7157   **St. Mary's RehabCare Center**
900 E Oak Hill Ave
Knoxville, TN 37917-4556   865-545-7962
FAX: 865-545-8133

Debbie Keeton, Director
Beth Greco, Executive Director
Provides comprehensive rehabilitation services for patients experiencing CVA, head trauma, orthopedic conditions, spinal cord injury or neurological impairment.

Texas

7158 Alpine Ridge and Brandywood
444 Devereux Drive
Victoria, TX 19085-2666

361-575-8271
800-345-1292
FAX: 361-575-6520
devereux.org

Robert Q. Kreider, President and CEO
Margaret McGill, SVP, Chief Operations Officer
Robert C. Dunne, SVP & Chief Financial Officer, Treasurer
Marilyn B. Benoit, M.D., SVP, Chief Clinical Officer, Chief Medical Officer

7159 Amity Lodge
Devereux Foundation
444 Devereux Drive
Victoria, TX 19085-2666

361-575-8271
800-345-1292
FAX: 361-575-6520
devereux.org

Robert Q. Kreider, President and CEO
Margaret McGill, SVP, Chief Operations Officer
Robert C. Dunne, SVP & Chief Financial Officer, Treasurer
Marilyn B. Benoit, M.D., SVP, Chief Clinical Officer, Chief Medical Officer

Offers residents a continuum of services ranging from minimal care and supervision to total physical and medical care.

7160 Baylor Institute for Rehabilitation
3500 Gaston Avenue
Dallas, TX 75246-2017

214-820-9300
800-4BA-YLOR
FAX: 214-841-2679
www.baylorhealth.com

Joel T. Allison, Chief Executive Officer
Gary Brock, President and Chief Operating Officer
LaVone Arthur, Vice President of Business Development
Wm. Stephen Boyd, Chief Legal Officer

A 92-bed specialty hospital offering comprehensive rehabilitation services for persons with spinal cord injury, traumatic brain injury, stroke, amputation, and other orthopedic and neurological disorders.

7161 Beneto Center
Devereux Foundation
444 Devereux Drive
Victoria, TX 19085-2666

361-575-8271
800-345-1292
FAX: 361-575-6520
devereux.org

Robert Q. Kreider, President and CEO
Margaret McGill, SVP, Chief Operations Officer
Robert C. Dunne, SVP & Chief Financial Officer, Treasurer
Marilyn B. Benoit, M.D., SVP, Chief Clinical Officer, Chief Medical Officer

Offers a continuum of services for residents requiring services ranging from minimal care and supervision to total physical and medical care.

7162 CORE Health Care
E&J Health Care
400 Highway 290
Bldg B, Suite. 205,
Dripping Springs, TX 78620

512-894-0801
866-683-1007
FAX: 512-858-4627
info@corehealth.com
www.corehealth.com

Eric Makowski, CEO
Kristi Jones, Marketing/Admissions Director
Erika Mountz, MBA, OTR/L, Director of Rehabilitation
Annie Freeman, MBA, PHR, Director of Huma Resources

Post acute and transitional rehabilitation, long-term care, community re-entry, for brain injury and complex psychiatric disorders.

7163 Center for Neuro Skills
1320 W Walnut Hill Ln
Irving, TX 75038-3007

972-580-8500
800-544-5448
FAX: 972-255-3162
srobinson@neuroskills.com
neuroskills.com

John Schultz, Administrator
Mark J. Ashley, President

Centre for Neuro Skills (CNS) seeks to provide medical rehabilitation programs, lifecare programs, advocacy, and research for people with brain injury in order to achieve a maximum quality of life.

7164 Dallas Services
4242 Office Pkwy
Dallas, TX 75204-3629

214-828-9900
FAX: 214-828-9901
www.dallasservices.org

Thomas . Turnage, Ph.D, Executive Director
Clark Thomas, Ph.D., Chair
Melissa Malonson, Vice-Chair
Cynthia O'Brien Robinson, Secretary

Offers four programs:1) an early education for children(6weeks-6yrs)with and without special needs.2)low vision clinic-provides low cost eye examsand glasses to low-income families as well as assistance to individuals who vision problems which cannot be corrected with glasses/surgery.3)mesquite day school- an early head start program for infants and toddlers of low-income families.4)special needs advocacy and inclusion program that offers families of special need children guidance and education.

7165 Daman Villa
Devereux Foundation
444 Devereux Drive
Victoria, TX 19085-2666

361-575-8271
800-345-1292
FAX: 361-575-6520
devereux.org

Robert Q. Kreider, President and CEO
Margaret McGill, SVP, Chief Operations Officer
Robert C. Dunne, SVP & Chief Financial Officer, Treasurer
Marilyn B. Benoit, M.D., SVP, Chief Clinical Officer, Chief Medical Officer

Offers residents a continuum of services ranging from minimal care and supervision to total physical and medical care.

7166 Devereux Advanced Behavioral Health Texas- League City Campus
1150 Devereux Dr.
League City, TX 77573

800-373-0011
www.devereux.org

7167 Devereux Advanced Behavioral Health Texas- Victoria Campus
120 David Wade Dr.
P.O. Box 2666
Victoria, TX 77902-2666

361-574-7208
800-345-1292
www.devereux.org

Pam Reed, Executive Director

Residential services for children, young adults and adults, foster care services for birth to 18, community based living program and vocational programs. Emotional/behavioral disorders, intellectual/developmental disabilities, dual diagnosis, and mild autism spectrum disorders.

7168 El Paso Lighthouse for the Blind
200 Washington St
El Paso, TX 79905-3897

915-532-4495
FAX: 915-532-6338
www.lighthouse-elpaso.com

Craig Hays, President
Lea Cochran, Vice President
Lola Dawkins, Secretary
Rusty Hooten, Chief Financial Officer

Enables people of all ages to embody blindness and vision impairment through training, rehabilitation, employment opportunity, advocacy and research. Provides access to opportunities and quality of life so that the blind and visually impaired can reach their fullest potential for self-sufficiency and independence.

7169   Harris Methodist Fort Worth/Mabee Rehabilitation Center
612 E. Lamar Boulevard
Arlington, TX 76011-2122   877-847-9355
                                        FAX: 817-882-2753
                                        www.texashealth.org

Louise Baldwin, President
Peggyo Ehrlich, Rehab Manager
Karen Mallett, Executive Director
Douglas D. Hawthorne, Chief Executive Officer
A hospital based inpatient rehab program and outpatient day programs in chronic pain management, work hardening and brain injury transitional services.

7170   HealthSouth Hospital of Cypress
13031 Wortham Center Dr
Houston, TX 77065   832-280-2500
                                feedback@healthsouth.com
                                    healthsouthcypress.com

Jerome Lengel, Executive Officer
Dewitt Hilton, Owner
Offers an individualized approach to the process of rehabilitation for severely injured or disabled individuals. The process begins with a pre-admissions assessment of each referred patient. The Center combines state-of-the-art technology and equipment with multi-disciplinary therapy and education in a cheerful, secure environment.

7171   Heights Hospital Rehab Unit
1917 Ashland St
Houston, TX 77008-3994   713-861-6161
                                        FAX: 713-802-8660
                                      www.selectmedical.com

Theresa Davis, CEO
Robert A. Ortenzio, Executive Chairman and Co-Founder
Rocco A. Ortenzio, Vice Chairman and Co-Founder
David S. Chernow, President and Chief Executive Officer
This program is designed to assist patients with physical disabilities achieve their maximum functional abilities.

7172   Hillcrest Baptist Medical Center
100 Hillcrest Medical Blvd
Waco, TX 76712   254-202-2000
                                        FAX: 254-202-5105
                                              www.sw.org

Anne Hott Kimberly, Program Director
Ann Gammel, Nurse Manager
Debbie Meurer, Manager
Designed to assist patients in adjustment to a physically limiting condition, utilizing interdisciplinary strategies to maximize each patient's ability and capability.

7173   Institute for Rehabilitation & Research
1333 Moursund St
Houston, TX 77030-3405   713-799-5000
                                           800-447-3422
                                        FAX: 713-797-5289
                                    tirr.memorialhermann.org

Carl Josehart, CEO
Jean Herzog, President
Gerard E. Francisco, M.D., Chief Medical Officer
Mary Ann Euliarte, CNO/COO
A national center for information, training, research, and technical assistance in independent living. The goal is to extend the body of knowledge in independent living and to improve the utilization of results of research programs and demonstration projects in this field. It has developed a variety of strategies for collecting, synthesizing, and disseminating information related to the field of independent living.

7174   Integrated Health Services of Amarillo
6141 Amarillo Blvd. West
Amarillo, TX 79106   806-356-0488
                                        FAX: 806-356-8074
                                  cheryl.studer@medcenter.org
                                        www.medcenter.org

Mary Bearden, Chairman
Jay L. Barrett, President
Marvin Franz, Executive Director & CEO
Provides acute, post acute, residential and outpatient health care services. IHS of Amarillo is a 153-bed facility with 120 beds licensed by The Texas Department of Health and Human Services, and is accredited by JCAHO. We serve urban and rural populations of over 500,000, drawing from a 5-state region.

7175   Kanner Center
Devereax Foundation
444 Devereux Drive
Victoria, TX 19085-2666   361-575-8271
                                           800-345-1292
                                        FAX: 361-575-6520
                                              devereux.org

Robert Q. Kreider, President and CEO
Margaret McGill, SVP, Chief Operations Officer
Robert C. Dunne, SVP & Chief Financial Officer, Treasurer
Marilyn B. Benoit, M.D., SVP, Chief Clinical Officer, Chief Medical Officer
A private nonprofit nationwide network of treatment services for individuals of all ages with emotional and/or developmental disabilities.

7176   Lighthouse of Houston
3602 W Dallas St
Houston, TX 77019-1704   713-527-9561
                                        FAX: 713-284-8451
                                  custserv@houstonlighthouse.org
                                      houstonlighthouse.org

Gibson DuTerroil, President
Shelagh Moran, VP/COO
Chelean Zander, VP Community Programs
Serves the blind, visually impaired, deaf-blind and multihandicapped blind. Provides workshops, vocational training and placement, low vision clinic, orientation and mobility, housing, Braille, volunteer services, senior center, visual aid sales, counseling and support, diabetic education and day health activity services and day summer camp, Summer Transition for Youth.

7177   Mainland Center Hospital RehabCare Unit
6801 Emmett F Lowry Expy
Texas City, TX 77591-2500   409-938-5000
                                        FAX: 409-938-5501
                                    www.mainlandmedical.com

Michael Ehrat, CEO
The RehabCare program is designed and staffed to assist functionally impaired patients improve to their maximum potential. The opportunities for improvement and adjustments are provided in a pleasant, supportive inpatient environment by therapists from the occupational, physical, recreational and speech therapy disciplines.

7178   North Texas Rehabilitation Center
1005 Midwestern Pkwy
Wichita Falls, TX 76302-2211   940-322-0771
                                        FAX: 940-766-4943
                                              ntrehab.org

Mike Castles, President/ CEO
Provides outpatient rehabilitation services to maximize independence or promote development to children and adults with disabilities. Programs include: physical, occupational, speech therapy, closed head injury, infant/child development, support groups, aquatics and wellness program and a child achievement program.

7179 **South Texas Lighthouse for the Blind**
PO BOX 9697
Corpus Christi, TX 78469-3321
361-883-6553
888-255-8011
FAX: 361-883-1041
Customer.service@stlb.net
www.stlb.net

Regis Barber, President
Nicky Ooi, Chief Operations Officer
Alana Manrow, Public Affairs Director
Their mission is to Employ, Educate and Empower their neighbors who are blind and visually impaired. They offer job opportunities in manufacturing, retail and administration, as well as orientation and mobility and adaptive technology training.

7180 **Texas Specialty Hospital at Dallas**
7955 Harry Hines Blvd
Dallas, TX 75235-3305
214-637-0000
FAX: 214-637-6512
Mary.Alexander@fundltc.com
www.texasspecialtydallas.com

Mary Alexander, CEO
Cathy Campbell, Chief Executive Officer
66 beds offering active/acute rehabilitation, brain injury day treatment, cognitive rehabilitation, complex care, extended rehabilitation and short term evaluation.

7181 **Transitional Learning Center at Gavelston and Lubbock**
1528 Post Office St
Galveston, TX 77550
409-762-6661
FAX: 409-763-3930
www.tlcrehab.org

Brent Masel, MD, President and Medical Director
Gary Seale, Ph.D., VP Clinical Programs
Jim Lovelace, MBA, VP of Operations
Shelley Kessler, CPA, Chief Financial Officer
Specializes solely in post-acute brain injury. A nationally known pioneer in the field and a not for profit with a three fold mission: treatment, research and education. Offers 6 hours of therapy a day from licensed/certified staff, on site physician and nursing services and long-term living for brian injured adults at Tideway on Gavelston Island. Accredited by CARF.
1982

7182 **Treemont Nursing And Rehabilitation Center**
5550 Harvest Hill Rd
Dallas, TX 75230-1684
972-661-1862
FAX: 972-788-1543
moreinfo@treemonthealthcare.com
treemonthealthcare.com

Bob Barker, Administrator
Postacute rehabilitation program.

7183 **West Texas Lighthouse for the Blind**
2001 Austin St
San Angelo, TX 76903-8796
325-653-4231
FAX: 325-657-9367
customerservice@lighthousefortheblind.org
www.lighthousefortheblind.org

David Wells, Executive Director
Stephen Horton, Operations Manager
Fonda V. Galindo, Finance & Human Resources Manager
Vickie Sanders, Sales & Marketing Manager
Offers services for the totally blind, legally blind, visually impaired, mentally retarded blind and more with health, counseling, educational, recreational, rehabilitation, computer training and professional training services.

Utah

7184 **Quincy Rehabilitation Institute of Holy Cross Hospital**
1050 E South Temple
Salt Lake City, UT 84102-1507
801-350-8140
FAX: 801-350-4791

Dave Jenson, President

Postacute rehabilitation program.

7185 **Wasatch Vision Clinic**
849 E 400 S
Salt Lake City, UT 84102-2928
801-328-2020
FAX: 801-363-2201
email@wasatchvision.com
eyeappointment.com

Craig Cutler, Owner
Camron Bateman OD, Doctor
Postacute rehabilitation program.

Vermont

7186 **Rutland Mental Health Services**
78 S Main St
Rutland, VT 05701-4594
802-775-2381
FAX: 802-775-4020
rmhsccn.org

Dan Quinn, President/ CEO
Scott Dikeman, Vice Chairman
Ron Holm, Secretary
Tom Pour, Treasurer
A private, non-profit comprehensive community mental health center. It provides services to individuals and families for mental health and substance abuse related problems and also to persons who are mentally retarded.

Virginia

7187 **Bay Pine-Virginia Beach**
680 South Fourth Street
Louisville, KY 40202
502-596-7300
TTY:800-545-0749
web_administrator@kindred.com
kindredhealthcare.com

Paul J. Diaz, President/ CEO
Postacute rehabilitation program.

7188 **Carilion Rehabilitation: New River Valley**
2013 S Jefferson Street
Roanoke, VA 24014
540-981-7377
FAX: 540-981-8233
www.carilionclinic.org

Nancy Howell Agee, President/ CEO
James A. Hartley, Chair
Briggs W. Andrews, Corporate Secretary
G. Robert Vaughan, Jr., Treasurer, SVP
CARF-accredited pain management program, work hardening program and comprehensive outpatient therapy clinic, massage therapy, outpatient programs and more. Program emphasis is on interdisiplinary behavioral rehab based pain management and functional restoration in conjunction with medical treatment. Work hardening is a transdisciplinary work simulation program taylored to the individual. Comprehensive outpatient program is multi-disciplinary with emphasis on manual treatment.

7189 **Faith Mission Home**
3540 Mission Home Ln
Free Union, VA 22940-1505
434-985-2294
FAX: 434-985-7633
www.beachyam.org

Paul Beiler, Manager
Reuben Yoder, Director
A Christian residential center that serves 60 mentally retarded children, including individuals with Down Syndrome, Cerebral palsy and other similar conditions. Children may be admitted from the time they are ambulatory until they reach 15 years of age. He or she may stay as long as it is in the child's best interests. The training program stresses the following areas: self-care, social, academic, vocational, crafts, speech and physical development.

7190 ManorCare Health Services-Arlington
333 N. Summit St.
Toledo, OH 43604

800-366-1232
CareLine@hcr-manorcare.com
hcr-manorcare.com

Marcia K Jarrell, Administrator
Ric Birch, Marketing Director
ManorCare-Arlington offers residents a full Continuum of Care in a caring environment. ManorCare's wide range of services includes subacute medical and rehabilitation programs for short term patients transitioning from hospital to home and Skilled Nursing Care.

7191 Pines Residential Treatment Center
825 Crawford Pkwy
Portsmouth, VA 23704-2301

757-393-0061
FAX: 757-393-1029

Lenard J Lexier, Medical Director
Judy Kemp, Admissions Director
A 310-bed residential treatment center in Portsmouth Virginia, providing a therapeutic environment for severely emotionally disturbed children and youth. Five unique programs meet behavioral, educational and emotional needs of males and females, five to twenty-two years of age. Multi-disciplinary teams devise individual service plans to enhance strengths and reverse self-defeating behavior. A highly effective positive reinforcement program with a proven track record.

7192 Resurrection Children's Center
2280 N Beauregard St
Alexandria, VA 22311-2200

703-998-0888
FAX: 703-820-2912
office@welcometoresurrection.org
www.welcometoresurrection.org

Jane McCabe, Parish Administrator
Deena Jaworski, Director of Music
Offers children ages 2-5 with varying disabilities academic education, parent education, opportunities including classes, workshops, support groups and individual counseling.

7193 Roanoke Memorial Hospital
Carilion Health System
2013 S Jefferson Street
Roanoke, VA 24014

540-981-7377
FAX: 540-981-8233
www.carilionclinic.org

Nancy Howell Agee, President/ CEO
James A. Hartley, Chair
Briggs W. Andrews, Corporate Secretary
G. Robert Vaughan, Jr., Treasurer, SVP
Carilion Health System exists to improve the health of the communities it serves. The vision is to assure accessible, affordable, high quality healthcare that meets the needs of the community. Motivate and educate individuals to improve their health. Champion community initiatives to reduce health risk

7194 Southside Virginia Training Center
P.O.Box 4030
Petersburg, VA 23803-30

804-524-7000
FAX: 804-524-7228
www.svtc.dbhds.virginia.gov

Bob Kaufman, Director, Administrative Service
Offers residential, vocational, occupational, physical, and speech therapies.

7195 Woodrow Wilson Rehabilitation Center
P.O.Box 1500
Fishersville, VA 22939-1500

540-332-7000
800-345-9972
FAX: 540-332-7132
colemawl@wwrc.state.va.lls
www.wwrc.net

Rick Sizemore, Executive Director
Amy Blalock, Admissions and Marketing Director
Comprehensive residential rehabilitation center offering complete medical and vocational rehabilitation services including: vocation evaluation, vocational training, transition from school to work, occupational therapy, physical therapy, speech, language and audiology, assistive technology, rehabilitation engineering, counseling/case management, behavioral health services, nursing and physician services, etc.

Washington

7196 Arden Rehabilitation And Healthcare Center
680 South Fourth Street
Louisville, KY 40202

502-596-7300
TTY:800-545-0749
web_administrator@kindred.com
kindredhealthcare.com

Paul J. Diaz, President/ CEO
Arden can accomodate 90 residents- post-acute/rehabilitation patients as well as long term residents. Medicare certified, the center also takes most managed healthcare insurance plans, as well as VA, respite and hospice patients.

7197 Bellingham Care Center
680 South Fourth Street
Louisville, KY 40202

502-596-7300
TTY:800-545-0749
web_administrator@kindred.com
kindredhealthcare.com

Paul J. Diaz, President/ CEO
Postacute rehabilitation program.

7198 Division of Vocational Rehabilitation Department of Social and Health Services
P.O.Box 45130
Olympia, WA 98504-5130

360-704-3560
800-737-0617
FAX: 360-570-6941
krulik@dshs.wa.gov
www1.dshs.wa.gov/dvr

Patrick Raines, Manager
Lynnea Ruttledge, Manager
Information on computers, supported employment, marketing rehabilitation facilities and transition.

7199 First Hill Care Center
1334 Terry Ave
Seattle, WA 98101

206-682-2661
FAX: 206-624-0188
www.khseattlefirsthill.com

7200 Harborview Medical Center, Low Vision Aid Clinic
Harborview Medical Center
325 9th Ave
Seattle, WA 98104-2499

206-744-3300
TTY:206-744-3246
comment@u.washington.edu
www.uwmedicine.org

Eileen Whalen, Executive director
J. Richard Goss, M.D.,, Medical director
Darcy Jaffe, Chief nursing officer and senior associate for patient care
Elise Chayet, Associate administrator, clinical support services and plan
Harborview Medical Center is the only designated Level 1 adult and pediatric trauma and burn center in the state of Washington and serves as the regional trauma and burn referral center for Alaska, Montana and Idaho. UW Medicine physicians and staff based at Harborview provide highly specialized services for vascular, orthopedics, neurosciences, ophthalmology, behavioral health, HIV/AIDS and complex critical care.

7201 Integrated Health Services of Seattle
820 NW 95th St
Seattle, WA 98117-2207

206-783-7649
FAX: 206-781-1448

Jerry Harvey, Administrator
Marlette Basada, Director Nursing
Flavia Lagrange, Director Admissions

Postacute rehabilitation program. IHS provides 24 hour subacute and long-term care. We can handle vent/trach/hemo andritoneal dialysis and provide a full scope of rehabilitation services.

7202 Lakeside Milam Recovery Centers (LMRC)
3315 S. 23rd Street
Ste 102
Tacoma, WA 98405 253-272-2242
800-231-4303
FAX: 253-272-0171
help@lakesidemilam.com
www.lakesidemilam.com

Michael Kinder, Administrator
LMRC was established in 1983 with a single mission, to help victims and families recover from the pain of drug/alcohol addiction. Enlightned by the work of Dr. James Milam in the 1960's and 70's, the founders of LMRC created a treatment system based on a bedrock set of principals.

7203 Lakewood Health Care Center
11411 Bridgeport Way SW
Lakewood, WA 98499-3047 253-581-9002
800-359-7412
FAX: 253-581-7016
www.lakewoodhc.com

Gwynn Rucker, Executive Director
Patty Wood, Administrator
Linda Doll, Social Services
Dr. Mian , Medical Director
Accomodates 80 residents. We offer 24 hour skilled nursing services, long-term care and rehab services which include Physical, Occupational and Speech Therapy.

7204 Manor Care Health Services-Tacoma
5601 S Orchard St
Tacoma, WA 98409-1371 253-474-8421
FAX: 253-471-8857
www.hcr-manorcare.com

Tina Irwin, Administrator
124-bed skilled nursing and rehabilitation center provides services for those seeking long term Skilled Nursing Care, short term subacute care, hospice services, Alzheimer's and respite care. Our Acadia Wing, a specialized Alzheimer's care unit, provides specialized programming and trained staff that truly makes us the leader in Alzheimers Services.

7205 ManorCare Health Services-Lynnwood
3701 188th St SW
Lynnwood, WA 98037-7626 425-775-9222
FAX: 425-712-3685
www.hcr-manorcare.com

Liza Loyet, Administrator
Our in-house therapists provide physical, occupational and speech therapies in our state-of-the-art therapy gym. Our team is goal oriented and focuses on producing positive outcomes for those recovering from illness, injury or surgery.

7206 ManorCare Health Services-Spokane
6025 N Assembly St
Spokane, WA 99205-7674 509-326-8282
FAX: 509-326-4790
www.hcrmanorcare.com

Cheri Kubu, Administrator
Sandra Hayes, Administrator
Provides skilled nursing and respite stays for those needing a break from care giving. We specialize in Rehabilitation Services provided by our in-house occupational, physical and speech therapists.

7207 Northwest Continuum Care Center
Kindred Health Care
128 Old Beacon Hill Dr
Longview, WA 98632-5859 360-423-4060
FAX: 360-636-0958
www.nwcontinuum.com

Steve M. Ross, Executive Director
Tami Wilson, Director of Nursing
Mary R., Activities Assistant
Kristen W., Health and Rehabilitation Center
Accomodates 69 residents. Employs the Angel Care Program designed to address any special needs that may arise during a resident's stay in our facility. The program focuses extra attention on residents and, in some cases, family members. The goal is to meet the special needs of the people we provide care to every day.

7208 Park Manor Convalescent Center
1710 Plaza Way
Walla Walla, WA 99362-4362 509-529-4218
FAX: 509-522-1729
egines@ensigngroup.net
www.parkmanorcare.com

Jed Gines, Administrator
Krista Maiuri, Directr Of Nursing
Sonya Taylor, Director of Rehabilitation
Mike Henckel, Admissions & Marketing Director
Residents of Park Manor enjoy a range of activities, developed to meet their needs, inculding excercise programs, social and recreational activities, arts and crafts, shopping trips and other excursions. We also offer religious services.

7209 Queen Anne Health Care
Queen Anne Health Care
2717 Dexter Ave N
Seattle, WA 98109-1914 206-284-7012
FAX: 206-283-3936
www.queenannehealthcare.com

Heather Eacker, Executive Director
Mary R., Activities Assistant
Kristen W., Health and Rehabilitation Center
Becky D., Activity Director
Our goal is to provide quality, compassionate care. Our cozy building accomodates 120 residents. We offer semi private rooms with space to add items from home for a special personalized touch

7210 Rainier Vista Care Center
920 12th Ave SE
Puyallup, WA 98372-4920 253-841-3422
FAX: 253-848-3937
www.rainiervistacc.com

Linda Larson, Administrator
Nancy L. Erckenbrack, Executive Director
Kristen W., Health and Rehabilitation Center
Becky D., Activity Director
Accomodates 120 residents. We are certified for Medicare and Medicaid and we offer a continuum of healthcare services from short-term or outpatient rehabilitation to long-term care. We offer semi-private and private rooms as well as rehabilitation and hospice suites. Rainier Vista Care Center is a recipient of the American Health Care Association Quality Award.

7211 Rehabilitation Enterprises of Washington
430 E Lauridsen Blvd
Port Angeles, WA 98362-7978 360-452-9789
FAX: 360-452-9700

Brett White, President
REW is the professional trade association representing community rehabilitation programs before government and other publics. These organizations provide a wide array of employment and training services for people with disabilities. The goal is to assist member organizations to provide the highest quality rehabilitative and employment services to their customers.

7212 Seattle Medical and Rehabilitation Center
Evergreen Healthcare
12040 NE 128th St
Kirkland, WA 98034-3013

425-899-3000
877-601-2271
TTY:425-899-2007
comment@evergreenhealthcare.org
evergreenhealthcare.org

Al DeYoung, Chair
Robert H. Malte, Chief Executive Officer
Neil Johnson, RN, MSA, Senior Vice President & Chief Operating Officer
Nancee Hofmeister, Vice President, Chief Nursing Officer
103 beds offering subacute rehabilitation, complex care, subacute treatment and short-term evaluation. Pulmonary unit offering long and short term care for ventilator dependent patients.

7213 Slingerland Institute for Literacy
Educators Publishing Service
12729 Northup Way
Suite 1
Bellevue, WA 98005

425-453-1190
FAX: 425-635-7762
mail@slingerland.org
www.slingerland.org

Bonnie Meyer, Executive Director
Elyce Newton, Program Support
A nonprofit public corporation founded in 1977 to carry on the work of Beth H. Slingerland in providing classroom teachers with the techniques, knowledge and understanding necessary for identifying and teaching children with Specific Language Disability. The main objective is to educate teachers in successful methods of identifying, diagnosing and instructing children and adults with SLD and to promote literacy through reading, writing and oral expression.

7214 Timberland Opportunities Association
400 W Curtis St
Aberdeen, WA 98520-7698

360-533-5823
FAX: 360-533-5848
jimeddy@techline.com
www.users.olynet.com/timberlandopp

Jim Eddy, Executive Director
Provides training and employment for disabled people.

7215 Vancouver Health and Rehabilitation Center
400 E 33rd St
Vancouver, WA 98663-2238

360-696-2561
FAX: 360-696-9275
www.vancouverhealthcare.com

Jody Wigen, Human Resources
Joe Joy, Executive Director
Kristen W., Health and Rehabilitation Center
Becky D., Activity Director
Postacute rehabilitation program.

Wisconsin

7216 Colonial Manor Medical And Rehabilitation Center
1010 E Wausau Ave
Wausau, WI 54403-3101

715-842-2028
FAX: 715-848-0510
www.colonialmanormrc.com

Ericca Ylitalo, Administrator
Shelley Solberg, Executive Director
Colonial Manor Medical and Rehabilitation Center is part of the Kindred Community and is located in Wausau, Wisconsin. The corporate headquarters are based in Louisville Kentucky. Our facility accomodates 150 residents.

7217 Waushers Industries
210 E Chicago Rd
Wautoma, WI 54982-6932

920-787-4696
FAX: 920-787-4698

Richard King, Human Resources

Provides various programming for individuals with disabilities in waushara county.

7218 Woodstock Health and Rehabilitation Center
3415 Sheridan Rd
Kenosha, WI 53140-1924

262-657-6175
FAX: 262-657-5756
www.woodstockhealth.com

Debra Lamb, Administrator
Darlene Einerson, Executive Director
Kristen W., Health and Rehabilitation Center
Becky D., Activity Director
Offers a full range of medical services to meet the individual needs of our residents, including short term rehabilitative services and long-tern skilled care.

Rehabilitation Facilities, Sub-Acute

Alabama

7219   UAB Spain Rehabilitation Center
1717 6th Ave S
Birmingham, AL 35233-7330   205-934-3450
www.uab.edu/medicine/physicalmedicine/
Tracy L Brewer, Administrative Manager
A 49-bed rehabilitation hospital featuring advanced, individualized care for adolescents and adult patients recovering from a broad variety of health problems. Patient care teams include physiatrists (doctors who specialized in rehabilitation medicine), nurses, nurse practitioners, physical therapists, occupational therapists, speech/language pathologists, psychologists, social workers, rehabilitation professionals and other health care professionals from all areas of the UAB Health System.

Alaska

7220   Fairbanks Memorial Hospital & DenaliCenter
1650 Cowles St
Fairbanks, AK 99701-5998   907-452-8181
FAX: 907-458-5324
www.fmhdc.com
Sheldon Stadnyk, MD, Interim Chief Executive Officer
The Denali Center offers the following rehabilitation services: Physical Therapy, Occupational Therapy, Speech Therapy, Sub-Acute Rehab.

Arizona

7221   Desert Life Rehabilitation & Care Center
Kindred Healthcare
1919 W Medical St
Tucson, AZ 85704-1133   520-297-8311
FAX: 520-544-0930
www.desertlifecc.com
Amad Nazifi, Executive Director
Jane Olmstead, Director of Nursing
Accomodates 240 residents. We provide skilled and intermediate nursing with occupational, physical, speech and respiratory therapy services. We offer special programs including an Alzheimer's Unit and a Young Adult Program, and are located in beautiful Southern Arizona where there is plenty of sunshine, mountains and desert views. Desert Life is a 2005 recipient of the American Health Care Association Quality Award.

7222   Hacienda Rehabilitation and Care Center
660 S Coronado Dr
Sierra Vista, AZ 85635-3386   520-459-4900
FAX: 520-458-4082
www.haciendarcc.com
Monica Vandivort, Medical Director
Kristen W., Health and Rehabilitation Center Executive Director
Becky D., Activity Director
Mary R., Activities Assistant
Accomodates 100 residents. We are located in Sierra Vista, near Kartchner Caverns, Fort Huachuca, Coronado National Forest and historic Tombstone. Serving the medical needs of the community since 1983, we strive to provide care with quality, compassion and integrity.

7223   Kachina Point Health Care & Rehabilitation Center
505 Jacks Canyon Rd
Sedona, AZ 86351-7856   928-284-1000
FAX: 928-284-0626
www.kindredkachinapoint.com
Michael Amadei, Medical Director
Accomodates 120 residents. We have met the healthcare needs of the community since 1984. Kachina Point is a 2004 recipient of the American Health Care Association's Quality Award.

7224   Mayo Clinic Scottsdale
13400 E Shea Blvd
Scottsdale, AZ 85259-5499   480-301-8000
800-446-2279
FAX: 480-301-9310
www.mayoclinic.org/arizona
Neena S. Abraham, Gastroenterology/ Hepatology
Roberta H. Adams, Hematology/Oncology
Charles H. Adler, Parkinson's Disease and Movement Disorders Center
Neera Agarwal, Hospital Internal Medicine
Mayo clinic is a not-for-profit medical practice dedicated to the diagnosis and treatment of virtually every type of complex illness. Mayo clinic staff members work together to meet your needs. You will see as many doctors, specialists, and other health care professionals as needed to provide comprehensive diagnosis, understandable answers and effective treatment.

7225   Sonoran Rehabilitation and Care Center
Kindred
4202 N 20th Ave
Phoenix, AZ 85015-5101   602-264-3824
FAX: 602-279-6234
Jeffrey Barrett, Executive Director
Offers the following rehabilitation services: Respiratory Therapy, Physical Therapy, Speech Therapy, Occupational Therapy, Restorative Therapy, Sub-Acute Rehabilitation, Wound Care.

7226   Valley Health Care and Rehabilitation Center
Kindred Health Care Center
5545 E Lee St
Tucson, AZ 85712-4205   520-296-2306
FAX: 520-296-4072
www.valleyhcr.com
Dale Pelton, Executive Director
Sandra Lewis, Administrator
Offers the following rehabilitation services: Physical Therapy, Occupational Therapy, Speech Therapy, Sub-Acute Rehab.

California

7227   Alamitos-Belmont Rehab Hospital
3901 E 4th St
Long Beach, CA 90814-1699   562-434-8421
FAX: 562-433-6732
www.alamitosbelmont.com
John L. Sorensen, Chairman of the Board of Directors.
Jonathan Sloey, Administrator
Offers the following rehabilitation services: Speech Therapy, Occupational Therapy, Physical Therapy, Sub-Acute Rehab.

7228   Bay View Nursing and Rehabilitation Center
Kindred Health Care
516 Willow St
Alameda, CA 94501-6132   510-521-5600
FAX: 510-865-9035
www.kindredhealthcare.com
Richard S Espinoza, Administrator
Say Silva, Assistant Executive Director
Accomodates 180 residents. Bay View is a 2004 recipient of the American Health Care Association's Quality Award. We provide short-term rehabilitative care, traditional long-term skilled care and Alzheimer's/dementia special care. Our combination of clinical skill and comprehensive rehabilitation services enables us to care for a variety of complex medical conditions.

7229 Foothill Nursing and Rehab Center
401 W Ada Ave
Glendora, CA 91741-4241
626-335-9810
FAX: 626-963-0720
www.foothillnursing.com

Arnie Shafer, Executive Director
Marianne Schultz, Administrator
Offers the following rehabilitation services: Physical Therapy, Occupational Therapy, Speech Therapy, In and Out Patient Rehab.

7230 Long Beach Memorial Medical Center Memorial Rehabilitation Hospital
2801 Atlantic Ave
Ground Floor
Long Beach, CA 90806-1701
562-933-9001
FAX: 562-933-9019
www.memorialcare.org/long_beach

Barry Arbuckle, President/CEO
The goal of the MemorialCare Rehabilitation Institute is to help persons with disabilities regain independence and rebuild their lives in an environment where loved ones are involved in the rehabilitation process. We are dedicated to the pursuit of our mission, vision and values.

7231 Mercy Medical Center Mt. Shasta
914 Pine St
Mount Shasta, CA 96067-2143
530-926-6111
FAX: 530-926-0517
www.mercymtshasta.org

Greg Lippert, Senior Director of Support and Information Services
Scott Foster, Director of Hospital Finance
Sister Anne Chester, Director of Mission Integration
Joyce Zwanziger, Director Marketing, Community Relations & Volunteer Services
Mercy Medical Center is committed to furthering the healing ministry of Jesus, and to provide high-quality, affordable healthcare to the communities we serve.

7232 Northridge Hospital Medical Center
18300 Roscoe Blvd
Northridge, CA 91328-4167
818-885-8500
www.northridgehospital.org

Michael Wall, CEO
Offers the following rehabilitation services: Physical Therapy, Occupational Therapy, Speech Therapy, Sub-Acute Rehab. As a member of the Catholic Heathcare West Northridge Hospital Medical Center is committed to serving the health needs of our communities with particular attention to the needs of the poor, the disadvantaged and vulnerable, and the comfort of the suffering and dying.

7233 Riverside Community Hospital
4445 Magnolia Ave
Riverside, CA 92501
951-788-3000
FAX: 630-792-5636
complaint@jointcommission.org
www.riversidecommunityhospital.com

Jaime Wesolowski, President/CEO
Patrick Brilliant, CEO
At Riverside Community Hospital, we are able to provide the healthcare services that you and your family will need through the many stages of your life. Services like Emergency/Trauma, Labor and Delivery, Cardiac Care, Orthopedics and Transplant are among our many Centers of Excellence.

7234 Saint Jude Medical Center
101 E Valencia Mesa Dr
Fullerton, CA 92835-3809
714-871-3280
800-870-7537
FAX: 714-992-3029
www.stjudemedicalcenter.org

April De Cou, Wellness Educator
Jane Wang, Wellness Programs Supervisor
Offers the following rehabilitation services: Out-patient Rehab, Sub-Acute Rehab, Occupational Therapy, Physical Therapy, Speech and Audiology Therapy, Pain Management Program.

7235 South Coast Medical Center
12 Mason
Suite A
Irvine, CA 92618-2733
714-669-4446
FAX: 714-669-4448
info@southcoastmedcenter.com
www.mission4health.com

Leigh Erin Connealy, Manager
Bruce Christian, President
Offers the following services: physical therapy, occupational therapy, speech therapy, cardica rehabilitation, incontinence program, sub-acute rehabilitation.

7236 Valley Garden Health Care and Rehabilitation Center
1517 Knickerbocker Dr
Stockton, CA 95210-3119
209-957-4539
FAX: 209-957-5831
www.valleygardenshealth.com

Dr. Alexande Chan, Medical Director
Accomodates 120 residents. Our center provides short-term nursing and rehabilitative care as well as traditional long-term skilled care. Our combination of clinical skill and comprehensive rehabilitation services enables us to care for a variety of complex medical conditions. Rehabilitative therapies are provided as needed by physical, occupational and speech therapists.

Colorado

7237 Boulder Community Hospital Mapleton Center
1100 Balsam
PO Box 9019
Boulder, CO 80301-9019
303-440-2273
info@bch.org
www.bch.org

Lou DellaCava, Chairman
Ric Porreca, Vice Chairman
Jean Dubofsky, Secretary
R. David Hoover, Treasurer
159-bed acute care hospital and 24-hour emergency department.

7238 Fairacres Manor
1700 18th Ave
Greeley, CO 80631-5152
970-353-3370
FAX: 970-353-9347
www.fairacresmanor.com

Kathy Gardner, Admissions/Marketing Director
Marla Trujillo, Director of Nursing
Ben Gonzales, Admissions/Marketing Assistant Director
Kathleen Mekelburg, Administrator
Offers the following rehabilitation services: Physical Therapy, Occupational Therapy, Speech Therapy, Restorative Therapy, Skilled Nursing, and Sub-Acute Rehabilitation.

7239 Rowan Community
4601 E Asbury Cir
Denver, CO 80222-4722
303-757-1228
FAX: 303-759-3390
tgleisner@pinonmgt.com
pinonmgt.com

Tammy Gleisner, Director/Admissions/Marketing Director
Jeff Jerebker, President/CEO
Bruce Odenthal, VP Operations
John D. Brammeier, CPA, FHFMA,, Chief Financial Officer
Rowan is a 70-bed community, small enough to support personal relationships between residents and caregivers. Our residents vary in age, reflecting the diversity of a much larger community. Rowan's focus is on a psycho-social model of care with a dynamic activities and social service program. Our staff is specially trained in behavior management and many are certified Eden AlternativeT associates and certifid Elder Care Specialists.

Connecticut

7240 Hamilton Rehabilitation and Healthcare Center
89 Viets St
New London, CT 6320-3355
860-447-1471
FAX: 860-439-0107

Steve Roizen, Executive Director
Offers the following rehabilitation services: Sub-Acute, Occupational Therapy, Speech Therapy, Physical Therapy.

7241 Hospital For Special Care (HSC)
2150 Corbin Ave
New Britain, CT 06053-2298
860-223-2761
FAX: 860-827-4849
info@hfsc.org
www.hfsc.org

John J. Votto, President/CEO
Paul J. Scalise, M.D., F.C.C.P, Senior Vice President
Thomas J. Soltis, M.D., M.P.H., Chief of Geriatrics
HSC is a private, not-for-profit 200-bed rehabilitation long-term acute and chronic care hospital, widely-known and respected for its expertise in physical rehabilitation, respiratory care, and medically-complex pediatrics. Special programs for spinal cord injuries, pulmonary rehabilitation, acquired brain injuries, stroke, ventilator management and geriatrics, make HSC an important regional resource for patients with special healthcare needs.

7242 Masonic Healthcare Center
MasoniCare Corporation
22 Masonic Ave
PO Box 70
Wallingford, CT 06492-3048
203-679-5900
877-424-3537
FAX: 203-679-6459
info@masonicare.org
www.masonicare.org

Stephen B. McPherson, President
Arthur Santilli, President
The states leading provider of healthcare and retirement living communities for seniors. We are not-for-profit and have more then 100 years of experience behind us. We're recognized for the quality, compassionate care and steadfast support we provide to our residents and patients.

7243 Stamford Hospital
30 Shelburne Rd
Stamford, CT 06904-3628
203-276-1000
FAX: 203-325-7905
info@stamhealth.org
www.stamfordhospital.org

Brian Grissler, President/CEO
Kathleen Silard, EVP/Chief Operating Officer
Kevin Gage, Senior Vice President, Finance/Chief Financial Officer
Sharon Kiely, MD, Senior Vice President, Medical Affairs/Chief Medical Officer
A not-for-profit, community teaching hospital that has been serving Stamford and surrounding communities for more then 100 years. We have 305 inpatient beds in medicine, surgery, obstetrics/gynecology, psychiatry, and medical and surgical critical care units and maintain an educational partnership with Columbia University College of Physicians and Surgeons for its teaching program in the internal medicine, family practice, obstetrics/gynecology and surgery

7244 Windsor Rehabilitation and Healthcare Center
581 Poquonock Ave
Windsor, CT 06095-2202
860-688-7211
FAX: 860-688-6715
www.windsorrehab.com

Jeffrey Robbins, Medical Director
Accomodates 116 residents. We offer private and semi-private rooms with access to private telephones and cable television. Our goal is to be a comprehensive, leading care center viewed by our community as an excellent resource for patients, families, and professionals.

Delaware

7245 Arbors at New Castle
32 Buena Vista Dr
New Castle, DE 19720-4660
302-328-2580
FAX: 302-326-4132
newcastle@extendicare.com
www.extendicareus.com/newcastle

Annette Moore, Administrator
A subacute and rehabilitation center offering skilled medical services, infusion therapies, cardiac recovery services, renal disease services, cancer services and digestive disease services. Skilled rehabilitation services include physical therapy, occupational therapy and speech therapy. Also provides case management and discharge planning, general nursing and restorative care and respite care.

Florida

7246 Avon Oaks Skilled Care Nursing Facility
37800 French Creek Rd
Avon, OH 44011-1763
440-934-5204
800-589-5204
jreidy@avonoaks.net
www.avonoaks.net

Natalie McIntyre, Human Resources Director
Stephanie Auvil, RN, BC, Director of Nursing
Joan Reidy, Administrator
Richard J. Reidy, Technologies & Information Manager
Oaks at Avon provides a full range of skilled nursing services including infusion therapy, enteral therapy, wound care, tracheotomy care, and portable diagnostics.

7247 Boca Raton Rehabilitation Center
755 Meadows Rd
Boca Raton, FL 33486-2384
561-391-5200
FAX: 561-391-0685

Stanley Mucinic, Administrator
Tracey Dougherty, Administrator
Offers the following rehabilitation services: Occupational Therapy, Speech Therapy, Physical Therapy, Sub-Acute Rehabilitation

7248 Cape Coral Hospital
636 Del Prado Blvd
Cape Coral, FL 33990
239-424-2000
FAX: 239-574-1935
www.leememorial.org

Richard Akin, Chairman
Sanford Cohen, MD, Vice Chairman
Marilyn Stout, Treasurer
Diane Champion, Secretary
A 291-bed acute care facility, Cape Coral Hospital features all private rooms. The hospital currently is undergoing a complete renovation, expansion and modernization of the Weigner-Taeni Center for Emergency Services, which will make the emergency department the largest in Lee County.

7249 Evergreen Woods Health and Rehabilitation Center
7045 Evergreen Woods Trl
Spring Hill, FL 34608-1306
352-596-8371
FAX: 352-596-8032

Janet Hanciles, Administrator
Offers the following rehabilitation services: Sub-Acute rehabilitation, Occupational therapy, Speech pathology therapy, Physical therapy.

7250 Healthcare and Rehabilitation Center of Sanford
950 Mellonville Avenue
Sanford, FL 32771-2237
407-322-8566
FAX: 407-322-0121
www.healthcareandrehabofsanford.com

Dr. S. Joshi, Medical Director
Kate Hilgar, Administrator
Vicky Smith, Director Admissions

We provide post-acute services, rehabilitative services, skilled nursing, short and long term care through Physical, Occupational, and Speech Therapists; Registered and Licensed Practical Nurses; and Certified Nursing Assistants. This is complemented by Social Services, Activities, Nutritional Services, Housekeeping and Laundry Services. With over 224 years of combined experience, our staff of professionals is here to meet the needs of each and every patient and resident.

7251 Highland Pines Rehabilitation Center
1111 S Highland Ave
Clearwater, FL 33756-4432
727-446-0581
FAX: 727-442-9425

Paula Anthony, Administrator
Offers the following rehabilitation services: Sub-Acute rehabilitation, Occupational Therapy, Speech Therapy, Physical Therapy.

7252 Jupiter Medical Center-Pavilion
1210 S Old Dixie Hwy
Jupiter, FL 33458-7205
561-747-2234
FAX: 561-744-4467
JCouris@jupitermed.com
www.jupitermed.com

John D. Couris, President/Chief Executive Officer
Dale Hocking, Vice President, Finance/Chief Financial Officer
Mike Fehr, Vice President, Information Services/Chief Information Offic
Steven Seeley, Vice President, Chief Operating Officer/Chief Nursing Office
Offers the following rehabilitation services: Sub-Acute Rehabilitation, Occupational Therapy, Speech Therapy, Physical Therapy.

7253 North Broward Medical Center
201 E Sample Rd
Deerfield Beach, FL 33064-4441
954-941-8300
FAX: 954-941-4233
www.browardhealth.org

Pauline Grant, CEO
Douglas Ford, Chief of Staff
Offers the following rehabilitation services: Sub-Acute rehabilitation, Physical Therapy, Occupational Therapy, Speech Therapy, Respiratory Therapy.

7254 Pompano Rehabilitation and Nursing Center
Senior Health Care Management
51 W Sample Rd
Pompano Beach, FL 33064-3542
954-942-5530
FAX: 954-942-0941

Jeff Nusbusn, Administrator
Offers the following rehabilitation services: Sub-Acute Rehabilitation, Physical Therapy, Occupational Therapy, Speech Therapy

7255 Rehabilitation Center of Palm Beach
300 Royal Palm Way
Palm Beach, FL 33480-4385
561-655-7266
FAX: 561-655-3269
info@rcca.org
www.rcca.org

Ellen O'Bannon, Manager
Pamela Henderson, Executive Director
Our mission is to improve the physical function, communication & independence of people with disabilities.

7256 Rehabilitation and Healthcare Center of Tampa
4411 N Habana Ave
Tampa, FL 33614-7211
813-872-2771
FAX: 813-871-2831
www.rehabilitationandhealthcarecenteroftampa.
Dr. Gustavo Barrazuetta, Medical Director
We provide post-acute services, rehabilitative services, skilled nursing, short and long term care through Physical, Occupational, and Speech Therapists; Registered and Licensed Practical Nurses; and Certified Nursing Assistants. This is complemented by Social Services, Activities, Nutritional Services, Housekeep-

ing and Laundry Services. With over 60 years of combined experience, our staff of professionals is here to meet the needs of each and every patient and resident.

7257 Shands Rehab Hospital
4101 NW 89th Blvd
Gainesville, FL 32606-3813
352-265-8938
FAX: 352-265-5420
www.ufhealth.org/shands-rehab-hospital
Tim Goldfarb,M.S., Chief Executive Officer
David S. Guzick, M.D., Ph.D., Senior Vice President
Ed . Jimenez, M.B.A, Senior Vice President/Chief Operating Officer
James Roberts, J.D., Senior Vice President/General Counsel
UF Health Shands Rehab Hospital is a 40-bed acute rehab hospital for patients who have suffered strokes, traumatic brain and spinal cord injuries, amputations, burns or major joint replacements.

7258 St. Anthony's Hospital
1200 7th Ave N
St Petersburg, FL 33705-1388
727-825-1100
www.stanthonys.com
William Ulbricht, President
Ron Colaguori, VP Operations
James McClintic, M.D., Vice President, Medical Affairs
Sr. Mary McNally, OSF, Vice President, Mission
We offer outstanding diagnostic and treatment options of all types of cancer. Our Susan Sheppard McGillicuddy Breast Center is unmatched in the community in diagnostic services and helping patients navigate their treatment options should they find a cancer diagnosis.

7259 Winkler Court
3250 Winkler Avenue Ext
Fort Myers, FL 33916-9414
239-939-4993
FAX: 239-939-1743
www.winklercourt.com
Michael Collier, Medical Director
Michael Stens, Medical Director
We provide post-acute services, rehabilitative services, skilled nursing, short and long term care through Physical, Occupational, and Speech Therapists; Registered and Licensed Practical Nurses; and Certified Nursing Assistants. This is complemented by Social Services, Activities, Nutritional Services, Housekeeping and Laundry Services. With over 100 years of combined experience, our staff of professionals is here to meet the needs of each and every patient and resident.

7260 Winter Park Memorial Hospital
Florida Hospital
200 N Lakemont Ave
Winter Park, FL 32792-3273
407-646-7000
FAX: 407-646-7639
healthcare@winterparkhospital.com
www.winterparkhospital.com
Ken Bradley, CEO
Nestled among the oak-shaded, brick-paved streets of one of the most picturesque hometowns in the country, Winter Park Memorial Hospital has continuously served the residents of Winter Park and its surrounding communities for more than 50 years.

Georgia

7261 Athena Rehab of Clayton
2055 Rex Rd
Lake City, GA 30260-3944
404-361-5144
FAX: 404-363-6366
Reginald Washington, Administrator
Offers the following rehabilitation services: Sub-Acute rehabilitation, Occupational therapy, Speech therapy, Physical therapy, Restorative care.

7262 Lafayette Nursing and Rehabilitation Center
110 Brandywine Blvd
Fayetteville, GA 30214-1500
770-461-2928
FAX: 770-461-8507
www.lafayetterehab.com

Wendy Goza, Medical Director
Lafayette Nursing and Rehab Center accomodates 179 residents. We are Medicare certified and our center also features a 25-bed postacute rehab unit and a 24-bed dementia unit. We have RN's LPN's and CNA's 24 hours a day. We also have physician services availiable seven days a week.

7263 Savannah Rehabilitation and Nursing Center
815 E 63rd St
Savannah, GA 31405-4499
912-352-8615
FAX: 912-355-4642
www.savannahrehab.com
Sandra Casper, Executive Director
At our facility, we provide quality care with modern rehabilitation and restorative nursing techniques. We aim to provide an atmosphere which encourages family involvement in the care-planning process, with the right mix of activities addressing the social, spiritual and intellectual needs of our residents.

7264 Specialty Hospital
PO Box 1566
Rome, GA 30162-1566
706-509-4100
FAX: 706-509-4159
www.thespecialtyhospital.com

7265 Walton Rehabilitation Health System
523 13th St.
Augusta, GA 30901-1037
706-823-8505
866-492-5866
FAX: 706-724-5752
postmaster@wrh.org
www.wrh.org
Dennis Skelley, President/CEO
Has Centers of Excellence in Stroke Brain Injury, Complex Orthopedics, Spinal Cord Injury and Pain Management. 58-bed nonprofit facility.

7266 Warner Robins Rehabilitation and Nursing Center
1601 Elberta Rd
Warner Robins, GA 31093-1393
478-922-2241
FAX: 478-328-1984
www.warnerrobinsrehabilitation.com
Laura Fergason, Administrator
Offers the following rehabilitation services: Sub-Acute rehabilitation, Physical Therapy, Occupational Therapy, Speech Therapy.

Hawaii

7267 Aloha Nursing and Rehab Center
45-545 Kamehameha Hwy
Kaneohe, HI 96744-1943
808-247-2220
FAX: 808-235-3676
info@alohanursing.com
alohanursing.com
Charles Harris, Executive Director
Amy Lee, Administrator
Our unique nursing care facility is nestled in the picturesque town of Kaneohe, Oahu, amid the towering Koolau Mountains and the panoramic vistas of Kaneohe Bay. In this tranquil setting, our 141-bed facility offers both long and short term care to residents who meet intermediate or skilled level of care criteria.

Idaho

7268 Boise Health And Rehabilitation Center
1001 S Hilton St
Boise, ID 83705-1925
208-345-4464
FAX: 208-345-2998
www.kindredboise.com

Jason Ludwig, Medical Director
Aaron Moorhouse, Medical Director
Debbie Mills, Executive Director
Offers the following rehabilitation services: Sub-acute rehabilitation, occupational therapy, speech therapy, physical therapy.

7269 Eastern Idaho Regional Medical Center
3100 Channing Way
Idaho Falls, ID 83404-7533
208-529-6111
FAX: 208-529-7021
www.eirmc.com
Cindy Smith-Putnam, Executive Director of Business Development, Marketing & Comm
Lou Fatkin, Executive Director of Risk Management, Physician Relations,
Matt Campbell, Director of Human Resources
Jared Rickabaugh, Director of Quality Management
The largest medical facility in the region, Eastern Idaho Regional Medical Center (EIRMC) is a modern, JCAHO-accredidted, full-service hospital. EIRMC serves as the region's healthcare hub, offering specialty services including open-heart surgery, leading-edge cancer treatment, trauma, neurosurgery, intensive care for adults and infants, and a helicopeter service.

7270 Kindred Transitional Care and Rehabilitation
3315 8th St
Lewiston, ID 83501-4966
208-743-9543
FAX: 208-746-8662
www.lewistonrehab.com
Debbie Freeze, Administrator
Lewiston Rehabilitation and Care Center has years of experience providing diversified healthcare services. We have our own staff of physical, occupational and speech therapists. Our therapy gym and rehab kitchen are a lovely atmosphere in which to work toward your therapy goals. We are an Eden Alternative Certified facility.

7271 Mountain Valley Care and Rehabilitation Center
601 West Cameron Avenue
PO Box 689
Kellogg, ID 83837- 2004
208-784-1283
FAX: 208-784-0151
www.mountainvalleycare.com
Maryruth Butler, Executive Director
Mountain Valley Care and Rehabilitation Center accomodates 68 residents. We are conveniently located in the heart of Kellogg Idaho. We strive to offer quality care and superior customer service in a home-like environment. Upon admission, you or your loved one is looked after by an assigned staff member. We call this our 'Angel Care' program. Our rehabilitation program focuses on meeting the individual needs of the resident so you or your loved one can see how they are going to progress.

7272 River's Edge Rehabilitation and Healthcare
Kindred Healthcare
714 N Butte Ave
Emmett, ID 83617-2799
208-365-4425
FAX: 208-365-6989
GDecker@ensigngroup.net
www.riversedgerehab.com
Janis Shields, Executive Director
Steve Balle, MPT, Director of Rehabilitation
Margaret Williams RN, BSN, Director of Nursing
Patty Alsup, Business Office Manager
Emmett Rehab & healthcare accomodates 95 residents. We are located in Emmett, Idaho, a rural community located an easy 30 minute drive from Boise. Emmett Rehab & 'healthcare has served the area for more then 40 years by providing healthcare for residents of Gem County.

Illinois

7273 Chevy Chase Nursing and Rehabilitation Center
3400 S Indiana Ave
Chicago, IL 60616-3841
312-842-5000
FAX: 312-842-3790

Tony Prather, Administrator
Our approach to care is multidisciplinary; our medical staff members work together as a team in a proactive fashion, challenging residents each and every day, in order to motivate them to rehabilitate and achieve their ultimate potential.

7274 Glenview Terrace Nursing Center
1511 Greenwood Rd
Glenview, IL 60026-1513
847-729-9090
FAX: 847-729-9135
www.glenviewterrace.com

Ian Crook, Administrator
We're best known as the industry leader in post-hospital rehabilitation, including orthopedic rehabilitation and stroke recovery. Our highly effective rehabilitation services feature one-on-one physical, occupational, speech and respiratory therapies up to seven days a week.

7275 Halsted Terrace Nursing Center
10935 S Halsted St
Chicago, IL 60628-3189
773-928-2000
FAX: 773-928-9154

Ted O'Brien, Administrator
Offers the following rehabilitation services: Sub-acute rehabilitation, physical therapy, occupational therapy, speech therapy, cardiac rehabilitation.

7276 Harmony Nursing and Rehabilitation Center
3919 W Foster Ave
Chicago, IL 60625-6056
773-588-9500
FAX: 773-588-9533
www.harmonychicago.com

John Sianghio, Administrator
Offers a friendly healthcare experience. You'll find compassionate experts who provide short-term rehabilitation and therapy, wound care, Alzheimer's and memory loss care, long-term nursing care and more.

7277 Imperial
1366 W Fullerton Ave
Chicago, IL 60614-2199
773-248-9300
FAX: 773-935-0036
www.imperialpavilion.com

David Hartman, Administrator
Mary Bangayan, M.D., Pulmonary Care Programme
Sanjay Gill, M.D., Cardiac Management Program
We offer a comprehensive approach to post acute care. One that takes into consideration our guests' unique needs, and utilizes a progressive healthcare model to provide them with a personalized rehabilitation program designed to offer them the fullest possible recovery.

7278 Jackson Square Nursing and Rehabilitation Center
5130 W Jackson Blvd
Chicago, IL 60644-4332
773-921-8000
FAX: 773-287-9302
www.jacksonsquarecare.com

Rick Walworth, Administrator
At Jackson Square, there is one primary goal: to help guests regain maximum independence and functioning so that they can safely, comfortably, and happily get their life back. Our physicians, therapists, and nurses use their experience, compassion, and skill-combined with the latest and best technology-to provide comprehensive rehabilitation for a wide range of physical disabilities and medical conditions.

7279 Renaissance at 87th Street
2940 W 87th St
Chicago, IL 60652-3832
773-434-8787
FAX: 773-434-8717
www.renaissanceat87.com

Juli Foy, Administrator
At Renaissance at 87th, there is one primary goal: to help guests regain maximum independence and functioning so that they can safely, comfortably, and happily get their life back. Our physicians, therapists, and nurses use their experience, compassion, and skill-combined with the latest and best technology-to provide comprehensive rehabilitation for a wide range of physical disabilities and medical conditions.

7280 Renaissance at Hillside
4600 N. Frontage Rd.
Hillside, IL 60162-1761
708-544-9933
FAX: 708-544-9966
www.ariapostacute.com

John Stare, Administrator
Utilizing a progressive healthcare model that takes into account each patient's individual needs, Aria Post Acute Care designs a personalized rehabilitation program offering guests the best chance at the fullest possible recovery.

7281 Renaissance at Midway
4437 S Cicero Ave
Chicago, IL 60632-4333
773-884-0484
FAX: 773-884-0485
www.renaissanceatmidway.com

Jeff Baker, Executive Director
At Renaissance at Midway, there is one primary goal: to help guests regain maximum independence and functioning so that they can safely, comfortably, and happily get their life back. Our physicians, therapists, and nurses use their experience, compassion, and skill-combined with the latest and best technology-to provide comprehensive rehabilitation for a wide range of physical disabilities and medical conditions.

7282 Renaissance at South Shore
2425 E 71st St
Chicago, IL 60649-2612
773-721-5000
FAX: 773-721-6850
www.rensouthshore.com

Dave Schechter, Administrator
The Renaissance at South Shore is a 248 bed skilled nursing facility with multiple services that include short-term rehabilitation, specialized dementia care and long-term care and hospice care. Our highly trained nursing professionals provide loving care in a home-like atmosphere.

7283 Schwab Rehabilitation Hospital
Mt. Sinai
1401 S California Ave
Chicago, IL 60608-1858
773-522-2010
schwabinquiries@sini.org
www.schwabrehab.org

Suzan Rayner, Medical Director
Lisa Thornton, Medical Staff President
Alan Channing, President/ Chief Executive Officer
Anita Halvorsen, Vice President of Schwab Rehabilitation Hospital
Schwab Rehabilitation Hospital is a freestanding, not-for-profit, 102-bed rehabilitation hospital located on Chicago's west side. It offers a therapeutic environment of comprehensive inpatient and outpatient rehabilitation, both for adults and children.

Indiana

7284 Angel River Health and Rehabilitation
5233 Rosebud Ln
Newburgh, IN 47630-9283
812-473-4761
FAX: 812-473-5190
HSDED0204@kindredhealthcare.com
www.angelriverhc.com

Kay Congleton, Executive Director

Our wide array of services enables our patients and residents to receive the medical care they need, the restorative therapy they require, and the support they and their families deserve. We serve many types of patient and resident needs - from short-term rehabilitation to traditional long-term care. Our resident council meets regularly to ensure that our residents' needs are being met to their satisfaction.

7285   Chalet Village Health and Rehabilitation Center
Magnolia Health Systems
1065 Parkway St
Berne, IN 46711-2366   260-589-2127
                                                FAX: 260-589-3521
                                        mwolfe@chalet-village.net
                                            www.chalet-village.net

Vicki Shepherd, Administrator
We provide dedicated, community-centered healthcare which was founded in Indiana, operates in Indiana, for people who live in Indiana.

7286   Columbus Health and Rehabilitation Center
2100 Midway St
Columbus, IN 47201-3722   812-372-8447
                                                FAX: 812-375-5117
                                              www.columbushrc.com

Sherry Harrison, Executive Director
William Lustig, Medical Director
Accomodates 235 residents. We offer a continuum of healthcare services. Our center also provides a Special Care Alzheimer's Unit. We are licensed by the Stat of Indiana and are Medicare and Medicaid approved provider. We are proud to offer a friendly home-like atmosphere while providing comprehensive healthcare services. These services include short-term medical and rehabilitation treatment, which is designed to address the individual needs of our residents and patients.

7287   Harrison Health and Rehabilitation Centre
150 Beechmont Drive
Corydon, IN 47112-1717   812-738-0550
                                                FAX: 812-738-6273
                                    HSDED0131@kindredhealthcare.com
                                              www.harrisonrehab.com

Sheila Bieker, Executive Director
Bruce Burton, Medical Director
We serve many types of patient and resident needs - from short-term rehabilitation to traditional long-term care. Working with your physician, our staff - including medical specialists, nurses, nutritionists, therapists, dietitians and social workers - establishes a comprehensive treatment plan intended to restore you or your loved one to the fullest practicable potential.

7288   Indian Creek Health and Rehabilitation Center
240 Beechmont Dr
Corydon, IN 47112-1718   812-738-8127
                                                      877-380-7211
                                                FAX: 812-738-2917
                                    HSDED0288@kindredhealthcare.com
                                             www.indiancreekhrc.com

Bonnie Fallin, Executive Director
Bruce Burton, Medical Director
140 bed facility offering the following rehabilitation services: Sub-Acute rehabilitation, Physical therapy, Occupational Therapy, Speech Therapy, pain management, Wound rehabilitation. Short and long term skilled nursing care certified for Medicare, Medicaid, Private Pay and Private Insurance. Hospice and respite care rated #1 in clinical care in southern Indiana district for 2002.

7289   Meadowvale Health and Rehabilitation Center
Kindred Health Care
1529 Lancaster St
Bluffton, IN 46714-1507   260-824-4320
                                                      800-743-3333
                                                FAX: 260-824-4689
                                    HSDED0269@kindredhealthcare.com
                                             www.meadowvalerehab.com

Todd Beaulieu, Executive Director
Yadagiri Jonna, Medical Director

Working with your physician, our staff - including medical specialists, nurses, nutritionists, therapists, dietitians and social workers - establishes a comprehensive treatment plan intended to restore you or your loved one to the fullest practicable potential.

7290   Muncie Health Care and Rehabilitation
680 South Fourth Street
Louisville, KY 40202   502-596-7300
                                                      800-545-0749
                                      web_administrator@kindred.com
                                            www.kindredhealthcare.com

Dee Harrold, Executive Director
Dr. Jeffery Hiltz, Medical Director
Offers the following rehabilitation services: Sub-Acute rehabilitation, physical therapy, occupational therapy, speech therapy.

7291   Rehabilitation Hospital of Indiana
4141 Shore Dr
Indianapolis, IN 46254-2607   317-329-2000
                                                FAX: 317-329-2104
                                                       www.rhin.com

Ian Worden, MHA, MBA, CPA, RHI Board Chair
James G. Terwilliger, MPH, Vice Chair/Secretary
Kyle Netter, MBA, PT, Executive Director of Corporate and Affiliate Relations
Larissa Swan, MS, OTR, Executive Director of Therapies
We approach every patient understanding that every diagnosis, every illness, and every injury are different. It's the collective effort of trained and compassionate team members who value the quality of life of every patient and their caregivers. It's the right kind of treatment- inpatient, outpatient, and follow-up services- provided under the same roof. It's one step closer to home. It's a continuum of care

7292   Sellersburg Health and Rehabilitation Centre
7823 Old State Road 60
Sellersburg, IN 47172-1858   812-246-4272
                                                FAX: 812-246-8160
                                            www.sellersburgrehab.com

Dave Powell, Administrator
Chris Hansen, Executive Director
Sellersburg is a modern healthcare center conveniently located on the edge of the community. Our center accomodates 110 residents and includes a rehabilitative program with a goal of returning residents home as quickly as possible. Sellersburg is a 2006 recipient of the American Health Care Association Quality Award.

7293   Westpark Rehabilitation Center
1316 N Tibbs Ave
Indianapolis, IN 46222-3024   317-634-8330
                                                FAX: 317-263-9442
                                            www.westparkhealthcare.com

Dave Mc Carroll, Owner
Offers the following rehabilitation services: Sub-acute rehabilitation, occupational therapy, physical therapy, speech therapy, respiratory therapy.

7294   Westview Nursing and Rehabilitation Center
1510 Clinic Dr
Bedford, IN 47421-3530   812-279-4494
                                                FAX: 812-275-8313
                            www.ascseniorcare.com/westview-nursing—rehab

Sholin Montgomery, Executive Director
Mike Spencer, Executive Director
Offers the following rehabilitation services: Sub-acute rehabilitation, physical therapy, occupational therapy, speech therapy.

7295   Windsor Estates Health and Rehab Center
429 W Lincoln Rd
Kokomo, IN 46902-3508   765-453-5600
                                                FAX: 765-455-0110
                                    HSDED0294@kindredhealthcare.com
                                             www.kindredkokomo.com

Brenda Alfrey, Administrator
Monica Martin, Executive Director

Our wide array of services enables our patients and residents to receive the medical care they need, the restorative therapy they require, and the support they and their families deserve. We serve many types of patient and resident needs - from short-term rehabilitation to traditional long-term care.

Iowa

7296 Madison County Rehab Services
Madison County Hospital
300 W Hutchings St
Winterset, IA 50273-2109   515-462-2373
FAX: 515-462-4492

Marcia Harris, CEO
Panndee Stebbins, Director
Offers the following rehabilitation services: Sub-acute rehabilitation, occupational therapy, physical therapy, speech therapy, home health rehab, wellness programs.

7297 Mercy Subacute Care
603 E 12th St
Des Moines, IA 50309-5515   515-247-4400
FAX: 515-643-0945

Bonnie Mc Coy, Manager
Pam Nelson, Intake Coordinator
Offers the following rehabilitation services: Sub-acute rehabilitation, physical therapy, speech therapy, occupational therapy.

Kentucky

7298 Danville Centre for Health and Rehabilitation
642 N 3rd St
Danville, KY 40422-1125   859-236-3972
FAX: 859-236-0703
HSDED0782@kindredhealthcare.com
www.danvillecentre.com

Debbie Gibson, Executive Director
We offer short-term rehabilitative care as well as long-term care. Our emphasis is on service excellence - providing quality care in a home-like environment to allow for independence and to enable our patients and residents to receive the medical care they need, the restorative therapy they require, and the support they and their families deserve.

7299 Fountain Circle Health & Rehabilitation
Kindred Healthcare
200 Glenway Rd
Winchester, KY 40391   859-744-1800
FAX: 859-744-0285
www.fountaincircle.com

William Whited, Executive Director
Kathryn Jones, Medical Director
Offers the following rehabilitation services: Sub-acute rehabilitation, speech therapy, physical therapy, occupational therapy.

7300 Lexington Center for Health and Rehabilitation
353 Waller Ave
Lexington, KY 40504-2974   859-252-3558
FAX: 859-233-0192

Karole Ward, Administrator
Offers the following rehabilitation services: Sub-acute rehabilitation, speech therapy, occupational therapy, physical therapy.

7301 Paducah Centre For Health and Rehabilitation
Wellsouth Health Systems
501 N 3rd St
Paducah, KY 42001-0749   270-444-9661
FAX: 270-443-9407
www.genesishcc.com/Paducah?

Jean Glisson, RN, Director of Nursing
Elizabeth Kay Chilton, Admissions Director
Tracy Summers, Rehab/Specialty Program Director
Cathy Ortega, Administrator

Paducah Center is an 86-bed skilled and long-term care facility with a 28-bed Alzheimer's secure unit. This unit has a private courtyard and structured activities throughout the day, and is the only true Alzheimer's secure unit in the area.

7302 Pathways Brain Injury Program
4200 Browns Ln
Louisville, KY 40220-1523   502-459-8900
FAX: 502-459-5026
www.hcr-manorcare.com

Pam Pearson, Manager
Offers the following rehabilitation services: Sub-acute rehabilitation, speech therapy, occupational therapy, physical therapy, recreational therapy.

Louisiana

7303 Guest House of Slidell Sub-Acute and Rehab Center
1051 Robert Blvd
Slidell, LA 70458-2011   985-643-5630
800-303-9872
FAX: 985-649-6065

Brandy Wheat, Administrator
116 bed healthcare center offering the following subacute services within the skilled nursing setting: physical, occupational, and speech therapies, infusion therapy, respiratory care, wound care, neurological rehabilitation, cardiac reconditioning, pain management, post surgical recovery, orthopedic rehabilitation.

7304 Irving Place Rehabilitation and Nursing Center
1736 Irving Pl
Shreveport, LA 71101-4606   318-631-9121
FAX: 318-222-2095

Webster Johnson, Administrator
Offers the following rehabilitation services: sub-acute rehabilitation, speech therapy, occupational therapy, physical therapy

Maine

7305 Augusta Rehabilitation Center
188 Eastern Ave
Augusta, ME 04330-5928   207-622-3121
800-457-1220
FAX: 207-623-7666
HSDED0544@kindredhealthcare.com
www.augustarehabcenter.com

Malcolm Dean, Executive Director
Cathleen O'Connor
From intensive short term rehabilitation therapy to longer-term restorative care, our Nursing and Rehabilitation Centers provide a full range of nursing care and social services to treat and support each of our patients and residents. Our clinical capabilities allow us to accept patients with greater medical complexity than a traditional nursing home. This is increasingly important as many patients require transitional care before they are ready to return home.

7306 Brentwood Rehabilitation and Nursing Center
370 Portland St
Yarmouth, ME 04096-8101   207-846-9021
800-457-1220
FAX: 207-846-1497
HSDED0555@kindredhealthcare.com
www.brentwoodrnc.com

Malcolm Dean, Executive Director
Daniel M. Pierce, Medical Director
Brentwood accomodates 82 residents. We are located at 370 Portland Street in Yarmouth, Maine. We strive to meet the healthcare needs of the greater Yarmouth community, including Portland and Brunswick, which are located within 10 miles of the center. In addition to Brentwood's rehabilitation and skilled nursing services, we also offer Alzheimer's specialty care in a comfortable setting.

7307   Den-Mar Rehabilitation and Nursing Center
44 South St
Rockport, MA 01966-1800   978-546-6311
                                                 800-439-2370
                                     FAX: 978-546-9185
                            HSDED0542@kindredhealthcare.com
                                     www.denmarrnc.com

Christine Marek, Executive Director
Den-Mar nursing and Rehab center accomodates 80 residents. We
provide skilled nursing and rehabilitation services as well as long
term care. We are certified for Medicare and Medicaid as well as
many insurance carriers. We offer semi-private and private
rooms, with many common areas for socializing.

7308   Eastside Rehabilitation and Living Center
516 Mount Hope Ave
Bangor, ME 04401-4215   207-947-6131
                                                 800-457-1220
                                     FAX: 207-942-0884
                            HSDED0545@kindredhealthcare.com
                                     www.eastsiderehab.com

Ryan Kelley, Executive Director
From intensive short term rehabilitation therapy to longer-term
restorative care, our Nursing and Rehabilitation Centers provide
a full range of nursing care and social services to treat and support
each of our patients and residents. Our clinical capabilities allow
us to accept patients with greater medical complexity than a traditional nursing home. This is increasingly important as many patients require transitional care before they are ready to return
home.

7309   Kennebunk Nursing & Rehabilitation Center
158 Ross Rd
Kennebunk, ME 04043-6532   207-985-7141
                                                 800-457-1220
                                     FAX: 207-985-0961
                            HSDED0549@kindredhealthcare.com
                                     www.kennebunknursing.com

Stephen Alaimo, Executive Director
We treat a variety of conditions and provide an array of services
including, but not limited to:Respiratory conditions such as
pneumonia and post-acute COPD episodes Cardiac conditions
and post surgical care (grafts, valves, stints) Wound Stroke Orthopedic Neurological illnesses Diabetes

7310   Norway Rehabilitation and Living Center
29 Marion Ave
Norway, ME 04268-5601   207-743-7075
                                                 800-457-1220
                                     FAX: 207-743-9269
                            info@norwayresidentialcare.com
                                     www.norwayresidentialcare.com

Carolyn Farley, Administrator
Norway Rehabilitation and Living Center has been a fixture in
the Norway community since 1976. We are a 70-bed facility offering short-term rehabilitation, skilled nursing services, long
term care and residential care services. Utilizing an interdisciplinary team led by a physician and consisting of qualified health
care specialists, we develop individualized plans of care for each
patient that are designed to restore maximum health and optimize
functional abilities and independence

7311   Shore Village Rehabilitation & Nursing Center
201 Camden St
\, ME 04841-2534   207-596-6423
                                                 800-457-1220
                                     FAX: 207-596-7235

Phyllis Nickerson, Administrator
Shore Village accomodates 60 residents and is located in the
mid-coast region of the state of Maine. We have a cozy size and a
primary goal for the staff is to ensure a home-like atmosphere for
all the residents. Shore Village provides skilled nursing and rehabilitation, respite care, and long term care. The facility is dually
certified for Medicare and Medicaid and accepts many commercial insurance plans.

Maryland

7312   Greater Baltimore Medical Center
6701 N Charles St
Baltimore, MD 21204-6881   443-849-2000
                                     FAX: 443-849-3024
                                     TTY:800-735-2258
                                     www.gbmc.org

John B. Chessare, M.D., President/Chief Executive Officer
Eric L. Melchior, Executive Vice President/Chief Financial Officer
Keith Poisson, Executive Vice President/Chief Operating Officer
*John W. Ellis, Senior Vice President/Corporate Strategy & Business
Developm*
The 281-bed medical center (acute and sub-acute care) is located
on a beautiful suburban campus and handles more than 26,700 in-
patient cases and approximately 60,000 emergency room visits
annually.

Massachusetts

7313   Bolton Manor Nursing Home
400 Bolton St
Marlborough, MA 01752-3912   508-481-6123
                                                 800-439-2370
                                     FAX: 508-481-6130
                                     www.boltonmanor.com

Michele Ricard, Medical Director
Thomas Sullivan, Executive Director
Bolton Manor accomodates 157 residents. We are located in
Marlboro, Massachusetts. We provide medical management and
long-term care through comprehensive skilled and post-acute
nursing services. We also provide physical, occupational, and
speech therapy services from an onsite dedicated staff of therapists. The facility is Joint Commission (formerly JCAHO) accredited and has an excellent survey history with the State
Department of Public Health.

7314   Brigham Manor Nursing and Rehabilitation Center
77 High St
Newburyport, MA 01950-3071   978-462-4221
                                                 800-439-2370
                                     FAX: 978-463-3297
                                     www.brighammanor.com

Stephen Cynewski, Executive Director
Brigham Manor accomodates 64 residents. We are a
Medicare-certified facility offering private, semi-private and
multi-bed suites. Our bright, formal dining room, with French
doors that open to a shaded courtyard, provides a warm atmosphere for entertaining family and friends. Each resident's personal tastes and medical needs are considered in the planning of
our weekly menus.

7315   Country Gardens Skilled Nursing and Rehabilitation Center
2045 Grand Army Hwy
Swansea, MA 02777-3932   508-379-9700
                                                 800-439-2370
                                     FAX: 508-379-0723
                            HSDED0534@kindredhealthcare.com
                                     www.cntrygrdns.com

Sandy Sarza, Executive Director
Country Gardens Skilled Nursing and Rehabilitation Center
accomodates 86 residents. We are located in a beautiful rural setting conveniently located about 15 minutes east of Providence
and 10 minutes west of Fall River. We have provided healthcare
service to the greater Swansea area for over 34 years.

7316   Country Manor Rehabilitation and Nursing Center
180 Low St
Newburyport, MA 01950-3519   978-465-5361
                                                 800-439-2370
                                     FAX: 978-463-9366
                                     www.countryrehab.com

Stephen Doyle, Executive Director
Country Rehabilitation and Nursing Center accomodates 123 residents. We are located in the quaint seaport town of Newburyport,

Massachusetts. We provide medical management and long-term care through comprehensive skilled and intermediate nursing services. We also provide physical, occupational, and speech therapy services from an onsite dedicated staff of therapists. The center offers an Alzheimer's special care unit with staff trained in dimentia care and dementia specific programs.

7317   Franklin Skilled Nursing and Rehabilitation Center
130 Chestnut St
Franklin, MA 02038-3903   508-528-4600
                                            800-439-2370
                                       FAX: 508-528-7976
                   HSDED0584@kindredhealthcare.com
                             www.franklinskilled.com
Paula Topijan, Executive Director
We treat a variety of conditions and provide an array of services including, but not limited to :Respiratory conditions such as pneumonia and post-acute COPD episodes,Cardiac conditions and post surgical care (grafts, valves, stints),Wound,Stroke,Orthopedic,Neurological illnesses,Diabetes

7318   Great Barrington Rehabilitation and Nursing Center
148 Maple Ave
Great Barrington, MA 01230-1906   413-528-3320
                                            800-439-2370
                                       FAX: 413-528-2302
                   HSDED0585@kindredhealthcare.com
                          www.greatbarringtonrnc.com
William Kittler, Executive Director
Andrew Potler, Medical Director
Great Barrington Rehabilitation and Nursing Center accomodates 106 residents. As part of a national network of long-term healthcare centers, we have the expertise and resources to provide care appropriate to the individual needs of each and every one of our residents. We provide personal care with minimal daily living assistance to the most skilled treatment for medically complex patients.

7319   Ledgewood Rehabilitation and Skilled Nursing Center
87 Herrick St
Beverly, MA 01915-2773   978-921-1392
                                            800-439-2370
                                       FAX: 978-927-8627
                             www.ledgewoodrehab.com
Frank Silvia, Executive Director
Ledgewood Rehabilitation and Skilled Nursing Center is a unique provider of healthcare services. We are part of a continuum of services that includes acute care services at Beverly Hospital, subacute care at Ledgewood, and care after discharge through Northeast Homecare. We believe this partnership offers the highest quality post-acute services north of Boston.

7320   Leo P La Chance Center for Rehabilitation and Nursing
59 Eastwood Cir
Gardner, MA 01440-3901   978-632-8776
                                       FAX: 978-632-5048
                        souellet@legendcenter.com
                             www.lachancecenter.com
Mark Alinger, Administrator
Leo P. LaChance, Founder
A privately owned facility, combines the best of medical technology with the ultimate in healing, compassionate rehabilitation and nursing care. Our goal is to help each client reach that ultimate goal of living life to the fullest.

7321   Oakwood Rehabilitation and Nursing Center
11 Pontiac Ave
Webster, MA 01570-1629   508-943-3889
                                            800-439-2370
                                       FAX: 508-949-6125
                   HSDED0517@kindredhealthcare.com
                             www.oakwoodrehab.com
Thomas Sullivan, Executive Director
Oakwood Rehabilitation and Nursing Center accomodates 81 residents. We offer 24-hour skilled nursing, inpatient rehabilitation, respite care, and hospice services. Our center has been successfully serving the greater Webster, Massachusetts, community for 35 years. We have a dedicated and caring staff and our com-

mon goal is to promote recovery and enhance quality of live whether your needs are short or long term.

7322   Walden Rehabilitation and Nursing Center
785 Main St
Concord, MA 01742-3310   978-369-6889
                                            800-439-2370
                                       FAX: 978-369-8392
                   HSDED0588@kindredhealthcare.com
                             www.waldenrehab.com
Ladan Azarm, Executive Director
Walden Rehabilitation and Nursing Center accomodates 123 residents. We are located in the quaint town of Concord, Massachusetts, across the street from Emerson Hospital and a short drive from the town center. Walden provides medical management and long-term care through comprehensive skilled and intermediate nursing services. We also provide physical, occupational, and speech therapy services from an onsite dedicated staff of therapists.

Michigan

7323   Boulder Park Terrace
14676 W Upright St
Charlevoix, MI 49720-1201   231-547-1005
                                       FAX: 231-547-1039
           www.mclaren.org/northernmichigan/northernmich
Reezie DeVet, President/CEO
Mary-Anne Ponti, COO
A partnership formed with Charlevoix Area Hospital, Boulder Park Terrace is a long-term care facility and Sub-acute Rehabilitation Center located in Chalrevoix near the shores of Lake Michigan. The Sub-acute Rehabilitation Center was created as a transition between an acute care hospital and home. Patients enter into the program to increase their strength, endurance and over-all functioning before returning home.

Minnesota

7324   Park Health And Rehabilitation Center
4415 W 36 1/2 St
St Louis Park, MN 55416-4890   952-927-9717
                                       FAX: 952-927-7687
                             park@extendicare.com
                             www.extendicare.com
Jennifer Kuhn, Administrator
Park Health & Rehabilitation Center is a leading provider of long-term skilled nursing care and short-term rehabilitation solutions. Our 93 bed facility offers a full continuum of services and care focused around each individual in today's ever-changing healthcare environment.

Missouri

7325   Barnes-Jewish Hospital Washington University Medical Center
1 Barnes Jewish Hospital Plz
Saint Louis, MO 63110-1003   314-747-3000
                                            866-867-3627
                                       FAX: 314-362-8877
                             www.barnesjewish.org
Richard Liekweg, President
John Beatty, Vice President of Human Resources
John Lynch, MD, Chief Medical Officer
David Jaques, MD, Vice President for Surgical Services
Barnes-Jewish Hospital at Washington University Medical Center is the largest hospital in Missouri and the largest private employer in the St. Louis region. An affiliated teaching hospital of Washington University School of Medicine, Barnes-Jewish Hospital has a 1,700 member medical staff with many who are recognized in the 'Best Doctors in America.

Montana

7326 Parkview Acres Care and Rehabilitation Center
200 N Oregon St
Dillon, MT 59725-3624
406-683-5105
866-253-4090
FAX: 406-683-6388
HSDED0433@kindredhealthcare.com
www.parkviewacres.com

Claire Miller, Executive Director
We are Medicare and Medicaid certified skilled nursing facility which accomodates 108 residents serving scenic Dillon and surrounding Montana communities.

Nebraska

7327 Homestead Healthcare and Rehabilitation Center
4735 S 54th St
Lincoln, NE 68516-1335
402-488-0977
800-833-0920
FAX: 402-488-4507
www.homesteadrehab.com

Matt Romshek, Executive Director
Gay Bate, RN, Director of Nursing
James Murray, Administrator
James Murray, LPN, Clinical Liaison/Admissions
Homestead Healthcare and Rehabilitation Center is one of the area's oldest providers of skilled nursing and rehabilitation services. We are a 163-bed skilled nursing and rehabilitation center nestled in a lovely, quiet established neighborhood in South Lincoln.

7328 Madonna Rehabilitation Hospital
5401 South St
Lincoln, NE 68506-2150
402-413-3000
800-676-5448
FAX: 402-486-5448
info@madonna.org
www.madonna.org

Marsha Lommel, CEO
Tom Stalder, VP Medical Affairs
Madonna provides intensive rehabilitation and expertise for a wide variety of conditions, such as: orthopedic injuries, work injuries, arthritis, amputation, neuromuscular diseases, cardiac conditions, pulmonary disease and conditions including those dependent upon a ventilator, cancer, lymphedema, osteoporosis, wounds, renal disorders, burns, fibromyalgia, multiple scelerosis, parkinson's disease and degenerative diseases.

7329 Mary Lanning Memorial Hospital
715 N Saint Joseph Ave
Hastings, NE 68901-4497
402-463-4521
866-460-5884
tanderson@mlmh.org
www.mlmh.org

Beth Schlichtman, Compensation/Benefit Services - Director
Lisa Brandt, Public Relations & Marketing Services - Director
Carrie Edwards, Home Care Services - Director
Chris Page, Ancillary Services - Director
Mary Lanning Healthcare is in its 95th year of providing quality healthcare for residents of the central Nebraska area. We continue to grow and expand, working to provide patient-centered care in a positive environment, while implementing some of the newest technologies available.

Nevada

7330 Las Vegas Healthcare and Rehabilitation Center
2832 S Maryland Pkwy
Las Vegas, NV 89109-1502
702-735-5848
800-326-6888
FAX: 702-735-6218
www.lasvegaskindred.com

Randall Fuller, Executive Director
Las Vegas Healthcare accomodates 79 residents. We have been serving the community for approximately 40 years. Located in close proximity to local hospitals and surrounded by medical complexes, our center offers both short-term rehabilitation and long-term care.

New Hampshire

7331 Dover Rehabilitation and Living Center
307 Plaza Dr
Dover, NH 03820-2455
603-742-2676
800-735-2964
FAX: 603-749-5375
www.doverrehab.com

Daniel Estee, Executive Director
Dover Rehab is a provider of postacute services in the greater New Hampshire Seacost area. We accomodate 112 residents and are licensed by the state of New Hampshire. We employ nearly 150 licensed nurses, therapists and other healthcare professionals, who strive to provide quality care. The goal of our patient service model is to bridge the gap between hospitalization and home so that recovery and physical functioning are maximized and hospital readmission is minimized.

7332 Northeast Rehabilitation Clinic
70 Butler St
Salem, NH 03079-3925
603-893-2900
800-825-7292
FAX: 603-893-1638
TTY: 800-439-2370
webmaster@northeastrehab.com
www.northeastrehab.com

John Prochilo, CEO/Administrator
Subacute rehabilitation at NRH was designed for people who have experienced an acutely disabling orthopedic, medical, or neurologic condition but who either do not require or are unable to participate in a full acute inpatient program. Impairment groups pertinent to this level of care include brain injury, spinal cord injury (traumatic/non-traumatic), stroke, orthopedic injury, amputation, and neurologic disorder.

New Jersey

7333 Atlantic Coast Rehabilitation & Healthcare Center
485 River Ave
Lakewood, NJ 08701-4720
732-364-7100
FAX: 732-364-2442
abby@atlanticcoastrehab.com
www.atlanticcoastrehab.com

Simon Shain, Administrator
Sharon Sckbower, Director of Nursing
Atlantic Coast is family owned and operated. It's a warm, friendly place where caregivers and patients know each other by first name. But it's also an innovative and energetic place, where the most advanced therapies and cutting edge techniques are offered. It's a comprehensive health care center that provides three distinct areas of care: Rehabilitative Therapy & Sub Acute Care, Long Term Care, Alzheimer's/Memory Impaired Care.

7334 Crestwood Nursing & Rehabilitation Center
101 Whippany Rd
Whippany, NJ 7981-1407
973-887-0311
FAX: 973-887-8355

Carol Shepard, Administrator

Sub-acute rehabilitation facility.

New York

7335 Lakeview Subacute Care Center
130 Terhune Dr
Wayne, NJ 7470-7104
973-839-4500
87-UBA-UTE
FAX: 973-839-2729
rgrossojr@lakeviewsubacute.com
www.lakeviewsubacute.com

Richard Grosso, Jr, Director
Sue Ahlers, Director of Admission
Kerry Iamurri, Director of Rehab
Nicole Iacolina, Director Social Services

Our comprehensive medical, nursing and rehabilitation services cater to a diverse patient population. In addition to long-term care, we offer exceptional inpatient subacute programs. We're proud to report that our average length of stay for subacute patients is a brief 14 days.

7336 Merwick Rehabilitation and Sub-Acute Care
79 Bayard Ln
Princeton, NJ 8540-3045
609-497-3000
FAX: 609-497-3024

Ryan Wismer, Administrator

76-bed skilled nursing and residential center as well as a separate 17-bed comprehensive rehabilitation center. Offers rehabilitation, physiatry, occupational therapy, respite care, speech/hearing therapy, sub-acute care.

7337 Seacrest Village Nursing Center
1001 Center St
Little Egg Harbor Twp, NJ 8087-1364
609-296-9292
FAX: 609-296-0508
info@seacrestvillagenj.com
seacrestvillagenj.com

Brian T Holloway, Administrator

Seacrest Village Nursing and Rehabilitation Center has specialized in quality rehabilitation, transitional and restorative care for more then a decade and is a perfect alternative for bridging the gap between hospital and home.

7338 St. Lawrence Rehabilitation Center
2381 Lawrenceville Rd
Lawrenceville, NJ 08648-2098
609-896-9500
FAX: 609-895-0242
epiechota@slrc.org
www.slrc.org

Kevin McGuigan, MD, Medical Director
Robyn F. Agri, MD, Doctor
Dr. Madhu Jain, Doctor
Charles Terry MD, Doctor

St. Lawrence Rehabilitation Center, a non-profit facility sponsored by the Roman Catholic Diocese of Trenton, is committed to maximizing the quality of human life by providing comprehensive physical rehabilitation and related programs to meet the healthcare needs of our communities.

7339 Summit Ridge Center Genesis Eldercare
20 Summit St
West Orange, NJ 07052-1501
973-736-2000
800-699-1520
FAX: 973-736-2764
info@genesishcc.com
www.genesishcc.com

Michele Cartagena, Director of Admissions
Elizabeth (L Orlando, Rehabilitation Program Director
Tsega Asefaha, LNHA, BS, MHA, Administrator
Elizabeth Martin, Customer Relations Manager

Summit Ridge Center provides skilled nursing, medical and rehabilitative care for patients requiring post-hospital, short stay rehabilitation and for longer term residents. Our Clinical Care Teams are focused on implementing your personalized care program to facilitate your recovery and improve your well-being.

7340 Beth Abraham Health Services
612 Allerton Ave
Bronx, NY 10467-7495
718-519-4037
888-238-4223
FAX: 718-547-1366
info@bethabe.org
www.bethabrahamhealthservices.org

Maria Provenzano, Program Director
Yolanda Lester, Director of Admissions
Rosalie Bernard, Director of Nursing Services
Vincent Bonadies, Director of Therapeutic Recreation

Offers the following rehabilitation services: Sub-Acute rehabilitation, brain injury rehabilitation, pain management, post-operative recovery. Home visits and a network of community-based programs help patients and their families with a successful transition home.

7341 Central Island Healthcare
825 Old Country Rd
Plainview, NY 11803-4913
516-433-0600
FAX: 516-868-7251
www.centralislandhealthcare.net

Michael Ostreicher, Administrator

Serving the community for over 33 years, Central Island Healthcare is Long Island's largest and most active sub-acute care provider. We offer comprehensive programs focused on restoring our patients to their maximum potential and returning home. Central Island's 202-bed facility provides top notch professionals and the latest in rehabilitation and therapeutic equipment in a beautiful and comfortable setting.

7342 Clove Lakes Health Care and Rehabilitation Center
25 Fanning St
Staten Island, NY 10314-5307
718-289-7900
FAX: 718-761-8701
info@clovelakes.com
www.clovelakes.com

Helene Demisay, CEO

Clove Lakes seeks to rehabilitate those who have sustained injury or illness to the highest level of independence possible and support those with disabling conditions to live meaningful and productive lives.

7343 Dr. William O Benenson Rehabilitation Pavilion
36-17 Parsons Blvd
Flushing, NY 11354-5931
718-961-4300
FAX: 718-939-5032
www.flushingmanors.com

Esther Benenson, Executive Director
Liza Marie Dowd, Director of Nursing
Erika Rossi, Director of Social Services
Diane Marron, Director of Admissions

The Dr. William O Benson Reahbilitation Pavilion is a subacute short-term rehabilitation center committed to the excellence of elevated health care for our patients. Through the use of the most comprehensive and specialized services available, our staff of dedicated professionals are devoted to putting patients back to the road to full recovery 24 hours a day.

7344 Flushing Manor Nursing and Rehab
35-15 Parsons Blvd
Flushing, NY 11354-4297
718-961-3500
FAX: 718-461-1784
www.flushingmanors.com

Esther Benenson, Executive Director
Dr. Ion Oltean, Medical Director
Myung Chung, Director of Nursing
Bridgett Brown, Director of Admissions

At the Flusing Manor Nursing and Rehabilitation, we stress the importance of family involvement because it is the true source of strength and stability in ones life...a tie that brings us all together as a team, enhancing the quality of life of the patients in our care.

7345 Glengariff Health Care Center
141 Dosoris Ln
Glen Cove, NY 11542
516-676-1100
FAX: 516-759-0216
info@glengariffcare.com
www.glenhaven.org

Jean Campo, Director Admissions
Michael Miness, President
Licensed skilled nursing and subacute medical and rehabilitation facility.

7346 Haym Salomon Home for The Aged
2340 Cropsey Ave
Brooklyn, NY 11214-5706
718-266-4063
FAX: 718-372-4781

Chain Lipschitz, Administrator
Religious nonmedical health care institution.

7347 Kings Harbor Multicare Center
2000 E Gun Hill Rd
Bronx, NY 10469-6016
718-320-0400
FAX: 718-671-5022
info@kingsharbor.com
www.kingsharbor.com

Morris Tenenbaum, Owner
Octavio Marin, Vice President
Kings Harbor Multicare Center provides long-term and short-term skilled nursing care for more then 700 residents. Kings Harbor is located in the Pelham Gardens neighborhood of Northeast Bronx, easily accessible to major highways and near public transportation. A 3 building campus facility with surrounding gardens ensures that residents with similar capabilities are grouped together.

7348 Northwoods of Cortland
28 Kellogg Rd
Cortland, NY 13045-3155
607-753-9631
FAX: 607-756-2968
www.northwoodshealth.net

Lawrence Mennig, Administrator
Subacute rehabilitation facility.

7349 Port Jefferson Health Care Facility
141 Dosoris Lane
Glen Cove, NY 11542
631-676-1100
FAX: 631-759-0216
info@glenhaven.org
www.glengariffcare.com

Ellen Harte, Administrator
Subacute medical and rehabilitative care and long term residential skilled nursing care.

7350 Rehab Institute at Florence Nightingale Health Center
1760 3rd Ave
New York, NY 10029-6810
212-410-8760
800-786-8968
FAX: 212-410-8792
info@rehabinstitute.org

7351 Schnurmacher Center for Rehabilitation and Nursing
Beth Abraham of Family Health Services
12 Tibbits Ave
White Plains, NY 10606-2438
914-287-7200
888-238-4223
FAX: 914-428-1824
info@schnurmacher.org
www.schnurmacher.org

Linda Murray, Executive Director
Thomas Camisa, Medical Director
Iryn Obaldo Fontanosa, Director of Rehabilitation
Filomena Cristo, Director of Therapeutic Recreation
The environment at Schnurmacher is tailored to the needs of patients who require medical and nursing services but who do not need the complexity of services associated with an acute-care hospital. And Schnurmacher Subacute Medical patients are out of bed more quickly and as often as possible, which helps them maintain functional status while recovery progresses.

7352 South Shore Healthcare
275 W Merrick Rd
Freeport, NY 11520-3346
516-623-4000
FAX: 516-223-4599
www.northshorelij.com

Winnie Mack, RN, BSN, MPA, Regional Executive Director
Gene Tangney, Senior Vice President/ Regional Executive Director
Michael J. Dowling, President/ CEO
David L. Battinelli, MD, Senior Vice President/Chief Medical Officer
North Shore-LIJ Health System includes 16 award-winning hospitals and nearly 400 physician practice locations throughout New York, including Long Island, Manhattan, Queens and Staten Island. Proudly serving an area of seven million people, North Shore-LIJ delivers world-class services designed for every step of your health and wellness journey.

7353 St. Camillus Health and Rehabilitation Center
813 Fay Rd
Syracuse, NY 13219-3009
315-488-2951
FAX: 315-488-3255
info@st-camillus.org
www.st-camillus.org

Aileen Balitz, President
Patrick VanBeveren, PT, DPT, M, Supervisor of Physical Therapy
Nancy , Pirro, RN, Case Manager
Kathy Walsh,PT, DPT, NCS, Designer/Facilitator
Since our founding in 1969, St. Camillus' mission has been to provide high-quality services and facilities emphasizing the rehabilitation of individuals to their maximum potential. The importance of the human spirit drives all we do. We are dedicated to caring for life and helping individuals achieve their highest possible level of independence.

North Carolina

7354 Chapel Hill Rehabilitation and Healthcare Center
1602 E Franklin St
Chapel Hill, NC 27514-2892
919-967-1418
800-735-8262
FAX: 919-918-3811
www.chapelhillhc.com

Turner Prichett, Executive Director
Chapel Hill Rehabilitation and Healthcare Center accomodates 120 residents. We are located in downtown Chapel Hill on Franklin Street and we provide roud the clock nursing care 365 days a year. Intensive rehabilitation services are administered by our licensed speech, occupational and physical therapists. Our staff is trained to care for medically complex patients such as those requiring intensive wound care, dialysis, and artificial nutrition.

7355 Cypress Pointe Rehabilitation and Healthcare Center
2006 S 16th St
Wilmington, NC 28401-6613
910-763-6271
800-735-8262
FAX: 910-251-9803
HSDED0188@kindredhealthcare.com
www.cypresspointehc.com

Sara Deiter, Executive Director
Dr. Jose Gonzalez, Medical Director
Cypress Pointe offers comprehensive physical, occupational, speech and respiratory therapy services. Following a physician's referral, patients are evaluated to determine their needs. Recommendations are then made for the appropriate interventions and rehabilitation. If therapy is required, a personalized care plan is developed.

7356 Pettigrew Rehabilitation and Healthcare Center
1551 W Pettigrew St
Durham, NC 27705-4821
919-286-0751
800-735-8262
FAX: 919-286-5992
HSDED0116@kindredhealthcare.com
www.pettigrewhc.com

La'Ticia Beatty, Executive Director

Pettigrew Rehabilitation and Healthcare Center accomodates 107 residents. Our healthcare center is certified by Medicare and Medicaid. We have experienced staff members who care for our residents. We strive to improve the quality of life our residents experience as a result of the services they receive from our nursing and therapy departments.

7357   Raleigh Rehabilitation and Healthcare Center
616 Wade Ave
Raleigh, NC 27605-1237   919-828-6251
                                                 800-735-8262
                                            FAX: 919-828-3294
                            HSDED0143@kindredhealthcare.com
                                        www.raleighrehabhc.com

Steven Jones, Executive Director
Raleigh Rehabilitation and Healthcare Center accomodates 172 residents. We provide short-term rehabilitation-including, physical, occupational, and speech therapies-as well as long-term nursing services. We specialize in neurological disorders, complex diabetes treatment, amputation recovery and pain management. We welcome short stays (respite care). Transportation services are avaliable for physician appointments and dialysis treatments.

7358   Rehabilitation and Healthcare Center of Monroe
1212 E Sunset Dr
Monroe, NC 28112-4318   704-283-8548
                                                 800-735-8262
                                            FAX: 704-283-4664
                            HSDED0707@kindredhealthcare.com
                                          www.monroehc.com

Judy Olson, Executive Director
We accomodate 159 residents and are certified for Medicare and Medicaid. We specialize in short-term rehabilitation as well as long-term care. Our therapists, wound nurse and dietician work closely to administer wound care. We hav 2 dialysis centers within a 10-block radius and gladly accpet their patients. We have an on-staff medical director as well as a psychiatrist.

7359   Winston-Salem Rehabilitation and Healthcare Center
1900 W 1st St
Winston Salem, NC 27104-4220   336-724-2821
                                                 800-735-8262
                                            FAX: 336-725-8314

Tom Bauer, Administrator
We accommodate 230 residents and we have approximately 250 employees. Our staffing ratio averages 1 licensed nurse for every 20 residents and 1 Certified Nursing Assistant for every 10 residents. We offer a wide range of services including but not limited to respiratory care, tracheotomy care and gastric tube feeding and we also feature an in house licensed therapy program.

Ohio

7360   Arbors East Subacute and Rehabilitation Center
5500 E Broad St
Columbus, OH 43213-1476   614-575-9003
                                            FAX: 614-575-9101
                                  arborseast@extendicare.com
                            www.arborseastskillednursing.com

7361   Arbors at Canton Subacute And Rehabilitation Center
2714 13th St NW
Canton, OH 44708-3121   330-456-2842
                                            FAX: 330-456-5343
                                      www.laurelsofcanton.com

Amy McDermand, Director of Marketing
Beth Jones, PT, DPT, Rehabilitation Services Director
Cindy Shingler, RN,, Director of Nursing
Jennifer Fess, Administrator
We provide individualized, quality care to guests staying short-term for rehabilitation services or long-term for extended care services. The highest level of independence for our guests is the creed of The Laurels of Canton.

7362   Arbors at Dayton
320 Albany St
Dayton, OH 45408-1402   937-496-6200
                                            FAX: 937-496-1990
                                     dayton@extendicare.com
                               www.extendicareus.com/dayton

Dave Maxwell, Administrator
Carlisa Pedalino, Administrator
Arbors at Dayton is a leading provider of long-term skilled nursing care and short-term rehabilitation solutions. Our 106 bed facility offers a full continuum of services and care focused around each individual in today's ever-changing healthcare environment.

7363   Arbors at Marietta
400 N 7th St
Marietta, OH 45750-2024   740-373-3597
                                            FAX: 740-376-0004
                                    marietta@extendicare.com
                             www.extendicareus.com/marietta

Joan Florence, Director of Nursing
Kenneth Leopold, Medical Director
Arbors at Marietta is a leading provider of long-term skilled nursing care and short-term rehabilitation solutions. Our 150 bed facility offers a full continuum of services and care focused around each individual in today's ever-changing healthcare environment.

7364   Arbors at Milford
5900 Meadow Creek Dr
Milford, OH 45150-5641   513-248-1655
                                            FAX: 513-248-7340
                                     milford@extendicare.com
                               www.extendicareus.com/milford

Bruce Yarwood, President/CEO
Mark Ostendorf, Administrator
Arbors at Milford is a leading provider of long-term skilled nursing care and short-term rehabilitation solutions. Our 139 bed facility offers a full continuum of services and care focused around each individual in today's ever-changing healthcare environment.

7365   Arbors at Sylvania
7120 Port Sylvania Dr
Toledo, OH 43617-1158   419-841-2200
                                            FAX: 419-841-2822
                                    sylvania@extendicare.com
                             www.extendicareus.com/sylvania

Sheril Flowers, Administrator
Graig Hopple, Medical Director
Arbors at Sylvania is a leading provider of long-term skilled nursing care and short-term rehabilitation solutions. Our 79 bed facility offers a full continuum of services and care focused around each individual in today's ever-changing healthcare environment.

7366   Arbors at Toledo Subacute and Rehab Centre
2920 Cherry St
Toledo, OH 43608-1716   419-242-7458
                                            FAX: 419-242-6514
                                        www.extendicare.com

Jill Schlievert, Administrator
Subacute rehabilitation services and facility.

7367   Bridgepark Center for Rehabilitation and Nursing Services
145 Olive St
Akron, OH 44310-3236   330-762-0901
                                                 800-750-0750
                                            FAX: 330-762-0905
                                      www.bridgeparkrehab.net

Joseph Burick, Medical Director
A skilled nursing and rehabilitation center located in Akron, Ohio, across the street from St. Thomas Hospital with a beautiful view of the Akron skyline. Access to Interstate 77 and State Route 8 is just minutes away. Our entire staff is committed to providing caring, customer-focused skilled nursing and rehabilitation. For

your convenience, we accept Medicare, Medicaid and most managed care and private insurance.

7368   Broadview Multi-Care Center
5520 Broadview Rd
Parma, OH 44134-1605   216-749-4010
                                     FAX: 216-749-0141
                              info@broadviewmulticare.com
                              www.broadviewmulticare.com

Harold Shachter, Owner
Mike Flank, VP
Broadview Multi-Care Center is a family run business with more than 40 years of experience providing quality care to the community. We are committed to meeting your needs and providing you with a warm, home-like environment. Our family is on-site and our doors are always open for your suggestions or to drop in and say hello. We always try to take and honor requests, whether it's a favorite food, an exciting activity or a particular room.

7369   Caprice Care Center
9184 Market St
North Lima, OH 44452-9558   330-965-9200
                                     FAX: 330-726-6097
                              capriceadm@chcccompanies.com
                              www.chcccompanies.com/CapriceMain.html

Lori Crowl, Owner
Becky Berger, Director of Nursin
Stacey Howell, Administrator
Valerie Conzett, Admission Liaison
A 106-bed skilled nursing, subacute and rehabilitation facility. Our goal is to provide comfortable living to all who are in our care. Caprice Health Care Center is a contemporary Medicare and Medicaid approved facility specializing in short-term rehabilitation services. The inpatient/outpatient rehab department includes physical, occupational, speech therapies, indoor aquatic therapy pool, as well as complimentary van transportation for outpatient services.

7370   Cleveland Clinic
9500 Euclid Ave
Cleveland, OH 44195-2   216-444-2200
                                     800-801-2273
                                     FAX: 216-444-7021
                              my.clevelandclinic.org/default.aspx

Gene Altus, Executive Director
Delos M. Cosgrove, MD, Chief Executive Officer, Preside
Joseph F. Hahn, MD, Chief of Staff, Vice Chairman of
David Bronson, MD, Chief Executive Officer, Clevela
A not-for-profit, multispecialty academic medical center that integrates clinical and hospital care with research and education. Cleveland clinic was founded in 1921 by 4 renowned physicians with a vision of providing outstanding patient care based upon the principals of cooperation, compassion and innovation. Today, Cleveland Clinic is one of the largest and most respected hospitals in the country.

7371   Columbus Rehabilitation And Subacute Institute
111 West Michigan Street
Milwaukee, WI 53203-2903
                                     800-395-5000
                              kschaewe@extendicare.com
                              www.extendicareus.com

Kelly Fligor, Administrator
Jillian Fountain, Secretary
Subacute rehabilitation programs and facility.

7372   LakeMed Nursing and Rehabilitation Center
70 Normandy Dr
Painesville, OH 44077-1616   440-357-1311
                                     800-750-0750
                                     FAX: 440-352-9977
                              www.lakemednursing.com

Connie Eyman, Administrator
Vesta Jones, Executive Director
Our goal is to provide you with quality care and we are known for our successful short-term rehab and care of the clinically complex. We also offer respite services to give caregivers a rest, and hospice services through our local hospice care provider. Our in-

terdisciplinary team works together as they strive to deliver quality care and responsive service to our residents.

7373   Oregon Nursing And Rehabilitation Center
904 Isaac Streets Dr
Oregon, OH 43616-3204   419-691-2483
                                     FAX: 419-697-5401
                              www.extendicareus.com/oregon

Mark Rogers, Administrator
Subacute rehabilitation facility and services.

7374   Sunset View Castle Nursing Homes Castle Nursing Homes
434 N Washington St
Millersburg, OH 44654-1188   330-674-0015
                                     FAX: 330-763-2238
                              info@castlenursinghomes.com
                              www.castlenursinghomes.com

Becky Snyder, Admissions Coordinator
Kathy Edwards, Admissions And Marketing
310 licensed, certified beds. Subacute rehabilitation facility and programs.

Oregon

7375   Care Center East Health & Specialty Care Center
Expendicare
11325 NE Weidler St
Portland, OR 97220-1950   503-253-1181
                                     FAX: 503-253-1871
                              www.extendicareus.com

Glydon Kimbrough, Administrator
Subacute rehabilitation facility and programs

7376   Medford Rehabilitation and Healthcare Center
Kindred Healthcare
625 Stevens St
Medford, OR 97504-6719   541-779-3551
                                     800-735-1232
                                     FAX: 541-779-3658
                              www.medfordrehab.com

Grant Gloor, Administrator
Dane Reeves, Executive Director
Kristen W., Health and Rehabilitation Center
Becky D., Activity Director
We strive to provide quality, compassionate care. Our cozy building accomodates 110 residents. Our smaller size creates an inviting and homelike environment. We offer semi-private rooms with space to add items from home for a special personalized touch.

Pennsylvania

7377   Dresher Hill Health and Rehabilitation Center
1390 Camp Hill Rd
Dresher, PA 19034-2805   215-643-0600
                                     FAX: 215-641-0628
                              www.dresherhillskillednursing.com

Earl Kimble, Administrator
Subacute rehabilitation facility and programs: physical/speech.

7378   Good Shepherd Rehabilitation
850 S 5th St
Allentown, PA 18103-3295   610-776-3586
                                     888-447-3422
                                     FAX: 610-776-8336
                              info@goodshepherdrehab.org
                              goodshepherdrehab.org

John Kristel, MBA, MPT, President & CEO
Mike Bonner, MBA, Vice President, Neurosciences
Ronald J. Petula, CPA, Senior Vice President, Finance and Chief Financial Officer
Joseph Shadid, Administrator, Good Shepherd Home-Bethlehem
A world class rehabilitation network, Good Shepherd provides comprehensive inpatient and outpatient services throughout Pennsylvania's Lehigh Valley. Founded in 1908, Good Shepherd

has steadily expanded over last 95 years. Good Shepherd is one of the most comprehensive rehabilitation institutes in the world.

7379 Statesman Health and Rehabilitation Center
2629 Trenton Rd
Levittown, PA 19056-1428 215-943-7777
FAX: 215-943-1240
www.statesmanskillednursing.com

Jamie Tanner, Administrator
Subacute rehabilitation facility and programs.

7380 UPMC Braddock
200 Lothrop St.
Pittsburgh, PA 15213-2582 412-647-8762
800-533-8762
FAX: 412-636-5398
hospitalbill@upmc.edu
upmc.com

Mark Sevco, Administrator
Rodney Jones, Vice President
With a team of more then 43,000 employees, UPMC serves the health needs of more then 4 million people each year, improving lives in western Pennsylvania-and beyond-through redefined models of health care delivery and superb clinical outcomes.

7381 UPMC McKeesport
Presby
1500 5th Ave
McKeesport, PA 15132-2422 412-664-2000
FAX: 412-664-2309
fisherpj@upmc.edu
upmc.com

Ronald H Ott, CEO
Offers 56 beds for patients who need skilled nursing care. Offers ongoing rehabilitation and educational programs to patients with cardiac, neurologic, and orthopaedic diagnosis.

7382 UPMC Passavant
9100 Babcock Blvd
Pittsburgh, PA 15237-5842 412-367-6700
800-533-8762
gloordc@ph.upmc.edu
upmc.com

William Kristan, Dir Inpatient Physical Therapy
Teresa Petrick, Chief Executive Officer
Patients who have had an acute illness, injury, or exacerbation of a disease and no longer need the intensity of services in the acute care setting, but still require some complex medical care or supervision and rehabilitation services, may be appropriate to be transferred into the Subacute Unit.

Rhode Island

7383 Kindred Heights Nursing & Rehabilitation Center
Kindred Healthcare
680 South Fourth Street
Louisville, KY 40202 502-596-7300
800-545-0749
web_administrator@kindred.com
www.kindredheights.com

Sandra Sarza, Manager
Jean Aubin, Director
Kindred Heights Nursing and Rehabilitation Center accomodates 58 residents and serves the needs of elders in the greater East Bay and Providence area. We are conveniently located on Wampanoag Trail in East Providence. Kindred Heights provides skilled nursing, short-term rehab and long-term care in a family environment, but we are large enough to manage the complex nursing and rehab care needs our residents may have.

7384 Oak Hill Nursing and Rehabilitation Center
Kindered Health Care
544 Pleasant St
Pawtucket, RI 02860-5776 401-725-8888
800-745-6575
FAX: 401-723-5720
www.oakhillrehab.com

Scott M. Sandborn, Executive Director
Heidi Capela, Director Nursing
Amybeth Almeida, Director Admissions
Aman Nanda, Medical Director
Accomodates 143 residents. Throughout our 40 year history, Oak Hill has developed a reputation as one of the finest healthcare centers in Rhode Island. Our center consists of 3 separate units. A 34-bed post-acute unit provides care to the medically complex and those in need of extensive rehabilitative services. A 20-bed Alzheimer's Special Care Unit provides a unique style of care utilizing habilitative therapy in comfortable, home-like surroundings.

7385 Southern New England Rehab Center
200 High Service Avenue
North Providence, RI 02904 401-456-3801
888-456-4501
FAX: 401-456-3784
www.snerc.com

Vivian Hagstrom, Manager
The Center's skilled staff of over 100 professionals provides a full range of coordinated rehabilitative care. Our clinical expertise and compassion make a big difference as we develop first-rate plans of care for the unique needs of each patient. Our medical staff is comprised of physicians board-certified in rehabilitation medicine and internal medicine.

South Carolina

7386 Tuomey Healthcare System
129 N Washington St
Sumter, SC 29150-4949 803-774-9000
FAX: 803-774-8737
www.tuomey.com

R Jay Cox, CEO
Here to anticipate the needs of the communities we serve, responding with proactive healthcare initiatives, providing expert rehabilitative services and delivering life-saving acute care.

Tennessee

7387 Camden Healthcare and Rehabilitation Center
680 South Fourth Street
Louisville, KY 40202 502-596-7300
800-545-0749
web_administrator@kindred.com
kindredhealthcare.com

Mark Walker, Administrator
Subacute rehabilitation products and services, nursing and life care homes.

7388 Centennial Medical Center Tri Star Health System
2300 Patterson St
Nashville, TN 37203-1538 615-342-1000
800-242-5662
FAX: 615-342-1045
Laurel.Haskamp@HCAHealthcare.com
tristarcentennial.com

Thomas L Herron, President/Chief Executive Office
Above all else we are committed to the care and improvement of human life by caring for those we serve with integrity, compassion, a positive attitude, respect and exceptional quality.

7389 Cordova Rehabilitation and Nursing Center
955 N Germantown Pkwy
Cordova, TN 38018-6215
901-754-1393
800-848-0299
FAX: 901-754-3332
cdadmi@gracehc.com
www.gracehccordova.com

John Palmer, Administrator
Renee Tutor, Executive Director
Our professional staff can help you make an informed decision. Upon admission, our interdisciplinary team develops a comprehensive care plan to meet not only physical and rehabilitative goals, but also social and emotional needs. We understand the importance of family and resident involvement and encourage participation in the development of a personalized plan of care.

7390 Erlanger Medical Center Baronness Campus
975 E 3rd St
Chattanooga, TN 37403-2147
423-778-7000
FAX: 423-778-7615
guestrelations@erlanger.org
www.erlanger.org

Kevin M. Spiegel, FACHE, President and CEO
James Creel, MD, Chief Medical Officer
Gregg T. Gentry, Chief Administrative Officer
Robert M. Brooks, FACHE, Executive Vice President and Chief Operating Officer
Our mission is to improve the health of the people we touch. Our vision is to be recognized locally, regionally, and and nationally, as a premiere healthcare system.

7391 Huntington Health and Rehabilitation Center
635 High St
Huntingdon, TN 38344-1703
731-986-8943
FAX: 731-986-3188
w.summers@huntingdonhealth.com
huntingdonhealth.com

Heidi Hawkins, Administrator
Windi Summers, Admissions Director
Subacute rehabilitation facility and programs.

7392 Madison Healthcare and Rehabilitation Center
431 Larkin Springs Rd
Madison, TN 37115-5005
615-865-8520
800-848-0299
FAX: 615-868-4455
www.madisonrehab.com

Phyllis Cherry, Executive Director
At our facility, we provide quality care with modern rehabilitation and restorative nursing techniques. We aim to provide an atmosphere which encourages family involvement in the care-planning process, with the right mix of activities addressing the social, spiritual and intellectual needs of our residents.

7393 Mariner Health of Nashville
3939 Hillsboro Cir
Nashville, TN 37215-2708
615-297-2100
FAX: 615-297-2197

David Reeves, Administrator
Amy Artrip, Director of Nursing
Religious nonmedical health care institution. 150-bed subacute rehabilitation facility

7394 Pine Meadows Healthcare and Rehabilitation Center
700 Nuckolls Rd
Bolivar, TN 38008-1531
731-658-4707
FAX: 731-658-4769
s.mckeen@pinemeadowshc.com
www.pinemeadowshc.com

Larry Shrader, Administrator
Sharon McKeen, Admissions Director
Our goal is to take care of your loved ones. Our professional team works with skilled hands, is directed by creative minds and is guided by compassionate hearts. Upon your admission, our interdisciplinary team develops a comprehensive care plan designed with a goal of meeting not only physical and rehabilitative objectives, but also social and emotional needs. We understand the importance of family and resident involvement and encourage participation in the development of a plan of care.

7395 Primacy Healthcare and Rehabilitation Center
Kindred Health Care
6025 Primacy Pkwy
Memphis, TN 38119-5763
901-767-1040
800-848-0299
FAX: 901-685-7362
www.primacyrehab.com

Donnie Dubert, Executive Director
Dr. Mark Hammond, Medical Director
Kristen W., Health and Rehabilitation Center
Becky D., Activity Director
Upon a resident's admission, our interdisciplinary team develops a comprehensive care plan with a goal of meeting not only physical and rehabilitative objectives but also social and emotional needs. We understand the importance of family and resident involvement and encourage participation in the development of a personalized plan of care.

7396 Ripley Healthcare and Rehabilitation Center
118 Halliburton St
Ripley, TN 38063-2011
731-635-5180
FAX: 731-635-0663
j.hodge@ripleyhc.com
www.ripleyhc.com

Johnny Rea, Executive Director
Brandon Whiteside, Executive Director
Jan Hodge, Admissions Directo
Jennifer Pitts, Administrator
Upon admission, our interdisciplinary team develops a comprehensive care plan to meet not only physical and rehabilitative goals, but also social and emotional needs. We understand the importance of family and resident involvement and encourage participation in the development of a personalized care plan. Our goal is to take care of your loved ones.

7397 Shelby Pines Rehabilitation and Healthcare Center
3909 Covington Pike
Memphis, TN 38135-2281
901-377-1011
FAX: 901-377-0032

Rene Tutor, Executive Director
Subacute rehabiltation facility and programs.

7398 Siskin Hospital for Physical Rehabilitation
1 Siskin Plz
Chattanooga, TN 37403-1306
423-634-1200
FAX: 423-634-4538
TTY:423-634-1201
info@siskinrehab.org
siskinrehab.org

Robert Main, CEO
Lindsay Wyatt, Media Coordinator, Marketing Co
Dedicated exclusively to physical rehabilitation and offers specialized treatment programs in brain injury, amputation, stroke, spinal cord injury, orthopeadics, and major multiple trauma.

Texas

7399 North Hills Hospital
4401 Booth Calloway Rd
North Richland Hills, TX 76180-7399
817-255-1000
FAX: 817-255-1991
northhillshospital.com

Randy Moresi, CEO
North Hills Hospital's services include a wide range of cardiovascular services, surgical services, emergency services, radiology, a rehabilitation unit, a senior health center, therapy services, and women's services.

7400 Valley Regional Medical Center
100 E Alton Gloor Blvd
Brownsville, TX 78526-3328   956-350-7000
                                    FAX: 956-350-7111
                            valleyregionalmedicalcenter.com

Susan Andrews, CEO
Francisco Javier Del Castillo, MD
Subramaniam Anandasivam, MD
Christopher Olson, MD
Above all else, we are committed to the care and improvement of
human life. In recognition of this committment, we strive to deliver high quality, cost effective healthcare in the communities
we serve. In persuit of our mission, we recognize and affirm the
unique and intrinsic worth of each individual. We treat all those
we serve with compassion and kindness. We act with absolute
honesty and integrity and fairness in the way we conduct our business and the way we live our lives.

Utah

7401 Crosslands Rehabilitation and Healthcare Center
680 South Fourth Street
Louisville, KY 40202   502-596-7300
                                            800-545-0749
                            web_administrator@kindred.com
                                    www.kindredhealthcare.com

John Williams, Executive Director
Lyle Black, Manager
Crossroads Rehabilitation and Healthcare accomodates 120 residents. We are fully Medicare and Medicaid certified. We are
proud of our reputation for providing quality, compassionate
care. Services availiable include in-house physical, occupational
and speech therapies, as well as 24-hour licensed nursing staff
coverage. We offer therapeutic recreation, in-house social services and registered dietician services, among many other
professional services.

7402 Federal Heights Rehabilitation and Nursing Center
Kindred Health Care
680 South Fourth Street
Louisville, KY 40202   502-596-7300
                                            800-545-0749
                            web_administrator@kindred.com
                                    www.kindredhealthcare.com

Pete Zeigler, Executive Director
Dr. Charles Canfield, Medical Director
Federal Heights accomodates 120 residents. We are located near
three major hospitals in the Salt Lake Valley. We specialize in
providing nursing services for complex medical and rehabilitation conditions. Our discharge planning works jointly with the
family and resident in determining the future needs and goals
upon discharge.

7403 St. George Care and Rehabilitation Center
Kindred Health Care Publications
1032 E 100 S
Saint George, UT 84770-3005   435-628-0488
                                            800-346-4128
                                    FAX: 435-628-7362
                                    www.stgeorgecare.com

John Larson, Plant Manager
Erin Hammon, Director of Nursing
Derrick Glum, Executive Director
St. George Care and Rehabilitation accomodates 95 residents. We
offer a 4,000 square foot rehabilitation gym with an indoor therapy pool for inpatient and outpatient services. Therapy is provided to meet specific needs seven days a week. There is a
dietitian on staff for individualized nutritional needs. We offer an
Alzheimer's unit with specialized staff. We provide compassionate health services including physicians, nurses, physical therapists, and occupational therapist and licensed aides.

7404 St. Mark's Hospital
1200 E 3900 S
Salt Lake City, UT 84124-1390   801-268-7111
                                    FAX: 801-270-3489
                                    www.stmarkshospital.com

Steve B. Bateman, CEO
Above all else we are committed to the care and improvement of
human life. In recognition of this commitment, we strive to deliver high quality, cost effective healthcare in the communities
we serve. We define quality as 'caring people with the commitment to a continuous process of improvement in the services provided, that will better enable the hospital to meet or exceed our
customer's needs and expectations.

7405 Wasatch Valley Rehabilitation
Kindred Healthcare
680 South Fourth Street
Louisville, KY 40202   502-596-7300
                                            800-545-0749
                            web_administrator@kindred.com
                                    www.kindredhealthcare.com

Alex Stevenson, Executive Director
Ric Toomer, Executive Director
Wasatch Valley accomodates 110 residents. We are licensed for
Medicare and Medicaid and we are conveniently located in the
heart of Salt Lake City with easy access from I-15 and I-215. We
are known by the area hospitals as a specialist in wound care and
for the care we provide to those with complex medical conditions.

Virginia

7406 Nansemond Pointe Rehabilitation and Healthcare Center
200 Constance Rd
Suffolk, VA 23434-4960   757-539-8744
                                            800-828-1140
                                    FAX: 757-539-6128
                                    www.nansemondhc.com

Mel Epelle, Executive Director
Mary R, Activities Assistant
Kristen W., Health and Rehabilitation Center
Becky D., Activity Director
Nansemond Pointe Rehabilitation and Healthcare Center
accomodates 160 residents in private and semi-private rooms. We
have been serving the needs of Suffolk, Virginia and the surrounding areas for over 38 years. We offer an entire continuum of
care from assisted living apartments to skilled nursing to
long-term care. Our licensed therapists, working with our dedicated nursing staff, share a common goal- to help our residents
improve their level of recovery and independence.

**7407 Rehabilitation and Research Center Virginia
Commonwealth University**
1250 East Marshall Street
Richmond, VA 23298   804-828-9000
                                    FAX: 804-828-5074
                                    www.vcuhealth.org

Michael Rao, Ph.D., VCU President & VCUHS President,
Sheldon M. Retchin, M.D., VP Health Sciences & CEO, VCUHS
John Duval, Chief Executive Officer MCV Hosp
Dominic J. Puleo, Executive VP Finance and CFO, VC
The Rehabilitation and Research Center is a collaborative effort
between the Department of Physical Medicine and Rehabilitation
and the Medical College of Virginia Hospitals. The goals of the
Rehabilitation and Research Center at the Medical College of
Virginia Hospitals (MCVH) are to provide highly-skilled, inter-
disciplinary, inpatient rehabilitative care to adults with complex
needs; to be an advocate and educator for patients and people
with disabilities.

7408   Warren Memorial Hospital
1000 N Shenandoah Ave
Front Royal, VA 22630-3598
540-636-0300
800-994-6610
FAX: 540-636-0258
complaint@jointcommission.org
www.valleyhealthlink.com
Mark H. Merrill, President & Chief Executive Officer
Tonya Smith, Vice President of Operations
Pete Gallagher, Senior Vice President & CFO
Joan Roscoe, Vice President of Information Sy
A nonprofit organization of health care providers, Valley Health offers a full spectrum of services in acute care, rehabilitation and extended care facilities, and outpatient and community settings to help the people of the region manage their health and enjoy a high quality of life. Valley Health has the resources to diagnose, treat and help patients manage virtually any medical problem that may be encountered.

7409   Winchester Rehabilitation Center
333 W Cork St
Suite 230
Winchester, VA 22601-3870
540-536-5114
800-994-6610
FAX: 540-536-1122
complaint@jointcommission.org
www.valleyhealthlink.com
Mark H. Merrill, President & Chief Executive Officer
Tonya Smith, Vice President of Operations
Pete Gallagher, Senior Vice President & CFO
Joan Roscoe, Vice President of Information Sy
Offers the following rehabilitation services: Sub-Acute inpatient rehabilitation, Speech therapy, Physical therapy, Occupational therapy, Disability evaluations. 30-bed inpatient center.

Washington

7410   Aldercrest Health and Rehabilitation Center
21400 72nd Ave W
Edmonds, WA 98026-7702
425-775-1961
FAX: 425-771-0116
aldercrest@extendicare.com
www.aldercrestskillednursing.com
Rick Milsow, Administrator
Aldercrest Health & Rehabilitation Center is a leading provider of long-term skilled nursing care and short-term rehabilitation solutions. Our 124 bed facility offers a full continuum of services and care focused around each individual in today's ever-changing healthcare environment.

7411   Arden Rehabilitation and Healthcare Center
16357 Aurora Ave N
Seattle, WA 98133-5651
206-542-3103
800-833-6384
FAX: 206-542-7192
www.ardenrehab.com
Matthew Preston, Administrator
Ann Zell, Executive Director
Kristen W., Health and Rehabilitation Center
Becky D., Activity Director
Arden Rehabilitation has been an integral part of the Shoreline community since 1953. It is a one-level building set on mature grounds with several beautiful courtyards for the residents to enjoy. Arden can accomodate 90 residents-post acute/rehabilitation patients as well as long-term residents. Medicare certified, the center also takes most managed healthcare insurance plans, as well as VA, respite and hospice patients.

7412   Bellingham Health Care and Rehabilitation Services
1200 Birchwood Ave
Bellingham, WA 98225-1302
360-734-9295
800-833-6384
FAX: 360-671-4368
www.avamererehabofbellingham.com
Melissa Nelson, Executive Director
Dr. Richard McClenahan, Medical Director
Kristen W., Health and Rehabilitation Center
Becky D., Activity Director
At Bellingham Health Care and Rehab, we strive to provide quality, compassionate care. Our cozy building accomodates 84 residents. Our smaller size creates an inviting and homelike environment for your loved one. We offer semi-private rooms with space to add items from home for a special personalized touch. Provides meals served restaurant style in our dinning room overlooking our beautiful grounds.

7413   Bremerton Convalescent and Rehabilitation Center
2701 Clare Ave
Bremerton, WA 98310-3313
360-377-3951
FAX: 360-377-5443
bremertonskillednursing.com
Stephanie Bonanzino, Administrator
Subacute rehabilitation facility and programs.

7414   Edmonds Rehabilitation & Healthcare Centerer
Kindred Healthcare
21008 76th Ave W
Edmonds, WA 98026-7104
425-778-0107
800-833-6384
FAX: 425-776-9532
www.edmondsrehab.com
Jane Davis, Executive Director
At Edmonds Rehabilitation and Healthcare, we strive to provide quality, compassionate care. Our center accomodates 91 residents. Our smaller size creates an inviting and homelike environment. We offer semi-private rooms with space to add items from home for a special personalized touch. Edmonds Rehabilitation and Healthcare provides delicious meals served restaurant style in our dinning room.

7415   Heritage Health and Rehabilitation Center
Kindred Health Care
3605 Y St
Vancouver, WA 98663-2647
360-693-5839
800-833-6384
FAX: 360-693-3991
www.heritagerehab.com
Michael Moses, Executive Director
Su Patchett, Director of Nursing
Heritage Health & Rehabilitation Center is the smallest free-standing healthcare center in southwest Washington with accomodations of 49, enabling more personal care and a more home-like environment. Heritage has licensed nursing staff, restorative aides, and certified nurses assistants, trained and experienced in providing Alzheimer's care, end of life/hospice care, psychiatric care, rehabilitative care, and respite care.

7416   North Auburn Rehabilitation And Health Center
111 West Michigan Street
Milwaukee, WI 53203-2903
800-395-5000
kschaewe@extendicare.com
extendicare.com
Allyson Jenkins, Administrator
Subacute rehabilitation facility and programs.

7417   Northwoods Lodge
2321 NW Schold Pl
Silverdale, WA 98383-9504
360-698-3930
FAX: 360-692-2169
mhalverson@encorecommunities.com
www.encorecommunities.com
Leslie Krueger, Owner
Debbie Griffin, Director of Rehab Services
Silverdale Campus, Executive Director

Provides you with a full-range of services from weekly house-keeping and laudry services, to grounds keeping and mainte-nance. Our monthy fee inculdes utilities and hot, delicious, nutritious meals served table side every day. We offer transporta-tion services, full-time activities directors, and numerous ameni-ties to add to your comfort and enjoyment.

7418   Pacific Specialty & Rehabilitation Center r
1015 N Garrison Rd
Vancouver, WA 98664-1313   360-694-7501
                                        FAX: 360-694-8148
                                www.pacificskillednursing.com
Rebecca Pruett, Administrator
Subacute rehabilitation facility and programs.

7419   Puget Sound Healthcare Center
4001 Capitol Mall Dr SW
Olympia, WA 98502-8657   360-754-9792
                                        FAX: 360-754-2455
                             www.pugetsoundskillednursing.com
Sheila Oberg, Administrator
Our goal is to provide excellence in patient care, veteran's bene-fits and customer satisfaction. We have reformed our department internally and are striving for high quality, prompt and seamless service to veterans. Our department employees continue to offer their dedication and commitment to help veterans get the services they have earned.

7420   Vancouver Health & Rhabilitation Center
400 E 33rd St
Vancouver, WA 98663-2238   360-696-2561
                                             800-833-6384
                                        FAX: 360-696-9275
                               www.vancouverhealthcare.com
Jody Wigen, Human Resources
Joe Joy, Executive Director
Kristen W., Health and Rehabilitation Center
Becky D., Activity Director
At Vancouver Health and Rehab Center we strive to provide qual-ity, compassionate care. Our cozy building accomodates 98 resi-dents. Our smaller size creates an inviting and homelike environment. We offer semi-private rooms with space to add items from home for a special personalized touch. Provides deli-cious meals served restaurant style in our dining room.

West Virginia

7421   War Memorial Hospital
1 Healthy Way
Berkeley Springs, WV 25411-1743   304-258-1234
                                        FAX: 304-258-5618
                               complaint@jointcommission.org
                                   www.valleyhealthlink.com
Mark H. Merrill, President & Chief Executive Officer
Tonya Smith, Vice President of Operations
Pete Gallagher, Senior Vice President & Chief Financial Officer
Joan Roscoe, Vice President of Information Systems
Offers physical therapy, occupational therapy, speech therapy, social services, and patient/family education for individuals who have experienced a recent physical disability due to disease, dys-function, or general debilitation. Helps patients to maximize their abilities through activities of daily living, mobility, self-medica-tion, and self-care and restore their ability to return to their previous lifestyle.

Wisconsin

7422   Cedar Spring Health and Rehabilitation Center
N27w5707 Lincoln Blvd
Cedarburg, WI 53012-2852   262-376-7676
                                        FAX: 262-376-7808
                                www.cedarspringsskillednursing.com
Mary Wirth, Executive Director
Subacute rehabilitation facility and programs.

7423   Clearview-Brain Injury Center
198 Home Rd
Juneau, WI 53039-1401   920-386-3400
                                             877-386-3400
                                        FAX: 920-386-3800
                                  lbertagnoli@co.dodge.wi.us
                                   co.dodge.wi.us/clearview
Jane E. Hooper, Administrator
Jacqueline Kuhl, Household Coordinator
Laura Bertagnoli
Kathy Lorenz, AFH Manager
A 30-bed, state certified, subacute neuro-rehabilitation program in Juneau, WI. We are located just 45 minutes northeast of Madi-son WI and 10 minutes east of Beaver Dam, WI. We are the first and longest standing of only 2 community re-entry programs in the state of Wisconsin providing subacute neuro-rehabilitation to teens and adults who have experienced a brain injury.

7424   Colonial Manor Medical and Rehabilitation Center
1010 E Wausau Ave
Wausau, WI 54403-3101   715-842-2028
                                             800-947-6644
                                        FAX: 715-848-0510
                                   www.colonialmanormrc.com
Ericca Ylitalo, Administrator
Shelley Solberg, Executive Director
Kristen W., Health and Rehabilitation Center
Becky D., Activity Director
Colonial Manor Medical and Rehabilitation Center is part of the Kindred Community and is located in Wausau, Wisconsin. The corporate headquarters are based in Louisville Kentucky. Our fa-cility accomodates 150 residents.

7425   Eastview Medical and Rehabilitation Center
729 Park St
Antigo, WI 54409-2745   715-623-2356
                                             800-947-6644
                                        FAX: 715-623-6345
                                   www.eastviewmedrehab.com
Wanda Hose, Administrator
Wanda Hose, Executive Director
Kristen W., Health and Rehabilitation Center
Becky D., Activity Director
Eastview Medical Center and Rehabilitation Center accomodates 165 residents. We are Medicare and Medicaid certified, as well as being Joint Commission accredited. Our 'TEAM' approach means specially trained staff work around the clock to assist in meeting rehabilitative goals established by our team of profes-sionals. We encourage family involvement in our rehabilitative process. The support of loved ones is a major key to a speedy recovery.

7426   Hospitality Nursing Rehabilitation Center
8633 32nd Ave
Kenosha, WI 53142-5187   262-694-8300
                                        FAX: 262-694-3622
                                www.hospitalityskillednursing.com
Marla Benson, Administrator
LaRae Nelson, President
Lisa Behling, Secretary
Scott Miller, Treasurer
Subacute rehabilitation facility and programs.

7427   Kennedy Park Medical Rehabilitation Center
Kindred Healthcare
6001 Alderson St
Schofield, WI 54476-3614   715-359-4257
                                             800-947-6644
                                        FAX: 715-355-4867
                                     info@kennedyparkrehab.com
                                   www.kennedyparkrehab.com
Judy Kowalski, Manager
Jim Torgerson, Executive Director
Kristen W., Health and Rehabilitation Center
Becky D., Activity Director
Kennedy Park Medical & Rehabilitation Center accomodates 154 residents. We are located in Schofield, WI. At Kennedy Park, we specialize in dementia care, with our Reflections and Passages

Units. Short-term rehabilitation and sub-acute care are provided in a setting conducive to meeting the individual needs of our residents and patients. We also provide general nursing care for persons with long-term care needs.

7428 Middleton Village Nursing & Rehabilitation
Kindred
6201 Elmwood Ave
Middleton, WI 53562-3319
608-831-8300
800-947-6644
FAX: 608-831-4253
www.middletonvillage.com
Nicholas Stamatas, Manager
Ashley Ostrowski, Executive Director
Kristen W., Health and Rehabilitation Center
Becky D., Activity Director
Middleton Village accomodates 97 residents. We specialize in post-surgical and post-acute rehabilitation and long-term care services.

7429 Mount Carmel Health & Rehabilitation Center
5700 W Layton Ave
Milwaukee, WI 53220-4099
414-281-7200
FAX: 414-281-4620
www.milwaukeemtcarmel.com
Mike Berry, Administrator
Darrin Hull, Executive Director
Kristen W., Health and Rehabilitation Center
Becky D., Activity Director
Subacute rehabilitation facility and programs.

7430 Mount Carmel Medical and Rehabilitation Center
680 South Fourth Street
Louisville, KY 40202
502-596-7300
800-545-0749
web_administrator@kindred.com
kindredhealthcare.com
Randy Nitschke, Administrator
Jeanne Piccioni, Executive Director
Mount Carmel Medical and Rehabilitation Center accomodates 155 residents. We are located in Burlington Wisconsin. Mount Carmel Medical and Rehabilitation center is a recipient of the American Health Care Association Quality Award.

7431 North Ridge Medical and Rehabilitation Center
1445 N 7th St
Manitowoc, WI 54220-2011
920-682-0314
800-947-6644
FAX: 920-682-0553
HSDED0769@kindredhealthcare.com
www.nrmrc.com
Jane Conway, Interim ED
Mary Ann Hamer, Executive Director
North Ridge Medical and Rehabiliation Center accomodates 110 residents. We have been serving the Manitowoc, Wisconsin area for over 25 years. Our goal is to provide services in a warm, homey environment. Many of our staff in all departments have a long history with North Ridge and have worked here for more then 20 years. We also take pride in the fact that we have all in-house staff. Our therapy team is availiable to provide physical, occupational and speech therapy 7 days a week.

7432 Oshkosh Medical and Rehabilitation Center
1580 Bowen St
Oshkosh, WI 54901
920-233-4011
FAX: 920-233-5177
www.northpointmedicalandrehab.com
Tom Wagner, President
Subacute rehabilitation facility and programs.

7433 San Luis Medical and Rehabilitation Center
680 South Fourth Street
Louisville, KY 40202
502-596-7300
800-545-0749
web_administrator@kindred.com
www.kindredhealthcare.com
Heather Dreier, Administrator
Tim Dietzen, Executive Director
Dr. John T. Warren, Medical Director
Kristen W., Health and Rehabilitation Center
San Luis Medical and Rehabilitation Center accomodates 126 residents. We are located in Green bay, WI. At San Luis, we strive to meet the needs of our residents and we specialize in dementia care, with our Reflections Unit. Our goal is to provide short-term rehabilitation and sub-acute care in a setting conducive to assisting the needs of our residents.

7434 Strawberry Lane Nursing & Rehabilitation Center
130 Strawberry Lane
Wisconsin Rapids, WI 54494-2156
715-424-1600
FAX: 715-424-4817
cglodoski@strawberrylanenursing.com
www.strawberrylanenursing.com
Cyndi Glodoski, Admissions Director
Carrie Russert, Administrator
Skilled nursing facility that provides both long term and short term care. Offer Alzheimer's and Dementia care units, as well as Hospice Care. Medicare and Medicaid certified.

Wyoming

7435 Mountain Towers Healthcare & Rehabilitation Center
3128 Boxelder Dr
Cheyenne, WY 82001-5808
307-634-7901
800-877-9975
FAX: 307-634-7910
www.mttowersrehab.com
Dan Stackis, Administrator
Toni Wyenn, Director of Nursing
Daniel G. Stackis, Executive Director
Dr. Kent Britton, Medical Director
Mountain Towers Healthcare and Rehabilitation Center accomodates 170 residents, including a 16-bed acute secure unit. We offer a full range of nursing and medical care to meet individual needs. We have a full staff to meet the needs of our residents.

7436 South Central Wyoming Healthcare and Rehabilitation
Kindred Healthcare
542 16th St
Rawlins, WY 82301-5241
307-324-2759
800-877-9975
FAX: 307-324-7579
www.kindredrawlins.com
Chris Tanner, Executive Director
Anthony Janusz, Administrator
Kristen W., Health and Rehabilitation Center
Becky D., Activity Director
South Central Wyoming Healthcare and Rehabilitation accomodates 52 residents. We are located in Rawlings, in south central Wyoming. We are Medicare and Medicaid certified by the State of Wyoming. We strive to provide quality personal services, long-term care or short-term rehabilitation to our residents in a comfortable home-like environment.

7437 Wind River Healthcare and Rehabilitation Center
Kindred Health Care
1002 Forest Dr
Riverton, WY 82501-2918
307-856-9471
800-877-9975
FAX: 307-856-1665
www.windriverhealthcare.com
Jo Ann Aldrich, Executive Director
Amelia Asay, Business Office Manager
Kristen W., Health and Rehabilitation Center
Becky D., Activity Director

Offers a full range of medical services to meet the individual needs of our residents, including short-term rehabilitative services and long-term skilled care. Working with the residents physician, our staff-including medical specialists, nurses, nutritionists, dietitians and social workers-establishes a comprehensive treatment plan intended to restore you or your loved one to the highest practicable potential.

Aging

Associations

7438 Aging Life Care Association
3275 W. Ina Road
Suite 130
Tucson, AZ 85741-2198 520-881-8008
FAX: 520-325-7925
www.aginglifecare.org

Kaaren Boothroyd, CEO
Amanda Mizell, Member Relations
Julie Wagner, Director of Administration
Chelsea Fouts, Administrative Assistant
A nonprofit association to create a world where adults and their families live well as they face the challenges of aging.

7439 Aging Services of California
1315 I St
Suite 100
Sacramento, CA 95814-2915 916-392-5111
FAX: 916-428-4250
info@aging.org
www.aging.org

Kay Kallander, Chair
Todd Murch, Chair Elect
Robert Edmondson, Vice Chair
Roberta Jacobsen, Vice Chair
The California Association of Homes and Services for the Aging (CAHSA) is the primary statewide association for not-for-profit organizations providing health care, housing and community services to older adults.

7440 Aging Services of Michigan
201 North Washington Square
Suite 920
Lansing, MI 48933 517-323-3687
FAX: 517-323-4569
info@leadingagemi.org
www.agingmi.org

David Herbel, President/CEO
Deanna Ludlow Mitchell, Senior Vice President for Perfor
Debra Danai, Director of Finance
Stephanie Shooks Winslow, Vice President for Government St
Aging Services of Michigan represents and promotes the common interests of its members through leadership, advocacy, education and other services in order to enhance members' ability to serve their constituencies.

7441 Aging Services of South Carolina
2711 Middleburg Dr
Suite 309-A
Columbia, SC 29204-2413 803-988-0005
FAX: 803-988-1017
information@leadingagesc.org
www.scanpha.org

Vickie Moody, President/CEO
Beth Bouknight, Education Coordinator
Aging Services of South Carolina represents not-for-profit organizations dedicated to providing high-quality health care, housing and services to the seniors of South Carolina.

7442 Aging Services of Washington
1495 Wilmington Driv
Ste 340
Dupont, WA 98327-8773 253-964-8870
FAX: 253-964-8876
info@leadingagewa.org
www.agingwa.org

Bonnie Blachly, Director of Clinical Services
Paul Montgomery, Director of Financial Services
Pat Sylvia, Director of Member Development
Julie Martin, Director of Senior Living & Community Services
Washington Association of Housing and Services for the Aging (WASHA) is the state association serving primarily not-for-profit organizations dedicated to providing quality housing, health, community and related services to older persons.

7443 Aging in America
1000 Pelham Pkwy South
Bronx, NY 10461-1198 718-824-4004
877-244-6469
FAX: 718-824-4242
admissiondept@aiamsh.org
www.aginginamerica.org

William T Smith, President/CEO
Research and services organization for professionals in gerontology. Objectives are: to produce, implement and share effective and affordable programs and services that improve the quality of life for the elderly community; to better prepare professionals and students interested in or currently involved with, aging and the aged. Conducts research projects, educational and training seminars, and in-service curricula for long-term and acute care facilities.

7444 Alliance for Aging Research
1700 K St., NW
Suite 740
Washington, DC 20006 202-293-2856
FAX: 202-955-8394
info@agingresearch.org
www.agingresearch.org

Allan M. Fox, Chair
James E. Eden, Chairmen Emeritus
Amye Leong, Treasurer
George Beach, Secretary
The leading nonprofit organization dedicated to accelerating the pace of scientific discoveries and their application to vastly improve the universal human experience of aging and health.

7445 Alliance for Retired Americans
815 16th Street, NW
Fourth Floor
Washington, DC 20006 202-637-5399
retiredamericans.org

Barbara Easterling, President
Richard Fiesta, Executive Director
Ruben Burks, Secretary-Treasurer
Liz Shuler, Executive Vice President
An alliance to ensure social and economic justice and full civil rights for all citizens so that they may enjoy lives of dignity, personal and family fulfillment and security.

7446 American Aging Association
PO Box 664236
Washington State University
Pullman, WA 99164-4236
Contact@AmericanAgingAssociation.org
www.americanagingassociation.org

Janko Nikolich-Zugich, Chair
Matt Kaeberlein, President-elect
James F. Nelson, President
Rochelle Buffenstein, Immediate Past President
It is a group of experts dedicated to understanding the basic mechanisms of aging and the development of interventions in age-related disease to increase healthy lifespan for all.

7447 American Association of Homes and Servicesfor the Aging
2519 Connecticut Ave NW
Washington, DC 20008-1520 202-783-2242
FAX: 202-783-2255
info@LeadingAge.org
www.leadingage.org

William L Minnix Jr, President/CEO
Katrinka Smith Sloan, Chief Operating Officer and Seni
Robyn I. Stone, Senior Vice President of Researc
Cheryl Phillips, Senior Vice President, Policy and Advocacy
The American Association of Homes and Services for the Aging (AAHS) represents not-for-profit organizations dedicated to providing high-quality health care, housing and services to the nation's elderly. AAHSA organizations serve more than one million older persons af all income levels, creeds and races.

7448 **American Association of Retired Persons**
601 E St NW
Washington, DC 20049-2

800-687-2277
TTY:877-434-7589
member@aarp.org
www.aarp.org

A Barry Rand, President/CEO
Hop Backus, Executive Vice President, State
Steve Cone, Executive Vice President of Integrated Value and Strategy
Lorraine Cort,s-V zquez, Executive Vice President, Multicultural Markets and Engageme
A nonprofit membership organization of persons 50 and older dedicated to addressing their needs and interests.

7449 **American Geriatrics Society**
40 Fulton St., 18th Floor
New York, NY 10038

212-308-1414
FAX: 212-832-8646
info.amger@americangeriatrics.org
www.americangeriatrics.org

Steven Counsell, President
Ellen Flaherty, President-Elect
Wayne C. McCormick, Chair
Debra Saliba, Secretary
A not-for-profit organization of more than 6,000 health professionals devoted to improving the health, independence and quality of life of all older people.

7450 **American Society on Aging**
575 Market St.
Suite 2100
San Francisco, CA 94105-2869

415-974-9600
800-537-9728
FAX: 415-974-0300
www.asaging.org

7451 **Arizona Association of Homes and Housing for the Aging**
3877 N 7th St
Ste 240
Phoenix, AZ 85014

602-230-0026
FAX: 602-230-0563
azaha@azaha.org
www.azaha.org

Genny Rose, Executive Director
Jon Scott Williams, Chair
The Arizona Association of Homes and Houses for the Aging is a not-for-profit trade association representing more than 100 facilities dedicated to providing quality health care, housing and services to over 12,000 elderly Arizona citizens. AzAHA is the only association in Arizona representing the full continuum of long term care, housing and services including: retirement communities, HUD subsidized senior housing, assisted living and nursing facilities.

7452 **Association for Gerontology in Higher Education**
1220 L Street NW
Suite 901
Washington, DC 20005

202-289-9806
www.aghe.org

Donna L. Wagner, President
Nina M. Silverstein, President-Elect
Christine A Fruhauf, Treasurer
Lydia Manning, Secretary
It is an association of diverse individuals bound by a common goal: to support the commitment and enhance the knowledge and skills of those who seek to improve the quality of life of older adults and their families.

7453 **Association of Ohio Philanthropic Homes, Housing and Services for the Aging**
855 S Wall St
Columbus, OH 43206-1921

614-444-2882
FAX: 614-444-2974
info@aopha.org
aopha.org

John Alfano, CEO

Founded in 1937, AOPHA, the advocate of not-for-profit services for older Ohioans, is a statewide nonprofit trade association representing over 335 not-for-profit senior housing apartments, home and community-based service providers, assisted living facilities, nursing homes and continuing care retirement communities (CCRCs).

7454 **Association on Aging with Developmental Disabilities**
2385 Hampton Ave.
St. Louis, MO 63139

314-647-8100
FAX: 314-647-8105
agingwithdd@msn.com
agingwithdd.org

7455 **Children of Aging Parents**
PO Box 167
Richboro, PA 18954-167

215-945-6900
800-227-7294
FAX: 215-945-8720
info@caps4caregivers.org
www.caps4caregivers.org

Karen Rosenberg, Director
A national clearinghouse for caregivers of the elderly. It provides information and referral, educational programs and materials and caregiver support groups. CAPS also produces a quarterly newsletter which is available through the organization. Individuals: $25.00. Organizational/Professional: $100.00.

7456 **Colorado Association of Homes and Services for the Aging**
303 E. 17th Ave.
Suite 502
Denver, CO 80203-1160

303-837-8834
FAX: 303-837-8836
Jennifer@LeadingAgeColorado.org
www.cahsa.org

Laura Landwirth, Executive Director
Michael Meehan, Secretary
Dan Stenersen, Treasurer
Jennifer Stone, Member Services Manager
The American Association of Homes and Services for the Aging (AAHS) represents nonprofit organizations dedicated to providing high quality health care, housing and services to the nation's elderly. AAHSA organizations serve more than one million older persons af all income levels, creeds and races.

7457 **Connecticut Association of Not-for-Profit Providers for the Aging**
1340 Worthington Rdg
Berlin, CT 06037-3208

860-828-2903
FAX: 860-828-8694
leadingagect@leadingagect.org
www.leadingagect.org

Andrea Bellofiore, Director of Member Programs & Services
Beth Ricker, Finance Manager & Membership Director
Mag Morelli, President
Nurka Carrero, Office Manager
LeadingAge Connecticut is a membership organization representing over 130 not-for-profit mission driven provider organizations serving elderly and disabled individuals across the continuum of care, including nursing homes, residential care homes, housing for the elderly, continuing care retirement communities, adult day centers, home care agencies and assisted living.

7458 **Georgia Association of Homes and Services for the Aging**
1440 Dutch Valley PL NE
Suite 120
Atlanta, GA 30324-5367

404-872-9191
FAX: 404-872-1737
selahi@leadingagega.org
www.centerforpositiveaging.org

Susan Watkins, Dir. of Member Services
Walter Coffey, President/C.E.O.
Jacque Thornton, Sr. Vice President
The Georgia Association of Homes and Services for the Aging (GAHSA) is an affiliated partner of the American Association of Homes and Services of the Aging (AASHA), which represents over 5,600 nonprofit facilities, over one million older adults in

the United States and maintains an impressive staff of 80 professionals at its headquarters in Washington, D.C.

7459 Gerontological Society of America
1220 L Street NW
Suite 901
Washington, DC 20005   202-842-1275
                                         www.geron.org

James Appleby, Executive Director/ CEO
Linda Krogh Harootyan, Senior Advisor
Judie Lieu, Sr. Director, Innovation
Rachel Whidden, Director of Meetings
The oldest and largest interdisciplinary organization devoted to research, education, and practice in the field of aging.

7460 Gulf States Association of Homes and Services for the Aging
PO Box 1748
Marrero, LA 70073-1748   504-442-0483
                                    FAX: 504-689-3982
                           kcontrenchis@gulfstatesahsa.org
                                   www.gulfstatesahsa.org

Cindy Ladnier, Chair
Dennis Adams, Vice-Chair
Scott Crabtree, Secretary/Treasurer
Karen Contrenchis, President
Along term care system which offers accessable, affordable, high-quality and innovative healthcare, housing and comminuty services. Provides value to the the senior population and their families through personal and professional commitment, in a compassionate manner, supported by benevolence and integrity. Socially resposible and accountable for promoting excellence in long-term care and support services.

7461 Healthy Aging Association
121 Downey Ave.
Suite 102
Modesto, CA 95354   209-523-2800
                              healthy.aging2000@gmail.com
                           www.healthyagingassociation.org

Marlyn Crawford, President
Lynne Sutton, Secretary
Mary Walton, Board Member
Marsha McNeill, Board Member
A Non-Profit Organization whose mission is to help older Americans live longer, healthier, more independent lives by promoting increased physical activity, and sound health, and nutrition practices.

7462 Indiana Association of Homes and Services for the Aging
PO Box 68829
Indianapolis, IN 46268-0829   317-733-2380
                                   FAX: 317-733-2385
                          jimleich@LeadingAgeIndiana.org
                                        www.iahsa.com

Emilie Perkins, CMP, Director of Training
Rebecca (Bec Carter, Director of Association Management
Jim Leich, President
Susan Darwent, Vice President of Operations
LeadingAge Indiana is an association representing not-for-profit services and facilities for the elderly. Members are non-profit organizations, providing high quality health care, services and housing for over 25,000 seniors throughout Indiana. Our members are sponsored by or affiliated with religious, fraternal, governmental, and community organizations.

7463 Iowa Association of Homes and Services forthe Aging
4200 University Ave.
Suite 305
West Des Moines, IA 50266-6723   515-440-4630
                                        888-440-4630
                                   FAX: 515-440-4631
                              info@leadingageiowa.org
                                  www.leadingageiowa.org

Bill Nutty, Director of Government Relations
Kathy Strang, Director of Professional Develop
Bill Nutty, Government Relations/Member Services Director
Shannon Strickler, President/CEO

LeadingAge Iowa is the state association serving not-for-profit and missiondriven organizations dedicated to providing quality housing, health, community, and related services to our state's seniors. LeadingAge Iowa represents and promotes the common interests of its members through advocacy, education and collaboration to enhance their ability to provide quality care and service within their community.

7464 Kentucky Association of Homes and Services for the Aging
2501 Nelson Miller Pkwy
Suite 200
Louisville, KY 40223- 2221   502-992-4380
                                   FAX: 502-992-4390
                                info@leadingageky.org
                                       www.kahsa.com

Timothy Veno, President
LeadingAge Kentucky (formerly Kentucky Association of Homes and Services for the Aging (KAHSA) was founded in 1977. The association represents not-for-profit community, church, proprietary and government sponsored health care facilities, retirement communities, assisted living, housing and service programs for the elderly and the disabled.

7465 Life Services Network of Illinois
1001 Warrenville Rd
Suite 150
Lisle, IL 60532   630-325-6170
                                   FAX: 630-325-0749
                                        info@lsni.org
                                        www.lsni.org

Kathy Burke, Director of Business Development
Suzanne Schemm, Director of Finance and Administration
Cathy Nelson RN, MS, LNHA, Director of Clinical Services
Karen Messer, Interim President
With over 500 partners in Illinois, Life Services Network is one of the largest and most respected associations of its type in the country. Founded in the early part of the 20th century by an ecumenical group of long term care providers, LSN has represented the complete continuum of services for older adults for over 75 years.

7466 LifeSpan Network: Maryland
10280 Old Columbia Road
Suite 220
Columbia, MD 21046- 2382   410-381-1176
                                   FAX: 410-381-0240
                              ifirth@lifespan-network.org
                                  www.lifespan-network.org

Kathy Bernetti, Director of Finance
Charlotte Eliopoulos, PULL Grant Program Director
Lisa Fichman, Director of Membership Services and Marketing
Isabella Firth, President
Senior care provider association representing more than 300 senior care provider organizations in Maryland and the District of Columbia. Lifespan members include non-profit and proprietary independent living, assisted living, continuing care retirement communities, nursing facilities, subsidized senior housing and community and hospital based services. Also provide education, advocacy and products and services, as well as networking for our members.

7467 Massachusetts Aging Services Association
246 Walnut Street
Suite 203
Newton, MA 02460-3328   617-244-2999
                                   FAX: 617-244-2995
                                office@LeadingAgeMA.org
                                     www.massaging.org

Sue Pouliot, Director of Education and Events
Don Powell, Director of Member Services
Elissa Sherman, President
Lisa Miano, Officer Manager
LeadingAge Massachusetts, formerly MassAging, is the only organization representing the full continuum of mission-driven, not-for-profit providers of health care, housing, and services for older persons in Massachusetts. Members of LeadingAge Massachusetts provide housing and services to more than 25,000 older persons in the Commonwealth each year.

7468 Missouri Association of Homes for the Aging
3412 Knipp Dr
Suite 102
Jefferson City, MO 65109   573-635-6244
                                        FAX: 573-635-6618
                                        diana@moaha.org
                                        www.moaha.org

Denise Clemonds, CEO
Diana Love
Patricia Hubbs
Patricia Hubbs
LeadingAge Missouri's work is dedicated to assisting its members to be the leaders in Missouri in the delivery of innovative, quality long-term health care, housing, and services for older adults. LeadingAge Missouri assists its members in providing quality services for the elderly

7469 National Association of Area Agencies on Aging
1730 Rhode Island Ave NW
Suite 1200
Washington, DC 20036-3109   202-872-0888
                                        FAX: 202-872-0057
                                        smarkwood@n4a.org
                                        www.n4a.org

Tom Endres, Director
Joanetta Bolden, Associate Director, Communications
Amy E. Gotwals, Senior Director, Public Policy and Advocacy
Virginia Dize, Program Manager/Assistant Director
The National Association of Area Agencies on Aging (n4a) is the leading voice on aging issues for Area Agencies on Aging and a champion for Title VI Native American aging programs. Through advocacy, training and technical assistance, we support the national network of 629 AAAs and 246 Title VI programs.

7470 National Association of Counties
25 Massachusetts Ave NW
Suite 500
Washington, DC 20001- 1430   202-393-6226
                                        888-407-6226
                                        888-407-6226
                                        FAX: 202-393-2630
                                        nacomeetings@naco.org
                                        naco.org
Maeghan Gilmore, Program Director, County Solutions & Innovation
Karon Harden, Director of Professional Development, Education and Training
Emilia Istrate, Director of Research
Kim Struble, Director of Conferences & Meetings
NACO represents elected officials and aging administrators who are interested in providing quality programs to their older constituents. NACO members work with Congress, the Administration on Aging, and other federal agencies to ensure that the nationa maintains an effective and efficient safety net of services for the elderly and their families.

7471 National Association of Home Care and Hospice
228 Seventh Street, SE
Washington, DC 20003   202-547-7424
                                        FAX: 202-547-3540
                                        www.nahc.org
Denise Schrader, Chair
Lucy Andrews, Vice Chair
Karen Thompson, Secretary
Walter W. Borginis, Treasurer
The largest and most respected professional association representing the interests of chronically ill, disabled, and dying Americans of all ages and the caregivers who provide them with in-home health and hospice services.

7472 National Association of Nutrition and Aging Services Programs
1612 K St NW
Suite 400
Washington, DC 20006-2829   202-682-6899
                                        FAX: 202-223-2099
                                        pcarlson@nanasp.com
                                        www.nanasp.org
Robert Blancato, Executive Director
Shannon Donahue, Associate
Pamela (Pam) Carlson, Membership & Education
Scott Carlson, Finance & Operations
A national membership organization for persons across the country working to provide older adults healthful food and nutrition through community-based services.

7473 National Association of State Units on Aging
1201 15th St NW
Suite 350
Washington, DC 20005-2842   202-898-2578
                                        FAX: 202-898-2583
                                        info@nasuad.org
                                        www.nasuad.org
Martha Roherty, Executive Director
Lindsey Copeland, Director of Policy and Legislative Affairs
Rachel Shiffrin Feldman, Director of Communications and Corporate Relations
John Michael Hall, Senior Director of Medicaid Policy and Planning
NASUAD represents the nation's 56 state and territorial agencies on aging and disabilities and supports visionary state leadership, the advancement of state systems innovation and the articulation of national policies that support home and community based services for older adults and individuals with disabilities.

7474 National Association on Area Agencies on Aging
1730 Rhode Island Avenue, NW
Suite 1200
Washington, DC 20036   202-872-0888
                                        FAX: 202-872-0057
                                        info@n4a.org
                                        www.n4a.org
Joseph Ruby, President
Mary Beals-Luedtka, 1st Vice President
Anne Hinton, 2nd Vice President
Odile Brunetto, Secretary
The National Association of Area Agencies on Aging (n4a) is a 501c(3) membership association representing America's national network of 618 Area Agencies on Aging (AAAs) and providing a voice in the nation's capital for the 246 Title VI Native American aging programs.

7475 National Council on Aging
1901 L St NW
4th Fl
Washington, DC 20036-3540   202-479-1200
                                        FAX: 202-479-0735
                                        TTY:202-479-6674
                                        membership@ncoa.org
                                        www.ncoa.org
James P Firman, EdD, President/CEO
Jay Robertson, Senior Vice President
Richard Birkel, PhD, MPA, Acting Senior Vice President, Ce
Nora Dowd Eisenhower, JD, Acting Senior Vice President, Ec
We are a national voice for older Americans and the community organizations that serve them. We bring together nonprofit organizations, businesses, and government to develop creative solutions that improve the lives of all older adults.

7476 National Gerontological Nursing Association
3493 Lansdowne Dr.
Suite 2
Lexington, KY 40517   859-977-7453
                                        800-723-0560
                                        FAX: 859-271-0607
                                        info@ngna.org
                                        www.ngna.org

7477   National Hispanic Council on Aging
734 15th St NW
Suite 1050
Washington, DC 20005-1038   202-347-9733
                                       FAX: 202-347-9735
                                       nhcoa@nhcoa.org
                                       www.nhcoa.org

Yanira Cruz, DrPH, President/CEO
Eric Rodriguez, Director
B rbara Robles, PhD, Director
Jorge Lambrinos, Director
To achieve its mission, NHCOA has developed a Hispanic Aging Network of community-based organizations across the continental U.S., the District of Columbia, and Puerto Rico that reaches millions of Latinos each year. NHCOA also works to ensure the Hispanic community is better understood and fairly represented in U.S. policies.

7478   National Indian Council on Aging
10501 Montgomery Blvd NE
Suite 210
Albuquerque, NM 87111-3851   505-292-2001
                                       FAX: 505-292-1922
                                       info@nicoa.org
                                       www.nicoa.org

Randella Bluehoose, Executive Director
Dorinda Fox, SCSEP Director
Jonnie Gilbert, Finance Director
Darrell Begay, Arizona Central Employment Speci
A non-profit organization, was founded by members of the National Tribal Chairmen's Association that called for a national organization to advocate for improved, comprehensive health and social services to American Indian and Alaska Native Elders.

7479   National Senior Citizens Law Center
1444 Eye Street NW
Suite 1100
Washington, DC 20005-6547   202-289-6976
                                       FAX: 202-289-7224
                                       nsclc@nsclc.org
                                       www.nsclc.org

Robert K. Johnson, Esq.,, Chair
Barrett S. Litt, Esq.,, Vice Chair
Paul Nathanson, Executive Director
Kevin Prindiville, Deputy Director
The National Senior Citizens Law Center is a non-profit organization whose principal mission is to protect the rights of low-income older adults. Through advocacy, litigation, and the education and counseling of local advocates, we seek to ensure the health and economic security of those with limited income and resources, and to preserve their access to the courts.

7480   Nebraska Association of Homes and Services for the Aging
900 North 90th Street
Suite 940
Omaha, NE 68114   402-990-2346
                                       kaminskij@leadingagene.org
                                       www.leadingagene.org

Julie Kaminski, Executive Director
Cheryl Wichman, Education Coordinator
LeadingAgeNebraska is the only State Association representing the full continuum of mission-driven, non-profit providers of health care, housing, and services for older adults in Nebraska. Members of LeadingAgeNebraska provide housing and services to more than 5,000 Nebraska seniors each year

7481   New Jersey Association of Homes and Services for the Aging
13 Roszel Rd
Suite C-200
Princeton, NJ 08540-6211   609-452-1161
                                       FAX: 609-452-2907
                                       mkent@leadingagenj.org
                                       www.leadingagenj.org

Amy S. Greenbaum, Director of Professional Develop
Michele M. Kent, President, CEO
Judy Collett-Miller, Executive Vice President
Darlene Arden, Executive Assistant

LeadingAge New Jersey represents not-for-profit nursing homes, assisted living residences, residential health care centers, independent senior housing, and continuing care retirement communities throughout the entire state of New Jersey. LeadingAge New Jersey serves over 140 member communities, many of which are supported through religious, fraternal and governmental sponsorship.

7482   New York Association of Homes and Services for the Aging
13 British American Blvd
Suite 2
Latham, NY 12110-1431   518-867-8383
                                       FAX: 518-867-8384
                                       info@leadingageny.org
                                       www.nyahsa.org

Ellen Quinn, SPHR, Director of Human Resources
Patrick Cucinelli, Sr. Director of Public Policy
Elliott Frost, Director of ProCare
Ami Schnauber, Director of Government Relations
Founded in 1961, LeadingAge New York, formerly the New York Association of Homes & Services for the Aging (NYAHSA), represents not-for-profit, mission-driven and public continuing care providers, including nursing homes, senior housing, adult care facilities, continuing care retirement communities, assisted living and community service providers. Leading Age New York's more than 600 members employ 150,000 professionals serving more than 500,000 New Yorkers annually.

7483   North Carolina Association of Non-Profit Homes for the Aging
100 Carolina Meadows
Chapel Hill, NC 27517   919-571-8333
                                       FAX: 919-571-1297
                                       info@leadingagenc.org
                                       www.leadingagenc.org

Tom Akins, President/CEO
Leslie Roseboro, Vice President
Anne Moffat, Chair
Kevin McLeod, Chair Elect
LeadingAge North Carolina is the state association of not-for-profit providers dedicated to providing quality care, housing, health, community and related services to the elderly. As the only Association in North Carolina exclusively representing not-for-profit long term care facilities, a primary goal is to support members in maintaining their 501(c)(3) status and promoting the not-for-profit philosophy of quality long term care and services for the elderly.

7484   Northern New England Association of Homes and Services for the Aging
PO Box 339
New Gretna, NJ 08224-0339   603-391-9881
                                       FAX: 603-391-9881
                                       rgoedtel@leadingagemenh.org
                                       www.leadingagemenh.org

Peter Warecki, Chair
Rebecca Smith, Vice Chair
Maureen Carland, Secretary
Lee Karker, Treasurer
The mission of LeadingAge Maine & New Hampshire is to promote the interests of its not-for-profit members in Maine and New Hampshire, which provide healthy, affordable and ethical long-term care to our older citizens through education, advocacy, representation and collaboration.

7485   Oklahoma Association of Homes and Services for the Aging
PO Box 1383
El Reno, OK 73036-1383   405-640-8040
                                       inquiry@LeadingAgeOK.org
                                       www.leadingageok.org

Mary Brinkley, Executive Director
Jessica Pfau, President
Lindsay Fick, Secretary
Jim O'Brien, Treasurer
LeadingAge Oklahoma represents an association of members who are forward-thinking in shaping the future of the long-term care profession. Our members lead in innovative practices that transform how we care for our aging population, cutting-edge ini-

tiatives to develop services that meet the needs and preferences of older adults and advocacy efforts to advance the interests of the aging consumer.

7486 Oregon Alliance of Senior and Health Services
7340 SW Hunziker St
Suite 104
Tigard, OR 97223-2303
503-684-3788
FAX: 503-624-0870
info@leadingageoregon.org
www.oashs.org

Ruth Gulyas, Executive Director
Margaret Cervenka, Deputy Director
Karen Nichols, Manager of Membership Services a
Denise Wetzel, Administrative Coordinator and B
Established in 1979, LeadingAge Oregon is the state association of not-for-profit, mission-directed organizations dedicated to providing quality housing, health, community and related services to the elderly and disabled. LeadingAge Oregon members set the standards for the field through service excellence and mission-driven objectives.

7487 Pennsylvania Association of Nonprofit Senior Services
1100 Bent Creek Blvd
Mechanicsburg, PA 17050-1872
717-763-5724
800-545-2270
FAX: 717-763-1057
info@leadingagepa.org
www.panpha.org

Ronald L Barth, President/CEO
Holly Rosini, Senior Vice President/Chief Operating Officer
Beth Greenberg, VP, Strategic Knowledge and Research
Heidi Geist, Communications Manager
LeadingAge PA's mission is to promote the interests of our members by enhancing their ability to provide quality services efficiently and effectively; and by representing our members through cooperative action.

7488 Quality Healthcare Foundation of Wyoming
6909 Foxglove Drive
Cheyenne, WY 82009
307-287-4594
800-773-2273
FAX: 307-638-8472
steve@qhcf.org
www.qhcf.org

Steve Bahmer, Executive Director
Eric Boley, President
Sandy Ward, Vice President
Jill Hult, Secretary/Treasurer
The American Association of Homes and Services for the Aging (AAHS) represents not-for-profit organizations dedicated to providing high-quality health care, housing and services to the nation's elderly. AAHSA organizations serve more than one million older persons af all income levels, creeds and races.

7489 Rhode Island Association of Facilities and Services for the Aging
225 Chapman St
2nd Floor
Providence, RI 02905-4533
401-490-7612
866-883-1631
FAX: 401-490-7614
TTY: 401-383-6578
info@leadingageri.org
www.leadingageri.org

James P Nyberg, Director
Matt Trimble, President
Sandra Cullen, Vice-President
Wendy Fargnoli, Treasurer
LeadingAge RI is committed to Expanding the World of Possibilities for Aging. As such, LeadingAge RI will continue its focus on advancing excellence in the field by fostering innovation, collaboration, and ethical leadership; advocating for sound public policy; providing education, collaboration, and professional development; valuing older people and their right to make choices; and promoting a continuum of services.

7490 Tennessee Association of Homes and Services for the Aging
5201 Virginia Way
Suite 325
Brentwood, TN 37027-4634
615-256-8240
FAX: 615-242-4803
webmaster@tha.com
www.tha.com

Patrick Turri, Senior Director Analysis/Information Technoloy
Joe Burchfield, Senior Director Operations and Member Services
Patrice Mayo, Vice President, Operations Director
Mary Ellen Mooney, Clinical Director
TNAHSA is an association of faclities and professionals providing quality housing, health, community and related services for the elderly. TNAHSA represents and promotes the common interest of its members through leadership, advocacy, education, communication and other services in order to enhance members' ability to serve their constituencies.

7491 Texas Association of Homes and Services for the Aging
2205 Hancock Dr
Austin, TX 78756-2508
512-467-2242
FAX: 512-467-2275
info@leadingagetexas.org
www.tahsa.org

Crystal Laza, CAE, Director of Member Services and Operations
Alyse Migliaro, Director of Public Policy
Claire Director of Education, Morris, CASP
George Linial, CAE, CASP, President/CEO
LeadingAge Texas (formerly the Texas Association of Homes and Services for the Aging - TAHSA) was established in 1959 as a Texas not-for-profit corporation. Its purpose is to provide leadership, advocacy, and education for not-for-profit retirement housing and nursing home communities that serve the needs of Texas retirees.

7492 Wisconsin Association of Homes and Services for the Aging
204 S Hamilton St
Madison, WI 53703-3212
608-255-7060
FAX: 608-255-7064
info@LeadingAgeWI.org
www.wahsa.org

John Sauer, President/CEO
Pam Walker, Executive Secretary
Janice Mashak, Vice President of Member Services & Innovation
Brian Schoeneck, Vice President of Financial & Regulatory Services
LeadingAge Wisconsin is committed to advancing the fields of long-term care, assisted living and retirement living. We strive to develop a continuum of elderly care and services that meets the holistic needs of seniors and individuals with a disability in order to encourage maximum independence and enhance quality of life. We serve as a resource for our members, assisting them in problem resolution and providing services and programs to meet their needs.

Print: Books

7493 Activities in Action
Routledge (Taylor & Francis Group)
270 Madison Ave
Fl 4 #4
New York, NY 10016-0601
212-695-6599
800-634-7064
FAX: 212-563-2269
www.routledgementalhealth.com/contact/
www.routledgementalhealth.com

Jeffrey Lim, Director
Francis Chua, Manager
Tamaryn Anderson, Marketing Manager
An invaluable resource which serves as a catalyst for professional and personal growth and provides a national forum on geriatric and activity issues. *$30.00*
116 pages Hardcover
ISBN 1-560241-32-4

7494 Activities with Developmentally Disabled Elderly and Older Adults
Routledge (Taylor & Francis Group)
270 Madison Ave
Fl 4 #4
New York, NY 10016-601
212-695-6599
800-637-7064
FAX: 212-563-2269
www.routledgementalhealth.com/contact/
www.routledgementalhealth.com

Jeffrey Lim, Director
Francis Chua, Manager
Tamaryn Anderson, Marketing Manager
Learn how to effectively plan and deliver activities for a growing number of older people with developmental disabilities. It aims to stimulate interest and continued support for recreation program development and implementation among developmental disability and aging service systems. *$42.00*
164 pages Hardcover
ISBN 1-560241-74-4

7495 Aging and Developmental Disability: Current Research, Programming, and Practice
Routledge (Taylor & Francis Group)
270 Madison Ave
Fl 4 #4
New York, NY 10016-601
212-695-6599
800-634-7064
FAX: 212-563-2269
www.routledgementalhealth.com/contact/
www.routledgementalhealth.com

Joy Hammel, Author
Susan Nochajski, Co-Author
Explores research findings and their implications for practice in relation to normative and disability-related aging experiences and issues. It discusses the effectiveness of specific intervention targeted toward aging adults with developmental disabilities such as Down's Syndrome, cerebral palsy, autism, and epilepsy, and offers suggestions for practice and future research in this area. *$48.00*
112 pages Hardcover
ISBN 0-789010-39-1

7496 Aging and Family Therapy: Practitioner Perspectives on Golden Pond
Routledge (Taylor & Francis Group)
270 Madison Ave
Fl 4 #4
New York, NY 10016-601
212-695-6599
800-634-7064
FAX: 212-563-2269
www.routledgementalhealth.com/contact/
www.routledgementalhealth.com

George Hughston, Author
Victor Christopherson, Co-Author
Marilyn Bojean, Co-Author
Here are creative strategies for use in therapy with older adults and their families. This significant new book provides practitioners with information, insight, reference tools, and other sources that will contribute to more effective intervention with the elderly and their families. *$48.00*
260 pages Hardcover
ISBN 0-866567-78-7

7497 Aging in Stride
IlluminAge Communications Partners
2200 1st Ave South
Suite 400
Seattle, WA 98134-1408
206-269-6363
888-620-8816
FAX: 206-269-6350
www.cobaltgroup.com/contact/
www.cobaltgroup.com

Dennis Kenny, Owner
Elizabeth N Oettinger, Co-Author
Dennis E Kenny JD, Co-Author
Guide to aging, the special needs of older adults, and the demands of providing care and support. Experts explain potential conflicts, planning opportunities and strategies for success. Six guides. *$24.95*
Paperback

7498 Aging in the Designed Environment
Routledge (Taylor & Francis Group)
270 Madison Ave
Fl 4 #4
New York, NY 10016-601
212-216-7800
800-634-7064
FAX: 212-563-2269
www.routledgementalhealth.com

Margaret Christenson, Author
Ellen D Taira, Co-Author
The key sourcebook for physical and occupational therapists developing and implementing environmental designs for the aging. *$30.00*
146 pages Hardcover
ISBN 1-560240-31-0

7499 Aging with a Disability
Special Needs Project
1405 Anderson Lane
Santa Barbara, CA 93111-2946
805-962-8087
800-333-6867
FAX: 805-962-5087
www.specialneeds.com

Hod Gray, Owner
Laura Mosqueda, Co-Author
Aging with a Disability provides clinicians with a complete guide to the care and treatment of persons aging with a disability. Divided into five parts, this book first addresses the perspective of the person with a disability and his or her family. *$24.95*
328 pages Paperback

7500 Assistive Technology for Older Persons: A Handbook
Idaho Assistive Technology Project
University of Idaho
1187 Altiras Dr.
Moscow, ID 83843
208-885-3557
800-432-8324
FAX: 208-885-6102
idahoat@uidaho.edu
www.idahoat.org

Ron Seiler, Project Director
This handbook is designed as a guide for Idaho's older citizens who, as they age, wish to preserve their independence, autonomy, productivity, and dignity. It is intended to provide information about assistive technology, home modifications, and the many service options available to older people in the mcomunities across the state.

7501 Caring for Those You Love: A Guide to Compassionate Care for the Aged
Horizon Publishers & Distributors
191 N 650 E
Bountiful, UT 84010-3628
801-295-9451
866-818-6277
FAX: 801-298-1305
www.duanescrowther.com

Duane S. Crowther, Author/President
Jean Crowther, Vice President/Sec
David Crowther, Vice President
This book is a practical guide to coping with special problems of the aged and infirm, and examines the many challenges of caring for the elderly on a personal and family level. *$12.98*
108 pages
ISBN 0-882902-70-9

7502   **Chronically Disabled Elderly in Society**
Greenwood Publishing Group
88 Post Rd W
Westport, CT 06880-4208   203-226-3571
                                       800-225-5800
                                   FAX: 877-231-6980
                          customer-service@greenwood.com
                                     www.greenwood.com

Merna J Alpert, Author
Lisa Scott, President
Herman Bruggink, CEO
This timely work increases awareness of and knowledge about
problems of societal living among the chronically disabled elderly, with implications for policy makers, educational institutions, advocacy groups, families and individuals. *$76.95*
160 pages Hardcover
ISBN 0-313291-09-8

7503   **Coping and Caring: Living with Alzheimer's Disease**
AARP Fulfillment
601 E St NW
Washington, DC 20049
                                       800-687-2277
                                   TTY:877-434-7589
                                      member@aarp.org
                                        www.aarp.org

Charles Leroux, Author
Steve Cone, Executive Vice President of Inte
Lorraine Cortes-Vazquez, Executive Vice President, Multic
Addresses the questions: What is Alzheimer's? How does the dis-
ease progress? How long does it last? How can families cope?
24 pages

7504   **Elder Abuse and Mistreatment**
Routledge (Taylor & Francis Group)
270 Madison Ave
Fl 4 #4
New York, NY 10016-601   212-695-6599
                                       800-634-7064
                                   FAX: 212-563-2269
                      www.routledgementalhealth.com/contact/
                           www.routledgementalhealth.com

Joanna Mellor, Author
Patricia Brownell, Co-Author
Elder Abuse and Mistreatment is a comprehensive overview of
current policy issues, new practice models, and up-to-date research on elder abuse and neglect. Experts in the field provide insight into elder abuse with newly examined populations to create
an understanding of how to design service plans for victims of
abuse and family mistreatment. The book addresses all forms of
abuse and neglect, examining the value issues and ethical dilemmas that social workers face in providing service to elderl
$120.00
284 pages Paperback
ISBN 0-789030-22-1

7505   **Explore Your Options**
Kansas Department on Aging
503 S Kansas Ave
New England Building
Topeka, KS 66603- 3404   785-296-4986
                                       800-432-3535
                                   FAX: 785-296-0256
                                   TTY: 785-291-3167
                               wwwmail@kdads.ks.gov
                                 www.agingKansas.org

Maria Russo, President
This book will help you through the maze of services available to
Kansas seniors. It is designed to help you take an active role in
making decisions that affect your health care and living situation.

7506   **Falling in Old Age**
Springer Publishing Company
11 W 42nd St
Fl 15 #15
New York, NY 10036-8002   212-431-4370
                                       877-687-7476
                                   FAX: 212-941-7842
                                    cs@springerpub.com
                                 www.springerjournals.com

Ursula Springer, President
Ted Nardin, CEO
Edie Lambiase, CFO
Presented are practical techniques for the prevention of falls and
for determining and correcting the causes. *$60.00*
412 pages Hardcover
ISBN 0-826152-91-6

7507   **Family Intervention Guide to Mental Illness**
New Harbinger Publications
5674 Shattuck Ave
Oakland, CA 94609-1662   510-652-0215
                                       800-748-6273
                                   FAX: 800-652-1613
                         customerservice@newharbinger.com
                               www.newharbinger.com

Matthew McKay, Owner
Kim T Mueser, Co-Author
Kirk Johnson, CFO
Bodie Morey, Co-Author
The Family Intervention Guide to Mental Illness outlines the nine
fundamental steps to recognizing, managing, and recovering
from mental illness. It provides both diagnostic information and
details about therapy options and useful medications. With the
right advice, determined effort, and a lot of love, you can make a
difference. *$17.95*
240 pages
ISBN 1-572245-06-8

7508   **Handbook of Assistive Devices for the Handicapped Elderly**
Routledge (Taylor & Francis Group)
270 Madison Ave
Fl 4 #4
New York, NY 10016-601   212-695-6599
                                       800-634-7064
                                   FAX: 212-563-2269
                           www.routledgementalhealth.com

Joseph A Breuer, Author
Jeffrey Lin, Director
Francis Chua, Manager
Tamaryn Anderson, Marketing Manager
Concise yet comprehensive reference of assistive devices for
handicapped elders. *$42.00*
77 pages Hardcover
ISBN 0-866561-52-5

7509   **Handbook on Ethnicity, Aging and Mental Health**
Greenwood Publishing Group
88 Post Rd W
Westport, CT 6880-4208   203-226-3571
                                       800-225-5800
                                   FAX: 877-231-6980
                          customer-service@greenwood.com
                                     www.greenwood.com

Deborah K Padgett, Author
Lisa Scott, President
Herman Bruggink, CEO
State-of-the-art reference by leading experts and first
book-length appraisal of research, practices and policies con-
cerning mental health needs of the ethnic elderly in America.
$141.95
376 pages Hardcover
ISBN 0-313282-04-8

7510 Health Care of the Aged: Needs, Policies, and Services
Routledge (Taylor & Francis Group)
270 Madison Ave
Fl 4 #4
New York, NY 10016-601

212-695-6599
800-634-7064
FAX: 212-563-2269
www.routledgementalhealth.com

Abraham Monk, Author
Jeffrey Lim, Director
Francis Chua, Manager
Tamaryn Anderson, Marketing Manager
Focusing on the need for developing new service delivery models for the aged, this book examines fiscal, political, and social criteria influencing this challenge of the 1990's. The aged are caught in the sweeping changes currently occurring in the financing, organizing and delivery of human health care services. *$36.00*
800 pages Hardcover
ISBN 1-560240-65-5

7511 Health Promotion and Disease Prevention in Clinical Practice
Lippincott, Williams & Wilkins
2001 Market Street
Two Commerce Square
Philadelphia, PA 19103-3603

215-521-8300
800-638-3030
FAX: 215-521-8902
customerservice@lww.com.
www.lww.com

Steven H Woolf MD, Co-Author
Steven Jonas MD, Co-Author
Evonne Kaplan-Liss, Co-Author
Rick Perry, CEO
Incorporating the latest guidelines from major organizations, including the U.S. Preventive Services Task Force, this book offers the clinician a complete overview of how to help patients adopt healthy behaviors and to deliver recommended screening tests and immunizations. *$52.95*
218 pages Softcover
ISBN 0-781775-99-1

7512 Life Planning for Adults with Developmental Disabilities
New Harbinger Publications
5674 Shattuck Ave
Oakland, CA 94609-1662

510-652-0215
800-748-6273
FAX: 800-652-1613
customerservice@newharbinger.com
www.newharbinger.com

Matthew McKay, Publisher
Kirk Johnson, CFO
Judith Greenbaum PhD, Author
The book begins by assessing the quality of life of the adult with a disability. It offers a wealth of suggestions for making that person's life even better. The book then focuses on long-term planning for the individual with a disability and helps answer the question, Who will take care of my child after I'm gone? *$19.95*
208 pages
ISBN 1-572244-51-1

7513 Long-Term Care: How to Plan and Pay for It
NOLO
950 Parker St
Berkeley, CA 94710-2524

510-549-1976
800-728-3555
FAX: 800-645-0895
www.nolo.com

Joseph L Matthews, Author
Ralph Warner, Chariman/CEO
Ann Heron, COO
Bob Dubow, CFO
This book helps you choose a nursing home, or find a viable alternative. Covers how to get the most out of Medicare and other benefit programs.
384 pages Paperback
ISBN 1-413305-21-0

7514 Mentally Impaired Elderly: Strategies and Interventions to Maintain Function
Routledge (Taylor & Francis Group)
270 Madison Ave
Fl 4 #4
New York, NY 10016-601

212-695-6599
800-634-7064
FAX: 212-653-2269
www.routledgementalhealth.com

Ellen D Taira, Author
Jeffrey Lim, Director
Francis Chua, Manager
Tamaryn Anderson, Marketing Manager
Provides effective support and sensitive care for the most vulnerable segment of the elderly population, those with mental impairment. *$34.00*
171 pages Hardcover
ISBN 1-560241-68-3

7515 Mirrored Lives: Aging Children and Elderly Parents
Praeger Publishers
88 Post Rd W
Westport, CT 06880-4208

203-226-3571
800-225-5800
FAX: 877-231-6980
customer-service@greenwood.com
www.greenwood.com

Tom Koch, Author
Lisa Scott, President
Herman Bruggink, CEO
Discusses geriatric decline connected to nonterminal illness in old age. Koch takes a sensitive but thorough look at the declining years of his father. *$117.95*
240 pages Hardcover
ISBN 0-275936-71-6

7516 Physical & Mental Issues in Aging Sourcebook
Omnigraphics
155 W Congree St
Suite 200 #200
Detroit, MI 48226-3261

313-961-1340
800-234-1340
FAX: 313-961-1383
info@omnigraphics.com
www.omnigraphics.com

Jennifer Swanson, Editor
Frederic Ruffner, Chairman
Kay Gill, Vice President
Laurie Harris, Manager
Basic information about maintaining health through the post-reproductive years. Includes stats, recommendations for lifestyle modifications, a glossary and resrouce information *$84.00*
660 pages Hard cover
ISBN 0-780802-33-9

7517 Prescriptions for Independence: Working with Older People Who are Visually Impaired
American Foundation for the Blind/AFB Press
11 Penn Plz
Suite 300
New York, NY 10001-2006

212-502-7600
800-232-3044
FAX: 212-502-7777
afborder@abdintl.com
www.afb.org

Carl Augusto, President
Gerda Groff, Co-Author
Richard Obnen, Chairman of the Board
Alan Lindroth, Principal
Easy-to-read manual on how older visually impaired persons can pursue their interests and activities in community residences, senior centers, long-term care facilities and other community settings. Paperback.
99 pages Paperback
ISBN 0-891282-44-0

7518 Sharing the Burden
Brookings Institution
1775 Massachusetts Ave NW
Washington, DC 20036-2188
202-797-6000
FAX: 202-797-6004
www.brookings.edu

Joshua N Weiner, Author
Laurel Hixon Illston, Co-Author
Raymond J Hanley, Co-Author
Strobe Talbott, President
The authors examine the cost of public and private initiatives and who would pay for them. Their answers emerge from a large computer simulation model that the authors developed. *$42.95*
342 pages Cloth
ISBN 0-815793-78-2

7519 Social Security, Medicare, and Government Pensions
NOLO
950 Parker St
Berkeley, CA 94710-2524
510-549-1976
800-728-3555
FAX: 800-645-0895
www.nolo.com

Joseph L Matthews, Author
Dorothy Matthews Berman, Co-Author
Ralph Warner, Chairman/CEO
Ann Heron, COO
Social Security, Medicare, SSI and more explained in this all-in-one resource that gets you the most out of your retirement benefits. *$24.95*
480 pages Paperback
ISBN 1-413307-53-5

7520 Successful Models of Community Long Term Care Services for the Elderly
Routledge (Taylor & Francis Group)
270 Madison Ave
Fl 4 #4
New York, NY 10016-601
212-695-6599
800-637-7064
FAX: 212-563-2269
www.routledgementalhealth.com

Eloise Killeffer, Author
Ruth Bennett, Co-Author
Jeffrey Lim, Director
Francis Chua, Manager
Experienced practitioners provide examples of successful community-based long term care service programs for the elderly. *$72.00*
174 pages Hardcover
ISBN 0-866569-87-3

7521 Therapeutic Activities with Persons Disabled by Alzheimer's Disease
Sage Publications
804 Anacapa Stree
Sanat Barbara, CA 93101-2212
805-899-8620
info@sagepub.com
www.sagepub.com

Sara Miller McCune, Founder, Publisher, Chairperson
Blaise Simqu, CEO
Tracey Ozmina, COO
Stephen Barr, Managing Director
A program of functional skills for activities of daily living. Hardcover. *$86.00*
432 pages
ISBN 0-834211-62-9

7522 Visually Impaired Seniors as Senior Companions: A Reference Guide
American Foundation for the Blind/AFB Press
11 Penn Plz
Suite 300
New York, NY 10001-2006
212-502-7600
800-232-3044
FAX: 212-502-7777
afborders@abdintl.com
www.afb.org

Carl Augusto, President
Alan Lindroth, Principal
Richard Obnen, Chairman of the Board
Michael Gilliam, Vice Chairman
This useful guide describes the Senior Companion Program that is intended to broaden opportunities for older persons with disabilities. Appendix includes training materials, evaluation forms, recruitment and public relations information. *$15.00*
108 pages Paperback
ISBN 0-891282-38-6

7523 Work, Health and Income Among the Elderly
Brookings Institution
1775 Massachusetts Ave NW
Washington, DC 20036-2188
202-797-6000
FAX: 202-797-6004
www.brookings.edu

Gary Burtless, Author
Strobe Talbott, President
Steven Bennett, Vice President/COO
Stewart Uretsky, Vice President/CFO
Employment, health and financial information for the elderly. *$26.95*
276 pages Cloth
ISBN 0-815711-76-6

Print: Journals

7524 Gerontology: Abstracts in Social Gerontology
National Council on the Aging
1901 L St NW
4th Floor
Washington, DC 20036-3506
202-479-1200
FAX: 202-479-0735
TTY:202-479-6674
info@ncoa.org
www.ncoa.org

James Firman, President/CEO
Jay Greenberg, ScD, Senior Vice President, Social Enterprise
Richard Birkel, PhD, MPA, Senior Vice President, Center for Healthy Aging and Director
Nora Dowd Eisenhower, JD, Senior Vice President, Economic Security and Director
Detailed abstracts are provided for recent major journal articles, books, reports and other materials on many facets of aging, including: adult education, demography, family relations, institutional care and work attitudes. Item No. AB100; Journals $114.00; Member Discount: $94.00.
Quarterly

7525 Physical & Occupational Therapy in Geriatrics
Taylor & Francis Group, LLC
325 Chestnut Street
Suite 800 #800
Philadelphia, PA 19106-2608
215-625-8900
800-354-1420
FAX: 215-625-2940
haworthpress@taylorandfrancis.com
www.tandf.co.uk

Ellen Dunleavey Taira, Editor
Barbara Pucher, CFO
Focuses on current practices and emerging issues in the care of the older client, including long-term care in institutional and community settings, crisis intervention, and innovative programming; the entire range of problems experienced by the elderly;

and the current skills needed for working with older clients.
$99.00
Quarterly

Print: Magazines

7526 **AARP Magazine**
American Association of Retired Persons
601 E St NW
Washington, DC 20049-3

202-434-7700
888-687-2277
FAX: 202-434-7710
TTY: 877-434-7598
member@aarp.org
www.aarp.org

A Barry Rand, President/CEO
Hop Backus, Executive Vice President, State
Steve Cone, Executive Vice President of Integrated Value
Lorraine Cort,s-V zquez, Executive Vice President, Multicultural
Markets
A nonprofit membership organization of persons 50 and older
dedicated to addressing their needs and interests.

Print: Newsletters

7527 **Aging & Vision News**
Lighthouse International
111 E 59th St
New York, NY 10022-1202

212-821-9216
800-829-0500
FAX: 212-821-9707
info@lighthouse.org
www.lightfair.com

Laurie A Silbersweig, Editorial Director
Intended for professionals engaged in research, education or service delivery in the field of vision and aging.
6-12 pages Newsletter

7528 **Aging News Alert**
C D Publications
8204 Fenton St
Silver Spring, MD 20910-4502

301-588-6380
800-666-6380
FAX: 301-588-6385
subscription@cdpublications.com
www.cdpublications.com/seniors/ana

Michael Gerecht, President
Ash Gerecht, Co-Owner
Reports on successful senior programs, funding opportunities,
and federal actions that effect the elderly. Available in 6, 12 or 24
month subscriptions online and online/print combinations.
$192.00
8 pages Monthly

7529 **Aging and Vision News**
Lighthouse International
111 E 59th St
New York, NY 10022-1202

212-821-9384
800-829-0500
FAX: 212-821-9707
TTY: 212-821-9713
info@lighthouse.org
www.lighthouse.org

Robert Rosenberg, Editor
Mark G. Ackermann, President/ Chief Executive Officer
Maura J. Sweeney, Senior Vice President/Chief Operating Officer
John Vlachos, Senior Vice President/Chief Financial Officer

Newsletter

7530 **Enabling News**
Access II Independent Living Centers
101 Industrial Parkway
Gallatin, MO 64640-1280

660-663-2423
888-663-2423
FAX: 660-663-2517
TTY: 660-663-2663
access@accessii.org
www.accessii.org

Debra Hawman, Executive Director
Gary Matticks, Owner
Debra Hawman, Executive Director
It is a newsletter published by Access II.
8 pages Quarterly

7531 **Part B News**
DecisionHealth
9737 Washingtonian Blvd
Two Washingtonian Center, Suite. 20
Gaithersburg, MD 20878-7364

301-287-2682
855-225-5341
FAX: 301-287-2535
customer@decisionhealth.com
www.decisionhealth.com

Scott Kraft, Editor
Scott Kraft, Director, Content Management
Steve Greenberg, President
Tonya Nevin, Vice President, New Business Development
Each week Part B News brings you comprehensive Medicare Part
B regulatory coverage, plain-English interpretive guidance, Fee
Schedule updates, claims filing strategies, coding, documenta-
tion and payment best practices, and the latest on Congressional
health care deliberations and how they affect your practice.
$519.00
Yearly

7532 **Social Security Bulletin**
US Social Security Administration
2100 M Street NW
Suite 829 #829
Washington, DC 20037- 0002

202-358-6066
800-772-1213
FAX: 202-282-7219
TTY: 800-325-0778
www.ssa.gov/policy

Karyn Tucker, Managing Editor
Richard Balkus, Assoc. Comm. Office Of Dis
Carolyn W. Colvin, Commissioner
James A. Kissko, Chief of Staff
Reports on results of research and analysis pertinent to the Social
Security and SSI programs. *$16.00*
Monthly

Non Print: Newsletters

7533 **AGRAM**
Assoc of Ohio Philanthropic Homes, Housing/Service
855 S Wall St
Columbus, OH 43206-1921

614-444-2882
FAX: 614-444-2974
info@aopha.org
www.aopha.org

John Alfano, CEO
Tim White, Executive Director
P Alfano, President/CEO

Weekly

7534 Aging News Alert
C D Publications
8204 Fenton Street
Silver Spring, MD 20910-4502   301-588-6380
                                            800-666-6380
                                    FAX: 301-588-6385
                    subscription@cdpublications.com
                            www.cdpublications.com

Ash Gerecht, Co-Owner
Sharon Livermore, Businesss Manager
Reports on successful senior programs, funding opportunities,
and federal actions that effect the elderly. Available in 6, 12 or 24
month subscriptions online and online/print combinations.
$192.00
8 pages Monthly

7535 CAHSA Connecting
Colorado Assoc of Homes and Services for the Aging
1888 Sherman St
Suite 610
Denver, CO 80203-1160   303-837-8834
                                    FAX: 303-837-8836
                                            info@cahsa.org
                            www.leadingagecolorado.org

Laura Landwirth, Executive Director
Elisabeth Borden, Director
Maureen Hewitt, President
Vennita Jenkins, Secretary
CAHSA Connecting is published monthly by the Colorado Asso-
ciation of Homes and Services for the Aging (CAHSA)

7536 CANPFA-Line
CT Assoc of Not-for-Profit Providers of the Aging
1340 Wilmington Rdg
Berlin, CT 6037   860-828-2903
                                    FAX: 860-828-8694
                        leadingagect@leadingagect.org
                            www.leadingagect.org

Mag Morelli, President
Nurka Carrero, Office Manager
Andrea Bellofiore, Director of Member Programs & Se
Beth Ricker, Finance Manager & Membership Dir
LeadingAge Connecticut promotes and advocates for a vision of
the world in which every community offers an integrated and co-
ordinated continuum of high quality, affordable health care,
housing and community based services.
Bi-Monthly

7537 Capitol Focus
Colorado Assoc of Homes and Services for the Aging
1888 Sherman St
Suite 610
Denver, CO 80203-1160   303-837-8834
                                    FAX: 303-837-8836
                                            info@cahsa.org
                            www.leadingagecolorado.org

Laura Landwirth, Executive Director
Elisabeth Borden, Director
Maureen Hewitt, President
Vennita Jenkins, Secretary
Capitol Focus is a weekly activities summary of the Colorado
Legislature for CAHSA members, provided by staff of the Colo-
rado Association of Homes and Services for the Aging.

7538 Capsule
Children of Aging Parents
P.O.Box 167
Richboro, PA 18954-167   215-945-6900
                                            800-227-7294
                                    FAX: 215-945-8720
                        info@caps4caregivers.org
                            www.caps4caregivers.org

Karen Rosenberg, Director
An informative newsletter for caregivers.
Quarterly

7539 Communique
Iowa Association of Homes & Services for the Aging

Bi-weekly

7540 Elder Visions Newsletter
National Indian Council on Aging
10501 Montgomery Blvd NE
Suite 210
Albuquerque, NM 87111-3832   505-292-2001
                                    FAX: 505-292-1922
                                            randella@nicoa.org
                                            www.nicoa.org

Traci Mc Clellan, Executive Director
James Delacruz, Chairman Of The Board
Phyllis Antone, Director
Provides information on issues affecting American Indian and
Alaska Native Elders.
Quarterly

7541 Innovations
National Council on Aging
1901 L Street NW
4th Floor
Washington, DC 20036-3506   202-479-1200
                                    FAX: 202-479-0735
                                    TTY:202-479-6674
                                            info@ncoa.org
                                            www.ncoa.org

Austin Han, Manager
James Firman, President/CEO
Donna Whitt, SVP/CFO
Nancy Whitelaw, SVP/Director
Explores significant developments in the field of aging, keeping
individuals informed on a broad range of topics.
Quarterly

7542 NASUA News
National Association of State Units on Aging
1201 15th Street NW
Suite 350
Washington, DC 20005-2842   202-898-2578
                                    FAX: 202-898-2583
                                            info@nasua.org
                                            www.nasuad.org

Martha Roherty, Executive Director
Peggie Rice, Director of Policy and Legislative Affairs
Eric Risteen, Chief Operating Officer
Kimberly Fletcher, Conference and Outreach Coordinator
It is the newsletter of the National Association of State Units on
Aging
Monthly

7543 NCOA Week
National Council on Aging
1901 L Street NW
4th Floor
Washington, DC 20036-3540   202-479-1200
                                    FAX: 202-479-0735
                                    TTY:202-479-6674
                                            info@ncoa.org
                                            www.ncoa.org

James P Firman, President/CEO
Donna Whitt, SVP/CFO
Nancy Whitelaw, SVP/Director
A concise e-newsletters focused on the issues you care about, in-
cluding policies that affect funding, grants and awards you can
apply for, and best practices you can adapt for your center.
Weekly

7544 NNEAHSA
Northn New England Assoc of Homes & Svcs for Aging
PO Box 1428
Standish, ME 04084-1428
207-773-4822
FAX: 207-773-0101
sderingis@nneahsa.org
www.agingservicesmenh.org

Sheila Deringis, Editor
Providing healthy, affordable and ethical long-term care to older citizens throughout Maine, New Hampshire and Vermont.

7545 NSCLC Washington Weekly
National Senior Citizens Law Center
1444 Eye St NW
Suite 1100
Washington, DC 20005-6547
202-289-6976
FAX: 202-289-7224
nscls@nsclc.org
www.nsclc.org

Paul Nathanson, Executive Director
Edward King, Executive Director
Edward Spurgeon, Executive Director
Provides the latest case information, administration and congressional developments of importance for the elderly.

7546 Quality First
American Assoc of Homes and Services for the Aging
2519 Connecticut Ave NW
Washington, DC 20008-1520
202-783-2242
FAX: 202-783-2255
www.leadingage.org

William L Minnix Jr, President
Features helpful tips for marketing services and earning the public's trust through the web site.
Quarterly

7547 Senior Focus
National Council on Aging
1901 L Street
4th Floor
Washington, DC 20036-3540
202-479-1200
FAX: 202-479-0735
TTY:202-479-6674
info@ncoa.org
www.ncoa.org

Austin Han, Manager
James Firman, President/CEO
Donna Whit, SVP/CFO
Nancy Whitelaw, SVP/Director
Contains health, financial, lifestyle tips written for seniors
Quarterly

Support Groups

7548 Area Agency on Aging of Southwest Arkansas
600 Columbia Road 11 East
PO Box 1863
Magnolia, AR 71753
870-234-7410
800-272-2127
FAX: 870-234-6804
inref@magnolia-net.com
www.agewithdignity.com

Janet Morrison, Executive Director
The Area Agency on Aging of Southwest Arkansas, Inc. is a non-profit organization serving adults age 60 or older, family caregivers, agencies and organizations working with seniors. It is part of a national network of more than 650 Area Agencies on Aging throughout the United States.

7549 Area Agency on Aging: Region One
1366 E Thomas Rd
Suite 108
Phoenix, AZ 85014-5739
602-264-2255
888-783-7500
FAX: 602-230-9132
www.aaaphx.org

Mary Lynn Kasunic, President
Jeannine Berg, Vice Chairman
Bobbie Garland, Vice Chairman
Richard Peitzmeier, Vice Chairman
We have a vast variety of programs and services to enhance the quality of life for residents of Maricopa County, Arizona. If you would like more information about services mentioned within the website please call.

7550 High Country Council of Governments Area Agency on Aging
468 New Market Blvd
Boone, NC 28607-1820
828-265-5434
FAX: 828-265-5439
breece@regiond.org
www.regiond.org

Robert L. Johnson, Chairman
Gary D. Blevins, Vice Chair
Brenda Lyerly, Secretary
Danny McIntosh, Treasurer
High Country Council of Governments is the multi-county planning and development agency for the seven northwestern North Carolina counties of Alleghany, Ashe, Avery, Mitchell, Watauga, Wilkes, and Yancey. The High Country region is a voluntary association of towns and counties located in the northern mountains of North Carolina.

7551 Institute on Aging
3575 Geary Blvd
San Francisco, CA 94118-3212
415-750-4111
877-750-4111
FAX: 415-750-5337
info@ioaging.org
www.ioaging.org

J. Thomas Briody, MHSc, President
Dustin Harper, Vice President, Community Living Services
Cindy Kauffman, MS, COO
Roxana Tsougarakis, MBA, Chief Financial Officer
Support Services for Elders (SSE) provides care coordination, household management, personal support, bookkeeping, and other assistance to help protect your financial affairs.

7552 Land-of-Sky Regional Council Area Agency on Aging
339 New Leicester Hwy
Suite 140
Asheville, NC 28806-2087
828-251-6622
FAX: 828-251-6353
info@landofsky.org
www.landofsky.org

LeeAnne Tucker, Aging & Volunteer Services Director
Terry Albrecht, Program Director
Joan Tuttle, Director
Joe Mc Kinney, Manager
Is the designated regional organization to meet the needs of persons over 60 in Buncombe, Henderson, Madison, and Transylvania counties, by the North Carolina Division of Aging and Adult Services.

7553 Lumber River Council of Governments Area Agency on Aging
30 Cj Walker Rd
COMtech Park
Pembroke, NC 28372-7340
910-618-5533
FAX: 910-521-7556
lrcog@mail.lrcog.dst.nc.us
www.lumberrivercog.org

Michelle Gaitley, Nutrition Program Director
Renee Cooper, Nutrition Program Assistant
Kristen Elk Maynor, Aging Program Coordinator
Margaret Lennon, Division Administrator

The Family Caregiver Support Program was created to assist family members, neighbors, and friends who help care for a person over the age of 60, or minor grandchildren being reared by a grandparent over 60.

7554   Mid-Carolina Area Agency on Aging
130 Gillespie Street
3rd Floor, Post Office Drawer 1510
Fayetteville, NC 28301-1510   910-323-4191
                                     FAX: 910-323-9330
                                     gdye@mccog.org
                                     www.mccog.org

James Caldwell, COG Executive Director
Glenda Dye, Aging Director
Lynda Barnett, Aging Care Manager
Carla Smith, Aging Program Specialist
The Mid-Carolina Area Agency on Aging is designated for planning, administration, and advocacy of services for persons aged 60 and older and their spouses who need assistance in order to remain as independent as possible.

7555   Piedmont Triad Council of Governments Area Agency on Aging
2216 W Meadowview Rd
Suite 201
Greensboro, NC 27407-3480   336-294-4950
                                     FAX: 336-632-0457
                                     acalhoun@ptcog.org
                                     www.ptcog.org

Blair Barton-Percival, Director
Adrienne Calhoun, Assistant Director
Bob Cleveland, Aging Program Planner
Joe Dzugan, Aging Systems Coordinator
Responsible for planning, developing, implementing, and coordinating aging services for seven counties in the Piedmont Triad (Alamance, Caswell, Davidson, Guilford, Montgomery, Randolph, and Rockingham) and their 185,00 residents age 60 and older.

7556   Southwestern Commission Area Agency on Aging
125 Bonnie Ln
Sylva, NC 28779-8552   828-586-1962
                                     FAX: 828-586-1968
                                     mary@regiona.org
                                     www.regiona.org

Ryan Sherby, Executive Director
Beth Cook, Workforce Development Director
Janne Mathews, Aging Program Coordinator
Sarajane Melton, Area Agency on Aging Administrator
The Area Agency on Aging (AAA) works on behalf of older adults and their caregivers in the seven southwestern counties of North Carolina. The Southwestern Commission Area Agency on Aging was established in 1980 as mandated by the 1977 Amendments of the Older Americans Act in order for a Planning and Service Area (PSA) to receive funds from the Act.

7557   Tompkins County Office for the Aging
214 W. Martin Luther King Jr./State
Ithaca, NY 14850-4299   607-274-5482
                                     FAX: 607-274-5495
                                     lholmes@tompkins-co.org
                                     www.tompkins-co.org

Lisa Holmes, Director
Lisa Lunas, Aging Services Planner
Katrina Schickel, Aging Services Specialist
David Stoyell, Aging Services Specialist
We provide objective and unbiased information regarding the array of services available for older adults and their caregivers. Established in 1975, our mission is to assist the senior population of Tompkins County to remain independent in their homes as long as is possible and appropriate, and with a decent quality of life and human dignity.

7558   Triangle J Council of Governments Area Agency on Aging
PO Box 12276
Research Triangle Park, NC 27709-2276   919-549-0551
                                         FAX: 919-549-9390
                                         ejones@tjcog.org
                                         www.tjaaa.org

Joan Pellettier, Director
Mary Warren, Assistant Director
Ashley Price, Program Associate
Jennifer Link, Regional Ombudsman for Long-Term Care
We serve to facilitate and support the development of programs to address the needs of older adults and to support investment in their talents and interests.

7559   University of California Memory and Aging Center
675 Nelson Rising Lane
Suite 190
San Francisco, CA 94143-1207   415-353-2057
                                    FAX: 415-476-5591
                                    webmaster@memory.ucsf.edu
                                    www.memory.ucsf.edu

Bruce L Miller, Director
Mary Koestler, Project Administrator
Carrie Cheung, Clinic Coordinator
Ken Edwards, Administrative Assistant
Provides support for patients and families affected by neurodegenerative diseases. In addition to our established support groups, we continue to develop new support groups.

7560   Upper Coastal Plain Council of Governments Area Agency on Aging
PO Box 9
Wilson, NC 27894-9   252-234-5952
                                    FAX: 252-234-5971
                                    helen.page@ucpcog.org
                                    www.ucpcog.org

Greg Godard, Executive Director
Jody Riddle, AAA Program Director
Helen Page, Aging Programs Specialist
Abigail W. Harper, Regional Ombudsman
The Upper Coastal Plain Area Agency On Aging is one of 16 Area Agencies on Aging across the state of NC, serving Region L. Counties include Edgecombe, Halifax, Nash, Northampton, and Wilson. The mission of the Area Agency on Aging is to empower senior adults, family caregivers, and individuals with disabilities residing in Edgecombe, Halifax, Nash, Northampton, and Wilson Counties to live independent, meaningful, healthy, and dignified lives.

Blind & Deaf

Associations

7561   American Association of the Deaf-Blind
8630 Fenton Street
PO Box 2831, Suite 121
Kensington, MD 20891-3803   301-495-4403
                                  FAX: 301-495-4404
                                  TTY: 301-495-4402
                                  aadb-info@aadb.org
                                  www.aadb.org

Jamie Pope, Executive Director
Elizabeth Spiers, Information Services Director
Jill Gaus, President

The American Association of the Deaf-Blind (AADB) is a non-profit 501(c)(3) national consumer organization of, by, and for deaf-blind Americans and their supporters. Deaf-Blind includes all types and degrees of dual vision and hearing loss. Our mission is to ensure that all deaf-blind persons achieve their maximum potential through increased independence, productivity, and integration into the community.
Membership dues

7562   American Society for Deaf Children
800 Florida Ave NE
Washington, DC 20002-3695   202-644-9204
                                  800-942-2732
                                  FAX: 410-795-0965
                                  asdc@deafchildren.org
                                  www.deafchildren.org

Jodee Crace, President

We believe deaf or hard-of-hearing children are entitled to full communication access in their home, school, and community. We also believe that language development, respect for the Deaf, and access to deaf and hard-of-hearing role models are important to assure optimal intellectual, social, and emotional development.

7563   Arena Stage
11101 Sixth St
Washington, DC 20024   202-554-9066
                                  FAX: 202-488-4056
                                  TTY: 202-484-0247
                                  arena@arenastage.org
                                  www.arenastage.org

David E. Shiffrin, Chair
Zelda Fichandler, Founding Director
Molly Smith, Artistic Director
Chad Bauman, Associate Executive Director

A pioneer in providing access to theater for people with disabilities and the birthplace of Audio Description. Offers infrared assistive listening devices (both loop and headset), program books in Braille, large print and wheelchair accessible seating with adjacent companion seating. Audio cassette format available upon request. Sign Interpretation and Audio Description are offered at selected performances. Cafe menus and shop lists in Braille. Wheelchair-accessible with lifts and ramps.

7564   Association of Late-Deafened Adults
8038 Macintosh Ln
Suite 2
Rockford, IL 61107-5300   815-332-1515
                                  866-402-2532
                                  TTY: 815-332-1515
                                  info@alda.org
                                  www.alda.org

Linda Drattell, President
Matt Ferrara, Region I Director
Marsha Kopp, Region II Directo
Dave Litman, Region III Director
Supports the empowerment of late-deafened people.

7565   Canadian Deafblind Association (CDBA) National Office
421 - 1860 Appleby Line
Suite 421
Burlington, ON, Canada L7L-7H7
                                  866-229-5832
                                  FAX: 905-319-2027
                                  info@cdbanational.com
                                  www.cdbanational.com

Carolyn Monaco, President
Suzanne McConnell, VP Administration
Ericka Dixon-Williams, VP Special Projects
Brad Ramey, Ontario Chapter Representative

The mission of the Canadian Deafblind Association's National organization is to promote and enhance the well-being of people who are deafblind through: advocacy, the development and dissemination of information, and the provision of support to our chapters, members, and community partners.

7566   Foundation Fighting Blindness
7168 Columbia Gateway Dr.
Ste 100
Columbia, MD 21046   410-423-0600
                                  800-683-5555
                                  FAX: 410-363-2393
                                  TTY: 800-683-5551
                                  info@fightblindness.org
                                  www.blindness.org

William T. Schmidt, Chief Executive Officer
Valerie Navy-Daniels, Chief Development Officer
Stephen M. Rose, Chief Research Officer
Rhea K. Farberman, Senior Director, Communications & Marketing

The foundation's mission is to drive the research that will provide preventions, treatments, and cures for people affected by retinitis pigmentosa, macular degeneration, Usher syndrome and the entire spectrum of retinal degenerative diseases.

7567   Hearing Loss Association of America
7910 Woodmont Ave
Suite 1200
Bethesda, MD 20814-7022   301-657-2248
                                  FAX: 301-913-9413
                                  TTY: 301-657-2248
                                  www.hearingloss.org

Brenda Battat, Executive Director
Barbara Kelley, Dep Exec Dir, Editor-In-Chief
Nancy Macklin, Director of Events & Marketing
Lise Hamlin, Director of Public Policy

The mission of the Hearing Loss Association of America is to open the world of communication to people with hearing loss through information, education, advocacy and support.

7568   Helen Keller National Center for Deaf- Blind Youths And Adults
141 Middle Neck Rd
Sands Point, NY 11050-1218   516-944-8900
                                  FAX: 516-944-7302
                                  TTY: 516-944-8637
                                  hkncinfo@hknc.org
                                  www.hknc.org

Joseph McNulty, Executive Director
Enables each person who is deaf/blind to live and work in his or her community of choice.

7569   Idaho Commission for the Blind and Visually Impaired
341 W. Washington St.
PO Box 83720
Boise, ID 83720-0012   208-334-3220
                                  800-542-8688
                                  FAX: 208-334-2963
                                  ajones@icbvi.idaho.gov
                                  www.icbvi.state.id.us

Angela Jones, Administrator
Raelene Thomas, Management Assistant
Bruce Christopherson, Rehabilitation Services Chief
Dana Ard, Vocational Rehabilitation Counse
Empowers persons who are blind or visually impaired by providing vocational rehabilitation training, skills training and educa-

tional opportunities to achieve self fulfillment through quality employment and independent living; to serve as a resource to families and employers and to expand public awareness regarding the potential of all persons who are blind or visually impaired.

7570 International Hearing Society
16880 Middlebelt Rd
Ste 4
Livonia, MI 48154-3374
734-522-7200
FAX: 734-522-0200
bdemicoli@ihsinfo.org
www.ihsinfo.org

Kathleen Mennillo MBA, Executive Director
Donna Kinnelly, Member Services Coordinator
Sandra den Boer, Communications Specialist
Marlene Deuby, Continuing Education Specialist
IHS members are engaged in the practice of testing human hearing and selecting, fitting and dispensing hearing instruments.

7571 Lilac Services for the Blind
1212 N Howard St
Spokane, WA 99201-2410
509-328-9116
800-422-7893
FAX: 509-328-8965
info@lilacblind.org
www.lilacblind.org

Cheryl Martin, Executive Director
Mathew Plank, Marketing Director
Peggy Swanson, Office Manager
Debbie Bowcutt, Rehabilitation Teacher & Low Vis
Lilac Services for the Blind provides independent living instruction, adaptive aids, counseling, low-vision evaluations, support groups, Braille transcription services, and much more for 14 counties in the inland Northwest.

7572 National Consortium on Deaf-Blindness
345 Monmouth Ave N
Monmouth, OR 97361-1329
800-438-9376
FAX: 503-838-8150
TTY:800-854-7013
info@nationaldb.org
www.nationaldb.org

D. Jay Gense, Director
Kathy McNulty, Associate Director
Joe Mcnulty, Co-Principal Investigator
Amy Parker, ED. D, Associate Director
Promotes academic achievement and results for children and youth who are deaf-blind, through technical assistanve, model demonstration, and information dissemination activities that are supported by evidence-based practices. Information about deaf-blindness is available free of charge through the Consortium's information services branch, DB-Link.

7573 National Family Association for Deaf-Blind
141 Middle Neck Rd
Sands Point, NY 11050-1218
516-944-8900
800-255-0411
FAX: 516-883-9060
TTY: 516-944-8637
NFADB@aol.com
www.nfadb.org

Susan Green, President
Janette Peracchio, Vice President
Cynthia Jackson-Glenn, Treasurer
Paddi Davies, Secretary
The National Family Association for Deaf-Blind (NFADB) is a non-profit, volunteer-based family association. Our philosophy is that individuals who are deaf-blind are valued members of society and are entitled to the same opportunities and choices as other members of the community. We are the largest national network of families focusing on issues surrounding deaf blindness.

7574 National Federation of the Blind
200 E. Wells St.
at Jernigan Place
Baltimore, MD 21230- 4998
410-659-9314
FAX: 410-685-5653
nfb@nfb.org
nfb.org

John Berggren, Executive Director, Operations
Anil Lewis, Executive Director, NFB Jernigan Institute
John G. Par, Jr., Executive Director, Advocacy & Policy
The National Federation of the Blind (NFB) is the largest organization of the blind in the world. The Federation's purpose is to help blind people achieve self-confidence, self-respect, and self-determination. Their goal is the complete integration of the blind into society on a basis of equality.

7575 National Information Center for Children and Youth with Disabilities (NICHCY)
1825 Connecticut Ave NW
Ste 700
Washington, DC 20009
202-884-8200
800-695-0285
FAX: 202-884-8441
TTY: 202-884-8200
nichcy@aed.org
www.nichcy.org

Suzanne Ripley, Manager
NICHCY is the center that provides information to the nation ondisabilities in children and youth; programs and services for infants, children, and youth with disabilities; IDEA, the nation's special education law; and research-based information on effective practices for children with disabilities.

7576 National Information Clearinghouse on Children who are Deaf-Blind
National Consortium on Deaf-Blindness
345 Monmouth Ave N
Monmouth, OR 97361-1329
503-838-8391
800-438-9376
877-877-1593
FAX: 503-838-8150
TTY:800-854-7013
dblink@tr.wou.edu
www.tr.wou.edu

Dr. Ella Taylor, Director
Nancy Ganson, Assistant to the Director
Mike Stewart, Grants Management Office
Cindi Mafit, Grants Management Office
Collects, organizes, and disseminates information related to children and youth of ages 0 to 21 who are deaf-blind and connects consumers of deaf-blind information to the appropriate resources. Publishes a number of topical papers and publishes Deaf-Blind Perspective.

7577 Ultratec
450 Science Dr
Madison, WI 53711-1166
608-238-5400
800-482-2424
FAX: 608-238-3008
TTY: 800-482-2424
www.ultratec.com

Jackie Morgan, Marketing Director
Ultratec works to make telephone access more convenient and reliable for people with hearing loss.

Camps

7578   Florida Lions Camp
Lions of Multiple District 35
2819 Tiger Lake Road
Lake Wales, FL 33898-9582   863-696-1948
                                        FAX: 863-696-2398
                                     bjcage@hotmail.com
                                      www.lionscampfl.org

Barbara Cage, Executive Director
Liz Cage, Program Director
Carissa Moen, Bookkeeping/Registrar
One-week sessions June-August for youths and adults with visual impairments and other challenging disabilities. Coed, ages 5 and up. A variety of traditional summer camp activities which include: swimming, canoeing, fishing, hiking, camping out and cooking over a fire, games, arts & crafts, singing & dancing, hay-wagon rides, challenge course and much more. Activities are adapted to the age and ability of each camper to ensure maximum participation, safety and fun.

7579   Florida School for the Deaf and Blind
207 San Marco Ave
St Augustine, FL 32084-2799   904-827-2200
                                             800-344-3732
                                        FAX: 904-827-2325
                                        info@fsdb.k12.fl.us
                                         www.fsdb.k12.fl.us
Dr. Jeanne Glidden Prickett, EdD, Shelter Administrator
Debbie Schuler, Administrator of Instructional S
Cindy Day, Executive Director of Parent Ser
Terri Wiseman, Administrator of Business Servic
Statewide public boarding school for eligible students who are deaf/hard-of-hearing or blind/visually impaired. FSDB serves children who are pre-k through high school.

Print: Books

7580   A Handbook for Writing Effective Psychoeducational Reports (2nd Edition)
PRO-ED Inc.
8700 Shoal Creek Blvd.
Austin, TX 78757-6897   512-451-3246
                                             800-897-3202
                                        FAX: 800-397-7633
                                    general@proedinc.com
                                        www.proedinc.com
Sharon Bradley-Johnson, Author
C. Merle Johnson, Author
This comprehensive book shows how to write useful reports once assessment information has been attained. It is a valuable resource for professionals working in school systems, as well as for those graduate students who are just learning to write reports. $32.00
134 pages Paperback
ISBN 1-416401-40-7

7581   Communicating with People Who Have Trouble Hearing & Seeing: A Primer
National Association for Visually Handicapped
22 W 21st St
Fl 6
New York, NY 10010-6943   212-255-2804
                                        FAX: 212-727-2931
                                         www.lighthouse.org
Roger O Goldman, Chairman Of The Board
Line drawings that depict problems for those with both deficiencies. $2.00

7582   Helen and Teacher: The Story of Helen & Anne Sullivan Macy
American Foundation for the Blind/AFB Press
11 Penn Plz
Suite 300
New York, NY 10001-2006   212-502-7600
                                             800-232-5463
                                        FAX: 212-502-7777
                                         afbinf@afb.net
                                            www.afb.org
Carl Augusto, President
Richard Obnen, Chairman Of The Board
Michael Gilliam, Vice Chairman
Alan Lindroth, Principal
A pictorial biography emphasizing Hellen Keller's accomplishments in public life over a period of more than 60 years. Traces Anne Sullivan's early years and her meeting with Helen Keller, and goes on to recount the joint events of their lives. A definitive biography. $29.95.
Paperback
ISBN 0-891282-89-0

7583   Independence Without Sight and Sound: Suggestions for Practitioners
American Foundation for the Blind/AFB Press
11 Penn Plz
Suite 300
New York, NY 10001-2006   212-502-7600
                                             800-232-8463
                                        FAX: 212-502-7777
                                         afbinfo@afb.net
                                            www.afb.org
Carl Augusto, President
Richard Obnen, Chairman Of The Board
Michael Gilliam, Vice Chairman
Alan Lindroth, Principal
This practical guidebook covers the essential aspects of communicating and working with deaf-blind persons. Includes useful information on how to talk with deaf-blind people, and adapt orientation and mobility techniques for deaf-blind travelers. $39.95
193 pages Paperback
ISBN 0-891282-46-7

7584   Reclaiming Independence: Staying in the Drivers Seat When You Are no Longer Drive.
American Printing House for the Blind
1839 Frankfort Ave
Louisville, KY 40206-3148   502-895-2405
                                             800-223-1839
                                        FAX: 502-899-2274
                                          info@aph.org
                                            www.aph.org
Tuck Tinsley, President
Joseph Paradis, Chairman
Kathleen Huebner, Vice Chairman
Jane Thompson, Executive Director
Useful for both individuals and professionals, this video/resource guide will help you successfuly use rehabilitation and transportation resources. $60.00

7585   Verbal View of the Web & Net
American Printing House for the Blind
1839 Frankfort Ave
Louisville, KY 40206-3148   502-895-2405
                                             800-223-1839
                                        FAX: 502-899-2274
                                          info@aph.org
                                            www.aph.org
Tuck Tinsley, President
Joseph Paradis, Chairman
Kathleen Huebner, Vice Chairman
Jane Thompson, Executive Director
One of a series of Verbal View titles, Verbal View of the Net & Web explains how to access information on the internet and teaches accessability features of Internet Explorer. $50.00

Print: Magazines

7586 Braille Montior
National Federation of the Blind Senior Division
200 E Wells St
Baltimore, MD 21230-4914   410-659-9314
                                  FAX: 410-685-5653
                                  nfbpublications@nfb.org
                                  www.nfb.org

Barbara Pierce, Editor
The Braille Monitor is the leading publication of the National Federation of the Blind. It covers the events and activities of the NFB and addresses the many issues and concerns of the blind.
11 times a year

7587 Deaf-Blind American
American Association of the Deaf-Blind (AADB)
8630 Fenton Street
PO Box 2831, Suite 121
Kensington, MD 20891-3803   301-495-4403
                                   FAX: 301-495-4404
                                   TTY:301-495-4402
                                   aadb-info@aadb.org
                                   www.aadb.org

Jamie Pope, Executive Director
Elizabeth Spiers, Information Services Director
Timothy Jackson, President
We are a consumer membership organization of, by and for people who have dual vision and hearing loss. Services we provide include an information clearinghouse on deaf blindness, a quarterly magazine (The Deaf Blind American), a newsletter, AADB news, a task force to improve interpreting for deaf-blind people, a listen for members, a partnership with the American Red Cross, and national conferences. $5.00
Quartlery

7588 Hearing Loss Magazine
HearingLoss Association of America
7910 Woodmont Ave
Ste 1200
Bethesda, MD 20814-7022   301-657-2248
                                 FAX: 301-913-9413
                                 www.hearingloss.org

Brenda Battat, Executive Director
Barbara Kelley, Editor-in-Chief/Deputy Executive Director of HLAA
Lisa Hamlin, Director Of Public Policy
Cindy Dyer, Graphic Design
Readers look to Hearing Loss Magazine to provide them with the latest information on products, services, research, and technology in the hearing health care field. They also look for personal stories of hard of hearing people to find encouragement, and give them the feeling that they're not alone in living with a hearing loss. They look for practical and useful information. Hearing Loss Magazine readers view the magazine as a lifeline to help them help themselves and live well with hearing loss.
Bi-Monthly

7589 Hearing Professional Magazine
International Hearing Society
Ste 4
16880 Middlebelt Rd
Livonia, MI 48154-3374   734-522-7200
                                FAX: 734-522-0200
                                knacarato@ihsinfo.org
                                www.ihsinfo.org

Scott Beall, Treasurer Director
Alan Lowell, President
Kathleen Mennillo, Executive Director
The Hearing Professional magazine is the official publication of the International Hearing Society. This quarterly publication includes industry news, membership highlights and best practices, hearing healthcare legislation, and other information and tools for hearing healthcare professionals.

Print: Newsletters

7590 Deaf-Blind Perspective
National Consortium on Deaf-Blindness
345 Monmouth Ave
Monmouth, OR 97361   503-838-8391
                            800-438-9376
                            FAX: 503-838-8150
                            TTY: 800-854-7013
                            dbp@wou.edu
                            www.tr.wou.edu/dblink

John Reiman PhD, Director
Peggy Malloy, Managing Editor
A free publication with articles, essays, and announcements about topics related to people who are deaf-blind. The primary focus is on the education of children and youth with deaf-blindness. Published two times a year (Spring and Fall) by the national consortium on Deaf-blindness at the Teaching Research Institute at Western Oregon University.

7591 InFocus
7168 Columbia Gateway Dri
Suite 100
Columbia, MD 21046   410-423-0600
                            800-683-5555
                            FAX: 410-363-2393
                            TTY: 800-683-5551
                            info@fightblindeness.org
                            www.blindness.org

Gordon Gund, Chairman
Edward H. Gollob, President
David Brint, VP
Haynes Lea, VP &Treasurer
Presents articles on coping, research updates, and Foundation news.
3x/year

7592 News from Advocates for Deaf-Blind
National Family Association for Deaf-Blind
141 Middle Neck Rd
Sands Point, NY 11050-1218   516-944-8900
                                    800-225-0411
                                    FAX: 516-883-9060
                                    TTY: 516-944-8637
                                    NFADB@gmail.com
                                    www.NFADB.org

Clara Berg, President
Edgenie Bellah, Affiliate Coordinator
Paddi Davies, Treasurer
Patti McGowan, Secretary
A membership organization which provide resources, education, advocacy, referrals and support for families with children who are deaf-blind; professionals in the field; and individuals who are deaf-blind.
20 pages TriAnnual

Non Print: Newsletters

7593 AADB E-News
American Association of the Deaf-Blind
8630 Fenton Street
Suite 121
Silver Spring, MD 20910- 3803   301-495-4403
                                        FAX: 301-495-4404
                                        aadb-info@aadb.org
                                        www.aadb.org

Jill Gaus, President
Lynn Jansen, VP
Debby Lieberman, Secretary
Mike Reese, Vice Treasurer
Contains information about the latest events occurring within AADB and in the deaf-blind community.

7594 ALDA Newsletter
ALDA
8038 Macintosh Ln
Suite 2
Rockford, IL 61107-5336

815-332-1515
866-402-2532
FAX: 877-907-1738
TTY: 815-332-1515
info@alda.org
www.alda.org

Mary Lou Mistretta, President
Dave Litman, President Elect
Brenda Estes, Past President
Articles, stories and poems by and about late-deafened adults.

7595 Beam
1850 W Roosevelt Rd
Chicago, IL 60608-1298

312-666-1331
FAX: 312-243-8539
TTY: 312-666-8874
www.chicagolighthouse.org

James Kesteloot, President
Terrence Longo, Assistant Director
Quarterly newsletter of the organization offering progressive programs for the blind, visually impaired, deaf-blind and multi-disabled children and adults, including vocational programs, computer and office skills training, job placement, independent living skills, orientation and mobility training, counseling and a low vision clinic.

7596 Endeavor
American Society for Deaf Children
800 Florida Ave NE
Washington, PA 20002-3695

717-703-0073
800-942-2732
FAX: 717-909-5599
TTY: 202-664-9204
asdc@deafchildren.org
www.deafchildren.org

Robert B Wells, Editor
Tami Hossler, Editor
ASDC's qurterly publication featuring committee reports, stories, and fun.
Quarterly

7597 HKNC Newsletter
Helen Keller National Center
141 Middle Neck Rd
Sands Point, NY 11050-1218

516-944-8900
FAX: 516-944-7302
TTY: 516-944-8637
hkncinfo@hknc.org
www.hknc.org

Joseph McNulty, Executive Director
Highlights recent activities at the national center.

7598 NAT-CENT
Helen Keller National Center
141 Middle Neck Rd
Sands Point, NY 11050-1218

516-944-8900
FAX: 516-944-7302
TTY: 516-944-8637
hkncinfo@hknc.org
www.hknc.org

Joseph McNulty, Executive Director
Contains articles on legislation, services, aids and devices, human interest and issues related to deaf-blindness.

Non Print: Software

7599 Braille + Mobile Manager
American Printing House for the Blind
1839 Frankfort Ave
Louisville, KY 40206-0085

502-895-2405
800-223-1839
FAX: 502-899-2284
info@aph.org
aph.org

Tuck Tinsley, President
Joseph Paradis, Chairman
Kathleen Huebner, Vice Chairman
Jane Thompson, Executive Director
Use it like a hand-held PDA or like a laptop. *$1395.00*

7600 MaximEyes
American Printing House for the Blind
1839 Frankfort Ave
Louisville, KY 40206-0085

502-895-2405
800-223-1839
FAX: 502-899-2284
info@aph.org
aph.org

Tuck Tinsley, President
Joseph Paradis, Chairman
Kathleen Huebner, Vice Chairman
Jane Thompson, Executive Director
MaximEyes is a plug-in for Internet Explorer that adds a toolbar that allows you to controll the size of website text and images. *$59.95*

Non Print: Video

7601 Getting in Touch
2612 N Mattis Ave
PO Box 7886
Champaign, IL 61826-1053

217-352-3273
800-519-2707
FAX: 217-352-1221
orders@researchpress.com
www.researchpress.com

Russell Pence, President
David Parkinson, Chairman
Cynthia Martin, Principal
Ann Parkinson, Principal

7602 Journey
Landmark Media
3450 Slade Run Dr
Falls Church, VA 22042-3940

703-241-2030
800-342-4336
FAX: 703-536-9540
info@landmarkmedia.com
landmarkmedia.com

Michael Hartogs, President
Richard Hartogs, VP Acquisitions
Peter Hartogs, VP New Business & Development
Eric Miller, Sales Representative
A moving portrayal of the extraordinary journey to Japan of 74-year-old Billie Sinclair, who is deaf, blind and mute. He funds his travels by weaving and selling baskets. In Japan he rides a roller coaster, tries judo and visits a deaf and blind acupuncturist. He demonstrates how it is possible to communicate by touch alone. *$195.00*
Video

Sports

7603 **ASD Athletics**
Alabama Institute for Deaf and Blind
205 South St E
Talladega, AL 35160-2411   256-761-3222
                       FAX: 256-761-3278
Ripley.Walter@aidb.state.al.us
aidb.org/alabama-school-for-the-deaf/athl etic
John Jernigan, Director, Student Development (ASD)
Walter Ripley, Director, Athletics & After-School Programs
Offers students opportunities to participate in a number of organizzed sports including basketball, volleyball, baseball, football, and cheerleading. Student athletes compete at national and international levels.

Support Groups

7604 **Aurora of Central New York**
518 James Street
Suite 100
Syracuse, NY 13203-2282   315-422-7263
                  FAX: 315-422-4792
                  TTY:315-422-9746
auroracny@auroracny.org
auroraofcny.org

John Scala, President
John McCormick, President
Ryan Emery, Treasurer
Leslie Rapson, Secretary
Professional counseling services to assist individuals and their families deal with the trauma of hearing or vision loss.

Cognitive

Associations

7605 ARC
1825 K St NW
Suite 1200
Washington, DC 20006

202-534-3700
800-433-5255
FAX: 202-534-3731
info@thearc.org
www.thearc.org

Nancy Webster, President
Ronald Brown, VP
Elise McMillan, Secretary
M. J. Bartelmay, Treasurer
The ARC promotes and protects the rights of people with intellectual and developmental disabilities and actively supports their inclusion and participation in the community throughout their lifetimes.

7606 Academy of Cognitive Therapy
245 N. 15th Street, MS 403
17 New College Building
Philadelphia, PA 19102

FAX: 215-537-1789
info@academyofct.org
www.academyofct.org

Aaron T. Beck, Honorary President
John P. Williams, President
Leslie Sokol, Secretary
James Korman, Treasurer
It is a non-profit organization, was founded in 1998 by a group of leading clinicians, educators, and researchers in the field of cognitive therapy.

7607 American Academy of Child & Adolescent Psychiatry
3615 Wisconsin Ave NW
Washington, DC 20016-3007

202-966-7300
FAX: 202-966-2891
communications@aacap.org
www.aacap.org

Elizabeth Hughes, Asst. Director of Education & Recertification
Alan Ezagui, Deputy Director of Development
Kristin Kroeger Ptakowski, Director & Sr. Deputy Executive Director
Michael Linskey, Assistant Director, Federal Government Affairs
Non-profit organization engaged in research and education specific to child and adolescent psychiatry. The AACAP aims to provide resources and knowledge beneficial to both patients and psychiatric professionals.

7608 American Delirium Society
1183 University Drive
Suite #105 - 106
Burlington, NC 27215

410-955-2343
www.americandeliriumsociety.org

7609 American Psychiatric Association
1000 Wilson Blvd
Ste 1825
Arlington, VA 22209-3901

703-907-7300
888-357-7924
FAX: 703-907-1085
apa@psych.org
www.psychiatry.org

Saul M. Levin, MD, Chief Executive Officer & Medical Director
Maria A. Oquendo, MD, President
The American Psychiatric Association is a medical specialty society recognized worldwide. Its over 35,000 U.S. and international member physicians work together to ensure humane care and effective treatment for all persons with mental disorders, including mental retardation and substance-related disorders.

7610 Association for Behavioral and Cognitive Therapies
305 7th Avenue, 16th Fl.
New York, NY 10001

212-647-1890
www.abct.org

Mary Jane Eimer, Executive Director
David Teisler, Director of Communications
Lisa Yarde, Membership Services Manager
Barbara Mazzella, Administrative Secretary
The ABCT is a multidisciplinary organization committed to the advancement of scientific approaches to the understanding and improvement of human functioning through the investigation and application of behavioral, cognitive, and other evidence-based principles to the assessment, prevention, treatment of human problems, and the enhancement of health and well-being.

7611 Association for Contextual Behavioral Science
1880 Pinegrove Dr.
Jenison, MI 49428

www.contextualscience.org

7612 Autism Research Institute
4182 Adams Ave
San Diego, CA 92116-2536

619-281-7165
866-366-3361
FAX: 619-563-6840
matt@autism.com
www.autismresearchinstitute.com

Steve Edelson Ph.D., Executive Director
Jane Johnson, Managing Director
Valerie Paradiz, Director
Anthony Morgali, Producer
Conducts research on the causes, diagnosis, and treatment of autism and publishes a quarterly newsletter that reviews worldwide research. Literature on causes and treatment available. Refers patients and families to health care professionals and clinics. Request publication list and sample newsletter, Autism Research Review International.

7613 Autism Services Center
929 4th Ave
PO Box 507
Huntington, WV 25701-1408

304-525-8014
FAX: 304-525-8026
www.autismservicescenter.org

Mike Grady, CEO
Jimmie Beirne, COO
Nathel Lewis, ASC Training Coordinator
Service agency for individuals with autism and developmental disabilities, and their families. Assists families and agencies attempting to meet the needs of individuals with autism and other developmental disabilities. Makes available technical assistance in designing treatment programs and more. The hotline provides informational packets to callers and assists via telephone when possible.

7614 Autism Treatment Center of America
2080 S Undermountain Rd
Sheffield, MA 01257-9643

413-229-2100
877-766-7473
FAX: 413-229-3202
correspondence@option.org
www.son-rise.org

Barry Kausman, Co-Founder/ Co-Originator/ Senio
Samahria Lyte Kaufman, Co-Founder/ Co-Originator/ Senio
Bryn Hogan, ATCA Senior Staff
William Hogan, ATCA Senior Staff
Since 1983, the Autism Treatment Center of America has provided innovative training programs for parents and professionals caring for children challenged by Autism, Autism Spectrum Disorders, Pervasive Developmental Disorders (PDD) and other development difficulties. The Son-Rise Program teaches a specific yet comprehensive system of treatment and education designed to help families and caregivers enable their children to dramatically improve in all areas of learning.

7615 **Beck Institute for Cognitive Therapy and Research**
1 Belmont Ave
Suite 700
Bala Cynwyd, PA 19004-1610   610-664-3020
                                    FAX: 610-709-5336
                                    info@beckinstitute.org
                                    www.beckinstitute.org

Aaron T Beck, President Emeritus
Judith S Beck PhD, President
Deborah Beck Busis, LSW, Diet Program Coordinator
Norman Cotterell, PhD, Senior Therapist and Clinical Co
Serves as a critically important training ground for cognitive
therapists/cognitive behavior therapists.

7616 **Best Buddies**
1243 Islington Ave
Suite 907
Toronto, ON, Canada M8X-1Y9   416-531-0003
                                     888-779-0061
                                     FAX: 416-531-0325
                                     info@bestbuddies.ca
                                     www.bestbuddies.ca

Steven Pinnock, Executive Director
Emily Bolyea-Kyere, Director of Program and Special
Amy Lynn Taylor, Program Manager
Gemma ', Program Manager
Our program gives people with intellectual disabilities the
chance to have experiences which most people take for granted.

7617 **Biologically Inspired Cognitive Architectures Society**
4450 Rivanna River Way
#3707
Fairfax, VA 22030-4441   703-910-3014
                                FAX: 877-532-0197
                                info@bicasociety.org
                                bicasociety.org

Alexei V. Samsonovich, President-Treasurer
Kamilla R. Johannsdottir, Secretary
Antonio Chella, Advisory Committee Chair
BICA Society shall bring together researchers from disjointed
fields and communities who devote their efforts to solving the
same challenge, despite that they may speak different languages.

7618 **Brain Injury Association of America**
1608 Spring Hill Rd
Suite 110
Vienna, VA 22182   703-761-0750
                          FAX: 703-761-0755
                          sconnors@biausa.org
                          www.biausa.org

Susan H Connors, President/CEO
Mary S. Ritter, Executive VP/COO
Marianna Abashian, Director of Professional Service
Gregory Ayotte, Director of Consumer Services
Creates a better future through brain injury prevention, research,
education and advocacy.

7619 **Brain Injury Association of New York State**
10 Colvin Ave
Albany, NY 12206-1242   518-459-7911
                               800-228-8201
                               FAX: 518-482-5285
                               President@bianys.org
                               bianys.org

Judith Avner, Executive Director
Marie Cavallo, Ph.D., President
Debbie Berenda, Director of Finance & Administra
Renee Bullis, Family Services Program Assistan
(BIANYS) is a statewide non-profit membership organization
that advocates on behalf of individuals with brain injury and their
families, and promotes prevention. Established in 1982,
BIANYS provides education, advocac, and community support
services that lead to improved outcomes for children and adults
with brain injuries and their families. BIANYS also offers chapters and support groups throughout the state, prevention programs, mentoring programs, speakers bureau and publications
library.

7620 **Brain Injury Association of Texas**
316 W 12th Street
Suite 405
Austin, TX 78701-1845   512-326-1212
                               800-392-0040
                               FAX: 512-478-3370
                               info@texasbia.com
                               www.texasbia.org

Judith Abner, Director
Penny Phillips, President
Donna Kuhlmann, Chairman
Kelly Ramsay, CFO
A online quarterly e-newsletter, as well as news and updates on
the Brain Injury Association of Texas.

7621 **Center Academy At Pinellas Park**
6710 86th Ave North
Pinellas Park, FL 33782-4502   727-541-5716
                                      FAX: 727-544-8186
                                      infopp@centeracademy.com
                                      www.centeracademy.com

Mack R. Hicks, Founder & CEO
Andrew P. Hicks, CEO & Clinical Director
Eric V. Larson, President & Chief Operating Officer
Steven Hicks, VP Operations
Since 1968, Center Academy has been specifically designed for
the learning disabled child and other children with difficulties in
concentration, social skills, impulsivity, distractibility and study
strategies. Programs offered include: academic day school and 5
week remedial summer program. 11 locations throughout
Florida.

7622 **Cerebral Palsy Associations of New York State**
330 W. 34th St
15th Floor
New York, NY 10001-2488   212-947-5770
                                 information@cpofnys.org
                                 www.cpofnys.org

Susan Constantino, President & CEO
Michael Alvaro, Executive Vice President
Judi Gerson, Vice President, Policy & Program Services
Al Shibley, Vice President, Communications
CP of NYS is a broad-based, multi-service organization encom-
passing 24 Affiliates who provide services and programs for indi-
viduals with cerebral palsy and developmental disabilities, as
well as resources for families.

7623 **Child Neurology Society**
1000 W. County Rd E.
Ste 290
Saint Paul, MN 55126   651-486-9447
                              FAX: 651-486-9436
                              nationaloffice@childneurologysociety.org
                              www.childneurologysociety.org

Roger Larson, Executive Director
Sue Hussman, Associate Director
Emily McConnell, Professional Development Manager
The CNS is designed for patiens, parents, and professionals alike,
with the aim of promoting continued research, providing support,
and offering informational resources and guidance. Members include over 180 child neurologists and related medical
professionals.

7624 **Cognitive Neuroscience Society**
267 Cousteau Place
Davis, CA 95618   916-850-0837
                         cnsinfo@cogneurosociety.org
                         www.cogneurosociety.org

Roberto Cabeza, Board Member
Marta Kutas, Board Member
Kate Tretheway, Executive Director
Sangay Wangmo, Administrative Assistant
It is committed to the development of mind and brain research
aimed at investigating the psychological, computational, and
neuroscientific bases of cognition.

7625   Cognitive Science Society
108 E. Dean Keeton, Stop A8000
Austin, TX 78712-1043   512-471-2030
                                     FAX: 512-471-3053
                                     cognitivesciencesociety.org

Richard Catrambone, Chair
Nora Newcombe, Chair Elect
Susan Trickett, Executive Officer
Susan Goldin-Meadow, Past Chair
It brings together researchers from around the world who hold a
common goal: understanding the nature of the human mind.

7626   Cognitive Science Student Association
University of California
Berkeley, CA

                                     cssa.berkeley@gmail.com
                                     cssa.berkeley.edu

Bridget MacDonald, President
Matthew Boggess, Internal Vice President
Matthew Shonman, Treasurer
Timothy Guan, Secretary
It support and enrich the academic life of anyone interested in the
interdisciplinary field of cognitive science.

7627   Dementia Society of America
PO Box 600
Doylestown, PA 18901

                                     844-336-3684
                                     www.dementiasociety.org

7628   Dynamic Learning Center
PO Box 112
Ben Lomond, CA 95005   831-336-3457
                                     FAX: 503-738-9546
                                     teresanlp@aol.com
                                     www.nlpu.com

Robert B Dilts, President
Teresa Epstein, Coordinator
The vision of NLP (neuro-lingusitic programming)University is
to create a context in which professionals of different backgrounds can develop fundamental and advanced NLP skills for
applications relevant to their profession. The mission of NLP
University is to provide the organizational structure through
which the necessary guidance, training, culture, and community
support can be brought to the people who are interested in exploring the global potential of Systemic NLP.

7629   Epilepsy Foundation
8301 Professional Place E.
Ste 200
Landover, MD 20785- 2353   301-459-3700
                                    800-332-1000
                                    866-330-2718
                                    FAX: 301-459-1569
                                    ContactUs@efa.org
                                    www.epilepsy.com

Philip M. Gattone, President & CEO
M. Vaneeda Bennett, Chief Development Officer
*Angela Ostrom, Chief Operating Officer & Vice President, Public
Policy*
The Epilepsy Foundation of America is the national voluntary
health agency dedicated solely to the welfare of the almost 3 million people with epilepsy in the U.S. and their families. The organization works to ensure that people with seizures are able to
participate in all life experiences; to improve how people with epilepsy are perceived, accepted and valued in society; and to
promote research for a cure.

7630   Focus Alternative Learning Center
126 Dowd Avenue
PO Box 452
Canton, CT 06019-452   860-693-8809
                                    FAX: 860-693-0141
                                    info@focuscenterforautism.org
                                    focusalternative.org

Marcia Bok, President
Claudia Godburn, Secretary
Rita Barredo, Treasurer

A private non profit, licensed clinical and learning center specialized in the treatment of creatively wired and socially challenged
kids. We treat kids on the autism spectrum who suffer from high
anxiety, experience processing difficulties and learning
problems.

7631   Lewy Body Dementia Association
912 Killian Hill Road, S.W.
Lilburn, GA 30047   404-935-6444
                                    FAX: 480-422-5434
                                    www.lbda.org

Mike Koehler, President
Shannon McCarty-Caplan, Vice President
Tamara Real, Secretary
Angela Herron, Treasurer
A nonprofit organization dedicated to raising awareness of the
Lewy body dementias (LBD), supporting people with LBD, their
families and caregivers and promoting scientific advances.

7632   Life Development Institute
18001 N 79th Ave
Suite E71
Glendale, AZ 85308-8396   866-736-7811
                                    FAX: 623-773-2788
                                    info@life-development-inst,org
                                    www.life-development-inst.org

Robert Crawford, CEO
Veronica Lieb (Crawford), President
Justin Coller, Manager of Marketing
Shirley Schroeder, CFO
Serves older adolescents and adults with learning disabilities,
ADD and related disorders. The purpose of the training is to enable program participants to pursue responsible independent living, enhance academic/workplace literacy skills and facilitate
placement in educational/employment opportunities, commensu-
rate with individual capabilities. Includes a stand alone,
regionally accredited 2-year college.

7633   Mental Health America
500 Montgomery St
Ste 820
Alexandria, VA 22314   703-684-7722
                                    800-969-6642
                                    FAX: 703-684-5968
                                    www.mentalhealthamerica.net

*Debbie Plotnick, Vice President for Mental Health & Systems Advo-
cacy*
*Danielle Fritze, Director of Public Education & Visual Communi-
cations*
*America Paredes, Senior Director of Community Outreach &
Partnerships*
Patrick Hendry, Vice President Of Consumer Advocacy
Nonprofit organization addressing all issues related to mental
health and mental illness. With more than 340 affiliates nationwide, NMHA works to improve the mental health of all Americans, especially the 54 million individuals with mental disorders,
through advocacy, education, research and service.

7634   Multiple Sclerosis Association of America
375 Kings Highway N.
Cherry Hill, NJ 08034   856-488-4500
                                    800-532-7667
                                    FAX: 856-661-9797
                                    msaa@mymsaa.org
                                    www.mymsaa.org

Cindy Richman, Senior Director of Patient & Healthcare Relations
Carla Foote, Director of Administrative Services
Susan Courtney, Senior Writer & Creative Director.
Kimberly Goodrich, CFRE, Senior Director of Development
a national non-profit organization dedicated to providing the
most up-to-date resources for those affected by MS, including research, public education, and best practices and policy for professionals working with MS patients.

7635 **NLP Comprehensive**
PO.Box 348
Indian Hills, CO 80454-648

303-987-2224
800-233-1657
FAX: 303-987-2228
learn@nlpco.com
www.nlpco.com

Tom Dotz, President
Sharon DeBault, Director of Community Relations
Jamie Reaser, PhD, Director of Professional Relatio
Christian Miller, Publishing Manager
An online e-newsletter on Neuro-linguistic programming.

7636 **National Alliance on Mental Illness(NAMI)**
3803 N Fairfax Dr
Ste 100
Arlington, VA 22203-3080

703-524-7600
800-950-6264
FAX: 703-524-9094
www.nami.org

Suzanne Vogel-Scibilia, President
Keris J,,n Myrick, Ph.Dc., First Vice President
Henry Acosta, M.A., M.S.W.,, Second Vice President
Ralph E. Nelson, Jr., M.D., Treasurer
Our mission is to provide you with the technical assistance, tools and referrals to resources you need to build organizational capacity and achieve the goals of the NAMI Standards of Excellence.

7637 **National Association for Down Syndrome**
PO Box 206
Wilmette, IL 60091-206

630-325-9112
FAX: 847-723-3138
info@nads.org
www.nads.org

Jackie Rotondi, President
Mary Lou Miller, 1st VP
Deanne Medina, 2nd VP
Beata McCann, Treasurer
Works for a strong network of support systems within their own organization and with medical, educational and school service professionals who work with children and adults with Down Syndrome. NADS serves the Chicago Metropolitan area.

7638 **National Association for the Dually Diagnosed**
132 Fair St
Kingston, NY 12401-4802

845-331-4336
800-331-5362
FAX: 845-331-4569
info@thenadd.org
www.thenadd.org

Robert J. Fletcher, Chief Executive Officer
Edward Seliger, Project Coordinator
Michelle Jordan, Office Manager
Cassie Lattin, Office Assistant
NADD is a not-for-profit membership association established for professionals, care providers and families to promote understanding of and services for individuals who have developmental disabilities and mental health needs. The mission of NADD is to advance mental wellness for persons with developmental disabilities through the promotion of excellence in mental health care.

7639 **National Association of Cognitive- Behavioral Therapists**
102 Gilson Ave
Weirton, WV 26062

304-224-2534
800-253-0167
FAX: 304-224-2584
nacbt@nacbt.org
www.nacbt.org

Dr. Aldo R. Pucci, President
An organization dedicated solely to the teaching and practice of cognitive-behavioral psychotherapy. The mission of the NACBT is two fold: to promote and support the teaching and practice of cognitive-behavioral psychotherapy and to support those professionals and students seeking to practice it; and to set standards for credentialing that enable the general public to be confident that they will receive quality CBT from our certified members.

7640 **National Association of Cognitive-Behavioral Therapists**
PO Box 2195
Weirton, WV 26062-1395

304-723-3982
800-853-1135
FAX: 304-723-3982
nacbt@nacbt.org?subject=General%20Message%20t
www.nacbt.org

Aldo R Pucci, President
Paul A. Hauck, Ph.D., Director
Michael R. Edelstein, Ph.D., Director
Bill Borcherdt, ACSW, BCD, Director
Dedicated exclusively to supporting, promoting, teaching, and developing cognitive-behavioral therapy.

7641 **National Association of Epilepsy Centers**
600 Maryland Ave SW
Ste 835W
Washington, DC 20024

202-524-6767
888-525-6232
FAX: 202-484-1244
info@naec-epilepsy.org
www.naec-epilepsy.org

Nathan B. Fountain, MD, President
Susan T. Herman, MD, Vice President
Jerry J. Shih, MD, Secretary/Treasurer
NAEC educates public and private policy makers and regulators about appropriate patient care standards, reimbusement and medical services policies. NAEC is designed to complement, not compete with, the efforts of existing scientific and charitable epilepsy organizations.

7642 **National Ataxia Foundation**
2600 Fernbrrok Ln
Ste 119
Minneapolis, MN 55447-4752

763-553-0020
FAX: 763-553-0167
naf@ataxia.org
www.ataxia.org

Michael Parent, Executive Director
Susan Hagen, Patient Services Director
Susan Perlman, MD, Medical Director
Harry T. Orr, PhD, Research Director
The National Ataxia Foundation is a non-profit, membership-supported organization established in 1957 to help ataxia families. The Foundation is dedicated to improving the lives of persons affected by ataxia through support, education, and research.

7643 **National Autism Association**
1 Park Ave
Ste 1
Portsmouth, RI 02871

401-293-5551
877-622-2884
FAX: 401-293-5342
naa@nationalautism.org
www.nationalautismassociation.org

Lori McIlwain, Board Chairperson
Wendy Fournier, President
Kelly Vanicek, Executive Director
Katie Wright-Hildebrand, Vice President
The mission of the National Autism Association is to educate and empower families affected by autism and other neurological disorders, while advocating on behalf of those who cannot fight for their own rights.

7644 **National Down Syndrome Congress**
30 Mansell Court
Suite 108
Roswell, GA 30076

770-604-9500
800-232-6372
FAX: 770-604-9898
info@ndsccenter.org
ndsccenter.org

Jim Faber, President
Marilyn Tolbert, 1st VP
Carole J. Guess, 2nd VP
Lori McKee, Treasurer

Provides information, advocacy and support concerning all aspects of life for individuals with Down syndrome. A world with equal rights and opportunitites for people with Down syndrome. It is the purpose of the NDSC to create a national climate in which all people will recognize and embrace the value and dignity of people with Down syndrome. That purpose is enhanced by the commitment of the NDSC to promote the accessability to a full range of opportunities that meet the needs of the individual.

7645 National Down Syndrome Society
666 Broadway
8th Floor
New York, NY 10012-2317   212-460-9330
                                                             800-221-4602
                                                        FAX: 212-979-2873
                                                             info@ndss.org
                                                                 ndss.org

Jon Colman, President
Patricia Baker, Program Manager
Madeline Alemar, Development Associate
Chris Burke, Goodwill Ambassador/Administrati

Not-for-profit organization increases public awareness about Down syndrome and works to discover its underlying causes through research, education and advocacy. Distributes timely and informative materials, encourages and supports the activities of local parent support groups, sponsors sonferences and scientific symposia and undertakes major advocacy efforts—all to increase awareness and acceptance of people with Down syndrome.

7646 National Hydrocephalus Foundation
12413 Centralia Rd
Lakewood, CA 90715-1653   562-924-6666
                                                             888-857-3434
                                                        info@nhfonline.org
                                                          www.nhfonline.org

Debbi Fields, Executive Director
Michael Fields, President
Jaynie Dunn, Secretary
Sarah Dunn, Junior Director

Assembles and disseminates information pertaining to hydrocephalus, its treatments and outcomes. Establishes and facilitates a communication network among affected families and individuals.

7647 National Institute on Deafness and Other Communication Disorder
Federal Government
31 Center Dr
MSC 2320
Bethesda, MD 20892-2320   301-496-7243
                                                             800-241-1044
                                                        FAX: 301-402-0018
                                                       nidcdinfo@nidcd.nih.gov
                                                         www.nidcd.nih.gov

James F Battey Jr. Dr., Director
Timothy J. Wheeles, Executive Officer and Chief
Chris Clements, Program Advisor
Chad Wysong, Deputy Executive Officer

The National Institute on Deafness and Other Communication Disorders (NIDCD) one of the National Institude of Health, supports and conducts research and research training on the normal and disordered processes of hearing, balance smell, taste, voice, speech and language.

7648 Oak Leyden Developmental Services
411 Chicago Ave
Oak Park, IL 60302   708-524-1050
                                                        FAX: 708-524-2469
                                                   batkinson@oak-leyden.org
                                                        www.oak-leyden.org

Bob Atkinson, President/CEO
Ken Cheatham, Division Chief of Facilities, Ma
Nancy Thomas, Director of Human Resources
Mary Taylor, Vice President of Finance

The mission of Oak-Leyden Developmental Services is to help people with developmental disabilities meet life's challenges and reach their highest potential. Our mission is to achieved through the following programs: Early Intervention Program, Vocational

Evaluation, Developmental Training Program, Supported Employment Program, Community Integrated Living Arrangements and Multi-disciplinary Clinic.

7649 Ontario Federation for Cerebral Palsy
104-1630 Lawrence Ave W
Toronto, ON, Canada M6L-1C5   416-244-9686
                                                             877-244-9686
                                                        FAX: 416-244-6543
                                                           info@ofcp.on.ca
                                                               www.ofcp.ca

Gordana Skrba, Interim Executive Director
Lynn Adae, Memebership Services Program Manager
Cindy DeGraaff, Planning Services Program Manager
Cathy Persons, Program Manager

Assisting individuals and member groups in the development and provision of services and programs including accommodation in all parts of the province of Ontario.

7650 Rettsyndrome.org
4600 Devitt Dr
Cincinnati, OH 45246-1104   513-874-3020
                                                             800-818-7388
                                                        FAX: 513-874-2520
                                                       admin@rettsyndrome.org
                                                        www.rettsyndrome.org

Gordon Rich, Chief Operating Officer
Mary Joyce Griffon, Director, Administration Officer
Steven Kaminsky, PhD, Chief Science Officer
Megan Betsch, Marketing Coordinator

The core mission of the IRSF is to fund research for treatments and a cure for Rett syndrome while enhancing the overall quality of life for those living with Rett syndrome by providing information, programs, and services.

7651 Society for Cognitive Rehabilitation
668 Exton Commons
Exton, PA 19341   276-472-369
                                              www.societyforcognitiverehab.org

Kit Malia, President
Rita Carroll, Secretary
Pat Benfield, Treasurer
Ron Savage, Board Member

SCR is a nonprofit, multidisciplinary, organization committed to the advancement of cognitive rehabilitation therapy across the globe.

7652 St. John Valley Associates
160 Main St
PO Box 419
Madawaska, ME 04756-1219   207-728-3336
                                                             800-339-9502
                                                        FAX: 207-728-3825
                                                       www.sjvalley-times.com

Megan Gendreau, Executive Director

A nonprofit association with the mission of empowering adult citizens with mental retardation to dignify themselves. Three broad-based programs and services (Independence Plus, Job Involvements, People Now) are designed to allow each individual to upgrade learning skills, assert rights, increase independence and accept new responsibilities. *$75.00*

7653 TEACCH
University of North Carolina at Chapel Hill
100 Renee Lynne Ct
Carrboro, NC 27510   919-966-2174
                                                        FAX: 919-966-4127
                                                           teacch@unc.edu
                                                            www.teacch.com

Dr. Laura Klinger, Director
Rebecca Mabe, Assistant Director of Business
Walter Kelly, Business Officer
Mark Klinger, Director of Research

Focus on the person with autism and the development of a program around this person's skills, interests and needs.

7654 **The Hemispherectomy Foundation**
8235 Lethbridge Rd
Millersville, MD 21108-1609
410-987-5221
FAX: 410-987-521
lynn@hemifoundation.org
hemifoundation.homestead.com

Kristi Hall, President, CEO, & Co-Founder
Cris A. Hall, Executive Director & Co-Founder
Lynn Miller, Specialty Director, Rasmussen's Encephalitis
National non-profit organization dedicated to providing emotional, financial, and educational support to individuals and their families who have undergone, or will undergo, a hemispherectomy or similar brain surgery. Dedicated to hemispherectomy education, awareness, fundraising, and research of the medical conditions causing intractable epilepsy that lead to surgery and the surgery itself.

7655 **Tourette Association of America**
Formerly Tourette Syndrome Association
42-40 Bell Blvd
Ste 205
Bayside, NY 11361-2874
718-224-2999
888-486-8758
FAX: 718-279-9596
support@tourette.org
www.tourette.org

John Miller, President & CEO
Kevin St. P. McNaught, Executive Vice President, Research & Medical Programs
Amanda Talty, Vice President, Development
Saskia Monteiro Thomson, Vice President, Marketing & Communcations
National, non-profit membership organization aiming to identify the cause for, find the cure for, and control the effects of Tourette syndrome. A growing number of local chapters nationwide provide educational materials, seminars, conferences and support groups for over 35,000 members. Publishes brochures, flyers, educational materials and papers on treatment and research. Offers videos for purchase through a catalog of publications.

7656 **United Cerebral Palsy**
1825 K St NW
Ste 600
Washington, DC 20006
202-776-0406
800-872-5827
FAX: 202-776-0414
info@ucp.org
www.ucp.org

Stephen Bennett, President & CEO
Ellie Collinson, Chief Program Officer
Kevin Sturtevant, Chief of Development
Jennifer McCue, Director, Advocacy
UCP educates, advocates, and provides support services to ensure a life without limits for people with a spectrum of disabilities. UCP works to advance the independence, productivity and full citizenship of people with disabilities through an affiliate network that has helped millions.

7657 **Younger Onset Dementia Association**
139 Cobham Ave
Melrose Park, IL 2114
youngeronset@yahoo.com.au
www.youngeronset.net

Camps

7658 **Adventure Learning Center at Eagle Village**
4507 170th Ave
Hersey, MI 49639-8785
231-832-2234
800-748-0061
FAX: 231-832-1468
alcinfo@eaglevillage.org
www.eaglevillage.org

Cathey Prudhomme, President/CEO
Jim McCain, Director of Support Services/CFO
Craig Weidner, Director of Advancement

Offers a variety of fun camp experiences with a low staff-to-camper ratio and exciting, challenging activities. This program accepts youth, ages 5-17, who are high risk or special needs - behavioral problems, emotionally unstable or Attention Deficit. The camping experience includes canoeing, hiking, swimming and high adventure activities. Half-week, one-week, and two-week sessions June-August. Coed.

7659 **CNS Camp New Connections**
Mclean Hospital Child/Adolescent Program
115 Mill St
Mailstop115
Belmont, MA 02478-1064
617-855-2000
800-333-0338
FAX: 617-855-2833
mcleaninfo@mclean.harvard.edu
www.mcleanhospital.org

Roya Ostovar PhD, Center Director
Scott L. Rauch, MD., President and Psychiatrist in Ch
Joseph Gold MD, Clinical Director
Cynthia Kaplan, CAP Administrative Director
Four-week summer day camp for children ages 7-17 who have pervasive developmental disorders, Asperger's Syndrome, autism spectrum disorders and non-verbal learning disabilities. The camp is designed to help children develop social skills through fun activities including: communication games, swimming, field trips, drama, and arts and crafts. *$4500.00*

7660 **Camp Baker**
Greater Richmond ARC
7600 Beach Rd
Chesterfield, VA 23838-6513
804-748-4789
FAX: 804-796-6880
campbaker@RichmondARC.org
richmondarc.org

Robert L. Sommerville, Chair - Officer
Thomas G. Haskins, Vice Chair - Officer
Chriss Mumford, Secretary Officer
Marshall W. Butler Jr., President
An organization created by families, for families that has grown to provide a continuum of programs and services for individuals with developmental disablties acroos the lifespan, helping each person achieve his or her potential and improving the quality of life for everyone in the community.

7661 **Camp Betsey Cox**
140 Betsey Cox Lane
Pittsford, VT 05763-9456
802-483-6611
info@campbetseycox.com
www.campbetseycox.com

Lorrie Byrom, Camp Director
Devri Byrom, Winter Office Director
Mike Byrom, Camp Director
Camp Betsey Cox is a summer camp with an educational mindset. Betsey Cox is a perfect setting to give children the chance to completely make their own choices in the course of the day. For many campers, this is the beggining of learning how to make intelligent and informed choices in life.

7662 **Camp Buckskin**
4124 Quebec Ave N
Suite 300, PO Box 389
Ely, MN 55731- 389
763-208-4805
FAX: 218-365-2880
info@campbuckskin.com
www.campbuckskin.com

Thomas R Bauer CCD, Camp Director
Mary Bauer, Co-Director
Jared Griffin, Program Director
Camp is located in Ely, Minnesota. Buckskin assists LD, AD/HD, Asperger's, and adopted individuals to realize and develop the potentials and abilities which they possess. Teaches a combination of traditional camp, academic activities and social skills so the campers experience success in many areas. Ages 6-18.

7663 Camp Candlelight
Epilepsy Foundation Arizona
3033A N. 7th Ave
Ste 104
Phoenix, AZ 85013   602-406-3581
                                     800-332-1000
                              info@epilepsyaz.org
              epilepsyaz.org/programs/camp-candlelight/
Suzanne Matsumori, Executive Director
Min Skivington, Program Manager
Camp Candlelight provides children ages 8 to 15 a unique camp
experience that mixes traditional summer camp with special sessions that teach campers about their seizures and gives them resources to manage the challenges that the seizures represent.
Staff includes a neurologist, several nurses and a school psychologist, in addition to traditional camp staff who are given specialized training in responding appropriately to the needs of kids with
epilepsy.

7664 Camp Evoked Potential @ Camp ASCCA
Epilepsy Foundation of Alabama
310-273 Azalea Rd
Office Park 3
Mobile, AL 36609-1970   251-341-0170
                                     800-626-1582
                                 ddodson@efala.org
               www.efala.org/camp-evoked-potential/
Donna Dodson, Executive Director
Paige Norris, Outreach/Program Director
Camp Evoked Potential is a 5-day overnight camp for children
and teens aged 6 to 18 years old living with epilepsy. The camp
provides a great opportunity for kids to experience the fun of
camp activities—swimming, fishing, sports, hiking and
more—in a safe, medically monitored setting. Camp activities are
designed to be accessible and adapted to campers' individual
needs and abilities.

7665 Camp Horizons
127 Babcock Hill Rd
PO Box 323
South Windham, CT 06266- 323   860-456-1032
                              FAX: 860-456-4721
                    scott.lambeck@camphorizons.org
                             www.camphorizons.org
Adam Milne, Chairman
L. Sanford Rice, Treasurer
Kathleen McNAboe, VP
Deirdhre Delaney, Board Secretary
Bordering Lake Probus, the facilities at the camp are equipped to
accomodate a wide range of activities and programs for campers
with developmental disabilities, or other challenging emotional
and social needs. There is a 5:1 camper-counselor ratio with a
schedule of three programs in the morning and four in the
afternoon.

7666 Camp Huntington
56 Bruceville St
PO Box 37
High Falls, NY 12440-37   845-687-7840
                                     855-707-2267
                              FAX: 845-213-4313
                    mbednarz@camphuntington.com
                             www.camphuntington.com
Michael Bednarz, Executive Director
Amber Allan-Latham, Camp Director
Stacy Kane Greenzeig, Visiting Prgm Supervisor Spec Ed
A co-ed residential summer camp specifically designed to focus
on Adaptive and Therapeutic Recreation. Campers include those
with learning and developmental disabilities, ADD/HD, Autism
Spectrum Disorders, Asperger's, PDD, and other special needs.
Three programs are offered that focus on: recreation and social
skills; independence; and participation.

7667 Camp Nissokone
YMCA Camping Services
1401 Broadway
Suite A
Detroit, MI 48226-8929   313-267-5300
                       office@ycampingservices.org
                             www.ymcadetroit.org
Doug Grimm, Vice President Camping Services
David Marks, Director
A six week summer resident camp program for boys and girls
whose learning and behavior styles have made successful participation in the traditional camp program difficult. All camp activities have a special emphasis on building self-esteem and peer
relationships. Strong in waterfront, nature, campcrafts and a
special arts program.

7668 Camp Northwood
132 State Route 365
Remsen, NY 13438-5700   315-831-3621
                              FAX: 315-831-5867
                    northwoodprograms@hotmail.com
                                   www.nwood.com
Gordon Felt, Camp Director
Donna Felt, International Counselor
Summer sessions for children with ADD. Coed, ages 8-18.

7669 Camp Nuhop
404 Hillcrest Dr
Ashland, OH 44805-4152   419-289-2227
                              FAX: 419-289-2227
                                        nuhop.org
Trevor Dunlap, Executive Director, CEO
Jim Machin, Director of Facilities and Maint
Terri Ru Lon, Office Manager
Terri Pringle, Director of Dining Services
A summer residential program for any youngster from 6 to 18
with a learning disability, behavior disorder or Attention Deficit
Disorder. 84 campers and 41 staff members live on site in groups
of to seven campers to every three counselors. Activities focus on
positive self-concept and behaviors and teaches children to learn
how to find their strengths, abilities and talents from a positive,
yet realistic viewpoint.

7670 Camp Ramapo
Route 52 Salisbury Turnpike
P.O.Box 266
Rt. 52 / Salisbury Turnpike
Rhinebeck, NY 12572-266   845-876-8403
                              FAX: 845-876-8414
                       office@ramapoforchildren.org
                           ramapoforchildren.org
Mike Kunin, Executive Director
Rachel Flynn, PhD, Senior Program Officer
Bruce Kuziola, Chief Financial and Administrative Officer
Adam Weiss, Chief Executive Officer
Ramapo's specific focus is adventure-based, experiential learn-
ing programs that promote positive character values in children
and teens with special needs.

7671 Camp Royall
Autism Society of North Carolina
505 Oberlin Road
Suite 230
Raleigh, NC 27605-1345   919-743-0204
                                     800-442-2762
                       info@autismsociety-nc.org
                           www.autismsociety-nc.org
Sharon Jeffries-Jones, Chair
Elizabeth Phillippi, Vice Chair
Darryl R. Marsch, Secretary
John Delaloye, Treasurer
The best source in North Carolina for connecting people who live
with autism (and those who care about them) with resources, sup-
port, advocacy and informantion tailored to thier unique needs.

7672 Camp Ruggles
PO Box 353
Chepachet, RI 02814
401-567-8914
info@ricamps.org
www.ricamps.org

Peter Swain, President
Jim Field, Camp Director
Mr. Robert Tyler, Treasurer
Ms. Nan Levine, Director
Camp Ruggles is located in Glocester, RI, and is a summer day camp for emotionally handicapped children. The Camp offers a 6 week co-ed summer session for 60 children ages 6-12.

7673 Camp Sisol
Jewish Community Center of Greater Rochester/JCC
1200 Edgewood Ave
Rochester, NY 14618-5408
585-461-2000
FAX: 585-461-0805
membership2@jccrochester.org
www.jccrochester.org

Leslie Berkowitz, Executive Director
Dan Irving, Children's Programs/Camp Sisol D
Bill Blodgett, Facilities Director
Anna Gossin, Librarian
Camp is located in Honeoye Falls, New York. Summer sessions for children with autism. Coed, ages 5-16.

7674 Camp World Light
Florida Baptist Convention
1230 Hendricks Ave
Jacksonville, FL 32207-8619
904-396-2351
800-226-8584
FAX: 904-396-6470
www.campworldlight.com

Anne Wilson, Camp Director
Delicia Garland, Ministry Assistant to Director
Camp is located in Marianna, Florida. One-week sessions June-July for girls with ADD. Ages 3-12. Activities include arts/crafts, challenge/rope courses, clowning, community service, dance, drama, drawing/painting, leadership development, performing arts and sailing.

7675 Camp-A-Lot And Leisure Express (PALS Program)
Arc of San Diego
3030 Market Street
San Diego, CA 92102
619-685-1175
FAX: 619-234-3759
pals@arc-sd.com
www.arc-sd.com

Lin Taylor, Camp Director
David W Schneider, President/CEO
Anthony J Desalis, Esq, Executive Vice President
Rich Coppa, Vice President Of Infrastructure
Offers one-week sessions for children and adults with attention deficit disorder, autism, mobility limitation and developmental disabilities.

7676 Carroll School Summer Programs
25 Baker Bridge Rd
Lincoln, MA 01773-3199
781-259-8342
FAX: 781-259-8842
admissions@carrollschool.org
carrollschool.org

Steve Wilkins, Head of School
Brad Watts, Treasurer
Sam Foster, Chair
Eileen Archambault, Technology Specialist
Academic and recreational programs designed to improve learning skills and build self-confidence. The school is a tutorial program for students not achieving their potential due to poor skills in reading, writing and math. The summer camp complements the summer school offering outdoor activities in a supportive, non-competitive environment.

7677 Casowasco Camp, Conference and Retreat Center
158 Casowasco Dr
Moravia, NY 13118-3498
315-364-8756
FAX: 315-364-7636
info@casowasco.org
www.casowasco.org

Mike Huber, Executive Director
Shelly Sherboneau, CRM Coordinating Registrar
Kevin Dunn, Casowasco Assistant Director
Roger Marshall, Property Manager
Camp is located in Moravia, New York. Summer sessions for children with ADD. Coed, ages 6-18 and families.

7678 Center Academy at Pinellas Park
6710 86th Ave North
Pinellas Park, FL 33782-4502
727-541-5716
FAX: 727-544-8186
infopp@centeracademy.com
www.centeracademy.com

Patricia Lambert, Principal
Mack R Hicks PhD, Founder/Chairman of the Board
Andrew P Hicks PhD, CEO/Clinical Director
Lisa Hartmann, Director Education
Specifically designed for the learning disabled child and other children with difficulties in concentration, strategy, social skills, impulsivity, distractibility and study strategies. Programs offered include: attention training, visual-motor remediation, socialization skills training, relaxation training, horseback riding and more. The day camp meets weekdays from 9-3 for 3,4 or 5 week sessions.

7679 Council for Extended Care of Mentally Retarded Citizens
11140 So. Towne Square
Ste. 101
Saint Louis, MO 63123
314-845-3900
FAX: 314-845-3901
info@sunnyhillinc.org
cecstl.org

Derrick Good, Chairman of the Board
Wes Burns, Vice Chairman
Vicky James, President/CEO
Sean King, Secretary
Services are provided to adults and children with developmental disabilities. Supported living arrangements are located in St. Louis city, St. Louis county and St. Charles County. Group home and camp services are located in Dittmer, MO. Travel program also available.

7680 Dallas Academy
950 Tiffany Way
Dallas, TX 75218-2743
214-324-1481
FAX: 214-327-8537
mail@dallas-academy.com
www.dallas-academy.com

Troy Sturrock, Chair
Terrence S. Welch, Vice Chair
Dallas Cothrum, Secretary
Redonna Higgins, Treasurer
7-week summer session for students who are having difficulty in regular school classes.

7681 Eagle Hill School: Summer Program
242 Old Petersham Road
P.O. Box 116
Hardwick, MA 01037- 0116
413-477-6000
FAX: 413-477-6837
admission@ehs1.org
www.ehs1.org

Peter J. Mc Donald, Headmaster
Marilyn Waller, President
Alden Bianchi, Vice President
Arthur Langhaus, Treasurer
For children ages 9-19 with specific learning (dis)abilities and/or Attention Deficit Disorder, this summer program is designed to remediate academic and social deficits while maintaining progress achieved during the school year. Electives and sports activities are combined with the academic courses to address the needs of the whole person in a camp-like atmosphere.

7682 Easter Seals Oklahoma
701 NE 13th St
Oklahoma City, OK 73104-5003
405-239-2525
FAX: 405-239-2278
sbusch@eastersealsoklahoma.org
www.eastersealsoklahoma.org

Paula K. Porter, President, CEO
Vida Wasinger, Director of Operations
Debora Baden, Activity Coordinator
Samantha Pascoe, Director, Child Development Center
Adult day health center, and child development center.

7683 Englishton Park Academic Remediation
Englishton Park Presbyterian
P.O.Box 228
Lexington, IN 47138-228
812-889-2046
ThomasLisaBarnett@etczone.com
www.englishtonpark.org

Lisa Barnett, Director
Thomas Barnett, Co-Director
Camp is located in Lexington, Indiana. Two-week sessions for children with ADD. Boys and girls, ages 7-12.

7684 Florida Sheriffs Caruth Camp
Florida Sheriffs Youth Ranches
2486 Cecil Webb Place
Boys Ranch, FL 32060
386-842-5501
800-765-3797
FAX: 386-842-2429
fsyr@youthranches.org
www.youthranches.org

Roger Bouchard, President
Bill Frye, Executive Vice President
Janet Bass, Vice President of Operations
Maria Knapp, Vice President of Donor Relation
Camp is located in Inglis, Florida. One-week sessions for children with ADD. Coed, ages 10-15.

7685 Gow School Summer Programs
2491 Emery Road
P.O. Box 85
South Wales, NY 14139-0085
716-652-3450
FAX: 716-652-3457
webmaster@gow.org
www.gow.org

Gayle Hutton, Director of Development
Robert Garcia, Director of Admissions
Eric Bray, Summer Program Director
Rosemary Shields, CPA, Director of Finance
Co-ed summer programs for students ages 8-16 with dyslexia or similar learning disabilities offer a balanced blend of morning academics, afternoon/evening traditional camp activities and weekend overnights. The primary purpose of these programs is to provide a positive experience while balancing these three elements. Committed to the creation of a positive and enjoyable experience for each participant by defining and merging the goals of the camp and the school, with those of camper students.

7686 Hill School of Fort Worth
4817 Odessa Ave
Fort Worth, TX 76133-1640
817-923-9482
FAX: 817-923-4894
hillschool@hillschool.org
www.hillschool.org

Roxann Breyer, Principal
Audrey Boda-Davis, Executive Director
Janet Smith, Account & Records Manager
Kathy Edwards, Principal, Grapevine campus
Provides an alternative learning environment for students having average or above-average intelligence with learning differences. Hill school is an established leader in North Texas with a 25 year history of effectively serving LD children. Beginning in 1961 as a tutorial service, Hill became a formal school in 1973. Our mission is to help those who learn differently develop skills and strategies to succeed. We do this by developing academic/study skills, and self-discipline.

7687 Indian Acres Camp for Boys
1712 Main St
Fryeburg, ME 04037-4327
207-935-2300
FAX: 954-349-7812
geoff@indianacres.com
www.indianacres.com

Michael Burness, Assistant Director
Mary Beth 'Bert' Wiig, Head Counselor, Camp Forest Acre
Lisa Newman, Director
Geoff Newman, Director
Camp is located in Fryeburg, Florida. Four and seven-week sessions June-August for boys with ADD ages 7-16.

7688 Lab School of Washington
4759 Reservoir Rd NW
Washington, DC 20007-1921
200-965-6600
labschool@webmail.org
www.labschool.org

Katherine Schantz, Head of School
Diana Meltzer, Associate Head of School
Laurelle Sheedy McCready, Associate Head of School for Fin
Bob Lane, Director of Admissions
The Lab School six week summer session includes individualized reading, spelling, writing, study skills and math programs. A multisensory approach addresses the needs of bright learning disabled children. Related services such as speech/language therapy and occupational therapy are integrated into the curriculum. Elementary/Intermediate; Junior High/High School.

7689 Lions Den Outdoor Learning Center
600 Kiwanis Dr
Eureka, MO 63025-2212
636-938-5245
FAX: 636-938-5289
info@wymancenter.org
www.wymancenter.org

David Hilliard, President
Theresa Mayberry, Executive VP
Kristine Ramsey, Sr. VP
Tony Etzkorn, VP
Varied programs for mentally retarded children, ages 6 and up, includes daily living, socialization and language skills. Sports, tent camping, crafts, and nature study are also offered. Sliding scale tuition for 2 weeks.

7690 Maplebrook School
5142 Route 22
Amenia, NY 12501-5357
845-373-9511
FAX: 845-373-7029
admin@maplebrookschool.org
www.maplebrookschool.org

Paul Scherer, Administrator
Donna Konkolics, Head Of School
A coeducational boarding school which offers a six week camp for children with learning differences and ADD.

7691 Marvelwood Summer
Marvelwood School
476 Skiff Mountain Road
PO Box 3001
Kent, CT 06757-3001
860-927-0047
FAX: 860-927-0021
summerschool@marvelwood.org
www.marvelwood.org

Alfred C Brooks, President
Arthur F Goodearl, Jr, Head Of School
The emphasis in this summer program is on diagnosis and remediation of individual reading, spelling, writing, mathematics and study problems. Offered to ages 12-16.

7692 New Horisons Summer Day Camp
YMCA
13821 Newport Avenue
Suite 200
Tustin, CA 92780-7803
714-549-9622
FAX: 714-838-5976
www.ymcaoc.org

Jeff Black, Vice Chair
Tom Reyes, Director
Christian Buell, Director
John Rochford, Director
One-week sessions for children with ADD and speech/communication impairment. Coed, ages 5-14.

7693 New Jersey YMHA/YWHA Camps Milford
21 Plymouth St
Fairfield, NJ 07004-1686
973-575-3333
800-776-5657
FAX: 973-575-4188
info@njycamps.org
www.njycamps.org

Leonard Robinson, President
Bruce Nussman, President
Camp is located in Milford, Pennsylvania. Summer sessions for children with ADD. Coed, ages 6-17 and families.

7694 Oakland School & Camp
Boyd Tavern
Keswick, VA 22947
434-293-9059
FAX: 434-296-8930
information@oaklandschool.net
www.oaklandschool.net

Carol Williams, School Director
Jamie Cato, Admissions Director
A highly individualized program stresses improving reading ability. Subjects taught are reading, English composition, math and word analysis. Recreational activities include horseback riding, sports, swimming, tennis, crafts, archery and camping. For girls and boys, ages 8-14.

7695 Outside In School Of Experiential Education, Inc.
P.O.Box 639
Greensburg, PA 15601-639
724-837-1518
FAX: 724-837-0801
administration@outsideinschool.com
myoutsidein.org

Michael C. Henkel, Executive Director
Camp is located in Bolivar, Pennsylvania. Sessions for children with ADD and substance abuse problems. Boys 11-18 and girls 13-18.

7696 Phelps School Summer School
583 Sugartown Rd
Malvern, PA 19355-2800
610-644-1754
FAX: 610-644-6679
admis@thephelpsschool.org
www.thephelpsschool.org

Christopher Chirieleison, Principal
Daniel E. Knopp, Head of School
Amy Anderson, Director of College Counseling
Janessa Davis, Director of Student Services
Open for grades 7-11 to make up academic deficiencies or complete studies in English, math and reading. Sports include riding, tennis and swimming. A program is also available to a limited number of international students in English as a Second Language.

7697 Quest Camp
2355 San Ramon Valley Blvd.
Suite 208
San Ramon, CA 94583-1763
925-743-2900
800-313-9733
FAX: 925-820-9761
questcamps@mac.com
www.questcamps.com

Robert Field, Founder/Executive Director
Debra Forrester-Field, M.A., Administrative Director
Adam Berman, Psy.D., Director
Aprilyn Artz, MA, Director
Camp is located in Alamo, California. Day camp offering three to eight-week sessions including psychological treatment for children with ADD and other mild to moderate psychological disorders. Coed, ages 6-15.

7698 Raven Rock Lutheran Camp
17912 Harbaugh Valley Road
P.O.Box 136
Sabillasville, MD 21780-136
410-303-2108
800-321-5824
ravenrock@innernet.net

Brenda Minnich, Executive Director
Christ-centered program for youth and mentally retarded adults.

7699 Rimland Services for Autistic Citizens
1265 Hartrey Ave
Evanston, IL 60202-1056
847-328-4090
877-395-6937
FAX: 847-328-8364
pwatson@rimland.org
www.rimland.org

Pamela Watson, CEO
Dave Work, Assoc Executive Director Program
Brendy Sims, Chief Operating Officer
Terrance Wimberly, Associate Executive Director of
An accessible camp facility that can be utilized by groups for day use or overnight camping experiences. Six winterized cabins, a meeting facility, indoor pool, full food service, and an excellent staff are available. Educational programs can be arranged or you can utilize the facility to manage your own programs.

7700 Rolling Hills Country Day Camp
P.O.Box 172
Marlboro, NJ 07746
732-308-0405
FAX: 732-780-4726
info@rollinghillsdaycamp.com
www.rollinghillsdaycamp.com

Billy Breitner, Director
Summer sessions for children with ADD. Coed, ages 3-12.

7701 SOAR Summer Adventures
NC Base Camp
226 SOAR Lane
P.O.Box 388
Balsam, NC 28707-0388
828-456-3435
FAX: 828-456-3449
admissions@soarnc.org
www.soarnc.org

John Willson, Executive Director
Catey Terry, CFO
Laura Pate, Director of Operations
Joe Geier, Director of the Academy at SOAR
A nonprofit adventure program working with disadvantaged youth diagnosed with learning disabilities in an outdoor, challenge based environment. Focuses on esteem building and social skills development through rock climbing, backpacking, whitewater rafting, mountaineering, sailing, snorkeling, and much more. Offers two week, one month, and semester programs available. SOAR programs utilize North Carolina, Florida, Colorado, American Southwest, Alaska, and Jamaica as program areas.

7702 Sherman Lake YMCA Outdoor Center
6225 N 39th St
Augusta, MI 49012-9722
269-731-3000
FAX: 269-731-3020
shermanlakeymca@ymcasl.org
www.shermanlakeymca.org

Luke Austenfeld, Executive Director
Jean Henderson, Business Manager
Lorrie Syverson, Director of Camping, Education &
Mark VanDaff, Facility Manager
Summer camping sessions for campers with ADD and spina bifida. Coed, ages 6-15 and families, seniors.

7703 Squirrel Hollow Summer Camp
The Bedford School
5665 Milam Rd
Fairburn, GA 30213-2851
770-774-8001
FAX: 770-774-8005
bbox@thebedfordschool.org
www.thebedfordschool.org

Betsy Box, Executive Director
Jeff James, Headmaster/Athletic Director./MS
Allisom DaY, Asst. Headmaster/MS Admin./ MS
Susan Blake, Art/After-School Care Coordinato
A remedial summer program for children with academic needs held on the campus of The Bedford School in Fairburn, Georgia. It is a five week day camp held from June 19 to July 21 and serves ages 6-16. For mor information contact Betsy Box at (770) 774-8001.

7704 Summit Camp
322 Route 46 West
Suite 210
Parsippany, NJ 07054
973-732-3230
800-323-9908
FAX: 973-732-3226
info@summitcamp.com
www.summitcamp.com

Mayer Stiskin, Owner
Eugene Bell, Senior Director
Debs Hugill, Head Counselor/Program Director
Maryann Santora, Clinical Social Worker & Admissi
Camp is located in Honesdale, Pennsylvania. Summer sessions for children with ADD. Coed, ages 8-17.

7705 Sunnyhill Adventure Center
Council for Extended Care
6555 Sunlit Way
Dittmer, MO 63023-3306
636-274-9044
314-781-4950
FAX: 636-285-1305
dropin4fun@aol.com
sunnyhilladventures.org

Victoria James, President/CEO
Kathleen Branson, Director of Finance
Donald Mitchell, Director of ISLA
Rob Darroch, Director of Sunnyhill Adventures
Camp is located in Dittmer, Missouri. Summer sessions for campers with developmental disabilities and autism. Coed, ages 8-99. Sunnyhill Adventures is program that offers campers fun, exciting, educational experiences in a beautiful outdoor setting. Our residential summer camp combines traditional camping activities plus specially selected and adapted events to meet the needs of each camper group.

7706 Talisman Summer Camp
64 Gap Creek Rd
Zirconia, NC 28790-8791
828-697-6249
855-588-8254
info@talismancamps.com
www.talismancamps.com

Linda Tatsapaugh, Operations Director & Owner
Robiyn Mims, Admissions Director
Doug Smathers, Summer Camps Director
Cory Greene, Program Manager
Camp is located in Black Mountain, North Carolina. Offers a program of hiking, rafting, climbing, and caving for learning disabled ADD/ADHD and autistic young people. Coed, ages 9-18.

7707 Timbertop Nature Adventure Camp
YMCA Camp Glacier Hollow
1000 Division St
Stevens Point, WI 54481-2724
715-342-2980
FAX: 715-342-2987
pmatthai@spymca.org
www.glacierhollow.com

Dave Morgan, Executive Director
Pete Matthai, Camp Director
Tiffany Praeger, Summer Camp Program Director
For children who can benefit from an individualized program of learning in a non-competitive outdoor setting under the skilled leadership of people who understand the environment and the unique potential of these children.

7708 Triangle Y Ranch YMCA
YMCA of Southern Arizona
PO Box 1111
Tucson, AZ 85702
520-623-5511
FAX: 520-624-1518
camp@tucsonymca.org
www.tucsonymca.org

Dane Woll, President and CEO
Kerry Dufour, V.P. Chief Development Officer
Cathy Scheirman, Chief Financial Officer
Amanda Thomas, Director of Communications and Special Projects
Summer camp programs for children and young adults ages 6-17. Camp offers horseback riding, sports, story telling, arts & crafts, swimming, archery and nature programs.

7709 Wendell Johnson Speech And Hearing Clinic
University Of Iowa
250 Hawkins Dr
Iowa City, IA 52242-1025
319-335-3500
FAX: 319-335-8851
dorothy-albright@uiowa.edu
www.uiowa.edu

Dorothy Albright, Department Administration
Lauren Eldridge, Undergraduate Academic Programs
Mary Jo Yotty, Graduate Programs
Lauren Eldridge, Clinic Appointments
The clinic offers assessment and remediation for communication disorders in adults and children. The clinic also offers a Intensive Summer Residential Clinic for school age children needing intervention services because of speech, language, hearing and/or reading problems.

Print: Books

7710 A Miracle to Believe In
Option Indigo Press
2080 S Undermountain Rd
Sheffield, MA 01257-9643
413-229-8727
800-714-2779
FAX: 413-229-8727
indigo@bcn.net
www.optionindigo.com

Barry Neil Kaufman, Author
A group of people from all walks of life come together and are transformed as they reach out, under the direction of the Kaufmans, to help a little boy the medical world had given up as hopeless. This heartwarming journey of loving a child back to life will not only inspire you, the reader, but presents a compelling new way to deal with life's traumas and difficulties.
379 pages
ISBN 0-449201-08-2

7711 ADD: Helping Your Child
Warner Books
1271 Avenue of the Americas
New York, NY 10020-1300
212-522-7200
FAX: 212-522-7989

Barbara Smalley, Author
Bruce Paonessa, Vice President
Elizabeth Nunuz, Manager

The definitive guide to helping children with AD/HD *$ 12.95*
224 pages Paperback
ISBN 0-446670-13-8

7712   ADHD Book of Lists: A Practical Guide for Helping Children and Teens with ADDs
Jossey-Bass
111 River St
Hoboken, NJ 7030-5773   201-748-6000
                                      FAX: 201-748-6008
                                      info@wiley.com
                                      www.wiley.com
Sandra F Rief, Author
Information about Attention Deficit/Hyperactivity Disorder including strategies, supports, and interventions that have been found to be the most effective. For teachers, parents, and counselors. *$29.95*
320 pages
ISBN 0-787965-91-X

7713   ADHD in the Schools: Assessment and Intervention Strategies
Guilford Press
72 Spring St
New York, NY 10012-4019   212-431-9800
                                      800-365-7006
                                      FAX: 212-966-6708
                                      info@guilford.com
                                      www.guilford.com
George J DuPaul, Author
Gary Stoner, Co-Author
This landmark volume emphasizes the need for a team effort among parents, community-based professionals, and educators. Provides practical information for educators that is based on empirical findings. Chapters focus on: how to identify and assess students who might have ADHD; the relationship between ADHD and learning disabilities; how to develop and implement classroom-based programs; communication strategies to assist physicians; and the need for community-based treatments. *$ 36.00*
269 pages Hardcover
ISBN 0-898622-45-X

7714   ADHD with Comorbid Disorders: Clinical Assessment and Management
Guilford Press
72 Spring St
New York, NY 10012-4019   212-431-9800
                                      800-365-7006
                                      FAX: 212-966-6708
                                      info@guilford.com
                                      www.guilford.com
Steven R Pliszka, MD, Author
Caryn Leigh Carlson, Co-Author
James M Swanson, Co-Author
$44.00
Cloth
ISBN 1-572304-78-2

7715   Adolescents with Down Syndrome: Toward a More Fulfilling Life
Brookes Publishing
P.O.Box 10624
Baltimore, MD 21285-624   410-337-9580
                                      800-638-3775
                                      FAX: 410-337-8539
                                      custserv@brookespublishing.com
                                      www.brookespublishing.com
Maria Sustrova, Author
Lauren Smith, Western Region Sales Representat
Jeannine Blimline, Central Region Sales Representat
Kevin Warg, Northeastern Region Sales Repres
Written for health care professionals, psychologists, other developmental disabilities practitioners, educators, and parents, it covers biomedical concerns; behavioral, psychological, and psy-

chiatric challenges; and education, employment, recreation, community, and legal concerns. *$35.95*
416 pages Paperback
ISBN 1-55766 -81-9

7716   Adult ADD: The Complete Handbook: Everything You Need to Know About How to Cope with ADD
Prima Publishing
P.O.Box 1260
Rocklin, CA 95677-1260   916-787-7000
                                      800-632-8676
                                      FAX: 916-787-7001
David B Sudderth, Author
In simple and friendly terms, the authors offer help to those leading frustrating lives. They provide coping mechanisms, both psychological and an up-to-date guide to the latest technology *$14.95*
272 pages
ISBN 0-761507-96-5

7717   All About Attention Deficit Disorders, Revised
Parent Magic
800 Roosevelt Rd
Glen Ellyn, IL 60137-5839   630-208-0031
                                      800-442-4453
                                      FAX: 630-208-7366
                                      custcare@parentmagic.com
                                      www.parentmagic.com
Thomas Phelan, Owner
A psychologist and expert on ADD outlines the symptoms, diagnosis and treatment of this neurological disorder. *$12.95*
248 pages Paperback
ISBN 1-889140-11-2

7718   Assistive Technology for Individuals withCognitive Impairments Handbook
Idaho Assistive Technology Project
University of Idaho
1187 Alturas Dr.
Moscow, ID 83843- 2268   208-885-3557
                                      800-432-8324
                                      FAX: 208-885-6102
                                      idahoat@uidaho.edu
                                      www.idahoat.org
Ron Seiler, Project Director
A handbook designed to provide resources and information on finding and acquiring assistive technology for individuals with cognitive impairments.

7719   Attention Deficit Disorder
Sage Publications
2455 Teller Road
Thousand Oaks, CA 91320
                                      800-818-7243
                                      FAX: 800-583-2665
                                      info@sagepub.com
                                      www.sagepub.com
Sara Miller McCune, Founder, Publisher, Chairperson
Blaise R Simqu, President & CEO
A book providing helpful suggestions for both home and classroom management of students with attention deficit disorder.

7720   Attention Deficit Disorder and Learning Disabilities
Books on Special Children
P.O.Box 305
Congers, NY 10920-305   845-638-1236
                                      FAX: 845-638-0847
                                      irene@boscbooks.com
Barbara Ingersoll, Author
Introduces ADD and learning disabilities. This is an easy reading book. Gives definitions and discusses some effective and controverial medication, dietary, biofeedback, cognitive therapy, and many more issues. *$15.95*
246 pages Softcover
ISBN 0-385469-31-4

7721 **Attention Deficit Disorder in Adults Workbook**
Taylor Publishing Company
7211 Circle S. Road
Austin, TX 78745-5007
214-637-2800
800-225-3687
FAX: 214-819-8220
Rings@balfour.com
www.balfour.com

Don Percenti, CEO
Workbook for adults with ADD. *$17.99*
192 pages Paperback
ISBN 0-878338-50-0

7722 **Attention Deficit Disorder: A Different Perception**
Underwood Books
PO Box 1919
Nevada City, CA 95959-1919
800-788-3123
rebecca@underwoodbooks.com
www.underwoodbooks.com

Thorn Hartmann, Author
Supports theory linking ADD to the genetic makeup of men and women who hunted for their food in prehestoric times. Also links second hand smoke to disruptive behavior. *$9.95*
180 pages Paperback
ISBN 0-887331-56-4

7723 **Attention Deficit Disorders: Assessment & Teaching**
Brooks/Cole Publishing Company
10650 Toebben Drive
Independence, KY 41051
859-525-2230
FAX: 859-282-5700
www.brookscole.com

Janet W Lerner, Author
A handy resource that offers teachers, school psychologists, councelors, social workers, administrators, and parents practical advice for working with children who have attention deficit disorders. *$18.95*
258 pages Paperback
ISBN 0-534250-44-0

7724 **Attention-Deficit Hyperactivity Disorder: Symptoms and Suggestons for Treatment**
Slosson Educational Publications Inc.
538 Buffalo Rd
East Aurora, NY 14052-280
716-652-0930
888-756-7766
FAX: 800-655-3840
slosson@slosson.com
www.slosson.com

Thomas W Phelan, Author
Steven Slosson, President
John Slosson, Vice President
David Slossan, Vice President
An exhaustive review of current research and decades of experience as practicing school-based professionals, as well as being a parent of an ADHD child, have culminated in this brief, to-the-point, and yet informed ADHD package which has recieved tremendous reviews. Well-grounded answers and suggestions which would facillitate behavior, learning, social-emotional functioning, and other factors in preschool and adolesence are discussed. Answers most commonly asked questions about ADHD/ADD. *$60.00*
61 pages

7725 **Attention-Deficit/Hyperactivity Disorder, What Every Parent Wants to Know**
Brookes Publishing
P.O.Box 10624
Baltimore, MD 21285-0624
410-337-9580
800-638-3775
FAX: 410-337-8539
custserv@brookespublishing.com
www.brookespublishing.com

Lauren Rohe, Regional Sales Consultant
Jeff Stickler, Educational Sales Representative
Sam Schissler, Educational Sales Representative
Dant Washington, Account Sales Manager
New easy-to-understand, non-technical edition helps teachers and parents get accessible answers to their ADHD. *$21.95*
304 pages Paperback
ISBN 1-557663-98-X

7726 **Augmenting Basic Communcation in Natural Contexts**
Brookes Publishing
P.O.Box 10624
Baltimore, MD 21285-0624
410-337-9580
800-638-3775
FAX: 410-337-8539
custserv@brookespublishing.com
www.brookespublishing.com

Lauren Rohe, Regional Sales Consultant
Jeff Stickler, Educational Sales Representative
Sam Schissler, Educational Sales Representative
Dant Washington, Account Sales Manager
Here you will find the techniques needed to establish a basic communication system for people of all ages with cognitive disabilities or motor sensory impairments. *$41.95*
304 pages Paperback
ISBN 1-55766 -43-6

7727 **Autism 24/7: A Family Guide to Learning at Home & in the Community**
Autism Society of North Carolina Bookstore
505 Oberlin Rd
Suite 230
Raleigh, NC 27605-1345
919-743-0204
800-442-2762
FAX: 919-743-0208
info@autismsociety-nc.org
www.autismsociety-nc.org

David Lax, Manager
Martina Ballen, Chair
Beverly Moore, Vice Chair
Elizabeth Phillippi, Secretary
Parents are encouraged to focus on skill sets and behaviors that most negatively affect family functioning, and replacing these behaviors with acceptable alternatives. *$19.95*

7728 **Autism Handbook: Understanding & Treating Autism & Prevention Development**
Oxford University Press
2001 Evans Rd
Cary, NC 27513-2010
919-677-0977
800-445-9714
FAX: 919-677-1303
custserv.us@oup.com
www.oup-usa.org

Thomas Carty, Senior Vice President
Simon Li, Regional Director
Adam Glazer, Director
Thomas McCarty, Manager/VP Operations
$25.00
320 pages
ISBN 0-195076-67-2

7729 Autism and Learning
Taylor & Francis
7625 Empire Dr
Florence, KY 41042-2919
212-695-6599
800-634-7064
FAX: 212-563-2269
orders@taylorandfrancis.com
www.taylorandfrancis.com

Rita Jordan, Author
Stuart Powell, Co-Author
This book is about how a cognitive perception on the way in which individuals with autism think and learn may be applied to particular curriculum areas.
160 pages Paperback
ISBN 1-853464-21-X

7730 Autism in Adolescents and Adults
Springer Publishing
11 W 42nd St
Floor 15
New York, NY 10036-8002
212-431-4370
FAX: 212-460-1575
service-ny@springer.com
www.springerjournals.com

Eric Schopler, Editor
$63.00
456 pages
ISBN 0-306410-57-5

7731 Autism...Nature, Diagnosis and Treatment
Autism Society of North Carolina Bookstore
505 Oberlin Rd
Suite 230
Raleigh, NC 27605-1345
919-743-0204
800-442-2762
FAX: 919-743-0208
jchampion@autismsociety-nc.com
www.autismbookstore.com

David Lax, Manager
Covers perspectives, issues, neurobiological issues and new directions in diagnosis and treatment. *$49.00*

7732 Autism: Explaining the Enigma
Wiley Publishers
111 River St
Suite 2000
Hoboken, NJ 7030-5773
201-748-6000
FAX: 201-748-6088
info@wiley.com
www.wiley.com

Uta Firth, Author
Explains the nature of autism. *$27.95*

7733 Autism: From Tragedy to Triumph
Branden Books
Po Box 812094
Wellesley, MA 02482
617-734-2045
FAX: 781-790-1056
www.brandenbooks.com

Carol Johnson, Author
Julia Crowder, Co-Author
A new book that deals with the Lovaas method and includes a foreward by Dr. Ivar Lovaas. The book is broken down into two parts — the long road to diagnosis and then treatment. *$12.95*

7734 Autism: Identification, Education and Treatment
Routledge (Taylor & Francis Group)
7625 Empire Dr
Florence, KY 41042-2919
212-695-6599
800-634-7064
FAX: 212-563-2269
orders@taylorandfrancis.com
www.routledge.com

Dianne Zager, Editor
Jeffrey Lin, Director
Francis Chua, Manager
Tamaryn Anderson, Marketing Manager

Chapters include medical treatments, early intervention and communication development in autism. *$36.00*

ISBN 0-805820-44-7

7735 Autism: The Facts
Oxford University Press
2001 Evans Rd
Cary, NC 27513-2010
919-677-0977
800-445-9714
FAX: 919-677-1303
custserv.us@oup.com
www.oup-usa.org

Simon Cohen, Author
Patrick Bolton, Co-Author
$22.50
128 pages
ISBN 0-192623-27-3

7736 Autistic Adults at Bittersweet Farms
Routledge (Taylor & Francis Group)
7625 Empire Dr
Florence, KY 41042-2919
212-695-6599
800-634-7064
FAX: 212-563-2269
orders@taylorandfrancis.com
www.routledge.com

Norman Giddan PhD, Author
Jane Giddan MA, Co-Author
Jefferey Lin, Director
Francis Chua, Manager
A touching view of an inspirational residential care program for autistic adolescents and adults. Also available in softcover. *$94.95*
Hardcover
ISBN 1-560240-42-3

7737 Be Quiet, Marina!
Star Bright Books
13 Landsdowne St
Cambridge, MA 02139
617-354-1300
FAX: 617-354-1399
orders@starbrightbooks.com
www.starbrightbooks.com

Kirsten Debear, Author
A noisy little girl with cerebral palsy and a quiet little girl with Down Syndrome learn to play together and eventually become best friends. *$16.95*
40 pages Hardcover
ISBN 1-887734-79-1

7738 Breakthroughs: How to Reach Students with Autism
Aquarius Health Care Media
30 Forest Road
PO Box 249
Millis, MA 02054
508-376-1244
FAX: 508-376-1245
aqvideos@tiac.net
www.aquariusproductions.com

Leslie Krussman, President/Producer
Joseph Wellington, Distribution Coordinator
Anne Baker, Billing & Accounting
Jane Hutchinson, Associate Director William Patte
A hands-on, how-to program for reaching students with autism, featuring Karen Sewell, Autism Society of America's teacher of the year. Here Sewell demonstrates the successful techniques she's developed over a 20-year career. A separate 250 page manual ($59) is also available which covers math, reading, fine motor, self help, social adaptive, vocational and self help skills as well as providing numerous plan reproducibles and an exhaustive listing of equipment and materials resources. Video. *$99.00*

7739 Bus Girl: Selected Poems
Brookline Books
8 Trumbull Rd
Suite B-001
Northampton, MA 01060
617-734-6772
800-666-2665
FAX: 617-734-3952
brbooks@yahoo.com
www.brooklinebooks.com

Gretchen Josephson, Author
Lula O Lubchenco, Editor
Poems written over several decades by a young woman with
Down Syndrome. *$14.95*
144 pages Paperback
ISBN 1-57129-41-9

**7740 Change Your Brain, Change Your Life: The Breakthrough
Program for Conquering Depression**
Three Rivers Press
3rd Floor
175 Broadway
New York, NY 10019
212-782-9000
FAX: 212-940-7860
www.randomhouse.com

Daniel G Amen MD, Author
Clinical neuroscientist and psychiatrist Amen uses nuclear brain
imaging to diagnose and treat behavioral problems. He explains
how the brain works, what happens when things go wrong, and
how to optimize brain function. Five sections of the brain are discussed, and case studies clearly illustrate possible problems.
$15.00
352 pages
ISBN 0-812929-98-5

**7741 Child and Adolescent Therapy: Cognitive-Behavioral
Procedures, Third Edition**
Guilford Press
72 Spring Street
New York, NY 10012-4019
212-431-9800
800-365-7006
FAX: 212-966-6708
info@guilford.com
www.guilford.com

Chris Jennison, Publisher Emeritus, Education
Seymour Weingarten, Editor-in-Chief
Jody Falco, Managing Editor: Periodicals
Natalie Graham, Editor: School Psychology, Liter
Incorporating significant developments in treatment procedures,
theory and clinical research, new chapters in this second edition
examine the current status of empirically supported interventions
and developmental issues specific to work with adolescents.
$45.00
432 pages Cloth
ISBN 1-572305-56-8

7742 Children with Mental Retardation
Woodbine House
6510 Bells Mill Rd
Bethesda, MD 20817-1636
301-897-3570
800-843-7323
FAX: 301-897-5838
info@woodbinehouse.com
www.woodbinehouse.com

Irv Shapell, Owner
A book for parents of children with mild to moderate mental retardation, whether or not they have a diagnosed syndrome or condition. It provides a complete and compassionate introduction to
their child's medical, therapeutic, and educational needs, and discusses the emotional impact on the family. New parents can rely
on Children with Mental Retardation to provide that solid foundation and confidence they need to help their child reach his or
her highest potential. *$14.95*
437 pages Paperback
ISBN 0-933149-39-5

**7743 Cognitive Behavioral Therapy for Adult Asperger
Syndrome**
Autism Society of North Carolina Bookstore
505 Oberlin Rd
Ste 230
Raleigh, NC 27605-1345
919-743-0204
800-442-2762
FAX: 919-743-0208
jchampion@autismsociety-nc.org
www.autismbookstore.com

David Lax, Manager
Text is prepared with case studies and examples from the author's
own experiences working as a cognitive-behavioral therapist
specializing in adults and adolescents with dual diagnosis, autism spectrum disorders, mood disorders, and anxiety disorders.

**7744 Communication Development in Children with Down
Syndrome**
Brookes Publishing
P.O.Box 10624
Baltimore, MD 21285-0624
410-337-9580
800-638-3775
FAX: 410-337-8539
custserv@brookespublishing.com
www.brookespublishing.com

Lauren Rohe, Regional Sales Consultant
Jeff Stickler, Educational Sales Representative
Sam Schissler, Educational Sales Representative
Dant Washington, Account Sales Manager
This book offers an extensive, detailed explanation of communi-
cation development in children with Down syndrome relative to
their advancing cognitive skills. It introduces a critical frame-
work for assessing and treating hearing, speech, and language
problems and provides explicit intervention methods and tested
clinical protocols.
Paperback
ISBN 1-55766-50-5

**7745 Comprehensive Guide to ADD in Adults: Research,
Diagnosis & Treatment**
ADD Warehouse
300 NW 70th Ave
Suite 102
Plantation, FL 33317-2360
954-792-8100
800-233-9273
FAX: 954-792-8545
websales@addwarehouse.com
www.addwarehouse.com

Harvey C Parker, Owner
The first to provide broad coverage of the burgeoning field. Written for professionals who diagnose and treat adults with ADD, it
provides information from psychologists and physicians on the
most current research and treatment issues *$50.95*
426 pages
ISBN 0-876307-60-8

7746 Concentration Cockpit: Explaining Attention Deficits
Educators Publishing Service
P.O.Box 9031
Cambridge, MA 02139-9031
617-367-2700
800-225-5750
FAX: 617-547-0412
CustomerService.EPS@schoolspecialty.com
eps.schoolspecialty.com

Rick Holden, President
Melvin D Levine, Author
This eight-page pamphlet explains the administration of The
Concentration Cockpit, a newly revised poster that helps children
with attention deficits gain insight into their problems and moni-
tor their progress in grappling with these problems. *$64.50*

ISBN 0-838820-59-X

7747 **Coping with ADD/ADHD**
Rosen Publishing Group
29 E 21st St
New York, NY 10010-6209
212-420-1600
800-237-9932
FAX: 888-436-4643
rosenpub@tribeca.ios.com
www.rosenpublishing.com

Jaydene Morrison, Author
At least 3.5 million American youngsters suffer from attention deficit disorder. This book defines the syndrome and provides specific information about treatment and counseling. *$16.95*

ISBN 0-823920-70-4

7748 **Count Us In**
Exceptional Parent Library
P.O.Box 1807
Englewood Cliffs, NJ 7632-1207
201-947-6000
800-535-1910
FAX: 201-947-9376
eplibrary@aol.com
www.eplibrary.com

Jason Kingsley, Author
Mitchell Levitz, Co-Author
Offers information on growing up with Downs Syndrome. *$9.95*

7749 **Culture and the Restructuring of Community Mental Health**
Greenwood Publishing Group
130 Cremona Drive
Santa Barbara, CA 93117
805-968-1911
800-368-6868
FAX: 866-270-3856
CustomerService@abc-clio.com
www.greenwood.com

William A Vega, Author
John W Murphy, Co-Author
Michael Millman, Editor, American History
Hilary Clagget, Editor, Business, Economics & Finance
Examines treatment, organizational planning and research issues and offers a critique of the theoretical and programmatic aspects of providing mental health services to traditionally underserved populations. $45.00-$52.95. *$95.00*
168 pages Hardcover
ISBN 0-313268-87-8

7750 **Difficult Child**
Bantam Books
1745 Broadway, 10th Floor
New York, NY 10019
212-782-9000
FAX: 212-302-7985
BBDPublicity@randomhouse.com
www.randomhouse.com/bantamdell

Stanley Turecki, Author
Leslie Tonner, Co-Author
The classic and definitive work on parenting hard-to-raise children with new sections on ADHD and the latest medications for childhood disorders. *$15.95*
302 pages Paperback
ISBN 0-553380-36-2

7751 **Disability Culture Perspective on Early Intervention**
Through the Looking Glass
3075 Adeline Street
Suite 120
Berkeley, CA 94703-2212
510-848-1112
800-644-2666
FAX: 510-848-4445
TTY: 510-848-1005
TLG@lookingglass.org
www.lookingglass.org

Megan Kirshbaum PhD, Author
For parents with physical or cognitive disabilities and their families. Available in braille, large print or cassette. *$2.00*
12 pages

7752 **Down Syndrome**
Aquarius Health Care Media
30 Forest Road
PO Box 249
Millis, MA 02054-1066
508-376-1244
888-440-2963
FAX: 508-376-1245
aqvideos@tiac.net
www.aquariusproductions.com

Lesile Kussmann, Owner
This is an excellent video for families who have just had a baby with Down Syndrome as well as professionals in the field of genetics and nursing. Through honest and open discussion, parents of children with Down Syndrome express the feelings and concerns they had during the early years of their child's life. Preview option available. *$150.00*
Video

7753 **Driven to Distraction**
Simon & Schuster/Touchstone Publishing
1230 Avenue of the Americas
Fl 11
New York, NY 10020- 1513
212-698-7000
FAX: 212-698-7009
www.simonsays.com

Edward M Hallowell, MD, Author
John J Ratey, MD, Co-Author
A practical book discussing adult as well as child attention deficit disorder (ADD). Non-technical, realistic and optimistic, it is an informative how-to manual for parents and consumers. *$23.00*

7754 **Dyslexia over the Lifespan**
Educators Publishing Service
PO Box 9031
Cambridge, MA 02139-9031
617-367-2700
800-225-5750
FAX: 617-547-0412
eps@schoolspecialty.com
www.epsbooks.com

Margaret B Rawston, Author
Discusses the educational and career development of 56 dyslexic boys from a private school that was one of the first to have a program to detect and treat developmental language disabilities. *$18.00*
224 pages
ISBN 0-838816-70-3

7755 **Embracing the Monster: Overcoming the Challenges of Hidden Disabilities**
Paul H Brookes Publishing Company
PO Box 10624
Baltimore, MD 21285-624
410-337-9580
800-638-3775
FAX: 410-337-8539
custserv@brookespublishing.com
www.brookespublishing.com

Veronica Crawford M.A., Author
Larry B Silver, MD, Foreword/Commentary
The author shares her experience of living with LD, ADHD and bipolar disorder to give readers an awareness of the challenges of living with hidden disabilities and what can be done to help *$24.95*
272 pages paperback
ISBN 1-557665-22-2

7756 **Encounters with Autistic States**
Jason Aronson
400 Keystone Industrial Park
Dunmore, PA 18512-1507
800-782-0015
FAX: 201-840-7242

Theodore Mitrani, Author
This book explores and explands the work of the late Frances Tustin, which was devoted to the psychoanalytic understanding of the bewildering elemental world of the autistic child. *$50.00*
448 pages Hardcover
ISBN 0-765700-62-

7757 Equal Treatment for People With Mental Retardation: Having and Raising Children
Harvard University Press
79 Garden St
Cambridge, MA 02138-1423

617-495-1000
800-405-1619
FAX: 617-495-5898
www.hup.harvard.edu

William Sisler, President
Valerie A Sanchez, Co-Author
Martha A Field, co-Author
A Harvard law professor and civil liberties practitioner provide a comprehensive examination of the reproductive and parental rights of mentally retarded citizens. *$19.95*
464 pages Paperback
ISBN 0-674006-97-6

7758 Families of Adults With Autism: Stories & Advice For the Next Generation
Autism Society of North Carolina Bookstore
505 Oberlin Road
Suite 230
Raleigh, NC 27605-1345

919-743-0204
800-442-2762
FAX: 919-743-0208
books@autismsociety-nc.org
www.autismbookstore.com

Tracey Sheriff, Chief Executive Officer
Paul Wendler, Chief Financial Officer
David Laxton, Director of Communications
Kristy White, Director of Development
This book's unique point of view is that of a parent who's been there and done that and is now willing to tell the reader what it was like. *$19.95*

7759 Family Therapy for ADHD: Treating Children, Adolescents and Adults
Guilford Press
72 Spring St
New York, NY 10012-4019

800-365-7006
www.guilford.com

Craig A Everett, Author
Sandra Volgy Everett, Co-Author
Presents an innovative approach to assesing and treating ADHD in the family context. *$29.00*
Paperback
ISBN 1-572304-38-3

7760 Fighting for Darla: Challenges for Family Care & Professional Responsibility
Teachers College Press
1234 Amsterdam Ave
New York, NY 10027-6602

212-678-3929
FAX: 212-678-4149
tcpress@tc.columbia.edu

Mary Lynch, Manager
Susan M Klein, Co-Author
Samuel Guskin, Co-Author
Samuel Guskin, Co-Author
Follows the story of Darla, a pregnant adolescent with autism. *$18.95*
161 pages
ISBN 0-807733-56-3

7761 Fragile Success
Brookes Publishing
PO Box 10624
Baltimore, MD 21285-624

410-337-9580
800-638-3775
FAX: 410-337-8539
www.brookespublishing.com

Virginia Walker Sperry, Author

A book about the lives of autistic children, whom the author has followed from their early years at the Elizabeth Ives School in New Haven, CT, through to adulthood. *$27.50*

ISBN 1-557664-58-7

7762 Getting Our Heads Together
Thoms Rehabilitation Hospital
68 Sweeten Creek Rd
Asheville, NC 28803-2318

828-274-2400
FAX: 828-274-9452

Kathi Petersen, Director Planning/Communication
Edgardo Diez MD, Medical Director Brain Injury
Kathy Price, Director Admissions
Chat Norvell, CEO
A handbook for families of head injured patients - available in Spanish as well as English. *$4.00*
40 pages Paperback

7763 Getting a Grip on ADD: A Kid's Guide to Understanding & Coping with ADD
Educational Media Corporation
1443 Old York Rd
Warmister, PA 18794

763-781-0088
800-448-9041
FAX: 215-956-9041
emedia@educationalmedia.com
www.educationalmedia.com

Kim Frank Ed.S., Author
Susan Smith-Rex Ed.D., Co-Author
Free catalog of resources.
64 pages Yearly

7764 Getting the Best for Your Child with Autism
Autism Society of North Carolina Bookstore
505 Oberlin Road
Suite 230
Raleigh, NC 27605-1345

919-743-0204
800-442-2762
FAX: 919-743-0208
books@autismsociety-nc.org
www.autismbookstore.com

Tracey Sheriff, Chief Executive Officer
Paul Wendler, Chief Financial Officer
David Laxton, Director of Communications
Kristy White, Director of Development
This treatment guide helps parents navigate the complex and overwhelming world of Autism. *$16.95*

7765 Group Activity for Adults with Brain Injury
Sage Publications
2455 Teller Road
Thousand Oaks, CA 91320

805-499-0721
800-818-7243
FAX: 805-499-0871
info@sagepub.com
www.sagepub.com

Sara Miller McCune, Founder, Publisher, Executive Chairman
Blaise R Simqu, President & CEO
Tracey A. Ozmina, Executive Vice President & Chief Operating Officer
Chris Hickok, Senior Vice President & Chief Financial Officer
This manual addresses attention, memory, reasoning, and language skills in group settings. *$53.00*

7766 Guide to Successful Employment for Individuals with Autism
Brookes Publishing
P.O. Box 10624
Baltimore, MD 21285-0624   410-337-9580
                                  800-638-3775
                             FAX: 410-337-8539
custserv@brookespublishing.com
www.brookespublishing.com

Marcia Daltow Smith, Author
Ronald G Belcher, Co-Author
Patricia D Juhrs, Co-Author
Lauren Smith, Western Region Sales Representat
Describing all aspects of job placement, this book details strategies for assessing workers, networking for job opportunities, and tailoring job supports to each individual. Also illustrates how to help individuals with autism become productive workers, and with detailed descriptions of specific jobs help provide ideas for employment. *$ 32.95*
336 pages Paperback
ISBN 1-55766-71-5

7767 Handbook of Autism and Pervasive Developmental Disorders
Autism Society of North Carolina Bookstore
505 Oberlin Road
Suite 230
Raleigh, NC 27605-1345   919-743-0204
                                 800-442-2762
                            FAX: 919-743-0208
books@autismsociety-nc.org
www.autismbookstore.com

David Laxton, Director of Communications
Paul Wendler, Chief Financial Officer
Tracey Sheriff, Chief Executive Officer
Kristy White, Director of Development
A list of contributors address such topics as characteristics of autistic syndromes and interventions. *$125.00*

7768 Helping People with Autism Manage Their Behavior
Indiana Resource Center For Autism
2853 E 10th St
Bloomington, IN 47408-2696   812-855-6508
                               FAX: 812-855-9630
prattc@indiana.edu
www.iidc.indiana.edu

David Mank, Executive Director
Scott Bellini, Assistant Director
Covers the broad topic of helping people with autism manage their behavior. *$7.00*

7769 Helping Your Child with Attention-Deficit Hyperactivity Disorder
Learning Disabilities Association of America
4156 Library Road
Pittsburgh, PA 15234-1349   412-341-1515
                               FAX: 412-344-0224
info@ldaamerica.org
www.ldaamerica.org

Nancie Payne, President
Ed Schlitt, First Vice President
Nanette Schweitzer, Second Vice President
Beth McGraw, Secretary
LDA is the largest non-profit volunteer organization advocating for individuals with learning disabilities

7770 Helping Your Hyperactive: Attention Deficit Child
Crown Publishing Company (Random House)
1745 Broadway
New York, NY 10019-4305   212-782-9000
                                  800-632-8676
                             FAX: 212-572-6066
websupportlife@primapub.com
crownpublishing.com

John Taylor, Author

$19.95

ISBN 1-559584-23-8

7771 Hidden Child: The Linwood Method for Reaching the Autistic Child
Woodbine House
6510 Bells Mill Road
Bethesda, MD 20817-1636   301-897-3570
                                  800-843-7323
                             FAX: 301-897-5838
info@woodbinehouse.com
www.woodbinehouse.com

Irv Shapell, Owner
Sabine Oishi, Co-Author
Chronicle of the Linwood Children's Center's successful treatment program for autistic children. *$17.95*
286 pages Paperback
ISBN 0-933149-06-9

7772 How To Reach and Teach Children and Teens with Dyslexia
Jossey-Bass
111 River St
Hoboken, NJ 7030-5773   201-748-6000
                           FAX: 201-748-6008
info@wiley.com
www.wiley.com

Cynthia M Stowe, Author
This practical resource gives educators at all levels essential information, techniques, and tolls for understanding dyslexia and adapting teaching methods in all subject areas to meet the learning style, social, and emotional needs of students who have dyslexia. *$ 22.95*
340 pages
ISBN 0-130320-18-8

7773 How to Own and Operate an Attention Deficit Disorder
Learning Disabilities Association of America
4156 Library Road
Pittsburgh, PA 15234-1349   412-341-1515
                               FAX: 412-344-0224
info@ldaamerica.org
www.ldaamerica.org

Nancie Payne, President
Ed Schlitt, First Vice President
Nanette Schweitzer, Second Vice President
Beth McGraw, Secretary
Clear, informative and sensitive introduction to ADHD. Packed with practical things to do at home and school, from a professional and mother of a son with ADHD. *$8.95*
43 pages

7774 Hyperactive Child, Adolescent, and Adult: ADD Through the Lifespan
Oxford University Press
198 Madison Ave
New York, NY 10016-4308   212-726-6000
www.us.oup.com/us

Paul H Wender, Author
Comprehensive general review. Update on previous research by the author, offering a basic text. Published by Connecticut Association for Children & Adults with Learning Disabilities (CACLD). *$8.75*
162 pages
ISBN 0-195113-49-7

7775   Hyperactivity, Attention Deficits, and School Failure: Better Ways
Learning Disabilities Association of America
4156 Library Road
Pittsburgh, PA 15234-1349

412-341-1515
FAX: 412-344-0224
info@ldaamerica.org
www.ldaamerica.org

Nancie Payne, President
Ed Schlitt, First Vice President
Nanette Schweitzer, Second Vice President
Beth McGraw, Secretary
LDA is the largest non-profit volunteer organization advocating for individuals with learning disabilities

7776   In Search of Wings: A Journey Back from Traumatic Brain Injury
Lash & Associates Publishing/Training
100 Boardwalk Drive, Suite 150
Youngsville, NC 27596

919-556-0300
FAX: 919-556-0900
orders@lapublishing.com
www.lapublishing.com

Marilyn Lash, President
Bob Cluett, CEO
Bill Herrin, Director of Graphics & Design
Nick Vidal, Director of IT
The true story of one woman coping with traumatic brain injury after a car accident that affected her cognitive skills and memory *$14.95*
233 pages
ISBN 1-882332-00-8

7777   In Their Own Way
Alliance for Parental Involvement in Education
375 Hudson Street
New York, NY 10014

212-366-2000
FAX: 212-366-2933
ecommerce@us.penguingroup.com
http://us.penguingroup.com

Thomas Armstrong, Author
John Makinson, Chairman and Chief Executive
Coram Williams, CFO
David Shanks, CEO
For the parents whose children are not thriving in school, Armstrong offers insight into individual learning styles. *$11.95*

7778   Increasing and Decreasing Behaviors of Persons with Severe Retardation and Autism
Research Press
PO Box 9177
Champaign, IL 61826-9177

217-352-3273
800-519-2707
FAX: 217-352-1221
rp@researchpress.com
www.researchpress.com

Dennis Wiziecki, Marketing
Richard M Fox, Author
These well-organized manuals are written for teachers, aides and persons responsible for designing or evaluating behavioral programs. Offers specific guidelines for arranging and managing the learning environment as well as standards for evaluating and maintaining success. In Volume Two of this series, chapters address more restrictive procedures including physical restraing, punishment, time-out and overcorrection. Set of two volumes. *$39.50*
230 pages Paperback
ISBN 0-878222-63-4

7779   Jumpin' Johnny Get Back to Work, A Child's Guide to ADHD/Hyperactivity
Ste 15-5
25 Van Zant St
Norwalk, CT 6855-1729

203-838-5010
FAX: 203-866-6108
CACLD@optonline.net
www.CACLD.org

Beryl Kaufman, Executive Director
Written primarily for elementary age youngsters with ADHD to help them understand their disability. Also valuable as an educational tool for parents, siblings, friends and classmates. Includes two pages on medication. *$12.50*
24 pages

7780   Keys to Parenting a Child with Attention Deficit Disorder
Barron's Educational Series
250 Wireless Blvd
Hauppauge, NY 11788-3924

631-434-3311
800-645-3476
FAX: 631-434-3723
barrons@barronseduc.com
barronseduc.com

Manuel H Barron, CEO
Francine McNamara MSW CSW, Co/Author
This book shows how to work with the child's school, effectively manage the child's behavior and act as the child's advocate. *$6.95*
160 pages Paperback
ISBN 0-812014-59-6

7781   Keys to Parenting a Child with Downs Syndrome
Barron's Educational Series
250 Wireless Blvd
Hauppauge, NY 11788-3924

631-434-3311
800-645-3476
FAX: 631-434-3723
barrons@barronseduc.com
barronseduc.com

Manuel H Barron, CEO
Lucy Guarino
Down Syndrome poses many challenges for children and their families. This book prepares parents and guardians to raise a child with Down Syndrome by discussing adjustment, advocacy, health and behavior, education and planning for greater independence. *$5.95*
160 pages Paperback
ISBN 0-812014-58-8

7782   Keys to Parenting the Child with Autism
Barron's Educational Series
250 Wireless Blvd
Hauppauge, NY 11788-3924

631-434-3311
800-645-3476
FAX: 631-434-3723
barrons@barronseduc.com
barronseduc.com

Manuel H Barron, CEO
Parents of children with autism will find a solid balance between home and practical information in this book. It explains what autism is and how it is diagnosed, then advises parents on how to adjust to their child and give the best care. *$6.95*
208 pages Paperback
ISBN 0-812016-79-3

7783   LD Child and the ADHD Child: Ways Parents & Professionals Can Help
1406 Plaza Dr
Winston Salem, NC 27103-1470

336-768-1374
800-222-9796
FAX: 336-768-9194
southern@blairpub.com
www.blairpub.com

Carolyn Sakowski, President
Susan H Stevens, Author
Book about learning disabilities available to parents. Stevens cuts through the jargon and complex theories which usually characterize books on the subject to present effective and practical

techniques that parents can employ to help their child succeed at home and at school. New edition adds information about ADHD children. *$12.95*
201 pages Paperback
ISBN 0-895871-42-4

7784 **Labeling the Mentally Retarded**
University of California Press
2120 Berkeley Way
Berkeley, CA 94704-1012   510-642-4247
                              FAX: 510-643-7127
                              www.ucpress.edu

Lynne Whity, Executive Director
Jane R Mercer, Author
Clinical and social system perspectives on mental retardation. *$12.95*
333 pages Paper

7785 **Let Community Employment be the Goal for Individuals with Autism**
Indiana Resource Center For Autism
2853 E 10th St
Bloomington, IN 47408-2601   812-855-9396
                              800-825-4733
                              FAX: 812-855-9630
                              prattc@indiana.edu
                              www.iidc.indiana.edu

David Mank, Executive Director
Scott Bellini, Assistant Director
A guide designed for people who are responsible for preparing individuals with autism to enter the work force. *$7.00*

7786 **Making the Writing Process Work**
Brookline Books
8 Trumbull Rd
Suite B-001
Northampton, MA 01060   617-734-6772
                              800-666-2665
                              FAX: 617-734-3952
                              brbooks@yahoo.com
                              www.brooklinebooks.com

Karen R Harris, Author
Steve Grahm, Co-Author
Making the Writing Process Work: Strategies for Composition and Self-Regulation is geared toward students who have difficulty organizing their thoughts and developing their writing. The specific strategies teach students how to approach, organize, and produce a final written product. *$24.95*
240 pages Paperback
ISBN 1-57129-10-9

7787 **Management of Autistic Behavior**
Sage Publications
2455 Teller Road
Thousand Oaks, CA 91320   805-499-0721
                              800-818-7243
                              FAX: 800-583-2665
                              info@sagepub.com
                              www.sagepub.com

Sara Miller McCune, Founder, Publisher, Executive Chairman
Blaise R Simqu, President & CEO
Tracey A. Ozmina, Executive Vice President & Chief Operating Officer
Stephen Barr, Managing Director/SAGE London
This excellent reference is a comprehensive and practical book that tells what works best with specific problems. *$41.00*
450 pages

7788 **Management of Children and Adolescents with AD-HD**
Learning Disabilities Association of America
4156 Library Road
Pittsburgh, PA 15234-1349   412-341-1515
                              FAX: 412-344-0224
                              info@ldaamerica.org
                              www.ldaamerica.org

Nancie Payne, President
Ed Schlitt, First Vice President
Nanette Schweitzer, Second Vice President
Beth McGraw, Secretary
LDA is the largest non-profit volunteer organization advocating for individuals with learning disabilities

7789 **Managing Attention Deficit Hyperactivity in Children: A Guide for Practitioners**
John Wiley & Sons Inc
111 River St
Hoboken, NJ 07030-5774   201-748-6000
                              800-825-7550
                              FAX: 201-748-6088
                              info@wiley.com
                              www.wiley.com

Warren J Baker, President
Michael Goldstein, Co-Author
Matthe S Kissner, CEO
Offers information about human personality, structure and dynamics, assessment and adjustment. *$27.50*
214 pages Hardcover
ISBN 0-471121-58-9

7790 **Mental Retardation**
McGraw-Hill, School Publishing
PO Box 182605
Columbus, OH 43218
                              800-338-3987
                              FAX: 609-308-4480
                              customer.service@mheducation.com
                              mcgraw-hill.com

David Levin, President and CEO
Patrick Milano, Chief Administrative Officer & CFO
Stephen Laster, Chief Digital Officer
David Stafford, SVP & General Counsel
Combines significant findings from the most current research, focusing on a unique relationship between the special educator and the learner with mental retardation.
656 pages Casebound

7791 **Mental Retardation: A Life-Cycle Approach**
Pearson Publishing
200 Old Tappan Rd
Old Tappan, NJ 07675-7033   201-785-2721
                              800-922-0579
                              FAX: 201-797-2993
                              www.pearsonhighered.com

Clifford J Drew, Author
Michael L Hardman, Co/Author
This text considers the needs of the retarded individual at every stage of life.
512 pages

7792 **Neurobiology of Autism**
Johns Hopkins University Press
2715 N Charles St
Baltimore, MD 21218-4363   410-516-6900
                              FAX: 410-516-6968
                              www.press.jhu.edu

William Brody, President
Thomas L Kemper, Co-Author
Margaret L Bauman, M.D., Co-Author
Thomas L Kemper, M.D., Co-Author
This book discusses recent advances in scientific research that point to a neurobiological basis for autism and examines the clinical implications of this research. *$28.00*
272 pages
ISBN 0-801880-47-5

7793 Out of the Fog: Treatment Options and Coping Strategies for ADD
Hyperion
1500 Broadway
3rd Floor
New York, NY 10036

212-563-6500
800-331-3761
FAX: 212-456-0176
www.hyperionbooks.com

Robert Miller, President
Suzanne Levert, Co-Author
Discusses the recent recognition of attention deficit disorder as a problem that is not outgrown in adolescence, and cogently summarizes the stumbling blocks this affliction creates in the pursuit of a career or attainment of a healthy family life *$14.95*
300 pages
ISBN 0-786880-87-2

7794 Overcoming Dyslexia
Vintage-Random House
3rd Fl
1745 Broadway
New York, NY 10019-4305

212-782-9000
FAX: 212-302-7985
www.randomhouse.com/vintage

Markus Dohle, CEO
Sally Shawitz, M.D., Author
Yale neuroscientist Shaywitz demystifies the roots of dyslexia (a neurologically based reading difficulty affecting one in five children) and offers parents and educators hope that children with reading problems can be helped. *$15.00*
432 pages
ISBN 0-679781-59-5

7795 Parent Survival Manual
Springer Publishing Company
11 W 42nd St
15th Floor
New York, NY 10036

212-431-4370
877-687-7476
FAX: 212-941-7842
cs@springerpub.com
www.springerpub.com

Ursula Springer, President
Ted Nardin, CEO
Edie Lambiase, CFO
A guide to crises resolution in autism and related developmental disorders. *$39.95*

7796 Parent's Guide to Down Syndrome: Toward a Brighter Future
Brookes Publishing
PO Box 10624
Baltimore, MD 21285-0624

410-337-9580
800-638-3775
FAX: 410-337-8539
custserv@brookespublishing.com
www.brookespublishing.com

Siegfried Pueschel MD PhD, Author
Highlights developmental stages and shows the advances that improve a child's quality of life. Includes discussions on easing the transition from home to school and choosing integration and curricular priorities, as well as guidelines for confronting adolescent and adult issues such as social and sexual needs and independent living and vocational options. *$21.95*
352 pages
ISBN 1-557664-52-8

7797 Parenting Attention Deficit Disordered Teens
CACLD
25 Van Zant Street
Norwalk, CT 06855-1729

203-838-5010
FAX: 203-866-6108
CACLD@optonline.net
cacld.org

Beryl Kaufman, Executive Director

Detailed outline of the various problems of adolescents with ADHD. Published by Connecticut Association for Children & Adults with Learning Disabilities (CACLD). *$3.25*
14 pages

7798 Parents Helping Parents: A Directory of Support Groups for ADD
Novartis Pharmaceuticals Division
59 State Route 10
East Hanover, NJ 7936-1005

862-778-7500
800-742-2422

Paulo Costa, CEO

7799 Please Don't Say Hello
Human Sciences Press
233 Spring St
New York, NY 10013-1522

212-229-2859
800-221-9369
FAX: 212-463-0742
http://isbndb.com

Charles Stenken, Author
Jaroslav Chobot, Author
Zirul Evany, Author
Bill Feldmaier, Author
Paul and his family moved into a new neighborhood. Paul's brother was autistic. The children thought that Eddie was retarded until they learned that there were skills that he could do better than they could. *$10.95*
47 pages Paperback
ISBN 0-89885 -99-8

7800 Preventable Brain Damage
Springer Publishing Company
11 W 42nd St
15th Floor
New York, NY 10036

212-431-4370
877-687-7476
FAX: 212-941-7842
cs@springerpub.com
www.springerpub.com

Donald L Templer, Author
Lawrence C Hartlage, Co-Author
Ursula Springer, President
Ted Nardin, CEO
Offers information on brain injuries from motor vehicle accidents, contact sports and injuries of children. *$35.95*
256 pages

7801 Reading, Writing and Speech Problems in Children
International Dyslexia Association
40 York Rd
4th Floor
Baltimore, MD 21204

410-296-0203
800-509-4980
FAX: 410-321-5069
info@idamd.org
www.interdys.org

Samuel Orton, Author
Steve Peregay, Executive Director
Kristin Penczek, Director Of Conferences
Kristi Bauman, Director Of Development
A tribute to the man who more than any other aroused the attention of the scientific community and who provided the sound educational principles on which much teaching of dyslexics today is based. *$27.00*

ISBN 0-89079 -79-1

7802 **Reality of Dyslexia**
Brookline Books
8 Trumbull Rd
Suite B-001
Northampton, MA 01060
617-734-6772
800-666-2665
FAX: 617-734-3952
brbooks@yahoo.com
www.brooklinebooks.com

John Osmond, Author
An informative and sensitive study of living with dyslexia which affects one in 25. He introduces the reader to the subject by sharing the difficulties of his dyslexic son. He then uses the personal accounts of other children and adult dyslexics, even entire dyslexic families, to illuminate the problems they encounter. *$14.95*
150 pages Paperback
ISBN 1-57129 -17-6

7803 **Relationship Development Intervention with Young Children**
Jessica Kingsley Publishers
400 Market St
Suite 400
Philadelphia, PA 19106
215-922-1161
FAX: 215-992-1417
orders@jkp.com
www.jkp.com

Steven E Gustein, Author
Rachelle Sheely, Co-Author
Social and emotional development activities for Asperger Syndrome, Autism, PDD and NLD. Comprehensive set of activities emphasizes foundation skills for younger children between the ages of two and eight. Covers skills such as social referencing, regulating behvior, conversational reciprocity, and synchronized actions. For use in therapeutic settings as well as schools and parents. *$22.95*
256 pages
ISBN 1-843107-14-7

7804 **Retarded Isn't Stupid, Mom!**
Brookes Publishing
4501 Forbes Blvd
Suite 200
Lanham, MD 20706
301-459-3366
800-638-3775
FAX: 301-429-5748
custserv@brookespublishing.com
www.pbrookescom/store/books/kaufman-3785
Sandra Z Kaufman, Author
Sandra Kaufman reveals the feelings of denial, guilt, frustration and eventual acceptance that resulted in a determination to help her daughter, Nicole, live an independent life. This edition, revised on the 10th anniversary of the book's original publication, adds a progress report that updates readers on Nicole's adult years and reflects on the revolutionary changes in society's attitudes toward people with disabilities since Nicole's birth. *$22.95*
272 pages Paperback
ISBN 1-557663-78-5

7805 **Rethinking Attention Deficit Disorder**
Brookline Books
8 Trumbull Rd
Suite B-001
Northampton, MA 01060-4533
617-734-6772
800-666-2665
FAX: 617-734-3952
brbooks@yahoo.com
www.brooklinebooks.com
Miriam Cherkes-Julkowski, Author
In contrast to the common focus on behavioral symptoms of attention disorders, this book emphasizes internal factors that make attention regulation difficult. In-depth discussions of social, emotional, and academic consequences and appropriate interventions are provided. *$27.95*
250 pages Paperback
ISBN 1-571290-30-7

7806 **Riddle of Autism: A Psychological Analysis**
Jason Aronson
4501 Forbes Blvd
Suite 200
Lanham, MD 20706-4346
301-459-3366
800-782-0015
FAX: 301-429-5746
www.rowmanlittlefield.com
Jason Aronson, Author
James Lyons, President/CEO
Stanley Plotnick, Chairman
Dr. Victor examines the myths that cloud an understanding of this disorder and describes the meanings of its specific behavioral symptoms. *$30.00*
356 pages Paperback
ISBN 1-568215-73-8

7807 **SCATBI: Scales Of Cognitive Ability for Traumatic Brain Injury**
Sage Publications
2455 Teller Road
Thousand Oaks, CA 91320
805-499-0721
800-818-7243
FAX: 805-499-0871
happiness@option.org
www.sagepub.com
Sara Miller McCune, Founder, Publisher, Executive Chairman
Blaise R Simqu, President & CEO
Tracey A. Ozmina, Executive Vice President & Chief Operating Officer
Stephen Barr, Managing Director/SAGE London
Assesses cognitive and linguistic abilities of adolescent and adult parents with head injuries. *$287.00*

7808 **Sex Education: Issues for the Person with Autism**
Indiana Resource Center For Autism
2853 E 10th St
Bloomington, IN 47408-2696
812-855-6508
800-825-4733
FAX: 812-855-9630
iidc@indiana.edu
www.iidc.indiana.edu
David Mank, Executive Director
Scott Bellini, Assistant Director
Discusses issues of sexuality and provides methods of instruction for people with autism. *$4.00*

7809 **Son-Rise: The Miracle Continues**
2080 South Undermountain Road
Sheffield, MA 01257
413-229-2100
800-562-7171
happiness@option.org
www.autismtreatmentcenter.org
Samahria Lyt Kaufman, Co-Founder and Co-Director
Dane Griffith, Director of Administrative Services
Bears Kaufman, Co-Founder and Co-Director
Raun Kaufman, Director of Global Education
Part One is the astonishing record of Raun Kaufman's development from an autistic and retarded child into a loving, brilliant youngster who shows no traces of his former condition. Part Two follows Raun's development after the age of four, teaching the limitless possibilities of the Son-Rise Program. Part Three shares moving accounts of five other ordinary families who became extraordinary when they used the Son-Rise Program to reach their own unreachable children. *$12.95*
343 pages
ISBN 0-915811-53-7

7810 **Soon Will Come the Light**
Future Horizons Inc
721 W Abram St
Arlington, TX 76013-6995
817-277-0727
800-479-0727
FAX: 817-277-2270
www.fhautism.com
Wayne Gilpin, Owner
Jennifer Gilpin, Vice President
Annette Vick, Manager

Offers new perspectives on the perplexing disability of autism. *$19.95*

7811 Successful Job Search Strategies for the Disabled: Understanding the ADA
Wiley Publishing
605 3rd Ave
New York, NY 10158-180
212-850-6000
FAX: 212-850-6088
www.wiley.com

Jeffrey G Allen, Author
Following a concise overview of the Americans with Disabilities Act (ADA), covers such topics as job identification, self-assessment, job leads, resumes, disability disclosure, interviewing, and accommodating specific disabilities. Includes dozen of relevant and instructive situation analyses, case examples, and answers to commonly asked questions. *$165.00*
229 pages

7812 Taking Charge of ADHD Complete Authoritative Guide for Parents
Guilford Press
72 Spring St
New York, NY 10012-4019
212-431-9800
800-365-7006
FAX: 212-966-6708
info@guilford.com
www.guilford.com

Russell A Barkley, Author
Revised and updated to incorporate the most current information on ADHD and its treatment. Provides parents with the knowledge, guidance and confidence they need to ensure that their child receives the best care possible. Also in cloth at $40.00 (ISBN# 1-57230-600-9 *$18.95*
331 pages Paperback
ISBN 1-572305-60-1

7813 Teaching Children with Autism: Strategies for Initiating Positive Interactions
Brookes Publishing
P.O.Box 10624
Baltimore, MD 21285-0624
410-337-9580
800-638-3775
FAX: 410-337-8539
custserv@brookespublishing.com
www.brookespublishing.com

Robert L. Koegel, Author
Lynn Kern Koegel, Co-Author
Robert Miller, Sales Director
Offers strategies for initiating positive interactions and improving learning opportunities. This guide begins with an overview of characteristics and long-term strategies and proceeds through discussions that detail specific techniques for normalizing environments, reducing disruptive behavior, improving language and social skills, and enhancing generalization. *$39.95*
256 pages Paperback
ISBN 1-557661-80-4

7814 Teaching and Mainstreaming Autistic Children
Love Publishing Company
9101 E Kenyon Ave
Suite 2200
Denver, CO 80237-1854
303-221-7333
FAX: 303-221-7444
lpc@lovepublishing.com
www.lovepublishing.com

Stan Love, Owner
Peter Knoblock, Author
Dr. Knoblock advocates a highly organized, structured environment for autistic children, with teachers and parents working together. His premise is that the learning and social needs of autistic children must be analyzed and a daily program designed with interventions that respond to this functional analysis of their behavior. *$24.95*

ISBN 0-89108-11-9

7815 Techniques for Aphasia Rehab: (TARGET) Generating Effective Treatment
Speech Bin
1965 25th Ave
Vero Beach, FL 32960-3062
772-770-0007
800-477-3324
FAX: 772-770-0006
store.schoolspecialty.com

Mary Jo Santo Pietro, Co-Author
Robert Goldfarb, Co-Author
TARGET is the kind of resource aphasia clinicians beg for. A practical resource that answers not only the what and how questions of treatment, but also the why. It describes dozens of treatment methods and gives you practical exercises and activities to implement each technique. It shows you how to treat all components of the disability, language disorder, overall impairment, communication problems, and the needs of the person with aphasia. *$45.00*
384 pages
ISBN 0-93785-50-5

7816 Teenagers with ADD
Woodbine House
6510 Bells Mill Rd
Bethesda, MD 20817-1636
301-897-3570
800-843-7323
FAX: 301-897-5838
info@woodbinehouse.com
www.woodbinehouse.com

Irv Shapell, Owner
Chris A Ziegler Dendy, M.S., Author
This best selling guide to understanding and coping with teenagers with attention deficit disorder (ADD) provides complete coverage of the special issues and challenges faced by these teens. Based on current diagnostic criteria and the latest literature and research in the field, the book discusses diagnosis, medical treatment, family and school life, intervention, advocacy, legal rights, and options after high school. Parents find strategies for dealing with their teen's difficult behaviors. *$18.95*
370 pages Paperback
ISBN 0-933149-69-7

7817 Understanding Down Syndrome: An Introduction for Parents
Brookline Books
8 Trumbull Rd
Suite B-001
Northampton, MA 01060-4533
617-734-6772
800-666-2665
FAX: 617-734-3952
brbooks@yahoo.com
www.brooklinebooks.com

Cliff Cunningham, Author
Using positive and readable language, this book helps parents understand Down Syndrome. Medical details are explained in lay terms, and advice is given on working with professionals, obtaining services, and treatment techniques that help the child. Cunningham alerts families to potential problems, the prospects for the child in schooling and the passage to adulthood. Revised 1996. *$14.95*
Softcover
ISBN 1-57129-09-5

7818 Valley News Dispatch
New York Families For Autistic Children
95-16 Pitkin Avenue
Ozone Park, NY 11417-2834
718-641-3441
FAX: 718-641-2228
help@nyfac.org
www.nyfac.org

Cheryl L. Marsh, Chairperson
Robert Burt, Treasurer
Education, recreation and support services for families and children with developmental disabilities.

7819 Verbal Behavior Approach: How to Teach Children with Autism & Related Disorders
Autism Society of North Carolina Bookstore
505 Oberlin Road
Suite 230
Raleigh, NC 27605-1345 919-743-0204
800-442-2762
FAX: 919-743-0208
books@autismsociety-nc.org
www.autismbookstore.com

David Laxton, Director of Communications
Paul Wendler, Chief Financial Officer
Tracey Sheriff, Chief Executive Officer
Kristy White, Director of Development
Provides full descriptions of how to teach the verbal operants that make up expressive language which include: manding, tacting, echoing and intraverbal skills. *$19.95*

7820 Without Reason: A Family Copes with two Generations of Autism
Books on Special Children
721 W Abram St
Arlington, TX 76013-6995 817-277-0727
800-489-0727
FAX: 817-277-2270
www.futurehorizons-autism.com

Wayne Tilton, President
The author discovers his son has autism. He delves into problems of the autistic person and explains reasons for their actions. *$20.95*
292 pages Hardcover

7821 Women with Attention Deficit Disorder: Embracing Disorganization at Home and Work
Underwood-Miller
708 Westover Dr
Lancaster, PA 17601-1242

288 pages
ISBN 1-887424-05-9

7822 You Mean I'm Not Lazy, Stupid or Crazy?!: A Self-Help Book for Adults with ADD
Simon & Schuster
1230 Avenue Of The Americas
11th Floor
New York, NY 10020-1513 212-698-7000
FAX: 212-698-7099
www.simonsays.com

Kate Kelly, Author
Peggy Ramundo, Co-Author
Practical advice on controlling adult ADD, a straightforward guide explains how to get along in groups, become organized, improve memory, and pursue professional help. *$15.00*
464 pages
ISBN 0-684815-31-1

7823 You and Your ADD Child
Nelson Publications
1 Gateway Plz
Port Chester, NY 10573-4674 914-481-5490
FAX: 914-937-8950

Paul Warren MD, Author
Jody Capehart M.Ed., Co-Author
$12.99
252 pages Paperback
ISBN 0-785278-95-8

Print: Journals

7824 American Journal on Mental Retardation
American Association on Mental Retardation
501 3rd Street NW
Suite 200
Washington, DC 20001 202-387-1968
800-424-3688
FAX: 202-387-2193
aamr@access.digex.net
www.aamr.org

Leonard Abbeduto, Editor
Articles cover biological, behavioral, and educational research: theory papers; and reviews of research literature on specific aspects of mental retardation. *$142.00*
112 pages BiMonthly

7825 Annals of Dyslexia
International Dyslexia Association
40 York Road
4th Floor
Baltimore, MD 21204 410-296-0232
800-ABC-D123
FAX: 410-321-5069
www.interdys.org

Hal Malchow, President
Ben Shifrin, Vice President
Elsa C. Hagen, Vice President
Suzanne Carreker, Secretary
IDA is a clearinghouse of scientific data and practice-based information related to dyslexia. Provides community-based referrals and information fact sheets in response to thousands of emails, calls & letters. Our annual conference attracts thousands of outstanding researchers, clinicians, parents, teachers, psychologists, educational therapists and people with dyslexia. *$15.00*
Paper

7826 Journal of Cognitive Rehabilitation
Neuroscience Publishers
6555 Carrollton Ave
Indianapolis, IN 46220-1664 317-257-9672
FAX: 317-257-9674
nsc@neuroscience.cnter.com
neuroscience.cnter.com

Odie L Bracy, Executive Director
Publication for therapists, family and patient, designed to provide information relevant to the rehabilitation of impairment resulting from brain injury. *$50.00*
36-48 pages Quarterly

Print: Magazines

7827 AWARE
National Fibromyalgia Association
1000 Bristol Street North
Suite 17-247
Irvine, CA 92660 714-921-0150
FAX: 714-921-6920
www.fmaware.org

Lynne Matallana, President/Founder
Mark Dobrilovic, Board of Director
John Fry, PhD, Board of Director
Michael Seffinger, DO, FAAFP, Board of Director
Magazine published three times a year with membership only.

7828 Attention
Children & Adults with ADHD
8181 Professional Place
Suite 150
Landover, MD 20785-2264 301-306-7070
800-233-4050
FAX: 301-306-7090
webmaster@chadd.org
www.chadd.org

Bryan Goodman, Director

A bi-monthly publication from CHADD. Free with membership.
Bi-monthly

Print: Newsletters

7829 **ADHD Report**
Guilford Press
72 Spring St
New York, NY 10012-4019   212-431-9800
                                           800-365-7006
                                    FAX: 212-966-6708
                                       info@guilford.com
                                         www.guilford.com

Russell A Barkley PhD, Editor
Presents the most up-to-date information on the evaluation, diagnosis and management of ADHD in children, adolescents and adults. This important newsletter is an invaluable resource for all professionals interested in ADHD. *$49.95*
16 pages BiMonthly
ISSN 1065-8025

7830 **Arc Connection Newsletter**
Arc of Tennessee
151 Athens Way
Suite 100
Nashville, TN 37228   615-248-5878
                                           800-835-7077
                                    FAX: 615-248-5879
                                       info@thearctn.org
                                            thearctn.org

John Lewis, President
John H. Shouse, VP,Planning & Rules committee Chair
Donna Lankford, Secretary
Ann Curl, Treasurer,Budget/Finance Committee Chair
Quarterly publication from the ARC of Tennessee. *$ 10.00*
12 pages Quarterly

7831 **Autism Research Review International**
Autism Research Institute
4182 Adams Ave
San Diego, CA 92116-2599   619-281-7165
                                    FAX: 619-563-6840
                            br@autismresearchinstitute.com
                                               autism.com

Steve Edelson, Executive Director
The Autism Research Institute has pubished this quarterly newsletter, Autism Research Review International (ARRI), since 1987. The ARRI has received worldwide praise for it's thoroughness and objectivity in reporting the current developments in biomedical and educational research. The latest findings are gleaned from a computer search of the 25,000 scientific and medical articles published every week. *$18.00*
8 pages Quarterly

7832 **Chadder**
Children & Adults with Attention Deficit Disorder
4601 Presidents Drive
Suite 300
Lanham, MD 20706   301-306-7070
                                    FAX: 301-306-7090
                                         www.chadd.org

Michael MacKay, President
Ruth Hughes, CEO
Susan Buning, Executive Editor
Christine hoch, Director of Development
Quarterly newsletter
Quarterly

7833 **Down Syndrome News**
National Down Syndrome Congress
30 Mansell Court
Suite 108
Roswell, GA 30076   770-604-9500
                                           800-232-6372
                                    FAX: 770-604-9898
                                        info@ndsccenter.org
                                          www.ndsccenter.org

Jim Faber, President
Marilyn Tolbert, 1st VP
Carole J. Guess, 2nd Vice President
Lori Mckee, Treasurer
Must become a member to receive the newsletter.

7834 **Farmington Valley ARC**
225 Commerce Dr
Canton, CT 06019-1099   860-693-6662
                                    FAX: 860-693-8662
                                               favarh.org

Diane Brown, President
Stephen Morris, Executive Director
The official newsletter containing information, new ideas, progress and more on the Farmington Valley Association for Retarded and Handicapped Citizens.

7835 **Imagine!**
Imagine!
1400 Dixon St
Lafayette, CO 80026-2790   303-665-7789
                                    FAX: 303-665-2648
                          gstebick@imaginecolorado.org
                                      imaginecolorado.org

John Taylor, President
Mark Emery, Executive Director
John Nevins, CFO
Susan LaHoda, Foundation Executive Director
For people of all ages with cognitive, developmental, physical & health related needs, so they may live lives of independence & quality in their homes and communities.
12-16 pages quarterly

7836 **Pure Facts**
Feingold Association of the US
11849 Suncatcher Dr
Fishers, IN 46037   631-369-9340
                                           800-321-3287
                                    FAX: 631-369-2988
                                        help@feingold.org
                                          www.feingold.org

Debbie Lehner, Manager
Relationship between foods, food additives and behavior/learning problems, including Attention Deficit Disorder (ADD) and hyperactivity. *$38.00*
10+ pages Monthly

Non Print: Newsletters

7837 **Arc Light**
Arc of Arizona
5610 S Central Ave
Phoenix, AZ 85040-3090   602-268-6101
                                           800-252-9054
                                    FAX: 602-268-7483
                                        thearcaz@gmail.com
                                          www.arcofarizona.org

Cindy Waymire, Editor
For people with intellectual and developmental disabilities.
Quarterly

7838 BIATX Newsletter
Brain Injury Association of Texas
316 W 12th Street
Suite 405
Austin, TX 78701-1845
512-326-1212
800-392-0040
FAX: 512-478-3370
info@texasbia.com
www.texasbia.org

Judith Abner, Director
Penny Phillips, President
Donna Kuhlmann, Chairman
Kelly Ramsay, CFO
A online quarterly e-newsletter, as well as news and updates on
the Brain Injury Association of Texas.

7839 BIAWV Newsletter
Brain Injury Association of America
PO Box 574
Institute, WV 25112-0574
304-766-4892
800-356-6443
FAX: 304-766-4940
biawv@aol.com
biawestvirginia.org

Peggy Brown, Director
Mike Davis, President

7840 Best Buddies Times
Best Buddies Times
907-1243 Islington Ave
Toronto, ON, Canada
416-531-0003
888-779-0061
FAX: 416-531-0325
info@bestbuddies.ca
www.bestbuddies.ca

Steven Pinnock, Director
Emily Bolyea-Kyere, Regional Program Manager
Bi-annual newsletter.

7841 Cognitive Therapy Today
Beck Institute for Cognitive Therapy & Research
One Belmont Avenue
Ste 700
Bala Cynwyd, PA 19004-1610
610-664-3020
FAX: 610-709-5336
info@beckinstitute.org
www.beckinstitute.org

Judith S Beck, Director
Aaron T Beck, President
Cognitive Therapy TodayT features articles on a wide range of
topics in CBT by leading clinicians from around the world. Articles have addressed evaluating psychotherapies; CBT and special populations, such as soldiers, the elderly, or diagnoses such
as schizophrenia; conceptualizing emotions; cross-cultural issues and many other issues of interest to clinicians. You will also
find information on workshops, speaking engagements by Beck
Institute faculty and more.

7842 Focus Times Newsletter
Focus Alternative Learning Center
126 Dowd Avenue
PO Box 452
Canton, CT 06019-0452
860-693-8809
FAX: 860-693-0141
info@focuscenterforautism.org
www.focus-alternative.org

Marcia Bok, President
Claudia Godburn, Secretary
Rita Barredo, Treasurer
Monthly online newsletter on autism.

7843 NAMI Advocate
National Alliance on Mental Illness
3803 N Fairfax Dr
Suite 100
Arlington, VA 22203-3080
703-524-7600
800-950-6264
FAX: 703-524-9094
www.nami.org

Suzanne Vogel-Scibilia, President
Our mission is to provide you with the technical assistance, tools
and referrals to resources you need to build organizational capacity and achieve the goals of the NAMI Standards of Excellence.

7844 NLP News
NLP Comprehensive
PO.Box 348
Indian Hills, CO 80454-648
303-987-2224
800-233-1657
FAX: 303-987-2228
learn@nlpco.com
www.nlpco.com

Christian Miller, Editor
Tom Dotz, President
Tom Hoobyar, Director Of Planning
Sharon DeBault, Director Of Community Relations
An online e-newsletter on Neuro-linguistic programming.

7845 REACH
TEACCH
100 Renee Lynn Ct
Carrboro, NC 27510
919-966-2174
FAX: 919-966-4127
teacch@unc.edu
www.teacch.com

Dr. Laura Klinger, Director
Walter Kelly, Business Officer
Rebecca Mabe, Assistant Director of Business
Mark Klinger, Director of Research
Free online newsletter.

7846 Weekly Wisdom
Autism Treatment Center of America
2080 S Undermountain Rd
Sheffield, MA 01257-9643
413-229-2100
877-766-7473
FAX: 413-229-3202
www.son-rise.org

Barry Kausman, Owner
Weekly Wisdom is available through a free email subscription.

Non Print: Software

7847 Cogrehab
Life Science Associates
1 Fenimore Rd
Bayport, NY 11705-2115
631-472-2111
FAX: 631-472-8146
lifesciassoc@pipeline.com
www.lifesciassoc.home.pipeline.com

Joann Mandriota, President
Divided into six groups for diagnosis and treatment of attention,
memory and perceptual disorders to be used by and under the
guidance of a professional. $95.-$1,950

Non Print: Video

7848 ADD, Stepping Out of the Dark
Child Development Media
5632 Van Nuys Blvd
Suite 286
Van Nuys, CA 91401-4602   818-989-7221
800-405-8942
FAX: 818-989-7826
info@childdevelopmentmedia.com
www.childdevelopmentmedia.com
Margie Wagner, Owner
A powerful, effective video, ideal for health professionals, educators and parents providing a visual montage designed to promote an understanding and awareness of attention deficit disorder. Based on actual accounts of those who have ADD, including a neurologist, an office worker, and parents of children with ADD. The DVD allows the viewer to feel the frustration and lack of attention that ADD brings to many. *$52.95*
Video

7849 ADHD in Adults
Guilford Press
72 Spring St
New York, NY 10012-4019   212-431-9800
800-365-7006
FAX: 212-966-6708
info@guilford.com
www.guilford.com
Russell A Barkley, Editor
This program integrates information on ADHD with the actual experiences of four adults who suffer from the disorder. Representing a range of professions, from a lawyer to a mother working at home, each candidly discusses the impact of ADHD on his or her daily life. These interviews are augmented by comments from family members and other clinicians who treat adults with ADHD. *$99.00*
DVD 1906
ISBN 0-898629-86-1

7850 ADHD: What Can We Do?
Guilford Press
72 Spring St
New York, NY 10012-4019   212-431-9800
800-365-7006
FAX: 212-966-6708
info@guilford.com
www.gulford.com
Russell A Barkley, Editor
A video program that introduces teachers and parents to a variety of the most effective technologies for managing ADHD in the classroom, at home, and on family outings. *$99.00*
DVD 1906
ISBN 0-898629-72-1

7851 ADHD: What Do We Know?
Guilford Press
72 Spring St
New York, NY 10012-4019   212-431-9800
800-365-7006
FAX: 212-966-6708
info@guilford.com
www.guilford.com
Bob Matloff, President
Russell A Barkley, Editor
An introduction for teachers and special education practitioners, school psychologists and parents of ADHD children. Topics outlined in this video include the causes and prevalence of ADHD, ways children with ADHD behave, other conditions that may accompany ADHD and long-term prospects for children with ADHD. *$99.00*
DVD 1906
ISBN 0-898629-71-3

7852 Around the Clock: Parenting the Delayed AD HD Child
Guilford Press
72 Spring St
New York, NY 10012-4019   212-431-9800
800-365-7006
FAX: 212-966-6708
info@guilford.com
Joan F Goodman, Editor
Susan Hoban, Editor
This videotape provides both professionals and parents a helpful look at how the difficulties facing parents of ADHD children can be handled. Video. *$150.00*
VHS 1994
ISBN 0-898629-68-3

7853 Attention Deficit Disorder: Adults
Aquarius Health Care Media
30 Forest Road
Millis, MA 02054   508-376-1244
888-440-2963
FAX: 508-376-1245
aqvideos@tiac.net
www.aquariusproductions.com
Lesile Kussmann, President/Owner
Joseph Wellington, Distribution Coordinator
Anne Baker, Billing & Accounting
Adults with ADD talk about how the disorder that went undiagnosed for so many years has affected their choice of spouses and work, and what they have found to help them. Biofeedback, which is growing as a treatment, is explained and demonstrated by its founder, Dr. Joel Lubar. Medical treatments like antidepressants and stimulants are also discussed, along with behavioral changes that can help the person with ADD and his or her spouse and family. *$149.00*
Video

7854 Attention Deficit Disorder: Children
Aquarius Health Care Media
30 Forest Rd
PO Box 249
Millisrn, MA 02054-7159   508-376-1244
888-440-2963
FAX: 508-376-1245
aqvideos@tiac.net
www.aquariusproductions.com
Lesile Kussmann, President/Owner
Everyone has been impulsive or easily distracted for different periods of time, so these symptoms that are hallmarks of Attention Deficit Disorder (ADD) have also led to criticism that too many people are being diagnosed with this biochemical brain disorder. This program examines who is being diagnosed, and what treatments are working. An innovative private school specializing in alternative education is profiled, and tips on structuring the school and home environment are included. *$149.00*
Video

7855 Autism: A World Apart
Fanlight Productions C/O Icarus Films
32 Court Street
Brooklyn, NY 11201-1731   718-488-8900
800-876-1710
FAX: 718-488-8642
info@fanlight.com
www.fanlight.com
Ben Achtenberg, Owner
Nicole Johnson, Publicity Coordinator
Anthony Sweeney, Marketing Director
In this documentary, three families show us what the textbooks and studies cannot: what it's like to live with autism day after day; to raise and love children who may be withdrawn and violent and unable to make personal connections with their families. 29 minutes. *$195.00*
VHS/DVD 1988
ISBN 1-572950-39-0

7856   **Autism: the Unfolding Mystery**
Aquarius Health Care Media
30 Forest Road
PO Box 249
Millis, MA 02054   508-376-1244
FAX: 508-376-1245
lkussmann@aquariusproductions.com
www.aquariusproductions.com

Lesile Kussmann, Owner
Explore what it means to be autistic, how you can recognize the signs of autism in your child, and hear about new treatments and programs to help children learn to deal with the disorder. *$145.00*
DVD 1905

7857   **Biology Concepts Through Discovery**
Educational Activities Software
5600 W 83rd Street
Suite 300, 8200 Tower
Bloomington, MN 55437
800-447-5286
FAX: 239-225-9299
info@edmentum.com
http://www.ea-software.com

Vin Riera, President/CEO
Rob Rueckel, CFO
Dave Adams, Chief Academic Officer
Paul Johansen, Chief Technology Officer
These videos, available in English and Spanish versions, encourage learning by presenting interactive problem solving in an effective VISUAL/AUDITORY style. *$89.00*
Video

7858   **Concentration Video**
Learning disAbilities Resources
6 E Eagle Road
Havertown, PA 19083   610-446-6126
800-869-8336
FAX: 610-525-8337
rcooper-ldr@comcast.net

Video

7859   **Educating Inattentive Children**
ADD Warehouse
300 Northwest 70th Avenue
Suite 102
Plantation, FL 33317-2360   954-792-8100
800-233-9273
FAX: 954-792-8545
websales@addwarehouse.com
www.addwarehouse.com

Harvey C Parker, Owner
Ideal for in-service to regular and special educators concerning the problems inattentive, elementarty and secondary students experience. *$49.00*
Video

7860   **Getting Started with Facilitated Communication**
Facilitated Communication Institute, Syracuse Univ
230 Huntington Hal
Syracuse, NY 13244-1   315-443-4752
FAX: 315-443-2258
http://thefci.syr.edu

Annegret Schubert, Director
Describes in detail how to help individuals with autism and/or severe communication difficulties to get started with facilitated communication.
Video

7861   **How to Cope with ADHD: Diagnosis, Treatment & Myths**
Aquarius Health Care Media
30 Forest Road
PO Box 249
Millis, MA 02054   508-376-1244
FAX: 508-376-1245
lkussmann@aquariusproductions.com
www.aquariusproductions.com

Lesile Kussmann, President/Owner

Learn how ADHD is diagnosed, clear up some of the myths, explain the treatmens that are availiable, and give you tips on how you can help your child at home. *$145.00*
DVD 1905

7862   **I Just Want My Little Boy Back**
Autism Treatment Center Of America
2080 South Undermountain Road
Sheffield, MA 01257   413-229-2100
800-714-2779
happiness@option.org
www.option.org

Samahria Lyt Kaufman, Co-Founder and Co-Director
Dane Griffith, Director of Administrative Services
Bears Kaufman, Co-Founder and Co-Director
Raun Kaufman, Director of Global Education
A great video for parents and professionals caring for children with special needs. Join one British family and their autistic son before, during and after their journey to America to attend The Son-Rise Program at The Autism Treatment Center of America. This informative, inspirational and deeply moving story not only captures the joy, tears, challenges and triumps of this amazing little boy and his family, but also serves as a powerful introduction to the attitude and principles of the program. *$25.00*

7863   **It's Just Attention Disorder**
Western Psychological Services
625 Alaska Avenue
Torrance, CA 90503-5124   424-201-8800
800-648-8857
FAX: 424-201-6950
customerservice@wpspublish.com
wpspublish.com

Gregg Gillmar, VP
This ground-breaking videotape takes the critical first steps in treating attention-deficit disorder: it enlists the inattentive or hyperactive child as an active participant in his or her treatment. *$99.50*
Video

7864   **Understanding ADHD**
Aquarius Health Care Videos
30 Forest Road
PO Box
Millis, MA 02054   508-376-1244
FAX: 508-376-1245
aqvideos@tiac.net
www.aquariusproductions.com

Leslie Kussmann, President/Owner
A look at some of the controversies surrounding Attention Deficit Hyperactivity Disorder. This video shows how the disorder is diagnosed and presents strategies for living with a child with the disorder. Diverse and candid opinions from teachers, social workers, a behavior specialist, a pediatrician and a parent with ADHD twins. Recommended for child development students, social workers, and caregivers. Preview option available. *$120.00*
Video

7865   **Understanding Attention Deficit Disorder**
CACLD
25 Van Zant Street
Norwalk, CT 6855-1713   203-838-5010
FAX: 203-866-6108
CACLD@optonline.net
www.CACLD.org

Beryl Kaufman, Executive Director
Helen Bosch, President
A video in an interview format for parents and professionals providing the history, symptoms, methods of diagnosis and three approaches used to ease the effects of attention deficit disorder. Published by Connecticut Association for Children & Adults with Learning Disabilities (CACLD). *$20.00*
45 Minutes VHS

7866 Understanding Autism
Fanlight Productions C/O Icarus Films
32 Court Street
Brooklyn, NY 11201

718-488-8900
800-876-1710
FAX: 718-488-8642
info@fanlight.com
www.fanlight.com

Ben Achtenberg, Owner
Susan Newman, Editor

Parents of children with autism discuss the nature and symptoms
of this lifelong disability and outline a treatment program based
on behavior modification principles. 19 minutes *$199.00*
VHS/DVD 1993
ISBN 1-572951-00-1

7867 We're Not Stupid
Media Projects Inc
5215 Homer St
Dallas, TX 75206-6623

214-826-3863
FAX: 214-826-3919
mail@mediaprojects.org
www.mediaprojects.org

Fonya Naomi Mondell, Producer

We're Not Stupid is an insightful and very personal video that
gives a voice to people who are struggling with learning disabilities. It was made by filmmaker Fonya Naomi Mondell, who is also
living with learning differences. The filmmaker camptures the
personal stories of young people from all walks of life who discuss what it's like to live with Attention Deficit Disorder and
Dyslexia. Their comments are open, honest and direct, and their
determination to manage their condition shines through. *$125.00*
Video

7868 Why Won't My Child Pay Attention?
ADD Warehouse
300 Northwest 70th Avenue
Suite 102
Plantation, FL 33317-2360

954-792-8100
800-233-9273
FAX: 954-792-8545
www.addwarehouse.com

Sam Goldstein, Ph.D, Author
Michael Goldstein, M.D., Co-Author

Practical and reassuring videotape, noted child psychologist tells
parents about two of the most common and complex problems of
childhood: inattention and hyperactivity. *$49.50*
224 pages Hardcover 1992
ISBN 0-471530-77-8

Support Groups

7869 Autism Society of America
4340 East-West Highway
Suite 350
Bethesda, MD 20814

301-657-0881
800-328-8476
FAX: 301-657-0869
info@autism-society.org
www.autism-society.org

Scott Badesch, President/CEO
Jennifer Repella, VP Programs
John Dabrowski, CFO
Doreen Allen, Marketing Manager

ASA is the largest and oldest grassroots organization within the
autism community, with more than 200 chapters and over 20,000
members and supporters nationwide. ASA is the leading source of
education, information and referral about autism and has been the
leader in advocacy and legislative initiatives for more than three
decades.

7870 National Autism Hotline
Autism Services Center
929 4th Ave
PO Box 507
Huntington, WV 25701-1408

304-525-8014
FAX: 304-525-8026
www.autismservicescenter.org

Mike Grady, CEO
Jimmie Beirne, COO
Nathel Lewis, ASC Training Coordinator

Service agency for individuals with autism and developmental
disabilities, and their families. Assists families and agencies attempting to meet the needs of individuals with autism and other
developmental disabilities. Makes available technical assistance
in designing treatment programs and more. The hotline provides
informational packets to callers and assists via telephone when
possible.

7871 National Health Information Center
Office Of Disease Prevention And Health Promotion
P.O.Box 1133
Washington, DC 20013-1133

301-565-4167
800-336-4797
301-468-7394
FAX: 301-984-4256
info@nhic.org
www.health.gov/nhic

Jessica Rowden, Sec Dept. Health Human Services
William Corr, J.D., Deputy Secretary

National health information center provides information referral
and support. NHIC links consumers and health professionals to
organizations that are best able to provide reliable health
information.

Dexterity

Associations

7872 American Amputee Foundation, Inc.
PO Box 94227
North Little Rock, AR 72190   501-835-9290
         FAX: 501-835-9292
        info@americanamputee.org
        www.americanamputee.org
Catherine J Walden LSW MPA CLCP, Executive Director
Serves primarily as a national information clearinghouse and referral center assisting mainly amputees and their families. AAF
researches and gathers information including studies, product information, services, self-help publications and review articles
written within the field. AAF has helped with claims, justifica-
tion letters to payers, testimony and life care planning. Free information packet for phone or letter inquiries.

**7873 American Board for Certification in Orthotics & Prosthetics
And Pedorthics, Inc.**
330 John Carlyle Street
Suite 210
Alexandria, VA 22314- 5760   703-836-7114
         FAX: 703-836-0838
         info@abcop.org
         www.abcop.org
Timothy E. Miller, CPO
Curt A. Bertram, President Elect
James H. Wynne, CPO
Donald D. Virostek, CPO/Past President
The American Board for Certification in Orthotics and Prosthet-
ics (ABC) is the national certifying and accrediting body for the
orthotic and prosthetic professions. The public requires and de-
serves assurance that the persons providing orthotic and prosthetic services and care are qualified to provide the appropriate
services, and it was on this basis that the ABC was established as a
credentialing organization.

7874 American Physical Therapy Association
1111 North Fairfax Street
Alexandria, VA 22314-1488   703-684-2782
         800-999-2782
         FAX: 703-684-7343
         TTY: 703-683-6748
         www.apta.org
J. Michael Bowers, Chief Executive Officer
Rob Batarla, EVP Financial & Business Affairs
Justin Moore, EVP Public Affairs
Bonnie Polvinale, EVP Member Affairs
It fosters advancements in physical therapy practice, research,
and education.

7875 American Stroke Association
American Heart Association
7272 Greenville Ave
Dallas, TX 75231-4596
         800-242-8721
         888-478-7653
         FAX: 214-706-5231
       strokeconnection@heart.org
    www.strokeassociation.org/STROKEORG/
Ralph L Sacco MS, President
Fifty-five state affiliates monitoring local chapters offering educational materials, seminars, conferences and transportation for
members nationwide. Maintains a listing of over 1,000 stroke
support groups across the nation for referral to stroke survivors,
their families, caregivers and interested professionals.

7876 Charcot-Marie-Tooth Association
PO Box 105
Glenolden, PA 19036   610-499-9264
         800-606-2682
        FAX: 610-499-9267
         info@cmtausa.org
         cmtausa.org
Herbert Beron, Chairman
Gary J. Gasper, Treasurer
Elizabeth Ouellette, Vice Chair
Patrick A. Livney, CEO
It support the development of new drugs to treat CMT, to improve
the quality of life for people with CMT, and, ultimately, to find a
cure.

7877 Dyspraxia Foundation
84 Westover Road
Highwood, IL 60040   847-780-3311
         www.dyspraxiausa.org

7878 Epilepsy Foundation
8301 Professional Place
Landover, MD 20785-2353   301-459-3700
         800-332-1000
         FAX: 301-577-2684
         ContactUs@efa.org
       www.epilepsyfoundation.org
Phil Gattone, President/CEO
Lee Gaston, Vice President Finance
Patty Dukes, VP Operations
Angela Ostrom, VP of Public Policy
The Epilepsy Foundation is the national voluntary agency solely
dedicated to the welfare of the 3 million people with epilepsy in
the U.S. and their families. The organization works to ensure that
people with seizures are able to participate in all life experiences;
and to prevent, control and cure epilepsy through research, education, advocacy and services.

7879 International Parkinson and Movement Disorder Society
555 East Wells Street
Suite 1100
Milwaukee, WI 53202- 3823   414-276-2145
         FAX: 414-276-3349
       info@movementdisorders.org
       www.movementdisorders.org
Matthew B. Stern, President
Oscar S. Gershanik, President-Elect
Francisco Cardoso, Secretary
Christopher Goetz, Treasurer
It is a professional society of clinicians, scientists, and other
healthcare professionals who are interested in Parkinson's dis-
ease, related neurodegenerative and neurodevelopmental disor-
ders, hyperkinetic movement disorders, and abnormalities in
muscle tone and motor control.

7880 Lewy Body Dementia Association
912 Killian Hill Road, S.W.
Lilburn, GA 30047   404-935-6444
         FAX: 480-422-5434
         www.lbda.org
Mike Koehler, President
Shannon McCarty-Caplan, Vice President
Tamara Real, Secretary
Angela Herron, Treasurer
A nonprofit organization dedicated to raising awareness of the
Lewy body dementias (LBD), supporting people with LBD, their
families and caregivers and promoting scientific advances.

7881 Multilingual Children's Association
20 Woodside Ave
San Francisco, CA 94127   415-690-0026
         FAX: 415-341-1137
      www.multilingualchildren.org

7882 **National Amputation Foundation**
40 Church St
Malverne, NY 11565-1735
516-887-3600
516-887-3600
FAX: 516-887-3667
amps76@aol.com
www.nationalamputation.org

Paul Bernacchio, President
William Sturges, 1st Vice President
Al Pennacchia, 2nd Vice President
Doanld A. Sioss, Executive Secretary
Information & resources for amputees. Scholarship programs for college students with major limb amputation. Free donated durable medical equipment open to anyone in need locally-as items need to be picked up.
Quarterly

7883 **National Commission on Orthotic and Prosthetic Education**
330 John Carlyle Street
Suite 200
Alexandria, VA 22314- 5760
703-836-7114
FAX: 703-836-0838
info@ncope.org
www.ncope.org

Robin C Seabrook, Executive Director
Jonathan D. Day, CPO
Dominique Mungo, Residency Program Manager
Joan M. Dallas, Accreditation Assistant
The mission of NCOPE is to be recognized authority for the development and accreditation of O&P education and residency standards leading to competent patient care in the changing healthcare environment. NCOPE develops, applies, and assures standards for orthotic and prosthetic education through accreditation and approval to promote exemplary patient care.

7884 **National Institute of Neurological Disorde Disorders & Stroke**
PO Box 5801
Bethesda, MD 20824-5801
301-496-5751
800-352-9424
FAX: 301-402-2186
www.ninds.nih.gov

Samahria Lyt Landis, Executive Director
Walter J Koroshetz MD, Deputy Director
Caroline Lewis, Executive Officer
Alfred W. Gordon, Ph.D., Associate Director for Special P
The mission of the National Institute of Neurological Disorders and Stroke is to reduce the burden of neurological disease.

7885 **National Stroke Association**
9707 E Easter Ln
Suite B
Centennial, CO 80112-3754
303-649-9299
800-787-6537
FAX: 303-649-1328
info@stroke.org
www.stroke.org

James Baranski, CEO
Sharon Jaunchowski, Executive VP
Teran Nash, Customer Relations
Carol Griffin, Development Manager
The only national health organization solely committed to stroke prevention, treatment, rehabilitation and community reintegration. Provides packaged training programs, on-site assistance, physician, patient and family education materials to acute and rehab hospitals. Develops workshops; operates the Stroke Information & Referral Center and produces professional publications such as Stroke: Clinical Updates and the Journal of Stroke and Cerebrovascular Diseases.

7886 **World Chiropractic Alliance**
2950 N Dobson Rd
Suite 3
Chandler, AZ 85224-1819
480-786-9235
800-347-1011
FAX: 480-732-9313
comments@worldchiropracticalliance.org
www.worldchiropracticalliance.org

Terry A Rondberg, Founder/CEO
Richard Barwell, President
Dedicated to protecting and strengthening chiropractic around the world. Serving as a watchdog and advocacy organization, we place our emphasis on education and political action.

Print: Books

7887 **Carpal Tunnel Syndrome**
Arthritis Foundation
1330 W Peachtree St
Suite 100
Atlanta, GA 30309
404-872-7100
800-283-7800
FAX: 404-872-0457
help@arthritis.org
www.arthritis.org

John H Klippel, President/CEO
Daniel T. McGowan, Chairman Of The Board
Rowland W. Chang, Vice Chair
Patricia Nov Nelson, Vice Chair
The Arthritis Foundation is committed to raising awareness and reducing the unacceptable impact of arthritis, a disease which must be taken as seriously as other chronic diseases because of its devastatng consequences.

7888 **Don't Feel Sorry for Paul**
Harper Collins Publishing
76 Ninth Ave
New York, NY 10011
800-843-2665
www.barnesandnoble.com

Bernard Wolf, Author
Ann Ledden, Vice President
Lorna Metzler, Manager
Paul is seven but was born with deformities of both hands and feet. Paul must wear a prosthesis on both feet so that he can walk. He has a third prosthesis for his right hand. The third prosthesis has a pair of hooks Paul uses as fingers.
94 pages Hardcover
ISBN 0-39731 -88-0

7889 **Functional Restoration of Adults and Children with Upper Extremity Amputation**
Demos Medical Publishing
11 West 42nd Street
15th Floor
New York, NY 10036-8804
212-683-0072
800-532-8663
FAX: 212-683-0118
orderdep@demospub.com
www.demosmedpub.com

Robert Meier III, Author
Diane Atkins, OTR, Co-Author
Provides a comprehensive reference to the surgery, prosthetic fitting, and rehabilitation of individuals sustaining an arm amputation. Covers the recent advancements in prosthetics and rehabilitation. *$165.00*
384 pages
ISBN 1-888799-73-0

Print: Magazines

7890   ABC Mark of Merit Newsletter
Amer Board for Cert in Otthotics & Prosthetics
330 John Carlyle St
Suite 210
Alexandria, VA 22314-5760   703-836-7114
                                             FAX: 703-836-0838
                                                  info@abcop.org
                                                  www.abcop.org

Timothy E. Miller, CPO
Curt A. Bertram, President Elect
James H. Wynne, CPO
Donald D. Virostek, CPO/Past President
An online bi-monthly newsletter.

7891   Active Living Magazine
American Amputee Foundation
PO Box 94227
North Little Rock, AR 72190   501-835-9290
                                             FAX: 501-835-9292
                                        info@americanamputee.org
                                        www.americanamputee.org

Catherine J Walden, Executive Director
A print magazine published four times a year.

7892   Stroke Connection Magazine
American Heart Association
7272 Greenville Ave
Dallas, TX 75231-5129   214-373-6300
                                                  888-478-7653
                                             FAX: 214-706-5231
                            www.strokeassociation.org/STROKEORG/

John Caswell, Editor
Debra Lockwood, Chairman
Nancy Brown, CEO
Ralph Sacco, President/Director
Free magazine for stroke survivors and their family caregivers.

Print: Newsletters

7893   NINDS Notes
Ntn'l Institute of Neurological Disorders & Stroke
P.O.Box 5801
Bethesda, MD 20284   301-496-5751
                                                  800-352-9424
                                             FAX: 202-944-3295
                                                   sbaa@sbaa.org
                                                 www.ninds.nih.gov

Caroline Lewis, Executive Officer
Story C. Landis, Director
Denise Dorsey, Chief Administrative Officer
Maryann Sofranko, Deputy Executive Officer
A print newsletter published three times a year.

Non Print: Newsletters

7894   Advocacy Pulse
American Stroke Association
7272 Greenville Ave
Dallas, TX 75231-5129   214-373-6300
                                                  888-478-7653
                                             FAX: 214-706-5231
                            www.strokeassociation.org/STROKEORG/
Ralph Sacco, President/Director
Debra Lockwood, Chairman
Nancy Brown, CEO

7895   Noteworthy Newsletter
Ntn'l Comm on Orthotic & Prosthetic Education
330 John Carlyle Street
Suite 200
Alexandria, VA 22314- 5760   703-836-7114
                                             FAX: 703-836-0838
                                                  info@ncope.org
                                                  www.ncope.org

Robin C Seabrook, Executive Director
Jonathan D. Day, CPO
Dominique Mungo, Residency Program Manager
Joan M. Dallas, Accreditation Assistant
The mission of NCOPE is to be recognized authority for the development and accreditation of O&P education and residency standards leading to competent patient care in the changing healthcare environment. NCOPE develops, applies, and assures standards for orthotic and prosthetic education through accreditation and approval to promote exemplary patient care.

7896   Stroke Smart Magazine
National Stroke Association
9707 E Easter Ln
Suite B
Centennial, CO 80112-3754   303-649-9299
                                                  800-787-6537
                                             FAX: 303-649-1328
                                                  info@stroke.org
                                                  www.stroke.org

James Baranski, CEO
Sharon Jaunchowski, Executive VP
Teran Nash, Customer Relations
Carol Griffin, Development Manager
The only national health organization solely committed to stroke prevention, treatment, rehabilitation and community reintegration. Provides packaged training programs, on-site assistance, physician, patient and family education materials to acute and rehab hospitals. Develops workshops; operates the Stroke Information & Referral Center and produces professional publications such as Stroke: Clinical Updates and the Journal of Stroke and Cerebrovascular Diseases.

Hearing

Associations

7897 Academy of Rehabilitative Audiology
PO Box 2323
Albany, NY 12220-0323

952-920-0484
FAX: 952-920-6098
ARA@audrehab.org
www.audrehab.org

Kathleen Cienkowski, President
Jan Moore, Ph.D, Treasurer
Kristin Vasil-Dilaj, Secretary
Sheila Pratt, Ph.D., JARA Editor
Provides professional education, research and interest in programs for hearing handicapped persons. The primary purpose of the ARAYis to promote excellence in hearing care through the provision of comprehensive rehabilitative and habilitative services.

7898 Alexander Graham Bell Association for the Deaf and Hard of Hearing
3417 Volta Pl NW
Washington, DC 20007-2737

202-337-5220
FAX: 202-337-8314
TTY:202-337-5221
info@agbell.org
agbell.org

Lyn Robertson, President
Steven W. Noyce, Secretary/Treasurer
Cheryl L. Dickson, Immediate Past President
Anita Bernstein, Director
The Alexander Graham Bell Association for the Deaf and Hard of Hearing (AG Bell) is the world's oldest and largest membership organization promoting the use of spoken language by children and adults who are hearing impaired. Members include parents of children with hearing loss, adults who are deaf or hard of hearing, educators, audiologists, speech-language pathologists, physicians and other professionals in fields related to hearing loss and deafness.

7899 American Association of People with Disabilities
2013 H Street, NW, 5th Floor
5th Floor, Suite 950
Washington, DC 20006

202-457-0046
800-840-8844
FAX: 866-536-4461
www.aapd.com

Mark Perriello, President/CEO
Henry Claypool, Executive VP
TaKeisha Walker, Director of Workplace & Leadership Initiatives
Adam Abosedra, Program Manager
Dedicated to ensuring economic self-sufficiency and political empowerment for more than 50 million Americans with disabilities.

7900 American Cochlear Implant Alliance
P.O. Box 103
McLEAN, VA 22101-103

703-534-6146
info@acialliance.org
www.acialliance.org

Craig A. Buchman, Chair
Teresa A. Zwolan, Vice Chair
Nancy M. Young, Secretary
Jill B. Firszt, Treasurer
A not-for-profit membership organization created with the purpose of eliminating barriers to cochlear implantation by sponsoring research, driving heightened awareness and advocating for improved access to cochlear implants for patients of all ages across the US.

7901 American Society for Deaf Children
800 Florida Ave NE
Suite 2047
Washington, DC 20002-3695

800-942-2732
866-895-4206
FAX: 410-795-0965
ascd@deafchildren.org
www.deafchildren.org

Beth S Benedict PhD, President
Supports and educates families of deaf and hard of hearing children and advocates for high quality programs and services.

7902 American Speech-Language-Hearing Association
2200 Research Blvd
Rockville, MD 20850-3289

301-296-5700
800-638-8255
FAX: 301-296-8255
actioncenter@asha.org
www.asha.org

Patricia A. Prelock, PhD, President
Elizabeth S. McCrea, President-Elect
Shelly S. Chabon, Immediate Past President
Perry F. Flynn, Chair
Provides information for both the general public and physicians in an easy-to-access manner, on speech, hearing and language disorders. Exhibits by companies specializing in alternative and augmentative communications products, publishers, software and hardware companies, and hearing aid testing equipment manufacturers.

7903 American Tinnitus Association
522 S W Fifth Ave
Suite 825
Portland, OR 97207-0005

503-248-9985
800-634-8978
FAX: 503-248-0024
tinnitus@ata.org
www.ata.org

Michael Manusevec, Executive Director
Katie Fuller, Director of Support
Jennifer Born, Director of Public Affairs
Cara James, Development Director
The American Tinnitus Association (ATA) is the national champion of tinnitus awareness, prevention, and treatment. Under its guiding principles—Education, Advocacy, Research and Support—the ATA offers prevention programs in schools, urges governmental and private organizations to support hearing conservation, funds the nation's brightest researchers, and facilitates self-help groups around the country.

7904 Association of Adult Musicians with Hearing Loss
P. O. Box 522
Rockville, MD 20848

info@aamhl.org
www.aamhl.org

Wendy Cheng, President
Jennifer Castellano, Secretary
Janice Rosen, Treasurer
Marshall Chasin, Board Member
It create opportunities for adult musicians with hearing loss to discuss the challenges they face in making and listening to music.

7905 Association of Late-Deafened Adults
8038 Macintosh Ln
Suite 2
Rockford, IL 61107-5336

815-332-1515
866-402-2532
FAX: 877-907-1738
TTY: 815-332-1515
info@alda.org
www.alda.org

Mary Lou Mistretta, President
Dave Litman, President Elect
Brenda Estes, Past President
Articles, stories and poems by and about late-deafened adults.

7906   **Better Hearing Institute**
1444 I St NW
Suite 700
Washington, DC 20005-6542   202-449-1100
800-327-9355
FAX: 202-216-9646
mail@betterhearing.org
www.betterhearing.org

Sergei Kochkin, Executive Director
Norm Crosby, Chairman
Shari Lewis, Chairman

The BHI is a not-for-profit corporation that educates the public
about the neglected problem of hearing loss and what can be done
about it. Founded in 1973 we are working to erase the stigma and
end the embarassment that prevents millions of people from seeking help for hearing loss and show the negative consequences of
untreated hearing loss for millions of Americans. And to promote
treatment and demonstrate that this is a national problem that can
be solved.

7907   **Center for Hearing and Communication**
50 Broadway
Fl 6
New York, NY 10004-3810   917-305-7700
FAX: 917-305-7888
TTY:917-305-7999
info@chchearing.org
www.chchearing.org

Laurie Hanin PhD CCC-A, Executive Director
Ellen Lafargue, Director of Audiology
Susan E. Adams, Coordinator
Anita Stein, Assistant Director

The Center for Hearing and Communication provides hearing
health services to people of all ages who have a hearing loss. With
offices in New York City and Florida, CHC meets all of your hearing and communication needs through professional services that
offer the highest level of clinical expertise and technical
know-how available in the hearing healthcare field. Visit us for a
wide array of services including free hearing screenings; complete hearing evaluations; pediatric services; hearing a

7908   **Communication Service for the Deaf**
3520 Gateway Lane
Sioux Falls, SD 57106
866-642-6410
FAX: 605-362-2806
TTY:866-273-3323
inquiry@c-s-d.org
www.c-s-d.org

Dr. Benjamin Soukup, Founder, Chairman & CEO
Christopher Soukup, President
Brad Hermes, CFO
Ann Marie Mickleson, VP, CSD Interpreting

CSD's mission is to create greater opportunities for Deaf and hard
of hearing individuals to reach their full potential. Through
global leadership and the development of innovative technologies, CSD provides tools conducive to a positive and fully
integrated life.

7909   **Conference of Educational Administrators of Schools and
Programs for the Deaf**
PO Box 1778
St Augustine, FL 32085-1778   904-810-5200
866-697-8805
FAX: 904-810-5525
nationaloffice@ceasd.org
www.ceasd.org

Joseph Finnegan, Executive Director
Ronald Stern, President
Nancy Hlibok Amann, Secretary
Peter L. Bailey, Treasurer

CEASD provides an opportunity for professional educators to
work together for the improvement of schools and educational
programs for individuals who are deaf or hard of hearing. The organization brings together a rich composite of resources and
reaches out to both enhance educational programs and influence
educational policy makers.

7910   **Council of American Instructors of the Deaf (CAID)**
PO Box 377
Bedford, TX 76095-0377   817-354-8414
FAX: 817-354-8414
caid@swbell.net
www.caid.org

Keith Mousley, President
Helen Lovato, Office Manager

The CAID continues to follow the tradition begun in 1850 and
recognizes the value of bringing fellow teaching professionals
together to share experiences and ideas for the purpose of improving learning opportunities for deaf and hard of hearing children,
adolescents and young adults.

7911   **Davis Center, The**
19 State Route 10 E
Suite 25
Succasunna, NJ 07876   862-251-4637
FAX: 862-251-4642
npdunn@thedaviscenter.com
www.thedaviscenter.com

Dorinne S Davis MA CCC-A FAAA, Director
Elizabeth Meade, Head Sound Therapist
Nancy Puckett-Dunn, Office Manager
Laura Darby, Part Time Sound Therapist

The Davis Center's Sound Therapy Programs make positive
changes for children and adults with autism, ADD/ADHD, auditory processing issues, Dyslexia, learning disabilities, and other
learning and wellness challenges. Our programs address issues
such as phonics, spelling, writing, reading comprehension, hearing only parts of words, following directions, discriminating between sounds, sound sensitivity, behavioral responses, focus,
attention, and more.

7912   **Deaf REACH**
3521 12th St NE
Washington, DC 20017-2545   202-832-6681
FAX: 202-832-8454
info@deaf-reach.org
deaf-reach.org

Sarah E. Brown, Executive Director
Annette Reichman, President
Jonathan Tomar, Vice-President
Myrene Sargent, Director of Administration

The psychosocial rehabilitation approach, ulitzed by all
Deaf-REACH programs, provides the solid foundation to member's success. Participants are activly involved in establishing
the format and level of highly individualized service delivery that
they receive. The concept, which has achieved national acclaim,
involves teaching members necessary life skills, thus minimizing
the need for assistance from a service professional. This is part of
what distinguishes the approach at Deaf-REACH.

7913   **Deaf Women United**
PO Box 61
South Barre, VT 5670
info@dwu.org
www.dwu.org

Alana Beal, President
Keri Darling, Vice President
Caroline Koo, Secretary
Amanda Tuite, Treasurer

It is committed to continuing a community of support of Deaf
women from all walks of life.

7914   **Deafness Research Foundation**
363 Seventh Avenue,
10th Floor
New York, NY 10001-3904   212-257-6140
866-454-3924
FAX: 212-257-6139
TTY: 888-435-6104
info@hearinghealthfoundation.org
www.drf.org

Shari Eberts, Chairman
Mark Angelo, President
Robert Boucai, Principal
Judy R. Dubno, Dept. of Otolaryngology-Head and Neck Surgery

Founded in 1958, the Deafness Research Foundation is the leading source of private funding for basic and clinical research in the hearing science. The DRF is committed to making lifelong hearing health a national priority by funding research and implementing education projects in both the government and private sectors.

7915 Dogs for the Deaf
10175 Wheeler Rd
Central Point, OR 97502-9360
541-826-9220
800-990-3647
FAX: 541-826-6696
TTY: 541-826-9220
info@dogsforthedeaf.org
dogsforthedeaf.org

Robin Dickson, CEO
Vaughan Maurice, General Manager
Janine Bol, Finance Director
John Drach, Training Dept. Manager
Rescues dogs from shelters and professionally trains them for people with special needs such as: deafness, autism for children, seniors, stroke victims, cerebral palsy, etc.

7916 Ear Foundation
1817 Patterson St
Nashville, TN 37203-2110
615-329-7849
800-545-4327
FAX: 615-329-7935
info@earfoundation.org
www.earfoundation.org

Suzanne Wyatt, Executive Director
National, nonprofit organization committed to integrating the hearing and balance impaired into the mainstream of society through public awareness and medical education. Also administers The Meniere's Network, a national network of patient support groups providing people with the opportunity to share experiences and coping strategies.

7917 Georgiana Institute
736 Harmony Street
New Orleans, LA 70115
203-994-8215
georgianainstitute@snet.net
www.georgianainstitute.org

Annabel Stehli, President
The information source for Auditory Integration Training (AIT)/Digital Auditory Aerobics (DAA).

7918 HEAR Center
301 E Del Mar Blvd
Pasadena, CA 91101-2714
626-796-2016
FAX: 626-796-2320
info@hearcenter.org
hearcenter.org

Ellen Simon, Executive Director
Deborah Lorino, Office Manager
Berenice Castro, Accounting Supervisor
Maline Medina, Accounts Receivable/Billing Cle
Auditory and verbal program designed to help hearing impaired children, infants and adults lead normal and productive lives. Seeks to develop auditory techniques to aid people who have communication problems due to deafness. Offers diagnostic evaluations for speech and hearing. Individual auditory, verbal training and speech-language therapy.

7919 Hearing Education and Awareness for Rockers
1405 Lyon St
San Francisco, CA 94115-2914
415-409-3277
FAX: 415-409-5683
info@hearnet.com
www.hearnet.com

Kathy Peck, Executive Director
Joseph Monatano, Chief of Audiology
Flash Gordon, Primary Care Physician
John Doyle, Secretary of the Board
H.E.A.R.'s mission is the prevention of hearing loss and tinnitus among musicians and music fans (especially teens) through education awareness and grassroots outreach advocacy.

7920 Hearing Industries Association
1444 I Street, N.W.
Suite 700
Washington, DC 20005
202-449-1090
FAX: 202-216-9646
mjones@bostrom.com
www.hearing.org

7921 Hearing Loss Association of America
7910 Woodmont Ave
Suite 1200
Bethesda, MD 20814-7022
301-657-2248
FAX: 301-913-9413
TTY:301-657-2248
hearingloss.org

Brenda Battat, Executive Director
Barbara Kelley, Dep Exec Dir, Editor-In-Chief
Nancy Macklin, Director of Events & Marketing
Lisa Hamlin, Director of Public Policy
The mission of the Hearing Loss Association of America is to open the world of communication to people with hearing loss through information, education, advocacy and support.

7922 Hearing, Speech and Deafness Center (HSDC)
1625 19th Ave
Seattle, WA 98122-2848
206-323-5770
888-222-5036
FAX: 206-328-6871
TTY: 206-388-1275
hsdc@hsdc.org
www.hsdc.org

Ken Block, Chairman
Norman Guadango, Managing Director
Robert Leining, Treasurer
Mike Redmond, President
Our mission is to enrich lives of all adults and children who experience hearing loss, speech and language impairments or who are deaf, by providing professional services and by promoting community awareness and accessibility.

7923 House Ear Institute
2100 W 3rd St
Los Angeles, CA 90057-1944
213-483-4431
800-388-8612
FAX: 213-484-8789
TTY: 213-484-2642
info@hei.org
www.hei.org

James Boswell, CEO
John.W House, M.D, President
Daniel. M Graham, Executive Vice President Develop
Neil Segil, Ph.D, Executive Vice President
Offers pediatric hearing tests, otologic and audiologic evaluation and treatment, rehabilitation, hearing aid dispensing, and cochlear implant services. Outreach programs focus on families with hearing impaired children.

7924 International Catholic Deaf Association
7202 Buchanan St
Landover Hills, MD 20784-2236
301-429-0697
FAX: 301-429-0698
homeoffice@icda-us.org
icda-us.org

Jean Cox, President
Kate Slosar, Vice President
T.K Hill, Secretary
Jimmy Kelly, Treasurer
An organization of Catholic deaf people and hearing people in the church working with the deaf in the united states of America.

7925 International Hearing Dog
5901 E 89th Ave
Henderson, CO 80640-8315
303-287-3277
FAX: 303-287-3425
info@hearingdog.org
www.pawsforsilence.org

Valerie Foss-Brugger, President
Robert Cooley, Field Representative
Andrea Paul, Vetinary Technician
Larry Norby, Accounting/HR
Trains and places Hearing dogs with deaf or hard-of-hearing persons, with or without multiple disabilities, nationwide, free of charge to the recipient.

7926 International Hearing Society
1688 Middlebelt Rd
Suite 4
Livonia, MI 48154-3374
734-522-7200
800-521-5247
FAX: 734-522-0200
chelms@ihsinfo.org
ihsinfo.org

Kathleen Mennillo, Executive Director
Joy Wilkins, Director of Education
Fran Vincent, Marketing Manager
Alissa Parady, Manager of Government Affairs
The IHS is the professional association that represents Hearing Instrument Specialists worldwide. IHS members are engaged in the practice of testing human hearing and selecting, fitting and dispensing hearing instruments. Founded in 1951, the Society continues to recognize the need for promoting and maintaining the highest possible standards for its members in the best interestof the hearing impaired it serves.

7927 League for the Hard of Hearing
50 Broadway
6th Fl
New York, NY 10004-3810
917-305-7700
TTY:917-305-7999
www.lhh.org

Laurie Hanin, Executive Director
Ellen Pfeffer Lafargue, Au.D, Director
Dorene Watkins, Coordinator
Anita Stein-Meyers, Au.D, C, Assistant Director
The Center for Hearing and Communication is a leading hearing center offering state-of-the-art hearing testing, hearing aid fitting, speech therapy and full range of services for people of all ages with hearing loss. Visit our offices in New York City and Florida for services that meet all of your hearing and communication needs.

7928 Lexington School for the Deaf: Center for the Deaf
30th Avenue and 75th St
Jackson Heights, NY 11370
718-350-3300
FAX: 718-899-9846
TTY:718-350-3056
generalinfo@lexnyc.org
www.lexnyc.org

Regina Carroll PhD, CEO/Executive Director
Philip W. Bravin, President
Gregory Hlibok, Vice President
Seth Bravin, Treasurer
Offers a comprehensive range of services to deaf, hard of hearing and speech impaired persons from infancy to elderly through its affiliate agencies: The Center for Mental Health Services; The Lexington Hearing and Speech Center, Lexington Vocational Services, and the Lexington School for the Deaf. The Lexington Center also provides services through its research division which houses the only federally funded Rehabilitation Engineering Center.

7929 Michigan Association for Deaf and Hard of Hearing
5236 Dumond Court
Suite C
Lansing, MI 48917-6001
517-487-0066
800-968-7327
FAX: 517-487-0202
info@madhh.org
www.madhh.org

Nancy Asher, Executive Director
Pat Walton, Office Manager
MADHH is a statewide collaboration agency dedicated to improving the lives of people who are deaf or hard of hearing through leadership in education, advocacy and services.

7930 National Alliance of Black Interpreters
P.O. Box 90532
Washington, DC 20090-532
202-810-4451
info@naobdic.org
www.naobidc.org

7931 National Association of Hearing Officials
PO Box 4999
Midlothian, VA 23112-17
www.naho.org

Bonny M Fetch CALJ, President
The mission of the National Association of Hearing Officials is to improve the administrative hearing process and thereby benefit hearing officials, their employing agencies, and the individuals they serve through promoting professionalism and by providing traininf, continuing education, a national forum for discussion of issues, and leadership concerning administrative harings.

7932 National Association of Parents with Children in Special Education
3642 E Sunnydale Drive
Chandler Heights, AZ 85142
800-754-4421
FAX: 800-424-0371
contact@napcse.org
www.napcse.org

George Giuliani, President
It is a national membership organization dedicated to rendering all possible support and assistance to parents whose children receive special education services, both in and outside of school.

7933 National Association of Special Education Teachers
1250 Connecticut Ave NW
Suite 200
Washington, DC 20036- 2643
202-296-7739
800-754-4421
FAX: 800-754-4421
contactus@naset.org
www.naset.org

Dr Roger Pierangelo, Executive Director
Dr. George Giuliani, Executive Director
The mission of NASET is to render all possible support and assistanve to professionals who teach children with special needs.

7934 National Association of the Deaf
8630 Fenton Street
Suite 820
Silver Spring, MD 20910- 3819
301-587-1788
FAX: 301-587-1791
TTY:301-587-1789
nadinfo@nad.org
www.nad.org

Howard A. Rosenblum, CEO
Shane H. Feldman, COO
Marc P. Charmatz, Staff Attorney
Lizzie Sorkin, Director of Communications
Nation's largest organization safeguarding the accessability and civil rights of 28 million deaf and hard of hearing Americans in education, employment, health care, and telecommunications. Focuses on grassroots advocacy and empowerment, captioned media deafness-related information and publications, legal assistance, and policy development.

7935 **National Black Association for Speech Language and Hearing**
700 McKnight Park Drive
Pittsburgh, PA 15237-1116
412-366-1177
FAX: 412-366-8804
nbaslh@nbaslh.org
www.nbaslh.org

Arnell Brady, Exec Board Chair
Carolyn Mayo, PhD, Secretary
Linda McCabe Smith, PhD, Treasurer
Rachel M. Williams, PhD, Convention Chair
The mission of the National Black Association of Speech-Language and Hearing is to maintain a viable mechanism through which the needs of black professionals, students and individuals with communication disorders can be met.

7936 **National Black Deaf Advocates**
PO Box 32
Frankfort, KY 40602
585-475-2411
800-421-1220
FAX: 585-475-6500
president@nbda.org
www.nbda.org

Benro Ogunyipe, President
Cory Parker, VP
Sharon.D White, Secretary
Betty Henderson, Treasurer
The Mission of the National Black Deaf Advocate is to promote the leadership development, economic and educational opportunities, social equality, and to safeguard the general health and welfare of Black deaf and hard of hearing people.

7937 **National Catholic Office of the Deaf**
7202 Buchanan St
Landover Hills, MD 20784-2299
301-577-1684
FAX: 301-577-1684
TTY:301-577-4184
info@ncod.org
www.ncod.org

Consuelo Martinez Wild, Executive Director
Helps coordinate efforts of deaf or hard of hearing people who are involved in the ministry, acts as a resource center, assists bishops and pastors become available to the deaf and hard of hearing.

7938 **National Cued Speech Association**
1300 Pennsylvania Avenue, NW
Suite 190-713
Washington, DC 20004
301-915-8009
800-459-3529
info@cuedspeech.org
www.cuedspeech.org

Amy Ruberl, Executive Director
Marah Baltzell, Executive Assistant
Shannon Howell, President
Champions effective communication, language development and literacy through the use of cued speech.

7939 **National Deaf Women's Bowling Association**
9244 E Mansfield Ave
Denver, CO 80237-1915
303-771-9018
ndwbast@gmail.com
www.ndwba.com

Gayle Willingham, President
Ali Martinez, VP
Holds world Deaf Bowling Torunament annually in July. Also holds Las Vegas Scratch Classic annually in October.

7940 **National Hearing Conservation Association**
3030 W 81st Ave
Westminster, CO 80031
303-224-9022
FAX: 303-458-0002
nhcaoffice@hearingconservation.org
www.hearingconservation.org

Jennifer Tufts, President
Beth Cooper, President Elect
Nancy Wojcik, Secretary/Treasurer
Cory Portnuff, Director of Communications

The mission of the NHCA is to prevent hearing loss due to noise and other environmental factors in all sectors of society.

7941 **National Student Speech Language Hearing Association**
2200 Research Blvd
Suite 450
Rockville, MD 20850-3289
301-296-5650
800-498-2071
FAX: 301-296-8580
TTY: 301-296-5650
nsslha@asha.org
www.nsslha.org

Patricia A. Prelock, PhD, President
Elizabeth S. McCrea, President-Elect
Shelly S. Chabon, Immediate Past President
Donna Fisher Smiley, Vice President for Audiology Practice
The American Speech-Language-Hearing Association is committed to ensuring that all people with speech, language, and hearing disorders receive services to help them communicate effectively.

7942 **Registry of Interpreters for the Deaf**
333 Commerce St
Alexandria, VA 22314-2801
703-838-0030
FAX: 703-838-0454
TTY:7038380459
ridinfo@rid.org
rid.org

Brenda Walke Prudhomme, President
Kelly L. Flores, VP
Dawn Whitcher, Secretary
Chris Grooms, Treasurer
The Registry of Interpreters for the Deaf, Inc. (RID), a national membership organization, plays a leading role in advocating for excellence in the delivery of interpretation and transliteration services between people who use sign language and people who use spoken language. In collaboration with the Deaf community, RID supports our members and encourages the growth of the profession through the establishment of a national standard for qualified sign language interpreters and transliterators, o

7943 **Sight & Hearing Association**
1246 University Ave. W.,
Suite #226
St. Paul, MN 55104- 4125
651-645-2546
800-992-0424
FAX: 651-645-2742
mail@sightandhearing.org
www.sightandhearing.org

Kathy Webb, Executive Director
Karen Klevar, Screening Director
Bernice Burgy, Program Assistant
Charles F. Barer, President
It is a nonprofit organization with a mission to enable lifetime learning by identifying preventable loss of vision and hearing in children.

7944 **Spring Dell Center**
6040 Radio Station Rd
La Plata, MD 20646-3368
301-934-4561
FAX: 301-870-2439
info@springdellcenter.org?subject=I'd like In
www.springdellcenter.org

Patsy Finch, President
Badgley CPA, Treasurer
Jean Hubbard, Secretary
Donna Rretzlaff, Executive Director
Since 1967, Spring Dell center has been, bridging the gap to enhance the lives of developmentally disabled people. Spring Dell's goal is to empower people in every aspect of their lives through the implementation of two programs, employment/vocational services and residential services including transportation. Spring Dell offers transportation door-to-door for persons with developmental disabilities, including day care programs, supportive environment, residential and any other transportation.

7945 **Starkey Hearing Foundation**
6700 Washington Ave S
Eden Prairie, MN 55344-3405

866-354-3254
FAX: 952-828-6900
hearingfoundation@starkey.com
www.starkeyhearingfoundation.org

Peter Lecy, President
Brady Forseth, Executive Director
Steven Sawalich, Executive Director
Dr.Paul Nash, Vice President
Continues to provide over 50,000 hearing aids per year to people
in the U.S. and all over the world.

7946 **Telecommunications for the Deaf and Hard of Hearing**
8630 Fenton St
Suite 121
Silver Spring, MD 20910-3803

301-563-9122
FAX: 301-589-3797
TTY:301-589-3006
info@tdi-online.org
tdiforaccess.org

Claude L Stout, Executive Director
James House, Director of Public Relations
John Skjeveland, Business Manager
Promoting equal access to telecommunications and media for
people who are deaf, late-deafened, hard of hearing or deaf-blind
through consumer education and involvement; technical assistance and consulting; applications of exisiting and emerging
technologies; networking and collaboration; uniformity of standards; and national policy development and advocacy.

7947 **United States Deaf Ski & Snowboard Association**
76 Kings Gate N
Rochester, NY 14617

585-286-2780
info@usdssa.org
usdssa.org

Anthony Di Giovani, Officer
It provides means for deaf people to get together to share their
love for skiing and sponsor races for deaf skiers.

7948 **Vestibular Disorders Association**
5018 NE 15th Ave
Portland, OR 97213-305

503-229-7705
800-837-8428
FAX: 503-229-8064
veda@vestibular.org
www.vestibular.org

Sue Hickey, President
Cynthia Ryan, MBA, Executive Director
Kerrie Denner, Outreach Coordinator
Karen Ilari, Administrative Support Coordinator
The mission of the Vestibular Disorders Association is to serve
people with vestibular disorders by providing access to informa-
tion, offering a support network, and elevating awareness of the
challenges associated with these disorders.

Camps

7949 **ASD Summer Camp**
Alabama Institute for Deaf & Blind
205 E South St
P.O. Box 698
Talladega, AL 35160

256-761-3214
FAX: 256-761-3278
TTY:256-761-3215
wiggins.lavina@aidb.state.al.us
www.aidb.org

Paul Millard, Principal
The Alabama School for the Deaf Summer Enrichment Camp is
designed especially for deaf and hard of hearing children ages
6-15. Recreation activities include swimming, skating, outdoor
games, horseback riding, field trips, arts and craft. Tuition is free.

7950 **Aspen Camp School for the Deafearing**
PO Box 1494
Aspen, CO 81612-1494

970-923-2511
FAX: 970-923-0643
info@aspencamp.org
www.aspencamp.org

Lesa Thompson, Camp Director
DJ Monahan, Program Coordinator
Katie Murch, Outreach Coordinator
Chelsea Bridges, Advocacy Coordinator
Aspen Camp's mission is to enrich the lives of Deaf and Hard of
Hearing individuals by providing experiential educational and
recreational activities which increase self-esteem, confidence,
and individual skills.

7951 **Aspen Camp of the Deaf & Hard of Hearing**
PO Box 1494
Aspen, CO 81612

970-923-2511
FAX: 970-923-0643
info@aspencamp.org
www.aspencamp.org

Lesa Thompson, Camp Director
Aspen Camp's mission is to enrich the lives of Deaf and Hard of
Hearing individuals by providing experiential educational and
recreational activities which increase self-esteem, confidence,
and individual skills.

7952 **CHAMP Camp**
1116 East Market St
Suite B-210
Indianapolis, IN 46202- 5629

317-679-1860
FAX: 317-245-2291
admin@champcamp.org
www.champcamp.org

Dave Carter, Co-Camp Director/Founder
Jamie Mitchell, Co-Camp Director
Nancy McCurdy, Camp Consultant/Founder
Kristina Watkins, Program Coordinator
We are an ACA accredited camp.

7953 **Camp Alexander Mack**
Indiana Deaf Camps Foundation
P.O.Box 158
Milford, IN 46542

574-658-4831
www.campmack.org

Galen Jay, Interim Executive Director
Lauren Carrick, Director of Development/Facility Manager
Amber Barrett, Food Service
Norma Miller, Ordained Minister
Our program is intentionally designed to provide campers with
life changing experiences that lead to a formation of personal
faith within a safe faith community.

7954 **Camp Bishopswood**
Diocese of Maine Episcopal
143 State St
Portland, ME 04101

207-772-1953
800-244-6062
FAX: 207-773-0095
mike@bishopswood.org
www.bishopswood.org

Laurie Kazilionis, President
Robert Johnston, VP
Jeff Mansir, Treasurer
Pam Waite, Secretary
Camp is located in Hope, Maine. One to seven-week sessions for
hearing impaired children June-August. Coed, ages 7-16.

7955 **Camp Capella**
8 Pearl Point Road
Dedham, ME 04429

207-843-5104
dana@campcabella.org
www.campcapella.org

Dana Mosher, Religious Leader
Provides an opportunity for children with disabilities to engage
in various recreational and social experiences.

7956   Camp Chris Williams
Lions 11 B-2 and MADHH
5236 Dumond Court
Suite C
Lansing, MI 48917-6001
                                    586-778-4188
                                    FAX: 586-285-1842
                                    TTY:586-285-1842
                                    info@madhh.org
                                    www.madhh.org

Nancy Asher, Executive Director
An exciting summer camp experience for deaf and hard of hearing youth and their siblings ages 8-14.

7957   Camp Comeca & Retreat Center
United Methodist Church
75670 Road 417
Conzad, NE 69130
                                    308-784-2808
                                    comeca@cozadtel.net
                                    www.campcomeca.com

John , Asst. Director
Camp is located in Cozad, Nebraska. Summer sessions for campers with diabetes and hearing impairment. Coed, ages 6-19, families, seniors, single adults.

7958   Camp Emanuel
P.O. Box 752343
Dayton, OH 45475
                                    937-477-5504
                                    crawford@campenamuel.org
                                    www.campemanuel.org

Stephanie Ackner, President
Brian Demarke, Vice President
Nan Crawford, Executive Director
Mary Foreman, Secretary
Camp for hearing impaired and normal hearing youth.

7959   Camp Grizzly
NorCal Services For Deaf & Hard Of Hearing, Inc.
4708 Roseville Road
Suite 112
North Highlands, CA 95660-5172
                                    916-349-7500
                                    FAX: 916-349-7580
                                    info@nocalcenter.org
                                    www.norcalcenter.org

Cheryl Bella, Chair
Sheri Farinah, CEO
Yim Orsi, Secretary
Andrew Metz, Treasurer
This camp is designed the deaf and hard of hearing youth or hearing youth with deaf or hard of hearing parent. The camp helps with social interaction, building self esteem, leadership skills while enriching the lives of the deaf and hard of hearing.

7960   Camp Isola Bella On Twin Lakes,Salisbury, Ct.
American School for the Deaf
139 N Main St
West Hartford, CT 06107-1264
                                    860-570-2300
                                    FAX: 860-570-2301
                                    TTY:860-570-2222
                                    Steve.Borsotti@asd-1817.org
                                    www.asd-1817.org

Alyssa Pecorino, Director
Edward Peltier, Executive Director
Steve Borsotti, Reunion Chairperson
Jenilee Terry, Camp Registrar
Hearing-impaired children, ages 6-19, blend educational instruction in communications with recreational activities. Qualified deaf and hearing staff members with experience in education, child care and counseling are employed at the camp.

7961   Camp Joy
3325 Swamp Creek Rd
Schwenksville, PA 19473-1518
                                    610-754-6878
                                    FAX: 610-754-7880
                                    campjoy@fast.net
                                    www.campjoy.com

Angus Murray, Camp Director

A special needs camp for kids and adults (ages 4-80+) with developmental disabilities such as: mental retardation, autism, brain injury, neurological disorder, visual and/or hearing impairments, Angelman and Down syndromes, and other developmental disabilities.

7962   Camp Juliena
Georgia Council for the Hearing Impaired
4151 Memorial Drive
Suite 103-B
Decatur, GA 30032
                                    404-292-5312
                                    800-541-0710
                                    FAX: 404-299-3642
                                    campjuliena@gmail.com
                                    www.gachi.org

Pat Ford, President
Jeanette Lorch, VP
Jimmy Peterson, Executive Director
Faithlyn Peart, Office Manager
A weeklong residential summer camp for youths and teens who are deaf or hard of hearing. Through challenging, team-oriented activities, campers form lasting friendships and acquire valuable leadership, social and communication skills.

7963   Camp Mark Seven
Mark Seven Deaf Foundation
144 Mohawk Hotel Rd
Old Forge, NY 13420
                                    315-357-6089
                                    FAX: 315-357-6403
                                    cm7campdirector@gmail.com
                                    www.campmark7.org

Dave Staehle, Camp Director
Chris McQuaid, Office Manager
Kelly Lange, Foundation director
Jenn Legg, KODA Programs Director
Adirondack Mountain camp for hard-of-hearing, deaf and hearing people. Coed, ages 1-99, families, seniors and single adults.

7964   Camp Pacifica, Inc.
California Lions Camp
45895 California Hwy. 49
Ahwahnee, CA 93601
                                    559-683-4660
                                    FAX: 209-543-9418
                                    webmaster@camppacifica.org
                                    www.camppacifica.org/

Ann Tognetti, President
Bob Ransom, Treasurer
Russ Custer, VP
Jill Loving, Secretary
Camp Pacifica is a camp for special needs children ages 7-15 years old. The camp offers outdoor recreational activities, along with promoting greater independence and self confidence among the children, and provides opportunities for social interaction, and further development of social skills.

7965   Camp Shocco for the Deaf
AL Baptist State Board of Missions
P.O. Box 6569
Talladega, AL 35161-886
                                    256-761-1100
                                    800-264-1225
                                    FAX: 256-761-1270
                                    campshocco@albcdeaf.org
                                    www.campshocco.org

Chad Fleming, Director
Matthew Dixon, Co-Director
Linnea Elliott, Assistant Director
Camp Shocco gives each child and teenager attending camp the opportunity to have an unforgettable one week of fun, games, and spiritual growth. Each camper also learns essence of teamwork, while developing their own unique abilities and talents that can often be overlooked.

7966 Camp Taloali
Lions Club of Oregon and Washington
15934 N Santiam Hwy
PO Box 32
Stayton, OR 97383-9619   971-239-8153
                                FAX: 503-769-6415
                          camptaloali@comcast.net
                              www.taloali.org

George Scheler, Chair
Sylvia Hall, Vice Chair
Rolland Hart, Executive Director
Dave Taylor, Secretary
Camp Taholi is a magic world of challenge and excitement where
campers learn new skills, goals, care, for the earth and share new
experience with both old and new friends.

7967 Camp Tekoa UMC
Western NC Conference/United Methodist Church
211 Thomas Rd.
Hendersonville, NC 28739   828-692-6516
                                FAX: 828-696-3699
                          director@camptekoa.org
                              www.camptekoa.org

James Johnson, Executive Director
John Isley, Asst. Director
Melisa Coates, Administrative Assistant
Karen Rohrer, Business Manager
Camping for children with asthma/respiratory ailments, hearing
impairment and developmental disabilities. Coed, ages 6-17.

7968 Deaf Kid's Kamp
Sproul Ranch, Inc.
42263 50th Street West
Suite 610
Quartz Hill, CA 93536   661-675-3323
                                          877-399-5449
                          deafkidskamp@earthlink.net
                              www.deafkidskamp.com

Buffy Sproul, Executive Director
Our purpose is to meet the needs of deaf children outside of the
classroom setting. These needs, as we have defined them, would
include but are not limited to: social contact with peers; contact
with the culture of the Deaf Community; educational and recreational programs not available in most school settings.

7969 Easter Seals Oklahoma
701 NorthEast 13th Street
Oklahoma City, OK 73104   405-239-2525
                                FAX: 405-239-2278
                          sbusch@eastersealsoklahoma.org
                              www.eastersealsoklahoma.org

Rodney Burgamy, Chairman
David Adams, Board Member
Kristen Sorocco, Secretary
Jeb Reid, Treasurer
Adult day health center, and child development center.

7970 Father Drumgoole Connelly Summer Camp
MIV: Mount Loretto
6581 Hylan Blvd
Staten Island, NY 10309-3830   718-317-2600
                                FAX: 718-317-2830
                              www.mountloretto.org

Stephen Rynn, Executive Director
Maryann Virga, Executive Assistant
Loretta Polanish, Executive Secretary
Ed Gani, Facilities Manager
Summer sessions for children with epilepsy, hearing impairment
and developmental disabilities. Coed, ages 5-13.

7971 Lions Camp Crescendo, Inc.
1480 Pine Tavern Road
P.O. Box 607
Lebanon Junction, KY 40150   502-833-3554
                                          888-879-8884
                                FAX: 502-833-4427
                          bjflannery@lions-campcrescendo.org
                              www.lions-campcrescendo.org

Major Wheat, Chairperson
Barbara Walker, Vice Chairperson
Billie J. Flannery, Administrator
Melinda Gilbert, Secretary
The enhancement of the quality of life for youth, especially those
with disabilities, through the delivery of a traditional camp experience by caring individuals and to enable others to use our camping and retreat facilities to serve the larger communities
humanitarian needs.

7972 Lions Camp Kirby
1735 Narrows Hill Rd
Upper Black Eddy, PA 18972-9712   610-982-5731
                          info@lionscampkirby.org
                              www.lionscampkirby.org

Bob Hunsberger, President
Alice Breon, Camp Director
Offers 4-week camps for deaf and hearing impaired children and
their siblings in eastern Pennsylvania.

7973 Lions Camp Merrick
Lions Clubs of District 22-C
P.O. Box 56
Nanjemoy, MD 20662   301-870-5858
                                FAX: 301-246-9108
                          info@LionsCampMerrick.org
                              lionscampmerrick.org

Wayne Magoon, President
Ray Shumaker, Vice President
Julie Andrew, Board Member
Frank Culhane, Treasurer
This recreational camp for special needs children offers a complete waterfront program including swimming, canoeing and
fishing for ages 6-16. Designed for children who are deaf and
hard of hearing, children of deaf parents, and children with diabetes. Also helps children to learn to deal with their special
conditions.

7974 Lions Wilderness Camp for Deaf Children, Inc.
Lions Clubs of California and Nevada
P.O.Box 195
Knightsen, CA 94548
                                          877-896-1598
                                          888-613-1557
                          campdirector@lionswildcamp.org
                              www.lionswildcamp.org

Richard A. Wilmot, President
Rachel Mix, Camp Program Director
Robin L. Nichol, Camp Manager
Dana Johnson, Secretary
A camp experience where a deaf child age 7 to 15 can learn out-
door skills and enjoy the wonder and beauty of nature to the full-
est extent.

7975 Meadowood Springs Speech and Hearing Camp
Oregon State Elks Association
P.O. Box 1025
Pendleton, OR 97801   541-276-2752
                                FAX: 541-276-7227
                          info@meadowoodsprings.org
                              www.meadowoodsprings.org

Michael Ashton, Executive Director
Kathy Hosek, Administrative Assistant
Patti Hall, Camp Staff Manager
On 143 acres in the Blue Mountains of Eastern Oregon, this camp
is designed to help young people who have diagnosed clinical disorders of speech, hearing or language. A full range of activities in
recreational and clinical areas is available.

7976 **Ramah in the Poconos**
2618 Upper Woods Road
Suite 734
Lakewood, PA 18439-3725   570-798-2504
FAX: 570-798-2049
info@ramahpoconos.org
www.ramahpoconos.org
Todd Zeff, Executive Director
Rabbi Joel Seltzer, Director
Bruce Lipton, Director of Finance & Operations
Deborah Jo Essrog, Development Director
Camp is located in Lake Como, Pennsylvania. Summer sessions
for children and adults with hearing impairment. Coed, ages
10-16, families and seniors.

7977 **Sandcastle Day Camp**
Children's Beach House
1800 Bay Ave
Lewes, DE 19958   302-645-9184
FAX: 302-645-9467
cterranova@cbhinc.org
www.cbhinc.org
Martha P. Tschantz, President
Maryann Helms, Vice President
Linda M. Fischer, Secretary
Charles H. Sterner, Treasurer
Camp is located in Lewes, Delaware. Four-week sessions
June-August for Delaware children with hearing impairment or
speech/communication impairment. Coed, ages 6-12.

7978 **Sertoma Camp Endeavor**
Sertoma Camp Endeavor
P.O.Box 910
Dundee, FL 33838-0910   863-439-1300
FAX: 863-439-1300
info@sertomacampendeavor.com
www.sertomacampendeavor.org
Jeff Nunemaker, Executive Director
The intergration of deaf, hard of hearing and hearing youngsters
is a unique characteristic of our camping program. Both hearing,
deaf and hard of hearing children have the opportunity to learn
about themselves and each other in an informal and empowering
setting.

7979 **Texas Lions Camp**
Lions Club of Texas
P.O.Box 290247
Kerrville, TX 78029   830-896-8500
FAX: 830-896-3666
smabry@lionscamp.com
www.lionscamp.com
Stephen Mabry, Executive Director
The primary purpose of the League shall be to provide, without
charge, a camp for physically disabled, hearing/vision impaired
and diabetic children from the State of Texas, regardless of race,
religion, or national origin. Our goal is to create an atmosphere
wherein campers will learn the can do philosophy and be allowed
to achieve maximum personal growth and self-esteem. The camp
welcomes boys and girls ages 7-16.

7980 **YMCA Camp Fitch**
The YMCA's Camp Fitch on Lake Erie
12600 Abels Rd
North Springfield, PA 16430-1014   814-922-3219
FAX: 814-922-7000
info@campfitchymca.org
www.campfitch.com
Brian Rupe, Executive Director
Greg Donahue, Assistant Camp Director
Dann Olin, Operations Director
Barb Olin, Senior Program Director
Camp is located in North Springfield, Pennsylvania. Camping
sessions for children and adults with diabetes, hearing impair-
ment, developmental disabilities, mobility limitation and
speech/communication impairment. Ages 8-16, families and
seniors.

7981 **YWCA Camp Westwind**
YWCA of Greater Portland
1111 SW 10th Ave
Portland, OR 97205   503-294-7400
FAX: 503-721-1751
connect@ywcapdx.org
http://www.ywcapdx.org
Susan Staoltenberg, Executive Director
Tracy Madsen, Development Director
Patricia Martin, Program Manager
*Rebecca Alexander, Foundation & Corporate Relations Program
Manager*
Promotes the understanding of racism and all forms of discrimi-
nation and fosters value, respect, and enjoyment of each person's
unique contribution.

7982 **Youth Leadership Camp**
National Association of the Deaf
8630 Fenton Street
Suite 820
Silver Spring, MD 20910   301-587-1788
FAX: 301-587-1791
info@nad.org
www.nad.org
Christopher Wagnor, President
Melissa S. Draganac-Hawk, VP
Howard A. Rosenblum, CEO
Joshua Beckman, Secretary
Sponsored by the National Association of the Deaf, this camp em-
phasizes leadership training for deaf teenagers and young adults.
In addition to many recreational activities and sports, there are
academic offerings and camp projects.

Print: Books

7983 **A Basic Course in American Sign Language**
TJ Publishers
2544 Tarpley Rd
Suite 108
Carrollton, TX 75006-2288   972-416-0800
800-999-1168
FAX: 972-416-0944
customerservice@tjpublishers.com
www.tjpublishers.com
Tom Humphries, Author
Carol Padden, Co-Author
Terrence J O'Rouke, Co-Author
Tanner Beach, Director
The first three DVDs in this series are designed to illustrate and
demonstrate each of the exercises and dialogues presented in A
Basic Course in American Sign Language. Four Deaf teachers
and three hearing students provide a variety of models for the ex-
ercises. $35.95
288 pages Spiral Bound
ISBN 0-932666-42-6

7984 **A Basic Course in Manual Communication**
Gallaudet University Bookstore
800 Florida Ave NE
Washington, DC 20002-3600   202-651-5855
866-204-0504
FAX: 773-660-2235
TTY: 202-651-5855
gupress@gallaudet.edu
www.clerccenter.gallaudet.edu
Terrence J O'Rourke, Author
T. Alan Hurwitz, President
Paul Kelly, Vice President Adm and Finance
Teach your students manual communication - that living, chang-
ing, growing language of signs.
161 pages Softcover

7985 **A Basic Vocabulary: American Sign Languagefor Parents and Children**
TJ Publishers
2544 Tarpley Rd
Suite 108
Carrollton, TX 75006-2288

972-416-0800
800-999-1168
FAX: 972-416-0944
customerservice@tjpublishers.com
www.tjpublishers.com

Terrence J O'Rouke, Author
Tanner Beach, Director
Carefully selected words and signs include those that children use every day. Alphabetically organized vocabulary incorporates developmental lists helpful to both deaf and hearing children and over 1000 clear sign language illustrations. *$9.95*
240 pages Softcover
ISBN 0-932666-00-0

7986 **A Loss for Words**
HarperCollins Publishers
10 E 53rd St
New York, NY 10022-5244

212-207-7901
800-242-7737
FAX: 212-702-2586
spsales@harpercollins.com
www.harpercollins.com

Lou Ann Walker, Author
From the time she was a toddler, Lou Ann Walker was the ears and voice for her deaf parents. Their family life was warm and loving, but outside the home, they faced a world that misunderstood and often rejected them. *$13.00*
224 pages Paperback 1987
ISBN 0-060914-25-4

7987 **Access for All: Integrating Deaf, Hard of Hearing and Hearing Preschoolers**
Gallaudet University Bookstore
800 Florida Avenue NorthEast
Washington, DC 20002-3600

202-651-5530
FAX: 202-651-5489
gupress@gallaudet.edu
http://www.gallaudet.edu

Stephanie Cawthon, Ph.D., Book Review Editor
Peter V. Paul, Ph.D., Editor, Literary Issues
Ye Wang, Ph.D., Senior Associate Editor
Feifei Ye, Ph.D., Associate Editor for Research Methodology
This exciting new 90 minute videotape and manual describes a model program for integrating deaf and hard of hearing children in early education.
169 pages Book & Video

7988 **Advanced Sign Language Vocabulary: A Resource Text for Educators**
Charles C. Thomas
2600 S First St
Springfield, IL 62704-4730

217-789-8980
800-258-8980
FAX: 217-789-9130
books@ccthomas.com
www.ccthomas.com

Michael P. Thomas, President
Elizabeth E Wolf, Co-Author
A resource text for educators, interpreters, parents and sign language instructors. *$53.95*
202 pages Spiral Paper
ISBN 0-398057-22-0

7989 **American Sign Language Handshape Dictionary**
Gallaudet University Press
800 Florida Ave NE
Washington, DC 20002-3600

773-568-1550
800-621-2736
FAX: 773-660-2235
TTY: 888-630-9347
gupress@gallaudet.edu
www.gupress.gallaudet.edu

Richard A Tennant, Author
Marianne Gluszak Brown, Co-Author
Valerie Nelson-Metlay, Illustrator
T. Alan Hurwitz, President
The new DVD shows how each sign is formed from beginning to end. Users can watch a sign at various speeds to learn precisely how to master it themselves. Together, the new edition of The American Sign Language Handshape Dictionary and its accompanying DVD presents students, sign language teachers, and deaf and hearing people alike with the perfect combination for enhancing communication skills in both ASL and English. *$45.00*
408 pages Hardcover
ISBN 1-563680-43-2

7990 **American Sign Language Phrase Book**
TJ Publishers
2544 Tarpley Rd
Suite 108
Carrollton, TX 75006-2288

972-416-0800
800-999-1168
FAX: 972-416-0944
customerservice@tjpublishers.com
www.tjpublishers.com

Lou Fant, Author
Terrence O'Rourke, Principal
Tanner Beach, Director
The author provides interesting, realistic and meaningful situations. Sign language is learned through novel remarks cleverly organized around everyday topics. *$18.95*
362 pages Softcover
ISBN 0-809235-00-5

7991 **American Sign Language: A Look at Its History, Structure & Community**
TJ Publishers
2544 Tarpley Rd
Suite 108
Carrollton, TX 75006-2288

972-416-0800
800-999-1168
FAX: 972-416-0944
customerservice@tjpublishers.com
www.tjpublishers.com

Charlotte Baker-Shenk, Author
Carol Padden, Co-Author
Terrence O'Rourke, Principal
Tanner Beach, Director
Answers basic questions about American Sign Language. What is it? What is its history? Who uses it? What is the Deaf community? Why is ASL important? What are the building blocks of ASL? What is the relationship between ASL and body language? What are examples of ASL -grammar? *$4.95*
22 pages Softcover
ISBN 0-93266 -01-9

7992 **At Home Among Strangers**
Gallaudet University Press
800 Florida Ave NE
Washington, DC 20002-3600

773-568-1550
800-621-2736
FAX: 773-660-2235
TTY: 888-630-9347
gupress@gallaudet.edu
www.gupress.gallaudet.edu

Jerome D Schein, Author
T. Alan Hurwitz, President
Paul Kelly, Vice President Adm And Finance

At Home Among Strangers presents an engrossing portrait of the Deaf community as a complex, nationwide social network that offers unique kinship to deaf people across the country. $36.95
264 pages Paperback
ISBN 1-563681-41-2

7993   BPPV: What You Need to Know
Vestibular Disorders Association
5018 NE 15th Ave
Portland, OR 97211-5331

503-229-7705
800-837-8428
FAX: 503-229-8064
veda@vestibular.org
www.vestibular.org

P J Haybach, Author
Lisa Haven, Executive Director
Jerry Underwood, Managing Director
Vincente Honrubia, Director
The aim of this book is to present basic information about benign paroxysmal positional vertigo (BPPV) including what it is, causes, how it is diagnosed, various treatments currently in use, and strategies for coping with the symptoms associated with BPPV. $29.95
207 pages Hardcover
ISBN 0-963261-14-2

7994   Ben's Story: A Deaf Child's Right to Sign
Gallaudet University Bookstore
800 Florida Avenue NorthEast
Washington, DC 20002-3600

202-651-5530
FAX: 202-651-5489
gupress@gallaudet.edu
http://www.gallaudet.edu

Stephanie Cawthon, Ph.D., Book Review Editor
Peter V. Paul, Ph.D., Editor, Literary Issues
Ye Wang, Ph.D., Senior Associate Editor
Feifei Ye, Ph.D., Associate Editor for Research Methodology
This is a mother's story of how she responded to the diagnosis of her son's deafness and how she struggled to have her son educated using sign language.
267 pages Softcover
ISBN 0-930323-47-5

7995   Book of Name Signs: Naming in American Sign Language
DawnSign Press
6130 Nancy Ridge Dr
San Diego, CA 92121-3223

858-625-0600
800-549-5350
FAX: 858-625-2336
info@dawnsign.com
www.dawnsign.com

Joe Dannis, President
Sam Supalla, Author
To explain how a name sign is chosen in the Deaf community, professor and researcher Sam Supalla wrote this valuable resource book. Revealing fascinating insights about the origins of ASL name signs, Supalla shows how they serve the same function as given names used in the hearing community. He also details how the history of the name sign system dates back to the early years of deaf education in America. Included for reference is a list of more than 500 name signs available for selection. $12.95
120 pages Paperback 1992
ISBN 0-915035-30-4

7996   Chelsea: The Story of a Signal Dog
Gallaudet University Bookstore
800 Florida Ave NE
Washington, DC 20002-3600

202-651-5855
866-204-0504
FAX: 773-660-2235
TTY: 202-651-5855
gupress@gallaudet.edu
www.clerccenter.gallaudet.edu

Paul Ogden, Author
T. Alan Hurwitz, President
Paul Kelly, Vice President Adm. And Finance

This is a story of a young deaf couple and their Belgian sheepdog, who acts as their ears. It explains how these dogs are trained and paired with their new owners.
169 pages

7997   Children of a Lesser God
Gallaudet University Bookstore
800 Florida Ave NE
Washington, DC 20002-3600

202-651-5855
866-204-0504
FAX: 773-660-2235
TTY: 202-651-5855
gupress@gallaudet.edu
www.clerccenter.gallaudet.edu

Mark Medoff, Author
T. Alan Hurwitz, President
Paul Kelly, Vice President Adm. And Finance
The movie that won the hearts of thousands. This is a story of a deaf woman who refuses to succumb to the hearing people's image of what a deaf person should be.
91 pages Softcover
ISBN 0-822202-03-4

7998   Choices in Deafness: A Parent's Guide to Communication Options
Woodbine House
6510 Bells Mill Rd
Bethesda, MD 20817-1636

301-897-3570
800-843-7323
FAX: 301-897-5838
info@woodbinehouse.com
www.woodbinehouse.com

Irv Shapell, Owner
Sue Schwartz, PhD., Editor
A useful aid in choosing the appropriate communication option for a child with a hearing loss. Experts present the following communication options: Auditory-Verbal Approach, Bilingual-Bicultural Approach, Cued Speech, Oral Approach, and Total Communication. This new edition explains medical causes of hearing loss, the diagnostic process, audiological assessment, and cochlear implants. Children and parents also offer their personal experiences. $24.95
400 pages Paperback
ISBN 1-890627-73-7

7999   Cochlear Implants for Kids
Alexander Graham Bell Association
3417 Volta Pl NW
Washington, DC 20007-2737

202-337-5220
FAX: 202-337-8314
info@agbell.org
www.listeningandspokenlanguage.org

Warren Estabrooks MEd, Editor
Alexander T. Graham, Executive Director
Susan Boswell, Director of Communications and Marketing
Judy Harrison, Director of Programs
Designed to educate readers about cochlear implants, including surgery, the importance of rehabilitation and the significance of parents' and professionals' roles. $12.49
404 pages Paperback
ISBN 0-882002-08-2

8000   Cognition, Education and Deafness: Directions for Research and Instruction
Gallaudet University Press
800 Florida Ave NE
Washington, DC 20002-3600

773-568-1550
800-621-2736
FAX: 773-660-2235
TTY: 888-630-9347
gupress@gallaudet.edu
www.gupress.gallaudet.edu

David S Martin, Editor
T. Alan Hurwitz, President
Paul Kelly, Vice President Adm. And Finance
This groundbreaking book integrates the work of 54 contributors to the 1984 symposium on cognition, education, and deafness. It

focuses on cognition and deaf students' growth and development, problem-solving strategies, thinking processes, language development, reading methodology, measurement of potential, and intervention programs. *$50.00*
248 pages Paperback
ISBN 1-563681-49-8

8001 College and University Programs for Deaf and Hard of Hearing Students
Gallaudet & NTID
800 Florida Avenue NE
Gallaudet University
Washington, DC 20002
    202-651-5000
    800-451-8834
    FAX: 202-651-5508
    www.lulu.com

S. Benaissa, & L. Dunning, Co-Authors
J. DeCaro, M. Karchmer, Co-Authors
J Hochgesang , Co-Author
T. Alan Hurwitz, President
Compiled by Gallaudet University and the National Technical Institute for the Deaf, this publication is a guide to accessibility for deaf and hard of hearing students in American colleges and universities. Available through LuLu Publishing. *$11.50*
240 pages Paperback
ISBN 9-998242-81-9

8002 Come Sign with Us
Gallaudet University Press
800 Florida Ave NE
Washington, DC 20002-3600
    773-568-1550
    800-621-2736
    FAX: 773-660-2235
    TTY: 888-630-9347
    gupress@gallaudet.edu
    www.gupress.gallaudet.edu

Jan C Hafer, Author
Robert M Wilson, Co-Author
T. Alan Hurwitz, President
Paul Kelly, Vice President Adm. And Finance
This fun guide for parents and educators on teaching hearing children how to sign has been thoroughly revised with completely new activities that provide contexts for practice. *$39.95*
160 pages Paperback
ISBN 1-563680-51-3

8003 Comprehensive Reference Manual for Signers and Interpreters
Charles C. Thomas
2600 S First St
Springfield, IL 62704-4730
    217-789-8980
    800-258-8980
    FAX: 217-789-9130
    books@ccthomas.com
    www.ccthomas.com

Michael P. Thomas, President
Cheryl M. Hoffman, Author
A classic in sign language literature since its introduction over two decades ago, this updated and expanded sixth edition of Comprehensive Reference Manual for Signers and Interpreters contains almost seven thousand entries, including vocabulary and idioms, with cross-references and sign descriptions. It is intended primarily for interpreters, but it can also be used effectively by signers who have at least a working knowledge of sign language. *$59.95*
404 pages Spiral Paper 1909
ISBN 0-398078-58-4

8004 Comprehensive Signed English Dictionary
Gallaudet University Press
800 Florida Ave NE
Washington, DC 20002-3600
    773-568-1550
    800-621-2736
    FAX: 773-660-2235
    TTY: 888-630-9347
    gupress@gallaudet.edu
    www.gupress.gallaudet.edu

Harry Bornstein, Editor
Karen L. Saulnier, Editor
Lillian B. Hamilton, Editor
T. Paul Hurwitz, President
The Comprehensive Signed English Dictionary is the premier volume of the Signed English series. This complete dictionary more than 3,100 signs, including signs reflecting lively, contemporary vocabulary. *$45.00*
464 pages Casebound
ISBN 0-913580-81-3

8005 Conversational Sign Language II: An Intermediate Advanced Manual
Gallaudet University Press
800 Florida Ave NE
Washington, DC 20002-3600
    773-568-1550
    800-621-2736
    FAX: 773-660-2235
    TTY: 888-630-9347
    gupress@gallaudet.edu
    www.gupress.gallaudet.edu

William J Madsen, Author
T. Alan Hurwitz, President
Paul Kelly, Vice President Adm. And Finance
This book presents English words and their American Sign Language (ASL) equivalents in 63 lessons. Part one covers 750 words and their signs. Part two deals with the interpretation of 220 English idioms (which have over 300 usages in ASL). Part three presents over 300 ASL idioms and colloquialisms prevalent in informal conversations. *$17.95*
236 pages Paperback
ISBN 0-913580-00-7

8006 Deaf Empowerment: Emergence, Struggle and Rhetoric
Gallaudet University Press
800 Florida Ave NE
Washington, DC 20002-3600
    773-568-1550
    800-621-2736
    FAX: 773-660-2235
    TTY: 888-630-9347
    gupress@gallaudet.edu
    www.gupress.gallaudet.edu

Katherine A Jankowski, Author
T. Alan Hurwitz, President
Paul Kelly, Vice President Adm. And Finance
Employing the methodology successfully used to explore other social movements in America, this meticulous study examines the rhetorical foundation that motivated Deaf people to work for social change during the past two centuries. *$49.95*
192 pages Hardcover
ISBN 1-563680-61-0

8007 Deaf History Unveiled: Interpretations from the New Scholarship
Gallaudet University Press
800 Florida Ave NE
Washington, DC 20002-3600
    773-568-1550
    800-621-2736
    FAX: 773-660-2235
    TTY: 888-630-9347
    gupress@gallaudet.edu
    www.gallaudet.edu

John Vickrey Van Cleve, Editor
T. Alan Hurwitz, President
Paul Kelly, Vice President Adm. And Finance
Deaf History Unveiled features 16 essays, including work by Harlan Lane, Renate Fischer, Margret Winzer, William McCagg, and other noted historians in this field. Readers will discover the new themes driving Deaf history, including a telling comparison

of the similar experiences of Deaf people and African Americans, both minorities with identifying characteristics that cannot be hidden to thwart bias. *$36.95*

316 pages Paperback
ISBN 1-563680-87-4

8008   Deaf Like Me
Gallaudet University Press
800 Florida Ave NE
Washington, DC 20002-3600

773-568-1550
800-621-2736
FAX: 773-660-2235
TTY: 888-630-9347
gupress@gallaudet.edu
www.gupress.gallaudet.edu

Thomas S Spradley, Author
James P Spradley, Co-Author
T. Alan Hurwitz, President
Paul Kelly, Vice President Adm. And Finance

Deaf Like Me is the moving account of parents coming to terms with their baby girl's profound deafness. The love, hope, and anxieties of all hearing parents of deaf children are expressed here with power and simplicity. *$16.95*

292 pages Paperback
ISBN 0-930323-11-4

8009   Deaf Parents and Their Hearing Children
Through the Looking Glass
3075 Adeline Street
Suite 120
Berkeley, CA 94703

510-848-1112
800-644-2666
FAX: 510-848-4445
tlg@lookingglass.org
www.lookingglass.org

Maureen Block, J.D., President
Thomas Spalding, Treasurer
Alice Nemon, Secretary
Mega Kirshbaum, Author

The focus of this review article is on families with Deaf parents and hearing children. We provide a brief description of the Deaf community, their language, and culture; describe communication patterns and parenting issues in Deaf-parented families, examine the role of the hearing child in a Deaf family and how that experience affects their functioning in the hearing world; and discuss important considerations and resources for families, educators, and health care and service providers. *$2.00*

8 pages

8010   Deaf in America: Voices from a Culture
TJ Publishers
2544 Tarpley Rd
Suite 108
Carrollton, TX 75006-2288

972-416-0800
800-999-1168
FAX: 972-416-0944
customerservice@tjpublishers.com
www.tjpublishers.com

Carol Padden, Author
Tom Humphries, Co-Author
Terrence O'Rourke, Principal
Tanner Beach, Director

Now available in paperback, this book opens deaf culture to outsiders, inviting readers to imagine and understand a world of silence. This book shares the joy and satisfaction many people have with their lives and shows that deafness may not be the handicap most hearing people think. *$15.95*

134 pages Softcover
ISBN 0-674194-24-1

8011   EASE Program: Emergency Access Self Evaluation
Telecommunications for the Deaf (TDI)
8630 Fenton St
Suite 604
Silver Spring, MD 20910-3822

301-589-3786
FAX: 301-589-3797
info@tdi-online.org
tdi-online.org

Claude L Stout, Executive Director
Gloria Carter, Executive Secretary
James House, Public Relations Director
Robert McConnell, Advertising Manager

A complete training, testing, maintenance and self evaluation program that helps emergency service providers prepare for emergency calls from TTY users and to comply with the American with Disabilities Act. *$35.00*

48 pages

8012   Encyclopedia of Deafness and Hearing Disorders
Powell's Books
1005 W Burnside St
Portland, OR 97209-3114

503-228-4651
800-873-7323
help@powells.com
www.powells.com

Carol Turkington, Author
Michael Powell, Owner

Presents the most current information on deafness and hearing disorders in an authoritative A-to-Z compendium. *$7.50*

294 pages Hardcover
ISBN 0-816056-15-3

8013   Expressive and Receptive Fingerspelling for Hearing Adults
Gallaudet University Bookstore
800 Florida Ave NE
Washington, DC 20002-3600

202-651-5855
866-204-0504
FAX: 773-660-2235
TTY: 202-651-5855
gupress@gallaudet.edu
www.clerccenter.gallaudet.edu

LaVera M Guillory, Author
T. Alan Hurwitz, President
Paul Kelly, Vice President Adm. And Finance

Here is a new and meaningful way for adults to increase their comfort with fingerspelling. The system is based on the principles of phonetics rather than letters of the English alphabet.

42 pages Softcover
ISBN 0-875110-55-X

8014   Eye-Centered: A Study of Spirituality of Deaf People
National Catholic Office for the Deaf
7202 Buchanan St
Hyattsville, MD 20784-2236

301-577-1684
FAX: 301-577-1684
info@ncod.org
www.ncod.org

Bill Key, Author
Arvilla Rank, Executive Director
Deacon Patrick Graybill, Vice President
Gregory Schott, Member at Large

The findings of the five-year De Sales Project conducted by The National Catholic Office for the Deaf. *$16.70*

167 pages

8015   For Hearing People Only
Harris Communications
15155 Technology Dr
Eden Prairie, MN 55344-2273

952-388-2152
800-825-6758
FAX: 952-906-1099
TTY: 800-825-9187
info@harriscomm.com
www.harriscomm.com

Robert Harris, Owner
Linda Levitan, Co-Author
Matthew S. Moore, Co-Author
Harlan Lane, Foreword
For Hearing People Only answers some of the most common
questions hearing people ask about Deaf culture and how Deaf
people communicate and live. *$35.95*
724 pages Paperback
ISBN 0-963401-63-7

8016   From Gesture to Language in Hearing and Deaf Children
Gallaudet University Press
800 Florida Ave NE
Washington, DC 20002-3600

773-568-1550
800-621-2736
FAX: 773-660-2235
TTY: 888-630-9347
gupress@gallaudet.edu
www.gupress.gallaudet.edu

Virginia Volterra, Editor
Carol J. Erting, Editor
In 21 essays on communicative gesturing in the first two years of
life, this vital collection demonstrates the importance of gesture
in a child's transition to a linguistic system. *$45.95*
358 pages Paperback
ISBN 1-563680-78-5

8017   From Mime to Sign Package
TJ Publishers
2544 Tarpley Rd
Suite 108
Carrollton, TX 75006-2288

972-416-0800
800-999-1168
FAX: 972-416-0944
customerservice@tjpublishers.com
www.tjpublishers.com

Gilbert C Eastman, Author
Terrence O'Rourke, Principal
Tanner Beach, Director
More than 1,000 photographs illustrate how natural gestures,
mime and facial expressions used every day can become the basis
for learning sign language. *$27.95*
183 pages Softcover
ISBN 0-932666-34-5

8018   GA and SK Etiquette
Telecommunications for the Deaf
8630 Fenton Street
Suite 604
Silver Spring, MD 20910- 3822

301-589-3786
FAX: 301-589-3797
info@tdi-online.org
www.tdi-online.org

Claude L Stout, Executive Director
Keith Cagle, Co-Author
Roy Miller, President
Gloria Carter, Administrator
Promoting equal access to telecommunications and media for
people who are deaf, late-deafened, hard-of-hearing or
deaf-blind through consumer education and involvement; technical assistance and consulting; applications of exisiting and
emerging technologies; networking and collaboration; uniformity of standards; and national policy development and advocacy. *$11.95*
54 pages Paperback
ISBN 0-961462-17-5

8019   Gallaudet Survival Guide to Signing
Gallaudet University Press
800 Florida Ave NE
Washington, DC 20002-3600

773-568-1550
800-621-2736
FAX: 773-660-2235
TTY: 888-630-9347
gupress@gallaudet.edu
www.gallaudet.edu

Jon Mitchiner, Manager
Leonard G. Lane, Author
Jan Skrobisz, Illustrator
T. Alan Hurwitz, President
Features 500 of the most frequently used signs with clear illustra-
tions and descriptions for each one. *$9.95*
218 pages Paperback
ISBN 0-930323-67-X

8020   Goldilocks and the Three Bears: Told in Signed English
Gallaudet University Press
800 Florida Ave NE
Washington, DC 20002-3600

773-568-1550
800-621-2736
FAX: 773-660-2235
TTY: 888-630-9347
gupress@gallaudet.edu
www.gupress.gallaudet.edu

Harry Bornstein, Author
Karen L Saulnier, Co-Author
T. Alan Hurwitz, President
Paul Kelly, Vice President Adm. And Finance
Goldilocks and the Three Bears offers children ages 3 - 8 all of the
fun their parents had when they first read about the little girl with
the golden curls who turned the Bears' house upside down. *$
21.95*
48 pages Hardcover
ISBN 1-563680-57-2

8021   Hearing Impaired Children and Youth with Developmental Disabilities
Gallaudet University Bookstore
800 Florida Ave NE
Washington, DC 20002-3600

202-651-5855
866-204-0504
FAX: 773-660-2235
TTY: 202-651-5855
gupress@gallaudet.edu
www.clerccenter.gallaudet.edu

Evelyn Cherow, Editor
T. Alan Hurwitz, President
Paul Kelly, Vice President Adm. And Finance
The insights of 24 experts help clarify relationships between
hearing impairment and developmental difficulties and propose
interdisciplinary cooperation as an approach to the problems created. *$29.95*
394 pages Hardcover
ISBN 0-913580-97-X

8022   Hollywood Speaks: Deafness and the Film Entertainment Industry
University of Illinois Press
1325 S Oak St
MC-566
Champaign, IL 61820-6903

217-333-0950
FAX: 217-244-8082
uipress@uillinois.edu
www.press.uillinois.edu

Willis G. Regier, Director
John S. Schuchman, Author
Kathy O'Neill, Assistant To The Director
Laurie Matheson, Editor-in-Chief
How deafness has been treated in movies and how it provides yet
another window onto social history in addition to a fresh angle
from which to view Hollywood. *$27.00*
200 pages Paperback 1999
ISBN 0-252068-50-8

8023 I Have a Sister, My Sister is Deaf
HarperCollins Publishers
10 E 53rd St
New York, NY 10022-5244
212-207-7901
800-242-7737
FAX: 212-702-2586
spsales@harpercollins.com
www.harpercollins.com

Jeanne Whitehouse Peterson, Author
Deborah Kogan Ray, Illustrator
Ann Ledden, Vice President
Lorna Metzler, Manager
An emphatic, affirmative look at the relationship between siblings, as a young deaf child is affectionately described by her older sister. This Coretta Scott King Honor Award winner helps young children develop an understanding that deaf children share the same interests as hearing children. *$6.99*
32 pages Paperback 1984
ISBN 0-064430-59-6

8024 Independence Without Sight or Sound
AFB Press
2 Penn Plaza
Suite 1102
New York, NY 10121-2006
212-502-7600
800-232-5463
FAX: 888-545-8331
afbweb@afb.net
www.afb.org

Richard Obnen, Chairman Of The Board
Carl Augusto, President and CEO
Rick Bozeman, Chief Financial Officer
Kelly Bleach, Chief Administrative Officer
This practical guidebook covers the essential aspects of communicating and working with deaf-blind persons. Full of valuable information on subjects such as how to talk with deaf-blind people, adapt orientation and mobility techniques for deaf-blind travelers, and interact with deaf-blind individuals socially, this useful manual also contains a substantial resource section detailing sources of information and adapted equipment. *$39.95*
193 pages Paperback
ISBN 0-891282-46-4

8025 Innovative Practices for Teaching Sign Language Interpreters
Gallaudet University Press
800 Florida Ave NE
Washington, DC 20002-3600
773-568-1550
800-621-2736
FAX: 773-660-2235
TTY: 888-630-9347
gupress@gallaudet.edu
www.gupress.gallaudet.edu
Cynthia B Roy, Editor
Researchers now understand interpreting as an active process between two languages and cultures, with social interaction, sociolinguistics, and discourse analysis as more appropriate theoretical frameworks. Roy's penetrating new book acts upon these new insights by presenting six dynamic teaching practices to help interpreters achieve the highest level of skill. *$45.95*
200 pages Hardcover
ISBN 1-563680-88-2

8026 Intermediate Conversational Sign Language
Gallaudet University Press
800 Florida Ave NE
Washington, DC 20002-3600
773-568-1550
800-621-2736
FAX: 773-660-2235
TTY: 888-630-9347
gupress@gallaudet.edu
www.gupress.gallaudet.edu
Willard J Madsen, Author
This fully illustrated text offers a unique approach to using American Sign Language (ASL) and English in a bilingual setting. Each of the 25 lessons involve sign language conversation using

colloquialisms that are prevalent in informal conversations. *$31.50*
400 pages Softcover
ISBN 0-913580-79-1

8027 Interpretation: A Sociolinguistic Model
Sign Media
4020 Blackburn Ln
Burtonsville, MD 20866-1167
301-421-0268
800-475-4756
FAX: 301-421-0270
info@signmedia.com
www.signmedia.com

Verden Ness, President
Dennis Cokely, Author
This text presents a sociolinguistically sensitive model of the interpretation process. The model applies to interpretation in any two languages although this one focuses on ASL and English. *$22.95*
199 pages
ISBN 0-932130-10-0

8028 Interpreting: An Introduction
Registry of Interpreters for the Deaf
333 Commerce St
Alexandria, VA 22314-2801
703-838-0030
FAX: 703-838-0454
TTY:703-838-0459
ridinfo@rid.org
www.rid.org

Nancy J Frishberg, Author
Shane Feldman, Executive Director
Don Roose, Director
Emil Ladner, Director
This text is written by a practicing interpreter and includes information on history, terminology, research, competence, setting and a comprehensive bibliography. *$24.95*
249 pages Softcover
ISBN 0-916883-07-8

8029 Joy of Signing
Gospel Publishing House
1445 N Boonville Ave
Springfield, MO 65802-1894
417-862-8000
800-641-4310
FAX: 417-862-5881
CustSrvOrders@ag.org
www.gospelpublishing.com

Lottie L Riekehof, Author
This manual on signing includes illustrations, information on sign origins, practice sentences, and step-by-step descriptions of hand positions and movements. *$23.99*
352 pages Hardcover
ISBN 0-882435-20-5

8030 Joy of Signing Puzzle Book
Harris Communications
15155 Technology Dr
Eden Prairie, MN 55344-2273
952-388-2152
800-825-6758
FAX: 952-906-1099
TTY: 800-825-9187
info@harriscomm.com
www.harriscomm.com

Robert Harris, Owner
Lottie L Riekehof, Co-Author
Whether you are learning sign language to communicate with a family member, co-worker, student or friend, this puzzle book makes the learning fun and interesting. *$4.50*
57 pages Softcover
ISBN 0-882436-76-7

8031 **Kid-Friendly Parenting with Deaf and Hard of Hearing Children**
Gallaudet University Press
800 Florida Ave NE
Washington, DC 20002-3600
773-568-1550
800-621-2736
FAX: 773-660-2235
TTY: 888-630-9347
gupress@gallaudet.edu
www.gupress.gallaudet.edu

Daria Medwid, Author
Denise Chapman Weston, Co-Author
At each chapter's beginning, experts (some deaf, some hearing), including I. King Jordan, Jack Gannon, Merv Garretson, and others, offer their insights on the subject discussed. Designed for parents with various styles, Kid-Friendly Parenting is a complete, step-by-step guide and reference to raising a deaf or hard of hearing child. *$35.95*
320 pages Paperback
ISBN 1-563680-31-9

8032 **Laurent Clerc: The Story of His Early Years**
Gallaudet University Press
800 Florida Ave NE
Washington, DC 20002-3600
773-568-1550
800-621-2736
FAX: 773-660-2235
TTY: 888-630-9347
gupress@gallaudet.edu
www.gupress.gallaudet.edu

Cathryn Carroll, Author
T. Alan Hurwitz, President
Paul Kelly, Vice President Adm. And Finance
In his own voice, Clerc vividly relates the experiences that led to his later progressive teaching methods. Especially influential was his long stay at the Royal National Institute for the Deaf in Paris, where he encountered sharply distinct personalities - the saintly, inspiring deaf teacher Massieu, the vicious Dr. Itard and his heartless experiments on deaf boys, and the Father of the Deaf, Abbe Sicard, who could hardly sign. *$13.95*
208 pages Paperback
ISBN 0-930323-23-8

8033 **Linguistics of American Sign Language: An Introduction**
Gallaudet University Press
800 Florida Ave NE
Washington, DC 20002-3600
773-568-1550
800-621-2736
FAX: 773-660-2235
TTY: 888-630-9347
gupress@gallaudet.edu
www.gupress.gallaudet.edu

Clayton Valli, Author
Ceil Lucas, Co-Author
Kristin J Mulrooney, Co-Author
Miako Villanueva, President
Completely reorganized to reflect the growing intricacy of the study of ASL linguistics, the 5th edition presents 26 units in seven parts. Part One: Introduction presents a revision of Defining Language and an entirely new unit, Defining Linguistics. Part Two: Phonology has been completely updated with new terminology and examples. *$75.00*
560 pages Hardcover
ISBN 1-563682-83-4

8034 **Literacy & Your Deaf Child: What Every Parent Should Know**
Gallaudet University Press
800 Florida Ave NE
Washington, DC 20002-3600
773-568-1550
800-621-2736
FAX: 773-660-2235
TTY: 888-630-9347
gupress@gallaudet.edu
www.gupress.gallaudet.edu

David A Stewart, Author
Bryan R Clarke, Co-Author
T. Alan Hurwitz, President
Paul Kelly, Vice President Adm. And Finance
Literacy and Your Deaf Child begins by introducing some common concepts, among them the importance of parental involvement in a deaf child's education. It outlines how children acquire language and describes the auditory and visual links to literacy. *$24.95*
240 pages Paperback
ISBN 1-563681-36-6

8035 **Mask of Benevolence: Disabling the Deaf Community, The**
DawnSign Press
6130 Nancy Ridge Dr
San Diego, CA 92121-3223
858-625-0600
800-549-5350
FAX: 858-625-2336
info@dawnsign.com
www.dawnsign.com

Joe Dannis, President
Harlan Lane, Author
Dr. Harlan Lane does not view deafness as a handicap but rather a different state from hearing. Deaf people are a societal minority and should be treasured, not eradicated. *$12.95*
360 pages Paperback 1992
ISBN 1-581210-09-5

8036 **Mother Father Deaf: Living Between Sound and Silence**
Harvard University Press
79 Garden St
Cambridge, MA 02138-1423
617-495-2600
800-405-1619
FAX: 617- 49- 589
contact_hup@harvard.edu
www.hup.harvard.edu

William Sisler, President
Paul Preston, Author
The book explores the intimate intersection of families like his own - families which embody the conflicts and resolutions of two often opposing world views, the Deaf and the Hearing. Although I have normal hearing, both of my parents are profoundly deaf. *$19.50*
278 pages Paperback
ISBN 0-674587-48-0

8037 **My First Book of Sign**
Gallaudet University Press
800 Florida Ave NE
Washington, DC 20002-3600
773-568-1550
800-621-2736
FAX: 773-660-2235
TTY: 888-630-9347
gupress@gallaudet.edu
www.gupress.gallaudet.edu

Pamela J Baker, Author
Patricia Bellan Gillen, Illustrator
T. Alan Hurwitz, President
Paul Kelly, Vice President Adm. And Finance
Full-color book gives alphabetically grouped signs for 150 words most frequently used by young children. *$22.95*
80 pages Hardcover
ISBN 0-930323-20-3

8038 **My Signing Book of Numbers**
Gallaudet University Press
800 Florida Ave NE
Washington, DC 20002-3600
773-568-1550
800-621-2736
FAX: 773-660-2235
TTY: 888-630-9347
gupress@gallaudet.edu
www.gupress.gallaudet.edu

Patricia Bellan Gillen, Author
This full-color book helps children learn their numbers in sign language. Each two-page spread of this delightfully illustrated book has the appropriate number of things or creatures for the numbers 0 through 20. *$22.95*
56 pages Hardcover
ISBN 0-930323-37-8

8039 **Nursery Rhymes from Mother Goose**
Gallaudet University Press
800 Florida Ave NE
Washington, DC 20002-3600
773-568-1550
800-621-2736
FAX: 773-660-2235
TTY: 888-630-9347
gupress@gallaudet.edu
www.gupress.gallaudet.edu

Harry Bornstein, Author
Karen L Saulnier, Co-Author
Patricia Peters, Illustrator
Linda Tom, Illustrator
Young readers, both hearing and deaf, will learn the special charm of rhyme while also discovering new vocabulary and new ways to experience English through signing. As they learn and memorize their favorite verses, children will also strengthen their language skills in a fun, entertaining way. *$21.95*
64 pages Hardcover
ISBN 0-930323-99-8

8040 **Outsiders in a Hearing World: A Sociology of Deafness**
Sage Publications
2455 Teller Rd
Thousand Oaks, CA 91320-2218
805-499-9774
800-818-7243
FAX: 805-499-0871
www.sagepub.com

Paul C Higgins, Author
An introduction to the social world of deaf people. The author gives a sociologists view of what it's like to be deaf. *$72.95*
208 pages Hardcover 1980
ISBN 0-803914-22-3

8041 **Perigee Visual Dictionary of Signing**
Harris Communications
15155 Technology Dr
Eden Prairie, MN 55344-2273
952-388-2152
800-825-6758
FAX: 952-906-1099
TTY: 800-825-9187
info@harriscomm.com
www.harriscomm.com

Robert Harris, Owner
Mickey Flodin, Co-Author
Rod R Butterworth, Co-Author
An A-to-Z guide to American Sign Language vocabulary. *$15.26*
450 pages Softcover
ISBN 0-399519-52-1

8042 **Phone of Our Own: The Deaf Insurrection Against Ma Bell**
Gallaudet University Press
800 Florida Ave NE
Washington, DC 20002-3600
773-568-1550
800-621-2736
FAX: 773-660-2235
TTY: 888-630-9347
gupress@gallaudet.edu
www.gupress.gallaudet.edu

Harry G Lang, Author
T. Alan Hurwitz, President
Paul Kelly, Vice President Adm. And Finance
A recount of the history of the teletypewriter, from the three deaf engineers who developed the acoustic coupler that made mass communication on TTY's feasible, through the deaf community's twenty-year struggle against the government and AT&T to have TTY's produced and distributed. *$36.50*
256 pages Hardcover
ISBN 1-563680-90-4

8043 **Place of Their Own: Creating the Deaf Community in America**
Gallaudet University Press
800 Florida Ave NE
Washington, DC 20002-3600
773-568-1550
800-621-2736
FAX: 773-660-2235
TTY: 888-630-9347
gupress@gallaudet.edu
www.gallaudet.edu

John V Van Cleve, Author
Barry A Crouch, Co-Author
T. Alan Hurwitz, President
Paul Kelly, Vice President Adm. And Finance
Traces development of American deaf society to show how deaf people developed a common language and sense of community. Views deafness as the distinguishing characteristic of a distinct culture. *$22.95*
224 pages Paperback
ISBN 0-930323-49-1

8044 **PreReading Strategies**
Gallaudet University Bookstore
800 Florida Ave NE
Washington, DC 20002-3600
202-651-5855
866-204-0504
FAX: 773-660-2235
TTY: 202-651-5855
gupress@gallaudet.edu
www.clerccenter.gallaudet.edu

David R Schleper, Author
T. Alan Hurwitz, President
Paul Kelly, Vice President Adm. And Finance
Here is a wealth of good advice for preparing students to understand what they read, building comprehension and enjoyment. *$14.95*
65 pages

8045 **Quad City Deaf & Hard of Hearing Youth Group: Tomorrow's Leaders for our Community**
Independent Living Research Utilization ILRU
2323 S Shepherd Dr
Houston, TX 77019-7019
713-520-9058
FAX: 713-520-5785
ilru@ilru.org

Lex Frieden, Director
Rose Sheperd, Manager
IICIL staff see this program as a way to develop young leaders for themovement. Emphasis is given to providing oppportunities for members of the youth group to develop skills in planning and organizing activities.

8046 Religious Signing: A Comprehensive Guide for All Faiths
TJ Publishers
P.O. Box 702701
Dallas, TX 75370

972-416-0800
800-999-1168
FAX: 972-416-0944
TTY: 301-585-4440
TJPubinc@aol.com
www.tjpublishers.com

Elaine Costello, Author
Terrence O'Rourke, Principal
Tanner Beach, Director
Contains over 500 religious signs for all denominations and their meanings illustrated by clear upper torso illustrations that show movements of hand, body and face. Includes a section on signing favorite verses, prayers and blessings. *$18.95*
219 pages Softcover
ISBN 0-553342-44-4

8047 Seeing Voices
Vintage and Anchor Books
1745 Broadway
3rd Floor
New York, NY 10019

212-782-9000
FAX: 212-572-6066
vintageanchor@randomhouse.com
www.randomhouse.com

Oliver Sacks, Author
Madeline McIntosh, President/Sales/Operations
Markus Dohle, Chairman/CEO
Andrew Weber, SVP Operations And Technology
Well known for his exploration of how people respond to neurological impairments, Dr Sacks explores the world of the deaf and discovers how deaf people respond to their loss of hearing and how they develop language. A highly readable introduction to deaf people, deaf culture and American Sign Language. *$13.95*
240 pages Softcover 2000
ISBN 0-375704-07-8

8048 Sign Language Interpreting and Interpreter Education
Oxford University Press
2001 Evans Rd
Cary, NC 27513-2009

919-677-0977
800-445-9714
FAX: 919-677-1303
custserv.us@oup.com
www.oup.com

Marc Marschark, Editor
Rico Peterson, Editor
Elizabeth A Winston, Editor
Patricia Sapere, Contributing Editor
Provides a coherent picture of the field as a whole, including evaluation of the extent to which current practices are supported by validating research. The first comprehensive source, suitable as both a reference book and a textbook for interpreter training programs and a variety of courses on bilingual education, psycholinguistics and translation, and cross-linguistic studies. *$65.00*
328 pages Hardcover
ISBN 0-195176-94-4

8049 Signed English Starter, The
Gallaudet University Press
800 Florida Ave NE
Washington, DC 20002-3600

773-568-1550
800-621-2736
FAX: 773-660-2235
TTY: 888-630-9347
gupress@gallaudet.edu
www.gupress.gallaudet.edu

Harry Bornstein, Author
Karen L Saulnier, Co-Author
T. Alan Hurwitz, President
Paul Kelly, Vice President Adm. And Finance
A first course in Signed English for adults and children, the book is fully illustrated (several figures per page), and it is organized in a way that leads to rewarding learning quite rapidly. The authors of this new and exciting text believe firmly that Signed English

must be made as easy as possible if it is going to be as useful (and used) as it can and should be. The book explains the rationale for the Signed English system and the conventions used to teach it. *$18.50*
232 pages Paperback
ISBN 0-913580-82-1

8050 Signing Family: What Every Parent Should Know About Sign Communication, The
Gallaudet University Press
800 Florida Ave NE
Washington, DC 20002-3600

773-568-1550
800-621-2736
FAX: 773-660-2235
TTY: 888-630-9347
gupress@gallaudet.edu
www.gupress.gallaudet.edu

David A Stewart, Author
Barbara Luetke-Stahlman, Co-Author
T. Alan Hurwitz, President
Paul Kelly, Vice President Adm. And Finance
This reader-friendly book shows parents how to create a set of goals around the communication needs of their deaf child. Describes in even-handed terms the major signing options available, from American Sign Language to Signed English. *$29.95*
192 pages Paperback
ISBN 1-563680-69-6

8051 Signing for Reading Success
Gallaudet University Press
800 Florida Ave NE
Washington, DC 20002-3600

773-568-1550
800-621-2736
FAX: 773-660-2235
TTY: 888-630-9347
gupress@gallaudet.edu
www.gupress.gallaudet.edu

Jan C Hafer, Author
Robert M Wilson, Co-Author
T. Alan Hurwitz, President
Paul Kelly, Vice President Adm. And Finance
This booklet provides summaries of four research students on the usefulness of signing for reading achievement. *$7.95*
24 pages Paperback
ISBN 0-930323-18-1

8052 Signing: How to Speak with Your Hands
TJ Publishers
2427 Bond Street
Suite 108
University Park, IL 60466- 2288

972-416-0800
800-999-1168
FAX: 972-416-0944
customerservice@tjpublishers.com
www.tjpublishers.com

Elaine Costello, Author
Terrence O'Rourke, Principal
Tanner Beach, Director
Presents 1,200 basic signs with clear illustrations in logical topical groupings. Linguistic principles are described at the beginning of each chapter, giving insight into the rules which govern American Sign Language. *$19.95*
248 pages Softcover
ISBN 0-553375-39-3

8053   Signs Across America
Gallaudet University Press
800 Florida Ave NE
Washington, DC 20002-3600   773-568-1550
                                   800-621-2736
                              FAX: 773-660-2235
                              TTY: 888-630-9347
                              gupress@gallaudet.edu
                              www.gupress.gallaudet.edu

Edgar H Shroyer, Author
Susan P Shroyer, Co-Author
T. Alan Hurwitz, President
Paul Kelly, Vice President Adm. And Finance
A look at regional variations in ASL. Signs for selected words
collected from 25 different states. More than 1,200 signs illus-
trated in the text. *$28.95*
304 pages Paperback
ISBN 0-913580-96-1

8054   Signs for Me: Basic Sign Vocabulary for Children, Parents
& Teachers
TJ Publishers
2427 Bond Street
Suite 108
University Park, IL 60466- 2288   972-416-0800
                                         800-999-1168
                                    FAX: 972-416-0944
                              customerservice@tjpublishers.com
                              www.tjpublishers.com

Ben Bahan, Author
Joe Dannis, Co-Author
Terrence O'Rourke, Principal
Tanner Beach, Director
Sign language vocabulary for preschool and elementary school
children introduces household items, animals, family members,
actions, emotions, safety concerns and other concepts. *$14.95*
112 pages Softcover
ISBN 0-915035-27-8

8055   Signs for Sexuality: A Resource Manual
Planned Parenthood of Western Washington
2001 E Madison St
Seattle, WA 98122-2959   206-328-7715
                           FAX: 206-328-6810
                           www.plannedparenthood.org

Marlyn Minken, Author
Laurie Rosen-Ritt, Co-Author
Cecile Richards, President
An important book for those who want to listen to and talk with
other people about feelings, loving and caring. *$40.00*
122 pages Softcover

8056   Signs of the Times
Gallaudet University Press
800 Florida Ave NE
Washington, DC 20002-3600   773-568-1550
                                   800-621-2736
                              FAX: 773-660-2235
                              TTY: 888-630-9347
                              gupress@gallaudet.edu
                              www.gupress.gallaudet.edu

Edgar H Shroyer, Author
Susan P Shroyer, Illustrator
T. Alan Hurwitz, President
Paul Kelly, Vice President Adm. And Finance
An excellent beginner's contact signing book that fills the gap be-
tween sign language dictionaries and American Sign Language
text. Designed for use as a classroom text. *$34.95*
448 pages Softcover
ISBN 0-913580-76-7

8057   Silent Garden, The
Gallaudet University Press
800 Florida Ave NE
Washington, DC 20002-3600   773-568-1550
                                   800-621-2736
                              FAX: 773-660-2235
                              TTY: 888-630-9347
                              gupress@gallaudet.edu
                              www.gupress.gallaudet.edu

Paul W Ogden, Author
T. Alan Hurwitz, President
Paul Kelly, Vice President Adm. And Finance
The author explain the broad range of hearing loss types, from minor to profound. Parents also are advised about what type of
school their child should attend and what kinds of professional
help will be best for the entire family. The book describes all
forms of communication, including choices in signing from
American Sign Language to the various manual systems based
upon English. Technological alternatives are presented also, including when and when not to consider cochler implants. *$34.95*
304 pages
ISBN 1-563680-58-0

8058   Sing Praise Hymnal for the Deaf
LifeWay Christian Resources
1 Lifeway Plz
MSN 146
Nashville, TN 37234-1001   615-251-2000
                                  800-458-2772
                             FAX: 615-251-3899
                             www.lifeway.com

Thom Rainer, President/CEO
Jerry Rhyne, CFO/ VP Finance And Buisness
Tim Vineyard, VP Technology And CIO
Designed to be used by interpreters to the deaf, sign-language
students, and deaf members of the congregation, this special
combined hymnal edition offers 234 of the most popular hymns.
$12.95
Hardcover 2000
ISBN 0-767314-09-3

8059   TDI National Directory & Resource Guide: Blue Book
Telecommunications for the Deaf
8630 Fenton Street
Suite 604
Silver Spring, MD 20910- 3822   301-589-3786
                                  FAX: 301-589-3797
                                  info@tdi-online.org
                                  www.tdi-online.org

Claude L Stout, Executive Director
Promoting Equal Access to Telecommunications and Media for
People who are Deaf, Late-Deafened, Hard-of-Hearing or
Deaf-Blind. *$ 20.00*
600 pages Annual

8060   Theoretical Issues in Sign Language Research
University of Chicago Press
1427 E 60th St
Chicago, IL 60637-2902   773-702-7700
                           FAX: 773-702-9756
                           sales@press.uchicago.edu
                           www.press.uchicago.edu

Donald A Collins, President
Susan D Fischer, Author
Patricia Siple, Co-Author
These volumes are an outgrowth of a conference held at the Uni-
versity of Rochester in 1986, dealing with the four traditional
core areas of phonology, morphology, syntax and semantics.
$29.95
348 pages Paperback 1990
ISBN 0-226251-52-7

8061 We CAN Hear and Speak
Alexander Graham Bell Association
3417 Volta Pl NW
Washington, DC 20007-2737

202-337-5220
FAX: 202-337-8314
info@agbell.org
www.agbell.org

Carol Flexer PhD, Author
Catherine Richards MA, Co-Author
K Houston PhD, Executive Director
John Wyant, Owner
Written by parents for families of children who are deaf or hard of hearing, this work describes auditory-verbal terminology and approaches and contains personal narratives written by parents and their children who are deaf or hard of hearing. *$6.98*
184 pages Softcover

8062 Week the World Heard Gallaudet, The
Gallaudet University Press
800 Florida Ave NE
Washington, DC 20002-3600

202-651-5000
800-621-2736
FAX: 202-651-5508
gupress@gallaudet.edu
www.gupress.gallaudet.edu

Jack R Gannon, Author
T. Alan Hurwitz, President
Paul Kelly, Vice President Adm. And Finance
This day-to-day description of the events surrounding the Deaf President Now movement at Gallaudet University includes full color and black and white photographs and interviews with people involved in the events of that week. *$49.95*
176 pages Hardcover
ISBN 0-930323-54-8

8063 What is Auditory Processing?
Abilitations - Speech Bin
P.O.Box 922668
Norcross, GA 30010-2668

770-449-5700
800-850-8602
FAX: 770-510-7290
info@speechbin.com
www.speechbin.com

Susan Bell, Author
What is Auditory Processing? It is and information-packed 16-page booklet created to explain auditory processing and it's disorders and offers practical suggestions for coping with this problem. It describes the listening process and tells how to help children with auditory processing problems. It shows what families and teachers can do to help children who have trouble remembering and understanding what they hear and offers easy-to-use activities and practical suggestions. *$ 22.69*
16 pages Softcover

8064 You and Your Deaf Child: A Self-Help Guidefor Parents of Deaf and Hard of Hearing Children
Gallaudet University Press
800 Florida Ave NE
Washington, DC 20002-3600

773-568-1550
800-621-2736
FAX: 773-660-2235
TTY: 888-630-9347
gupress@gallaudet.edu
www.gupress.gallaudet.edu

John W Adams, Author
T. Alan Hurwitz, President
Paul Kelly, Vice President Adm. And Finance
Eleven chapters focus on such topics as feelings about hearing loss, the importance of communication in the family, and effective behavior management. Many chapters contain practice activities and questions to help parents retain skills taught in the chapter and check their grasp of the material. Four appendices provide references, general resources, and guidelines for evaluating educational programs. *$29.95*
224 pages Paperback
ISBN 1-563680-60-2

Print: Journals

8065 American Journal of Audiology
American Speech-Language-Hearing Association
2200 Research Blvd
Rockville, MD 20850-3289

240-632-2081
800-638-8255
FAX: 301-296-8580
actioncenter@asha.org
www.asha.org

Gary Dunham, Editor-in-Chief
Bridget Murray Law, Managing Editor
Carol Polovoy, Assistant Managing Editor
Kellie Rowden-Racette, Print and Online Writer/Editor
Articles concern screening, assesment, and treatment techniques; prevention; professional issues; supervision; administration. Includes clinical forums, clinical reviews, letters to the editor, or research reports that emphasize clinical practice.
2 x year

8066 Hearing Professional
International Hearing Society
16880 Middlebelt Rd
Ste 4
Livonia, MI 48154-3374

734-522-7200
800-521-5247
FAX: 734-522-0200
akovach@ihsinfo.org
www.ihsinfo.org

Kathleen Mennillo, MBA, Executive Director
Kara Nacarato, Editor & Mgr Of Strgc. Alliances
Scott Beall, Treasurer Director
Alan Lowell, President
Provides authoritative technical and business information that will help hearing aid specialists serve the hearing impaired.
bi-monthly

8067 JADARA
ADARA National Office
12461 Stottlemeyer Rd
Myersville, MD 21773-9620

301-293-8969
FAX: 301-293-9698
adaraorg@comcast.net
www.adara.org

Gary Dunham, Editor-in-Chief
Bridget Murray Law, Managing Editor
Carol Polovoy, Assistant Managing Editor
Kellie Rowden-Racette, Print and Online Writer/Editor
A professional journal sharing new procedures, thoughts, and research with application to the working professional.

8068 Journal of Speech, Language and Hearing Research
American Speech-Language-Hearing Association
2200 Research Blvd
Rockville, MD 20850-3289

301-296-5700
800-638-8255
FAX: 301-296-8580
actioncenter@asha.org
www.asha.org

Gary Dunham, Editor-in-Chief
Bridget Murray Law, Managing Editor
Carol Polovoy, Assistant Managing Editor
Kellie Rowden-Racette, Print and Online Writer/Editor
Pertains broadly to studies of the processess and disorders of hearing, language, and speech diagnosis and treatment of such disorders.

8069 Journal of the Academy of Rehabilitative Audiology
Academy of Rehabilitative Audiology
PO Box 2323
Albany, NY 12220-0323
952-920-0484
FAX: 952-920-6098
ara@audrehab.org
www.audrehab.org

Linda Thibodeau, President
Laura A. Wilber, Parlamentarian
Kristin V. Dilaj, Secretary
Sherri Smith, Treasurer
A peer-reviewed journal published annually. *$25.00*

8070 Literature Journal, The
Gallaudet University
800 Florida Ave NE
Washington, DC 20002-3695
202-651-5488
800-621-2736
FAX: 202-651-5508
Oluyinka.Fakunle@gallaudet.edu
www.clerccenter.gallaudet.edu

Charles C Welsh-Charrier, Author
T. Alan Hurwitz, President
Paul Kelly, Vice President Adm. And Finance
This book includes extensive examples of student and teacher entries taken from actual journals of deaf high school students. *$12.95*
44 pages Spiral Bound

8071 Sign Language Studies
Gallaudet University Press
800 Florida Ave NE
Washington, DC 20002-3695
202-651-5488
800-621-2736
FAX: 202-651-5508
gupress@gallaudet.edu
www.gupress.gallaudet.edu

Ceil Lucas, Editor
T. Alan Hurwitz, President
Paul Kelly, Vice President Adm. And Finance
Presents a unique forum for revolutionary papers on signed languages and other related disciplines, including linguistics, anthropology, semiotics, and deaf studies, history, and literature. *$ 55.00*
Quarterly

8072 Volta Review
Alexander Graham Bell Association
3417 Volta Pl NW
Washington, DC 20007-2778
202-337-5220
FAX: 202-337-8314
mfelzien@agbell.org
www.agbell.org

Jackson Roush, PhD, Editor
K Houston, PhD, Executive Director
John Wyant, Owner
Professionally refereed journal that publishes articles and research on education, rehabilitation and communicative development of people who have hearing impairments. Also includes subscription to Volta Voices, up-to-date magazine, bimonthly. *$60.00*
Quarterly

8073 Endeavor Magazine
American Society for Deaf Children
800 Florida Avenue NorthEast
#2047
Washington, Dc 20002-3695
717-703-0073
866-942-2732
800-942-ASDC
FAX: 410-795-0965
asdc@deafchildren.org
www.deafchildren.org

Beth Benedict, President
Avonne Rutowski, VP
Timothy Frelich, Treasurer
Tami Hossler, Executive Secretary

8074 Hearing Health Magazine
Deafness Research Foundation
363 Seventh Avenue
10th Floor
New York, NY 10001-3904
212-257-6140
866-454-3924
FAX: 212-257-6139
info@drf.org
www.drf.org

Andrea Boidman, Executive Director
Andrea Delbanco, Senior Editor
Yishane Lee, Editor
Julie Grant, Art Director
Serves as a source of quality information and provides the tools and resources to help people seek treatment for and manage hearing loss. Each issue features relevant and timely information on the latest research, articles written by leading authorities in the field, news about the latest technology, and human interest stories about those living with hearing loss.

8075 Hearing Loss Magazine
Hearing Loss Association of America
7910 Woodmont Ave
Ste 1200
Bethesda, MD 20814-7022
301-657-2248
FAX: 301-913-9413
info@hearingloss.org
www.hearingloss.org

Barbara Kelley, Editor-In-Chief/Deputy Ex. Dir.
Cindy Dyer, Graphic Design
Provides the latest information on products, services, research, and technology in the hearing health care field. *$35.00*
40 pages BiMonthly

8076 Tinnitus Today
American Tinnitus Association
PO Box 5
Portland, OR 97207-5
503-493-2550
800-634-8978
FAX: 503-248-0024
tinnitus@ata.org
www.ata.org

Nina Rogozen, Editor
Michael Malusevic, Executive Director
The magazine contains up-to-date medical and research news, feature articles on urgent tinnitus issues, questions and answers, self-help suggestions and letters to the editor from others with tinnitus. *$35.00*
28 pages 3 x year

8077 Volta Voices
Alexander Graham Bell Association
3417 Volta Pl NW
Washington, DC 20007-2737
202-337-5220
FAX: 202-337-8314
mfelzien@agbell.org
www.agbell.org

Melody Felzien, Editor
K Houston, Executive Director
John Wyant, Owner
Covers a variety of topics, including hearing aids and cochlear implants, early intervention and education, professional guidance, legislative updates and perspectives from individuals from across the United States and around the world. *$60.00*
Bi-Monthly

Print: Newsletters

8078 AAPD Newsletter
American Association of People with Disabilities
1629 K Street NW
Suite 950
Washington, DC 20006-1634
202-457-0046
800-840-8844
www.aapd.com

Mark Perriello, President/CEO
Helena Berger, COO
Robin Shaffert, Senior Director
Provides latest information on a variety of national disability policies and issues.

8079 ASHA Leader, The
American Speech-Language-Hearing Association
2200 Research Blvd
Rockville, MD 20850-3289
301-215-6710
800-638-8255
FAX: 301-296-8580
leader@asha.org
www.asha.org

Gary Dunham, Editor-in-Chief
Bridget Murray Law, Managing Editor
Carol Polovoy, Assistant Managing Editor
Kellie Rowden-Racette, Print and Online Writer/Editor
Association publication containing news, notices of events and activities and information for members on issues facing the profession of audiology and speech-language pathology. *$80.00*
35 pages 2 x month

8080 American Annals of the Deaf
Gallaudet University Press
800 Florida Ave NE
Washington, DC 20002-3600
202-651-5000
800-621-2736
FAX: 202-651-5508
paul.3@osu.edu
www.gupress.gallaudet.edu

Peter V. Paul, Editor, Literary Issues
T. Alan Hurwitz, President
Paul Kelly, Vice President Adm. And Finance
Quarterly publication from the Conference of Educational Administrators Serving the Deaf. *$55.00*
Quarterly

8081 CommuniquŠ
Michigan Assoc for the Deaf and Hard of Hearing

Quarterly

8082 Connect - Commmunity News
Hearing, Speech & Deafness Center (HSDC)
1625 19th Ave
Artz Communication Center
Seattle, WA 98122-2848
206-323-5770
888-222-5036
FAX: 206-328-6871
TTY:206-388-1275
admin@hsdc.org
www.hsdc.org

David Delmar, Editor
Connect is the quarterly eNews of the Hearing, Speech & Deafness Center.
8 pages Annual

8083 Deaf Catholic
International Catholic Deaf Association
7202 Buchanan St
Landover Hills, MD 20784-2236
301-429-0697
FAX: 301-429-0698
homeoffice@icda-us.org
www.icda-us.org

Jean Cox, President
Kate Slosar, Vice President
TK Hill, Treasurer
Aline Shaw, Secretary
Newsletter reporting the news of the Archdiocese, Deaf Apostolate and each of the Catholic Deaf Organizations. *$20.00*
16 pages Quarterly

8084 Hearing, Speech & Deafness Center (HSDC)
1625 19th Ave
Artz Communication Center
Seattle, WA 98122-2848
206-323-5770
888-222-5036
FAX: 206-328-6871
TTY:206-388-1275
admin@hsdc.org
www.hsdc.org

David Webster, Director of Finance
Cherylyn McRae, Director of Development
Roger Mauldin, Interim CEO
Gordon Braun, CFO
Newsletter with information on Center services, activities, news, helpful articles.
10 pages Quarterly

8085 League Letter
Center for Hearing and Communication
50 Broadway
6th Floor
New York, NY 10004-3810
917-305-7700
FAX: 917-305-7888
TTY:917-305-7999
info@chchearing.org
www.lhh.org

Laurie Hanin, Executive Director
Ellen Lafargue, Au.D., CCC, Director, Hearing Technology
Lois Kam Heymann, M.A., CCC, Director, Communication
Linda Kessler, M.A., CCC-SLP, Assistant Director, Communication

Quarterly

8086 NAHO News
National Association of Hearing Officials
PO Box 4999
Midlothian, VA 23112-17
701-328-3260
jwezelman.wezelmanlaw@midconectwork.com
www.naho.org

Joy Wezelman, Editor
Janice Deshais, Editor
National Association of Hearing Officials newsletter.

8087 Newsletter Bulletin
John Tracy Clinic
806 W Adams Blvd
Los Angeles, CA 90007-2505

213-748-5481
800-522-4582
FAX: 213-749-1651
ealaniz@jtc.org
www.jtc.org

Gaston Kent, President Director
Blythe Maling, Vice President Of Development
A newsletter for our friends and families.
8 pages Bi-annually

8088 On the Level
Vestibular Disorders Association
5018 NE 15th Ave
Portland, OR 97211-5331

503-229-7705
800-837-8428
FAX: 503-229-8064
veda@vestibular.org
www.vestibular.org

Lisa Haven PhD, Executive Director
Jerry Underwood, Director
Vincente Honrubia, Director
Contents of each issue include information about local support
groups, a calendar of conferences and training opportunities for
health professionals, a list of donors, and special items indexed
below. *$5.00*
12 pages Quarterly

8089 Paws for Silence
International Hearing Dog
5901 E 89th Ave
Henderson, CO 80640-8315

303-287-3277
FAX: 303-287-3425
info@hearingdog.org
www.ihdi.org

Valerie Foss-Brugger, Executive Director
Robert Cooley, Field Representative/Placement Counselor
Andrea Paul, Veterinary Technician/Hd Trainer
Cindy Horn, Kennel Technician & Assistant Trainer
Paws for Silence is our quarterly newsletter. In this publication
you will find up-to-date information on what's going on at IHDI,
future plans and in-depth stories.
4-8 pages Quarterly

8090 Soundings Newsletter
American Hearing Research Foundation
8 South Michigan Avenue
Suite 1205
Chicago, IL 60603- 4539

312-726-9670
FAX: 312-726-9695
ahrf@american-hearing.org
www.american-hearing.org

Sharon Parmet, Executive Director
Promote, conduct and furnish financial assistance for medical research into the cause, prevention and cure of deafness, impaired
hearing and balance disorders; encourage the collaboration of
clinical and laboratory research; encourage and improve teaching
in the medical aspects of hearing problems; and disseminate the
most reliable scientific knowledge to physicians, hearing
professionals and the public.
Quarterly

8091 Spring Dell Center Newsletter
Spring Dell Center
6040 Radio Station Rd
La Plata, MD 20646-3368

301-934-4561
FAX: 301-870-2439
donnaretzlaf@springdellcenter.org
www.springdellcenter.org

Donna Retzlaff, Executive Director
Jody Loper, President
Brett Hamorsky, Vice President
Jeff Hubbard, Treasurer

Quarterly

Non Print: Newsletters

8092 Canine Listener
Dogs for the Deaf
10175 Wheeler Rd
Central Point, OR 97502

541-826-9220
800-990-3647
800-990-3647
FAX: 541-826-6696
TTY:541-826-9220
info@dogsforthedeaf.org
dogsforthedeaf.org

Marvin Rhodes, Chair
Susan Bahr, Vice Chair
Kelly Gonzales, Development Director
Janine Bol, Finance Director
Provides information on Hearing Dogs, placements, dog training,
and other news about happenings at Dogs for the Deaf.
Quarterly

8093 Cochlear Implants In Children: Ethics and Choices
Gallaudet University Press
800 Florida Ave NE
Washington, DC 20002-3600

202-651-5000
800-621-2736
FAX: 202-651-5508
gupress@gallaudet.edu
www.gupress.gallaudet.edu

John B Christiansen, Author
Irene W Leigh, Co-Author
T. Alan Hurwitz, President
Paul Kelly, Vice President Adm. And Finance
Designed to educate readers about cochlear implants, including
surgery, the importance of rehabilitation and the significance of
parents' and professionals' roles. *$55.00*
340 pages Casebound
ISBN 1-563681-16-1

8094 Communique
Michigan Association for Deaf Hard of Hearing
5236 Dumond Court
Suite C
Lansing, MI 48917-6001

517-487-0066
800-968-7327
FAX: 517-487-2586
info@madhh.org
www.madhh.org

Nancy Asher, Executive Director
Pat Walton, Office Manager
Provides leadership through advocacy and education. The association conducts leadership training for youth, information and referral services, interpreter referral, legislative advocacy, and a
variety of other services.
4-8 pages Bi-annually

8095 Listner
HEAR Center
301 E Del Mar Blvd
Pasadena, CA 91101-2714

626-796-2016
FAX: 626-796-2320
info@hearcenter.org
www.hearcenter.org

Ellen Simon, Executive Director
Berenice Castro, Accounting Supervisro
Debbie Lorino, Office Manager
Chronicals current events, spotlights pediatric and adult clients
as well as community outreach events.
Semi-Quarterly

8096 NAD E-Zine
National Association of the Deaf
8630 Fenton Street
Suite 820
Silver Spring, MD 20910- 3819   301-587-1788
                                  FAX: 301-587-1791
                                  TTY:301-587-1789
                                      nadinfo@nad.org
                                          www.nad.org

Bobbie Beth Scoggins, President
Christopher Wagner, Vice President
Includes up-to-the-minute information about the NAD, including
Board news, advocacy, outreach and community activities, as
well as NAD Conference and other information.

8097 Pinnacle Newsletter
Academy of Rehabilitative Audiology
PO Box 26532
Minneapolis, MN 55426-532   952-920-0484
                              FAX: 952-920-6098
                                  sherri.smith@va.gov
                                      www.audrehab.org

John Greer Clark, Editor
Diana Derry, Co-Editor
Sherri Smith, Ph.D.,, Content Editor
Academy of Rehabilitative Audiology newsletter.

8098 So the World May Hear
Starkey Hearing Foundation
6700 Washington Ave S
Eden Prairie, MN 55344-3405   952-941-6401
                                      866-354-3254
                                  FAX: 952-828-6900
                          info@StarkeyFoundation.org
                              www.sotheworldmayhear.org

Brady Forseth, Executive Director
Steven Sawalich, Senior Executive Director
Ann Spilker, Director of Operations
Frederic Rondeau, International Director
Our mission, So the World May Hear, is about bringing under-
standing between people through caring and sharing. We believe
caring develops trust and by sharing we find our humanity.
Quarterly

8099 Vision Magazine
National Catholic Office of the Deaf
7202 Buchanan St
Hyattsville, MD 20784-2236   301-577-1684
                              FAX: 301-577-1684
                                      info@ncod.org
                                          www.ncod.org

Arvilla Rank, Editor/Executive Director
Published as a pastoral service for the deaf and hard of hearing.
Provides information to members and others working in ministry.
$15.00
Quarterly

Non Print: Video

8100 Christmas Stories
Video Learning Library
15838 N 62nd St
Scottsdale, AZ 85254-1988   480-596-9970
                                      800-383-8811
                                  FAX: 480-596-9973
                              info@videolearning.com
                                  www.videolearning.com

Jim Spencer, Owner
Told by popular deaf story-tellers, the stories included are A
Christmas Carol, Night Before Christmas, Story of the First
Christmas Tree, Birth of Christ, The Great Walled City, and Little
Match Girl. *$29.95*
Video/80 Mins 1986
ISBN 1-882257-02-2

8101 Fantastic Series Videotape Set
Gallaudet University Press
800 Florida Ave NE
Washington, DC 20002-3695   202-651-5488
                                      800-621-2736
                                  FAX: 202-651-5489
                                  gupress@gallaudet.edu
                                  www.gupress.gallaudet.edu

Rita Corey, Director
T. Alan Hurwitz, President
Paul Kelly, Vice President Adm. And Finance
These videotapes offer a blend of entertainment and information
to both deaf and hearing children ages 6-10. A total of eight tapes
in the series. *$254.00*
Video 8 VHS
ISBN 1-563680-12-2

8102 Fantastic: Colonial Times, Chocolate, and Cars
Gallaudet University Press
800 Florida Ave NE
Washington, DC 20002-3695   202-651-5488
                                      800-621-2736
                                  FAX: 202-651-5489
                                  gupress@gallaudet.edu
                                  www.gupress.gallaudet.edu

Rita Corey, Director
T. Alan Hurwitz, President
Paul Kelly, Vice President Adm. And Finance
Young viewers visit Colonial Williamsburg in Virginia to see var-
ious crafts. Other parts show chocolate being made, and films of
old cars. *$39.95*
Video
ISBN 1-563680-06-8

8103 Fantastic: Dogs at Work and Play
Gallaudet University Press
800 Florida Ave NE
Washington, DC 20002-3695   202-651-5488
                                      800-621-2736
                                  FAX: 202-651-5489
                                  gupress@gallaudet.edu
                                  www.gupress.gallaudet.edu

Rita Corey, Director
T. Alan Hurwitz, President
Paul Kelly, Vice President Adm. And Finance
See how dogs are trained, including Fantastic's own hearing-ear
dog, police dogs, plus puppies, and dogs in space? *$39.95*
Video
ISBN 1-563680-03-3

8104 Fantastic: Exciting People, Places and Things!
Gallaudet University Press
800 Florida Ave NE
Washington, DC 20002-3695   202-651-5488
                                      800-621-2736
                                  FAX: 202-651-5489
                                  gupress@gallaudet.edu
                                  www.gupress.gallaudet.edu

Rita Corey, Director
T. Alan Hurwitz, President
Paul Kelly, Vice President Adm. And Finance
Welcomes young viewers for a trip to a crayon factory, a jump
rope tournament, and mime by actor Bernard Bragg. *$39.95*
Video
ISBN 1-563680-01-7

8105 Fantastic: From Post Offices to Dairy Goats
Gallaudet University Press
800 Florida Ave NE
Washington, DC 20002-3695   202-651-5488
                                      800-621-2736
                                  FAX: 202-651-5489
                                  gupress@gallaudet.edu
                                  www.gupress.gallaudet.edu

Rita Corey, Director
T. Alan Hurwitz, President
Paul Kelly, Vice President Adm. And Finance

In this video children follow the route of a letter from the mailbox through the post office to its final destination. Also, they visit dairy goats and other animals. *$39.95*
Video
ISBN 1-563680-05-X

8106   Fantastic: Imagination, Actors, and 'Deaf Way'
Gallaudet University Press
800 Florida Ave NE
Washington, DC 20002-3695   202-651-5488
                                   800-621-2736
                                   202-651-5508
                                   FAX: 202-651-5489
                                   gupress@gallaudet.edu
                                   www.gupress.gallaudet.edu

Rita Corey, Director
T. Alan Hurwitz, President
Paul Kelly, Vice President Adm. And Finance
Deaf clowns, mimes, and actors display the wonders of imagination, along with performances at the international cultural celebration 'Deaf Way.' *$39.95*
Video
ISBN 1-563680-04-1

8107   Fantastic: Roller Coasters, Maps, and Ice Cream!
Gallaudet University Press
800 Florida Ave NE
Washington, DC 20002-3695   202-651-5488
                                   800-621-2736
                                   FAX: 202-651-5489
                                   gupress@gallaudet.edu
                                   www.gupress.gallaudet.edu

Rita Corey, Director
T. Alan Hurwitz, President
Paul Kelly, Vice President Adm. And Finance
In this program Mike Montangino leads the way on rides at Kings Dominion, and also to see how maps are drawn, and how ice cream is made. *$39.95*
Video
ISBN 1-563680-07-6

8108   Fantastic: Skiing, Factories, and Race Hores
Gallaudet University Press
800 Florida Ave NE
Washington, DC 20002-3695   202-651-5488
                                   800-621-2736
                                   FAX: 202-651-5489
                                   gupress@gallaudet.edu
                                   www.gupress.gallaudet.edu

Rita Corey, Director
T. Alan Hurwitz, President
Paul Kelly, Vice President Adm. And Finance
Snow Skiing starts this program, which continues in a factory where 'who-knows-what' is made. Also, young viewers learn about horse care, and also about the making of Oreos. *$39.95*
Video
ISBN 1-563680-08-4

8109   Fantastic: Wonderful Worlds of Sports and Travel
Gallaudet University Press
800 Florida Ave NE
Washington, DC 20002-3695   202-651-5488
                                   800-621-2736
                                   FAX: 202-651-5489
                                   gupress@gallaudet.edu
                                   www.gupress.gallaudet.edu

Rita Corey, Director
T. Alan Hurwitz, President
Paul Kelly, Vice President Adm. And Finance
In this program, young viewers ride on a train, watch deaf athletes compete, and see actor Bernard Bragg perform 'The Lion and the Mouse.' *$39.95*
Video
ISBN 1-563680-02-5

8110   Fingerspelling: Expressive and Receptive Fluency
DawnSign Press
6130 Nancy Ridge Dr
San Diego, CA 92121-3223   858-625-0600
                                  800-549-5350
                                  FAX: 858-625-2336
                                  info@dawnsign.com
                                  www.dawnsign.com

Joe Dannis, President
Joyce Linden Groode, Fingerspelling Teacher
Improve your fingerspelling with this new video guide. A 24-page instructional booklet is included with fingerspelling practice suggestions. *$29.95*
120 Minutes
ISBN 1-581210-46-9

8111   Getting Better
Vestibular Disorders Association
5018 NE 15th Ave
Portland, OR 97211-5331   503-229-7705
                                 800-837-8428
                                 FAX: 503-229-8064
                                 veda@vestibular.org
                                 www.vestibular.org

Cynthia Ryan MBA, Executive Director
Tony Staser,, Development Director
Vicente Honrubia, Director
Joel A. Goebel, MD, FACS, Director, Vestibular & Oculomotor Laboratory
Interviews with physicians, physical therapists, psychologists, social workers, and patients on Managing Symptoms, Diagnosis & Treatment, and Cognitive/Psychological Impacts. *$24.95*
Video

8112   Helping the Family Understand
Vestibular Disorders Association
5018 NE 15th Ave
Portland, OR 97211-5331   503-229-7705
                                 800-837-8428
                                 FAX: 503-229-8064
                                 veda@vestibular.org
                                 www.vestibular.org

Cynthia Ryan MBA, Executive Director
Tony Staser,, Development Director
Vicente Honrubia, Director
Joel A. Goebel, MD, FACS, Director, Vestibular & Oculomotor Laboratory
Interviews with physicians, physical therapists, psychologists, social workers, and patients on Managing Symptoms, Diagnosis & Treatment and Cognitive/Psychological Impacts. *$24.95*
Video

8113   Managing Your Symptoms
Vestibular Disorders Association
5018 NE 15th Ave
Portland, OR 97211-5331   503-229-7705
                                 800-837-8428
                                 FAX: 503-229-8064
                                 veda@vestibular.org
                                 www.vestibular.org

Cynthia Ryan MBA, Executive Director
Tony Staser,, Development Director
Vicente Honrubia, Director
Joel A. Goebel, MD, FACS, Director, Vestibular & Oculomotor Laboratory
Interviews with physicians, physical therapists, psychologists, social workers, and patients. on Managing Symptoms, Diagnosis & Treatment, and Cognitive/Psychological Impacts. *$24.95*
Video

Sports

8114   American Hearing Impaired Hockey Association
4214 W. 77th Place
Chicago, IL 60652-1618

978-922-0955
FAX: 312-829-2098
kkmm2won@aol.com
www.ahiha.org

Stan Mikita, President
Cheryl Hager, General Manager
Helen Tovey, Registrar, USA Hockey Reg.

The American Hearing Impaired Hockey Association provides deaf and hard of hearing hockey players the opportunity to learn about and improve their hockey skills through our program. We offer these hockey players the opportunity to be coached by a coaching staff with college, national and international experience.

8115   USA Deaf Sports Federation
102 N Krohn Pl
PO Box 910338
Lexington, KY 40591-0338

605-367-5760
FAX: 605-782-8441
TTY:605-367-5761
homeoffice@usadeafsports.org
www.usdeafsports.org

Jack C Lamberton, President
Mark Apodaca, VP Of Financial Affairs
William J Bowman, VP Of International Affairs
Jeffrey L. Salit?, Vice-President of NSO Affairs

The USA Deaf Sports Federation's purpose was to foster and regulate uniform rules of competition and provide social outlets for deaf members and their friends; serve as a parent organization for regional sports organizations; conduct annual athletic competitions; and assist in the participation of U.S. teams in international competition.

Support Groups

8116   Dial-a-Hearing Screening Test
Occupational Hearing Services Inc.
300 S Chester Rd
Suite 301
Swarthmore, PA 19081-1800

610-544-7700
800-622-3277
FAX: 610-543-2802
DAHST@aol.com

George Biddle, President/Owner
James Biddle, Vice President
Phyllis Biddle, Treasurer

A national telephone resource providing information about hearing impairments and deafness. Dial-A-Hearing Screening Test: national test number for free telephone hearing test: 1-800-222-EARS, MON-FRI: 9:00 AM to 5:00 PM Eastern time.

Mobility

Associations

8117 Academy of Spinal Cord Injury Professionals
206 S. 6th St
Springfield, IL 62701   217-753-1190
                                    FAX: 217-525-1271
                                www.academyscipro.org
Destiny Nance-Evans, Director Of Memebership Services
Kim Ruff, Director Of Education
An interdisciplinary organization dedicated to advancing the care of people with spinal cord injury/dysfunction, providing resources, research, and insights for SCI/D professionals.

8118 Acid Maltase Deficiency Association
P.O. Box 700248
San Antonio, TX 78270-248   210-494-6144
                                    FAX: 210-490-7161
                                TiffanyLHouse@aol.com
                                www.amda-pompe.org
Tiffany House, President
The Acid Maltase Deficiency Association offers resource materials to help raise awareness and provide education and insight into Pompe disease (a.k.a. Acid Maltase Deficiency), a rare genetic disease derived from the family of Lysosomal Storage Disease. The association offers information for patients, their families, as well as medical professionals.

8119 American Academy of Osteopathy
The Pyramids
3500 Depauw Blvd.,
Ste 1080
Indianapolis, IN 46268-1174   317-879-1881
                                    FAX: 317-879-0563
                        dcole@academyofosteopathy.org
                            www.academyofosteopathy.org
Sherri Quarles, Interim Executive Director & Accountant
Laura E. Griffin, D.O.; FAAO, President
The mission of the American Academy of Osteopathy is to teach, advocate, and research the science, art and philosophy of osteopathic medicine, emphasizing the integration of osteopathic principles, practice and manipulative treatment in patient care.

**8120 American Association of Neuromuscular &
Electrodiagnostic Medicine**
2621 Superior Drive NW
Rochester, MN 55901   507-288-0100
                                    FAX: 507-288-1225
                                    aanem@aanem.org
                                    www.aanem.org
Shirlyn A. Adkins, JD, Executive Director
Patrick Aldrich, CPA, Finance Director
Lori Nierman, Office Manager
Amy White, Education Coordinator
The American Association of Neuromuscular & Electrodiagnostic Medicine (AANEM) is a nonprofitmembership association dedicated to the advancement of neuromuscular (NM), musculoskeletal, and electrodiagnostic (EDX) medicine.

**8121 American Association of Spinal Cord Injury Psychologists
& Social Workers**
75-20 Astoria Boulevard
Jackson Heights, NY 11370-1138   718-803-3782
                                    FAX: 718-803-0414
                                info@unitedspinal.org
                        www.unitedspinal.org/donations/online-
Lex Frieden, Chairman of the Board
Paul Tobin, President and Chief Executive Officer
Michael B. Kinne, Secretary
Janeen Earwood, Treasurer
Organized and operated for scientific and educational purposes to advance and improve the psychosocial care of persons with spinal cord impairment, develop and promote education and re-search related to the psychosocial care of persons with spinal cord injury, recognize psychologists and social workers whose careers are devoted to the problems of spinal cord impairment.

8122 American Back Society
2648 International Blvd
Ste 502
Oakland, CA 94601-1537   510-536-9929
                                    FAX: 510-536-1812
                                info@americanbacksoc.org
                                www.americanbacksoc.org
James W Simmons M.D. F.A.C.S., President
Ronald G Donelson M.D. M.S, Vice President
Carol McFarland, Secretary
Thomas E Dreisinger PhD, Treasurer
The American Back Society is a non-profit organization dedicated to providing an interdisciplinary educational forum for healthcare professionals committed to relieving pain and diminishing impairment in patients suffering from neck and back conditions through proper diagnosis and treatment.

8123 American Dystonia Society
17 Suffolk Lane
Princeton Junction, NJ 8550   310-237-5478
                                    FAX: 609-275-5663
                                info@dystonia.us
                                www.dystoniasociety.org

8124 American Parkinson Disease Association
135 Parkinson Avenue
Staten Island, NY 10305   718-981-8001
                                        800-223-2732
                                    FAX: 718-981-4399
                                apda@apdaparkinson.org
                                www.apdaparkinson.org
Leslie A. Chambers, President & CEO
Stephanie Paul, VP Development and Marketing
Robin Kornhaber, MSW, VP of Programs and Services
Julie Sacks, MSW, LCSW, Sr Director Programs & Services
APDA was founded in 1961 with the dual purpose to find the Curefor Parkinson's disease.

8125 American Stroke Association
7272 Greenville Ave
Dallas, TX 75231-4596
                                        800-242-8721
                                        888-478-7653
                                    FAX: 214-706-5231
                                strokeconnection@heart.org
                                www.strokeassociation.org
Ralph Sacco, President/Director
Donna Arnett, Ph.D., President
Debra Lockwood, Chairman
Nancy Brown, CEO
Fifty-five state affiliates monitoring local chapters offering educational materials, seminars, conferences and transportation for members nationwide. Maintains a listing of over 1,000 stroke support groups across the nation for referral to stroke survivors, their families, caregivers and interested professionals.

8126 Amytrophic Lateral Sclerosis Association
27001 Agoura Rd
Ste 250
Calabasas Hills, CA 91301-5104   818-880-9007
                                        800-782-4747
                                    FAX: 818-880-9006
                                alsinfo@alsa-national.org
                                www.alsa.org
Janes H Gilbert, President/CEO
Michelle Powers Keegan, Chief Development Officer
Daniel M. Reznikov, CFO
Lance Slaughter, Chief Chapter Relations Officer
The ALS association is the only national not-for-profit health organization dedicated soley to lead the fight against ALS. The Association covers all the bases-research, patient and community services, public education, and advocacy-in providing help and hope to those facing the disease. The mission is to lead the fight to cure and treat ALS through global cutting edge research, and to

empower people with Lou Gehrig's disease to live fuller lives & provide them with compassion care and support.

8127   Arthritis Foundation
PO Box 932915
Atlanta, GA 31193-2915   404-872-7100
                                          800-283-7800
                                          FAX: 404-872-0457
                                          aforders@arthritis.org
                                          www.arthritis.org

Daniel T. McGowan, Chair
Rowland W. (Bing) Chang, Vice Chairs
Patricia Novak Nelson, Vice Chairs
Michael V. Ortman, Treasurer
Offers information and referrals regarding educational materials and programs, fund-raising, support groups, seminars and conferences offered by 55 local chapters across the United States.

8128   Association for Neurologically Impaired Brain Injured Children
61-35 220th St
Oakland Gardens, NY 11364   718-423-9550
                                          FAX: 718-423-9838
                                          mail@anibic.org
                                          www.anibic.org

Gerard Smith, Executive Director
John F DeBiase, Associate Executive Director
Rachel Plakstis, MSC Director
Gail Baquero, Residential Director
ANIBIc is a voluntary, multi-service organization that is dedicated to serving individuals with severe learning disabilities, neurological impairments and other developmental disabilities. Services include: residential, vocational, family support services, recreation (children and adults), respite (adult), in home support services, counseling and tramatic brain injury services (adults).

8129   Capital Area Parkinsons Society
PO Box 27565
Austin, TX 78755-2565   512-371-3373
                                          www.capitalareaparkinsons.org
Tereasa Ford, President
Dr. Nina Mosier, Vice-president
Lina Supnet-Zapata, Secretary
Alex Andron, Treasurer
Founded in 1984, the Capital Area Parkinson's Society addresses the needs for those impacted by Parkinson's disease in central Texas. The organization offers a multitude of support groups, resources, monthly meetings, exercise programs and a community for people afflicted by Parkinson's and their care partners.

8130   Children's Hemiplegia & Stroke Association
4101 W. Green Oaks Blvd
Ste 305-149
Arlington, TX 76016   817-478-0861
                                          info437@chasa.org
                                          www.chasa.org
Nancy Atwood, Executive Director & Founder
Jana Smoot White, President
Julie Ring, Vice President
Jackie Haley, Treasurer
Offering support and information to families of infants, children and young adults who have hemiplegia or hemiplegic cerebral palsy.

8131   Christopher & Dana Reeve Paralysis Resource Center
636 Morris Turnpike
Suite 3A
Short Hills, NJ 07078-2608   973-379-2690
                                          800-225-0292
                                          FAX: 973-912-9433
                                          information@christopherreeve.org
                                          www.christopherreeve.org
John M. Hughes, Chairman
Arnold H. Snider, Vice Chairman
Henry G. Stifel, III, Vice Chairman
Joel M. Faden, Chairman, Executive Committee

Our goal is to provide you with the information you need to live a healthy life, make informed decisions, and better understand paralysis, spinal cord injury and other conditions.

8132   Consortium of Multiple Sclerosis Centers
3 University Plaza Dr.
Ste 116
Hackensack, NJ 07601   201-487-1050
                                          FAX: 862-772-7275
                                          www.mscare.org

June Halper, Chief Executive Officer
Gary Cutter, PhD, President
Lisa Skutnik, Chief Operating Officer
Marguerite Herman, Executive Assistant
CMSC provides leadership in clinical research and education; develops vehicles to share information and knowledge among members; disseminates information to the health care community and to persons affected by Multiple Sclerosis; and develops and implements mechanisms to influence health care delivery.

8133   Cure SMA
Formerly: Families of Spinal Muscular Atrophy
925 Busse Rd
P.O. Box 196
Elk Grove Village, IL 60007   847-367-7620
                                          800-886-1762
                                          FAX: 847-367-7623
                                          info@curesma.org
                                          www.curesma.org

Jill Jarecki, Research Director
Kenneth Hobby, President
Karen O'Brien, Membership
Colleen McCarthy O'Toole, Senior Director, Family Support & Development
Cure SMA is the largest international organization dedicated solely to eradicating spinal muscular atrophy (SMA) by promoting and supporting research, helping families cope with SMA through informational programs and support, and educating the public and professional community about SMA.

8134   Dystonia Advocacy Network
One East Wacker Drive
Suite 2810
Chicago, IL 60601

                                          dystonia-advocacy.org

8135   Epilepsy Foundation
8301 Professional Pl
Landover, MD 20785-2353
                                          800-332-1000
                                          866-330-2718
                                          FAX: 301-459-1569
                                          ContactUs@efa.org
                                          www.epilepsyfoundation.org
Diane Rubinstein, Senior Director Finance/Controller
Ken Lowenberg, Senior Director Marketing and Communications
Chad Hartman, Senior Director of Development
Adina Frazier, Director of Special Events
The organization works to ensure that people with seizures are able to participate in all life experiences; to improve how people with epilepsy are perceived, accepted and valued in society; and to promote research for a cure. In addition to programs conducted at the national level, epilepsy clients throughout the United States are served by 48 Epilepsy Foundation affiliates around the country.

8136   Friends of Disabled Adults and Children
4900 Lewis Rd
Stone Mountain, GA 30083-1104   770-491-9014
                                          866-977-1204
                                          chrisbrand@fodac.org
                                          www.fodac.org
Chris Brand, President
FODAC's mission is to provide durable medical equipment (DME) such as wheelchairs and hospital beds at little or no cost to the disabled and their families. We seek to enhance the quality of life for people of all ages who have any type of illness or physical

disability. Since 1986, FODAC has collected and distributed more than 29,000 wheelchairs!

8137 Head Injury Rehabilitation And Referral Service, Inc. (HIRRS)
11 Taft Court
Suite 100
Rockville, MD 20850-4162 301-309-2228
FAX: 301-309-2278
tbi@headinjuryrehab.org
www.headinjuryrehab.org
Maggie Hunter, Director of Admissions and Quality Assurance
Robert Cousland, Director of Rehabilitation
Debbie Jones, Director of Individual Support
Janet McCloskey, Director of Community Living Services
Head Injury Rehabilitation and Referral Services, Inc. (HIRRS) is a private not-for-profit agency that provides comprehensive brain injury support including long-term living, daily programs, vocational supports and services to individuals that live in the community. The agency is located in Rockville, MD, but serves the DC Metropolitan area.

8138 International Parkinson and Movement Disorder Society
555 East Wells Street
Suite 1100
Milwaukee, WI 53202- 3823 414-276-2145
FAX: 414-276-3349
info@movementdisorders.org
www.movementdisorders.org
Matthew B. Stern, MD, President
Francisco Cardoso, MD, PhD, Secretary
Christopher Goetz, MD, Treasurer
The International Parkinson and Movement Disorder Society (MDS) is a professional society of clinicians, scientists, and other healthcare professionals who are interested in Parkinson's disease, related neurodegenerative and neurodevelopmental disorders, hyperkinetic movement disorders, and abnormalities in muscle tone and motor control.

8139 Lewy Body Dementia Association
912 Killian Hill Road S.W.
Lilburn, GA 30047 404-935-6444
800-539-9767
FAX: 480-422-5434
www.lbda.org
Mike Koehler, President
Angela Herron, Treasurer
Mark Wall, Director of Operations
Angela Taylor, Director of Programs
The Lewy Body Dementia Association (LBDA) is a nonprofit organization dedicated to raising awareness of the Lewy body dementias (LBD), supporting people with LBD, their families and caregivers and promoting scientific advances.

8140 Mobility International USA
132 E. Broadway
Suite 343
Eugene, OR 97401-2767 541-343-1284
FAX: 541-343-6812
info@miusa.org
www.miusa.org
Susan Sygall, Executive Director
Alison Ecker, Project Assistant
Cerise Roth Vinson, Chief Operating Officer
Cindy Lewis, Director of Programs
A US based national nonprofit organization dedicated to empowering people with disabilities around the world through leadership development, training and international exchange to ensure inclusion of people with disabilities in international exchange and development programs. The National Clearinghouse on Disability & Exchange, a joint project managed by MIUSA provides free information and referrals.

8141 Multiple Sclerosis Association of America
706 Haddonfield Rd
Cherry Hill, NJ 08002-2652 856-488-4500
800-532-7667
FAX: 856-488-8257
northeast@mymsaa.org
www.msassociation.org
Robert Manley, Chair
Sue Rehmu, Vice Chair
William Saunders, Treasurer
Monica Derbes Gibson, Secretary
MSAA is a national non-profit organization dedicated to enriching the quality of life for evryone affected by multiple sclerosis.

8142 Multiple Sclerosis Foundation
6350 N. Andrews Ave
Fort Lauderdale, FL 33309-2132 954-776-6805
800-225-6495
FAX: 954-938-8708
admin@msfocus.org
www.msfocus.org
Jules Kuperberg, Executive Director
Alan Segaloff, Co- Executive Director
Kasey Minnis, Director, Operations & Communications
Natalie Blake, Director, Programs & Services
Contemporary national, nonprofit organization that provides free support services and public education for persons with Multiple Sclerosis, newsletters, toll-free phone support, information, referrals, home care, assitive technology, and support groups.

8143 NBIA Disorders Association
2082 Monaco Ct.
El Cajon9, CA 92019-4235 619-588-2315
FAX: 619-588-4093
info@NBIAdisorders.org
www.nbiadisorders.org
Patricia Wood, President
Marsha Bryan, Development Director
Melissa Woods, Social Media Director
Mike Cohn, Director of Adult Programs
NBIA provides support to families, educate the public and accelerate research with collaborators from around the world.

8144 National Association for Continence
P.O. Box 1019
Charleston, SC 29402-1019 843-377-0900
800-252-3337
FAX: 843-377-0905
memberservices@nafc.org
www.nafc.org
Katherine F. Jeter, EdD, Founder
Steven G. Gregg, PhD, Executive Director
Meghan Hansen, Membership and Fund Development
NAFC's mission is to educate the public about the causes, diagnosis, categories, treatment options and management alternatives for incontinence, voiding dysfunction and related pelvic floor disorders; to network with other organizations and agencies; to elevate the visibility and priority given to these areas; and to advocate on behalf of consumers who suffer from such symptoms as a result of disease or other illness.

8145 National Coalition for Assistive and Rehab Technology
54 Towhee Court
East Amhurst, NY 14051 716-839-9728
FAX: 716-839-9624
info@ncart.us
www.ncart.us
Don Clayback, Executive Director
Gary Gilberi, President
Doug Westerdahl, Treasurer
Bob Gouy, Executive Committee Member
The coalition's mission is to ensure proper and appropriate access to complex rehab and assistive technologies.

8146   National Council on Independent Living
1710 Rhode Island Ave NW
5th Floor
Washington, DC 20036-3007
202-207-0334
877-525-3400
FAX: 202-207-0341
TTY: 202-207-0340
ncil@ncil.org
www.ncil.org

Kelly Buckland, Executive Director
Tim Fuchs, Operations Director
Dan Kessler, President
Lou Ann Kibbee, Vice President
NCIL advances independent living and the rights of people with disabilities through consumer-driven advocacy.

8147   National Fibromyalgia Association
2121 S Towne Centre Place
Ste 300
Anaheim, CA 92806-6124
714-921-0150
FAX: 714-921-6920
fmaware.org
www.fmaware.org

Lynne Matallana, President
Mark Dobrilovic, Board of Director
John Fry, PhD, Board of Directors
Michael Seffinger, DO, FAAFP, Board of Directors
National Fibromyalgia Association's mission is to develop and execute programs dedicated to improving the quality of life for people with fibromyalgia.

8148   National Mobility Equipment Dealers Association
3327 West Bearss Avenue
Tampa, FL 33618
813-264-2697
866-948-8341
FAX: 813-962-8970
info@nmeda.org
www.nmeda.com

8149   National Spasmodic Dysphonia Association
300 Park Boulevard
Suite 335
Itasca, IL 60143
800-795-6732
FAX: 630-250-4505
nsda@dysphonia.org
www.dysphonia.org

8150   National Spasmodic Torticollis Association
9920 Talbert Avenue
Fountain Valley, CA 92708
714-378-9837
800-487-8385
NSTAmail@aol.com
www.torticollis.org

8151   Paralyzed Veterans of America
801 18th St NW
Washington, DC 20006-3517
202-872-1300
800-424-8200
888-888-2201
FAX: 202-785-4432
TTY:800-795-4327
info@pva.org
www.pva.org

Homer S. Townsend, Jr., Executive Director
Larry Dodson, National Secretary
Bill Lawson, National President
Al Kovach, Jr, Natonal Senior Vice President
A congressionally chartered veterans service organization, has developed a unique expertise on a wide variety of issues involving the special needs of our members— veterans of the armed forces who have experienced spinal cord injury or dysfunction.

8152   Parkinson's Disease Research Society
25 N. Winfield Road
4 North Tower
Winfield, IL 60190
630-933-4384
630-933-3077
FAX: 630-933-3077
info@parkinsonsprogress.org
parkinsonsprogress.org

Michael Rezak, M.D., Ph.D., Medical Director
The PDRS mandate is to mount a concerted effort to intensify the research, both in the basic science laboratory as well as with clinical trials, to advance the diagnosis, treatment and prevention of Parkinson's disease.

8153   Post-Polio Health International
4207 Lindell Blvd
Ste 110
Saint Louis, MO 63108-2930
314-534-0475
FAX: 314-534-5070
info@post-polio.org
www.post-polio.org

Joan L Headley, Executive Director
Gayla Hoffman, Editor
Sheryl R. Rudy, Editor
Judith Raymond Fischer, MSLS, Editor
Educates, advocates and networks the survivors of polio and the health professionals who treat them. Funds a research grant, publishes Post Polio Health (Quarterly, 12 page newsletter).

8154   Simon Foundation for Continence
P.O. Box 815
Wilmette, IL 60091-815
847-864-3913
800-237-4666
FAX: 847-864-9758
info@simonfoundation.org
www.simonfoundation.org

Cheryl B. Gartley, Founder/President
Elizabeth A. LaGro, Vice President, Communications & Education Services
Twila Yednock, Director of Special Events
The Simon Foundation is known throughout the world for its innovative educational projects and tireless efforts on behalf of people with loss of bladder and bowel control. Simon has led the way forward with many groundbreaking projects, for example: the first book written for laypersons, Managing Incontinence: A Guide to Living with the Loss of Bladder Control.

8155   Society for Progressive Supranuclear Palsy
30 E. Padonia Road,
Suite 201
Timonium, MD 21093
800-457-4777
FAX: 410-785-7009
info@curepsp.org
www.psp.org

Janet Edmunson, Med, Chair
Dan Johnson, Vice-Chair
George S. Jankiewicz, CPA, CFP,, Treasurer
John T. Burhoe, Secretary
Members of the Board of Directors of CurePSP accept the major responsibility of implementing the mission of the Foundation for PSP | CBD and Related Brain Diseases. Board members are actively involved in continually defining and redefining the mission and participating in strategic planning to review purposes, programs, priorities, funding needs, and levels of achievement.

8156   United Spinal Association
120-34 Queens Blvd
Ste 320
Kew Gardens, NY 11415
718-803-3782
FAX: 718-803-0414
www.unitedspinal.org

8157 **Vermont Back Research Center**
1 S Prospect St
Burlington, VT 05405

802-656-3131
FAX: 802-660-9243
learn@uvm.edu
www.uvm.edu

8158 **World Chiropractic Alliance**
2683 Via De La Valle
Suite G 629
Del Mar, CA 92014

480-786-9235
866-789-8073
FAX: 480-732-9313
comments@worldchiropracticalliance.org
www.worldchiropracticalliance.org

Linda Bevel, Manager
Terry A Rondberg DC, Founder/CEO
The World Chiropractic Alliance was founded in 1989 as a non-profit organization dedicated to protecting and strengthening chiropractic around the world. Since its inception, the WCA has played an important role in the global chiropractic community. In 1998, it was granted status as a Non-Governmental Organization (NGO) associated with the United Nations Department of Public Information.

Camps

8159 **Autism Day Camp**
Hillcroft Services: Isanogel
114 E. Streeter Avenue
Muncie, IN 47304

765-288-1073
FAX: 765-288-3101
TTY:765-288-1073
demcintosh@bsu.edu
www.hillcroft.org

Ted Baker, Chair
Brenda Llyod, Vice Chair
Bruce Baldwin, Director
Julie Bering, Secretary/ Treasurer
The camp is designed to improve the academic, social skills, and behaviors of children with autism spectrum disorders. The day camp is an 8-week intensive experience for children classified with autism spectrum disorders.

8160 **Camp Esperanza**
Southern California Chapter
West 6th Street
Suite 1250
Los Angeles, CA 90017

323-954-5760
800-954-2873
FAX: 213-954-5790
jziegler@arthritis.org
www.arthritis.org

Jennifer Ziegler, Camp Director
Lindsey Gonzales, Regional Director, Human Resources
Manuel Loya, Chief Executive Officer
Teri Lim, Chief Marketing Officer
A one-week camp in August that allows children with arthritis to participate in such activities as horseback riding, swimming, etc. in a fun-filled environment.

8161 **Camp Oakhurst**
New York Service for the Handicapped
111 Monmouth Rd
Oakhurst, NJ 7755-1514

732-531-0215
FAX: 732-531-0292
info@nysh.org
www.nysh.org

Robert Pacenza, Executive Director:
Charles Sutherland, Camp Director
Camp Oakhurst, established in 1906, is operated by New York Service for the Handicapped (NYSH), an independent non-profit social service agency with offices in New York City and Oakhurst, New Jersey.

8162 **Easter Seals Camp Stand by Me**
Easter Seal Society of Washington
17809 S. Vaughn Road KPN
PO Box 289
Vaughn, WA 98394-313

253-884-2722
FAX: 253-590-0594
camp@wa.easterseals.com
www.wa.easterseals.com

Cathy Bisaillon, President/Camp Director
Jennifer Ting, Board Chair
Dr. Tim Johnson, Vice Chair
Charissa Manglona, Secretary
Camp Stand By Me provides a safe, barrier-free environment for children and adults to experience all aspects of camp without limitations.

8163 **Summer Wheelchair Sports Camp**
University of Illinois
1207 S Oak St
Champaign, IL 61820-6901

217-333-4606
FAX: 217-244-0014
TTY:217-244-9738
sportscamp@illinois.edu
www.disability.illinois.edu

Brian Walsh, Camp Director
Kim Collins, Asst. Dir., Academic Disability Support Services
Pat Malik, Asst. Dir., Non-Academic Disability Support Services
Angella Anderson, Disability Specialist, Accessible Media
Rigorous camps designed for individuals with lower extremity physical disabilities. Camp attendees will spend an average of 8-9 hours a day, focusing on development and refinement of fitness, techniques and strategies. Strength training, nutrition and mental training sessions will also be included in all camps. The camp staff is comprised of athletic staff and faculty front, the Division of Rehabilitation Education Services and local wheelchair athletes with coaching experience.

8164 **Twin Lakes Camp**
1451 E Twin Lakes Rd
Hillsboro, IN 47949-8004

765-798-4000
outdoors@twinlakescamp.com
www.twinlakescamp.com

Jon Beight, Executive Director
Duane Bush, Guest Service
Dan Daily, Program Director
Donna Beight, Secretary
Provides a summer camp program for special needs children and young adults. Campers suffer from a wide range of maladies including crippling accidents, Spina Bifida, epilepsy, Cerebral Palsy, Muscular Dystrophy, Quadriplegia, Paraplegia, and other disabling diseases. Campers range in age from 8 to 27.

8165 **YMCA Camp Fitch**
Youngstown YMCA
17 N Champion St
P.O. Box 1287
Youngstown, OH 44501

330-744-8411
FAX: 330-744-8415
info@campfitchymca.com
www.youngstownymca.org

Thomas Fleming, Chair/ CVO
James B. Greene, 1st Vice chiar
Thomas Gacse, 2nd Vice chiar
Donald Harrison, 3rd Vice chiar
Camp is located in North Springfield, Pennsylvania. Camping sessions for children and adults with diabetes, hearing impairment, developmental disabilities, mobility limitation and speech/communication impairment. Ages 8-16, families and seniors.

Print: Books

8166 **Adapted Physical Education and Sport**
Human Kinetics, Inc.
1607 N Market Street
Champaign, IL 61820-2220

217-351-5076
800-747-4457
FAX: 217-351-1549
info@naspem.org
www.naspem.org

Joseph P Winnick EdD, Author
Scott Kimberly, Owner
Rainer Martens, President/Treasurer
Jill Wikgren, COO
Designed as a resource for both present and future physical education leaders, this book is an exceptional book for teaching exceptional children. It emphasizes the physical education of young people with disabilities. *$68.00*
592 pages Hardcover
ISBN 0-736052-16-X

8167 **Arthritis Bible**
Inner Traditions - Bear & Company
PO Box 388
Rochester, VT 05767-0388

802-767-3174
800-246-8648
FAX: 802-767-3726
customerservice@innertraditions.com
www.innertraditions.com

Craig Weatherby, Author
Leonid Gordin MD, Co-Author
A comprehensive guide to the alternative therapies and conventional treatments for Arthritic diseases including Osteoarthritis, Rheumatoid Arthritis, Gout, Fibromyalgia and more. *$16.95*
272 pages Paperback 1999
ISBN 0-892818-25-5

8168 **Arthritis Helpbook: A Tested Self Management Program for Coping with Arthritis**
Da Capo Press
44 Farnsworth Street,
Boston, MA 02210

617-252-5200
FAX: 617-252-5265
www.dacapopress.com

Kate Lorig, Author
James Fries, Co-Author
The Arthritis Helpbook is the world's leading guide to coping with joint pain, and has been used by more than 600,000 readers over its twenty years in print. It succeeds because of its tested advice, its hundreds of useful hints, and its emphasis on self-management-helping people with arthritis and fibromyalgia to achieve their own health goals. *$18.95*
Paperback
ISBN 0-738210-38-2

8169 **Arthritis Sourcebook**
McGraw-Hill Professional
7500 Chavenelle Rd
Dubuque, IA 52002-9655

563-584-6000
877-833-5524
FAX: 614-759-3749
pbg.ecommerce_custserv@mcgraw-hill.com
www.mhprofessional.com

Earl J Brewer Jr MD, Author
Kathy Cochran Angel, Co-Author
A comprehensive guide to the latest information on treatments, medications, and alternative therapies for arthritis. *$ 16.95*
272 pages Paperback
ISBN 0-737303-81-6

8170 **Arthritis, What Exercises Work: Breakthrough Relief for the Rest of Your Life**
MacMillan - St. Martin's Press
175 5th Ave
New York, NY 10010-7703

646-307-5151
FAX: 212-420-9314
press.inquiries@macmillanusa.com
www.us.macmillan.com

Dava Sorbel, Author
Arthur C Klein, Co-Author
What is the most powerful arthritis treatment ever developed to help restore you to a healthy, pain-free, and vigorous life—for the rest of your life? It's exercise. Here are the right exercised for your kind of arthritis, pain-level, age, occupation, and hobbies. *$14.99*
200 pages Paperback 1995
ISBN 0-312130-25-2

8171 **Arthritis: A Take Care of Yourself Health Guide**
Da Capo Press
44 Farnsworth Street,
Boston, MA 02210

617-252-5200
FAX: 617-252-5265
www.dacapopress.com

James F Fries, Author
Donald M Vickery, Co-Author
In this updated book the author draws on new research to recommend exercises and new pain medications for both arthritis and fibromyalgia. *$18.95*
Paperback 1909
ISBN 0-738202-25-8

8172 **Disability and Sport**
Human Kinetics, Inc.
1607 N Market Street
Champaign, IL 61820-2220

217-351-5076
800-747-4457
FAX: 217-351-1549
info@hkusa.com
www.naspem.org

Karen P DePauw, Author
Susan J Gavron, Co-Author
Scott Kimberley, Owner
Rainer Martens, President/Treasurer
Provides a comprehensive and practical look at the past, present, and future of disability sport. Topics covered are inclusive of youth through adult participation with in-depth coverage of the essential issues involving athletes with disabilities. This new edition has updated references and new chapter-opening outlines that assist with individual study and class discussions. *$48.00*
408 pages Hardcover
ISBN 0-736046-38-0

8173 **Fitness Programming for Physical Disabilities**
Human Kinetics, Inc.
1607 N Market Street
Champaign, IL 61820-2220

217-351-5076
800-747-4457
FAX: 217-351-1549
info@hkusa.com
www.naspem.org

Patricia D Miller, Editor
Scott Kimberley, Owner
Rainer Martens, President/Treasurer
Jill Wikgren, COO
A book offering information for developing and conducting exercise programs for groups that included people with physical disabilities. A dozen authorities in exercise science and adapted exercise programming explain how to effectively and safely modify existing programs for individuals with physical disabilities. *$42.00*
232 pages Paperback
ISBN 0-873224-34-5

8174 **Freedom from Arthritis Through Nutrition**
Tree of Life Publications
PO Box 126
Joshua Tree, CA 92252-0126

760-366-2937
FAX: 760-366-2937
office@booxr.us
www.treelifebooks.com

Philip J Welsh DDS ND, Author
Bianca Leonardo ND, Co-Author
Reveals the results of 60 years of research on arthritis by noted nutritionist, Dr. Philip J. Welsh, D.D.S. N.D. Here you will find simple, natural, inexpensive, tested ways of coping with the various forms of arthritis, using only nutrition and other natural methods. There are no drugs or gadgets in this program. *$24.95*
255 pages Softcover

8175 **Functional Electrical Stimulation for Ambulation by Paraplegics**
Krieger Publishing Company
1725 Krieger Drive
PO Box 9542
Malabar, FL 32950

321-724-9542
800-724-0025
FAX: 321-951-3671
info@krieger-publishing.com
www.krieger-publishing.com

Daniel Graupe, Author
Kate H Kohn, Co-Author
FES is employed to enable spinal cord injury patients who are complete paraplegics to stand and ambulate without bracing. The text covers 12 years of amulation experience. *$49.50*
210 pages Paperback 1994
ISBN 0-894648-45-4

8176 **Guide to Managing Your Arthritis**
Arthritis Foundation
1330 W. Peachtree St
Suite 100
Atlanta, GA 30309

404-872-7100
800-283-7800
FAX: 404-237-8153
AFOrders@pbd.com
www.arthritis.org

Mary Anne Dunkin, Author
John Klippel, President/CEO
Cecile Perich, Chairman
William Brackney, Vice Chair
Expert reviewers answer questions about basic arthritis facts, treatments, research, surgery and more. Also, specific information about six common conditions: rheumatoid arthritis, osteoarthritis, osteoporosis, fibromyalgia, lupus and gout. *$9.95*
193 pages Paperback
ISBN 0-912423-28-5

8177 **How to Deal with Back Pain and Rheumatoid Joint Pain: A Preventive and Self Treatment Manua**
Global Health Solutions
2146 Kings Garden Way
Falls Church, VA 22043-2593

703-848-2333
800-759-3999
FAX: 703-848-0028
information@watercure.com
www.watercure.com

Fereydoon Batmanghelidj, Author
Xiaopo Batmanjhelidj, President
Kristin Swan, Administrator
The physiology of pain production and its direct relationship to chronic regional dehydration of some joint spaces is explained: Special movements that would create vacuum in the disc spaces and draw water and the displaced discs into the vertebral joints are demonstrated. *$14.95*
100 pages Paperback
ISBN 0-962994-20-0

8178 **Inclusive Games**
Human Kinetics
1607 N Market Street
PO Box 5076
Champaign, IL 61825- 5076

217-351-5076
800-747-4457
FAX: 217-351-1549
info@hkusa.com
www.humankinetics.com

Susan L Kasser, Author
Scott Kimberley, Owner
Rainer Martens, President/Treasurer
Jill Wikgren, COO
Features more than 50 games, helpful illustrations, and hundreds of game variations. The book shows how to adapt games so that children of every ability level can practice, play and improve their movement skills together. The game finder makes it easy to locate an appropriate game according to its name, approximate grade level, difficulty within the grade level, skills required/developed, and number of players. *$17.95*
120 pages Paperback
ISBN 0-873226-39-9

8179 **Inside The Halo and Beyond: The Anatomy of a Recovery**
WW Norton & Company
500 5th Ave
New York, NY 10110-2

212-354-5500
FAX: 212-869-0856
www.wwnorton.com

Maxine Kumin, Author
W Drake McFeely, Chairman/President
Stephen King, VP Finance/CFO
Robert Weil, VP/Executive Editor
A skilled horsewoman and lifelong athlete, poet Kumin was 73 when a riding accident left her with two broken vertebrae in her neck. Kumin survived in the face of overwhelming odds that she would be paralyzed for the rest of her life. Miraculously, however, she was walking again within weeks of the accident; now, though one hand and an arm remain partially immobilized, her life has largely resumed its normal course. Here is the journal of her first nine months of recovery. *$13.95*
192 pages Softcover
ISBN 0-393049-00-0

8180 **Life on Wheels: For the Active Wheelchair User**
Patient-Centered Guides
1005 Gravenstein Hwy North
Sebastopol, CA 95472-2811

707-827-7000
800-998-9938
FAX: 707-829-0104
order@oreilly.com
www.oreilly.com

Gary Karp, Author
For 1.5 million Americans, life includes a wheelchair for mobility. Life on Wheels is for people who want to take charge of their life experience. Author Gary Karp describes medical issues (paralysis, circulation, rehab, cure research); day-to-day living (exercise, skin, bowel and bladder, sexuality, home access, maintaining a wheelchair); and social issues (self-image, adjustment, friends, family, cultural attitudes, activism). *$24.95*
565 pages Paperback 1999
ISBN 1-565922-53-0

8181 **Paralysis Resource Guide**
Christopher and Dana Reeve Paralysis Resource Ctr
636 Morris Turnpike
Suite 3A
Short Hills, NJ 07078

973-467-8270
800-539-7309
FAX: 973-912-9433
information@christopherreeve.org
www.paralysis.org

John M. Hughes, Chairman
John E. McConnell, Vice Chair
Matthew Reeve, Vice Chair
Peter T. Wilderotter, President

A comprehensive information tool for people affected by paralysis and for those who care for them. English or Spanish.
336 pages

8182 Primer on the Rheumatic Diseases
Arthritis Foundation
1330 W. Peachtree St
Suite 100
Atlanta, GA 30309-2111
404-872-7100
800-933-7023
FAX: 404-237-8153
AFOrders@pbd.com
www.arthritis.org

Rob Shaw, President
Patience White M.D., Editor
John H. Klippel, Editor
The leading professional book about arthritis and related diseases, the Primer is published by Springer and the Arthritis Foundation. *$79.95*
724 pages Softcover
ISBN 0-387356-64-8

8183 Sport Science Review: Adapted Physical Activity
Human Kinetics
1607 N Market Street
Champaign, IL 61820-2220
217-351-5076
800-747-4457
FAX: 217-351-1549
info@hkusa.com
www.naspem.org

Rainer Martens, President/Treasurer
Scott Kimberley, Owner
Jill Wikgren, COO
This issue of Sport Science Review examines the newly emerging academic discipline of adapted physical activity. Researchers from diverse academic backgrounds and parts of the world review the issues and controversies surrounding inclusion in physical education and sport. *$15.00*
96 pages Paperback
ISBN -073602-07-9

8184 Still Me
Random House
1745 Broadway
3rd Floor
New York, NY 10019-4305
212-782-9000
FAX: 212-572-6066
vintageanchor@randomhouse.com
www.randomhouse.com

Christopher Reeve, Author
Markus Dohle, Chairman/CEO
Madeline McIntosh, President
Andrew Weber, SVP Operations
The man who was Superman begins with his debilitating riding accident, then weaves back and forth between past and present, creating a thorough biography of Reeve's life. *$7.99*
336 pages Paperback 1999
ISBN 0-345432-41-4

8185 When Your Student Has Arthritis
Arthritis Foundation
2970 Peachtree Rd NW
PO Box 932915, Ste 200
Atlanta, GA 31193-2915
404-237-8771
800-933-7023
FAX: 404-237-8153
aforders@arthritis.org
www.afstore.org

Rob Shaw, President
An overview of arthritis, including juvenile rheumatoid arthritis and treatment. Also includes a school activities checklist for students, education rights, and how teachers can help.
28 pages

8186 Yoga for Fibromyalgia: Move, Breathe, and Relax to Improve Your Quality of Life
Mobility Limited
PO Box 838
Morro Bay, CA 93443-0838
805-772-3560
800-366-6038
FAX: 805-772-4717
shsh@mobilityltd.com
www.mobilityltd.com

Shoosh Lettick Crotzer, Director
The first book devoted exclusively to managing the symptoms of fibromyalgia; the comprehensive program of 26 illustrated poses, breathing techniques, and guided visualization and relaxation sessions can be practiced regardless of age or experience. The Living with Fibromyalgia section discusses lifestyle concerns. *$14.95*
128 pages 1908

Print: Magazines

8187 Arthritis Today
Arthritis Foundation
1330 W. Peachtree St.
Suite 100
Atlanta, GA 30309
404-872-7100
800-933-7023
FAX: 404-237-8153
info.ga@arthritis.org
www.arthritis.org

Dan McGowan, Chairman
Rowland W. Chang, Vice Chair
Ann M. Palmer, President and CEO
Patricia N. Nelson, Secretary
Magazine for patients, physicians, public authorities and others with an interest in the field of arthritis. (Price noted paid for yearly subscription) *$12.95*
Bi-Monthly

8188 Fibromyalgia AWARE Magazine
National Fibromyalgia Association
2121 S Towne Centre Pl
suite 30
Orange, CA 92865-6124
714-921-0150
FAX: 714-921-6920
paird@fmaware.org
fmaware.org

Lynne Matallana, Editor In Chief
Malina Anderson, CFO
Eroll Landy, Treasurer
Addresses the needs and concerns of people affected by fibromyalgia and overlapping conditions. *$35.00*
3 times a year

8189 New Mobility
Leonard Media Group
75-20 Astoria Blvd.
East Elmhurst, NY 11370-2068
215-675-9133
888-850-0344
FAX: 215-675-9376
jeff@leonardmedia.com
www.newmobility.com

Amy Blackmore, Vice President Sales
Jean Dobbs, Editorial Director
Tim Gilmer, Editor
Josie Byzek, Managing Editor
The full-service, full-color lifestyle magazine for the disability community. The award-winning magazine is contemporary, witty and candid. Produced by professional journalists and visual artists, the magazine's voice is uncompromising and unsentimental, yet practical, knowing and friendly. The magazine covers issues that matter to readers: medical news, and cure research; jobs, benefits and civil rights; sports, recreation and travel; product news, technology and innovation. *$27.95*
Monthly

8190 **PALAESTRA: Forum of Sport, Physical Education and Recreation for Those with Disabilities**
Challenge Publications Limited
1807 N. Federal Drive
Urbana, IL 61801

217-359-5940
800-327-5557
FAX: 217-359-5975
challpub@macomb.com
www.palaestra.com

David P Beaver EdD, Fonding Editor
Martin.E Block, Editor-in-Chief
Julian U. Stein, Associate Editor
Kathleen Stanton, Asst. Editors

The most comprehensive resource on sport, physical education and recreation for individuals with disabilities, their parents and professionals in the field of adapted physical activity. Published in cooperation with US Paralympics and AAHPERD's Adapted Physical Activity Council. Informative yet entertaining and delivers valuable insights for consumers, families and professionals in the field. Published quarterly.

8191 **PN/Paraplegia News**
PVA Publications
2111 E Highland Ave
Suite 180
Phoenix, AZ 85016-4702

602-224-0500
888-888-2201
FAX: 602-224-0507
info@pnnews.com
www.pn-magazine.com

Richard Hoover, Editor
Ann Santos, Assistant Editor

Packed with timely information on spinal-cord-injury research, new products, legislation that impacts people with disabilities, accessible travel, computer options, car/van adaptations, news for veterans, housing, employment, health care and all issues affecting wheelers and caregivers around the world.

8192 **Spirit Magazine**
Special Olympics International
1133 19th St NW
Washington, DC 20036-3604

202-628-3630
FAX: 202-824-0200
info@specialolympics.org
www.specialolympics.org

Kathy Smallwood, Editor
Timothy P Shriver PhD, Chariman/CEO
J Brady Lum, President/COO

This magazine reflects the power of Special Olympics to build bridges between people with and without intellectual disabilities and spark personal insight, compassion and gratitude for life.
Quarterly

8193 **Strides Magazine**
North American Riding for the Handicapped Assoc
7475 Dakin Street
Suite 600
Denver, CO 80221-6920

303-452-1212
800-369-7433
FAX: 303-252-4610
narha@narha.org
www.narha.org

Carol Nickell, CEO
Sheila Dietrich, Executive Director
William Scebbi, CEO

This engaging magazine is a non-technical, yet accurate journal that focuses on the work of NARHA. Rider profiles, how-to articles, editorials and instructional columns seek to educate a general readership of the diverse aspects of equine facilitated therapy and activities. Each seasonal issue carries a theme.
Quarterly

8194 **Stroke Connection Magazine**
American Stroke Association
7272 Greenville Ave
Dallas, TX 75231-5129

214-373-6300
888-478-7653
FAX: 214-706-1191
www.strokeassociation.org

Ralph Sacco, President/Director
Nancy Brown, CEO
Debra Lockwood, Chairman

From in-depth information on conditions such as aphasia, central pain, high blood pressure and depression, to tips for daily living from healthcare professionals and other stroke survivors. Stroke Connection keeps you abreast of how to cope, how to reduce your risk of stroke and how to make the most of each day.
6 issues

Print: Newsletters

8195 **Arthritis Foundation Great West Region**
Arthritis Foundation
115 N.E. 100th St
Suite 350
Seattle, WA 98125

206-547-2707
888-391-9389
FAX: 206-547-2805
tzuehl@arthritis.org
www.arthritis.org

Scott Weaver, CEO
Kelsey Birnbaum, Vice President, Development
Deborah Genge, Vice President, Development
Duane Hille, Development Coordinator

Offers regional updates, information on activities and events, resources and medical research for members.
Newsletter

8196 **Arthritis Update**
Arthritis Foundation
1330 W. Peachtree St.
Suite 100
Atlanta, GA 30309

404-872-7100
info.uny@arthritis.org
www.arthritis.org

Dan McGowan, Chairman
Rowland W. Chang, Vice Chair
Ann M. Palmer, President and CEO
Patricia N. Nelson, Secretary

Offers chapter updates, information on activities and events, resources and medical research for members.
Newsletter

8197 **Focus**
Arthritis Foundation
1330 W. Peachtree St.
Suite 100
Atlanta, GA 30309

404-872-7100
info.coh@arthritis.org
www.arthritis.org

Dan McGowan, Chairman
Rowland W. Chang, Vice Chair
Ann M. Palmer, President and CEO
Patricia N. Nelson, Secretary

Offers chapter updates, information on activities and events, resources and medical research for members.
Newsletter

8198   Joint Efforts
Arthritis Foundation
1330 W. Peachtree St.
Suite 100
Atlanta, GA 30309
404-872-7100
800-464-6240
FAX: 415-356-1240
info.nca@arthritis.org
www.arthritis.org

Dan McGowan, Chairman
Rowland W. Chang, Vice Chair
Ann M. Palmer, President and CEO
Patricia N. Nelson, Secretary
Offers chapter updates, information on activities and events, resources and medical research for members.
Newsletter

8199   Post-Polio Newsletter
Post-Polio Health International
4207 Lindell Blvd
Ste 110
Saint Louis, MO 63108-2930
314-534-0475
FAX: 314-534-5070
info@post-polio.org
www.post-polio.org

Joan Headley, Executive Director
Gayla Hoffman, Editor
Contains current information about the late effects of polio, updates about post-polio related and neuromuscular respiratory research, as well as articles that offer practical and useful advice by experienced survivors and health care professionals. Available with membership.
12 pages Quarterly

8200   SCILIFE
National Spinal Cord Injury Association
75-20 Astoria Blvd
East Elmhurst, NY 11370
718-803-3782
800-404-2898
FAX: 718-803-0414
info@spinalcord.org
www.unitedspinal.org

David C. Cooper, Chairman
Patrick W. Maher, Vice Chairman
Joseph Gaskins, President and CEO
Denise A. McQuade, Secretary
Filled with issue-driven articles, and news of interest to the SCI community and the larger disability community.
Bi-monthly

Non Print: Newsletters

8201   A World Awaits You
Mobility International USA
132 E Broadway
Suite 343
Eugene, OR 97401-3155
541-343-1284
FAX: 541-343-6812
clearinghouse@miusa.org
www.miusa.org

Susan Sygall, Executive Director
Includes interviews with people with disabilities who have participated in a wide range of international exchange programs.

8202   ABS Newsletter
American Back Society
2648 International Blvd
Suite 502
Oakland, CA 94601-1547
510-536-9929
FAX: 510-536-1812
info@americanbacksoc.org
www.americanbacksoc.org

Scott Haldeman, President
Aubrey Swartz MD, Executive Director

Keeps subscribers current with timely topics on the diagnosis and treatment of a wide spectrum of painful and disabling conditions of the spine.

8203   CurePSP Magazine
Society for Progressive Supranuclear Palsy
2648 International Blvd
Suite 502
Hunt Valley, MD 21031-1002
410-785-7004
800-457-4777
FAX: 410-785-7009
info@curepsp.org
www.psp.org

Richard Gordon Dyne DMin, President
Janet Edmunson, Chair
Dan Johnson, Vice Chair
Informs readers of findings in the area of PSP.

8204   EpilepsyUSA Magazine
Epilepsy Foundation of America
8301 Professional Pl
Landover, MD 20785-2237
301-459-3700
FAX: 301-577-2684
www.epilepsyfoundation.org

Brien J Smith Md, Chair
Mark E Nini, Senior Vice Chair
Richard P Denness, President/CEO
Alexandra K Finucane Esq, Executive Vice President
The Epilepsy Foundation's award-winning magazine, epilepsyUSA, is published online four times a year. The magazine is one of the only publications of its kind devoted entirely to news and up-to-the-minute information about epilepsy.

8205   Exchange
ALS Association
27001 Agoura Rd
Suite 250
Agoura Hills, CA 91301-5105
818-340-0182
800-782-4747
FAX: 818-880-9006
webmaster@alsa.org
www.alsa.org

Gary A Leo, CEO
Morton Charlestein, Chairman
Andrew Soffel, Chairman
Julie Sharpe, Executive Director
Covers a broad range of subjects including stories about the lives of ALS patients, special events, research and public policy in the ALS community.
4-6 times/year

8206   Fibromyalgia Online
National Fibromyalgia Association
2121 S Towne Centre Pl
suite 300
Ornage, CA 92865-6124
714-921-0150
FAX: 714-921-6920
www.fmaware.org

Lynne Matallana, President/Editor In Chief
Malina Anderson, CFO
Eroll Landy, Treasurer
An educational resource for patients and healthcare professionals that brings the latest news on fibrmyalgia and overlapping conditions.
Monthly

8207   MIUSA's Global Impact Newsletter
Mobility International USA
132 E. Broadway
Suite 343
Eugene, OR 97401-2767
541-343-1284
FAX: 541-343-6812
info@miusa.org
www.miusa.org

Susan Sygall, Executive Director
Cindy Lewis, Director
Olivia Hardin, Information Services Coordinator

Each issue features photos, alumni updates, highlights from recent activities, and new publications.
semi-annually

8208 Motivator
Multiple Sclerosis Association of America
706 Haddonfield Rd
Cherry Hill, NJ 8002-2652

856-488-4500
800-532-7667
FAX: 856-661-9797
jmasino@mymsaa.org
www.msassociation.org

Andrea L GriesS, Editor
Susan W Courtney, Sr Writer & Creative Director
Amanda Bednar, Contributing Writer
MSAA's 48-plus page magazine highlights and explains many vital issues of importance to our readers affected by MS. These include cover and feature stories about a variety of topics such as depression, assistive technology, the role of pets and service animals, parents with MS, and clinical trials, to name a few.
48 pages Quarterly

8209 New York Arthritis Reporter
New York Chapter of the Arthritis Foundation
122 East 42nd Street
New York, NY 10168-1898

212-984-8700
FAX: 212-878-5960
info.ny@arthritis.org
www.arthritis.org

Phyllis Geraghty, Editor
Ross Alfieri, President
Daniel T. McGowan, Chair
Provides public access to current arthritis information and resources on important health issues.
Quarterly

8210 SCI Psychosocial Process
American Assoc of Spinal Cord Injury Psych/Soc Wor
75-20 Astoria Blvd
East Elmhurst, NY 11370

718-803-3782
800-404-2898
FAX: 718-803-0414
info@unitedspinal.org
www.unitedspinal.org

David C. Cooper, Chairman
Patrick W. Maher, Vice Chairman
Joseph Gaskins, President and CEO
Denise A. McQuade, Secretary
The purpose of this e journal is disseminating information of value to psychologists, social workers and other psychological caring for spinal cord injured persons.
2 time a year

Non Print: Video

8211 A Wheelchair for Petronilia
Fanlight Productions C/O Icarus Films
32 Court St.
21st Floor
Brooklyn, NY 11201-1731

718-488-8900
800-876-1710
FAX: 718-488-8642
info@fanlight.com
www.fanlight.com

Bob Gliner, Director
Jonathan Miller, President
Meredith Miller, Sales Manager
Anthony Sweeney, Acquisitions
Profiles a program, organized and run by Guatemalans with disabilities, which trains them to manufacture and repair cheap, sturdy wheelchairs designed for conditions in developing countries. 28 Minutes.
VHS/DVD
ISBN 1-572953-98-5

8212 Beyond the Barriers
Aquarius Health Care Videos
30 Forest Road
PO Box 249
Millis, MA 02054

508-376-1244
888-440-2963
FAX: 508-376-1245
www.aquariusproductions.com

Mark Wellman, Director
Leslie Kussmann, President/Producer
For too many years, paraplegics, amputees, quadraplegics and the blind have felt trapped by their disabilities. No more! Mark Wellman and other disabled adventurers, rock climb the desert towers of Utah, sail in British Columbia, body-board the big waves of Pipeline and Waimea Bay, scuba dive with sea lions in Mexico and hand glide the California coast. This film delivers the simple message: Don't give up, and never give in. If you can't ever lose, then you can't ever win. Preview option.
Video/47 Mins

8213 Breathing Lessons: The Life and Work of Mark O'Brien
Fanlight Productions C/O Icarus Films
32 Court St.
21st Floor
Brooklyn, NY 11201-1731

718-488-8900
800-876-1710
FAX: 718-488-8642
info@fanlight.com
www.fanlight.com

Jessica Yu, Director
Jonathan Miller, President
Meredith Miller, Sales Manager
Anthony Sweeney, Acquisitions
Breathing Lessons breaks down barriers to understanding by presenting an honest and intimate portrait of a complex, intelligent, beautiful and interesting person, who happens to be disabled.
$225.00
Video/35 Mins 1996
ISBN 1-572958-41-3

8214 Complete Armchair Fitness
CC-M Productions
7755 16th St NW
Washington, DC 20012-1460

202-882-7432
800-453-6280
FAX: 202-882-7432
info@armchairfitness.com
www.armchairfitness.com

Robert Mason, Manager
Armchair Fitness video series. 4 DVDs: Armchair Fitness Aerobic, Armchair Fitness Gentle, Armchair Fitness Strength and Armchair Fitness Yoga. *$120.00*
Video

8215 How Come You Walk Funny?
Fanlight Productions C/O Icarus Films
32 Court St.
21st Floor
Brooklyn, NY 11201-1731

718-488-8900
800-876-1710
FAX: 718-488-8642
info@fanlight.com
www.fanlight.com

Tina Hahn, Director
Jonathan Miller, President
Meredith Miller, Sales Manager
Anthony Sweeney, Acquisitions
Profiles a unique experiment in reverse integration: a school where non disabled kids attend a kindergarten designed for children with physical disabilities. The kids and families tackle their differences and discover common ground through finding a way that all can play. *$ 179.00*
Video/47 Mins 2004
ISBN 1-572958-84-7

8216 Key Changes: A Portrait of Lisa Thorson
Fanlight Productions C/O Icarus Films
32 Court St.
21st Floor
Brooklyn, NY 11201-1731

718-488-8900
800-876-1710
FAX: 718-488-8642
info@fanlight.com
www.fanlight.com

Cindy Marshall, Director
Jonathan Miller, President
Meredith Miller, Sales Manager
Anthony Sweeney, Acquisitions

A documentary profiling Lisa Thorson, a gifted vocalist who uses a wheelchair. Ms. Thorson defines herself as a performer first, a person with a disability second, and this thoughtful portrait respects that distinction. Her work as a jazz singer is at the heart of the film, reflecting her philosophy that the biggest contribution that she can make to the struggle for the rights of people with disabilities is doing her art the best way she can. *$149.00*
Video/28 Mins 1993
ISBN 1-572959-30-4

8217 Wheelchair Bowling
American Wheelchair Bowling Association
PO Box 69
Clover, VA 24534-69

434-454-2269
FAX: 434-454-6276
garyryan210@gmail.com
www.awba.org

Dick Schaaf, Author
Dave Roberts, Executive Secretary Treasurer

In addition to providing historical background, it includes principles of the game from keeping score through ball drilling for the wheelchair bowler. Through profiles of wheelchair bowlers, the text covers ball delivery, spare making techniques and special equipment that can be used. *$9.95*
96 pages

8218 Yoga for Arthritis
Mobility Limited
601 Morro Bay Blvd
Suite E
Morro Bay, CA 93442-2000

805-772-3560
800-366-6038
FAX: 805-772-4717
shsh@mobilityltd.com
www.mobilityltd.com

Shoosh Crotzer, Owner/Executive Director

A yoga-based program with five separate segments, which includes breathing and relaxation techniques, stretching and strengthening routines, and aerobic exercises. This 52-minute program can also be performed seated. Available on DVD or VHS; DVD includes Spanish version. *$19.95*
Video

8219 Yoga for MS and Related Conditions
Mobility Limited
601 Morro Bay Blvd
Suite E
Morro Bay, CA 93442-2000

805-772-3560
800-366-6038
FAX: 805-772-4717
shsh@mobilityltd.com
www.mobilityltd.com

Shoosh Crotzer, Owner/Executive Director

A yoga-based program. Shows assisted versions of each exercise for those who require it; is available with an optional Instructional Guidebook with illustrations, alternative positions, and hints. This 48-minute program can also be performed seated. Available on DVD or VHS; DVD includes Spanish version. *$19.95*
Video

Sports

8220 Access to Sailing
423 E Shoreline Village Drive
Long Beach, CA 90802

562-901-9999
info@accesstosailing.org
www.accesstosailing.org

Duncan Milne, Founder/Executive Director
Cliff Larson, Director
Gaile Oslapas, Assistant Director

Provides therapeutic rehabilitation to disabled and disadvantaged children and adults, through interactive sailing outings.

8221 Achilles Track Club
42 West 38th Street
Suite 400
New York, NY 10018-6241

212-354-0300
FAX: 212-354-3978
info@achillestrackclub.org
www.achillestrackclub.org

Richard Traum PhD, President/Founder
Mary Bryant, Vice President
Kathleen Bateman, Director

Organization whose goal is to guide disabled athletes into the able-bodied community.

8222 Adaptive Sports Center
PO Box 1639
Crested Butte, CO 81224-1639

970-349-2296
866-349-2296
FAX: 970-349-2077
info@adaptivesports.org
www.adaptivesports.org

Christopher Hensley, Executive Director
Chris Read, CTRS Program Director
Ella Fahrlander, Development Director
Erin English, Marketing/Communications Dir.

Year round adaptive, adventure recreation program located at the base of Crested Butte Mountain Resort, Crested Butte ,CO. The Adaptive Sports Centers provides adaptive downhill and cross country ski lessons, ski rentals and snowboarding lessons in the winter. Offers a variety of wilderness based programs in the summer including multi-day trips into the back country, extensive cycling programs, canoeing, and white water rafting.

8223 American Wheelchair Bowling Association
PO Box 69
Clover, VA 24534-69

434-454-2269
FAX: 434-454-6276
garyryan210@gmail.com
www.awba.org

Joseph L. Fox, Chairman
Wayne Webber, Vice Chairperson
Paul Kenney, Treasurer
Gary Rayan, Secretary

A non-profit organization, composed of wheelchair bowlers, dedicated to encouraging, developing, and regulating wheelchair bowling and wheelchair bowling leagues.

8224 Bold Tracks
Big Earth Publishing
3005 Center Green Drive
Suite 225
Boulder, CO 80301

800-258-5830
FAX: 303-443-9687
books@bigearthpublishing.com
www.bigearthpublishing.com

Hal O'Leary, Author
Janet Heisz, Sales Manager

This guide is essential for instructor and student alike. It covers skiing for the visually and hearing impaired as well as the physically and developmentally disabled. *$24.95*
156 pages Paperback
ISBN 1-555661-14-4

8225 Chesapeake Region Accessible Boating
PO Box 6564
Annapolis, MD 21401-564

410-626-0273
FAX: 410-626-6070
info@crabsailing.org
www.crab-sailing.org

Daniel Jarzynski, President
Lance Hinrichs, Vice President
Ernie Shineman, Treasurer
Loren Barnett, Secretary
Provides opportunities for the disabled and their friends to sail the Chesapeake Bay. Day sails, lessons, organized races. Call for charter information. Sail for free on the fourth Sunday of each month, May through October.

8226 Disabled Sports Program Center
Disabled Sports USA Far West
PO Box 9780
Truckee, CA 96162-7780

530-581-4161
FAX: 530-581-3127
dsusa@disabledsports.net
www.dsusafw.org

Doug Pringle, President
Marilyn Cummings,, Office Manager
Haakon Lang-Ree, Manager
Founded in 1967, Disabled Sports USA Far West is dedicated to innovative programs that provide an environment with positive therapeutic and psychological outcomes. Individuals are empowered to reach their full potential. Our programs allow individuals of all abilities to discover their own strengths and interests.

8227 Disabled Sports USA
451 Hungerford Dr
Suite 100
Rockville, MD 20850-5102

301-217-0960
FAX: 301-217-0968
information@dusa.org
www.disabledsportsusa.org

Kirk Bauer, Executive Director
Kathy Chandler, Executive Director
Kathy Celo, Operations
Kathy Laffey, Special Projects Manager
Provides year-round sports and recreation opportunities for people with physical disabilities, veterans and non-veterans alike, such as sanctioned regional and national events in alpine and Nordic skiing, cycling, shooting swimming, table tennis, track and field, volleyball, and weightlifting. The organization handles physical disabilities which restrict mobility, including amputations paraplegia, quadriplegia, cerebral palsy, head injury, mulitple sclerosis, muscular dystrophy, and more.

8228 Disabled Watersports Program
Mission Bay Aquatic Center
1001 Santa Clara Pl
San Diego, CA 92109

858-488-1000
FAX: 858-488-9625
mbac@sdsu.edu
www.missionbayaquaticcenter.com

Kevin Starw, Director
Kevin Waldick, Asst. director
Eric Fehrs, Maintenance Director
Amanda Burgess, Office Supervisor
Devoted to providing accessible water sports and recreational opportunities for individuals with disabilities. Specially designed equipment makes water skiing, wake boarding, keelboat sailing, windsurfing, rowing, surfing, and kayaking possible for people with varying levels of mobility and ability.

8229 Galvin Health and Fitness Center
Rehabilitation Institute of Chicago
345 East Suuperior St.
Chicago, IL 60611

312-238-1000
800-354-7342
800-354-REHA
FAX: 312-238-5017
sports@ric.org
http://www.ric.org

Jude Reyes, Chair
Mike P. Kransy, Vice Chair
Thomas Reynolds III, Vice Chair
Joanne C. Smith, President & CEO
The RIC Sports and Fitness Program offers people with physical disabilities an on-site fitness center, specialized exercise classes and services, and adult and junior competitive and recreational sports opportunities, including the recreational/social Caring for Kids program for youth ages 7-17. Most programs are provided free of charge or for a nominal fee.

8230 Guide to Wheelchair Sports and Recreation
Paralyzed Veterans of America
801 18th St NW
Washington, DC 20006-3517

202-872-1300
800-424-8200
888-888-2201
FAX: 202-785-4432
TTY:800-795-4327
info@pva.org
www.pva.org

Homer S. Townsend, Jr., Executive Director
Larry Dodson, National Secretary
Bill Lawson, National President
Al Kovach, Jr, Natonal Senior Vice President
This guide is published to introduce and increase awareness of people with disabilities to the many sports and recreational opportunities available. It lists descriptions of adaptive sports and recreation, activity and equipment directories, and additional resources for people with disabilities.
28 pages Booklet

8231 Handicapped Scuba Association International
Handicapped Scuba Association
1104 El Prado
San Clemente, CA 92672-4637

949-498-4540
FAX: 949-498-6128
hsa@hsascuba.com
www.hsascuba.com

Jim Gatacre, President
Patricia Derk, Vice President
A nonprofit volunteer organization dedicated to improving the physical and social well being of those with special needs through the exhilarating sport of scuba diving. An educational program for able bodied scuba instructors to learn to teach and certify people with special needs. Accessible travel opportunities.

8232 Lakeshore Foundation
4000 Ridgeway Dr
Birmingham, AL 35209-5563

205-313-7400
FAX: 205-313-7475
information@lakeshore.org
www.lakeshore.org

Jeff Underwood, President & CEO
Beth Curry, Chief Program Officer
Jen Remick, Director, Communications & Membership
Damian Veazey, Associate Director, Communications
Promotes independence for persons with physically disabling conditions and provides opportunities to pursue active, healthy lifestyles.

8233 National Disability Sports Alliance
25 W Independence Way
Kingston, RI 02881-1124

401-792-7130
FAX: 401-792-7132
info@ndsaonline.org
http://nationaldisabilitysportsalliance.webs.

Jerry McCole, Executive Director

Serves to present disabled athletes with the opportunity to perform in many different sports. Participants range from the beginning athlete to the elite, international caliber athlete.

8234   National Skeet Shooting Association
5931 Roft Rd
San Antonio, TX 78253-9261
                                   210-688-3371
                                   800-877-5338
                                   FAX: 210-688-3014
                                   nsca@nssa-nsca.com
                                   www.mynssa.com

Michael Hampton, Jr., Executive Director
Royce Graff, NSSA Director
Amber Schwarz, NSC Assistant Director
Linda Mayes, NSSA Director
Offers information on sporting clay targets for the disabled hunter.

8235   National Sports Center for the Disabled
33 Parsenn Road
PO Box 1290
Winter Park, CO 80482-1290
                                   303-316-1518
                                   FAX: 970-726-4112
                                   info@nscd.org
                                   www.nscd.org

Diane Eustace, Marketing Director
Beth Fox, Operations Director,
Erica Mays, Human Resources Director
Ellen White, Finance Director/CFO
Our mission is to provide quality outdoor sports and therapeutic recreation programs that positively impact the lives of people with physical, cognitive, emotional, or behavioral challenges.
6-8 pages Quarterly

8236   National Wheelchair Poolplayers Association
90 Flemons Dr
Somerville, AL 35670
                                   256-778-0449
                                   FAX: 703-817-1215
                                   www.nwpainc.org

Jeffrey Dolezal, President
Bob Calderon, Secretary
Ken Force, Editor
Works together with other groups, organizations, and tournaments to update rules to include wheelchair players.

8237   North American Riding for the Handicapped Association
7475 Dakin Street
Suite 600
Denver, CO 80221-6920
                                   303-452-1212
                                   800-369-7433
                                   FAX: 303-252-4610
                                   narha@narha.org
                                   www.pathintl.org

Sheila Dietrich, Executive Director
Carolyn Malcheski,, Director of Finance and Human Resources
Kaye Marks, Director of Marketing and Communications
Kay Green, Chief Executive Officer
Professional Association of Therapeutic Horsemanship International (PATH Intl.), a federally-registered 501(c3) nonprofit, was formed in 1969 as the North American Riding for the Handicapped Association to promote equine-assisted activities and therapies (EAAT) for individuals with special needs. *$35.00*
42 pages Quarterly

8238   Ontario Cerebral Palsy Sports Association
P.O. Box 60082
Ottawa, ON, Canada K1T-0K9
                                   613-723-1806
                                   866-286-2772
                                   FAX: 613-723-6742
                                   www.ocpsa.on.ca

Amanda Fader, Executive Director
Don Sinclair, President
Lorette Dupuis, Vice President
Sue Bartol, Development Director
Organization that provides, promotes and coordinates competitive opportunities as well as encourages individual excellence through sport for athletes within the cerebral palsy family. To that

end, OCPSA recruits, develops and supports athletes, coaches and volunteers.

8239   Special Olympics
1133 19th St NW
Washington, DC 20036-3604
                                   202-393-1251
                                   FAX: 202-715-1146
                                   info@specialolympics.org
                                   www.specialolympics.org

Timothy P Shriver PhD, Chariman/CEO
J Brady Lum, President/COO
Stephen M Carter, Lead Director/CEO/Vice Chair
A year-round worldwide program that promotes physical fitness, sports training and athletic competition for children and adults with intellectual disabilities.

8240   Special Olympics International
1133 19th St NW
Washington, DC 20036-3604
                                   202-393-1251
                                   FAX: 202-715-1146
                                   info@specialolympics.org
                                   www.specialolympics.org

Timothy P Shriver PhD, Chariman/CEO
J Brady Lum, President/COO
Stephen M Carter, Lead Director/CEO/Vice Chair
Provides year-round training and athletic competition in a variety of well-coached, Olympic-type sparts for persons with mental retardation. Offers opportunities to develop physical fitness, prepare for entry into school and community sports programs. Athletes express courage, experience joy and participate in gifts, skills and friendship with their families and other Special Olympics athletes. Local information can be provided by regional offices.

8241   United Foundation for Disabled Archers
20 NE 9th Ave. Glenwood,
PO Box 251
Glenwood, MN 56334- 251
                                   320-634-3660
                                   info@uffdaclub.com
                                   www.uffdaclub.com

Daniel James Hendricks, President
Russ Kalk, Vice President
Debbie Kalk, Treasurer
It is the mission of the United Foundation for Disabled Archers to promote and provide a means to practice all forms of archery for any physically challenged person.

8242   Wheelchair Sports, USA
PO Box 5266
Kendall Park, NJ 08824-5266
                                   732-266-2634
                                   FAX: 732-355-6500
                                   office@wsusa.org
                                   www.wsusa.org

Kelly Behlmann, Owner
Gregg Baumgraten, Chairperson
Denise Hutchins, Vice-Chairperson
Jessica Galli, Secretary
Initiates, stimulates and promotes the growth and development of wheelchair sports.

Support Groups

8243   Information Hotline
Arthritis Foundation, Southeast Region Inc
1330 W. Peachtree St.
Suite 100
Atlanta, GA 30309
                                   404-872-7100
                                   800-933-7023
                                   FAX: 404-237-8153
                                   info.ga@arthritis.org
                                   www.arthritis.org

Dan McGowan, Chairman
Rowland W. Chang, Vice Chair
Ann M. Palmer, President and CEO
Patricia N. Nelson, Secretary

The mission of the Arthritis Foundation is to improve lives through leadership in the prevention, control and cure of arthritis and related diseases.

8244 **Kids on the Block Programs**
9385 Gerwig Lane
Suite C
Maryland, MD 21157-2893

410-290-9095
800-368-5437
FAX: 410-290-9358
kob@kotb.com
www.kotb.com

Aric Darroe, President
Jane Thuman, Vice President
Christina Grogan, Marketing Manager
Features life-size puppets in educational programs that enlighten children and adults on the issues of disability awareness, medical and educational differences, and social concerns.

General Disorders

Associations

8245 **AIDS United**
1424 K Street, N.W.
Ste 200
Washington, DC 20005-1511 202-408-4848
888-234-2437
FAX: 202-408-1818
info@aidsunited.org
www.aidsunited.org

Jesse Milan Jr., JD, Interim President & CEO
Matthew J. Kessler, Vice President, Operations
Cody Barnett, Commuications Coordinator
Monique Tula, Vice President, Programs
AIDS United advocates for people living with or affected by HIV/AIDS and the organizations that serve them. AIDS United's mission is to end the AIDS epidemic in the United States through strategic grantmaking, capacity building, policy/advocacy, technical assistance and formative research.

8246 **American Academy of Allergy, Asthma & Immunology**
555 E Wells St.
Ste 1100
Milwaukee, WI 53202-3823 414-272-6071
FAX: 414-272-6070
info@aaaai.org
www.aaaai.org

Thomas A. Fleisher, M.D.; FAAAAI, President
An association of medical professionals and specialists that places focus on research and treatment for allergic and immunologic diseases, as well as improved patient care.

8247 **American Academy of Otolaryngology - Head and Neck Surgery**
1650 Diagonal Rd
Alexandria, VA 22314-2857 703-836-4444
FAX: 703-683-5100
TTY:703-519-1585
www.entnet.org

James c. Denneny III, M.D., Executive Vice President & CEO
Sujana S. Chandrasekhar, M.D., President
Carol R. Bradford, Director, Academic
Michael D. Seidman, Director, Academic
The American Academy of Otolaryngology-Head and Neck Surgery (AAO-HNS) is an organization representing specialists who treat the ear, nose, throat, and related structures of the head and neck.

8248 **American Academy of Physical Medicine and Rehabilitation**
9700 W Bryn Mawr Ave
Ste 200
Rosemont, IL 60018-5701 847-737-6000
877-227-6799
FAX: 847-737-6001
info@aapmr.org
www.aapmr.org

Thomas E. Stautzenbach, Executive Director & Chief Executive Officer
Gregory M. Worsowicz, President
Darryl L. Kaelin, Vice President
This national medical specialty society represents more than 6,500 physical medicine and rehabilitation physicians, whose patients include people with physical disabilities and chronic, disabling illnesses. The academy's mission is to maximize quality of life, minimize the incidence and prevalence of impairments and disability, promote societal health and enhance the understanding and development of the specialty. The organization offers information, referrals, and patient materials.

8249 **American Association for Respiratory Care**
9425 N. MacArthur Blvd.
Ste 100
Irving, TX 75063-4706 972-243-2272
FAX: 972-484-2720
info@aarc.org
www.aarc.org

Tom Kallstrom, Executive Director
Steve Bowden, IT, General Inquiries
AARC's mission is to advance the science, technology, ethics and art of respiratory care through research and education for its members and to teach the general public about pulmonary health and disease prevention.

8250 **American Association of Cardiovascular and Pulmonary Rehabilitation**
330 N. Wabash Avenue
Suite 2200
Chicago, IL 60611 312-321-5146
FAX: 312-673-6924
aacvpr@aacvpr.org
www.aacvpr.org

Adam T. deJong, President
Megan Cohen, Executive Director
Jessica Eustice, Director Of Corporate Relations
Abigail Lynn, Operations Senior Manager
The mission of American Association of Cardiovascular and Pulmonary Rehabilitation is to reduce morbidity, mortality, and disability from cardiovascular and pulmonary diseases through education, prevention, rehabilitation, research, and aggressive disease management.

8251 **American Brain Tumor Association**
8550 W. Bryn Mawr Ave
Ste 550
Chicago, IL 60631-4106 773-577-8750
800-886-2282
FAX: 773-577-8738
info@abta.org
www.abta.org

Elizabeth Wilson, President & CEO
Martha Carlos, Chief Communications Officer
Kerri Mink, Chief Operating Officer
Sandy Abraham, Director, Marketing & Communications
A non-profit organization founded in 1973 dedicated to the elimination of brain tumors through research and patient education services.

8252 **American Diabetes Association**
1701 N Beauregard St
Alexandria, VA 22311-1733 703-549-1500
800-342-2383
FAX: 703-836-7439
askada@diabetes.org
www.diabetes.org

Kevin L. Hagan, Chief Executive Officer
Margaret Powers, PhD; RD; CDE, President, Health Care & Education
Provides diabetes research, information and advocacy. The mission of the Association is to prevent and cure diabetes and to improve the lives of all people affected by diabetes.

8253 **American Group Psychotherapy Association**
25 E. 21st St.
6th Floor
New York, NY 10010-6207 212-477-2677
877-668-2472
FAX: 212-979-6627
info@agpa.org
www.agpa.org

Marsha S. Block, Chief Executive Officer
Eleanor F. Counselman, EdD; CGP, President
Nina Brown, Secretary
AGPA serves as the national voice specific to the interests of group psychotherapy. Its 4,100 members and 31 affiliate societies provide a wealth of professional, educational and social support for group psychotherapists in the United States and around the world.

8254 American Head and Neck Society
11300 W. Olympic Blvd
Ste 600
Los Angeles, CA 90064-1663   310-437-0559
                                FAX: 310-437-0585
                                admin@ahns.info
                                www.ahns.info

Dennis Kraus, MD, President
Jonathan Irish, MD, Vice President
Brian B. Burkey, MD; MEd, Secretary
Ehab Hanna, Treasurer
AHNS is a professional organization, formed in 1998 to promote research and education in head and neck oncology. The AHNS offers clinical practice guidelines, details of events, grants, and patient information. It aims to promote and advance the knowledge of prevention, diagnosis, treatment, and rehabilitation of neoplasms and other diseases of the head and neck.

8255 American Lung Association
55 W. Wacker Dr.
Ste 1150
Chicago, IL 60601   312-781-1100
                                    800-548-8252
                                FAX: 202-452-1085
                                    info@lung.org
                                    www.lung.org

Harold P. Wimmer, President & CEO
Sue . Swan, National Chief Development Officer
Sally Draper, National Vice President, Development
Kim Lacina, National Vice President, Marketing & Communications
The ALA is an organization dedicated to combating tobacco use, eliminating lung diseases, and improving air quality through research, education, and advocacy. The association provides knowledge beneficial to patients, patients' families, and medical professionals and specialists.

8256 American SIDS Institute
528 Raven Way
Naples, FL 34110   239-431-5425
                                FAX: 239-431-5536
                                    prevent@sids.org
                                    www.sids.org

Marc Peterzell, JD, Chairman
Betty McEntire, PhD, Executive Director & CEO
Nicole Dobson, MD, Board Member
Alfred Steinschneider, MD, President Emeritus
American SIDS Institute is a national nonprofit health care organization that is dedicated to the prevention of sudden infant death and the promotion of infant health through an aggressive, comprehensive nationwide program of research, clinical services, education and family support.

8257 American Sexual Health Association
P.O. Box 13827
Research Triangle Park, NC 27709-3827   919-361-8400
                                     FAX: 919-361-8425
                                     info@ashasexualhealth.org
                                     www.ashastd.org
Lynn Barclay, President & CEO
Deborah Arrindell, Vice President, Health Policy
The American Sexual Health Association is a trusted source of information on sexual health, relationships, and measures to prevent adverse sexual health

8258 American Society of Pediatric Hematology/Oncology
8735 West Higgins Rd.
Ste. 300
Chicago, IL 60631   847-375-4716
                                FAX: 847-375-6483
                                    info@aspho.org
                                    www.aspho.org

Sally Weir, Executive Director
Steve Biddle, Education Consultant
Jackie Holcomb, Education Manager
Sergio Miranda, Memeber Services
ASPHO is multidisciplinary organization dedicated to promoting optimal care of children and adolescents with blood disorders and

cancer by advancing research, education, treatment and professional practice.

8259 American Thoracic Society
25 Broadway
18th Floor
New York, NY 10004-2755   212-315-8600
                                FAX: 212-315-6498
                                    atsinfo@thoracic.org
                                    www.thoracic.org
Steve Crane, Executive Director
Nicola Black, Associate Director, Governance Activities
Jennifer A. Ian, Director, Member Services & Chapter Relations
Eileen Larsson, Chief Program Officer
The American Thoracic Society is dedicated to research, public health education, and patient care in relation to pulmonary disease, critical illness, and sleep disorders.

8260 Aplastic Anemia and MDS International Foundation
100 Park Ave
Ste 108
Rockville, MD 20850   301-279-7202
                                    800-747-2820
                                FAX: 301-279-7205
                                    help@aamds.org
                                    www.aamds.org

John Huber, Executive Director
Angie Onofre, Director of Patient Programs and Services
Leigh Clark, Patient Educator
Benita Marcus, Senior Director Of Operations
This organization, formerly known as Aplastic Anemia Foundation of America, provides a resource directory for patient assistance, produces educational material and supports research into AA and MDS.

8261 Canadian Cancer Society
55 St. Clair Avenue W.
Ste 300
Toronto, ON, Canada M4V- 2Y7   416-961-7223
                                    888-939-3333
                                FAX: 416-961-4189
                                TTY:866-786-3934
                                    ccs@cancer.ca
                                    www.cancer.ca

Anne V,zina, Interim President & CEO
Martin Kabat, Chief Executive Officer
Lesley Ring, Vice President, Development & Marketing
A national community-based organization of volunteers whose mission is the eradication of cancer and the enhancement of the quality of life for people living with cancer.

8262 Canadian Diabetes Association
1400-522 University Ave
Toronto, ON, Canada M5G-2R5   416-363-3373
                                    800-226-8464
                                FAX: 416-408-7015
                                    info@diabetes.ca
                                    www.diabetes.ca

Doug Macnamara, President & CEO
Paul Kilbertus, Senior Director, Strategic Communications
The mission of the Canadian Diabetes Association is to promote the health of Canadians through diabetes research, education, service and advocacy.

8263 Canadian Lung Association
1750 Courtwood Cres
Ottawa, ON, Canada K2C-2B5   613-569-6411
                                    888-566-5864
                                FAX: 613-569-8860
                                    info@lung.ca
                                    www.lung.ca

Debra Lynkowksi, President & CEO
Anne Van Dam, Director, Research & Knowledge Translation
Amy Henderson, Manager, Public Policy & Health Communications
Janis Hass, Director, Marketing & Communications
The Canadian Lung Association is a non-profit and volunteer-based health charity, dedicated to improving lung health in

the Canadian community through research, education, prevention and advocacy.

8264 Childhood Cancer Canada Foundation
21 St. Clair Ave E
Ste 801
Toronto, ON, Canada M4T-1L9 416-489-6440
800-363-1062
FAX: 416-489-9812
info@childhoodcancer.ca
www.childhoodcancer.ca

Clare Davenport, President & CEO
Natasha Bowes, Senior Manager, Fund Development
Patricia Zareba, Fund Development Manager
Jessica MacInnis, Manager of Marketing & Communications
A national, volunteer governed, charitable organization dedicated to improving the quality of life for children with cancer. The foundation raises funds to assist with cancer research undertakings across Canada.

8265 Childhood Leukemia Foundation
807 Mantoloking Rd
Brick, NJ 08723 732-920-8860
888-253-7109
www.clf4kids.org

Barbara Haramis, Executive Director & Founder
Barb Estelle, Chief Operating Officer
Kim Wetmore, Director, Development
Kate Booth, Program Services Coordinator
The CLF is a national, non-profit organization providing education, information, support, and advocacy for patients of cancer and their families. the foundation works closely with health professionals, social workers, and specialists to offer a variety of programs that aim to enrich the lives of children living with cancer.

8266 Division for Physical, Health & Multiple Disabilities
Council for Exceptional Children
2900 Crystal Dr.
Ste 1000
Arlington, VA 22202 888-232-7733
FAX: 703-264-9494
TTY:866-915-5000
www.community.cec.sped.org/dphmd/home

Pat Kuntzler, President
Angie Juarez, Vice President
Mari Beth Coleman, Communications
Laura Clarke, Policy & Advocacy Committee
This division of the CEC advocates for the provision of quality education for individuals with physical disabilities, multiple disabilities, and special health care needs served in schools, hospitals, or home settings. DPHMD's members include classroom teachers, administrators, related service personnel, hospital/homebound teachers, and parents.

8267 Emphysema Foundation for Our Right to Survive
PO Box 20241
Kansas City, MO 64119-0241 866-363-2673
FAX: 816-413-0176
efforts-request@effortslist.org
www.emphysema.net

Linda Watson, President
Debbie Snodell, Secretary
EFFORTS is a non-profit organization that takes an active role in promoting research for more effective treatments and perhaps a cure for emphysema and related lung diseases. It also works to further education about the disease and provides a support mailing list for members.

8268 Environmental Health Center: Dallas
8345 Walnut Hill Lane
Ste 220
Dallas, TX 75231-4205 214-368-4132
FAX: 214-691-8432
contact@ehcd.com
www.ehcd.com

William J Rea, Director
Chris Rea, Business Manager
Yaqin Pan, M.D., Research Physician
Bertie Griffiths, Ph.D., Microbiologist/Immunologist
Clinic providing patient care in the areas of Immunotherapy, Nutrition, Physical Therapy, Chemical Depuration, Energy Balancing, Electromagnetic Sensitivity Testing, Psychological Support Services, Family Practice Medicine and Internal Medicine. Provides services for individuals whose diseases are caused by environmental factors.

8269 Eunice Kennedy Shriver National Institute of Child Health and Human Development (NICHD)
National Institutes of Health (NIH)
31 Center Dr.
Bldg 31, Rm 2A32
Bethesda, MD 20892-2425 301-496-5097
800-370-2943
FAX: 866-760-5947
TTY: 888-320-6942
nichdinformationresourcecenter@mail.nih.gov
www.nichd.nih.gov

Catherine Y. Spong, MD, Acting Director
The NICHD, part of the federal National Institutes of Health, conducts and supports research topics related to the health of children, adults, families, and populations, including growth and development; parenting; learning and reading; and mental retardation, autism, and developmental disabilities, and provides information on these topics.

8270 Herpes Resource Center
American Social Health Association
P.O. Box 13827
Research Triangle Park, NC 27709-3827 919-361-8400
800-227-8922
FAX: 919-361-8425
customerservice@ashastd.org
www.ashastd.org/stdsstis/herpes/

Lynn Barclay, President & CEO
The Herpes Resource Center (HRC) focuses on increasing education, public awareness, and support to anyone concerned about herpes.

8271 International Academy of Biological Dentistry and Medicine
19122 Camellia Bend Circle
Ste 101
Spring, TX 77379 281-651-1745
FAX: 281-440-1258
drdawn@drdawn.net
www.iabdm.org

Dr. Dawn Ewing, Executive Director
Felix Liao, President
Toby Ewing, Assistant Director
The IABDM promotes non-toxic diagnostic and therapeutic approaches in dentistry and hosts seminars on biological diagnosis and therapy.

8272 International Academy of Oral Medicine & Toxicology
8297 ChampionsGate Blvd
Ste 193
ChampionsGate, FL 33896-8387 863-420-6373
FAX: 863-419-8136
info@iaomt.org
www.iaomt.org

Mark Wisniewski, President
Tammy DeGregorio, Executive Vice President
Kym Smith, Executive Director
A non-profit organization dedicated to funding solid peer-reviewed scientific research in the area of toxic substances used in dentistry as well as providing continuing education and carefully

reviewed procedures, protocols, and methodologies to reduce the risk for patients and professionals.

8273 International Association for Cancer Victors & Friends
P.O. Box 745
Lakeport, CA 95453
408-834-5300
FAX: 408-264-9659
contact@cancervictors.net
www.cancervictors.net

a.k.a. Cancer Victors & Friends

8274 International Association of Hygienic Physicians
4620 Euclid Blvd
Youngstown, OH 44512-1633
330-788-0526
FAX: 330-788-0093
www.iahp.net

Alec Burton, Co-Founder
Mark A. Huberman, Secretary/Treasurer

The International Association of Hygienic Physicians (IAHP) is a professional association for licensed, primary care physicians (Medical Doctors, Osteopaths, Chiropractors, and Naturopaths) who specialize in Therapeutic Fasting Supervision as an integral part of Hygienic Care.

8275 International Medical and Dental Hypnotherapy Association
8852 SR 3001
RR 2
Laceyville, PA 18623-9417
570-869-1021
800-553-6886
FAX: 570-869-1249
www.hypnosisalliance.com/imdha

Linda Otto, Executive Director
Robert Otto, President & CEO
Christie Boecker, Membership Services Coordinator

The association provides and encourages education programs to further, the knowledge, understanding, and application of hypnosis in complementary healthcare; encourages research and scientific publication in the field of hypnosis; and advocates for further recognition and acceptance of hypnosis as an important tool in healthcare and focus for scientific research.

8276 International Myeloma Foundation
12650 Riverside Dr
Ste 206
North Hollywood, CA 91607- 3421
818-487-7455
800-452-2873
FAX: 818-487-7454
theimf@myeloma.org
www.myeloma.org

David Girard, Executive Director
Susie Novis, President
Diane Moran, Senior Vice President, Strategic Planning
Selma Plascencia, Director of Operations

The IMF serves myeloma patients, family members, and the medical community, offering a wide range of programs in the areas of Research, Education, Support, and Advocacy.

8277 Leukemia & Lymphoma Society
3 International Dr
Ste 200
Rye Brook, NY 10573
914-949-5213
800-955-4572
FAX: 914-949-6691
supportservices@lls.org
www.lls.org

Louis DeGennaro, President & CEO
Piper Medcalf, Executive Director
Nancy Hallberg, Chief Marketing Officer
Marcie Klein, Senior Vice President, Communications

The Leukemia and Lymphoma Society is the world's largest voluntary health organization dedicated to funding blood cancer research, education and patient services. The society offers information and support for patients of various blood cancer types, including leukemia, lymphoma, Hodgkin's disease and myeloma. It also offers services and resources to help improve the quality of life of patients and their families.

8278 Little People of America
250 El Camino Real
Ste 218
Tustin, CA 92780
714-368-3689
888-572-2001
FAX: 714-368-3367
info@lpaonline.org
www.lpaonline.org

Joanna Campbell, Executive Director
Gary Arnold, President
April Brazier, Senior Vice President
Mark Povinelli, Membership Director

Little People of America is a national non-profit organization that provides support and information to people of short stature and their families. Short stature is generally caused by one of the more than 200 medical conditions known as dwarfism. LPA offers information on employment, education, disability rights, adoption, medical issues, clothing, adaptive products, and the many stages of parenting a short-statured child - from birth to adult.

8279 Lymphoma Canada
Formerly The Lymphoma Foundation Canada
6860 Century Ave
Ste 202
Mississauga, ON, Canada L5N-2W5
905-858-5967
866-659-5556
info@lymphoma.ca
www.lymphoma.ca

Robin Markowitz, Chief Executive Officer
Lorna Warwick, National Director, Education & Services
Charlene Ragin, Marketing & Communications
Anwar Knight, Director, Mississauga, ON

Lymphoma Canada provides, at no cost and in both official languages: electronic and print materials on the Hodgkin lymphoma, non-Hodgkin lymphoma and CLL, peer and caregiver support groups, educational forums and advocacy on behalf of patients. Lymphoma Canada also funds Canadian research.

8280 Myositis Association
1737 King Street
Ste 600
Alexandria, VA 22314
703-299-4850
800-821-7356
FAX: 703-535-6752
tma@myositis.org
www.myositis.org

Bob Goldberg, Executive Director
Theresa Reynolds Curry, Communications Manager
Aisha Morrow, Operations Manager
Charlia Sanchez, Member Services Coordinator

The aim of TMA's programs and services is to provide information, support, advocacy and research for those concerned about myositis, as well as serving those affected by these diseases. Support groups offer members the chance to share and discuss their concerns with people in similar situations.

8281 National Association for Children of Alcoholics
10920 Connecticut Ave
Ste 100
Kensington, MD 20895-3007
301-468-0985
888-554-2627
FAX: 301-468-0987
nacoa@nacoa.org
www.nacoa.org

Sis Wenger, President & CEO
Steve Hornberger, Program Director

National non-profit membership and affiliate organization working on behalf of children of alcohol and drug dependent parents to help eliminate the adverse impact of drug use on children through public awareness, policy, advocacy, education, and support.

8282   National Association for Home Care & Hospice
228 7th St SE
Washington, DC 20003-4306   202-547-7424
FAX: 202-547-3540
webmaster@nahc.org
www.nahc.org

Val J. Halamandris, President
Lucy Andrews, Vice Chair
Karen Marshall Thompson, Secretary
Thomas Moreland, Treasurer
This is a non-profit trade association representing various home care, hospice and health aid organizations. With services aimed at assiting the chronically ill and disabled, the NAHC offers information on how to choose a home care provider and a zip code driven locator for home care and hospice.

8283   National Association for Medical Direction of Respiratory Care
8618 Westwood Center Dr
Ste 210
Vienna, VA 22182-2273   703-752-4359
FAX: 703-752-4360
execoffice@namdrc.org
www.namdrc.org

Phillip Porte, Executive Director
Vickie Parshall, Director, Member Services
Karen Lui, RN, Associate Executive Director
NAMDRC's primary mission is to improve access to quality care for patients with respiratory disease by removing regulatory and legislative barriers to appropriate treatment.

8284   National Association for Proton Therapy
1155 15th St NW
Ste 500
Washington, DC 20005   202-495-3133
FAX: 202-530-0659
info@proton-therapy.org
www.proton-therapy.org

Leonard Arzt, Executive Director
The National Association for Proton Therapy (NAPT) is registered as an independent, non-profit, public benefit corporation providing education and awareness for the public, professional and governmental communities. It promotes the therapeutic benefits of proton therapy for cancer treatment in the U.S. and abroad.

8285   National Association of Anorexia Nervosa and Associated Disorders
750 E Diehl Road
Ste 127
Naperville, IL 60563   630-577-1333
FAX: 847-433-4632
anadhelp@anad.org
www.anad.org

Laura Zinger, Executive Director
Deb Prinz, Director, Community Relations
A non-profit organization that seeks to alleviate the problems of eating disorders, especially anorexia nervosa and bulimia nervosa, by promoting eating disorder awareness, prevention and recovery through supporting, educating, and connecting individuals, families and professionals.

8286   National Association of Chronic Disease Directors
2200 Century Parkway
Ste 250
Atlanta, GA 30345   770-458-7400
FAX: 770-458-7401
jrobitscher@chronicdisease.org
www.chronicdisease.org

John w. Robitscher, Chief Executive Officer
Namvar Zohoori, President
John Patton, Director, Communications
Margaret Gillan Ritchie, Communications & Member Services Coordinator
A national public health association founded in 1988 to link the chronic disease program directors of each state and U.S. territory to provide a national forum for chronic disease prevention and control efforts. NACDD aims to mobilize national efforts to reduce chronic diseases and the associated risk factors.

8287   National Association to Advance Fat Acceptance
P.O. Box 4662
Foster City, CA 94404-0662   916-558-6880
FAX: 916-558-6881
www.naafaonline.com

8288   National Cancer Institute
National Institutes Of Health
9609 Medical Center Drive
Ste 300
Rockville, MD 20850   301-496-0909
800-422-6237
TTY:800-332-8615
cancergovstaff@mail.nih.gov
www.cancer.gov

Douglas R. Lowy, Acting Director
The National Cancer Institute coordinates the National Cancer Program, which conducts and supports research, training, health information dissemination, and other programs with respect to the cause, diagnosis, prevention, and treatment of cancer, rehabilitation from cancer, and the continuing care of cancer patients and the families of cancer patients.

8289   National Diabetes Information Clearinghouse
National Institutes of Health
1 Information Way
Bethesda, MD 20892-3560   800-860-8747
FAX: 703-738-4929
TTY:866-569-1162
ndic@info.niddk.nih.gov
www.diabetes.niddk.nih.gov

Griffin Rodgers, Director
Gregory Germino, Deputy Director
An information and referral service of the National Institute of Diabetes and Digestive and Kidney Diseases, one of the National Institutes of Health. The clearinghouse responds to written inquiries, develops and distributes publications about diabetes, and provides referrals to diabetes organizations, including support groups. The NDIC maintains a database of patient and professional education materials, from which literature searches are generated.

8290   National Digestive Diseases Information Clearinghouse
National Institutes of Health
2 Information Way
Bethesda, MD 20892-3570   301-654-3810
800-891-5389
FAX: 703-738-4929
TTY: 866-559-1162
nddic@info.niddk.nih.gov
www.digestive.niddk.nih.gov

Griffin Rodgers, Director
Information and referral service of the National Institute of Diabetes and Digestive and Kidney Diseases. A central information resource on the prevention and management of digestive diseases, the clearinghouse responds to written inquiries, develops and distributes publications about digestive diseases, provides referrals to digestive disease organizations and support groups, and maintains a database of patient and professional education materials from which literature searches are generated.

8291   National Fibromyalgia Association
1000 Bristol St N.
Ste 17-247
Newport Beach, CA 92660   949-734-0195
nfa@fmaware.org
www.fmaware.org

Lynne Matallana, Founder
Richard Matallana, Board of Director
Craig Kennedy, Board of Director
Michael Seffinger, DO, FAAFP, Board of Director
National Fibromyalgia Association's mission is to develop and execute programs dedicated to improving the quality of life for people with fibromyalgia.

855

8292 **National Hemophilia Foundation**
7 Penn Plaza
Ste 1204
New York, NY 10001

212-328-3700
800-424-2634
FAX: 212-328-3777
handi@hemophilia.org
www.hemophilia.org

Val Bias, Chief Executive Officer
Neil Frick, Vice President, Research & Medical Information
Joseph Kleiber, Chief Strategy Officer
Mady J. Schuman, Vice President, Development

The National Hemophilia Foundation is dedicated to finding better treatments and cures for bleeding and clotting disorders and to preventing the complications of these disorders through education, advocacy and research. Established in 1948, The National Hemophilia Foundation has chapters throughout the country.

8293 **National Kidney and Urologic Diseases Information Clearinghouse**
National Institutes of Health
3 Information Way
Bethesda, MD 20892-3560

800-860-8747
TTY:866-569-1162
nkudic@info.niddk.nih.org
www.kidney.niddk.nih.gov

Griffin Rodgers, Director
Gregory Germino, Deputy Director

NKUDIC was established in 1987 to increase knowledge and understanding about diseases of the kidneys and urologic system among people with these conditions and their families, health care professionals, and the general public.

8294 **National Organization for Albinism and Hypopigmentation**
P.O. Box 959
East Hampstead, NH 03826-0959

603-887-2310
800-473-2310
FAX: 800-648-2310
info@albinism.org
www.albinism.org

Michael McGowan, Executive Director
Diana McCown, Vice-chair
Kris Baker, Secretary
Kathi O'Donnell, Administration

Organization offering information and support to people with albinism, their families and the prodessionals who work with them.

8295 **National Organization on Fetal Alcohol Syndrome**
1200 Eton Ct NW
3rd Fl
Washington, DC 20007-3239

202-785-4585
800-666-6327
FAX: 202-466-6456
information@nofas.org
www.nofas.org

Tom Donaldson, President
Kathleen Tavenner Mitchell, Vice President
Andy Kachor, Communications Director
Katelyn Reitz, Development Director

Dedicated to eliminating birth defects caused by alcohol consumption during pregnancy and improving the qualtiy of life for those individuals and families affected.

8296 **Overeaters Anonymous World Service Office**
6075 Zenith Crt NE
Rio Rancho, NM 87144-6424

505-891-2664
FAX: 505-891-4320
info@oa.org
www.oa.org

Naomi Lippel, Manager

OA aims to provide physical, emotional, and practical support for those seeking to improve their dietary habits. OA encourages members to develop a food plan with a health care professional and a sponsor.

8297 **Prader-Willi Syndrome Association USA**
8588 Potter Park Dr
Ste 500
Sarasota, FL 34238

941-312-0400
800-926-4797
FAX: 941-312-0142
pwsausa@pwsausa.org
www.pwsausa.org

Ken Smith, Executive Director
Jack Hannings, Development Director
Donny Moore, Development & Communications Specialist

National, nonprofit public charity that works for the benefit of individuals with Prader-Willi syndrome and their families. Dedicated to serving individuals affected by Prader-Willi syndrome (PWS) their families, and interested professionals, providing information, education, and support services to its members.

8298 **Simonton Cancer Center**
P.O. Box 6607
Malibu, CA 90264-6607

818-879-7904
800-459-3424
FAX: 310-457-0421
simontoncancercenter@msn.com
www.simontoncenter.com

Dr. O. Carl Simonton, Founder
Edward Gilbert, MD, Medical Director
Karen Smith Simonton, Executive / Program Director
Jessica Jedvaj, Administrative Assistant

The Simonton Cancer Center is a non-profit organization dedicated to improving the health and lives of cancer patients and their families through psycho-social oncology.

8299 **Special Care Dentistry Association**
330 N. Wabash Avenue
Ste 2000
Chicago, IL 60611-4245

312-527-6764
FAX: 312-673-6663
scda@scdaonline.org
www.scdaonline.org

Kristin Dee, Executive Director
Miriam Robbins, President
Jeffrey Hicks, President-Elect
Sam Zwetchkenbaum, Vice President

The Special Care Dentistry Association serves as a resource to all oral health care professionals who serve or are interested in serving patients with special needs through education and networking to increase access to oral healthcare for patients with special needs.

8300 **Spina Bifida Association**
1600 Wilson Blvd
Ste 800
Arlington, VA 22209

202-944-3285
800-621-3141
FAX: 202-944-3295
sbaa@sbaa.org
www.spinabifidaassociation.org

Sara Struwe, President & CEO
Lee Towns, National Director, Communications & Outreach
Elizabeth Merck, National Director, Development
Nora Beierwaltes, Marketing Coordinator

Non-profit organization whose mission is to promote the prevention of spina bifida and to enhance the lives of all affected. Addresses the specific needs of the spina bifida community and serves as the national representative of almost 60 chapters. Services include Toll free 800 information and referral service, as well as legislative updates.

8301 Spina Bifida and Hydrocephalus Association of Canada
167 Lombard Ave
Ste 647
Winnipeg, MB, Canada R3B-0v3   204-925-3650
                                      800-565-9488
                                 FAX: 204-925-3654
                                      info@sbhac.ca
                                      www.sbhac.ca

Susana Scott, President
Linda Randall, Vice President
Bonnie Hidlebaugh, National Manager, Communications & Development Coordinator
Cindy Garofalo, Administrative Assistant
The Spina Bifida and Hydrocephalus Association of Canada has been working on behalf of people with spina bifida and/or hydrocephalus and their families.

8302 Taking Control of Your Diabetes (TCOYD)
1110 Camino Del Mar
Ste B
Del Mar, CA 92014-2649   858-755-5683
                                     800-998-2693
                                FAX: 858-755-6854
                                     info@tcoyd.org
                                     www.tcoyd.org

Steve Edelmant, Founder & Director
Sandra Bourdette, Co-Founder & Executive Director
Jennifer Braidwood, Vice Executive Director
Jill Yapo, Director, Operations
Taking Control of Your Diabetes works to educate and motivate people with diabetes to take a more active role in their condition and to provide innovative and integrative continuing diabetes education to medical professionals caring for people with diabetes.

8303 United Brachial Plexus Network, Inc.
32 William Rd
Reading, MA 01867   781-315-6161
                                      ubpn@ubpn.org
                                      www.ubpn.org

Richard Looby, President
Dan Aldrich, Co- Vice President & Traumatic BPI Group
The United Brachial Plexus Network, Inc. provides education, information, and assistance for those affected by Brachial Plexus Palsy by offering information, contacts, resources, parent matching, and assistance developing chapters or support groups throughout the United States and the world.

Camps

8304 ADA Camp Grenada
American Diabetes Association
1701 N. Beauregard St.
Alexandria, VA 22311   217-875-9011
                                     800-DIA-ETES
                                     800-342-2383
                                FAX: 217-726-2260
                                volunteerupdates@diabetes.org.
                                     diabetes.org

Dwight Holing, Chair
Larry Hausner, CEO
Debbie Johnson, CFO
Greg Elfers, Chief Field Development Officer
Camp Granada is an American Diabetes Association resident Camp located in Monticello, Illinois at the 4H Memorial Camp owned by the University of Illinois. For children with diabetes, ages 8-16. Activities include swimming, canoeing, wall climbing, tie-dying shirts, arts & crafts and fun filled evening programs.

8305 ADA Camp Kushtaka
American Diabetes Association
8216 Princeton-Glendale Rd.
PMB200
West Chester, OH 45069-1675   907-272-1424
                                     800-342-2383
                                FAX: 907-272-1428
                                     pbell@diabetes.org
                                     www.childrenwithdiabetes.com

Lori Cowie, Executive Director
Pam Bell, Organizer
Katherine Swartz, Program Director
ADA Camp Kushtaka is for children ages 7-17 with diabetes and their family (space permitting) and is located on the shores of Kenai Lake on the Kenai Peninsula in Cooper Landing. Camp is held in June and combines ongoing and informal diabetes management and education along with the fun of outdoor activities such as hiking, canoeing, crafts and swimming.

8306 ADA Camp Needlepoint
American Diabetes Association
1701 N. Beauregard St.
Alexandria, VA 22311   763-593-5333
                                     800-DIA-ETES
                                     800-342-2383
                                FAX: 952-582-9000
                                     cholten@diabetes.org
                                     www.diabetes.org

Dwight Holing, Chair
Larry Hausner, CEO
Debbie Johnson, CFO
Greg Elfers, Chief Field Development Officer
Camping for children who have type 1 diabetes. Coed, ages 5-16.

8307 ADA Camp for Kids
American Diabetes Association
1701 N. Beauregard St.
Alexandria, VA 22311-3649   505-266-5716
                                     888-342-2383
                                     800-DIA-ETES
                                FAX: 505-268-4533
                                     lbrown@diabetes.org
                                     www.diabetes.org/adacampnm

Dwight Holing, Chair
Larry Hausner, CEO
Debbie Johnson, CFO
Greg Elfers, Chief Field Development Officer
One-week camping session for children with diabetes. Coed, ages 8-13. Camp will be held at Manzano Mountain Retreat, one hour from Albuquerque, New Mexico. Please call for exact dates.

8308 ADA Teen Adventure Camp
American Diabetes Association
1701 N. Beauregard St.
Alexandria, VA 22311   312-346-1805
                                     888-342-2383
                                     800-DIA-ETES
                                FAX: 312-346-5342
                                     mejohnson@diabetes.org
                                     www.diabetes.org/adacampteenadventure

Dwight Holing, Chair
Larry Hausner, CEO
Debbie Johnson, CFO
Greg Elfers, Chief Field Development Officer
Camping for teenagers with diabetes. Coed, ages 14 to 18. Camp dates are early in August. Located at the YMCA Camp Duncan in Ingleside, Illinois. Featured activities include archery and crafts, singing, outdoor movie night, and roller skating.

8309 ADA Triangle D Camp
American Diabetes Association
1701 N. Beauregard St.
Alexandria, VA 22311
312-346-1805
888-342-2383
800-DIA-ETES
FAX: 312-346-5342
mejohnson@diabetes.org
www.diabetes.org/adacamptriangled

Dwight Holing, Chair
Larry Hausner, CEO
Debbie Johnson, CFO
Greg Elfers, Chief Field Development Officer
Triangle D Camp is a resident camp program located at the YMCA Camp Duncan in Ingleside, Illinois. Activities include swimming, row boating, canoeing, high ropes (11-13 yr. olds), climbing tower (9-10 yr. olds), Camp games, singing, archery, campfires, soccer, basketball, volleyball and diabetes education.

8310 ASCCA
Alabama Easter Seal Society
5278 Camp Ascca Dr
P.O. Box 21
Jacksons Gap, AL 36861
256-825-9226
800-843-2267
FAX: 256-825-8332
info@campascca.org
www.campascca.org

John Stephenson, Administrator
Matt Rickman, Camp Director
Dana Rickman, Director, Marketing Communications
Allison Wetherbee, Director, Community Relations
Camp ASCCA is for children and adults with disabilities or health impairments. Camp ASCCA strives to help these individuals achieve equality, independence and dignity in a safe environment.

8311 Adventure Day Camp
3480 Commission Ct
Lake Ridge, VA 22192
703-491-1444
office@princewilliamacademy.com
www.princewilliamacademy.com
Dr. Samia Harris, Founder & Executive Director
Rebecca Nykwest, Communications Director
Lindsay Chickering, Office Manager
Shiree Slade, Principal
Camping for children with asthma/respiratory ailments and cancer. Coed, ages 2-13.

8312 Agassiz Village
238 Bedford St
Suite B
Lexington, MA 02420-3477
781-860-0200
FAX: 781-860-0352
csimmonds@agassizvillage.org
www.agassizvillage.org
Cliff Simmonds, Executive Director
Thomas Semeta, Camp Director
Warren Soar, Facility Director
Warren H Burroughs, Honorary Chairman
Agassiz Village offers a variety of activities for all campers, boys and girls, younger camper and teens, and programs for physically challenged children and teens. By participating in daily activities, campers build a cooperative and positive community of different races, ages, ethnic and cultural backgrounds while enhancing confidence and individuality. Camp is located in Poland, Maine. For ages 8-17.

8313 Arizona Camp Sunrise
American Cancer Society
PO Box 27872
Tempe, AZ 85285
602-952-7550
800-865-1582
FAX: 602-404-1118
barb.nicholas@cancer.org
www.azcampsunrise.org

Barbara Nicholas, Director
Leigh Ansley, Manager
Melissa Lee, Camp Director
Jason Poulter, Technical Media Director
Provides one-week summer camping sessions to children aged 8-16 who have had, or currently have, cancer. The classes range from sports and outdoor games to dance and drama, arts, crafts, and cooking. Other activities planned for the campers include horseback riding, a trip to a lake, a dance, and learning to make friendship bracelets.

8314 Bearskin Meadow Camp
Diabetic Youth Foundation
5167 Clayton Road
Suite F
Concord, CA 94521
925-680-4994
FAX: 925-680-4863
info@dyf.org
www.dyf.org

Mark McComb, President
Paula Gogin, Development Director
Janet Kramschuster, Interim Executive Director
Jennifer Goerzen, Resident Camp manager
Bearskin Meadow Camp is for children, teens and their families who are affected by diabetes. Bearskin teaches skills for blook glucose checking and techniques for adjusting insulin, food choices and how to have a fun, active life while living with diabetes.

8315 Becket Chimney Corners YMCA Camps and Outdoor Center
748 Hamilton Rd
Becket, MA 01223
413-623-8991
FAX: 413-623-5890
cburke@bccymca.org
www.bccymca.org

Drew Lipsher, Chair
David Smith, Vice Chair
Christine Kalakay, Chief Financial Officer
Phil Connor, CEO
Half-week and one-week sessions for campers with asthma/respiratory ailments. Coed, ages 3 and up, families, seniors, single adults.

8316 Bright Horizons Summer Camp
Sickle Cell Disease Association of Illinois
8100 S. Western Avenue
Chicago, IL 60620
773-526-5016
866-798-1097
FAX: 773-526-5012
sicklecelldisease-illinois@scdai.org
sicklecelldisease-illinois.org

Darryl H. Armstrong, Chair
TaLana Hughes, Executive Director
Anquineice Brown, Outreach Coordinator
Alana Burke, Case Manager
Camping for children with blood disorders, ages 7-13. The joys of learning include instruction in first aid, swimming and water safety, boating, horseback riding and bowling plus arts and crafts. In addition, there is a traditional menu of camp pleasures, like hayrides, cookouts, nature hikes and sing-a-longs.

8317 **Camp Alpine**
Alpine Alternatives
2518 E. Tudor Road
Ste 105
Anchorage, AK 99507-1105 907-561-6655
800-361-4174
FAX: 907-563-9232
alpinealternatives@arctic.net
www.alpinealternatives.org/programs.html
Margaret Webber, Executive Director
LaVerne Lee, Day Outings Director & Camp Alpine Director
Offers programs aimed at helping disabled youth expand their horizons, master new skills, make new friends, and increase motor coordination. Most importantly, participants experience growth in self-confidence and independence that affects all aspects of an individual's life. Camp services are open to all, regardless of type of disability or age. Activities include canoeing, hiking, swimming, outdoor games, sports, nature identification and much more.

8318 **Camp Anuenue**
250 Williams St. NW
Atlanta, GA 30303 808-595-7500
888-227-2345
FAX: 808-595-7502
debra.glowik@cancer.org
www.cancer.org

Pamela K. Meyerhoffer, Chair
Robert E. Youle, Vice Chairman
Douglas K. Kelsey, Board Scientific Officer
Daniel P. Heist, Secretary/Treasurer
(1 week) June, children with or recovered from cancer.

8319 **Camp Birchwood**
Muscular Dystrophy Association
171 David Blackburn Rd
Chugiak, AK 99567 907-688-2734
info@birchwoodcamp.prg
www.birchwoodcamp.org
Marie Sweezey, Camp Director
Stephen Sweezey, Program Director & Camp Manager
Summer camp at Birchwood Camp in Chugiak, Alaska for individuals ages 6-21 who are affected by any of the 40-plus neuromuscular diseases in MDA's program. Common activities include: swimming, hockey, baseball, soccer, football, boating, horseback riding, fishing, music, cooking, arts and crafts, movies, dancing, talent shows, Harley-Davidson motorcycle sidecar or three-wheeled cycle rides, a visit from fire fighters and time for socializing and laughing.

8320 **Camp Boggy Creek**
30500 Brantley Branch Rd
Eustis, FL 32736 352-483-4200
866-462-6449
FAX: 352-483-0589
info@campboggycreek.org
www.boggycreek.org

J. Patterson Cooper, Chair
Wendy Durden, Vice Chair
June Clark, President/CEO
Paul Newman, Founder
Year-round sessions for children with a variety of chronic or life-threatening illnesses including cancer, hemophila, epilepsy, heart defects, HIV, spina bifida and asthma/respiratory ailments. Coed, ages 7-16.

8321 **Camp Bon Coeur**
Bon Coeur, Inc.
405 West Main St.
Lafayette, LA 70505-3765 337-233-8437
FAX: 337-233-4160
info@heartcamp.com
www.heartcamp.com

Susannah Craig, Executive Director
Antonio Conner, MBA, President
Susan Randol, RN, MSN, Vice-President
Martha Wyatt, CPA, Treasurer

Two-week sessions June-July for children with heart defects. Coed, ages 8-16.

8322 **Camp Breathe Easy**
American Lung Association
404-231-9887
annie@camptwinlakes.org
campbreatheeasy.com
Annie Garrett, Camp Director
Camp Breathe Easy is a seven-day, six-night overnight camp for children, ages 7-13, with asthma who need medication and are limited in summer camping opportunities. The children learn asthma self-management techniques and coping strategies to better handle their illness. Campers swim, repel off trees, fish, canoe, play soccer, basketball and miniature golf, and participate in ceramics and arts and crafts.

8323 **Camp Can Do**
3 Unami Trail
Chalfont, PA 18914
info@campcandoforever.com
campcandoforever.org
Tom Prader, Board
Sharon Maerten, Board
Stephanie Cole, Board
Amy McGonigal, Board
Camp Can Do is for children, ages 8-17, who have been diagnosed with cancer in the last 5 years.

8324 **Camp Carefree**
American Diabetes Association
1846 West Seventh Street
Piscataway, NJ 08850-1918 732-752-1715
director@campcarefreekids.org
www.campcarefreekids.org
Phyllis Woestemeyer, Director
Katie Nitchie, Camp Coordinator
Camp is located in Wolfeboro, New Hampshire. Sessions for campers with diabetes.

8325 **Camp Catch-a-Rainbow**
American Cancer Society
250 Williams St. NW
Atlanta, GA 30303 808-595-7500
888-227-2345
FAX: 808-595-7502
debra.glowik@cancer.org
www.cancer.org

Pamela K. Meyerhoffer, Chair
Robert E. Youle, Vice Chairman
Douglas K. Kelsey, Board Scientific Officer
Daniel P. Heist, Secretary/Treasurer
Camp Catch-a-Rainbow's programs are available completely free to any child in MI or IN who has or has had cancer, between the ages of 4 and 20, with their doctor's approval. Family Camp is reserved for those campers who have attended camp during that year's summer sessions and their families. Day, week, adult retreat, and family camp are available options.

8326 **Camp Cheerful**
Achievement Centers For Children
15000 Cheerful Ln
Strongsville, OH 44136-5420 440-238-6200
FAX: 440-238-1858
www.achievementcenters.org

Tim Fox, Executive Director
Bonnie Boenig, OTR/L, Director Therapy Services & Intensive Therapy Clinic
Donna Hefner McClure, M.S., Director of Education
Darla Motil, R.N., Director of Community Relations
Sessions for campers with developmental disabilities, mobility limitation and speech/communication impairment. Coed, ages 7-99.

8327   **Camp Christmas Seal**
American Lung Association of Oregon
102 W McDowell Rd
Phoenix, AZ 85003-1213   602-258-7505
                                  FAX: 202-452-1805
                                  info@lungoregon.org
                                  www.lungoregon.org

Kathryn A. Forbes, Chairman
John F. Emanuel, Vice Chair
Harold Wimmer, President/CEO
Penny J. Siewert, Secretary/Treasurer
Camp is located in Sisterhood, Oregon. Sessions for children
with asthma/respiratory ailments. Coed, ages 8-15.

8328   **Camp Classen YMCA**
YMCA of Greater Oklahoma City
10840 Main Camp Rd
Davis, OK 73030   580-369-2272
                                  FAX: 580-369-2284
                                  www.itsmycamp.org

Ford C. Price, Chair
Tricia Everest, Vice Chairman
Mike Grady, President & CEO
Don Harris, Vice President & CFO
Camp is located in Davis, Oklahoma. Sessions for children and
adults with diabetes. Coed, ages 8-17, families, seniors and sin-
gle adults.

8329   **Camp Conrad-Chinnock**
Diabetic Youth Services
12045 E. Waterfront Drive
Playa Vista, CA 90094   310-751-3057
                                  FAX: 888-800-4010
                                  www.dys.org

Rocky Wilson, Executive and Camp Director
Dale Lissy, Camp Manager
Ryan Martz, Program Director
Tom Jenkins, Chief Operating Officer
Camp Conrad-Chinnock offers many recreational programs such
as swimming, canoeing, arts & crafts to young adults and their
families with diabetes. Dietary education programs and diabetes
management are also available.

8330   **Camp Courage North**
Courage Center
3915 Golden Valley Rd
Golden Valley, MN 55422   763-588-0811
                                      888-846-8253
                                  FAX: 763-520-0577
                          Information@CourageCenter.org
                                  www.couragecenter.org

Jan Malcolm, CEO
Pamela J. Lindemoen, Executive Vice President of Oper
Stephen Bariteau, Chief Development Officer
Alice Johnson, Chief Financial Officer
Courage Center Camps - Camp Courage & Camp Courage North -
are part of Courage Center, a non-profit rehabilitation and resource center for people of all ages and abilities who are experiencing barriers to health & independence. For more than 50 years,
Courage Center camps have served children and adults with physical disabilities and those who are deaf and hard of hearing. In
2008, more than 800 people attended a Courage Center camp session. For more information, visit our web-site.

8331   **Camp Del Corazon**
11615 Hesby St
North Hollywood, CA 91601-3620   818-754-0312
                                      888-621-4800
                                  FAX: 818-754-0842
                          information@campdelcorazon.org
                                  www.campdelcorazon.org

Kevin Shannon, Co-Founder/President/Medical Director
Dan Levi, Board Member
Joel McHale, Board Member
Tom Arnold, Board Member
Active program for campers with heart disease, Camp del
Corazon provides summer activities free of charge that include

hiking and archery, arts and crafts, court and field games, waterfront activities and a beach barbecue.

8332   **Camp Discovery**
American Diabetes Association
1168 K-157 Hwy
Junction, KS 35804   316-684-6091
                                  FAX: 316-941-5699
                                  abowman@diabetes.org
                                  www.diabetes.org

Mark Moyer, President
Terry Ackley, Executive Director
Anne Bowman, Camp Director
Camp is located in Junction City, Kansas. Offers young people
with diabetes a week of fun at rock springs 4-H Center. Special attention to diabetes makes Camp Discovery a safe environment for
active youth while providing valuable diabetes managment education. Call the American Diabetes Association Kansas area office for more information. Coed, ages 8-17.

8333   **Camp Discovery - Illinois**
American Diabetes Association
875 Roosevelt Rd
Health Track
Glen Ellyn, IL 60137   312-346-1805
                                  FAX: 312-346-5342
                          illinoiscamps@diabetes.org
                  diabetes.org/in-my-community/diabetes-camp
Kalina Gurovski, Camp Director
The purpose of the American Diabetes Association, Northern Illinois Area Day Camp is to provide a unique recreational and educational experience for children with diabetes. With guidance
from the camp staff, day campers can to participate in various
camping activities and develop independence and confidence in
caring for their diabetes. Diabetes education sessions teach
campers about nutrition, exercise, insulin, highs and lows and
blood sugar testing.

8334   **Camp Eden Wood**
Friendship Ventures
10509 108th St NW
Annandale, MN 55302   952-852-0101
                                      800-450-8376
                                  FAX: 952-852-0123
                          info@friendshipventures.org
                                  friendshipventures.org

Floyd Adelman, Chair
Jeff Bangsberg, Board Member
Robert Harnett, Board Member
Jerry Caruso, Board Member
Camp is located in Eden Prairie, Minnesota. Offers resident camp
programs for children, teenagers and adults with developmental,
physical or multiple disabilities, Down Syndrome, special medical conditions, Williams Syndrome, autism and/or other conditions. Fishing, creative arts, golf, sports and other activities are
available. Respite care weekend camps year round for children,
teenagers and adults. Guided vacations for teens and adults with
developmental disabilities or other unique needs.

8335   **Camp Floyd Rogers**
Floyd Rogers Foundation
P.O.Box 31536
Omaha, NE 68131   402-341-0866
                                  FAX: 402-341-0866
                                  www.campfloydrogers.com

Buzz Wheeler, Camp Director
A camp for diabetic children. Coed, ages 8-18. 100 children come
to Camp Floyd Rogers each summer. They come to enjoy activities, participate in special events, engage in innovative evening
programs, and they meet other children their own age with diabetes. Camp Floyd Rogers offers young people an opportunity to
share some of life's adventures with others who also happen to
have diabetes.

8336 Camp Fun in the Sun
Inland NorthWest Health Services
P.O.Box 469
Spokane, WA 99210-0469
509-232-8138
www.campfuninthesun.org

Debbie Belknap, Registered Nurse
Colleen Carey, Endocrinologist
Joan Milton, Registered Dietitian
Laurie Payne, Registered Dietitian
Summer camp for children ages 8-18 whom have diabetes.

8337 Camp Glengarra
Girl Scouts - Foothills Council
33 Jewett Pl
Utica, NY 13501-4715
315-733-1909
FAX: 315-733-1909
nbrown@girlscoutsfoothills.org
www.girlscoutsfoothills.org

Natalie Brown, Executive Director
Karen Lubecki, Director
Camp Glengarra is located on 500+ acres of fields and forests, about eight miles west of Camden. This Girl Scout Camp hosts a myriad of programs throughout the year as well as summer day and resident camp. Summer sessions for girls 5-17 with ADD or asthma/respiratory ailments.

8338 Camp Glyndon
American Diabetes Association
800 Wyman Park Dr
Suite 110
Baltimore, MD 21211-2837
410-265-0075
800-342-2383
FAX: 410-235-4048
askada@diabetes.org
www.childrenwithdiabetes.com

Heather Magoon, Director
Camp is located in Nanjemoy, Maryland. One and two-week sessions July-August for children with diabetes and their families. Coed, ages 8-16.

8339 Camp Harkness
Arc of New London County
125 Sachem St
Norwich, CT 06360
860-889-4435
FAX: 860-889-4662
TTY:860-859-5493
info@thearcnlc.org
www.thearcnlc.org/

Enrico DeMatto, President
Linda Rhodse, VP
Alan Messier, Treasurer
Wendy Mis, Secretary
In 1991 a group of parents and adults with spina bifida, were brought together with the mission to educate the public about spina bifida and issues affecting people who have this disability in addition To providing support and information and promoting programs that will help people with spina bifida. Since then SBAC has worked hard to support parents, adults with spina bifida and families

8340 Camp Hertko Hollow
101 Locust St
Des Moines, IA 50309
515-471-8523
888-437-8652
FAX: 515-288-2531
a.wolf@camphertkohollow.com
www.camphertkohollow.com

Troy Norman, President
Brant Ausenhus, VP
Vicki Hertko, Treasurer
Steve Roy, Legal Counsel
Camp Hertko Hollow is a resident camp held at the Des Moines YMCA Camp site, located along the Des Moines River north of Boone, Iowa. Activities include horseback riding, swimming, canoeing, rappelling, crafts, ropes course, archery and riflery to name a few, plus special activities for different ages. Half-week and one-week sessions for children with diabetes. Coed, ages 6-16.

8341 Camp Hickory Hill
Central Missouri Diabetic Childrens Camp
P.O.Box 1942
Columbia, MO 65205
573-445-9146
CampHickoryHill@gmail.com
www.camphickoryhill.com

David Bernhardt, President
Lisa Bernhardt, Camp Director
Nate Wisdom, Program Director
Frank La Mantia, Development Director
Educates diabetic children concerning diabetes and its care. In addition to daily educational sessions on some aspects of diabetes, campers participate in swimming, sailing, arts and crafts and overnight camping. Coed, ages 8-17.

8342 Camp Ho Mita Koda
Diabetes Association Of Greater Cleveland
3601 South Green Road
Suite 100
Cleveland, OH 44122
216-591-0800
FAX: 216-591-0320
information@diabetespartnership.org
www.dagc.org

Roger Ruch, Chair
William Murman, Vice Chair
Christina R. Milano, President/CEO
Kyle Chones, Camp Director
Camp is located in Newbury, Ohio. Summer sessions for children with type 1 diabetes. Coed, ages 6-15. Type 2 diabetes, coed, ages 12-17. Bicycle adventure, coed, ages 13-19. Mini-day camp, ages 4-7, coed.

8343 Camp Hodia
1701 N 12th Street
Boise, ID 83702
208-891-1023
FAX: 208-891-1023
alan@hodia.org
www.hodia.org

Natalie B. DelRio, Chair
Richard Christensen, Vice Chair
lLisa Gier, Executive Director
Vicki Cutshall, R.N., Director, Hodia Kids Camp
Camp is located in Alturas Lake, Idaho. One-week sessions for children with diabetes. Coed, ages 8-18. Ski Camp in Sun Valley in January, ages 12-18.

8344 Camp Honor
Hemophilia Association
826 N. 5th Ave.
Phoenix, AZ 85003
602-955-3947
888-754-7017
FAX: 602-955-1962
info@hemophiliaz.org
www.hemophiliaz.org

Steven Helm, President
Jim Drurr, Vice President
Cindy Komar, CEO
Lindsey Bogard, Communications Director
Camp is located in Payson, Arizona at the Whispering Hope Ranch. One-week sessions for children with hemophilia or HIV and their siblings, as well as children of hemophiliacs. Coed, ages 7-17. Activities include swimming, canoeing, sports, archery and arts and crafts (to name a few fun things).

8345 Camp Independence
National Kidney Foundation
30 East 33rd Street
New York, NY 10016
770-452-1539
800-622-9010
FAX: 212-689-9261
info@kidney.org
www.kidneyga.org

Gregory W. Scott, Chair
Beth Piraino, President
Bruce Skyer, CEO
Joseph Vassalotti, Chief Medical Officer
Camp Independence is Georgia's a overnight, week-long summer camp providing essential medical care, treatment & fun for kids

with kidney disease and transplants. Camp Independence recognizes that campers are normal children but have special needs providing these children with opportunities for development & individual growth, peer support & normal life experiences. Activities include swimming, arts & crafts, fishing and horsebackriding, in addition to archery, games and sports, and ceramics.

8346   Camp Jened
United Cerebral Palsy Association New York
P.O.Box 483
Rock Hill, NY 12775-483   845-434-2220
                                        FAX: 845-434-2253
                                        www.campjened.org
Michael Branam, Executive Director
Camp is located in Rock Hill, New York. Sessions for adults with severe developmental and physical disabilities. Coed, ages 18-99.

8347   Camp John Warvel
American Diabetes Association
1701 N. Beauregard St.
Alexandria, VA 22311   312-346-1805
                                        888-342-2383
                                        800-DIA-ETES
                                        FAX: 317-594-0748
                                        www.diabetes.org
Dwight Holing, Chair
Larry Hausner, CEO
Debbie Johnson, CFO
Greg Elfers, Chief Field Development Officer
Camp is located in North Webster, Indiana. Provides an enjoyable, safe and educational out-of-doors experience for children with insulin-dependent diabetes. A unique learning atmosphere for children to acquire new skills in caring for their disease. The camp experience instills confidence for the child's self-management of diabetes. Offers one-week sessions and can accommodate 200 campers, boys and girls aged 7-16.

8348   Camp Joslin
Barton Center for Diabetes Education
30 Ennis Road
PO Box 356
North Oxford, MA 01537-0356   508-987-2056
                                        FAX: 508-987-2002
                                        info@bartoncenter.org
                                        www.bartoncenter.org
Thomas C. Lynch, Chair
John Peri-Okonny, 1st Vice chiar
Kristin Dyer, 2nd Vice Chair
Mark W. Fuller, Treasurer
Camp is located in Charlton, Massachusetts. For boys, ages 7-16, with diabetes. This program offers active summer sports and activities, supplemented by medical treatment and diabetes education. Coed Winter Camp and Coed Weekend Retreats are offered during the school year.

8349   Camp Joy
3325 Swamp Creek Rd
Schwenksville, PA 19473-1518   610-754-6878
                                        FAX: 610-754-7880
                                        campjoy@fast.net
                                        www.campjoy.com
Robert G Griffith, President
A special needs camp for kids and adults (ages 4-80+) with developmental disabilities such as: mental retardation, autism, brain injury, neurological disorder, visual and/or hearing impairments, Angelman and Down syndromes, and other developmental disabilities.

8350   Camp Ko-Man-She
American Diabetes Association
2555 S Dixie Drive
Suite 112
Dayton, OH 45409   937-220-6611
                                        FAX: 937-224-0240
                                        dada@diabetesdayton.org
                                        www.diabetesdayton.org
Terry Fague, President
Tyler Starline, VP
Susan McGovern, Executive Director
Robin Robertson, Administrative Assistant
Camp is located in Bellefontaine, Ohio. Summer sessions for children with diabetes. Coed, ages 8-17. Held in July.

8351   Camp Kweebec
157 Game Farm Rd.
Schwenksville, PA 19473   610-667-2123
                                        FAX: 610-667-6376
                                        info@kweebec.com
                                        www.kweebec.com
Les Weiser, Owner/Director
Maddy Weiser, Owner/Director
Rachel Weiser, Associate Director, Director of
Josh Weiser, Associate Director
Camp is located in Schwenksville, Pennsylvania. Sessions for children and adults with diabetes. Coed, ages 6-16, families, seniors and single adults.

8352   Camp L-Kee-Ta
940 Golden Valley Drive
Bettendorf, IA 52722   319-752-3639
                                        800-798-0833
                                        FAX: 319-753-1410
                                        www.gseiwi.org
Teresa Colgan, Chair
Jill Dashner, 1st Vice chiar
Anna Gibney, Development Manager
Ann Hulett, Business Operations Coordinator
Camp is located in Danville, Iowa. Half-week and one-week sessions June-August for children with asthma/respiratory ailments. Girls, ages 7-18 and families.

8353   Camp Latgawa
Oregon-Idaho Conference Center
13250 S Fork Little Butte Creek Rd
Eagle Point, OR 97524- 5593   541-826-9699
                                        camplatgawa@hotmail.com
                                        www.latgawa.gocamping.org
Eva LaBonty, Director
Camp Latgawa provides year round hospitality for groups up to 90 people. The bunk/dormitory style facilities are heated and have restrooms and showers either in the cabin or nearby.

8354   Camp Libbey
Maumee Valley Girl Scout Center
2244 Collingwood Blvd
Toledo, OH 43620-1147   419-243-8216
                                        800-860-4516
                                        FAX: 419-245-5357
                                        KelleeChancellor@girlscoutsofwesternohio.org
                                        www.girlscoutsofwesternohio .org
Jody Wainscott, Chair
Ellen Iobst, 1st Vice Chair
Susan Gantz Matz, 2nd Vice Chair
Jerry Brose, Secretary
Camp for girls 7-18 with asthma/respiratory ailments, diabetes, epilepsy and muscular dystrophy is located in Defiance, Ohio.

8355 Camp MITIOG
Share, Inc
7615 N. Platte Purchase Drive
Kansas City, MO 64118

816-221-4450
877-221-4450
FAX: 816-221-1420
midlands@midlandsmc.org
www.midlandsmc.org

Mike Hale, President/Financial Officer
Pam Mathena, Adm. Assistant to MMC Financial Officer
Donna Fletcher, Congregational Consultant
Don McLaughlin, Outreach Coordinator

Camp is located in Excelsior Springs, Missouri. One-week summer sessions for children with spina bifida. Coed, ages 6-16.

8356 Camp Magruder
Oregon-Idaho Conference Center
17450 Old Pacific Hwy
Rockaway Beach, OR 97136

503-355-2310
FAX: 503-355-8701
director@campmagruder.org
www.campmagruder.org

Steve Rumage, Camp Director
Amy Wood, Program Services Director
Diana Gutzke, Reservations/ Guest Services
Mark Burley Manager, Maintenance Team

Camp is located in Rockaway Beach, Oregon. Sessions for children and adults with cancer and developmental disabilities. Coed, ages 9-18, families, seniors and single adults.

8357 Camp Nejeda
Camp Nejeda Foundation
910 Saddlebrook Road
P.O. Box 156
Stillwater, NJ 07875

973-383-2611
FAX: 973-383-9891
information@campnejeda.org
www.campnejeda.org

Henry Anhalt, President
Scott Ross, VP
Denise Dadika, Board Member
William Curcio, Board Member

For children with diabetes, ages 7-15. Provides an active and safe camping experience which enables the children to learn about and understand diabetes. Activities include boating, swimming, fishing, archery, as well as camping skills.

8358 Camp Not-A-Wheeze
American Lung Association In Arizona
102 W McDowell Rd
Phoenix, AZ 85003-1213

602-258-7505
FAX: 202-452-1805
info@lungoregon.org
www.lungarizona.org

Kathryn A. Forbes, Chairman
John F. Emanuel, Vice Chair
Harold Wimmer, President/CEO
Penny J. Siewert, Secretary/Treasurer

Camp Not-A-Wheeze is designed especially for kids ages 7-14 with moderate to severe asthma and was created to provide a traditional residential camp experience and teach children how to manage their asthma.

8359 Camp Okizu
Okizu Foundation
16 Digital Dr
Suite 130
Novato, CA 94949

415-382-9083
FAX: 415-382-8384
info@okizu.org
www.okizu.org

John H. Bell, Chair
Michael D. Amylon, Vice Chair
Suzie Randall, Executive Director/Camp Director
Beth Dekker, Assistant Camp Director

Camp Okizu offers a place where children struggling with a life threatening illness and thier families can come to explore and enjoy a normal life experience. The camp also provides peer support, respite, mentoring, and a variety of other programs designed to help members of families affected by childhood cancer. The camp is open from April through October

8360 Camp Pelican
Louisiana Lions Camp
P.O.Box 290247
Kerrville, TX 78029

830-896-8500
FAX: 830-896-3666
tlc@ktc.com
www.lionscamp.org

Tim Matakas, President
Kim Breaux, Vice President
Tessie Guillory, Treasurer
Autumn Gaspard, Secretary

Camp Pelican is an overnight residential camp for children with moderate to severe asthma or other pulmonary problems. Founded in 1977, Camp Pelican is jointly sponsored by the Louisiana Pulmonary Disease Camp Inc and the Louisiana Lions Camp. Over 100 children attend annually and participate in education, sports, arts and crafts, swimming and other camping activities. Medical staff including physicians, nurses, respiratory therapists and social workers participate in camp. Coed, ages 5-17.

8361 Camp Rainbow
Phoenix Childrens Hospital
1919 East Thomas Road
Phoenix, AZ 85016

602-933-1000
888-908-5437
888-908-KIDS
FAX: 602-546-0276
rlyddon@phoenixchildrens.com
www.phoenixchildrens.org/

Jon Hulburd, Chair
Jacque Sokolov, MD, Vice Chair
Robert Meyer, President/CEO
David Lenhardt, Director

Camp is located in Prescott, Arizona. Offers one-week sessions for children who have had, or currently have, cancer. Boys and girls ages 7-17. Camp activities include swimming, horseback riding, arts and crafts, canoeing, performing arts, archery, rollerskating, fishing, an overnight camping trip and much more! It's a week filled with laughter, new experiences and new friends.

8362 Camp Rap-A-Hope
2701 Airport Blvd
Mobile, AL 36606

251-476-9880
FAX: 251-476-9495
info@camprapahope.org
www.camprapahope.org

Melissa McNichol, Executive Director
Roz Dorsett, Assistant Director
Cecy Lowell, Development Director

Camp Rap-A-Hope is a one-week summer camp for children and teenagers who are battling cancer or have ever been diagnosed with cancer and are 7 to 17 years of age. It is free of charge. Camp Rap-A-Hope strives to make sure every camper gets the opportunity to develop new skills and self-confidence. Camp activities are appropriate for our campers' ages and abilities and include, but are not limited to: swimming, music, arts and crafts, archery, fishing, canoeing and horseback riding.

8363 Camp Ronald McDonald for Good Times
Ronald McDonald House For Charities-Southern Calif
1250 Lyman Place
Los Angeles, CA 90029

310-268-8488
800-625-7295
FAX: 310-473-3338
www.campronaldmcdonald.org

Edward Lodgen, President
Jodi Lesh, Vice President
Sarah Orth, Executive Director
Ken Teasdale, Treasurer

Free year-round residential camping for children with cancer and their families.

8364 Camp Sawtooth
Oregon-Idaho Conference Center
P.O.Box 68
Fairfield, ID 83327-68

800-593-7539
sawtooth@gocamping.org
www.gocamping.org

David Hargreaves, Director
Camp located 35 miles north of fairfield, centrally located for all of southern Idaho.

8365 Camp Seale Harris
Southeastern Diabetes Education Services
500 Chase Park S
Ste 104
Birmingham, AL 35244

205-402-0415
FAX: 205-402-0416
info@campsealeharris.org
www.campsealeharris.org

Tip McAlpin, Chair
David Jamieson, Vice Chair
Rhonda McDavid, Executive Director
John Latimer, Camp & Community Programs Director
Camp Seale Harris is a medically-supervised, fun camp experience and family connection to year-round support that helps them fight diabetes every day.

8366 Camp Setebaid
Setebaid Services
PO Box 196
Winfield, PA 17889-196

570-524-9090
866-738-3224
FAX: 570-523-0769
info@setebaidservices.org
www.setebaidservices.org

Mark A. Moyer, President
David Langdon, VP
Peggy Coleman, Secretary
Jane Evans, Treasurer
Camping sessions for children with diabetes. Coed, ages 3-18 years. Family retreat for children with diabetes and their families.

8367 Camp Smile-A-Mile
1510 5th Ave S
P.O. Box 550155
Birmingham, AL 35255

205-323-8427
888-500-7920
FAX: 205-323-6220
info@campsam.org
www.campsam.org

Bruce Hooper, Executive Director
Jennifer Amundsen, Program Director
Savannah Lanler, Development Director
Katie Langley, Administrative & Development Assistant
Camp Smile-A-Mile is a non-profit organization for children in Alabama who have or had cancer. Camp Smile-A-Mile's mission is to provide challenging, unforgettable recreational and educational experiences for young cancer patients from across Alabama at no cost to their families. The camp provides these children with avenues for fellowship, to help them cope with their disease, and to prepare them for life.

8368 Camp Sunrise
Johns Hopkins Hospital
600 North Wolfe Street
CMSC 800
Baltimore, MD 21287-5904

410-955-5311
www.campsunrisemd.org

Sherryce Robinson, Mission Delivery Manager
Kira Elring, Regional Mission Director
Gloria Jetter, Regional Executive Director
Jack Shipkoski, CEO
Week long summer camp in White Hall, MD., for children ages 6-18 who have been diagnosed with or have survived cancer. Camp sunrise also has a 'day camp' program available for children ages 4-5. Camp activities include sports & games, swimming, arts & crafts, and nature hikes.

8369 Camp Sweeney
Southwestern Diabetic Fund
P.O.Box 918
Gainesville, TX 76241

940-665-2011
FAX: 940-665-9467
info@campsweeney.org
www.campsweeney.org

Ernie Fernandez, Executive Director
Teaches self-care and self-reliance to children ages 7-18 with diabetes. Campers participate in such activities such as swimming, fishing, horseback riding and arts and crafts while learning about how to self manage their diabetes.

8370 Camp Tall Turf
816 Madison SE
Grand Rapids, MI 49507

616-452-7906
FAX: 616-452-7907
info@tallturf.org
www.tallturf.org

Eric Brown, Chair
Ed Van Poolen, Vice Chair
Miriam DeJong, Director of Programs
Victoria P. Gibbs, Interim Executive Director
Camp is located in Walkerville, Michigan. Summer camping sessions for youth with asthma/respiratory ailments and ADD. Coed, ages 8-16.

8371 Camp Taylor, Inc.
5424 Pirrone Road
Salida, CA 95368

209-545-4715
FAX: 209-543-1861
kimberlie@kidsheartcamp.org
www.kidsheartcamp.org

Kimberlie Gamino, Board Member
Rollin A. Podwys, Board Member
Steven Barbieri, Board Member
Charlie Liamos, Board Member
Camp Taylor is a place where children and young adults with heart disease and thier families can come for recreational activities and programs. The camp is open from May through September.

8372 Camp Vacamas
256 Macopin Rd
West Milford, NJ 07480

973-838-0942
877-428-8222
info@vacamas.org
www.vacamas.org

Felix A. Urrutia, Executive Director
Kristin Short, Camp Director
Karen Wendolowski, Executive Secretary
Seth Friedman, MPA, Program Director
Disadvantaged children with asthma or sickle cell anemia, ages 8-16, are offered special programs in canoeing, backpacking, camping, music and leadership training. Sliding scale tuition. Year round programs for youth at risk groups. Conference center facility open for group rentals.

8373 Camp Waziyatah
530 Mill Hill Rd
Waterford, ME 04088-4011

207-583-2267
FAX: 509-357-2267
info@wazi.com
wazi.com

Gregg Parker, Owner/Director
Mitch Parker, Owner/Director
Camp is located in Waterford, Massachusetts. Three, four and seven-week sessions June-August for campers with cancer and diabetes. Coed, ages 8-15 and families, single adults.

8374   Camp WheezeAway
YMCA Camp Chandler
1240 Jordan Dam Rd
Wetumpka, AL 36092   334-229-0035
                        jreynolds@ymcamontgomery.org
                        ymcamontgomery.org/camp/wheezeaway
Jeff Reynolds, Executive Director
Art Mason, Operations Director
Suzy Stewart, Program Director
Kids age 8-12 suffering from moderate to severe asthma can apply for this FREE summer camp program offered at YMCA Camp Chandler. Kids experience all the fun of summer camp while learning confidence building skills in asthma management from medical professionals.

8375   Camps for Children & Teens with Diabetes
Diabetes Society
1165 Lincoln Ave
Suite 300
San Jose, CA 95125-3052   408-287-3785
                                                      800-989-1165
                                            FAX: 408-287-2701
                                      info@diabetessociety.org
                                      www.diabetessociety.org/camps
Sharon Ogbor, Executive Director
Thomas Smith, Director
Since 1974, sponsors up to 20 day camps, family camps and resident camps for children 4 through 17. These camps provide an opportunity for children with diabetes to go to camp, meet other children and gain a better understanding of their diabetes. The total experience can help campers develop more confidence in their abilities to control their diabetes effectively while enjoying the traditional camp experience. Camps are located throughout CA and parts of Nevada.

8376   Cedar Ridge Camp
4120 Old Routt Road
Louisville, KY 40299   502-267-5848
                                            FAX: 502-267-0116
                                      info@cedarridgecamp.com
                                      www.cedarridgecamp.com
Andrew Hartmans, Executive Director
Half-week, one and two-week sessions for children with diabetes, developmental disabilities and muscular dystrophy. Coed, ages 6-17.

8377   Champ Camp
American Lung Association In Alaska
7420 SW Bridgeport Road
Suite 200
Tigard, OR 97224   503-294-4094
                                                      800-586-4872
                                            FAX: 503-294-4120
                                      info@lungmtpacific.org
                                      www.aklung.org
Kathryn A. Forbes, Chairman
John F. Emanuel, Vice Chair
Harold Wimmer, President and CEO
Penny J. Siewert, Secretary/Treasurer
Champ Camp is a week long summer recreation and asthma education program at Camp Kushtaka on the beautiful shores of Kenai Lake. Campers are able to explore their skills in outdoor activities including canoeing, hiking, swimming, archery, and arts and crafts. More importantly, Champ Camp boosts self-confidence and instills a sense of responsibility. It teaches preventive measures to improve asthma management, and avoid asthmatic episodes as well as increases a camper's sense of independence.

8378   Clara Barton Diabetes Camp
Clara Barton for Girls with Diabetes
30 Ennis Road
PO Box 356
North Oxford, MA 01537-0356   508-987-2056
                                            FAX: 508-987-2002
                                      info@bartoncenter.org
                                      www.bartoncenter.org
Kevin Wilcoxen, Executive Director
Jesse Welch, Site & Facilities Director
Thomas Racine, Facilities Assistant
Brendan Duffy, Facilities Assistant
Girls, ages 3-17, with diabetes participate in a well-rounded camp program with special education in diabetes, health and safety. Activities include swimming, boating, sports, dance, music and arts and crafts. Two week adventure camp for high school girls offering camping, hiking, canoeing, etc. Also a minicamp (one week) for girls 6-12. Day camps are offered in Worcester, Boston, and New York City.

8379   Diabetes Camp
Tanager Place
1614 W Mount Vernon Road
Mount Vernon, IA 52314   319-363-0681
                                            FAX: 319-365-6411
                                      dpirrie@tanagerplace.org
                                      www.camptanager.org
Donald Pirrie, Camp Director
Provides children and adolescents with Diabetes a safe and healthy environment and healthy environment to enjoy a variety of recreational activities designed for fun and fitness. The camp held each July has an on-site 24-hour physician and nursing staff. Ages 6-13.

8380   EDI Camp
Wyman Center
600 Kiwanis Dr
St. Louis, MO 63025-2212   636-938-5245
                                            FAX: 636-938-5289
                                      info@wymancenter.org
                                      www.wymancenter.org
David Hilliard, President
Theresa Mayberry, Senior Vice President
Youngsters with diabetes learn how to care for themselves while participating in a wide variety of outdoor activities and trips. The camp, managed and financed by the American Diabetes Association Greater St. Louis Affiliate, offers camperships to children from the Greater St. Louis area, ages 7-16, but nonresidents may also apply.

8381   Echoing Hills
36272 County Road 79
Warsaw, OH 43844   740-327-2311
                                                      800-419-6513
                                            FAX: 740-327-6371
                                      info@echoinghillsvillage.org
                                      www.echoinghillsvillage.org
Buddy Busch, President/CEO
Summer camp for children and adults with cerebral palsy. Coed, ages 7-70.

8382   Edward J Madden Open Hearts Camp
250 Monument Valley Road
Great Barrington, MA 01230   413-528-2229
                                      hearts@openheartscamp.org
                                      www.openheartscamp.org
Rick Farrell, President
David Zaleon, Executive Director
Jacqueline Reasor, Counselor
Jill Helme, Asst. Director
Eight week program for children who have had and are fully recovered from open heart surgery or a heart transplant. Four two week sessions by age group. Small camp - 25 campers per session.

8383 **FCYD Camp**
Foundation for Children and Youth with Diabetes
1995 W 9000 S
West Jordan, UT 84084   801-566-6913
                                          www.fcydcamp.org
Nathan Gedge, Chair
David Okubo, President/Co-Founder
Elizabeth Elmer, Vice President
Sherrie Hardy, Director
Camping for children with diabetes. Coed, ages 1-18 and families.

8384 **Father Drumgoole Connelly Summer Camp**
MIV Mount Loretto
6581 Hylan Blvd
Staten Island, NY 10309-3830   718-317-2600
                                    FAX: 718-317-2830
                                          www.mountloretto.org
Stephen Rynn, Executive Director
Maryann Virga, Executive Assistant
Loretta Polanish, Executive Secretary
Ed Gani, Facilities Manager
Summer sessions for children with epilepsy, hearing impairment
and developmental disabilities. Coed, ages 5-13.

8385 **Florida Diabetes Camp**
P.O. Box 14136
Gainesville, FL 32604   352-334-1321
                                    FAX: 352-334-1326
                              fccyd@floridadiabetescamp.org
                                    www.floridadiabetescamp.org
Gary Cornwell, Executive Director
Chris Satkely, Assistant Director
Amy Soileau, Outreach Director
Robena Cornwell, Finance
Camp is located in Florida. One and two-week sessions June-August
for children with diabetes. Coed, ages 6-18 and families.
Camps throughout the year.

8386 **Friends Academy Summer Camps**
Duck Pond Rd
Locust Valley, NY 11560   516-393-4207
                                    FAX: 516-465-1720
                                          camp@fa.org
                                          www.fasummercamp.org
Rich Mack, Camp Director
Summer sessions for children with diabetes. Coed, ages 3-14,
families.

8387 **God's Camp**
Episcopal Church of Hawaii
68-729 Farrington Hwy
Waialua, HI 96791-9314   808-637-6241
                                          808-637-5505
                                    FAX: 808-637-5505
                              info@campmokuleia.com
                                    www.campmokuleia.org
Debbie Alemeda, Manager
Episcopal Church tent camping, 5 nights, July. Church groups,
family reunions, weddings, other organizations.

8388 **Growing Together Diabetes Camp**
ETMC
1000 S. Beckham
Tyler, TX 75701   903-597-0351
                                          800-232-8318
                                          info@etmc.org
                                          www.etmc.org
Marty Wiggins, Development Director
Vicki Jowell, Director
Elmer G. Ellis, President
Jerry Massey, Senior Vice President
A summer camp for youths ages 6 to 15 with Type 1 or Type 2 diabetes.

8389 **Happiness Is Camping**
2169 Grand Concourse
Bronx, NY 10453-2201   718-295-3100
                                    FAX: 718-295-0406
                              hicoffice@happinessiscamping.org
                                    www.happinessiscamping.org
Kurt Struver, Executive Director
Richard G. Gorlick, M.D, Medical Director
Louis D'Agostino, President Of The Board
Antonio Dominiguez, Secretary
Happiness Is Camping, for children with cancer, was founded in
1980. About 400 children, girls and boys aged 6-15 years, attend
the overnight camp, staying from one to all of the sessions, depending on their health.

8390 **Hemophilia Camp**
Tanager Place
1614 W Mount Vernon Road
Mount Vernon, IA 52314   319-363-0681
                                    FAX: 319-365-6411
                              dpirrie@tanagerplace.org
                                    www.camptanager.org
Donald Pirrie, Camp Director
During the six-day camp children with Hemophilia and their siblings
participate in individual and group activities designed for
fun and fitness. The camp held each year in mid-June has a
24-hour physician and nursing staff. Ages 5-16.

8391 **Hole in the Wall Gang Camp**
565 Ashford Center Rd
Ashford, CT 06278   860-429-3444
                                    FAX: 860-429-7295
                              ashford@holeinthewallgang.org
                                    www.holeinthewallgang.org
Raymond Lamontagne, Chairman
Ken Alberti, Chief Development Officer
James H. Canton, Chief Executive Officer
Kevin M. Magee, Chief Financial Officer
Low-cost eight-week sessions June-August for children with
cancer and HIV. Coed, ages 7-15.

8392 **Kiwanis Camp Wyman**
Wyman Center
600 Kiwanis Dr
Eureka, MO 63025-2212   636-938-5245
                                    FAX: 636-938-5289
                              info@wymancenter.org
                                    www.wymancenter.org
Keat Wilkins, Chairman
Dave Hilliard, President/CEO
Tom Etzkorn, VP,Executive Resource Officer

Mindy Sharp, MBA, SVP, Finance & Administration

Summer sessions for youth with diabetes. Coed, ages 8-16, run in
conjunction with the American Diabetes Association. Call for
program description.

8393 **Makemie Woods Camp**
Presbytery of Eastern Virginia
P.O.Box 39
Barhamsville, VA 23011   757-566-1496
                                          800-566-1496
                                    FAX: 757-566-8803
                              makwoods@makwoods.org
                                    www.makwoods.org
Mike Burcher, Director
Sherri Egerton, Program Director
Karen Broughman, Office Manager
Anthony Burcher, Storyteller in Residence
Residential Christian camp that tailors each group and individual
goals. Counselors serve as teachers, friends and activity leaders.
For children 8-18 with diabetes.

8394   Makemie Woods Camp/Conference Retreat
Presbytery of Eastern Virginia
P.O.Box 39
Barhamsville, VA 23011   757-566-1496
                                          800-566-1496
                                     FAX: 757-566-8803
                                  makwoods@makwoods.org
                                     www.makwoods.org

Mike Burcher, Director
Sherri Egerton, Program Director
Karen Broughman, Office Manager
Anthony Burcher, Storyteller in Residence
Counselors serve as teachers, friends and activity leaders. The individual is important within the small group. No camper is lost in the crowd, but is an integral partner in the group process. Residential Christian Camp and conference center. Summer camp for children 8-18 and special camp for children with diabetes.

8395   Marist Brothers Mid-Hudson Valley Camp
PO Box 197
Esopus, NY 12429   212- 55- 123
                             info@maristbrotherscenter.org
                              www.maristretreathouse.net

Don Nugent, Property Director
Qwen Ormsby, Executive Director
Matt Falon, Director of Operations
Mike Trainor, Facilities Director
Serves special people: children who have cancer or who are HIV positive, deaf or mentally retarded.

8396   Med-Camps of Louisiana
102 Thomas Road
Suite 615
West Monroe, LA 71291   318-329-8405
                                          877-282-0802
                                     FAX: 318-329-8407
                                  infos@medcamps.com
                                     www.medcamps.com

Caleb Seney, Executive Director
Bethany Gerfers, Administrative Assistant
Kacie Hobson, Events & Volunteer Coordinator
Serves children with severe asthma and allergies and many more.

8397   Mountaineer Spina Bifida Camp
909 N. Sepulveda Blvd.
11th Floor
El Segundo, CA 90245   304-558-7098
                                          877-242-9330
                                     FAX: 310-280-5177
                                  info@kidscamps.com
                                     www2.kidscamps.com

Milisa Galazzi, Director
Joey Waldman, Owner
Karen T. Safran, VP of Marketing
Is a non profit organization which pursues education and training and focuses on activities that promote independence and those that facilitate everyday life. The objectives are to build self esteem, promote independence and enhance the development of social skills.

8398   Muscular Dystrophy Association Free Camp
222 S. Riverside Plaza
Suite 1500
Chicago, IL 60606   907-276-2131
                                          800-572-1717
                                     FAX: 907-276-0946
                                     www.mdausa.org

R. Rodney Howell, MD, Chairman
Steven M. Derks, President/CEO
Julie Faber, EVP/CFO
Pete Morgan, EVP/COO
MDA Camp provides a wide range of activities for those who have limited mobility or are in wheelchairs. The camp offers may outdoor sporting activities, art's & crafts and talent shows.

8399   NeSoDak
Lutherans Outdoors in South Dakota
3285 Camp Dakota Dr.
Waubay, SD 57273-1   605-947-4440
                                          800-888-1464
                                     FAX: 605-274-5024
                                     nesodak@losd.org
                                        www.losd.org

Teri Gayer, Director
Layne Nelson, Executive Director
Nathan Skadsen, Program Director
Doug Nelson, Maintenance Director
NeSoDak provides a safe place for youth to build relationship, develop new skills, and live in a grace-filled community as they learn about Christ's love for them-all while enjoying time at the lake with a caring, well trained, energetic, and fun loving staff.

8400   Northwest Kiwanis Camp
P.O.Box 1227
Port Hadlock, WA 98339   360-732-7222
                                     nwkc@earthlink.net
                       weareugn.org/community-services/nw-kiwanis-ca

Kim Hammers, President
Carla Caldwell, Executive Director
Nikki Russell, Director, Development & Community Engagement
Debbie Reid, Administrative Assistant
Campers range from 6-60 in age, and includes those with developmental disabilities, cerebral palsy, autism, downs syndrome, and other physical and/or mental handicaps.

8401   Phantom Lake YMCA Camp
S110 W30240 YMCA Camp Road
Mukwonago, WI 53149   262-363-4386
                                     FAX: 262-363-4351
                                office@phantomlakeymca.org
                                  www.phantomlakeymca.org

Ray Gooden, Chair
James Scharine, Vice Chair
Jodi Jacobsen, Secretary
Mike Hase, Treasurer
Summer camping for children with epilepsy, ages 7-15.

8402   Shady Oaks Camp
16300 Parker Road
Homer Glen, IL 60491   708-301-0816
                                     FAX: 708-301-5091
                                  soc16300@sbcglobal.net
                                     shadyoakscamp.org

Harry Burroughs, Chairman
Robert Szajkovics, President
Lori McAleavy, Vice President
Scott Steele, Executive Director
Shady Oaks Camp provides outdoor fun and recreation for children and adults with cerebral palsy and similar disabilities. Our camp is organized with the goal of providing stimulating life experiences that our campers may not have the opportunity to engage in elsewhere.

8403   Sherman Lake YMCA Summer Camp
Sherman Lake YMCA Outdoor Center
6225 N 39th St
Augusta, MI 49012   269-731-3000
                                     FAX: 269-731-3020
                               shermanlakeymca@ymcasl.org
                                  www.shermanlakeymca.org

Luke Austenfeld, Executive Director
Jean Henderson, Business Manager
Lorrie Syverson, Director,Camping, Education & Retreat Services
Mark VanDaff, Facility Manager
Summer camping sessions for campers with ADD and spina bifida. Coed, ages 6-15 and families, seniors.

8404 **Strength for the Journey**
Oregon-Idaho Conference Center
1505 SW 18th Ave
Portland, OR 97201

503-802-9210
800-593-7539
FAX: 503-228-3196
geneva@umoi.org
www.gocamping.org

Lisa Jean Hoefner, Executive Director
Geneva Cook, Camping Registrar
Eric Conklin, Office Assistant
Jennifer Aldrich, Assistant Treasurer
Camp is located near Sisters, Oregon. For adults living with HIV/AIDS.

8405 **Summer Camp for Children with Muscular Dystrophy**
Muscular Dystrophy Association - USA
222 S. Riverside Plaza
Suite 1500
Chicago, IL 60606

520-529-2000
800-572-1717
FAX: 520-529-5300
mda@mdausa.org
www.mdausa.org

R. Rodney Howell, MD, Chairman
Steven M. Derks, President/CEO
Pete Morgan, EVP/COO
Julie Faber, EVP/CFO
Offers a wide range of activities such as adaptive sports, swimming, fishing, archery, scavenger hunts, dances & talent shows, art's & crafts, karaoke, and campfires.

8406 **Summer Camp for Physically & Mentally Challenged Children & Adults**
Kansas Jaycees' Cerebral Palsy Foundation
P.O.Box 267
Augusta, KS 67010

316-775-2421
FAX: 316-775-2421
execdirector@cpranch.org
www.cpranch.org

Cheryl Schmeidler, Executive Director
Sarah Walker, Camp Director
Our mission is to provide a program which will allow individuals to enjoy their highest level of functioning and independence, consistant with their abilities, in a summer camp setting.

8407 **Suttle Lake Camp**
Oregon/Idaho Conference Center
The United Methodist Church
475 Riverside Drive
New York, NY 10115

541-595-6663
800-UMC-GBGM
800-862-4246
FAX: 541-595-2818
info@umcmission.org
www.gbgm-umc.org

Deborah Mahaney, Executive Secretary
Denise Honeycutt, Deputy General Secretary
Roland Fernandes, Finance & Administration, General Treasurer
Rev. Shawn Bakker, Communications & Development
Camp is located in Sisters, Oregon. Camping sessions for children and adults with HIV. Coed, ages 6-18, families, seniors and single adults.

8408 **TSA CT Kid's Summer Event**
Tourette Syndrome Association of Connecticut (TSA)
c/o Massachusetts Chapter
39 Godfrey Street
Taunton, MA 02780

617-277-7589
info@tsa-ma.org
www.tsact.org

Tom Meehan, Chairman
Peter Tavolacci, Vice-Chairman
Paul Nazario, Treasurer
TSA of Connecticut sponsors summer events for children with TS/Tourette Syndrome activities of which include minature golf in addition to an Annual Conference. The kids' program at this annual conference provides children who have TS a unique opportunity to meet other children like them who also struggle with TS. Entertainment includes puppeteers, magicians, learning karate from the experts, getting face paintings and more.
uniqu pages

8409 **Texas Lions Camp**
Lions Club Of Texas
P.O.Box 290247
Kerrville, TX 78029

830-896-8500
FAX: 830-896-3666
tlc@ktc.com
www.lionscamp.com

Stephen Mabry, Executive Director
The primary purpose of the League shall be to provide, without charge, a camp for physically disabled, hearing/vision impaired and diabetic children from the State of Texas, regardless of race, religion, or national origin. Our goal is to create an atmosphere wherein campers will learn the can do philosophy and be allowed to achieve maximum personal growth and self-esteem. The camp welcomes boys and girls ages 7-16.

8410 **Twin Lakes Camp**
1451 E Twin Lakes Rd
Hillsboro, IN 47949-8004

765-798-4000
outdoors@twinlakescamp.com
www.twinlakescamp.com

Jon Beight, Executive Director
Dan Daily, Program Director
Duane Bush, Guest Service
Donna Beight, Secretary
Provides a summer camp program for special needs children and young adults. Campers suffer from a wide range of maladies including crippling accidents, Spina Bifida, epilepsy, Cerebral Palsy, Muscular Dystrophy, Quadriplegia, Paraplegia, and other disabling diseases. Campers range in age from 8 to 27.

8411 **VACC Camp**
Miami Childrens Hospital
3200 W.W. 60 Ct
Suite 203
Miami, FL 33155-4076

305-662-8222
FAX: 786-268-1765
bela.florentin@mch.com
www.vacccamp.com

Bela Florentin, Camp Coordinator
Ivette Hidalgo, MSN, ARNP, Camp Clinical Coordinator
Rose Ann Farrell, LCSW, Volunteer Assistant Coordinator
Javier Hern ndez, RRT, Volunteer Respiratory Therapist
VACC Camp gives families a fun opportunity to socialize with peers and enjoy activities not readily accessible to technology dependent children. The program includes swimming, field trips to local attractions, campsite entertainment, structured games, free play, and more - all to promote family growth and development while enhancing individual self-esteem and social skills. Parents have formal and informal opportunities to network among themselves.

8412 **Wallowa Lake Camp**
Oregon-Idaho Conference Center
84522 Church Ln
Joseph, OR 97846

541-432-1271
wallowa@gocamping.org
www.wallowalakecamp.org

David Lovegren, Manager
Peggy Lovegren, Manager
Camp offers volleyball, badminton, horseshoes, baseball, crafts and wildlife viewing.

8413 Wisconsin Lions Camp
Wisconsin Lions Foundation
3834 County Road A
Rosholt, WI 54473
715-677-4969
FAX: 715-677-3297
info@wisconsinlionscamp.com
wisconsinlionscamp.com

Evett J. hartvig, Executive Director
Elizabeth shelley, Administrative Assistant
Dale Schroeder, Facility Director
Meghan Postelnik, Office Asst.

Serves children who have either a visual, hearing or mild cognitive disability, as well as diabetes types I and II. Program activities include sailing, ropes course, hiking and canoe trips, environmental education, swimming, camping, canoeing, outdoor living skills and handicrafts. ACA accredited, located in central Wisconsin, near Stevens Point.

8414 Y Camp
YMCA of Greater Des Moines
1192 166th Drive
Boone, IA 50036
515-432-7558
FAX: 515-432-5414
ycamp@dmymca.org
www.y-camp.org

David Sherry, Executive Director
Mike Havlik, Program Director- Environmental
Alex Kretzinger, Program Director- Summer Camp
Amy Joanning, Development Coordinator/Registrar

Camp is located in Boone, Iowa. Year-round one and two-week sessions for boys and girls with cancer, diabetes, asthma, cystic fibrosis, hearing impaired and other disabilities. Coed, ages 6-16 and families.

8415 YMCA Camp Fitch
The YMCA Of Youngstown - Metro Office
17 N Champion St
P.O. Box 1287
Youngstown, OH 44501
330-744-8411
FAX: 330-744-8415
info@campfitchymca.com
www.youngstownymca.org

Thomas Fleming, Chair/ CVO
James B. Greene, 1st Vice chiar
Thomas Gacse, 2nd Vice chiar
Donald Harrison, 3rd Vice chiar

Camp is located in North Springfield, Pennsylvania. Camping sessions for children and adults with diabetes, hearing impairment, developmental disabilities, mobility limitation and speech/communication impairment. Ages 8-16, families and seniors.

8416 YMCA Camp Horseshoe
Ohio-West Virginia YMCA
PO Box 239
Point Pleasant, WV 25550-9408
304-675-5899
FAX: 304-478-4446
horseshoe@hi-y.org
www.yla-youthleadership.org

David King, Executive Director
Summer camping for children with cancer, ages 7-18.

8417 YMCA Camp Ihduhapi
Minneapolis YMCA Camping Services
15200 Hanson Blvd.
Andover, MN 55304
763-230-9622
info@campihduhapi.org
campihduhapi.org

Kerry Pioske, Camp Executive
Josh Cobb, Overnight Camp Director
Devin Hanson, Day Camp Director
Eric Wobschall, Building Superintendent

Camp is located in Loretto, Minnesota. Summer sessions for campers with asthma/respiratory ailments and epilepsy. Coed, ages 7-16.

8418 YMCA Camp Kitaki
Lincoln YMCA
570 Fallbrook Blvd.
Suite 210
Lincoln, NE 68521
402-434-9200
FAX: 402-434-9208
info@ymcalincoln.org
www.ymcalincoln.org

Barb Bettin, President/CEO
J.P. Lauterbach, COO
Misty Muff, Chief Administrative Officer
Renee Yost, CFO

Camp is located in Louisville, Nebraska. Summer sessions for children with cystic fibrosis. Coed, ages 7-17 and families.

8419 YMCA Camp Orkila
YMCA of Greater Seattle
909 4th Ave
Seattle, WA 98104
206-382-5010
FAX: 206-382-4920
dstankevich@seattleymca.org
www.seattleymca.org

John F. Vynne, Chair
David H. Wright, Vice Chair
Molly B. Stearns, Secretary
Nathaniel T. Brown, Treasurer

Camping for children with blood disorders and diabetes, ages 8-18.

8420 YMCA Camp Shady Brook
YMCA of the Pikes Peak Region (PPYMCA)
316 N. Tejon Street
Colorado Springs, CO 80903
719-329-7227
FAX: 719-272-7026
campinfo@ppymca.org
www.campshadybrook.org

Sonny Adkins, Executive Director
Laura Petersen, Program Director
Patrick Casey, Facility Director
Michaela Eddleston, Conference & Retreat Director

Camp is located in Sedalia, Colorado. One-week sessions for campers with HIV. Boys and girls 7-16. Also families, seniors and single adults.

8421 YMCA Camp Weona
YMCA of Greater Buffalo
301 Cayuga Rd
Suite 100
Buffalo, NY 14225
716-565-6000
FAX: 716-565-6007
contactus@ymcabuffaloniagra.org
www.ymcabuffaloniagara.org

John D. Murray, President/CEO

Camp is located in Gainesville, New York. Camping sessions for children and adults with epilepsy. Coed, ages 7-16, families and single adults. Nestled in 1,000 acres of hardwood and pine forests, Weona has miles of picturesque hiking trails, brooks, a heated outdoor pool and a world class adventure ropes course. Our indoor facilities include arts and crafts studios, environmental classrooms and a challenging rock climbing wall. It is the ideal setting for hands-on fun, adventure and learning.

8422 YMCA Camp jewell
YMCA of Greater Hartford
6 Prock Hill Road
P.O. Box 8
Colebrook, CT 06021
860-379-2782
888-412-2267
FAX: 860-379-8715
camp.jewell@ghymca.org
www.ghymca.org

Eric Tucker, Executive Director
Camp is located in Colebrook, Connecticut. Two-week sessions for children with cancer. Coed, ages 8-16. Also families.

8423 YMCA Camp of Maine
305 Winthrop Center Rd
P.O. Box 446
Winthrop, ME 04364

207-395-4200
FAX: 207-395-7230
info@maineycamp.org
www.maineycamp.org

Tom Christensen, CVO
Rebecca Henry, Vice CVO
Marty Allen, Treasurer
Heather Priest, Secretary
Activities include arts and crafts, nature study, hiking, and over-
night camping, dancing, and singing. Summer session dates run
from June through August; for ages 8-16.

8424 YMCA Outdoor Center Campbell Gard
4803 Augspurger Road
Hamilton, OH 45011

513-867-0600
877-224-9622
FAX: 513-867-0127
camp@gmvymca.org
www.ccgymca.org

Pete Fasano, Executive Director
Darren Corns, Program Director
Tom Andrews, Facilities and Properties Manager
Wendi Moore, Office Manager
Camp is located in Hamilton, Ohio. Camping sessions for chil-
dren with ADD, autism, developmental disabilities and blind-
ness/visual impairment. Coed, ages 6-17 and families.

Print: Books

8425 A Woman's Guide to Living with HIV Infection
Johns Hopkins University Press
2715 N Charles St
Baltimore, MD 21218-4363

410-516-6900
800-548-1784
FAX: 410-516-6998
jwehmueller@press.jhu.edu
www.press.jhu.edu

Rebecca A Clark M.D., PhD, Author
Robert T Maupin Jr. M.D. FACOG, Co-Author
Jill Hayes Hammer PhD, Co-Author
A resource for women with HIV that discusses coping with the diagnosis, finding a physician, recognizing symptoms, and preventing complications. Explains the latest treatment options and
advice on coping with gynecologic infections. *$18.00*
328 pages Hardback

8426 ABC of Asthma, Allergies & Lupus
Global Health Solutions
2146 Kings Garden Way
PO Box 3189
Falls Church, VA 22043-2593

703-848-2333
800-759-3999
FAX: 703-848-0028
information@watercure.com
www.watercure.com

Fereydoon Batmanghelidj MD, Author
Xiaopo Batmanghelidj, President
Kristin Swan, Administrator
This book introduces new approaches in preventing and treating
asthma, allergies and lupus without toxic chemicals. It also offers
new insight on how to prevent and treat children's asthma. *$
17.00*
240 pages
ISBN 0-962994-26-x

8427 AIDS Sourcebook
Omnigraphics, Inc.
PO Box 31-1640
Detroit, MI 48231-8002

610-461-3548
800-234-1340
FAX: 610-532-9001
info@omnigraphics.com
www.omnigraphics.com

Sandra J Judd, Editor
Basic consumer health information about the Human Immunodeficiency Virus (HIV) and Acquired Immunodeficiency Syndrome
(AIDS), including facts about its origins, stages, types, transmission, risk factors, and prevention, and featuring details about diagnostic testing, antiretroviral treatments, and co-occurring
infections. *$ 85.00*
600 pages 5th Edition 1911
ISBN 0-780811-47-8

8428 AIDS and Other Manifestations of HIV Infection
Elsevier Inc
30 Corporate Dr
Suite 400
Burlington, MA 01803-4252

781-313-4700
800-545-2522
FAX: 800-568-5136
usbkinfo@elsevier.com
www.elsevier.com

Gary Wormser MD, Editor
A comprehensive overview of the biological properties of this
etiologic viral agent, its clinicopathological manifestations, the
epidemiology of its infection, and present and future therapeutic
options. *$249.95*
1000 pages 2004
ISBN 0-127640-51-7

**8429 AIDS in the Twenty-First Century: Disease and
Globalization**
Palgrav Macmillan
175 5th Ave
New York, NY 10010-7703

888-330-8477
FAX: 800-672-2054
onlinesupportusa@palgrav.com
www.palgrave-usa.com

Gabriella Georgiades, Editor
Alan Whiteside, Author
Tony Barnett, Co-Author
The authors — exprets in the field for over 15 years — argue that
it is vital to not only look at AIDS in terms of prevention and treatment, but to also consider consequences which affect households, communities, companies, governments, and countries.
This is a major contribution toward understanding the global public health crisis, as well as the relationship between poverty, inequality, and infectious diseases. *$32.00*
464 pages
ISBN 1-403997-68-5

**8430 Adult Leukemia: A Comprehensive Guide for Patients and
Families**
O'Reilly Media Inc
1005 Gravenstein Hwy N
Sebastopol, CA 95472-2811

707-827-7000
800-998-9938
FAX: 707-829-0104
order@oreilly.com
www.oreilly.com

Linda Lamb, Editor
Barb Lackritz, Author
For the tens of thousands of Americans with adult leukemia,
Adult Leukemia: A Comprehensive Guide for Patients and Families addresses diagnosis, medical tests, finding a good
oncologist, treatments, side effects, getting emotional and other
support, resources for further study, and much more. The book includes real-life stories from those who have battled leukemia
themselves. *$29.95*
536 pages Paperback
ISBN 0-596500-01-7

8431 Advanced Breast Cancer: A Guide to Living with Metastic Disease
O'Reilly Media Inc
1005 Gravenstein Hwy N
Sebastopol, CA 95472-2811

707-827-7000
800-998-9938
FAX: 707-829-0104
order@oreilly.com
www.oreilly.com

Linda Lamb, Editor
Musa Mayer, Author
This is the only book on breast cancer that deals honestly with the realities of living with metastic disease, yet offers hope and comfort. All aspects of facing the disease are covered, including: coping with the shock of recurrence, seeking information and making treatment decisions, communicating effectively with medical personnel finding support, and handling disease progression and end-of-life issues. A comprehensive guide, it also provides updated resources and treatment developments. *$24.95*
532 pages Paperback 1998
ISBN 1-565925-22-X

8432 Allergies & Asthma: What Every Parent Needs To Know (2nd Edition)
American Academy of Pediatrics
141 Northwest Point Blvd
Elk Grove Village, IL 60007-1019

847-434-4000
800-433-9016
FAX: 847-434-8000
newpubs@aap.org
www.aap.org

Bernard P. Dreyer, MD; FAAP, President
Karen Remley, MD; MBA; MPH, Executive Director & CEO
Consumer resource for parents who need answers and information about their children's allergies and asthma. Covers advice on identifying allergies and asthma, preventing attacks, minimizing triggers, understanding medications, explaining allergies to young children, and helping children manage symptoms. *$14.95*
174 pages Paperback; eBook available 1910
ISBN 1-581104-45-6

8433 Allergies Sourcebook
PO Box 31-1640
Detroit, MI 48231-8002

610-461-3548
800-234-1340
FAX: 610-532-9001
info@omnigraphics.com
www.omnigraphics.com

Amy L Sutton, Editor
Basic comsumer health information about the immune system and allergic disorders, including rhinitis (hay fever), sinusitis, conjunctivitis, asthma, atopic dermatitis, and anaphylaxis, and allergy triggers such as pollen, mold, dust mites, animal dander, chemicals, foods and additives, and medications; along with facts about allergy diagnosis and treatment, tips on avoiding triggers and preventing symptoms, a glossary of related terms, and directories of resources for additional help and info. *$95.00*
608 pages 4th Edition 1911

8434 Alternative Approach to Allergies
Harper Collins Publishers
10 E 53rd St
New York, NY 10022-5244

212-207-7901
800-242-7737
FAX: 212-702-2586
spsales@harpercollins.com
www.harpercollins.com

Theron G Randolph M.D., Author
Ralph W Moss PhD, Co-Author
Here is the book that revolutionized the way allergies and other common illnesses were diagnosed and treated.

ISBN 0-060916-93-1

8435 Alzheimer Disease Sourcebook
Omnigraphics
PO Box 8002
Aston, PA 19014-8002

800-234-1340
FAX: 800-875-1340
info@omnigraphics.com
www.omnigraphics.com

Amy L. Sutton, Editor
Alzheimer Disease Sourcebook, Fifth Edition provides updated information about causes, symptoms, and stages of AD and other forms of dementia, including mild cognitive impairment, corticobasal degeneration, dementia with Lewy bodies, frontotemporal dementia, Huntington disease, Parkinson disease, and dementia caused by infections. *$95.00*
600 pages 1911
ISBN 0-780811-50-8

8436 Alzheimer Disease Sourcebook, 4th Edition
Omnigraphics
PO Box 8002
Aston, PA 19014-8002

610-461-3548
800-234-1340
FAX: 800-875-1340
customerservice@omnigraphics.com
www.omnigraphics.com

Peter Ruffner, President, Co-Founder
Fred Ruffner, Founder
Basic consumer health information about alzheimer disease, other dementias, and related disorders, including multi-infarct dementia, dementia with lewy bodies, frontotemporal dementia (pick disease), Wernicke-Korsakoff syndrome (alcohol-related dementia), AIDS dementia complex, Huntington disease, Creutzfeldt-Jacob disease, and delirium. *$84.00*
603 pages
ISBN 0-780810-01-3

8437 Amyotrophic Lateral Sclerosis: A Guide for Patients and Families
Demos Medical Publishing
11 West 42nd Street
15th Floor
New York, NY 10036

212-683-0072
800-532-8663
FAX: 212-683-0118
support@demosmedical.com
www.demosmedpub.com

Richard Winters, Executive Editor
Beth Kaufman Barry, Publisher
Noreen Henson, Executive Director of Demos Heal
Reina Santana, Director of Special Sales & Righ
This comprehensive guide covers every aspect of the management of ALS. Beginning with discussions of its clinical features of the disease, diagnosis, and an overview of symptom management, major sections deal with medical and rehabilitative management, living with ALS, managing advanced disease and end-of-life issues, and reources that can provide support and assistance. *$29.95*
470 pages 2001
ISBN 1-888799-28-5

8438 Arthritis Sourcebook.
Omnigraphics
PO Box 31-1640
Detroit, MI 48231-8002

610-461-3548
800-234-1340
FAX: 610-532-9001
info@omnigraphics.com
www.omnigraphics.com

Amy L Sutton, Editor
Basic consumer health information about osteoarthritis, rheumatoid arthritis, other rheumatic disorders, infectious forms of arthritis, and diseases with symptoms linked to arthritis, and facts about diagnosis, pain management, and surgical therapies. *$84.00*
567 pages 2nd Edition
ISBN 0-780806-67-2

8439 **Asthma Sourcebook.**
Omnigraphics
PO Box 31-1640
Detroit, MI 48231-8002
610-461-3548
800-234-1340
FAX: 610-532-9001
info@omnigraphics.com
www.omnigraphics.com

Karen Bellenir, Editor
Provides information about asthma, including symptoms, remedies and research updates. *$84.00*
581 pages 2nd Edition
ISBN 0-780808-66-9

8440 **Asthma and Allergy Answers: A Patient Education Library**
Asthma and Allergy Foundation of America
8201 Corporate Dr
Suite 1000
Landover, MD 20785
202-466-7643
800-727-8462
FAX: 202-466-8940
info@aafa.org
www.aafa.org

Amy Patterson, Senior Director of Administration & Governance
Jacqui Vok, Director of Programs and Services
William McLin, M.Ed., President/CEO
This resource contains 50 reproducible fact sheets for patients on a variety of popular asthma and allergy topics. Information is written in a patient-friendly question and answer format and packaged in a durable binder for easy storage and use. *$50.00*

8441 **Back & Neck Sourcebook.**
Omnigraphics
PO Box 31-1640
Detroit, MI 48231-8002
610-461-3548
800-234-1340
FAX: 610-532-9001
info@omnigraphics.com
www.omnigraphics.com

Amy L Sutton, Editor
Basic consumer health information about back and neck pain, spinal cord injuries, and related disorders, such as degenerative disk disease, osteoarthritis, scoliosis, sciatica, spina bifida, and spinal stenosis, and featuring facts about maintaining spinal health, self-care, rehabilitative care, chiropractic care, spinal surgeries, and complementary therapies. *$84.00*
607 pages 2nd Edition
ISBN 0-780807-38-9

8442 **Being Close**
National Jewish Health
1400 Jackson St
Denver, CO 80206-2761
303-398-1002
877-225-5654
FAX: 303-398-1125
allstetterw@njc.org
www.nationaljewish.org

Michael Salem M.D., President/CEO
William Allstetter, Director Media/External Relation
A booklet offering information to patients suffering from a respiratory disorder such as emphysema, asthma or tuberculosis, that discusses sexual problems and feelings.

8443 **Bittersweet Chances: A Personal Journey o f Living and Learning in the Face of Illness**
PublishAmerica
PO Box 151
Frederick, MD 21705-151
301-695-1707
FAX: 301-631-9073
support@publishamerica.com
www.publishamerica.com

Dana Selenke Broehl, Author
Recounts Doug and Dana Broehl's journey of growth through the darkness of cystic fibrosis and the renewed hope of a double lung transplant. *$24.95*
189 pages Softcover
ISBN 1-413713-24-6

8444 **Blood and Circulatory Disorders Sourcebook**
Omnigraphics
PO Box 31-1640
Detroit, MI 48231-8002
610-461-3548
800-234-1340
FAX: 610-532-9001
info@omnigraphics.com
www.omnigraphics.com

Amy L Sutton, Editor
Sandra J. Judd, Editor
Blood and Circulatory Disorders Sourcebook, Third Edition offers facts about blood function and composition, the maintenance of a healthy circulatory system, and the types of concerns that arise when processes go awry. It discusses the diagnosis and treatment of many common blood cell disorders, bleeding disorders, and circulatory disorders, including anemia, hemochromatosis, leukemia, lymphoma, hemophilia, hypercoagulation, thrombophilia, atherosclerosis, blood pressure irregularities, coronary *$84.00*
634 pages 2nd Edition
ISBN 0-780807-46-4

8445 **Blooming Where You're Planted: Stories From The Heart**
Meeting Life's Challenges
9042 Aspen Grove Lane
Madison, WI 53717-2700
608-824-0402
FAX: 608-824-0403
help@MeetingLifesChallenges.com
www.makinglifeeasier.com

Shelley Peterman Schwatz, Editor
Author Shelley Peterman Schwarz takes you on her journey of self-discovery and change following her diagnosis of multiple sclerosis in 1979. Her personal stories are warm and humorous, and insightful. This 138-page book will motivate and inspire you to rise above life's challenges and live life to its fullest. *$12.95*
138 pages 1998
ISBN 0-891854-01-1

8446 **Brain Allergies: The Psychonutrient and Magnetic Connections**
McGraw-Hill
www.allergiesshop.com

William Philpott PhD, Author
Dwight Keating PhD, Author
Linus Pauling PhD, Author
A complete overview of the concept of brain allergies - the theory that exposure to certain foods and other substances triggers mental disorders in people so predisposed, and that such disturbances can be cured by eliminating these substances. *$16.95*

ISBN 0-658003-98-1

8447 **Brain Disorders Sourcebook**
Omnigraphics
PO Box 31-1640
Detroit, MI 48231-8002
610-461-3548
800-234-1340
FAX: 610-532-9001
info@omnigraphics.com
www.omnigraphics.com

Sandra J Judd, Editor
Joyce Brennfleck Shannon, Editor
Brain Disorders Sourcebook, Third Edition provides readers with updated information about brain function, neurological emergencies such as a brain attack (stroke) or seizure, and symptoms of brain disorders. It describes the diagnosis, treatment, and rehabilitation therapies for genetic and congenital brain disorders, brain infections, brain tumors, seizures, traumatic brain injuries, and degenerative neurological disorders such as Alzheimer disease and other dementias, Parkinson disease, and am *$84.00*
600 pages 2nd Edition
ISBN 0-780807-44-0

8448   **Breast Cancer Sourcebook**
Omnigraphics
PO Box 31-1640
Detroit, MI 48231-8002
610-461-3548
800-234-1340
FAX: 610-532-9001
info@omnigraphics.com
www.omnigraphics.com

Sandra J Judd, Editor
Amy L. Sutton, Editor
Breast Cancer Sourcebook, Fourth Edition, provides updated information about breast cancer and its causes, risk factors, diagnosis, and treatment. Readers will learn about the types of breast cancer, including ductal carcinoma in situ, lobular carcinoma in situ, invasive carcinoma, and inflammatory breast cancer, as well as common breast cancer treatment complications, such as pain, fatigue, lymphedema, hair loss, and sexuality and fertility issues. Information on preventive therapies, nutrition *$84.00*
600 pages 3rd Edition
ISBN 0-780810-30-3

8449   **Breathe Free**
Lotus Press
P.O.Box 325
Twin Lakes, WI 53181
262-889-8561
800-824-6396
FAX: 262-889-8591
lotuspress@lotuspress.com
www.lotuspress.com

D Gagnon, Author
A Morningstar, Co-Author
A nutritional and herbal medicine self-help guide to treating a full range of respiratory conditions, including colds and flu. *$14.95*
179 pages
ISBN 0-914955-07-1

8450   **Cancer Sourcebook**
Omnigraphics
PO Box 31-1640
Detroit, MI 48231-8002
610-461-3548
800-234-1340
FAX: 610-532-9001
info@omnigraphics.com
www.omnigraphics.com

Karen Bellenir, Editor
Cancer Sourcebook, Sixth Edition provides updated information about common types of cancer affecting the central nervous system, endocrine system, lungs, digestive and urinary tracts, blood cells, immune system, skin, bones, and other body systems. It explains how people can reduce their risk of cancer by addressing issues related to cancer risk and taking advantage of screening exams. *$84.00*
1105 pages 5th Edition
ISBN 0-780809-47-5

8451   **Cancer Sourcebook for Women**
Omnigraphics
PO Box 31-1640
Detroit, MI 48231-8002
610-461-3548
800-234-1340
FAX: 610-532-9001
info@omnigraphics.com
www.omnigraphics.com

Amy L Sutton, Editor
Karen Bellenir, Editor
Cancer Sourcebook for Women, Fourth Edition offers updated information about gynecologic cancers and other cancers of special concern to women, including breast cancer, cancers of the female reproductive organs, and cancers responsible for the highest number of deaths in women. It explains cancer risks-including lifestyle factors, inherited genetic abnormalities, and hormonal medications-and methods used to diagnose and treat cancer. *$84.00*
687 pages 5th Edition
ISBN 0-780808-67-6

8452   **Cardiovascular Diseases and Disorders Sourcebook, 3rd Edition**
Omnigraphics
PO Box 8002
Aston, PA 19014-8002
610-461-3548
800-234-1340
FAX: 800-875-1340
customerservice@omnigraphics.com
www.omnigraphics.com

Peter Ruffner, President, Co-Founder
Fred Ruffner, Founder
Cardiovascular Diseases and Disorders Sourcebook, Third Edition, provides information about the symptoms, diagnosis, and treatment heart diseases and vascular disorders. It includes demographic and statistical data, an overview of the cardiovascular system, a discussion of risk factors and prevention techniques, a look at cardiovascular concerns specific to women, and a report on current research initiatives. *$84.00*
687 pages Hard cover
ISBN 0-780807-39-6

8453   **Childhood Cancer Survivors: A Practical Guide to Your Future**
O'Reilly Media Inc
1005 Gravenstein Hwy N
Sebastopol, CA 95472-2811
707-827-7000
800-998-9938
FAX: 707-829-0104
order@oreilly.com
www.oreilly.com

Linda Lamb, Editor
Nancy Keene, Author
Wendy Hobbie, Co-Author
Kathy Ruccione, Co-Author
More than 250,000 people have survived childhood cancer - a cause for celebration. Authors Keene, Hobbie, and Ruccione chart the territory of long-term survivorship: relationships; overcoming employment or insurance discrimination; maximizing health; follow-up schedules; medical late effects. The stories of over sixty survivors - their challenges and triumphs - are told. Includes medical history record-keeper. *$27.95*
464 pages Paperback 1906
ISBN 0-596528-51-5

8454   **Childhood Cancer: A Parent's Guide to Solid Tumor Cancers**
O'Reilly Media Inc
1005 Gravenstein Highway North
Sebastopol, CA 95472
707-827-7000
800-889-8969
FAX: 707-829-0104
order@oreilly.com
www.oreilly.com

560 pages Paperback
ISBN 0-596500-14-9

8455   **Childhood Diseases and Disorders Sourcebook, 2nd Edition**
Omnigraphics
PO Box 8002
Aston, PA 19014-8002
610-461-3548
800-234-1340
FAX: 800-875-1340
customerservice@omnigraphics.com
www.omnigraphics.com

Peter Ruffner, President, Co-Founder
Fred Ruffner, Founder
Sandra J Judd, Editor
Basic consumer health information about medical problems often encountered in pre-adolescent children, including respiratory tract ailments, ear infections, sore throats, disorders of the skin and scalp, digestive and genitourinary diseases, infectious diseases, inflammatory disorders, chronic physical and developmental disorders, allergies, and more. *$84.00*
600 pages Hard cover
ISBN 0-780810-31-0

8456 **Childhood Leukemia: A Guide for Families, Friends & Caregivers**
O'Reilly Media Inc
1005 Gravenstein Hwy N
Sebastopol, CA 95472-2811

707-827-7000
800-998-9938
FAX: 707-829-0104
order@oreilly.com
www.oreilly.com

Linda Lamb, Editor
Nancy Keene, Author
The second edition of this comprehensive guide offers detailed and precise medical information for parents that includes day-to-day practical advice on how to cope with procedures, hospitalization, family and friends, school, and social, emotional, and financial issues. It features a wealth of tools for prents and contains significant updates on treatments and procedures. *$29.95*
528 pages 4th Edition 1910
ISBN 0-596500-15-7

8457 **Children with Cerebral Palsy: A Parents' Guide**
Woodbine House
6510 Bells Mill Road
Bethesda, MD 20817-1636

301-897-3570
800-843-7323
FAX: 301-897-5838
info@woodbinehouse.com
www.woodbinehouse.com

Irvin Shapell, Owner
Beth Binns, Special Marketing Manager
Sarah Glenner, Office Receptionist;
Fran Marinaccio, Marketing Manager
A classic primer for parents that provides a complete spetrum of information and compassionate advice about cerebral palsy and its effect on their child's development and education. *$18.95*
481 pages
ISBN 0-933149-82-4

8458 **Chronic Fatigue Syndrome: Your Natural Gu ide to Healing with Diet, Herbs and Other Methods**
Random House Publishing
1745 Broadway
3rd Floor
New York, NY 10019-4305

212-782-9000
FAX: 212-572-6066
ecustomerservice@randomhouse.com
www.randomhouse.com

Susanna Porter, Editor
Michael T Murray N.D.
Explains specific measures sufferers can take to improve stamina, mental energy, and physical abilities. *$15.00*
208 pages
ISBN 1-559584-90-6

8459 **Coffee in the Cereal: The First Year with Multiple Sclerosis**
Pathfinder Publishing

520-647-0158
800-977-2282
bill@pathfinderpublishing.com
www.pathfinderpublishing.com

96 pages
ISBN 0-934793-07-7

8460 **Colon & Rectal Cancer: A Comprehensive Guide for Patients & Families**
O'Reilly Media Inc
1005 Gravenstein Hwy N
Sebastopol, CA 95472-2811

707-827-7000
800-998-9938
FAX: 707-829-0104
order@oreilly.com
www.oreilly.com

Linda Lamb, Editor
Lorraine Johnston, Author
The fourth most common cancer, colon and rectal cancer is diagnosed in 130,000 new cases in the United States each year. Pa-

tients and families need uo-to-date and in-depth information to participate wisely in treatment decisions (e.g., knowing what sexual and fertility issues to discuss with the doctor before surgery). This book covers coping with tests and treatment side effects, caring for ostomies, finding supportt, and other practical issues. *$24.95*
544 pages Paperback 1999
ISBN 1-565926-33-1

8461 **Colon Health: Key to a Vibrant Life**
Norwalk Press
P.O.Box 190526
Boise, ID 83719-526

928-445-5567
FAX: 928-445-5567
info@drnormanwalker.com
www.drnormanwalker.com

Norman Walker MD, Editor
Includes complete glossary of terms and index of referrals.

8462 **Complementary Alternative Medicine and Multiple Sclerosis**
Demos Medical Publishing
11 West 42nd Street
15th Floor
New York, NY 10036

212-683-0072
800-532-8663
FAX: 212-683-0118
support@demosmedical.com
www.demosmedpub.com

Richard Winters, Executive Editor
Beth Kaufman Barry, Publisher
Noreen Henson, Executive Director of Demos Heal
Reina Santana, Director of Special Sales & Righ
Offers reliable information on the relevance, safety, and effectiveness of various alternative therapies that are not typically considered in discussions of MS management, yet are in widespread use. *$24.95*
304 pages
ISBN 1-932603-54-9

8463 **Conquering the Darkness: One Story of Recovering from a Brain Injury**
Paragon House
1925 Oakcrest Avenue
Suite 7
Saint Paul, MN 55113-2619

651-644-3087
800-447-3709
FAX: 651-644-0997
info@paragonhouse.com
www.paragonhouse.com

Rosemary Yokoi, Publicity Director
Gordon Anderson, Executive Director
Deborah Quinn, Author
The course of recovery from a brain injury by a woman who lived through it. *$15.95*
276 pages 1998
ISBN 1-557787-63-8

8464 **Coping with Cerebral Palsy**
Rosen Publishing
29 East 21st Street
New York, NY 10010

800-237-9932
FAX: 888-436-4643
www.rosenpublishing.com

Laura Anne Gilman, Author
This second edition book provides parents of children and adults with cerebral palsy the answers to more than 300 questions that have been carefully researched. It represents 40 years of experience by the author and is presented in a highly readable, jargon-free manner. *$31.95*

ISBN 0-823931-50-1

8465 **Curing MS: How Science is Solving the Mysteries of Multiple Sclerosis**
Random House Publishing
1745 Broadway
3rd Floor
New York, NY 10019-4305   212-782-9000
                                 FAX: 212-572-6066
                    ecustomerservice@randonhouse.com
                             www.randomhouse.com

Howard L Weiner M.D., Author
Founder-director of the Multiple Sclerosis Center at Mass General Hospital discusses what ends up as a deconstruction of the last 30 years of his own and general MS research and of experience in treating patients with the puzzling disorder. Weiner summarizes what is currently known about treatments and the potential for a cure. *$14.95*
352 pages 1905
ISBN 0-307236-04-8

8466 **Cystic Fibrosis: A Guide for Patient and Family**
Lippincott Williams & Wilkins
16522 Hunters Green Parkway
PO Box 1620
Hagerstown, MD 21741-1620   301-223-2300
                                    800-638-3030
                              FAX: 301-223-2400
                                 orders@lww.com
                                  www.lww.com

David M Orenstein MD, Author
Text is designed specifically for patients with cystic fibrosis and their families. Explains the disease process, outlines the fundamentals of diagnosing and screening, and addresses the challenges of treatment for those living with CF. Includes new material on carrier testing, infection control, and more. *$51.50*
448 pages 3rd Edition
ISBN 0-781741-52-1

8467 **Diabetes Sourcebook.**
Omnigraphics
PO Box 31-1640
Detroit, MI 48231-8002   610-461-3548
                                    800-234-1340
                              FAX: 610-532-9001
                            info@omnigraphics.com
                             www.omnigraphics.com

Karen Bellenir, Editor
Diabetes Sourcebook, Fourth Edition contains updated information for people seeking to understand the risk factors, complications, and management of diabetes. It discusses medical interventions, including the use of insulin and oral diabetes medications, self-monitoring of blood glucose, and complementary and alternative therapies. *$84.00*
627 pages 4th Edition
ISBN 0-780810-05-1

8468 **Digestive Diseases & Disorders Sourcebook**
Omnigraphics
PO Box 8002
Aston, PA 19014-8002   610-461-3548
                                    800-234-1340
                              FAX: 800-875-1340
                      customerservice@omnigraphics.com
                             www.omnigraphics.com

Peter Ruffner, President, Co-Founder
Fred Ruffner, Founder
Digestive Diseases and Disorders Sourcebook provides basic information for the layperson about common disorders of the upper and lower digestive tract. It also includes information about medications and recommendations for maintaining a healthy digestive tract in addition to a glossary of important terms and a directory of digestive diseases organizations are also provided. *$84.00*
323 pages Hard cover
ISBN 0-780803-27-5

8469 **Duchenne Muscular Dystrophy**
Oxford University Press
198 Madison Ave
New York, NY 10016-4308   212-726-6000
                                    800-445-9714
                              FAX: 919-677-1303
                              custserv.us@oup.com
                              www.global.oup.com

William Lamsback, Editor
Alan Emery, Author
Francesco Muntoni, Co-Author
Identification of the genetic defect responsible for Duchenne Muscular Dystrophy and isolation of the protein dystrophin have led to the development of new theories for the disease's pathogenesis. This title incorporates these advances from the field of molecular biology, and describes the resultant opportunities for screening, prenatal diagnosis, genetic counselling and management. *$135.00*
282 pages 3rd Edition 2003
ISBN 0-198515-31-6

8470 **Ear, Nose, and Throat Disorders Sourcebook**
Omnigraphics
PO Box 31-1640
Detroit, MI 48231-8002   610-461-3548
                                    800-234-1340
                              FAX: 610-532-9001
                            info@omnigraphics.com
                             www.omnigraphics.com

Sandra J Judd, Editor
Ear, Nose and Throat Disorders Sourcebook, Second Edition, provides consumers with updated health information on the most common disorders of the ear, nose, and throat. The book also includes descriptions of current diagnostic tests, discussion of common surgical procedures, including cosmetic surgery on the nose and ears, a glossary of related medical terms, and a directory of sources for further help and information. *$84.00*
631 pages 2nd Edition
ISBN 0-780808-72-0

8471 **Eating Disorders Sourcebook.**
Omnigraphics
PO Box 31-1640
Detroit, MI 48231-8002   610-461-3548
                                    800-234-1340
                              FAX: 610-532-9001
                            info@omnigraphics.com
                             www.omnigraphics.com

Joyce Brennfleck Shannon, Editor
Provides general imformation, causes and treatments of eating disorders. *$84.00*
557 pages 2nd Edition
ISBN 0-780809-48-2

8472 **Educational Issues Among Children with Spina Bifida**
Spina Bifida Association of America
1600 Wilson Boulevard
Suite 800
Arlington, VA 22209   202-944-3285
                                    800-621-3141
                              FAX: 202-944-3295
                                 sbaa@sbaa.org
                                  www.sbaa.org

Ana Ximenes, Chair
Sara Struwe, President & CEO
Mark Bohay, National Web Initiatives & Development Manager
Elizabeth Merck, Development Manager
Children with spina bifida/ hydrocephalus often show unique learning strengths and weaknesses that affect their schoolwork. Parents and schools need to work together to help the young people meet their physical, social, emotional, and academic goals.

8473 Epilepsy, 199 Answers: A Doctor Responds to His Patients' Questions

Demos Medical Publishing
11 West 42nd Street
15th Floor
New York, NY 10036

212-683-0072
800-532-8663
FAX: 212-683-0118
support@demosmedical.com
www.demosmedpub.com

Richard Winters, Executive Editor
Beth Kaufman Barry, Publisher
Noreen Henson, Executive Director of Demos Heal
Andrew N. Wilner MD, FACP, FAAN, Author

An epilepsy specialist answers questions about the causes, diagnosis, and treatments, and how to live and work with this brain disorder. Includes an epilepsy history timeline, patient health record form, resources, and a glossary. *$19.95*
180 pages
ISBN 1-932603-35-2

8474 Epilepsy: Patient and Family Guide

Demos Medical Publishing
11 West 42nd Street
15th Floor
New York, NY 10036

212-683-0072
800-532-8663
FAX: 212-683-0118
support@demosmedical.com
www.demosmedpub.com

Richard Winters, Executive Editor
Beth Kaufman Barry, Publisher
Noreen Henson, Executive Director of Demos Heal
Orrin Devinsky, MD, Author

A guide for adults with epilepsy and for parents of children with the disorder explains the nature and diversity of seizures, the risks and benefits of the various antiepileptic drugs, and medical and surgical therapies. *$16.95*
408 pages
ISBN 1-932603-41-7

8475 Ethnic Diseases Sourcebook

Omnigraphics
PO Box 8002
Aston, PA 19014-8002

610-461-3548
800-234-1340
FAX: 800-875-1340
customerservice@omnigraphics.com
www.omnigraphics.com

Peter Ruffner, President, Co-Founder
Fred Ruffner, Founder

Ethnic Diseases Sourcebook provides health information about genetic and chronic diseases that affect ethnic and racial minorities in the United States. Information about mental health services, women's health, and tips for improving health are also included, along with a glossary and a list of resources for additional help and informatio methods, treatment options, and current research initiatives. *$84.00*
648 pages Hard cover
ISBN 0-780803-36-7

8476 From Where I Sit: Making My Way with Cerebral Palsy

Scholastic
557 Broadway
New York, NY 10012-3962

124-484-2800
FAX: 212-343-6934
contact@scholastic.co.in
www.scholastic.com

Dick Robinson, Chairman & CEO
Maureen O'Connell, Executive Vice President, Chief
Kyle Good, Senior Vice President, Corporate
Shelley Nixon, Author

An autobiographical account of a young woman explores how it feels to live with cerebral palsy while struggling to have a full life despite the challenges facing her every day. *$13.00*
136 pages
ISBN 0-590395-84-X

8477 Genetics and Spina Bifida

Spina Bifida Association of America
1600 Wilson Boulevard
Suite 800
Arlington, VA 22209

202-944-3285
800-621-3141
FAX: 202-944-3295
sbaa@sbaa.org
www.sbaa.org

Ana Ximenes, Chair
Sara Struwe, President & CEO
Mark Bohay, National Web Initiatives & Development Manager
Elizabeth Merck, Development Manager

Spina bifida is a birth defect involving incomplete formation of the spine.

8478 Growing Up with Epilepsy: A Pratical Guide for Parents

Demos Medical Publishing
11 West 42nd Street
15th Floor
New York, NY 10036

212-683-0072
800-532-8663
FAX: 212-683-0118
support@demosmedical.com
www.demosmedpub.com

Richard Winters, Executive Editor
Beth Kaufman Barry, Publisher
Noreen Henson, Executive Director of Demos Heal
Lynn Bennett Blackburn, PhD, Author

Developed to help parents with the uniques challenges that this disorder presents *$19.95*
168 pages
ISBN 1-888799-74-9

8479 Guide to Living with HIV Infection: Developed at the Johns Hopkins AIDS Clinic

Johns Hopkins Universty Press
2715 N Charles St
Baltimore, MD 21218-4363

410-516-6900
800-548-1784
FAX: 410-516-6998
webmaster@jhupress.jhu.edu
www.press.jhu.edu

William Brody, President
John G Bartlett, M.D., Author
Ann K Finkbeiner, Co-Author

A handbook and reference for people living with HIV infection and their families, friends, and caregivers. *$19.95*
408 pages 6th Edition
ISBN 0-801884-85-6

8480 Handbook of Chronic Fatigue Syndrome

John Wiley & Sons
1 Wiley Drive
Somerset, NJ 08875-1272

732-469-4400
800-225-5945
FAX: 732-302-2300
custserv@wiley.com
www.as.wiley.com

Leonard A Jason, Editor
Patricia A Fennell, Editor
Renee R Taylor, Editor

Discusses diagnosis and treatment as well as the history, phenomenology, symptomatology, assessment, and pediatric and community issues. Introduces phase-based therapy and nutritional approaches. *$ 110.00*
794 pages 2003
ISBN 0-471415-12-1

8481 Handbook of Epilepsy

Lippincott, Williams & Wilkins
Philadelphia, PA 19106-3713

215-521-8300
800-777-2295
FAX: 301-824-7390
www.lpub.com

J Lippincott, CEO

Pocket-sized reference provides concise, up-to-date, clinically oriented reviews of each of the major areas of diagnosis and management of epilepsy. *$42.95*

272 pages
ISBN 0-781743-52-4

8482 Healthy Breathing
National Jewish Health
1400 Jackson St
Denver, CO 80206-2761

303-270-2708
877-225-5654
FAX: 303-398-1125
physicianline@njhealth.org
www.nationaljewish.org

Richard A. Schierburg, Chair
Robin Chotin, Vice Chair
Don Silversmith, Vice Chair
Michael Salem, CEO
Offers patients with lung or respiratory disorders information on exercise and healthy breathing.

8483 Heart of the Mind
New World Library
14 Pamaron Way
Novato, CA 94949

415-884-2100
800-972-6657
FAX: 415-884-2199
ami@newworldlibrary.com
www.newworldlibrary.com

208 pages
ISBN 1-577311-56-6

8484 Hepatitis Sourcebook
Omnigraphics
PO Box 8002
Aston, PA 19014-8002

610-461-3548
800-234-1340
FAX: 800-875-1340
customerservice@omnigraphics.com
www.omnigraphics.com

Peter Ruffner, President, Co-Founder
Fred Ruffner, Founder
Hepatitis Sourcebook provides basic consumer health information about hepatitis A, hepatitis B, hepatitis C, and other types of hepatitis, including autoimmune hepatitis, alcoholic hepatitis, nonalcoholic steatohepatitis, and toxin-induced hepatitis. It gives the facts about risk factors, prevention, transmission, screening and diagnostic methods, treatment options, and current research initiatives. *$84.00*

570 pages Hard cover
ISBN 0-780807-49-5

8485 Hip Function & Ambulation
Spina Bifida Association of America
1600 Wilson Boulevard
Suite 800
Arlington, VA 22209

202-944-3285
800-621-3141
FAX: 202-944-3295
sbaa@sbaa.org
www.sbaa.org

Ana Ximenes, Chair
Sara Struwe, President & CEO
Mark Bohay, National Web Initiatives & Development Manager
Elizabeth Merck, Development Manager
The ability to walk is important in our society, despite recent advances in wheelchair design and wheelchair accessibility. It also is a desire of children with spina bifida.

8486 Hydrocephalus: A Guide for Patients, Families & Friends
O'Reilly Media Inc
1005 Gravenstein Hwy N
Sebastopol, CA 95472-2811

707-827-7000
800-998-9938
FAX: 707-829-0104
order@oreilly.com
www.oreilly.com

Linda Lamb, Editor
Chuck Toporek, Author
Kellie Robinson, Author
Hydrocephalus is a life-threatening condition often referred to as, water on the brain, that is treated by surgical placement of a shunt system. Hydrocephalus: A Guide for Patients, Families and Friends educates families so they can select a skilled neurosurgeon, understand treatments, participate in care, know what symptoms need attention, discover where to turn for support, keep records needed for follow-up treatments, and make wise lifestyle choices. *$19.95*

379 pages Paperback 1999
ISBN 1-565924-10-X

8487 Hypertension Sourcebook
Omnigraphics
PO Box 8002
Aston, PA 19014-8002

610-461-3548
800-234-1340
FAX: 800-875-1340
customerservice@omnigraphics.com
www.omnigraphics.com

Peter Ruffner, President, Co-Founder
Fred Ruffner, Founder
This Sourcebook describes the known causes and risk factors associated with essential (or primary) hypertension, secondary hypertension, prehypertension, and other hypertensive disorders. The book also provides information about blood pressure management strategies, including dietary changes, weight loss, exercise, and medications. *$ 84.00*

588 pages Hard cover
ISBN 0-780806-74-0

8488 Immune System Disorders Sourcebook.
Omnigraphics
PO Box 31-1640
Detroit, MI 48231-8002

610-461-3548
800-234-1340
FAX: 610-532-9001
info@omnigraphics.com
www.omnigraphics.com

Joyce Brennfleck Shannon, Editor
Immune System Disorders Sourcebook provides information about inherited, acquired, and autoimmune diseases including primary immune deficiency, acquired immunodeficiency syndrome (AIDS), lupus, multiple sclerosis, type one diabetes, rheumatoid arthritis, and Graves' disease. Tips for coping with an immune disorder, caregiving, and treatments are presented along with a glossary and directory of additional resourcesories of additional resources. *$84.00*

643 pages 2nd Edition
ISBN 0-780807-48-8

8489 Informed Touch; A Clinician's Guide To TheEvaluation Of Myofascial Disorders
Inner Traditions/Bear And Company
One Park Street
PO Box 388
Rochester, VT 05767-0388

802-767-3174
800-246-8648
FAX: 802-767-3726
customerservice@innertraditions.com
www.innertraditions.com

Rob Meadows, VP Sales/Marketing
Jessica Arsenault, Sales Associate
Donna Finando, LAc, LMT, Author
Steven Finando, PhD, LAc, Co-Author

A Clinician's guide to the evaluation and treatment of myofascial disorders. *$30.00*
224 pages
ISBN 0-892817-40-5

8490 Injured Mind, Shattered Dreams: Brian's Survival from a Severe Head Injury
Brookline Books
8 Trumbull Rd,
Northampton, MA 01060-4533
413-584-0184
800-666-2665
FAX: 413-584-6184
brbooks@yahoo.com
www.brooklinebooks.com
Paperback
ISBN 0-91479-95-6

8491 Interdisciplinary Clinical Assessment of Young Children with Developmental Disabilities
Brookes Publishing
P.O.Box 10624
Baltimore, MD 21285-0624
410-337-9580
800-638-3775
FAX: 410-337-8539
custserv@brookespublishing.com
www.brookespublishing.com

Paul H. Brookes, Chairman
Jeffrey D. Brookes, President
Melissa A. Behm, Executive Vice President
George S. Stamathis, Vice President & Publisher
Offers insight from veteran team members on interdisciplinary team assessments. Professionals organizing a team as well as students preparing for practice will find advice on how practitioners gather information, approach assessment, make decisions, and face the challenges of their individual fields. Includes case studies and appendix of photocopiable questionnaires for clinicians and parents. *$44.95*
796 pages Hardcover
ISBN 1-557664-50-1

8492 Introduction to Spina Bifida
Spina Bifida Association of America
1600 Wilson Boulevard
Suite 800
Arlington, VA 22209
202-944-3285
800-621-3141
FAX: 202-944-3295
sbaa@sbaa.org
www.sbaa.org

Ana Ximenes, Chair
Sara Struwe, President & CEO
Mark Bohay, National Web Initiatives & Development Manager
Elizabeth Merck, Development Manager
An aid for parents, family and nonmedical people who care for a child with spina bifida. *$7.00*

8493 It's All in Your Head: The Link Between Mercury Amalgams and Illness
Avery Publishing Group
299 W. Houston Street
New York, NY 10014
212-859-1100
FAX: 212-859-1150
info@programexchange.com
programexchange.com
208 pages

8494 Joslin Guide to Diabetes: A Program for Managing Your Treatment
Joslin Diabetes Center
1 Joslin Pl
Boston, MA 02215-5306
617-732-2400
FAX: 617-732-2452
www.joslin.org

Richard S Beaser, M.D., Author
Amy Campbell,Ms, RD, CDE, Co-Author
Ralph M. James, Chairperson of the Board
John L. Brooks III, President/CEO

Discusses the causes of diabetes, the role of diet and exercise, meal planning and complications. Also provide information on drawing blood, mixing and injecting insulin, special challenges, living with diabetes. *$16.95*
352 pages Revised Edition

8495 Journey to Well: Learning to Live After Spinal Cord Injury
Altarfire Publishing
1835 Oak Terrace
Newcastle, CA 95658
www.altarfire.com

Margie Williams, Author
The author's close-up view of what life is like during and after such an incident, including her experience with institutional medicine and insurance companies (for better and for worse), and her determined - and ultimately successful - effort to rehabilitate herself and reconstruct her life. *$15.95*
251 pages
ISBN 0-965555-82-8

8496 Ketogenic Diet: A Treatment for Children and Others with Epilepsy
Demos Medical Publishing
11 West 42nd Street
15th Floor
New York, NY 10036
212-683-0072
800-532-8663
FAX: 212-683-0118
support@demosmedical.com
www.demosmedpub.com

Richard Winters, Executive Editor
Beth Kaufman Barry, Publisher
Noreen Henson, Executive Director of Demos Heal
John M. Freeman, MD, Co Author
Patient education reference on the use of the ketogenic diet to conrol epilepsy in children. *$24.95*
328 pages Paperback
ISBN 1-932603-18-2

8497 Latex Allergy in Spina Bifida Patients
Spina Bifida Association of America
1600 Wilson Boulevard
Suite 800
Arlington, VA 22209
202-944-3285
800-621-3141
FAX: 202-944-3295
sbaa@sbaa.org
www.sbaa.org

Ana Ximenes, Chair
Sara Struwe, President & CEO
Mark Bohay, National Web Initiatives & Development Manager
Elizabeth Merck, Development Manager
The Spina Bifida Association (SBA) serves adults and children who live with the challenges of Spina Bifida.

8498 Learning Among Children with Spina Bifida
Spina Bifida Association of America
1600 Wilson Boulevard
Suite 800
Arlington, VA 22209
202-944-3285
800-621-3141
FAX: 202-944-3295
sbaa@sbaa.org
www.sbaa.org

Ana Ximenes, Chair
Sara Struwe, President & CEO
Mark Bohay, National Web Initiatives & Development Manager
Elizabeth Merck, Development Manager
The Spina Bifida Association (SBA) serves adults and children who live with the challenges of Spina Bifida.

8499 **Let's Talk About Having Asthma**
Rosen Publishing
29 E 21st St
New York, NY 10010-6209
212-420-1600
800-237-9932
FAX: 888-436-4643
www.rosenpublishing.com

Marianna Johnstone, Co-Author
Elizabeth Weitzman, Co-Author
Kelly Chambers, Marketing Assistant
Many kids suffer from asthma, which can overtake them suddenly, causing them terror as they struggle for breath. This book talks about the causes and treatments for asthma, as well as precautions sufferers should take. *$21.95*

ISBN 0-823950-32-8

8500 **Leukemia Sourcebook**
Omnigraphics
PO Box 8002
Aston, PA 19014-8002
610-461-3548
800-234-1340
FAX: 800-875-1340
customerservice@omnigraphics.com
www.omnigraphics.com

Peter Ruffner, President, Co-Founder
Fred Ruffner, Founder
This Sourcebook provides health information about adult and childhood leukemias focusing on the diagnosis and treatments for leukemia, including chemotherapy, radiation, drug therapy, and transplantation of peripheral blood stem cells or marrow. Also included are tips for nutrition, pain and fatigue control, and recognizing possible long-term and late effects of leukemia treatment, along with a glossary and directories of additional resources. *$84.00*
564 pages Hard cover
ISBN 0-780806-27-6

8501 **Life After Trauma: A Workbook for Healing**
Guilford Press
72 Spring St
New York, NY 10012-4019
212-431-9800
800-365-7006
FAX: 212-966-6708
info@guilford.com
www.guilford.com

Denaour Rosenbloom, Author
Mary Beth Williams, Co-Author
Barbar E Watkins, Co-Author
Laurie Anne Pearlman, Foreword
A self-help book on how to deal with trauma. *$19.95*
300 pages Paperback 1910
ISBN 1-606236-08-6

8502 **Life Line**
National Hydrocephalus Foundation
12413 Centralia St
Lakewood, CA 90715-1653
562-402-3523
888-857-3434
888-260-1789
FAX: 562-924-6666
debbifields@nhfonline.org
www.nhfonline.org

Debbi Fields, Executive Director
Michael Fields, President/Treasurer
Jaynie Dunn, Secretary
Sarah Dunn, Junior Director
National Hydrocephalus Foundation quarterly newsletter.
$35.00
12 pages Quarterly

8503 **Lipomas & Lipomyelomeningocele**
Spina Bifida Association of America
1600 Wilson Boulevard
Suite 800
Arlington, VA 22209
202-944-3285
800-621-3141
FAX: 202-944-3295
sbaa@sbaa.org
www.sbaa.org

Ana Ximenes, Chair
Sara Struwe, President & CEO
Mark Bohay, National Web Initiatives & Development Manager
Elizabeth Merck, Development Manager
The Spina Bifida Association (SBA) serves adults and children who live with the challenges of Spina Bifida.

8504 **Liver Disorders Sourcebook**
Omnigraphics
PO Box 8002
Aston, PA 19014-8002
610-461-3548
800-234-1340
FAX: 800-875-1340
customerservice@omnigraphics.com
www.omnigraphics.com

Peter Ruffner, President, Co-Founder
Fred Ruffner, Founder
Liver Disorders Sourcebook contains basic consumer health information about the liver, how it works, and how to keep it healthy through diet, vaccination, and other preventive care measures. Readers will learn about the symptoms and treatment options for such diseases as hepatitis, primary biliary cirrhosis, Wilson's disease, hemochromatosis, liver failure, cancer of the liver, and disorders related to drugs and other toxins. *$84.00*
580 pages Hard cover
ISBN 0-780803-83-1

8505 **Living Beyond Multiple Sclerosis: A Woman's Guide**
Hunter House
PO Box 2914
Alameda, CA 94501-914
510-865-5282
800-266-5592
FAX: 510-865-4295
ordering@hunterhouse.com
www.hunterhouse.com

Judith Lynn Nichols, Author
Lily Jung, Foreword
This collection of e-mail conversations provides anecdotal and personal information contributed by women with multiple sclerosis. *$14.95*
256 pages
ISBN 0-897932-93-6

8506 **Living Well with Asthma**
Guilford Press
72 Spring St
New York, NY 10012-4019
212-431-9800
800-365-7006
FAX: 212-966-6708
info@guilford.com
www.guilford.com

Cynthia L Divino, Author
Michael R Freedman, Co-Author
Samuel J Rosenberg, Co-Author
James D Crapo, Foreword
Meeting the needs of a growing clinical population, this reader-friendly, practical book offers a lifeline to asthma patients attempting to understand and cope with the psychological ramifications of their illness and its treatment. *$15.95*
213 pages Paperback
ISBN 1-572300-51-4

8507 Living Well with Chronic Fatigue Syndrome and Fibromyalgia
Harper Collins Publishers
10 E 53rd St
New York, NY 10022-5244
212-207-7901
800-242-7737
FAX: 212-702-2586
spsales@harpercollins.com
www.harpercollins.com

Mary J Shomon, Author
From the author of Living Well With Hypothyroidism, a comprehensive guide to the diagnosis and treatment of chronic fatigue syndrome and fibromyalgia—vital help for the millions of people suffering from pain, fatigue, and sleep problems. *$14.95*
416 pages 2004
ISBN 0-060521-25-2

8508 Living Well with HIV and AIDS
Bull Publishing
PO Box 1377
Boulder, CO 80306-1377
303-545-6350
800-676-2855
FAX: 303-545-6354
www.bullpub.com

David Sobel, MPH, Author
Virginia Gonzalez MPH, Co-Author
Daina Laurent MPH, Co-Author
Kate Lorig RN, Co-Author
New drugs and drug combinations have turned HIV/AIDS into a long-term illness rather than a death sentence. Practical advice on mental adjustments and physical vigilance is outlined. *$18.95*
245 pages 3rd Edition
ISBN 0-923521-52-6

8509 Living With Spinal Cord Injury Series
Fanlight Productions C/O Icarus Films
32 Court St.
21st Floor
Brooklyn, NY 11201
718-488-8900
800-876-1710
FAX: 718-488-8642
info@fanlight.com
www.fanlight.com

Barry Corbet, Producer
Jonathan Miller, President
Meredith Miller, Sales Manager
Anthony Sweeney, Acquisitions
The producer, himself injured in a helicopter crash, brings a unique perspective to this classic three-part series on coming to terms with spinal cord injury. These films offer enduring proof that a tough break doesn't have to mean a ruined life. *$210.00*
VHS 1973

8510 Living with Brain Injury: A Guide for Families
Delmar Cengage Learning
PO Box 6904
Florence, KY 41022-6904
800-354-9706
FAX: 800-487-8488
esales@cengage.com
www.cengagesites.com

Richard C Senelick MD, Author
Karla Dougherty, Co-Author
A consumer text to aid people living with brain-injured survivors, includes facts on neuroplasticity, experimental rehabilitation research, and the process of rehabilitation itself. *$19.95*
225 pages Softcover 2001
ISBN 1-891525-09-3

8511 Living with Spina Bifida: A Guide for Families and Professionals
University of North Carolina at Chapel Hill
116 S Boundary St
Chapel Hill, NC 27514-3808
919-966-3561
800-848-6224
FAX: 919-962-2704
uncpress@unc.edu
www.uncpress.unc.edu

Adrian Sandler MD, Author
A handbook that addresses patients' biopsychosocial and developmental needs from birth through adolescence and into adulthood. Sandler's holistic approach encourages families to focus more on the child and less on the disability while providing abundant information about this condition. *$20.95*
296 pages 2004
ISBN 0-807855-47-8

8512 Lung Cancer: Making Sense of Diagnosis, Treatment, and Options
O'Reilly Media Inc
1005 Gravenstein Hwy N
Sebastopol, CA 95472-2811
707-827-7000
800-998-9938
FAX: 707-829-0104
order@oreilly.com
www.oreilly.com

Linda Lamb, Editor
Lorraine Johnston, Author
Straightforward language and the words of patients and their families are the hallmarks of this book on the number one cancer killer in the US. Written by a widely respected author and patient advocate, Lung Cancer: Making Sense of Diagnosis, Treatment, & Options has been meticulously reviewed by top medical experts and physicians. Readers will find medical facts simply explained, advice to ease their daily life, and tools to be strong advocates for themselves or a family member. *$ 27.95*
530 pages Paperback 2001
ISBN 0-596500-02-5

8513 Lung Disorders Sourcebook
Omnigraphics
PO Box 8002
Aston, PA 19014-8002
610-461-3548
800-234-1340
FAX: 800-875-1340
customerservice@omnigraphics.com
www.omnigraphics.com

Peter Ruffner, President, Co-Founder
Fred Ruffner, Founder
Lung Disorders Sourcebook offers information about specific types of lung disorders, including diagnosis, treatment, and prevention issues. The book offers advice for preventing some types lung disorder that are acquired by asbestos, radon, and other environmental exposures. *$84.00*
657 pages Hard cover
ISBN 0-780803-39-8

8514 Lupus: Alternative Therapies That Work
Inner Traditions
PO Box 388
Rochester
VT, 05 0388-802-
800-246-8648
802-767-3726
TTY:customerserv
info@innertraditions.com
www.innertraditions.com

Sharon Moore, Author
A comprehensive guise to noninvasive, nontoxic therapies for lupus - written by a lupus survivor. *$14.95*
256 pages 2000
ISBN 0-892818-89-1

8515 MAGIC Touch
MAGIC Foundation for Children's Growth
6645 North Ave
Oak Park, IL 60302-1057

708-383-0808
800-362-4423
FAX: 708-383-0899
mary@magicfoundation.org
www.magicfoundation.org

Mary Andrews, CEO
Dianne Kremidas, Executive Director
Pam Pentaris, Office Manager
Jamie Harvey, Technical Education Teacher
Provides support and education regarding growth disorders in children and related adult disorders, including adult GHD. Dedicated to helping children whose physical growth is affected be a medical problem by assisting families of afflicted children through local support groups, public education/awareness, newsletters, specialty divisions and programs for the children.
36-40 pages Quarterly

8516 Management of Autistic Behavior
Sage Publications
2455 Teller Road
Thousand Oaks, CA 91320

805-499-0721
800-818-7243
FAX: 805-499-0871
info@sagepub.com
www.sagepub.com

Sara Miller McCune, Founder, Publisher, Executive Chairman
Blaise R Simqu, President & CEO
Tracey A. Ozmina, Executive Vice President & Chief Operating Officer
Stephen Barr, Managing Director/SAGE London, President of SAGE Internation
Comprehensive and practical book that tells what works best with specific problems. *$51.00*
450 pages Paperback
ISBN 0-890791-96-1

8517 Management of Genetic Syndromes
John Wiley & Sons
111 River St
Hoboken, NJ 07030-5774

201-748-6000
201-748-6088
info@wiley.com
www.as.wiley.com

Suzanne B Cassidy, Editor
Judith E Allanson, Editor
Edited by two of the field's most highly esteemed experts, this landmark volume provides: A precise reference of the physical manifestations of common genetic syndromes, clearly written for professionals and families, Extensive updates, particularly in sections on diagnostic criteria and diagnostic testing, pathogenesis, and management, A tried-and-tested, user-friendly format, with each chapter including information on incidence, etiology and pathogenesis, diagnostic criteria and testing, and d *$204.95*
720 pages 3rd Edition
ISBN 0-470191-41-5

8518 Managing Post Polio: A Guide to Living Well with Post Polio
ABI Professional Publications
PO Box 149
St Petersburg, FL 33731-149

727-556-0950
800-551-7776
FAX: 727-556-2560
webmaster@vandamere.com
www.abipropub.com

Lauro S Halstead MD, Editor
Edited by Lauro S. Halstead, M.D., Managing Post-Polio, 2nd Edition, provides a comprehensive overview dealing with the medical, psychological, vocational, and many other challenges of living with post-polio syndrome. With contributions from over 15 healthcare professionals, the majority of whom are polio survivors themselves, Managing Post-Polio distills and summarizes

the wealth of information presented from over the past 20 plus years.
256 pages
ISBN 1-886236-17-8

8519 Meniere's Disease
Vestibular Disorders Association
5018 NE 15th Avenue
Portland, OR 97211

800-837-8428
FAX: 503-229-8064
info@vestibular.org
www.vestibular.org

P. Ashley Wackym, Chair
Cynthia Ryan MBA, Executive Director
Tony Staser, Development Director
Kerrie Denner, Outreach Coordinator
VEDA's website contains a wealth of information on the symptoms, diagnosis and treatment of various types of vestibular disorders. *$5.00*

8520 Menopause without Medicine
Hunter House
PO Box 2914
Alameda, CA 94501-914

510-865-5282
800-266-5592
FAX: 510-865-4295
ordering@hunterhouse.com
www.hunterhouse.com

Linda Ojeda PhD, Author
Menopause Without Medicine provides complete information on the symptoms of menopause - hot flashes, fatigue, sexual changes, depression and osteoporosis - and how to alleviate them. *$18.95*
304 pages 5th Edition
ISBN 0-897934-05-3

8521 Movement Disorders Sourcebook
Omnigraphics
PO Box 8002
Aston, PA 19014-8002

610-461-3548
800-234-1340
FAX: 800-875-1340
customerservice@omnigraphics.com
www.omnigraphics.com

Peter Ruffner, President, Co-Founder
Fred Ruffner, Founder
This Sourcebook provides health information about neurological movement disorders, their symptoms, causes, diagnostic tests, and treatments. Readers will learn about Essential Tremor, Parkinson's Disease, Dystonia, and many other early-onset and adult-onset movement disorders. Information about mobility and assistive technology aids is included, along with a glossary and a listing of additional resources. *$84.00*
600 pages Hard cover
ISBN 0-780810-34-1

8522 Multiple Sclerosis and Having a Baby
Inner Traditions
PO Box 388
Rochester, VT 05767-0388

802-767-3174
800-246-8648
FAX: 802-767-3726
customerservice@innertraditions.com
www.innertraditions.com

Judy Graham, Author
Everything you need to know about conception, pregnancy and parenthood. *$12.95*
160 pages 2001
ISBN 0-892817-88-7

8523 Multiple Sclerosis: 300 Tips for Making Life Easier
Demos Medical Publishing
11 West 42nd Street
15th Floor
New York, NY 10036   212-683-0072
                                            800-532-8663
                                      FAX: 212-683-0118
                              support@demosmedical.com
                                    www.demosmedpub.com

Richard Winters, Executive Editor
Beth Kaufman Barry, Publisher
Noreen Henson, Executive Director of Demos Heal
Shelley Peterman Schwarz, Author
This latest book in the Making Life Easier series features tip,
techniques and shortcuts for conserving time and energy so you
can do more of the things you want to do. These tips should help
increase the number of good days you have while encouraging
you to develop your own techniques for making life easier.
$16.95
128 pages
ISBN 1-932603-21-2

8524 Multiple Sclerosis: A Guide for Families
Demos Medical Publishing
11 West 42nd Street
15th Floor
New York, NY 10036   212-683-0072
                                            800-532-8663
                                      FAX: 212-683-0118
                              support@demosmedical.com
                                    www.demosmedpub.com
Richard Winters, Executive Editor
Beth Kaufman Barry, Publisher
Noreen Henson, Executive Director of Demos Heal
Rosalind C. Kalb, Ph.D., Author
Guide for living and coping with multiple sclerosis. *$24.95*
256 pages
ISBN 1-932603-10-7

8525 Multiple Sclerosis: A Guide for the Newly Diagnosed
Demos Medical Publishing
11 West 42nd Street
15th Floor
New York, NY 10036   212-683-0072
                                            800-532-8663
                                      FAX: 212-683-0118
                              support@demosmedical.com
                                    www.demosmedpub.com
Richard Winters, Executive Editor
Beth Kaufman Barry, Publisher
Noreen Henson, Executive Director of Demos Heal
Nancy J. Holland, RN, EdD,, Co Author
A must-have title for anyone who has recently been diagnosed
with MS and a good idea for family members and friends. *$19.95*
256 pages
ISBN 1-932603-27-1

**8526 Multiple Sclerosis: The Guide to Treatment and
Management**
Demos Medical Publishing
11 West 42nd Street
15th Floor
New York, NY 10036   212-683-0072
                                            800-532-8663
                                      FAX: 212-683-0118
                              support@demosmedical.com
                                    www.demosmedpub.com
Richard Winters, Executive Editor
Beth Kaufman Barry, Publisher
Noreen Henson, Executive Director of Demos Heal
Chris H. Polman, MD, FRCP, Co Author
A current guide to modern therapies. *$24.95*
216 pages
ISBN 1-932603-15-4

8527 Muscular Dystrophies
Oxford University Press
198 Madison Avenue
New York, NY 10016   212-726-6000
                                            800-445-9714
                                      FAX: 919-677-1303
                                  custserv.us@oup.com
                                        www.oup.com
Alan E.H. Emery, Author
Describes the opportunities for management of more than 30
types of MD through respiratory care, physiotherapy and surgical
correction of contractures, and examines the potential for effective treatment utilizing the new techniques of gene and cell therapy *$ 165.00*
330 pages
ISBN 0-192632-91-4

8528 Muscular Dystrophy in Children: A Guide for Families
Demos Medical Publishing
11 West 42nd Street
15th Floor
New York, NY 10036   212-683-0072
                                            800-532-8663
                                      FAX: 212-683-0118
                              support@demosmedical.com
                                    www.demosmedpub.com
Richard Winters, Executive Editor
Beth Kaufman Barry, Publisher
Noreen Henson, Executive Director of Demos Heal
Defines the available medical options at every stage of the disease and offers guidance even when it may seem that little or noth-
ing can be done. Includes a glossary and suggestions for furhter
reading. *$19.95*
144 pages Paperback
ISBN 1-888799-33-1

8529 Muscular Dystrophy: The Facts
Oxford University Press
198 Madison Avenue
New York, NY 10016   212-726-6000
                                            800-445-9714
                                      FAX: 919-677-1303
                                  custserv.us@oup.com
                                        www.oup.com
Peter Harper, Author
A good first book for individuals and families faced with the like-
lihood or reality of a muscular dystrophy diagnosis. *$22.50*
178 pages
ISBN 0-192632-17-5

**8530 My House is Killing Me! The Home Guide for Families with
Allergies and Asthma**
Johns Hopkins University Press
2175 N Charles St
Baltimore, MD 21218-4363   410-516-6900
                                             800-548-1784
                                       FAX: 410-516-6968
                               webmaster@jhupress.jhu.edu
                                     www.press.jhu.edu
Jeffrey C May, Author
Jonathan M Samet, M.D., Foreword
Kathleen Keane, Director
Chemical consultant May describes where and how the various
parts of a residence can cause temporary or chronic illness for
those with allergies or other sensitivities. *$20.95*
352 pages
ISBN 0-801867-30-9

8531 Neuropsychiatry of Epilepsy
Cambridge University Press
100 Brookhill Dr
West Nyack, NY 10994   845-353-7500
                                             845-353-4141
                                       www.cambridge.org
Michael R Trimble, Editor
Bettina Schmitz, Editor

Covers the practical implications of ongoing research, and offers a diagnostic and management perspective. Topics include cognitive aspects, nonepileptic attacks, and clinical aspects. For professionals treating epileptic patients. *$104.00*
232 pages 2nd Edition 1911
ISBN 0-521154-69-7

8532   Nick Joins In
Spina Bifida Association of America
1600 Wilson Boulevard
Suite 800
Arlington, VA 22209   202-944-3285
                                     800-621-3141
                            FAX: 202-944-3295
                                  sbaa@sbaa.org
                                  www.sbaa.org

Ana Ximenes, Chair
Sara Struwe, President & CEO
Mark Bohay, National Web Initiatives & Development Manager
Elizabeth Merck, Development Manager
When Nick, who is in a wheelchair, enters a regular classroom for the first time, he realizes that he has much to contribute. *$17.00*

8533   No More Allergies
Random House
1745 Broadway
3rd Floor
New York, NY 10019-4305   212-782-9000
                            FAX: 212-572-6066
                   ecustomerservice@randonhouse.com
                            www.randomhouse.com

Markus Dohle, CEO
Gary Null PhD, Author
Null redefines a health problem that afflicts 40 million Americans: More than mere hay fever, contemporary allergic reactions include chronic fatigue syndrome, Alzheimer's disease, and even HIV infection. These conditions, he explains, occur when our immune systems break down. This ground-breaking book now prescribes effective solutions. *$23.00*
464 pages 1992
ISBN 0-679743-10-1

8534   No Time for Jello: One Family's Experience
Brookline Books
8 Trumbull Rd,
Northampton, MA 01060-4533   413-584-0184
                                     800-666-2665
                            FAX: 413-584-6184
                               brbooks@yahoo.com
                            www.brooklinebooks.com

Softcover
ISBN 0-91479-56-5

8535   Nocturnal Asthma
National Jewish Health
1400 Jackson Street
Denver, CO 80206   303-270-2708
                                     877-225-5654
                            FAX: 303-398-1125
                                allstetterw@njc.org
                                nationaljewish.org

Rich Schierburg, Chair
Robin Chotin, Vice Chair
Michael Salem, M.D., President and CEO
Christine Forkner, CFO and Executive Vice President
Offers information to patients about how to understand and manage asthma at night.

8536   Obesity
Spina Bifida Association of America
1600 Wilson Boulevard
Suite 800
Arlington, VA 22209   202-944-3285
                                     800-621-3141
                            FAX: 202-944-3295
                                  sbaa@sbaa.org
                                  www.sbaa.org

Ana Ximenes, Chair
Sara Struwe, President & CEO
Mark Bohay, National Web Initiatives & Development Manager
Elizabeth Merck, Development Manager
The Spina Bifida Association (SBA) serves adults and children who live with the challenges of Spina Bifida. *$8.00*

8537   Obesity Sourcebook
Omnigraphics
PO Box 8002
Aston, PA 19014-8002   610-461-3548
                                     800-234-1340
                            FAX: 800-875-1340
                   customerservice@omnigraphics.com
                            www.omnigraphics.com

Peter Ruffner, President, Co-Founder
Fred Ruffner, Founder
Discusses diseases and other problems associated with obesity. *$78.00*
376 pages
ISBN 0-780803-33-6

8538   Occulta
Spina Bifida Association of America
1600 Wilson Boulevard
Suite 800
Arlington, VA 22209   202-944-3285
                                     800-621-3141
                            FAX: 202-944-3295
                                  sbaa@sbaa.org
                                  www.sbaa.org

Ana Ximenes, Chair
Sara Struwe, President & CEO
Mark Bohay, National Web Initiatives & Development Manager
Elizabeth Merck, Development Manager
The Spina Bifida Association (SBA) serves adults and children who live with the challenges of Spina Bifida. *$8.00*

8539   Official Patient's Sourcebook on Bell's Palsy
Icon Group International
9606 Tierra Grande Street
Suite 205
San Diego, CA 92126
                            FAX: 858-635-9414
                         orders@icongroupbooks.com
                            www.icongroupbooks.com

ISBN 0-597835-20-9

8540   Official Patient's Sourcebook on Cystic Fibrosis
Icon Group International
9606 Tierra Grande Street
Suite 205
San Diego, CA 92126
                            FAX: 858-635-9414
                         orders@icongroupbooks.com
                            icongroupbooks.com

356 pages
ISBN 0-597831-46-7

8541 Official Patient's Sourcebook on Muscular Dystrophy
Icon Group International
9606 Tierra Grande Street
Suite 205
San Diego, CA 92126

FAX: 858-635-9414
orders@icongroupbooks.com
icongroupbooks.com

268 pages
ISBN 0-597832-10-2

8542 Official Patient's Sourcebook on Osteoporosis
Icon Group International
9606 Tierra Grande Street
Suite 205
San Diego, CA 92126

FAX: 858-635-9414
orders@icongroupbooks.com
icongroupbooks.com

ISBN 0-597833-04-4

8543 Official Patient's Sourcebook on Post-Polio Syndrome: A Revised and Updated Directory
Icon Group International
9606 Tierra Grande Street
Suite 205
San Diego, CA 92126

FAX: 858-635-9414
orders@icongroupbooks.com
icongroupbooks.com

124 pages
ISBN 0-597835-31-4

8544 Official Patient's Sourcebook on Primary Pulmonary Hypertension
Icon Group International
9606 Tierra Grande Street
Suite 205
San Diego, CA 92126

FAX: 858-635-9414
orders@icongroupbooks.com
icongroupbooks.com

ISBN 0-597831-54-8

8545 Official Patient's Sourcebook on Pulmonary Fibrosis
Icon Group International
9606 Tierra Grande Street
Suite 205
San Diego, CA 92126

FAX: 858-635-9414
orders@icongroupbooks.com
icongroupbooks.com

ISBN 0-597831-65-3

8546 Official Patient's Sourcebook on Scoliosis
Icon Group International
9606 Tierra Grande Street
Suite 205
San Diego, CA 92126

FAX: 858-635-9414
orders@icongroupbooks.com
icongroupbooks.com

ISBN 0-597829-90-X

8547 Official Patient's Sourcebook on Sickle Cell Anemia
Icon Group International
9606 Tierra Grande Street
Suite 205
San Diego, CA 92126

FAX: 858-635-9414
orders@icongroupbooks.com
icongroupbooks.com

ISBN 0-597831-57-2

8548 Official Patient's Sourcebook on Ulcerative Colitis
Icon Group International
9606 Tierra Grande Street
Suite 205
San Diego, CA 92126

FAX: 858-635-9414
orders@icongroupbooks.com
icongroupbooks.com

ISBN 0-597834-09-1

8549 One Day at a Time: Children Living with Leukemia
Gareth Stevens Publishing
111 East 14th Street
Suite #349
New York, NY 10003

800-542-2595
FAX: 877-542-2596
customerservice@gspub.com
www.garethstevens.com

56 pages Hardcover
ISBN 1-55532-13-6

8550 Options: Revolutionary Ideas in the War on Cancer
People Against Cancer
P.O.Box 10
604 East Street
Otho, IA 50569

515-972-4444
800-662-2623
FAX: 515-972-4415
info@PeopleAgainstCancer.org
www.peopleagainstcancer.com

Frank D. Wiewel, Executive Director/Founder
Publication of People Against Cancer, a nonprofit, grassroots public benefit organization dedicated to 'New Directions in the War on Cancer.' We help people to find the best cancer treatment. We are a democratic organization of people with cancer, their loved ones and citizens working together to protect and enhance medical freedom of choice.

8551 Osteoporosis Sourcebook
Omnigraphics
PO Box 8002
Aston, PA 19014-8002

313-961-1340
800-234-1340
FAX: 800-875-1340
customerservice@omnigraphics.com
www.omnigraphics.com

Peter Ruffner, President, Co-Founder
Fred Ruffner, Founder
Discusses causes, risk factors, treatments and traditional and non-traditional pain management issues concerning osteoporosis. $ 84.00
568 pages Hard cover
ISBN 0-780802-39-1

8552 Parent's Guide to Allergies and Asthma
Allergy & Asthma Network Mothers of Asthmatics
Ste 150
PO Box 7474
Fairfax Station, VA 22039-7474

703-323-9170
800-756-5525
FAX: 703-323-9173
custsvc@parent-institute.com
www.parent-institute.com

John H Wherry, Ed.D, President

A up-to-date, easy-to-read resource offering essential information on asthma and allergies.

8553   Partial Seizure Disorders: A Guide for Patients and Families
O'Reilly Media Inc
1005 Gravenstein Hwy N
Sebastopol, CA 95472-2811   707-827-7000
                                             800-998-9938
                                             FAX: 707-829-0104
                                             order@oreilly.com
                                             www.oreilly.com

Linda Lamb, Editor
Mitzi Waltz, Author
Partial Seizure Disorders helps patients and families get an accurate diagnosis of this condition, understand medications and their side effects, and learn coping skills and other adjuncts to medication. It walks readers through developmental and school issues for young children; adult issues such as employment and driving; working with an existing health plan; and getting further help through advocacy and support organizations, articles, and online resources. *$19.95*
288 pages Paperback
ISBN 0-596500-03-3

8554   Penitent, with Roses: An HIV+ Mother Reflects
University Press of New England
1 Court St
Ste 250
Lebanon, NH 03766-1358   603-448-1533
                                             800-421-1561
                                             FAX: 603-448-7006
                                             www.upne.com

Paula W Peterson, Author
Peterson, a married, middle-class, Jewish mother, was diagnosed with full-blown AIDS four years into her marriage and 11 months after her son was born. In seven poignant autobiographical essays and a collection of letters to her uninfected, four-year-old son, the author maintains an upbeat tone and describes her unsuccessful attempts to find the source of her infection (her husband tested negative), her relationships with her doctors, and her work as an HIV activist. *$26.95*
256 pages 2001
ISBN 1-584651-28-4

8555   Plan Ahead: Do What You Can
Spina Bifida Association of America
1600 Wilson Boulevard
Suite 800
Arlington, VA 22209   202-944-3285
                                             800-621-3141
                                             FAX: 202-944-3295
                                             sbaa@sbaa.org
                                             www.sbaa.org

Ana Ximenes, Chair
Sara Struwe, President & CEO
Mark Bohay, National Web Initiatives & Development Manager
Elizabeth Merck, Development Manager
Folic aciid information for women at risk for recurrence. *$15.00*

8556   Post-Polio Syndrome: A Guide for Polio Survivors and Their Families
Yale University Press
PO Box 209040
New Haven, CT 6520-9040   203-432-0960
                                             203-432-0948
                                             language.yalepress@yale.edu
                                             www.yalepress.yale.edu

Julie K Silver M.D., Author
Laro S Halstead, M.D., Foreword
A guide for polio survivors, their families, and their health care providers offers expert advice on all aspects of post-polio syndrome. Based on the author's experience treating post-polio patients, Silver discusses issues of critical importance, including how to find the best medical care, deal with symptoms, sustain

mobility, manage pain, approach insurance issues, and arrange a safe living environment. *$19.50*
304 pages 2002
ISBN 0-300088-08-3

8557   Prader-Willi Syndrome: Development and Manifestations
Cambridge University Press
32 Avenue of the Americas
New York, NY 10013-2473   212-924-3900
                                             212-691-3239
                                             www.cambridge.org

Joyce Whittington, Author
Tony Holland, Co-Author
Seeks to identify and provide the latest findings about how best to manage the complex medical, nutritional, psychological, educational, social and therapeutic needs of people with PWS. *$130.00*
230 pages 2004
ISBN 0-521840-29-3

8558   Preventing Secondary Conditions Associated with Spina Bifida or Cerebral Palsy
Spina Bifida Association of America
1600 Wilson Boulevard
Suite 800
Arlington, VA 22209   202-944-3285
                                             800-621-3141
                                             FAX: 202-944-3295
                                             sbaa@sbaa.org
                                             www.sbaa.org

Ana Ximenes, Chair
Sara Struwe, President & CEO
Mark Bohay, National Web Initiatives & Development Manager
Elizabeth Merck, Development Manager
This report is for health professionals, parents and teachers. *$3.00*

8559   Prostate and Urological Disorders Sourcebook
Omnigraphics
PO Box 8002
Aston, PA 19014-8002   313-961-1340
                                             800-234-1340
                                             FAX: 800-875-1340
                                             customerservice@omnigraphics.com
                                             www.omnigraphics.com

Peter Ruffner, President, Co-Founder
Fred Ruffner, Founder
Peter Ruffner, Co-Founder
Prostate and Urological Disorders Sourcebook provides information about prostate cancer and other prostate problems, such as prostatitis and benign prostatic hyperplasia. A glossary of andrological terms and a directory of resources for additional help and information are also included. *$84.00*
604 pages Hard cover
ISBN 0-780807-97-6

8560   Protecting Against Latex Allergy
Spina Bifida Association of America
1600 Wilson Boulevard
Suite 800
Arlington, VA 22209   202-944-3285
                                             800-621-3141
                                             FAX: 202-944-3295
                                             sbaa@sbaa.org
                                             www.sbaa.org

Ana Ximenes, Chair
Sara Struwe, President & CEO
Mark Bohay, National Web Initiatives & Development Manager
Elizabeth Merck, Development Manager
Because awareness and proper action may help prevent an allergic reation, learning about latex allergy is especially important for parents, health care workers and anyone who is exposed to latex regulary. *$20.00*

8561 Questions and Answers: The ADA and Personswith HIV/AIDS
US Department of Justice
950 Pennsylvania Ave NW
Washington, DC 20530-9

202-307-0663
800-514-0301
FAX: 202-307-1197
TTY: 800-514-0383
www.ada.gov

Joanne Graham, Manager
Rebecca B. Bond, Chief
Zita Johnson Betts, Deputy Chief
James Bostrom, Deputy Chief

A 16-page publication explaining the requirements for employers, businesses and nonprofit agencies that serve the public, and state and local governments to avoid discriminating against persons with HIV/AIDS.

8562 Raynaud's Phenomenon
Arthritis Foundation
1330 W. Peachtree Street
Suite 100
Atlanta, GA 30309

404-872-7100
800-283-7800
FAX: 404-872-0457
arthritis.org

Daniel T. McGowan, Chair
Michael V. Ortman, Vice Chair
Ann M. Palmer, CEO/President
Peter W.C. Barnhart, Treasurer

The Arthritis Foundation is the largest national nonprofit organization that supports the more than 100 types of arthritis and related conditions. Founded in 1948, with headquarters in Atlanta, the Arthritis Foundation has multiple service points located throughout the country.

8563 Reaching the Autistic Child: A Parent Training Program
Brookline Books
8 Trumbull Rd,
Northampton, MA 01060-4533

413-584-0184
800-666-2665
FAX: 413-584-6184
brbooks@yahoo.com
www.brooklinebooks.com

Softcover
ISBN 1-571290-56-7

8564 Respiratory Disorders Sourcebook
Omnigraphics
PO Box 8002
Aston, PA 19014-8002

313-961-1340
800-234-1340
FAX: 800-875-1340
customerservice@omnigraphics.com
www.omnigraphics.com

Peter Ruffner, President, Co-Founder
Fred Ruffner, Founder
Sandra J Judd, Editor

Respiratory Disorders Sourcebook provides up-to-date information about infectious, inflammatory, occupational, and other types of respiratory disorders. Tips for managing chronic respiratory diseases and suggestions for ways to promote lung health are presented, and the book concludes with a glossary of related terms and a list of additional resources. *$84.00*
638 pages Hard cover
ISBN 0-780810-07-5

8565 SPINabilities: A Young Person's Guide to Spina Bifida
Spina Bifida Association of America
1600 Wilson Boulevard
Suite 800
Arlington, VA 22209

202-944-3285
800-621-3141
FAX: 202-944-3295
sbaa@sbaa.org
www.sbaa.org

Ana Ximenes, Chair
Sara Struwe, President & CEO
Mark Bohay, National Web Initiatives & Development Manager
Elizabeth Merck, Development Manager

A cool and practical book for young adults becoming independent. *$22.30*

8566 Seizures and Epilepsy in Childhood: A Guide
John Hopkins University Press
2715 N Charles St
Baltimore, MD 21218-4363

410-516-6900
800-548-1784
FAX: 410-516-6998
webmaster@jhupress.jhu.edu
www.press.jhu.edu

Kathleen Keane, Director
Eileen P G Vining MD, Co-Author
Diana J Pillas, Co-Author
John M Freeman, M.D., Co-Author

The award-winning Seizures and Epilepsy in Childhood is the standard resource for parents in need of comprehensive medical information about their child with epilepsy. *$54.00*
432 pages 3rd Edition
ISBN 0-801870-51-4

8567 Sexuality and the Person with Spina Bifida
Spina Bifida Association of America
1600 Wilson Boulevard
Suite 800
Arlington, VA 22209

202-944-3285
800-621-3141
FAX: 202-944-3295
sbaa@sbaa.org
www.sbaa.org

Ana Ximenes, Chair
Sara Struwe, President & CEO
Mark Bohay, National Web Initiatives & Development Manager
Elizabeth Merck, Development Manager

Dr Sloan foucuses on sexual development, sexual activity and other important issues. *$11.00*

8568 Sinus Survival: A Self-help Guide
Penguin Group
375 Hudson St
New York, NY 10014-3658

212-366-2372
FAX: 212-366-2933
insidesales@penguingroup.com
us.penguingroup.com

Robert S Ivker, Author

Self-help manual for sufferers of bronchitis, sinusitis, allergies, and colds. *$15.95*
336 pages Paperback 2000
ISBN 1-101798-02-6

8569 Social Development and the Person with Spina Bifida
Spina Bifida Association of America
1600 Wilson Boulevard
Suite 800
Arlington, VA 22209

202-944-3285
800-621-3141
FAX: 202-944-3295
sbaa@sbaa.org
www.sbaa.org

Ana Ximenes, Chair
Sara Struwe, President & CEO
Mark Bohay, National Web Initiatives & Development Manager
Elizabeth Merck, Development Manager

Examines how spina bifida and hydrocephalus may influence development and learning social skills.

8570 Solving the Puzzle of Chronic Fatigue
Essential Science Publishing
1216 S 1580 W
Ste A
Orem, UT 84058-4906
801-224-6228
800-336-6308
FAX: 801-224-6229
info@essentialscience.net
www.essentialsciencepublishing.com

Michael Rosenbaum, Author
Murray Susser, Co-Author
Although primarily a book about CFS, this comprehensive study also provides a detailed overview of candidiasis, including its causes and best approaches for treatment. *$14.95*
190 pages
ISBN 0-943685-11-7

8571 Son Rise: The Miracle Continues
New World Library
14 Pamaron Way
Novato, CA 94949
415-884-2100
800-972-6657
FAX: 415-884-2199
ami@newworldlibrary.com
www.newworldlibrary.com

Barry Neil Kaufman, Author
Documents Raun Kaufman's astonishing development from a lifeless, autistic, retarded child into a highly verbal, lovable youngster with no traces of his former condition. Details Raun's extraordinary progress from the age of four into young adulthood, also shares moving accounts of five families that successfully used the Son-Rise Program to reach their own special children. *$14.96*
372 pages
ISBN 0-915811-53-7

8572 Steps to Independence: Teaching Everyday Skills to Children with Special Needs
Spina Bifida Association of America
1600 Wilson Boulevard
Suite 800
Arlington, VA 22209
202-944-3285
800-621-3141
FAX: 202-944-3295
sbaa@sbaa.org
www.sbaa.org

Ana Ximenes, Chair
Sara Struwe, President & CEO
Mark Bohay, National Web Initiatives & Development Manager
Elizabeth Merck, Development Manager
A guide to help parents teach life skills to their disabled child. *$34.25*

8573 Stroke Sourcebook
PO Box 8002
Aston, PA 19014-8002
313-961-1340
800-234-1340
FAX: 800-875-1340
customerservice@omnigraphics.com
www.omnigraphics.com

Peter Ruffner, President, Co-Founder
Fred Ruffner, Founder
Peter Ruffner, Co-Founder
Basic Consumer Health Information about Stroke, Including Ischemic, Hemorrhagic, and Mini Strokes, as Well as Risk Factors, Prevention Guidelines, Diagnostic Tests, Medications and Surgical Treatments, and Complications of Stroke.

8574 Stroke Sourcebook, 2nd Edition
Omnigraphics
PO Box 8002
Aston, PA 19014-8002
313-961-1340
800-234-1340
FAX: 800-875-1340
customerservice@omnigraphics.com
www.omnigraphics.com

Peter Ruffner, President, Co-Founder
Fred Ruffner, Founder
Peter Ruffner, Co-Founder
Stroke Sourcebook, Second Edition provides updated information about stroke, its causes, risk factors, diagnosis, acute and long-term treatment, and recent innovations in poststroke care. Information on rehabilitation therapies, prevention strategies, and tips on caring for a stroke survivor is also included, along with a glossary of related terms and a directory of organizations that offer additional information to stroke survivors and their families. *$84.00*
626 pages Hard cover
ISBN 0-780810-35-8

8575 Succeeding With Interventions For Asperger Syndrome Adolescents
Autsim Society of North Carolina Bookstore
505 Oberlin Road
Suite 230
Raleigh, NC 27605-1345
919-743-0204
800-442-2762
FAX: 919-743-0208
books@autismsociety-nc.org
www.autismbookstore.com

Tracey Sheriff, Chief Executive Officer
David Laxton, Director of Communications
Paul Wendler, Chief Financial Officer
Kristy White, Director of Development
This book includes a very useful outline of all the therapy sessions, which can be used as a template by a practitioner for creating their own interaction therapy intervention for adolescents.

8576 Symptomatic Chiari Malformation
Spina Bifida Association of America
1600 Wilson Boulevard
Suite 800
Arlington, VA 22209
202-944-3285
800-621-3141
FAX: 202-944-3295
sbaa@sbaa.org
www.sbaa.org

Ana Ximenes, Chair
Sara Struwe, President & CEO
Mark Bohay, National Web Initiatives & Development Manager
Elizabeth Merck, Development Manager
The Spina Bifida Association (SBA) serves adults and children who live with the challenges of Spina Bifida.

8577 Taking Charge
Spina Bifida Association of America
1600 Wilson Boulevard
Suite 800
Arlington, VA 22209
202-944-3285
800-621-3141
FAX: 202-944-3295
sbaa@sbaa.org
www.sbaa.org

Ana Ximenes, Chair
Sara Struwe, President & CEO
Mark Bohay, National Web Initiatives & Development Manager
Elizabeth Merck, Development Manager
Teenagers talk about life and physical disabilities. *$7.95*

8578 **Ten Things I Learned from Bill Porter**
New World Library
14 Pamaron Way
Novato, CA 94949 415-884-2100
800-972-6657
FAX: 415-884-2199
ami@newworldlibrary.com
www.newworldlibrary.com

Shelly Ackerman, Author
Bill Porter worked for the Watkins Corp, selling household products door-to-door in one of Portland's worst neighborhoods. Afflicted with cerebral palsy and burdened with continual pain, Porter was determined not to live on government disability and went on to become Watkin's top-grossing salesman in Portland, the Northwest, and the US. This book was written by the woman who worked as Porter's typist and driver and later became his friend and cospeaker. $20.00
192 pages
ISBN 1-577312-03-1

8579 **Thyroid Disorders Sourcebook**
Omnigraphics
PO Box 8002
Aston, PA 19014-8002 313-961-1340
800-234-1340
FAX: 800-875-1340
customerservice@omnigraphics.com
www.omnigraphics.com

Peter Ruffner, President, Co-Founder
Fred Ruffner, Founder
Thyroid Disorders Sourcebook provides essential information about thyroid and parathyroid function, diseases, and treatments. Also presented are symptoms, risk factors, diagnosis, treatments, thyroid effects on the body, and the impact of environmental conditions on the thyroid. $84.00
573 pages Hard cover
ISBN 0-780807-45-7

8580 **Tourette Syndrome: The Facts**
Oxford University Press
198 Madison Avenue
New York, NY 10016 212-726-6000
800-445-9714
FAX: 919-677-1303
custserv.us@oup.com
www.oup.com

Mary Robertson, Co-Editor
Andrea Cavanna, Co-Editor
Johnathan Keats, Author
Jim Cullen, Author
The causes of the syndrome, how it is diagnosed, and the ways in which it can be treated. $35.00
122 pages
ISBN 0-198523-98-X

8581 **Tourette's Syndrome: Finding Answers and Getting Help**
O'Reilly Media Inc
1005 Gravenstein Hwy N
Sebastopol, CA 95472-2811 707-827-7019
800-889-8969
FAX: 707-824-8268
order@oreilly.com
www.oreilly.com

416 pages Paperback
ISBN 0-596500-07-6

8582 **Tourette's Syndrome: Tics, Obsessions, Compulsions: Developmental Psychopathology**
John Wiley & Sons
111 River Street
Hoboken, NJ 07030-5774 201-748-6000
FAX: 201-748-6088
info@wiley.com
www.wiley.com

Peter Booth Wiley, Chairman
Stephen M. Smith, President & CEO
John Kitzmacher, EVP, CFO
Ellis E. Cousens, Executive Vice President, COO
Contains 21 contributions compromising the work of researchers associated with the Yale Child Study Center, which has been at the forefront of research on Tourette's syndrome and associated disorders. $85.00
600 pages
ISBN 0-471113-75-1

8583 **Treating Epilepsy Naturally: A Guide to Alternative and Adjunct Therapies**
McGraw-Hill Company
P.O.Box 182605
Columbus, OH 43218 800-338-3987
FAX: 609-308-4480
customer.service@mheducation.com
www.mcgraw-hill.com

David Levin, President and CEO
Patrick Milano, Chief Administrative Officer & CFO
Stephen Laster, Chief Digital Officer
David Stafford, SVP & General Counsel
Offers alternative treatments to replace and to complement traditional therapies and sound advice to find the right health practitioner. $15.95
288 pages
ISBN 0-658013-79-3

8584 **Understanding Asthma**
National Jewish Health
1400 Jackson Street
Denver, CO 80206 303-270-2708
877-225-5654
FAX: 303-398-1125
allstetterw@njc.org
nationaljewish.org

Rich Schierburg, Chair
Robin Chotin, Vice Chair
Michael Salem, M.D., President and CEO
Christine Forkner, CFO and Executive Vice President
Offers a brief introduction to asthma and then goes into the physiology of asthma, the triggers of asthma, and diagnosis and monitoring of asthma.
27 pages

8585 **Understanding Asthma: The Blueprint for Breathing**
Allergy & Asthma Network Mothers of Asthmatics
8229 Boone Boulevard
Suite 260
Vienna, VA 22182 800-878-4403
FAX: 703-288-5271
www.aanma.org

Michael Amato, Chair
Tonya Winders, President & CEO
Brenda Silvia-Torma, Project Manager
Gary Fitzgerald, Managing Editor
A layman's guide to asthma facts based on a presentation from the first national asthma patient conference.

8586   **Understanding Cystic Fibrosis**
University Press of Mississippi
3825 Ridgewood Road
Jackson, MS 39211-6492   601-432-6205
                                          800-737-7788
                                          FAX: 601-432-6217
                                          press@ihl.state.ms.us
                                          www.upress.state.ms.us

Leila W. Salisbury, Director
Craig Gill, Assistant Director/Editor-in-Chief
Anne Stascavage, Managing Editor
Vijay Shah, Acquiring Editor
A reference for CF patients and their families. *$14.00*
128 pages
ISBN 0-878059-67-9

8587   **Understanding Multiple Sclerosis**
University Press of Mississippi
3825 Ridgewood Road
Jackson, MS 39211-6492   601-432-6205
                                          800-737-7788
                                          FAX: 601-432-6217
                                          press@ihl.state.ms.us
                                          www.upress.state.ms.us

Melissa Stauffer, Author
Craig Gill, Assistant Director/Editor-in-Chief
Anne Stascavage, Managing Editor
Vijay Shah, Acquiring Editor
Two psychologists discuss their roles with a member who has multiple sclerosis. Includes chapters on adolescents with multiple sclerosis, employment, and research. *$14.00*
136 pages
ISBN 1-578068-03-7

8588   **Urologic Care of the Child with Spina Bifida**
Spina Bifida Association of America
1600 Wilson Boulevard
Suite 800
Arlington, VA 22209   202-944-3285
                                          800-621-3141
                                          FAX: 202-944-3295
                                          sbaa@sbaa.org
                                          www.sbaa.org

Ana Ximenes, Chair
Sara Struwe, President & CEO
Mark Bohay, National Web Initiatives & Development Manager
Elizabeth Merck, Development Manager
The Spina Bifida Association (SBA) serves adults and children who live with the challenges of Spina Bifida.

8589   **Usher Syndrome**
National Institute on Deafness & Other Communicati
31 Center Drive MSC 2320
Bethesda, MD 20892-2320   301-496-7243
                                          800-241-1044
                                          FAX: 301-770-8977
                                          nidcdinfo@nidcd.nih.gov
                                          www.nidcd.nih.gov

James F Battey Jr MD PhD, Director
Judith A. Cooper, Deputy Director
Timothy J. Wheeles, Executive Officer
Tanya Brown, Executive Assistant
Explains what is Usher Syndrome, who is affected by Usher syndrome, what causes Usher syndrome, how is Usher syndrome treated, and what research is being conducted on Usher syndrome.

8590   **What Everyone Needs to Know About Asthma**
Allergy & Asthma Network Mothers of Asthmatics
8229 Boone Boulevard
Suite 260
Vienna, VA 22182   800-878-4403
                                          FAX: 703-288-5271
                                          www.aanma.org

Michael Amato, Chair
Tonya Winders, President & CEO
Brenda Silvia-Torma, Project Manager
Gary Fitzgerald, Managing Editor
Offers information and facts on gaining control of asthma, asthma triggers and monitoring asthma disorders.

8591   **When the Road Turns: Inspirational Stories About People with MS**
Health Communications
3201 SouthWest 15th Street
Deerfield Beach, FL 33442   954-360-0909
                                          800-441-5569
                                          FAX: 954-360-0034
                                          www.hci-online.com

300 pages
ISBN 1-558749-07-1

8592   **Young Person's Guide to Spina Bifida**
Spina Bifida Association of America
1600 Wilson Boulevard
Suite 800
Arlington, VA 22209   202-944-3285
                                          800-621-3141
                                          FAX: 202-944-3295
                                          sbaa@sbaa.org
                                          www.sbaa.org

Ana Ximenes, Chair
Sara Struwe, President & CEO
Mark Bohay, National Web Initiatives & Development Manager
Elizabeth Merck, Development Manager
Gives practical tips and suggestions for becoming independent and managing your health. *$19.00*

8593   **Your Child and Asthma**
National Jewish Health
1400 Jackson Street
Denver, CO 80206   303-270-2708
                                          877-225-5654
                                          FAX: 303-398-1125
                                          allstetterw@njc.org
                                          nationaljewish.org

Rich Schierburg, Chair
Robin Chotin, Vice Chair
Michael Salem, M.D., President and CEO
Christine Forkner, CFO and Executive Vice President
A booklet offering information to parents and family about their child with asthma. Offers information on diagnosis, treatments, triggers and family concerns.

8594   **Your Cleft Affected Child**
Hunter House Inc. Publisher
PO Box 2914
Alameda, CA 94501-914   510-865-5282
                                          800-266-5592
                                          FAX: 510-865-4295
                                          ordering@hunterhouse.com
                                          www.hunterhouse.com

Carrie T Gruman Trinker, Author
The book also provides in-depth information, guidance, and support on a wide variety of relevant topics, from feeding to surgery to helping a child cope until his/her cleft has been fully corrected. *$16.95*
288 pages Paperback
ISBN 0-897931-85-4

8595 Your Guide to Bowel Cancer
Oxford University Press
2001 Evans Road
Cary, NC 27513

919-677-0977
800-445-9714
FAX: 919-677-1303
custserv.us@oup.co
www.us.oup.com

ISBN 0-340927-46-1

Print: Journals

8596 AIDS: The Official Journal of the International AIDS Society
Lippincott Williams & Wilkins
2 Commerce Square
2001 Market St.
Philadelphia, PA 19103

215-521-8300
FAX: 215-521-8902
customerservice@lww.com
lww.com

JA Levy, Co Editor
B. Autran, Co Editor
R. A Coutinho, Co Editor
J. P Phair, Co Editor
The latest groundbreaking research on HIV and AIDS. *$ 433.00*
18 per year

8597 American Journal of Orthopsychiatry
American Psychological Association
750 1st Street NorthEast
Washington, DC 20002-4242

202-336-5500
800-374-2721
FAX: 202-336-5502
TTY: 202-336-6123
www.apa.org

Nadine J. Kaslow, President
Norman B. Anderson, PhD, CEO & EVP
Bonnie Markham, Treasurer
Jennifer F. Kelly, Recording Secretary
Mental health issues from multidisciplinary and interprofessionals perspectives: clinical, research and expository approaches. *$45.00*
160 pages Quarterly

8598 Annals of Otology, Rhinology and Laryngology
Annals Publishing Company
4507 Laclede Ave
Saint Louis, MO 63108-2103

314-367-4987
FAX: 314-367-4988
manager@annals.com
www.annals.com

Ken Cooper, President
Richard J. Smith, Editor
Monica L. Bergers, Editor's Assistant
Jim Cunningham, Advertising Representative
Original, peer-reviewed articles in the fields of otolaryngology - head and neck medicine and surgery, broncho-esophagology, audiology, speech, pathology, allery, and maxillofacial surgery. Official journal of the American Laryngological Association/American Broncho-Esophagological Association. *$170.00*
112 pages Monthly

8599 Archives of Neurology
American Medical Association
P.O.Box 10946
Chicago, IL 60654

312-670-7827
800-262-2350
FAX: 312-464-4184
subscriptions@jamanetwork.com
archpsyc.jamanetwork.com/public/contact.as px

Margaret Vanner, Manager
Mission is to publish scientific information primarily important to those physicians caring for people with neurologic disorders,

but also for those interested in the structure and function of the normal and diseased nervous system. *$235.00*
198 pages Monthly

8600 Cleft Palate-Craniofacial Journal
Cleft Palate Foundation
810 E. 10th Street
Ste 102
Lawrence, NC 27514-2820

785-843-1234
800-242-5338
FAX: 785-843-1274
membership@acpa-cpf.org
www.cpcjournal.org

Howard M. Saal, MD, President
Mark P. Mooney, PhD, President-Elect
Helen M. Sharp, PhD, CCC-SLP, Vice President
Ronal Reed Hathaway, DDS, MS, Vice President-Elect
A peer reviwed international multidisciplinary journal dedicated to current research on the care and treatment of children born with cleft lip and palate and other craniofacial anomalies. 6 issues/year

8601 Journal of Head Trauma Rehabilitation
Lippincott, Williams & Wilkins
P.O.Box 1620
Hagerstown, MD 21740

301-223-2300
800-638-3030
FAX: 301-223-2400
orders@lww.com
www.lww.com

John D Corrigan PhD, ABPP, Editor
Scholarly journal designed to provide information on clinical management and rehabilitation of the head-injured for the practicing professional. Published bimonthly. *$113.96*

Print: Magazines

8602 Coping with Cancer Magazine
Media America
P.O.Box 682268
Franklin, TN 37068-2268

615-790-2400
FAX: 615-794-0179
copingmag.com

53 pages 6 x year

8603 CurePSP Magazine
Society for Progressive Supranuclear Palsy
Suite 201
30 E. Padonia Road
Timonium, MD 21093

410-785-7004
800-457-4777
FAX: 410-785-7009
info@curepsp.org
www.psp.org

John T. Burhoe, Chair
Everett R. Cook, Vice Chair
Richard Gordon Zyne, President-CEO
Kathleen Matarazzo Speca, VP, Development & Donor Relations
Quarterly newsletter. The society's mission is to promote and fund research into finding the cause and cure for progressive supranuclear palsy (PSP). Provides information, support and advocacy to persons diagnosed with PSP, their families and caregivers. Educates physicians and allied health professionals on PSP and how to improve patient care.

8604 EpilepsyUSA
Epilepsy Foundation
8301 Professional Place
Landover, MD 20785-2353
301-459-3700
800-332-1000
FAX: 301-459-1569
ContactUs@cfa.org
epilepsyfoundation.org

Warren Lammert, Chair
Phil Gattone, President and CEO
May J. Liang, Secretary
Roger Heldman, Treasurer
Magazine reporting on issues of interest to people with epilepsy
and their families. *$15.00*
22 pages Bi-Monthly

8605 MSFOCUS Magazine
Multiple Sclerosis Foundation
6520 North Andrews Avenue
Fort Lauderdale, FL 33309-2130
954-776-6805
888-MSF-CUS
888-225-6495
FAX: 954-938-8708
support@msfocus.org, admin@msfocus.org

www.msfocus.org

Eric Schenck, President, Director
Charles Eader, Vice President, Treasurer
Jules Kuperberg, Executive Director
Alan Segaloff, Co- Executive Director
Contemporary national, nonprofit organization that provides free
support services and public education for persons with Multiple
Sclerosis, newsletters, toll-free phone support, information, re-
ferrals, home care, assitive technology and support groups.
48 pages Quarterly

8606 Orthotics and Prosthetics Almanac
American Orthotic & Prosthetics Association
330 John Carlyle Street
Suite 200
Alexandria, VA 22314
571-431-0876
FAX: 571-431-0899
info@aopanet.org
www.aopanet.org

Anita L. Lampear, President
Charles H. Dankmeyer, Vice President
Thomas F. Fise, JD, Executive Director
Don DeBolt, Chief Operating Officer
Features articles covering current professional, patient care, gov-
ernment, business and National Office activities affecting the
orthotics and prosthetics profession and industry. *$40.00*
80 pages Monthly
ISSN 1061-46 1

8607 PDF News
Parkinson's Disease Foundation
1359 Broadway
Suite 1509
New York, NY 10018
212-923-4700
800-457-6676
FAX: 212-923-4778
info@pdf.org
www.pdf.org

Howard D. Morgan, Chair
Woodruff Atwell, Ph.D., Vice Chair
Stephen Ackerman, Treasurer
Isobel Robins Konecky, Secretary

8-12 pages Quarterly

8608 POZ Magazine
Smart + Strong
462 Seventh Ave
19th Floor
New York, NY 10018-7424
212-242-2163
800-973-2376
FAX: 212-675-8505
webmaster@poz.com
www.poz.com

Megan Strub, Publisher
Oriol Gutierrez, Editor In-Chief
Jennifer Morton, Managing Editor
Kate Ferguson, Senior Editor
A health title written for individuals who are HIV+, their friends
and families. POZ provides the latest treatment information, in-
vestigative journalism and survivor profiles.

8609 SCI Life
National Spinal Cord Injury Association
11300 Rockville Pike
Suite 803
Rockville, MD 20852
301-468-3902
FAX: 301-468-3904
info@ilcreations.com
ilcreations.com

Quarterly/Free

8610 Spine
Lippincott, Williams & Wilkins
530 Walnut St
Philadelphia, PA 19106-3603
215-521-8300
FAX: 215-521-8411
customerservice@lww.com
lww.com

James N Weinstein DO MSc, Editor
Publishes original papers on theoretical issues and research concerning the spine and spinal cord injuries. *$9.00*
26 Issues Year

8611 Ventilator-Assisted Living
International Ventilator Users Network
4207 Lindell Blvd
Suite 110
Saint Louis, MO 63108-2930
314-534-0475
FAX: 314-534-5070
info@ventusers.org
www.ventusers.org

William G. Stothers, President/Chairperson
Saul J. Morse, Vice President
Joan L. Headley,MS, Editor
Marny E. Eulberg, Secretary
To enhance the lives and independence of ventilator-assisted liv-
ing by promoting education, networking, and advocacy among
these individuals and healthcare providers. Ventilator-Assisted
Living supports Post-Polio Health International's educational,
research, and advocacy efforts. Offers information about
relevant events.
Quarterly

Print: Newsletters

8612 ACPOC News
Assoc of Children's Prosthetic-Orthotic Clinics
6300 N River Rd
Suite 727
Rosemont, IL 60018-4226
847-698-1637
FAX: 847-823-0536
acpoc@aaos.org
www.acpoc.org

David B. Rotter,CPO, President
Jorge A. Fabregas, Vice President
Hank White,PT,PhD, Secretary-Treasurer
Anna Cuomo, Director
Quarterly publication from the Association of Children's Pros-
thetic/Orthotic Clinics. Included with membership.
40 pages Quarterly

8613   AID Bulletin
Project AID Resource Center
P.O. Box 5190
Kent, OH 44242-0001
330-672-3000
FAX: 330-672-4724
info@kent.edu
www.kent.edu/

Beverly Warren, President
Todd A. Diacon, Provost & SVP
Gregg S. Floyd, Sr. Vice President
Greg Jarvie, Vice President
Has the latest news on upcoming conferences, literature, developments in programs and/or services for disabled persons who are substance abusers. Offers articles on their experiences, ideas and questions of others in this field which includes providers and consumers. *$7.50*

8614   AIDS Alert
AHC Media LLC
PO Box 550669
Atlanta, GA 30355
404-262-5436
800-688-2421
FAX: 404-262-5560
www.ahcpub.com/

Joy Daughtery Dickinson, Senior Managing Editor
Source of AIDS news and advice for health care professionals. Covers up-to-the-minute developments and guidance on the entire spectrum of AIDS challenges, including treatment, education, precautions, screening, diagnosis and policy. *$499.00*
Monthly

8615   Adaptive Tracks
Adaptive Sports Center
P.O.Box 1639
Crested Butte, CO 81224
970-349-2296
866-349-2296
FAX: 970-349-2077
info@adaptivesports.org
www.adaptivesports.org

Christopher Hensley, Executive Director
Chris Read, CTRS, Program Director
Ella Fahrlander, Development Director
Mike Neustedter, Marketing Director
The Adaptive Sports Center (ASC) of Crested Butte, Colorado is a non-profit organization that provides year-round recreation activities for people with disabilities and their families. The ASC provides adaptive snowboarding downhill skiing, cross country skiing as well as backcountry trips. Summer activities include a variety of wilderness-based programs, multi-day trips into the back country, extensive cycling programs, canoeing, and white water rafting.
6 pages Quarterly

8616   Arthritis Self-Management
Rapaport Publishing, Inc.
150 W 22nd St
Ste 800
New York, NY 10011-2421
212-989-0200
FAX: 212-989-4786
ASMcustserv@cdsfulfillment.com
www.arthritisselfmanagement.com

Richard A Rapaport, President
Maryanne Schott Turner, Director of Manufacturing
Richard Boland, Art Director
James Moorehead, Circulation Director
Arthritis Self-Management publishes practical 'how-to' information for the growing number of people with arthritis who want to know more about managing their condition. We focus on the day-to-day and long-term aspects of arthritis in a positive and upbeat style, giving our subscribers up-to-date news, facts, and advice to help them make informed decisions about their health.
$9.97
BiMonthly

8617   Breaking Ground
Tennessee Council on Developmental Disabilities
404 James Robertson Pkwy
Suite 130
Nashville, TN 37243- 0228
615-532-6615
FAX: 615-532-6964
TTY:615-741-4562
tnddc@tn.gov
www.tn.gov/cdd

Stephanie Brewer cook, Chair
Roger D. Gibbens,, Vice Chair
Wanda Willis, Executive Director
Errol Elshtain, Director of Development
Newsletter
20 pages 6 x Year

8618   Breaking New Ground News Note
Purdue University
225 West University Street
West Lafayette, IN 47907
765-494-4600
800-825-4264
FAX: 765-496-1356
engineering.purdue.edu/

Paul Jones, Project Manager
Bill Field, Project Director
Denise Heath, Project Asst.
Robert Stuthridge, Project Ergonomist
News, practical ideas and success stories of and for farmers and other agricultural workers with physical disabilities.
2 pages Quarterly

8619   Diabetes Self-Management
Rapaport Publishing, Inc.
150 W 22nd St
Ste 800
New York, NY 10011-2421
212-989-0200
FAX: 212-989-4786
webeditor@diabetes-self-mgmt.com
www.diabetesselfmanagement.com

Richard A Rapaport, President
Maryanne Schott Turner, Director of Manufacturing
Richard Boland, Art Director
James Moorehead, Circulation Director
Publishes practical how-to information, focusing on the day-to-day and long-term aspects of diabetes in a positive and upbeat style. Gives subscribers up-to-date news, facts and advice to help them maintain their wellness and make informed decisions regarding their health. *$9.97*
BiMonthly

8620   Directions
Families of Spinal Muscular Dystrophy
925 Busse Road
Elk Grove Village, IL 60007
847-367-7620
800-886-1762
FAX: 847-367-7623
info@fsma.org
www.fsma.org

Richard Rubenstein, Chair
Kenneth Hobby, President
Sue Kovach, Director of Finance
Megan Lenz, Communications Manager
$35.00
60-70 pages Quarterly

8621   IAL News
International Association of Laryngectomees
925B Peachtree Street NE
Suite 316
Atlanta, GA 30309
866-425-3678
www.larynxlink.com

Wade Hampton, President
Susan Reeves, Administrative Manager
Jodi Knott, Director, Voice Institute
Charles Rusky, Treasurer

Focuses on rehabilitation and well-being of persons who have had laryngectomy surgery.

8622 Informer
Simon Foundation
P.O.Box 815
Wilmette, IL 60091

847-864-3913
800-237-4666
FAX: 847-864-9758
info@simonfoundation.org
simonfoundation.org

Cheryle Gartley, President and Founder
Elizabeth T. LaGro, VP, Communications & Education
Twila Yednock, Director of Special Events
Monica Liebert, Scientific Liason
Publishes items of interest to people with bladder or bowel incontinence, including medical articles, helpful devices, publications and a pen pal list. Quarterly newsletter.
Quarterly

8623 Moisture Seekers
Sjogren's Syndrome Foundation
6707 Democracy Boulevard
Suite 325
Bethesda, MD 20817

301-530-4420
800-475-6473
FAX: 301-530-4415
tms@sjogrens.org
www.sjogrens.org

Kenneth Economou, Chair
Steven Taylor, CEO
Sheriese DeFruscio, VP of Development
Elizabeth Trocchio, Director of Marketing
Newsletter of the organization for lay people and professionals interested in Sjogren's Syndrome. Contains medical news, current research, and essential tips for daily living. *$25.00*
15-16 pages Monthly

8624 Momentum
National Multiple Sclerosis Society
Ste 6
421 New Karner Rd
Albany, NY 12205-3838

518-464-0850
800-344-4867
FAX: 518-464-1232
nyr@nmss.org
www.nationalmssociety.org

Eli Rubenstein, Chair
Cynthia Zagieboylo, President & CEO
Sherri Giger, EVP, Marketing
Jennifer Douglas, EVP,Technology
News and information on research progress, medical treatments, patient services, therapeutic claims and activities.

8625 Options
People Against Cancer
P.O.Box 10
604 East Street
Otho, IA 50569

515-972-4444
800-662-2623
FAX: 515-972-4415
info@PeopleAgainstCancer.org
www.peopleagainstcancer.com

Frank D. Wiewel, Executive Director/Founder
Publication of People Against Cancer, a nonprofit, grassroots public benefit organization dedicated to 'New Directions in the War on Cancer.' We help people to find the best cancer treatment. We are a democratic organization of people with cancer, their loved ones and citizens working together to protect and enhance medical freedom of choice.
8 pages Quarterly

8626 PDF Newsletter
Parkinson's Disease Foundation
1359 Broadway
Suite 1509
New York, NY 10018

212-923-4700
800-457-6676
FAX: 212-923-4778
info@pdf.org
www.pdf.org

Howard D. Morgan, Chair
Woodruff Atwell, Ph.D., Vice Chair
Stephen Ackerman, Treasurer
Isobel Robins Konecky, Secretary
The Parkinson's Disease Foundation (PDF) is a leading national presence in Parkinson's disease research, education and public advocacy.
12-16 pages Quarterly

8627 Parkinsons Report
National Parkinson Foundation
200 SE 1st Street
Suite 800
Miami, FL 33131

305-243-6666
800-473-4636
800-4PD-INFO
FAX: 305-537-9901
contact@parkinson.org
www.parkinson.org

John W. Kozyak, Chairman
Andrew B. Albert, Vice Chairman
Joyce Oberdorf, President and CEO
Leilani Pearl, VP,Marketing & Communications
Articles, reports and news on Parkinson's disease and the activities of the National Parkinson Foundation.
32 pages Qarterly

8628 Post-Polio Health
Post-Polio Health International
Ste 110
4207 Lindell Blvd
Saint Louis, MO 63108-2930

314-534-0475
FAX: 314-534-5070
info@post-polio.org
www.post-polio.org

William G. Stothers, President
Saul J. Morse, Vice President
Joan L. Headley,MS, Executive Director
Marny E. Eulberg, Secretary
To enhance the lives and independence of polio survivors by promoting education, networking, and advocacy among these individuals and healthcare providers. Post-Polio Health supports Post-Polio Health International's educational, research, and advocacy efforts. Offers information about relevant events. *$30.00*
12 pages quarterly

8629 Prader-Willi Alliance of New York Newsletter
244 5th Avenue
Suite D-110
New York, NY 10001

716-276-2211
800-442-1655
FAX: 585-271-2782
alliance@prader-willi.org
www.prader-willi.org

Amy McDougall, President
Rachel Johnson, Vice President
Nancy Finegold, Vice President
Nina Roberto, Executive Director
The Prader-Willi Foundation is a national, nonprofit public charity that works for the benefit of individuals with Prader-Willi syndrome and their families. *$20.00*
Quarterly

8630 **Quality Care Newsletter**
National Association for Continence
P.O.Box 1019
Charleston, SC 29402-1019 843-352-2559
800-BLA-DER
FAX: 843-352-2563
memberservices@nafc.org
www.nafc.org

Donna Deng, Chairman
Nancy Hicks, Vice Chaiperson
Steven Gregg, Executive Director
Wendy Pokoski, Financial Administrator
Newsletter from NAFC. By donating $25 and becomming a Quality Care donor, you may receive our quarterly newsletter. *$25.00*
14-16 pages Quarterly

8631 **Rasmussen's Syndrome and Hemispherectomy Support Network Newsletter**
55 Kenosia Avenue
Danbury, CT 06810 203-744-0100
FAX: 203-798-2291
rssnlynn@aol.com
http://www.rarediseases.org/rare-disease-info
Ronald J. Bartek, Chair
Sheldon M. Schuster, Vice Chair
Peter L. Saltonstall, President & CEO
Pamela Gavin, COO
National, not-for-profit organization dedicated to providing information and support to individuals affected by Rasmussen's Syndrome and hemispherectomy. Publishes a periodic newsletter and disseminates reprints of medical journal articles concerning Rasmussen's Syndrome and its treatments. Maintains a support network that provides encouragement and information to individuals affected by Rasmussen's Syndrome and their families.

8632 **SCI Psychosocial Process**
Amer Assn of Spinal Cord Injury Psych & Soc Wks
75-20 Astoria Blvd
East Elmhurst, NY 11370 718-803-3782
800-404-2898
FAX: 718-803-0414
info@unitedspinal.org
http://www.unitedspinal.org/
David C. Cooper, Chairman
Patrick W. Maher, Vice Chairman
Joseph Gaskins, President and CEO
Denise A. McQuade, Secretary
Quarterly newsletter.

8633 **Special Care in Dentistry**
Blackwell Publishing
350 Main St
Malden, MA 02148 781-388-0200
FAX: 781-388-8210
www.blackwellpublishing.com

Peter Booth Wiley, Chairman
Stephen M. Smith, President & CEO
John Kitzmacher, EVP, CFO
Ellis E. Cousens, Executive Vice President, COO
$125.00
48 pages BiMonthly

8634 **TSA Newsletter**
Tourette Syndrome Association
42-40 Bell Boulevard
Bayside, NY 11361 718-224-2999
800-237-0717
FAX: 718-279-9596
ts@tsa-usa.org
www.tsa-usa.org

Stephen M. McCall, President
National non-profit membership organization whose mission is to identify the cause of, find the cure for, and control the effects of this disorder. A growing number of local chapters nationwide provide educational materials, seminars, conferences and support groups for over 35,000 members.
Quarterly

8635 **Tethering Cord**
Spina Bifida Association of America
PO Box 5801
Bethesda, MD 20284 301-496-5751
800-352-9424
FAX: 202-944-3295
sbaa@sbaa.org
www.ninds.nih.gov/

Caroline Lewis, Executive Officer
Story C. Landis, Director
Denise Dorsey, Chief Administrative Officer
Maryann Sofranko, Deputy Executive Officer
Tethered spinal cord syndrome is a neurological disorder caused by tissue attachments that limit the movement of the spinal cord within the spinal column. Attachments may occur congenitally at the base of the spinal cord (conus medullaris) or they may develop near the site of an injury to the spinal cord.

8636 **Tourette Syndrome Association Children's Newsletter**
42-40 Bell Boulevard
Bayside, NY 11361 718-224-2999
800-237-0717
FAX: 718-279-9596
ts@tsa-usa.org
tsa-usa.org

Stephen M. McCall, President
National, nonprofit membership organization. Mission is to identify the cause of, find the cure for, and control the effects of this disorder. A growing number of local chapters nationwide provide educational materials, seminars, conferences and support groups for over 35,000 members.

8637 **Voice of the Diabetic**
NFB Diabetes Action Network
200 East Wells Street
Baltimore, MD 21230-4914 410-659-9314
888-581-4741
FAX: 410-685-5653
editor@diabetes.nfb.org
www.nfb.org

Elizabeth Lunt, Editor
Marc Maurer, President
Fredric Schroeder, First Vice President
Ron Brown, Second Vice President
Newsletter containing personal stories and practical guidelines by blind diabetics and medical professionals, medical news, resource column and a recipe corner. We are a support and information network for all diabetics.
28 pages Quarterly

Non Print: Newsletters

8638 **Teens & Asthma**
American Lung Association
530 7th St SE
Washington, DC 20003 202-546-5864
FAX: 202-546-5607
randrewn@aladc.org
www.epa.gov/

Rolando E Bates Jr, CEO
Tips from other teens with asthma to help those having it get on with the serious business of having fun with the rest of their lives.
Online/Free

Non Print: Video

8639 **Fragile X Family**
Fanlight Productions
c/o Icarus Films
32 Court Street, 21st Floor
Brooklyn, NY 11201
718-488-8900
800-876-1710
FAX: 718-488-8642
info@fanlight.com, sales@icarusfilms.com
www.fanlight.com

Ben Achtenberg, Founder, Owner
Eric Kutner, Producer
Fragile X Family takes viewers inside the lives of a developmentally disabled family who are affected by Fragile X Syndrome, an inherited chromosomal disorder which is the second most common cause of mental retardation. *$149.00*
VHS/VIDEO
ISBN 1-572954-14-0

8640 **In the Middle**
Fanlight Productions
c/o Icarus Films
32 Court Street, 21st Floor
Brooklyn, NY 11201
718-488-8900
800-876-1710
FAX: 718-488-8642
info@fanlight.com, sales@icarusfilms.com
www.fanlight.com

Ben Achtenberg, Founder, Owner
Documents the problems and joys shared by Ryanna, who has Spina Bifida, and her parents, teachers and classmates during her first year of being mainstreamed in a Head Start Program. *$99.00*

8641 **Narcolepsy**
Fanlight Productions
c/o Icarus Films
32 Court Street, 21st Floor
Brooklyn, NY 11201
718-488-8900
800-876-1710
FAX: 718-488-8642
info@fanlight.com, sales@icarusfilms.com
www.fanlight.com

Ben Achtenberg, Founder, Owner
Jason Margolis, Producer
Presents the experiences of three individuals who lives and relationships have been disrupted by narcolepsy. Rental $50/day. *$199.00*
VHS/25 Minutes

8642 **Twitch and Shout**
Fanlight Productions
c/o Icarus Films
32 Court Street, 21st Floor
Brooklyn, NY 11201
718-488-8900
800-876-1710
FAX: 718-488-8642
info@fanlight.com, sales@icarusfilms.com
www.fanlight.com

Ben Achtenberg, Founder, Owner
Laurel Chitden, Producer
This documentary provides an intimate journey into the startling world of Tourette Syndrome (TS), a genetic disorder that can cause a bizarre range of involuntary movements, vocalizations, and compulsions. Through the eyes of a photojournalist with TS, the film introduces viewers to others who have this puzzling disorder. This is an emotionally absorbing, sometimes, unsettling, and finally uplifting program about people who must contend with a society that often sees them as crazy or bad. *$225.00*

Sports

8643 **National Sports Center for the Disabled**
P.O.Box 1290
33 Parsenn Road
Winter Park, CO 80482
970-726-1518
FAX: 970-726-4112
volunteer@nscd.org
www.nscd.org

Becky Zimmermann, President/CEO
Greg Voss, CFO
Diane Eustace, Marketing Director
Beth Fox, Operations Director
Innovative non-profit organization that provides year-round recreation for children and adults with disabilities. The world's largest adaptive ski program, teaching 25,000 lessons per winter at Winter Park Resort, Colorado. Also snowboarding, ski racing, showshoeing, cross-country skiing. Summer sports: rafting, sailing, camping, hiking, hand cycling, mountain biking, tandem biking, in-line skating, horseback riding, fishing, rock climbing. Sports symposium and clinics.

8644 **Rehabilitation Institute of Chicago's Virginia Wadsworth Sports Program**
345 East Suuperior St.
Chicago, IL 60611
312-238-1000
800-354-7342
800-354-REHA
FAX: 312-238-5017
sports@ric.org
www.ric.org

Jude Reyes, Chair
mike P. Kransy, Vice Chair
Thomas Reynolds III, Vice Chair
Joanne C. Smith, President & CEO
RIC's Center for Health and Fitness is a full service fitness center for individuals with disablilties and the administrative offices for RIC's Wirtz Sports Program. Eighteen different sport and recreation programs are offered free of charge. The facility is adjacent to RIC's main building and also is the location of a branch of The National Center for Physical Activity and Disability (NCPAD), a joint project operated by the University of Illinois-Chigcago.

8645 **US Paralympics**
1 Olympic Plaza
Colorado Springs, CO 80901
719-866-2030
888-222-2313
FAX: 719-866-2029
customerservice@donorsupportusoc.org
www.usparalympics.org

Jessica Galli, Track & Field
Derek Arneaud, Soccer
Willie Steward, Nordic Skiing
Muffy Davis, Alpine Skiing
A division of the US Olympic Committee focused on enhancing programs, funding and opportunities for persons with physical disabilities to participate in Paralymic sports.

Support Groups

8646 **AAN's Toll-Free Hotline**
Allergy and Asthma Network Mothers of Asthmatics
8229 Boone Boulevard
Suite 260
Vienna, VA 22182
800-878-4403
FAX: 703-288-5271
www.aanma.org

Michael Amato, Chair
Tonya Winders, President & CEO
Brenda Silvia-Torma, Project Manager
Gary Fitzgerald, Managing Editor
Offers answers to questions regarding allergies and asthma, provides referrals and support to assist the patient and his or her family.

8647 Breaking New Ground Resource Center
Purdue University
225 S University St
West Lafayette, IN 47907

765-494-5088
800-825-4264
FAX: 765-496-1356
bng@ecn.purdue.edu
engineering.purdue.edu/

Bill Field, Project Director
Paul Jones, Project Manager
Steve Swain, Rural Rehab Specialist
Robert Stuthridge, Project Ergonomist

A resource center devoted to helping farmers and ranchers with physical disabilities. Resource materials and a free newsletter are available to anyone.

8648 Cancer Information Service
National Cancer Institute
BG 9609 MSC 9760
9609 Medical Center Drive
Bethesda, MD 20892-9760

301-496-8531
800-422-6237
800-4 C-NCER
FAX: 304-402-0181
cancergovstaff@mail.nih.gov
www.cancer.gov

Barbara K. Rimer, Chairperson
Harold Varmus,MD, Director
Abby Sandler, Executive Secretary
Bruce A. Chabner, Chair

A nationwide network of 19 regional field offices supported by the National Cancer Institute which provides accurate, up-to-date information on cancer to patients and their families, health professionals and the general public. The CIS can provide specific information in understandable language about particular types of cancer, as well as information on second opinions and the availability of clinical trials.

8649 Clearinghouse on Disability Information: Office Special Education & Rehabilitative Service
U S Department of Education
400 Maryland Ave SW
Washington, DC 20202-1

202-245-7549
800-872-5327
FAX: 202-245-7614
www.ed.gov

Arne Duncan, Secretary Of Education
Tony Miller, Deputy Secretary
Martha Kanter, Under Secretary
Jo Anderson, Senior Advisor

Provides information to people with disabilities or anyone requesting information, by doing research and providing documents in response to inquiries. The information provided includes areas of federal funding for disability-related programs. Information provided may be useful to disabled individuals and their families, schools and universities, teacher's and/or school administrators, and organizations who have persons with disabilities as clients.

8650 Compassionate Friends, The
P.O.Box 3696
Oak Brook, IL 60522

630-990-0010
877-969-0010
FAX: 630-990-0246
nationaloffice@compassionatefriends.org
compassionatefriends.org

Patrick O'Donnell, President
Georgia Cockerham, Vice President
Lisa Corrao, COO
Alan Pedersen, Executive Director

Peer support for bereaved parents, grandparents and siblings, offering over 600 chapters in the United States. The organization also offers a quarterly magazine, We Need Not Walk Alone, and TCF resources of brochures, DVDs, and memorial wristbands for the bereaved parent, grandparent and sibling.

8651 Cornerstone Services
777 Joyce Rd
Joliet, IL 60436

815-741-7600
FAX: 815-723-1177
jhogan@cornerstoneservices.org
cornerstoneservices.org

John R. Rogers, Chair
Vincent A. Benigni, Vice Chairperson
Ben Stortz, President/CEO
Don Hospell, Vice President/COO

Cornerstone Services provides progressive, comprehensive services for people with disabilities, promoting choice, dignity and the opportunity to live and work in the community. Established in 1969, the agency provides developmental, vocational, residential and behavior health services.

8652 Disability Network
Ste 54
3600 S Dort Hwy
Flint, MI 48507

810-742-1800
FAX: 810-742-2400
TTY:810-742-7647
tdn@disnetwork.org
www.disnetwork.org

Bruce Chargo, Chairman
Diane Brown, Treasurer/ Vice Chairman
Mike Zelley, President & CEO
Linda F, Director, Finance, Operations

The Disability Network's mission is to realize consumer empowerment, self determination, full inclusion and participation of all people in the communities through independent living philosophy and the unequivocal implementation of the Americans with Disabilities Act

8653 Disability and Health: National Center for Birth Defects and Developmental Disabilities
Centers for Disease Control and Prevention
1600 Clifton Road
Atlanta, GA 30333

404-498-3012
800-232-4636
800-CDC-INFO
FAX: 404-498-3060
cdcinfo@cdc.gov
www.cdc.gov/ncbddd/dh

Dr. Tom Frieden, Director
Sherri A. Berger, COO
Carmen Villar, Chief of Staff
Ileana Arias, Principal Deputy Director

Located within the new CDC, National Center for Birth Defects and Developmental Disabilities, the Disability and Health section, operates a relatively small program that primarily supports: data collection on the prevalence of people with disabilities & their health status and risk factors for poor health and well-being; research on measures of disability, functioning and health; health promotion intervention studies; and dissemination of health information.

8654 Easter Seals
233 South Wacker Drive
Suite 2400
Chicago, IL 60606

312-726-6200
800-221-6827
FAX: 312-726-1494
www.easterseals.com

Richard W. Davidson, Chairman
Sandra L Bouwman, 1st Vice Chairman
Joseph G. Kern, 2nd Vice Chairman
Eileen H. Boone, Secretary

Easter Seals has been helping individuals with disabilities and special needs, and their families, live better lives for over 80 years. From child development centers to physical rehabilitation and job training for people with disabilities, Easter Seals offers a variety of services to help people with disabilities address life's challenges and achieve personal goals.

8655 Epilepsy Foundation
8301 Professional Place
Landover, MD 20785-2353
301-459-3700
800-332-1000
FAX: 301-459-1569
ContactUs@efa.org
epilepsyfoundation.org

Warren Lammert, Chair
Phil Gattone, President and CEO
May J. Liang, Secretary
Roger Heldman, Treasurer
Offers information and referrals, support groups for dually diagnosed persons.

8656 Family Support Project for the Developmentally Disabled
3424 Kossuth Ave
Bronx, NY 10467-2410
718-519-5000
FAX: 718-519-4902
www.nyc.gov/html/hhc/ncbh/home.html

William Walsh, Vice President
Sheldon McLeod, COO

8657 Head Injury Hotline
Brain Injury Resource Center
P.O.Box 84151
Seattle, WA 98124-5451
206-621-8558
FAX: 206-329-0912
brain@headinjury.com
www.headinjury.com

Hugh R. MacMahon, Neurology
Constance Miller, Founder
Paul M. Kuroiwa, Performance management consultant
B. Parker Lindner, Communications specialist
Disseminates head injury information and provides referrals to facilitate adjustment to life following head injury. Organizes seminars for professionals, head injury survivors, and their families.

8658 International Braille and Technology Center for the Blind
National Federation of the Blind
200 East Wells Street
Baltimore, MD 21230-4914
410-659-9314
FAX: 410-685-5653
access@nfb.org
www.nfb.org

Marc Maurer, President
Fredric Schroeder, First Vice President
Ron Brown, Second Vice President
Marc Maurer, CEO
World's largest and most complete evaluation and demonstration center of all assistive technology used by the blind from around the world. Includes all braille, synthetic speech, print-to-speech scanning, internet and portable devices and programs. Available for tours by appointment to blind persons, employers, technology manufacturers, teachers, parents and those working in the assistive technology field.

8659 Lung Line Information Service
National Jewish Health
1400 Jackson Street
Denver, CO 80206
877-225-5654
877-225-5654
FAX: 303-398-1125
allstetterw@njc.org
nationaljewish.org

Rich Schierburg, Chair
Robin Chotin, Vice Chair
Michael Salem, M.D., President & CEO
Christine Forkner, CFO and Executive Vice President
A free information service answering questions, sending literature and giving advice to patients with immunologic or respiratory illnesses. The Line is an educational service and not a substitute for medical care. Diagnosis or suggested treatment will not be provided for a caller's specific condition.

8660 National AIDS Hotline
Centers for Disease Control and Prevention
1600 Clifton Road
Atlanta, GA 30333
404-639-3311
800-232-4636
800-CDC-INFO
FAX: 404-498-3060
cdcinfo@cdc.gov
www.cdc.gov

Dr. Tom Frieden, Director
Sherri A. Berger, COO
Carmen Villar, Chief of Staff
Ileana Arias, Principal Deputy Director
Offers free confidential information and publications on HIV infection and AIDS.

8661 PALS Support Groups
Parent Professional Advocacy League
10th Fl
45 Bromfield St
Boston, MA 02108
866-815-8122
FAX: 617-542-7832
info@ppal.net
ppal.net

Earl N. Stuck, Chair
Lisa Lambert, Executive Director
Deborah A Fauntleroy, Associate Director
Meri Viano, Senior Regional Manager
Offers emotional support to parents and families of disabled children.

8662 PXE International
Ste 404
4301 Connecticut Ave NW
Washington, DC 20008- 2369
202-362-9599
FAX: 202-966-8553
info@pxe.org
www.pxe.org

Patrick F. Terry, President
Sharon Terry, CEO
Terry M. Dermaid, Executive Director
Ian Terry, Webmaster
Provides support for individuals and families affected by psukdoxanthoma elasticum (PXE), and resources for healthcare professionals. PXE causes select elastic tissue to mineralize, and effects the skin, eyes, cardiovascular, and GI systems.

8663 Parent Assistance Network
Good Samaritan Hospital
10 E. 31st Street
Kearney, NE 68847
308-865-7100
800-235-9905
FAX: 308-865-2924
sheilameyer@catholichealth.net
www.gshs.org

Randy DeFreece, President
Kent Barney, Chairman
Mary Henning, Vice Chairman
Julie Speirs, Secretary
Provides information and emotional support to all parents and especially to parents of children with disabilities in the central Nebraska area. Ongoing activities include parent support group meetings, parent-to-parent networking and referrals and Respite Care provider trainings.

8664 Post-Polio Support Group
Adventist Hinsdale Hospital
120 N Oak St
Hinsdale, IL 60521-3829
630-856-9000
FAX: 630-856-6000
www.keepingyouwell.com

David Crane, President
Information and support for polio patients and their families; meets the fourth Wednesday of each month.

8665 Prevent Child Abuse America
288 South Wabash Avenue
10th floor
Chicago, IL 60604

312-663-3520
800-244-5373
800-CHI-DREN
FAX: 312-939-8962
mailbox@preventchildabuse.org
preventchildabuse.org

Fred M. Riley, Chair
David Rudd, Vice Chair
James Hmurovich, President & CEO
Robert Allen, Sr. Director, Administration
Through public education, community partnerships and support services, PCAMW helps everyone play a role in prevention. We share information on prevention stategies and effective parenting at community forums and events and advocate for polices and services that keep children safe. We operate PhoneFriend, a telephone support line for children at home without adult supervision and conduct personal safety workshops in schools, camps and libraries.

8666 Son-Rise Program
Option Institute
2080 South Undermountain Road
Sheffield, MA 01257

413-229-2100
877-766-7473
happiness@option.org
www.autismtreatmentcenter.org

Samahria Lyt Kaufman, Co-Founder and Co-Director
Dane Griffith, Director of Administrative Services
Bears Kaufman, Co-Founder and Co-Director
Raun Kaufman, Director of Global Education
Internationally renowned and highly effective method for working with children challenged by autism, autism spectrum disorders, PDD and all other developmental difficulties. The program teaches parents, relatives, volunteers and professionals how to design and implement a child-centered, home-based educational program. Modality comprises an innovative and comprehensive system for learning and growth with specific impact in areas including eye contact, speech and communication and more.

8667 Special Children
1306 Wabash Ave
Belleville, IL 62220-3370

618-234-6876
FAX: 618-234-6150
kathleencullan@sbcglobal.net
specialchildren.net

Kathleen Cullen, Administrator
A nonprofit agency serving children with developmental disabilities ages birth to 6 years

8668 Support Works
1607 Dilworth Rd W
Charlotte, NC 28203-5213

704-331-9500
feedback@supportworks.org
www.supportworks.org

Joel Fisher, Manager
SupportWorks helps people find and form support groups. An 8 page publication Power Tools, clearly walks new group leaders through steps of putting together a healthy self-help group. SupportWorks also has a telephone conference program which allows people with similar diseases or other nonprofit issues to meet by phone conference for free or at very low cost.

8669 Toll-Free Information Line
Asthma and Allergy Foundation of America
8201 Corporate Drive
Suite 1000
Landover, MD 20785

202-466-7643
800-727-8462
800-7 A-THMA
FAX: 202-466-8940
info@aafa.org
aafa.org

Lynn Hanessian, Chair
Yolanda Miller, SVP & COO
Lynda Mitchell, VP, Food Allergies
Nancy Kercher, Secretary
The Asthma and Allergy Foundation of America (AAFA) provides practical information, community based services and support through a national network of chapters and support groups. AAFA develops health education, organizes state and national advocacy efforts and funds research to find better treatments and cures.

8670 Visiting Nurse Association of America
2121 Crystal Drive
Suite 750
Arlington, VA 22202

571-527-1520
888-866-8773
FAX: 571-527-1527
webadmin@vnaa.org
vnaa.org

Mary B. DeVeau, Chair
Linnea Windel, Vice Chair
Tracey Moorhead, President & CEO
Magaret Terry, VP of Quality & Innovation
The VNAA is the official national association for not-for-profit, community based home health organizations known as the Visiting Nurse Associations (VNA's). They created the profession of home health care more then 100 years ag. They have a united mission to bring compassionate, high-quality and cost-effective home care to individuals in their communities.

Speech & Language

Associations

8671 Academic Language Therapy Association
14070 Proton Road
Suite 100, LB 9
Dallas, TX 75244
972-233-9107
FAX: 972-490-4219
office@altaread.org
www.altaread.org

Marilyn Mathis, President
Jo Ann Handy, VP Membership
Lynne Fitzhugh, VP Public Relations
Suzanne Crawford, VP Programs
The Academic Language Therapy Associationr (ALTA) is a non-profit national professional organization incorporated in 1986 for the purpose of establishing, maintaining, and promoting standards of education, practice and professional conduct for Certified Academic Language Therapists. Academic Language Therapy is an educational, structured, comprehensive, phonetic, multisensory approach for the remediation of dyslexia and/or written-language disorders.

8672 American Speech-Language-Hearing Association
2200 Research Blvd
Rockville, MD 20850-3289
301-296-5700
800-638-8255
FAX: 301-296-8580
TTY: 301-296-5650
actioncenter@asha.org
www.asha.org

Patricia A. Prelock, PhD, CCC-SLP, President
Elizabeth S. McCrea, PhD, CCC-SLP, President-Elect
Donna Fisher Smiley, PhD, CC, Vice President for Audiology Practice
Howard Goldstein, PhD, CCC-SL, Vice President for Science and Research
The American Speech-Language Association is the professional, scientific, and credentialing association for 135,000 members and affiliates who are speech-language pathologists, audiologists, and speech, language, and hearing scientists in the United States and internationally. ASHA provides information for the public, professionals, students, and the research community related to hearing, balance, speech, language and swallowing disorders.

8673 Aphasia Hope Foundation
PO Box 26304
Shawnee, KS 66225-6304
913-839-8083
855-764-4673
sandycaudell@aphasiahope.org
www.aphasiahope.org

Sandy Caudell, Program Diretor
Judi Stradinger, Executive Director
Aphasia Hope Foundation is a nonprofit foundation with a two-fold mission: 1.to promote research into the prevention and cure of aphasia and 2. to ensure that all survivors of aphasia and their caregivers are aware of and have access to the best possible tratments.

8674 Association of Language Companies
9707 Key West Avenue
Suite 100
Rockville, MD 20850
240-404-6511
FAX: 301-990-9771
info@alcus.org
www.alcus.org

Camilo Muñoz, President
Douglas J. Strock, Vice President
Julie Hill, Marketing Director
Morgan Wisher, Meeting Planner
The Association of Language Companies (ALC) is a national trade association representing businesses that provide translation, interpretation, localization, and language training services.

8675 Atlanta Aphasia Association
1811 Windemere Drive
Atlanta, GA 30324
404-413-8299
jlaures@gsut.edu
www.atlantaaphasia.org

Nancy Morris, President
Jacqueline Laures-Gore PhD, Co-President
Alan Morris, Secretary/Treasurer
The Altanta Aphasia Association has several purposes: to organize and provide resources to individuals with aphasia and those involved with aphasia at vaious levels; to educate the community about aphasia through resources, discussions and communication about research advances in stroke and aphasia; to promote socialization of those with aphasia through various functions; to provide support and training for the vocational needs of those with aphasia.

8676 Autism Research Institute
4182 Adams Ave
San Diego, CA 92116-2599
619-281-7165
866-366-3361
FAX: 619-563-6840
www.autism.com

Stephen Edelson, Executive Director
Jane Johnson, Managing Director
Valerie Paradiz, Director
Rebecca McKenney, Office Manager
Conducts research on the causes, diagnosis, and treatment of autism and publishes a quarterly newsletter that reviews worldwide research. Literature on causes and treatment available. Refers patients and families to health care professionals and clinics. Request publication list and sample newsletter, Autism Research Review.

8677 Autism Services Center
929 4th Ave
PO Box 507
Huntington, WV 25701-0507
304-525-8014
FAX: 304-525-8026
candy@autismwv.org
www.autismservicescenter.org

Jimmie Moss, Director
Jodi Fields, Director
Barbara Bragg, Director
David Finley, Director
Provides developmental disabilities services with a specialty in autism. Services include case management, residential, personal care, assessments and evaluations, supported employment, independent living and family support.

8678 Autism Treatment Center of America
2080 S Undermountain Rd
Sheffield, MA 1257-9643
413-229-2100
877-766-7473
correspondence@option.org
www.autismtreatmentcenter.org

Barry Neil Kaufman, Co-Founder/ Co-Originator/Senior Teacher/Trainer
Samahria Lyte Kaufman, Co-Founder/ Co-Originator/Senior Teacher/Trainer
Bryn Hogan, ATCA Senior Staff
William Hogan, ATCA Senior Staff
Since 1983, the Autism Treatment Center of America has provided innovative training programs for parents and professionals caring for children challenged by Autism, Autism Spectrum Disorders, Pervasive Developmental Disorders (PDD) and other development difficulties. The Son-Rise Program teaches a specific yet comprehensive system of treatment and education designed to help families and caregivers enable their children to dramatically improve in all areas of learning.

8679   Childhood Apraxia of Speech Association
416 Lincoln Avenue
2nd Fl.
Pittsburgh, PA 15209

www.apraxia-kids.org

Mary Sturm, President
Sharon Gretz, M.Ed, Executive Director
Earnie Sotirokos, Digital Media Specialist
Kathy Hennessy, Education Director

The Childhood Apraxia of Speech Association is a 501(c)(3) non-profit publicly funded charity whose mission is to strengthen the support systems in the lives of children with apraxia so that each child is afforded their best opportunity to develop speech and communication.

8680   Communication Help, Education, Research, Apraxia Base (CHERAB)
PO Box 8524
PSL, FL 34952-8524

772-335-5135
help@cherab.org
www.cherab.org

Lisa Geng, Founder, President

The Cherab Foundation is a world-wide nonprofit organization working to improve the communication skills and education of all children with speech and language delays and disorders. Their area of emphasis is verbal and oral apraxia, severe neurologically-based speech and language disorders that hinder children's ability to speak.

8681   Communication in Autism
Federal Government
1 Communication Avenue
Bldg 1
Bethesda, MD 20892-3456

800-241-1044
FAX: 310-770-8977
TTY:800-241-1055
nidcdinfo@nidcd.nih.gov
www.nidcd.nih.gov

James M. Anderson, M.D., Ph.D., Chairperson
James F. Battey, Jr. M.D., Ph., Director
Judith A. Cooper, Ph.D., Deputy Director
Timothy J. Wheeles, Executive Officer

The National Institute on Deafness and Other Communication Disorders (NIDCD) one of the National Institute of Health, supports and conducts research and research training on the normal and disordered processes of hearing, balance smell, taste, voice, speech and language.

8682   Davis Center, The
19 State Route 10 E
Ste 25
Succasunna, NJ 07876

862-251-4637
FAX: 862-251-4642
npdunn@thedaviscenter.com
www.thedaviscenter.com

Dorinne S Davis MA CCC-A FAAA, Director
Elizabeth Meade, Head Sound Therapist
Nancy Puckett-Dunn, Office Manger
Donna Warr, Office Assistant

The Davis Center's Sound Therapy Programs make positive changes for children and adults with autism, ADD/ADHD, auditory processing issues, Dyslexia, learning disabilities, and other learning and wellness challenges. Our programs address issues such as phonics, spelling, writing, reading comprehension, hearing only parts of words, following directions, discriminating between sounds, sound sensitivity, behavioral responses, focus, attention, and more.

8683   Deafness and Communicative Disorders Branch of Rehab Services Administration Office
Special Education And Rehab Services
400 Maryland Ave SW
Washington, DC 20202-1

202-245-7489
800-872-5327
FAX: 202-245-7614
TTY: 800-437-0833
customerservice@inet.ed.gov
www.ed.gov

Arne Duncan, Secretary Of Education
Tony Miller, Deputy Secretary
Martha Kanter, Under Secretary
Jo Anderson, Senior Advisor

Promotes improved rehabilitation services for deaf and hard of hearing people and individuals with speech or language impairments. Provides technical assistance to public and private agencies and individuals.

8684   Dysphagia Research Society
4550 Post Oak Place
Suite 342
Houston, TX 77027

713-965-0566
FAX: 713-960-0488
drs@meetingmanagers.com
www.dysphagiaresearch.org

Douglas J. Van Daele, MD, President
Lynne Tiras, CMP, Executive Director
Lauren Wood, Association Manager
Angie Guy, MPA, Meeting and Events Manager

The Dysphagia Research Society is organized exclusively for charitable, educational and scientific purposes.

8685   Hearing, Speech and Deafness Center (HSDC)
Hearing, Speech & Deafness Center (HSDC)
1625 19th Ave
Seattle, WA 98122-2848

206-323-5770
888-222-5036
FAX: 206-328-6871
TTY: 206-388-1275
hsdc@hsdc.org
www.hsdc.org

Cherylyn McRae, Director of Development
David Webster, Director of Finance
Roger Mauldin, Interim CEO
Bryan Bullock, Billing Specialist & Facilities Manager

Our mission is to enrich lives of all adults and children who experience hearing loss, speech and language impairments or who are deaf, by providing professional services and by promoting community awareness and accessibility.

8686   International Cluttering Association
705 Tilbury Court
Sun City Center, FL 33573

elanouette@tampabay.rr.com
associations.missouristate.edu/ica

Charley Adams, Ph.D., Chair
Kathleen Scaler Scott, Coordinator
Klaas Bakker, Webmaster
Ellen Bennett, Membership

They work to increase awareness of the communication disorder of cluttering worldwide among speech-language therapists/logopedists, healthcare professionals, people with cluttering, and the public.

8687   International Fluency Association
Northern Illinois University
Dept. of Communicative Disorders
DeKalb, IL 60115-2899

msugarman1@aol.com
www.theifa.org

David Shapiro, President
Manon Abbink-Spruit, Vice-President
Dorothy Ross, Treasurer
Norimune Kawai, Secretary

The International Fluency Association is a not-for-profit, international, interdisciplinary organization devoted to the understanding and management of fluency disorders, and to the improvement in the quality of life for persons with fluency disorders.

8688   Lindamood-Bell Home Learning Process
416 Higuera Street
San Luis Obispo, CA 93401   805-541-3836
                                             800-233-1819
                                        FAX: 805-541-8756
                                        www.lindamoodbell.com

Nanci Bell, Founder/Director
Patricia C. Lindamood, Founder/Director
Founded in 1986 by Nanci Bell and Patricia Lindamood, Lindamood-Bell Learning Process is dedicated to enhancing human learning. Our critically acclaimed instructional programs teach children and adults to read, spell, comprehend, and express language.

8689   Myositis Association, The
1737 King Street
Suite 600
Alexandria, VA 22314   703-299-4850
                                             800-821-7356
                                        FAX: 703-535-6752
                                        TMA@myositis.org
                                        www.myositis.org

Bob Goldberg, Executive Director
Theresa E. Curry, Communications Manager
Aisha Morrow, Operations Manager
Charlia Sanchez, Member Services Manager
They work to provide support to myositis patients and their families.

8690   National Aphasia Association
350 Seventh Avenue
Suite 902
New York, NY 10001
                                             800-922-4622
                                        naa@aphasia.org
                                        www.aphasia.org

Donald Weinstein, Ph.D, Board President
Darlene S. Williamson, M.S., Vice President Programs
Daniel Martin, Vice President Strategic Planning
J. Tyler Entwistle, Treasurer/Vice President Budget & Finance
The National Aphasia Association (NAA) is a nonprofit organization that promotes public education, research, rehabilitation and support services to assist people with aphasia and their families.

8691   National Association of Special Education Teachers
1250 Connecticut Ave NW
Ste 200
Washington, DC 20036- 2643   202-296-7739
                                             800-754-4421
                                        FAX: 800-754-4421
                                        contactus@naset.org
                                        www.naset.org

Dr Roger Pierangelo, Executive Director
Dr George Giuliani, Executive Director
The National Association of Special Education Teachers (NASET) is a national membership organization dedicated to rendering all possible support and assistance to those preparing for or teaching in the field of special education. NASET was founded to promote the profession of special education teachers and to provide a national forum for their ideas.

8692   National Black Association for Speech-Language and Hearing
700 McKnight Park Drive
Pittsburgh, PA 15237   412-366-1177
                                        FAX: 412-366-8804
                                        nbaslh@nbaslh.org
                                        www.nbaslh.org

Arnell Brady, Chair
Carolyn Mayo, Secretary
Linda McCabe Smith, Treasurer
The mission of the National Black Association of Speech-Language and Hearing is to maintain a viable mechanism through which the needs of black professionals, students and individuals with communication disorders can be met.

8693   National Center for Accessible Media
WGBH Educational Foundation
1 Guest St
Boston, MA 02135-2016   617-300-3400
                                        FAX: 617-300-1035
                                        TTY:617-300-2489
                                        access@wgbh.org
                                        www.ncam.wgbh.org

Larry Goldberg, Director of Media Access and oversees
Geoff Freed, Director of technology projects and Web media standards
Madeleine Rothberg, Project Director
Bryan Gould, Project Manager of NCAM's Effective Practices for Describing
The Carl and Ruth Shapiro Family National Center for Accessible Media (NCAM) at Boston public broadcaster WGBH is a research and development facility dedicated to addressing barriers to media and emerging technologies for people with disabilities in their homes, schools, workplaces, and communities..

8694   National Cued Speech Association
Information Service
1300 Pennsylvania Avenue
Suite 190-713
Washington, DC 20004-1021   301-915-8009
                                             800-459-3529
                                        FAX: 301-915-8009
                                        TTY: 800-459-3529
                                        sroffe@cuedspeech.org
                                        www.cuedspeech.org

Shannon Howell, President
Penny Hakim, First Vice President
John Brubaker, VP Fundraising
Doug Dawson, Treasurer
The NCSA champions effective communication, language development and literacy through the use of cued speech. The NCSA envisions that individuals communicate effectively in the languageof their family and society. Families are informed about Cued Speech along with other communication options. Their rights are respected and instruction is provided to facilitate the use of cued languages. Students achieve literacy through full access to language and education.

8695   National Fragile X Foundation
2100 M St NW
Ste 170, P.O. Box 302
Washington, DC 20037-1233   202-747-6208
                                             800-688-8765
                                        FAX: 925-938-9315
                                        natlfx@fragilex.org
                                        www.fragilex.org

Robert Miller, Executive Director
Linda Sorensen, MS, Chief Operating Officer
Jeffrey Cohen, Director, Public Policy & Government Affairs
David Salomon, Communications Manager
Unites the fragile X community to enrich lives through educational and emotional support, promote public and professional awareness and advance research toward improvemed treatments and cure for fragile X syndrome.

8696   National Spasmodic Dysphonia Association
300 Park Boulevard
Suite 335
Itasca, IL 60143
                                             800-795-6732
                                        FAX: 630-250-4505
                                        NSDA@dysphonia.org
                                        www.dysphonia.org

Charlie Reavis, President
Marcia Sterling, Treasurer
Kimberly Kuman, Executive Director
Elaine Beamer, Program Coordinator
The National Spasmodic Dysphonia Association (NSDA) is a not-for-profit 501c(3) organization dedicated to advancing medical research into the causes of and treatments for SD, promoting

physician and public awareness of the disorder, and providing support to those affected by SD through symposiums, support groups, and on-line resources.

8697   National Student Speech Language Hearing Association
2200 Research Blvd
Rockville, MD 20850-3289   301-296-5700
                                              800-498-2071
                                         FAX: 301-296-8580
                                         TTY: 301-296-5650
                                            nsslha@asha.org
                                          www.asha.org/nsslha

Patricia A. Prelock, PhD, CCC-SLP, President
Elizabeth S. McCrea, PhD, CCC-SLP, President-Elect
Carlin F. Hageman, PhD, CCC-SLP, National Student Speech Language Hearing Association (NSSLHA
Lauren Zanfardino, Council Member
Founded in 1972, NSSLHA is the national organization for graduate and undergraduate students interested in the study of normal and disordered human communication. NSSLHA is the only official national student association recognized by the American Speech Language Hearing Association (ASHA).

8698   National Stuttering Association
119 W 40th St
Fl 14
New York, NY 10018-2514   212-944-4050
                                              800-937-8888
                                         FAX: 212-944-8244
                                           info@westutter.org
                                            www.westutter.org

Sheryl Hunter, Esquire, Chairwoman
Kenny Koroll, Vice-Chairman
Bob Wellington, Treasurer and Chairman of the Finance Committee
Pattie Wood, Chair Family Programs
A nonprofit organization dedicated to bringing hope, dignity, support, education, and empowerment to children and adults who stutter and their families, and the professionals who serve them.

8699   National Tourette Syndrome Association
42-40 Bell Boulevard
Bayside, NY 11361   718-224-2999
                                         FAX: 718-279-9596
                                             www.tsa-usa.org

8700   Providence Speech and Hearing Center
1301 W Providence Ave
Orange, CA 92868-3892   714-923-1521
                                         FAX: 714-639-2593
                                              pshc@pshc.org
                                                www.pshc.org

Bruce May, President
Kevin Timone, Vice President - Fund Development
Randy Free, Vice President - Finance
Casey Immel, Treasurer
Mission is to provide the highest quality services available in the identification, diagnosis, treatment and prevention of speech, language and hearing disorders for persons of all ages.

8701   Scottish Rite Center for Childhood Language Disorders
Seattle Clinic
1207 North 152nd St
PO Box 4144
Olympia, WA 98501-144   360-357-5933
                                         FAX: 206-324-3332
                                          hfray@ritecarewa.org
                                            www.scottishrite.org

Jacqueline Brown, Clinical Director
Offers speech-language evaluations and treatment, hearing screening and consultations to children ages birth through adolescence. Bilingual services are also available.

8702   Stern Center
183 Talcott Road
Suite 101
Williston, VT 05495-9209   802-878-0230
                                         FAX: 802-878-0230
                                           www.sterncenter.org

Blanche Podhajski PhD, President
Edward R. Wilkens, Ed.D., Vice President for Development
Janna Osman, M.Ed., Vice President for Programs
Michael Shapiro, M.B.A., Chief Financial Officer
The Stern Center was founded as a nonprofit learning center dedicated to helping children and adults reach their full potential. Stern Center professionals evaluate and teach all kinds of learners, including those with learning disabilities such as dyslexia or attention deficit disorders. We evaluate and teach over 1,000 children and adults each year including those with learning disabilities, dyslexia, language disorders, autism, attention deficit disorders, and learning style differences.

8703   Stuttering Foundation of America
1805 Moriah Woods Blvd,
PO Box 11749, Suite 3
Memphis, TN 38111-0749   901-761-0343
                                              800-992-9392
                                         FAX: 901-761-0484
                                         info@stutteringhelp.org
                                          www.stutteringhelp.org

Jane Fraser, President
Dennis Drayna, Director
Joseph R. G. Fulcher, Director
Frances Cook, Director
Provides resources, services, and support to those who stutter and their families, as well as support for research into the causes of stuttering.

8704   Texas Speech-Language-Hearing Association
2025 M Street NW,
Suite 800
Washington, DC 20036-2342   855-330-8742
                                              888-729-8742
                                         FAX: 512-494-1129
                                          tsha@assnmgmt.com
                                               www.txsha.org

Judith Keller, President
Larry Higdon, Director
Melanie McDonald, President Elect
Tori Gustafson, Vice President
Mission is to encourage and promote the role of the speech-language pathologist and audiologist as a professional in the delivery of clinical services to persons with communications disorders. Encourages basic scientific study of processes of individual human communication with reference to speech, hearing and language.

8705   Wendell Johnson Speech And Hearing Clinic
University Of Iowa
116 Wendell Johnson Speech and Hear
Iowa City, IA 52242- 1025   319-335-8736
                                         FAX: 319-335-8851
                                         linda-louka@uiowa.edu
                                                www.uiow.edu

Ruth Bentler, Professor & Department Chair
Dorothy Albright, Secretary
Kathy Miller, Clerk
Elizabeth Walker, Audiologist
The clinic offers assessment and remediation for communication disorders in adults and children. The clinic also offers a Intensive Summer Residential Clinic for school age children needing intervention services because of speech, language, hearing and/or reading problems.

Camps

8706 CNS Camp New Connections
Mclean Hospital Child/Adolescent Program
Mailstop115
115 Mill Street
Belmont, MA 02478

617-855-2000
800-333-0338
FAX: 617-855-2833
mcleaninfo@partners.org
mcleanhospital.org

Scott L. Rauch, MD, President & Chief Psychiatrist
Blaise Aguirre, Clinical Staff
Alan Barry, Clinical Staff
Susan L. Andersen, Research Staff

Four-week summer day camp for children ages 7-17 who have pervasive developmental disorders, Asperger's Syndrome, autism spectrum disorders and non-verbal learning disabilities. The camp is designed to help children develop social skills through fun activities including: communication games, swimming, field trips, drama, and arts and crafts. *$4500.00*

8707 Camp Royall
Autism Society of North Carolina
Ste 230
505 Oberlin Rd
Raleigh, NC 27605-1345

919-743-0204
800-442-2762
FAX: 919-743-0208
jchampion@autismsociety-nc.com
www.autismsociety-nc.org

Sharon Jeffries-Jones, Chair
Elizabeth Phillippi, Vice Chair
Paul Wendler, Chief Financial Officer
David Laxton, Director of Communications

The best source in North Carolina for connecting people who live with autism (and those who care about them) with resources, support, advocacy and informantion tailored to thier unique needs.

8708 Camp Sisol
Jewish Community Center of Greater Rochester/JCC
1200 Edgewood Ave
Rochester, NY 14618

585-461-2000
membership2@jccrochester.org
www.jccrochester.org

Marshall Lesser, Chair
Jeremy Wolk, President
Dan Goldstein, VP & Secretary
Leslie Berkoitz, Executive Director

Camp is located in Honeoye Falls, New York. Summer sessions for children with autism. Coed, ages 5-16.

8709 Childrens Beach House
100 West 10th Street
Suite 411
Wilmington, DE 19801-1674

302-655-4288
FAX: 302-655-4216
inquiry@cbhinc.org
www.cbhinc.org

Martha P. Tschantz, President
Mary Helms, Vice President
Richard T Garrett, Executive Director
Nicholas Imhoff, Business Manager

Camp is located in Lewes, Delaware. Four-week sessions June-August for Delaware children with hearing impairment or speech/communication impairment. Coed, ages 6-12.

8710 Easter Seals Oklahoma
701 NorthEast 13th Street
Oklahoma City, OK 73104

405-239-2525
FAX: 405-239-2278
sbusch@eastersealsoklahoma.org
www.eastersealsoklahoma.org

Rodney Burgamy, Chairman
David Adams, Board Member
Kristen Sorocco, Secretary
Jeb Reid, Treasurer

Adult day health center, and child development center.

8711 Meadowood Springs Speech and Hearing Camp
Institute for Rehab., Research, & Recreation Inc
P.O. Box 1025
Pendleton, OR 97801

541-276-2752
FAX: 541-276-7227
info@meadowoodsprings.org
www.meadowoodsprings.com

Michael Ashton, Executive Director
Cliff Story, Property Manager
Missy Newcomb, Clinical Director
Audrey Black, Program Director

On 143 acres in the Blue Mountains of Eastern Oregon, this camp is designed to help young people who have diagnosed clinical disorders of speech, hearing or language. A full range of activities in recreational and clinical areas is available.

8712 New Horizons Summer Day Camp
YMCA
13821 Newport Avenue
Suite 200
Tustin, CA 92780

714-549-9622
FAX: 714-838-5976
www.ymcaoc.org

Robert Traut, Chair
Jeff Black, Vice Chair
Jeff McBride, President/CEO
Cara Owens, COO/VP, Operations

One-week sessions for children with ADD and speech/communication impairment. Coed, ages 5-14.

8713 Sequanota Lutheran Conference Center and Camp
P.O. Box 245
Jennerstown, PA 15547

814-629-6627
FAX: 814-629-0128
contact@sequanota.com
www.sequanota.com

Carol Custead, President
David Shoemaker, Vice President
Nathan Pile, Executive Director
Loren Kurtz, Maintenance Director

Summer sessions for adults with developmental disabilities and speech/communication impairment.

8714 Talisman Summer Camp
64 Gap Creek Rd
Zirconia, NC 28790

828-697-6313
855-588-8254
855-LUV-TALI
info@talismancamps.com
www.talismancamps.com

Doug Smathers, Camp Director/Owner
Linda Tatsapaugh, Operations Director/Owner
Robiyn Mims, Admissions Coordinator
Cory Greene, Program Manager

Camp is located in Black Mountain, North Carolina. Offers a program of hiking, rafting, climbing, and caving for learning disabled ADD/ADHD and autistic young people. Coed, ages 9-18.

8715 Wendell Johnson Speech & Hearing Clinic
University Of Iowa
250 Hawkins Dr
Iowa City, IA 52242-1025

319-335-8736
FAX: 319-335-8851
kathy-miller@uiowa.edu
www.uiowa.edu

Chuck Wieland, President
Hans Hoerschelman, Vice President
Josh Smith, Budget Officer
Shannon Lizakowski, Secretary

The clinic offers assessment and remediation for communication disorders in adults and children. The clinic also offers a Intensive Summer Residential Clinic for school age children needing intervention services because of speech, language, hearing and/or reading problems.

8716 **YMCA Camp Fitch**
The YMCA Of Youngstown - Metro Office
17 N Champion St
P.O. Box 1287
Youngstown, OH 44501

330-744-8411
FAX: 330-744-8415
info@campfitchymca.org
www.youngstownymca.org

Thomas Fleming, Chair/CVO
James B. Greene, 1st Vice Chair
Thomas Gacse, 2nd Vice Chairman
Timothy M. Hilk, President/CEO
Camp is located in North Springfield, Pennsylvania. Camping sessions for children and adults with diabetes, hearing impairment, developmental disabilities, mobility limitation and speech/communication impairment. Ages 8-16, families and seniors.

Print: Books

8717 **Autism 24/7: A Family Guide to Learning at Home & in the Community**
Autism Society of North Carolina Bookstore
Ste 230
505 Oberlin Rd
Raleigh, NC 27605-1345

919-743-0204
800-442-2762
FAX: 919-743-0208
jchampion@autismsociety-nc.org
http://www.autismsociety-nc.org/

Sharon Jeffries-Jones, Chair
Elizabeth Phillippi, Vice Chair
Tracey Sheriff, Chief Executive Officer
Paul Wendler, Chief Financial Officer
Parents are encouraged to focus on skill sets and behaviors that most negatively affect family functioning, and replacing these behaviors with acceptable alternatives. *$19.95*

8718 **Autism Handbook: Understanding & Treating Autism & Prevention Development**
Oxford University Press
2001 Evans Road
Cary, NC 27513

919-677-0977
800-445-9714
FAX: 919-677-1303
custserv.us@oup.co
http://www.oup.com/us/

320 pages
ISBN 0-195076-67-2

8719 **Autism and Learning**
Taylor & Francis
37-41 Mortimer St
London, UK W1T 3

http://www.informatandm.com

Stuart Powell, Author
Rita Jordan, Editor
This book is about how a cognitive perception on the way in which individuals with autism think and learn may be applied to particular curriculum areas.
160 pages Paperback
ISBN 1-853464-21-X

8720 **Autism in Adolescents and Adults**
Springer Publishing
233 Spring St
New York, NY 10013

877-283-3229
ainy@aveda.com
http://aveda.edu/new-york

Eric Schopler, Editor
Gary B. Mesibov, Editor
This book is a great history lesson in the development of understanding about autism spectrum disorders, and is a testament to how far research and services in the field have come. This book contains lots of information about what general thinking and ser-

vices used to be like, in an era when still little was understood about these disorders. *$63.00*
456 pages
ISBN 0-306410-57-5

8721 **Autism...Nature, Diagnosis and Treatment**
Autism Society of North Carolina Bookstore
Ste 230
505 Oberlin Rd
Raleigh, NC 27605-1345

919-743-0204
800-442-2762
FAX: 919-743-0208
jchampion@autismsociety-nc.com
http://www.autismsociety-nc.org/

Sharon Jeffries-Jones, Chair
Elizabeth Phillippi, Vice Chair
Paul Wendler, Chief Financial Officer
David Laxton, Director of Communications
Covers perspectives, issues, neurobiological issues and new directions in diagnosis and treatment. *$49.00*

8722 **Autism: Explaining the Enigma**
Wiley Publishers
111 River Street
Hoboken, NJ 07030-5774

201-748-6000
FAX: 201-748-6088
info@wiley.com
http://as.wiley.com

Peter Booth Wiley, Chairman
Stephen M. Smith, President & CEO
John Kitzmacher, EVP, CFO
Ellis E. Cousens, Executive Vice President, COO
Explains the nature of autism. *$27.95*

8723 **Autism: From Tragedy to Triumph**
Branden Publishing Company
17 Station St
Brookline, MA 2445-7995

617-730-5757
branden@branden.com
http://www.yogainthevillage.com

Karen Wenc, Teaching Staff
Veronica Wolff, Teaching Staff
Annie Hoffman, Teaching Staff
Keith Beasley, Teaching Staff
A new book that deals with the Lovaas method and includes a foreward by Dr. Ivar Lovaas. The book is broken down into two parts — the long road to diagnosis and then treatment. *$12.95*

8724 **Autism: Identification, Education and Treatment**
Routledge (Taylor & Francis Group)
270 Madison Ave
New York, NY 10016-601

212-576-1411
http://books.google.co.in/books/about/Autism.

Dianne Zager, Editor
Chapters include medical treatments, early intervention and communication development in autism. *$36.00*

ISBN 0-805820-44-7

8725 **Autism: The Facts**
Oxford University Press
2001 Evans Road
Cary, NC 27513

919-677-0977
800-445-9714
FAX: 919-677-1303
custserv.us@oup.co
http://www.oup.com/us/corporate/contact/?view

Simon Baron-Cohen, Co-Author
Patrick Bolton, Co-Author
$22.50
128 pages
ISBN 0-192623-27-3

8726   Autistic Adults at Bittersweet Farms
Routledge (Taylor & Francis Group)
12660 Archbold-Whitehouse Rd.
Whitehouse, OH 43571   419-875-6986
                            mtilkins@bittersweetfarms.org.
                            http://www.bittersweetfarms.org/
Robert St. Clair, President
Matt Anderson, VP
Jan Toczynski, Secretary
Jon Ahlberg, Board Member
A touching view of an inspirational residential care program for autistic adolescents and adults. Also available in softcover. *$94.95*
Hardcover
ISBN 1-560240-42-3

8727   Beyond Baby Talk: From Sounds to Sentences, a Parent's Guide to Language Development
Prima Publishing
P.O.Box 1260
Rocklin, CA 95677-1260   916-787-7000
                                             800-632-8676
                                        FAX: 916-787-7001
                                        www.primapublishing.com
Fernando Bueno, Editor in Chief
Julie Asbury, Managing Editor
Christopher Buffa, Sr. Editor
Andrea Hill, Community Manager
The authors discuss the best ways to help your child develop the all-important skill of communication and to recognize the signs of language development problems. *$15.95*
224 pages
ISBN 0-761526-47-1

8728   Breaking the Speech Barrier: Language Develpment Through Augmented Means
Brookes Publishing
P.O.Box 10624
Baltimore, MD 21285-0624   410-337-9580
                                             800-638-3775
                                        FAX: 410-337-8539
                                        custserv@brookespublishing.com
                                        readplaylearn.com
Paul Brookes, Owner
This resource describes the creation of the System for Augmenting Language (SAL) for school-age youth with mental retardation and offers important insights into the language development of children who are not learning to communicate typically. *$39.95*
224 pages Paperback
ISBN 1-557663-90-0

8729   Breakthroughs: How to Reach Students with Autism
Aquarius Health Care Media
Ste 230
505 Oberlin Rd
Raleigh, NC 27605-1345   919-743-0204
                                             800-442-2762
                                        FAX: 919-743-0208
                                        jchampion@autismsociety-nc.org
                            http://www.autismtreatmentcenter.org/cont ents
Sharon Jeffries-Jones, Chair
Elizabeth Phillippi, Vice Chair
Tracey Sheriff, CEO
Paul Wendler, CFO
A hands-on, how-to program for reaching students with autism, featuring Karen Sewell, Autism Society of America's teacher of the year. Here Sewell demonstrates the successful techniques she's developed over a 20-year career. A separate 250 page manual ($59) is also available which covers math, reading, fine motor, self help, social adaptive, vocational and self help skills as well as providing numerous plan reproducibles and an exhaustive listing of equipment and materials resources. Video. *$99.00*

8730   Childhood Speech, Language & Listening Problems
Wiley Publishing
605 3rd Ave
New York, NY 10158-180   212-850-6000
                                        FAX: 212-850-6088
                            http://books.google.co.in/books/about/Childho
Patricia McAleer Hamaguchi
Language pathologist Hamaguchi employs her 15 years of experience to show parents how to recognize the most common speech, language, and listening problems. *$16.95*
224 pages Paperback
ISBN 0-471387-53-3

8731   Cognitive Behavioral Therapy for Adult Asperger Syndrome
Autism Society of North Carolina Bookstore
Ste 230
505 Oberlin Rd
Raleigh, NC 27605-1345   919-743-0204
                                             800-442-2762
                                        FAX: 919-743-0208
                                        jchampion@autismsociety-nc.org
                                        http://www.autismsociety-nc.org
Sharon Jeffries-Jones, Chair
Elizabeth Phillippi, Vice Chair
Tracey Sheriff, CEO
Paul Wendler, CFO
Text is prepared with case studies and examples from the author's own experiences working as a cognitive-behavioral therapist specializing in adults and adolescents with dual diagnosis, autism spectrum disorders, mood disorders, and anxiety disorders.

8732   Communication Development and Disorders in African American Children
Brookes Publishing
P.O.Box 10624
Baltimore, MD 21285-0624   410-337-9580
                                             800-638-3775
                                        FAX: 410-337-8539
                                        custserv@brookespublishing.com
                                        readplaylearn.com
Paul Brooks, Owner
Research, Assessment, and Intervention. This text presents research on communication disorders and language development in African American children. Also addresses multicultural aspects of service delivery and intervention and discusses issues in assessing, diagnosing, and treating communication disorders. *$39.00*
400 pages Paperback
ISBN 1-55766 -53-3

8733   Communication Development in Children with Down Syndrome
Brookes Publishing
P.O.Box 10624
Baltimore, MD 21285-0624   410-337-9580
                                             800-638-3775
                                        FAX: 410-337-8539
                                        custserv@brookespublishing.com
                                        readplaylearn.com
Paul Brooks, Owner
This book offers an extensive, detailed explanation of communication development in children with Down syndrome relative to their advancing cognitive skills. It introduces a critical framework for assessing and treating hearing, speech, and language problems and provides explicit intervention methods and tested clinical protocols.
Paperback
ISBN 1-55766 -50-5

8734 Coping for Kids Who Stutter
Speech Bin
P.O.Box 1579
Appleton, WI 54912

419-589-1425
888-388-3224
FAX: 888-388-6344
info@speechbin.com
www.speechbin.com

James R. Henderson, Chairman
Joseph M. Yorio, President & CEO
Rick Holden, EVP, Educators Publishing Service
Patrick T. Collins, EVP, Distribution
Informative book for children and adults about stuttering and
how to manage it. *$15.95*
32 pages
ISBN 0-93785 -43-2

**8735 Disorders of Motor Speech: Assessment, Treatment, and
Clinical Characterization**
Brookes Publishing
P.O.Box 10624
Baltimore, MD 21285-0624

410-337-9580
800-638-3775
FAX: 410-337-8539
custserv@brookespublishing.com
readplaylearn.com

Paul Brooks, Owner
This book provides a probing examination of normal, dysarthric,
and apraxic speech. Great for speech-language pathologists, neurologists, physical or occupational therapists, and physiatrists.
$47.00
400 pages Hardcover
ISBN 1-55766 -23-1

**8736 Employment for Individuals with Asperger Syndrome or
Non-Verbal Learning Disability**
Jessica Kingsley Publishers
400 Market Street
Suite 400
Philadelphia, PA 19106-2513

215-922-1161
866-416-1078
FAX: 215-922-1474
orders@jkp.com
www.jkp.com

Laurie Schlesinger, Vp Of Sales & Marketing
Yvona Fast, Author
Most people with Non-Verbal Learning Disorder (NLD) or
Asperger Syndrome (AS) are underemployed. This book sets out
to change this. With practical and technical advice on everything
from job hunting to interview techniques, from 'fitting in' in the
workplace to whether or not to disclose a diagnosis, this book
guides people with NLD or AS successfully through the employment mine field. There is also information for employers, agencies and careers counsellors on AS and NLD as 'invisible'
disabili *$22.95*
272 pages
ISBN 1-843107-66-X

8737 Encounters with Autistic States
Jason Aronson
400 Keystone Industrial Park
Dunmore, PA 18512-1507

800-782-0015

448 pages Hardcover
ISBN 0-765700-62-

8738 Kitten Who Couldn't Purr
William Morrow & Company
1350 Avenue of the Americas
New York, NY 10019-4702

212-261-6500
FAX: 212-261-6925
http://www.goodreads.com/book/show/2319648.Th

Otis Chandler, CEO & Co-Founder
Eve Titus, Author
Jonathan the kitten doesn't know how to purr to say thank you, so
he sets off to find someone to teach him. *$12.95*
32 pages

8739 Language Disabilities in Children and Adolescents
McGraw-Hill School Publishing
PO Box 182605
Columbus, OH 43218

800-338-3987
FAX: 609-308-4480
customer.service@mheducation.com
mcgraw-hill.com

David Levin, President and CEO
Patrick Milano, Chief Administrative Officer & CFO
Stephen Laster, Chief Digital Officer
David Stafford, SVP & General Counsel
A comprehensive review of research in language disabilities.

8740 Language and the Developing Child
International Dyslexia Association
40 York Road
4th Floor
Baltimore, MD 21204

410-296-0232
800-ABC-D123
FAX: 410-321-5069
www.interdys.org

Hal Malchow, President
Ben Shifrin, Vice President
Elsa C. Hagen, Vice President
Suzanne Carreker, Secretary
This collection of papers introduces a new generation of teachers,
clinicians and parents to the work of one of the key figures in the
search for the causes and treatment of dyslexia. *$15.00*

8741 Late Talker: What to Do If Your Child Isn't Talking Yet
St Martin's Griffin
175 5th Ave
New York, NY 10010-7703

646-307-5151
888-330-8477
FAX: 212-674-6132
customerservice@mpsvirginia.com
www.us.macmillan.com

Marilyn C Agin, Author
This handbook offers advice on ways to identify the warning
signs of a speech disorder, information on how to get the right
kind of evaluations and therapy, ways to obtain appropriate services through the school system and health insurance, at-home
activities that parents can do with their child to stimulate speech,
benefits of nutritional supplementation, and advice from experienced parents who've been there on what to expect and what you
can do to be your child's best advocate. *$13.95*
256 pages Paperback
ISBN 0-312309-24-4

**8742 Let Community Employment be the Goal for Individuals
with Autism**
Indiana Resource Center For Autism
1905 North Range Road
Bloomington, IN 47408-9801

812-855-6508
800-825-4733
FAX: 812-855-9630
iidc@indiana.edu
www.iidc.indiana.edu/irca

Cathy Pratt, Director
Catherine Davies, Educational Consultant
Pamela Anderson, Outreach/Resource Specialist
Melissa Dubie, Research Associate
A guide designed for people who are responsible for preparing in-
dividuals with autism to enter the work force. *$7.00*

8743 Lollipop Lunch
Speech Bin-Abilitations
P.O.Box 1579
Appleton, WI 54912-1579

419-589-1425
888-388-3224
FAX: 888-388-6344
info@speechbin.com
www.speechbin.com

James R. Henderson, Chairman
Joseph M. Yorio, President & CEO
Rick Holden, EVP, Educators Publishing Service
Patrick T. Collins, EVP, Distribution

Cleverly illustrated stories and activities for phonological and language development. *$19.95*
128 pages
ISBN 0-937857-54-8

8744 Management of Autistic Behavior
Sage Publications
2455 Teller Road
Thousand Oaks, CA 91320
805-499-0721
800-818-7243
FAX: 805-499-0871
info@sagepub.com
www.sagepub.com

Sara Miller McCune, Founder, Publisher, Chairperson
Blaise R Simqu, President & CEO
Tracey A. Ozmina, Executive Vice President & Chief Operating Officer
Stephen Barr, Managing Director/SAGE London, President of SAGE Internation
This excellent reference is a comprehensive and practical book that tells what works best with specific problems. *$41.00*
450 pages

8745 Motor Speech Disorders
WB Saunders Company
14 Main Street
Southampton, NY 11968-2822
631-283-5050
800-523-1649
FAX: 631-283-2290
info@saunders.com
www.wbsaunders.com

Joseph R Duffy PhD, Author
Professional text on rehabilitation techniques for motor speech disorders. *$74.00*
592 pages
ISBN 0-323024-52-5

8746 Neurobiology of Autism
Johns Hopkins University Press
National Library of Medicine
Building 38A
Bethesda, MD 20894
410-516-6900
888-346-3656
888-FIN- NLM
FAX: 410-516-6998
info@ncbi.nlm.nih.gov
http://www.ncbi.nlm.nih.gov/pubmed/17919129

Pardo CA, Co-Author
Ebarhat CG, Co-Author
This book discusses recent advances in scientific research that point to a neurobiological basis for autism and examines the clinical implications of this research. *$28.00*
272 pages
ISBN 0-801880-47-5

8747 Nonverbal Learning Disabilities at Home: A Parent's Guide
Jessica Kingsley Publishers
400 Market Street
Suite 400
Philadelphia, PA 19106
215-922-1161
866-416-1078
FAX: 215-922-1474
hello.usa@jkp.com
www.jkp.com

Jessica Kingsley, Chairman & Managing Director
Jemima Kingsley, Director
Octavia Kingsley, Production Director
Lisa Clark, Sr. Commissioning Editor
Explores the variety of daily life problems children with NLD may face, and provides practical strategies for parents to help them cope and grow, from preschool age through their challenging adolescent years. *$19.95*
272 pages Paperback
ISBN 1-853029-40-0

8748 Parent Survival Manual
Springer Publishing Company
11 West 42nd Street
8th Floor
New York, NY 10036
212-355-1501
FAX: 212-355-7370
christieseducation@christies.edu
http://www.christieseducation.com

Craig Lickliter, Manager
A guide to crises resolution in autism and related developmental disorders. *$39.95*

8749 Perspectives: Whole Language Folio
Gallaudet University Bookstore
PO Box 35009
Charlotte, NC 28235-5009
202-651-5750
800-995-0550
FAX: 202-651-5744
http://www.cpcc.edu/disabilities/student-clas

Edwin A. Dalrymple, Chairman
Judith N. Allison, Vice Chair
Tony Zeiss, President
Ellen Zaremba, Administrative Assistant to the President
The 19 articles in this collection offer practical help to teachers seeking to emphasize whole language strategies in their classroom. *$9.95*
64 pages

8750 Please Don't Say Hello
Human Sciences Press
233 Spring St
New York, NY 10013
877-283-3229
ainy@aveda.com
http://aveda.edu/new-york

Phyllis Terri Gold, Author
Paul and his family moved into a new neighborhood. Paul's brother was autistic. The children thought that Eddie was retarded until they learned that there were skills that he could do better than they could. *$10.95*
47 pages Paperback
ISBN 0-89885 -99-8

8751 Promoting Communication in Infants and Young Children: 500 Ways to Succeed
Speech Bin-Abilitations
P.O.Box 1579
Appleton, WI 54912-1579
419-589-1425
888-388-3224
FAX: 888-388-6344
info@speechbin.com
www.speechbin.com

James R. Henderson, Chairman
Joseph M. Yorio, President & CEO
Rick Holden, EVP, Educators Publishing Service
Patrick T. Collins, EVP, Distribution
This practical reference for parents, caregivers and professional service providers how to promote communication development in infants and young children. Gives down-to-earth information and activities to help your youngest children succeed. It provides step-by-step suggestions for stimulationg children's speech and language skills. Paperback. *$14.95*

ISBN 0-937857-72-6

8752 Reading, Writing and Speech Problems in Children
International Dyslexia Association
40 York Road
4th Floor
Baltimore, MD 21204
410-296-0232
800-ABC-D123
FAX: 410-321-5069
www.interdys.org

Hal Malchow, President
Ben Shifrin, Vice President
Elsa C. Hagen, Vice President
Suzanne Carreker, Secretary

A tribute to the man who more than any other aroused the attention of the scientific community and who provided the sound educational principles on which much teaching of dyslexics today is based. *$27.00*

ISBN 0-89079 -79-1

8753 Relationship Development Intervention with Young Children
Taylor & Francis Group
73 Collier St.
London, N1 9BE
44- 0 -0 78
FAX: 44- 0 -0 78
hello.usa@jkp.com
http://www.jkp.com/jkp/distributors.php

Jessica Kingsley, Chairman
Jemima Kingsley, Director
Octavia Kingsley, Production Director
Lisa Clark, Sr. Commissioning Editor

Social and emotional development activities for Asperger Syndrome, Autism, PDD and NLD. Comprehensive set of activities emphasizes foundation skills for younger children between the ages of two and eight. Covers skills such as social referencing, regulating behvior, conversational reciprocity, and synchronized actions. For use in therapeutic settings as well as schools and parents. *$22.95*
256 pages
ISBN 1-843107-14-7

8754 Riddle of Autism: A Psychological Analysis
Jason Aronson
Ste 200
4501 Forbes Blvd
Lanham, MD 20706
301-459-3366
800-462-6420
FAX: 301-429-5746
customercare@nbnbooks.com
http://www.nbnbooks.com

Jason Brockwell, Sales Staff
Michael Sullivan, Sales
Mark Cozy, Sales Staff
Dennis Hayes, Director of Special Markets

Dr. Victor examines the myths that cloud an understanding of this disorder and describes the meanings of its specific behavioral symptoms. *$30.00*
356 pages Paperback
ISBN 1-568215-73-8

8755 Self-Therapy for the Stutterer
Stuttering Foundation of America
1805 Moriah Woods Blvd.
Suite 3
Memphis, TN 38117
901-761-0343
800-992-9392
FAX: 901-761-0484
info@stutteringhelp.org.
www.stutterhelp.org

Jane Fraser, President
Jean Gruss, Journalist
Robert M. Kurtz, Chairman & CEO
Malcolm Houg Fraser, Founder

A guide to help adults who stutter overcome the problem on their own. *$3.00*
191 pages Paperback
ISBN 0-933388-32-2

8756 Sex Education: Issues for the Person with Autism
Indiana Resource Center For Autism
1905 North Range Road
Bloomington, IN 47408-9801
812-855-6508
800-825-4733
FAX: 812-855-9630
iidc@indiana.edu
www.iidc.indiana.edu/irca

Cathy Pratt, Director
Catherine Davies, Educational Consultant
Pamela Anderson, Outreach/Resource Specialist
Melissa Dubie, Research Associate

Discusses issues of sexuality and provides methods of instruction for people with autism. *$4.00*

8757 Son-Rise: The Miracle Continues
2080 South Undermountain Road
Sheffield, MA 01257
413-229-2100
800-714-2779
sonrise@option.org
http://www.option.org

Samahria Lyt Kaufman, Co-Founder and Co-Director
Dane Griffith, Director of Administrative Services
Bears Kaufman, Co-Founder and Co-Director
Raun Kaufman, Director of Global Education

Part One is the astonishing record of Raun Kaufman's development from an autistic and retarded child into a loving, brilliant youngster who shows no traces of his former condition. Part Two follows Raun's development after the age of four, teaching the limitless possibilities of the Son-Rise Program. Part Three shares moving accounts of five other ordinary families who became extraordinary when they used the Son-Rise Program to reach their own unreachable children. *$12.95*
343 pages
ISBN 0-915811-53-7

8758 Sound Connections for the Adolescent
Speech Bin
P.O.Box 1579
Appleton, WI 54912-1579
419-589-1425
888-388-3224
FAX: 888-388-6344
info@speechbin.com
www.speechbin.com

James R. Henderson, Chairman
Joseph M. Yorio, President & CEO
Rick Holden, EVP, Educators Publishing Service
Patrick T. Collins, EVP, Distribution

A resource to help older elementary and secondary students understand their sound systems an how it functions. It targets skills critical for academic achievement: phonological awareness, phonemic relationships, phonemic processing, listening and memory and teaches linguistic rules they need to succeed. *$19.95*
Paperback

8759 Talkable Tales
Speech Bin-Abilitations
P.O.Box 1579
Appleton, WI 54912-1579
419-589-1425
888-388-3224
FAX: 888-388-6344
info@speechbin.com
www.speechbin.com

James R. Henderson, Chairman
Joseph M. Yorio, President & CEO
Rick Holden, EVP, Educators Publishing Service
Patrick T. Collins, EVP, Distribution

Read-a-rebus stories and pictures targeting most consonant phonemes for K-5 children. *$25.95*
128 pages
ISBN 0-93783 -44-0

8760 **Teaching Children with Autism: Strategies for Initiating Positive Interactions**
Brookes Publishing
P.O. Box 10624
Baltimore, MD 21285-0624
410-337-9585
888-337-8808
FAX: 410-337-8539
custserv@healthpropress.com
http://www.healthpropress.com

Melissa A. Behm, President
Mary Magnus, Director
Stategies for initiating positive interactions and improving learning opportunities. This guide begins with an overview of characteristics and long-term strategies and proceeds through discussions that detail specific techniques for normalizing environments, reducing disruptive behavior, improving language and social skills, and enhancing generalization. *$32.95*
256 pages Paperback
ISBN 1-55766-80-4

8761 **Teaching and Mainstreaming Autistic Children**
Love Publishing Company
9101 East Kenyon Avenue
Suite 2200
Denver, CO 80237
303-221-7333
FAX: 303-221-7444
lpc@lovepublishing.com
http://www.lovepublishing.com/

Peter Knoblock, Author
Dr. Knoblock advocates a highly organized, structured environment for autistic children, with teachers and parents working together. His premise is that the learning and social needs of autistic children must be analyzed and a daily program designed with interventions that respond to this functional analysis of their behavior. *$24.95*

ISBN 0-89108-11-9

8762 **Techniques for Aphasia Rehab: (TARGET) Generating Effective Treatment**
Speech Bin
P.O. Box 1579
Appleton, WI 54912-1579
419-589-1425
888-388-3224
FAX: 888-388-6344
info@speechbin.com
www.speechbin.com

James R. Henderson, Chairman
Joseph M. Yorio, President & CEO
Rick Holden, EVP, Educators Publishing Service
Patrick T. Collins, EVP, Distribution
Practical treatment manual for use by aphasia clinicians. *$45.00*
384 pages
ISBN 0-93785-50-5

8763 **Understanding & Controlling Stuttering: A Comprehensive New Approach Based on the Valsa Hyp**
National Stuttering Association
119 West 40th Street
14th Floor
New York, NY 10018
212-944-4050
800-937-8888
FAX: 212-944-8244
info@westutter.org
www.nsastutter.org

Kenny Koroll, Chair
Tammy Flores, Executive Director
Stephanie Coopen, Family Programs Administrator
Mandy Finstad, Editor/Webmaster
Demonstrates how physical and psychological factors may interact to stimulate and perpetuate stuttering through a Valsalva-Stuttering cycle. *$25.00*
176 pages
ISBN 7-929773-01-3

8764 **Verbal Behavior Approach: How to Teach Children with Autism & Related Disorders**
Autism Society of North Carolina Bookstore
Ste 230
505 Oberlin Rd
Raleigh, NC 27605-1345
919-743-0204
800-442-2762
FAX: 919-743-0208
jchampion@autismsociety-nc.com
http://www.autismsociety-nc.org

Sharon Jeffries-Jones, Chair
Elizabeth Phillippi, Vice Chair
Tracey Sheriff, CEO
Paul Wendler, CFO
Provides full descriptions of how to teach the verbal operants that make up expressive languate which include: manding, tacting, echoing and intraverbal skills. *$19.95*

8765 **Without Reason: A Family Copes with two Generations of Autism**
Books on Special Children
721 W Abram St
Arlington, TX 76013-6995
817-277-0727
800-489-0727
FAX: 817-277-2270
http://www.fhautism.com/

R. Wayne Gilpin, President
Jennifer Gilpin Yacio, Vice President and Editorial Director
David Reasor, CPA and Administrative Director
Teresa Corey, Conference Administrator
The author discovers his son has autism. He delves into problems of the autistic person and explains reasons for their actions. *$20.95*
292 pages Hardcover

Print: Journals

8766 **American Journal of Speech-Language Pathology**
American Speech-Language-Hearing Association
2200 Research Boulevard
Rockville, MD 20850-3289
301-296-5700
800-638-8255
FAX: 301-296-8580
nsslha@asha.org, productsales@asha.org
www.asha.org

Elizabeth S. McCrea, PhD, CCC-SLP, President
Barbara K. Cone, PhD, CCC-A, Vice President for Academic Affairs in Audiology
Carolyn W. Higdon, EdD, CCC-SLP, Vice President for Finance
Kaci Roger, Council Member
This is a quarterly journal of clinical practice for speech-language pathologists and language researchers. This journal will be online only beginning January 2010.

8767 **Journal of Speech, Language and Hearing Research**
American Speech-Language-Hearing Association
2200 Research Boulevard
Rockville, MD 20850-3289
301-296-5700
800-638-8255
FAX: 301-296-8580
nsslha@asha.org, productsales@asha.org
www.asha.org

Elizabeth S. McCrea, PhD, CCC-SLP, President
Barbara K. Cone, PhD, CCC-A, Vice President for Academic Affairs in Audiology
Carolyn W. Higdon, EdD, CCC-SLP, Vice President for Finance
Kaci Roger, Council Member
This bimonthly journal contains basic, as well as applied research in normal and disordered communication processes. It will be available online only beginning January 2010.

8768 Language, Speech, and Hearing Services in Schools
International Fluency Association
Northern Illinois University
Dept. of Communicative Disorders
DeKalb, IL 60115-2899

www.theifa.org

David Shapiro, President
Norimune Kawat, Secretary
Rachel Everard, Treasurer
Shelley Brundage, Membership
This is a quarterly journal focusing on research appropriate to speech-language pathologists and audiologists in schools. The journal will only be available online beginning in January 2010.

Print: Magazines

8769 Communication Outlook
Artificial Language Laboratory
220 Trowbridge Road
East Lansing, MI 48824

517-353-8332
FAX: 517-353-4766
artling@msu.edu
www.msu.edu

Lou Anna K. Simon, President
Satish Udpa, EVP for Administrative Services
Bill Beekman, VP & Secretary
Mark P. Haas, VP for Finance & Treasurer
Communication Outlook (CO) is an international quarterly magazine, which focuses on the techniques and technology of augmentative and alternative communication. CO provides information on technological developments for persons experiencing communication handicaps due to neurological, sensory or neuromuscular conditions. *$18.00*
32 pages Quarterly

Print: Newsletters

8770 Access Audiology
American Speech-Language-Hearing Association
2200 Research Boulevard
Rockville, MD 20850-3289

301-296-5700
800-638-8255
FAX: 301-296-8580
nsslha@asha.org, productsales@asha.org
www.asha.org

Elizabeth S. McCrea, PhD, CCC-SLP, President
Barbara K. Cone, PhD, CCC-A, Vice President for Academic Affairs in Audiology
Carolyn W. Higdon, EdD, CCC-SLP, Vice President for Finance
Kaci Roger, Council Member
Dedicated to the specific needs of all professionals interested in hearing, balance, and the field of audiology. Each issue spotlights a specific topic of interest and relevance to audiologists.

8771 Autism Research Review International
Autism Research Institute
4182 Adams Avenue
San Diego, CA 92116-2599

619-281-7165
866-366-3361
FAX: 619-563-6840
br@autismresearchinstitute.com
autism.com

Stephen Edelson, Executive Director
Jane Johnson, Managing Director
Valerie Paradiz, Director
Anthony Morgali, Producer
Provides clearly written summaries of articles selected from computer searches. *$18.00*
8 pages Quarterly

8772 Communicologist
Texas Speech-Language-Hearing Association
Ste 200
918 Congress Ave
Austin, TX 78701-2342

512-494-1128
888-729-8742
FAX: 512-494-1129
tsha@assnmgmt.com
cisaustin.org

Judith Keller, President
Larry Higdon, Director
Melanie McDonald, President Elect
Tori Gustafson, Vice President
A forum for distributing current information relevant to the practices of speech-language pathology and audiology across the state. Provides TSHA membership with the latest news from the Executive Board and Task Forces, as well as information about regional associations, distinguished service providers, the TSHA Annual Convention, and committee honors and nominations. Also contains advertisements of interest to the field.

8773 Connect
Hearing, Speech & Deafness Center (HSDC)
1625 19th Avenue
Seattle, WA 98122

206-323-5770
888-222-5036
FAX: 206-328-6871
hsdc@hsdc.org
www.hsdc.org

Pamela Anderson, President
Ken Block, VP
David Webster, Director of Finance
Brayde Williamson, Director of Education
A newsletter that addresses concerns of those affected by speech and language disorders.
8 pages Quarterly

8774 NSSLHA Now
Ntn'l Student Speech Language Hearing Association
2200 Research Boulevard
Rockville, MD 20850-3289

301-296-5700
800-638-8255
FAX: 301-296-8580
nsslha@asha.org, productsales@asha.org
www.asha.org

Elizabeth S. McCrea, PhD, CCC-SLP, President
Barbara K. Cone, PhD, CCC-A, Vice President for Academic Affairs in Audiology
Carolyn W. Higdon, EdD, CCC-SLP, Vice President for Finance
Kaci Roger, Council Member
Published three times per year.

8775 On Cue
National Cued Speech Association
1300 Pennsylvania Avenue, NW
Suite 190-713
Washington, DC 20004

301-915-8009
800-459-3529
www.cuedspeech.org

Shannon Howell, President
Penny Hakim, 1st Vice President
John Brubaker, VP Fundraising
Doug Dawson, Treasurer
Published several times a year and mailed to members of the Association.

8776 **Stuttering & Your Child: Help For Parents**
Stuttering Foundation of America
18005 Moriah Woods Blvd
PO Box 11749, Suite 3
Memphis, TN 38111-0749
901-761-0343
800-992-9392
FAX: 901-761-0484
info@stutteringhelp.org
www.StutteringHelp.org

Jane Fraser, President
Dennis Drayna, Director
Joseph R. G. Fulcher, Director
Frances Cook, Director

The Stuttering Foundation provides resources, services and support to those who stutter and their families, as well as support research into the cause of stuttering. The Stuttering Foundation provides a referral list of speech-language pathologists and referrals to other information including research on stuttering, intensive workshops and camps. *$10.00*

8777 **Stuttering Foundation Newsletter**
Stuttering Foundation of America
P.O.Box 11749
Memphis, TN 38111-0749
901-761-0343
800-992-9392
FAX: 901-761-0484
info@stutteringhelp.org
www.stutteringhelp.org

Jane Fraser, President
Jean Gruss, Journalist
Robert M. Kurtz, Chairman & CEO
Malcolm Houg Fraser, Founder

8778 **Voice**
Providence Speech and Hearing Association
1301 Providence Avenue
Orange, CA 92868
714-923-1521
855-901-7742
FAX: 714-744-3841
pshc@pshc.org
www.pshc.org

Lewis Jaffe, President
Bret Rathwick, Vice President - Finance
Casey Immel, Treasurer
Marlene Woodworth, Secretary

People of all ages with speech and hearing problems by providing specialized products and services.

Non Print: Newsletters

8779 **Access Academics & Research**
American Speech-Language-Hearing Association
2200 Research Boulevard
Rockville, MD 20850-3289
301-296-5700
800-638-8255
FAX: 301-296-8580
nsslha@asha.org, productsales@asha.org
www.asha.org

Elizabeth S. McCrea, PhD, CCC-SLP, President
Barbara K. Cone, PhD, CCC-A, Vice President for Academic Affairs in Audiology
Carolyn W. Higdon, EdD, CCC-SLP, Vice President for Finance
Kaci Roger, Council Member

Dedicated to the specific needs of academic and clinical faculty, PhD students and researchers. The e-newsletter was developed as part of the Focused Initiative on the PhD Shortage in Higher Education.

8780 **Access SLP Health Care**
American Speech-Language-Hearing Association
2200 Research Boulevard
Rockville, MD 20850-3289
301-296-5700
800-638-8255
FAX: 301-296-8580
nsslha@asha.org, productsales@asha.org
www.asha.org

Elizabeth S. McCrea, PhD, CCC-SLP, President
Barbara K. Cone, PhD, CCC-A, Vice President for Academic Affairs in Audiology
Carolyn W. Higdon, EdD, CCC-SLP, Vice President for Finance
Kaci Roger, Council Member

An e-newsletter dedicated to the specific needs of speech-language pathologists in healthcare settings. Each issue of Access SLP Health Care features recent legislative activity impacting SLPs and provides information on clinical issues, continuing education opportunities, and ASHA web-based resources.

8781 **Access Schools**
American Speech-Language-Hearing Association
2200 Research Boulevard
Rockville, MD 20850-3289
301-296-5700
800-638-8255
FAX: 301-296-8580
nsslha@asha.org, productsales@asha.org
www.asha.org

Elizabeth S. McCrea, PhD, CCC-SLP, President
Barbara K. Cone, PhD, CCC-A, Vice President for Academic Affairs in Audiology
Carolyn W. Higdon, EdD, CCC-SLP, Vice President for Finance
Kaci Roger, Council Member

Dedicated to the specific needs of school-based speech-language pathologists. Each Access Schools e-newsletter features recent legislative activity impacting school SLPs and provides information on clinical issues, continuing education opportunities, and ASHA web-based resources.

8782 **Stuttering**
Federal Government
31 Center Drive MSC 2320
Bethesda, MD 20892-2320
301-496-7243
800-241-1044
FAX: 301-402-0018
nidcdinfo@nidcd.nih.gov
www.nidcd.nih.gov

James F. Battey, Director
Judith A. Cooper, Deputy Director
Timothy J. Wheeles, Executive Officer
Tanya Brown, Executive Assistant

Describes how speech is produced, treatments for stuttering and research supported by the federal government.

Non Print: Video

8783 **Autism: A World Apart**
Fanlight Productions
c/o Icarus Films
32 Court Street, 21st Floor
Brooklyn, NY 11201
718-488-8900
800-876-1710
FAX: 718-488-8642
info@fanlight.com, sales@icarusfilms.com
www.fanlight.com

Ben Achtenberg, Owner, Founder
Nicole Johnson, Publicity Coordinator
Anthony Sweeney, Marketing Director

In this documentary, three families show us what the textbooks and studies cannot: what it's like to live with autism day after day; to raise and love children who may be withdrawn and violent and unable to make personal connections with their families. 29 minutes.
VHS/DVD
ISBN 1-572950-39-0

8784 Autism: the Unfolding Mystery
Aquarius Health Care Media
18 N Main St
Sherborn, MA 1770-1066   508-650-1616
                                 lkussmann@aquariusproductions.com
Lesile Kussmann, Owner
Explore what it means to be autistic, how you can recognize the signs of autism in your child, and hear about new treatments and programs to help children learn to deal with the disorder. *$145.00 DVD*

8785 Getting Started with Facilitated Communication
Facilitated Communication Institute, Syracuse Univ
370 Huntington Hall
Syracuse, NY 13244-1   315-443-9657
                               FAX: 315-443-9218
                               fcstaff@syr.edu
                               www.thefci.syr.edu
Annegret Schubert, Producer
Describes in detail how to help individuals with autism and/or severe communication difficulties to get started with facilitated communication.
Video

8786 I Just Want My Little Boy Back
Autism Treatment Center Of America
2080 South Undermountain Road
Sheffield, MA 01257   413-229-2100
                             800-714-2779
                             happiness@option.org
                             http://www.option.org
Samahria Lyt Kaufman, Co-Founder and Co-Director
Dane Griffith, Director of Administrative Services
Bears Kaufman, Co-Founder and Co-Director
Raun Kaufman, Director of Global Education
A great video for parents and professionals caring for children with special needs. Join one British family and their autistic son before, during and after their journey to America to attend The Son-Rise Program at The Autism Treatment Center of America. This informative, inspirational and deeply moving story not only captures the joy, tears, challenges and triumps of this amazing little boy and his family, but also serves as a powerful introduction to the attitude and principles of the program. *$25.00*

8787 Understanding Autism
Fanlight Productions
c/o Icarus Films
32 Court Street, 21st Floor
Brooklyn, NY 11201   718-488-8900
                            800-876-1710
                            FAX: 718-488-8642
                            info@fanlight.com, sales@icarusfilms.com
                            www.fanlight.com
Ben Achtenberg, Owner, Founder
Nicole Johnson, Publicity Coordinator
Anthony Sweeney, Marketing Director
Parents of children with autism discuss the nature and symptoms of this lifelong disability and outline a treatment program based on behavior modification principles. 19 minutes
VHS/DVD
ISBN 1-572951-00-1

Support Groups

8788 Autism Society of America
4340 East West Highway
Suite 350
Bethesda, MD 20814-3067   301-657-0881
                                 800-328-8476
                                 FAX: 301-657-0869
                                 dallen@autism-society.org
                                 www.autism-society.org
Mary Beth Collins, Director of Programs
Tonia Ferguson, Senior Director of Content
Scott Badesch, President/Chief Executive Officer
John Dabrowski, Chief Financial Officer

ASA is the largest and oldest grassroots organization within the autism community, with a nationwide network of chapters and over 20,000 members and supporters nationwide. ASA is the leading source of education, information and referral about autism and has been the leader in advocacy and legislative initiatives for more than four decades.

8789 Cherab Foundation
P.O.Box 8524
Port St Lucie, FL 34985-8524   772-335-5135
                                       FAX: 772-337-4812
                                       help@cherab.org
                                       www.cherab.org
Marilyn Agin, MD
Lisa Geng, Co Author
Helps to start, supports, and works together with other support groups and nonprofits (such as ECHO, VOICES, and Apraxia Network) that have mutual goals for helping children with apraxia and other speech disorders.

8790 Friends: National Association of Young People who Stutter
38 S Oyster Bay Rd
Syosset, NY 11791-5033
                                       866-866-8335
                                       lcaggiano@aol.com
                                       www.friendswhostutter.org
Lee Caggiano, President
A national organization created to provide a network of love and support for children and teenagers who stutter, their families, and the professionals who work with them.

8791 National Health Information Center
US Department of Health
P.O.Box 1133
Washington, DC 20013-1133   301-565-4167
                                    800-336-4797
                                    301-468-7394
                                    FAX: 301-984-4256
                                    healthypeople@hhs.gov
                                    http://www.healthypeople.gov
Jonathan Fielding, Chair
Shirika Kumanyika, Vice Chair
A health information referral service that puts health professionals and consumers who have health questions in touch with those organizations that are best able to provide answers.

8792 Speech Pathways
410 Meadow Creek Drive
Suite 206
Westminster, MD 21158   410-374-0555
                                800-961-2724
                                FAX: 410-374-8620
                                kim.bell@speechpathways.net
                                speechpathways.net
Kimberly A. Bell, Owner
Karie Hadley, Therapist
Erica Hamilton, Therapist
Julie Kumpar, Therapist
We realize that parent and family support is critical to a child's success, in therapy as well as in life. We offer support at local and regional levels along with traditional speech and language services, and a wide variety of specialized pediatric programs. Our support groups/services are open to the larger community as well as to our clients.

Visual

Associations

8793 ACB Government Employees
American Council of the Blind
2200 Wilson Blvd
Ste 650
Arlington, VA 22201-3354
202-467-5081
800-424-8666
FAX: 703-465-5085
info@acb.org
www.acb.org

Sarah Presley, President
Kim Charlson, Vice President
Marliana Lieberg, Secretary
Carla Ruschival, Treasurer
Members are present, former and retired employees of federal, state and local government agencies. Concerns of the organization include recruitment, placement and advancement of blind and visually impaired employees.

8794 ACB Radio Amateurs
American Council of the Blind
167 Green St
Reading, MA 01867
202-467-5081
800-424-8666
FAX: 202-467-5085
acbra@acb.org
www.acbhams.org

Steve Dresser, President
Mike Duke, Vice President
Robert Rogers, Treasurer
Robert Spangler, Secretary
ACBRA is an organization of blind and sighted licensed radio amateurs who work together to make the hobby more accessible to people who are blind

8795 ACB Social Service Providers
American Council of the Blind
2200 Wilson Blvd
Ste 650
Arlington, VA 22201-3354
202-467-5081
800-424-8666
FAX: 703-465-5085
info@acb.org
www.acb.org

Mitch Pomerantz, President
Kim Charlson, Vice President
Marliana Lieberg, Secretary
Carla Ruschival, Treasurer
Blind and visually impaired social workers, social service professionals, students pursuing careers in social work and other interested persons are members of this organization. ACBSSP works to promote full participation by visually impaired social services professionals in the field of social welfare.

8796 Achromatopsia Network
PO Box 214
Berkeley, CA 94701-214
510-540-4700
FAX: 510-540-4767
achromatopsia@cox.net
www.achromat.org

Frances Futterman, President
The Achromatopsia Network is a nonprofit organization for individuals concerned with achromatopsia. It is committed to sharing information about achromatopsia and providing resources to meet the special needs of those affected by this eye condition; helping individuals and families concerned with achromatopsia to connect with one another; and promoting awareness and educating with a special emphasis on accomplishing this goal among those who provides services to the visually impaired.

8797 American Academy of Ophthalmology
655 Beach St.
PO Box 7424
San Francisco, CA 94120-7424
415-561-8500
866-561-8558
FAX: 415-561-8533
customer_service@aao.org
www.aao.org

Randy Johnston, President
The American Academy of Ophthalmology is the largest national membership association of Eye M.D.s. Eye M.D.s are ophthalmologists, medical and osteopathic doctors who provide comprehensive eye care, including medical, surgical and optical care. More than 90 percent of practicing U.S. Eye M.D.s are Academy members, and the Academy has more than 7,000 international members.

8798 American Action Fund for Blind Children and Adults
1800 Johnston St
Ste 100
Baltimore, MD 21230-4914
410-659-9315
FAX: 410-685-5653
actionfund@actionfund.org
www.actionfund.org

Barbara Loos, President
Ramona Walhof, Vice President
Sandra Halverson, Second Vice President/Medical Transcriptionist
James Omvig, Treasurer
A service agency which specializes in providing to blind people help which is not readily available to them from government programs or other existing service systems. The services are planned especially to meet the needs of blind children, the elderly blind, and the deaf-blind.

8799 American Council of Blind Lions
148 Vernon Avenue
Suite 650
Louisville, KY 40206-3354
502-897-1472
800-424-8666
FAX: 703-465-5085
info@acb.org
www.acb.org/acbl

Mitch Pomerantz, President
Kim Charlson, First Vice President
Brenda Dillon, Second Vice President
Marlaina Lieberg, Secretary
A wonderful combination of Lionism and visual impairment nurtures the American Council of Blind Lions. ACBL's mission is awareness and highlights the great activities of the Knights of the Blind. The goals are to assist all clubs in their understanding of issues surrounding blind and visually impaired individuals.

8800 American Council of the Blind
2200 Wilson Blvd
Ste 650
Arlington, VA 22201-3354
202-467-5081
800-424-8666
FAX: 703-465-5085
ebridges@acb.org
www.acb.org

Mitch Pomerantz, President
Kim Charlson, Vice President
Marliana Lieberg, Secretary
Carla Ruschival, Treasurer
A national membership organization whose members are visually impaired and fully sighted individuals who are concerned about the dignity and well-being of blind people throughout America. Formed in 1961, the Council has become the largest organization of blind people in the US with over 70 state affiliates and special interest chapters.

8801 American Foundation for the Blind
11 Penn Plz
Suite 300
New York, NY 10121-2018

212-502-7600
800-232-5463
FAX: 212-502-7777
afbinfo@afb.net
www.afb.org

Carl Augusto, President/CEO
Paul Schroeder, Vice President
Rick Bozeman, Director
Scott Truax, Manager
The organizaton to which Helen Keller devoted her life, is a national nonprofit organization whose mission is to ensure that the ten million Americans who are blind or visually impaired enjoy the same rights and opportunities as other citizens.

8802 American Optometric Association
243 N Lindbergh Blvd
Saint Louis, MO 63141-7881

314-991-4100
800-365-2219
FAX: 314-991-4101
MDJones@aoa.org
www.aoa.org

Ronald L Hopping, President
Mitchell Munson, President-Elect
David A. Cockrell, Vice President
Steven Loomis, Secretary-Treasurer
the AOA is the acknowledged leader and recognised authority for the eye and vision care in the world. The objectives of the AOA are centered on improving the quality and availiability of eye and vision care. The AOA fulfills its missions in accordance with health care and public policy related to eye care will uniformly recognise optometrists as primary health care providers and ensure the public has acess to the full scope of optometric care.

8803 American Printing House for the Blind
1839 Frankfort Avenue
PO Box 6085
Louisville, KY 40206- 0085

502-895-2405
800-223-1839
FAX: 502-899-2284
info@aph.org
www.aph.org

Charles Barr, Chairman
The world's largest nonprofit organization creating educational, workplace and independent living products and services for people who are visually impaired. Also promotes independence of the blind and visually impaired persons by providing specialized materials, products, and services needed for educationand life.

8804 Associated Blind

212-683-4950
FAX: 212-683-4975
memberservices@esightcareers.net
www.tabinc.org

Nancy O'Connell, Executive Director
Privately funded, non-profit agency, that was founded by a group of blind individuals as an organization promoting autonomy and self-determination. The mission is to assist individuals who are blind, visualy impaired or who have physical disabilities to become self-reliant and achieve financial independence through mainstream employment.

8805 Associated Services for the Blind
919 Walnut St
Philadelphia, PA 19107-5287

215-627-0600
FAX: 215-922-0692
asbinfo@asb.org
www.asb.org

Patricia C. Johnson, President/Chief Executive Officer
Derby Ewing, Director, Human Services
Richard Forsythe, Director, Braille Division and Custom Audio
Linda Gaffney, Coordinator, Volunteer Services
ASB, a non-private, non-profit organization, promotes self esteem, independence, and self-determination in people who are blind or visually impaired. ASB accomplishes this by providing support through education, training and resources, as well as through community action and public education, serving as a voice and advocate for the rights of all people who are blind or visually impaired.

8806 Association for Education & Rehabilitationof the Blind & Visually Impaired
1703 N Beauregard St
Suite 440
Alexandria, VA 22311-1744

703-671-4500
877-492-2708
FAX: 703-671-6391
jgandorf@aerbvi.org
www.aerbvi.org

Mr. Jim Adams, President
Ms. Christy Shepard, President-elect
Dr. Susan Jay Spungin, Secretary
Mr. Cliff Olstrom, Treasurer
The mission of AER is to support professionals who provide education and rehabilitation services to people with visual impairments, offering professional development opportunities, publications, and public advocacy.

8807 Association for Macular Diseases
210 E 64th St
8th Fl
New York, NY 10065-7471

212-605-3719
800-622-8524
FAX: 212-605-3795
association@retinal-research.org
www.macula.org

Bernard Landou, President
Mary Fern Breheney, Board Member
Fern Breheney, Board Member
Joan R. Daly, Board Member
The Macula Foundation, Inc., a not-for-profit organization was established in 1978 to support basic and clinical research in vitreous retinal and macular diseases, a major cause of blindness of all age groups. Since it was formed, the Foundation has distributed grants and awards of approximately 15 million dollars earmarked for important clinical and scientific research and related teaching programs. Numerous research projects have been successful as a result of the Foundation.

8808 Association for Research in Vision and Ophthalmology
1801 Rockville Pike,
Suite 400
Rockville, MD 20852-5622

240-221-2900
FAX: 240-221-0370
www.arvo.org

Iris M. Rush, CAE, Executive Director
Joanne Olson, Deputy Executive Director
Loren Malaney, Director, Human Resources
Betsy Clarke, Manager, Executive Operations
ARVO advances research worldwide into understanding the visual system and preventing, treating and curing its disorders

8809 Association for Vision Rehabilitation andEmployment
174 Court St
Binghamton, NY 13901

607-724-2428
FAX: 607-771-8045
avreinfo@avreus.org
www.avreus.org

Shawnna Armstrong, Vision Rehabilitation Therapist
John Martin, Chair
Kelly Storm, Vice Chair
Brian Kessler, Secretary
A private, non-profit organization that serves people with sustained and severe vision loss. People of all ages, from infants to seniors, can and do benefit from our services.

8810 Association of Blind Citizens
PO Box 246
Holbrook, MA 2343

781-961-1023
FAX: 781-961-0004
president@blindcitizens.org
www.blindcitizens.org

8811 Blind Childrens Center
4120 Marathon St
Los Angeles, CA 90029-3584
323-664-2153
800-222-3566
FAX: 323-665-3828
info@blindchildrenscenter.org
www.blindchildrenscenter.org

Lena French, Executive Director
Fernanda Armenta-Schmitt, PhD, Director of Education & Family
Services/Assistant Executive
Muriel Scharf, Director of Development
Ross Vergara, Director of Finance

A family centered agency which serves children with visual impairments from birth to school-age. The center-based and home-based programs and services help the children aquire skills and build their independence. The center utilizes its expertise and experience to serve families and professionals worldwide through support services, education, and research.

8812 Blind Information Technology Specialists
American Council of the Blind
2200 Wilson Blvd
Ste 650
Arlington, VA 22201-3354
703-841-0048
800-424-8666
202-465-5085
FAX: 703-465-5085
president@bits-acb.org
www.bits-acb.org

Richard Villa, President
Renee Zelickson, Vice President
Tom L. Jones, Secretary
Lynne Koral, Treasurer

BITS is a non profit organization which fosters the career development of blind computer professionals, promotes the use of computer technology by blind persons to improve the qualtiy of their personal and professional lives, and advocate for improved information access for all visually impaired people.

8813 Blinded Veterans Association
477 H St NW
Washington, DC 20001-2694
202-371-8880
800-669-7079
FAX: 202-371-8258
bva@bva.org
www.bva.org

Samuel Huhn, President
Mark Cornell, Vice President
Robert Dale Stamper, Secretary
Roy Young, Treasurer

BVA locates blinded veterans who need assistance, guides them through the rehabilitation process, and acts as advocates for them before Congress and the Department of Veterans Affairs in the securing of all the benefits they have earned throught their service to the nation. Promotes access to technology and the practical use of the latest research. Its Field Service Program provides encouragement and emotional support through role models, who can demonstrate that the challenges can be overcome.

8814 Books for Blind and Physically Handicapped Individuals
Library of Congress
1291 Taylor St NW
Washington, DC 20011
202-707-5100
888-657-7323
FAX: 202-707-0712
TTY: 202-707-0744
nls@loc.gov
www.loc.gov/nls

Frank Cylke, Director

Administers a national library service that provides braille and recorded books and magazines on free loan to anyone who cannot read standard print because of visual of physical disabilities who are eligible residents of the Unites States of America citizens living abroad.

8815 Braille Institute of America
741 N Vermont Ave
Los Angeles, CA 90029-3594
323-663-1111
800-272-4553
FAX: 323-663-0867
tours@brailleinstitute.org
www.brailleinstitute.org

Lester M. Sussman, Chair
Percy Duran, Audit
Richard Larson, Development
Harvey Strode, Finance

Provides an environment of hope and encouragement for people who are blind and visually impaired through integrated educational, social and recreational programs and services. Provides assistance at 5 regional centers in Southern California and through 200 community outreach programs. In 2005-06, the Institute provided these services to more than 55,000 people. The Institute is operated and funded almost entirely through private individual and foundation sources.

8816 California State Library Braille and Talking Book Library
PO Box 942837
Sacramento, CA 94237-0001
916-634-0640
800-952-5666
FAX: 916-654-1119
btbl@library.ca.gov
www.btbl.ca.gov

Mike Marlin, Director

The State Library stands as one of California's great public research institutions with a five-fold mission:serving the needs of elected officials and state agency employees;preserving the state's cultural heritage by collecting historic materials on California and the West;assisting public libraries through financial aid and consulting services;offering special services to disadvantaged and handicapped clients;ensuring that the general public has convenient and consistent access to resources.

8817 Canine Helpers for the Handicapped
5699 Ridge Rd
Lockport, NY 14094-9408
716-433-4035
FAX: 716-439-0822
chhdogs@aol.com
www.caninehelpers.netfirms.com

Beverly Underwood, Executive Director
Laura Gates, Trainer

A nonprofit organization devoted to custom training Assistance Dogs to assist people with disabilities to lead more independent, secure lives.

8818 Caption Center
125 Western Ave
Boston, MA 02134
617-300-3600
FAX: 617-300-1020
TTY:617-300-3600
access@wgbh.org
www.mattapanchc.org

Cristopher Brandon, Chair
Glenola Mitchell, Vice Chair
Dale L. Kurtz, Treasurer
Nelda M. Headley, Secretary

Has been pioneering and delivering accessible media to disabled adults, students and their families, teachers and friends for over 30 years. Each year, the Center captions more than 10,000 hours worth of broadcast and cable programs, feature films, large-format and IMAX films, home videos, music videos, DVDs, teleconferences and CD-Roms.

8819 Central Association for the Blind & Visually Impaired
507 Kent St.
Utica, NY 13501
315-797-2233
877-719-9996
www.cabvi.org

Edward P. Welsh, Chair
Kenneth C. Thayer, Vice Chair
Richard Evans, Treasurer
Marie Bord, Secretary

It assists people who are blind or visually impaired to achieve their highest levels of independence.

8820 Chicago Lighthouse for People who are Blind and Visually Impaired
1850 W Roosevelt Rd
Chicago, IL 60608-1298
312-666-1331
FAX: 312-243-8539
TTY:312-666-8874
support@chicagolighthouse.org
www.chicagolighthouse.org

Bruce R. Hague, Chairman
Sandra C. Forsythe, Vice Chairman
Janet P. Szlyk, President
David Huber, Treasurer

A non profit agency committed to providing the highest quality educational, clinical, vocational, and rehabilitation services for children, youth and adults who are blind or visually impaired, including deaf blind and multi disabled. Also respects personal dignity and partners with individuals to enhance independent living and self sufficiency. This agency is a leader, innovator and advocate for people who are blind or visually impaired, enhancing the quality of life for all individuals.

8821 Clovernook Center for the Blind and Visually Impaired
7000 Hamilton Ave
Cincinnati, OH 45231-5240
513-522-3860
888-234-7156
FAX: 513-728-3946
TTY:513-522-3860
contact@clovernook.org
www.clovernook.org

Alfred J. Tuchfarber, Chair
Wilbert F. Schwartz, Vice Chair
Mark Jackson, Treasurer
Thomas R. Flottman, Secretary

Mission is to promote independence and foster the highest quality of life for people with visual impairments, including those with additional disabilities. We provide comprehensive program services including training and support for independent living, orientation and mobility instruction, vocational training, job placement, counseling, recreation, and youth services. Meaningful employment opportunities are also provided to individuals who are blind or visually impaired.

8822 Clovernook Printing House, The Clovernook Center for the Blind and Visually Impaired
7000 Hamilton Ave
Cincinnati, OH 45231-5240
513-522-3860
888-234-7156
FAX: 513-728-3946
contact@clovernook.org
www.clovernook.org

Alfred J. Tuchfarber, Chair
Wilbert F. Schwartz, Vice Chair
Mark Jackson, Treasurer
Thomas R. Flottman, Secretary

Clovernook also offers Braille Transcription Services including: Literary Books, Literary Magazines, Religious Materials, Instructional Manuals, ADA Conformance Materials, Literary Textbook Materials, Menus, Braille Alphabet Cards, and Forms. In addition, our Business Operations provide meaningful employment opportunities for individuals who are blind or visually impaired, while at the same time manufacturing high-quality products for customers across the country. *$145.00*
591 pages
ISBN 1-930956-48-7

8823 College of Optometrists in Vision Development
215 W Garfield Rd
Ste 200
Aurora, OH 44202-7884
330-995-0718
888-268-3770
FAX: 330-995-0719
info@covd.org
www.covd.org

David A. Damari, President
Kara Heying, Vice President
Christine Allison, Secretary-Treasurer
Pamela R. Happ, Executive Director

The College of Optometrists in Vision Development (COVD) is an international membership association of eye care professionals including optometrists, optometry students, and vision therapists. Members of COVD provide developmental vision care, vision therapy and vision rehabilitation services for children and adults.

8824 College of Syntonic Optometry
2052 W. Morales Drive
Pueblo West, CO 81007-4202
719-547-8177
877-559-0541
FAX: 719-547-3750
Syntonics@q.com
www.collegeofsyntonicoptometry.com

Larry Wallace, O.D., FCSO, Education Director
Mary Van Hoy, O.D., FCOVD,, President
Stefan Collier, F.O., FCSO, Vice President
John Pulaski, O.D., FCSO, Treasurer

An active and growing post-graduate educational organization. Established in 1933 its members include optometrists and other health professionals and supporters from around the world. Those who achieve a clinical level of experience and mastery are awarded the status of Fellow. Today, scientific as well as clinical verification of light's impact on health and healing and a growing public demand for functional and rehabilitative vision therapy continue to vitalise the college and its mission.

8825 Columbia Lighthouse for the Blind
1825 K St NW
Suite 1103
Washington, DC 20910-1261
301-589-0894
877-324-5252
FAX: 202-955-6401
info@clb.org
www.clb.org

Tony Cancelosi, President
Anthony J. (Cancelosi, K.M., President/CEO

Offer programs that enable individuals who are blind or visually impaired to obtain and maintain independence at home, school, work and in the community. The programs and services include asistive technology training, career services, rehabilitation services, comprehensive low vision care and a wide range of children's programs.

8826 Council of Families with Visual Impairments
American Council of the Blind
1155 15th St NW
Ste 1004
Washington, DC 20005-2706
202-467-5081
800-424-8666
FAX: 202-467-5085
cindy.vw@msn.com
www.acb.org

Jill Gaus, President
Lynn Jansen, Vice President
Debby Lieberman, Secretary
Mike Reese, Treasurer

A network of parents with blind or visually impaired children that offers support and outreach, shares experiences in parent/child relationships, exchanges educational, cultural and medical information about child development and more.

8827 Deaf-Blind Division of the National Federation of the Blind
200 East Wells Street
Baltimore, MD 21230-4914
410-659-9314
FAX: 410-685-5653
nfb@nfb.org
www.nfb.org

Marc Maurer, CEO

The nation's largest and most influential membership organization of blind persons, with a two-fold purpose: to help blind persons achieve self-confidence and self respect and to act as a vehicle for collective self-expression by the blind. The NFB improves blind people's lives through advocacy, education, research, technology, and programs encouraging independence and self-confidence. It is the leading force in the blindness field today and is the voice of the nations blind.

8828   **Desert Blind and Handicapped Association**
777 E Tahquitz Canyon Way
Suite 200-48
Palm Springs, CA 92262   760-969-5025
                                      info@desertblind.org
                                      www.desertblind.org

Mike Carson, President
Karen Travaglino, Vice President
Diane Stielstra, Secretary
George Holliday, Treasurer
It helps people to remain independent for as long as practical by
providing the transportation they need.

8829   **Eye Bank Association of America**
1015 18th St NW
Suite 1010
Washington, DC 20036-5223   202-775-4999
                                       FAX: 202-429-6036
                                      info@restoresight.org
                                      www.restoresight.org

David Korroch, Chair
David Glasser, Chair-Elect
Donna Drury, Secretary
Woodford Van Meter, Treasurer
Established in 1961 by the American Academy of Ophthalmology's Committee on Eye Banks, the EBAA is a not-for-profit organization of eye banks dedicated to the restoration of sight
through the promotion and advancement of eye banking. The
EBAA has lead the transplantation field with the establishment of
medical standards for the procurement and distribution of corneal
tissue, accreditation of eye banks, and comprehensive education
programs for doctors, technicians, and administrators.

8830   **Fidelco Guide Dog Foundation**
103 Vision Way
Bloomfield, CT 06002-1424   860-243-5200
                                       FAX: 860-243-7215
                                       info@fidelco.org
                                       www.fidelco.org

Stephen H. Matheson, Chairman
John H. Gotta, Vice Chairman
Glynis Cassis, Secretary
Mary P. CraigCraig, DVM, MBA,, Treasurer
The Fidelco Guide Dog Foundation, located in Bloomfield,
Conn., is dedicated to providing increased freedom and inde-
pendence to men and women who are blind by providing them
with the highest quality guide dogs. We rely solely on the gifts
and the generosity of individuals, foundations, corporations and
organizations that partner with Fidelco to 'Share the Vision.'

8831   **Fight for Sight**
381 Park Ave S
Suite 809
New York, NY 10016-8806   212-679-6060
                                       FAX: 212-679-4466
                                      info@fightforsight.com
                                      www.fightforsight.com

Norman J. Kleiman, Ph.D., Board President
Gaby Kressly, BoardSecretary/Treasurer
Janice Benson, Asst Director
Amanda Angulo, Board Member
The mission is to support vision research, to find causes and cures
for blindness, and to help save the sight of children through sup-
port of pediatric eye centers.

8832   **Foundation Fighting Blindness**
7168 Columbia Gateway Dr
Ste 100
Columbia, MD 21046   410-423-0600
                                           800-683-5555
                                       FAX: 410-363-2393
                                       TTY: 800-683-5551
                                      info@fightblindness.org
                                      www.blindness.org

William T. Schmidt, Chief Executive Officer
Valerie Navy-Daniels, Chief Development Officer
Stephen M. Rose, Chief Research Officer
Rhea K. Farberman, Senior Director, Communications &
Marketing
The aim of the Foundation Fighting Blindness, Inc. is to drive the
research that will provide preventions, treatments and cures for
people affected by the entire spectrum of retinal degenerative
diseases.

8833   **Guide Dog Users**
4851 N. Cedar Ave.
Apt 119
Fresno, CA 93726-2245   301-598-2131
                                           866-799-8436
                                       FAX: 301-871-7591
                                       treasurer@gdui.org
                                       www.gdui.org

Laurie Mehta, President
Mary Beth Randall, First Vice President
Charles Crawford, Second Vice President
Sarah Calhoun, Secretary
Guide Dog Users Inc, (GDUI) an affiliate of the American Council of the Blind, is the largest guide dog consumer driven group in
the world. Since 1972, members can excercise the privilege of
shaping the initiatives and issues that most profoundly affect
guide dog handlers. GDUI has 19 affiliate organizations throughout the US where members can personally interact and work together on local as well as global issues.

8834   **Guide Dogs for the Blind**
PO Box 151200
San Rafael, CA 94915-1200   415-499-4000
                                           800-295-4050
                                       FAX: 415-499-4035
                                      information@guidedogs.com
                                      www.guidedogs.com

Bob Burke, Chair
Paul A. Lopez, President & CEO
George Kercher, Vice Chair
Stuart Odell, Vice Chair, Finance
A nonprofit, charitable organization with a mission to provide
Guide Dogs and training in their use to visually impaired people
throughout the United States and Canada.

8835   **Guiding Eyes for the Blind**
611 Granite Springs Rd
Yorktown Heights, NY 10598-3499   914-245-4024
                                           800-942-0149
                                       FAX: 914-245-1609
                                       info@guidingeyes.org
                                       guidingeyes.org

Wendy Aglietti, Chairman
Mary J. Conway, Vice Chair
Curt J. Landtroop, Vice Chair/Treasurer
Lorraine Miller, Secretary
An internationally recognized guide dog school that is dedicated
to enriching the lives of blind and visually impaired men and
women by providing them with the freedom to travel safely,
thereby assuring greater independence, dignity and new horizons
of opportunity

8836   Guiding Eyes for the Blind: Breeding and Placement Center
Guiding Eyes for the Blind
611 Granite Springs Rd
Yorktown Heights, NY 10598-3499   914-245-4024
                                        800-942-0149
                                   FAX: 914-245-1609
                                   infor@guidingeyes.org
                                   www.guidingeyes.org

Bill Badger, President/CEO
Sue Dishart, Vice President
Carolyn Kihm, Director
Jerry Attard, Comptroller
Provides the means for blind and visually impaired individuals to
achieve mobility, independence and companionship through the
use of our professionally bred and trained guide dogs. Each
month Guiding Eyes graduates approximately 12 guide dog/stu-
dent teams from all over the US, Canada, and internationally. The
guide dogs, 26 day residential training program, special needs
program and lifetime follow-up services are offered at no cost to
the students. Also provides at home training at no cost.

8837   Horizons for the Blind
125 Erick Street
A103
Crystal Lake, IL 60014-4404   815-444-8800
                                     800-318-2000
                                FAX: 815-444-8830
                                TTY: 815-444-8800
                                mail@horizons-blind.org
                                www.horizons-blind.org

Camille Caffarelli, Executive Director
Jeff T. Thorsen, First Vice President/Treasurer
Keith Myers, Second Vice President
Maryann Bartkowski, Secretary
Horizons for the Blind is a 501(c)(3) nonprofit organization dedi-
cated to improving the quality of life for people who are blind or
visually impaired, through our consumer products and services,
the cultural arts, education and recreation.

8838   Independent Visually Impaired Enterprisers
American Council of the Blind
1155 15th St NW
Ste 1004
Washington, DC 20005-2706   202-467-5081
                                   800-424-8666
                              FAX: 202-467-5085
                                   info@acb.org
                                   www.ivie-acb.org

Jill Gaus, President
Lynn Jansen, Vice President
Debby Lieberman, Secretary
Mike Reese, Treasurer
Strives to broaden vocational opportunities in business for the vi-
sually impaired. Works to improve rehabilitation facilities for all
types of business enterprises and publicizes the capabilities of
blind and visually impaired business persons.

8839   Institute for Families
4650 Sunset Blvd
Mail Stop 111
Los Angeles, CA 90027- 6062   323-361-4649
                                FAX: 323-665-7869
                                info@instituteforfamilies.org
                                www.instituteforfamilies.org

Margaret Yoshina, Executive Director
Jazmin Asbun, Administrative Assistant
Institute for Families offers counseling and support to families
whose child has been diagnosed with cancer or other diseases that
may impact vision. In addition to the counseling services, we provide books and videos to families and healthcare professionals as
an additional resource to assist them during the difficult days
after diagnosis.

**8840   International Association of Audio Information Services
(IAAIS)**
P.O.Box 847
Lawrence, KS 66044   412-434-6023
                            800-280-5325
                            lrk@ku.edu
                            www.iaais.org

Stuart Holland, President
Marjorie Williams, First Vice President
Jennifer Nigro, Secretary
Amy Hatter, Treasurer
A volunteer driven membership organization of services that turn
text into speech for people who cannot see, hold or comprehend
the printed word and who may be unable to access information
due to a disability or health condition. IAAIS shall encourage and
support the establishment and maintenance of audio information
services that provide access to printed information for individuals who cannot read conventional print because of blindess or any
other visual, physical or learning disability.

8841   Jewish Braille Institute International
110 E 30th St
New York, NY 10016-7393   212-889-2525
                                 800-433-1531
                            FAX: 212-689-3692
                                 library@jbilibrary.org
                                 www.jbilibrary.org

Judy E. Tenney, Chairman of the Board
Dr. Ellen Isler, President and CEO
Israel A. Taub, Vice President and CFO
Frances Brandt, Treasurer
JBI International is a non-profit organization dedicated to meeting the Jewish and general cultural needs of the visually impaired, blind, physically handicapped and reading disabled - of
all ages and backgrounds - worldwide. For nearly 80 years, JBI
has provided people of all ages who are blind, visually impaired
or reading disabled with books, magazines, and special publications in Braille, Large Print and in Audio format.

8842   Keystone Blind Association
1230 Stambaugh Ave.
Sharon, PA 16146   724-347-5501
                     FAX: 724-347-2204
                          info@keystoneblind.org
                          www.keystoneblind.org

Jonathan Fister, President/ CEO
Karen Anderson, Board Member
Sam Bellich, Board Member
Al Boland, Board Member
It changes people's lives for the better and empower, educate, and
employ individuals with vision loss or other disabilities.

8843   Lighthouse International
111 E 59th St
New York, NY 10022-1202   212-821-9200
                                 800-829-0500
                            FAX: 212-821-9707
                            TTY: 212-821-9713
                                 info@lighthouse.org
                                 www.lighthouse.org

Ralph Caprio, Director, Facilities
Leslie Jones, Executive Director, Music School
William H. Seiple, PhD, Vice President of Research
Mark G. Ackermann, President and Chief Executive Officer
Since 1905, Lighthouse International has led the charge in the
fight against vision loss through prevention, treatment and empowerment. Our founders, Winifred and Edith Holt, blazed a trail
of firsts and opened up new doors of opportunity for people without sight. Today, we're proud to continue the Holt legacy on behalf of all those who look to the Lighthouse as a beacon of hope
today - and will for many years to come.

8844   Lions Clubs International
300 W 22nd St
Oak Brook, IL 60523-8842
                                        630-571-5466
                                        FAX: 630-571-8890
                                        TTY:630-571-6533
                                        lions@lionsclubs.org
                                        www.lionsclubs.org
Benedict Ancar, Director
Jui-Tai Chang, Director
Jaime Garcia Cepeda, Director
Kalle Elster, Director
Our 46,000 clubs and 1.35 million members make us the world's largest service club organization. We're also one of the most effective. Our members do whatever is needed to help their local communities. Everywhere we work, we make friends. With children who need eyeglasses, with seniors who don't have enough to eat and with people we may never meet.

8845   Macular Degeneration Foundation
PO Box 531313
Henderson, NV 89053-1313
                                        702-450-2908
                                        888-633-3937
                                        liz@eyesight.org
                                        www.eyesight.org
Liz Trauernicht, President/Director of Communications
Julie Zavala, VP/Asst Director of Operations
David Seftel, M.D., MBA, Executive Vice President/Director of Research Development
Ron Gallemore, Board Of Scientific Advisors
The Macular Degeneration Foundation is dedicated to those who have and will develop macular degeneration. We offer this growing community the latest information, news, hope and encouragement.

8846   National Alliance of Blind Students NABS Liaison
American Council of the Blind
1155 15th St NW
Ste 1004
Washington, DC 20005-2706
                                        202-467-5081
                                        800-424-8666
                                        FAX: 202-467-5085
                                        info@acb.org
                                        www.acb.org
Jill Gaus, President
Lynn Jansen, Vice President
Debby Lieberman, Secretary
Mike Reese, Treasurer
A student affiliate of the American Council of the Blind which is a national organization of blind and visually impaired high school and college students who believe that every blind and visually impaired student has the right to an equal and accessible education. Also encourages blind and visually impaired students to challenge their limits and reach their potential.

8847   National Association for Parents of Children with Visual Impairments (NAPVI)
PO Box 317
Watertown, MA 02471-317
                                        617-972-7441
                                        800-562-6265
                                        FAX: 617-972-7444
                                        spedex.com@gmail.com
                                        www.spedex.com/napvi
Susan LaVenture, Executive Director
Julie Urban, President
Venetia Hayden, Vice President
Kim Alfonso, Treasurer
A non profit organization of, by and for parents committed to providing support to the parents of children who have visual impairments . Also a national organization that enables parents to find information and resources for their children who are blind or visually impaired including those with additional disabilities. NAPVI also provides leadership, support, and training to assist parents in helping children reach their potential.

8848   National Association for Visually Handicapped (NAVH)
111 E 59th S
Fl 6
New York, NY 10022-1202
                                        212-889-3141
                                        800-829-0500
                                        FAX: 212-821-9707
                                        TTY: 212-821-9713
                                        info@lighthouse.org
                                        www.lighthouse.org/navh
Mark G Ackerman, President & CEO
Barbara Gyde, Vice President
Ralph Caprio, Director
Karen Campbell, LCSW, Director of Social Services
NAVH is unique in the services it offers to the hard of seeing™ worldwide and is the only non-profit organization solely dedicated to providing assistance to this population. NAVH runs senior support groups, provides individual consultations, informational materials, training in the use of visual aids, and numerous other tools to ensure that the visually impaired can remain independent and lead fulfilling lives.

8849   National Association of Blind Educators
National Federation of the Blind
200 East Wells St
Baltimore, MD 21230-4914
                                        410-659-9314
                                        FAX: 410-685-5653
                                        nfb@nfb.org
                                        www.nfb.org
Marc Maurer, CEO
Membership organization of blind teachers, professors and instructors in all levels of education. Provides support and information regarding professional responsibilities, classroom techniques, national testing methods and career obstacles. Publishes The Blind Educator, national magazine specifically for blind educators.

8850   National Association of Blind Lawyers
National Federation of the Blind
1660 South Albion Street
Denver, CO 80222-4046
                                        303-504-5979
                                        FAX: 303-757-3640
                                        slabarre@labarrelaw.com
                                        www.nfb.org
Scott LaBarre, President
Membership organization of blind attorneys, law students, judges and others in the law field. Provides support and information regarding employment, techniques used by the blind, advocacy, laws affecting the blind, current information about the American Bar Association and other issues for blind lawyers.

8851   National Association of Blind Merchants
National Federation of the Blind
1837 S.Nevada Avenue
PMB #243
Colorado Springs, CO 80905-4286
                                        719-423-2384
                                        888-691-1819
                                        866-543-6808
                                        kevanwirkey@blindmerchants.org
                                        www.blindmerchants.org
Kevan Worley, President
Membership organization of blind persons employed in either self-employment work or the Randolph-Sheppard vending program. Provides information regarding rehabilitation, social security, tax and other issues which directly affect blind merchants. Serves as advocacy and support group.

8852   National Association of Blind Secretaries and Transcribers
National Federation of the Blind
200 East Wells St
Baltimore, MD 21230-4914
                                        410-659-9314
                                        FAX: 410-685-5653
                                        nfb@nfb.org
                                        www.nfb.org
Marc Maurer, CEO
Membership organization of blind secretaries and transcribers at all levels, including medical and paralegal transcription, office workers, customer-service personnel and many other similar

fields. Addresses issues such as technology, accomodation, career planning and job training.

8853   National Association of Blind Students
National Federation of the Blind
200 East Wells St
Baltimore, MD 21230-4914   410-659-9314
FAX: 410-685-5653
nfb@nfb.org
www.nfb.org

Marc Maurer, CEO
For over 30 years this national organization of blind students has provided support, information, and encouragement to blind college and university students. NABS leads the way in offering resources in issues such as national testing, accessible textbooks and materials, overcoming negative attitudes about blindness from school personnel, developing new techniques of accomplishing laboratory or field assignments, and many other college experiences.

8854   National Association of Blind Teachers
American Council of the Blind
1155 15th St NW
Ste 1004
Washington, DC 20005-2706   202-467-5081
800-424-8666
FAX: 202-467-5085
johnbuckley25@hotmail.com
www.blindteachers.net

Jill Gaus, President
Lynn Jansen, Vice President
Debby Lieberman, Secretary
Mike Reese, Treasurer
Works to advance the teaching profession for blind and visually impaired people, protects the interest of teachers, presents discussions and solutions for special problems encountered by blind teachers and publishes a directory of blind teachers in the US.

8855   National Association of Blind Veterans
PO Box 784957
Winter Garden, FL 34778   321-948-1466
president@nabv.org
www.nabv.org

Dwight Sayer, President
Gene Huggins, 1st Vice President
Larry Ball, 2nd Vice President
Patty Sayer, Secretary
A nationwide organization of blind and visually impaired veterans striving to serve fellow veterans who have lost their sight in the service of country or have lost their sight after serving country.

8856   National Association of Guide Dog Users
National Federation of the Blind
1003 Papaya Dr
Tampa, FL 33619-4629   813-626-2789
800-558-8261
888-624-3841
president@nagdu.org
www.nagdu.org

Marion Gwizdala, President
Provides information and support for guide dog users and works to secure high standards in guide dog training. Addresses issues of discrimination of guide dog users and offers public education about guide dog use. Biennial newsletter available: Harness Up!

8857   National Association to Promote the Use of Braille
National Federation of the Blind
39481 Gallaudet Dr
Apt 127
Fremont, CA 94538   510-248-0100
877-558-6524
FAX: 818-344-7930
mwillows@sbcglobal.net
www.nfbcal.org

Nadine Jacobson, President
Robert Jaquiss, Vice President
Linda Mentink, Second Vice President
Jennifer Dunnam, Secretary
Dedicated to securing improved Braille instruction, increasing the number of braille materials available to the blind and providing information of braille in securing independence, education and employment for the blind.

8858   National Beep Baseball Association
1501 41st NW
Apt G1
Rochester, MN 55901   866-400-4551
www.nbba.org

Stephen A. Guerra, Secretary
It facilitates and provides the adaptive version of America's favorite pastime for the blind, low vision and legally blind.

8859   National Braille Association
95 Allens Creek Rd
Bldg 1 Ste 202
Rochester, NY 14618- 3252   585-427-8260
FAX: 585-427-0263
nbaoffice@nationalbraille.org
www.nationalbraille.org

David Shaffar, Executive Director
Jan Carroll, President
Whitney Gregory-Williams, Vice President
Heidi Lehmann, Secretary
The only national organization dedicated to the professional development of individuals who prepare and produce braille materials.

8860   National Braille Press
88 Saint Stephen St
Boston, MA 02115-4312   617-266-6160
888-965-8965
888-965-8965
FAX: 617-437-0456
contact@nbp.org
www.nbp.org

Brian A. Mac Donald, President
Kimberley Ballard, Vice President
Tony Grima, Vice President of Braille Publications
Diane L. Croft, Publisher
The guiding purposes of National Braille Press are to promote the literacy of blind children through braille, and to provide access to information that empowers blind people to actively engage in work, family, and commuity affairs.

8861   National Center for Vision and Child Development
Lighthouse International
111 E 59th St
New York, NY 10022-1202   212-821-9200
800-829-0500
FAX: 212-821-9707
TTY: 212-821-9713
info@lighthouse.org
www.lighthouse.org

Mark G Ackerman, President/CEO
Barbara Gyde, Vice President
Ralph Caprio, Director
The worldwide leader in helping people of all ages who are blind or partially sighted overcome the challenges of vision loss.

8862 **National Diabetes Action Network for the Blind**
National Federation of the Blind
1212 London Dr
Columbia, MO 65203-2012

573-875-8911
ebryant@socket.net
www.nfb.org

Ed Bryant, Manager
Leading support and information organization of persons losing vision due to diabetes. Provides personal contact and resource information with other blind diabetics about non-visual techniques of independently managing diabetes, monitoring glucose levels, measuring insulin and other matters concerning diabetes. Publishes Voice of the Diabetic, the leading publication about diabetes and blindness.

8863 **National Eye Institute**
31 Center Drive MSC 2510
Bethesda, MD 20892-2510

301-496-5248
FAX: 301-402-1065
2020@nei.nih.gov
www.nei.nih.gov

Paul A Sieving MD PhD, Director
To conduct and support research for blinding eye diseases, visual disorders, mechanisms of visual function, and the preservation of sight.

8864 **National Federation of the Blind**
200 E. Wells St.
at Jernigan Place
Baltimore, MD 21230- 4998

410-659-9314
FAX: 410-685-5653
nfb@nfb.org
nfb.org

John Berggren, Executive Director for Operation
John G. Paré Jr., Executive Director for Strategic Initiatives
Mark Riccobono, Executive Director, NFB Jernigan Institute
Joanne Wilson, Executive Director for Affiliate Action
The National Federation of the Blind (NFB) is the largest organization of the blind in the world. The Federation's purpose is to help blind people achieve self-confidence, self-respect, and self-determination. Their goal is the complete integration of the blind into society on a basis of equality.

8865 **National Industries for the Blind**
1310 Braddock Pl
Alexandria, VA 22314-1691

703-310-0500
FAX: 703-998-8268
info@nib.org
www.nfb.org

Gary J. Krump, Chairperson
Ronald Tascarella, Vice Chairperson
Kristin Graham Koehler, Secretary
A nonprofit organization that represents over 100 associated industries serving people who are blind in thirty-six states. These agencies serve people who are blind or visually impaired and help them to reach their full potential. Services include job and family counseling, job skills training, instruction in Braille and other communication skills, children's programs and more.

8866 **National Library Services for the Blind& Physically Handicapped**
Library of Congress
1291 Taylor Street North West
Washington, DC 20011

202-707-5100
FAX: 202-707-0712
TTY:202-707-0744
nls@loc.gov
www.loc.gov/nls

Karen Keninger, Director
NLS is responsible for the selection, copyright clearance, and procurement of reading materials for blind and physically handicapped individuals. Distribution of the materials and relevant bibliographic information either directly or through cooperating state and local network libraries. Design, development, and procurement of sound reproduction equipment and its distribution either directly or through cooperating agencies.

8867 **National Organization of Parents of Blind Children**
National Federation of the Blind
200 East Wells St
Baltimore, MD 21230-4914

410-659-9314
FAX: 410-685-5653
jim@riversedgehomes.com
www.nfb.org

Carlton Walker,, President
Barbara Cheadle,, President Emerita
Stephanie Kieszak-Holloway, First Vice-President
Andrea Beasley, Secretary
Support information and advocacy organization of parents of blind or visually impaired children. Addresses issues ranging from help to parents of a newborn blind infant, mobility and braille instruction, education, social and community participation, development of self confidence and other vital factors involved in growth of a blind child.

8868 **New Eyes for the Needy**
549 Millburn Avenue
PO Box 332
Short Hills, NJ 07078-332

973-376-4903
FAX: 973-376-3807
neweyesfortheneedy@verizon.net
www.neweyesfortheneedy.org

Susan Dyckman, Executive Director
Marianne Muench Busby, Vice President
Barbara Daney, Treasurer
Suzanne Escousee, Secretary
New Eyes provides new prescription glasses for poor children and adults in the U.S. through a voucher system.

8869 **Prevent Blindness America**
211 W Wacker Drive
Suite 1700
Chicago, IL 60606

312-363-6001
800-331-2020
FAX: 312-363-6052
info@preventblindness.org
www.preventblindness.org

James E. Anderson, Chair
Kira Baldanado, Director
Arzu Bilazer, Creative Director
Mary Bregantini, Senior Director
The nation's leading volunteer eye health and safety organization dedicated to fighting blindness and saving sight. Also touches the lives of millions of people each year through public and professional education, advocacy, certified vision screening training, community and patient service programs and research.

8870 **Seeing Eye, The**
10 Washington Valley Rd
PO Box 375
Morristown, NJ 07963-0375

973-539-4425
FAX: 973-539-0922
info@seeingeye.org
www.seeingeye.org

Peggy Gibbon,, Director of Canine Development
James A Kutsch Jr, President/CEO
Dolores Holle, VMD,, Director of Canine Medicine & Surgery
Randall Ivens, Director of Human Resources
An organization that concentrates on its mission to enhance the independence, dignity, and self confidence of blind people through the use of seeing eye dogs. The Seeing Eye will be an organization that concentrates on its mission to enhance the independence, dignity, and self confidence of blind people through the use of Seeing Eye dogs, and on improving its ability to fulfill this mission. We will maintain and nuture the spirit of our founders and adhere to the highest standards of respect

8871 Services for the Visually Impaired
8720 Georgia Ave
Suite 210
Silver Spring, MD 20910-3614   301-589-0894
                                 FAX: 301-589-0884
                                      info@clb.org
                                       www.clb.org

Ann Cook, Executive Director
Anthony J. (Cancelosi, CEO
Provides skills and resources to DC area residents who are blind
or experiencing vision loss, and are also committed to helping
people regain their indepence and maintaining it.

8872 Society for the Blind
1238 S St.
Sacramento, CA 95811   916-452-8271
                                 FAX: 916-492-2483
                           info@societyfortheblind.org
                                societyfortheblind.org

Shari Roeseler, Executive Director
Shane Snyder, Director of Programs
Serving 26 counties in Northern California, Society for the Blind
is a full service, nonprofit, agency providing services and programs for people who are blind or have low vision. services include the Low Vision Clinic, Braille Classes, computer training,
support groups, living skills instruction, mobility training, and
the Products for Independence Store.

8873 United States Association of Blind Athletes
1 Olympic Plaza
Colorado Springs, CO 80909-3508   719-866-3224
                                 FAX: 719-866-3400
                                   mlucas@usaba.org
                                     www.usaba.org

Mark A. Lucas, Executive Director
Ryan Ortiz, Assistant Executive Director
John Potts, Goalball High Performance Director
Lacey Markle, Public Relations and Events Coordinator
USABA is a Colorado-based 501(c) (3) organization that provides life-enriching sports opportunities for every individual
with a visual impairment. A member of the U.S. Olympic Committee, USABA provides athletic opportunities in various sports
including, but not limited to track and field, nordic and alpine skiing, biathlon, judo, wrestling, swimming, tandem cycling,
powerlifting and goalball (a team sport for the blind and visually
impaired).

8874 United States Blind Golfers Association
125 Gilberts Hill Rd
Lehighton, PA 18235   615-679-9629
                                  info@usblindgolf.com
                                   www.usblindgolf.com

Jim Baker, President
Diane Wilson, Vice President
Tony Schiros, Board Member
Alan Hooper, Board Member
It encourages and enhances opportunities of blind and visually
impaired golfers to compete in golf.

8875 United States Braille Chess Association
1881 N. Nash St.
Unit 702
Arlington, VA 22209   516-223-8685
                               jaylev7@verizon.net
                           www.americanblindchess.org

LA Pietrolungo, President
Alan Dicey, Vice President
Jay Leventhal, Secretary
Alan Schlank, Treasurer
It is dedicated to encourage and assist in the promotion and ad-
vancement of correspondence and over-the board chess among
chess enthusiasts who are blind or visually impaired.

8876 Vermont Association for the Blind and Visually Impaired
60 Kimball Ave
South Burlington, VT 05403   802-863-1358
                                     800-639-5861
                                 FAX: 802-863-1481
                                   general@vabvi.org
                                      www.vabvi.org

James Mooney, President
Thomas Chase, Vice President
Debbie Balserus, Secretary
Patricia Henderson, Treasurer
The Vermont Association for the Blind and Visually Impaired
(VABVI), a non-profit organization founded in 1926, is the only
private agency to offer free training, services and support to visu-
ally impaired Vermonters. Each year we serve hundreds of chil-
dren from birth to age 22 and adults age 55 and over.

8877 Vision Forward Association
912 N. Hawley Road
Milwaukee, WI 53213   414-615-0100
                                     855-878-6056
                                 FAX: 414-256-8748
                                www.vision-forward.org

Terri Davis, Executive Director
Jacci Borchardt, Program Director
Jacque Cline, Human Resources Director
Dena Fellows, Marketing Director
Its mission is to empower, educate, and enhance the lives of indi-
viduals impacted by vision loss through all of life's transitions.

8878 Vision World Wide
Apt 302
5707 Brockton Dr
Indianapolis, IN 46220-5481   317-254-1332
                                     800-431-1739
                                 FAX: 317-251-6588
                                   info@visionww.org
                                    www.visionww.org

Patricia L Prince, President
A non profit organization dedicated to improving the lives of the
vision impaired through direct interaction and indirectly through
the caregiving community. Also serve both the totally blind and
those with various degrees and forms of vision loss.

8879 Visions Center on Blindness (VCB)
111 Summit Park Rd
Spring Valley, NY 10977-1221   212-625-1616
                                     888-245-8333
                                 FAX: 845-354-5130
                                   info@visionsvcb.org
                                    www.visionsvcb.org

Nancy T. Jones, President
Richard P. Simon, Vice President
Burton M. Strauss, Treasurer
Carol Spawn Desmond, Secretary
VISIONS VCB is a 35-acre year round residential rehabilitation
and training center in Rockland County, New York, 35 miles
north of New York City in the Village of New Hempstead. Since
it's founding over 85 years ago, VCB has become one of the largest and most comprehensive overnight training and vision rehabilitation facilities in the United States. Year round on weekends
and during summer sessions, VCB serves 600 people of all ages.

8880 Visually Impaired Veterans of America
American Council of the Blind
1155 15th St NW
Ste 1004
Washington, DC 20005-2706   202-467-5081
                                     800-424-8666
                                 FAX: 202-467-5085
                              bj2kiowa@worldnet.att.net
                                       www.acb.org

Jill Gaus, President
Lynn Jansen, Vice President
Debby Lieberman, Secretary
Mike Reese, Treasurer
Maintain, promote and foster the well bring and rehabilitation of
all visually Impaired Veterans of the Armed Forces of the United

States of America who are eligible to receive from the Veterans Administration; develops and encourages the practice of high standards of personal professional conduct among Visually Impaired Veterans; maintain, promote, and foster public confidence and awareness In Visually Impaired Veterans.

8881 Washington Ear
12061 Tech Rd
Ste B
Silver Spring, MD 20904-7826   301-681-6636
FAX: 301-625-1986
information@washear.org
www.washear.org

George Long, Chairman
Neely Oplinger, Executive Director
Freddie L. Peaco, President
Paul D'Addario, President-Elect
A non profit organization providing reading and information services for blind, visually impaired and physically disabled people who cannot effectively read print, see plays, watch television programs and films, or view museum exhibits. Ear free services strive to substitute hearing for seeing, improving the lives of people with limited or no vision by enabling them to be well-informed, fully productive members of their families, their communities and the working world.

Camps

8882 Camp Barakel
P.O.Box 159
Fairview, MI 48621-0159   989-848-2279
FAX: 989-848-2280
info@campbarakel.org
www.campbarakel.org

Paul Gardner, Camp Director
Hannah Gardner, Music Coordinator
Jon Ford, Head Lifeguard
Stacy Ford, Adult Program Staff
Five-day Christian camp experience in mid-August for campers ages 18-55 who are physically disabled, visually impaired, upper trainable mentally impaired or educable mentally impaired, bus transportation provided from locations in Lansing, Flint and Bay City, Michigan.

8883 Camp Challenge
8914 US Highway 50 East
Bedford, IN 47421   812-834-5159
info@gocampchallenge.com
www.gocampchallenge.com

Maria , Director of Engagement
One and two-week sessions for campers with developmental and or physical disabilities, hearing impairment and the blind/visually impaired. Ages 6-99 and families.

8884 Camp Lawroweld
Northern New England Conference
228 West Side Road
Weld, ME 04285   207-585-2984
FAX: 207-585-2985
camplawroweld@gmail.com
www.lawroweld.org

Harry Sabnani, Executive Director
Camp is located in Weld, Maine. Week sessions July for campers who are blind or visually impaired, all ages. Other camps coed, ages 9-16 and families, single adults, June - September.

8885 Camp Lou Henry Hoover
Girl Scouts of Washington Rock Council
201 East Grove Street
Westfield, NJ 07090   908-518-4400
FAX: 908-232-4508
girlscouts@gshnj.org
www.gshnj.org

Samantha Basek, Field Executive
Susan Brooks, CEO

Camp is located in Middleville, New Jersey. Sessions for girls who are blind/visually impaired, ages 7-18.

8886 Camp Merrick
PO Box 56
Nanjemoy, MD 20662   301-870-5858
FAX: 301-246-9108
info@LionsCampMerrick.org
lionscampmerrick.org

Wayne Magoon, President
Ray Shumaker, Vice President
Julie Andrew, Board Member
Frank Culhane, Treasurer
Programs offered April-January for children who are blind/visually impaired, hearing impaired or diabetic. Coed, ages 6-15.

8887 Camp Winnekeag
257 Ashby Road
Ashburnham, MA 01430   978-827-4455
FAX: 978-827-4551
sneconference@sneconline.org
www.campwinnekeag.com

Frank Tochterman, Religious Leader
Camp is located in Ashburnham, Massachusetts. Camping sessions for blind/visually impaired children. Coed, ages 8-16.

8888 Columbia Lighthouse for the Blind Summer Camp
Columbia Lighthouse for the Blind
1825 K Street NorthWest
Suite 1103
Washington, DC 20006   202-454-6400
FAX: 877-595-9228
info@clb.org
clb.org

Tony Cancelosi, President
Anthony Cancelosi, CEO
Helps enable the blind or visually impaired to obtain and maintain independence at home, school, work and in the community. Programs and services include early intervention services, training and consultation in assistive technology, career placement services, comprehensive low vision care and a wide range of rehabilitation services. Highly acclaimed summer camp, picnics and holiday activities encourage blind and visualy impaired children to make new friends and experience the joys of childhood.

8889 Easter Seals Oklahoma
701 NorthEast 13th Street
Oklahoma City, OK 73104   405-239-2525
FAX: 405-239-2278
sbusch@eastersealsoklahoma.org
www.eastersealsoklahoma.org

Rodney Burgamy, Chairman
David Adams, Board Member
Kristen Sorocco, Secretary
Jeb Reid, Treasurer
Adult day health center, and child development center.

8890 Enchanted Hills Camp for the Blind
Lighthouse for the Blind
214 Van Ness Avenue
San Francisco, CA 94102   415-431-1481
888-400-8933
FAX: 415-863-7568
info@lighthouse-sf.org
lighthouse-sf.org

Joshua A. Miele, President
Chris Downey, 1st Vice President
Gena Harper, Secretary
Joseph Chan, Treasurer
Camp is located in Napa, California. Half-week, one and two-week sessions for blind, deaf/blind children and adults, ages 5 and up. This program offers a basic camping experience. Activities include music, art, dance, hiking and riding. Camperships are available to California residents.

8891 Highbrook Lodge
PO Box 1988
1909 East 101st Street
Cleveland, OH 44106- 8696
216-791-8118
FAX: 216-791-1101
www.clevelandsightcenter.org

William L. Spring, Chair
Thomas P. Furnas, 1st Vice Chair
Gary W. Poth, Treasurer
Sheryl King Benford, Secretary
Camp is located in Chardon, Ohio. Summer sessions for children, adults and familieswho are blind or have low vision. There are seven sessions held annually through June, July and August with an wide range of outdoor camp activities. Camp activities focus on gaining independent skills, mobility, orientation and self confidence in an accessable and traditional camp setting.
220-660/session

8892 Indian Creek Camp
Kentucky Tennessee Conference
150 Cabin Circle Drive
Liberty, TN 37095
615-548-4411
FAX: 615-548-4029
info@indiancreekcamp.com
www.indiancreekcamp.com

Ken Wetmore, Director
Marty Sutton, Asst. Director
Toni Stephens, Program Director
Stephanie Rufo, Public Relations Director
Camp is located in Liberty, Tennessee. Summer sessions for children and adults who are blind/visually impaired. Coed, ages 7-17, families and seniors.

8893 Kamp A-Komp-Plish
9035 Ironsides Rd
Nanjemoy, MD 20662-3432
301-870-3226
301-934-3590
FAX: 301-870-2620
recreation@melwood.org
www.kampakomplish.org

Jonathan Rondeau, Chief Program Officer
Bekah Carmichael, Director
Doria Fleisher, Associate Director
Marisa Cucuzella, Assistant Director
Camp is located in Nanjemoy, Maryland. Half-week, one-week and two-week sessions for blind/visually impaired children and those with developmental disabilities and mobility limitation. Coed, ages 8-16.

8894 Kamp Kaleo
46872 Willow Springs Road
Burwell, NE 68823
308-346-5083
kampkaleo@gmail.com
www.kampkaleo.com

Gaylene O'Brien, Administrator
Sandy Denton, Minister Of Faith Development
Camp is located in Burwell, Nebraska. Summer sessions for campers who are blind/visually impaired or have developmental disabilities. Coed, ages 9-18 and families, seniors, single adults.

8895 National Camp for Blind Children
Christian Record Services
P.O. Box 6097
Lincoln, NE 68506-0097
402-488-0981
FAX: 402-488-7582
infochristianrecord.org
www.christianrecord.org

Dan Jackson, Chair
Tom Lemon, Vice Chair
Larry Pitcher, President, Secretary
Al Burdick, Board Member
To enrich lives of those who are blind, visually impaired or physically challenged regardless of race, creed, economic status or gender. Also encourages each camper to achieve greater self-esteem and self confidence while seeking to excel in the use of his/her physical , mental, and spiritual capacities. Provides fee Christian publications and programs for people with visual impairments.
Monthly

8896 National Camps for Blind Children
Christian Record Services
P.O. Box 6097
Lincoln, NE 68506-0097
402-488-0981
FAX: 402-488-7582
info@christianrecord.org
blindcamps.com

Dan Jackson, Chair
Tom Lemon, Vice Chair
Larry Pitcher, President, Secretary
Al Burdick, Board Member
Provides free Christian publications and programs, as well as new opportunities for people with visual impairments. Free services include subscription magazines available in braille, large print and audio cassette, full-vision books combining braille and print, lending library, gift bibles and study guides in braille, large print and audio cassette, national camps for blind children and scholarship assistance for blind young people trying to obtain a college education.

8897 Texas Lions Camp
Lions Club Of Texas
P.O.Box 290247
Kerrville, TX 78029
830-896-8500
FAX: 830-896-3666
tlc@ktc.com
www.lionscamp.com

Stephen Mabry, Executive Director
The primary purpose of the League shall be to provide, without charge, a camp for physically disabled, hearing/vision impaired and diabetic children from the State of Texas, regardless of race, religion, or national origin. Our goal is to create an atmosphere wherein campers will learn the can do philosophy and be allowed to achieve maximum personal growth and self-esteem. The camp welcomes boys and girls ages 7-16.

8898 VISIONS Vacation Camp for the Blind
VISIONS Center on Blindness
111 Summit Park Road
Spring Valley, NY 10977
212-625-1616
888-245-8333
FAX: 845-354-5130
cthorne@visionsvcb.org
www.visionsvcb.org

Nancy T. Jones, President
Richard P. Simon, Vice President
Burton M. Strauss, Treasurer
Carol Spawn Desmond, Secretary
Is a non profit agency that promotes the independence of people of all ages who are blind or visually imparied. Camp offers braille classes, computers with large print and voice output, support groups, discussions, mobility lessions, cooking classes, personal and home management training, large print and Braille books.

8899 Wendell Johnson Speech And Hearing Clinic
University Of Iowa
250 Hawkins Dr
Iowa City, IA 52242-1025
319-335-8736
FAX: 319-335-8851
kathy-miller@uiowa.edu
www.uiowa.edu

Chuck Wieland, President
Hans Hoerschelman, Vice President
Josh Smith, Budget Officer
Shannon Lizakowski, Secretary
The clinic offers assessment and intervention for communication disorders in adults and children as well as an audiology clinic. The clinic also offers several summer programs for children with hearing, speech, language, autism and/or reading disorders, including a summer residential program for teens who stutter.

8900 **YMCA Camp Chingachgook on Lake George**
Capital District YMCA
1872 Pilot Knob Road
Kattskill Bay, NY 12844
518-656-9462
FAX: 518-656-9362
chingachgook@cdymca.org
www.cdymca.org

George Painter, Executive Director
Billy Rankin, Senior Program Director
Dan Poole, Adventure Trip Director
Carol Lewis, Office Manager
Sailing programs for people with disabilities. Sessions for campers who are blind/visually impaired. Coed, ages 7-16, families, seniors and single adults.

Print: Books

8901 **A Christian Approach to Overcoming Disability: A Doctor's Story**
Routledge (Taylor & Francis Group)
711 Third Ave.
New York, NY 10017
212-216-7800
FAX: 212-564-7854
orders@taylorandfrancis.com
www.routledge.com

Dr. Elaine Leong Eng, M.D.
A personal account of Dr. Elaine Leong Eng and her career move from obstetrician/gynecologist to full-time mom, as she faces the diagnosis of impending visual impairment. Dr. Eng offers personal experience and faith-based, psychological techniques for coping with disability.
142 pages Hardcover

8902 **AFB Directory of Services for Blind and Visually Impaired Persons in the US and Canada**
American Foundation for the Blind/AFB Press
2 Penn Plaza
Suite 1102
New York, NY 10121
212-502-7600
800-232-5463
FAX: 888-545-8331
afbinfo@afb.net
www.afb.org

Carl Augusto, President & Chief Executive Officer
Rick Bozeman, Finance Director, Chief Financial Officer
Kelly Bleach, Chief Administrative Officer
Stacy Rollins, Executive Administrative Assistant to the President
Comprehensive print resource containing more that 2,500 local, state, regional, and national services throughout the US and Canada for persons who are blind or visually impaired. *$79.95*
624 pages Paperback/onlin
ISBN 0-891288-05-3

8903 **About Children's Eyes**
National Association for Visually Handicapped
111 East 59th Street
New York, NY 10022-1202
212-821-9384
800-829-0500
FAX: 212-821-9707
info@lighthouse.org
lighthouse.org/navh

Mark G. Ackermann, President / CEO
How to identify the child with a visual problem. LightHouse acquired NAVH.

8904 **About Children's Vision: A Guide for Parents**
National Association for Visually Handicapped
111 East 59th Street
New York, NY 10022-1202
212-821-9384
800-829-0500
FAX: 212-821-9707
info@lighthouse.org
lighthouse.org/navh

Mark G. Ackermann, President / CEO

Offers a better understanding of the normal and possible abnormal development of a child's eyesight. LightHouse acquired NAVH. *$.50*

8905 **Access to Art: A Museum Directory for Blind and Visually Impaired People**
American Foundation for the Blind/AFB Press
2 Penn Plaza
Suite 1102
New York, NY 10121
212-502-7600
800-232-5463
FAX: 888-545-8331
afbinfo@afb.net
www.afb.org

Carl R. Augusto, President & Chief Executive Officer
Rick Bozeman, Finance Director, Chief Financial Officer
Kelly Bleach, Chief Administrative Officer
Stacy Rollins, Executive Administrative Assistant to the President
Details the access facilities of over 300 museums, galleries and exhibits in the United States. Also included are organizations offering art-related resources such as, art classes, competitions and traveling exhibits. *$19.95*
144 pages Large Print
ISBN 0-891281-56-8

8906 **African Americans in the Profession of Blindness Services**
Mississippi State University
P.O.Box 6189
Mississippi State, MS 39762
662-325-2001
FAX: 662-325-8989
TTY:662-325-2694
nrtc@colled.msstate.edu
www.blind.msstate.edu

Jacqui Bybee, Research Associate II
Douglas Bedsaul, Research and Training Coordinator
Anne Carter, Research and Training Coordinator
Brenda Cavenaugh, Ph.D., Research Professor
This study investigated the level of participation by African Americans in vocational rehab. (VR) services to persons who are visually impaired. Using surveys and interviews with all state VR directors, national census data and national RSA data, it was found nationally that African Americans are substantially under-represented in the service provider ranks, yet over-represented as clients. *$20.00*
61 pages Paperback

8907 **Age-Related Macular Degeneration**
National Association for Visually Handicapped
111 East 59th Street
New York, NY 10022-1202
212-821-9384
800-829-0500
FAX: 212-821-9707
info@lighthouse.org
lighthouse.org/navh

Mark G. Ackermann, President / CEO
A large booklet offering information and up-to-date research on Macular Degeneration. Also available in Russian. Revised in 2007. LightHouse acquired NAVH. *$5.00*

8908 **American Anals of the Deaf Reference**
800 Florida Ave NE
Washington, DC 20002-3600
202-651-5530
FAX: 202-651-5489
gupress@gallaudet.edu
gupress.gallaudet.edu/annals

Stephanie Cawthon, Ph.D., Book Review Editor
Peter V. Paul, Ph.D., Editor, Literary Issues
Ye Wang, Ph.D., Senior Associate Editor
Feifei Ye, Ph.D., Associate Editor for Research Methodology
The controlled scope of GUPress operations allows the continuance of a highly focused commitment to individual titles that has contributed significantly to its 20 years of leadership in publishing on Deaf issues. Gallaudet University Press brings unmatched experience and knowledge to the marketplace for books on and for the Deaf community, its advocates, and scholars invested in the study of deaf society.

8909 Americans with Disabilities Act Guide for Places of Lodging: Serving Guests Who Are Blind
US Department of Justice
950 Pennsylvania Avenue NorthWest
Washington, DC 20530
202-307-0663
800-574-0301
FAX: 202-307-1197
TTY: 800-514-0383
www.ada.gov

Rebecca B. Bond, Chief
Zita Johnson Betts, Deputy Chief
Sally Conway, Deputy Chief
James Bostrom, Deputy Chief
A 12-page publication explaining what hotels, motels, and other places of transient lodging can do to accommodate guests who are blind or have low vision.

8910 Art and Science of Teaching Orientation and Mobility to Persons with Visual Impairments
American Foundation for the Blind/AFB Press
2 Penn Plaza
Suite 1102
New York, NY 10121
212-502-7600
800-232-5463
FAX: 888-545-8331
afbinfo@afb.net
www.afb.org

Carl R. Augusto, President & Chief Executive Officer
Rick Bozeman, Finance Director, Chief Financial Officer
Kelly Bleach, Chief Administrative Officer
Stacy Rollins, Executive Administrative Assistant to the President
Comprehensive description of the techniques of teaching orientation and mobility, presented along with considerations and strategies for sensitive and effective teaching. Hardcover. Paperback also available. *$48.00*
200 pages
ISBN 0-891282-45-9

8911 Awareness Training
Landmark Media
3450 Slade Run Drive
Falls Church, VA 22042
703-241-2030
800-342-4336
FAX: 703-536-9540
info@landmarkmedia.com
landmarkmedia.com

Michael Hartogs, President
Peter Hartogs, VP New Business & Development
Richard Hartogs, VP Acquisitions
Beverly Weisenberg, Sales Representative
Covers disabilities of various types — vision, hearing, speech disorders, loss of limbs, loss of mobility, or mental/emotional limitations and how to integrate such individuals into various business and educational settings. It is a 4-part series designed to identify and enable others to interact effectively with those suffering such disabilities. *$495.00*
Set of 4

8912 Babycare Assistive Technology
Through the Looking Glass
3075 Adeline Street
Suite 120
Berkeley, CA 94703
510-848-1112
800-644-2666
FAX: 510-848-4445
tlg@lookingglass.org
www.lookingglass.org

Maureen Block, J.D., President
Thomas Spalding, Treasurer
Alice Nemon, Secretary
Mega Kirshbaum, Author
Available in braille, large print or cassette. Provides an overview of the baby care assistive technology work at Through The Looking Glass including a discussion of TLG's intervention model, the impact of babycare equipment and guidelines for equipment development print. *$2.00*
8 pages

8913 Babycare Assistive Technology for Parents with Physical Disabilties
Through the Looking Glass
3075 Adeline Street
Suite 120
Berkeley, CA 94703
510-848-1112
800-644-2666
FAX: 510-848-4445
tlg@lookingglass.org
www.lookingglass.org

Maureen Block, J.D., President
Thomas Spalding, Treasurer
Alice Nemon, Secretary
Mega Kirshbaum, Author
Examines the provision of babycare equipment through the lens of ithe infant/parent relationship, the lens of the family system, and through the lens of culture. Availiable in braille, large print or cassette. *$2.00*
7 pages

8914 Basic Course in American Sign Language
TJ Publishers
P.O. Box 702701
Dallas, TX 75370
972-416-0800
800-999-1168
FAX: 972-416-0944
TTY: 301-585-4440
TJPubinc@aol.com
www.tjpublishers.com/

Tom Humphries, Author
Carol Padden, Co-Author
Terrance J O'Rourke, Co-Author
Accompanying videotapes and textbooks include voice translations. Hearing students can analyze sound for initial instruction, or opt to turn off the sound to sharpen visual acuity. Package includes the Basic Course in American Sign Language text, Student Study Guide, the original four 1-hour videotapes plus the ABCASI Vocabulary videotape. *$139.95*
280 pages

8915 Behavioral Vision Approaches for Persons with Physical Disabilities
Optometric Extension Program Foundation
7754 Braegger Road
Three Lakes, WI 54562
714-250-0176
Info@depf.org
www.depf.org

Kristin R. Jungbluth, President
Eric J. Lindberg, VP
Barbara Kuntz, Secretary
Patricia S. Lindberg, Treasurer
A discussion of the behavioral vision/neuro-motor approach to providing directions for prescriptive and therapeutic services for the visually handicapped child or adult. *$49.50*
197 pages

8916 Belonging
Dial Books
375 Hudson St
New York, NY 10014-3657
212-366-2000
FAX: 212-414-3394
www.penguin.com/

Deborah Kent, Author
Meg attended special schools for the blind until she was ready for high school. She decided that she wanted to go to a regular high school. She and her mother practiced her walks to school and studied the layout of the building prior to school starting, but Meg was unprepared for the trip when there were 1,500 students. She adjusted quickly to the crowds and the pace of the new school.
200 pages Hardcover
ISBN 0-80370 -30-1

8917 Berthold Lowenfeld on Blindness and Blind People
American Foundation for the Blind/AFB Press
2 Penn Plaza
Suite 1102
New York, NY 10121   212-502-7600
                                                 800-232-5463
                                            FAX: 888-545-8331
                                            afbinfo@afb.net
                                            www.afb.org

Carl R. Augusto, President & Chief Executive Officer
Rick Bozeman, Finance Director, Chief Financial Officer
Kelly Bleach, Chief Administrative Officer
Stacy Rollins, Executive Administrative Assistant to the President
These writings of the pioneering educator, author and advocate
range over a forty-year period include various ground-breaking
papers for the blind educator, a remembrance of Helen Keller
and other essays on education, sociology and history. *$21.95*
254 pages Paperback
ISBN 0-891281-01-0

8918 Blind and Vision-Impaired Individuals
Mainstream
Ste 830
3 Bethesda Metro Ctr
Bethesda, MD 20814-6301   301-961-9299
                                                 800-247-1380
                                            FAX: 301-654-6714
                                            info@mainstreaminc.org

Charles Moster
Mainstreaming blind individuals into the workplace. *$ 2.50*
12 pages

**8919 Blindness and Early Childhood Development Second
Edition**
American Foundation for the Blind/AFB Press
2 Penn Plaza
Suite 1102
New York, NY 10121   212-502-7600
                                                 800-232-5463
                                            FAX: 888-545-8331
                                            afbinfo@afb.net
                                            afb.org

Carl R. Augusto, President & Chief Executive Officer
Rick Bozeman, Finance Director, Chief Financial Officer
Kelly Bleach, Chief Administrative Officer
Stacy Rollins, Executive Administrative Assistant to the President
A review of current knowledge on motor and locomotor develop-
ment, perceptual development, language and cognitive pro-
cesses, and social, emotional and personality development.
Paperback. *$34.95*
384 pages
ISBN 0-891281-23-8

8920 Blindness: What it is, What it Does and How to Live with it
American Foundation for the Blind/AFB Press
2 Penn Plaza
Suite 1102
New York, NY 10121   212-502-7600
                                                 800-232-5463
                                            FAX: 888-545-8331
                                            afbinfo@afb.net
                                            www.afb.org

Carl R. Augusto, President & Chief Executive Officer
Rick Bozeman, Finance Director, Chief Financial Officer
Kelly Bleach, Chief Administrative Officer
Stacy Rollins, Executive Administrative Assistant to the President
A classic work on how blindness affects self-perception and so-
cial interaction and what can be done to restore basic skills, mo-
bility, daily living and an appreciation of life's pleasures. *$15.95*
396 pages Paperback
ISBN 0-891282-05-

8921 Books are Fun for Everyone
Nat'l Lib Svc/Blind And Physically Handicapped
1291 Taylor Street North West
Washington, DC 20011   202-707-5100
                                            FAX: 202-707-0712
                                            TTY:202-707-0744
                                            nls@loc.gov
                                            www.loc.gov/nls

Karen Keninger, Director

8922 Books for Blind & Physically Handicapped Individuals
Nat'l Lib Svc/Blind And Physically Handicapped
1291 Taylor Street North West
Washington, DC 20011   202-707-5100
                                            FAX: 202-707-0712
                                            TTY:202-707-0744
                                            nls@loc.gov
                                            www.loc.gov/nls

Karen Keninger, Director
A free national library program of braille and recorded materials
for blind and physically handicapped persons.

8923 Books for Blind and Physically Handicapped Individuals
Nat'l Lib Svc/Blind And Physically Handicapped
1291 Taylor Street North West
Washington, DC 20011   202-707-5100
                                            FAX: 202-707-0712
                                            TTY:202-707-0744
                                            nls@loc.gov
                                            www.loc.gov/nls

Karen Keninger, Director
A free national library program of braille and recorded materials
for blind and physically handicapped persons is administered by
the National Library Service for the Blind and Physically Handicapped Library of Congress.
Annual

8924 Braille Book Bank, Music Catalog
National Braille Association
95 Allens Creek Road
Building 1, Suite 202
Rochester, NY 14618   585-427-8260
                                            FAX: 585-427-0263
                                            nbaoffice@nationalbraille.org
                                            www.nationalbraille.org

Jan Carroll, President
Cindi Laurent, Vice President
David Shaffer, Executive Director
Heidi Lehmann, Secretary
Offers hundreds of musical titles in print form, braille and on cas-
sette.
62 pages

8925 Braille: An Extraordinary Volunteer Opportunity
Nat'l Lib Svc/Blind And Physically Handicapped
1291 Taylor Street North West
Washington, DC 20011   202-707-5100
                                            FAX: 202-707-0712
                                            TTY:202-707-0744
                                            nls@loc.gov
                                            www.loc.gov/nls

Karen Keninger, Director

8926 Burns Braille Transcription Dictionary
American Foundation for the Blind/AFB Press
2 Penn Plaza
Suite 1102
New York, NY 10121   212-502-7600
                                      800-232-5463
                                 FAX: 888-545-8331
                                 afbinfo@afb.net
                                      afb.org

Carl R. Augusto, President & Chief Executive Officer
Rick Bozeman, Finance Director, Chief Financial Officer
Kelly Bleach, Chief Administrative Officer
Stacy Rollins, Executive Administrative Assistant to the President
A handy, portable guide that is a quick reference for anyone who needs to check print-to-braille and braille-to-print meanings and symbols. Paperback. *$21.95*
96 pages 96 pages
ISBN 0-891282-32-7

8927 Can't Your Child See? A Guide for Parents of Visually Impaired Children
Sage Publications
2455 Teller Road
Thousand Oaks, CA 91320   805-499-0721
                                      800-818-7243
                                 FAX: 805-499-0871
                                 info@sagepub.com
                                 www.sagepub.com
Sara Miller McCune, Founder, Publisher, Executive Chairman
Blaise R Simqu, President & CEO
Tracey A. Ozmina, Executive Vice President & Chief Operating Officer
Stephen Barr, Managing Director/SAGE London, President of SAGE Internation
This second edition offers parents optimistic, practical guidelines for helping visually impaired children reach their full potential. *$26.00*
279 pages Paperback

8928 Career Perspectives: Interviews with Blindand Visually Impaired Professionals
American Foundation for the Blind/AFB Press
2 Penn Plaza
Suite 1102
New York, NY 10121   212-502-7600
                                      800-232-5463
                                 FAX: 888-545-8331
                                 afbinfo@afb.net
                                      afb.org

Carl R. Augusto, President & Chief Executive Officer
Rick Bozeman, Finance Director, Chief Financial Officer
Kelly Bleach, Chief Administrative Officer
Stacy Rollins, Executive Administrative Assistant to the President
Profiles of 20 successful archivers who describe in their own words what it takes to pursue and attain professional success in a sighted world. Available in large print, cassette and braille. *$19.95*
96 pages
ISBN 0-891281-70-2

8929 Careers in Blindness Rehabilitation Services
Mississippi State University
P.O.Box 6189
Mississippi State, MS 39762   662-325-2001
                                 FAX: 662-325-8989
                                 TTY:662-325-2694
                                 nrtc@colled.msstate.edu
                                 www.blind.msstate.edu
Jacqui Bybee, Research Associate II
Douglas Bedsaul, Research and Training Coordinator
Anne Carter, Research and Training Coordinator
Brenda Cavenaugh, Ph.D., Research Professor
In a follow-up study in a series examining the substantial under-representation of African Americans as professionals in blindness services, researchers questioned college students about their knowledge, opinions and interests in blindness services. *$15.00*
54 pages Paperback

8930 Cataracts
National Association for Visually Handicapped
111 East 59th Street
New York, NY 10022-1202   212-821-9384
                                      800-829-0500
                                 FAX: 212-821-9707
                                 info@lighthouse.org
                                 lighthouse.org/navh
Mark G. Ackermann, President / CEO
A booklet offering information about Cataracts, diagnosis and treatment of this common condition. LightHouse acquired NAVH. *$ 4.00*

8931 Characteristics, Services, & Outcomes of Rehab. Consumers who are Blind/Visually Impaired
Mississippi State University
P.O.Box 6189
Mississippi State, MS 39762   662-325-2001
                                 FAX: 662-325-8989
                                 TTY:662-325-2694
                                 nrtc@colled.msstate.edu
                                 www.blind.msstate.edu
Jacqui Bybee, Research Associate II
Douglas Bedsaul, Research and Training Coordinator
Anne Carter, Research and Training Coordinator
Brenda Cavenaugh, Ph.D., Research Professor
Issues regarding the efficacy of separate state agencies providing specialized vocational rehabilitation (VR) services to consumers who are blind have generated spirited discussions within the rehabilitation community throughout the history of the state-federal program. In this monograph, RRTC researches report results of their investigation of services provided to blind consumers in separate and general (combined) rehabilitation agencies. *$20.00*
45 pages Paperback

8932 Childhood Glaucoma: A Reference Guide for Families
NAPVI
1 North Lexington Avenue
White Plains, NY 10601   617-972-7441
                                      800-562-6265
                                 FAX: 617-972-7444
                                 napvi@guildhealth.org
                                 www.napvi.org
Julie Urban, President
Venetia Hayden, Vice President
Susan LaVenture, Executive Director
Randi Sher, Secretary
A vaulable tutorial and resource covering all aspects from genetics through diagnosis, sibling relationships and more.
36 pages

8933 Children with Visual Impairments: A Guide For Parents
American Foundation for the Blind/AFB Press
105 East 22nd Street
New York, NY 10010   212-949-4800
                                 childrensaidsociety.org
William D. Weisberg, Ph.D., President & CEO
Drema Brown, VP of Education
Katherine Eckstein, Chief of Staff
Beverly Colon, VP for Health & Wellness
Written by parents and professional, this book presents a comprehensive overview of the issues that are crucial to the healthy development of children with mild to severe visual impaiments. It also offers insight from parents about coping with the emotional aspects of raising a child with special needs. *$16.95*
416 pages
ISBN 0-933149-36-0

8934 Classification of Impaired Vision
National Association for Visually Handicapped
111 East 59th Street
New York, NY 10022-1202   212-821-9384
                                      800-829-0500
                                 FAX: 212-821-9707
                                 info@lighthouse.org
                                 lighthouse.org/navh
Mark G. Ackermann, President / CEO

Designed to provide a foundation for a better understanding of teaching reading, writing, and listning skills to students with visual impairments from preschool age through adult levels. Light-House acquired NAVH. *$57.95*
322 pages
ISBN 0-398066-93-2

8935   Communication Skills for Visually Impaired Learners
Charles C. Thomas
2600 S First St
Springfield, IL 62704-4730   217-789-8980
                                            800-258-8980
                                       FAX: 217-789-9130
                                       books@ccthomas.com
                                          www.ccthomas.com

Michael P. Thomas, President
Randall Harley, Author
Mila Truan, Author
LaRhea Sanford, Author
This book has been designed to provide a foundation for a better understanding of teaching reading, writing, and listening skills to students with visual impairments from preschool age through adult levels. The plan of the book incorporates the latest research findings with the practical experiences learned in the classroom. *$57.95*
322 pages Paperback
ISBN 0-398066-93-2

8936   Comprehensive Examination of Barriers to Employment Among Persons who are Blind or Impaire
Mississippi State University
P.O.Box 6189
Mississippi State, MS 39762   662-325-2001
                                       FAX: 662-325-8989
                                       TTY:662-325-2694
                                     nrtc@colled.msstate.edu
                                       www.blind.msstate.edu

Jacqui Bybee, Research Associate II
Douglas Bedsaul, Research and Training Coordinator
Anne Carter, Research and Training Coordinator
Brenda Cavenaugh, Ph.D., Research Professor
A multi-phase research project designed to: identify barriers to employment; identify and develop innovative successful strategies to overcome these barriers; develop methods for others to utilize these strategies; disseminate this information to rehabilitation providers; replicate the use of selected strategies in other settings. *$20.00*
90 pages Paperback

8937   Contrasting Characteristics of Blind and Visually Impaired Clients
Mississippi State University
P.O.Box 6189
Mississippi State, MS 39762   662-325-2001
                                       FAX: 662-325-8989
                                       TTY:662-325-2694
                                     nrtc@colled.msstate.edu
                                       www.blind.msstate.edu

Jacqui Bybee, Research Associate II
Douglas Bedsaul, Research and Training Coordinator
Anne Carter, Research and Training Coordinator
Brenda Cavenaugh, Ph.D., Research Professor
This report examines cases in the National Blindness and Low Vision Employment Database to identify and profile environmental and personal characteristics of clients who are blind or visually impaired and who were achieving successful and unsuccessful retention of competitive jobs. A total of 787 cases were analyzed. *$15.00*
44 pages Paperback

8938   Dancing Cheek to Cheek
Blind Children's Center
4120 Marathon Street
Los Angeles, CA 90029-3584   323-664-2153
                                            800-222-3567
                                       FAX: 323-665-3828
                                   info@blindchildrenscenter.org
                                   www.blindchildrenscenter.org

Scott E. Schaldenbrand, President
Mark Correa, Board Member
Midge Horton, Executive Director
Pamela Lansky, Co-Author
Beginning social, play and language interactions. *$ 10.00*
23 pages

8939   Development of Social Skills by Blind and Visually Impaired Students
American Foundation for the Blind/AFB Press
2 Penn Plaza
Suite 1102
New York, NY 10121   212-502-7600
                                            800-232-5463
                                       FAX: 888-545-8331
                                          afbinfo@afb.net
                                            www.afb.org

Carl R. Augusto, President & Chief Executive Officer
Rick Bozeman, Finance Director, Chief Financial Officer
Kelly Bleach, Chief Administrative Officer
Stacy Rollins, Executive Administrative Assistant to the President
Offers an examination of the social interactions of blind and visually impaired children in mainstreamed settings and the community that highlights the need to teach social interaction skills to children and provide them with support. Paperback. *$45.95*
232 pages
ISBN 0-891282-17-4

8940   Diabetic Retinopathy
National Association for Visually Handicapped
111 East 59th Street
New York, NY 10022-1202   212-821-9384
                                            800-829-0500
                                       FAX: 212-821-9707
                                          info@lighthouse.org
                                         lighthouse.org/navh

Mark G. Ackermann, President / CEO
A booklet offering information about Diabetic Retinopathy. LightHouse acquired NAVH.

8941   Diversity and Visual Impairment: The Influence of Race, Gender, Religion and Ethnicity
American Foundation for the Blind
2 Penn Plaza
Suite 1102
New York, NY 10121   212-502-7600
                                            800-232-5463
                                       FAX: 888-545-8331
                                          afbinfo@afb.net
                                            www.afb.org

Carl R. Augusto, President & Chief Executive Officer
Rick Bozeman, Finance Director, Chief Financial Officer
Kelly Bleach, Chief Administrative Officer
Stacy Rollins, Executive Administrative Assistant to the President
Cultural, social, ethnic, gender, and religious issues can influence the way an individual perceives and copes with a visual impairment. *$45.95*
480 pages
ISBN 0-891283-83-8

8942   Do You Remember the Color Blue: The Questi Ons Children Ask About Blindness
Viking Books
375 Hudson Street
New York, NY 10014-3657   212-366-2000
                                       FAX: 212-366-2933
                                 ecommerce@us.penguingroup.com
                                     www.us.penguingroup.com

John Makinson, Chairman & CEO

The author answers thirteen thought-provoking questions that children have asked her over the years about being blind.
78 pages
ISBN 0-670880-43-4

8943 Don't Lose Sight of Glaucoma
National Eye Institute
2020 Vision Place
Building 31 Room 6a32
Bethesda, MD 20892-3655

301-496-5248
800-869-2020
FAX: 301-402-1065
2020@nei.nih.gov
www.nei.nih.gov

8944 Early Focus: Working with Young Children Who Are Blind or Visually Impaired & Their Families
American Foundation for the Blind/AFB Press
2 Penn Plaza
Suite 1102
New York, NY 10121

212-502-7600
800-232-5463
FAX: 888-545-8331
afbinfo@afb.net
www.afb.org

Carl R. Augusto, President & Chief Executive Officer
Rick Bozeman, Finance Director, Chief Financial Officer
Kelly Bleach, Chief Administrative Officer
Stacy Rollins, Executive Administrative Assistant to the President
Describes early intervention techniques used with blind and visually impaired children and stresses the benefits of family involvement and transdisciplinary teamwork. Paperback. *$32.95*
176 pages
ISBN 0-891282-15-7

8945 Encyclopedia of Blindness and Vision Impairment Second Edition
Facts on File
132 West 31st Street
17th Floor
New York, NY 10001

800-322-8755
FAX: 800-678-3633
CustServ@InfobaseLearning.com
www.factsonfile.com

Jill Sardenga, Author
Susan Shelly, Co-Author
Alan Shelly MD, Co-Author
Scott M Steidl MD, Co-Author
Designed to provide both laymen and professionals with concise, practical information on the second most common disability in the U.S. *$65.00*
340 pages Hardcover
ISBN 0-816042-80-2

8946 Equals in Partnership: Basic Rights for Families of Children with Blindness
NAPVI
1 North Lexington Avenue
White Plains, NY 10601

617-972-7441
800-562-6265
FAX: 617-972-7444
napvi@guildhealth.org
www.napvi.org

Julie Urban, President
Venetia Hayden, Vice President
Susan LaVenture, Executive Director
Randi Sher, Secretary
A comprehensive compilation of educational advocacy materials to help parents better understand the special needs of their children with visual impairments and to assist them in accessing appropriate services for their children.

8947 Eye Research News
Research to Prevent Blindness
645 Madison Avenue
Floor 21
New York, NY 10022-1010

212-752-4333
800-621-0026
FAX: 212-688-6231
inforequest@rpbusa.org
www.rpbusa.org

Diane S. Swift, Chair
Brian F. Hofland, PhD, President
David H. Brenner, VP & Secretary
Richard E. Baker, Treasurer & Asst. Secretary
Yearly publication from Research to Prevent Blindness. Free.
4 pages Yearly

8948 Eye and Your Vision
National Association for Visually Handicapped
111 East 59th Street
New York, NY 10022-1202

212-821-9384
800-829-0500
FAX: 212-821-9707
info@lighthouse.org
lighthouse.org/navh

Mark G. Ackermann, President / CEO
A large booklet offering information, with illustrations, on the eye. Includes information on protection of eyesight, how the eye works and vision disorders. Available in Russian and Spanish also. LightHouse acquired NAVH. *$5.00*

8949 Eye-Q Test
National Association for Visually Handicapped
111 East 59th Street
New York, NY 10022-1202

212-821-9384
800-829-0500
FAX: 212-821-9707
info@lighthouse.org
lighthouse.org/navh

Mark G. Ackermann, President / CEO
Five questions and answers to assist in knowing more about vision. Also available in Spanish and Russian. LightHouse acquired NAVH.

8950 Family Context and Disability Culture Reframing: Through the Looking Glass
Through the Looking Glass
3075 Adeline Street
Suite 120
Berkeley, CA 94703

510-848-1112
800-644-2666
FAX: 510-848-4445
tlg@lookingglass.org
www.lookingglass.org

Maureen Block, J.D., President
Thomas Spalding, Treasurer
Alice Nemon, Secretary
Mega Kirshbaum, Author
This article provides an overview of the issues and guiding perspectives underlying 'Through the Lookinglass' eighteen years of work with families. Available in braille, large print or cassette. *$2.00*
5 pages

8951 Family Guide to Vision Care (FG1)
American Optometric Association
243 North Lindbergh Boulevard
Floor 1
Saint Louis, MO 63141-7881

800-365-2219
aoa.org

David A. Cockrell, OD, President
Andrea P. Thau, OD, Vice President
Barry Barresi, Executive Director
Christopher Quinn, OD, Secretary-Treasurer
Offers information on the early developmental years of your vision, finding a family optometrist and how to take care of your eyesight through the learning years, the working years and the mature years.

8952 **Family Guide: Growth & Development of the Partially Seeing Child**
National Association for Visually Handicapped
111 East 59th Street
New York, NY 10022-1202

212-821-9384
800-829-0500
FAX: 212-821-9707
info@lighthouse.org
lighthouse.org/navh

Mark G. Ackermann, President / CEO
Offers information for parents and guidelines in raising a partially seeing child. LightHouse acquired NAVH. *$.60*

8953 **Fathers: A Common Ground**
Blind Children's Center
4120 Marathon Street
Los Angeles, CA 90029-3584

323-664-2153
800-222-3567
FAX: 323-665-3828
info@blindchildrenscenter.org
www.blindchildrenscenter.org

Scott E. Schaldenbrand, President
Mark Correa, Board Member
Midge Horton, Executive Director
Fernanda Schmitt PhD, Co-Author
Exploring the concerns and roles of fathers of children with visual impairments. *$10.00*
50 pages

8954 **Fighting Blindness News**
Foundation Fighting Blindness
7168 Columbia Gateway Drive
Suite 100
Columbia, MD 21046

410-423-0600
800-683-5555
FAX: 410-363-2393
TTY: 800-683-5551
info@FightBlindness.org
www.blindness.org

Gordon Gund, Chair
David Brent, Vice Chair of Research
Edward H. Gollob, President
Steve Alper, Director
Offers information on medical updates, donor programs, assistive devices, resources and clinical trial information for persons with visual imparments, blindness and retinal degenerative diseases.
2x Year

8955 **First Steps**
Blind Children's Center
4120 Marathon Street
Los Angeles, CA 90029-3584

323-664-2153
800-222-3567
FAX: 323-665-3828
info@blindchildrenscenter.org
www.blindchildrenscenter.org

Scott E. Schaldenbrand, President
Mark Correa, Board Member
Midge Horton, Executive Director
Ferdinand Schmitt PhD, Co-Author
A handbook for teaching young children who are visually impaired. Designed to assist students, professionals and parents working with children who are visually impaired. Visit our website for many publications addressing training very young children who are blind or visually impaired. *$35.00*
203 pages

8956 **Foundations of Orientation and Mobility**
American Foundation for the Blind/AFB Press
2 Penn Plaza
Suite 1102
New York, NY 10121

212-502-7600
800-232-5463
FAX: 888-545-8331
afbinfo@afb.net
www.afb.org

Carl R. Augusto, President & Chief Executive Officer
Rick Bozeman, Finance Director, Chief Financial Officer
Kelly Bleach, Chief Administrative Officer
Stacy Rollins, Executive Administrative Assistant to the President
This text has been updated and revised and includes current research from a variety of disciplines, an international perspective, and expanded contents on low vision, aging, multiple disabilities, accessibility, program design and adaptive technology from more that 30 eminent subject experts. *$79.95*
775 pages
ISBN 0-891289-46-3

8957 **Foundations of Rehabilitation Counseling with Persons Who Are Blind r Visually Impaired**
American Foundation for the Blind/AFB Press
2 Penn Plaza
Suite 1102
New York, NY 10121

212-502-7600
800-232-5463
FAX: 888-545-8331
afbinfo@afb.net
www.afb.org

Carl R. Augusto, President & Chief Executive Officer
Rick Bozeman, Finance Director, Chief Financial Officer
Kelly Bleach, Chief Administrative Officer
Stacy Rollins, Executive Administrative Assistant to the President
Rehabilitation professionals have long recognized that the needs of people who are blind or visually impaired are unique and requie a special knowledge and expertise to provide and corrdinate rehabilitation services. *$59.95*
477 pages
ISBN 0-891289-45-3

8958 **General Facts and Figures on Blindness**
Prevent Blindness America
211 West Wacker Drive
Suite 1700
Chicago, IL 60606

800-331-2020
info@preventblindness.org
www.preventblindness.org

Paul G. Howes, Chairman
Hugh R. Parry, President & CEO,Prevent Blindness America
Jerome Desserich, Vice President & Chief Financial Officer
Danielle Disch, Development Manager

8959 **Get a Wiggle On**
American Alliance for Health, Phys. Ed. & Dance
1900 Association Drive
Reston, VA 20191-1598

703-476-3400
800-213-7193
FAX: 703-476-9527
aapar@aahperd.org
aahperd.org

Dolly D. Lambdin, President
E. Paul Roetert, CEO
Marybell Avery, Director
Frances E. Cleland, Director
Gives teachers and parents practical suggestions for helping blind and visually impaired infants grow and learn like other children. *$5.00*
80 pages
ISBN 0-88314 -77-2

8960 Gift of Sight
RP Foundation Fighting Blindness
1401 W Mount Royal Ave
Baltimore, MD 21217-4245
410-225-9409
800-683-5555
FAX: 410-225-3936

8961 Glaucoma
Glaucoma Research Foundation
251 Post Street
Suite 600
San Francisco, CA 94108
415-986-3162
800-826-6693
FAX: 415-986-3763
question@glaucoma.org
glaucoma.org

Andrew L. Iwach, MD, Chair
Robert L. Stamper, MD, Vice Chair
Thomas M. Brunner, President and CEO
Bill Stewart, Secretary
Offers information on what glaucoma is, the causes, treatments, types of glaucoma, eye exams and prevention.

8962 Glaucoma: The Sneak Thief of Sight
National Association for Visually Handicapped
Fl 6
22 W 21st St
New York, NY 10010-6943
212-242-4438
800-3 C-NCOS
FAX: 631-736-0371
customerservice@cancos.com
cancos.com

Denise Green, Owner
A pamphlet describing the disease, treatment and medications. Also available in Russian and Spanish. Revised in 1999. *$3.50*

8963 Guidelines and Games for Teaching Efficient Braille Reading
American Foundation for the Blind/AFB Press
2 Penn Plaza
Suite 1102
New York, NY 10121
212-502-7600
800-232-5463
FAX: 888-545-8331
afbinfo@afb.net
www.afb.org

Carl R. Augusto, President & Chief Executive Officer
Rick Bozeman, Finance Director, Chief Financial Officer
Kelly Bleach, Chief Administrative Officer
Stacy Rollins, Executive Administrative Assistant to the President
Based on research in the areas of rapid reading and precision teaching, these guidelines represent a unique adaptation of a general reading program to the needs of braille readers. Paperback. *$24.95*

116 pages Paperback
ISBN 0-891281-05-4

8964 Guidelines for Comprehensive Low Vision Care
National Association for Visually Handicapped
111 East 59th Street
New York, NY 10022-1202
212-821-9384
800-829-0500
FAX: 212-821-9707
info@lighthouse.org
lighthouse.org/navh

Mark G. Ackermann, President / CEO
A description of the proper method to conduct a low vision evaluation.LightHouse acquired NAVH. *$.50*

8965 Handbook for Itinerant and Resource Teachers of Blind Students
National Federation of the Blind
200 East Wells St
Baltimore, MD 21230-4914
410-659-9314
nfb@iamdigex.net

Doris Willoughby, Author
Sharon L Monthei, Co-Author

The Handbook provides help to teachers, school administrators or other school personnel that have experience with blind or visually impaired students. The Handbook devotes 45 pages to Braille and how to teach Braille for parents and teachers. There are other chapters offering information on the law, physical education, fitting in socially, testing and evaluation, home economics, daily living skills and more. *$23.00*
533 pages Softcover
ISBN 0-962412-20-1

8966 Handbook of Information for Members of the Achromatopsia Network
P.O.Box 214
Berkeley, CA 94701-214
510-540-4700
FAX: 510-540-4767
futterman@achromat.org
www.achromat.org

8967 Health Care Professionals Who Are Blind or Visually Impaired
American Foundation for the Blind
2 Penn Plaza
Suite 1102
New York, NY 10121
212-502-7600
800-232-5463
FAX: 888-545-8331
afbinfo@afb.net
afb.org

Carl R. Augusto, President & Chief Executive Officer
Rick Bozeman, Finance Director, Chief Financial Officer
Kelly Bleach, Chief Administrative Officer
Stacy Rollins, Executive Administrative Assistant to the President
This resource is essential reading for older students and young adults who are blind or visually impaired, their families, and the professionals who work with them. *$21.95*
160 pages
ISBN 0-891283-88-9

8968 Heart to Heart
Blind Children's Center
4120 Marathon Street
Los Angeles, CA 90029-3584
323-664-2153
800-222-3567
FAX: 323-665-3828
info@blindchildrenscenter.org
www.blindchildrenscenter.org

Scott E. Schaldenbrand, President
Mark Correa, Board Member
Midge Horton, Executive Director
Dori Hayashi MA, Co-Author
Parents of children who are blind and partially sighted talk about their feelings. *$10.00*
12 pages

8969 Heartbreak of Being A Little Bit Blind
National Association for Visually Handicapped
111 East 59th Street
New York, NY 10022-1202
212-821-9384
800-829-0500
FAX: 212-821-9707
info@lighthouse.org
lighthouse.org/navh

Mark G. Ackermann, President / CEO
Summary of what it means to have impaired vision; includes illustrations. LightHouse acquired NAVH.

8970 Helen Keller National Center Newsletter
141 Middle Neck Road
Sands Point, NY 11050
516-944-8900
800-225-0411
FAX: 516-944-7302
hkncinfo@hknc.org
www.hknc.org

Joseph McNulty, Executive Director
The center provides evaluation and training in vocational skills, adaptive technology and computer skills, orientation and mobil-

ity, independent living, communication, speech-language skills, creative arts, fitness and leisure activities.

8971 Helping the Visually Impaired Child with Developmental Problems
Teachers College Press
1234 Amsterdam Avenue
New York, NY 10027

212-678-3929
800-575-6566
FAX: 212-678-4149
tcpress@tc.columbia.edu
www.teacherscollegepress.com

Mary Lynch, Manager
Brian Ellerbeck, Executive Acquisitions Editor
Marie Ellen Larcada, Senior Acquisitions Editor
Emily Spangler, Acquisitions Editor

This book aims to explore the human consequences of severe visual problems combined with other handicaps. The application of child development research to educational interventions, the need for educational and rehabilitative services that serve the human and the special needs of children and their families and the promise of technology in helping to expand communicative possibilities are also discussed. *$18.95*

216 pages Paperback
ISBN 0-807729-02-7

8972 History and Use of Braille
American Council of the Blind
2200 Wilson Boulevard
Suite 650
Arlington, VA 22201-3354

202-467-5081
800-424-8666
FAX: 703-465-5085
info@acb.org
acb.org

Kim Charlson, President
Jeff Thom, 1st Vice President
Melanie Brunson, Executive Director

A system of touch reading and writing for blind persons in which raised dots represent the letters of the alphabet.

8973 How to Thrive, Not Just Survive
American Foundation for the Blind/AFB Press
2 Penn Plaza
Suite 1102
New York, NY 10121

212-502-7600
800-232-5463
FAX: 888-545-8331
afbinfo@afb.net
www.afb.org

Carl R. Augusto, President & Chief Executive Officer
Rick Bozeman, Finance Director, Chief Financial Officer
Kelly Bleach, Chief Administrative Officer

Practical, hands-on guide for parents, teachers, and everyone involved in helping children develop the skills necessary for socialization, orientations and mobility, and leisure and recreational activities. Some of the subjects covered are eating, dressing, personal hygiene, self-esteem and etiquette. *$24.95*

104 pages Paperback
ISBN 0-89128 -48-7

8974 Hub
SPOKES Unlimited
1006 Main Street
Klamath Fals, OR 97601

541-883-7547
FAX: 541-885-2469
spokes@internetcds.com
spokesunlimited.org

Wendy Howard, Executive Director
Celeste Wolf, Clerical Support Specialist II

Newsletter on rehabilitation, peer counseling, blindness, visual impairments, information and referral.

8975 If Blindness Comes
National Federation of the Blind
200 East Wells St
Baltimore, MD 21230-4914

410-659-9314
FAX: 410-685-5653
nfb@iamdigex.net
www.nfb.org

Kenneth Jerrigan, Editor

An introduction to issues relating to vision loss and provides a positive, supportive philosophy about blindness. It is a general information book which includes answers to many common questions about blindness, information about services and programs for the blind and resource listings. Contact the Materials Center.

8976 If Blindness Strikes Don't Strike Out
2600 South 1st Street
Springfield, IL 62704

217-789-8980
800-258-8980
FAX: 217-789-9130
books@ccthomas.com
www.ccthomas.com

Bob Stork, Owner

8977 Imagining the Possibilities: Creative Approaches to Orientation and Mobility Instructio
American Foundation for the Blind
2 Penn Plaza
Suite 1102
New York, NY 10121

212-502-7600
800-232-5463
FAX: 888-545-8331
afbinfo@afb.net
afb.org

Carl R. Augusto, President & Chief Executive Officer
Rick Bozeman, Finance Director, Chief Financial Officer
Kelly Bleach, Chief Administrative Officer

Innovative and varied approaches to O&M techniques and teaching and dynamic suggestions on how to analyze learning styles are just some of the important topics included. *$49.95*

378 pages
ISBN 0-891283-82-X

8978 Increasing Literacy Levels: Final Report
Mississippi State University
P.O.Box 6189
Mississippi State, MS 39762

662-325-2001
FAX: 662-325-8989
TTY:662-325-2694
nrtc@colled.msstate.edu
www.blind.msstate.edu

Jacqui Bybee, Research Associate II
Douglas Bedsaul, Research and Training Coordinator
Anne Carter, Research and Training Coordinator
Brenda Cavenaugh, Ph.D., Research Professor

This study is composed of three research projects to identify and analyze the appropriate use of and instruction in Braille, optical devices and other technologies as they relate to literacy and employment of individuals who are blind or visually impaired. *$20.00*

148 pages Paperback

8979 Information Access Project
National Federation of the Blind
200 East Wells St
Baltimore, MD 21230-4914

410-659-9314
FAX: 410-685-5653
nfb@nfb.org
nfb.org

Marc Maurer, President

Assists entities covered by the ADA in finding methods for converting visually displayed information, such as flyers, brochures and pamphlets, to formats accessible to individuals who are visually impaired.

8980 Information on Glaucoma
Glaucoma Research Foundation
251 Post Street
Suite 600
San Francisco, CA 94108 415-986-3162
800-826-6693
FAX: 415-986-3763
question@glaucoma.org
www.glaucoma.org

Andrew L. Iwach, MD, Chair
Robert L. Stamper, MD, Vice Chair
Thomas M. Brunner, President and CEO
Bill Stewart, Secretary

8981 Intervention Practices in the Retention of Competitive Employment
Mississippi State University
P.O.Box 6189
Mississippi State, MS 39762 662-325-2001
FAX: 662-325-8989
TTY:662-325-2694
nrtc@colled.msstate.edu
www.blind.msstate.edu

Jacqui Bybee, Research Associate II
Douglas Bedsaul, Research and Training Coordinator
Anne Carter, Research and Training Coordinator
Brenda Cavenaugh, Ph.D., Research Professor
This study investigated the methods by which an individual can retain competitive employment after the onset of a significant vision loss. Interviews were conducted with 89 rehabilitation counselors across the US Strategies that contribute to successful job retention were identified as well as best rehabilitation practices in job retention. *$15.00*
60 pages Paperback

8982 Know Your Eye
American Council of the Blind
2200 Wilson Boulevard
Suite 650
Arlington, VA 22201-3354 202-467-5081
800-424-8666
FAX: 703-465-5085
info@acb.org
acb.org

Kim Charlson, President
Jeff Thom, 1st Vice President
Melanie Brunson, Executive Director

8983 Large Print Loan Library
National Association for Visually Handicapped
111 East 59th Street
New York, NY 10022-1202 212-821-9384
800-829-0500
FAX: 212-821-9707
info@lighthouse.org
lighthouse.org/navh

Mark G. Ackermann, President / CEO
A huge large print catalog of all the publications, fiction and non-fiction, cassette tapes, books-on-tape and videos available for the visually impaired from the loan library of the National Association for the Visually Handicapped. LightHouse acquired NAVH.

8984 Large Print Loan Library Catalog
National Association for Visually Handicapped
111 East 59th Street
New York, NY 10022-1202 212-821-9384
800-829-0500
FAX: 212-821-9707
info@lighthouse.org
lighthouse.org/navh

Mark G. Ackermann, President / CEO
Listing of over 7,000 commercially published and NAVH large print books available through NAVH on a loan basis. Includes a limited selection of titles available for purchase. LightHouse acquired NAVH.

8985 Large Print Recipies for a Healthy Life
123601 Wilshire
Los Angeles, CA 90025 310-826-8280
800-481-EYES
FAX: 310-458-8179

Judith Caditz PhD, Author
$21.95
283 pages
ISBN 0-962236-82-9

8986 Learning to Play
Blind Children's Center
4120 Marathon Street
Los Angeles, CA 90029-3584 323-664-2153
800-222-3567
FAX: 323-665-3828
info@blindchildrenscenter.org
www.blindchildrenscenter.org

Scott E. Schaldenbrand, President
Mark Correa, Board Member
Midge Horton, Executive Director
Presenting play activities to the pre-school child who is visually impaired. *$10.00*
12 pages

8987 Let's Eat
Blind Children's Center
4120 Marathon Street
Los Angeles, CA 90029-3584 323-664-2153
800-222-3567
FAX: 323-665-3828
info@blindchildrenscenter.org
www.blindchildrenscenter.org

Scott E. Schaldenbrand, President
Mark Correa, Board Member
Midge Horton, Executive Director
Feeding a child with visual impairment. *$10.00*
28 pages

8988 Library Services for the Blind
South Carolina State University
300 College Street NorthEast
P.O. Box 7491
Orangeburg, SC 29117 803-536-7045
FAX: 803-536-8902
reference@scsu.edu
library.scsu.edu

Adrienne C. Webber, Dean, Library/Information Services
Ramona S. Evans, Administrative Specialist
Ruth A. Hodges, Reference & Information Specialist
Wanda L. Priester, Library Technical Asst.
News and information on developments in library services for readers who are blind and physically disabled.

8989 Lifestyles of Employed Legally Blind People
Mississippi State University
P.O.Box 6189
Mississippi State, MS 39762 662-325-2001
FAX: 662-325-8989
TTY:662-325-2694
nrtc@colled.msstate.edu
www.blind.msstate.edu

Jacqui Bybee, Research Associate II
Douglas Bedsaul, Research and Training Coordinator
Anne Carter, Research and Training Coordinator
Brenda Cavenaugh, Ph.D., Research Professor
Results from a telephone survey show that visually impaired respondents are involved in a wide variety of activities with little restrictions on their range of activities. Sighted respondents tended to spend more time in child care, obtaining goods and services, attending to self-care activities and engaging in social activities, while visually impaired respondents spent more time in education and passive activities. This report is a study of expenditures and time use. *$ 10.00*
193 pages Paperback

8990 **Lion**
Lion's Clubs International
300 West 22nd Street
Oak Brook, IL 60523-8842
630-571-5466
FAX: 630-571-8890
TTY:630-571-6533
www.lionsclubs.org/

Joseph Preston, International President
Jitsuhiro Yamada, 1st Vice President
Robert E. Corlew, 2nd Vice President
Peter Lynch, Executive Director
Publication for the blind.

8991 **Living with Achromatopsia**
P.O.Box 214
Berkeley, CA 94701-214
510-540-4700
FAX: 510-540-4767
futterman@achromat.org
www.achromat.org

Frances Futterman, Author
Consists entirely of comments from persons who know firsthand about living with achromatopsia.

8992 **Low Vision Questions and Answers: Definitions, Devices, Services**
American Foundation for the Blind/AFB Press
2 Penn Plaza
Suite 1102
New York, NY 10121
212-502-7600
800-232-5463
FAX: 888-545-8331
afbinfo@afb.net
afb.org

Carl R. Augusto, President & Chief Executive Officer
Rick Bozeman, Chief Financial Officer
Kelly Bleach, Chief Administrative Officer
Stacy Rollins, Executive Administrative Assistant to the President
What does low vision mean? What do low vision services cost? What diseases cause low vision? Answers to these and other questions are presented in a comprehensive format with accompanying photographs. $50.00/pack of 25.
21 pages Pamphlet
ISBN 0-891281-96-7

8993 **Low Vision: Reflections of the Past, Issues for the Future**
American Foundation for the Blind/AFB Press
2 Penn Plaza
Suite 1102
New York, NY 10121
212-502-7600
800-232-5463
FAX: 888-545-8331
afbinfo@afb.net
www.afb.org

Carl R. Augusto, President & Chief Executive Officer
Rick Bozeman, Chief Financial Officer
Kelly Bleach, Chief Administrative Officer
Stacy Rollins, Executive Administrative Assistant to the President
Background papers and a strategies section are used to identify the shifting needs of visually impaired persons and the resources that may be needed to address them. Paperback. $34.95
Paperback
ISBN 0-891282-18-1

8994 **Mainstreaming and the American Dream**
American Foundation for the Blind/AFB Press
2 Penn Plaza
Suite 1102
New York, NY 10121
212-502-7600
800-232-5463
FAX: 888-545-8331
afbinfo@afb.net
www.afb.org

Carl R. Augusto, President & Chief Executive Officer
Rick Bozeman, Chief Financial Officer
Kelly Bleach, Chief Administrative Officer
Stacy Rollins, Executive Administrative Assistant to the President

Based on in-depth interviews with parents and professionals, this research monograph presents information on the needs and aspirations of parents of blind and visually impaired children. Paperback. $34.95
256 pages Paperback
ISBN 0-891281-91-7

8995 **Mainstreaming the Visually Impaired Child**
NAPVI
1 North Lexington Avenue
White Plains, NY 10601
617-972-7441
800-562-6265
FAX: 617-972-7444
napvi@guildhealth.org
www.napvi.org

Julie Urban, President
Venetia Hayden, Vice President
Susan LaVenture, Executive Director
Randi Sher, Secretary
A unique, informative guide for teachers and educational professionals that work with the visually impaired. $10.00
121 pages Paper

8996 **Making Life More Livable**
American Foundation for the Blind
2 Penn Plaza
Suite 1102
New York, NY 10121
212-502-7600
800-232-5463
FAX: 888-545-8331
afbinfo@afb.net
www.afb.org

Carl R. Augusto, President & Chief Executive Officer
Rick Bozeman, Chief Financial Officer
Kelly Bleach, Chief Administrative Officer
Stacy Rollins, Executive Administrative Assistant to the President
Shows how simple adaptations in the home and environment can make a big difference in the lives of blind and visually impaired older persons. The suggestions offered are numerous and specific, ranging from how to mark food cans for greater visibility to how to get out of the shower safley. Large print. $24.95
128 pages
ISBN 0-891283-87-0

8997 **Meeting the Needs of People with Vision Loss: Multidisciplinary Perspective**
Resources for Rehabilitation
22 Bonad Road
Winchester, MA 01890
781-368-9080
FAX: 781-368-9096
orders@rfr.org
www.rfr.org

Susan L Greenblatt, Editor
Written by rehabilitation professionals, physicians, and a sociologist, this book discusses how to provide appropriate information and how to serve special populations. Chapters on the role of the family, diabetes and vision loss, special needs of children and adolescents, adults with hearing and vision loss. $29.95

ISBN 0-929718-07-0

8998 **Model Program Operation Manual: Business Enterprise Program Supervisors**
Mississippi State University
P.O.Box 6189
Mississippi State, MS 39762
662-325-2001
FAX: 662-325-8989
TTY:662-325-2694
nrtc@colled.msstate.edu
www.blind.msstate.edu

Jacqui Bybee, Research Associate II
Douglas Bedsaul, Research and Training Coordinator
Anne Carter, Research and Training Coordinator
Brenda Cavenaugh, Ph.D., Research Professor
This monograph serves as a Model Program Operation Manual for Business Enterprise Program Supervisors who administer Randolph-Sheppard vending facilities under the

Randolph-Sheppard Act. A wide variety of topics are covered including the role of the State Committee of Blind Venders, the role and responsibilities of the Vending Facility Operator, model qualification, for potential Facility Managers, guidelines for location of vending facilities and policies for closing vending facilities. *$20.00*
199 pages Paperback

8999   More Alike Than Different: Blind and Visually Impaired Children
American Foundation for the Blind/AFB Press
2 Penn Plaza
Suite 1102
New York, NY 10121
212-502-7600
800-232-5463
FAX: 888-545-8331
afborders@abdintl.com
www.afb.org

Carl R. Augusto, President & Chief Executive Officer
Rick Bozeman, Chief Financial Officer
Kelly Bleach, Chief Administrative Officer
Stacy Rollins, Executive Administrative Assistant to the President
Offers photographs of blind and visually impaired children around the world learning to read and write, travel independently and performing basic living skills. Covers the most recent technological advances and demonstrates the universality of educational needs and goals. Paperback. $100.00/pack of 25.

ISBN 0-891281-69-0

9000   Mothers with Visual Impairments who are Raising Young Children
American Foundation for the Blind/AFB Press
2 Penn Plaza
Suite 1102
New York, NY 10121
212-502-7600
800-232-5463
FAX: 888-545-8331
afbinfo@afb.net
www.afb.org

Carl R. Augusto, President & Chief Executive Officer
Rick Bozeman, Chief Financial Officer
Kelly Bleach, Chief Administrative Officer
Stacy Rollins, Executive Administrative Assistant to the President
Available in braille, large print or cassette. *$2.00*
16 pages

9001   Move With Me
Blind Children's Center
4120 Marathon Street
Los Angeles, CA 90029-3584
323-664-2153
800-222-3567
FAX: 323-665-3828
info@blindchildrenscenter.org
www.blindchildrenscenter.org

Scott E. Schaldenbrand, President
Mark Correa, Board Member
Midge Horton, Executive Director
Nancy Chernus-Mansfield MA, Co-Author
A parent's guide to movement development for babies who are visually impaired. *$10.00*
12 pages

9002   National Eye Institute
National Institute of Health
31 Center Drive MSC 2510
Bethesda, MD 20892-2510
301-496-5248
FAX: 301-402-1065
2020@nei.nih.gov
www.nei.nih.gov

9003   Orientation and Mobility Primer for Families and Young Children
American Foundation for the Blind/AFB Press
2 Penn Plaza
Suite 1102
New York, NY 10121
212-502-7600
800-232-5463
FAX: 888-545-8331
afbinfo@afb.net
www.afb.org

Carl R. Augusto, President & Chief Executive Officer
Rick Bozeman, Chief Financial Officer
Kelly Bleach, Chief Administrative Officer
Stacy Rollins, Executive Administrative Assistant to the President
Practical information for helping a child learn about his or her environment right from the start. Covers sensory training, concept development and orientation skills. Paperback. *$14.95*
48 pages
ISBN 0-891281-57-6

9004   Out of the Corner of My Eye: Living with Vision Loss in Later Life
American Foundation for the Blind/AFB Press
2 Penn Plaza
Suite 1102
New York, NY 10121
212-502-7600
800-232-5463
FAX: 888-545-8331
afbinfo@fb.net
www.afb.org

Carl R. Augusto, President & Chief Executive Officer
Rick Bozeman, Chief Financial Officer
Kelly Bleach, Chief Administrative Officer
Stacy Rollins, Executive Administrative Assistant to the President
A personal account of students' vision loss and subsequent adjustment that is full of practical advice and cheerful encouragement, told by an 87 year old retired college teacher who has maintained her independence and zest for life. Available in paperback or on audio cassette. *$23.95*
120 pages
ISBN 0-891281-82-1

9005   Out of the Corner of My Eye: Living with Macular Degeneration
American Foundation for the Blind/AFB Press
2 Penn Plaza
Suite 1102
New York, NY 10121
212-502-7600
800-232-5463
FAX: 888-545-8331
afbinfo@afb.net
www.afb.org

Carl R. Augusto, President & Chief Executive Officer
Rick Bozeman, Chief Financial Officer
Kelly Bleach, Chief Administrative Officer
Stacy Rollins, Executive Administrative Assistant to the President
A personal account of students' vision loss and subsequent adjustment that is full of practical advice and cheerful encouragement, told by an 87 year old retired college teacher who has maintained her independence and zest for life. *$29.95*
168 pages Paperback
ISBN 0-891238-31-2

9006   Pain Erasure: the Bonnie Prudden Way
Ballantine Books
1540 Broadway
New York, NY 10036-4039
212-751-2600
FAX: 212-572-4949

Bonnie Prudden, Author
Revolutionary breakthrough in pain relief involves trigger points-tender areas where muscles have been damaged from falls, childhood ailments, poor posture, and the stresses of daily life.

9007 **Patient's Guide to Visual Aids and Illumination**
National Association for Visually Handicapped
111 East 59th Street
New York, NY 10022-1202

212-821-9384
800-829-0500
FAX: 212-821-9707
info@lighthouse.org
lighthouse.org/navh

Mark G. Ackermann, President / CEO
A reference booklet offering information on aids for the visually
impaired. LightHouse acquired NAVH. *$.75*

9008 **Pediatric Visual Diagnosis Fact Sheets**
Blind Children's Center
4120 Marathon Street
Los Angeles, CA 90029-3584

323-664-2153
800-222-3567
FAX: 323-665-3828
info@blindchildrenscenter.org
blindchildrenscenter.org

Scott E. Schaldenbrand, President
Mark Correa, Board Member
Midge Horton, Executive Director
Collection of fact sheets addressing commonly encountered eye
conditions, diagnostic tests and materials. *$10.00*
10 pages

9009 **Perkins Activity and Resource Guide: A Handbook for
Teachers**
Perkins School for the Blind
175 North Beacon Street
Watertown, MA 02472

617-924-3434
FAX: 617-972-7363
info@perkins.org
www.perkins.org

Frederic M. Clifford, Chair of the Board
Philip L. Ladd, Vice Chair of the Board
Leslie Nordon, Secretary
Charles C.J. Platt, Treasurer
This is a comprehensive, two volume guide with over 1,000 pages
of activities, resources and instructional strategies for teachers
and parents of students with visual and multiple disabilities.
$80.00

9010 **Personal Reader Update**
Personal Reader Department
9 Centennial Dr
Peabody, MA 01960-7906

978-977-2000
800-343-0311
FAX: 978-977-2409

9011 **Preschool Learning Activities for the Visually Impaired
Child**
NAPVI
1 North Lexington Avenue
White Plains, NY 10601

617-972-7441
800-562-6265
FAX: 617-972-7444
napvi@guildhealth.org
www.napvi.org

Julie Urban, President
Venetia Hayden, Vice President
Susan LaVenture, Executive Director
Randi Sher, Secretary
This guide for parents offers games and activities to keep visually
impaired children active during the preschool years. *$8.00*
91 pages Paperback

9012 **Reaching, Crawling, Walking....Let's Get Moving**
Blind Children's Center
4120 Marathon Street
Los Angeles, CA 90029-3584

323-664-2153
800-222-3567
FAX: 323-665-3828
info@blindchildrenscenter.org
www.blindchildrenscenter.org

Scott E. Schaldenbrand, President
Mark Correa, Board Member
Midge Horton, Executive Director
Orientation and mobility for preschool children who are visually
imapired. *$10.00*
24 pages

9013 **Reading Is for Everyone**
Nat'l Lib Svc/Blind And Physically Handicapped
1291 Taylor Street North West
Washington, DC 20011

202-707-5100
FAX: 202-707-0712
TTY:202-707-0744
nls@loc.gov
www.loc.gov/nls

Karen Keninger, Director

9014 **Reading with Low Vision**
Nat'l Lib Svc/Blind And Physically Handicapped
1291 Taylor Street North West
Washington, DC 20011

202-707-5100
FAX: 202-707-0712
TTY:202-707-0744
nls@loc.gov
www.loc.gov/nls

Karen Keninger, Director

9015 **Recording for the Blind & Dyslexic**
20 Roszel Road
Princeton, NJ 08540

800-221-4792
FAX: 609-987-8116
Custserv@LearningAlly.org
www.learningally.org/

Brad Grob, Chairman
Harold J. Logan, Vice Chairman
Andrew Friedman, President & CEO
Jim Halliday, Executive Vice President
Provides recorded and computerized textbooks, library services
and other educational resources to people who cannot effectively
read standard print because of visual impairment, dyslexia or
other physical disability. RFB&D is now Learning Ally.

9016 **Reference and Information Services From NLS**
Nat'l Lib Svc/Blind And Physically Handicapped
1291 Taylor Street North West
Washington, DC 20011

202-707-5100
FAX: 202-707-0712
TTY:202-707-0744
nls@loc.gov
www.loc.gov/nls

Karen Keninger, Director

9017 **Resource List for Persons with Low Vision**
American Council of the Blind
2200 Wilson Boulevard
Suite 650
Arlington, VA 22201-3354

202-467-5081
800-424-8666
FAX: 703-465-5085
info@acb.org
acb.org

Kim Charlson, President
Jeff Thom, 1st Vice President
Melanie Brunson, Executive Director

9018 Rose-Colored Glasses
Human Sciences Press
233 Spring St
New York, NY 10013-1522

212-229-2859
800-221-9369
FAX: 212-463-0742

30 pages Hardcover
ISBN 0-87705-08-8

9019 Say it with Sign
Harris Communications
15155 Technology Drive
Eden Prairie, MN 55344

952-388-2152
800-825-6758
FAX: 952-906-1099
info@harriscomm.com
harriscomm.com

Robert Harris, Owner
Contains both the serious and fun side of signing and provides the basic signs that might be needed in an emergency situation. *$299.50*
10-DVD set

9020 See A Bone
Facts on File
132 West 31st Street
14th Floor
New York, NY 10001

212-967-8800
800-683-5433
FAX: 212-760-0862
info@northernleasing.com
northernleasing.com

Mark Donnell, President
$65.00
352 pages
ISBN 0-816042-80-2

9021 See What I Feel
Britannica Film Company
345 4th Street
San Francisco, CA 94107

415-928-8466
FAX: 415-928-5027
pacbikes.com

Dave Bekowich, Owner
A blind child tells her friends about her trip to the zoo. Each experience was explained as a blind child would experience it. A teacher's guide comes with this video.
Film

9022 Selecting a Program
Blind Children's Center
4120 Marathon Street
Los Angeles, CA 90029-3584

323-664-2153
800-222-3567
FAX: 323-665-3828
info@blindchildrenscenter.org
www.blindchildrenscenter.org

Scott E. Schaldenbrand, President
Mark Correa, Board Member
Midge Horton, Executive Director
A guide for parents of infants and preschoolers with visual impairments. *$10.00*
28 pages

9023 Show Me How: A Manual for Parents of Preschool Blind Children
American Foundation for the Blind/AFB Press
2 Penn Plaza
Suite 1102
New York, NY 10121

212-502-7600
800-232-5463
FAX: 888-545-8331
afbinfo@afb.net
www.afb.org

Carl R. Augusto, President & Chief Executive Officer
Rick Bozeman, Chief Financial Officer
Kelly Bleach, Chief Administrative Officer
Stacy Rollins, Executive Administrative Assistant to the President
A practical guide for parents, teachers and others who help preschool children attain age-related goals. Covers issues on playing precautions, appropriate toys and facilitating relationships with playmates. Paperback. *$12.95*
56 pages
ISBN 0-891281-13-4

9024 Sign of the Times
Fanlight Productions
c/o Icarus Films
32 Court Street, 21st Floor
Brooklyn, NY 11201

718-488-8900
800-876-1710
FAX: 718-488-8642
info@fanlight.com, sales@icarusfilms.com
www.fanlight.com

Ben Achtenberg, Owner, Founder
Profiles a public school in the heart of Los Angeles - an American microcosm where over 300 languages are spoken, and where cultures and races collide. Fairfax High, publicized as the site of gang activity and murder, has long been a focus for bad press. But something very right is going on in this school. A Sign of the Times offers a positive example of how the American dream and American education are still alive

9025 Special Technologies Alternative Resources
210 McMorran Boulevard
Port Huron, MI 48060

810-987-7323
877-987-READ
star@sccl.lib.mi.us
www.sccl.lib.mi.us/star.html

Arnold H. Larson, Chairman
Kathleen J. Wheelihan, Vice Chairman
Arlene M. Marcetti, Board Member
Stan Arnetti, Director
Addresses the needs of a very unique diverse group of people by offering a full range of library services for people who cannot read standard print. Provides reading material in specialized formats that permit individuals with disabilities to have access to the written word, delivering to customer's mailboxes free of charge. Talking Book Machines, recorded books and magazines, descriptive videos, large print editions and braille books and magazines.

9026 Standing on My Own Two Feet
Blind Children's Center
4120 Marathon Street
Los Angeles, CA 90029-3584

323-664-2153
800-222-3567
FAX: 323-665-3828
info@blindchildrenscenter.org
www.blindchildrenscenter.org

Scott E. Schaldenbrand, President
Mark Correa, Board Member
Midge Horton, Executive Director
A guide to constructing mobility devices for children who are visually impaired. *$10.00*
38 pages

9027　**Starting Points**
Blind Children's Center
4120 Marathon Street
Los Angeles, CA 90029-3584　　　　　323-664-2153
　　　　　　　　　　　　　　　　　　　800-222-3567
　　　　　　　　　　　　　　　　FAX: 323-665-3828
　　　　　　　　　　　info@blindchildrenscenter.org
　　　　　　　　　　　www.blindchildrenscenter.org

Scott E. Schaldenbrand, President
Mark Correa, Board Member
Midge Horton, Executive Director
Basic information for the classroom teacher of 3 to 8 year olds
whose multiple disabilities include visual impairment. *$35.00*
157 pages
ISBN 0-891280-61-8

9028　**Step-By-Step Guide to Personal Management for Blind**
Persons
American Foundation for the Blind/AFB Press
2 Penn Plaza
Suite 1102
New York, NY 10121　　　　　　　　212-502-7600
　　　　　　　　　　　　　　　　　　800-232-5463
　　　　　　　　　　　　　　　　FAX: 888-545-8331
　　　　　　　　　　　　　　　　　afbinfo@afb.net
　　　　　　　　　　　　　　　　　　www.afb.org

Carl R. Augusto, President & Chief Executive Officer
Rick Bozeman, Chief Financial Officer
Kelly Bleach, Chief Administrative Officer
Stacy Rollins, Executive Administrative Assistant to the President
A manual of techniques in the areas of hygiene, grooming, cloth-
ing, shopping and child care. *$19.95*
136 pages Spiralbound
ISBN 0-891280-61-8

9029　**Student Teaching Guide for Blind and Visually Impaired**
College Students
American Foundation for the Blind/AFB Press
2 Penn Plaza
Suite 1102
New York, NY 10121　　　　　　　　212-502-7600
　　　　　　　　　　　　　　　　　　800-232-5463
　　　　　　　　　　　　　　　　FAX: 888-545-8331
　　　　　　　　　　　　　　　　　afbinfo@afb.net
　　　　　　　　　　　　　　　　　　www.afb.org

Carl R. Augusto, President & Chief Executive Officer
Rick Bozeman, Chief Financial Officer
Kelly Bleach, Chief Administrative Officer
Stacy Rollins, Executive Administrative Assistant to the President
A comprehensive resource designed to enable the student to enter
the classroom of a university or college with confidence. Large
print. *$14.95*
52 pages
ISBN 0-891281-42-8

9030　**Survey of Direct Labor Workers Who Are Blind &**
Employed by NIB
Mississippi State University
P.O.Box 6189
Mississippi State, MS 39762　　　　　662-325-2001
　　　　　　　　　　　　　　　　FAX: 662-325-8989
　　　　　　　　　　　　　　　TTY:662-325-2694
　　　　　　　　　　　nrtc@colled.msstate.edu
　　　　　　　　　　　www.blind.msstate.edu

Jacqui Bybee, Research Associate II
Douglas Bedsaul, Research and Training Coordinator
Anne Carter, Research and Training Coordinator
Brenda Cavenaugh, Ph.D., Research Professor
This report is a follow-up to surveys by National Industries for
the Blind in 1983 and 1987 and summarizes the results of a national survey of approximately 500 legally blind direct labor
workers. *$10.00*
101 pages Paperback

9031　**Talk to Me**
Blind Children's Center
4120 Marathon Street
Los Angeles, CA 90029-3584　　　　　323-664-2153
　　　　　　　　　　　　　　　　　　　800-222-3567
　　　　　　　　　　　　　　　　FAX: 323-665-3828
　　　　　　　　　　　info@blindchildrenscenter.org
　　　　　　　　　　　www.blindchildrenscenter.org

Scott E. Schaldenbrand, President
Mark Correa, Board Member
Midge Horton, Executive Director
A language guide for parents of children who are visually im-
paired. *$10.00*
11 pages

9032　**Talk to Me II**
Blind Children's Center
4120 Marathon Street
Los Angeles, CA 90029-3584　　　　　323-664-2153
　　　　　　　　　　　　　　　　　　　800-222-3567
　　　　　　　　　　　　　　　　FAX: 323-665-3828
　　　　　　　　　　　info@blindchildrenscenter.org
　　　　　　　　　　　www.blindchildrenscenter.org

Scott E. Schaldenbrand, President
Mark Correa, Board Member
Midge Horton, Executive Director
a sequel to Talk to Me *$10.00*
15 pages

9033　**Talking Books & Reading Disabilities**
Nat'l Lib Svc/Blind And Physically Handicapped
1291 Taylor Street North West
Washington, DC 20011　　　　　　　202-707-5100
　　　　　　　　　　　　　　　　FAX: 202-707-0712
　　　　　　　　　　　　　　　TTY:202-707-0744
　　　　　　　　　　　　　　　　　　nls@loc.gov
　　　　　　　　　　　　　　　　www.loc.gov/nls

Karen Keninger, Director

9034　**Talking Books for People with Physical Disabilities**
Nat'l Lib Svc/Blind And Physically Handicapped
1291 Taylor Street North West
Washington, DC 20011　　　　　　　202-707-5100
　　　　　　　　　　　　　　　　FAX: 202-707-0712
　　　　　　　　　　　　　　　TTY:202-707-0744
　　　　　　　　　　　　　　　　　　nls@loc.gov
　　　　　　　　　　　　　　　　www.loc.gov/nls

Karen Keninger, Director

9035　**Teaching Orientation and Mobility in the Schools: An**
Instructor's Companion
American Foundation for the Blind
2 Penn Plaza
Suite 1102
New York, NY 10121　　　　　　　　212-502-7600
　　　　　　　　　　　　　　　　　　800-232-5463
　　　　　　　　　　　　　　　　FAX: 888-545-8331
　　　　　　　　　　　　　　　　　afbinfo@afb.net
　　　　　　　　　　　　　　　　　　www.afb.org

Carl R. Augusto, President & Chief Executive Officer
Rick Bozeman, Chief Financial Officer
Kelly Bleach, Chief Administrative Officer
Stacy Rollins, Executive Administrative Assistant to the President
This book, with its useful forms, checklists, and tips, will help
O&M instructors and teachers of visually impaired students mas-
ter the arts of planning schedules, organizing equipment and
work routines, working with school personnel and educational
team members, and effectively providing instruction to children
with diverse needs. *$ 45.95*
176 pages
ISBN 0-891283-91-1

9036   Teaching Visually Impaired Children
Charles C. Thomas
2600 S First St
Springfield, IL 62704-4730   217-789-8980
                                              800-258-8980
                                         FAX: 217-789-9130
                                       books@ccthomas.com
                                          www.ccthomas.com

Michael P. Thomas, President
A comprehensive resource for the classroom teacher who is working with a visually impaired child for the first time, as well as a
systematic overview of education for the specialist in visual disabilities. It approaches instructional challenges with clear explanations and practical suggestions, and it addresses common
concerns of teachers in a reassuring and positive manner. Also
available in cloth. *$49.95*
352 pages Paper 2004
ISBN 0-398074-77-7

9037   Textbook Catalog
National Braille Association
95 Allens Creek Road
Building 1, Suite 202
Rochester, NY 14618   585-427-8260
                                         FAX: 585-427-0263
                                 nbaoffice@nationalbraille.org
                                       www.nationalbraille.org

Jan Carroll, President
Cindi Laurent, Vice President
David Shaffer, Executive Director
Heidi Lehmann, Secretary
Lists hundreds of scholarly, college and professional textbooks
offered in large print, braille or on cassette for visually impaired
readers.
80 pages

9038   Three Rivers News
Carnegie Library of Pitts. Library for the Blind
4724 Baum Boulevard
Pittsburgh, PA 15213   412-687-2440
                                              800-242-0586
                                         FAX: 412-687-2442
                                           clbph@clpgh.org
                                            www.clpgh.org

Kathleen Kappel, Executive Director
Loans recorded books/magazines and playback equipment, large
print books and described videos to western PA residents unable
to use standard printed materials due to a visual, physical, or
physically-based reading disability.
12 pages Quarterly

9039   To Love this Life: Quotations by Helen Keller
American Foundation for the Blind/AFB Press
2 Penn Plaza
Suite 1102
New York, NY 10121   212-502-7600
                                              800-232-5463
                                         FAX: 888-545-8331
                                           afbinfo@afb.org
                                              www.afb.org

Carl R. Augusto, President & Chief Executive Officer
Rick Bozeman, Chief Financial Officer
Kelly Bleach, Chief Administrative Officer
Stacy Rollins, Executive Administrative Assistant to the President
Inspirational work that offers the penetrating observations of
Helen Keller, the beloved deaf-blind champion of the rights of
people with disabilities. Also available on cassette at $21.95
(ISBN# 0-89128-348-X) *$21.95*
144 pages Hardcover
ISBN 0-891283-47-1

**9040   Touch the Baby: Blind & Visually Impaired Children As
Patients**
American Foundation for the Blind/AFB Press
2 Penn Plaza
Suite 1102
New York, NY 10121   212-502-7600
                                              800-232-5463
                                         FAX: 888-545-8331
                                           afbinfo@afb.net
                                              www.afb.org

Carl R. Augusto, President & Chief Executive Officer
Rick Bozeman, Chief Financial Officer
Kelly Bleach, Chief Administrative Officer
Stacy Rollins, Executive Administrative Assistant to the President
A how-to manual for health care professionals working in hospitals, clinics and doctors' offices. Teaches the special communication and touch-related techniques needed to prevent blind and
visually impaired patients from withdrawing from the healthcare
workers and the outside world. $25.00/pack of 25.
13 pages
ISBN 0-891281-97-5

**9041   Transition Activity Calendar for Students with Visual
Impairments**
Mississippi State University
P.O.Box 6189
Mississippi State, MS 39762   662-325-2001
                                         FAX: 662-325-8989
                                         TTY:662-325-2694
                                   nrtc@colled.msstate.edu
                                     www.blind.msstate.edu

Jacqui Bybee, Research Associate II
Douglas Bedsaul, Research and Training Coordinator
Anne Carter, Research and Training Coordinator
Brenda Cavenaugh, Ph.D., Research Professor
The Transition Activity Calendar guides the student with a visual
disability through the maze of college preparation. Beginning in
junior high school, clearly written steps are listed for each grade
level. Students planning to enter college after high school gradu-
ation can check-off their accomplishments each step of the way.
The calendar helps students focus on their goals while providing
reminders of tasks yet to be completed. It can be used in a self-directed manner or in a group format. *$4.25*
16 pages Paperback

**9042   Transition to College for Students with Visual Impairments:
Report**
Mississippi State University
P.O.Box 6189
Mississippi State, MS 39762   662-325-2001
                                         FAX: 662-325-8989
                                         TTY:662-325-2694
                                   nrtc@colled.msstate.edu
                                     www.blind.msstate.edu

Jacqui Bybee, Research Associate II
Douglas Bedsaul, Research and Training Coordinator
Anne Carter, Research and Training Coordinator
Brenda Cavenaugh, Ph.D., Research Professor
A report offering results from telephone interviews of college
students with visual impairments and mail surveys of college officials which examines the transition experience of successful
college students. General domains in the study include demographics, educational history, computers, specialized and adaptive equipment, resources, college preparation, problems
adjusting to college and O&M skills. A literature review covers
preparing for college, task timelines, and classroom, labs and
tests. *$20.00*
151 pages Paperback

9043 **Unseen Minority: A Social History of Blindness in the United States**
American Foundation for the Blind/AFB Press
2 Penn Plaza
Suite 1102
New York, NY 10121
212-502-7600
800-232-5463
FAX: 888-545-8331
abfinfo@abf.org
www.afb.org

Carl R. Augusto, President & Chief Executive Officer
Rick Bozeman, Chief Financial Officer
Kelly Bleach, Chief Administrative Officer
Stacy Rollins, Executive Administrative Assistant to the President
A lively narrative, with anecdotes, that recounts how the blind overcame discrimination to gain full participation in the social, educational, economic and legislative spheres. Hardcover. *$59.95*
573 pages Paperback
ISBN 0-891288-96-1

9044 **Vision Enhancement**
UN Printing
122
1790 E 54th St
Indianapolis, IN 46220-3454
317-254-1332
800-431-1739
FAX: 317-251-6588
info@visionenhancement.org
www.visionww.org

Patricia L Price, Managing Editor
Designed to encourage and support individuals with vision loss, family members, and caregivers. *$25.00*
72-78 pages Quarterly

9045 **Visual Impairment: An Overview**
American Foundation for the Blind/AFB Press
2 Penn Plaza
Suite 1102
New York, NY 10121
212-502-7600
800-232-5463
FAX: 888-545-8331
afbinfo@afb.net
www.afb.org

Carl R. Augusto, President & Chief Executive Officer
Rick Bozeman, Chief Financial Officer
Kelly Bleach, Chief Administrative Officer
Stacy Rollins, Executive Administrative Assistant to the President
An overall look at the most common forms of vision loss and their impact on the individual. Includes drawings as well as photographs that stimulate how people with vision loss see. Paperback. *$19.95*
56 pages
ISBN 0-891281-74-0

9046 **Visual Impairments And Learning**
Sage Publications
2455 Teller Road
Thousand Oaks, CA 91320
805-499-0721
800-818-7243
FAX: 805-499-0871
info@sagepub.com
www.sagepub.com

Sara Miller McCune, Founder, Publisher, Executive Chairman
Blaise R Simqu, President & CEO
Tracey A. Ozmina, Executive Vice President & Chief Operating Officer
Stephen Barr, Managing Director/SAGE London, President of SAGE Internation
The major focus of this new, third edition is to present a new way of thinking about individuals with visual impairment so that they are viewed as participating members of a seeing world despite their reduced visual functioning. *$40.00*
213 pages
ISBN 0-890798-68-3

9047 **Walking Alone and Marching Together**
National Federation of the Blind
200 East Wells St
Baltimore, MD 21230-4914
410-659-9314
FAX: 410-685-5653
nfb@iamdigex.net
www.nfb.org

Floyd Matson, Author
The history of the organized blind movement, this book spans more than 50 years of civil rights, social issues, attitudes and experiences of the blind. Published in 1990, it has been read by thousands of blind and sighted persons and is used in colleges, libraries and programs across the country as an important tool in understanding blindness and it's impact on both personal lives and the society at large. Braille $130, 2 track or 4 track cassette $40, Print $33.00. Contact Materials Center.

9048 **What Do You Do When You See a Blind Person- and What Don't You Do?**
American Foundation for the Blind/AFB Press
2 Penn Plaza
Suite 1102
New York, NY 10121
212-502-7600
800-232-5463
FAX: 888-545-8331
afbinfo@afb.net
afb.org

Carl R. Augusto, President & Chief Executive Officer
Rick Bozeman, Chief Financial Officer
Kelly Bleach, Chief Administrative Officer
Stacy Rollins, Executive Administrative Assistant to the President
Examples of real-life situations that teach sighted persons how to interact effectively with blind persons. Topics covered include how to help someone across the street, how not to distract a guide dog and how to take leave of a blind person. *$25.00*
8 pages
ISBN 0-891281-95-5

9049 **What Museum Guides Need to Know: Access for the Blind and Visually Impaired**
American Foundation for the Blind/AFB Press
2 Penn Plaza
Suite 1102
New York, NY 10121
212-502-7600
800-232-5463
FAX: 888-545-8331
afbinfo@afb.net
www.afb.org

Carl R. Augusto, President & Chief Executive Officer
Rick Bozeman, Chief Financial Officer
Kelly Bleach, Chief Administrative Officer
Stacy Rollins, Executive Administrative Assistant to the President
Explains how blind and visually impaired museum-goers experience art and offers pointers on greeting people, asking if help is needed and teaching about a specific work of art. Contains information on access laws, resources, training guides and guidelines for preparing large print, cassette and braille materials. *$14.95*
64 pages Paperback
ISBN 0-891281-58-4

9050 **Work Sight**
Lighthouse International
111 East 59th Street
New York, NY 10022-1202
212-821-9384
800-829-0500
FAX: 212-821-9707
info@lighthouse.org
www.lighthouse.org

Mark G. Ackermann, President / CEO
Intended for employers and employees who have concerns about vision loss and job performance. *$25.00*

9051 **World Through Their Eyes**
Lighthouse International
111 East 59th Street
New York, NY 10022-1202

212-821-9384
800-829-0500
FAX: 212-821-9707
info@lighthouse.org
www.lighthouse.org

Mark G. Ackermann, President / CEO
Intended to help nursing home staff understand how residents
with impaired vision perceive the world. Concrete suggestions
help staff provide better care to visually impaired residents.
$25.00

9052 **You Seem Like a Regular Kid to Me**
American Foundation for the Blind/AFB Press
2 Penn Plaza
Suite 1102
New York, NY 10121

212-502-7600
800-232-5463
FAX: 888-545-8331
afbinfo@afb.net
www.afb.org

Carl R. Augusto, President & Chief Executive Officer
Rick Bozeman, Chief Financial Officer
Kelly Bleach, Chief Administrative Officer
Stacy Rollins, Executive Administrative Assistant to the President
An interview with Jane, a blind child, tells other children what it's
like to be blind. Jane explains how she gets around, takes care of
herself, does her school work, spends her leisure time and even
pays for things when she can't see money.
16 pages
ISBN 0-891289-21-6

Print: Journals

9053 **Journal of Visual Impairment and Blindness**
Sheridan Press,
450 Fame Ave
Hanover, PA 17331-1585

717-632-3535
800-352-2210
FAX: 717-633-8929
pubsvc@tsp.sheridan.com
www.sheridanreprints.com

Sharon Shively, Editor
Published in braille, regular print and on ASC II disk and cassette,
this journal contains a wide variety of subjects including rehabilitation, psychology, education, legislation, medicine, technology,
employment, sensory aids and childhood development as they relate to visual impairments. $130 annual individual subscription,
$180 annual institutional subscription.
64 pages Monthly
ISSN 0145-48 x

Print: Magazines

9054 **Blind Educator**
National Organization of Blind Educators
200 East Wells Street
Jernigan Place
Baltimore, MD 21230

410-659-9314
FAX: 410-685-5653
nfb@nfb.org
www.nfb.org

Marc Mauer, President
Magazine specifically for blind educators.

9055 **Braille Forum**
American Council of the Blind
2200 Wilson Boulevard
Suite 650
Arlington, VA 22201-3354

202-467-5081
800-424-8666
FAX: 703-465-5085
info@acb.org
www.acb.org

Kim Charlson, President
Jeff Thom, 1st Vice President
Melanie Brunson, Executive Director
Offered in print, braille, cassette, IBM computer disk and e-mail.
$25 per format per year for companies and non-US residents.
48 pages Magazine

9056 **Braille Monitor**
Deaf-Blind Division of the Ntn'l Fed of the Blind
200 East Wells St
Baltimore, MD 21230-4914

410-659-9314
FAX: 410-685-5653
nfbpublications@nfb.org
www.nfb.org

Marc Maurer, CEO
Barbara Pierce, Editor
The Braille Monitor is the leading publication of the National
Federation of the Blind. It covers the events and activities of the
NFB and addresses the many issues and concerns of the blind.

9057 **Dialogue Magazine**
Blindskills Inc.
P.O. Box 5181
Salem, OR 97304-0181

503-581-4224
800-860-4224
FAX: 503-581-0178
info@blindskills.com
www.blindskills.com

Marja Byers, Executive Director
B.T. Kimbrough, Editor
Publishes quarterly magazine in braille, large-type, cassette and
email of news items, technology and articles of special interest to
visually impaired youth and adults. Annual subscription cost $35
for braille, large print or cassette, $20 for email. *$35.00*
Quarterly

9058 **Future Reflections**
Deaf-Blind Division of the Ntn'l Fed of the Blind
200 East Wells Street
Baltimore, MD 21230-4914

410-659-9314
FAX: 410-685-5653
www.nfb.org

Marc Maurer, President
A magazine for parents and teachers of blind children.

9059 **Guide Magazine**
The Seeing Eye
P.O. Box 375
10 Washington Valley Road
Morristown, NJ 7963

973-539-4425
FAX: 973-539-0922
info@seeingeye.org
seeingeye.org

James A. Kutsch, Jr., Ph.D., President & CEO
Robert Pudlak, CFO & Director of Administration & Finance
Glenn Cianci, Director of Facilities Management
Jean Thomas, Director of Donor & Public Relations
The Guide offers stories of inspiration from our graduates and
news of the latest program developments.

9060   JBI Voice
Jewish Braille Institute of America
110 Est 30th Street
New York, NY 10016

212-889-2525
800-433-1531
FAX: 212-689-3692
admin@jbilibrary.org
www.jbilibrary.org

Judy E. Tenney, Chairman
Thomas G. Kahn, Viec Chairman
Dr. Ellen Isler, President and CEO
Israel A Taub, Vice President and CFO
Monthly recorded magazine emphasizing Jewish current events and culture.

9061   Jewish Braille Review
Jewish Braille Institute of America
110 Est 30th Street
New York, NY 10016

212-889-2525
800-433-1531
FAX: 212-689-3692
admin@jbilibrary.org
www.jbilibrary.org

Judy E. Tenney, Chairman
Thomas G. Kahn, Viec Chairman
Dr. Ellen Isler, President and CEO
Israel A Taub, Vice President and CFO
The JBI seeks the integration of Jews who are blind, visually impaired and reading disabled into the Jewish community and society in general. More than 20,000 men, women and children in 50 countries receive a broad variety of JBI services.

9062   Merchant Messenger
National Association of Blind Merchants
1837 South Nevada avenue
PMB #243
Colorado Springs, CO 80905

719-423-4384
888-691-1819
FAX: 719-527-0129
markharris1222@sbcglobal.net
www.blindmerchants.org

Kevin Worley, President

9063   Musical Mainstream
Nat'l Lib Svc/Blind And Physically Handicapped
1291 Taylor Street North West
Washington, DC 20011

202-707-5100
FAX: 202-707-0712
TTY:202-707-0744
nls@loc.gov
www.loc.gov/nls

Karen Keninger, Director
Articles selected from print music magazines.
Quarterly

9064   Opportunity
National Industries for the Blind
1310 Braddock Place
Alexandria, VA 22314-1691

703-310-0500
FAX: 703-998-8268
services@nib.org
www.nib.org

The Honorabl Krump, Esq., Chairman
Louis J. Jablonski, Jr., Vice Chairman
Kevin A. Lynch, President and Chief Executive Officer
James M Kesteloot, Director
Offers information and articles on the newest technology, equipment, services and programs for blind and visually impaired persons.
Quarterly

9065   Providing Services for People with Vision Loss:
Multidisciplinary Perspective
Resources for Rehabilitation
22 Bonad Road
Winchester, MA 01890-1302

781-368-9080
FAX: 781-368-9096
orders@rfr.org
www.rfr.org

Susan L Greenblatt, Editor
A collection of articles by ophthalmologists and rehabilitation professionals, including chapters on operating a low vision service, starting self-help programs, mental health services, aids and techniques that help people with vision loss. *$19.95*
136 pages
ISBN 0-929718-02-0

Print: Newsletters

9066   AFB News
American Foundation for the Blind/AFB Press
2 Penn Plaza
Suite 1102
New York, NY 10121

212-502-7600
800-232-5463
FAX: 888-545-8331
afbinfo@afb.net
www.afb.org

Carl R. Augusto, President & Chief Executive Officer
Rick Bozeman, Chief Financial Officer
Kelly Bleach, Chief Administrative Officer
Stacy Rollins, Executive Administrative Assistant to the President
National newsletter for general readership about blindness and visual impairments featuring people, programs, services and activities.
12 pages Quarterly

9067   ASB Visions Newsletter
Associated Services for the Blind
919 Walnut Street
Philadelphia, PA 19107

215-627-0600
FAX: 215-922-0692
asbinfo@asb.org
www.asb.org

Patricia C. Johnson, President and CEO
Tim McGovern, Human Relations
Brian Rusk, Public Relations Officer
Derby Ewing, Director, Human Services
Newsletter associated services for the blind and visually impaired.

9068   Adaptive Services Division
District of Columbia Public Library
901G St NW,
Rm 215
Washington, DC 20001-4531

202-727-2142
FAX: 202-727-0322
TTY:202-559-5368
lbph.dcpl@dc.gov
www.dclibrary.org

Venetia Demson, Chief, Adaptive Services
DC Regional Library for the blind, deaf and physically handicapped. Provides adaptive technology and training programs.
8 pages Quarterly

9069   Alumni News
Guide Dogs for the Blind
P.O.Box 151200
San Rafael, CA 94915-1200

415-499-4000
800-295-4050
FAX: 415-499-4035
guidedogs.com

Bob Burke, Chairman
Stuart Odell, Vice Chairman
Chris Benninger, President and CEO
Jay Harris, Secretary
Restricted to graduates only.

9070 Annual Report/Newsletter
National Accreditation Council for Agencies/Blind
Rm 1004
15 E 40th St
New York, NY 10016-401 212-683-5068
FAX: 212-683-4475
Ruth Westman, Executive Director
Provides standards and a program of accreditation for schools and organizations which serve children and adults who are blind or vision impaired.

9071 Association for Macular Diseases Newsletter
210 East 64th Street
New York, NY 10065 212-605-3719
FAX: 212-605-3795
association@retinal-research.org
macula.org

Bernard Landou, President
Mary Fern Breheny, Board Member
Patricia Dahl, Board Member
Walter Ross, Editor-In-Chief
Not-for-profit organization promotes education and research in this scarcely explored field. Acts as a nationwide support group for individuals and their families endeavoring to adjust to the restrictions and changes brought about by macular disease. Offers hotline, educational materials, quarterly newsletter, support groups, referrals and seminars for persons and families affected by macular disease.

9072 Awareness
NAPVI
1 North Lexington Avenue
White Plains, NY 10601 617-972-7441
800-562-6265
FAX: 617-972-7444
napvi@guildhealth.org
www.napvi.org

Julie Urban, President
Venetia Hayden, Vice President
Susan LaVenture, Executive Director
Randi Sher, Secretary
Newsletter offering regional news, sports and activities, conferences, camps, legislative updates, book reviews, audio reviews, professional question and answer column and more for the visually impaired and their families.
Quarterly

9073 BTBL News
Braille and Talking Book Library
P.O. Box 942837
Sacramento, CA 94237-0001 916-654-0261
800-952-5666
FAX: 916-654-1119
btbl@library.ca.gov
www.btbl.ca.gov

Janet Coles, Editor
Christopher Berger, Senior Librarian
Olena Bilyk, Web Developer
Kim Brown, Communications Officer
BTBL News, the quarterly newsletter of the California Braille and Talking Book Library, features articles on topics of interest to library customers, including information about new services, existing services, events, staff and more.

9074 Canes and Trails
Guide Dogs for the Blind
P.O.Box 151200
San Rafael, CA 94915-1200 415-499-4000
800-295-4050
FAX: 415-499-4035
guidedogs.com

Bob Burke, Chairman
Stuart Odell, Vice Chairman
Chris Benninger, President and CEO
Jay Harris, Secretary
A quarterly newsletter for orientation and mobility specialists, rehabilitation professionals, teachers, and service providers in the field of blindness and visual impairment.

9075 Community Connection
Guide Dogs for the Blind
P.O.Box 151200
San Rafael, CA 94915-1200 415-499-4000
800-295-4050
FAX: 415-499-4035
guidedogs.com

Bob Burke, Chairman
Stuart Odell, Vice Chairman
Chris Benninger, President and CEO
Jay Harris, Secretary
A newsletter produced for our volunteers and other friends of Guide Dogs.

9076 DVH Quarterly
University of Arkansas at Little Rock
2801 S University Ave
Little Rock, AR 72204-1000 501-569-3000

Bob Brasher, Editor
Mary Boaz, Manager
Offers information on upcoming events, conferences and workshops on and for visual disabilities. Book reviews, information on the newest resources and technology, educational programs, want ads and more.
Quarterly

9077 Deaf-Blind Perspective
National Consortium on Deaf-Blindness
345 North Monmouth Avenue
Monmouth, OR 97361 503-838-8391
800-438-9376
FAX: 503-838-8150
TTY: 800-854-7013
info@teachingresearchinstitute.org
www.tr.wou.edu

Ingrid Amerson, Child Development Center
Lyn Ayer, Center on Deaf & Blindness
Robert Ayres, Evaluation and Research
Cori Brownell, Center on Early Learning
A free publication with articles, essays, and announcements about topics related to people who are deaf-blind. Published two times a year (Spring and Fall) by the Teaching Research Institute of Western Oregon University, its purpose is to provide information and serve as a forum for discussion and sharing ideas.

9078 Fidelco
Fidelco Guide Dog Foundation
103 Vision Way
Bloomfield, CT 06002 860-243-5200
FAX: 860-769-0567
info@fidelco.org
fidelco.org

Karen C. Tripp, Chairman
G. Kenneth Bernhard, Vice Chairman
Eliot D. Matheson, CEO
Diane R. Lindeland, VP, Finance
A newsletter published by Fidelco Guide Dog Foundation.

9079 Focus
Visually Impaired Center
1422 W Court St
Flint, MI 48503-5008 810-767-4014
FAX: 810-767-0020
www.vcflint.org

Charles Tommasulo, Executive Director
Newsletter offering information for the visually impaired person in the forms of legislative and law updates, ADA information, support groups, hotlines, and articles on the newest technology in the field.
Quarterly

9080 Gleams Newsletter
Glaucoma Research Foundation
2345 Yale Street
2nd Floor
Palo Alto, CA 94306
650-328-3388
800-826-6693
FAX: 415-986-3763
info@glaucoma.org
auorthodontics.com

Tom Brunner, CEO
Offers updated medical & research information on glaucoma. Included are glaucoma treatmant and coping tips, legsilative information, professional articles and book reviews.
6 pages Quarterly

9081 Guide Dog News
Guide Dogs for the Blind
P.O.Box 151200
San Rafael, CA 94915-1200
415-499-4000
800-295-4050
FAX: 415-499-4035
guidedogs.com

Bob Burke, Chairman
Stuart Odell, Vice Chairman
Chris Benninger, President and CEO
Jay Harris, Secretary
Read about changes to our teaching techniques, our new Adult Learning Program, vet tips, and find news about our graduates.

9082 Guideway
Guide Dog Foundation for the Blind
371 East Jericho Turnpike
Smithtown, NY 11787-2976
631-930-9000
800-548-4337
FAX: 631-930-9009
info@guidedog.org
www.guidedog.org

James C. Bingham, Chairman
Alphonce J. Brown, Jr., Vice Chairman
Wells B. Jones, CEO
Jack Sage, Secretary
Offers updates and information on the foundation's activities and guide dog programs. In print form but is also available on cassette.
Monthly

9083 Guild Briefs
Catholic Guild for The Blind
65 East Wacker Place
Suite 1010
Chicago, IL 60601
312-236-8569
FAX: 312-236-8128
info@guildfortheblind.org
www.guildfortheblind.org

Brett Christenson, President
Laura Rounce, Vice President
David Tabak, Executive Director
Toria Emas, Secretary
Monthly publication for individuals who are blind or visually impaired. It contains articles on topics such as service programs, scholarships, education, seniors, research, and government.
12 pages monthly

9084 IAAIS Report
Int'l Association of Audio Information Services
3920 Willshire Dr
Lawrence, KS 66049-3673
412-434-6023
800-280-5325
aiblink@ak.net
www.iaais.org

Stuart Holland, President
Marjorie Williams, 1st Vice President
Linda Hynson, Secretary
Andrea Pasquale, Treasurer
Newsletter for persons interested in radio reading services. *$7.00*
Quarterly

9085 Insight
United States Association of Blind Athletes
1 Olympic Plaza
Colorado Springs, CO 80909
719-630-0422
FAX: 719-630-0616
media@usaba.org
www.usaba.org

Mark A. Lucas, MS, Executive Director
Ryan Ortiz, Assistant Executive Director
John Potts, Goalball High Performance director
Matt Simpson, Membership & Outreach Coordinator
Covers news, announcements and activities of the association.
20 pages Quarterly

9086 LampLighter
Columbia Lighthouse for the Blind
1825 K Street NorthWest
Suite 1103
Washington, DC 20006
202-454-6400
FAX: 877-595-9228
info@clb.org
clb.org

Tony Cancelosi, President
Anthony Cancelosi, CEO
Dedicated to helping the blind or visually impaired population.

9087 Library Users of America Newsletter
American Council of the Blind
2200 Wilson Boulevard
Suite 650
Arlington, VA 22201-3354
202-467-5081
800-424-8666
FAX: 703-465-5085
info@acb.org
www.acb.org

Kim Charlson, President
Jeff Thom, 1st Vice President
Melanie Brunson, Executive Director
Published twice yearly, the newsletter contains much information about library services of particular interest to blind and visually impaired patrons, and is available in the following formats: Braille, audiocassette, large print and e-mail.

9088 Light the Way
Blind Children's Center
4120 Marathon Street
Los Angeles, CA 90029-3584
323-664-2153
800-222-3567
FAX: 323-665-3828
info@blindchildrenscenter.org
blindchildrenscenter.org

Scott E. Schaldenbrand, President
Mark Correa, Board Member
Midge Horton, Executive Director
Newsletter of the Blind Childrens Center, a family-centered agency which serves young children with visual impairments. The center-based and home-based services help the children to acquire skills and build their independence. The center utilizes its expertise and experience to serve families and professionals worldwide through support services, education and research.

9089 Lighthouse Publication
Chicago Lighthouse
1850 West Roosevelt Road
Chicago, IL 60608-1298
312-666-1331
FAX: 312-243-8539
TTY:312-666-8874
publications@chicagolighthouse.org
www.thechicagolighthouse.org

Janet P. Szlyk, Ph.D., President & Chief Executive Officer
Mary Lynne Januszewski, Executive Vice President/CFO
Melanie M. Hennessy, SVP
Terrence J. longo, Executive Vice President/COO

9090 **Lights On**
Fight for Sight
Ste 809
391 Park Ave S
New York, NY 10016-8806
212-679-6060
FAX: 212-679-4466
www.fightforsight.com

Mary Prudden, Executive Director
A newsletter published by Fight for Sight.

9091 **Long Cane News**
American Foundation for the Blind/AFB Press
2 Penn Plaza
Suite 1102
New York, NY 10121
212-502-7600
800-232-5463
FAX: 888-545-8331
afbinfo@afb.net
www.afb.org

Carl R. Augusto, President & Chief Executive Officer
Rick Bozeman, Chief Financial Officer
Kelly Bleach, Chief Administrative Officer
Stacy Rollins, Executive Administrative Assistant to the President

SemiAnnual

9092 **Magnifier**
Macular Degeneration Foundation
P.O.Box 531313
Henderson, NV 89053
702-450-2908
888-633-3937
liz@eyesight.org
www.eyesight.org

Liz Trauernicht, President & Director of Communications
Julie Zavala, VP & Asst. Director of Operations
David Seftel, EVP & Dircetor, R & D
Ron Gallamore, Board of Scientific Advisors
The Magnifier is the distributed without charge via email and by regular mail to those without access to the Internet. It features breaking news, clinical trails, clarifies recent reports in the media, announces new Internet resources and informs the public of important additions to the web site.

9093 **NAVH Update**
National Association of Visually Handicapped
111 East 59th Street
New York, NY 10022-1202
212-821-9384
800-829-0500
FAX: 212-821-9707
info@lighthouse.org
lighthouse.org/navh

Mark G. Ackermann, President / CEO
A newsletter published by the National Association of Visually Impaired. LightHouse acquired NAVH.

9094 **NBA Bulletin**
National Braille Association
95 Allens Creek Road
Building 1, Suite 202
Rochester, NY 14618
585-427-8260
FAX: 585-427-0263
nbaoffice@nationalbraille.org
www.nationalbraille.org

Jan Carroll, President
Cindi Laurent, Vice President
David Shaffer, Executive Director
Heidi Lehmann, Secretary
Published quarterly and included int he price of the regular and student NBA membership.

9095 **NLS News**
Nat'l Lib Svc/Blind And Physically Handicapped
1291 Taylor Street North West
Washington, DC 20011
202-707-5100
FAX: 202-707-0712
TTY:202-707-0744
nls@loc.gov
www.loc.gov/nls

Karen Keninger, Director
Newsletter on current program developments.
Quarterly

9096 **NLS Newsletter**
Nat'l Lib Svc/Blind And Physically Handicapped
1291 Taylor Street North West
Washington, DC 20011
202-707-5100
FAX: 202-707-0712
TTY:202-707-0744
nls@loc.gov
www.loc.gov/nls

Karen Keninger, Director
Newsletter on the service's volunteer activities.
Quarterly

9097 **PBA News**
Prevent Blindness America
211 West Wacker Drive
Suite 1700
Chicago, IL 60606
800-331-2020
info@preventblindness.org
www.preventblindness.org

Paul G. Howes, Chairman
Hugh R. Parry, President & CEO,Prevent Blindness America
Jerome Desserich, Vice President & Chief Financial Officer
Danielle Disch, Development Manager
Newsletter is filled with the information you need to protect your eyes, preserve your sight, and educate yourself about your own eye condition or that of a family member. Publication offered three times yearly.
3 times yearly

9098 **Planned Giving Department of Guide Dogs for the Blind**
Guide Dogs for the Blind
P.O.Box 151200
San Rafael, CA 94915-1200
415-499-4000
800-295-4050
FAX: 415-499-4035
guidedogs.com

Bob Burke, Chairman
Stuart Odell, Vice Chairman
Chris Benninger, President and CEO
Jay Harris, Secretary
A newsletter published by Guide Dogs for the Blind.

9099 **Playback**
Recording for the Blind & Dyslexic
20 Roszel Road
Princeton, NJ 08540
800-221-4792
FAX: 609-987-8116
Custserv@LearningAlly.org
www.learningally.org/

Brad Grob, Chairman
Harold J. Logan, Vice Chairman
Andrew Friedman, President & CEO
Jim Halliday, Executive Vice President
A publication dedicated to our unit's family of members, volunteers, supporters and staff. RFB&D is now Learning Ally.
3x Year

9100 Quarterly Update
National Association for Visually Handicapped
111 East 59th Street
New York, NY 10022-1202
212-821-9384
800-829-0500
FAX: 212-821-9707
info@lighthouse.org
lighthouse.org/navh

Mark G. Ackermann, President / CEO
Quarterly newsletter offering information on new products for the visually impaired, advances in medical treatments, new books available in the NAVH large print loan library and any new/updated booklets. Free. LightHouse acquired NAVH.

9101 RP Messenger
Texas Association of Retinitis Pigmentosa
P.O.Box 8388
Corpus Christi, TX 78468-8388
361-852-8515
FAX: 361-852-8515
tarp@homebiz101.com
www.geocities.com

Dorothy Steifel, Executive Director
A bi-annual newsletter offering information on Retinitis Pigmentosa. *$15.00*
BiAnnual

9102 SCENE
Braille Institute
527 North Dale Avenue
Anaheim, CA 92801
714-821-5000
800-272-4553
FAX: 714-527-7621
oc@brailleinstitute.org
brailleinstitute.org

Lester M. Sussman, Chairman
Peter A. Mindnich, President
Jon K. Hayashida, OD, FAAO, Vice President, Programs & Services
Rezaur Rehman, Vice President, Finance
Offers information on the organization, question and answer column, articles on the newest technology and more for visually impaired persons.

9103 STAR
Special Technologies Alternative Resources
210 McMorran Boulevard
Port Huron, MI 48060
810-987-7323
877-987-READ
star@sccl.lib.mi.us
www.sccl.lib.mi.us

Arnold H. Larson, Chairman
Kathleen J. Wheelihan, Vice Chairman
Arlene M. Marcetti, Board Member
Stan Arnetti, Director
A newsletter published by Special Technologies Alternative Resources.

9104 Seeing Eye Guide
The Seeing Eye
P.O.Box 375
10 Washington Valley Road
Morristown, NJ 07963
973-539-4425
FAX: 973-539-0922
info@seeingeye.org
seeingeye.org

James A. Kutsch, Jr., Ph.D., President & CEO
Randall Ivens, Director of Human Resources
Robert Pudlak, CFO & Director of Administration & Finance
David Johnson, Director of Instruction & Training
A quarterly publication from Seeing Eye.
Quarterly

9105 Shared Visions
Vista Center for the Blind & Visually Impaired
413 Laurel St
Santa Cruz, CA 95060-4904
831-458-9766
800-705-2970
FAX: 831-426-6233
information@vistacenter.org
doranblindcenter.org

Pam Brandin, Executive Director
A quarterly publication for Blind and Visually Impaired individuals from Vista Center for the Blind and Visually Impaired.

9106 Sharing Solutions: A Newsletter for Support Groups
Lighthouse International
111 East 59th Street
New York, NY 10022-1202
212-821-9384
800-829-0500
FAX: 212-821-9707
info@lighthouse.org
www.lighthouse.org

Mark G. Ackermann, President / CEO
A newsletter for members and leaders of support groups for older adults with impaired vision. The letter provides a forum for support groups members to network and share information, printed in a very large type format.

9107 Sightings Newsletter
Schepens Eye Research Institute
20 Staniford Street
Boston, MA 02114
617-912-0100
FAX: 617-912-0110
www.schepens.harvard.edu

Michael Gilmore, Director
Mary E. Leach, Director of Public Affairs
Frances Ng, Director of Human Resources
Ojas P. Mehta, Director, Intellectual Property & Commercial Ventures
Publication of prominent center for research on eye, vision, and blinding diseases; dedicated to research that improves the understanding, management, and prevention of eye diseases and visual deficiencies; fosters collaboration among its faculty members; trains young scientists and clinicians from around the world; promotes communication with scientists in allied fields; leader in the worldwide dispersion of basic scientific knowledge of vision.

9108 Smith Kettlewell Rehabilitation Engineering Research Center
2318 Fillmore Street
San Francisco, CA 94115
415-345-2000
FAX: 415-345-8455
rerc@ski.org
ski.org/rerc

John Brabyn, Ph.D., CEO/Executive Director
Ruth S. Poole, COO
Arthur Jampolsky, Director
Arthur Jampolsky, M.D., Founder
Reports on technology and devices for persons with visual impairments.

9109 Student Advocate
National Alliance of Blind Students NABS Liaison
Ste 1004
1155 15th St NW
Washington, DC 20005-2706
202-467-5081
800-424-8666
FAX: 202-467-5085
www.blindstudents.org

Melanie Brunson, Executive Director
A newsletter created by members of NABS and for any interested parties.

9110 TBC Focus
Chicago Public Library Talking Books Center
400 South State Street
Chicago, IL 60605   312-747-4300
                          800-757-4654
                    FAX: 312-747-1609
                    www.chipublib.org

Linda Johnson Rice, President
Christopher Valenti, VP
Christina Benitez, Secretary
Karim Adib, Director
Published quarterly by the Chicago Public Library Talking Book Center. Free of charge.
4 pages Quarterly

9111 Talking Books Topics
Nat'l Lib Svc/Blind And Physically Handicapped
1291 Taylor Street North West
Washington, DC 20011   202-707-5100
                        FAX: 202-707-0712
                        TTY:202-707-0744
                             nls@loc.gov
                          www.loc.gov/nls

Karen Keninger, Director
New recorded books and program news
Bi-monthly

9112 Upstate Update
New York State Talking Book & Braille Library
222 Madison Avenue
Albany, NY 12230-1   518-474-5935
                          800-342-3688
                    FAX: 514-474-5786
                    TTY: 518-474-7121
                   nyslweb@mail.nysed.gov
                      www.nysl.nysed.gov

Bernard A. Margolis, State Librarian & Asst. Commissioner for Libraries
Loretta Ebert, Research Library Director
Liza Duncan, Technical Services & Systmes
Books on audio cassette, cassette players, braille books, summer reading programs, braille writer, magnifiers, closed-circuit T.V., large-print photocopier, cassette books and magazines, children's books on cassette, reference materials on blindness and other handicaps.
4 pages Quarterly

9113 Visual Aids and Informational Material
National Association for Visually Handicapped
111 East 59th Street
New York, NY 10022-1202   212-821-9384
                            800-829-0500
                      FAX: 212-821-9707
                      info@lighthouse.org
                      lighthouse.org/navh

Mark G. Ackermann, President / CEO
A complete listing of the visual aids NAVH carries such as magnifiers, talking clocks, large print playing cards, etc. LightHouse acquired NAVH. *$2.50*
65 pages

9114 Voice
Vermont Assn for the Blind & Visually Impaired
60 Kimball Avenue
South Burlington, VT 05403   802-863-1358
                              800-639-5861
                        FAX: 802-863-1481
                        General@vabvi.org
                              vabvi.org

Thomas Chase, President
Stephen Pouliot, Executive Director
Kathleen Quinlan, Director of Operations
Lori Newsome, Office Manager
The Voice is a newsletter published by Vermont Association for the Blind and Visually Impaired.

9115 Voice of Vision
GW Micro
725 Airport North Office Park
Fort Wayne, IN 46825   260-489-3671
                        FAX: 260-489-2608
                        sales@gwmicro.com
                          www.gwmicro.com

Dan Weirich, Owner
Offers product reviews, product announcements, tips for making systems or applications more accessible, or explanations of concepts of interest to any computer user or would-be computer user. This association newsletter is available in braille, in large print, on audio cassette and on 3.5 or 5.25 IBM format diskette.
Quarterly

Non Print: Newsletters

9116 Insight
Eye Bank Association of America
Ste 1010
1015 18th Street NorthWest
Washington, DC 20036   202-775-4999
                        FAX: 202-429-6036
                      info@restoresight.org
                      www.restoresight.org

David Glasser, Chairman
Kevin Corcoran, President & Chief Executive Officer
Molly Georgakis, VP of Member Services
Patricia Hardy, Manager of Communications
An electronic newsletter.

9117 Listen Up
Recording for the Blind & Dyslexic
20 Roszel Rd
Princeton, NJ 8540-6206   609-452-0606
                              866-732-3585
                        FAX: 609-520-7990
                        www.learningally.org

John Kelly, CEO
RFB&D's bi-monthly electronic newsletter for members.

Non Print: Video

9118 Aging and Vision: Declarations of Independence
American Foundation for the Blind/AFB Press
2 Penn Plaza
Suite 1102
New York, NY 10121   212-502-7600
                          800-232-5463
                    FAX: 888-545-8331
                    afbinfo@afb.net
                          www.afb.org

Carl R. Augusto, President & Chief Executive Officer
Rick Bozeman, Chief Financial Officer
Kelly Bleach, Chief Administrative Officer
Stacy Rollins, Executive Administrative Assistant to the President
A very personal look at five older people who have successfully coped with visual impairmant and continue to lead active, satisfying lives. Their stories are not only inspirational, but also provide practical, down-to-earth suggestions for adapting to vision loss later in life. 18 minute video tape. Also available in PAL, $52.95, 0-89128-276-9. *$42.95*
VHS
ISBN 0-891282-20-3

9119   Blindness, A Family Matter
American Foundation for the Blind/AFB Press
2 Penn Plaza
Suite 1102
New York, NY 10121   212-502-7600
                                      800-232-5463
                                 FAX: 888-545-8331
                                   afbinfo@afb.net
                                      www.afb.org

Carl R. Augusto, President & Chief Executive Officer
Rick Bozeman, Chief Financial Officer
Kelly Bleach, Chief Administrative Officer
Stacy Rollins, Executive Administrative Assistant to the President
A frank exploration of the effects of an individual's visual impairment on other members of the family and how those family members can play a positive role in the rehabilitation process. Features interviews with three families whose 'success stories' provide advice and encouragement, as well as interviews with newly blinded adults currently involved in a rehabilitation program. 23 minute video tape. Also available in PAL, $49.95, 0-89128-271-8. *$43.95*
VHS
ISBN 0-891282-22-X

9120   Building Blocks: Foundations for Learning for Young Blind and Visually Impaired Children
American Foundation for the Blind/AFB Press
2 Penn Plaza
Suite 1102
New York, NY 10121   212-502-7600
                                      800-232-5463
                                 FAX: 888-545-8331
                                   afbinfo@afb.net
                                      www.afb.org

Carl R. Augusto, President & Chief Executive Officer
Rick Bozeman, Chief Financial Officer
Kelly Bleach, Chief Administrative Officer
Stacy Rollins, Executive Administrative Assistant to the President
Presents the essential components of a successful early intervnetion program, including collaboration with family members, positive relationships between parents and professionals, public education, and attention to important programming components such as space exploration, braille readiness, orientation and mobility, play, cooking and music. Includes interviews with parents. Available in English or Spanish. 10 minute video tape. Also available in PAL, $33.95, 0-89128-268-8. *$26.95*
VHS
ISBN 0-891282-14-9

9121   Choice Magazine Listening
85 Channel Drive
Port Washington, NY 11050   516-883-8280
                                      888-724-6423
                                      888-724-6423
                                 FAX: 516-944-5849
                                  choicemag@aol.com
                          www.choicemagazinelistening.org

Pamela Loeser, Editor in Chief
Ann Schlegel-Kyrkostas, Associate Editor
David Graham Pade, Associate Editor
Michael Tedeschi, Webmaster
A free audio anthology is available bi-monthly to visually impaired/physically disabled or dislexic persons nationwide. Playable on the special free 4-track cassette playback equipment which is provided by the Library of Congress through the National Library Service. Each issue features eight hours of unabridged magazine articles, short stories, poetry and media selections from over 100 sources. College level and older. Bimonthly distribution.
Bi-Monthly

9122   Juggler
Beacon Press
24 Farnsworth Street
Boston, MA 02210   617-742-2110
                                 FAX: 617-723-3097
                                       beacon.org

Helene Atwan, Executive Director

Andre was the young son of a wealthy, early Quebec fur trader. Because he was almost totally blind, he was overly protected by his family, and his movement outside his home was very limited.
Film

9123   Let's Eat Video
Blind Children's Center
4120 Marathon Street
Los Angeles, CA 90029-3584   323-664-2153
                                      800-222-3567
                                 FAX: 323-665-3828
                          info@blindchildrenscenter.org
                             blindchildrenscenter.org

Scott E. Schaldenbrand, President
Mark Correa, Board Member
Midge Horton, Executive Director
Babies and toddlers with visual impairments lack one major avenue of exploration, and this significantly infuleces their awareness, perceptions, and anticipation of the food which is presented to them. *$35.00*
VHS/DVD

9124   Look Out for Annie
Lighthouse International
111 East 59th Street
New York, NY 10022-1202   212-821-9384
                                      800-829-0500
                                 FAX: 212-821-9706
                                  info@lighthouse.org
                                    www.lighthouse.org

Mark G. Ackermann, President / CEO
Depicts an older woman coping with her vision loss. It focuses on the emotional issues surrounding vision loss and conveys the idea that both the person with the vision disorder and their family and friends will need to make adjustments. *$25.00*
Video

9125   Not Without Sight
American Foundation for the Blind/AFB Press
PO Box 1020
Sewickley, PA 15143-920   412-741-1142
                                      800-232-3044
                                 FAX: 412-741-0609
                                afborders@abdintl.com
                                      www.afb.org

Carl R Augusto, President/CEO
Tracy Charlovich, Css
This video describes the major types of visual impairment and their causes and effects on vision, while camera simulations approximate what people with each impairmant actually see. Also demonstrates how people with low vision make the best use of the vision they have. 20 minute video tape, $49.95. *$42.95*
VHS 17 min
ISBN 0-891282-27-3

9126   Out of Left Field
American Foundation for the Blind/AFB Press
2 Penn Plaza
Suite 1102
New York, NY 10121   212-502-7600
                                      800-232-5463
                                 FAX: 888-545-8331
                                   afbinfo@afb.net
                                          afb.org

Carl R. Augusto, President & Chief Executive Officer
Rick Bozeman, Chief Financial Officer
Kelly Bleach, Chief Administrative Officer
Stacy Rollins, Executive Administrative Assistant to the President
Illustrates how youngsters who are blind or visually impaired integrated with their sighted peers in a variety of recreational and athletic activities. 17 minute video tape. Also available in PAL, $33.95, 0-89128-270-X. *$29.95*
VHS 17 minutes
ISBN 0-891282-28-0

9127 See What I'm Saying
Fanlight Productions
c/o Icarus Films
32 Court Street, 21st Floor
Brooklyn, NY 11201   718-488-8900
                                       800-876-1710
                                 FAX: 718-488-8642
          info@fanlight.com, sales@icarusfilms.com
                                    www.fanlight.com

Ben Achtenberg, Founder, Owner
The documentary follows Patricia, who is deaf and from a Spanish-speaking family, through her first year at the Kendall Demonstration Elementary School of Gallaudet University.
VHS/DVD

9128 See for Yourself
Lighthouse International
111 East 59th Street
New York, NY 10022-1202   212-821-9384
                                       800-829-0500
                                 FAX: 212-821-9706
                                 info@lighthouse.org
                                    www.lighthouse.org

Mark G. Ackermann, President / CEO
This video features older adults with impaired vision who have been helped by vision rehabilitation. *$50.00*

9129 Shape Up 'n Sign
Harris Communications
15155 Technology Dr
Eden Prairie, MN 55344-2273   952-906-1180
                                       800-825-6758
                                 FAX: 952-906-1099
                                 info@harriscomm.com

Robert Harris, Owner
An aerobic exercise tape introducing the basic sign language for deaf and hearing children ages six to ten. *$29.95*
30 Minutes DVD

9130 Sight by Touch
Landmark Media
3450 Slade Run Drive
Falls Church, VA 22042   703-241-2030
                                       800-342-4336
                                 FAX: 703-536-9540
                                 info@landmarkmedia.com
                                    landmarkmedia.com

Michael Hartogs, President
Peter Hartogs, VP New Business & Development
Beverly Weisenberg, Sales Rep
Richard Hartogs, VP Acquisitions
This video features the life and importance of Louis Braille. Vision-impaired performers and teachers demonstrate how Braille has benefitted their lives, and how improvements are constantly being made. *$195.00*
Video

9131 Taping for the Blind
3935 Essex Lane
Houston, TX 77027   713-622-2767
                                 FAX: 713-622-2772
                                 info@tapingfortheblind.org
                                    www.afb.org

Carl R. Augusto, President & Chief Executive Officer
Rick Bozeman, Chief Financial Officer
Robin Vogel, VP, Resource Development
Cynthia Fanzetti, Executive Director
An independent non profit educational organization funded by corporations, listeners and individuals, with a mission to turn sight into sound, enriching the lives of individuals with visual, physical and learning disabilities. Founded in 1967 to read materials not availiable through other sources onto standard audio cassettes in our custom recording division. In 1978, Houston Taping fFor The Blind signed on the air. Reading several dozen popular magazines and best selling books on the air.

9132 We Can Do it Together!
American Foundation for the Blind/AFB Press
2 Penn Plaza
Suite 1102
New York, NY 10121   212-502-7600
                                       800-232-5463
                                 FAX: 888-545-8331
                                 afbinfo@afb.net
                                    afb.org

Carl R. Augusto, President & Chief Executive Officer
Rick Bozeman, Chief Financial Officer
Kelly Bleach, Chief Administrative Officer
Stacy Rollins, Executive Administrative Assistant to the President
This video illustrates a transdisciplinary team orientation and mobility program for students with severe visual and multiple impairments, covering both adapted communication systems used to teach mobility skills and basic indoor mobility in the school. For mobility instructors, administrators, teachers of the visually and severely handicapped, occupational, physical and speech therapists and parents. Discussion guide included. 10 minute video tape. Also available in PAL, $33.95, 0-89128-267-X. *$26.95*
VHS
ISBN 0-891282-13-0

Sports

9133 American Blind Bowling Association
1209 Somerset Road
Raleigh, NC 27610   919-755-0700
                          www.abba1951.org/contact.htm

Thomas Lester, President
A.J. Inglesby, 1st Vice President
James Benton, 2nd Vice President
Judy Mandelkow, Tournament Director
Promotes blind bowling throughout the US and Canada by sanctioning blind bowling leagues and conducting a National Tournament. Current membership exceeds 2,000 people in the United States and Canada.

9134 Basketball: Beeping Foam
Maxi Aids
42 Executive Boulevard
Farmingdale, NY 11735   631-752-0521
                                       800-522-6294
                                 FAX: 631-752-0689
                                 TTY: 631-752-0738
                                 sales@maxiaids.com
                                    www.maxiaids.com

Elliot Zaretsky, President
This sound making basketball enables the visually impaired to play basketball or other games. *$29.95*

9135 Blind Outdoor Leisure Development
P.O.Box 6639
Snowmass Village, CO 81615   970-923-0578
                                 FAX: 970-923-7338
                          possibilities@challengeaspen.com
                                    challengeaspen.org

Jimmy Yeager, President
Jack Kennedy, VP
Grayson Stover, Secretary
Kevin Berg, Director
Outdoor recreation for the blind. Winter program of skiing with guides plus numerous summer programs for the visually impaired.

9136 Challenge Golf
otivation Media
1245 Milwaukee Ave
Glenview, IL 60025-2400   847-827-9057
                                 FAX: 847-297-6829

Dorothy Bauer, Coordinator
A plain-language video, Challenge Golf is packed with information for beginners or veterans. Peter Longo covers 5 handicaps (one-arm, one-leg, in a seated position, blind, and arthritis)

clearly and concisely, on how to play golf with a physical disability. In color, complete with special effects, graphs and real handicapped golfers at play. *$38.95*
Home Edition

9137   US Association of Blind Athletes
1 Olympic Plaza
Colorado Springs, CO 80909
719-630-0422
FAX: 719-630-0616
media@usaba.org
www.usaba.org

Mark A. Lucas, MS, Executive Director
Ryan Ortiz, Assistant Executive Director
John Potts, Goalball High Performance director
Matt Simpson, Membership & Outreach Coordinator
Provides athletic opportunities and training in competitive sports for visually impaired and blind individuals throughout the US Competitions indlcude local, regional and national events, internation events, and the Winter and Summer Paralympic Games.

9138   United States Blind Golf Association
3094 Shamrock St N
Tallahassee, FL 32309-2735
864-987-9688
info@usblindgolf.com
www.blindgolf.com

Jim Baker, President
Mike McKone, Vice President
Bill McMahon, Board Member
Jack Rupert, Board Member
Provides blind and vision impaired gold tournaments to members.

Support Groups

9139   Braille Institute Orange County Center
527 North Dale Avenue
Anaheim, CA 92801
714-821-5000
800-272-4553
FAX: 714-527-7621
oc@brailleinstitute.org
brailleinstitute.org

Lester M. Sussman, Chairman
Peter A. Mindnich, President
Jon K. Hayashida, OD, FAAO, Vice President, Programs & Services
Rezaur Rehman, Vice President, Finance
Offers services, publications, information and programs free of charge to blind and visually impaired persons of all ages.

9140   Consumer and Patient Information Hotline
Prevent Blindness America
211 West Wacker Drive
Suite 1700
Chicago, IL 60606
800-331-2020
info@preventblindness.org
www.preventblindness.org/

Paul G. Howes, Chairman
Hugh R. Parry, President & CEO,Prevent Blindness America
Jerome Desserich, Vice President & Chief Financial Officer
Danielle Disch, Development Manager
A toll-free line offering free information on a broad range of vision, eye health and safety topics including sports eye safety, diabetic retinopathy, glaucoma, cataracts, children's eye disorders and more.

9141   Department of Ophthalmology Information Line
Eye & Ear Infirmary
1855 W Taylor St
Chicago, IL 60612-7242
312-996-6590
FAX: 312-996-7770
eyeweb@uic.edu
www.uic.edu

Jospeh White, President

Offers eye clinic and physician referrals to persons suffering from vision disorders as well as offers emergency information.

9142   Lighthouse International Information and Resource Service
111 East 59th Street
New York, NY 10022-1202
212-821-9384
800-829-0500
FAX: 212-821-9707
info@lighthouse.org
lighthouse.org

Mark G. Ackermann, President / CEO
Provides information about eye diseases, low vision, age-related vision loss, adaptive technology, optical devices, large print and braille publishers, helps people find low vision services, vision rehabilitation services, and support groups across the U.S.; offers large selection of consumer products.

9143   National Association for Parents of Children with Visual Impairments (NAPVI)
1 North Lexington Avenue
White Plains, NY 10601
617-972-7441
800-562-6265
FAX: 617-972-7444
napvi@guildhealth.org
www.napvi.org

Julie Urban, President
Venetia Hayden, Vice President
Susan LaVenture, Executive Director
Randi Sher, Secretary
In 1979, a group of parents responding to their own needs founded NAPVI, the National Association for Parents of the Visually Impaired, Inc. Never before was there a self-help organization specific to the needs of families of children with visual impairments. Since that time, NAPVI has grown and helped families across the US and in other countries.

9144   VUE: Vision Use in Employment
Carroll Center for the Blind
770 Centre Street
Newton, MA 02458-2597
617-969-6200
800-852-3131
FAX: 617-969-6204
info@carrol.org
www.carroll.org

Joseph Abely, President
Brian Charlson, Director of Technology
Diane M. Newark, Chief Development Officer
Janet Perry, Human Resources Director
Provides engineering solutions plus training to help people keep jobs despite their vision loss.

9145   Washington Connection
American Council of the Blind
1703 N. Beauregard St
Ste 420
Alexandria, VA 22311
202-467-5081
800-424-8666
FAX: 703-465-5085
info@acb.org
www.acb.org/wc

Kim Charlson, President
Jeff Thom, 1st Vice President
Eric Bridges, Executive Director
Coverage of issues affecting blind people via legislative information, participates in law-making, legislative training seminars and networking of support resources across the US.

A

A I Squared, 1628
A-Solution, 548
A4 Tech (USA) Corporation, 1606
AACRAO, 2181
AACRC Annual Meeting, 1827
AADB E-News, 7593
AADB National Conference, 1828
AAIDD Annual Meeting, 1829
AAN's Toll-Free Hotline, 8646
AAO Annual Meeting, 1830
AAPD Newsletter, 8078
AARP, 2195
AARP Fulfillment, 5092, 5124, 5212, 7503
AARP Magazine, 7526
ABA Commission on Mental & Physical Disability Law, 4596, 4624
ABA Commission on Mental and Physical Disability, 2465
ABC Mark of Merit Newsletter, 7890
ABC Union, ACE, ANLV, Vegas Western Cab, 5540
ABC of Asthma, Allergies & Lupus, 8426
ABC-CLIO, 2428
ABD Winter Conference, 1831
ABDA/ABMPP Annual Conference, 4578
ABI Professional Publications, 8518
ABLE Center for Independent Living, 4466
ABLE Industries, 5833
ABLE Program MCC-Longview, 2659
ABLEDATA, 1553
ABS Newsletter, 8202
ACA Annual Conference, 1832
ACB Annual Convention, 1833
ACB Government Employees, 8793
ACB Radio Amateurs, 8794
ACB Social Service Providers, 8795
ACES/ACCESS Inclusion Program, 6694
ACLD/An Association for Children and Adult s with Learning Disabilities: Greater Pittsburgh, 6168
ACM Lifting Lives Music Camp, 1373
ACPOC News, 8612
ACS Federal Healthcare, 759
ACT Assessment Test Preparation Reference Manual, 6012
AD/HD and the College Student: The Everyth ing Guide to Your Most Urgent Questions, 2275
ADA Annual Scientific Sessions, 1834
ADA Camp Grenada, 1412, 8304
ADA Camp Kushtaka, 947, 8305
ADA Camp Needlepoint, 8306
ADA Camp Sunshine, 1256
ADA Camp for Kids, 8307
ADA Guide for Small Businesses, 4993
ADA Hotel Built-In Alerting System, 198
ADA Information Services, 4994
ADA Pipeline, 4995
ADA Questions and Answers, 4996, 5378
ADA Tax Incentive Packet for Business, 4997
ADA Technical Assistance Program, 3416
ADA Teen Adventure Camp, 937, 8308
ADA Triangle D Camp, 938, 8309
ADA and City Governments: Common Problems, 4998
ADA-TA: A Technical Assistance Update from the Department of Justice, 4999
ADARA National Office, 8067
ADD Challenge: A Practical Guide for Teachers, 2276
ADD Warehouse, 7745, 7859, 7868
ADD, Stepping Out of the Dark, 7848
ADD-SOI Center, The, 2583
ADD: Helping Your Child, 7711
ADDitude Directory, 2054
ADEC Resources for Independence, 5989
ADHD Book of Lists: A Practical Guide for Helping Children and Teens with ADDs, 7712
ADHD Coaching: A Guide for Mental Health P rofessionals, 2277
ADHD Report, 7829
ADHD in Adults, 7849

ADHD in the Classroom: Strategies for Teachers, 2278
ADHD in the Schools: Assessment and Intervention Strategies, 2279, 7713
ADHD with Comorbid Disorders: Clinical Assessment and Management, 7714
ADHD: What Can We Do?, 7850
ADHD: What Do We Know?, 7851
ADRS Lakeshore, 5792
AEPS Child Progress Record: For Children Ages Three to Six, 1903
AEPS Child Progress Report: For Children Ages Birth to Three, 2584
AEPS Curriculum for Birth to Three Years, 2280
AEPS Curriculum for Three to Six Years, 1904
AEPS Data Recording Forms: For Children Ages Birth to Three, 2585
AEPS Data Recording Forms: For Children Ages Three to Six, 1905
AEPS Family Interest Survey, 1906
AEPS Family Report: Birth to Three Years, 5190
AEPS Family Report: For Children Ages Birth to Three, 5000
AEPS Family Report: For Children Ages Three to Six, 5191
AEPS Measurement for Birth to Three Years, 2586
AEPS Measurement for Three to Six Years, 2587
AER Annual International Conference, 1835
AFB Center on Vision Loss, 3188
AFB Directory of Services for Blind and Visually Impaired Persons in the US and Canada, 8902
AFB News, 9066
AFB Press, 2076, 8024
AG Bell Convention, 1836
AGRAM, 7533
AGS, 1926, 1952, 1978, 1994, 2009, 2614, 2615, 2616, 2618, 2626, 2628, 2629, 2630, 2646
AHC Media LLC, 8614
AHEAD, 1837, 2209, 5156
AHEAD Association, 760
AI Squared, 1626
AID Bulletin, 8613
AIDS Alert, 8614
AIDS Legal Council of Chicago, 4555
AIDS Sourcebook, 8427
AIDS Treatment Data Network, 2268
AIDS United, 8245
AIDS and Other Manifestations of HIV Infec tion, 8428
AIDS in the Twenty-First Century: Disease and Globalization, 8429
AIDS: The Official Journal of the Internat ional AIDS Society, 8596
AIDSLAW of Louisiana, 4556
AIM Independent Living Center: Corning, 4334
AIM Independent Living Center: Elmira, 4335
AIMS Multimedia, 1640
AIR: Assessment of Interpersonal Relations, 2588
AJ Pappanikou Center, 2261, 2262
AL Baptist State Board of Missions, 943, 7965
ALDA, 7594
ALDA Newsletter, 7594
ALS Association, 8205
ALST: Adolescent Language Screening Test, 2589
AMC Cancer Research Center, 4683
AMI, 307
APA Access, 2228
APSE, 761
APSE Conference: Revitalizing Supported Employment, Climbing to the Future, 1838
APT Technology, 514
ARC, 7605
ARC Fresno-Kelso Activity Center, 6541
ARC Gateway, 3399
ARC Of San Diego-ARROW Center, The, 6542
ARC Of San Diego-East County Training Center, The, 6543
ARC Of San Diego-Rex Industries, The, 6544
ARC Of San-Diego-South Bay, 6545
ARC Of Southeast Los Angeles-Southeast Industries, 6546
ARC of Allen County, 5990
ARC of Gloucester, 1247
ARC of Gloucester County, 6095

ARC of Hunterdon County, The, 6096
ARC of Mercer County, 6097
ARC of Monmouth, 6098
ARC of Somerset County, 1241
ARC's Government Report, 5001
ARC-Adult Vocational Program, 5834
ARC: VC Community Connections West, 6547
ARC: VC Ventura, 6548
ARCA - Dakota County Technical College, 5002
ARCA Newsletter, 5002
ARISE, 4336
ARISE: Oneida, 4337
ARISE: Oswego, 4338
ARISE: Pulaski, 4339
ARJO Inc., 152
ASB Visions Newsletter, 9067
ASCCA, 963, 8310
ASD Athletics, 7603
ASD Summer Camp, 7949
ASHA Convention, 1839
ASHA Leader, The, 8079
ASIA Annual Scientific Meeting, 1840
ASL Camp, 1146
ASSIST! to Independence, 3885
ASSISTECH, 195, 196, 239
ASSISTECH Special Needs, 183
AT&T Foundation, 3023
ATIA Conference, 1841
ATLA, 3321
ATTAIN, 1554, 6315
ATV Solutions, 596, 602, 606
AUCD, 802
AV Hunter Trust, 2797
AVKO Educational Research Foundation, 2016, 1946, 1948, 1992, 2008, 2427, 2456, 2647
AWARE, 7827
Abacus, 1607
Abbot and Dorothy H Stevens Foundation, 2939
Abell-Hangar Foundation, 3189
Abilitations, 1996
Abilitations - Speech Bin, 8063
Abilities Center of New Jersey, 6099
Abilities Expo, 1842
Abilities Unlimited of Western New England, 1179
Abilities Without Boundaries, 5893
Abilities in Motion, 4414
Abilities of Florida: An Affiliate of Service Source, 5919
Abilities of Northwest New Jersey, 6100
Abilities!, 762
Abilitree, 4406
Ability 1st, 3998
Ability Center, 71, 4328
Ability Center of Greater Toledo, 1608, 4389
Ability Center of Greater Toledo: Defiance, 4390
Ability Center of Greater Toledo: Port Cli nton, 4391
Ability Jobs, 5379
Ability Magazine, 5295, 5379
Ability Research, 1504
Ability Resources, 4402
Ability Works Incorporated, 6073
AbilityFirst, 5835, 6549, 979
Abingdon Press, 5264
Able Trek Tours, 5515
Able Trust, 2833
Able Trust, The, 5920
Able to Laugh Fanlight Productions/Icarus Films, 5305
AbleApparel Affordable Adaptive Clothing and Accessories, 5380
AbleArts, 1
AbleNet, 207, 231, 235, 303, 331, 350, 367, 370, 512, 513, 518, 538, 543, 1511, 1520, 1530, 1540, 1634, 1939, 2319, 5480
AbleNet, Inc., 5457
Abledata, 5381
Ablenet, 238
Ablex Publishing Corporation, 2560
About Children's Eyes, 8903
About Children's Vision: A Guide for Parents, 8904
About Special Kids, 6316
Academic Language Therapy Association, 8671
Academic Press, Journals Division, 2214

Academic Software, 1507, 1528, 1541, 1682, 1695, 1716
Academic Software Inc, 1505
Academic Therapy Publications, 2077, 2323
Academy Eye Associates, 7075
Academy for Guided Imagery, 2660
Academy of Cognitive Therapy, 7606
Academy of Rehabilitative Audiology, 7897, 8069, 8097
Academy of Spinal Cord Injury Professionals, 8117
Acc-u-trol, 72
Accent Books & Products, 1898, 5090, 5091, 5093, 5119, 5135, 5155, 5168, 5224, 5491
Accent Special Publications, 1889
Accent on Living Magazine, 5003
Accentcare, 6550
Access Academics & Research, 8779
Access Alaska: ADA Partners Project, 3873
Access Alaska: Fairbanks, 3874
Access Alaska: Mat-Su, 3875
Access America, 5498
Access Audiology, 8770
Access Center for Independent Living, 4392
Access Center of San Diego, 3900
Access Control Systems: NHX Nurse Call System, 199
Access Currents, 1886
Access Design Services: CILs as Experts, 5004
Access Equals Opportunity, 1887
Access II Independent Living Center, 4271
Access II Independent Living Centers, 7530
Access Independence, 4504
Access Living of Metropolitan Chicago, 4057
Access Mobility Systems, 118
Access SLP Health Care, 8780
Access Schools, 8781
Access Services, 4918
Access Store Products for Barrier Free Environments, 439
Access Store.Com, 439
Access To Independence Inc., 5005
Access To Recreation, 650, 691
Access Travel: Airports, 5487
Access Unlimited, 5382
Access Utah Network, 3797
Access Yosemite National Park, 5499
Access for 911 and Telephone Emergency Services, 5006
Access for All, 1888
Access for All: Integrating Deaf, Hard of Hearing and Hearing Preschoolers, 7987
Access for Disabled Americans, 5485
Access to Art: A Museum Directory for Blind and Visually Impaired People, 8905
Access to Health Care: Number 3&4, 2281
Access to Independence, 3901, 5005
Access to Independence of Cortland County , Inc., 4340
Access to Independence of Imperial Valley, 3902
Access to Independence of North County, 3903
Access to Recreation, 440, 234, 421
Access to Sailing, 8220
Access with Ease, 348, 612
Access-USA, 501, 610
Access-USA: Transcription Services, 502
AccessText Network, 2078
AccessToThePlanet, 5516
Accessibility Lift, 377
Accessible Home of Your Own, 1889
Accessible Journeys, 5517, 5516
Accessible Space, Inc., 4243
Accessible Vans Of America, 5541
Accessnorth CIL of Northeastern MN: Aitkin, 4244
Accessnorth CIL of Northeastern MN: Duluth, 4245
Achieva, 1337
Achievement Centers For Children, 1299, 8326
Achievement House & NCI Affiliates, 5836
Achievement Products, 441
Achieving Diversity and Independence, 5007
Achilles Track Club, 8221
Achromatopsia Network, 8796
Acid Maltase Deficiency Association, 8118

Acrontech International, 1759
Acting Blind Fanlight Productions/Icarus Films, 5306
Action Products, 270
Action Toward Independence: Middletown, 4341
Action Toward Independence: Monticello, 4342
Active Citizenship and Disability: Impleme nting the Personalization of Support, 4973
Active Living Magazine, 7891
Active Re-Entry, 4489
Active Re-Entry: Vernal, 4490
Activities in Action, 7493
Activities with Developmentally Disabled Elderly and Older Adults, 7494
Activity-Based Approach to Early Intervention, 2nd Edition, 2282
Activity-Based Intervention: 2nd Edition, 5008
Acupressure Institute, 763
Ad Lib Drop-In Center: Consumer Management, Ownership and Empowerment, 5009
Ada S McKinley Vocational Services, 5965
Adam's Camp, 1006
Adams Media, 4956
Adaptable Housing: A Technical Manual for Implementing Adaptable Dwelling, 1890
Adaptations by Adrian, 1460
Adapted Physical Activity, 5192
Adapted Physical Activity Programs, 2172
Adapted Physical Education and Sport, 8166
Adapted Physical Education for Students with Autism, 2283
Adaptek Systems, 200
Adapting Early Childhood Curricula for Children with Special Needs (9th Edition), 2284
Adapting Instruction for the Mainstream: A Sequential Approach to Teaching, 2285
Adaptivation, 1506
Adaptive Baby Care, 5307
Adaptive Baby Care Equipment Video and Book Through the Looking Glass, 5308
Adaptive Clothing: Adults, 442, 1461
Adaptive Education Strategies Building on Diversity, 2286
Adaptive Environments Center, 1877, 1891
Adaptive Mainstreaming: A Primer for Teachers and Principals, 3rd Edition, 2590
Adaptive Services Division, 9068
Adaptive Sports Center, 8222, 8615
Adaptive Technology Catalog, 443
Adaptive Tracks, 8615
Adaptivemall.com, 1907
Addictive & Mental Disorders Division, 3573
Addie McBryde Rehabilitation Center for the Blind, 7016
Addison Point Specialized Services, 6037
Addison-Wesley Publishing Company, 5044
Address Book, 611
Adelante Development Center, 6128
Adjustable Bath Seat, 153
Adjustable Bed, 184
Adjustable Chair, 249
Adjustable Clear Acrylic Tray, 250
Adjustable Incline Board, 378
Adjustable Raised Toilet Seat & Guard, 154
Adjustable Rigid Chair, 251
Adjustable Tee Stool, 252
Adjustable Wedge, 271
Adjustment Training Center, 4451
Adlib, 4195
Administration Building D HS S Campus, 3382
Administration for Children & Families, 2047
Administration for Community Living, 2117
Administration on Aging, 3287
Administration on Children, Youth and Families, 3288
Administration on Developmental Disabilities, 3289
Administrative Office, 6518, 6519
Adobe News, 5010
Adolescents and Adults with Learning Disab ilities and ADHD, 2287
Adolescents with Down Syndrome: Toward a More Fulfilling Life, 7715
Adolph Coors Foundation, 2798

Adult ADD: The Complete Handbook: Everyt hing You Need to Know About How to Cope with ADD, 7716
Adult Absorbent Briefs, 1495
Adult Day Training, 3999
Adult Lap Shoulder Bodysuit, 1496
Adult Leukemia: A Comprehensive Guide for Patients and Families, 8430
Adult Long Jumpsuit with Feet, 444
Adult Short Jumpsuit, 445, 1462
Adult Sleeveless Bodysuit, 1497
Adult Swim Diaper, 1498
Adult Tee Shoulder Bodysuit, 1499
Adult Waterproof Overpant, 1500
Advance for Providers of Post-Acute Care, 2173
Advanced Breast Cancer: A Guide to Living with Metastic Disease, 8431
Advanced Language Tool Kit, 1908
Advanced Sign Language Vocabulary: A Resource Text for Educators, 7988
Advanced Sign Language Vocabulary: A Resource Text for Educators, 2288
Advances in Cardiac and Pulmonary Rehabilitation, 2289
Advantage Wheelchair & Walker Bags, 671
Adventist HealthCare, 2661
Adventist Hinsdale Hospital, 8664
Adventure Camp, 1413
Adventure Day Camp, 1414, 8311
Adventure Learning Center at Eagle Village, 7658
Adventures Without Limits, 1323
Adventures in Musicland, 1662
Advocacy, 3791
Advocacy Center, 764, 3493
Advocacy Center for Persons with Disabilities, 3400
Advocacy Center for Persons with Disabilit ites, 765
Advocacy Pulse, 7894
Advocacy Services of Alaska, 3330
Advocado Press, 4620
The Advocado Press, 4986
Advocate, 5011
Advocate Christ Hospital and Medical Center, 6810
Advocate Christ Medical Center & Advocate Hope Children's Hospital, 6811
Advocate Illinois Masonic Medical Center, 6812
Advocates for Better Living For Everyone (A.B.L.E.), 4117
Advocates for Children of New York, 766
Aerie Experiences, 1048, 1048
Aerospace America, 570
Aerospace Compadre, 570
Aetna Foundation, 2805
African Americans in the Profession of Blindness Services, 8906
Agassiz Village, 8312
Agassiz Village Camp, 1164
Age Appropriate Puzzles, 5456
Age-Related Macular Degeneration, 8907
Agency for Healthcare Research and Quality, 2131
Agency of Human Services, 1605, 6201
Agency of Human Svcs Dept Disabilities, Aging & IL, 3818
Ages & Stages Questionnaires, 2591
Aging & Vision News, 7527
Aging Brain, 2290
Aging Life Care Association, 7438
Aging News Alert, 7528, 7534
Aging Services of California, 7439
Aging Services of Michigan, 7440
Aging Services of South Carolina, 7441
Aging Services of Washington, 7442
Aging and Developmental Disability: Current Research, Programming, and Practice, 7495
Aging and Disabilities, 3815
Aging and Disability Services Division, 3593
Aging and Disability: Crossing Network Lin es, 2291
Aging and Family Therapy: Practitioner Perspectives on Golden Pond, 7496
Aging and Rehabilitation II: The State of the Practice, 2292

Aging and Vision News, 7529
Aging and Vision: Declarations of Independence, 9118
Aging in America, 7443
Aging in Stride, 7497
Aging in the Designed Environment, 7498
Aging with a Disability, 7499
Agnes M Lindsay Trust, 3003
Ahmanson Foundation, 2737
Ahnafield Corporation, 72, 78, 81, 89, 90, 105, 109, 121, 123, 124, 130, 135, 147, 148, 149, 151
Ai Squared, 1663, 5383
Aiphone Corporation, 199
Air Lift Oxygen Carriers, 641
Air Lift Unlimited, 641
Air Products Foundation, 3137
Akron Area YMCA, 1316
Akron Community Foundation, 3103
Akron Resources, 201
Alabama Council For Developmental Disabilities, 3309
Alabama Department Of Rehabilitation Services, 5792, 5801
Alabama Department of Education: Division of Special Education Services, 2109
Alabama Department of Labor, 5798
Alabama Department of Public Health, 3310
Alabama Department of Rehabilitation Services, 3311, 6489
Alabama Department of Rehabilitation Services, 5799, 5800, 5804, 5805, 5806, 5807, 5808, 5809, 5810, 5811, 5812, 5813, 5814, 5815, 5816, 6494
Alabama Department of Senior Services, 3312
Alabama Disabilities Advocacy Program, 3313
Alabama Division of Rehabilitation and Crippled Children, 3314
Alabama Easter Seal Society, 963, 8310
Alabama Goodwill Industries, 5793
Alabama Governor's Committee on Employment of Persons with Disabilities, 3315
Alabama Institute for Deaf & Blind, 7949
Alabama Institute for Deaf and Blind, 7603
Alabama Institute for Deaf and Blind Library and Resource Center, 4646
Alabama Power Foundation, 2726
Alabama Public Library Service, 4648
Alabama Radio Reading Service Network (ARRS), 4647
Alabama Regional Library for the Blind and Physically Handicapped, 4648
Alabama State Department of Human Resources, 3316
Alabama VA Benefits Regional Office - Montgomery, 5562
Alabama VA Medical Center - Birmingham, 5563
Alamitos-Belmont Rehab Hospital, 7227
Alante, 571
Alaska Center for the Blind and Visually Impaired, 6511
Alaska Commission on Aging, 3322
Alaska Department of Education: Special Education, 2110
Alaska Department of Handicapped Children, 3323
Alaska Department of Labor & Workforce Development, 5821
Alaska Division of Vocational Rehabilitati on, 5819
Alaska Division of Vocational Rehabilitati on:, 3324
Alaska Fair Employment Practice Agency, 5820
Alaska Job Center Network, 5821
Alaska SILC, 3876
Alaska State Commission for Human Rights, 5820
Alaska State Library Talking Book Center, 4653
Alaska VA Healthcare System - Anchorage, 5566
Albany County Department for Aging and Alb any Social Services, 3637
Albany VA Medical Center: Samuel S Stratton, 5695
Albany Vet Center, 5696
Albert & Bessie Mae Kronkosky Charitable Foundation, 3190
Albert G and Olive H Schlink Foundation, 3104
Aldercrest Health and Rehabilitation Center, 7410

Aleda E Lutz VA Medical Center, 5656
Alert, 2229
Alex Stern Family Foundation, 3100
Alexander Graham Bell Association, 1836, 1915, 1922, 1923, 2032, 2313, 2426, 2481, 2528, 5325, 7999, 8061, 8072, 8077
Alexander Graham Bell Association for the Deaf and Hard of Hearing, 7898
Alexander and Margaret Stewart Trust, 2821
Alexandria Community Y Head Start, 6204
Alexandria Library Talking Book Service, 4919
Alexandria VA Medical Center, 5639
Alexian Brothers Medical Center, 6813
Alfred I DuPont Hospital for Children, 6709
Alfred I. duPont Hospital for Children, 4693
AliMed, 446
Alice Tweed Touhy Foundation, 2738
Alinna Health, 6362
All About Attention Deficit Disorders, Revised, 7717
All About Attention Deficit Disorders, Rev ised, 5309
All About You: Appropriate Special Interactions and Self-Esteem, 1664
All Days Are Happy Days Summer Camp, 1374
All Garden State Physical Therapy, 7040
All Kinds of Minds, 1909
All Star Review, 1665
All View Mirror, 73
All-Turn-It Spinner, 5457
Allen County Public Library, 4751
Allen P & Josephine B Green Foundation, 2984
Allergies & Asthma: What Every Parent Need s To Know (2nd Edition), 8432
Allergies Sourcebook, 8433
Allergy & Asthma Network, 5255
Allergy & Asthma Network Mothers of Asthmatics, 8552, 8585, 8590
Allergy & Asthma Today, 5255
Allergy and Asthma Network Mothers of Asthmatics, 8646
Alliance Center for Independance, 4312
Alliance House, 6924
Alliance for Aging Research, 7444
Alliance for Disabled in Action, 4312
Alliance for Disabled in Action New Jersey, 6101
Alliance for Parental Involvement in Education, 2017
Alliance for Parental Involvement in Education, 5241, 7777
Alliance for People with Disabilities: Sea ttle, 4526
Alliance for Retired Americans, 7445
Alliance for Technology Access, 767, 1566
Alliance of People with Disabilities: Redmond, 4527
Allied Community Services, 5894
Allied Enterprises of Tupelo, 6073
Allied Services John Heinz Institute of Rehabilitation Medicine, 6409
Allied Services Rehabilitation Hospital, 6410
Allyn & Bacon, 1641, 2432, 2436, 2441, 2442, 2443, 2447, 2460, 2492, 2524, 2527, 2533, 2549, 2558, 2562, 2595, 2658
Allyn & Bacon Longman College Faculty, 2556
Aloha Nursing and Rehab Center, 7267
Aloha Special Technology Access Center, 1555
Alpha Home Royal Maid Association for the Blind, 4260
Alpha One: Bangar, 4182
Alpha One: South Portland, 4183
Alphabetic Phonics Curriculum, 2293
Alpine Alternatives, 948, 8317
Alpine North Nursing and Rehabilitation Center, 7018
Alpine Nursing and Rehabilitation Center of Hershey, 7132
Alpine Ridge and Brandywood, 7158
Alta Bates Medical Center, 4676
Altarfire Publishing, 8495
Alternating Hemiplegia of Childhood Foundation, 2739
Alternative Approach to Allergies, 8434
Alternative Educational Delivery Systems, 2294
Alternative Teaching Strategies, 2295
Alternative Work Concepts, 2018

Alternatives for Growth: New Jersey, 6102
Alternatives in Education for the Hearing Impaired (AEHI), 5384
Altimate Medical, 393
Altman Foundation, 3024
AlumiRamp, 379
Aluminum Adjustable Support Canes for the Blind, 622
Aluminum Crutches, 642
Aluminum Walking Canes, 643
Alumni News, 9069
Alvin C York VA Medical Center, 5752
Alzheimer Disease Sourcebook, 8435
Alzheimer Disease Sourcebook, 4th Edition, 8436
Alzheimer's Association, 2864
Alzheimer's Store, 672
Amarillo VA Healthcare System, 5757
Amarillo Vet Center, 5758
Ambrose Monell Foundation, 3025
Ambulatory Cosmetology Technicians, 173
Amer Assn of Spinal Cord Injury Psych & Soc Wks, 8632
Amer Board for Cert in Otthotics & Prosthetics, 7890
American Academy Of Dermatology, 1066
American Academy Of Opthamology, 1830
American Academy for Cerebral Palsy and Developmental Medicine Annual Conference, 1843
American Academy of Allergy, Asthma & Immu nology, 8246
American Academy of Audiology, 5385
American Academy of Child & Adolescent Psychiatry, 7607
American Academy of Disability Evaluating Physicians, 768
American Academy of Environmental Medicine, 769
American Academy of Ophthalmology, 8797
American Academy of Osteopathy, 8119
American Academy of Otolaryngology - Head and Neck Surgery, 8247
American Academy of Pediatrics, 770, 8432
American Academy of Physical Medicine & Rehab, 5286
American Academy of Physical Medicine and Rehabilitation, 8248
American Action Fund for Blind Children and Adults, 8798
American Advertising Dist of Northern Virginia, 2180
American Aging Association, 7446
American Alliance for Health, Phys. Ed. & Dance, 8959
American Amputee Foundation, 7891
American Amputee Foundation, Inc., 7872
American Anals of the Deaf Reference, 8908
American Annals of the Deaf, 8080
American Art Therapy Association, 5274
American Art Therapy Association (AATA), 2
American Assn. of Children's Residential Centers, 1827
American Assoc of Homes and Services for the Aging, 7546
American Assoc of Spinal Cord Injury Psych/Soc Wor, 8210
American Association for Respiratory Care, 8249
American Association of Cardiovascular and Pulmonary Rehabilitation, 8250
American Association of Children's Residential Centers, 771
American Association of Homes and Services for the Aging, 7447
American Association of Neuromuscular & El ectrodiagnostic Medicine, 8120
American Association of Oriental Medicine, 772
American Association of People with Disabilities, 773, 5386, 7899
American Association of People with Disabilities, 5178, 8078
American Association of Retired Persons, 7448, 7526
American Association of Spinal Cord Injury Psychologists & Social Workers, 8121

American Association of University Affilia ted Programs for Persons with Dev Disabilities, 2079

American Association of the Deaf-Blind, 7561, 1828, 7593

American Association of the Deaf-Blind (AADB), 7587

American Association on Health and Disabil ity, 774

American Association on Mental Retardation, 1829, 7824

American Back Society, 8122, 8202

American Baptist Churches Rhode Island, 1363

American Bar Association, 4622, 4626, 4632

American Blind Bowling Association, 9133

American Board for Certification in Orthotics & Prosthetics And Pedorthics, Inc., 7873

American Board of Clinical Metal Toxicology, 775

American Board of Disability Analysts, 1831, 1859, 4578, 5281

American Board of Disability Analysts Annual Conference, 1844

American Board of Professional Disability Consultants, 776

American Botanical Council, 777, 5387

American Brain Tumor Association, 8251

American Camping Association, 778

American Cancer Society, 950, 1059, 1185, 8313, 8325

American Cancer Society c/o CR4TS, 983

American Chai Trust, 3026

American Chemical Society, 5302

American Chiropractic Association, 779

American Cochlear Implant Alliance, 7900

American College Testing Program, 2592, 2420, 2636, 6012

American College of Advancement in Medicine, 780

American College of Nurse Midwives, 781

American College of Rheumatology, Research and Education Foundation, 5388

American Counceling Association, 2473

American Council for Headache Education (ACHE), 2019

American Council for the Blind, 1833

American Council of Blind Lions, 8799

American Council of the Blind, 3, 8800, 8793, 8794, 8795, 8812, 8826, 8838, 8846, 8854, 8880, 8972, 8982, 9017, 9055, 9087, 9145

American Counseling Association, 782, 2080, 1832, 2185, 2202, 2232, 2233

American Counselling Association, 2020

American Dance Therapy Association (ADTA), 4

American Delirium Society, 7608

American Diabetes Association, 8252, 937, 938, 947, 1116, 1148, 1255, 1256, 1287, 1296, 1304, 1318, 1379, 1412, 1435, 1834, 8304, 8305, 8306, 8307, 8308, 8309, 8324, 8332, 8333, 8338, 8347, 8350

American Disability Association, 783

American Disabled Golfers Association, 784

American Discount Medical, 447

American Dystonia Society, 8123

American Express Foundation, 3027

American Falls Office: Living Independently for Everyone (LIFE), 4043

American Foundation Corporation, 3105

American Foundation for the Blind, 3028, 8801, 2579, 3188, 8941, 8967, 8977, 8996, 9035

American Foundation for the Blind / AFB Press, 2076

American Foundation for the Blind/ AF B Press, 1586

American Foundation for the Blind/AFB Press, 7517, 7522, 7582, 7583, 8902, 8905, 8910, 8917, 8919, 8920, 8926, 8928, 8933, 8939, 8944, 8956, 8957, 8963, 8973, 8992, 8993, 8994, 8999, 9000, 9003, 9004, 9005, 9023, 9028, 9029, 9039, 9043, 9045, 9048, 9049, 9052, 9066, 9091, 9118, 9119, 9120, 9125, 9126, 9132

American Geriatrics Society, 7449

American Group Psychotherapy Association, 8253

American Head and Neck Society, 8254

American Health Assistance Foundation, 2920

American Health Care Association, 5287

American Hearing Impaired Hockey Associati on, 8114

American Hearing Research Foundation, 8090

American Heart Association, 7875, 7892

American Herb Association Newsletter, 5012

American Herbalists Guild, 785

American Holistic Medical Association, 786

American Hotel and Lodging Foundation, 5500

American Institute for Foreign Study, 2693

American Journal of Audiology, 8065

American Journal of Orthopsychiatry, 8597

American Journal of Physical Medicine & Rehabilitation, 5271

American Journal of Psychiatry, 5272

American Journal of Public Health, 5273

American Journal of Speech-Language Pathology, 8766

American Journal on Intellectual and Devel opmental Disabilities, 2174

American Journal on Mental Retardation, 7824

American Liver Foundation, 5389

American Lung Association, 8255, 955, 1014, 1049, 8322, 8638

American Lung Association In Alaska, 8377

American Lung Association In Arizona, 8358

American Lung Association of Oregon, 1065, 8327

American Massage Therapy Association, 787

American Medical Association, 5105, 8599

American Medical Industries, 308

American Mobility: Personal Mobility Solutions, 5390

American Music Therapy Association (AMTA), 5

American National Bank and Trust Company, 2865

American Network of Community Options & Resource, 5110

American Network of Community Options & Resources, 5059

American Occupational Therapy Association, 788, 5300

American Occupational Therapy Association (AOTA), 5049

American Occupational Therapy Foundation, 2921

American Optometric Association, 8802, 8951

American Organization for Bodywork Therapies of Asia, 789

American Orthopsychiatric Association, 2224

American Orthotic & Prosthetic Association, 2254

American Orthotic & Prosthetics Association, 8606

American Parkinson Disease Association, 8124

American Physical Therapy Association, 7874, 1873

American Printing House for the Blind, 8803, 7584, 7585, 7599, 7600

American Psychiatric Association, 7609, 5272

American Psychological Association, 2184, 8597

American Public Health Association, 790, 5273

American Red Cross, 791

American SIDS Institute, 8256

American School for the Deaf, 1025

American School Counselor Association, 2020

American School for the Deaf, 7960

American Self-Help Clearinghouse, 792

American Sexual Health Association, 8257

American Sign Language Handshape Dictionary, 7989

American Sign Language Handshape Cards, 1910

American Sign Language Phrase Book, 7990

American Sign Language: A Look at Its Hist ory, Structure & Community, 7991

American Social Health Association, 8270

American Society for Deaf Children, 7562, 7901, 7596, 8073

American Society for the Alexander Technique, 793

American Society of Bariatric Physicians, 794

American Society of Clinical Hypnosis, 795

American Society of Pediatric Hematology/O ncology, 8258

American Society on Aging, 7450

American Speech-Language and Hearing Association, 5391

American Speech-Language-Hearing Association, 8672

American Speech-Language-Hearing Associati on, 7902

American Speech-Language-Hearing Association, 1839, 1956, 8065, 8068, 8079, 8766, 8767, 8770, 8779, 8780, 8781

American Spinal Injury Association, 1840

American Stroke Association, 7875, 8125, 7894, 8194

American The Beautiful; National Parks & Federal Recreation Lands, 5518

American Thermoform Corporation, 1544

American Thoracic Society, 8259

American Tinnitus Association, 7903, 8076

American Universities International Programs, 2694

American Wheelchair Bowling Association, 8223, 8217

American-Scandinavian Foundation, 2695

Americans with Disabilities Act Informationn, 3290

Americans with Disabilities Act Checklist for New Lodging Facilities, 5013

Americans with Disabilities Act Guide for Places of Lodging: Serving Guests Who Are Blind, 8909

Americans with Disabilities Act Handbook, 5014

Americans with Disabilities Act Manual, 4579

Americans with Disabilities Act: ADA Home Page, 5392

Americans with Disabilities Act: Selected Resources for Deaf, 4580

Amerock Corporation, 2866

Amigo Mobility International, 572, 410, 572

Amigo Mobility International Inc., 573

Amity Lodge, 7159

Amplified Handsets, 202

Amplified Phones, 203

Amplified Portable Phone, 204

Amputee Coalition, 5294

Amputee Coalition Of America, 1383, 1413

Amtrak, 5501

Amyotrophic Lateral Sclerosis: A Guide for Patients and Families, 8437

Amytrophic Lateral Sclerosis Association, 8126

Anaheim Veterans Center, 6551

Analog Switch Pad, 1507

Andalusia Health Services, 2727

Anderson Woods, 1083

Andrew Heiskell Braille and Talking Book Library, 4857

Angel River Health and Rehabilitation, 7284

Angel View Crippled Children's Foundation, 973

Anglo California Travel Service, 5519

Anheuser-Busch, 2985

Anixter Center, 5966

Ann Arbor Area Community Foundation, 2955

Ann Arbor Center for Independent Living, 4213, 6067

Annals Publishing Company, 8598

Annals of Dyslexia, 7825

Annals of Otology, Rhinology and Laryngolo gy, 8598

Annandale Village, 6788

Anne and Henry Zarrow Foundation, 3131

Annual Conference on Dyslexia and Related Learning Disabilities, 1845

Annual Report Sarkeys Foundation, 5016

Annual Report/Newsletter, 9070

Annual TASH Conference, The, 1846

Antecedent Control: Innovative Approaches to Behavioral Support, 2296

Anthony Brothers Manufacturing, 5458

Anthracite Region Center for Independent Living, 4415

Antioch College, 2696

Anxiety-Free Kids: An Interactive Guide for Parents and Children, 2297

Aphasia Hope Foundation, 8673

Aplastic Anemia and MDS International Foundation, 8260

Appalachian Center for Independent Living, 4533

Appalachian Center for Independent Living: Spencer, 4534
Appalachian Independence Center, 4505
Appliance 411, 5393
Applied Kinesiology: Muscle Response in Diagnosis, Therapy and Preventive Medicine, 5017
Applied Rehabilitation Counseling (Springer Series on Rehabilitation), 2298
Approaching Equality, 4581
Apria Healthcare, 448, 6695
Aquarius Health Care Media, 5310, 7738, 7752, 7853, 7854, 7856, 7861, 8729, 8784
Aquarius Health Care Videos, 5074, 5240, 5343, 5344, 5345, 5346, 5349, 5350, 5359, 5362, 5364, 5368, 5369, 7864, 8212
Aquatic Access, 411
Arbors East Subacute and Rehabilitation Center, 7360
Arbors at Canton Subacute And Rehabilitation Center, 7361
Arbors at Dayton, 7362
Arbors at Marietta, 7363
Arbors at Milford, 7364
Arbors at New Castle, 7245
Arbors at Sylvania, 7365
Arbors at Toledo Subacute and Rehab Centre, 7366
The Arc, 1847
Arc Bridges, 5991
Arc Connection Newsletter, 5018, 7830
Arc Light, 7837
Arc Massachusetts, 5011
Arc Michigan, 4214
Arc National Convention, The, 1847
Arc Of Alabama, The, 2728
Arc Of Georgia, 2847
Arc Of Meriden-Wallingford, Inc., 6696
Arc Of West Virginia, The, 3243
Arc South County Chapter, 3161
Arc of Alaska, 2729
The Arc of Anchorage, 2729
Arc of Anderson County, 3176
Arc of Arizona, 7837
The Arc of Arizona, 2731
Arc of Arkansas, 2735
Arc of Bergen and Passaic Counties, 6103
Arc of Blackstone, 4440
Arc of Blackstone Valley, 3162
Arc of California, 2740
Arc of Cape Cod, 4196
Arc of Colorado, 2799
Arc of Connecticut, 2806
Arc of Davidson County, 3177
Arc of Delaware, 2819, 3387
Arc of Dunn County, 3245
Arc of Eau Claire, 3246
Arc of Florida, 2834
Arc of Fox Cities, 3247
Arc of Hamilton County, 3178
Arc of Hawaii, 2858
Arc of Illinois, 2867
Arc of Indiana, 2902
Arc of Iowa, 2906
Arc of Jefferson County, 5794
Arc of Kansas, 2911
Arc of Kentucky, 2914
Arc of Louisiana, 2915
Arc of Maryland, 2922
Arc of Massachusetts, The, 2940
Arc of Michigan, 2956
Arc of Minnesota, 2973
Arc of Mississippi, 2983
Arc of Natrona County, 3259
Arc of Nebraska, 2994
Arc of New Jersey, 3005
The Arc of New Jersey, 1250
Arc of New London County, 1022, 8339
Arc of New Mexico, 3019
Arc of North Carolina, 3092
Arc of North Dakota, 3101
Arc of Northern Bristol County, 2941
Arc of Northern Rhode Island, 3163
Arc of Ohio, 3106
Arc of Oregon, 3133
Arc of Pennsylvania, 3138

Arc of Racine County, 3248
Arc of San Diego, 991, 7675
Arc of South Carolina, 3173
Arc of Tennessee, 3179, 5018, 7830
Arc of Texas, The, 3191
Arc of Utah, 3222
Arc of Virginia, 3226
Arc of Washington County, 3180
Arc of Washington State, 3233
Arc of Williamson County, 3181
Arc of Wisconsin Disability Association, 3249
Arc of the District of Columbia, 2822, 5001
Arc of the Farmington Valley, 6697
Arc of the US Missouri Chapter, 2986
Arc of the United States, 5394
Arc-Dane County, 3250
Arc-Diversified, 3182
Arc/Muskegon, 4215
Arcadia Foundation, 3139
Arcadia University, 2700
Architectural Barriers Action League, 5488
Archives of Neurology, 8599
Arcoa Travel Chair, 694
Arcola Bus Sales, 115, 117
Arcola Mobility, 74
Arctic Access, 3877
Arden Rehabilitation And Healthcare Center, 7196
Arden Rehabilitation and Healthcare Center, 7411
Ardence, 6382
Ardmore Developmental Center, 6045
Area Access, 380
Area Agency on Aging of Southwest Arkansas, 7548
Area Agency on Aging: Region One, 7549
Area Cooperative Educational Services (ACES), 5895
Arena Stage, 6, 7563
Arista Surgical Supply Company, 642
Arista Surgical Supply Company/AliMed, 153, 161, 180, 649, 659, 730
Arizona State Department of Health Services, 2273
Arizona Association of Homes and Housing for the Aging, 7451
Arizona Autism Resources, 2731
Arizona Braille and Talking Book Library Arizona State Library, 4654
Arizona Bridge to Independent Living, 3886, 5034
Arizona Bridge to Independent Living: Phoenix, 3887
Arizona Bridge to Independent Living: Mesa, 3888
Arizona Camp Sunrise, 950, 8313
Arizona Center for Disability Law, 3339
Arizona Center for the Blind and Visually Impaired, 6512
Arizona Civil Rights Division, 5823
Arizona Community Foundation, 2732
Arizona Department of Economic Security, 3332
Arizona Department of Health Services, 3333, 2274, 2399
Arizona Division of Aging and Adult Services, 3334
Arizona Industries for the Blind, 6513
Arizona Instructional Resource Center for Students who are Blind or Visually Impaired, The, 2733
Arizona Lions Clubs Multiple District 21, 957
Arizona Rehabilitation State Services for the Blind and Visually Impaired, 3335
Arjo Inc, 168, 174, 255, 256, 413, 418, 419
Arkansas Assistive Technology Projects, 3342
Arkansas Department of Human Services, 5832
Arkansas Department of Special Education, 2111
Arkansas Division of Aging & Adult Services, 3343
Arkansas Division of Developmental Disabilities Services, 3344
Arkansas Division of Services for the Blind, 3345
Arkansas Employment Security Department, 5828
Arkansas Employment Service Agency and Job Training Program, 5828
Arkansas Governor's Developmental Disabilities Council, 3346
Arkansas Independent Living Council, 3894
Arkansas Lighthouse for the Blind, 6534

Arkansas Regional Library for the Blind and Physically Handicapped, 4662
Arkansas School for the Blind, 4663
Arkasas Rehab Services, 5830
Arkenstone: The Benetech Initiative, 1508
Arlington County Department of Libraries, 4920
Arlington County Library, 4920
Arms Wide Open, 4027
Armstrong Medical, 449
Army and Air Force Exchange Services, 2697
Arnold A Schwartz Foundation, 3006
Aromatherapy Book: Applications and Inhalations, 5019
Aromatherapy for Common Ailments, 5020
Around the Clock: Parenting the Delayed ADHD Child, 7852
Arrowhead West, 6905
Art Therapy, 5274
Art Therapy SourceBook, 7
Art and Disabilities, 8
Art and Healing: Using Expressive Art to Heal Your Body, Mind, and Soul, 9
Art and Science of Teaching Orientation and Mobility to Persons with Visual Impairments, 8910
Art for All the Children: Approaches to Art Therapy for Children with Disabilities, 10
Art-Centered Education and Therapy for Children with Disabilities, 2299
Arthritis Bible, 8167
Arthritis Foundation, 8127, 5127, 5128, 7887, 8176, 8182, 8185, 8187, 8195, 8196, 8197, 8198, 8562
Arthritis Foundation Distribution Center, 5354
Arthritis Foundation Great West Region, 8195
Arthritis Foundation, Southeast Region Inc, 8243
Arthritis Helpbook: A Tested Self Management Program for Coping with Arthritis, 8168
Arthritis Self-Management, 8616
Arthritis Sourcebook, 8169
Arthritis Sourcebook., 8438
Arthritis Today, 8187
Arthritis Update, 8196
Arthritis, What Exercises Work: Breakthrough Relief for the Rest of Your Life, 8170
Arthritis: A Take Care of Yourself Health Guide, 8171
Arthur C. Luf Children's Burn Camp, 1021
Arthur Ross Foundation, 3029
Artic Business Vision (for DOS) and Artic WinVision (for Windows 95), 1629
Artic Technologies, 1629
Artificial Language Laboratory, 4810, 8769
Artificial Larynx, 205
Artists Fellowship, 3030
Arts Unbound, 11
The Arts of Life, 66
As I Am, 5021
Ascension Health, 6361
Asheville VA Medical Center Charles George, 5711
Ashton Memorial Nursing Home and Chemical Dependency Center, 6806
Aspen Camp School for the Deaf earing, 7950
Aspen Camp of the Deaf & Hard of Hearing, 1007, 7951
Aspen Publishers, 5014, 5175
Aspire of Western New York, 7055
Assemblies of God Center for the Blind, 4837
Assessing Students with Special Needs, 2593
Assessing the Handicaps/Needs of Children, 2300
Assessment & Management of Mainstreamed Hearing-Impaired Children, 2301
Assessment Log & Developmental Progress Charts for the CCPSN, 2302, 2594
Assessment and Remediation of Articulatory and Phonological Disorders, 2303
Assessment in Mental Handicap: A Guide to Assessment Practices & Tests, 2304
Assessment of Children and Youth, 2305
Assessment of Individuals with Severe Disabilities, 2306
Assessment of Learners with Special Needs, 2595
Assessment of the Feasibility of Contracting with a Nominee Agency, 4582

Assessment of the Technology Needs of Vending Facilitiy Managers In Tennessee, 2307
Assessment: The Special Educator's Role, 2308
Assets School, 5954
Assist. Tech. Resources for Children & Adults, 1854
Assistech, 560
Assistive Technology, 206, 175
Assistive Technology Educational Network of Florida, 3401
Assistive Technology Industry Association, 1841
Assistive Technology Journal, 450
Assistive Technology Resource Centers of Hawaii (ATRC), 4733
Assistive Technology Resource Centers of Hawaii, 3428
Assistive Technology Sourcebook, 451
Assistive Technology Training and Informat ion Center (ATTIC), 4096
Assistive Technology for Individuals with Cognitive Impairments Handbook, 7718
Assistive Technology for Infants and Toddl ers with Disabilities Handbook, 4951
Assistive Technology for Older Persons: A Handbook, 7500
Assistive Technology for Parents with Disa bilities Handbook, 5193
Assistive Technology for School-Age Children with Disabilities - Handbook, 4952
Assistive Technology in the Schools: A Guide for Idaho Educators, 2309
Assoc of Children's Prosthetic-Orthotic Clinics, 8612
Assoc of Ohio Philanthropic Homes, Housing/Service, 7533
Assoc. for Educ. & Rehab of the Blind/Vis. Imp., 1835
Assoc. on Handicapped Student Service Program, 5036
Associated Blind, 8804
Associated Services For The Blind & Visually Impaired, 4895
Associated Services for the Blind, 8805, 9067
Association For Individual Development Elgin Area, 6837
Association for Applied Psychophysiology and Biofeedback, 796
Association for Behavioral and Cognitive T herapies, 7610
Association for Contextual Behavioral Scie nce, 7611
Association for Driver Rehabilitation Spec ialists, 2021
Association for Education & Rehabilitation of the Blind & Visually Impaired, 8806
Association for Gerontology in Higher Educ ation, 7452
Association for International Practical Training, 2698
Association for Macular Diseases, 8807
Association for Macular Diseases Newsletter, 9071
Association for Neurologically Impaired Brain Injured Children, 8128
Association for Persons in Supported Employment, 797
Association for Persons in Supported Employment, 1838
Association for Persons with Severe Handicaps (TASH), 798
Association for Research in Vision and Oph thalmology, 8808
Association for Retarded Citizens: Alameda County, 6552
Association for Vision Rehabilitation and Employment, 8809
Association for the Blind, 7149
Association for the Cure of Cancer of the Prostate (CaP CURE)-Prostate Cancer Foundation, 5395
Association of Adult Musicians with Hearin g Loss, 7904
Association of Assistive Technology Act Pr ograms, 799
Association of Blind Citizens, 8810

Association of Disability Advocates, The, 800
Association of Educational Therapists, 801
Association of Language Companies, 8674
Association of Late-Deafened Adults, 7564, 7905
Association of Mouth and Foot Painting Art ists (AMPFA), 12
Association of Ohio Philanthropic Homes, H ousing and Services for the Aging, 7453
Association of Schools & Programs of Public Health, 5288
Association of University Centers on Disabilities, 802
Association on Aging with Developmental D isabilities, 7454
Association on Handicapped Student Service Program, 2229
Association on Higher Education And Disability, 1837
Association on Higher Education and Disability, 2022
Association on Higher Education and Disability (AHEAD), 803
Assumption Activity Center, 6925
Asthma & Allergy Education for Worksite Clinicians, 2662
Asthma & Allergy Essentials for Children's Care Provider, 2663
Asthma Action Cards: Child Care Asthma/Allergy Action Card, 1911
Asthma Action Cards: Student Asthma Action Card, 1912
Asthma Care Training for Kids (ACT), 2664
Asthma Management and Education, 2310
Asthma Sourcebook., 8439
Asthma and Allergy Answers: A Patient Educ ation Library, 8440
Asthma and Allergy Foundation of America, 5396, 1911, 1912, 1973, 1983, 2310, 2662, 2663, 2664, 8440, 8669
Aston-Patterning, 2311
At Home Among Strangers, 7992
Athena Rehab of Clayton, 7261
Athens Talking Book Center-Athens-Clarke County Regional Library, 4718
Atherton Family Foundation, 2859
Atkinson Foundation, 2741
Atlanta Aphasia Association, 8675
Atlanta Institute of Medicine and Rehabilitation, 6789
Atlanta Regional Office, 5609
Atlanta VA Medical Center, 5610
Atlantic Coast Rehabilitation & Healthcare Center, 7333
Atlantis Community, 3966
Attainment Company, 1666, 463
Attention, 7828
Attention Deficit Disorder, 7719
Attention Deficit Disorder and Learning Disabilities, 7720
Attention Deficit Disorder in Adults Workbook, 7721
Attention Deficit Disorder in Children, 2312
Attention Deficit Disorder: A Different Perception, 7722
Attention Deficit Disorder: Adults, 7853
Attention Deficit Disorder: Children, 7854
Attention Deficit Disorders Association, Southern Region: Annual Conference, 1848
Attention Deficit Disorders: Assessment & Teaching, 7723
Attention Getter, 1667
Attention Teens, 1668
Attention-Deficit Hyperactivity Disorder: Symptoms and Suggestons for Treatment, 7724
Attention-Deficit/Hyperactivity Disorder, What Every Parent Wants to Know, 7725
Attitudes Toward Persons with Disabilities, 5022
Attorney General's Office: Disability Rights Bureau & Health Care Bureau, 3448
Audio Book Contractors, 623
Audiogram/Clinical Records Manager, 1556
Auditech: Classroom Amplification System Focus CFM802, 1913
Auditech: Personal FM Educational System, 1914

Auditech: Personal PA Value Pack System, 329
Auditech: Pocketalker Pro, 330
Auditory-Verbal International AG Bell, 5397
Auditory-Verbal Therapy for Parents and Professionals, 1915
Augmentative Communication Systems (AAC), 1509
Augmenting Basic Communciation in Natural Contexts, 7726
Augusta Rehabilitation Center, 7305
Augusta Talking Book Center, 4719
Augusta VA Medical Center, 5611
Aural Habilitation, 2313
Aurora of Central New York, 7604
Austin Resource Center for Independent Living, 4467
Austin Resource Center: Round Rock, 4468
Austin Resource Center: San Marcos, 4469
Authoritative Guide to Self- Help Resource in Mental Health, 5023
Autism 24/7: A Family Guide to Learning at Home & in the Community, 7727, 8717
Autism Aquarius Health Care Media, 5310
Autism Community Store, 1916
Autism Day Camp, 1084, 8159
Autism Handbook: Understanding & Treating Autism & Prevention Development, 7728, 8718
Autism Research Institute, 7612, 8676, 7831, 8771
Autism Research Review International, 7831, 8771
Autism Services Center, 7613, 8677, 7870
Autism Society of America, 7869, 8788
Autism Society of North Carolina, 1289, 7671, 8707
Autism Society of North Carolina Bookstore, 7727, 7731, 7743, 7758, 7764, 7767, 7819, 8717, 8721, 8731, 8764
Autism Treatment Center Of America, 7862, 8786
Autism Treatment Center of America, 7614, 8678, 7846
Autism and Learning, 7729, 8719
Autism in Adolescents and Adults, 7730, 8720
Autism-Products.com, 1917
Autism...Nature, Diagnosis and Treatment, 7731, 8721
Autism: A World Apart, 7855, 8783
Autism: Explaining the Enigma, 7732, 8722
Autism: From Tragedy to Triumph, 7733, 8723
Autism: Identification, Education and Treatment, 7734, 8724
Autism: The Facts, 7735, 8725
Autism: the Unfolding Mystery, 7856, 8784
Autistic Adults at Bittersweet Farms, 7736, 8726
Automatic Card Shuffler, 5459
Automatic Wheelchair Anti-Rollback Device, 672
Automobile Lifts for Scooters, Wheelchairs and Powerchairs, 75
Automobility Program, 2961
Autsim Society of North Carolina Bookstore, 8575
Avery Publishing Group, 8493
Avis Rent A Car, 5542
Avon Oaks Skilled Care Nursing Facility, 7246
Awakenings Project, The, 13
AwareNews, 5024
Awareness, 9072
Awareness Training, 8911
Away We Ride, 1669
Away We Ride IntelliKeys Overlay, 1510
Ayer Company Publishers, 2489
Ayurvedic Institute, 2665
Azure Acres Recovery Center, 6553

B

BA and Elinor Steinhagen Benevolent Trust, 3192
BCR Foundation, 2918
BDRC Newsletter, 5398
BG Industries, 193
BI-County Services, 5992
BIATX Newsletter, 7838
BIAWV Newsletter, 7839
BIGmack Communication Aid, 1511
BIPAP S/T Ventilatory Support System, 309
BOSC: Directory of Facilities for People with Learning Disabilities, 2055

BPPV: What You Need to Know, 7993
BTBL News, 9073
Babycare Assistive Technology, 8912
Babycare Assistive Technology for Parents with
    Physical Disabilties, 8913
Babyface: A Story of Heart and Bones, 5194
Bach Flower Therapy: Theory and Practice, 5025
Back & Neck Sourcebook., 8441
Back in the Saddle, 6554
Back in the Saddle Hippotherapy Program, 6814
Back-Huggar Pillow, 272
BackSaver, 253
BackSaver Products Company, 253
Backgammon Set: Deluxe, 5460
Backyards and Butterflies: Ways to Include
    Children with Disabilities in Outdoor Activities,
    5195
Bad Axe: Blue Water Center for Independent
    Living, 4216
Bagel Holder, 345
Bahmann Foundation, 3107
Bailey, 452
Bailey Manufacturing, 452
Bailey Manufacturing Company, 249, 250, 252,
    266, 271, 378, 437, 509, 510, 511, 520, 521, 526,
    536, 692
Bain, Inc. Center For Independent Living, 4028
Bainbridge Subregional Library for the Blind &
    Physically Handicapped, 4720
Baker Commodities Corporate Giving Program,
    2742
Bakersfield ARC, 5837
Bakersfield Regional Rehabilitation Hospital,
    6241
Balance Centers of America, 5993
Ball Brothers Foundation, 2903
Ball Memorial Hospital, 6879
Ballantine Books, 5138, 9006
Ballard Rehabilitation Hospital, 6555
Baltimore Community Foundation, 2923, 2925
Baltimore Regional Office, 5644
Baltimore VA Medical Center, 5645
Bancroft, 7041
Bancroft Rehabilitation Living Centers, 6926
Bangor Public Library, 4780
Bangor Veteran Center: Veterans Outreach Center,
    6038
Bank of America, 3207
Bank of America Client Foundation, 2835
Bank of America Foundation, 2743
Bank of Hawaii, 2860
Bankers Trust Company, 2816
Banner Good Samaritan Medical Center, 6514
Bantam Books, 5170, 7750
Baptist Health Rehabilitation Institute, 3347
Baptist Heath, 3347
Barbara Chambers Children's Center, 6719
Barbara Olson Center of Hope, 6815
Bariatric Wheelchairs Regency FL, 695
Barnes-Jewish Hospital Washington University
    Medical Center, 7325
Baroco Corporation, 6960
Barrier Free Education, 1918
Barrier Free Travel: A Nuts and Bolts Guid e for
    Wheelers and Slow Walkers (3rd Edition), 5026
Barron Collier Jr Foundation, 2836
Barron's Educational Series, 4955, 7780, 7781,
    7782
Barrow Neurological Institute Rehab Center, 6236
Bartholomew County Public Library, 4752
Bartolucci Center, The- ILC Enterprises, 6816
Barton Center for Diabetes Education, 1169, 8348
Baruch College, 1568
Basement Motorhome Lift By Handicaps, Inc., 381
A Basic Course in American Sign Language, 7983
Basic Course in American Sign Language, 8914
Basic Course in American Sign Language (B100)
    Harris Communications, Inc., 5311
A Basic Course in Manual Communication, 7984
Basic Facts on Study Abroad, 2699
Basic Math: Detecting Special Needs, 1641
Basic Rear Closure Sweat Top, 1485
A Basic Vocabulary: American Sign Language for
    Parents and Children, 7985
Basketball: Beeping Foam, 9134

Bastyr University Natural Health Clinic, 804
Bath Fixtures, 155
Bath Products, 156
Bath Shower & Commode Chair, 157
Bath VA Medical Center, 5697
Bath and Shower Bench 3301B, 158
BathEase, 159
Bathroom Transfer Systems, 160
Bathtub Safety Rail, 161
Baton Rouge Area Foundation, 2916
Battenberg & Associates, 1670
Battery Device Adapter, 331
Battery Operated Cushion, 673
Battle Creek VA Medical Center, 5657
Baxter Healthcare Corporation, 6817, 318
Bay Area Coalition for Independent Living, 4217
Bay Pine-Virginia Beach, 7187
Bay Pines VA Medical Center, 5603
Bay View Nursing and Rehabilitation Center, 7228
Bayfront Medical Center, 6726
Bayfront Rehabilitation Center, 6726
Baylor College of Medicine, 4907, 4909
Baylor College of Medicine Birth Defects Center,
    4906
Baylor College of Medicine: Cullen Eye Institute,
    4907
Baylor Institute for Rehabilitation, 7160
Bayshore Medical Center: Rehab, 6440
Bayview Nursing and Rehabilitation, 6556
Be Quiet, Marina!, 7737
BeOK Key Lever, 503
Beach Center on Families and Disability, 805, 3478
Beacon Foundation for the Mentally Retarded,
    6515
Beacon Group SW Inc, 5825
Beacon Press, 9122
Beacon Therapeutic Diagnostic and Treatment
    Center, 6818
Beam, 7595
Bearskin Meadow Camp, 964, 8314
Beaumont Senior Center: Community Access
    Center, 3904
Beaver College, 2700
Beck Institute for Cognitive Therapy & Research,
    7841
Beck Institute for Cognitive Therapy and R
    esearch, 7615
Becket Chimney Corners YMCA Camps and
    Outdoor Center, 1165, 8315
Bed Rails, 310
The Bedford School, 1058, 7703
Beechwood Rehabilitation Services A Community
    Integrated Brain Injury Program, 7133
Before and After Zachariah, 5262
Beginning ASL Video Course Harris
    Communications, Inc., 5312
Beginning Reasoning and Reading, 1919
Behavior Analysis in Education: Focus on
    Measurably Superior Instruction, 2314
Behavior Modification, 2315
Behavior Skills: Learning How People Should
    Act, 1671
Behavioral Disorders, 2316
Behavioral Vision Approaches for Persons with
    Physical Disabilities, 8915
Behind Special Education, 2317
Being Close, 8442
Belden Center, 6557
Beliefs, Values, and Principles of Self Advocacy,
    5027
Beliefs: Pathways to Health and Well Being, 5028
Believable Hope Conference, 1849
Bellefaire Jewish Children's Bureau, 7088
Bellingham Care Center, 7197
Bellingham Health Care and Rehabilitation
    Services, 7412
Belonging, 8916
Ben B Cheney Foundation, 3234
Ben's Story: A Deaf Child's Right to Sign, 7994
Bench Marks, 5029
Benchmark Measures, 2596
Bend Work Activity Center, 6163
Benefis Healthcare, 7028
Beneto Center, 7161
Benjamin Benedict Green-Field Foundation, 2868

Benwood Foundation, 3183
Berklee Press Publications, 54
Berkley Publishing Group, 5234
Berkshire Meadows, 6961
Bernard McDonough Foundation, 3244
Berrien Community Foundation, 2957
Berthold Lowenfeld on Blindness and Blind
    People, 8917
Best 25 Catalog Resources for Making Life Easier,
    453
Best Buddies, 7616
Best Buddies Times, 7840, 7840
Beth Abraham Health Services, 7340
Beth Abraham of Family Health Services, 7351
Bethany House Publishers (Baker Publishing
    Group), 5261
Bethel Mennonite Camp, 1119
Bethy and the Mouse: A Father Remembers His
    Children with Disabilities, 5263
Better Back, 254
Better Hearing Institute, 7906
Better Sleep, 297
Betty Bacharach Rehabilitation Hospital, 6374
Beverly Enterprises Network, 6535
Beyond Baby Talk: From Sounds to Sentence s, a
    Parent's Guide to Language Development, 8727
Beyond Sight, 624
Beyond Tears: Living After Losing a Child, 5196
Beyond the Barriers, 8212
Big Bold Timer Low Vision, 346
Big Earth Publishing, 8224
Big Lakes Developmental Center, 6906
Big Lamp Switch, 504
Big Number Pocket Sized Calculator, 625
Big Print Address Book, 612
Big Red Switch, 207
Big Sky Kids Cancer Camps, 1222
Bill Rice Ranch, 1375
The Billings Lions Club, 1224
Biloxi/Gulfport VA Medical Center, 5667
BioMedical Life Systems, 315, 603
Biologically Inspired Cognitive Architectu res
    Society, 7617
Biology Concepts Through Discovery, 7857
Biomedical Concerns in Persons with Down's
    Syndrome, 2318
Birdie Thornton Center, 3867
Birmingham Alliance for Technology Access
    Center, 1557
Birmingham Independent Living Center, 1557
Birth Defect Research for Children, 806, 5398
Bittersweet Chances: A Personal Journey o f
    Living and Learning in the Face of Illness, 8443
Black Hawk Center for Independent Living, 4109
Black Hills Workshop, 4452
Black Hills Workshop & Training Center, 4452
Blackwell Publishing, 8633
Blazing Toward a Cure Annual Conference, 1850
Blind & Vision Rehabilitation Services Of
    Pittsburgh, 7134
Blind Babies Foundation, 2744, 6558
Blind Children's Center, 5333, 8938, 8953, 8955,
    8968, 8986, 8987, 9001, 9008, 9012, 9022,
    9026, 9027, 9031, 9032, 9088, 9123
Blind Children's Fund, 2958, 2269
Blind Childrens Center, 8811, 1851
Blind Childrens Center Annual Meeting, 1851
Blind Educator, 9054
Blind Industries and Services of Maryland, 6949
Blind Information Technology Specialists, 8812
Blind Outdoor Leisure Development, 9135
Blind Service Association, 6819
Blind and Physically Handicapped Library
    Services, 4834
Blind and Vision-Impaired Individuals, 8918
Blinded Veterans Association, 8813, 1852
Blinded Veterans Association National
    Convention, 1852
Blindness Landmark Media, Inc., 5313
Blindness and Early Childhood Development
    Second Edition, 8919
Blindness, A Family Matter, 9119
Blindness: What it is, What it Does and How to
    Live with it, 8920
Blindskills Inc., 9057

Blinker Buddy II Electronic Turn Signal, 76
Blocks in Motion, 1672
Blood and Circulatory Disorders Sourcebook, 8444
Blooming Where You're Planted: Stories Fro m The Heart, 8445
Blowitz-Ridgeway Foundation, 2869
Blue Chip II, 474
Blue Peaks Developmental Services, 5878
Blue Ridge Independent Living Center, 4506
Blue Ridge Independent Living Center: Christianburg, 4507
Blue Ridge Independent Living Center: Low Moor, 4508
Blueberry Hill Healthcare, 6962
Bluebook: Explanation of the Contents of the ADA, 4583
Bluegrass Technology Center, 1558
Board Games: Snakes and Ladders, 5461
Board Games: Solitaire, 5462
Bob & Kay Timberlake Foundation, 3093
Bobby Dodd Institute (BDI), 6790
Boca Raton Rehabilitation Center, 7247
Bodie, Dolina, Smith & Hobbs, P.C., 5030
Bodman Foundation, 3031
Body Reflexology: Healing at Your Fingertips, 5031
Body Silent: The Different World of the Disabled, 5032
Body Suits, 454, 1463
Body of Knowledge/Hellerwork, 5033
Bodyline Comfort Systems, 272
Boise Health And Rehabilitation Center, 7268
Boise Regional Office, 5617
Boise VA Medical Center, 5618
Bold Line Paper, 613
Bold Tracks, 8224
Bolton Manor Nursing Home, 7313
Bon Coeur, Inc., 1126, 8321
Bonfils-Stanton Foundation, 2800
Bonnie Prudden Myotherapy, 807
Book of Name Signs: Naming in American Sig n Language, 7995
Bookholder: Roberts, 505
Books are Fun for Everyone, 8921
Books for Blind & Physically Handicapped Individuals, 8922
Books for Blind and Physically Handicapped Individuals, 8814, 8923
Books for the Blind of Arizona, 4655
Books on Special Children, 2055, 2075, 2300, 6387, 7720, 7820, 8765
Bootheel Area Independent Living Services, 4272
Booties with Non-Skid Soles, 1454
Boston Center for Independent Living, 4197
Boston Foundation, 2942
Boston Globe Foundation, 2943
Boston University, 4797, 6967
Boston University Arthritis Center, 4797
Boston University Center for Human Genetics, 4798
Boston University Hospital Vision Rehabilitation Services, 6963
Boston University Robert Dawson Evans Memorial Dept. of Clinical Research, 4799
Boston VA Regional Office, 5650
Bothin Foundation, 2745
Botsford Center For Rehabilitation & Health Improvement-Redford, 6992
Boulder Community Hospital Mapleton Center, 7237
Boulder Park Terrace, 7323
Boulder Public Library, 4684
Boulder Vet Center, 5588
Bounder Plus Power Wheelchair, 742
Bounder Power Wheelchair, 743
Box Top Opener, 347
Boxlight, 1624
Boxlight Corporation, 1624
Boy Inside, The Fanlight Productions/Icarus Films, 5314
Brachial Plexus Palsy Foundation, 3140
Bradford Regional Medical Center, 7135
Bradford Woods: Camp Riley, 1085
Braille + Mobile Manager, 7599

Braille Book Bank, Music Catalog, 8924
Braille Circulating Library for the Blind, 4921
Braille Compass, 626
Braille Documents, 5315
Braille Forum, 9055
Braille Institute, 9102
Braille Institute Library, 4667
Braille Institute Orange County Center, 9139
Braille Institute Santa Barbara Center, 4668
Braille Institute Sight Center, 4669
Braille Institute of America, 8815
Braille Keyboard Labels, 1543
Braille Monitor, 9056
Braille Montior, 7586
Braille Notebook, 614
Braille Plates for Elevator, 627
Braille Playing Cards: Plastic, 5463
Braille Touch-Time Watches, 628
Braille and Talking Book Library, 9073
Braille and Talking Book Library, Perkins School for the Blind, 4800
Braille and Talking Book Library: California, 4670
Braille: An Extraordinary Volunteer Opportunity, 8925
Braille: Bingo Cards, Boards and Call Numbers, 5464
Braille: Desk Calendar, 615
Braille: Greeting Cards, 616
Braille: Rook Cards, 5465
Brailon Thermoform Duplicator, 1544
Brain Allergies: The Psychonutrient and Magnetic Connections, 8446
Brain Clinic, The, 2597
Brain Disorders Sourcebook, 8447
Brain Injury Association of America, 808, 7618, 5291, 7839
Brain Injury Association of New York State, 7619
Brain Injury Association of Texas, 7620, 7838
Brain Injury Rehabilitation Center Dr. P. Phillips Hospital, 6727
Brain Injury Rehabilitation Center Dr. P. Phillips, 6727
Brain Injury Resource Center, 8657
Brandecker Rehabilitation Center, 6820
Branden Books, 7733
Branden Publishing Company, 8723
Brandt Industries, 506
Braun Corporation, 77, 162, 85, 162
Braun Corporation, The, 382
Brave Heart's Camp, 1086
Bravo! + Three-Wheel Scooter, 574
Brawner Building, 2821
Brazoria County Center For Independent Living, 4470
Breaking Barriers, 2319
Breaking Ground, 8617
Breaking New Ground News Note, 8618
Breaking New Ground Resource Center, 8647
Breaking the Speech Barrier: Language Develpment Through Augmented Means, 8728
Breakthroughs: How to Reach Students with Autism, 7738, 8729
Breast Cancer Sourcebook, 8448
Breathe Free, 8449
Breathing Lessons: The Life and Work of Mark O'Brien, 8213
Breckenridge Outdoor Education Center, 1008
Breez 1025, 744
Breezy, 696
Bremerton Convalescent and Rehabilitation Center, 7413
Brentwood Rehabilitation and Nursing Cente r, 7306
Brentwood Subacute Healthcare Center, 6821
Brevard County Libraries, 4700
Brevard County Library System, 4714
Brevard County Talking Books Library, 4700
Brewer Rehab and Living Center, 6350
Brian's House, 4416
Briarcliff Nursing Home & Rehab Facility, 6490
The Bridge Center, 1178
Bridge Newsletter, 5034

Bridge Pointe Services & Goodwill of Southern Indiana, Inc, 5994
Bridgepark Center for Rehabilitation and Nursing Services, 7367
Bridgeport Art Center, 60
Bridging the Gap: A National Directory of Services for Women & Girls with Disabilities, 5035
Briefs, 1501
Briggs Foundation, 2746
Brigham Manor Nursing and Rehabilitation Center, 7314
Brigham and Women s Hospital, 4802
Brigham and Women's Hospital: Asthma and Allergic Disease Research Center, 4801
Brigham and Women's Hospital: Robert B Brigham Multipurpose Arthritis Center, 4802
Bright Horizons Summer Camp, 1166, 8316
Brighten Place, 6411
Brike International, 553
Bringing Out the Best, 5316
Britannica Film Company, 5326, 5374, 9021
Broadmead, 4186
Broadview Multi-Care Center, 7368
Broken Dolls: Gathering the Pieces: Caring for Chronically Ill Children, 5197
Bronx Continuing Treatment Day Program, 7056
Bronx Independent Living Services, 4343
Bronx VA Medical Center, 5698
Brooke Publishing, 2547
Brookes Publishing, 1903, 1904, 1905, 1906, 1979, 2003, 2280, 2282, 2296, 2302, 2325, 2326, 2329, 2333, 2336, 2344, 2346, 2360, 2361, 2363, 2380, 2381, 2383, 2398, 2409, 2415, 2431, 2433, 2450, 2458, 2471, 2514, 2534, 2538, 2553, 2577, 2584, 2585, 2586, 2587, 2591, 2594, 2599, 2610, 2612, 4958, 4987, 4989, 5000, 5008, , 5052, 5058, 5071, 5073, 5114, 5151, 5172, 5176, 5190, 5191, 5199, 5202, 5203, 5204, 5220, 5230, 5236, 5246, 5256, 5257, 5276, 5282, 5298, 5299, 5329, 5361, 5367, 7715, 7725, 7726, 7744, 7761, 7766, 7766, 7796
Brookes Publishing Company, 2081, 2286, 2306, 2308, 2314, 2343, 2384, 2418, 2488, 2581
Brookings Institution, 4584, 7518, 7523
Brookline Books, 14, 2082, 8, 23, 1962, 1965, 1966, 2005, 2006, 2304, 2322, 2342, 2358, 2362, 2367, 2392, 2429, 2515, 2518, 2536, 2539, 2544, 2546, 2559, 2564, 5027, 5063, 5068, 5116, 5120, 5122, 5160, 5195, 5198, 5201, 5211, 5226, 5243, 5260, 5263, 7739, 7786, 7802, 7805, 7817, 8490, 8534, 8563
Brookline Books Publications, 2379
Brooklyn Bureau of Community Service, 7057
Brooklyn Campus of the VA NY Harbor Healthcare System, 5699
Brooklyn Center for Independence of the Disabled, 4344
Brooks / Cole Publishing Company, 2354
Brooks Memorial Hospital Rehabilitation Center, 6728
Brooks Rehabilitation Hospital, 2666
Brooks/Cole Publishing Company, 2083, 7723
Brotman Medical Center, 6559
Brotman Medical Center: RehabCare Unit, 6242, 6559
Broward County Talking Book Library, 4701
Brown County Library, 4945
Brown Foundation, 3193
Brown-Heatly Library, 4908
Bruno Independent Living Aids, 383, 75, 387, 395, 396, 407, 417, 429, 430, 434, 594
Bryn Mawr Rehabilitation Hospital, 7136
Buck & Buck, 1446, 1447, 1448, 1449, 1450, 1451, 1452, 1453, 1454, 1455, 1456, 1458, 1459, 1468, 1475, 1476, 1477, 1480, 1482, 1483, 1484, 1485, 1486, 1487, 1488, 1489, 1490, 1492, 1493, 1494, 1502
Buck and Buck Clothing, 1464
Budget Cotton/Poly Open Back Gown, 1446
Budget Flannel Open Back Gown, 1447
Buffalo Hearing and Speech Center, 7058

Buffalo Regional Office Department of Veterans Affairs, 5700
Buffalo State (SUNY), 2701
Build Rehabilitation Industries, 6560
Builders of Skills, 6308
Building Blocks: Foundations for Learning for Young Blind and Visually Impaired Children, 9120
Building Bridges: Including People with Disabilities in International Programs, 2702
Building Owners and Managers Association International, 1878
Building Skills for Independence in the Ma instream, 2320
Building Skills for Success in the Fast-Pa ced Classroom, 2321
Building the Healing Partnership: Parents, Professionals and Children, 2322, 5198
Bull Publishing, 8508
Bulletin of the Association on the Handicapped, 5036
Burbank Rehabilitation Center, 6964
Bureau Of Exceptional Education And Student Services, 3402
Bureau of Elderly & Adult Services, 3611
Bureau of Employment Programs Division of Workers' Compensation, 3841
Bureau of Rehabilitations Services, 4690
Burger School for the Autistic, 4811
Burke Rehabilitation Hospital, 6383
Burn Institute, 965
Burnett Foundation, 3194
Burns Braille Transcription Dictionary, 8926
Burns-Dunphy Foundation, 2747
BurnsBooks Publishing, 2084
Burnt Gin Camp, 1365
Bus Girl: Selected Poems, 7739
Bus and Taxi Sign, 507
Bushrod H Campbell and Ada F Hall Charity Fund, 2944
Business Publishers, 3285, 4618, 4625
Business as Usual Fanlight Productions/Icarus Films, 5317
Butler Adult Training Center, 6491
Butler VA Medical Center, 5733
Butlers Wheelchair Lifts, 384
Button Aid, 298
Buy!, 1920
Buying Time: The Media Role in Health Care Fanlight Productions/Icarus Films, 5318
Bye-Bye Decubiti (BBD), 273
Bye-Bye Decubiti Air Mattress Overlay, 185

C

C D Publications, 7528, 7534
C&C Software, 1647
C-4 Work Center, 5967
C-CAD Center of United Cerebral Palsy of Metropolitan Dallas, 6192
CA Health and Human Services Agency Dept of Rehab, 3357
CACLD, 5336, 7797, 7865
CAHSA Connecting, 7535
CAI, Career Assessment Inventories for the Learning Disabled, 2323
CANPFA-Line, 7536
CAPCO Capability Corporation, 1764
CAPP National Parent Resource Center Federation for Children with Special Needs, 809
CAREERS & the disABLED Magazine, 5275
CARF International, 2023
CARF International (Commission on Accredit ation of Rehabilitation Facilities), 2023
CARF Rehabilitation Accreditation Commission, 810
CASA Inc., 4329
CC-M Productions, 8214
CD Publications, 3262
CDR Reports, 5037
CEC Catalog, 2175
CEC-Division for Early Childhood, 2024
CH Foundation, 3195
CHAMP Camp, 1087, 7952

CHOICES Center for Independent Living, 4330
CIL of Central Florida, 4000
CINTEX: Speak to Your Appliances, 1673
CITE: Lighthouse for Central Florida, 1559
CNI Cochlear Kids Camp, 1009
CNS Camp New Connections, 7659, 8706
CORE Health Care, 7162
CPB/WGBH National Center for Access Media, 6965
CQL Accreditation, 1853
CRC Press, 2509
CREVT: Comprehensive Receptive and Expressive Vocabulary Test, 2598
CT Assoc of Not-for-Profit Providers of the Aging, 7536
CV Mosby Company, 2246
CW Resources, 5896
CYO Day Camp: Wickliffe, 1297
Cabell County Public Library/Talking Book Department/Subregional Library for the Blind, 4937
Cabinet for Health Services, 3489
Caddo-Bossier Association for Retarded Citizens, 6927
Cadinal Hill Medical Center, 6915
Caglewood, Inc., 1050
Cahaba Media Group, 2194
California Community Care News, 4974
California Community Foundation, 2748
California Department of Aging, 3351
California Department of Education: Special Education Division, 2112
California Department of Fair Employment & Housing, 5838, 4599, 4600, 4603
California Department of Handicapped Children, 3352
California Department of Rehabilitation, 3353
California Elwyn, 6561
California Endowment, 2749
California Eye Institute, 6562
California Financial Power of Attorney, 5038
California Foundation For Independent Living Centers, 3905
California Foundation for Independent Living Centers, 3906
California Governor's Committee on Employment of People with Disabilities, 3354
California Lions Camp, 978, 7964
California Protection & Advocacy: (PAI) A Nonprofit Organization, 3355
California School of Professional Psychology, 4679
California State Council on Developmental Disabilities, 3356
California State Independent Living Counci l (SILC), 3907
California State Library Braille and Talking Book Library, 4671, 8816
Cambridge Career Products Catalog, 455
Cambridge Educational, 455, 1722
Cambridge University Press, 4973, 8531, 8557
Camden City Independent Living Center, 4313
Camden Healthcare and Rehabilitation Center, 7387
Camiccia-Arnautou Charitable Foundation, 2837
Camp Waban, 1134
Camp AIM, 1338
Camp Abilities Brockport, 1257
Camp Abilities Tucson, 951
Camp About Face, 1088
Camp Adam Fisher, 1366
Camp Akeela, 1339
Camp Albrecht Acres, 1104
Camp Aldersgate, 959
Camp Aldersgate, Inc., 959
Camp Alexander Mack, 1089, 7953
Camp Allen, 1236
Camp Allyn, 1298
Camp Alpine, 948, 8317
Camp Amigo Burn Camp, 1035
Camp Anuenue, 1059, 8318
Camp Baker, 7660
Camp Barakel, 1183, 8882
Camp Barefoot, 1184
Camp Barnabas, 1209

Camp Be An Angel, 1384
Camp Benedict, 1198
Camp Betsey Cox, 1409, 7661
Camp Beyond The Scars, 965
Camp Birchwood, 949, 8319
Camp Bishopswood, 1135, 7954
Camp Bloomfield, 966
Camp Boggy Creek, 1036, 8320
Camp Bon Coeur, 1126, 8321
Camp Brave Eagle, 1090
Camp Breathe Easy, 1049, 8322
Camp Buck, 1232
Camp Buckskin, 1199, 7662
Camp CAMP, 1385
Camp Caglewood, 1050
Camp Callahan, 1064
Camp Callahan, Inc., 1064
Camp Can Do, 1340, 8323
Camp Candlelight, 952, 7663
Camp Capella, 1136, 7955
Camp Carefree, 1286, 8324
Camp Carolina Trails, 1287
Camp Catch-a-Rainbow, 1185, 8325
Camp Challenge, 1037, 1091, 1127, 8883
Camp Chatterbox, 1239
Camp Cheerful, 1299, 8326
Camp Chris Williams, 1186, 7956
Camp Christian Berets, 967
Camp Christmas Seal, 1065, 8327
Camp Civitan, 953
Camp Classen YMCA, 1320, 8328
Camp Coelho, 968
Camp Comeca & Retreat Center, 1225, 7957
Camp Confidence, 1200
Camp Conrad-Chinnock, 969, 8329
Camp Costanoan, 970
Camp Courage North, 1201, 8330
Camp Courageous, 1300
Camp Courageous of Iowa, 1105
Camp Cpals, 1386
Camp Crosley YMCA, 1092, 1093
Camp Debbie Lou, 1367
Camp Del Corazon, 971, 8331
Camp Dickenson, 1415
Camp Discovery, 1066, 1376, 8332
Camp Discovery - Illinois, 8333
Camp Discovery - Kansas, 1116
Camp Dream, 1051
Camp Dream Foundation, 1051
Camp Dream Street, 1208, 1240
Camp Dream Street, MS, 1208
Camp Dunmore ia, 1341
Camp Easter Seals, 1067
Camp Easter Seals Virginia, 1416
Camp Eden Wood, 8334
Camp Emanuel, 1301, 7958
Camp Encourage, 1210
Camp Esperanza, 1052, 8160
Camp Evoked Potential @ Camp ASCCA, 939, 7664
Camp Fairlee Manor, 1029, 1147
Camp Fire USA, 1426
Camp Firefly, 972
Camp Floyd Rogers, 1226, 8335
Camp Forrest, 973
Camp Foundation, 3227
Camp Friendship, 1202, 1370
Camp Fun in the Sun, 1425, 8336
Camp Funshine, 960
Camp Funshine Foundation, Inc., 960
Camp Giddy-Up, 1400
Camp Gilbert, 1371
Camp Glengarra, 1258, 8337
Camp Glyndon, 1148, 8338
Camp Good Days and Special Times, 1259
Camp Grace Bentley, 1187
Camp Gravatt, 1368
Camp Grizzly, 974, 7959
Camp Happiness, 1302
Camp Harkness, 1022, 8339
Camp Hawkins, 1053
Camp Heartland, 1203
Camp Hemlocks, 1023
Camp Hertko Hollow, 1106, 8340
Camp Hickory Hill, 1211, 8341

Camp Ho Mita Koda, 1303, 8342
Camp Hobe, 1401
Camp Hodia, 1061, 8343
Camp Holiday Trails, 1417
Camp Honor, 954, 8344
Camp Hope, 1444
Camp Horizons, 1024, 7665
Camp Howe, 1167
Camp Hug The Bear, 1068
Camp Huntington, 1260, 7666
Camp I Am Me, 1069
Camp Independence, 1261, 8345
Camp Isola Bella, 1025
Camp Isola Bella On Twin Lakes, Salisbury, Ct., 7960
Camp J CC, 2683
Camp JCC, 1149
Camp Jabberwocky, 1168
Camp Jened, 1262, 8346
Camp John Marc, 1387
Camp John Warvel, 1093, 8347
Camp Joslin, 1169, 8348
Camp Jotoni, 1241
Camp Joy, 1150, 7961, 8349
Camp Juliena, 1054, 7962
Camp Kee-B-Waw, 1434
Camp Killoqua, 1426
Camp Kindle, 975, 1227
Camp Knutson, 1204
Camp Knutson And Knutson Point Retreat Center, 1204
Camp Ko-Man-She, 1304, 8350
Camp Koinonia, 1377
Camp Kostopulos, 1402
Camp Kota, 961
Camp Krem, 976
Camp Kudzu, 1055
Camp Kudzu, Inc., 1055
Camp Kweebec, 1342, 8351
Camp L-Kee-Ta, 1107, 8352
Camp Latgawa, 8353
Camp Latgawa Special Needs, Inc., 1324
Camp Lawroweld, 1137, 8884
Camp Lee Mar, 1343
Camp Libbey, 1305, 8354
Camp Little Giant, 1070
Camp Little Red Door, 1094
Camp Lotsafun, 1233
Camp Lou Henry Hoover, 1242, 8885
Camp Loud And Clear, 1418
Camp MITIOG, 1212, 8355
Camp Magruder, 1325, 8356
Camp Mak-A-Dream, 1223
Camp Manito/Camp Lenape, 1030
Camp Mark Seven, 1263, 7963
Camp Mauchatea, 1361
Camp Merrick, 8886
Camp Merrimack, 940
Camp Merry Heart, 1243
Camp Milldale, 1151
Camp Millhouse, 1095
Camp Nah-Nah-Mah, 1403
Camp Needlepoint, 1435
Camp Nejeda, 1244, 8357
Camp Nejeda Foundation, 1244, 8357
Camp Neuron, 1388
Camp New Connections, 1170
Camp New Hope, 1071, 1288
Camp Nissokone, 1188, 7667
Camp No Limits, 1138
Camp Northwood, 1264, 7668
Camp Not-A-Wheeze, 955, 8358
Camp Nuhop, 1306, 7669
Camp Oakhurst, 1245, 8161
Camp Okawehna, 1378
Camp Okizu, 977, 8359
Camp Pacifica, Inc., 978, 7964
Camp Paha Rise Above, 1010
Camp Paivika, 979
Camp Pelican, 1128, 8360
Camp Perfect Wings, 1321
Camp Pinecone, 1139
Camp Prime Time, 1427
Camp Quality Arkansas, 962

Camp Quality Central Missouri, 1213
Camp Quality George Washington University, 1152
Camp Quality Greater Kansas City, 1214
Camp Quality Heartland, 1108
Camp Quality Illinois, 1072
Camp Quality Kansas, 1117
Camp Quality Kentuckiana, 1120
Camp Quality Louisiana, 1129
Camp Quality Michigan, 1189
Camp Quality New Jersey, 1246
Camp Quality Northwest Missouri, 1215
Camp Quality Ohio, 1307
Camp Quality Ozarks, 1216
Camp Quality Texas, 1389
Camp Quest, 980
Camp Rainbow, 956, 8361
Camp Rainbow Gold, 1062
Camp Ramah In California, 981
Camp Ramah in New England, 1171
Camp Ramah in the Poconos Education, Inc., 1344
Camp Ramapo, 1265, 7670
Camp Rap-A-Hope, 941, 8362
Camp ReCreation, 982
Camp Reach for the Sky, 983
Camp Recovery Center, 6563
Camp Red Cedar, 1096
Camp Riley, 1190
Camp Riley/Riley's Children Foundation, 1097
Camp Rocky Mountain Village, 1011
Camp Roehr, 1153
Camp Roger, 1190
Camp Ronald McDonald for Good Times, 984, 8363
Camp Ronald McDonald® at Eagle Lake, 985
Camp Royall, 1289, 7671, 8707
Camp Rubber Soul, 986
Camp Ruggles, 1362, 7672
Camp Sawtooth, 1063, 8364
Camp Seale Harris, 942, 8365
Camp Sertoma, 1290
Camp Setebaid, 1345, 8366
Camp Shocco for the Deaf, 943, 7965
Camp SignShine, 1234
Camp Sioux, 1296
Camp Sisol, 1266, 7673, 8708
Camp Sky Ranch, 1291
Camp Smile-A-Mile, 944, 8367
Camp Sno Mo, 1237
Camp Spearhead, 1369
Camp Spike 'n' Wave, 1390
Camp Starfish, 1172
Camp Starlight, 1326
Camp Stepping Stone, 1308
Camp Sugar Falls, 1379
Camp Summit, 1391
Camp Sun'N Fun, 1247
Camp Sunburst, 987
Camp Sunnyside, 1109
Camp Sunrise, 1154, 8368
Camp Sunshine, 1056, 1140
Camp Sunshine Dreams, 988
Camp Superkids, 1155
Camp Surefoot Center, 1346
Camp Sweeney, 1392, 8369
Camp Tall Turf, 1191, 8370
Camp Taloali, 1327, 7966
Camp Tanager, 1110
Camp Taylor, Inc., 989, 8371
Camp Tekoa UMC, 1292, 7967
Camp Thorpe, 1410
Camp Thunderbird, 1038
Camp Tova, 1267
Camp Trinity, 990
Camp Twin Lakes, 1057
Camp Vacamas, 1248, 8372
Camp Venture, Inc., 1268
Camp Victory, 1130, 1347
Camp Virginia Jaycee, 1419
Camp Virginia Jaycee Newsletter, 2230
Camp Vision, 1404
Camp Volasuca, 1428
Camp Wapiyapi, 1012
Camp Waziyatah, 1141, 8373

Camp Wee-Kan-Tu, 1173
Camp Wesley Woods: Northeastern Pennsylvan, 1348
Camp WheezeAway, 945, 8374
Camp Whitman on Seneca Lake, 1269
Camp Winnebago, 1142
Camp Winnekeag, 8887
Camp Woodlands, 1349
Camp World Light, 7674
Camp Wyoming, 1111
Camp X-Treme, 1405
Camp for All, 1393
Camp for All Foundation, 1393
Camp for Kids With Diabetes, 1255
Camp-A-Lot And Leisure Express (PALS Program), 991, 7675
CampCare, 1235
Campaign Math, 1642
Campbell Soup Foundation, 3007
Camping Unlimited, 992, 976
Camping Unlimited for Children & Adults, 993
Camping Unlimited-Camp Krem, 993
Campobello Chemical Dependency Recovery Center, 6564
Camps for Children & Teens with Diabetes, 1420, 8375
Can America Afford to Grow Old?, 4584
Can't Your Child See? A Guide for Parents of Visually Impaired Children, 8927
Can-Do Products Catalog, 163
Canadian Cancer Society, 8261
Canadian Deafblind Association (CDBA) National Office, 7565
Canadian Diabetes Association, 8262
Canadian Lung Association, 8263
Canandiagua VA Medical Center, 5701
Cancer Care, 3033
Cancer Clinical Trials: A Commonsense Guide to Experimental Cancer Therapies and Trials, 5247
Cancer Immunology Research Foundation (CIRF) Cancer Research Institute National Headquar, 5399
Cancer Immunotherapy and Gene Therapy, 5400
Cancer Information Service, 8648
Cancer Research Institute, 5401
Cancer Sourcebook, 8450
Cancer Sourcebook for Women, 8451
Candlelighters Childhood Cancer Foundation, 2924
Candler General Hospital: Rehabilitation Unit, 6301
Canes and Trails, 9074
Canine Companions for Independence, 811
Canine Helpers for the Handicapped, 812, 8817
Canine Listener, 8092
Canonicus Camp, 1363
Cape Coral Hospital, 7248
Cape Organization for Rights of the Disabled (CORD), 813
Cape Organization for Rights of the Disabl ed (CORD), 4198
Capital Area Center for Independent Living, 4218
Capital Area Parkinsons Society, 8129
Capital District Center for Independence, 4345
Capital District YMCA, 1284, 8900
Capitol Focus, 7537
Caprice Care Center, 7369
Capron Rehabilitation Center, 6677
Capscrew, 348
Capsule, 7538
Caption Center, 4803, 8818
Captus Press, 4982
Car Builder Deluxe, 1674
Card Holder Deluxe, 5466
Cardinal Hill Rehabilitation Hospital, 6338, 6915
Cardiovascular Diseases and Disorders Sour cebook, 3rd Edition, 8452
Cards: Musical, 5467
Cards: UNO, 5468
Care Center East Health & Specialty Care Center, 7375
Care Electronics, 508
Care Master Medical Services, 6798
Care-One, 7051
Career Assessment & Planning Services, 5921

Career Connection Transition Program, 5839
Career Connections, 6213
Career Development Program (CDP), 5840
Career Development and Transition for Exce ptional Individuals, 2176
Career Opportunity Development of New Jersey, 6104
Career Perspectives: Interviews with Blind and Visually Impaired Professionals, 8928
Career Success for Disabled High-Flyers, 4984
Careers in Blindness Rehabilitation Services, 8929
Caremark Healthcare Services, 6822
Carendo, 255
Carex Health Brands, 456
Carey Services, 5995
Carilion Health System, 7193
Carilion Rehabilitation: New River Valley, 7188
Caring and Sharing Center for Independent Living, 4001
Caring and Sharing Center: Pasco County, 4002
Caring for America's Heroes, 5039
Caring for Children with Chronic Illness, 2324
Caring for Persons with Developmental Disabilities, 5319
Caring for Those You Love: A Guide to Compassionate Care for the Aged, 7501
Carl T Hayden VA Medical Center, 5569
Carl Vinson VA Medical Center, 5612
Carnegie Library of Pitts. Library for the Blind, 9038
Carnegie Library of Pittsburgh Library for the Blind & Physically Handicapped, 4896
Caro: Blue Water Center for Independent Li ving, 4219
Carolina Computer Access Center, 1560
Carolina Curriculum for Infants and Toddlers with Special Needs (3rd Edition), 2325, 5256
Carolina Curriculum for Preschoolers with Special Needs, 2326, 2599
Carolyn's Catalog, 1465
Carolyn's Low Vision Products, 457
Carondelet Brain Injury Programs and Services (Bridges Now), 6516
Carpal Tunnel Syndrome, 7887
Carrie Estelle Doheny Foundation, 2750
Carroll Center for the Blind, 6966, 9144
Carroll School Summer Programs, 1174, 7676
Carson City Center for Independent Living, 4306
Cary Library, 4781
Casa Colina Center for Rehabilitation, 6567
Casa Colina Centers for Rehabilitation, 6565
Casa Colina Padua Village, 6566
Casa Colina Residential Services: Rancho Pino Verde, 6567
Casa Colina Transitional Living Center, 6568
Casa Colina Transitional Living Center: Pomona, 6569
Casa Colinas Centers for Rehabilitation, 6243
Case Management Society of America, 814
Case Manager Magazine, 2177
Case Western Reserve University, 4882
Case Western Reserve University Northeast Ohio Multipurpose Arthritis Center, 4883
Casey Eye Institute, 4892
Casowasco Camp, Conference and Retreat Center, 1270, 7677
Casper Vet Center, 5788
Castle Point Campus of the VA Hudson Valley Healthcare System, 5702
Catalog for Teaching Life Skills to Persons with Development Disability, 1921
Catalyst, 2178
The Catalyst, 2178
Cataracts, 8930
Catholic Charities, 6928
Catholic Charities Health & Human Services, 1302
Catholic Charities Health and Human Services, 1297
Catholic Guild for The Blind, 9083
Catholic Medical Center, 7037
Catholic Southwest, 6756
Catskill Center for Independence, 4346
Cave Spring Rehabilitation Center, 6791
Cecil R Bomhr Rehabilitation Center of Nacogdoches Memorial Hospital, 6441

Cedar Ridge Camp, 1121, 8376
Cedar Spring Health and Rehabilitation Cen ter, 7422
Cedars of Marin, 6570
Cengage Learning, 2423, 4978
Centegra Northern Illinois Medical Center, 6823
Centennial Medical Center Tri Star Health System, 7388
Center Academy At Pinellas Park, 7621
Center Academy at Pinellas Park, 1039, 7678
The Center For Courageouos Kids, 1125
Center For Courageous Kids, The, 1122
Center For Independent Living- Kauai, 4038
Center For Personal Development, 2600
Center for Accessible Living, 4165
Center for Accessible Living: Murray, 4166
Center for Accessible Technology, 1561
Center for Applied Special Technology, 1562
Center for Assistive Technology & Inclusive Education Studies, 1563
Center for Assistive Technology & Env Access, 1918
Center for Assistive Technology and Environmental Access, 815, 6792
Center for Best Practices in Early Childhood, 1675
Center for Community Alternatives, 4347
Center for Comprehensive Services, 6824
Center for Disabilities Studies, 3793
Center for Disabilities and Development, 3471
Center for Disability Resources, 816, 3174, 2159
Center for Disability Rights, 3982
Center for Disability Services, 1271
Center for Disability and Elder Law, Inc., 4557
Center for Educational Advancement New Jersey, 6105
Center for Health Research: Eastern Washin gton University, 5040
Center for Hearing and Communication, 7907, 8085
Center for Human Potential, 2601
Center for Independence, 3967
Center for Independence of the Disabled, 3908
Center for Independence of the Disabled of New York, 4348
Center for Independence of the Disabled of New York, 4349
Center for Independence of the Disabled- Daly City, 3909
Center for Independent Living, 3910
Center for Independent Living Options, 4393
Center for Independent Living SC, 3983
Center for Independent Living SW Kansas: L iberal, 4118
Center for Independent Living Southwest Kansas, 4119
Center for Independent Living Southwest Ka nsas: Dodge City, 4120
Center for Independent Living in Central Florida, 4003
Center for Independent Living of Mid-Michigan, 4220
Center for Independent Living of Broward, 4004
Center for Independent Living of Central Nebraska, 4299
Center for Independent Living of Florida Keys, 4005
Center for Independent Living of Middle Tennessee, 4460
Center for Independent Living of N Florida, 4006
Center for Independent Living of NE Minnesota, 4246
Center for Independent Living of NW Florid a, 4007
Center for Independent Living of North Central Florida, 4008
Center for Independent Living of North Cen tral Florida, 4009
Center for Independent Living of S Florida, 4010
Center for Independent Living of SW Florida, 4011
Center for Independent Living of Western Wisconsin, 4538
Center for Independent Living: East Oakland, 3911

Center for Independent Living: Kentucky Department for the Blind, 4167
Center for Independent Living: Long Branch, 4314
Center for Independent Living: Oakland, 3912
Center for Independent Living: South Jersey, 4315
Center for Independent Living: Tri-County, 3913
Center for Independent Living:Fresno, 3914
Center for Independent Living:Oakland, 3915
Center for Interdisciplinary Research on Immunologic Diseases, 4804
Center for Learning, 6309
Center for Libraries and Educational Improvement, 5041
Center for Living & Working: Fitchburg, 4199
Center for Living & Working: Framingham, 4200
Center for Living & Working: Worcester, 4201
Center for Mental Health Services, 2132
Center for Mind/Body Studies, 817
Center for Neuro Skills, 6571, 7163
Center for Neuro-Rehabilitation, 6950
Center for Neuropsychology, Learning & Dev elopment, 2602
Center for Pain Control and Rehabilitation, 6729
Center for Parent Information and Resource s, 2667
Center for People with Disabilities, 3968
Center for People with Disabilities: Pueblo, 3969
Center for People with Disabilities: Bould er, 3970
Center for Psychiatric Rehabilitation, 6967
Center for Public Representation, 3520, 4634
Center for Rehabilitation Technology, 549
Center for Rehabilitation at Rush Presbyterian: Johnston R Bowman Health Center, 6825
Center for Research on Women with Disabilities, 4909
Center for Spinal Cord Injury Recovery, 2668
Center for Spine, Sports & Occupational Rehabilitation, 6826
Center for Student Health and Counseling, 2603
Center for Universal Design, 818
Center for Vision Rehabilitation, 7075
Center for the Improvement of Human Functioning, 4763
Center for the Partially Sighted, 6572
Center for the Visually Impaired, 6793
Center of Independent Living: Visalia, 3916
Center on Deafness, 4058
Center on Evaluation of Assistive Technology, 1564
Center on Human Policy: School of Educatio n, 4858
Center on the Social & Emotional Foundations for Early Learning (CSEFEL), 5402
Centering Corporation, 5083, 5215
Centering Corporation Grief Resources, 5042
Centers for Disease Control and Prevention, 5043, 4727, 8653, 8660
Centers for Medicare & Medicaid Services, 2133
Centers for The Developmentally Disabled North Central Alabama, 6492
Central Alabama Veterans Healthcare System, 5564
Central Arkansas Rehab Hospital, 6232
Central Association for the Blind & Visual ly Impaired, 8819
Central Coast Center for IL: San Benito, 3917
Central Coast Center for Independent Living, 3918
Central Coast Center: Independent Living - Santa Cruz Office, 3919
Central Coast Neurobehavioral Center OPTIONS, 6573
Central Coast for Independent Living, 3920
Central Coast for Independent Living: Watsonville, 3921
Central Connecticut Association For Retarded Citizens, 5897
Central Iowa Center for Independent Living, 4110, 5060
Central Island Healthcare, 7341
Central Kansas Library Systems Headquarter s (CSLS), 4764
Central Library Downtown, 4945
Central Louisiana State Hospital Medical and Professional Library, 4776
Central Missouri Diabetic Childrens Camp, 1211, 8341

Central Rappahannock Regional Library, 4922

Central Utah Independent Living Center, 4491

Centre, The, 4471

Century 50/60XR Sit, 256

Century College, 4829

Cerebral Palsy Association of Middlesex County, 6106

Cerebral Palsy Associations of New York St ate, 7622

Cerebral Palsy of Colorado, 6678

Cerebral Palsy: North County Center, 6574

Ceres Press, 1901

Cervical Support Pillow, 186

Chadder, 7832

Chaddick Institute for Metropolitan Development, 2870

Chalet Village Health and Rehabilitation C enter, 7285

Challenge Aspen, 1013

Challenge Golf, 9136

Challenge Magazine, 2179

Challenge Publications Limited, 8190

Challenge of Educating Together Deaf and Hearing Youth: Making Manistreaming Work, 2327

Challenged Scientists: Disabilities and the Triumph of Excellence, 2328

Chamberlain Group, 2875

Champ Camp, 1014, 8377

Champion 1000, 697

Champion 2000, 698

Champion 3000, 699

Champlin Foundations, 3164

Change, 819

Change Your Brain, Change Your Life: The Breakthrough Program for Conquering Depression, 7740

Chapel Haven, 3984

Chapel Hill Rehabilitation and Healthcare Center, 7354

Characteristics, Services, & Outcomes of Rehab. Consumers who are Blind/Visually Impaired, 8931

Charcot-Marie-Tooth Association, 7876

Charles C Thomas Publisher LTD, 2085

Charles C. Thomas, 10, 24, 37, 2283, 2288, 2299, 2312, 2327, 2337, 2353, 2385, 2387, 2393, 2417, 2419, 2424, 2525, 2551, 2557, 2582, 5171, 5216, 5231, 5283, 5289, 5481, 7988, 8003, 8935, 9036

Charles Campbell Childrens Camp, 1224

Charlotte Vet Center, 5712

Charlotte White Center, 6944

Chase Bank of Texas, 3192

Chatlos Foundation, 2838

Cheaha Regional Mental Health Center, 6493

Checker Set: Deluxe, 5469

Cheever Publishing, 5003

Cheley/Children's Hospital Burn Camps Program, 1015

Chelsea Community Hospital Rehabilitation Unit, 6993

Chelsea: The Story of a Signal Dog, 7996

Cherab Foundation, 8789

Cherry Hills Health Care Center, 6679

Chesapeake Region Accessible Boating, 8225

Chess Set: Deluxe, 5470

Chestnut Hill Rehabilitation Hospital, 6412

Chevy Chase Nursing and Rehabilitation Cen ter, 7273

Chevy Lowered Floor, 78

Cheyenne VA Medical Center, 5789

Cheyenne Village, 5879

Chi Medical Library, 4812

Chicago Community Trust, 2871

Chicago Community Trust and Affiliates, 2872

Chicago Lawyers' Committee for Civil Rights Under Law, 4558

Chicago Lighthouse, 9089

Chicago Lighthouse for People who are Blind and Visually Impaired, 8820

Chicago Public Library Talking Book Center, 4737

Chicago Public Library Talking Books Center, 9110

Chicago Review Press, 5262

Child Care and the ADA: A Handbook for Inclusive Programs, 2329

Child Convertible Balance Beam Set, 509

Child Development Media, 7848

Child Find/Early Childhood Disabilities Unit Montgomery County Public Schools, 6951

Child Neurology Society, 7623

Child Variable Balance Beam, 510

Child With Special Needs: Encouraging Inte llectual and Emotional Growth, 5044

Child and Adolescent Therapy: Cognitive-Be havioral Procedures, Third Edition, 7741

Child and Parent Resource Institute, 820

Child with Disabling Illness, 2330

Child's Mobility Crawler, 511

Childcare Services Division, 3316

Childcare and the ADA, 4585

Childhood Apraxia of Speech Association, 8679

Childhood Behavior Disorders: Applied Research & Educational Practice, 2331

Childhood Cancer Canada Foundation, 8264

Childhood Cancer Guides/O'Reilly Media, 5254

Childhood Cancer Survivors: A Practical Guide to Your Future, 8453

Childhood Cancer: A Parent's Guide to Solid Tumor Cancers, 8454

Childhood Disablty and Family Systems (Routledge Library Editions) (Volume 5), 2332

Childhood Diseases and Disorders Sourceboo k, 2nd Edition, 8455

Childhood Glaucoma: A Reference Guide for Families, 8932

Childhood Leukemia Foundation, 8265

Childhood Leukemia: A Guide for Families, Friends & Caregivers, 8456

Childhood Speech, Language & Listening Pro blems, 8730

Children & Adults with ADHD, 7828

Children & Adults with Attention Deficit Disorder, 7832

Children and Youth Assisted by Medical Technology in Educational Settings, 2nd Edition, 2333

Children of Aging Parents, 7455, 7538

Children of a Lesser God, 7997

Children s Hospital Boston, 3522

Children s Medical Program, 3565

Children with Cerebral Palsy: A Parents' G uide, 8457

Children with Disabilities, 5199

Children with Mental Retardation, 7742

Children with Special Health Care Needs, 3847

Children with Visual Impairments: A Guide For Parents, 8933

Children's Aid Society, 1283

Children's Alliance, 821

Children's Assessment Center, The, 2604

Children's Association for Maximum Potenti al Summer Camp, 1394

Children's Beach House, 1032, 7977

Children's Burn Camp Of North Florida, Inc., 1035

Children's Center for Neurodevelopmental Studies, 4656

Children's Fresh Air Society Fund, 2925

Children's Healthcare of Atlanta at Egleston, 6302

Children's Hemiplegia & Stroke Association, 8130

Children's Home and Aid Society of Illinois, 6827

Children's Hopes & Dreams Wish Fulfillment Foundation, 3008

The Children's Hospital, 1015

Children's Hospital Central California Reh abilitation Center, 6575

Children's Hospital Los Angeles Rehabilitation Program, 6576

Children's Hospital Rehabilitation Center, 6272

Children's Medical Services, 3348

Children's Mental Health and EBD E-news, 2231

Children's National Medical Center, 822

Children's Needs Psychological Perspective, 2334

Children's Press, 5061

Children's Rehabilitation Service - District Office, Montgomery, 6494

Children's Special Health Services Program, 3750

Children's Specialized Hospital, 6375

Children's Specialized Hospital Medical Library - Parent Resource Center, 4850

Children's Therapy Center, 6577

Children's Tumor Foundation, 3034

Children's Understanding of Disability, 4953

Childrens Beach House, 1031, 8709

Childrens Hospital Medical Center, 4804

Chiles Foundation, 3134

Chillicothe VA Medical Center, 5719

Chilton-Shelby Mental Health Center, 6495

Chinese Herbal Medicine, 5045

Choice Magazine Listening, 9121

Choice Switch Latch and Timer, 512

Choices in Deafness: A Parent's Guide to C ommunication Options, 7998

Choices to Work Program, 5922

Choices, Choices 5.0, 1774

Choices: A Guide to Sex Counseling with Physically Disabled Adults, 2335

Choosing Options and Accommodations for Children, 2336

Choosing Outcomes and Accommodations for Children (COACH) (2nd Edition), 5257

Choosing a Wheelchair: A Guide for Optimal Independence, 700

Christ Hospital Rehabilitation Unit, 7089

A Christian Approach to Overcoming Disability: A Doctor's Story, 8901

Christian Approach to Overcoming Disabilit y: A Doctor's Story, 5046

Christian Berets, Inc., 967

Christian Education for the Blind, 4910

Christian Hospital Northeast, 7019

Christian Record Services, 1230, 8895, 8896

Christmas Stories, 8100

Christopher & Dana Reeve Foundation Resour ce Center, 4851

Christopher & Dana Reeve Paralysis Resourc e Center, 8131

Christopher and Dana Reeve Paralysis Resource Ctr, 8181

Chronic Fatigue Syndrome: Your Natural Gu ide to Healing with Diet, Herbs and Other Methods, 8458

Chronically Disabled Elderly in Society, 7502

Chronicle Guide to Grants, 3260

Church of the Nazarene, 4838

Cincinnati Children's Hospital Medical Center, 4884

Cincinnati VA Medical Center, 5720

Circline Illuminated Magnifier, 629

Cirriculum Development for Students with Mild Disabilities, 2337

City of Lakewood, 1010

Civil Rights Division/Disability Rights Se ction, 3291

Civitan Acres for the Disabled, 1421

Civitan Foundation, 953

Clara Barton Diabetes Camp, 1175, 8378

Clara Barton for Girls with Diabetes, 1175, 8378

Clare Branch, 6994

Clark House Nursing Center At Foxhill Village, 6968

Clark Memorial Hospital: RehabCare Unit, 6317

Clark-Winchcole Foundation, 2926

Clarke Health Care Products, 164

Clarke Healthcare Products, Inc., 164

Clarkston Spec Healthcare Center, 6995

Classic, 79

Classification of Impaired Vision, 8934

Classique, 385

Classroom GOAL: Guide for Optimizing Auditory Learning Skills, 1922

Classroom Notetaker: How to Organize a Program Serving Students with Hearing Impairments, 1923

Classroom Success for the LD and ADHD Child, 2338

Clausen House, 6578

Clay Center Adult Training Center, 6022

Clay Tree Society, 823

Clearbrook, 5968

Clearinghouse for Specialized Media and Translations, 4672

Clearinghouse on Disability Information: Office Special Education & Rehabilitative Service, 8649

Clearview-Brain Injury Center, 7423

Cleft Palate Foundation, 8600

Cleft Palate-Craniofacial Journal, 8600

Clement J Zablocki VA Medical Center, 5784

Cleveland Clinic, 7370

Cleveland FES Center, 4885

Cleveland Foundation, 3108

Cleveland Public Library, 4886

Cleveland Regional Office, 5721

Cleveland Sight Center, 1310, 7090

Cleveland Society for the Blind, 7090

Client Assistance Program (CAP), 3449

Client Assistance Program: Alabama, 3317

Client Assistance Program: Alaska, 3325

Client Assistance Program: California, 3357

Clinch Independent Living Services, 4509

Clinical Alzheimer Rehabilitation, 2339

Clinical Applications of Music Therapy in Developmental Disability, Pediatrics and Neurolog, 15

Clinical Connection, 2180

Clinical Management of Childhood Stuttering, 2nd Edition, 2340

Clinician's Practical Guide to Attention-Deficit/Hyperactivity Disorder, 5276

Clinton County Rehabilitation Center, 6828

Clip Board Notebook, 617

Clipper Ship Foundation, 2945

Clock, 1676

Clockworks, 5320

Close Encounters of the Disabling Kind, 5321

Close-Up 6.5, 1512

Closing the Gap, 5047

Closing the Gap's Annual Conference, 1854

Clove Lakes Health Care and Rehabilitation Center, 7342

Clover Patch Camp, 1271

Clovernook Center for the Blind and Visually Impaired, 8821

Clovernook Printing House, The Clovernook Center for the Blind and Visually Impaired, 8822

Co: Writer, 1775

Coalition for Independence, 4121

Coalition for Independence: Missouri Branch Office, 4273

Coalition for Independent Living Options: Fort Pierce, 4013

Coalition for Independent Living Options, 4014

Coalition for Independent Living Options: Stuart, 4015

Coalition for Independent Living Options: Okeechobee, 4012

Coalition for the Education of Disabled Children, 5076

Coalition of Responsible Disabled, 4528

Coast to Coast Home Medical, 311

Coatesville VA Medical Center, 5734

Cobb Hospital and Medical Center: Rehab Care Center, 6303

Cochlear Implants In Children: Ethics and Choices, 8093

Cochlear Implants for Kids, 7999

Cockrell Foundation, 3196

Coeta and Donald Barker Foundation, 2751

Coffee County Training Center, 5795

Coffee in the Cereal: The First Year with Multiple Sclerosis, 8459

Cognition, Education and Deafness: Directions for Research and Instruction, 8000

Cognitive Approaches to Learning Disabilities, 2341

Cognitive Behavioral Therapy for Adult Asperger Syndrome, 7743, 8731

Cognitive Neuroscience Society, 7624

Cognitive Science Society, 7625

Cognitive Science Student Association, 7626

Cognitive Solutions Learning Center, 2605

Cognitive Strategy Instruction That Really Improves Children's Academic Skills, 2342

Cognitive Therapy Today, 7841

Cogrehab, 7847

Coleman Tri- County Services, 4059

Collaborating for Comprehensive Services for Young Children and Families, 2343

Collaborative Teams for Students with Severe Disabilities, 2344

The College At Brockport, State Univ Of New York, 1257

College Board, 2049

College Internship Program at the Berkshire Center, 6969

College Student's Guide to Merit and Other No-Need Funding, 3261

College and University, 2181

College and University Programs for Deaf and Hard of Hearing Students, 8001

College of Optometrists in Vision Development, 8823

College of Syntonic Optometry, 8824

Colleton Regional Hospital: RehabCare Unit, 6427

Colmery-O'Neil VA Medical Center, 5632

Colon & Rectal Cancer: A Comprehensive Guide for Patients & Families, 8460

Colon Health: Key to a Vibrant Life, 8461

Colonial Life and Accident Insurance Company Contributions Program, 3175

Colonial Manor Medical And Rehabilitation Center, 7216

Colonial Manor Medical and Rehabilitation Center, 7424

Colorado Assoc of Homes and Services for the Aging, 7535, 7537

Colorado Association of Homes and Services for the Aging, 7456

Colorado Civil Rights Divsion, 5880

Colorado Department of Aging & Adult Services, 3366

Colorado Department of Education, 2113

Colorado Department of Education: Special Education Service Unit, 2113

Colorado Developmental Disabilities Council, 3367

Colorado Division of Mental Health, 3368

Colorado Employment Service, 5881

Colorado Health Care Program for Children with Special Needs, 3369

Colorado Lions Camp, 1016

Colorado Neurological Institute, 1009

Colorado Springs Independence Center, 3971

Colorado Talking Book Library, 4685

Colorado/Wyoming VA Medical Center, 5589

Colton-Redlands-Yucaipa Regional Occupational Programs, 5841

Columbia Disability Action Center, 4446

Columbia Foundation, 2927

Columbia Gas of Pennsylvania Corporate Giving, 3141

Columbia Lighthouse for the Blind, 8825, 1033, 8888, 9086

Columbia Lighthouse for the Blind Summer Camp, 1033, 8888

Columbia Medical Center: Peninsula, 6744

Columbia Medical Manufacturing, 160

Columbia Regional Hospital: RehabCare Unit, 6363

Columbia Regional Office, 5747

Columbus Foundation and Affiliated Organizations, 3109

Columbus Health and Rehabilitation Center, 7286

Columbus McKinnon Corporation, 386

Columbus Rehab & Subacute, 6391

Columbus Rehabilitation And Subacute Institute, 7371

Columbus Speech and Hearing Center, 7091

Columbus Subregional Library For The Blind And Physically Handicapped, 4721

Combination File/Reference Carousel, 549

Come Sign with Us, 8002

Committee for Purchase from People Who Are Blind or Severely Disabled, 3292

Commode, 165

Common ADA Errors and Omissions in New Construction and Alterations, 4586

Commonly Asked Questions About Child Care Centers and the Americans with Disabilities Act, 4587

Commonly Asked Questions About Title III of the ADA, 4588

Commonly Asked Questions About the ADA and Law Enforcement, 4589

Commonwealth Fund, 3035

Communi Care Health Services, 7092

CommuniCare of Clifton Nursing and Rehabilitation Center, 7092

Communicating with Parents of Exceptional Children, 2345

Communicating with People Who Have Trouble Hearing & Seeing: A Primer, 7581

Communication & Language Acquisition: Discoveries from Atypical Development, 2346

Communication Aids for Children and Adults, 458

Communication Center/Minnesota State Services for the Blind, 4830

Communication Development and Disorders in African American Children, 8732

Communication Development in Children with Down Syndrome, 7744, 8733

Communication Disorders Quarterly, 2182

Communication Help, Education, Research, A praxia Base (CHERAB), 8680

Communication Outlook, 8769

Communication Service for the Deaf, 7908

Communication Service for the Deaf: Rapid City, 4453

Communication Skills for Visually Impaired Learners, 8935

Communication Skills for Working with Elders, 2347

Communication Unbound, 2348

Communication in Autism, 8681

Communicologist, 8772

Communique, 7539, 8094

CommuniquŠ, 8081

Communities Actively Living Independent and Free, 3922

Communities Foundation of Texas, 3197

Community Access Center, 3923

Community Access Center: Indio Branch, 3924

Community Access Center: Perris, 3925

Community Connection, 9075

Community Connections of Southwest Michigan, 4221

Community Disability Services: An Evidence -Based Approach to Practice, 4975

Community Enterprises, 824, 5898

Community Exploration, 1776

Community Foundation for Greater Buffalo, 3036

Community Foundation for Greater Atlanta, 2848

Community Foundation of Boone County, 2904

Community Foundation of Champaign County, 2873

Community Foundation of Greater Chattanooga, 3184

Community Foundation of Herkimer & Oneida Counties, 3037

Community Foundation of Monroe County, 2959

Community Foundation of New Jersey, 3009

Community Foundation of North Central Washington, 3235

Community Foundation of North Texas, 3198

Community Foundation of Richmond & Central Virginia, 3228

Community Foundation of Shreveport-Bossier, 2917

Community Foundation of Southeastern Connecticut, 2807

Community Foundation of Western Massachusetts, 2946

Community Foundation of the Capitol Region, 3038

Community Gatepath, 6579

Community Health Funding Report, 3262

Community Health Network, 6880

Community Hospital Back and Conditioning Clinic, 6680

Community Hospital and Rehabilitation Center of Los Gatos-Saratoga, 6580

Community Hospital of Los Gatos Rehabilitation Services, 6244
Community Opportunities of East Ascension, 6032
Community Outpatient Rehabilitation Center, 5842
Community Outreach Program for the Deaf, 3889
Community Rehabilitation Services, 3926
Community Residential Alternative, 4059
Community Residential Care Association of CA, 4974
Community Resource Directory, 2056
Community Resources for Independence, 4417
Community Resources for Independence, Inc., Bradford, 4418
Community Resources for Independence: Lewistown, 4419
Community Resources for Independence: Mendocino/Lake Branch, 3927
Community Resources for Independence: Alto ona, 4420
Community Resources for Independence: Clar ion, 4421
Community Resources for Independence: Clea rfield, 4422
Community Resources for Independence: Herm itage, 4423
Community Resources for Independence: Lewi sburg, 4424
Community Resources for Independence: Napa, 3928
Community Resources for Independence: Oil City, 4425
Community Resources for Independence: Warr en, 4426
Community Resources for Independence: Well sboro, 4427
Community Resources for Independent Living: Hayward, 3929
Community Resources for Independent Living, 3930
Community Services for the Blind and Partially Sighted Store: Sight Connection, 1924
Community Services for the Blind and Parti ally Sighted Store: Sight Connection, 4529
Community Signs, 1925
Community Skills: Learning to Function in Your Neighborhood, 1677
Community Supports for People with Disabilities (CSP), 2139
Community Systems Inc., 6710
Commuter & Kid's Commuter, 732
Compact Folding Travel Rollator, 644
Companion Activities, 1678
Compass Learning, 1661, 1676, 1712, 1736, 1748, 1749, 1750, 1754, 1776, 1782, 1806, 1807, 1808
Compassionate Friends, The, 8650
Complementary Alternative Medicine and Mul tiple Sclerosis, 8462
Complete Armchair Fitness, 8214
Complete Directory for Pediatric Disorders, 2057
Complete Directory for People with Chronic Illness, 2058
The Complete Guide to Creating a Special Needs Life Plan, 5238
Complete Handbook of Children's Reading Disorders: You Can Prevent or Correct LDs, 2349
Complete IEP Guide: How to Advocate for Yo ur Special Ed Child (8th Edition), 4954, 5258
Complete Learning Disabilities Directory, 2059
Complete Mental Health Directory, 2060
Complying with the Americans with Disabili s Act, 4590
Comprecare Foundation, 2801
Comprehensive Assessment of Spoken Language (CASL), 1926
Comprehensive Care Coordination for Chroni cally Ill Adults, 4976
Comprehensive Examination of Barriers to Employment Among Persons who are Blind or Impaire, 8936
Comprehensive Guide to ADD in Adults: Research, Diagnosis & Treatment, 7745
Comprehensive Pain Management Associates, 7071

Comprehensive Reference Manual for Signers and Interpreters, 8003
Comprehensive Rehabilitation Center at Lee Memorial Hospital, 6730
Comprehensive Rehabilitation Center of Naples Community Hospital, 6731
Comprehensive Signed English Dictionary, 8004
Compuserve: Handicapped Users' Database, 1565
Computer & Web Resources for People With Disabilities, 1566
Computer Access Center, 1567
Computer Access/Computer Learning, 2350
Computer Center for Visually Impaired People: Division of Continuing Studies, 1568
Computer Paper for Brailling, 1545
Computer Resources for People with Disabilities, 1569
Computer-Enabling Drafting for People with Physical Disabilities, 1570
Computerized Speech Lab, 1630
Comsearch: Broad Topics, 3039
Concentration Cockpit: Explaining Attention Deficits, 7746
Concentration Video, 7858
Concepts on the Move Advanced Overlay CD, 1513
Concepts on the Move Advanced Preacademics, 1679
Concepts on the Move Basic Overlay CD, 1514
Concern Foundation, 5399
Concerned Care, Inc., 1217
Conditional Love: Parents' Attitudes Toward Handicapped Children, 5200
Conference Department, 1866
Conference of Educational Administrators of Schools and Programs for the Deaf, 7909
Confidence Learning Center, 1205, 1205
Conklin Center for the Blind, 6732
Connect, 8773
Connect - Commmunity News, 8082
Connecticut Association of Not-for-Profit Providers for the Aging, 7457
Connecticut Board of Education and Service for the Blind, 3374
Connecticut Braille Association, 4687
Connecticut Burns Care Foundation, 1021
Connecticut Commission on Aging, 3375
Connecticut Department of Children and Youth Services, 3376
Connecticut Department of Education: Bureau of Special Education, 2114
Connecticut Developmental Disabilities Council, 3377
Connecticut Governor's Committee on Employment of People With Disabilities, 5899
Connecticut Library for the Blind and Phys ically Handicapped, 4688
Connecticut Mutual Life Foundation, 2808
Connecticut Office of Protection and Advocacy for Persons with Disabilities, 3378
Connecticut State Government, 4689
Connecticut State Library, 4689
Connecticut Subacute Corporation, 6698
Connecticut Tech Act Project: Connecticut Department of Social Services, 4690
Connections for Independent Living, 3972
Connelly Foundation, 3142
Conover Company, 1812, 1814
Conquering the Darkness: One Story of Recovering from a Brain Injury, 8463
Conrad N Hilton Foundation, 2999
Consortium of Multiple Sclerosis Centers, 8132
Constellations, 5048
Consulting & Engineering for the Handicapp ed (CEH), 5543
Consulting Psychologists Press, 2351
Consumer Buyer's Guide for Independent Living, 5049
Consumer Care Products, 278, 658, 664
Consumer Information Center, 5487
Consumer and Patient Information Hotline, 9140
Consumer's Guide to Home Adaptation, 1891
Contact Technologies, 71, 126
Contemporary Art Therapy with Adolescents, 16

Continucare, A Service of the Rehab Institute of Chicago, 6829
Continuing Care, 2183
Contra Costa ARC, 6581
Contrasting Characteristics of Blind and Visually Impaired Clients, 8937
Convaid, 701, 733
Convaid Products, 267, 575
Conversational Sign Language II: An Interm ediate Advanced Manual, 8005
Conversations, 1777
Convert-Able Table, 257
Convert-O-Bike, 5458
Cooking Class: Learning About Food Preparation, 1680
Cool Handle, 349
Cooper Foundation, 2995
Coordinacion De Servicios Centrado En La Familia, 5201
Coping and Caring: Living with Alzheimer's Disease, 7503
Coping for Kids Who Stutter, 8734
Coping with ADD/ADHD, 7747
Coping with Cancer Magazine, 8602
Coping with Cerebral Palsy, 8464
Coping+Plus: Dimensions of Disability, 5050
Cora Hoffman Center Day Program, 7059
Corcoran Physical Therapy, 6814
Cordless Big Red Switch, 513
Cordless Receiver, 350
Cordova Rehabilitation and Nursing Center, 7389
Core-Reading and Vocabulary Development, 1778
Corflex, 282
Cornelia de Lange Syndrome Foundation, 2809
Cornell Communications, 208
Cornerstone Services, 5969, 8651
Cornucopia, 6153
Cornucopia Software, 1810
Corona Regional Medical Center- Rehabiltation Center, 6582
Corporate Giving Program, 2928
Corporate Office, 6390, 6735
Corwin Press Inc., 2566
Cottage Health System, 6605
Cottage Rehabilitation Hospital, 2669
Cotton Full-Back Vest, 1486
Cotton/Poly House Dress, 1448
Council For Exceptional Children, 825, 928
Council News, 5051
Council On International Educational Exchange, 5497
Council for Disability Rights, 5037
Council for Exceptional Children, 2025, 4923, 2024, 2088, 2175, 2191, 2227, 2316, 2621, 8266
Council for Exceptional Children (CEC), 2026
Council for Exceptional Children Annual Convention and Expo, 1855
Council for Extended Care, 1220, 7705
Council for Extended Care of Mentally Retarded Citizens, 7679
Council of American Instructors of the Dea f (CAID), 7910
Council of B BB s Foundation, 1887
Council of Families with Visual Impairments, 8826
Council on Quality and Leadership, 1853
Counseling Parents of Children with Chronic Illness or Disability, 5277
Counseling Persons with Communication Disorders and Their Families, 2352
Counseling Psychologist, 2184
Counseling Today, 2232
Counseling and Values, 2185
Counseling in Terminal Care & Bereavement, 5052
Counseling in the Rehabilitation Process, 2353
Counselor Education and Supervision, 2233
Count Us In, 7748
Country Gardens Skilled Nursing and Rehabilitation Center, 7315
Country Manor Rehabilitation and Nursing C enter, 7316
County College of Morris, 1570
County of Santa Clara, 6263
Courage Center, 4247, 1201, 1206, 8330

Courage Center Camps, 1206
Courage Kenny Rehabilitation Institute, 2670
Court-Related Needs of the Elderly and Persons with Disabilities, 4591
Covenant Health, 6435
Covenant Health Systems Owens White Outpatient Rehab Center, 6442
Covenant Healthcare Rehabilitation Program, 6357
Cowan Slavin Foundation, 2960
Cowley County Developmental Services, 4122
Craig Hospital, 6273
Crane Plumbing/Fiat Products, 155
CranstonArc, 3165
CreateSpace, an Amazon Company, 5265
Creating Options for Family Recovery: A Pr ovider's Guide to Promoting Parental Mental Health, 5278
Creating Positive Classroom Environments: Strategies for Behavior Management, 2354
Creating Wholeness: Self-Healing Workbook Using Dynamic Relaxation, Images and Thoughts, 5053
Creative Arts Resources Catalog, 17
Creative Arts Therapy Catalogs, 1927
Creative Designs, 1479
Creative Growth Art Center, 18
Creative Work Systems, 6039
Creativity Explored, 19
Crescent Porter Hale Foundation, 2752
Crestwood Communication Aids, 458
Crestwood Nursing & Rehabilitation Center, 7334
Criminal Law Handbook on Psychiatric & Psychological Evidence & Testimony, 4592
Cristo Rey Handicappers Program, 4222
Critical Air Medicine, 6583
Critical Voices on Special Education: Prob lems & Progress Concerning the Mildly Handicapped, 2355
Crockett Resource Center for Independent Living, 4472
Crosslands Rehabilitation and Healthcare Center, 7401
Crossroads Industrial Services, 6881
Crossroads of Western Iowa, 6888
Crotched Mountain Adult Brain Injury Center, 7032
Crotched Mountain Foundation, 7032
Crown Publishing Company (Random House), 7770
Cruiser Bus Buggy 4MB, 575
Crutcher's Serenity House, 6584
Crutches, 645
Cub, SuperCub and Special Edition Scooters, 576
Cullen Foundation, 3199
Cultural Diversity, Families and the Special Education System, 2356
'Cultural Life,' Disability, Inclusion, and Citizenship: Moving Beyond Leisure in Isolation, 4972
Culture, 5101
Culture and the Restructuring of Community Mental Health, 7749
Cunard Line, 5520
Curb-Sider, 387
Curb-Sider Super XL, 388
Cure SMA, 8133
CurePSP Magazine, 8203, 8603
Curing MS: How Science is Solving the Myst eries of Multiple Sclerosis, 8465
Curriculum Decision Making for Students with Severe Handicaps, 2357
Cursive Writing Skills, 1928
Curtis & Doris K Hankamer Foundation, 3200
Curtis Instruments, Inc., 684
Custom, 702
Custom Durable, 703
Custom Earmolds, 332
Custom Lift Residential Elevators, 389
Cypress Pointe Rehabilitation and Healthca re Center, 7355
Cystic Fibrosis Foundation, 2929
Cystic Fibrosis: Medical Care, 5279
Cystic Fibrosis: A Guide for Patient and F amily, 8466

D

D AR S, 3784
D C General Hospital, 3390
D C Office of Human Rights, 5913
DA Schulman, 673
DAMAR Services, 4097
DARCI, 1820
DAV Department of Alaska, 5567
DAV National Service Headquarters, 5553
DAWN Center for Independent Living, 4316
DAYS: Depression and Anxiety in Youth Scale, 2606
DB-Link, 826
DBTAC-Great Lakes ADA Center, 6310
DD Center/St Lukes: Roosevelt Hospital Center, 4350
DDDS/Georgetown Center, 6711
DE French Foundation, 3040
DEUCE Environmental Control Unit, 514
DHHARC, 1234
DIRECT Center for Independence, 3890
DIRLINE, 1571
DMC Health Care Center-Novi, 6996
DNA People's Legal Services, 4559
DOCS: Developmental Observation Checklist System, 2607
DPS with BCP, 1760
DRAIL (Disability Resource Agency for Independent Living), 3931
DREAMMS for Kids, 4859, 1683
DRS Connection, 5054
DRTAC: Southeast ADA Center, 4995
DSHS/Aging & Adult Disability Services Administration, 3829
DVH Quarterly, 9076
DW Auto & Home Mobility, 80
Da Capo Press, 8168, 8171
Da Capo Press/ Perseus Books Group, 4970
Dade County Talking Book Library, 4702
Daimler Chrysler, 2961
Dakota Center for Independent Living: Dickinson, 4384
Dakota Center for Independent Living: Bism arck, 4385
Dallas Academy, 1395, 7680
Dallas Foundation, 3201
Dallas Services, 7164
Damaco, 745
Damaco D90, 745
Daman Villa, 7165
Damon Runyon Cancer Research Foundation, 5403
Dana Alliance for Brain Initiatives, 3041
Dana Foundation, 3041
Dancing Cheek to Cheek, 8938
Dancing from the Inside Out, 20
Daniel Freeman Rehabilitation Centers, 6585
Daniels and Fisher Tower, 2800
Danmar Products, 459
Danville Centre for Health and Rehabilitat ion, 7298
Dapper Folding Adustable Cane, 646
Dapper Walking Stick, 647
Darci Too, 1515
Darden Rehabilitation Center, 6496
Dare Care Charity, 2230
Datahr Rehabilitation Institute, 6699
Daughters of Miriam Center/The Gallen Institute, 7042
David D & Nona S Payne Foundation, 3202
David Fulton Publishers (Routledge), 2565
David J Green Foundation, 3042
David and Lucile Packard Foundation, 2753
Davidson College, 2703
Davidson College, Office of Study Abroad, 2703
Davis Center, 209
Davis Center for Rehabilitation Baptist Hospital of Miami, 6733
Davis Center, The, 827, 7911, 8682
Dawn Enterprises, 4044
DawnSign Press, 7995, 8035, 8110
Dayle McIntosh Center: Laguna Niguel, 3932
Dayspring Associates, 460
Dayton VA Medical Center, 5722

Dazor Manufacturing Corporation, 515, 629, 638
Deaf Action Center Of Greater New Orleans, 6928
Deaf Camp, 1156
Deaf Catholic, 8083
Deaf Children Signers, 5322
Deaf Culture Series, 5323
Deaf Education Center/Gallaudet University, 893
Deaf Empowerment: Emergence, Struggle and Rhetoric, 8006
Deaf History Unveiled: Interpretations from the New Scholarship, 8007
Deaf Kid's Kamp, 994, 7968
Deaf Like Me, 8008
Deaf Mosaic, 5324
Deaf Parents and Their Hearing Children, 8009
Deaf REACH, 7912
Deaf West Theatre, 21
Deaf Women United, 7913
Deaf in America: Voices from a Culture, 8010
Deaf-Blind American, 7587
Deaf-Blind Division of the National Federa tion of the Blind, 8827
Deaf-Blind Division of the Ntn'l Fed of the Blind, 9056, 9058
Deaf-Blind Perspective, 7590, 9077
Deafness Research Foundation, 7914, 8074
Deafness and Communicative Disorders Branch of Rehab Services Administration Office, 8683
Dean A McGee Eye Institute, 7120
Deciphering the System: A Guide for Families of Young Disabled Children, 2358
DecisionHealth, 7531
Defining Rehabilitation Agency Types, 2359
Delano Regional Medical Center, 6586
Delaware Assistive Technology Initiative (DATI), 4693
Delaware Assistive Technology Initiative (DATI), 3380
Delaware Association for the Blind, 6712
Delaware Client Assistance Program, 3381
Delaware Department of Health and Social Services, 3382
Delaware Department of Labor, 5907, 5908
Delaware Department of Public Instructing, 3383
Delaware Developmental Disability Council, 3384
Delaware Division for the Visually Impaire d, 3385
Delaware Division of Vocational Rehabilita tion, 5907
Delaware Fair Employment Practice Agency, 5908
Delaware Industries for the Blind, 3386
Delaware Job Training Program Liaison, 5909
Delaware Library for the Blind and Physically Handicapped, 4694
Delaware Protection & Advocacy for Persons with Disabilities, 3387
Delaware VA Regional Office, 5596
Delaware Veterans Center, 6713
Delaware Workers Compensation Board, 3388
Dell Rapids Sportsmens Club, 5521
Delmar Cengage Learning, 8510
Delta Center, 6830
Delta Center for Independent Living, 4274
Delta Resource Center for Independent Living, 3895
Delta Society National Service Dog Center, 531
Deluxe Bath Bench with Adjustable Legs, 166
Deluxe Convertible Exercise Staircase, 390
Deluxe Corporation, 2974
Deluxe Corporation Foundation, 2974
Deluxe Long Ring Low Vision Timer, 351
Deluxe Nova Wheeled Walker & Avant Wheeled Walker, 648
Deluxe Roller Knife, 352
Deluxe Signature Guide, 618
Deluxe Sock and Stocking Aid, 299
Deluxe Standard Wood Cane, 649
Demand Response Transportation Through a Rural ILC, 5055
Dementia Society of America, 7627
Demos Health Publishing, 5026
Demos Medical Publishing, 5102, 7889, 8437, 8462, 8473, 8474, 8478, 8496, 8523, 8524, 8525, 8526, 8528

Demystifying Job Development: Field-Based Approaches to Job Development for the Disabled, 5296
Den-Mar Rehabilitation and Nursing Center, 7307
Dennis Developmental Center, 2608
Dental Amalgam Syndrome (DAMS) Newsletter, 4673
Denver CIL, 3973
Denver Foundation, 2802
Denver VA Medical Center, 5590
Department Human Services, 3621
Department Of Health and Human Services, 3345
Department Of Health& Social Services Division Of Behaviorial Health, 3326
Department Of Human Services, 6062
Department Of Ophthalmalogy, 4715
Department Of Rehabilitative Services, 6205
Department Of Workforce Development, 6055
Department of Heath Education, 3646
Department of Aging and Independent Living, 4500
Department of Blind Rehabilitation, 3528
Department of Education, 2116, 3592, 3605, 4832, 6094
Department of Employment Security, 5972
Department of Health, 3432
Department of Health & Rehabilitative Services, 3403
Department of Health and Human Services, 3590, 3606, 6142
Department of Housing & Urban Development (HUD), 5098
Department of Human Rights, 3470
Department of Human Services, 3343, 4060, 4063, 6116, 6186
Department of Justice ADA Mediation Program, 4593
Department of Labor, 3701, 3820, 6084, 6117
Department of Labor & Workforce Development, 3331, 5819
Department of Labor and Employment, 5881
Department of Labor and Industrial Realtions, 3572
Department of Medicine and Surgery Veterans Administration, 5554
Department of Mental Health, Retardation and Hospitals of Rhode Island, 3729
Department of Ophthalmology Information Line, 9141
Department of Ophthalmology and Visual Science, 4738
Department of Pennsylvania, 3720
Department of Physical Medicine & Rehabilitation at Sinai Hospital, 828
Department of Physical Medicine and Rehabilitation, 7033
Department of Physical Medicine and Rehabilitation, 6725
Department of Public Health Human Services, 2143
Department of Public Instruction: Exceptional Children & Special Programs Division, 2116
Department of Rehabilitation Services & Bureau of Education And Services for the Blind, 2115
Department of Services for the Blind, 6214
Department of Services for the Blind National Business & Disability Council, 6214
Department of Social Services, 3500, 5906
Department of Social and Health, 6218
Department of Social and Health Services, 3835
Department of Veteran s Affairs, 5581
Department of Veterans Affairs, 5639, 5758
Department of Veterans Affairs Vet Center #418, 6882
Department of Veterans Affairs Regional Office - Vocational Rehab Division, 5555
Department of Veterans Affairs of Washington DC, 6539
Department of Veterans Benefits, 5556
Dept of Labor & Workforce Development, 3768
Des Moines Division-VA Central Iowa Health Care System, 6889
Des Moines VA Medical Center, 5627
Des Moines VA Regional Office, 5628
Desert Area Resources and Training, 6591

Desert Blind and Handicapped Association, 8828
Desert Haven Enterprises, 5843
Desert Life Rehabilitation & Care Center, 6517, 7221
Desert Regional Medical Center, 6587
Design for Accessibility, 1892
Designing and Using Assistive Technology: The Human Perspective, 2360
Designs for Comfort, 1467
Detroit Center for Independent Living, 4223
Deutsch Foundation, 2754
Developing Cross-Cultural Competence:Guide to Working with Young Children & Their Families, 2361
Developing Individualized Family Support Plans: A Training Manual, 2362
Developing Organized Coalitions and Strategic Plans, 5056
Developing Personal Safety Skills in Children with Disabilities, 5202
Developing Staff Competencies for Supporting People with Disabilities, 2363
Development of Language, 2364
Development of Social Skills by Blind and Visually Impaired Students, 8939
Developmental Disabilities Council, 1572
Developmental Disabilities Planning Council, 6318
Developmental Disabilities in Infancy and Childhood, 5203
Developmental Disabilities of Learning, 2365
Developmental Disabilities: A Handbook for Occupational Therapists, 2366
Developmental Disabilities: A Handbook for Interdisciplinary Practice, 2367
Developmental Disability Council: Arizona, 3336
Developmental Disability Services Section, 3670
Developmental Evaluation and Adjustment Fa cilities, 4202
Developmental Services Center, 2609
Developmental Services of Northwest Kansas, 6907
Developmental Training Services, 5882
Developmental Variation and Learning Disorders, 2368
Devereax Foundation, 7175
Devereux Advanced Behavioral Health - Florida, 6735
Devereux Advanced Behavioral Health - National Office, 7137
Devereux Advanced Behavioral Health Arizon a - Tucson, 6519
Devereux Advanced Behavioral Health Arizona - Scottsdale, 6518
Devereux Advanced Behavioral Health California, 6588
Devereux Advanced Behavioral Health Colorado - Cleo Wallace Center, 6681
Devereux Advanced Behavioral Health Connecticut, 2687
Devereux Advanced Behavioral Health Flori da - Orlando Campus, 6736
Devereux Advanced Behavioral Health Florid a - Viera Campus, 6737
Devereux Advanced Behavioral Health Florida, 6738
Devereux Advanced Behavioral Health Florida - Titusville Campus, 6734
Devereux Advanced Behavioral Health Georgi a, 6794
Devereux Advanced Behavioral Health Massachusetts & Rhode Island, 6970
Devereux Advanced Behavioral Health New Jersey, 7043
Devereux Advanced Behavioral Health New York, 7060
Devereux Advanced Behavioral Health Texas - League City Campus, 7166
Devereux Advanced Behavioral Health Texas- Victoria Campus, 7167
Devereux Foundation, 7159, 7161, 7165
Devereux Pennsylvania, 7138
Devereux Threshold Center for Autism, 6738
DiaMedica Inc., 5247

Diabetes Association Of Greater Cleveland, 1303, 8342
Diabetes Camp, 1112, 8379
Diabetes Network of East Hawaii, 3429
Diabetes Self-Management, 8619
Diabetes Society, 1420, 8375
Diabetes Sourcebook., 8467
Diabetic Cruise Desk, 5522
Diabetic Retinopathy, 8940
Diabetic Youth Foundation, 964, 8314
Diabetic Youth Services, 969, 8329
Diagnostic Report Writer, 1761
Dial Books, 8916
Dial-a-Hearing Screening Test, 8116
Dial: Disabled Information Awareness & Liv ing, 4317
Dialog Corporation, 1581
Dialogue Magazine, 9057
Dialysis at Sea Cruises, 5523
Dice: Jumbo Size, 5471
Dictionary of Congenital Malformations & Disorders, 5057
Dictionary of Developmental Disabilities Terminology, 5058, 5204
Didlake, 6206
Diestco Manufacturing Company, 688
Different Dream Parenting: A Practical Guide to Raising a Child with Special Needs, 5248
Different Roads to Learning, 1929
Difficult Child, 7750
Digest of Neurology and Psychiatry, 2369
Digestive Diseases & Disorders Sourcebook, 8468
Digi-Flex, 516
Digital Hearing Aids, 333
Dilemma, 1681
Dimensions of State Mental Health Policy, 4594
Dino-Games, 1682
Diocese of Maine Episcopal, 1135, 7954
Dionysus Theatre, 22
Directions, 8620
Directions Unlimited Acccessible Tours, 5524
Directions: Technology in Special Education, 1683
Directory Of Services For People With Disa bilities, 2061
Directory for Exceptional Children, 2062
Directory of Accessible Building Products, 1893
Directory of Financial Aids for Women, 3263
Directory of Members, 5059
Directory of Travel Agencies for the Disabled, 5489
disABILITY LINK: Rome, 4037
disAbility Connections, 4242
DisAbility Information and Resources, 5404
DisAbility LINK, 829
DisAbility Resource Center: Knoxville, 4461
DisAbility Resource Connection: Everett, 4530
disAbility Solutions for Independent Livin g, 4026
Disabilities Network of Eastern Connecticu t, 3985
Disabilities Rights Center, Inc, 3613
Disabilities Sourcebook, 461
Disability & Rehabilitation Journal, 5280
Disability & Society, 2186
Disability Action Center, 4447
Disability Action Center NW, 4045
Disability Action Center NW: Coeur D'Alene, 4046
Disability Action Center NW: Lewiston, 4047
Disability Advocates of Kent County, 4224
Disability Analysis Handbook: Tools for Independent Practice, 5281
Disability Analyst, 1844
Disability Awareness Guide, 5060
Disability Awareness Network, 4376
Disability Bookshop Catalog, 462
Disability Center for Independent Living, 3974
Disability Coalition of Northern Kentucky, 4168
Disability Compliance for Higher Education, 2234, 4595
Disability Connection, 4225
Disability Connections, 4029
Disability Culture Perspective on Early Intervention, 7751
Disability Determination Section, 3842

Disability Determination Service: Birmingham, 3318

Disability Discrimination Law, Evidence an d Testimony, 4596

Disability Funders Network, 830

Disability Funding News, 2370, 3264

Disability Law Center, 3807

Disability Law Center of Alaska, 3329

Disability Law Project, 3808

Disability Law in the United States, 4597

Disability Matters, 1856

Disability Ministries at St. Augustine Parish, 1317

Disability Net, 5405

Disability Network, 8652

Disability Network Southwest Michigan, 4226

Disability Network of Mid-Michigan, 4227

Disability Network of Oakland & Macomb, 4228

Disability Network/Lakeshore, 4229

Disability Policy Consortium, 3769

Disability Pride Newsletter, 2235

Disability Resource Agency for Independent Living: Modesto, 3933

Disability Resource Association, 4275

Disability Resource Center, 4016, 4510

Disability Resource Center of Fairfield County, 3986

Disability Resource Initiative, 4169

Disability Resources, 2236

Disability Resources Monthly, 2236

Disability Rights & Resources, 4377

Disability Rights Activist, 5406

Disability Rights Bar Association, 831

Disability Rights Center of Kansas, 3484

Disability Rights Education and Defense Fund, 4560

Disability Rights Education and Defense Fn, 4583

Disability Rights Education and Defense Fund, 4598, 5348

Disability Rights Montana, 3574

Disability Rights Movement, 5061

Disability Rights New Jersey, 4318

Disability Rights Now, 4598

Disability Rights Texas, 4561

Disability Rights Vermont, 3809

Disability Rights Wisconsin: Milwaukee Office, 3851

Disability Rights: Washington, 3830

Disability Services & Legal Center, 3934

Disability Services Division of Montana, 7029

Disability Studies Quarterly, 2187

Disability Studies and the Inclusive Class room, 2371

Disability Under the Fair Employment & Housing Act: What You Should Know About the Law, 4599

Disability and Communication Access Board, 3430

Disability and Health Journal, 2188

Disability and Health: National Center for Birth Defects and Developmental Disabilities, 8653

Disability and Medical Resources Mall, 5407

Disability and Rehabilitation, 2372

Disability and Social Performance: Using Drama to Achieve Successful Acts, 23

Disability and Sport, 8172

Disability, Sport and Society, 2373

DisabilityResources.org, 5408

Disabled & Alone/Life Services for the Handicapped, 5113, 5213

Disabled American Veterans, 5557

Disabled American Veterans, National Service & Legislative Headquarters, 5599

Disabled American Veterans: Ocean County, 5689

Disabled Athlete Sports Association, 832

Disabled Businesspersons Association, 833

Disabled Children's Relief Fund, 834

Disabled Drummers Association, 835

Disabled God: Toward a Liberatory Theology of Disability, 5264

Disabled People's International Fifth World Assembly as Reported by Two US Participants, 5062

Disabled Resource Services, 3975, 5054

Disabled Resources Center, 3935

Disabled Rights: American Disability Polic y and the Fight for Equality, 2374

Disabled Sports Program Center, 8226

Disabled Sports USA, 8227

Disabled Sports USA Far West, 8226

Disabled Watersports Program, 8228

Disabled We Stand, 5063

Disabled and Alone/Life Services for the Handicapped, 836

Disabled, the Media, and the Information Age, 5064

Disbled Resource Services, 3976

Discount School Supply, 1930

Discover Technology, 5409

Discovery Camps, 1406

Discovery Education, 1640

Discovery House Publishers, 5248

Discovery Newsletter, 5065

Discrimination is Against the Law, 4600

Discriptive Language Arts Development, 1762

Disorders of Motor Speech: Assessment, Treatment, and Clinical Characterization, 8735

District of Columbia Center for Independen t Living, 3996

District of Columbia Department of Employment Services, 5911

District of Columbia Department of Handicapped Children, 3390

District of Columbia Dept. of Employment Services: Office of Workforce Development, 5912

District of Columbia Fair Employment Practice Agencies, 5913

District of Columbia General Hospital Physical Medicine & Rehab Services, 6720

District of Columbia Office on Aging, 3391

District of Columbia Public Library, 4696, 9068

District of Columbia Public Library: Services for the Deaf Community, 4696

District of Columbia Public Schools: Special Education Division, 2118

District of Columbia Regional Library for the Blind and Physically Handicapped, 4697

Diversified Opportunities, 7076

Diversity and Visual Impairment: The Influ ence of Race, Gender, Religion and Ethnicity, 8941

Divided Legacy: A History of the Schism in Medical Thought, The Bacteriological Era, 2375

Division Of Workforce Development, 6140

Division for Physical, Health & Multiple Disabilities, 2026, 8266

Division for the Blind and Visually Impaired, 6044

Division of Birth Defects and Developmental Disabilities, 3417

Division of Blind Services, 6739

Division of Developmental Disabilities, 3616

Division of Developmental Disabilities: De partment of Social & Health Services, 6215

Division of Disability Aging & Rehab Services, 1554

Division of Employment & Rehabilitation Services, 5826

Division of Employment & Training, 5909

Division of Graham-Field, 467

Division of Labor and Management, 3751

Division of Mental Health and Substance Abuse, 3680

Division of Physical Medicine and Rehabilitation, 6589

Division of Rehabilitation, 6709

Division of Rehabilitation Services, 4030, 4060, 3419, 6959

Division of Rehabilitation Services (DI RS), 6050

Division of Rehabilitation Services: Staff Library, 4938

Division of Rehabilitation-Education Services, University of Illinois, 6831

Division of Rehabilitative Services, 6189

Division of Special Education, 3770

Division of Vocational Rehabilitation Department of Social and Health Services, 7198

Division of Vocational Rehabilitation (DVR), 3327

Division of Vocational Rehabilitation of Wyoming, 6223

Division of Workers Compensation, 3404

Division of Workers' Compensation Department of Labor & Employment, 3370

Dixie EMS, 424

Do You Hear That?, 5325

Do You Remember the Color Blue: The Questi Ons Children Ask About Blindness, 8942

Do-Able Renewable Home, 1894

Do2learn, 1931

Doctor Yvonne Jones and Associates, 2027

Doctors Hospital, 7093

Dodd Hall at the Ohio State University Hospitals, 7094

Dodge Lowered Floor, 81

Dogs for the Deaf, 7915, 8092

Doing Things Together, 5326

Dolfinger-McMahon Foundation, 3143

Dolphin Computer Access, 2086

Don Johnston, 550, 1932, 1672, 1700, 1739, 1756, 1757, 1763, 1771, 1775, 1785, 1794, 1797, 1800, 1801, 1826

Don't Call Me Special: A First Look at Dis ability, 4955

Don't Feel Sorry for Paul, 7888

Don't Lose Sight of Glaucoma, 8943

Donaldsville Association for Retarded Citizens, 6929

Doorbell Signalers, 334

Dorma Architectural Hardware, 517

Dothan Houston County Library System, 4649

Double Gong Indoor/Outdoor Ringer, 335

Double H Ranch, 1272

Dover Rehabilitation and Living Center, 7331

Down Syndrome, 7752

Down Syndrome News, 7833

Down Syndrome Society of Rhode Island, 3166

Downtown Neighborhood Learning Center, 5822

Doylestown Hospital Rehabilitation Center, 6413

Dr Scholl Foundation, 2874

Dr. Karen H Chao Developmental Optometry Karen H. Chao. O.D., 6590

Dr. William O Benenson Rehabilitation Pavilion, 7343

Draft: Builder, 1763

Dragonfly Forest Summer Camp, 1350

Dream Oaks Camp, 1040

Dream Street Camp, 995

Dream Street Foundation, 995

Dreamer, 1609

Dresher Hill Health and Rehabilitation Cen ter, 7377

Dressing Stick, 300

Dressing Tips and Clothing Resources for Making Life Easier, 463

Drew Karol Industries, 312

Drive Master Company, 82, 88, 103, 114, 140, 143

Driven to Distraction, 7753

Driving Systems Inc., 83

DuPage Center for Independent Living, 4061

Dual Brake Control, 84

Dual Brush with Suction Base, 353

Dual Relationships in Counseling, 2376

Dual Security Bed Rail, 187

Dual Switch Latch and Timer, 518

Dual-Mode Charger, 674

Duane Morrs Llt, 3158

Duchenne Muscular Dystrophy, 8469

Duchossois Foundation, 2875

Duke Endowment, 3094

Duke Medical Center, 4879

Duke University Medical Center, 6389

Duluth Public Library, 4831

Duracell & Rayovac Hearing Aid Batteries, 336

Duraline Medical Products Inc., 313

Durham VA Medical Center, 5713

Duro-Med Industries, 314

Dusters, 1449

Dutch Neck T-Shirt, 1487

Duxbury Braille Translator, 1546

Duxbury Systems, 1546

Duxbury Systems Incorporated, 1551

Dvorak Expeditions, 5525

Dwight D Eisenhower VA Medical Center, 5633

Dyna Vox Technologies, 1631

DynaVox Technologies Speech Communication Devices, 1631

Dynamic Dimensions, 5883

Dynamic Learning Center, 7628

Dynamic Living, 5410
Dynamic Systems, 274, 296
Dyslexia Training Program, 1933
Dyslexia over the Lifespan, 7754
Dysphagia Research Society, 8684
Dyspraxia Foundation, 7877
Dystonia Advocacy Network, 8134

E

E VA S, 1637
E&J Health Care, 7162
E-Z Access Van Ramp, 391
EASE Program: Emergency Access Self Evalua
tion, 8011
ECHO Housing: Recommended Construction and
Installation Standards, 1895
EDI Camp, 8380
EL Wiegand Foundation, 3000
ENDependence Center of Northern Virginia, 4511
ENVISION, 6908
EP Resource Guide, 5066
ERIC Clearinghouse on Disabilities and Gifted
Education, 2087
ESCIL Update Newsletter, 5067
ESI Master Resource Guide, 1684
ESS Work Center, 5844
ESpecial Needs, 1934
ETMC, 8388
EZ Dot, 1764
EZ Keys, 1685
EZ Keys for Windows, 1765
EZ-International, 574, 578, 583, 599, 608, 609
Eagle Hill School: Summer Program, 1176, 7681
Eagle Mount-Bozeman, 1222
Eagle Pond Rehabilitation and Living Cente r,
6971
Eagle Sportschairs, LLC, 755
Eagle View Ranch, 1445
Ear Foundation, 7916
Ear, Nose, and Throat Disorders Sourcebook, 8470
Early Childhood Connection, 2237
Early Childhood E-News, 2238
Early Childhood Intervention Clearinghouse, 2189
Early Childhood Reporter, 2239
Early Childhood Services, 6591
Early Communication Skills for Children wi th
Down Syndrome, 2377
Early Focus: Working with Young Children W ho
Are Blind or Visually Impaired & Their
Families, 8944
Early Games for Young Children, 1686
Early Intervention, 2189
Early Intervention Program, 6836
Early Intervention: Implementing Child & Family
Services for At-Risk Infants and Toddlers, 2378
Early Learning 1, 5472
Early Music Skills, 1687
East Bay Community Foundation, 2755
East Jefferson General Hospital Rehab Center,
6930
East King County Office, 4527
East Los Angeles Doctors Hospital, 6592
East Orange Campus of the VA New Jersey
Healthcare System, 5690
East Penn Manufacturing Company, 756, 756
Easter Seal Camp Wawbeek, 1436
Easter Seal Society of Mahoning, 7095
Easter Seal Society of New Jersey Highlands
Workshop, 6107
Easter Seal Society of Washington, 1429, 8162
Easter Seal Work Center, 5829
Easter Seal of Greater Dallas, TX, 3771
Easter Seal of Ocean County, 6108
Easter Seals, 837, 6832, 8654, 946, 5095, 5126,
5145, 6107
Easter Seals Broward County, 6740
Easter Seals Camp ASCCA, 946
Easter Seals Camp Harmon, 996
Easter Seals Camp Stand by Me, 1429, 8162
Easter Seals Camp Sunnyside, 1073
Easter Seals Central Alabama, 6497
Easter Seals Central California, 996
Easter Seals Colorado, 1011, 1018

Easter Seals DE/MD Eastern Shore, 1029
Easter Seals Delaware & Maryland's Eastern
Shore, 6714
Easter Seals Disability Svcs: Bay Area, 6593
Easter Seals DuPage And The Fox Valley Region,
6833
Easter Seals East Georgia, 6795
Easter Seals Gilchrist-Marchman Rehab Center,
6834
Easter Seals Greater NW Texas, 3772
Easter Seals Iowa, 6890, 1073
Easter Seals Jayne Shover Center, 6835
Easter Seals Joliet Region, 6832
Easter Seals National, 6743, 6807, 6890
Easter Seals Nebraska, 1228, 1228, 5099
Easter Seals New Jersey, 6109
Easter Seals New York, 3043
Easter Seals Northwest Alabama, 6498
Easter Seals Of Delaware, 1147
Easter Seals Of Florida, 1037
Easter Seals Of Iowa, 1109
Easter Seals Oklahoma, 1322, 7682, 7969, 8710,
8889
Easter Seals Project ACTION, 5502
Easter Seals South Florida, 6741
Easter Seals Southwest Flordia, 6742
Easter Seals Superior California, 6594
Easter Seals Tennessee - State Headquarters, 1380
Easter Seals Tennessee Camping Program, 1380
Easter Seals UCP, 1081
Easter Seals Wayne/Union Counties, 6319
Easter Seals West Alabama, 6499
Easter Seals West Central Alabama Rehabili tation
Center, 6500
Easter Seals of Alabama, 5796
Easter Seals-Goodwill Northern Rocky Mountains,
6807
Easter Seals: Achievement Center, 5796
Easter Seals: Arkansas, 6536
Easter Seals: Connecticut, 1023
Easter Seals: Massachusetts, 1164
Easter Seals: New Hampshire, 1237
Easter Seals: New Jersey, 1243
Easter Seals: Opportunity Center, 5797
Easter Seals: Oregon, 1067
Easter Seals: Southeastern Pennsylvania, 1341,
1346
Easter Seals: Virginia, 1416
Easter Seals: Volusia and Flagler Counties , FL,
6743
Easter Seals: Wisconsin, 1436
Eastern Blind Rehabilitation Center, 6700
Eastern Colorado Services for the Disabled, 3371
Eastern Idaho Regional Medical Center, 7269
Eastern Oregon Center for Independent Living,
4407
Eastern Shore Center for Independent Living,
4187
Eastern Shore Center for Independent Living, 5067
Eastern Washington University, 4585
Eastside Rehabilitation and Living Center, 7308
Eastview Medical and Rehabilitation Center, 7425
Easy Pivot Transfer Machine, 392
Easy Ply, 315
Easy Pour Locking Lid Pot, 354
Easy Stand, 393
Easy Things to Make Things Simple: Do It
Yourself Modifications for Disabled Persons,
5068
EasyStand 6000 Glider, 650
Eating Disorders Sourcebook., 8471
Eating Skills: Learning Basic Table Manners,
1688
Echo Grove Camp, 1192
Echoing Hills, 1309, 8381
Ecology of Troubled Children, 2379
Econo-Float Water Flotation Cushion, 275
Econo-Float Water Flotation Mattress, 276
Economical Liberty, 394
Eden Acres Administrative Services, 6110
Edge, 704
Edgemoor Day Program, 6715
Edison Sheltered Workshop, 6111

Edith Nourse Rogers Memorial Veterans Hospital,
5651
Edmonds Rehabilitation & Healthcare Center er,
7414
Edna McConnel Clark Foundation, 3044
Educating Children with Disabilities: A
Transdisciplinary Approach, 2380
Educating Children with Multiple Disabilities: A
Transdisciplinary Approach, 2381
Educating Inattentive Children, 7859
Educating Individuals with Disabilities: IDEIA
2004 and Beyond (1st Edition), 2382
Educating Students Who Have Visual Impairments
with Other Disabilities, 2383
Educating all Students in the Mainstream, 2384
Education and Auditory Research Foundation,
3185
The Education of Children with Acquired Brain
Injury, 2565
Education of the Handicapped: Laws, Legislative
Histories and Administrative Document, 4601
Educational Accessibility Services, 838
Educational Activities, 1778
Educational Activities Software, 1643, 1649, 1681,
1697, 1762, 1777, 1780, 1792, 1798, 1816, 7857
Educational Audiology for the Limited Hearing
Infant and Preschooler, 2385
Educational Care, 2386
Educational Equity Concepts, 1947, 2430, 5035
Educational Intervention for the Student, 2387
Educational Issues Among Children with Spi na
Bifida, 8472
Educational Media Corporation, 7763
Educational Prescriptions, 2388
Educational Productions, 5304, 5363, 5372
Educational Referral Service, 2027
Educational Services for the Visually Impaired,
4664
Educational Software Institute, 1684
Educational Tutorial Consortium, 2011
Educators Publishing Service, 1951, 1964, 1976,
1980, 1986, 2293, 2368, 2386, 2388, 2422,
2491, 2493, 2596, 2631, 2632, 2633, 2634,
2635, 2642, 7213, 7746, 7754
Educators Resource Directory, 2063
Edward Hines Jr Hospital, 5619
Edward J Madden Open Hearts Camp, 1177, 8382
Edward John Noble Foundation, 3045
Edwin Mellen Press, 2412, 5227
Edyth Bush Charitable Foundation, 2839
Effective Instruction for Special Education, 2389
Effectively Educating Handicapped Students, 2390
Eggleston Services, 1421
Ehrman Medical Library, 4860
Eight CAP, Inc. Head Start, 6997
El Paso Lighthouse for the Blind, 7168
El Paso Natural Gas Foundation, 3203
El Paso VA Healthcare Center, 5759
El Pomar Foundation, 2803
El Valle Community Parent Resource Center, 3773
El Valor Corporation, 6836
Elastic Shoelaces, 301
Elder Abuse and Mistreatment, 7504
Elder Visions Newsletter, 7540
ElderLawAnswers.com, 4602, 5411
Elderly Guide to Budget Travel/Europe, 5490
Eleanora CU Alms Trust, 3110
Electra-Ride, 395
Electra-Ride Elite, 396
Electra-Ride III, 397
Electric Can Opener & Knife Sharpener, 355
Electric Leg Bag Emptier and Tub Slide Shower
Chair, 167
Electric Mobility Corporation, 577, 592, 593
Electro Kinetic Technologies, 744
Electronic Courseware Systems, 1689, 1662, 1687,
1703, 1704, 1737
Electronic House, 1896
Electronic House: Enhanced Lifestyles with
Electronics, 1896
Electronic Speech Assistance Devices, 1632
Electronic Stethoscopes, 316
Elgin Training Center, 6837

Elkhart Public Library for the Blind and Physiclly Handicapped, 4753
Elling Camps, 1351
Elmhurst Hospital Center, 7061
Elsevier Health, 2177
Elsevier Inc, 8428
Elwyn, 839
Elwyn Delaware, 4695, 6716
Embracing the Monster: Overcoming the Challenges of Hidden Disabilities, 7755
Emerging Horizon, 2190
Emerging Leaders, 5327
Emory Autism Resource Center, 4722
Emory University, 4722
Emory University Laboratory for Ophthalmic Research, 4723
Emotional Problems of Childhood and Adolescence, 2391
Emotorsports, 554
Emphysema Foundation for Our Right to Survive, 8267
Employment Development Department, 3354, 5845, 5851
Employment Discrimination Based on Disability, 4603
Employment Options Inc., 5278
Employment Resources Program, 1573
Employment Service: California, 5845
Employment Standards Administration Department of Labor (ESA), 4604
Employment and Training Division, Region B, 5948
Employment for Individuals with Asperger Syndrome or Non-Verbal Learning Disability, 8736
Empress Travel, 5524
EnTech: Enabling Technologies of Kentuckiana, 4773
Enable America Inc., 840
Enabling & Empowering Families: Principles & Guidelines for Practice, 2392
Enabling Devices, 519, 5473
Enabling News, 7530
Enabling Romance: A Guide to Love, Sex & Relationships for the Disabled, 5069
Enabling Technologies Company, 1547
Enchanted Hills Camp for the Blind, 997, 8890
Encounters with Autistic States, 7756, 8737
Encyclopedia of Basic Employment and Daily Living Skills, 1935
Encyclopedia of Blindness and Vision Impairment Second Edition, 8945
Encyclopedia of Deafness and Hearing Disorders, 8012
Encyclopedia of Disability, 5070
Encyclopedia of Genetic Disorders & Birth Defects, 5205
Endeavor, 7596
Endeavor Magazine, 8073
Enforcing the ADA: A Status Report from the Department of Justice, 4605
Englishton Park Academic Remediation, 1098, 7683
Englishton Park Presbyterian, 1098, 7683
Enhancer Cushion, 277
Enhancing Everyday Communication for Children with Disabilities, 5282
Enrichments Catalog, 464
Entervan, 85
Environmental Health Center: Dallas, 8268
Environmental Traveling Companions, 5526
Epilepsy Council of Greater Cincinnati, 3688
Epilepsy Foundation, 7629, 7878, 8135, 8655, 4791, 8604
Epilepsy Foundation Arizona, 952, 7663
Epilepsy Foundation Greater Southern Illinois, 1153
Epilepsy Foundation Of Northern California, 968
The Epilepsy Foundation Of Northern California, 980
Epilepsy Foundation of Alabama, 939, 7664
Epilepsy Foundation of America, 8204
Epilepsy Foundation of Long Island, 3046
Epilepsy Foundation of Southeast Texas, 3204

Epilepsy Foundation: Central and South Texas, 3205
Epilepsy, 199 Answers: A Doctor Responds to His Patients' Questions, 8473
Epilepsy: Patient and Family Guide, 8474
EpilepsyUSA, 8604
EpilepsyUSA Magazine, 8204
Episcopal Charities, 3047
Episcopal Church of Hawaii, 8387
Equal Access Center for Independence, 4512
Equal Employment Advisory Council, 4562
Equal Opportunity Employment Commission, 3293
Equal Opportunity Publications, 5275
Equal Treatment for People With Mental Retardation: Having and Raising Children, 7757
Equalizer 1000 Series, 675
Equalizer 5000 Home Gym, 676
Equals in Partnership: Basic Rights for Families of Children with Blindness, 8946
Equip for Equality, 3450
Equip for Equality - Carbondale Office, 3451
Equip for Equality - Moline Office, 3452
Equip for Equality - Springfield Office, 3453
Equipment Shop, 465
Eric Clearinghouse on Disabilities and Gifted Education, 2088
Erie VA Medical Center, 5735
Erlanger Medical Center Baronness Campus, 7390
Ernest Health, 6463
Esalen Institute, 841
Escort II XL, 86
The Essential Brain Injury Guide (5th Edition), 5291
Essential First Steps for Parents of Children with Autism, 5249
Essential Medical Supply, Inc., 466
Essential Science Publishing, 8570
Esther A & Joseph Klingenstein Fund, 3048
Esu Memorial Union, 4765
Etac USA: F3 Wheelchair, 705
Ethical Issues In Home Health Care (2nd Edition), 5283
Ethnic Diseases Sourcebook, 8475
Eugene J Towbin Healthcare Center, 5572
Eugene and Agnes E Meyer Foundation, 2823
Eunice Kennedy Shriver National Institute of Child Health and Human Development (NICHD), 8269
Eva L And Joseph M Bruening Foundation, 3111
Evac + Chair Emergency Evacuation Chair, 258
Evac + Chair North America LLC, 258
Evacu-Trac, 706
Evaluation and Educational Programming of Students with Deafblindness & Severe Disabilities, 2393
Evaluation and Treatment of the Psychogeriatric Patient, 2394
Evans Newton, 2052
Evansville Association for the Blind, 5996
Evelyn and Walter Hans Jr Haas Jr, 2756
Evenston Community Foundation, 2876
Everest & Jennings, 467, 708
Evergreen Healthcare, 7212
Evergreen Woods Health and Rehabilitation Center, 7249
Evert Conner Rights & Resources CIL, 4111
EveryBody's Different: Understanding and Changing Our Reactions to Disabilities, 5071
Everybody Counts Center for Independent Living, 4098
Everybody's Guide to Homeopathic Medicines, 5072
Everyday Social Interaction: A Program for People with Disabilities, 5073
Everything Parent's Guide to Special Education, 4956
Evio Plastics, 356
Exceed: A Division of Valley Resource Center, 6595
Exceptional Children, 2191
Exceptional Children in Focus, 2395
Exceptional Education, 1969, 1970, 1971, 1972, 2495
Exceptional Lives: Special Education in Today's Schools, 4th Edition, 2396

Exceptional Parent Library, 4619, 5066, 5232, 5235, 5237, 5340, 5355, 7748
Exceptional Parent Magazine, 5206
Exceptional Student in the Regular Classroom (6th Edition), 5259
Exceptional Teaching Inc, 1936, 1936
Exchange, 8205
Exeter Hospital, 7033
Expendicare, 7375
Explode the Code, 1937
Explore Your Options, 7505
Explorer+ 4-Wheel Scooter, 578
Exploring Autism: A Look at the Genetics of Autism, 5412
Express Medical Supply, 468
Expressive Arts for the Very Disabled and Handicapped of All Ages, 24
Expressive and Receptive Fingerspelling for Hearing Adults, 8013
Exquisite Egronomic Protective Wear, 1466
Extendicare Health Services, Inc., 6485
Extensions for Independence, 551
Extra Loud Alarm with Lighter Plug, 630
Eye & Ear Infirmary, 9141
Eye Bank Association of America, 8829, 1857, 9116
Eye Bank Association of America Annual Meeting, 1857
Eye Foundation of Kansas City, 7026
Eye Institute of New Jersey, 4852
Eye Institute of the Medical College of Wisconsin and Froedtert Clinic, 4946
Eye Medical Center, 6596
Eye Medical Center of Fresno, 6596
Eye Relief Word Processing Software, 1821
Eye Research News, 8947
Eye and Your Vision, 8948
Eye-Centered: A Study of Spirituality of Deaf People, 8014
Eye-Q Test, 8949
Eyegaze Computer System, 1516

F

FAVRAH Senior Adult Enrichment Program, 6701
FC Search, 3265
FCYD Camp, 1407, 8383
FDR Series of Low Vision Reading Aids, 1625
FHI 360, 5413
FM Kirby Foundation, 3010
FOR Community Services, 6972
FPL Group Foundation, 2840
FREED Center for Independent Living, 3936
FREED Center for Independent Living: Marysville, 3937
FSSI, 2611
FYI, 2240
Face First Fanlight Productions/Icarus Films, 5328
Face of Inclusion, 5207
Facilitated Communication Institute, Syracuse Univ, 7860, 8785
Facilitating Self-Care Practices in the Elderly, 2397
Facts on File, 5205, 8945, 9020
Fair Employment Practice Agency: Arizona, 5823
Fair Housing Design Guide for Accessibility, 1897
Fair Housing and Equal Employment, 5949
Fairacres Manor, 7238
Fairbanks Memorial Hospital & Denali Center, 7220
Fairfax County Public Library, 4918
Fairfield Center for Disabilities and Cerebral Palsy, 4394
Fairlawn Rehabilitation Hospital, 6973
Fairway Golf Cars, 552
Fairway Spirit Adaptive Golf Car: Model 4852, 552
Faith Mission Home, 7189
Fall Fun, 1690
Falling in Old Age, 7506
Families Magazine, 5208
Families of Adults With Autism: Stories & Advice For the Next Generation, 7758
Families of Spinal Muscular Dystrophy, 8620

Families, Illness & Disability, 5209
Family Caregiver Alliance, 2757
Family Challenges: Parenting with a Disability, 5074
Family Context and Disability Culture Reframing: Through the Looking Glass, 8950
Family Counseling Center, 6838
Family Guide to Vision Care (FG1), 8951
Family Guide: Growth & Development of the Partially Seeing Child, 8952
Family Intervention Guide to Mental Illness, 7507
Family Interventions Throughout Disability, 5210
Family Matters, 6839
Family Resource Associates, 4319, 4963
Family Resource Center on Disabilities, 842
Family Service Society, 6931
Family Support Project for the Developmentally Disabled, 8656
Family Therapy for ADHD: Treating Children, Adolescents and Adults, 7759
Family Voices, 843
Family-Centered Early Intervention with Infants and Toddlers, 2398
Family-Centered Service Coordination: A Manual for Parents, 5211
Family-Guided Activity-Based Intervention for Toddlers & Infants, 5329
Fanlight Productions, 25, 20, 70, 4959, 5021, 5187, 5239, 5305, 5306, 5314, 5317, 5318, 5328, 5334, 5337, 5347, 5351, 5352, 5353, 5356, 5371, 5373, 5375, 5376, 8639, 8640, 8641, 8642, 8783, 8787, 9024,
Fanlight Productions C/O Icarus Films, 7855, 7866, 8211, 8213, 8215, 8216, 8509
Fannie E Rippel Foundation, 3011
Fantastic Series Videotape Set, 8101
Fantastic: Colonial Times, Chocolate, and Cars, 8102
Fantastic: Dogs at Work and Play, 8103
Fantastic: Exciting People, Places and Thi ngs!, 8104
Fantastic: From Post Offices to Dairy Goat s, 8105
Fantastic: Imagination, Actors, and 'Deaf Way', 8106
Fantastic: Roller Coasters, Maps, and Ice Cream!, 8107
Fantastic: Skiing, Factories, and Race Hor es, 8108
Fantastic: Wonderful Worlds of Sports and Travel, 8109
Farewell, My Forever Child, 5265
Fargo VA Medical Center, 5717
Farmington Health Care Center, 6358
Farmington Valley ARC, 7834
Farnum Rehabilitation Center, 7034
Fashion Collection, 1469
Father Drumgoole Connelly Summer Camp, 1273, 7970, 8384
Fathers: A Common Ground, 8953
Favarh/Farmington Valley ARC, 844
Fay J Lindner Foundation, 3049
Faye McBeath Foundation, 3251
Fayetteville VA Medical Center, 5573, 5714
Feather River Industries, 5846
Featherlite, 579
Featherspring, 677
Featherweight Reachers, 302
Fedcap Rehabilitation Services, 845
Federal Aviation Administration, 3296
Federal Benefits for Veterans and Dependents, 5558
Federal Communications Commission, 3294
Federal Emergency Management Agency, 2119
Federal Government, 3510, 7647, 8681, 8782
Federal Grants & Contracts Weekly, 3266
Federal Heights Rehabilitation and Nursing Center, 7402
Federal Laws of the Mentally Handicapped: Laws, Legislative Histories and Admin. Documents, 4606
Federal Student Aid Information Center, 2824
Federation Employment And Guidance Service (F-E-G-S), 7062
Federation for Children with Special Needs, 846, 5219

Federation of Families for Children's Mental Health, 847
Feeding Children with Special Needs, 2399
Feingold Association of the US, 848, 7836
Feldenkrais Guild of North America (FGNA), 849
Fellow Insider, 2241
Fibromyalgia AWARE Magazine, 8188
Fibromyalgia Online, 8206
Fidelco, 9078
Fidelco Guide Dog Foundation, 2810, 8830, 9078
Field Foundation of Illinois, 2877
Field Notes, 2242
Fifth Third Bank, 3110
Fight for Sight, 8831, 9090
Fighting Blindness News, 8954
Fighting for Darla: Challenges for Family Care & Professional Responsibility, 7760
Filmakers Library, 5330
Filmakers Library: An Imprint Of Alexander Street Press, 5331
Films & Videos on Aging and Sensory Change, 5332
Films Media Group, 1811, 5357
Final Report: Challenges and Strategies of Disabled Parents: Findings from a Survey (1997), 5250
Financial Aid for Asian Americans, 3267
Financial Aid for Hispanic Americans, 3268
Financial Aid for Native Americans, 3269
Financial Aid for Research and Creative Ac tivities Abroad, 3270
Financial Aid for Veterans, Military Personnel and their Dependents, 3271
Financial Aid for the Disabled and Their F amilies, 2758, 3272
Finger Lakes Developmental Disabilities Service Office, 4861
Finger Lakes Independence Center, 4351
Fingerspelling: Expressive and Receptive Fluency, 8110
Firefighters Burn Institute, 998
Firefighters Kids Camp, 998
The Firefly Foundation, 972
Firemans Fund Foundation, 2759
Firemans Fund Insurance Companies, 2759
First Descents, 1017
First Hill Care Center, 7199
First Manhattan Company, 3064
First Occupational Center of New Jersey, 6112
First State Senior Center, 6717
First Step Independent Living, 3938
First Steps, 8955
First Union Foundation, 3095
Fit for Work at Exeter Hospital, 6090
Fit to Work, 5847
Fite Center for Independent Living, 4062
Fitness Programming for Physical Disabilit ies, 8173
Five Green & Speckled Frogs, 1691
Five Green & Speckled Frogs IntelliKeys Overlay, 1517
Five Star Industries, 6840
FlagHouse Rehab Resources, 469
FlagHouse Special Populations, 470
Flagstaff City-Coconino County Public Library, 4657
Flannel Gowns, 1450
Flannel Pajamas, 1480
Flashing Lamp Telephone Ring Alerter, 210
FlexShield Keyboard Protectors, 1610
Flinchbaugh Company, 384
Flint Osteopathic Hospital: RehabCare Unit, 6359
Float Dress, 1451
Florence C and Harry L English Memorial Fund, 2849
Florida Adult Services, 3405
Florida Baptist Convention, 7674
Florida CORF, 6744
Florida Commission on Human Relations, 5924
Florida Community College at Jacksonville/ Services for Students with Disabilities, 6745
Florida Department of Education: Bureau of Exceptional Education And Student Services, 2121

Florida Department of Handicapped Children, 3406
Florida Department of Mental Health and Rehabilitative Services, 3407
Florida Developmental Disabilities Council, 3408
Florida Diabetes Camp, 1041, 8385
Florida Division of Blind Services, 4703
Florida Division of Vocational Rehabilitation, 3409, 5923
Florida Fair Employment Practice Agency, 5924
Florida Hospital, 6300, 7260
Florida Hospital Rehabilitation Center, 6279
Florida Institute Of Rehabilitation Education (FIRE), 6746
Florida Institute for Neurologic Rehabilitation, Inc, 6747
Florida Instructional Materials Center for the Visually Impaired (FIMC-VI), 4704
Florida Lions Camp, 1042, 7578
Florida School for the Deaf and Blind, 7579
Florida Sheriffs Caruth Camp, 1043, 7684
Florida Sheriffs Youth Ranches, 1043, 7684
Florida's Protection and Advocacy Programs for Persons with Disabilities, 3410
Floyd Healthcare Resources, 6305
Floyd Rogers Foundation, 1226, 8335
Flushing Hospital, 7063
Flushing Manor Nursing and Rehab, 7344
Flying Wheels Travel, 5527
Foam Decubitus Bed Pads, 188
Focal Group Psychotherapy, 2400
Focus, 8197, 9079
Focus Alternative Learning Center, 850, 7630, 7842
Focus Times Newsletter, 7842
Focus on Autism and Other Developmental Disabilities, 2192
Focus on Exceptional Children, 2193
Fold-Down 3-in-1 Commode, 317
Folding Chair with a Rigid Feel, 707
Fontana Rehabilitation Workshop, 6597
Food Markers/Rubberbands, 357
Food!, 1938
Foot Inversion Tread, 520
Foot Pedal Extensions, 87
Foot Placement Ladder, 521
Foot Snugglers, 1455
Foot Steering, 88
Foot Steering System, 89
Foothill Nursing and Rehab Center, 7229
Foothill Vocational Opportunities, 6598
For Hearing People Only, 8015
Force A Miracle, 5075
Ford Foundation, 3050
Ford Lowered Floor, 90
Formed Families: Adoption of Children with Handicaps, 4607
Formerly Adaptive Environments, 1879
Formerly Houston-Love Memorial Library, 4649
Formerly Resources for Children with Special Needs, 5421
Formerly The Lymphoma Foundation Canada, 8279
Formerly Tourette Syndrome Association, 7655
Formerly: Families of Spinal Muscular Atrophy, 8133
Formula Series Active Mobility Wheelchairs, 708
Forsyth Medical Center, 7077
Fort Howard VA Medical Center, 5646
Fort Lauderdale Veterans Medical Center, 6748
Fortis Foundation, 3051
Fortress, 681, 702, 704, 709, 715, 732, 735, 736, 737, 740, 750
Forum, 5076
Fotheringhay Farms, 5900
Foundation & Corporate Grants Alert, 3273
Foundation 1000, 3274
Foundation Center, 3052, 3039, 3053, 3265, 3274, 3275, 3276, 3278, 3280, 3284, 5077
Foundation Center Library Services, 3053
Foundation Directories, 3275
Foundation Fighting Blindness, 2930, 5414, 7566, 8832, 8954
Foundation For Blind Children, 2733

Foundation For Dreams, Inc., 1040
Foundation Fundamentals for Nonprofit Organizations, 5077
Foundation Grants to Individuals, 3276
Foundation Industries, 6932
Foundation Management Services, 3111
Foundation for Advancement in Cancer Therapy, 3054
Foundation for Children and Youth with Diabetes, 1407, 8383
Foundation for Seacoast Health, 3004
Foundation for the Carolinas, 3096
Foundations of Orientation and Mobility, 8956
Foundations of Rehabilitation Counseling with Persons Who Are Blind r Visually Impaired, 8957
Fountain Circle Health & Rehabilitation, 7299
Fountain Hills Lioness Braille Service, 4658
Fountain House Gallery, 26
Four Oaks Center, 7096
Four Rivers Resource Services, 4099, 5997
Four-Ingredient Cookbook, 5078
The Fowler Center For Outdoor Learning, 1184
Fox Subacute Center, 7139
Fox Subacute at Clara Burke, 7140
Fraction Factory, 1644
Fragile Success, 7761
Fragile X Family, 8639
Frames of Reference for the Assessment of Learning Disabilities, 2610
Francis Beidler Charitable Trust, 2878
Frank & Mollie S VanDervoort Memorial Foun dation, 2962
Frank Mobility Systems, 679
Frank Olean Center, 3167
Frank R and Elizabeth Simoni Foundation, 2947
Frank Stanley Beveridge Foundation, 2948
Franklin County Work Activity Center, 6013
Franklin Court Assisted Living, 4441
Franklin Skilled Nursing and Rehabilitation Center, 7317
Fraser, 4386
Frasier Rehabilitation Center Division of Clark Memorial Hospital, 6883
Frazier Rehab Institute, 6916
Fred & Lillian Deeks Memorial Foundation, 3112
Fred Finch Youth Center, 6599
Fred Gellert Foundation, 2760
Fred J Brunner Foundation, 2879
Free Appropriate Public Education: The Law and Children with Disabilities, 4608
Free Hand: Enfranchising the Education of Deaf Children, 2401
Free Library of Philadelphia: Library for the Blind and Physically Handicapped, 4897
Free and User Supported Software for the IBM PC: A Resource Guide, 1692
Freedom Bath, 168
Freedom Center, 4188
Freedom Center for Independent Living, 3990
Freedom Resource Center for Independent Living: Fergus Falls, 4248
Freedom Resource Center for Independent Li ving: Fargo, 4387
Freedom Rider, 471, 471
Freedom Ryder Handcycles, 553
Freedom Scientific, 5415, 1786
Freedom Scientific Blind/Low Vision Group, 1548
Freedom Three Wheel Walker, 651
Freedom Valley Disability Center, 4428
Freedom Wheels, 398
Freedom from Arthritis Through Nutrition, 8174
Freestone Rehabilitation Center, 6520
Freestyle II, 709
Fremont Area Community Foundation, 2963
Frequently Asked Questions About Multiple Chemical Sensitivity, 5079
Fresno City College, 5848
Fresno City College: Disabled Students Programs and Services, 5848
Fresno County Free Library Blind and Handicapped Services, 4674
Friday Afternoon, 1779
Friendly Ice Cream Corp Contributions Prog ram, 2949

Friends Academy Summer Camps, 1274, 8386
Friends In Art (FIA), 27
Friends of Disabled Adults and Children, 8136
Friends of Libraries for Deaf Action, 4794
Friends: National Association of Young Peo ple who Stutter, 8790
Friendship 101, 2402
Friendship Circle Summer Camp, 1275
Friendship Press, 4971
Friendship Ventures, 1202, 8334
FriendshipVentures, 1288
Frohock-Stewart, 154, 172, 176, 269
From Gesture to Language in Hearing and Deaf Children, 8016
From Mime to Sign Package, 8017
From Where I Sit: Making My Way with Cereb ral Palsy, 8476
From the State Capitals: Public Health, 3277
Frost Foundation, 3020
Fulton County Rehab Center, 5970
Fun for Everyone, 1939
Functional Assessment Inventory Manual, 2403
Functional Electrical Stimulation for Ambu lation by Paraplegics, 8175
Functional Forms, 278
Functional Literacy System, 1812
Functional Resources, 1574
Functional Restoration of Adults and Child ren with Upper Extremity Amputation, 7889
Functional Skills Screening Inventory, 1574
Fund for New Jersey, 3012
Fundamentals of Autism, 1940
The Fundamentals of Special Education: A Practical Guide for Every Teacher, 2566
Future Choices Independent Living Center, 4100
Future Horizons, 28
Future Horizons Inc, 7810
Future Horizons, Inc., 39, 62, 64
Future Reflections, 9058

G

G W Micro, 1639
GA Baptist Childrens Homes & Family Ministries,Inc, 1053
GA and SK Etiquette, 8018
GAR Foundation, 3113
GE Foundation, 2811
GEICO Philanthropic Foundation, 2825
GM Mobility Program, 5503
GN Wilcox Trust, 2860
GO-MO Articulation Cards- Second Edition, 1941
GW Micro, 1518, 9115
Gadabout Wheelchairs, 710, 710
Gainesville Division, North Florida/South Georgia Veterans Healthcare System, 5604
Gales Creek Camp Foundation, 1328
Gales Creek Diabetes Camp, 1328
Gallaudet & NTID, 8001
Gallaudet Survival Guide to Signing, 8019
Gallaudet University, 8070
Gallaudet University Bookstore, 2446, 2459, 2568, 4580, 7984, 7987, 7994, 7996, 7997, 8013, 8021, 8044, 8749
Gallaudet University Press, 2089, 5416, 2455, 2522, 7989, 7992, 8000, 8002, 8004, 8005, 8006, 8007, 8008, 8016, 8019, 8020, 8025, 8026, 8031, 8032, 8033, 8034, 8037, 8038, 8039, 8042, 8043, 8049, 8050, 8051, 8053, 8057, 8062, 8064, 8071, 8080, 8093, 8101, 8102, 8103, 8104, 8105, 8106, 8107, 8108, 8109
Gallery Bookshop, 2349, 2365, 2440, 2462, 2470
Gallo Foundation, 2761
Galvin Health and Fitness Center, 8229
Garaventa Canada, 706
Gareth Stevens Publishing, 8549
Garfield Medical Center, 6245
Garten Services, 7125
Gateway Arts Center: Studio, Craft Store & Gallery, 6056
Gateway Center of Monterey County, 6600
Gateway Community Industries Inc.,, 7064
Gateway Industries: Castroville, 6601
Gateway Services/JCARC, 5998

Gaylord Hospital, 6702
Gaymar Industries, 279, 279, 713
Gazette International Networking Institute, 5163
Gear Shift Adaptor By Handicaps, Inc., 91
Geer Adult Training Center, 6501
Gem Wheelchair & Scooter Service: Mobility & Homecare, 678, 711, 746
Gendron, 712, 695
General Electric Company, 2811
General Facts and Figures on Blindness, 8958
General Mills Foundation, 2975
General Motors Mobility Program for Persons with Disabilities, 5503
Genesis Health System, 6891
Genesis Healthcare System, 7097
Genesis Regional Rehabilitation Center, 6891
Genetic Disorders Sourcebook, 5080
Genetic Nutritioneering, 5081
Genetics and Spina Bifida, 8477
Genova Diagnostics, 4877
Geo-Matt for High Risk Patients, 280
George A Martin Center, 7098
George Gund Foundation, 3114
George Hegyi Industrial Training Center, 5901
George M Eisenberg Foundation for Charities, 2880
George Washington University Health Resource Center, 851
George Washington University Medical Center, 6721
George Washington University Medical Center, 6721
George Wasserman Family Foundation, 2931
Georgetown University, 889
Georgetown University Center for Child and Human Development, 4698
Georgia Advocacy Office, 3418
Georgia Association of Homes and Services for the Aging, 7458
Georgia Client Assistance Program, 3419
Georgia Commission on Equal Opportunity, 5949
Georgia Council On Developmental Disabilities, 3420
Georgia Council On Developmental Disabilities, 5125
Georgia Council for the Hearing Impaired, 1054, 7962
Georgia Department of Aging, 3421
Georgia Department of Handicapped Children, 3422
Georgia Department of Labor, 4030, 6791
Georgia Division of Mental Health, Developmental Disabilities & Addictive Diseases, 3423
Georgia Industries for the Blind, 6796
Georgia Library for the Blind and Physically Handicapped, 4724
Georgia Power, 2850
Georgia Public Library, 4724
Georgia State Board of Workers' Compensation, 3424
Georgiana Institute, 7917
Gerontological Society of America, 7459
Gerontology: Abstracts in Social Gerontology, 7524
Get Ready for Jetty!: My Journal About ADH D and Me, 2404
Get a Wiggle On, 8959
Getting Around Town, 2405
Getting Better, 8111
Getting Our Heads Together, 7762
Getting Ready for the Outside World (G.R.O.W.), 2129
Getting Started with Facilitated Communication, 7860, 8785
Getting a Grip on ADD: A Kid's Guide to Understanding & Coping with ADD, 7763
Getting in Touch, 7601
Getting the Best for Your Child with Autism, 7764
Giant Food Foundation, 2932
Gift of Sight, 8960
Gillingham Manaual, 1942
Gilroy Workshop, 6602

Girl Scouts - Foothills Council, 1258, 8337
Girl Scouts of Washington Rock Council, 1242, 8885
Gladys Brooks Foundation, 3056
Glaser Progress Foundation, 3236
Glaucoma, 8961
Glaucoma Laser Trial, 4813
Glaucoma Research Foundation, 2762, 4675, 5417, 8961, 8980, 9080
Glaucoma: The Sneak Thief of Sight, 8962
Gleams Newsletter, 9080
Glendale Adventist Medical Center, 6603
Glendale Memorial Hospital and Health Center Rehabilitation Unit, 6604
Glendale Memorial Hospital and Health Center, 6604
Glengariff Health Care Center, 7345
The Glenholme School, 2687
Glenkirk, 5971
Glenview Terrace Nursing Center, 7274
Glickenhaus Foundation, 3057
Global Assistive Devices, Inc., 189
Global Health Solutions, 8177, 8426
Global Perspectives on Disability: A Curriculum, 2406
Glossary of Terminology for Vocational Assessment/Evaluation/Work, 2407
GoalView: Special Education and RTI Student Management Information System, 1693
Goals and Objectives, 1766
Goals and Objectives IEP Program Curriculum Associates LLC, 1767
God's Camp, 8387
Going to School with Facilitated Communication, 5082
Gold Violin, 662
Golden Technologies, 259, 184, 571, 595, 598
Goldilocks and the Three Bears: Told in Signed English, 8020
Goleta Valley Cottage Hospital, 6605
Golf Xpress, 554
Gonzales Warm Springs Rehabilitation Hospital, 6443
Good Grips Cutlery, 358
Good Samaritan Health System, 7141
Good Samaritan Healthcare Physical Medicine and Rehabilitation, 6478
Good Samaritan Hospital, 6478, 7142, 8663
Good Samaritan Hospital-Health System Center, 7142
Good Shepherd Rehabilitation, 7378
A Good and Perfect Gift: Faith, Expectations, and a Little Girl Named Penny, 5261
Goodwill Easter Seals of the Gulf Coast, 6502
Goodwill Industries - Suncoast, 3999, 5934, 5944
Goodwill Industries - Suncoast Incorporated, 5921
Goodwill Industries International, 852
Goodwill Industries of Central Indiana, 5999
Goodwill Industries of New Mexico, 6129
Goodwill Industries of North Georgia, 5948
Goodwill Industries of RI, 6176
Goodwill Industries of Southern New Jersey, 6113
Goodwill Industries- Suncoast, 5931, 5932, 5933, 5937
Goodwill Industries-Suncoast, 5922
Goodwill Industries-Suncoast Adult Day Training, 5925
Goodwill Industries-Suncoast Inc. Adult Day Training, 5926
Goodwill Industries-Suncoast Inc. Adult Day Training, 5927
Goodwill Industries-Suncoast Non-Residential Supports And Services Program, 5928
Goodwill Industries-Suncoast Supported Living, 5929
Goodwill Industries-Suncoast,Adult Day Training, 5930
Goodwill International, 5994
Goodwill Temporary Staffing, 5931
Goodwill of Greater Washington, 5914
Gospel Publishing House, 8029
Govennor's Council on Developmental Disabilities, 5029
Goverment of Rhode Isalnd, 3729

Government, 4694
Government Printing Office, 5558
Governor's Committee on Employment and Rehabilitation of People with Disabilities, 3327
Governor's Council on Developmental Disabilities, 3337
Governor's Council on Disabilities and Spe cial Education, 3328
Governor's Developmental Disability Council, 3467
Governor's Office oe Executive Policy & Programs, 3744
Gow School Summer Programs, 1276, 7685
Gpk, 263, 535
Graduate Technological Education and the Human Experience of Disability, 2408
Grady Memorial Hospital, 7099
Graham Street Community Resources, 4448
Graham-Field, 689
Graham-Field Health Products, 262, 284, 420, 720
Gram Newsletter, The, 2243
Grand Island VA Medical System, 5678
Grand Junction VA Medical Center, 5591
Grand Rapids Foundation, 2964
Grand Traverse Area Community Living Management Corporation, 4230
Grand Traverse Area Library for the Blind and Physically Handicapped, 4814
Grandmar, 666
Granger Foundation, 2965
Granite State Independent Living Foundation, 4311
Grant Guides, 3278
Grassroots Consortium, 3774
Gray Street Workcenter, 5884
Grayson Foundation, 2851
Great Barrington Rehabilitation and Nursing Center, 7318
Great Big Safety Tub Mat, 169
Great Lakes Regional Rehabilitation Center, 6392
Great Lakes/Macomb Rehabilitation Group, 4231
Great Oaks Joint Vocational School, 6154
Greater Baltimore Medical Center, 6952, 7312
Greater Cincinnati Foundation, 3115
Greater Detroit Agency for the Blind and Visually Impaired, 6998
Greater Kansas City Community Foundation & Affiliated Trusts, 2987
Greater Milwaukee Area Health Care Guide for Older Adults, 2064
Greater Milwaukee Area Senior Housing Options, 2065
Greater Richmond ARC, 7660
Greater St Louis Community Foundation, 2988
Greater Tacoma Community Foundation, 3237
Greater Worcester Community Foundation, 2950
Greeley Center for Independence, 3977
Green County Independent Living Resource Center, 4403
Green Door, 5915
Greenery Extended Care Center: Worcester, 6974
Greenery Rehabilitation & Skilled Nursing Center, 6975
Greenroots Consortium, 3774
Greenville County Recreation District, 1369
Greenwood Publishing Group, 2090, 2328, 2414, 2452, 4590, 4594, 4611, 4612, 4623, 4630, 5050, 5064, 5085, 5100, 5166, 5183, 5200, 5223, 5228, 7502, 7509, 7749
Gresham Driving Aids, 92, 95, 96, 98, 107, 110, 113, 120, 128, 131, 132, 133, 134, 141
Grey House Publishing, 2091
Grief: What it is and What You Can Do, 5083
Griffin Area Resource Center Griffin Community Workshop Division, 5950
Groden Center, 6177
Grossberg Company, 2931
Grossmont Hospital Rehabilitation Center, 6246
Group Activity for Adults with Brain Injury, 7765
Grover Hermann Foundation, 2881
Growing Readers, 2244
Growing Together Diabetes Camp, 1396, 8388
Growing Up with Epilepsy: A Pratical Guide for Parents, 8478

Guardianship Services Associates, 4563
Guest House of Slidell Sub-Acute and Rehab Center, 7303
Guide Dog Foundation for the Blind, 3058, 9082
Guide Dog News, 9081
Guide Dog Users, 8833
Guide Dogs for the Blind, 8834, 9069, 9074, 9075, 9081, 9098
Guide Magazine, 9059
Guide Service of Washington, 5528
A Guide for the Wheelchair Traveler, 5485
A Guide to Disability Rights Laws, 4990
Guide to Funding for International and Foreign Programs, 3279
A Guide to International Educational Excha nge, 2692
Guide to Living with HIV Infection: Develo ped at the Johns Hopkins AIDS Clinic, 8479
Guide to Managing Your Arthritis, 8176
Guide to Successful Employment for Individuals with Autism, 7766
Guide to Teaching Phonics, 1943
A Guide to Teaching Students With Autism S pectrum Disorders, 2271
Guide to US Foundations their Trustees, Officers and Donors, 3280
Guide to Wheelchair Sports and Recreation, 8230
Guide to the Selection of Musical Instruments, 29
Guided Tour for Persons 17 & Over with Developmental and Physical Challenges, 5529
Guidelines and Games for Teaching Efficient Braille Reading, 8963
Guidelines for Comprehensive Low Vision Care, 8964
Guidelines on Disability, 5084
Guideway, 9082
Guiding Eyes for the Blind, 8835, 8836
Guiding Eyes for the Blind: Breeding and Placement Center, 8836
Guild Briefs, 9083
Guild for the Blind, 4739
Guilford Press, 5023, 5292, 7713, 7714, 7741, 7759, 7812, 7829, 7849, 7850, 7851, 7852, 8501, 8506
Guilford Publication, 2278
Gulf Coast Independent Living Center, 4261
Gulf States Association of Homes and Servi ces for the Aging, 7460

H

H UD U SE R, 1890
H&R Block Foundation, 2989
H.E.L.P. Knife, 359
HAC Hearing Aid Centers of America: HARC Mercantile, 472
HANDYBAR, The, 93
HARC Mercantile, 76, 198, 202, 203, 204, 205, 211, 216, 221, 222, 223, 224, 226, 227, 230, 232, 233, 237, 240, 241, 242, 246, 247, 316, 323, 334, 335, 338, 339, 340, 341, 539, 540, 547, 630
HASL Independent Abilities Center, 4408
HCR Health Care Services, 6393
HCR Manor Care Foundation, 3116
HEAL: Health Education AIDS Liaison, 2028
HEALTH E-News, 2245
HEAR Center, 7918, 8095
HELP, 1694
HIV Infection and Developmental Disabilities, 2409
HKNC Newsletter, 7597
HRSA Information Center, 853
HSC Pediatric Center, The, 6722
HSI Austin Center For Development, 6841
Hacienda La Puente Unified School District, 6610
Hacienda Rehabilitation and Care Center, 7222
Hackett Hill Nursing Center and Integrated Care, 7035
Haldimand-Norfolk Resource Education and C ounseling, 854
Halifax Hospital Medical Center Eye Clinic Professional Center, 6749
Hall County Library: East Hall Branch and Special Needs Library, 4725

Hall-Perrine Foundation, 2907
Hallmarks and Features of High-Quality Community-Based Services, 4977
Halsted Terrace Nursing Center, 7275
Hamilton Adult Center, 7100
Hamilton Rehabilitation and Healthcare Center, 7240
Hammill Institute on Disabilities, 2092
Hampton VA Medical Center, 5770
Hand Brake Control Only, 94
Hand Dimmer Switch, 95
Hand Dimmer Switch with Horn Button, 96
Hand Gas & Brake Control, 97
Hand Operated Parking Brake, 98
Hand Parking Brake, 99
Handbook About Care in the Home, 5212
Handbook for Implementing Workshops for Siblings of Special Children, 2410
Handbook for Itinerant and Resource Teachers of Blind Students, 8965
Handbook for Speech Therapy, 2411
A Handbook for Writing Effective Psychoeducational Reports (2nd Edition), 7580
Handbook for the Special Education Administrator, 2412
Handbook of Acoustic Accessibility, 2413
Handbook of Adaptive Switches and Augmentative Communication Devices, 1695
Handbook of Assistive Devices for the Handicapped Elderly, 7508
Handbook of Autism and Pervasive Developmental Disorders, 7767
Handbook of Career Planning for Students with Special Needs, 6193
Handbook of Chronic Fatigue Syndrome, 8480
Handbook of Developmental Education, 2414
Handbook of Epilepsy, 8481
Handbook of Information for Members of the Achromatopsia Network, 8966
Handbook of Services for the Handicapped, 5085
Handbook on Ethnicity, Aging and Mental Health, 7509
Handbook on Supported Education for People with Mental Illness, 2415
Handi Camp, 1352
Handi Home Lift, 399
Handi Kids, 1178
Handi Lift, 400
Handi Prolift, 401
Handi Vangelism Ministries International, 1352
Handi-Lift, 385, 394, 399, 401, 409
Handi-Ramp, 402, 402
Handi-Works Productions, 6933
HandiWARE, 1696
Handicapped Driving Aids, 100
Handicapped Driving Aids of Michigan, 100
Handicapped Scuba Association, 8231
Handicapped Scuba Association International, 8231
Handicaps, 142
Handicaps, Inc., 101
Hands To Love, 1044
Hands-Free Controller, 5474
Handy-Helper Cutting Board, 360
Happiness Bag, 1099
Happiness Is Camping, 1249, 8389
Harbor House Law Press, 2093
Harborview Medical Center, 7200
Harborview Medical Center, Low Vision Aid Clinic, 7200
Harc Mercantile Ltd., 211
Hard Manufacturing Company, 190
Harden Foundation, 2763
Harlem Independent Living Center, 4352
Harmony Nursing and Rehabilitation Center, 7276
Harper Collins Publishers, 38, 8434, 8507
Harper Collins Publishers/Basic Books, 5088
Harper Collins Publishing, 7888
HarperCollins Publishers, 7986, 8023
Harriet & Robert Heilbrunn Guild School, 2671
Harriet McDaniel Marshall Trust in Memory of Sanders McDaniel, 2852
Harrington House Nursing And Rehabilitation Center, 6976
Harris Communicatin, 5323

Harris Communications, 337, 229, 337, 1957, 1993, 5311, 5312, 5322, 5324, 8015, 8030, 8041, 9019, 9129
Harris Methodist Fort Worth Hospital Mabee Rehabilitation Center, 6444
Harris Methodist Fort Worth/Mabee Rehabilitation Center, 7169
Harris and Eliza Kempner Fund, 3206
Harrison Center for the Arts, 6334
Harrison Health and Rehabilitation Centre, 7287
Harry C Moores Foundation, 3117
Harry S Truman Memorial Veterans' Hospital, 5669
Harry and Jeanette Weinberg Foundation, 2933
Hartford Foundation for Public Giving, 2812
Hartford Holidays, 5522
Hartford Insurance Group, 2813
Hartford Regional Office, 5592
Hartford Vet Center, 5593
Harvard University Howe Laboratory of Ophthalmology, 4805
Harvard University Press, 7757, 8036
Harvey Randall Wickes Foundation, 2966
Hasbro Children's Hospital Asthma Camp, 1364
Hausmann Industries, 6114
Havirmill Foundation, 2967
Hawaii Assistive Technology Training and, 3431
Hawaii Center For Independent Living, 4039
Hawaii Center for Independent Living-Maui, 4040
Hawaii Centers for Independent Living, 4041
Hawaii Community Foundation, 2861
Hawaii Department for Children With Special Needs, 3432
Hawaii Department of Education, 2122
Hawaii Department of Education: Special Needs, 2122
Hawaii Department of Health, Adult Mental Health Division, 3433
Hawaii Department of Human Serv, 3434
Hawaii Department of Human Services, 3434
Hawaii Disability Compensation Division Department of Labor and Industrial Relations, 3435
Hawaii Disability Rights Center, 3436
Hawaii Executive Office on Aging, 3437
Hawaii Fair Employment Practice Agency, 5955
Hawaii State Council on Developmental Disabilities, 3438
Hawaii State Library for the Blind and Physically Handicapped, 4734
Hawaii Vocational Rehabilitation Division, 5956
Haworth Press, 2201, 2207, 2255, 2289, 2366, 2394, 2397, 2408, 2474, 2480, 2506, 4607, 5046, 5108, 5169, 6384
Haym Salomon Home for The Aged, 7346
Head Injury Hotline, 8657
Head Injury Rehabilitation And Referral Service, Inc. (HIRRS), 8137
Head Injury Rehabilitation: Children, 2416
Head Injury Treatment Program at Dover, 6370
The Head's Up Foundation, 1088
Headlight Dimmer Switch, 102
Headliner Hats, 1467
Healing Dressing for Pressure Sores, 318
Healing Herbs, 5086
Health Action, 855
Health Alliance, 6400
Health Care Corporation of America, 6767
Health Care Financing Administration, 3295
Health Care Management in Physical Therapy, 2417
Health Care Professionals Who Are Blind or Visually Impaired, 8967
Health Care Quality Improvement Act of 1986, 4609
Health Care Solutions, 6414
Health Care for Students with Disabilities, 2418
Health Care of the Aged: Needs, Policies, and Services, 7510
Health Communications, 8591
Health KiCC, 3752
Health Promotion and Disease Prevention in Clinical Practice, 7511
Health Resource Center for Women with Disabilities, 856

Health Resources & Services Administration : State Bureau of Health, 3510
Health South Cane Creek Rehabilitation Center, 6430
Health South Corporation, 6337, 6430, 6606
Health South Corporation in Burmingham Alabama, 6754
Health South Corporation of Alabama, 6284
Health South Tustin Rehabilitation Hospita, 6247
Health South of Nittany Valley, 6416
Health and Rehabilitation Products, 473
Health and Wellfare, 3443
HealthCare Solutions, 474
HealthCraft SuperPole Traveller, 522
HealthQuest Subacute and Rehabilitation Programs, 6750
HealthSouth Central Georgia Rehabilitation Hospital, 6304
HealthSouth Chattanooga Rehabilitation Hospital, 6431
HealthSouth Corporation, 6503, 6274
HealthSouth Deaconess Rehabilitation Hospital, 6884
HealthSouth Emeral Coast Sports & Rehabilitation Center, 6751
HealthSouth Harmarville Rehabilitation Hospital, 6415
HealthSouth Hospital of Cypress, 7170
HealthSouth Lakeshore Rehabilitation Hospital, 6227
HealthSouth Mountain View Regional Rehab Hospital, 6483
HealthSouth Nittany Valley Rehabilitation Hospital, 6416
HealthSouth Northern Kentucky Rehabilitation Hospital, 6917
HealthSouth Plano Rehabilitation Hospital, 6445
HealthSouth Regional Rehab Center/Florida, 6280
HealthSouth Rehab Hospital Of Arlington, 6446
HealthSouth Rehab Hospital Of Austin, 6447
HealthSouth Rehab Hospital Of Erie, 6417
HealthSouth Rehab Hospital Of Utah, 6469
HealthSouth Rehab Hospital: Largo, 6281
HealthSouth Rehab Hospital: South Carolina, 6428
HealthSouth Rehabilitation Center of Humble Texas, 6448
HealthSouth Rehabilitation Center: New Mexico, 6381
HealthSouth Rehabilitation Cntr/Tennessee, 6432
HealthSouth Rehabilitation Hospital, 6233, 6376, 6449
HealthSouth Rehabilitation Hospital of Tallahassee, 6752
HealthSouth Rehabilitation Hospital Of Fort Smith, 6537
HealthSouth Rehabilitation Hospital Of Miami, 6753
HealthSouth Rehabilitation Hospital Of Western Massachusetts, 6977
HealthSouth Rehabilitation Hospital of Altoona, 6418
HealthSouth Rehabilitation Hospital of Beaumont, 6450
HealthSouth Rehabilitation Hospital of Colorado Springs, 6274
HealthSouth Rehabilitation Hospital of North Alabama, 6228
HealthSouth Rehabilitation Hospital of Sarasota, 6754
HealthSouth Rehabilitation Institute Of San Antonio (RIOSA), 6451
HealthSouth Rehabilitation of Louisville, 6339
HealthSouth Sea Pines Rehabilitation Hospital, 6755
HealthSouth Specialty Hospital Of North Louisiana, 6342
HealthSouth Sports Medicine & Rehabilitation Center, 6282
HealthSouth Sports Medicine Center, 6237
HealthSouth Sports Medicine and Rehabilitation Center, 6283
HealthSouth Treasure Coast Rehabilitation Hospital, 6284
HealthSouth Tustin Rehabilitation Hospital, 6606

HealthSouth Valley Of The Sun Rehabilitation Hospital, 6521
HealthSouth Western Hills Regional Rehab Hospital, 6484
Healthcare and Rehabilitation Center of Sanford, 7250
Healthline, 2246
Healthsouth Corporation, 6752
Healthsouth Rehab Institute of Tucson, 6238
Healthsouth Rehabilitation Hospital of Greater Pittsburgh, 6419
Healthsouth Rehabilitation Hospital of Mechanicsburg, 6420
Healthsouth Rehabilitation Hospital of York, 6421
Healthwin Specialized Care, 6885
Healthy Aging Association, 7461
Healthy Breathing, 8482
Hear You Are, 475
Hearing Aid Batteries, 338
Hearing Aid Battery Testers, 339
Hearing Aid Dehumidifier, 340
Hearing Center, 472
Hearing Education and Awareness for Rockers, 7919
Hearing Health Magazine, 8074
Hearing Impaired Children and Youth with Developmental Disabilities, 8021
Hearing Industries Association, 7920
Hearing Loss Association of America, 7567, 7921, 8075
Hearing Loss Magazine, 7588, 8075
Hearing Professional, 8066
Hearing Professional Magazine, 7589
Hearing, Speech & Deafness Center (HDSC), 496
Hearing, Speech & Deafness Center (HSDC), 8084, 8082, 8685, 8773
Hearing, Speech and Deafness Center (HSDC), 7922, 8685
HearingLoss Association of America, 7588
Hearst Foundations, 3059
Heart of the Mind, 8483
Heart to Heart, 8968
Heart to Heart Blind Childrens Center, Inc, 5333
Heartbreak of Being A Little Bit Blind, 8969
Hearth Day Treatment and Vocational Services, 6155
Heartland Opportunity Center, 5849
Heartspring, 6909
Heather Hill, 6394
Heather Hill Rehabilitation Hospital, 6394
Heightened Independence and Progress: Hack ensack, 4320
Heightened Independence and Progress: Jers ey City, 4321
Heights Hospital Rehab Unit, 7171
Heinz Endowments, 3144
Heldref Publications, 2206
Helen Bader Foundation, 3252
Helen Beebe Speech and Hearing Center, 5418
Helen K and Arthur E Johnson Foundation, 2804
Helen Keller International, 4862
Helen Keller National Center, 7597, 7598
Helen Keller National Center Newsletter, 8970
Helen Keller National Center for Deaf - Blind Youths And Adults, 4863
Helen Keller National Center for Deaf- Blind Youths And Adults, 5087, 7568
Helen Steiner Rice Foundation, 3118
Helen and Teacher: The Story of Helen & Anne Sullivan Macy, 7582
Helm Distributing, 675, 676
Help Newsletter, 2247
Helping Hands Fanlight Productions/Icarus Films, 5334
Helping Learning- Disabled Gifted Children Learn Through Compensatory Active Play, 2419
Helping People with Autism Manage Their Behavior, 7768
Helping Students Grow, 2420
Helping Your Child with Attention-Deficit Hyperactivity Disorder, 7769
Helping Your Hyperactive: Attention Deficit Child, 7770
Helping the Family Understand, 8112

Helping the Visually Impaired Child with Developmental Problems, 8971
Hemisphere Publishing Corporation, 2211
The Hemispherectomy Foundation, 7654
Hemophilia Association, 954, 8344
Hemophilia Camp, 1277, 8390
Henkind Eye Institute Division of Montefiore Hospital, 7065
Henry Ford Health System, 7011
Henry J Kaiser Family Foundation, 2764
Henry L Hillman Foundation, 3145
Henry Nias Foundation, 2814
Henry W Bull Foundation, 2765
Henry and Lucy Moses Fund, 3060
Hepatitis Sourcebook, 8484
Herb Research Foundation, 5419
Herbert W Hoover Foundation, 3119
Heritage Health and Rehabilitation Center, 7415
Herman Goldman Foundation, 3061
Herpes Resource Center, 8270
Herrick Health Sciences Library, 4676
Hi-Desert Medical Center, 6607
HiRider, 713
Hidden Child: The Linwood Method for Reaching the Autistic Child, 7771
Hig's Manufacturing, 476
High Country Council of Governments Area A gency on Aging, 7550
High Profile Single Compartment Cushion, 281
High School Senior's Guide to Merit and Ot her No-Need Funding, 3281
High School Students Guide to Study, Travel, and Adventure Abroad, 2704
High Tech Center, 1575
High-Low Chair, 260
Highbrook Lodge, 1310, 8891
Highland Pines Rehabilitation Center, 7251
Highland Unlimited Business Enterprises of CRI, 6156
Highlighter and Note Tape, 619
Hilcrest Medical Center: Kaiser Rehab Cent er, 6402
Hill School of Fort Worth, 1397, 7686
Hillcrest Baptist Medical Center, 7172
Hillcrest Baptist Medical Center: Rehab Care Unit, 6452
Hillcrest Foundation, 3207
Hillcroft Services: Isanogel, 1084, 1102, 8159
Hillhaven Rehabilitation, 6797
Hillsborough County Talking Book Library Tampa-Hillsborough County Public Library, 4705
Hilo Vet Center, 5614
Hip Function & Ambulation, 8485
Hiring Idahoans with Disabilities, 5297
His & Hers, 1481
History and Use of Braille, 8972
Hitchcock Rehabilitation Center, 7150
Hoblitzelle Foundation, 3208
Hockanum Greenhouse, 6703
Hockanum Industry, 6703
Hoffmann + Krippner Inc., 1633
A Hole In The Wall Camp, 1272
Hole in the Wall Gang Camp, 1026, 8391
Holiday Inn Boxborough Woods, 6978
Holiday Lake 4-H Educational Center, 1418
Hollister Workshop, 5850
Hollywood Speaks: Deafness and the Film En tertainment Industry, 8022
Holston Conference of United Methodist Church, 1415
Holt Paperbacks (Macmillan Publishers), 5270
Holy Cross Comprehensive Rehabilitation Center, 6248
Holy Cross Hospital, 6756
Holzer Clinic, 7101
Holzer Clinic Sycamore, 7102
Holzer Medical Center, 7102
Home Bed Side Helper, 523
Home Health Care Provider: A Guide to Esse ntial Skills, 2421
Home is in the Heart: Accommodating People with Disabilities in the Homestay Experience, 5335
Home of the Guiding Hands, 6608

HomeCare Magazine, 2194
Homelink, 6892
Homemade Battery-Powered Toys, 1944
Homeopathic Educational Services, 857
The Homestead Group Administrative Offices, 3163
Homestead Healthcare and Rehabilitation Ce nter, 7327
Homewaiter, 403
Honolulu VBA Regional Office, 5615
Hooleon Corp, 1521
Hooleon Corporation, 1549, 1543, 1552, 1610
Hoosier Burn Camp, 1100
Hope Center, 5885
Hope Community Resources, 3878
Hope Haven, 4112
Hope Network, 6999
Hope Network Rehabilitation Services, 6999
Hope Rehabilitation Services, 5850
Horace A Kimball and S Ella Kimball Foundation, 3168
Horcher Lifting Systems, 404
Horizon Publishers & Distributors, 7501
Horizon Rehabilitation Center, 6388
Horizons for the Blind, 4740, 8837
Horizontal Steering, 103
Horn Control Switch, 104
Hornch Lifting Systems, 404
Hospice Alternative, 5088
Hospital Audiences, 1888
Hospital Environmental Control System, 524
Hospital For Special Care (HSC), 7241
Hospital of the Good Samaritan Acute Rehabilitation Unit, 6609
Hospitality Nursing Rehabilitation Center, 7426
Hospitalized Veterans Writing Project, 5559
Hostelling International, 5530
Hostelling North America, 5530
House Ear Institute, 7923
Housing Unlimited, 4189
Housing and Transportation of the Handicapped, 4610
Houston Center for Independent Living, 4473
Houston Endowment, 3209
Houston Public Library: Access Center, 4911
Houston Regional Office, 5760
How Come You Walk Funny?, 8215
How Difficult Can This Be ? (Fat City) Rick Lavoie, 5336
How To Reach and Teach Children and Teens with Dyslexia, 7772
How We Play Fanlight Productions/Icarus Films, 5337
How to Conduct an Assessment, 2611
How to Cope with ADHD: Diagnosis, Treatment & Myths, 7861
How to Deal with Back Pain and Rheumatoid Joint Pain: A Preventive and Self Treatment Manua, 8177
How to File a Title III Complaint, 5089
How to Live Longer with a Disability, 5090
How to Own and Operate an Attention Deficit Disorder, 7773
How to Pay for Your Degree in Business & Related Fields, 3282
How to Pay for Your Degree in Education & Related Fields, 3283
How to Read for Everyday Living, 1780
How to Teach Spelling/How to Spell, 2422
How to Thrive, Not Just Survive, 8973
How to Write for Everyday Living, 1697
Howard Heinz Endowment, 3144
Howard School, The, 2672
Howard University Child Development Center, 6723
Hub, 8974
Hugh J Andersen Foundation, 2976
Hull Park, 1329
Human Ecology Action League (HEAL), 858
Human Exceptionality: School, Community, and Family (12th Edition), 2423, 4978
Human Kinetics, 2172, 5192, 8178, 8183
Human Kinetics, Inc., 8166, 8172, 8173
Human Resource Management and the Americans with Disabilities Act, 4611

Human Rights Commission, 6191
Human Sciences Press, 2485, 7799, 8750, 9018
Human Services Building, 3554
Human Ware, 1627
Humana Hospital: Morristown RehabCare, 7152
Hunter Holmes McGuire VA Medical Center, 5771
Hunter House, 8505, 8520
Hunter House Inc. Publisher, 8594
Hunter House Publishers, Inc, 1569
Huntington Health and Rehabilitation Cente r, 7391
Huntington Regional Office, 5779
Huntington VA Medical Center, 5780
Huntleigh Healthcare, 477
Huntsville Subregional Library for the Blind &
   Physically Handicapped, 4650
Huntsville-Madison County Public Library, 4650
Hutchinson Community Foundation, 2912
Hyams Foundation, 2951
Hyde Park-Woodlawn, 6842
Hydrocephalus: A Guide for Patients, Families &
   Friends, 8486
Hyperactive Child, Adolescent, and Adult: ADD
   Through the Lifespan, 7774
Hyperactivity, Attention Deficits, and School
   Failure: Better Ways, 7775
Hyperion, 7793
Hypertension Sourcebook, 8487
Hypokalemic Periodic Paralysis Resource Page,
   5420

I

I Can't Hear You in the Dark: How to Lean and
   Teach Lipreading, 2424
I ET Resources, 1666
I Have a Sister, My Sister is Deaf, 8023
I Heard That!, 2425
I Heard That!2, 2426
I Just Want My Little Boy Back, 7862, 8786
I KNOW American History, 1698
I KNOW American History Overlay CD, 1699
I Wonder Who Else Can Help, 2195
I'm Not Disabled Landmark Media, Inc., 5338
IAAIS Report, 9084
IAL News, 8621
IBM Corporation, 2853
IBM National Support Center, 5951
IDEAMATICS, 212
IDF National Conference, 1858
IKRON Institute for Rehabilitative and
   Psychological Services, 7103
IN-SIGHT Independent Living, 4442
IN-SOURCE, 6320
INCLUDEnyc, 5421
IOS Press, 4980, 4988
IPACHI, 3392
IRET Corporate Services Division, 6138
ISC, 5134
Iberville Association for Retarded Citizens, 6934
Icon Group International, 8539, 8540, 8541, 8542,
   8543, 8544, 8545, 8546, 8547, 8548
Idaho Assistive Technology Project, 1576, 1945,
   4735, 2309, 4951, 4952, 5193, 5297, 7500, 7718
Idaho Commission for Libraries: Talking Book
   Service, 4736
Idaho Commission for the Blind & Visually
   Impaired, 5964
Idaho Commission for the Blind and Visually
   Impaired, 7569
Idaho Commission on Aging, 3442
Idaho Council on Developmental Disabilities,
   3443
Idaho Council on Developmental Disabilities, 5185
Idaho Department of Employment, 5960
Idaho Department of Handicapped Children, 3444
Idaho Disability Determinations Service, 3445
Idaho Elks Rehabilitation Hospital, 6808
Idaho Employment Service and Job Training
   Program Liaison, 5960
Idaho Fair Employment Practice Agency, 5961
Idaho Falls Office: Living Independently for
   Everyone (LIFE), 4048
Idaho Governor's Committee on Employment of
   People with Disabilities, 5962

Idaho Human Rights Commission, 5961
Idaho Industrial Commission, 3446
Idaho Mental Health Center, 3447
Idaho Vocational Rehabilitation Agency, 5963
Ideal-Phone, 212
Ideas for Easy Travel, 5491
Ideas for Kids on the Go, 5091
Ideas for Making Your Home Accessible, 1898
If Blindness Comes, 8975
If Blindness Strikes Don't Strike Out, 8976
If I Only Knew What to Say or Do, 5092
If It Is To Be, It Is Up To Me To Do It!, 1946
If It Is To Be, It Is Up To Us To Help!, 2427
If it Weren't for the Honor: I'd Rather Have
   Walked, 5093
Illinois Assistive Technology Project, 3454
Illinois Center for Autism, 6843
Illinois Council on Developmental Disability,
   3455
Illinois Department of Mental Health and
   Developmental Disabilities, 3456
Illinois Department of Rehab Services, 4063
Illinois Department of Rehabilitation, 3457
Illinois Department on Aging, 3458
Illinois Early Childhood Intervention
   Clearinghouse, 4741
Illinois Employment Service, 5972
Illinois Fire Safety Alliance, 1069
The Illinois Life Span Project, 2867
Illinois Machine Sub-Lending Agency, 4742
Illinois Regional Library for the Blind and
   Physically Handicapped, 4743
Illinois State Board of Education, 3449
Illinois State Board of Education: Department of
   Special Education, 2123
Illinois Valley Center for Independent Living,
   4064
Illinois and Iowa Center for Independent L iving,
   4065
IlluminAge Communications Partners, 7497
Imagery Procedures for People with Special
   Needs, 5339
Imagery in Healing Shamanism and Modern
   Medicine, 5094
Images of the Disabled, Disabling Images, 2428
Imagine!, 7835, 7835
Imagine: Innovative Resources for Cognitive &
   Physical Challenges, 5886
Imagining the Possibilities: Creative Approaches
   to Orientation and Mobility Instructio, 8977
Immune Deficiency Foundation, 1858
Immune System Disorders Sourcebook., 8488
Imp Tricycle, 734
Impact Center for Independent Living, 4066
Impact: Ocala Vocational Services, 5932
Imperial, 7277
Implementing Family-Centered Services in Early
   Intervention, 2429
In Search of Wings: A Journey Back from T
   raumatic Brain Injury, 7776
In Their Own Way, 7777
In Time and with Love: Caring for the Spec ial
   Needs Infant and Toddler, 5266
In Touch Systems, 1617, 1618
In the Ear Hearing Aid Battery Extractor, 341
In the Middle, 8640
In-Definite Arts Society, 30
In-Home Medical Care, 6798
In-Sight, 7147
InFocus, 1626, 7591
inMotion Magazine, 5294
Incite Learning Series, 1700
Inclinator Company of America, 377, 403, 405,
   425, 428
Inclinette, 405
Include Us, 5340
Including All of Us: An Early Childhood
   Curriculum About Disability, 2430
Including Students with Severe and Multiple
   Disabilites in Typical Classrooms, 2431
Including Students with Special Needs: A Practical
   Guide for Classroom Teachers, 2432
Inclusion, 2196

Inclusive & Heterogeneous Schooling:
   Assessment, Curriculum, and Instruction, 2433,
   2612
Inclusive Games, 8178
Inclusive Leisure Services (3rd Edition), 4979
Inclusive Play People, 1947
Increasing Capabilities Access, 3342
Increasing Capabilities Access Network, 1577
Increasing Literacy Levels: Final Report, 8978
Increasing and Decreasing Behaviors of Per sons
   with Severe Retardation and Autism, 2066, 7778
Independence, 4123, 5095
Independence Associates, 4203
Independence CIL, 5152
Independence Council for Economic
   Development, 4564
Independence Empowerment Center, 4513
Independence First, 4539
Independence First: West Bend, 4540
Independence Northwest Center for Independent
   Living, 3987
Independence Now, 4190
Independence Now: Silver Spring, 4191
Independence Place, 4170
Independence Resource Center, 4514
Independence Unlimited, 3988
Independence Without Sight and Sound:
   Suggestions for Practitioners, 7583
Independence Without Sight or Sound, 8024
Independent Connection, 4124
Independent Connection: Abilene, 4125
Independent Connection: Beloit, 4126
Independent Connection: Concordia, 4127
Independent Driving Systems, 406
Independent Life Center, 3978
Independent Life Styles, 4474
Independent Living, 3991, 4353
Independent Living Aids, 163, 177, 210, 563, 564,
   567, 568, 620, 621, 625, 628, 634, 639, 640
Independent Living Approach to Disability Policy
   Studies, 2434
Independent Living Center Network: Department
   of the Visually Handicapped, 4515
Independent Living Center of Eastern Indiana
   (ILCEIN), 4101
Independent Living Center of Kern County, 3939
Independent Living Center of Lancaster, 3940
Independent Living Center of Mobile, 3868
Independent Living Center of Southeast Missouri,
   4276
Independent Living Center of Stavros: Gree nfield,
   4204
Independent Living Center of Stavros: Spri ngfield,
   4205
Independent Living Center of the North Sho re &
   Cape Ann, 4206
Independent Living Centers and Managed Care:
   Results of an ILRU Study on Involvement, 5096
Independent Living Challenges the Blues, 5097
Independent Living Office, 5098, 4167
Independent Living Research Utilization, 5104
Independent Living Research Utilization Project,
   4475
Independent Living Research Utilization (ILRU),
   4977
Independent Living Research Utilization ILRU,
   4575, 5004, 5007, 5009, 5055, 5056, 5062,
   5079, 5096, 5097, 5117, 5146, 5147, 5148,
   5150, 5181, 5189, 5222, 8045
Independent Living Resource Center, 3941, 4128
Independent Living Resource Center: Santa
   Barbara, 3942
Independent Living Resource Center: San Fr
   ancisco, 3943
Independent Living Resource Center: Santa Maria
   Office, 3944
Independent Living Resource Center: Ventur a,
   3945
Independent Living Resource of Contra Coast,
   3946
Independent Living Resource of Fairfield, 3947
Independent Living Resource: Antioch, 3948
Independent Living Resource: Concord, 3949
Independent Living Resources, 4409
Independent Living Resources (ILR), 3950

Independent Living Resources Of Greater Birmingham: Alabaster, 3869
Independent Living Resources of Greater Birmingham: Jasper, 3870
Independent Living Resources of Greater Birmingham, 3871
Independent Living Service Northern California: Redding Office, 3951
Independent Living Services of Northern California, 3952
Independent Living for Persons with Disabilities and Elderly People, 4980
Independent Living for Physically Disabled People, 4981
Independent Mobility Systems, 129
Independent Newsletter, 5099
Independent Resource Georgetown, 3992
Independent Resources: Dover, 3993
Independent Resources: Wilmington, 3994
Independent Visually Impaired Enterprisers, 8838
Indian Acres Camp for Boys, 1143, 7687
Indian Creek Camp, 1381, 8892
Indian Creek Health and Rehabilitation Center, 7288
Indian Creek Nursing Center, 6910
Indian Rivers Mental Health Center - Bibb, 6504
Indian Rivers Mental Health Center - Pickens, 6505
Indian Rivers Mental Health Center - Tuscaloosa, 6506
Indian Summer Camp, 1123
Indian Trails Camp, 1193
Indiana Association of Homes and Services for the Aging, 7462
Indiana Children's Deaf Camp, 1101
Indiana Civil Rights Commission, 6000
Indiana Client Assistance Program, 3462
Indiana Congress of Parent and Teachers, 6321
Indiana Deaf Camps Foundation, 1089, 7953
The Indiana Deaf Camps Foundation, Inc., 1101
Indiana Department of Education, 2124, 6328
Indiana Department of Education: Special Education Division, 2124
Indiana Developmental Disability Council, 3463
Indiana Directory of Disability Resources, 2067
Indiana Employment Services and Job Training Program Liaison, 6001
Indiana Hemophilia And Thrombosis Center, 1090
Indiana Protection & Advocacy Services Commission, 3464
Indiana Protection and Advocacy Services Commission, 6322
Indiana Resource Center For Autism, 7768, 7785, 7808, 8742, 8756
Indiana Resource Center for Autism, 4754
Indiana Resource Center for Families with Special, 6320
Indiana State Commission for the Handicapped, 3465
Indiana State Department of Health, 6329
Indiana University, 1085
Indiana University: Multipurpose Arthritis Center, 4755
Indianapolis Regional Office, 5623
Indianapolis Resource Center for Independent Living, 4102
Individualized Keyboarding, 1948
Industrial Accident Board de dept, 3388
Industrial Support Systems, 6597
Industries for the Blind of New York State, 7066
Industries of the Blind, 7078
Industries: Cambridge, 7012
Industries: Mora, 7013
Infant & Toddler Convection of Fairfield: Falls Church, 2613
Infinity Dance Theater, 31
Infirmary Health, 6229
Inflatable Back Pillow, 282
Infobase Publishing, 1811
Infogrip: AdjustaCart, 555
Infogrip: BAT Personal Keyboard, 556
Infogrip: King Keyboard, 1611
Infogrip: Large Print Keyboard, 1612

Infogrip: Large Print/Braille Keyboard Labels, 1550
Infogrip: OnScreen, 1613
Informa Healthcare, 5057
Information & Referral Center, 2435
Information & Referral Services, 1645
Information + Referral Services, 1645
Information Access Project, 8979
Information Hotline, 8243
Information Service, 8694
Information Services for People with Developmental Disabilities, 5100
Information from HEATH Resource Center, 2094
Information on Glaucoma, 8980
Information, Protection & Advocacy for Persons with Disabilities, 3392
Information, Protection and Advocacy Center for Handicapped Individuals, 3393
Informed Touch; A Clinician's Guide To The Evaluation Of Myofascial Disorders, 8489
Informer, 8622
Ingham Regional Medical Center, 4812
Injured Mind, Shattered Dreams: Brian's Survival from a Severe Head Injury, 8490
Inland NorthWest Health Services, 1425, 8336
Inland Northwest Community Foundation, 3238
Innabah Camps, 1353
Inner Traditions, 5017, 5025, 8514, 8522
Inner Traditions - Bear & Company, 8167
Inner Traditions/Bear And Company, 8489
Innerlip Plates, 361
Innovation Management Group, 1701, 5422
Innovations, 7541
Innovative Industries, 6014
Innovative Practices for Teaching Sign Language Interpreters, 8025
Innovative Products, 714
Innovative Programs: An Example of How CILs Can Put Their Work in Context, 5101
Innovative Rehabilitation Services, 6610
Innoventions, 632
Inova Mount Vernon Hospital Rehabilitation Program, 6476
Inova Rehabilitation Center, 6476
Inpatient Pain Rehabilitation Program, 7067
Inside The Halo and Beyond: The Anatomy of a Recovery, 8179
Insight, 9085, 9116
Insights, 2248
Inspiration Ministries, 4541
Institute For Rehabilitation & Research, 4475
Institute On Disability/UCED, 6230
Institute for Basic Research in Developmental Disabilities, 4864
Institute for Families, 8839
Institute for Human Centered Design, 1879
Institute for Human Development, 3567, 6522
Institute for Rehab., Research, & Recreation Inc, 1330, 8711
Institute for Rehabilitation & Research, 6453, 7173
Institute for Scientific Research, 859
Institute for Visual Sciences, 4865
Institute of Living: Hartford Hospital, 2369
Institute of Physical Medicine and Rehabilitation, 6311
Institute of Transpersonal Psychology, 860
Institute on Aging, 7551
Institute on Disabilities At Temple Univ., 4429
Institute on Disability, 2148
Instruction of Persons with Severe Handicaps, 1949
Instructional Methods for Students, 2436
Instrumental Music for Dyslexics: A Teaching Handbook, 32
Insurance Solutions: Plan Well, Live Better, 5102
Int'l Association of Audio Information Services, 9084
Integrated Health Services at Waterford Commons, 7104
Integrated Health Services of Amarillo, 7174
Integrated Health Services of Durham, 6389
Integrated Health Services of Michigan at Clarkston, 6360
Integrated Health Services of Seattle, 7201

Integrated Health Services of St. Louis at Gravois, 7020
Intellectual and Developmental Disabilities, 2197
Intelli Tools, 1614, 1615, 1620, 1702, 1822, 1825
IntelliKeys, 213, 1614
IntelliKeys USB, 1615
IntelliPics Studio 3, 1702
IntelliTalk, 1822
IntelliTools, 213
Intensive Early Intervention and Beyond, 5341
Interact Center, 33
Interact Center for the Visual and Performing Arts, 33
Interactions: Collaboration Skills for School Professionals, 2437
Interdisciplinary Clinical Assessment of Young Children with Developmental Disabilities, 8491
An Interdisciplinary Journal for the Social Study of Health, Illness and Medicine, 5015
Intermediate Conversational Sign Language, 8026
International Academy of Biological Dentistry and Medicine, 8271
International Academy of Oral Medicine & Toxicology, 8272
International Association for Cancer Victors & Friends, 8273
International Association of Audio Information Services (IAAIS), 8840
International Association of Hygienic Physicians, 8274
International Association of Laryngectomees, 8621
International Association of Machinists, 861
International Association of Parents and Professionals for Safe Alternatives in Childbirth, 2029
International Association of Yoga Therapists, 862
International Braille and Technology Center for the Blind, 8658
International Catholic Deaf Association, 7924, 8083
International Center for the Disabled, 1578
International Childbirth Education Association, 2030
International Chiropractors Association, 863
International Christian Youth Exchange, 2705
International Clinic of Biological Regeneration, 864
International Cluttering Association, 8686
International Directory of Libraries for the Disabled, 5103
International Dyslexia Association, 2031, 3511, 3547, 3635, 3708, 7801, 7825, 8740, 8752
International Dyslexia Association of DC, 3394
International Dyslexia Association of NY: Buffalo Branch, 3638
International Dyslexia Association of New England, 3521
International Dyslexia Association: Arizona Branch, 3338
International Dyslexia Association: Austin Branch, 3775
International Dyslexia Association: Central California Branch, 3358
International Dyslexia Association: Central Ohio Branch, 3689
International Dyslexia Association: Florida Branch, 3411
International Dyslexia Association: Georgia Branch, 3425
International Dyslexia Association: Hawaii Branch, 3439
International Dyslexia Association: Illinois Branch, 3459
International Dyslexia Association: Indiana Branch, 3466
International Dyslexia Association: Kansas/West Missouri Branch, 3479
International Dyslexia Association: Maryland Branch, 3511
International Dyslexia Association: Minnesota Branch, 3547
International Dyslexia Association: Mississippi Branch, 3559

International Dyslexia Association: Nebraska Branch, 3583
International Dyslexia Association: Oregon Branch, 3708
International Dyslexia Association: Pennsylvania Branch, 3717
International Dyslexia Association: Rocky Mountain Branch, 3372
International Dyslexia Association: Tennessee Branch, 3759
International Dyslexia Association: Virginia Branch, 3821
International Dyslexia Association: Washington State Branch, 3831
International Dyslexia Association: Wisconsin Branch, 3852
International Dyslexia Association: Iowa Branch, 3468
International Dyslexia Association: New Jersey Branch, 3617
International Dyslexia Association: North Carolina Branch, 3671
International Education, 2699
International Fluency Association, 8687, 8768
International Handbook on Mental Health Policy, 4612
International Hearing Dog, 7925, 8089
International Hearing Society, 7570, 7926, 7589, 8066
International Journal of Arts Medicine, 2438
International Medical and Dental Hypnotherapy Association, 8275
International Myeloma Foundation, 8276
International Organization for the Education of the Hearing Impaired, 2032
International Paper Company Foundation, 3186
International Parkinson and Movement Disorder Society, 7879, 8138
International Partnership for Service-Learning and Leadership, 2706
International Rehabilitation Review, 2198
International Rolf Institute, 2249
International Student Exchange Programs (I SEP), 2707
International University Partnerships, 2708
International Ventilator Users Network, 8611
International Women's Health Coalition, 865
Interpretation: A Sociolinguistic Model, 8027
Interpreting Disability: A Qualitative Reader, 2439
Interpreting: An Introduction, 8028
Interstitial Cystitis Association, 5423
Intervention Practices in the Retention of Competitive Employment, 8981
Intervention Research in Learning Disabilities, 2440
Intervention in School and Clinic, 2199
Introduction to Learning Disabilities, 2441
Introduction to Mental Retardation, 2442
Introduction to Special Education: Teaching in an Age of Challenge, 4th Edition, 2443
Introduction to Spina Bifida, 8492
Introduction to the Profession of Counseling, 2444
Invacare Corporation, 319, 478, 423, 580, 724
Invacare Fulfillment Center, 580
Invacare IVC Tracer EX2 Wheelchair with Le grest, 748
Invacare Lynx L-3 Scooter, 581
Invacare Top End, 757
Invacare Top End Excelerator XLT Gold Hand cyle, 758
Invisible Children, 5342
Invisible Disabilities Association, 866
InvoTek, Inc., 1519
Iowa Association of Homes & Services for the Aging, 7539
Iowa Association of Homes and Services for the Aging, 7463
Iowa Central Industries, 6893
Iowa Child Health Specialty Clinics, 3469
Iowa City VA Medical Center, 5629
Iowa Civil Rights Commission, 6015
Iowa Commission of Persons with Disabilities, 3470
Iowa Compass, 3471
Iowa Conference United Methodist, 1114

Iowa Department for the Blind, 3472
Iowa Department for the Blind Library, 4760
Iowa Department of Economic Development, 6017
Iowa Department of Human Services, 3473
Iowa Department of Public Instruction: Bureau of Special Education, 2125
Iowa Department on Aging, 3474
Iowa Employment Service, 6016
Iowa Job Training Program Liaison, 6017
Iowa Protection & Advocacy for the Disabled, 3475
Iowa Registry for Congenital and Inherited Disorders, 4761
Iowa Valley Community College, 6018
Iowa Vocational Rehabilitation Services, 6019
Iredell Vocational Workshop, 6141
Iris Network for the Blind, 6945
Iron Horse Productions, 731
Iron Mountain VA Medical Center, 5658
Irvine Health Foundation, 2766
Irving Place Rehabilitation and Nursing Ce nter, 7304
Issues and Research in Special Education, 2445
Issues in Independent Living, 5104
It isn't Fair!: Siblings of Children with Disabilities, 4957
It's All in Your Head: The Link Between Mercury Amalgams and Illness, 8493
It's Just Attention Disorder, 7863

J

J E Stewart Teaching Tools, 1975
J.L. Bedsole/Rotary Rehabilitation Hospita l, 6229
JADARA, 8067
JAMA: The Journal of the American Medical Association, 5105
JARC, 4232
JBI Voice, 9060
JCIL Advocate Times, 5106
JCYS Camp Red Leaf, 1074
JE Stewart Teaching Tools, 1766, 1920, 1925, 1938, 1974, 1982, 2014
JFK Johnson Rehab Institute, 6377
JGB Audio Library for the Blind, 2048, 2671
JGB Cassette Library International, 4866
JOBS Administration Job Opportunities & Basic Skills, 5824
JOBS VI and SAGE, 6135
Jack C. Montgomery VA Medical Center, 5724
Jack C. Montomery VA Medical Center, 5725
Jackson Center for Independent Living, 4462, 5106
Jackson Cervipillo, 191
Jackson Foundation, 3135
Jackson Independent Living Center, 4262
Jackson Regional Office, 5668
Jackson Square Nursing and Rehabilitation Center, 7278
Jacksonville Area CIL: Havana, 4067
Jacksonville Area Center for Independent Living, 4068
Jacksonville Public Library: Talking Books /Special Needs, 4706
Jacob and Charlotte Lehrman Foundation, 2826
James A Haley VA Medical Center, 5605
James Branch Cabell Library, 4924
James E Van Zandt VA Medical Center, 5736
James H And Cecile C Quillen Rehabilitation Hospital, 6433
James L. Maher Center, 3169
James Lawrence Kernan Hospital, 6953
James R Thorpe Foundation, 2977
James S McDonnell Foundation, 2990
Jane Coffin Childs Memorial Fund for Medical Research, 2815
Jane Phillips Medical Center, 6403, 7121, 6403
Janus of Santa Cruz, 6611
Jason & Nordic Publishers, Inc., 5107
Jason Aronson, 7756, 7806, 8737, 8754
Jawonio, 3639
Jawonio Vocational Center, 3640
Jay and Rose Phillips Family Foundation, 2978
Jefferson Industries, 275, 276, 295
Jefferson Lee Ford III Memorial Foundation, 2841

Jelly Bean Switch, 1520
Jennifer Roberts Building, 3952
Jeremy P Tarcher, 5072
Jerry L Pettis Memorial VA Medical Center, 5576
Jersey Cape Diagnostic Training & Opportunity Center, 6115
Jessica Kingsley Publishers, 42, 43, 59, 4983, 4984, 4985, 5238, 7803, 8736, 8747
Jessie Ball duPont Fund, 2842
Jet 3 Ultra Power Wheelchair, 749
Jewish Braille Institute International, 8841
Jewish Braille Institute of America, 9060, 9061
Jewish Braille Review, 9061
Jewish Community Center, 1151
Jewish Community Center of Greater Columbus, 1311
Jewish Community Center of Greater Rochester/JCC, 1266, 7673, 8708
Jewish Community Center of Greater Washington, 1149
Jewish Council for Youth Services, 1074
Jewish Guild for the Blind, 2033
Jewish Healthcare Foundation of Pittsburgh, 3146
Jewish Hospital of St. Louis: Department of Rehabilitation, 6364
Jewish Vocational Service of Jewish Family and Children's Services, 6068
Jewish Vocational Services, 5973
Jim Thorpe Rehabilitation Center at Southwest Medical Center, 6404
JoDavies Workshop, 5974
Job Accommodation Network, 867, 2034
The Job Developer's Handbook: Practical Ta ctics for Customized Employment, 4989
Job Hunting Tips for the So-Called Handicapped, 6249
Job Opportunities for the Blind, 6046
Job Service North Dakota, 6151
Job Success for Persons with Developmental Disabilities, 4985
Job Training Program Liaison: California, 5851
JobWorks NISH Food Service, 5933
JobWorks NISH Postal Service, 5934
Jobri, 283
Joey Interior Platform Lift, 407
John C Lincoln Hospital North Mountain, 6523
John D Dingell VA Medical Center, 5659
John D and Catherine T MacArthur Foundation, 2882
John Edward Fowler Memorial Foundation, 2827
John F. Blair Publishing, 2338
John G & Marie Stella Kennedy Memorial Foundation, 3210
John H and Ethel G Nobel Charitable Trust, 2816
John H and Wilhelmina D Harland Charitable Foundation, 2854
John Hopkins Bayview Medical Center, 1155
John Hopkins Hospital, 1154
John Hopkins University Press, 8566
John J Pershing VA Medical Center, 5670
John L McClellan Memorial Hospital, 5574
John Muir Medical Center Rehabilitation Services, Therapy Center, 6612
John O Pastore Center, 3734
John Randolph Foundation, 3229
John S Dunn Research Foundation, 3211
John Tracy Clinic, 8087
John W Anderson Foundation, 2905
John Wiley & Sons, 8480, 8517, 8582
John Wiley & Sons Inc, 7789
Johns Hopkins Hospital, 8368
Johns Hopkins University Dana Center for Preventive Ophthalmology, 4787
Johns Hopkins University Press, 5290, 7792, 8425, 8530, 8746
Johns Hopkins University: Asthma and Allergy Center, 4788
Johns Hopkins Universty Press, 8479
Johnson Controls Foundation, 3253
Johnson County Developmental Supports, 6911
Johnston County Industries, 7079
Joint Conference with ABMPP Annual Conference, 1859
Joint Efforts, 8198

Jonathan M Wainwright Memorial VA Medical Center, 5775
Joni and Friends, 868
Joseph Drown Foundation, 2767
Joseph P Kennedy Jr Foundation, 2828
Joseph Willard Health Center, 2613
Joslin Diabetes Center, 8494
Joslin Guide to Diabetes: A Program for Managing Your Treatment, 8494
Jossey-Bass, 7712, 7772
Journal for Vocational Special Needs Education, 2200
Journal of Applied School Psychology, 2201
Journal of Cognitive Rehabilitation, 7826
Journal of Counseling & Development, 2202
Journal of Disability & Religion, 5267
Journal of Disability Policy Studies, 2203
Journal of Emotional and Behavioral Disorders, 2204
Journal of Head Trauma Rehabilitation, 8601
Journal of Learning Disabilities, 2205
Journal of Motor Behavior, 2206
Journal of Musculoskeletal Pain, 2207
Journal of Positive Behavior Interventions, 2208
Journal of Postsecondary Education & Disability, 2209
Journal of Prosthetics and Orthotics, 2210
Journal of Public Health, 5284
Journal of Reading, Writing and Learning Disabled International, 2211
Journal of School Health Association, 2212
Journal of Social Work in Disabilty & Rehabilitation, 5108
Journal of Special Education, 2213
Journal of Speech, Language and Hearing Re search, 8068, 8767
Journal of Visual Impairment and Blindness, 9053
Journal of Vocational Behavior, 2214
Journal of the Academy of Rehabilitative A udiology, 8069
Journey, 7602
Journey to Well: Learning to Live After S pinal Cord Injury, 8495
Joy of Signing, 8029
Joy of Signing Puzzle Book, 8030
Joy: A Shabazz Center for Independent Living, 4378
Joystick Driving Control, 105
Judevine Center for Autism, 4839
Judge David L Bazelon Center for Mental Health Law, 4565
Judson Press, 5269
Juggler, 9122
Juliet L Hillman Simonds Foundation, 3147
Julius and Betty Levinson Center, 6844
Jumpin' Johnny Get Back to Work, A Child's Guide to ADHD/Hyperactivity, 7779
Jumpsuits, 1491
Junction Center for Independent Living, 4516
Junction Center for Independent Living: Du ffield, 4517
Junior Blind of America, 2768, 966
Junior League Of Little Rock, 961
Jupiter Medical Center-Pavilion, 7252
Just Like Everyone Else, 5109
Just One Break (JOBS), 6136
Juvenile Diabetes Research Foundation International, 869

K

The K&W Guide to Colleges for Students with Learning Disabilties (13th Edition), 2567
K-BIT: Kaufman Brief Intelligence Test, 2614
K-FAST: Kaufman Functional Academic Skills Test, 2615
K-SEALS: Kaufman Survey of Early Academic and Language Skills, 2616
KG Saur/Division of RR Bowker, 5103
KIDS (Keyboard Introductory Development Series), 1703
KLST-2: Kindergarten Language Screening Test Edition, 2nd Edition, 2617

Kachina Point Health Care & Rehabilitation Center, 7223
Kaleidoscope: Exploring the Experience of Disability through Literature & the Fine Arts, 34
Kamp A-Komp-Plish, 1157, 8893
Kamp Kaleidoscope, 1398
Kamp Kaleo, 1229, 8894
Kamp Kiwanis, 1278
Kamp for Kids: Camp Togowauk, 1179
Kanawha County Public Library, 4939
Kanner Center, 7175
Kansas Advocacy and Protective Services, 3480
Kansas City VA Medical Center, 5671
Kansas Client Assistance Program, 3481
Kansas Commission on Disability Concerns, 3482
Kansas Department on Aging, 3483, 7505
Kansas Developmental Disability Council, 3484
Kansas Fair Employment Practice Agency, 6023
Kansas Jaycees' Cerebral Palsy Foundation, 1118, 8406
Kansas Rehabilitation Hospital, 6336
Kansas Services for the Blind & Visually Impaired, 4129
Kansas State Board of Education: Special Education Services, 2126
Kansas State Library, 4765
Kansas Talking Books Regional Library, 4766
Kansas VA Regional Office, 5634
Kansas Vocational Rehabilitation Agency, 6024
Kaplan Early Learning Company, 1950
Kaplen JCC On The Palisades, 1240
Kate B Reynolds Charitable Trust, 3097
Kauai Center for Independent Living, 4042
Kaufman Test of Educational Achievement (K-TEA), 2618
Kay Elemetrics Corporation, 1630, 1768
Kayelemetrics Corporation, 1773
Keats Publishing, 5139
Keep the Promise: Managed Care and People with Disabilities, 5110
Keeping Ahead in School, 1951
Keeping Our Families Together, 5111
Kelley Diversified, 5952
Kelly Services Foundation, 2968
Ken McRight Supplies, 185, 273
Kenai Peninsula Independent Living Center, 3879
Kenai Peninsula Independent Living Center: Seward, 3880
Kendall Demonstration Elementary School Curriculum Guides, 2446
Keni Peninsula Independent Living Center: Central Peninsula, 3881
Kennebunk Nursing & Rehabilitation Center, 7309
Kennedy Center, 5902
Kennedy Job Training Center, 5975
Kennedy Krieger Institute, 2673, 2934
Kennedy Park Medical Rehabilitation Center, 7427
Kenneth & Evelyn Lipper Foundation, 3062
Kenneth T and Eileen L Norris Foundation, 2769
Kenny Foundation, 5504
Kensington Publishing, 5245
Kent County Arc, 3170
Kent District Library for the Blind and Physically Handicapped, 4815
Kentfield Rehabilitation Hospital & Outpatient Center, 6250
Kentucky Assistive Technology Service Network, 1579
Kentucky Association of Homes and Services for the Aging, 7464
Kentucky Committee on Employment of People with Disabilities, 6025
Kentucky Council on Developmental Disability, 3485
Kentucky Department for Employment Service and Job Training Program Liaison, 6026
Kentucky Department for Mental Health and Mental Retardation Services, 3486
Kentucky Department for Mental Health:, 3487
Kentucky Department for the Blind, 3488, 6027
Kentucky Department of Education: Division of Exceptional Children's Services, 2127
Kentucky Office for the Blind, 6028
Kentucky Office of Aging Services, 3489

Kentucky Protection & Advocacy, 3490
Kentucky Talking Book Library Kentucky Dept. for Libraries and Archives, 4774
Kentucky Tennessee Conference, 1381, 8892
Kentucky Vocational Rehabilitation Agency, 6029
Keshet Dance Company, 35
Kessler Institute for Rehabilitation, 106
Kessler Institute for Rehabilitation, Welkind Facility, 6378
Kessler Rehabilitation Corporation, 2674
Ketch Industries, 6912
Ketogenic Diet: A Treatment for Children and Others with Epilepsy, 8496
Key Changes: A Portrait of Lisa Thorson, 8216
Key Holders, Ignition & Door Keys, 107
Key Tronic KB 5153 Touch Pad Keyboard, 1616
KeyMath Teach and Practice, 1952
KeyTronic, 1616
Keyboard Tutor, Music Software, 1704
Keyboarding by Ability, 1705
Keyboarding for the Physically Handicapped, 1706
Keyboarding with One Hand, 1707
Keys to Parenting a Child with Attention Deficit Disorder, 7780
Keys to Parenting a Child with Downs Syndrome, 7781
Keys to Parenting the Child with Autism, 7782
Keystone Blind Association, 8842
The Keystone Group, 3165
Keywi, 1633
Kid's Custom, 735
Kid's Edge, 736
Kid's Liberty, 737
Kid-Friendly Chairs, 738
Kid-Friendly Parenting with Deaf and Hard of Hearing Children, 8031
Kids on the Block Programs, 8244
Kindered Health Care, 7384
Kindred, 6679, 7225, 7428
Kindred Health Care, 7207, 7228, 7289, 7395, 7402, 7415, 7437
Kindred Health Care Center, 7226
Kindred Health Care Publications, 7403
Kindred Healthcare, 6968, 7221, 7272, 7299, 7376, 7383, 7405, 7414, 7427, 7436
Kindred Healthcare, Inc., 6674
Kindred Heights Nursing & Rehabilitation Center, 7383
Kindred Hospital-La Mirada, 6613
Kindred Transitional Care and Rehabilitati on, 7270
King's Daughter's Medical Center's Rehab Unit/Work Hardening Program, 6918
King's Rehabilitation Center, 5852
King's Rule, 1646
King's View Work Experience Center- Atwater, 6614
Kings Harbor Multicare Center, 7347
Kiplinger Foundation, 2829
Kitsap Community Resources, 4531
Kitten Who Couldn't Purr, 8738
Kiwanis Camp Wyman, 1218, 8392
Kiwanis Club of Montavilla, 1331
Kleinert's, 479
Kluge Children's Rehabilitation Center, 6477
Knee Socks, 1468
Kneelkar, 108
Knock Light, 525
Know Your Eye, 8982
Knowing Your Rights, 4613
Knox County Council for Developmental Disabilities, 5976
Knoxville VA Medical Center, 5630
Koala Miniflex, 739
Koicheff Health Care Center, 7068
Kokomo Rehabilitation Hospital, 6323
Koret Foundation, 2770
Kostopulos Dream Foundation, 1402
Kreider Services, 5977
Kresge Foundation, 2969
Krieger Publishing Company, 2335, 2541, 8175
Kris' Camp, 1045
Kroepke Kontrols, 84, 94, 97, 99, 102, 104, 111
Kuhn Employment Oppurtunities, 6704

Kuschall North America, 251
Kuschall of America, 697, 698, 699, 707
Kuzell Institute for Arthritis and Infectious Diseases, 4677

L

LA Lions League for Crippled Children, 1131
LA84 Foundation, 2771
LC Technologies Inc, 1516
LD Child and the ADHD Child: Ways Parents & Professionals Can Help, 7783
LD Monthly Report, 2250
LD OnLine WETA Public Television, 5424
LDS Hospital Rehabilitation Center, 6470
LIFE Center for Independent Living, 4069
LIFE of Mississippi, 4263
LIFE of Mississippi: Biloxi, 4264
LIFE of Mississippi: Greenwood, 4265
LIFE of Mississippi: Hattiesburg, 4266
LIFE of Mississippi: McComb, 4267
LIFE of Mississippi: Meridian, 4268
LIFE of Mississippi: Oxford, 4269
LIFE of Mississippi: Tupelo, 4270
LIFE/ Run Centers for Independent Living, 4476
LIFE: Fort Hall, 4049
LINC-Monroe Randolph Center, 4070
LINK: Colby, 4130
LJ Skaggs and Mary C Skaggs Foundation, 2772
LK Whittier Foundation, 2773
LPB Communications, 214
LPDOS Deluxe, 1708
LRP Publications, 2234, 2239, 2264, 3266, 3273, 4595, 4617, 4965, 6297
LS&S, 480, 492
La Frontera Center, 6524
La-Z-Boy, 408
LaBac Systems, 753
LaFayette-Walker Public Library, 4728
LaPalma Intercommunity Hospital, 6615
LaRabida Children's Hospital and Research Center, 6312
Lab School of Washington, 1034, 7688
Labeling the Mentally Retarded, 7784
Laboure College Library, 4806
Ladacain Network, 7044
Ladybug Corner Chair, 261
Lafayette Nursing and Rehabilitation Center, 7262
Lake County Center for Independent Living, 4071
Lake County Health Department, 6845
Lake County Public Library Talking Books Service, 4756
Lake Erie College, 2709
Lake Michigan Academy, 2675
LakeMed Nursing and Rehabilitation Center, 7372
Lakeland Adult Day Training, 4017
Lakeland Center, 7000
Lakemary Center, 6913
Lakeshore Foundation, 8232
Lakeshore Learning Materials, 1953
Lakeside Milam Recovery Centers (LMRC), 7202
Lakeview NeuroRehabilitation Center, 6371
Lakeview Rehabilitation Hospital, 6340
Lakeview Subacute Care Center, 7335
Lakewood Health Care Center, 7203
Lambs Farm, 5978
Lambton County Developmental Services, 870
LampLighter, 9086
Lamplighter's Work Center, 6063
Lanakila Rehabilitation Center, 5957
Land of Lincoln Goodwill Industries, 5979
Land-of-Sky Regional Council Area Agency on Aging, 7552
Landmark Media, 5313, 5338, 5366, 7602, 8911, 9130
Lane Community College, 2710
Language Arts: Detecting Special Needs, 2447
Language Disabilities in Children and Adolescents, 8739
Language Learning Practices with Deaf Children, 2448
Language Parts Catalog, 1954
Language Tool Kit, 1955

Language and Communication Disorders in Children, 2449
Language and the Developing Child, 8740
Language, Learning & Living, 215
Language, Speech and Hearing Services in School, 1956
Language, Speech, and Hearing Services in Schools, 8768
Lanting Foundation, 2970
Lapeer: Blue Water Center for Independent Living, 4233
Laradon Hall Society for Exceptional Children and Adults, 6682
Large Button Speaker Phone, 216
Large Print DOS, 1709
Large Print Keyboard Labels, 1521
Large Print Loan Library, 8983
Large Print Loan Library Catalog, 8984
Large Print Recipies for a Healthy Life, 8985
Large Print Telephone Dial, 217
Large Print Touch-Telephone Overlays, 218
Large Type, 1823
Las Animas County Rehabilitation Center, 5887
Las Vegas Healthcare And Rehabilitation Center, 7030
Las Vegas Healthcare and Rehabilitation Center, 7330
Las Vegas Veterans Center, 5682
Las Vegas-Clark County Library District, 4847
Lash & Associates Publishing/Training, 7776
Latchloc Automatic Wheelchair Tiedown, 109
Late Talker: What to Do If Your Child Isn't Talking Yet, 8741
Latex Allergy in Spina Bifida Patients, 8497
Laureate Learning Systems, 1710
Laurel Designs, 671, 5078
Laurel Grove Hospital: Rehab Care Unit, 6251
Laurel Hill Center, 4410
Laurent Clerc: The Story of His Early Years, 8032
Law Center Newsletter, 4614
LeBonheur Cardiac Kids Camp, 1382
LeBonheur Children's Hospital, 1382
League Letter, 8085
League at Camp Greentop, 1158
The League for People with Disabilities, 1158
League for the Blind and Disabled, 4103
League for the Hard of Hearing, 7927
League of Human Dignity, Center for Independent Living, 4113
League of Human Dignity: Lincoln, 4300
League of Human Dignity: Norfolk, 4301
League of Human Dignity: Omaha, 4302
Learn About the ADA in Your Local Library, 5112
Learning About Numbers, 1647
Learning Activity Packets, 1813
Learning American Sign Language, 1957
Learning Among Children with Spina Bifida, 8498
Learning Company, 1711, 1648, 1795
Learning Corporation of America, 5320, 5342
Learning Disabilities Association of America, 871
Learning Disabilities Association of America, 872, 2216, 7769, 7773, 7775, 7788
Learning Disabilities Association of Arkansas, 2247
Learning Disabilities Association of New York State, 872
Learning Disabilities Consultants, 2251
Learning Disabilities Consultants Newsletter, 2251
Learning Disabilities Sourcebook, 3rd Ed., 36
Learning Disabilities Worldwide, 873
Learning Disabilities, Literacy, and Adult Education, 2450
Learning Disabilities: A Contemporary Journal, 2215
Learning Disabilities: A Multidisciplinary Journal, 2216
Learning Disabilities: Concepts and Characteristics, 2451
Learning Disability Quarterly, 2217
Learning Disability: Social Class and the Cons of Inequality In American Education, 2452
Learning English: Primary, 1781
Learning English: Rhyme Time, 1782
Learning House, 2619
Learning Independence Through Computers, 1580

Learning Resources, 1958
Learning Services Corporation, 6390
Learning Services of Northern California, 6616
Learning Services: Bear Creek, 6683
Learning Services: Carolina, 7080
Learning Services: Harris House Program, 6799
Learning Services: Morgan Hill, 6617
Learning Services: Shenandoah, 6207
Learning Services: Supported Living Programs, 6618
Learning Tools International, 1693
Learning and Individual Differences, 2453
Learning disAbilities Resources, 7858
Learning to Feel Good and Stay Cool: Emotional Regulation Tools for Kids With AD/HD, 2454
Learning to Play, 8986
Learning to See: American Sign Language as a Second Language, 2455
Learning to Sign in My Neighborhood, 1959
LearningRx, 2620
Lebanon VA Medical Center, 5737
Lectra-Lift, 408
Ledgewood Rehabilitation and Skilled Nursing Center, 7319
Lee County Library System: Talking Books Library, 4707
Lee Memorial Hospital, 6757
Left Foot Accelerator, 110
Left Foot Gas Pedal, 111
Left Foot Gas Pedal by Handicaps, Inc., 112
Left Hand Shift Lever, 113
Leg Elevation Board, 526
Legacy Emanuel Rehabilitation Center, 7126
Legal Action Center, 4566
Legal Center for People with Disabilities & Older People, 3373, 4567, 4615
Legal Right: The Guide for Deaf and Hard of Hearing People, 4616
Legal Rights of Persons with Disabilities, 4617
Legislative Handbook for Parents, 4568
Legislative Network for Nurses, 4618
Legler Benbough Foundation, 2774
Lehigh Valley Center for Independent Living, 4430
Lehigh Valley Center for Independent Living, 5115
Leisure Lift, 582, 582
Leisure-Lift, 586
Leo P La Chance Center for Rehabilitation and Nursing, 7320
Leo Yassenoff JCC Specialty Day Camp, 1311
Leon S Peters Rehabilitation Center, 6619
Leonard Media Group, 8189
Les Turne Amyotrophic Laterial Sclerosis Foundation, 2883
Leslie G Ehmann Trust, 3136
Lester Electrical, 674
Lester H Higgins Adult Center, 7105
Let Community Employment be the Goal for Individuals with Autism, 7785, 8742
Let's Count Braille and Tactile Numbers Poster, 5475
Let's Eat, 8987
Let's Eat Video, 9123
Let's Talk About Having Asthma, 8499
Let's Write Right: Teacher's Edition, 2456
Letter Writing Guide, 620
Lettering Guide Value Pack, 621
Lettie Pate Whitehead Foundation, 2855
Leukemia & Lymphoma Society, 8277
Leukemia Sourcebook, 8500
Levenger, 633
Leveron, 527
Levi Strauss Foundation, 2775
Levindale Hebrew Geriatric Center, 6954
Levinson Medical Center, 2676
Lewiston Public Library, 4782
Lewy Body Dementia Association, 7631, 7880, 8139
Lexia I, II and III Reading Series, 1783
Lexia Learning Systems, 1783, 1791
Lexington Center for Health and Rehabilitation, 7300
Lexington School for the Deaf: Center for the Deaf, 7928
Lexington VA Medical Center, 5636

Liberator, 219
Liberty, 715
Liberty LT, 409
Liberty Lightweight Aluminum Stroll Walker, 652
Liberty Resources, 4431
Library Commission for the Blind, 4762
Library Cooperative/ Library for the blind, 4821
Library Manager's Guide to Hiring and Serving
    Disabled Persons, 2457
Library Services for the Blind, 8988
Library Users of America Newsletter, 9087
Library for the Blind & Physically Handicapped,
    4901
Library for the Blind and Physically Handicapped
    SW Region of Arkansas, 4665
Library of Congress, 8814, 8866
Library of Michigan Service for the Blind, 4816
Life After Trauma: A Workbook for Healing, 8501
Life Beyond the Classroom: Transition Strategies
    for Young People with Disabilities, 4958
Life Beyond the Classroom: Transition Strategies
    for Young People with Disabilities, 5298
Life Center for Independent Living: Pontiac, 4072
Life Centered Career Education: A Contemporary
    Based Approach, 4th Edition, 2621
Life Development Institute, 7632
Life Line, 8502
Life Planning for Adults with Developmental
    Disabilities, 7512
Life Science Associates, 7847
Life Services Network of Illinois, 7465
Life Skills Foundation, 4277
Life Skills Laundry Division, 6894
Life Way Christian Resources Southern Baptist
    Conv, 2576
Life and Independence for Today, 4432
Life on Wheels: For the Active Wheelchair User,
    8180
Life-Span Approach to Nursing Care for
    Individuals with Developmental Disabilities,
    2458
LifeLines, 5113, 5213
LifeSkills Industries, 6919
LifeSpan, 7081
LifeSpan Network: Maryland, 7466
LifeWay Christian Resources, 8058
LifeWay Christian Resources Southern Baptist
    Conv., 2526
Lifelong Leisure Skills and Lifestyles for Persons
    with Developmental Disabilities, 5114
Lifestand, 679, 726
Lifestyles of Employed Legally Blind People,
    8989
Lifeworks Employment Services, 6979
Lift-All, 410
Lifts for Swimming Pools and Spas, 411
Light the Way, 9088
Lighthouse Central Florida, 4018, 5935
Lighthouse International, 8843, 481, 5332, 7527,
    7529, 8861, 9050, 9051, 9106, 9124, 9128
Lighthouse International Information and
    Resource Service, 9142
Lighthouse Low Vision Products, 481
Lighthouse Publication, 9089
Lighthouse for the Blind, 997, 8890
Lighthouse for the Blind in New Orleans, 6935
Lighthouse for the Blind of Palm Beach, 6758
Lighthouse for the Visually Impaired and Blind,
    6759
Lighthouse of Houston, 7176
Lights On, 9090
Lightweight Breezy, 716
Lilac Services for the Blind, 7571
Lincoln County Health System, 7154
Lincoln Regional Office, 5679
Lincoln VA Medical Center, 5680
Lincoln YMCA, 1231, 8418
Lindamood-Bell Home Learning Process, 8688
Lindustries, 527
Linguistics of American Sign Language: An
    Introduction, 8033
Linking Employment, Abilities and Potential,
    4395
Lion, 8990

Lion's Blind Center of Diablo Valley, Inc. Lions
    Center For The Visually Impaired, 6620
Lion's Blind Center of Oakland, 6621
Lion's Clubs International, 8990
Lions 11 B-2 and MADHH, 1186, 7956
Lions Camp Crescendo, Inc., 1124, 7971
Lions Camp Kirby, 1354, 7972
Lions Camp Merrick, 1159, 7973
Lions Camp Tatiyee, 957
Lions Club And American Diabetes Association,
    1130
Lions Club Industries for the Blind, 7082
Lions Club Of Louisiana, 1132
Lions Club Of Texas, 1399, 8409, 8897
Lions Club of Oregon and Washington, 1327, 7966
Lions Club of Texas, 7979
Lions Clubs International, 2711, 8844
Lions Clubs of District 22-C, 1159, 7973
Lions Clubs of California and Nevada, 999, 7974
Lions Den Outdoor Learning Center, 1219, 7689
Lions Services Inc., 7083
Lions Wilderness Camp for Deaf Children, Inc.,
    999, 7974
Lions World Services for the Blind, 6538
Lions of Multiple District 35, 1042, 7578
Lipomas & Lipomyelomeningocele, 8503
Lippincott Williams And Wilkins, 2479
Lippincott Williams & Wilkins, 8466, 8596
Lippincott, Williams & Wilkins, 2330, 2463, 2466,
    2467, 2499, 5271, 5279, 7511, 8481, 8601, 8610
Lisle, 2712
Listen Up, 9117
Listner, 8095
Literacy & Your Deaf Child: What Every Parent
    Should Know, 8034
Literacy Program, 1960
Literature Based Reading, 1961
Literature Journal, The, 8070
Little City Foundation, 2884
Little Friends, Inc., 6846
Little Mack Communicator, 1634
Little People of America, 8278
Little Red Door Cancer Agency, 1094
Little Red Hen, 1712
Little Rock Vet Center #0713, 6539
Live Independently Networking Center, 4379
Live Independently Networking Center: Hickory,
    4380
Live Oaks Career Development Campus, 7106
Liver Disorders Sourcebook, 8504
Livin', 5115
Living Beyond Multiple Sclerosis: A Woman's
    Guide, 8505
Living Independence Network Corporation, 4050
Living Independence Network Corporation: Twin
    Falls, 4051
Living Independence Network Corporation: C
    aldwell, 4052
Living Independence for Everyone (LIFE), 4031
Living Independent for Everyone (LIFE):
    Pocatello Office, 4053
Living Independently Now Center (LINC), 4073
Living Independently Now Center: Sparta, 4074
Living Independently Now Center: Waterloo, 4075
Living Independently for Everyone (LIFE):
    Blackfoot Office, 4054
Living Independently for Everyone (LIFE): Pocate,
    4054
Living Independently for Everyone: Burley, 4055
Living Independently for Today and Tomorrow,
    4292
Living Independently in Northwest Kansas: Hays,
    4131
Living Skills Center for the Visually Impaired,
    6622
Living Well with Asthma, 8506
Living Well with Chronic Fatigue Syndrome and
    Fibromyalgia, 8507
Living Well with HIV and AIDS, 8508
Living With Spinal Cord Injury Series, 8509
Living an Idea: Empowerment and the Evolution
    of an Alternative School, 1962
Living in a State of Stuck, 5116
Living in the Community, 5117

Living with Achromatopsia, 8991
Living with Brain Injury: A Guide for Families,
    8510
Living with Spina Bifida: A Guide for Families
    and Professionals, 8511
Living with a Brother or Sister with Special
    Needs: A Book for Sibs, 5214
Livingston Center for Independent Living, 4234
Lloyd Hearing Aid Corporation, 332, 333, 336, 343
LoSeCa Foundation, 874
Lodi Memorial Hospital, 6252
Lodi Memorial Hospital West, 6252
Lola Wright Foundation, 3212
Lollipop Lunch, 8743
Loma Linda University Orthopedic and
    Rehabilitation Institute, 6623
Long Beach Department of Health and Human
    Services, 3359
Long Beach Memorial Medical Center Memorial
    Rehabilitation Hospital, 6253, 7230
Long Beach VA Medical Center, 5577
Long Cane News, 9091
Long Handled Bath Sponges, 170
Long Island Alzheimer's Foundation, 3063
Long Island Center for Independent Living, 4354
Long Island Talking Book Library System, 4873
Long Oven Mitts, 362
Long-Term Care: How to Plan and Pay for It, 7513
Longman Education/Addison Wesley, 2305, 2437
Longman Group, 2535
Longman Publishing Group, 2390, 2503, 2590,
    2593
Longreach Reacher, 528
Longwood Foundation, 2820
Look Out for Annie, 9124
Look Who's Laughing Aquarius Health Care
    Media, 5343
Looking Good: Learning to Improve Your
    Appearance, 1713
Loop Scissors, 529
Los Angeles County Department of Health
    Services, 3360
Los Angeles Regional Office, 5578
A Loss for Words, 7986
Lost Tree Village Charitable Foundation, 2843
Lotus Press, 8449
Loud, Proud and Passionate, 5118
Loudoun County Local Government, 1422
Loudoun County Special Recreation Programs,
    1422
Louis A Johnson VA Medical Center, 5781
Louis R Lurie Foundation, 2776
Louis Stokes VA Medical Center Wade Park
    Campus, 5723
Louis and Anne Abrons Foundation, 3064
Louis de la Parte Florida Mental Health Institute
    Research Library, 4708
Louisiana Assistive Technology Access Network,
    3494
Louisiana Center for Dyslexia and Related
    Learning Disorders, 3495
Louisiana Center for the Blind, 6936
Louisiana Department of Aging, 3496
Louisiana Department of Education, 2128
Louisiana Department of Education: Office of
    Special Education Services, 2128
Louisiana Developmental Disability Council, 3497
Louisiana Division of Mental Health, 3498
Louisiana Employment Service and Job Training
    Program Liaison, 6033
Louisiana Learning Resources System, 3499
Louisiana Lions Camp, 1131, 1128, 8360
Louisiana Lions Camp - Camp Pelican, 1132
Louisiana State Library, 4777
Louisiana State University Eye Center, 6937
Louisiana State University Genetics Section of
    Pediatrics, 4778
Louisiana Vocational Rehabilitation Agency, 6034
Louisville Free Public Library, 4775
Louisville VA Medical Center, 5637
Louisville VA Regional Office, 5638
Lourdes Regional Rehabilitation Center, 7045
Lousiana State University, 6937

Love Publishing Company, 2193, 2317, 2345, 2552, 2561, 4608, 7814, 8761
Love: Where to Find It, How to Keep It, 5119
Loving & Letting Go, 5215
Loving Justice, 4619
Low Effort and No Effort Steering, 114
Low Tech Assistive Devices: A Handbook for the School Setting, 1963
Low Vision Questions and Answers: Definitions, Devices, Services, 8992
Low Vision Services of Kentucky, 6920
Low Vision Telephones, 631
Low Vision: Reflections of the Past, Issues for the Future, 8993
Lowe's Syndrome Association, 1860
Lowe's Syndrome Conference, 1860
Loyola Press, 5268
Lucy Lee Hospital, 7023
Luke B Hancock Foundation, 2777
Lumber River Council of Governments Area Agency on Aging, 7553
Lumex Cushions and Mattresses, 284
Lumex Recliner, 262
Luminaud, 482, 473, 1632
Lung Cancer: Making Sense of Diagnosis, Treatment, and Options, 8512
Lung Disorders Sourcebook, 8513
Lung Line Information Service, 8659
Lupus: Alternative Therapies That Work, 8514
Lutheran Blind Mission, 4840
Lutheran Charities Foundation of St Louis, 2991
Lutherans Outdoors in South Dakota, 1372, 8399
Lutherdale Bible Camp, 1437
Lutherdale Ministries, 1437
Lyme Disease Foundation, 5425
Lymphoma Canada, 8279
Lynchburg Area Center for Independent Living, 4518
Lynde and Harry Bradley Foundation, 3254
Lynne Rienner Publishers, 2095
Lyons Campus of the VA New Jersey Healthcare System, 5691

M

M ER S Goodwill, 7021
M Evans and Company, 5221
M&M Health Care Apparel Company, 1469
MA Report, 2252
MAClown Vocational Rehabilitation Workshop, 5936
MADAMIST 50/50 PSI Air Compressor, 320
MAGIC Foundation for Children's Growth, 2885, 8515
MAGIC Touch, 8515
MAP Training Center, 6847
MAPCON Technologies, 2096
MCC Supportive Care Services, 875
MDA Newsmagazine, 2218
MEDLINE, 1581
MIUSA's Global Impact Newsletter, 8207
MIV Mount Loretto, 1273, 8384
MIV: Mount Loretto, 7970
MIW, 6895
MMB Music, 17, 29, 45, 65, 1927, 2002, 2438
MN Governor's Council on Development Disabilities, 5144
MOMS Catalog, 483
MOOSE: A Very Special Person, 5120
MOSAIC In Colorado Springs MOSAIC, 6684
MSFOCUS Magazine, 8605
MTA Readers, 1964
MVP+ 3-Wheel Scooter, 583
Mac's Lift Gate, 412
MacDonald Training Center, 6760
MacMillan - St. Martin's Press, 8170
Macomb Library for the Blind & Physically Handicapped, 4817
Macon Library for the Blind and Physically Handicapped, 4726
Macon Resources, 6848
Macular Degeneration Foundation, 8845, 9092
Mad Hatters: Theatre That Makes a World of Difference, 2677

Mada Medical Products, 158, 310, 317, 320, 328, 645, 651, 652, 655, 656, 657, 660, 665, 719, 727
Maddak Inc., 484
Madison County Hospital, 7296
Madison County Rehab Services, 7296
Madison Healthcare and Rehabilitation Center, 7392
Madonna Rehabilitation Hospital, 6368, 7328
Magee Rehabilitation Hospital, 6422
Magic Wand Keyboard, 1617
Magnetic Card Reader, 363
Magni-Cam & Primer, 632
Magnifier, 9092
Magnifier Bookweight, 633
Magnolia Health Systems, 7285
Maine Assistive Technology Projects, 3502
Maine Association of Non Profits, 2919
Maine Bureau of Elder and Adult Services, 3503
Maine CITE, 1582
Maine Department Of Labor, 6040
Maine Department of Health and Human Services, 3504
Maine Developmental Disabilities Council, 3505
Maine Division for the Blind and Visually Impaired, 3506
Maine Governor's Committee on Employment of the Disabled, 6041
Maine Human Rights Commission, 6042, 6042
Maine Office of Elder Services, 3507
Maine State, 4783
Maine State Library, 4783
Maine VA Regional Office, 5642
Maine Workers' Compensation Board, 3508
Mainland Center Hospital RehabCare Unit, 7177
Mainstay Life Services Summer Program, 1355
Mainstream, 876, 3896, 6047, 2468, 5321, 6053, 8918
Mainstream Living, 5426
Mainstream Magazine, 5121
Mainstream Online Magazine of the Able-Disabled, 5427
Mainstreaming Deaf and Hard of Hearing Students: Questions and Answers, 2459
Mainstreaming Exceptional Students: A Guide for Classroom Teachers, 2460
Mainstreaming and the American Dream, 8994
Mainstreaming the Visually Impaired Child, 8995
Mainstreaming: A Practical Approach for Teachers, 2461
Majors Medical Equipment, 717
Makemie Woods Camp, 1423, 8393
Makemie Woods Camp/Conference Retreat, 8394
Making Changes: Family Voices on Living Disabilities, 5122
Making Choices for Independent Living, 4192
Making Informed Medical Decisions: Where to Look and How to Use What You Find, 5123
Making Life More Livable, 8996
Making News: How to Get News Coverage of Disability Rights Issues, 4620
Making News: How to Get News Coverage of Disability Rights Issues, 4986
Making School Inclusion Work: A Guide to Everyday Practice, 1965
Making Self-Employment Work for People with Disabilities, 4987
Making Wise Decisions for Long-Term Care, 5124
Making a Difference, 5125
Making a Difference: A Wise Approach, 5126
Making the Writing Process Work, 7786
Making the Writing Process Work: Strategies for Composition and Self-Regulation, 1966
Man's Low-Vision Quartz Watches, 634
Management of Autistic Behavior, 7787, 8516, 8744
Management of Children and Adolescents with AD-HD, 7788
Management of Genetic Syndromes, 8517
Managing Attention Deficit Hyperactivity in Children: A Guide for Practitioners, 7789
Managing Diagnostic Tool of Visual Perception, 2462
Managing Post Polio: A Guide to Living Well with Post Polio, 8518

Managing Your Activities, 5127
Managing Your Health Care, 5128
Managing Your Symptoms, 8113
Manatee Springs Care & Rehabilitation Center, 6285
Manchester Regional Office, 5686
Manchester VA Medical Center, 5687
Manhattan Public Library, 4767
Manor Care Health Services- Citrus Heights, 6624
Manor Care Health Services- Palm Desert, 6625
Manor Care Health Services-Fountain Valley, 6626
Manor Care Health Services-Hemet, 6627
Manor Care Health Services-Sunnyvale, 6628
Manor Care Health Services-Tacoma, 7204
Manor Care Health Services-Walnut Creek, 6629
Manor Care Nursing and Rehab Center: Tucson, 6525
Manor Care Nursing and Rehabilitation Center: Boulder, 6685
Manor Care Nursing: Denver, 6686
Manor Care Ohio, 6685
ManorCare Health Services-Arlington, 7190
ManorCare Health Services-Lynnwood, 7205
ManorCare Health Services-Spokane, 7206
Manual Alphabet Poster, 1967
Manual of Sequential Art Activities for Classified Children and Adolescents, 37
Many Faces of Dyslexia, 1968
Maplebrook School, 1279, 7690
Mapleton Center, 6275
MarbleSoft, 5472, 5479
March of Dimes Birth Defects Foundation, 877
Margaret L Wendt Foundation, 3065
Margaret T Morris Foundation, 2734
Marianjoy Rehabilitation Hospital and Clinics, 6313
Marin Center for Independent Living, 3953
Marin Community Foundation, 2778
Mariner Health Care: Connecticut, 6277
Mariner Health of Nashville, 7393
Mariner Shower and Commode Chair, 171
Marion VA Medical Center, 5620
Marist Brothers Mid-Hudson Valley Camp, 1280, 8395
Mark Elmore Associates Architects, 1880
Mark Seven Deaf Foundation, 1263, 7963
Marriner S Eccles Foundation, 3223
Marshall & Ilsley Trust Company, 3258
Marshall & Ilsley Trust of Florida, 2913
Marshall University College Of Educational & Human, 4942
Martin Luther Homes of Indiana, 4104
Martin Luther Homes of Iowa, 4114
Martin Technology, 663
Martinez Outpatient Clinic, 5579
Martinsburg VA Medical Center, 5782
Marvelwood School, 1027, 7691
Marvelwood Summer, 1027, 7691
Mary A Crocker Trust, 2779
Mary Bryant Home for the Blind, 6849
Mary Free Bed Rehabilitation Hospital, 7001
Mary Lanning Memorial Hospital, 7329
Mary Reynolds Babcock Foundation, 3098
Maryland Client Assistance Program Division of Rehabilitation Services, 3512
Maryland Department of Aging, 3513
Maryland Department of Disabilities, 1583
Maryland Department of Handicapped Children, 3514
Maryland Developmental Disabilities Council, 3515
Maryland Division of Mental Health, 3516
Maryland Employment Services and Job Training Program Liaison, 6048
Maryland Fair Employment Practice Agency, 6049
Maryland State Department of Education, 6050, 4789
Maryland State Department of Education: Division of Special Education, 2134
Maryland State Library for the Blind and Physically Handicapped, 4789
Maryland Technology Assistance Program, 1583
Maryland Veterans Centers, 5647
Mask of Benevolence: Disabling the Deaf Community, The, 8035

MasoniCare Corporation, 7242
Masonic Healthcare Center, 7242
Massachusetts Aging Services Association, 7467
Massachusetts Assistive Technology Partnership, 3522
Massachusetts Client Assistance Program, 3523
Massachusetts Department of Education, 2130
Massachusetts Department of Education: Program Quality Assurance, 2130
Massachusetts Department of Mental Health, 3524
Massachusetts Developmental Disabilities Council, 3525
Massachusetts Eye & Ear Infirmary, 4805
Massachusetts Eye and Ear Infirmary & Vision Rehabilitation Center, 6980
Massachusetts Fair Employment Practice Agency, 6057
Massachusetts Governor's Commission on Employment of Disabled Persons, 6058
Massachusetts Office on Disability, 3523
Massachusetts Rehabilitation Commission, 4807
Massena Independent Living Center, 4355
Mat Factory, 680, 683, 685
Match-Sort-Assemble Job Cards, 1969
Match-Sort-Assemble Pictures, 1970
Match-Sort-Assemble SCHEMATICS, 1971
Match-Sort-Assemble TOOLS, 1972
Math Rabbit, 1648
Math for Everyday Living, 1649
Math for Successful Living, 1650
Maumee Valley Girl Scout Center, 1305, 8354
Maxi Aids, 485, 93, 165, 166, 169, 171, 179, 181, 187, 217, 218, 298, 300, 305, 306, 326, 327, 345, 346, 349, 351, 354, 355, 357, 359, 360, 363, 364, 371, 391, 504, 522, 523, 557, 559, 561, 562, 565, 566, 569, 581, 589, 614, 615, 618, 622, 626, 627, 635, 636, , 637, 643, 644, 646, 647, 653, 667, 669, 694, 728, 748, 749, 758, 1545, 5459, 5460, 5461, 5462, 5463, 5464, 5465, 5466, 5468, 5469, 5470, 5475, 5483, 5484, 9134
Maxi Marks, 557
Maxi Superior Cane, 653
Maxi-Aids Braille Timer, 364
MaximEyes, 7600
Maynord's Chemical Dependency Recovery Centers, 6630
Maynord's Ranch for Men, 6631
Mayo Clinic Scottsdale, 7224
Mayor of the West Side, 4959
Mc Graw- Hill, School Publishing, 2545
McAlester Regional Health Center RehabCare Unit, 7122
McCune Charitable Foundation, 3021
McDonald's Corporation Contributions Program, 2886
McFarland & Company, 1692, 2457
McGraw-Hill, 8446
McGraw-Hill Company, 2097, 7, 2487, 5081, 8583
McGraw-Hill Professional, 8169
McGraw-Hill School Publishing, 1949, 2285, 2303, 2391, 2395, 2444, 2451, 2461, 2486, 2529, 2532, 2554, 8739
McGraw-Hill School Publishn, 2449
McGraw-Hill, School Publishing, 2004, 2364, 7790
McInerny Foundation Bank Of Hawaii, Corporate Trustee, 2862
McKey Mouse, 1618
McLean Hospital, 1170
Mclean Hospital Child/Adolescent Program, 7659, 8706
The Mead Center for American Theater, 6
Meadowbrook Manor, 6632
Meadowood Springs Speech and Hearing Camp, 1330, 7975, 8711
Meadows Foundation, 3213
Meadowvale Health and Rehabilitation Cente r, 7289
Meadowview Manor, 6633
Measure of Cognitive-Linguistic Abilities (MCLA), 2622
Measurement and Evaluation in Counseling, 2219
Mecalift Sling Lifter, 413
Med Covers, 690

Med-Camps of Louisiana, 1133, 8396
MedDev Corporation, 321
MedEscort International, 5505
MedStar National Rehabilitation Network, 2678
Medford Rehabilitation and Healthcare Cent er, 7376
Medi-Grip, 322
Media America, 8602
Media Foundation, 3239
Media Projects Inc, 7867
MedicAlert Foundation International, 5455
Medical Aspects of Disability: A Handbook For The Rehabilitation Professional, 5129
Medical Camping, 1125
Medical Rehabilitation, 2463
Medical Research Institute Of San Francisco, 4677
Medical University of South Carolina Arthritis Clinical/Research Center, 4902
Medicare and Medicaid Patient and Program Protection Act of 1987, 4621
Medicenter of Tampa, 6761
Medina Foundation, 3239
Mediplex Rehab: Camden, 6379
Mediplex Rehab: Denver, 6276
Mediplex of Colorado, 6687
Mednet, 108
Medpro, 285, 286, 292, 293
Medpro Static Air Chair Cushion, 285
Medpro Static Air Mattress Overlay, 286
Meeting Life's Challenges, 453, 8445
Meeting the ADD Challenge: A Practical Guide for Teachers, 2464
Meeting the Needs of Employees with Disabilities, 5130
Meeting the Needs of People with Vision Loss: Multidisciplinary Perspective, 8997
Meeting-in-a-Box, 1973
Mega Wolf Communication Device, 1635
Melwood, 6051
Member Update, 2253
Memorial Hospital of Gardenia, 6634
Memorial Regional Rehabilitation Center, 6324, 6886
Memory Castle, 1784
Memphis Center for Independent Living, 4463
Memphis VA Medical Center, 5753
Men's/Women's Low Vision Watches & Clocks, 635
Meniere's Disease, 8519
Menopause without Medicine, 8520
Mental & Physical Disability Law Reporter, 4622
Mental & Physical Disability Law Digest, 2465
Mental Disabilities and the Americans with Disabilities Act, 4623
Mental Disability Law, Evidence and Testimony, 4624
Mental Health America, 878, 7633
Mental Health Association in Pennysylvania, 3718
Mental Health Center: Riverside Courtyard, The, 7036
Mental Health Commission, 4591
Mental Health Concepts and Techniques for the Occupational Therapy Assistant, 2466
Mental Health Law Reporter, 4625
Mental Health Unit, 6865
Mental Health and Mental Illness, 2467
Mental Retardation, 7790
Mental Retardation: A Life-Cycle Approach, 7791
Mental and Physical Disability Law Reporter, 4626
Mentally Disabled and the Law, 4627
Mentally Ill Individuals, 2468
Mentally Impaired Elderly: Strategies and Interventions to Maintain Function, 7514
Mentor Network, 6824
Mentor Network, The, 7151
Merchant Messenger, 9062
Merck Company Foundation, 3013
Mercy Dubuque Physical Rehabilitation Unit, 6896
Mercy Hospital, 6635
Mercy Medical Center Mt. Shasta, 7231
Mercy Medical Center-Pain Services, 6897
Mercy Medical Group, 6635
Mercy Memorial Health Center-Rehab Center, 6405

Mercy Subacute Care, 7297
Meridan Medical Center For Subacute Care, 6955
Meridian Valley Clinical Laboratory, 4934
Merion Publications, 2173
Merrill Lynch & Company Foundation, 3066
Merrimack Hall Performing Arts Center, 940
Merwick Rehabilitation and Sub-Acute Care, 7336
MessageMate, 1522
Metametrix Clinical Laboratory, 879
Metamorphous Press, 5028
Methodist Hospital Rehabilitation Institute, 6325
Metro Health: St. Luke's Medical Center Pain Management Program, 7107
MetroHealth Medical Center, 7108
MetroWest Center for Independent Living, 4207
Metrolina Association for the Blind, 5315
Metropolitan Center for Independent Living, 4249
Metropolitan Employment & Rehabilitation Service, 7021
Metropolitan Washington Ear, 220
Metzger-Price Fund, 3067
The Meyer Foundation, 2823
Miami Childrens Hospital, 1047, 8411
Miami Dade Public Library System, 4702
Miami Foundation, The, 2844
Miami Heart Institute Adams Building, 6762
Miami Lighthouse for the Blind, 6763
Miami VA Medical Center, 5606
Miami-Dade County Disability Services and Independent Living (DSAIL), 4019
Michael E. Debakey VA Medical Center, 5761
Michael Reese Health Trust, 2887
Michigan Assoc for the Deaf and Hard of Hearing, 8081
Michigan Association for Deaf Hard of Hearing, 8094
Michigan Association for Deaf and Hard of Hearing, 3529, 7929
Michigan Association for Deaf, and Hard of Hearing, 3530
Michigan Career And Technical Institute, 7002
Michigan Client Assistance Program, 3531
Michigan Coalition for Staff Development and School Improvement, 3532
Michigan Commission for the Blind - Gaylord, 3533
Michigan Commission for the Blind, 3534
Michigan Commission for the Blind Training Center, 3535, 7003
Michigan Commission for the Blind: Independent Living Rehabilitation Program, 4235
Michigan Commission for the Blind: Detroit, 4236
Michigan Commission for the Blind: Escanab a, 3536
Michigan Commission for the Blind: Flint, 3537
Michigan Commission for the Blind: Grand Rapids, 3538
Michigan Council of the Blind and Visually Impaired (MCBVI), 3539
Michigan Department of Civil Rights, 6064
Michigan Department of Education: Special Education Services, 2137
Michigan Department of Handicapped Children, 3540
Michigan Dept Of Energy, Labor & Economic Growth, 3534
Michigan Developmental Disabilities Council, 3541
Michigan Employment Service, 6065
Michigan Office of Services to the Aging, 3542
Michigan Protection & Advocacy Service, 3543
Michigan Psychological Association, 2035
Michigan Rehabilitation Services, 3544
Michigan Rehabilitation Services: Dept of Labor & Regulatory Affairs, 6066
Michigan Resources, 6002
Michigan State University, 4810
Michigan VA Regional Office, 5660
Michigan's Assistive Technology Resource, 4818
Micro Audiometrics Corporation, 342
Microcomputer Evaluation of Careers & Academics (MECA), 1814
Microsoft Accessibility Technology for Everyone, 5428
Microsystems Software, 1696

Mid-America Rehabilitation Hospital HealthSouth, 6337
Mid-Carolina Area Agency on Aging, 7554
Mid-Illinois Talking Book Center, 4744
Mid-Iowa Health Foundation, 2908
Mid-Michigan Industries, 7004
Mid-Ohio Board for an Independent Living Environment (MOBILE), 4396
Mid-State Independent Living Consultants: Wausau, 4542
Mid-state Independent Living Consultants: Stevens Point, 4543
Middleton Village Nursing & Rehabilitation, 7428
Middletown Regional Hospital: Inpatient Rehabilitation Unit, 7109
Mideastern Michigan Library Co-op, 4819
Midland Empire Resources for Independent Living (MERIL), 4278
Midland Memorial Hospital & Medical Center, 6454
Midland Treatment Furniture, 2469
Milbank Foundation for Rehabilitation, 3068
Milwaukee Foundation, 3255
Mind, Body, Health Sciences, 880
Mindplay, 1642, 1793
Mini Teleloop, 221
Mini-Bus and Mini-Vans, 115
Mini-Max Cushion, 287
Mini-Rider, 116
Minneapolis Foundation, 2979
Minneapolis VA Medical Center, 5663
Minneapolis YMCA Camping Services, 1207, 8417
Minnesota Assistive Technology Project, 3548
Minnesota Association of Centers for Independent Living, 4250
Minnesota Board on Aging, 3549
Minnesota Children with Special Needs, Minnesota Department of Health, 3550
Minnesota Department of Employment and Economic Development - Vocational Rehab Services, 6069
Minnesota Department of Labor & Industry Workers Compensation Division, 3551
Minnesota Dept. Of Human Rights, 6070
Minnesota Disability Law Center, 3552, 3555
Minnesota Employment Practice Agency, 6070
Minnesota Governor's Council on Developmental Disabilities GCDD, 3553
Minnesota Library for the Blind and Physically Handicapped, 4832
Minnesota Mental Health Division, 3554
Minnesota Protection & Advocacy for Persons with Disabilities, 3555
Minnesota STAR Program, 1584, 5048
Minnesota State Council on Disability (MSCOD), 3556
Minnesota State Services for the Blind, 3557
A Miracle to Believe In, 7710
Miracle-Ear Children's Foundation, 2935
Miriam, 2623
Mirror Go Lightly, 303
Mirrored Lives: Aging Children and Elderly Parents, 7515
Mission Bay Aquatic Center, 8228
Mississippi Assistive Technology Division, 3560
Mississippi Bureau of Mental Retardation, 3561
Mississippi Client Assistance Program, 3562
Mississippi Department Of Human Services, 3564
Mississippi Department of Education: Office of Special Services, 2142
Mississippi Department of Mental Health, 3563
Mississippi Department of Rehabilitation Services, 6074
Mississippi Department of Rehabilitation Services, 3562
Mississippi Division of Aging and Adult Services, 3564
Mississippi Employment Security Commission, 6075
Mississippi Library Commission, 4835, 4834
Mississippi Library Commission\Talking Book and Braille Services, 4836
Mississippi Methodist Rehabilitation Center, 7017
Mississippi Project START, 1585

Mississippi State Department of Health, 3565
Mississippi State University, 2307, 2359, 2435, 4582, 6076, 8906, 8929, 8931, 8936, 8937, 8978, 8981, 8989, 8998, 9030, 9041, 9042
Mississippi: Workers Compensation Commission, 3566
Missouri Association of Homes for the Agin g, 7468
Missouri Commission on Human Rights, 6077
Missouri Department Of Mental Health, 3568
Missouri Department of Elementary and Secondary Education: Special Education Programs, 2141
Missouri Division Of Developmental Disabilities, 3568
Missouri Easter Seal Society: Southeast Region, 7022
Missouri Governor's Council on Disability, 6078
Missouri Job Training Program Liaison, 6079
Missouri Protection & Advocacy Services, 3569
Missouri Rehabilitation Center, 2679
Missouri Rehabilitation Services for the Blind, 3570
Missouri Vocational Rehabilitation Agency, 6080
Mobile ARC, 6507
Mobile Care, 5544
Mobility International U SA, 2406
Mobility International USA, 8140, 2692, 2702, 2724, 4992, 5118, 5327, 5335, 5486, 8201, 8207
Mobility Limited, 8186, 8218, 8219
Mobility Training for People with Disabilities, 5216
Mobility Vehicle Stairlifts and Ramps, 117
Model Program Operation Manual: Business Enterprise Program Supervisors, 8998
Modular QuadDesk, 263
Modular Wall Grab Bars, 172
Moisture Seekers, 8623
Molded Sock and Stocking Aid, 304
Momentum, 8624
MonTECH, 3575
MonTECH, Montana's Statewide Assistive Tec hnology Program, 4843
Monarch Mark 1-A, 118
Monkeys Jumping on the Bed, 1714
Monmouth Vans, Access and Mobility, 119
MonoMouse Electronic Magnifiers, 636
Monroe Center for Independent Living, 4237
Montana Blind & Low Vision Services, 3576
Montana Council on Developmental Disabilit ies, 3577
Montana Department of Aging, 3578
Montana Department of Handicapped Children, 3579
Montana Fair Employment Practice Agency, 6082
Montana Governor's Committee on Employment of Disabled People, 6083
Montana Independent Living Project, Inc., 4293
Montana Protection & Advocacy for Persons with Disabilities, 3580
Montana State Fund, 3581
Montana State Library-Talking Book Library, 4844
Montana VA Regional Office, 5674
Montgomery Career Center: Alabama Employme nt Services Division, 5798
Montgomery Center for Independent Living, 3872
Montgomery County Arc, 3187
Montgomery County Department of Public Libraries/Special Needs Library, 4790
Montgomery Field, 6583
Moody Foundation, 3214
More Alike Than Different: Blind and Visually Impaired Children, 8999
More Food!, 1974
More Than Just a Job, 6230
More Than a Job: Securing Satisfying Caree rs for People with Disabilities, 5299
More Work!, 1975
Morgan Stanley Foundation, 3069
Morongo Basin Work Activity Center, 5853
Morris and Gwendolyn Cafritz Foundation, 2830
Morse Code WSKE, 1715
Mosaic, 2996, 4104
Mosaic Of De, 3995
Mosaic of Axtell Bethpage Village, 4303

Mosaic of Beatrice, 4304
Mosaic: Pontiac, 4076
Mosiac: York, 4305
Moss Rehabilitation Hospital, 6423, 5494
MossRehab ResourceNet, 5429
Mother Father Deaf: Living Between Sound a nd Silence, 8036
Mother Lode Independent Living Center (DRAIL: Disability Resource Agency for Independent, 3954
Mother Lode Rehabilitation Enterprises, 5854
Mother to Be, 5217
Mothers with Visual Impairments who are Raising Young Children, 9000
Motion Design, 716
Motivational Services, 4184
Motivator, 8208
Motor Speech Disorders, 8745
Motorhome Lift By Handicaps, Inc., 414
Mott Respiratory Care, 1196
Mount Carmel Health & Rehabilitation Center, 7429
Mount Carmel Medical and Rehabilitation Center, 7430
Mount Sinai Medical Center, 3070
Mount Sinai Medical Center Rehabilitation Unit, 6764
Mountain Home VA Medical Center James H Quillen VA Medical Center, 5754
Mountain State Center for Independent Living, 4535
Mountain State Center for Independent Living, 4536
Mountain Towers Healthcare & Rehabilitation Center, 7435
Mountain Valley Care and Rehabilitation Ce nter, 7271
Mountaineer Spina Bifida Camp, 1432, 8397
Mouthsticks, 1523
Move With Me, 9001
Movement Disorders, 2220
Movement Disorders Sourcebook, 8521
Moxie, 584
Mozart Effect: Tapping the Power of Music to Heal the Body, Strengthen the Mind, 38
Mt Hood Kiwanis Camp, 1331
Mt Sinai Medical Center, 4710
Mt. Carmel Guild, 7046
Mt. Sinai, 7283
Mt. Washington Pediatric Hospital, 6352
Muhlenberg County Opportunity Center, 6921
Mulholland Positioning Systems, 264
Multi Resource Centers, 6071
Multi-Cultural Independent Living Center of Boston, 4208
Multi-Scan Single Switch Activity Center, 1716
Multidisciplinary Assessment of Children With Learning Disabilities and Mental Retardation, 2470
Multilingual Children's Association, 7881
Multiple Choices Center for Independent Living, 4032
Multiple Phone/Device Switch, 222
Multiple Sclerosis Association of America, 7634, 8141, 8208
Multiple Sclerosis Foundation, 8142, 8605
Multiple Sclerosis National Research Institute, 5430
Multiple Sclerosis and Having a Baby, 8522
Multiple Sclerosis: 300 Tips for Making Life Easier, 8523
Multiple Sclerosis: A Guide for Families, 8524
Multiple Sclerosis: A Guide for the Newly Diagnosed, 8525
Multiple Sclerosis: The Guide to Treatment and Management, 8526
Multisensory Teaching Approach, 1976
Multisensory Teaching of Basic Language Skills: Theory and Practice, 2471
Muncie Health Care and Rehabilitation, 7290
Muppet Learning Keys, 1717
Muscular Dystrophies, 8527
Muscular Dystrophy Association, 949, 2218, 8319
Muscular Dystrophy Association - USA, 881, 1079, 8405

Muscular Dystrophy Association Free Camp, 1075, 8398
Muscular Dystrophy in Children: A Guide fo r Families, 8528
Muscular Dystrophy: The Facts, 8529
Mushroom Inserts, 343
Music Therapy, 39
Music Therapy and Leisure for Persons with Disabilities, 40
Music Therapy for the Developmentally Disa bled, 41
Music Therapy in Dementia Care, 42
Music Therapy, Sensory Integration and the Autistic Child, 43
Music and Dyslexia: A Positive Approach, 44
Music for the Hearing Impaired, 45
Music, Disability, and Society, 2472
Music: Physician for Times to Come, 46
Musical Mainstream, 9063
Muskegon Area District Library for the Bli nd and Physically Handicapped, 4820
Muu Muu, 1452
My Body is Not Who I Am Aquarius Health Care Media, 5344
My Country Aquarius Health Care Media, 5345
My First Book of Sign, 8037
My House is Killing Me! The Home Guide for Families with Allergies and Asthma, 8530
My Own Pain, 1718
My Signing Book of Numbers, 8038
Mycoclonus Research Foundation, 4853
Myositis Association, 8280
Myositis Association, The, 8689
Myths and Facts, 4628

N

N AH B Research Center, 1893
NACDD Annual Conference, 1861
NAD Broadcaster, 4629
NAD E-Zine, 8096
NADD, 1862
NADR Conference, 1863
NAHO News, 8086
NAMI Advocate, 7843
NAMI Indiana, 6326
NAMI Texas, 3776
NAPVI, 4568, 8932, 8946, 8995, 9011, 9072
NASPAC Annual Conference Association Annual Convention/Expo, 1864
NASUA News, 7542
NASW, 1865
NASW-NYS Chapter, 1865
NAT-CENT, 7598
NAVH Update, 9093
NBA Bulletin, 9094
NBIA Disorders Association, 8143
NC Base Camp, 1293, 7701
NC Department Of Commerce, 6140
NC State University, 818
NCD Bulletin, 5131
NCDE Survival Strategies for Oversease Liv ing for People with Disabilities, 5132
NCOA Week, 7543
NEXUS Wheelchair Cushioning System, 288
NFB Diabetes Action Network, 8637
NHeLP, 4569
NINDS Notes, 7893
NISH, 6208
NLP Comprehensive, 7635, 7844
NLP News, 7844
NLS News, 9095
NLS Newsletter, 9096
NNEAHSA, 7544
NOD E-Newsletter, 5133
NOLO, 4631, 5038, 7513, 7519
NOLO (Internet Brands), 4954, 5258
NORESCO Workshop, 5888
NSCLC Washington Weekly, 7545
NSSLHA Now, 8774
NYS Commission on Quality of Care & Advocacy for Persons with Disabilities, 3641
NYS Independent Living Council, 4356
NYSARC, 3642

Nabisco Foundation, 3014
NanoPac, 1673
Nansemond Pointe Rehabilitation and Health care Center, 7406
Nantahala Outdoor Center, 5506
Napa County Mental Health Department, 6636
Napa Valley PSI Inc., 5855
Napa Valley Support Systems, 6637
Narcolepsy, 8641
Nasheville Regional Office, 5755
Nashville Rehabilitation Hospital, 6434
Nashville VA Medical Center, 5756
Nasometer, 1768
Nassau County Office for the Physically Challenged, 4357
Nassau Library System, 4867
Nat l Council for Community Behavioral Healthcare, 2223
Nat'l Council for Community Behavioral Healthcare, 2519
Nat'l Lib Svc/Blind And Physically Handicapped, 8921, 8922, 8923, 8925, 9013, 9014, 9016, 9033, 9034, 9063, 9095, 9096, 9111
National 4-H Council, 2713
National AIDS Hotline, 8660
National Accreditation Council for Agencies/Blind, 9070
National Allergy and Asthma Network, 2252
National Alliance of Black Interpreters, 7930
National Alliance of Blind Students NABS Liaison, 8846
National Alliance of Blind Students NABS Liaison, 9109
National Alliance of the Disabled (NAOTD), 5431
National Alliance on Mental Illness, 7843
National Alliance on Mental Illness (NAMI), 7636
National Alliance on Mental Illness of New York State, 3643
National Amputation Foundation, 7882
National Aphasia Association, 8690
National Arts and Disability Center (NADC), 47
National Assoc of State Directors of DD Services, 5154
National Assoc. of Subacute and Post Acute Care, 1864
National Association for Adults with Speci al Learning Needs, 2036
National Association for Children of Alcoholics, 8281
National Association for Continence, 8144, 8630
National Association for Down Syndrome, 7637
National Association for Drama Therapy, 48
National Association for Holistic Aromatherapy, 882
National Association for Home Care & Hospice, 8282
National Association for Medical Direction of Respiratory Care, 8283
National Association for Parents of Children with Visual Impairments (NAPVI), 8847, 9143
National Association for Proton Therapy, 8284
National Association for Visually Handicapped (NAVH), 8848
National Association for Visually Handicap ped Lighthouse International, 5432
National Association for Visually Handicapped, 7581, 8903, 8904, 8907, 8930, 8934, 8940, 8948, 8949, 8952, 8962, 8964, 8969, 8983, 8984, 9007, 9100, 9113
National Association for the Dually Diagnosed, 7638
National Association for the Dually Diagnosed, 1862
National Association for the Education of African American Children with LD, 2037
National Association of Anorexia Nervosa and Associated Disorders, 8285
National Association of Area Agencies on Aging, 7469
National Association of Blind Educators, 8849
National Association of Blind Lawyers, 8850
National Association of Blind Merchants, 883, 8851, 9062

National Association of Blind Secretaries and Transcribers, 8852
National Association of Blind Students, 8853
National Association of Blind Teachers, 8854
National Association of Blind Veterans, 8855
National Association of Chronic Disease Directors, 8286
National Association of Cognitive- Behavioral Therapists, 7639
National Association of Cognitive-Behavior al Therapists, 7640
National Association of Colleges and Employers, 2038
National Association of Councils on Develo pmental Disabilities, 884
National Association of Counties, 7470
National Association of Developmental Disabilities Councils, 885
National Association of Disability Represe ntatives, 886
National Association of Epilepsy Centers, 7641
National Association of Guide Dog Users, 8856
National Association of Hearing Officials, 7931, 8086
National Association of Home Care and Hosp ice, 7471
National Association of Nutrition and Aging Services Programs, 7472
National Association of Parents with Child ren in Special Education, 2039, 7932
National Association of Private Special Education Centers, 2040
National Association of School Psychologists, 2098
National Association of School Psychologists, 2294, 2334, 2453, 2637
National Association of Special Education Teachers, 7933, 8691
National Association of State Directors of Developmental Disabilities Services (NASDDDS), 887
National Association of State Directors of Special Education, 2041
National Association of State Units on Aging, 7473
National Association of State Units on Aging, 7542
National Association of Visually Handicapped, 9093
National Association of the Deaf, 7934, 1163, 4616, 4629, 7982, 8096
National Association on Area Agencies on A ging, 7474
National Association to Advance Fat Acceptance, 8287
National Association to Promote the Use of Braille, 8857
National Ataxia Foundation, 7642
National Autism Association, 7643
National Autism Hotline, 7870
National Autism Resources, 1977
National Beep Baseball Association, 8858
National Black Association for Speech Language and Hearing, 7935
National Black Association for Speech-Lang uage and Hearing, 8692
National Black Deaf Advocates, 7936
National Braille Association, 4868, 8859, 8924, 9037, 9094
National Braille Press, 8860
National Brain Tumor Foundation National Brain Tumor Society, 5433
National Business & Disability Council, 888, 5434
National Camp for Blind Children, 8895
National Camps for Blind Children, 1230, 8896
National Cancer Institute, 8288, 8648
National Car Rental System, 5545
National Catholic Office for the Deaf, 8014
National Catholic Office of the Deaf, 7937, 8099
National Center for Accessible Media, 8693
National Center for Education in Maternal and Child Health, 889
National Center for Homeopathy, 2042
National Center for Learning Disabilities, 2221

National Center for Vision and Child Development, 8861
National Center on Birth Defects and Developmental Disabilities, 4727
National Center on Caregiving at Family Caregiver Alliance (FCA), 2780
National Cerebral Palsy of American, 3796
National Clearinghouse for Professions, 2043
National Clearinghouse on Disability and Exchange, 5132
National Clearinghouse on Family Support and Children's Mental Health, 2120
National Clearinghouse on Postsecondary Education, 2094
National Coalition for Assistive and Rehab Technology, 8145
National Coalition of Federal Aviation Employees with Disabilities, 3296
National College of Naturopathic Medicine, 890
National Commission on Orthotic and Prosth etic Education, 7883
National Conference on Building Codes and Standards, 1881
National Consortium on Deaf-Blindness, 7572, 826, 7576, 7590, 9077
National Council of Architectural Registration Boards (NCARB), 1882
National Council on Aging, 7475, 7541, 7543, 7547
National Council on Disability, 891, 3297, 4639, 5131
National Council on Independent Living, 892, 3997, 8146
National Council on Multifamily Housing Industry, 1897
National Council on Rehabilitation Education (NCRE), 2044
National Council on the Aging, 7524
National Council on the Aging Conference, 1866
National Cued Speech Association, 7938, 8694, 8775
National Deaf Education Network and Clearinghouse/Info To Go, 893
National Deaf Women's Bowling Association, 7939
National Diabetes Action Network for the Blind, 8862
National Diabetes Information Clearinghouse, 8289
National Digestive Diseases Information Clearinghouse, 8290
National Directory of Corporate Giving, 3284
National Disability Rights Network, 894
National Disability Sports Alliance, 8233
National Dissemination Center for Children and Youth with Disabilities (NICHCY), 895
National Division of the Blind and Visually Impaired, 3298
National Down Syndrome Congress, 7644, 7833
National Down Syndrome Society, 7645
National Early Childhood Technical Assistance Center, 896
National Easter Seal Society, 897
National Easter Seals Chicago, 7095
National Education Association of the United States, 2045
National Endowment for the Arts Office, 1892
National Endowment for the Arts: Office for AccessAbility, 49
National Epilepsy Library (NEL), 4791
National Eye Institute, 8863, 9002, 8943
National Eye Research Foundation, 2888
National Eye Research Foundation (NERF), 4745
National Family Association for Deaf-Blind, 7573, 7592
National Federation of the Blind, 2936, 7574, 8864, 6046, 6658, 8849, 8850, 8851, 8852, 8853, 8856, 8857, 8862, 8867, 8965, 8975, 8979, 9047
National Federation of the Blind Jernigan Institute, 4792
National Federation of the Blind Senior Division, 7586
National Fibromyalgia Association, 8147, 8291, 7827, 8188, 8206

National Foundation for Ectodermal Dysplasias, 2889
National Foundation for Facial Reconstruction, 3071
National Foundation of Wheelchair Tennis, 2781
National Fragile X Foundation, 8695
National Gerontological Nursing Associatio n, 7476
National Guild of Hypnotists, 898
National Headache Foundation, 2890
National Health Information Center, 7871, 8791
National Hearing Conservation Association, 7940
National Hemophilia Foundation, 3072, 8292
National Hispanic Council on Aging, 7477
National Hookup, 5134
National Human Genome Research Institute, 2135
National Hydrocephalus Foundation, 7646, 8502
National Indian Council on Aging, 7478, 7540
National Industries for the Blind, 8865, 9064
National Information Center for Children, 899
National Information Center for Children and Youth with Disabilities (NICHCY), 7575
National Information Clearinghouse on Children who are Deaf-Blind, 7576
National Institue Health, 4796
National Institute of Art and Disabilities, 50
National Institute of Environmental Health Sciences, 2144
National Institute of General Medical Scie nces, 2136
National Institute of Health, 9002
National Institute of Neurological Disorde Disorders & Stroke, 7884
National Institute on Deafness & Other Communicati, 8589
National Institute on Deafness and Other Communication Disorder, 7647
National Institute on Disability and Rehabilitation Research, 900, 4699
National Institutes Of Health, 8288
National Institutes of Health, 2135, 8289, 8290, 8293
National Institutes of Health (NIH), 8269
National Institutes of Health: National Eye Institute, 3299
National Jewish Health, 8442, 8482, 8535, 8584, 8593, 8659
National Jewish Medical & Research Center, 4686
National Kidney Foundation, 1261, 8345
National Kidney and Urologic Diseases Information Clearinghouse, 8293
National Lekotek Center, 4746, 5476
National Library Office, 4887
National Library Service for the Blind And Physically Handicapped, 51
National Library Service in Washington, 4888
National Library Services for the Blind & Physically Handicapped, 8866
National Library of Medicine, 1571
National Maternal and Child Health Bureau, 3517
National Mobility Equipment Dealers Associ ation, 8148
National Multiple Sclerosis Society, 5916, 8624
National Offices, 811
National Organization for Albinism and Hypopigmentation, 8294
National Organization of Blind Educators, 9054
National Organization of Parents of Blind Children, 8867
National Organization on Disability, 901, 5435, 5133
National Organization on Fetal Alcohol Syndrome, 8295
National Parkinson Foundation, 2845, 1850, 8627
National Parkinson Foundation & ADPF, 1876
National Parks Service, 5518
National Rehabilitation Association (NRA), 902, 5285
National Rehabilitation Association Annual Report, 5285
National Rehabilitation Hospital, 6278, 1564
National Rehabilitation Information Center, 5436
National Rehabilitation Information Center (NARIC), 903, 4793

National Right to Work Legal Defense and Education Foundation, 4570
National Science Foundation, 2167
National Senior Citizens Law Center, 7479, 7545
National Skeet Shooting Association, 8234
National Society for Experiential Education, 2046
National Spasmodic Dysphonia Association, 8149, 8696
National Spasmodic Torticollis Association, 8150
National Spinal Cord Injury Association, 8200, 8609
National Sports Center for the Disabled, 8235, 8643
National Stroke Association, 7885, 7896
National Student Speech Language Hearing A ssociation, 7941, 8697
National Stuttering Association, 8698, 8763
National Technology Database, 1586
National Theatre Workshop of the Handicapp ed (NTWH), 52
National Theatre of the Deaf, 53
National Tourette Syndrome Association, 8699
National Vaccine Information Center, 904
National Wheelchair Poolplayers Association, 8236
National Women's Health Network, 905
National Women's Health Resource Center, 5437
National-Louis University, 6309
Nationwide Foundation, 3120
Native American Advocacy Program for Perso ns with Disabilities, 4454
Native American Protection and Advocacy, 906
Natl. Clearinghouse for Alcohol & Drug Information, 2580
Natural Access, 718
Navarro Hospital, 6455
Navarro Regional Hospital: RehabCare Unit, 6455
Nazarene Publishing House, 4838
NeSoDak, 1372, 8399
Neal Freeling, 3539
Nebraska Advocacy Services, 3584
Nebraska Assistive Technology Partnership Nebraska Department of Education, 4845
Nebraska Association of Homes and Services for the Aging, 7480
Nebraska Client Assistance Program, 3585
Nebraska Commission for the Blind & Visually Impaired, 3586
Nebraska Department of Education: Special Populations Office, 2147
Nebraska Department of Health & Human Services of Medically Handicapped Children's Prgm, 3587
Nebraska Department of Health and Human Services, Division of Aging Services, 3588
Nebraska Department of Mental Health, 3589
Nebraska Employment Services, 6084
Nebraska Fair Employment Practice Agency, 6085
Nebraska Library Commission: Talking Book and Braille Service, 4846
Nebraska Planning Council on Developmental Disabilities, 3590
Nebraska Vocational Rehabilitation Agency, 6086
Nebraska Workers' Compensation Court, 3591
NeckEase, 192
Neisloss Family Foundation, 3073
Nell J Redfield Foundation, 3001
Nelson Publications, 7823
NeuroControl Corporation, 5438
Neurobehavioral Medicine Center, 6765
Neurobiology of Autism, 7792, 8746
Neuropsychiatry of Epilepsy, 8531
Neuropsychology Assessment Center, 2624
Neuroscience Publishers, 7826
Neuroxcel, 2680
Nevada Assistive Technology Project, 3594
Nevada Bureau of Vocational Rehabilitation, 3595
Nevada Community Enrichment Program (NCEP), 3596
Nevada Department of Education: Special Eduction Branch, 2152
Nevada Developmental Disability Council, 3597
Nevada Diabetes Association, 1232
Nevada Disability Advocacy and Law Center -Sparks/Reno Office, 3598

Nevada Division for Aging: Las Vegas, 3599
Nevada Division of Mental Health and Devel opmental Services, 3600
Nevada Equal Rights Commission Department Of Employment, Training & Rehabilitation, 6087
Nevada Governor's Committee on Employment of Persons with Disabilities, 6088
Nevada State Library and Archives, 4848
Nevada's Care Connection, 2068
New Bedford Rehabilitation Hospital, 6353
New Beginnings: The Blind Children's Center, 4678
New Courier Travel, 5531
New Directions For People With Disabilitie s, Inc., 5532
New Directions for People with Disabilities, 2714
New England Center for Children, 6981
New England Eye Center, Tufts Medical Cent er, 6982
New England Regional Genetics Group, 4784
New England Rehabilitation Hospital of Portland, 6351
New England Rehabilitation Hospital: Massachusetts, 6354
New Eyes for the Needy, 8868
New Focus, 6020
New Hampshire Workers Compensation Board, 3604
New Hampshire Assistive Technology Partnership Project, 3605
New Hampshire Bureau of Developmental Services, 3606
New Hampshire Client Assistance Program, 3607
New Hampshire Commission for Human Rights, 3608
New Hampshire Department of Education: Bureau for Special Education Services, 2149
New Hampshire Department of Mental Health, 3609
New Hampshire Developmental Disabilities Council, 3610
New Hampshire Division of Elderly and Adult Services, 3611
New Hampshire Employment Security, 6091
New Hampshire Fair Employment Practice Agency, 6092
New Hampshire Governor's Commission on Disability, 3612
New Hampshire Job Training Program Liaison, 6093
New Hampshire Protection & Advocacy for Persons with Disabilities, 3613
New Hampshire Rehabilitation and Sports Medicine, 7037
New Hampshire State Library: Talking Book Services, 4849
New Hampshire Veterans Centers, 5688
New Harbinger Publications, 2400, 7507, 7512
New Hope Services, 6003
New Horisons Summer Day Camp, 7692
New Horizons Independent Living Center, 4960
New Horizons Independent Living Center: Prescott Valley, 3891
New Horizons Rehabilitation, 6004
New Horizons Summer Day Camp, 1000, 8712
New Horizons Village, 3989
New Horizons in Sexuality, 5135
New Horizons: Central Louisiana, 4173
New Horizons: Northeast Louisiana, 4174
New Horizons: Northwest Louisiana, 4175
New Jersey Association of Homes and Servic es for the Aging, 7481
New Jersey Camp Jaycee, 1250
New Jersey Center for Outreach and Service s for the Autism Community (COSAC), 4854
New Jersey Commission for the Blind and Visually Impaired, 3618, 6116
New Jersey Council on Developmental Disabilities, 5149
New Jersey Department of Aging, 3619
New Jersey Department of Education, 2150
New Jersey Department of Education: Office of Special Education Program, 2150

New Jersey Department of Health and Senior Service, 3620
New Jersey Department of Health/Special Child Health Services, 3620
New Jersey Department of Labor & Workforce Development, 1587
New Jersey Developmental Disabilities Council, 5208
New Jersey Division of Mental Health Services, 3621
New Jersey Employment Service and Job Training Program Services, 6117
New Jersey Governor's Liaison to the Office of Disability Employment Policy, 3622
New Jersey Library for the Blind and Handicapped, 4855
New Jersey Medical School, 4852
New Jersey Protection & Advocacy for Persons with Disabilities, 3623
New Jersey Protection and Advocacy, 4318
New Jersey YMHA/YWHA Camps Milford, 1251, 7693
New Language of Toys: Teaching Communicati on Skills to Children with Special Needs, 5218, 5477
New Medico Community Re-Entry Service, 7005
New Medico Rehabilitation and Skilled Nursing Center at Lewis Bay, 6983
New Medico, Highwatch Rehabilitation Center, 7038
New Mexico Aging and Long-Term Services Department, 3626
New Mexico Client Assistance Program, 3627
New Mexico Commission for the Blind, 3628
New Mexico Department of Health: Children's Medical Services, 3629
New Mexico Employment Services and Job Training Liaison, 6130
New Mexico Governor's Committee on Concerns of the Handicapped, 3630
New Mexico Protection & Advocacy for Persons with Disabilities, 3631
New Mexico State Department of Education, 2151
New Mexico State Library for the Blind and Physically Handicapped, 4856
New Mexico State Veterans' Home, 5693
New Mexico Technology Assistance Program, 1588, 3632, 4331
New Mexico VA Healthcare System, 5694
New Mexico Workers Compensation Administration, 3633
New Mobility, 8189
New Music Therapist's Handbook, 2nd Ed. Berklee School of Music, 54
New Orleans Resources for Independent Living, 4176
New Orleans Speech and Hearing Center, 6938
New Orleans VA Medical Center, 5640
New Quad Grip, 120
New State Office of Mental Health Agency, 3644
New Ventures, 5953
New Vision Enterprises, 6922
New Vision Store, 486, 5471
New Vistas, 4332
New Voices: Self Advocacy By People with Disabilities, 5136
New World Library, 8483, 8571, 8578
New York Arthritis Reporter, 8209
New York Association of Homes and Services for the Aging, 7482
New York Branch International Dyslexia Association, 1845
New York Chapter of the Arthritis Foundation, 8209
New York City Bar, 4592
New York City Campus of the VA NY Harbor Healthcare System, 5703
New York Client Assistance Program, 3645
New York Community Trust, 3074
New York Department of Handicapped Children, 3646
New York District Kiwanis Foundation, 1278
New York Families For Autistic Children, 7818
New York Foundation, 3075

New York Public Library, 4857
New York Regional Office, 5704
New York Service for the Handicapped, 1245, 8161
New York State Commisionon Qualityof Careand Advoc, 3652
New York State Commission for the Blind, 3647
New York State Commission on Quality of Care, 3648
New York State Congress of Parents and Teachers, 3649
New York State Department of Labor, 6137
New York State Education Department, 2153, 3666
New York State Library and Education, 4869
New York State Office of Advocates for Persons with Disabilities, 3650
New York State Office of Mental Health, 3651
New York State TRAID Project, 3652
New York State Talking Book & Braille Library, 4869
New York State Talking Book & Braille Library, 9112
New York State Talking Book and Braille Library, 4966
New York Therapeutic Riding Center-Equestr ia, 907
New York University Medical Center, 4860
New York-Presbyterian Hospital, 7069
Newark Healthcare Center, 7110
Newark Regional Office, 5692
Newport County Chapter of Retarded Citizens, 6178
Newport Hospital, 7148
Newport News Public Library System, 4925
News from Advocates for Deaf-Blind, 7592
NewsLine, 5219
Newsletter Bulletin, 8087
Newsletter of PA's AT Lending Library, 5439
Nexus Health Systems, 6467
Nick Joins In, 8532
Nightshirts, 1482
Nintendo, 5474
Nishna Productions-Shenandoah Work Center, 6898
No Barriers Aquarius Health Care Media, 5346
No Boundaries, 579, 584
No Limits, 55
No Limits Communications & New Mobility, 541
No Limits Limb Loss Foundation, 1138
No Longer Disabled: the Federal Courts & the Politics of Social Security Disability, 4630
No Longer Immune: A Counselor's Guide to AIDS, 2473
No More Allergies, 8533
No Time for Jello: One Family's Experience, 8534
Noble Of Indiana, 6005
Noble, Inc., 6005
Nocturnal Asthma, 8535
Nolo's Guide to Social Security Disability Getting and Keeping Your Benefits, 4631
Non-Traditional Casting Project, 56
Nonverbal Learning Disabilities at Home: A Parent's Guide, 8747
NorCal Services For Deaf & Hard Of Hearing, Inc., 974, 7959
Norcliffe Foundation, 3240
Nordson Corporate Giving Program, 3121
Norfolk Foundation, 3230
Norman Marcus Pain Institute, 7070
North America Riding for the Handicapped Association, 908
North American Riding for the Handicapped Association, 8237
North American Riding for the Handicapped Assoc, 8193
North Atlantic Books, 2375, 5019
North Auburn Rehabilitation And Health Center, 7416
North Broward Medical Center, 7253, 6766
North Broward Rehab Unit, 6766
North Carolina Workers Compensation Board, 3672
North Carolina Accessibility Code, 1899

North Carolina Assistive Technology Project, 3673
North Carolina Association of Non-Profit Homes for the Aging, 7483
North Carolina Children & Youth Branch, 3674
North Carolina Client Assistance Program, 3675
North Carolina Department of Insurance, 1899
North Carolina Department of Public Instruction: Exceptional Children Division, 2145
North Carolina Developmental Disabilities, 3676
North Carolina Division of Aging, 3677
North Carolina Division of Services for the Blind, 6142
North Carolina Industrial Commission, 3678
North Carolina Library for the Blind and Physically Handicapped, 4878
North Carolina Publc of Health, 3674
North Central Independent Living Services, 4294
North Chicago VA Medical Center, 5621
North Coast Rehabilitation Center, 6254
North Country Center for Independent Livin g, 4358
North Country Independent Living, 4544
North Country Independent Living: Ashland, 4545
North Dakota Workers Compensation Board, 3681
North Dakota Client Assistance Program, 3682
North Dakota Community Foundation, 3102
North Dakota Department of Education: Special Education, 2146
North Dakota Department of Human Resources, 3683
North Dakota Department of Human Services, 3684
North Dakota Department of Labor, Human Ri ghts Division, 6150
North Dakota Employment Service and Job Training Program Liaison, 6151
North Dakota State Library Talking Book Services, 4881
North Dakota State Library Talking Book Services, 5065
North Dakota VA Regional Office Fargo Regional Office, 5718
North Dakota Vocational Rehabilitation Agency, 6152
North District Independent Living Program, 4033
North Georgia Talking Book Center, 4728
North Hastings Community Integration Association, 909
North Hills Hospital, 7399
North Little Rock Regional Office, 5575
North Ridge Medical and Rehabilitation Cen ter, 7431
North Star Community Services, 5137
North Texas Rehabilitation Center, 7178
North Valley Services, 6638
Northampton VA Medical Center, 5652
Northeast Independent Living Program, 4209
Northeast Independent Living Services, 4279
Northeast Occupational Exchange, 6043
Northeast Rehabilitation Clinic, 7332
Northeast Rehabilitation Hospital, 6372
Northeast Wisconsin Directory of Services for Older Adults, 2069
Northeastern Pennsylvania Center for Independent Living, 4433
Northern Arizona University, 6522
Northern Arizona VA Health Care System, 5570
Northern Cartographic, 5498
Northern Illinois Center for Adaptive Technology, 1589
Northern Illinois Special Recreation Association (NISRA), 6850
Northern Nevada Center for Independent Liv ing: Fallon, 4307
Northern Nevada Center for Independent Living, 5051
Northern New England Association of Homes and Services for the Aging, 7484
Northern New England Conference, 1137, 8884
Northern New Hampshire Mental Health and Developmental Services, 7039
Northern New York Community Foundation, 3076
Northern Regional Center for Independent Living: Watertown, 4359

Northern Regional Center for Independent L iving: Lowville, 4360
Northern Suburban Special Recreation Association, 1068
Northern Utah Center for Independent Living, 4492
Northern Virginia Resource Center for Deaf and Hard of Hearing Persons, 4926
Northern West Virginia Center for Independent Living, 4537
Northland Library Cooperative, 4821
Northn New England Assoc of Homes & Svcs for Aging, 7544
Northport VA Medical Center, 5705
Northridge Hospital Medical Center, 6255, 7232
Northridge Hospital Medical Center Rehabiltation Medicine, 6639
Northridge Hospital Medical Center: Center for Rehabilitation Medicine, 6640
Northstar Community Services, 6899
Northview Developmental Services, 6914
Northwest Arkansas Rehabilitation Hospital, 6234
Northwest Continuum Care Center, 7207
Northwest Hospital Center for Medical Rehabilitation, 6479
Northwest Kansas Library System Talking Books, 4768
Northwest Kiwanis Camp, 1430, 8400
Northwest Limousine Service, 5546
Northwest Medical Center, 6767
Northwest Ozarks Regional Library for the Blind and Handicapped, 4666
Northwestern Mutual Life Foundation, 3256
Northwestern University Multipurpose Arthritis & Musculoskeletal Center, 4747
Northwoods Lodge, 7417
Northwoods of Cortland, 7348
Norton- Lambert Corporation, 1512
Norwalk Hospital Section Of Physical Medicine And Rehabilitation, 6705
Norwalk Press, 8461
Norway Rehabilitation and Living Center, 7310
Norwegian Cruise Line, 5533
Nosey Cup, 365
Not Without Sight, 9125
Noteworthy Newsletter, 7895
Nothing is Impossible: Reflections on a N ew Life, 5138
Nova Care, 6526
Novartis Pharmaceuticals Division, 7798
Ntn'l Comm on Orthotic & Prosthetic Education, 7895
Ntn'l Institute of Neurological Disorders & Stroke, 7893
Ntn'l Student Speech Language Hearing Association, 8774
Nurse Healers: Professional Associates International, 910
Nursery Rhymes from Mother Goose, 8039
Nutritional Desk Reference, 5139
Nutritional Influences on Illness:, 5140
Nuvisions For Disabled Artists, Inc., 57

O

O&P Almanac, 2254
O'Reilly Media Inc, 8430, 8431, 8453, 8454, 8456, 8460, 8486, 8512, 8553, 8581
OASYS, 1815
OCCK, 1590
ODHH Directory of Resources and Services, 2070
OMRON Foundation OMRON Electronics, 2891
ONLINE, 2625
OPTIONS, 4251
OPTIONS for Independence, 4492
OPTIONS for Independence: Brigham Satellit e, 4493
OT Practice Magazine, 5300
OWLS: Oral and Written Language Scales LC/OE & WE, 2626
Oak Forest Hospital of Cook County, 6851
Oak Hill Nursing and Rehabilitation Center, 7384
Oak Leyden Developmental Services, 7648
Oakcrest Care Center, 7127

Oakhill-Senior Program, 7128
Oakland County Library for the Visually & Physically Impaired, 4822
Oakland School & Camp, 1424, 7694
Oakland VA Regional Office, 5580
Oakland Work Activity Area, 5856
Oakwood Rehabilitation and Nursing Center, 7321
Oberkotter Foundation, 3148
Obesity, 8536
Obesity Sourcebook, 8537
Ocala Adult Day Training, 4020
Occulta, 8538
Occupational Center of Hudson County, 6118
Occupational Center of Union County, 6119
Occupational Hearing Services Inc., 8116
Occupational Therapy Across Cultural Boundaries, 2474
Occupational Therapy Approaches to Traumatic Brain Injury, 2475
Occupational Therapy Strategies and Adaptations for Independent Daily Living, 6384
Occupational Therapy and Vocational Rehabi litation, 5301
Occupational Therapy in Health Care, 2255
Occupational Training Center of Burlington County, 6120
Occuptational Training Center of Camden County, New Jersey, 6121
Ocean State Center for Independent Living, 4443
Oconee Regional Library, 4729
Office Of Disease Prevention And Health Promotion, 7871
Office Of Library & Information Services for the Blind and Physically Handicapped, 4900
Office for Students with Disabilities, University of Texas at Arlington, 4477
Office of Disability and Employment Policy, 2034
Office of Elderly Affairs, 3496
Office of Grants Management, 2882
Office of Juvenile Justice and Delinquency Prevention, 5440
Office of Mental Health, 3644
Office of Policy, 3300
Office of Rehabilitation Services, 4444, 6179
Office of Special Education Programs: Department of Education, 3301
Office of State Coordinator of Vocational Education for Students with Disability, 6006
Office of Vocational Rehabilitation, 6169
Office of Vocational Rehabilitation Servic es (OVRS), 3709
Office of the Commissioner, 1587
Office of the Governor, 3748
Official Patient's Sourcebook on Bell's Pa lsy, 8539
Official Patient's Sourcebook on Cystic Fi brosis, 8540
Official Patient's Sourcebook on Muscular Dystrophy, 8541
Official Patient's Sourcebook on Osteoporo sis, 8542
Official Patient's Sourcebook on Post-Poli o Syndrome: A Revised and Updated Directory, 8543
Official Patient's Sourcebook on Primary Pulmonary Hypertension, 8544
Official Patient's Sourcebook on Pulmonary Fibrosis, 8545
Official Patient's Sourcebook on Scoliosis, 8546
Official Patient's Sourcebook on Sickle Ce ll Anemia, 8547
Official Patient's Sourcebook on Ulcerativ e Colitis, 8548
Ohio Bureau for Children with Medical Hand icaps, 3690
Ohio Bureau of Worker's Compensation, 3691
Ohio Civil Rights Commission, 6157
Ohio Client Assistance Program, 3692
Ohio Coalition for the Education of Children with Disabilities, 2256
Ohio Commission On Minority Health, 6158
Ohio County Public Library Services for the Blind and Physically Handicapped, 4940
Ohio Department of Aging, 3693
Ohio Department of Education, 2154

Ohio Department of Education: Division of Special Education, 2154
Ohio Department of Health, 3690
Ohio Department of Mental Health, 3694
Ohio Developmental Disabilities Council, 3695
Ohio Developmental Disability Council (ODD C), 3696
Ohio Governor's Council on People with Disabilities, 3697
Ohio Regional Library for the Blind and Physically Handicapped, 4887
Ohio Rehabilitation Services Commission, 3698
Ohio Statewide Independent Living Council, 4397
Ohio Women, Infants, & Children Program Ohio Department of Health, 3699
Ohio-West Virginia YMCA, 1433, 8416
Okizu Foundation, 977, 8359
Oklahoma Workers Compensation Board, 3701
Oklahoma Association of Homes and Services for the Aging, 7485
Oklahoma City VA Medical Center, 5726, 5039
Oklahoma Client Assistance Program/Office of Disability Concerns, 3702
Oklahoma Department of Human Services Aging Services Division, 3703
Oklahoma Department of Labor, 3704
Oklahoma Department of Mental Health & Substance Abuse Services, 3705
Oklahoma Department of Rehabilitation Services, 3706, 6160
Oklahoma Employment Services and Job Training Program Liaison, 6161
Oklahoma Governor's Committee on Employment of People with Disabilities, 6162
Oklahoma League for the Blind, 7123
Oklahoma Library for the Blind & Physically Handicapped, 4889
Oklahoma Medical Research Foundation, 4890
Oklahoma State Department of Education, 2155
Oklahoma Veterans Centers Vet Center, 5727
Oklahomans for Independent Living, 4404
Old Adobe Developmental Services, 6641, 6648
Old Adobe Developmental Services-Rohnert Park Services (Behavioral), 6642
Old MacDonald's Farm Deluxe, 1719
Old MacDonald's Farm IntelliKeys Overlay, 1524
Older Americans Report, 3285
Omnigraphics, 36, 461, 5080, 7516, 8435, 8436, 8438, 8439, 8441, 8444, 8447, 8448, 8450, 8451, 8452, 8455, 8467, 8468, 8470, 8471, 8475, 8484, 8487, 8488, 8500, 8504, 8513, 8521, 8537, 8551, 8559, 8574, 8579
Omnigraphics, Inc., 8427
On Cue, 8775
On My Own, 4280
On The Spectrum Fanlight Productions/Icarus Films, 5347
On a Green Bus: A UKanDu Little Book, 1785
On the Level, 8088
On the Road to Autonomy: Promoting Self-Competence in Children & Youth with Disabilities, 5220
One Day at a Time: Children Living with Leukemia, 8549
One Heartland, 1203
One Step At A Time Camp, 1076
One Thousand FS, 681, 750
One for All Lift All, 415
One-Stop Service, 5937
Ontario Cerebral Palsy Sports Association, 8238
Ontario Federation for Cerebral Palsy, 7649
Open Back Nightgowns, 1483
Open Book, 1786
Open Circle Theatre, 58
Open for Business, 5348
Open to the Public Aquarius Health Care Media, 5349
Opening the Courthouse Door: An ADA Access Guide for State Courts, 4632
Operation Job Match, 5916
Ophthalmic Research Laboratory Eye Institute/First Hill Campus, 4935
Opportunities for Access: A Center for Independent Living, 4077

Opportunities for the Handicapped, 5857
Opportunity, 9064
Opportunity East Rehabilitation Services for the Blind, 7153
Optelec U S, 1625, 1708, 1709
Optimum Resource, 1655, 1656, 1657, 1658, 1659, 1660, 1674, 1720, 1731, 1732, 1733, 1734, 1735, 1788, 1790, 1796, 1799, 1802, 1803, 1804, 1805, 1809, 1817
Optimum Resource Educational Software, 1720
Optimum Resource Software, 1787
Optimum Resources/Stickybear Software, 1721
Option Indigo Press, 5365, 7710
Option Institute, 8666
Options, 8625
Options Center for Independent Living: Bourbonnais, 4078
Options Center for Independent Living: Watseka, 4079
Options Interstate Resource Center for Independent Living, 4252
Options for Independence: Auburn, 4361
Options for Independent Living, 4546
Options for Independent Living: Fox Valley, 4547
Options of Linn County, 6900
Options: Revolutionary Ideas in the War on Cancer, 8550
Optometric Extension Program Foundation, 2937, 8915
Orange County ARC, 5858
Orange County Library System: Audio-Visual Department, 4709
Orchard Village, 5980
Ordean Foundation, 2980
Oregon Advocacy Center, 3710
Oregon Alliance of Senior and Health Services, 7486
Oregon Bureau of Labor & Industry, 6164
Oregon Client Assistance Program, 3711
Oregon Commission for the Blind, 3712
Oregon Council on Developmental Disabilities, 5141
Oregon Department of Education:, 2156
Oregon Department of Education: Office of Special Education, 2156
Oregon Department of Mental Health, 3713
Oregon Fair Employment Practice Agency, 6164
Oregon Health Sciences University, 5728
Oregon Health Sciences University, Elks' Children's Eye Clinic, 4892
Oregon Nursing And Rehabilitation Center, 7373
Oregon Perspectives, 5141
Oregon State Elks Association, 7975
Oregon Talking Book & Braille Services, 4893
Oregon Technology Access for Life, 3714
Oregon-Idaho Conference Center, 1063, 1324, 1325, 1332, 1335, 8353, 8356, 8364, 8404, 8412
Oregon/Idaho Conference Center, 1333, 8407
Organ Transplants: Making the Most of Your Gift of Life, 5142
Orientation and Mobility Primer for Families and Young Children, 9003
Origin Instruments Corporation, 1525
Orthopedic Products Corporation, 254
Orthotics and Prosthetics Almanac, 8606
Oryx Press, 1961
Osborn Medical Corporation, 325
Oshkosh Medical and Rehabilitation Center, 7432
Ostberg Foundation, 3015
Osteogenesis Imperfecta Foundation, 5441
Osteoporosis Sourcebook, 8551
Osterguard Enterprises c/o Jim's Shop, 686
Otto Bremer Foundation, 2981
Our Lady of Lourdes Medical Center, 7045
Our Lady of Lourdes Rehabilitation Center, 6343
Our Own Road Aquarius Health Care Media, 5350
Our Way: The Cottage Apt Homes, 3897
Our World, 2221
Out of Left Field, 9126
Out of the Corner of My Eye: Living with Vision Loss in Later Life, 9004
Out of the Corner of My Eye: Living with Macular Degeneration, 9005

Out of the Fog: Treatment Options and Coping Strategies for ADD, 7793
Out-N-About American Walker, 654
Out-Sider III, 416
Out-Sider Meridian, 417
Outdoor Independence, 585
Outside In School Of Experiential, 1356
Outside In School Of Experiential Education, Inc., 7695
Outsider: The Life and Art of Judith Scott Fanlight Productions/Icarus Films, 5351
Outsiders in a Hearing World: A Sociology of Deafness, 8040
Oval Window Audio, 344
Over the Rainbow Disabled Travel Services & Wheelers Accessible Van Rentals, 5547
Overcoming Dyslexia, 7794
Overcoming Dyslexia in Children, Adolescents and Adults, 2476
Overcoming Mobility Barriers International, 1883
Overeaters Anonymous World Service Office, 8296
Overnight Camps, 1408
Oxford Journals, Oxford University Press, 5284
Oxford Textbook of Geriatric Medicine, 2477
Oxford University Press, 2477, 2516, 2530, 5167, 7728, 7735, 7774, 8048, 8469, 8527, 8529, 8580, 8595, 8718, 8725
Ozark Independent Living, 4281

P

P A Department of Labor and Industry, 6170
P CI Educational Publishing, 1664
P ES CO International, 6135
PAC Unit, 121
PACE Center for Independent Living, 4080
PACER Center (Parent Advocacy Coalition for Educational Rights), 911
PACER E-News, 2257
PACER Partners, 2258
PACESETTER, 2259
PAL News, 4633
PALAESTRA: Forum of Sport, Physical Education and Recreation for Those with Disabilities, 8190
PALS Support Groups, 8661
PARC, 6852
PARI Independent Living Center, 4445
PAT-3: Photo Articulation Test, 2627
PBA News, 9097
PCI, 5478
PCI Education Publishing, 1671, 1688, 1921
PDF News, 8607
PDF Newsletter, 8626
PEAK Parent Center, 912, 2099, 5143
PECO Energy Company Contributions Program, 3149
PEERS Program, 6256
PIRS Hotsheet, 6257
PKU Camp, 1180
PKU for Children: Learning to Measure, 2478
PM&R Journal, 5286
PN/Paraplegia News, 8191
PNC Bank Foundation, 3150
POZ Magazine, 8608
PRIDE Industries, 5859, 6643
PRO-ED, 2100
PRO-ED Inc., 2378, 5303, 7580
PSS CogRehab Software, 1769
PVA Publications, 8191
PVA Sports and Recreation Program, 5600
PVA Summit & Expo, 1867
PWI Forum, 6071
PWI Profile, 6052
PWSA (USA) Conference, 1868
PXE International, 8662
Pac-All Carriers, 682
Pac-All Wheelchair Carrier, 682
Pace Saver Plus II, 586
Pacific Hospital Of Long Beach-Neuro Care Unit, 6644
Pacific Institute of Aromatherapy, 913
Pacific Islands Health Care System, 5616

Pacific Rim International Conference on Disability And Diversity, 1869
Pacific Specialty & Rehabilitation Center r, 7418
Pacific Spine and Pain Center, 7129
Paddy Rossbach Youth Camp, 1383
Paducah Centre For Health and Rehabilitati on, 7301
Pain Alleviation Center, 7071
Pain Centers: A Revolution in Health Care, 2479
Pain Control & Rehabilitation Institute of Georgia, 6800
Pain Erasure, 5221
Pain Erasure: the Bonnie Prudden Way, 9006
Pain Institute of Tampa, 6768
Pain Treatment Center, Baptist Hospital of Miami, 6769
Painted Turtle, The, 1001
Palestine Resource Center for Independent Living, 4478
Palgrav Macmillan, 8429
Palm Beach County Library, 4713
Palm Beach Habilitation Center, 5938
Palmer & Dodge, 2944
Palmer Independence, 587
Palmer Industries, 585, 587, 588
Palmer Twosome, 588
Panhandle Action Center for Independent Living Skills, 4479
Panties, 1502
Paradigm Design Group, 1884
Paradise Vally Hospital-South Bay Rehabilitation Center, 6645
Paragon House, 8463
Parallels in Time, 5144
Paralysis Resource Guide, 8181
Paralysis Society of America, 5507
Paralyzed Veterans Of America, 1867
Paralyzed Veterans of America, 8151, 1884, 5492, 5507, 5600, 8230
Paraquad, 4282
Parent Assistance Network, 8663
Parent Centers and Independent Living Centers: Collectively We're Stronger, 5222
Parent Connection, 3777
Parent Magic, 5309, 7717
Parent Professional Advocacy League, 914, 4633, 8661
Parent Survival Manual, 7795, 8748
Parent to Parent of New York State, 3653
Parent's Guide to Allergies and Asthma, 8552
Parent's Guide to Down Syndrome: Toward a Brighter Future, 7796
Parent-Child Interaction and Developmental Disabilities, 5223
Parental Concerns in College Student Mental Health, 2480
Parenting, 5224
Parenting Attention Deficit Disordered Teens, 7797
Parenting with a Disability, 5225
Parents Helping Parents (PHP), 915
Parents Helping Parents: A Directory of Support Groups for ADD, 7798
Parents Supporting Parents Network, 3778
Parents and Friends, 6646
Parents and Friends, Inc, 5860
Parents and Teachers, 2481
Parents, Let's Unite for Kids, 1591
Paring Boards, 366
Park Brake Extension By Handicaps, Inc., 122
Park DuValle Community Health Center, Inc., 6923
Park Health And Rehabilitation Center, 7324
Park Manor Convalescent Center, 7208
Parker Bath, 418
Parker Foundation, 2782
Parker Publishing Company, 5031
Parker-Hannifin Foundation, 3122
Parkinson's Disease Foundation, 2892, 3077, 8607, 8626
Parkinson's Disease Research Society, 8152
Parkinsons Report, 8627
Parkview Acres Care and Rehabilitation Cen ter, 7326
Parkview Regional Rehabilitation Center, 6327

Parma Community General Hospital Acute Rehabilitation Center, 6395, 7111
Parrot Easy Language Simple Anaylsis, 1770
Parrot Software, 1761, 1770, 1789
Part B News, 7531
Part of the Team, 5145
Partial Seizure Disorders: A Guide for Patients and Families, 8553
Partnering with Public Health: Funding & Advocacy Opportunities for CILs and SILCs, 5146
Partners Resource Network, 3779
Parts of Speech, 1788
Pasadena Foundation, 2783
Passion for Justice, 5352
PathPoint, 5861
Pathfinder Publishing, 8459
Pathfinder Village, 7072
Pathfinders for Independent Living, 4171
Pathways Brain Injury Program, 7302
Pathways To Inclusion (2nd Edition), 4982
Pathways for the Future Center for Indepen dent Living, 4381
Pathways to Independence, Inc., 6122
Patient Lifting & Injury Prevention, 419
Patient Transport Chair, 719
Patient and Family Education, 2482
Patient's Guide to Visual Aids and Illumination, 9007
Patient-Centered Guides, 700, 5123, 5142, 8180
Patient-Centered Guides/O'Reilly Media, 5251
Patricia Neal Rehab Center : Ft. Sanders R egional Medical Center, 6435
Patrick Rehab Wellness Center, 7154
Patrick and Anna M Cudahy Fund, 3257
Patriot Extra Wide Folding Walkers, 655
Patriot Folding Walker Series, 656
Patriot Reciprocal Folding Walkers, 657
Patterson Medical, 487
Paul H Brookes Publishing Company, 2318, 2483, 7755
Paul and Annetta Himmelfarb Foundation, 2831
Paws for Silence, 8089
Peabody Articulation Decks, 1978
Peabody Early Experiences Kit (PEEK), 2628
Peabody Individual Achievement Test-Revised Normative Update (PIAT-R-NU), 2629
Peabody Language Development Kits (PLDK), 2630
Pearle Vision Foundation, 3215
Pearlman Biomedical Research Institute, 4710
Pearson, 2657, 5259
Pearson Education, 2396
Pearson Higher Education, 2284
Pearson Performance Solutions, 488
Pearson Publishing, 7791
Pearson Reid London House, 489
Pedal Ease, 123
Pedal-in-Place Exerciser, 530
Pediatric Center at Plymouth Meeting Integrated Health Services, 7143
Pediatric Early Elementary (PEEX II) Examination, 2631
Pediatric Exam of Educational-PEERAMID Readiness at Middle Childhood, 2632
Pediatric Examination of Educational Readiness, 2633
Pediatric Extended Examination at-PEET Three, 2634
Pediatric Rehabilitation Department, JFK Medical Center, 7047
Pediatric Rheumatology Clinic, 4879
Pediatric Seating System, 289
Pediatric Visual Diagnosis Fact Sheets, 9008
Pediatrics, School Of Medicine,Univ Of S. Carolina, 816
Peer Counseling: Roles, Functions, Boundaries, 5147
Peer Mentor Volunteers: Empowering People for Change, 5148
Pegasus LITE, 1824
Peidmont Independent Living Center, 4519
Pencil/Pen Weighted Holders, 558
Penguin Books USA, 5194
Penguin Group, 8568

Peninsula Center for Independent Living, 4520
Penitent, with Roses: An HIV+ Mother Refle cts, 8554
Penn State Milton S. Hershey Medical Center College Of Medicine, 7144
Pennstate, 7132
Pennsylvania Workers Compensation Board, 3719
Pennsylvania Association of Nonprofit Senior Services, 7487
Pennsylvania Bureau of Blindness & Visual Services, 3720
Pennsylvania Client Assistance Program, 3721
Pennsylvania College of Optometry Eye Institute, 4898
Pennsylvania Council on Independent Living, 4415
Pennsylvania Department of Aging, 3722
Pennsylvania Department of Children with Disabilities, 3723
Pennsylvania Department of Education: Bureau of Special Education, 2157
Pennsylvania Developmental Disabilities Council, 3724
Pennsylvania Employment Services and Job Training, 6170
Pennsylvania Governor's Committee on Employment of Disabled Persons, 6171
Pennsylvania Human Relations Commission Agency, 6172
Pennsylvania Pain Rehabilitation Center, 7145
Pennsylvania Protection & Advocacy for Persons with Disabilities, 3725
Pennsylvania Veterans Centers, 5738
Pennsylvania's Initiative on Assistive Technology, 1592
Penrose Hospital/ St. Francis Healthcare System, 6677
People & Families, 2222
People Against Cancer, 8550, 8625
People First of Canada, 916
People First of Oregon, 917
People Services, 6647
People Services, Inc, 5862
People With Disabilities Press (iUniverse), 4981
People and Families, 5149
People to People International, 2715
People with Disabilities & Abuse: Implications for Center for Independent Living, 5150
People with Disabilities Who Challenge the System, 5151
The People's Burn Foundation, 1086
People's Voice, 5152
People-to-People Committee on Disability, 918
People-to-People International: Committee for the Handicapped, 919
Peoria Area Blind People's Center, 6853
Peoria Area Community Foundation, 2893
Perfect Solutions, 1526
Perigee Visual Dictionary of Signing, 8041
Perkins Activity and Resource Guide: A Handbook for Teachers, 9009
Perkins Brailler, 559
Perkins School for the Blind, 9009
Permaflex Home Care Mattress, 193
Permobil, 751, 752
Permobil Max 90, 751
Permobil Super 90, 752
Permobil USA, 739
Perry Health Facility, 6286
Perry Point VA Medical Center, 5648
Perry Rehabilitation Center, 6527
Perry River Home Care, 4253
Person to Person: Guide for Professionals Working with the Disabled, 2483
Personal FM Systems, 223
Personal Infrared Listening System, 224
Personal Perspectives on Personal Assistance Services, 5153
Personal Reader Department, 9010
Personal Reader Update, 9010
Personality and Emotional Disturbance, 2484
Perspectives, 5154
Perspectives on a Parent Movement, 5226
Perspectives: Whole Language Folio, 8749
Pervasive Developmental Disorders: Finding a Diagnosis and Getting Help, 5251

Pet Partners, 531
Petaluma Recycling Center, 6648
Peter A Towne Physical Therapy Center, 7112
Pettigrew Rehabilitation and Healthcare Center, 7356
Peytral Publications, 2101
Phantom Compact Size Scooter, 589
Phantom Lake YMCA Camp, 1438, 8401
PharmaThera, 7155
Phelps School Summer School, 1357, 7696
Phenomenology of Depressive Illness, 2485
Philadelphia Foundation, 3151
Philadelphia Regional Office and Insurance Center, 5739
Philadelphia VA Medical Center, 5740
Phillip Roy, 1527
Phillip Roy, Inc., 1935
Philomatheon Society of the Blind, 7113
Phoenix Childrens Hospital, 956, 8361
Phoenix Dance Fanlight Productions/Icarus Films, 5353
Phoenix Veterans Center, 6528
Phone of Our Own: The Deaf Insurrection Against Ma Bell, 8042
PhoneMax Amplified Telephone, 560
Phonemic Awareness in Young Children: A Classroom Curriculum, 1979
Phonics for Thought, 1980
Phonological Awareness Training for Reading, 1981
Physical & Mental Issues in Aging Sourcebook, 7516
Physical & Occupational Therapy in Geriatrics, 7525
Physical Disabilities and Health Impairments: An Introduction, 2486
Physical Education and Sports for Exceptional Students, 2487
Physical Management of Multiple Handicaps: A Professional's Guide, 2488
Physically Handicapped in Society, 2489
Physically Impaired Association of Michigan, 4818
Piece of Cake Math, 1651
Pied Piper: Musical Activities to Develop Basic Skills, 59
Piedmont Independent Living Center, 4521
Piedmont Living Center, 4519
Piedmont Triad Council of Governments Area Agency on Aging, 7555
Pilgrim Pines Camp & Conference Center, 1002
Pillow Talk, 197
Pilot Books, 5490
Pilot Industries: Ellenville, 7073
Pine Castle, 6770
Pine Meadows Healthcare and Rehabilitation Center, 7394
Pine Tree Camp, 1144
Pine Tree Society, 1139, 1144
Pinecrest Rehabilitation Hospital and Outpatient Centers, 6287
Pinellas Park Adult Day Training, 4021
Pinellas Talking Book Library for the Blind and Physically Handicapped, 4711
Pines Residential Treatment Center, 7191
Pinnacle Newsletter, 8097
Pioneer Center of McHenry County, 6854
Pioneer Vocational/Industrial Services, 6030
Pittsburgh Foundation, 3152
Pittsburgh Regional Office, 5741
A Place for Me Educational Productions, 5304
Place of Their Own: Creating the Deaf Community in America, 8043
Place to Live, 5155
Placer Independent Resource Services, 3955, 6257
Places for People, 4283
Plan Ahead: Do What You Can, 8555
Planned Giving Department of Guide Dogs for the Blind, 9098
Planned Parenthood of Western Washington, 8055
Plastic Card Holder, 532
Platte River Industries, 6688
Play!, 1982
Playback, 9099
Please Don't Say Hello, 7799, 8750

Please Understand Me: Software Program and Books, 1722
Plenum Publishing Corporation, 5053
Plum Enterprises, 534, 1466
Pocatello Regional Medical Center, 6307
Pocket Guide to the ADA: Accessibility Guidelines for Buildings and Facilities, 4571
Pocket Otoscope, 323
Polaris Industries, 590
Polaris Trail Blazer, 590
Polk Brothers Foundation, 2894
Polk County Association for Handicapped Citizens, 6771
Polyester House Dress, 1453
Pomerado Rehabilitation Outpatient Service, 6649
Pomona Valley Workshop, 5863
Pompano Rehabilitation and Nursing Center, 7254
Pond, 1723
Pool Exercise Program Arthritis Water Exercise / Arthritis Foundation, 5354
Poplar Bluff RehabCare Program, 7023
Port City Enterprises, 6939
Port Huron: Blue Water Center for Independent Living, 4238
Port Jefferson Health Care Facility, 7349
PortaPower Plus, 1619
Portable Hand Controls, 124
Portable Hand Controls By Handicaps, Inc., 125
Portable Large Print Computer, 1627
Portable Shampoo Bowl, 173
Portable Vehicle Controls, 126
Porterville Sheltered Workshop, 5864
Portland Public Library, 4785
Portland Regional Office, 5729
Portland VA Medical Center, 5730
Portneuf Medical Center Rehabilitation, 6809
Post-Polio Health, 8628
Post-Polio Health International, 8153, 8199, 8628
Post-Polio Newsletter, 8199
Post-Polio Support Group, 8664
Post-Polio Syndrome: A Guide for Polio Survivors and Their Families, 8556
Postgraduate Center for Mental Health, 4870
Posture-Glide Lounger, 720
Potomac Technology, 490
Potty Learning for Children who Experience Delay, 5355
Powell's Books, 8012
Power Breathing Program, 1983
Power Door, 533
Power Seat Base (6-Way), 127
Power Wheelchairs, 753
Power for Off-Pavement, 754
Power of Attorney for Health Care, 4634
PowerLink 2 Control Unit, 367
A Practical Guide to Art Therapy Groups, 4991
Practicing Rehabilitation with Geriatric Clients, 2490
Prader-Willi Alliance Of New York, 1868
Prader-Willi Alliance of New York Newsletter, 8629
Prader-Willi Syndrome Association USA, 8297
Prader-Willi Syndrome: Development and Manifestations, 8557
Praeger - ABC-CLIO, 4957
Praeger Publishers, 7515
Pragmatic Approach, 2491
Prairie Cruiser, 721
Prairie Freedom Center for Independent Living: Sioux Falls, 4455
Prairie Freedom Center for Independent Living: Madison, 4456
Prairie Freedom Center for Independent Living: Yankton, 4457
Prairie IL Resource Center, 4132
Prairie Independent Living Resource Center, 4133
Pre-Reading Screening Procedures, 2635
PreReading Strategies, 8044
Prelude, 174
Prentke Romich Company, 225, 215, 219, 244, 245, 248, 524, 1755
Prentke Romich Company Product Catalog, 491
Preparing for ACT Assessment, 2636
Presby, 7381

Presbyterian Church USA, 1111, 1269
Presbytery of Eastern Virginia, 1423, 8393, 8394
Preschool Learning Activities for the Visually Impaired Child, 9011
Preschoolers with Special Needs: Children At-Risk, Children with Disabilities, 2492
Prescott Public Library, 4659
Prescriptions for Independence: Working with Older People Who are Visually Impaired, 7517
President's Committee for People with Intellectual Disabilities, 2047
President's Committee on Employment of Employment of the Disabled, 5981
President's Committee on People with Disabilities: Arkansas, 3349
President's Committee on People with Intellecutual Disabilities, 3302
Prevent Blindness America, 8869, 8958, 9097, 9140
Prevent Blindness Connecticut, 4691
Prevent Child Abuse America, 8665
Preventable Brain Damage, 7800
Preventing Academic Failure - Teachers Handbook, 2493
Preventing School Dropouts, 2494
Preventing Secondary Conditions Associated with Spina Bifida or Cerebral Palsy, 8558
Prevocational Assessment, 2495
Pride Industries: Grass Valley, 6650
Prima Publishing, 7716, 8727
Primacy Healthcare and Rehabilitation Center, 7395
Primary Children's Medical Center, 6471
Primary Phonics, 1984
Primary Special Needs and the National Curriculum, 2496
Prime Engineering, 265, 265
Primer on the Rheumatic Diseases, 8182
Primrose Supported Employment Programs, 5939
The Princeton Review - Penguin Random House, 2567
Print, Play & Learn #1 Old Mac's Farm, 1724
Print, Play & Learn #7: Sampler, 1725
Printed Rear Closure Sweat Top, 1488
Pro-Ed Publications, 2505, 2607, 2649, 2654, 6193
Pro-Max/ Division Of Bow-Flex Of America, 436
Proceedings, 5156
Products for People with Disabilities, 492
Professional Development Programs, 2140
Professional Fit Clothing, 1470
Profex Medical Products, 188
Programming Concepts, 1677, 1680, 1713, 1758, 1819
Programs for Aphasia and Cognitive Disorders, 1789
Programs for Children with Disabilities: Ages 3 through 5, 6328
Programs for Children with Special Health Care Needs, 6329
Programs for Infants and Toddlers with Disabilities: Ages Birth through 2, 6330
Progress Center for Independent Living, 4081
Progress Center for Independent Living: Blue Island, 4082
Progress Valley: Phoenix, 6529
Progress Without Punishment: Approaches for Learners with Behavior Problems, 2497
Progressive Center for Independent Living, 4322
Progressive Center for Independent Living: Flemington, 4323
Progressive Independence, 4405
Progressive Options, 4411
Project AID Resource Center, 8613
Project Freedom, 4324
Project Freedom: Hamilton, 4325
Project Freedom: Lawrence, 4326
Project Independence, 5865
Project Kindle/Camp Kindle, 1227
Project LINK, 6053
Project Onward Gallery, 60
Projects W Industry Goodwill Industries of America, 6052

Promoting Communication in Infants and Young Children: 500 Ways to Succeed, 8751
Promoting Postsecondary Education for Students with Learning Disabilities, 2498
Prone Support Walker, 658
Propet Leather Walking Shoes, 1456
Prorter Sargent, 2062
Prostate and Urological Disorders Sourcebo ok, 8559
Prosthetics and Orthotics Center in Blue Island, 6855
ProtectaCap, ProtectaCap+PLUS, ProtectaChin Guard and ProtectaHip, 534
Protecting Against Latex Allergy, 8560
Protection & Advocacy Project, 3685
Protection & Advocacy System: Alaska, 3329
Protection & Advocacy for People with Disabilities, 3741
Protection & Advocacy for Persons with Developmental Disabilities: Alaska, 3330
Protection & Advocacy for Persons with Disabilities: Arizona, 3339
Protection and Advocacy (PA I), 3355
Protection and Advocacy Agency of NY, 3654
Protection and Advocacy System, 3863
Protestant Guild Learning Center, 6984
Providence Health System, 6258
Providence Holy Cross Medical Center, 6258
Providence Hospital Work, 7114
Providence Medical Center, 6480
Providence Regional Office, 5745
Providence Rehabilitation Services, 6481, 6481
Providence Speech and Hearing Association, 8778
Providence Speech and Hearing Center, 8700
Providence VA Medical Center, 5746
Provider Magazine, 5287
Providing Services for People with Vision Loss: Multidisciplinary Perspective, 9065
Prudential Financial, 3016
Prudential Foundation, 3016
Prufrock Press, 2102, 2297, 2542, 2643
Psy-Ed Corporation, 5206
Psychiatric Institute of Washington, 6724
Psychiatric Mental Health Nursing, 2499
Psychiatric Staffing Crisis in Community Mental Health, 2223
Psycho-Educational Assessment of Preschool Children, 2637
Psychoeducational Assessment of Visually Impaired and Blind Students, 2500
Psychological & Educational Publications, 2411, 2645
Psychological & Social Impact of Disabilit y, 5157
Psychological Software Services, 1769
Psychological and Social Impact of Illness and Disability, 2501
Psychology and Health, 5158
Psychology of Disability, 5159
Public Health Reports, 5288
Public Interest Law Center of Philadelphia, 3726, 4614
Public Law 101-336, 4572
Public Library Of Anniston-Calhoun County, 4651
Public Radio WBHM 90.3 FM, 4647
Public Technology, 5548
Public Welfare Foundation, 2832
PublishAmerica, 8443
Publix Super Market Corporation Office, 2846
Publix Super Markets Charities, 2846
Pueblo Diversified Industries, 6689
Pueblo Goodwill Industries, 3979
Puget Sound Healthcare Center, 7419
Punctuation Rules, 1790
Purdue University, 8618, 8647
Purdue University Press, 4975
Pure Facts, 7836
Pure Vision Arts, 61
Push to Talk Amplified Handset, 226
Push-Button Quad Cane, 659
Pushin' Forward Fanlight Productions/Icarus Films, 5356
Putnam County Comprehensive Services, 6007
Putnam Independent Living Services, 4362
Puzzle Games: Cooking, Eating, Community and Grooming, 5478

Puzzle Power: Sampler, 1726
Puzzle Power: Zoo & School Days, 1727
Puzzle Tanks, 1652
The Pyramids, 8119

Q

Quad Canes, 660
Quad City Deaf & Hard of Hearing Youth Group: Tomorrow's Leaders for our Community, 8045
Quad Commander, 535
Quad Grip with Pin, 128
Quadtro Cushion, 290
Quaezar, 5903
Quality Care Newsletter, 8630
Quality First, 7546
Quality Healthcare Foundation of Wyoming, 7488
Quality of Life for Persons with Disabilities, 5160
Quan Yin Healing Arts Center, 920
Quantum Books, 5186
Quantum Technologies, 5442
Quarterly Update, 9100
Queen Anne Health Care, 7209, 7209
Queen of Angels/Hollywood Presbyterian Medical Center, 6259
Queen of the Valley Hospital, 6260
Quest, 5940, 6772
Quest - Tampa Area, 5941, 6773
Quest Books, 46
Quest Camp, 1003, 7697
Quest, Inc., 1038
Questar Corporation Contributions Program, 3224
Questions and Answers: The ADA and Hiring Police Officers, 4573
Questions and Answers: The ADA and Persons with HIV/AIDS, 8561
Queue, 1644
Queue Inc, 1651
Queue Incorporated, 1686
Quick Reading Test, Phonics Based Reading, Reading SOS (Strategies for Older Students), 1791
Quick Talk, 1792
Quickie 2, 591
Quincy Rehabilitation Institute of Holy Cross Hospital, 7184

R

RA Bloch Cancer Foundation, 2992
RAIL, 4284
RB King Counseling Center, 6856
RC Baker Foundation, 2784
A RC Community Support Systems, 6839
RCI, 6131
RD Equipment, 167, 182
REACH, 7845
REACH Rehabilitation Program: Leader Nursing and Rehabilitation Center, 7048
REACH Rehabilitation and Catastrophic Long-Term Care, 7049
REACH of Dallas Resource Center on Independent Living, 4480
REACH of Dallas Resource on Independent Living, 5161
REACH of Denton Resource Center on Independent Living, 4481
REACH of Fort Worth Resource Center on Ind ependent Living, 4482
REACH/Resource Centers on Independent Livi ng, 4574
REACHing Out Newsletter, 5161
REAL Design, 257
REHAB Products and Services, 6857
RENEW: Gillette, 4551
RENEW: Rehabilitation Enterprises of North Eastern Wyoming, 4552
RESNA Annual Conference, 1870
RI Services for the Blind and Visually Impaired, 6180
RIC Northshore, 6858
RIC Prosthetics and Orthotics Center, 6859
RIC Windermere House, 6860
RISE, 6901

RISE-Resource: Information, Support and Empowerment, 4483
ROHO, 287, 288, 289, 290
ROHO Group, 277, 281
ROW Adventures, 5534
RP Foundation Fighting Blindness, 8960
RP Messenger, 9101
RSA Union Building, 3309
RTC Connection, 5162
RULES: Revised, 2638
Race the Clock, 1793
Ragtime Industries, 6902
Rainier Vista Care Center, 7210
Raised Dot Computing, 1551
Raised Line Drawing Kit, 561
Raleigh Rehabilitation and Healthcare Cent er, 7357
Ralph H Johnson VA Medical Center, 5748
Ralph M Parsons Foundation, 2785
Ramah in the Poconos, 7976
Ramapo Training, 2681
Ramapo for Children, 2681
Ramplette Telescoping Ramp, 420
Rampvan, 129
Rancho Adult Day Care Center, 6651
Rancho Los Amigos Medical Center, 6651
Rancho Los Amigos National Rehabilitation Center, 6261
Rand-Scot, 661, 392
Random House, 8184, 8533
Random House Publishing, 8458, 8465
Ranger All Seasons Corporation, 597, 600
Rapaport Publishing, Inc., 8616, 8619
Rascal 3-Wheeler, 592
Rascal ConvertAble, 593
Rasmuson Foundation, 2730
Rasmussen's Syndrome and Hemispherectomy Support Network Newsletter, 8631
Rational Effectiveness Training Systems, 6138
Raven Rock Lutheran Camp, 1160, 7698
Ray Graham Association for People with Disabilities, 6861
Raynaud's Phenomenon, 8562
Raytheon Company Contributions Program, 2952
Reach Rehabilitation Program: Americana Healthcare, 6862
Reaching the Autistic Child: A Parent Trai ning Program, 8563
Reaching the Child with Autism Through Art, 62
Reaching, Crawling, Walking....Let's Get Moving, 9012
Read How You Want Large Print Books, 5179
Read: Out Loud, 1794
Reader Rabbit, 1795
Reader's Digest Foundation, 3078
Readers Digest Association, 3078
Reading Comprehension Series, 1796
Reading Is for Everyone, 9013
Reading Rehabilitation Hospital, 4899
Reading and Deafness, 2502
Reading for Content, 1985
Reading from Scratch, 1986
Reading in the Workplace, 1816
Reading with Low Vision, 9014
Reading, Writing and Speech Problems in Children, 7801, 8752
Readings on Research in Stuttering, 2503
Readings: A Journal of Reviews and Commentary in Mental Health, 2224
Readjustment Counciling Service Western Mountain Re, 5677
Reality of Dyslexia, 7802
Rear Closure Shirts, 1489
Rear Closure T-Shirt, 1490
Rebound: Northeast Methodist Hospital, 6456
Rebsamen Rehabilitation Center, 6235
Receptive-Expressive Emergent-REEL-2 Language Test, 2nd Edition, 2639
Recipe for Reading, 1987
Reclaiming Independence: Staying in the Dr ivers Seat When You Are no Longer Drive., 7584
Recognizing Children with Special Needs, 5357
Recording for the Blind & Dyslexic, 9015, 9099, 9117
Recreation Activities for the Elderly, 2504

Recreation Unlimited Foundation, 1312, 1313, 1314, 1315
Recreation Unlimited: Day Camp, 1312
Recreation Unlimited: Residential Camp, 1313
Recreation Unlimited: Respite Weekend Camp, 1314
Recreation Unlimited: Specialty Camp, 1315
Red Notebook, 4794
Red Rock Center for Independence, 4494
Redman Apache, 722
Redman Crow Line, 723
Redman Powerchair, 268, 722, 723, 747, 754
Reduced Effort Steering, 130
Reference Manual for Communicative Sciences and Disorders, 2505
Reference Service Press, 2758, 3261, 3263, 3267, 3268, 3269, 3270, 3271, 3272, 3281, 3282, 3283
Reference and Information Services From NLS, 9016
Regal Research & Manufacturing Company, 601
Regal Scooters, 594
Regent, 595
Regenta Park, 6750
Regents' Center for Learning Disorders, 2640
Regional ADA Technical Assistance Center, 3624
Regional Access & Mobilization Project, 4083
Regional Access & Mobilization Project: Be lvidere, 4084
Regional Access & Mobilization Project: De Kalb, 4085
Regional Access & Mobilization Project: Fr eeport, 4086
Regional Assessment and Training Center, 5889
Regional Center for Independent Living, 4363
Regional Center for Rehabilitation, 6652
Regional Early Childhood Director Center, 3655
Regional Library, 4703
Regional Rehabilitation Center Pitt County Memorial Hospital, 7084
Regional Resource Centers Program, 5443
Regis College, 1182
Registry of Interpreters for the Deaf, 7942, 8028
Rehab Care, 6940, 7121
Rehab Engineering & Assistive Tech. North America, 1870
Rehab Home Care, 7085
Rehab Institute at Florence Nightingale He alth Center, 7350
Rehab Pro, 2225
Rehab and Educational Aids for Living, 260, 261
RehabCare, 6941
Rehabiliation Engineering Center for Personal Licensed Transportation, 5549
Rehabilitation & Nursing Center at Greater Pittsburgh, The, 7146
Rehabilitation Achievement Center, 6863
Rehabilitation Associates, Inc., 6706
Rehabilitation Center Baptist Hospital, 6436
Rehabilitation Center at McFarland Hospital, 6437
Rehabilitation Center at Thibodeaux Regional, 6940
Rehabilitation Center for Children and Adults, 6774
Rehabilitation Center of Lake Charles Memorial Hospital, 6344
Rehabilitation Center of Palm Beach, 7255
Rehabilitation Engineering & Assistive Technology Society of North America (RESNA), 1593
Rehabilitation Engineering and Assistive Technology Society of North America (RESNA), 493
Rehabilitation Enterprises of North Easter n Wyoming: Newcastle, 4553
Rehabilitation Enterprises of Washington, 7211
Rehabilitation Gazette, 5163
Rehabilitation Hospital of Indiana, 7291
Rehabilitation Hospital of the Pacific, 6805
Rehabilitation Institute of Chicago, 856, 6858, 6859, 8229
Rehabilitation Institute of Chicago's Virginia Wadsworth Sports Program, 8644
Rehabilitation Institute of Chicago: Alexian Brothers Medical Center, 6864

Rehabilitation Institute of Ohio at Miami Valley Hospital, 6396
Rehabilitation Institute of Santa Barbara, 6653
Rehabilitation Institute of Sarasota, 6288
Rehabilitation Institute of Southern California, 6654
Rehabilitation International, 921, 1871, 2198
Rehabilitation Interventions for the Institutionalized Elderly, 2506
Rehabilitation Nursing for the Neurological Patient, 2507
Rehabilitation Opportunities, 6956
Rehabilitation Research Library, 4871
Rehabilitation Research and Development Center, 5581
Rehabilitation Resource Manual: VISION, 2508
Rehabilitation Resource University, 2407
Rehabilitation Service of North Central Oh io, 4398
Rehabilitation Services, 922, 7097
Rehabilitation Services Administration, 5917, 6530
Rehabilitation Specialists, 7050
Rehabilitation Technology, 2509
Rehabilitation Technology Association Conference, 1872
Rehabilitation and Healthcare Center of Mo nroe, 7358
Rehabilitation and Healthcare Center of Ta mpa, 7256
Rehabilitation and Research Center Virginia Commonwealth University, 7407
Rehabilitative Services Administration, 3303
Reinberger Foundation, 3123
Reizen Braille Labeler, 562
Relationship Development Intervention with Young Children, 7803, 8753
Relaxation Techniques for People with Special Needs, 5358
Relaxation: A Comprehensive Manual for Adults and Children with Special Needs, 5164
Reliance House, 6707
Religious Signing: A Comprehensive Guide for All Faiths, 8046
Remedial and Special Education, 2226
Removing the Barriers: Accessibility Guidelines and Specifications, 1900
Renaissance Center, 6775
Renaissance Clubhouse, 4210
Renaissance at 87th Street, 7279
Renaissance at Hillside, 7280
Renaissance at Midway, 7281
Renaissance at South Shore, 7282
Reno Regional Office, 5683
Report Writing in Assessment and Evaluation, 2510
Research & Training Center on Mental Health for Hard of Hearing Persons, 4679
Research Press, 2103, 2066, 2464, 5164, 5339, 5358, 7778
Research Press Company, 2104
Research and Training Center, 5162
Research to Prevent Blindness, 3079, 8947
Research!America, 5444
Residential Camp, 1102
Resource Center for Accessible Living, 4364
Resource Center for Independent Living, 4134, 4365
Resource Center for Independent Living (RCIL), 1594
Resource Center for Independent Living, In c. (RCIL), 4135
Resource Center for Independent Living: Emporia, 4136
Resource Center for Independent Living: Minot, 4388
Resource Center for Independent Living: Ar kansas City, 4137
Resource Center for Independent Living: Bu rlington, 4138
Resource Center for Independent Living: Co ffeyville, 4139
Resource Center for Independent Living: El Dorado, 4140

Resource Center for Independent Living: Ft Scott, 4141
Resource Center for Independent Living: Ot tawa, 4142
Resource Center for Independent Living: Ov erland Park, 4143
Resource Center for Independent Living: To peka, 4144
Resource List for Persons with Low Vision, 9017
Resource Room, The, 2511
Resources for Independence, 4193
Resources for Independent Living, 3956, 4522
Resources for Independent Living: Baton Rouge, 4176
Resources for Independent Living: Metairie, 4177
Resources for People with Disabilities and Chronic Conditions, 5165
Resources for Rehabilitation, 2512, 2508, 5130, 5165, 8997, 9065
Resources in Special Education, 2263
Respiratory Disorders Sourcebook, 8564
Respironics, 309
Responding to Crime Victims with Disabilit ies, 2071
Restructuring High Schools for All Students: Taking Inclusion to the Next Level, 2513
Restructuring for Caring and Effective Education: Administrative Guide, 2514
Resurrection Children's Center, 7192
Retarded Isn't Stupid, Mom!, 7804
Rethinking Attention Deficit Disorder, 7805
Retirement Research Foundation, 2895
Rettsyndrome.org, 7650
Rewarding Speech, 1988
Rhode Island Arc, 3171
Rhode Island Association of Facilities and Services for the Aging, 7489
Rhode Island Department Health, 3730
Rhode Island Department of Education: Office of Special Needs, 2158
Rhode Island Department of Elderly Affairs, 3731
Rhode Island Department of Mental Health, 3732
Rhode Island Developmental Disabilities Council, 3733
Rhode Island Disability Law Center, 3736
Rhode Island Foundation, 3172
Rhode Island Governor's Commission on Disabilities, 3734
Rhode Island Lions Sight Foundation, Inc., 1361
Rhode Island Parent Information Network, 3735
Rhode Island Protection & Advocacy for Persons with Disabilities, 3736
Rhode Island Services for the Blind and Visually Impaired, 3737
Rich Foundation, 2856
Richard L Roudebush VA Medical Center, 5624
Richard W Higgins Charitable Foundation, 2913
Richmond Research Training Center, 6209
Rickshaw Exerciser, 421
Ricon, 79, 116, 127
Ricon Corporation, 422
Riddle of Autism: A Psychological Analysis, 7806, 8754
Rifin Family/Daughters of Israel, 2048
Right Hand Turn Signal Switch Lever, 131
Right Turn, 1653
Right at Home Aquarius Health Care Media, 5359
Rigid Aluminum Cane with Golf Grip, 637
Riley Child Development Center, 6331
Rimland Services for Autistic Citizens, 1077, 7699
Rio Vista Rehabilitation Hospital, 6457
Ripley Healthcare and Rehabilitation Cente r, 7396
Rita J and Stanley H Kaplan Foundation, 3080
River's Edge Rehabilitation and Healthcare, 7272
Riverdeep Incorporated, 1752
Riverside Community Hospital, 7233
Riverside Medical Center, 6865
Riverview School, 2129
Road Ahead: Transition to Adult Life for Persons with Disabilities (3rd Edition), 4988
Roadster 20, 596
Roanoke City Public Library System, 4927
Roanoke Memorial Hospital, 7193
Roanoke Regional Office, 5772

Robert Campeau Family Foundation, 3124
Robert Ellis Simon Foundation, 2786
Robert J Dole VA Medical Center, 5635
Robert Sterling Clark Foundation, 3081
Robert Wood Johnson Foundation, 3017
Robert Young Mental Health Center Division of Trinity Regional Haelth System, 6866
Robey W Estes Family Foundation, 3231
Robey W Estes Jr, 3231
RoboMath, 1654
Rochester Area Foundation, 2982
Rochester Institute Of Technology, 4875
Rochester Rotary Club, 1281
Rocker Balance Square, 536
Rockland Independent Living Center, 4366
Rocky Mountain Resource & Training Institute, 6231
Rocky Mountain Village, 1018
Rodale Press, 5086
Rodeo, 1728
Roger Randall Center, 6946
Role Portrayal and Stereotyping on Television, 5166
Rolf Institute, 923
Roll Chair, 266
Rollin M Gerstacker Foundation, 2971
Rolling Along with Goldilocks and the Three Bears, 4961
Rolling Hills Country Day Camp, 1252, 7700
Rolling Start, 3957
Rolling Start: Victorville, 3958
Rolls 2000 Series, 724
Rome Subregional Library for the Blind and Physically Handicapped, 4730
Ronald McDonald House, 924
Ronald McDonald House Charities - Southern Calif., 984
Ronald McDonald House For Charities-Southern Calif, 8363
Room Valet Visual-Tactile Alerting System, 227
Rosalind Russell Medical Research Center for Arthritis, 4680
Rose-Colored Glasses, 9018
Roseburg VA Medical Center, 5731
Rosen Publishing, 8464, 8499
Rosen Publishing Group, 7747
Rosewood Center, 6957
Rosomoff Comprehensive Pain Center, The, 6776
Rotary Camp, 1316
Rotary International, 2716
Rotary Youth Exchange, 2716
Round Lake Camp, 1253
Roundup River Ranch, 1019
Route 52 Salisbury Turnpike, 1265, 7670
Routledge (Taylor & Francis Group), 2332, 2475, 4953, 4972, 4991, 5267, 5293, 7493, 7494, 7495, 7496, 7498, 7504, 7508, 7510, 7514, 7520, 7734, 7736, 8724, 8726, 8901
Rowan Community, 7239
Rowan County Vocational Workshop, 6143
Royal C Johnson Veterans Memorial Medical Center, 5750
Ruben Center for Independent Living, 4105
Rubicon Programs, 6655
Rural Center for Independent Living, 4308
Rush Copley Medical Center-Rehab Neuro Physical Unit, 6314
Rusk Institute of Rehabilitation Medicine, 6385
Rutherford Vocational Workshop, 6144
Rutland Mental Health Services, 7186
Ryland Group, 2928

S

S W Georgia Regional Library, 4720
SACC Assistive Technoloy Center, 1595
SAGE Publications, 2540
SAILS, 4484
SAMHSA News, 2260
SAYdee Posters, 1989
SB Waterman & E Blade Charitable Foundation, 3258
SC Department of Health and Environmental Control, 1365

SCARC, Inc Evaluation, Training + Emploment Center, 5942
SCATBI: Scales Of Cognitive Ability for Traumatic Brain Injury, 7807
SCCIL at Titusville, 4022
SCENE, 9102
SCI Life, 8609
SCI Psychosocial Process, 8210, 8632
SCILIFE, 8200
SEMO Alliance for Disability Independence, 4285
SHALOM Denver, 6690
SILC Department of Vocational Rehabilitation, 4172
SILC, Indiana Council on Independent Living (ICOIL), 4106
SIU:Carbondale Therapeutic Recreation Prgm, 1070
SJR Rehabilitation Hospital, 7053
SL Start and Associates, 6216
SLIDER Bathing System, 175
SMILES, 4254
SMILES: Mankato, 4255
SOAR, 1445
SOAR Summer Adventures, 1293, 7701
SOLO Literacy Suite, 1771
SPIN Early Childhood Care & Education Cntr, 6691
SPINabilities: A Young Person's Guide to Spina Bifida, 8565
SPOKES Unlimited, 4412, 8974
SS-Access Single Switch Interface for PC's with MS-DOS, 1528
SSD (Services for Students with Disabilities), 2049
STAR, 9103, 3548
Sacramento Center & Regional Offices, 6594
Sacramento Medical Center, 5582
Sacramento Vocational Services, 5866
Sacremento State, 1575
Safari Scooter, 597
Safari Tilt, 267
Safety Deck II, 683
Sagamore Publishing, 40
Sage Publications, 2105, 41, 1941, 1981, 2192, 2199, 2204, 2205, 2213, 2226, 2267, 2301, 2315, 2331, 2340, 2341, 2352, 2389, 2448, 2476, 2494, 2498, 2500, 2502, 2543, 2548, 2555, 2571, 2572, 2574, 2588, 2598, 2606, 2617, 2627, 2639, 2648, 2650, 2651, 2652, 2653, 5015, 5070, 7521, 7719, 7765, 7787, 7807, 8040, 8516, , 8744, 8927, 9046
Saint Joseph Regional Medical Center- South Bend, 6887
Saint Jude Medical Center, 7234
Salem VA Medical Center, 5773
Salvation Army, 1192
Sammons Preston Enrichments Catalog, 494
Sammons Preston Rolyan, 368, 347, 352, 353, 362, 374, 375, 390, 464, 494, 503, 648, 670, 1523, 2469
Sampson-Katz Center, 6867
Samuel W Bell Home for Sightless, 4399
San Antonio Area Foundation, 3216
San Antonio Warm Springs Rehabilitation Hospital, 6458
San Bernardino Valley Lighthouse for the Blind, 6656
San Diego VA Regional Office, 5583
San Francisco Foundation, 2787
San Francisco Public Library for the Blind and Print Handicapped, 4681
San Francisco Vocational Services, 5867
San Joaquin General Hospital, 6589
San Joaquin Valley Rehabilitation Hospital, 6262
San Jose State University Library, 4682
San Juan Center for Independence, 4333
San Luis Medical and Rehabilitation Center, 7433
Sandcastle Day Camp, 1032, 7977
Sandhills School, 2682
Sandusky: Blue Water Center for Independent Living, 4239
Sanford Children's Specialty Clinic, 1371
Sanilac County Community Mental Health, 7006
Santa Barbara Bank & Trust, 2765
Santa Barbara Foundation, 2788, 5010

Santa Clara Valley Blind Center, Inc., 6657
Santa Clara Valley Medical Center, 6263
Santa Fe Community Foundation, 3022
Sarasota Memorial Hospital/Comprehensive Rehabilitation Unit, 6777
Sarkeys Foundation, 3132
Savannah Association for the Blind, 6801
Savannah Rehabilitation and Nursing Center, 7263
Say What, 305
Say it with Sign, 9019
Scandinavian Exchange, 2717
Scanning WSKE, 1621
Schaefer Enterprises, 6692
Schepens Eye Research Institute, 4808, 9107
Scheuer Associates Foundation, 2817
Schmieding Developmental Center, 2641
Schnurmacher Center for Rehabilitation and Nursing, 7351
Scholastic, 8476
School Of Medicine, Rheumatology Division, 4755
School Specialty, 1908, 1909, 1919, 1928, 1933, 1937, 1942, 1943, 1954, 1955, 1960, 1984, 1985, 1987, 1995, 1998, 1999, 2000, 2001, 2013
School of Piano Technology for the Blind, 6217
Schools And Services For Children With Autism Spectrum Disorders., 3656
Schroth School & Technical Education Center, 7044
Schwab Rehabilitation Hospital, 7283
Scoffolding Student Learning, 2515
Scoota Bug, 598
Scooter & Wheelchair Battery Fuel Gauges and Motor Speed Controllers, 684
Scott Sign Systems, 537
Scottish Rite Center for Childhood Language Disorders, 8701
Scottsdale Healthcare, 6239
Screening in Chronic Disease, 5167
Scripps Memorial Hospital at La Jolla, 6264
Scripps Memorial Hospital: Pain Center, 6658
Sea Pines Rehabilitation Hospital, 6289, 6755
Seacrest Village Nursing Center, 7337
Seagull Industries for the Disabled, 5943
Sears-Roebuck Foundation, 2896
Seat-A-Robics, 5360
Seattle Clinic, 8701
Seattle Medical and Rehabilitation Center, 7212
Seattle Regional Office, 5776
Sebasticook Farms-Great Bay Foundation, 6947
Second Time Around, 6021
Secret Agent Walking Stick, 662
Secretary State Office, 4842
Sedgwick County Workshop, 5890
Sedgwick Press/Grey House Publishing, 2057, 2058, 2059, 2060, 2063
See A Bone, 9020
See What I Feel, 9021
See What I'm Saying, 9127
See for Yourself, 9128
The Seeing Eye, 9059, 9104
Seeing Eye Guide, 9104
Seeing Eye, The, 8870
Seeing Voices, 8047
Seersucker Shower Robe, 1484
Seizures and Epilepsy in Childhood: A Guide, 8566
Selecting a Program, 9022
Selective Nontreatment of Handicapped, 2516
Selective Placement Program Coordinator Directory, 2072
Self Reliance, 4023
Self-Therapy for the Stutterer, 8755
Sellersburg Health and Rehabilitation Centre, 7292
Semiotics and Dis/ability: Interogating Categories of Difference, 2517
Senior Focus, 7547
Senior Health Care Management, 7254
Senior Program for Teens and Young Adults with Special Needs, 2683
Sensation Products, 1990
Sense-Sations, 544, 611, 613, 616, 617, 5467
Sensory University Toy Company, The, 1991
Sequanota Lutheran Conference Center and Camp, 1358, 8713

Sequential Spelling: 1-7 with 7 Student Re sponse Books, 1992
Series Adapter, 538
Sertoma Camp Endeavor, 1046, 7978, 1046, 7978
Sertoma Centre, 5982
Service Coordination for Early Intervention: Parents and Friends, 2518
Service Source, 5910
ServiceSource, 6210
Services Center For Independent Living, 3959
Services Maximizing Independent Living and Empowerment (SMILE), 3892
Services for Independent Living, 4286, 4400, 5024
Services for Students with Disabilities, 2138
Services for the Blind, 4830
Services for the Blind and Visually Impaired, 3738
Services for the Seriously Mentally Ill: A Survey of Mental Health Centers, 2519
Services for the Visually Impaired, 8871
Setebaid Services, 1345, 8366
Seven Fifty-Five FS, 740
7 Steps for Success, 2270
Sex Education: Issues for the Person with Autism, 7808, 8756
Sexual Adjustment, 5168
Sexuality and Disabilities: A Guide for Human Service Practitioners, 5169
Sexuality and Disability, 2520
Sexuality and the Developmentally Handicapped, 5227
Sexuality and the Person with Spina Bifida, 8567
Shady Oaks Camp, 1078, 8402
Shalom House, 4185
Shambhala Publications, 5045, 5094
Shands Rehab Hospital, 7257
Shannon Medical Center: RehabCare Unit, 6459
Shape Up 'n Sign, 9129
Share, Inc, 1212, 8355
Shared Visions, 9105
Sharing Solutions: A Newsletter for Support Groups, 9106
Sharing the Burden, 7518
Sharp Calculator with Illuminated Numbers, 563
Sharp Coronado Hospital, 6659
Shasta County Opportunity Center, 5868
Shattered Dreams-Lonely Choices: Birth Parents of Babies with Disabilities, 5228
Shaughnessy-Kaplan Rehabilitation Hospital, 6985
Shawmut Bank, 2818
Shelby County Community Services, 6868
Shelby Pines Rehabilitation and Healthcare Center, 7397
Shell Oil Company Foundation, 3217
Sheltered Occupational Center of Virginia, 6211
Shenandoah Valley Workforce Investment Board, 4523
Shenango Valley Foundation, 3153
Shepherd Center for Treatment of Spinal Injuries, 6802
Sheridan Press,, 9053
Sheridan VA Medical Center, 5790
Sherman Lake YMCA Outdoor Center, 1194, 7702, 8403
Sherman Lake YMCA Summer Camp, 8403
The Shield Institute, 61
Shilo Inns & Resorts, 5508
Shining Bright: Head Start Inclusion, 5361
Shoe and Boot Valet: Decreased Mobility Ai d, 306
Shop Talk, 2521
Shop Til You Drop, 1729
Shore Community Services, 5983
Shore Training Center, 5983
Shore Village Rehabilitation & Nursing Center, 7311
Show Me How: A Manual for Parents of Preschool Blind Children, 9023
Shreveport VA Medical Center, 5641
Shriner's Hospitals for Children Newslette r, 4962
Shriners Burn Institute: Cincinnati Unit, 6397
Shriners Burn Institute: Galveston Unit, 6460
Shriners Burns Hospital: Boston, 6355
Shriners Hospital Springfield Unit Springfield Unit for Crippled Children, 6356
Shriners Hospital for Children-Shreveport, 6345

Shriners Hospital for Children: Honolulu, 6306
Shriners Hospitals, 6482
Shriners Hospitals For Children-Northern California, 6660
Shriners Hospitals for Children St. Louis, 7024
Shriners Hospitals for Children Cincinnati, 6397
Shriners Hospitals for Children, Greenville, 6429
Shriners Hospitals for Children, Philadelphia, 6424
Shriners Hospitals for Children, Erie, 6425
Shriners Hospitals for Children, Houston, 6461
Shriners Hospitals for Children, Lexington, 6341
Shriners Hospitals for Children: Intermountain, 6472
Shriners Hospitals for Children: Los Angel es, 6661
Shriners Hospitals for Children: Portland, 6408
Shriners Hospitals for Children: Spokane, 6482
Shriners Hospitals for Children: Tampa, 6290
Shriners Hospitals for Children: Twin Cities, 7014
Shriners Hospitals, Philadelphia Unit, for Crippled Children, 6426
Shrinners Hospitals for Children, 6424
Sibling Forum: A FRA Newsletter, 4963
Sibling Information Network Newsletter, 2261
The Sibling Slam Book: What It's Really Li ke To Have a Brother or Sister with Special Needs, 4967
Sibling Support Project, 4967, 4968, 4969, 5214
Sibling Supporting Project, 4964
The Sibling Survival Guide, 4968
Siboney Learning Group, 1650
Sibpage, 2262
Sibshops: Workshops for Siblings of Children with Special Needs, 4964
Sickened: The Memoir of a Muchausen by Pro xy Childhood, 5170
Sickle Cell Disease Association of Illinois, 1166, 8316
Side Velcro Slacks, 1492
Side-Zip Sweat Pants, 1493
Sidney Stern Memorial Trust, 2789
Sierra 3000/4000, 599
Sierra Health Foundation, 2790
Sierra Pain Institute, 7031
Sight & Hearing Association, 7943
Sight by Touch, 9130
Sightings Newsletter, 9107
Sign Language Interpreting and Interpreter Education, 8048
Sign Language Studies, 8071
Sign Media, 8027
Sign of the Times, 9024
Signaling Wake-Up Devices, 539
Signature and Address Self-Inking Stamps, 564
Signed English Schoolbook, 2522
Signed English Starter, The, 8049
Signing Family: What Every Parent Should Know About Sign Communication, The, 8050
Signing Naturally Curriculum, 1993
Signing for Reading Success, 8051
Signing: How to Speak with Your Hands, 8052
Signs Across America, 8053
Signs for Me: Basic Sign Vocabulary for Children, Parents & Teachers, 8054
Signs for Sexuality: A Resource Manual, 8055
Signs of the Times, 8056
Silent Call Communications, 228
Silent Garden, The, 8057
Silicon Valley Community Foundation, 2791
Silicon Valley Independent Living Center, 3960
Silicon Valley Independent Living Center: South County Branch, 3961
Silicone Padding, 291
Silver Towers Camp, 1411
Silvercrest Center for Nursing & Rehabilitation, 6386
Simon & Schuster, 5020, 7822
Simon & Schuster/Touchstone Publishing, 7753
Simon Foundation, 8622
Simon Foundation for Continence, 8154
Simon SIO, 1797
Simonton Cancer Center, 8298
Simplicity, 1529

Sinai Hospital of Detroit: Dept. of Opthalmology, 4813
Since Owen, A Parent-to-Parent Guide for Care of the Disabled Child, 5229
Sing Praise Hymnal for the Deaf, 8058
Singeria/Metropolitan Parent Center, 3657
Single Switch Games, 5479
Single Switch Latch and Timer, 5480
Sinus Survival: A Self-help Guide, 8568
Sioux Falls Regional Office, 5751
Siouxland Community Foundation, 2910
Siragusa Foundation, 2897
Siskin Hospital For Physical Rehabilitation, 7156
Siskin Hospital for Physical Rehabilitation, 7398
Sisler McFawn Foundation, 3125
Sister Cities International, 2718
Six County, Inc., 7115
Sjogren's Syndrome Foundation, 2938, 8623
Skadden Fellowship Foundation, 3082
SkiSoft Publishing Corporation, 1821
Skills Inc., 5984
Skills Unlimited, 7074
Skokie Accessible Library Services, 4748
Skokie Public Library, 4748
Skyway, 725
Skyway Machine, 725
Sleep Better! A Guide to Improving Sleep for Children with Special Needs, 5230
SleepSafe Beds, 194
Slicing Aid, 369
Slim Armstrong Mounting System, 1530
Slim Line Brake Only, 132
Slim Line Control, 133
Slim Line Control: Brake and Throttle, 134
Slingerland Institute for Literacy, 7213
Slingerland Screening Tests, 2642
Slosburg Family Charitable Trust, 2997
Slosson Educational Publications, 2537
Slosson Educational Publications Inc., 1940, 7724
Small Appliance Receiver, 370
Small Business Development Center, 6067
Small Differences Aquarius Health Care Media, 5362
Small Wonder, 1994
Smart + Strong, 8608
Smart Kitchen/How to Design a Comfortable, Safe & Friendly Workplace, 1901
Smart Leg, 423
Smith Kettlewell Rehabilitation Engineering Research Center, 9108
Smoke Detector with Strobe, 540
Smooth Mover, 424
Snug Seat, 156, 369
So the World May Hear, 8098
Social Development and the Person with Spi na Bifida, 8569
Social Learning Center, 6948
Social Security, 3362, 3413, 3414, 3440, 3491, 3492, 3739, 3760, 3798, 3832, 3843, 3860
Social Security Administration, 3304, 3412, 3545, 3625, 3679, 3300, 3415, 3476
Social Security Admission, 3340
Social Security Bulletin, 7532
Social Security Library, 4795
Social Security Online, 5445
Social Security, Medicare, and Government Pensions, 7519
Social Security: Albany Disability Determination, 3658
Social Security: Arkansas Disability Determination Services, 3350
Social Security: Atlanta Disability Determination, 3426
Social Security: Austin Disability Determination, 3780
Social Security: Baltimore Disability Determination, 3518
Social Security: Baton Rouge Disability Determination, 3500
Social Security: Bismarck Disability Determination, 3686
Social Security: Boston Disability Determination, 3526

Social Security: California Disability Determination Services, 3361
Social Security: Carson City Disability Determination, 3601
Social Security: Charleston Disability Determination, 3843
Social Security: Cheyenne Disability Determination, 3860
Social Security: Columbus Disability Determination, 3700
Social Security: Concord Disability Determination, 3614
Social Security: Decatur Disability Determination, 3427
Social Security: Des Moines Disability Determination, 3476
Social Security: Frankfort Disability Determination, 3491
Social Security: Fresno Disability Determination Services, 3362
Social Security: Harrisburg Disability Determination, 3727
Social Security: Hartford Area Office, 3379
Social Security: Helena Disability Determination, 3582
Social Security: Honolulu Disability Determination, 3440
Social Security: Jefferson City Disability Determination, 3571
Social Security: Lincoln Disability Determination, 3592
Social Security: Louisville Disability Determination, 3492
Social Security: Madison Field Office, 3853
Social Security: Maine Disability Determination, 3509
Social Security: Miami Disability Determination, 3413
Social Security: Mobile Disability Determination Services, 3319
Social Security: Nashville Disability Determination, 3760
Social Security: Oakland Disability Determination Services, 3363
Social Security: Olympia Disability Determination, 3832
Social Security: Orlando Disability Determination, 3414
Social Security: Phoenix Disability Determination Services, 3340
Social Security: Providence Disability Determination, 3739
Social Security: Sacramento Disability Determination Services, 3364
Social Security: Salem Disability Determination, 3715
Social Security: Salt Lake City Disability Determination, 3798
Social Security: San Diego Disability Determination Services, 3365
Social Security: Santa Fe Disability Determination, 3634
Social Security: Springfield Disability Determination, 3460
Social Security: St. Paul Disability Determination, 3558
Social Security: Tampa Disability Determination, 3415
Social Security: Tucson Disability Determination Services, 3341
Social Security: Vermont Disability Determination Services, 3810
Social Security: West Columbia Disability Determination, 3742
Social Security: Wilmington Disability Determination, 3389
Social Skills for Students With Autism Spectrum Disorders and Other Dev Disabilities, 2523
Social Studies: Detecting and Correcting Special Needs, 2524
Social Vocational Services, 5869
Social and Emotional Development of Exceptional Students: Handicapped, 2525
Socialization Games for Persons with Disabilities, 5171, 5481

Society for Cognitive Rehabilitation, 7651
Society for Disability Studies, 2050
Society for Equal Access: Independent Living Center, 4401
Society for Progressive Supranuclear Palsy, 8155, 8203, 8603
Society for Rehabilitation, 7116
Society for the Blind, 6662, 8872
Society for the Study of Disability in the Middle Ages, 2051
Society's Assets: Elkhorn, 4548
Society's Assets: Kenosha, 4549
Society's Assets: Racine, 4550
Sociopolitical Aspects of Disabilities (2nd Edition), 5289
Soft Touch, 1531, 1532, 1536, 1537, 1538, 1667, 1668, 1669, 1678, 1679, 1690, 1691, 1698, 1699, 1714, 1718, 1719, 1725, 1726, 1727, 1728, 1729, 1730, 1738, 1746, 1747, 1751, 1753
Soft Touch Inc, 1510, 1513, 1514, 1517, 1524
Soft Touch Incorporated, 1724
Soft-Touch Convertible Flotation Mattress, 292
Soft-Touch Gel Flotation Cushion, 293
SoftTouch, 1535, 1740, 1741, 1742, 1743, 1744, 1745
SoftTouch Incorporated, 1534
Softfoot Ergomatta, 685
Solo Scooter, 600
SoloRider Industries, 601
Solutions at Santa Barbara: Transitional Living Center, 6663
Solving Language Difficulties, 1995
Solving the Puzzle of Chronic Fatigue, 8570
Someday's Child Educational Productions, 5363
Somerset Training and Employment Program, 6123
Somerset Valley Rehabilitation and Nursing Center, 7051
Something's Wrong with My Child!, 5231
Sometimes I Get All Scribbly, 5232
Sometimes You Just Want to Feel Like a Human Being, 5172
Son Rise: The Miracle Continues, 8571
Son-Rise Program, 6986, 8666
Son-Rise: The Miracle Continues, 5233, 7809, 8757
Songs I Sing at Preschool, 1730
Songs I Sing at Preschool IntelliKeys Overlay, 1531
Sonic Alert, 229
Sonic Alert Bed Shaker, 195
Sonora Area Foundation, 2792
Sonoran Rehabilitation and Care Center, 7225
Soon Will Come the Light, 7810
Sophie Russell Testamentary Trust Bank Of Hawaii, 2863
Sound & Fury Aquarius Health Care Media, 5364
Sound Connections for the Adolescent, 8758
Sound Induction Receiver, 230
Sound Sentences, 1798
Soundings Newsletter, 8090
Source-APTA Audio Conference, 1873
Sources for Community IL Services, 3898
South Arlington Medical Center: Rehab Care Unit, 6462
South Bay Vocational Center, 5870
South Carolina Assistive Technology Program (SCATP), 2159
South Carolina Assistive Technology Project, 3743
South Carolina Assistive Technology Program, 5173
South Carolina Client Assistance Program, 3744
South Carolina Commission for the Blind, 3745
South Carolina Department of Children with Disabilities, 3746
South Carolina Department of Education: Office of Exceptional Children, 2160
South Carolina Department of Mental Health and Mental Retardation, 3747
South Carolina Developmental Disabilities Council, 3748
South Carolina Employment Security Commission South Carolina Center, 6181
South Carolina Governor's Committee on Employment of the Handicapped, 6182

South Carolina Independent Living Council, 4449
South Carolina State Library, 4903
South Carolina State University, 8988
South Carolina Vocational Rehabilitation Department, 6183
South Central Alabama Mental Health, 6491
South Central Iowa Center for Independent Living, 4115
South Central Kansas Library System, 4769
South Central Pennsylvania Center for Independence Living, 4434
South Central Technical College (SCTC), 2139
South Central Wisconsin Directory of Services for Older Adults, 2073
South Central Wyoming Healthcare and Rehabilitation, 7436
South Coast Medical Center, 6265, 7235
South Dakota Advocacy Services, 3753
South Dakota Assistive Technology Project: DakotaLink, 4458
South Dakota Department of Aging, 3754
South Dakota Department of Education & Cultural Affairs: Office of Special Education, 2161
South Dakota Department of Health, 3752
South Dakota Department of Human Services: Computer Technology Services, 1596
South Dakota Department of Human Services Division of Community Behavioral Health, 3755
South Dakota Department of Labor, 3751
South Dakota Developmental Disability Council, 3756
South Dakota Division of Rehabilitation, 3757
South Dakota Governor's Advisory Committee on Employment of the Disabled, 6185
South Dakota State Library, 4904
South Dakota State Vocational Rehabilitation, 6186
South Dakota Workforce Investment Act Training Programs, 6187
South Dakota of Human Services, 3755
South Georgia Regional Library-Valdosta Talking Book Center, 4731
South Hills YMCA, 1338
South Louisiana Rehabilitation Hospital, 6346
South Miami Hospital, 6291
South Shore Healthcare, 7352
South Texas Charitable Foundation, 3218
South Texas Lighthouse for the Blind, 7179
South Texas Rehabilitation Hospital, 6463
South Texas Veterans Healthcare System, 5762
Southeast Alaska Independent Living, 3882
Southeast Alaska Independent Living: Ketchikan, 3883
Southeast Alaska Independent Living: Sitka, 3884
Southeast Center for Independent Living, 4211
Southeast Disability & Business Technical Assist., 3416
Southeast Kansas Independent Living (SKIL), 4145
Southeast Kansas Independent Living: Independence, 4146
Southeast Kansas Independent Living: Chanute, 4147
Southeast Kansas Independent Living: Columbus, 4148
Southeast Kansas Independent Living: Fredonia, 4149
Southeast Kansas Independent Living: Hays, 4150
Southeast Kansas Independent Living: Pittsburg, 4151
Southeast Kansas Independent Living: Sedan, 4152
Southeast Kansas Independent Living: Yates Center, 4153
Southeast Ohio Sight Center, 7117
Southeast Wisconsin Directory of Services for Older Adults, 2074
Southeastern Blind Rehabilitation Center, 6508
Southeastern Diabetes Education Services, 942, 8365
Southeastern Michigan Commission for the Blind, 4240
Southeastern Minnesota Center for Independent Living: Red Wing, 4256
Southeastern Minnesota Center for Independent Living: Rochester, 4257

Southeastern Paralyzed Veterans of America (PVA), 5613
Southern Adirondack Independent Living, 4367
Southern Adirondack Independent Living Center, 4368
Southern Arizona Association For The Visually Impaired, 6531
Southern Arizona VA Healthcare System, 5571
Southern California Chapter, 1052, 8160
Southern California Rehabilitation Services, 3962
Southern Indiana Center for Independent Living, 4107
Southern Indiana Resource Solutions, 6008
Southern Maryland Center for LIFE, 4194
Southern Nevada Center for Independent Living: North Las Vegas, 4309
Southern Nevada Center for Independent Living: Las Vegas, 4310
Southern New England Rehab Center, 7385
Southern Oregon Rehabilitation Center & Clinics, 5732
Southern Tier Independence Center, 4369
Southern Worcester County Rehabilitation Inc. D/B/A Life-Skills, Inc., 6987
Southside Virginia Training Center, 7194
Southwest Branch of the International Dyslexia Association, 3635
Southwest Center for Independence, 3980
Southwest Center for Independence: Cortez, 3981
Southwest Center for Independent Living (SCIL), 4287
Southwest Communication Resource, 7054
Southwest Conference On Disability, 1874
Southwest District Independent Living Program, 4034
Southwest Louisiana Independence Center: Lake Charles, 4178
Southwest Louisians Independence Center: Lafayette, 4179
Southwest Medical Center, 6404
Southwestern Center for Independent Living, 4258
Southwestern Commission Area Agency on Aging, 7556
Southwestern Diabetic Fund, 1392, 8369
Southwestern Idaho Housing Authority, 4056
Southwestern Independent Living Center, 4370
Soyland Access to Independent Living (SAIL), 4087
Soyland Access to Independent Living: Charleston, 4088
Soyland Access to Independent Living: Shelbyville, 4089
Soyland Access to Independent Living: Sullivan, 4090
Spa Area Independent Living Services, 3899
Space Coast CIL News, 5174
Space Coast Center for Independent Living, 4024, 5174
Spalding Rehab Hospital West Unit, 6693
Spalding Rehabilitation Hospital at Memorial Hospital of Laramie, 6488
Span-America Medical Systems, 280
Spatial Tilt Custom Chair, 268
Spaulding University, 4773
SpeakEasy Communication Aid, 231
Spec-L Clothing Solutions, 1471
Special Camp For Special Kids, 1004
Special Camps for Special Kids, 1387
Special Care Dentistry Association, 8299
Special Care in Dentistry, 8633
Special Children, 8667
Special Children/Special Solutions, 5365
Special Clothes, 442, 444, 445, 454, 1461, 1462, 1463, 1472, 1473, 1491, 1495, 1496, 1497, 1498, 1499, 1500, 1501
Special Clothes Adult Catalogue, 1472
Special Clothes for Children, 5446
Special Clothes for Special Children, 1473
Special Edge, 2263
Special Education And Rehab Services, 8683
Special Education Report, 2264, 4965
Special Education Today, 2526
Special Education and Vocational Rehabilitation Agency: New York, 6139

Special Education for Today, 2527
Special Format Books for Children and Youth Ages 3-19, 4966
Special Kids Need Special Parents: A Resource for Parents of Children With Special Needs, 5234
Special Needs Advocacy Resource Book, 2643
Special Needs Center/Phoenix Public Library, 4660
Special Needs Project, 2106, 451, 1944, 2295, 2350, 2410, 5207, 5229, 5499, 6249, 7499
Special Needs Systems, 5951
Special Needs Trust Handbook, 5175
Special Olympics, 8239
Special Olympics International, 8240, 8192
Special Parent, Special Child, 5235
Special Services Division: Indiana State Library, 4757
Special Siblings: Growing Up With Someone with A Disability, 5176
Special Technologies Alternative Resources, 9025, 9103
Special Tree Rehabilitation System, 7007
Special U, 4833
Specialty Care Shoppe, 1474
Specialty Hospital, 6305, 7264
SpectraLift, 425
Spectrum Aquatics, 426
Spectrum Products, 427
Spectrum Products Catalog, 427
Speech Bin, 1996, 2644, 1988, 1989, 2622, 2638, 5482, 7815, 8734, 8758, 8762
Speech Bin-Abilitations, 8743, 8751, 8759
Speech Discrimination Unit, 232
Speech Pathways, 8792
Speech and the Hearing-Impaired Child, 2528
Speech-Language Delights, 1997
Speech-Language Pathology and Audiology: An Introduction, 2529
Speechmaker-Personal Speech Amplifier, 233
Spell of Words, 1998
Spellbound, 1999
Spelling Dictionary, 2000
Spelling Rules, 1799
Spenco Medical Group, 294, 291
Spina Bifida Association, 8300
Spina Bifida Association of America, 5188, 5218, 5477, 8472, 8477, 8485, 8492, 8497, 8498, 8503, 8532, 8536, 8538, 8555, 8558, 8560, 8565, 8567, 8569, 8572, 8576, 8577, 8588, 8592, 8635
Spina Bifida Program of DC Children's Hospital, 6725
Spina Bifida and Hydrocephalus Association of Canada, 8301
Spinal Cord Dysfunction, 2530
Spinal Cord Injury Center, 2684
Spinal Network: The Total Wheelchair Resource Book, 541
Spine, 8610
Spirit Magazine, 8192
The Spiritual Art of Raising Children with Disabilities, 5269
Spiritually Able: A Parents Guide to Teaching Faith To Children with Special Needs, 5268
Spokane VA Medical Center, 5777
Sport Science Review: Adapted Physical Activity, 8183
Sportaid, 495
Sports n' Spokes Magazine, 5492
Sportster 10, 602
Spring Dell Center, 7944, 8091
Spring Dell Center Newsletter, 8091
Springboard Consulting, 1856
Springer Publishing, 2291, 2339, 2421, 2501, 2520, 7730, 8720
Springer Publishing Company, 2292, 2298, 2347, 2382, 2482, 2490, 2504, 2507, 2563, 2573, 5022, 5129, 5157, 5158, 5159, 5210, 7506, 7795, 7800, 8748
Springfield Center for Independent Living, 4091
Sproul Ranch, Inc., 994, 7968
Square D Foundation, 2898
Squirrel Hollow Summer Camp, 1058, 7703
St Frances Cabrini Hospital, 6347

St George's Society of New York, 3083
St Lukes Roosevelt, 4350
St Martin's Griffin, 8741
St. Anne's Nursing Center, 6292
St. Anthony Hospital, 6406
St. Anthony Hospital: Rehabilitation Unit, 6406
St. Anthony Memorial Hospital: Rehab Unit, 6332
St. Anthony's Hospital, 6293, 7258
St. Anthony's Rehabilitation Hospital, 6294
St. Augustine Rainbow Camp, 1317
St. Camillus Health and Rehabilitation Center, 7353
St. Catherine's Hospital, 6486
St. Catherine's Rehabilitation Hospital and Villa Maria Nursing Center, 6295
St. Clair County Library Special Technologies Alternative Resources (S.T.A.R.), 4823
St. Cloud VA Medical Center, 5664
St. Davids Medical Center, 6464
St. David's Rehabilitation Center, 6464
St. Frances Cabrini Hospital: Rehab Unit, 6347
St. Francis Camp On The Lake, 1195
St. Francis Health Care Centre, 6398
St. Francis Rehabilitation Hospital, 7118
St. George Care and Rehabilitation Center, 7403
St. James Association for Retarded Citizens, 6035
St. John Hospital: North Shore, 6361
St. John Valley Associates, 7652
St. John of God Community Services Vocational Rehabilitation, 6124
St. John's Nursing Center, 6296
St. John's Pleasant Valley Hospital Neuro Care Unit, 6664
St. John's Regional Medica Center- Industrial Therapy Center, 6665
St. Joseph Health System, 6266
St. Joseph Hospital, 6487
St. Joseph Hospital Rehabilitation, 6373
St. Joseph Hospital Rehabilitation Center, 4758
St. Joseph Hospital and Medical Center, 6240
St. Joseph Rehabilitation Center, 6266
St. Joseph Rehabilitation Hospital and Outpatient Center, 6382
St. Jude Brain Injury Network, 6267
St. Jude Hospital, 6267
St. Jude Medical Center, 6268
St. Lawrence Rehabilitation Center, 7338
St. Louis Regional Office, 5672
St. Louis Society for the Blind and Visually Impaired, 7025
St. Louis VA Medical Center, 5673
St. Mark's Hospital, 7404
St. Martin's Griffin (Macmillan Publishers), 5196
St. Mary Medical Center, 6269
St. Mary's Medical Center: RehabCare Center, 6438
St. Mary's Regional Rehabilitation Center, 6365
St. Mary's RehabCare Center, 7157
St. Patrick Hospital: Rehab Unit, 6348
St. Patrick RehabCare Unit, 6941
St. Paul Abilities Network, 925
St. Paul Press, 5197
St. Paul Regional Office, 5665
St. Petersburg Regional Office, 5607
St. Rita's Medical Center Rehabilitation Services, 6399
St. Vincent Hospital and Health Center, 6367
Stae Agency, 3828
StairClimber, 663
StairLIFT SC & SL, 428
Stairway Elevators, 429
Stamford Hospital, 7243
Stand-Up Wheelchairs, 726
Standard 3-in-1 Commode, 324
Standard Touch Turner Sip & Puff Switch, 234
Standard Wheelchair, 727
Standing Aid Frame with Rear Entry, 664
Standing on My Own Two Feet, 9026
Stanford Health Care, 2685
Stanley W Metcalf Foundation, 3084
Star Bright Books, 7737
Star Center, 1597
Stark Community Foundation, 3126
Starkey Hearing Foundation, 7945, 8098

Start-to-Finish Library, 1800
Start-to-Finish Literacy Starters, 1801
Starting Over, 2001
Starting Points, 9027
Starting and Sustaining Genetic Support Groups, 5290
State Agency for the Blind and Visually Impaired, 3659
State Department of Wyoming, 3864
State Division of Vocational Rehabilitation, 6333
State Education Agency Rural Representative, 3660
State Library of Louisiana: Services for the Blind and Physically Handicapped, 4779
State Library of Ohio: Talking Book Program, 4888
State Mental Health Representative for Children and Youth, 3661
State Mental Retardation Program, 3662
State Of Iowa, 3472, 4760, 4762
State Office Building, 3513
State Office of Wisconsin, 3856
State Planning Council on Developmental Disabilities, 3441
State University of New York, 2719
State University of New York Health Sciences Center, 4872
State University of New York Press, 2355, 2511, 2517
State of Alaska, 2110, 4653
State of Connecticut Agency, 2115
State of Illinois Center, 3455
State of Maine, 3507
State of Massachusetts, 6055
State of Michigan, 2956
State of Michigan Workers' Compensation Agency, 3546
State of Nebraska, 3591
State of Nevada, 6089
State of Nevada Client Assistance Program, 3602
State of Oregon Office of Vocational Rehabilitation Service, 6165
State of Vermont Department of Disabilities, Aging and Independent Living, 6201
State of Washington, 3840
State of West Virginia, 3841
Staten Island Center for Independent Living, Inc., 4371
Statesman Health and Rehabilitation Center, 7379
Statewide Independent Living Council of Georgia, 4035
Statewide Information at Texas School for the Deaf, 3781
Staunton Farm Foundation, 3154
Staunton Public Library Talking Book Center, 4928
Steady Write, 565
Steel Food Guard, 371
Steelcase Foundation, 2972
Steele, 542
SteeleVest, 542
Steering Backup System, 135
Steering Device By Handicaps, Inc., 136
Stella B Gross Charitable Trust C/O Bank of The West Trust Department, 2793
Step-By-Step Guide to Personal Management for Blind Persons, 9028
Step-by-Step Communicator, 235
Stepping Stones Center, 1298, 1308
Steps to Independence: Teaching Everyday Skills to Children with Special Needs, 8572
Steps to Success: Scope & Sequence for Skill Development, 2531
Sterling Ranch, 3893
Sterling Ranch: Residence for Special Women, 3893
Sterling-Turner Foundation, 3219
Stern Center, 8702
Stevens Publishing Corporation, 2183
Stewardship Foundation, 3241
Stewart Huston Charitable Trust, 3155
Stewart Rehabilitation Center: McKay Dee Hospital, 6473
Stick Canes, 665
Stickybear Early Learning Activities, 1731

Stickybear Kindergarden Activities, 1732
Stickybear Math I Deluxe, 1655
Stickybear Math II Deluxe, 1656
Stickybear Math Splash, 1657
Stickybear Math Word Problems, 1658
Stickybear Money, 1659
Stickybear Numbers Deluxe, 1660
Stickybear Reading Comprehension, 1802
Stickybear Reading Fun Park, 1803
Stickybear Reading Room Deluxe, 1804
Stickybear Science Fair Light, 1733
Stickybear Spelling, 1805
Stickybear Town Builder, 1734
Stickybear Typing, 1735, 1817
Still Me, 8184
Stocker Foundation, 3127
Stone-Hayes Center for Independent Living, 4092
Stonewall Community Foundation, 3085
Stop-Leak Gel Flotation Mattress, 295
Store @ HDSC Product Catalog, 496
Storybook Maker Deluxe, 1736
Stout Vocational Rehab Institute, 2403, 2510, 2575
Straight and Custom Curved Stairlifts, 430
Strategies for Teaching Learners with Special Needs, 2532
Strategies for Teaching Students with Learning and Behavior Problems, 2533
Strategies for Working with Families of Young Children with Disabilities, 5236
Strawberry Lane Nursing & Rehabilitation Center, 7434
Streator Unlimited, 6869
Strength for the Journey, 1332, 8404
Strengthening the Roles of Independent Living Centers Through Implementing Legal Service, 4575
Stretch-View Wide-View Rectangular Illuminated Magnifier, 638
Strider, 325
Strides Magazine, 8193
Strive Physical Therapy Centers, 6778
Strobe Light Signalers, 236
Stroke Connection Magazine, 7892, 8194
Stroke Smart Magazine, 7896
Stroke Sourcebook, 8573
Stroke Sourcebook, 2nd Edition, 8574
Student Advocate, 9109
Student Disability Services, 926
Student Guide, 3286
Student Independent Living Experience Massachusetts Hospital School, 4212
Student Teaching Guide for Blind and Visually Impaired College Students, 9029
Students with Acquired Brain Injury: The School's Response, 2534
Students with Disabilities Office, 1598
Students with Mild Disabilities in the Secondary School, 2535
Studio 49 Catalog, 2002
Study Power Workbook: Exercises in Study Skills to Improve Your Learning and Your Grades, 5260
Stuttering, 8782
Stuttering & Your Child: Help For Parents, 8776
Stuttering Foundation Newsletter, 8777
Stuttering Foundation of America, 8703, 8755, 8776, 8777
Stuttering Severity Instrument for Children and Adults, 2645
Sub-Acute Saratoga Hospital, 6666
Succeeding With Interventions For Asperger Syndrome Adolescents, 8575
Successful Job Accommodation Strategies, 6297
Successful Job Search Strategies for the Disabled: Understanding the ADA, 7811
Successful Models of Community Long Term Care Services for the Elderly, 7520
Suffolk Cooperative Library System: Long Island Talking Book Library, 4873
Suffolk Independent Living Organization (SILO), 4372
Summaries of Legal Precedents & Law Review, 4576
Summer Camp for Children with Muscular Dystrophy, 1079, 8405

Summer Camp for Physically & Mentally Challenged Children & Adults, 1118, 8406
Summer Wheelchair Sport Camps, 1080
Summer Wheelchair Sports Camp, 8163
Summit Camp, 1254, 7704
Summit Independent Living Center: Kalipsell, 4295
Summit Independent Living Center: Hamilton, 4296
Summit Independent Living Center: Missoula, 4297
Summit Independent Living Center: Ronan, 4298
Summit Ridge Center, 7052
Summit Ridge Center Genesis Eldercare, 7339
Sumner Regional Medical Center, 6439
Sun Trust Bank Atlanta, 2849, 2852, 2857
Sun-Mate Seat Cushions, 296
SunTrust Bank, Atlanta Foundation, 2857
Sunbridge Care and Rehabilitation, 6779
Sunburst Projects, 987
Suncoast Center for Independent Living, Inc., 4025
Sundial Special Vacations, 5535
Sunnyhill Adventure Center, 1220, 7705
Sunnyside Nursing Center, 6270
Sunrise Medical/Quickie Designs, 591, 696
Sunset View Castle Nursing Homes Castle Nursing Homes, 7374
Sunshine Campus, 1281
Sunshine Services, 6903
Super Challenger, 1737
Super Grade 4 Hand Controls By Handicaps, Inc., 137
Super Grade IV Hand Controls, 138
Super Light Folding Transport Chair with Carry Bag, 728
Super Stretch Socks, 1475
Superarm Lift for Vans By Handicaps, Inc., 431
Superintendent of Documents, 5495
Superintendent of Public Instruction: Special Education Section, 2169
Superior Alliance for Independent Living (SAIL), 4241
Support Plus, 1503
Support Works, 8668
Supported Employment Program, 5944
A Supported Employment Workbook: Individual Profiling and Job Matching, 4983
Supporting Success for Children with Hearing Loss, 2107
Supporting and Strengthening Families, 2536
Surdna Foundation, 3086
SureHands Lift & Care Systems, 432
Suregrip Bathtub Rail, 176
Surf Chair, 729
Survey of Direct Labor Workers Who Are Blind & Employed by NIB, 9030
Survival Strategies for Going Abroad, A Guide for People with Disabilites, 5493
Survivors Art Foundation, 63
Suttle Lake Camp, 1333, 8407
Swedish Covenant Hospital Rehabilitation Services, 6870
Swindells Charitable Foundation Trust, 2818
Switch Basics, 1738
Switch Basics IntelliKeys Overlay, 1532
Switch Interface Pro 5.0, 1739
Sycamore Rehabilitation Services, 6009
Symptomatic Chiari Malformation, 8576
Synapse Adaptive, 443
Synergos Neurological Center: Hayward, 6667
Synergos Neurological Center: Mission Hills, 6668
Syracuse Community-Referenced Curriculum Guide for Students with Disabilties, 2003
Syracuse University, 4858
Syracuse University, School of Education, 5082
Syracuse VA Medical Center, 5706
System 2000/Versa, 1622
Systems 2000, 603
Systems Unlimited/LIFE Skills, 5370

T

T AF KI D, 5707
T HI Brentwood, 6821
T J Publishers, 1959, 4581
T J Publishers, Distributor, 1910
TAC Enterprises, 7119
TASH, 1846
TASH Connections, 4577
TASK Team of Advocates for Special Kids, 1599
TBC Focus, 9110
TCRC Sight Center, 6871
TDI National Directory & Resource Guide: Blue Book, 8059
TEACCH, 7653, 7845
TERI, 5177
TERRA-JET USA, 604
TESTS, 2537
TETRA Services, 5825
TJ Publishers, 1967, 2401, 7983, 7985, 7990, 7991, 8010, 8017, 8046, 8052, 8054, 8914
TJX Companies, 2953
TJX Foundation, 2953
TLC's Summer Programs, 1161
TLC: Treatment and Learning Centers, 6958
TLL Temple Foundation, 3220
TMX Tricycle, 741
TOVA, 1772
TRIAID, 605, 607, 734, 741
TRU-Mold Shoes, 1457
TS Micro Tech, 1609
TSA CT Kid's Summer Event, 1181, 8408
TSA National Conference, 1875
TSA Newsletter, 8634
TTY's: Telephone Device for the Deaf, 237
TV & VCR Remote, 543
Tacoma Area Coalition of Individuals with Disabilities, 4532
Taconic Resources for Independence, 4373
Tactile Thermostat, 544
Take a Chance, 5482
Taking Charge, 8577
Taking Charge of ADHD Complete Authoritative Guide for Parents, 7812
Taking Control of Your Diabetes (TCOYD), 8302
Taking Part: Introducing Social Skills to Young Children, 2646
Talisman Summer Camp, 1294, 7706, 8714
Talk to Me, 9031
Talk to Me II, 9032
TalkTrac Wearable Communicator, 238
Talkable Tales, 8759
Talking Bathroom Scale, 177
Talking Book & Braille Services Oregon State Library, 4894
Talking Book Center Brunswick-Glynn County Regional Library, 4732
Talking Book Department, Parkersburg and Wood County Public Library, 4941
Talking Book Library at Worcester Public Library, 4809
Talking Book Program, 4912
Talking Book Program/Texas State Library, 4912
Talking Book Service: Mantatee County Central Library, 4712
Talking Book and Braille Service, 4846
Talking Books & Reading Disabilities, 9033
Talking Books Library for the Blind and Physically Handicapped, 4713
Talking Books Plus, 4901
Talking Books Service Evansville Vanderburgh County Public Library, 4759
Talking Books Topics, 9111
Talking Books for People with Physical Dis abilities, 9034
Talking Books/Homebound Services, 4714
Talking Calculators, 239
Talking Clinical Thermometer, 326
Talking Clocks, 240
Talking Desktop Calculators, 566
Talking Electronic Organizers, 567
Talking Screen, 1636
Talking Thermometers, 327
Talking Watches, 241

Tampa Bay Academy, 6780
Tampa General Rehabilitation Center, 6298, 6781
Tampa Lighthouse for the Blind, 6782
Tanager Place, 1110, 1112, 1277, 8379, 8390
Taping for the Blind, 9131
Target Teach, 2052
Tarjan Center at UCLA, 47
Taylor & Francis, 15, 16, 2372, 2416, 2484, 7729, 8719
Taylor & Francis Group, 2290, 8753
Taylor & Francis Group, LLC, 7525
Taylor & Francis Online, 5280
Taylor Publishing Company, 7721
Tazewell County Resource Center, 6872
Teach Me Phonemics Blends Overlay CD SoftTouch Inc., 1533
Teach Me Phonemics Medial Overlay CD, 1534
Teach Me Phonemics Overlay Series Bundle, 1535
Teach Me Phonemics Series Bundle, 1740
Teach Me Phonemics Super Bundle, 1741
Teach Me Phonemics: Blends, 1742
Teach Me Phonemics: Final, 1743
Teach Me Phonemics: Initial, 1744
Teach Me Phonemics: Medial, 1745
Teach Me to Talk, 1746
Teach Me to Talk Overlay CD, 1536
Teach Me to Talk: USB-Overlay CD, 1537
Teacher Preparation and Special Education, 927
Teacher of Students with Visual Impairment s, 2686
Teacher's Guide to Including Students with Disabilities in Regular Physical Education, 2538
A Teacher's Guide to Isovaleric Acidemia, 2272
A Teacher's Guide to Methylmalonic Acidemia, 2273
A Teacher's Guide to PKU, 2274
Teachers Institute for Special Education, 1707
Teachers College Press, 2348, 2356, 2357, 2439, 2445, 2497, 2569, 7760, 8971
Teachers Institute for Special Education, 1705, 1706
Teachers Working Together, 2539
Teachig Students with Special Needs in Inclusive Classrooms, 2540
Teaching Adults with Learning Disabilities, 2541
Teaching Asperger's Students Social Skills Through Acting, 64
Teaching Basic Guitar Skills to Special Learners, 65
Teaching Chemistry to Students with Disabi lities: A Manual, 5302
Teaching Children With Autism in the General Classroom, 2542
Teaching Children with Autism: Strategies for Initiating Positive Interactions, 7813, 8760
Teaching Children with Down Syndrome about Their Bodies, Boundaries, and Sexuality, 5252
Teaching Disturbed and Disturbing Students: An Integrative Approach, 2543
Teaching Every Child Every Day: Integrated Learning in Diverse Classrooms, 2544
Teaching Exceptional Children, 2227
Teaching Individuals with Physical and Multiple Disabilities, 2004
Teaching Infants and Preschoolers with Handicaps, 2545
Teaching Language-Disabled Children: A Communication/Games Intervention, 2546
Teaching Learners with Mild Disabilities: Integrating Research and Practice, 2547
Teaching Mathematics to Students with Learning Disabilities, 2548
Teaching Mildly and Moderately Handicapped Students, 2549
Teaching Orientation and Mobility in the Schools: An Instructor's Companion, 9035
Teaching Reading to Children with Down Syndrome: A Guide for Parents and Teachers, 2550
Teaching Reading to Disabled and Handicapped Learners, 2551
Teaching Reading to Handicapped Children, 2552
Teaching Self-Determination to Students with Disabilities, 2553

Teaching Special Students in Mainstream, 2075
Teaching Students Ways to Remember, 2005
Teaching Students with Learning Problems, 2554
Teaching Students with Learning and Behavi or Problems, 2555
Teaching Students with Mild and Moderate Learning Problems, 2556
Teaching Students with Moderate/Severe Disabilities, Including Autism, 2557
Teaching Students with Special Needs in Inclusive Settings, 2558
Teaching Test-Taking Skills: Helping Students Show What They Know, 2006
Teaching Visually Impaired Children, 9036
Teaching Young Children to Read, 2559
Teaching and Mainstreaming Autistic Children, 7814, 8761
Teaching of Reading: A Continuum from Kindergarten through College, The, 2647
Teaching the Bilingual Special Education Student, 2560
Teaching the Learning Disabled Adolescent: Strategies and Methods, 2561
Teaching the Mentally Retarded Student: Curriculum, Methods, and Strategies, 2562
Tech Connection, 1600
Tech Notes, 2265
Tech-Able, 1601
Techniques for Aphasia Rehab: (TARGET) Generating Effective Treatment, 7815, 8762
Technology Access Center of Tucson, 1602
Technology Assistance for Special Consumers, 1603, 4652
Technology and Handicapped People, 2563
Technology and Media Division, 928
Technology for the Disabled Landmark Media, Inc., 5366
Teen Tunes Plus, 1747
Teen Tunes Plus IntelliKeys Overlay, 1538
Teenagers with ADD, 7816
Teens & Asthma, 8638
Teichert Foundation, 2794
Telecaption Adapter, 242
Telecommunications for the Deaf, 8018, 8059
Telecommunications for the Deaf (TDI), 8011
Telecommunications for the Deaf and Hard o f Hearing, 7946
Teleflex Foundation, 3156
Television Remote Controls with Large Numbers, 568
Temple Community Hospital, 6669
Temple University, 1592, 4429
Temple University Institute on Disabilities, 5439
Ten Things I Learned from Bill Porter, 8578
Tenco Industries, 6904
Tenet South Florida, 6287
Tennessee Assistive Technology Projects, 3761
Tennessee Association of Homes and Service s for the Aging, 7490
Tennessee Client Assistance Program, 3762
Tennessee Commission on Aging and Disability, 3763
Tennessee Council on Developmental Disabilities, 3764
Tennessee Council on Developmental Disabilities, 8617
Tennessee Department Human Services, 6189
Tennessee Department of Children with Disabilities, 3765
Tennessee Department of Education, 2162
Tennessee Department of Labor: Job Training Program Liaison, 6190
Tennessee Department of Mental Health, 3766
Tennessee Division of Rehabilitation, 3767
Tennessee Fair Employment Practice Agency, 6191
Tennessee Jaycees and Tennessee Jaycee Foundation, 1376
Tennessee Library for the Blind and Physically Handicapped, 4905
Tennessee Protection and Advocacy, 3762
Tennessee State Library Archives, 4905
Tennessee Technology Access Program (TTAP), 4464

Terra-Jet: Utility Vehicle, 604

Terrier Tricycle, 605
Terry-Wash Mitt: Medium Size, 178
Test Critiques: Volumes I-X, 2648
Test of Early Reading Ability Deaf or Hard of Hearing, 2649
Test of Language Development: Primary, 2650
Test of Mathematical Abilities, 2nd Editio n, 2651
Test of Nonverbal Intelligence, 3rd Editio n, 2652
Test of Phonological Awareness, 2653
Test of Written Spelling, 3rd Edition, 2654
Tethering Cord, 8635
Texas Advocates Supporting Kids with Disabilities, 3782
Texas Association of Homes and Services for the Aging, 7491
Texas Association of Retinitis Pigmentosa, 9101
Texas Commission for the Blind, 3783
Texas Commission for the Deaf and Hard of Hearing, 3784
Texas Council for Developmental Disabilities, 3785
Texas Department of Assistive and Rehabili tative Services, 4485
Texas Department of Human Services, 3786
Texas Department of Mental Health & Mental Retardation, 3787
Texas Department on Aging, 3788
Texas Education Agency, 2163
Texas Education Agency: Special Education Unit, 2164
Texas Employment Services and Job Training Program Liaison, 6194
Texas Federation of Families for Children's Mental Health, 3789
Texas Governor's Committee on People with Disabilities, 3790
Texas Lions Camp, 1399, 7979, 8409, 8897
Texas NeuroRehab Center, 6465
Texas Protection & Advocacy Services for Disabled Persons, 3791
Texas Respite Resource Network, 3792
Texas School of the Deaf, 2165
Texas Scottish Rite Hospital for Children, 2655
Texas Specialty Hospital at Dallas, 6466, 7180
Texas Speech-Language-Hearing Association, 8704, 8772
Texas Technology Access Project, 3793
Texas UAP for Developmental Disabilities, 3794
Texas Workers Compensation Commission, 3795
Texas Workforce Commission, 6194
Textbook Catalog, 9037
Textbooks and the Student Who Can't Read Them: A Guide for Teaching Content, 2564
That All May Worship: An Interfaith Welcom e to People with Disabilities, 5178
That's My Child, 5237
Theatre Without Limits, 67
Theoretical Issues in Sign Language Research, 8060
Therapeutic Activities with Persons Disabled by Alzheimer's Disease, 7521
Therapeutic Nursery Program, 2609
Therapro, Inc., 170, 178, 299, 301, 302, 304, 322, 358, 361, 365, 366, 372, 373, 376, 505, 516, 528, 529, 532, 545, 558, 619, 1963
Therapy Putty, 545
Therapy Shoppe, 2007
There are Tyrannosaurs Trying on Pants in My Bedroom, 1748
There's a Hearing Impaired Child in My Class, 2568
They Don't Come with Manuals, 5239
They're Just Kids, 5240
Thibodaux Regional Medical Center, 6349
Thick-n-Easy, 372
Thigh-Hi Nylon Stockings, 1476
Thinking Differently: An Inspiring Guide for Parents of Children with Learning Disabilities, 5253
Third Line Press, 5140
Thoele Manufacturing, 530
Thoms Rehabilitation Hospital, 7086, 7086, 7762
Three Billy Goats Gruff, 1749
Three Little Pigs, 1750

Three R's for Special Education: Rights, Resources, Results, 5367
Three Rivers Center for Independent Living: New Castle, 4435
Three Rivers Center for Independent Livi ng: Washington, 4436
Three Rivers Center for Independent Living, 4116, 4437
Three Rivers Health Care, 6366
Three Rivers Independent Living Center, 4154
Three Rivers Independent Living Center: Clay, 4155
Three Rivers Independent Living Center: Ma nhattan, 4156
Three Rivers Independent Living Center: Se neca, 4157
Three Rivers Independent Living Center: To peka, 4158
Three Rivers News, 9038
Three Rivers Press, 7740
Three Rivers Press/Crown Publishing-Random House, 9
Thresholds AMISS, 5985
Thresholds Bridge Deaf North Program, 6873
Thresholds Psychiatric Rehabilitation Centers, 929
Thresholds Psychiatric Rehabilitation Centers, 6873
Thresholds South Suburbs, 6874
Through the Looking Glass, 3963, 4576, 5111, 5209, 5217, 5225, 5244, 5250, 5307, 5308, 7751, 8009, 8912, 8913, 8950
Thumb Industries, 7008
Thumbs Up Cup, 373
Thyroid Disorders Sourcebook, 8579
Thyssen Krupp Access, 433
Tic Tac Toe, 5483
Tidewater Center for Technology Access Special Education Annex, 1604
Tilt-N-Table, 686
Tim's Trim, 139
Timber Pointe Outdoor Center, 1081
Timber Ridge Ranch NeuroRestorative Services, 6540
Timberland Opportunities Association, 7214
Timbertop Nature Adventure Camp, 1439, 7707
Timex Easy Reader, 639
Tinnitus Today, 8076
Tiny Tech, 2266
Tisch Foundation, 3087
Title II & III Regulation Amendment Regarding Detectable Warnings, 4635
Title II Complaint Form, 4636
Title II Highlights, 4637
Title III Technical Assistance Manual and Supplement, 4638
To Live with Grace and Dignity, 5180
To Love this Life: Quotations by Helen Keller, 9039
To Teach a Dyslexic, 2008
To a Different Drumbeat, 5241
Togus VA Medical Center, 5643
Tohatchi Area of Opportunity & Services, 6132
Toilet Guard Rail, 179
Toledo Community Foundation, 3128
Toll-Free Information Line, 8669
Tom Snyder Productions, 1665, 1774
Tomah VA Medical Center, 5785
Tomorrow's Promise: Language Arts, 1806
Tomorrow's Promise: Mathematics, 1661
Tomorrow's Promise: Reading, 1807
Tomorrow's Promise: Spelling, 1808
Tompkins County Office for the Aging, 7557
Tools for Students Aquarius Health Care Media, 5368
Tools for Transition, 2009
Topeka & Shawnee County Public Library Talking Books Service, 4770
Topeka Independent Living Resource Center, 4159
Topics in Early Childhood Special Education, 2267
Torah Alliance of Families of Kids with Disabilities, 5707
Torso Support, 666
Total Living Center, 4327
Touch Turner Company, 243

Touch Turner-Page Turning Devices, 243
Touch the Baby: Blind & Visually Impaired Children As Patients, 9040
Touch/Ability Connects People with Disabilities & Alternative Health Care Pract., 5181
TouchCorders, 1751
TouchWindow Touch Screen, 1752
Touchdown Keytop/Keyfront Kits, 1552
Touchstone Neurorecovery Center, 6467
Tourette Association of America, 7655
Tourette Syndrome Association, 1875, 8634
Tourette Syndrome Association Children's Newsletter, 8636
Tourette Syndrome Association of Connecticut (TSA), 1181, 8408
Tourette Syndrome: The Facts, 8580
Tourette's Syndrome: Finding Answers and Getting Help, 8581
Tourette's Syndrome: Tics, Obsessions, Com pulsions: Developmental Psychopathology, 8582
Touro Rehabilitation Center LCMC (Louisiana Children's Medical Center), 6942
Toward Effective Public School Program for Deaf Students, 2569
Toward Independence, 4639
Tower Program at Regis College, 1182
Toyei Industries, 6532
Trace Research and Development Center, 4947
Trail's Edge Camp, 1196
Training Resource Network, 5296
Training, Resource & Assistive-Technology, 6943
Trans Health Incorporated, 6388
Transfer Bench, 328
Transfer Bench with Back, 269
Transfer Tub Bench, 180
Transition Activity Calendar for Students with Visual Impairments, 9041
Transition to College for Students with Visual Impairments: Report, 9042
Transitional Hospitals Corporation, 6803
Transitional Learning Center at Gavelston and Lubbock, 7181
Transportation Equipment for People with Disabilities, 140
Transylvania Vocational Services, 6145
Travel Information Service/Moss Rehab Hospital, 5494
Travelers Aid International, 5509
Treating Adults with Disabilities: Access and Communication, 2570
Treating Cerebral Palsy for Clinicians by Clinicians, 2571
Treating Disordered Speech Motor Control, 2572
Treating Epilepsy Naturally: A Guide to Al ternative and Adjunct Therapies, 8583
Treating Families of Brain Injury Survivors, 2573
Treatment Review, 2268
Treatment and Learning Centers, 2656
Treatment and Learning Centers (TLC), 6054
Tree of Life Publications, 8174
Treemont Nursing And Rehabilitation Center, 7182
Trekker 40, 606
Tri-County Center for Independent Living, 4288
Tri-County Independent Living Center, 3964, 4495, 5871
Tri-County Patriots for Independent Living, 4438
Tri-Grip Bathtub Rail, 181
Tri-Lo's, 607
Tri-Post Steering Wheel Spinner, 141
Tri-State Resource and Advocacy Corporation, 4465
Triangle Community Foundation, 3099
Triangle D Camp, 1318
Triangle J Council of Governments Area Age ncy on Aging, 7558
Triangle Y Ranch YMCA, 958, 7708
Trinity Health Foundation, 6866
Trips Inc., 5536
Triumph 3000/4000, 608
Triumph Scooter, 609
Truman Medical Center Low Vision Rehabilitation Program, 7026
Truman Neurological Center, 7027
Trumbull Park, 6875
Trunks, 1494

Tub Slide Shower Chair, 182
Tulsa City-County Library System: Outreach Services, 4891
Tulsa City: County Library System, 4891
Tunnell Center for Rehab, 6670
Tuolumne Trails, 1005
Tuomey Healthcare System, 7386
Turn Signal Adapter By Handicaps, Inc., 142
Turnabout Game, 5484
Turning Automotive Seating (TAS), 434
Turnkey Computer Systems for the Visually, Physically, and Hearing Impaired, 1637
Turtle Teasers, 1753
Tuscaloosa VA Medical Center, 5565
Twin Lakes Camp, 1103, 8164, 8410
Twin Peaks Press, 5489
Twin-Rest Seat Cushion & Glamour Pillow, 297
Twitch and Shout, 8642
21st Century Scientific, Inc. Bounder Power Wheelchair, 693

U

U CL A Medical Center, 6271
U S Department of Education/ NI DR R, 6315
U S Department of Education, 4699, 8649
U S Department of Health and Human Services, 2260, 3289, 3389
U S Department of Justice, 4635, 4638
U S Social Security Administration, 4795
U-Control III, 1539
U-Step Walking Stabilizer: Walker, 667
U.S. Department of Justice, 4990
U.S. Department of Justice, Civil Rights Division, 4993, 4994, 4996, 5378
U.S. Department of Veteran Affairs, 5562, 5568, 6508
UAB Eye Care, 6509
UAB Spain Rehabilitation Center, 2688, 7219
UCLA Medical Center: Department of Anesthesiology, Acute Pain Services, 6271
UCP Huntsville, 4652
UCP Washington Wire, 4640
UN Printing, 9044
UNUM Charitable Foundation, 2919
UPMC Braddock, 7380
UPMC McKeesport, 7381
UPMC Passavant, 7382
US Airways/America West Airlines, 5510
US Association of Blind Athletes, 9137
US Department Of Justice, 3291
US Department Veterans Affairs Beckley Vet Center, 5783
US Department of Education, 2824, 3286
US Department of Education: Office of Civil Rights, 3305
US Department of Health, 8791
US Department of Health and Human Services Office for Civil Rights, 4641
US Department of Health and Human Services, 5043
US Department of Housing & Urban Development, 5084
US Department of Justice, 3290, 4572, 4573, 4579, 4586, 4587, 4588, 4589, 4593, 4605, 4628, 4636, 4637, 4997, 4998, 4999, 5006, 5013, 5089, 5112, 8561, 8909
US Department of Labor, 4642, 3395
US Department of Labor Office of Federal Contract Compliance Programs, 4643
US Department of Labor: Office of Federal Contract Programs, 3306
US Department of Transportation, 3307, 5548
US Department of Veterans Affairs National Headquarters, 5560
US Healthworks, 6173
US Office of Personnel Management, 3308
US Paralympics, 8645
US Role in International Disability Activities: A History, 5182
US Servas, 5511
US Social Security Administration, 7532
US Veteran's Affairs, 5561
USA Deaf Sports Federation, 8115

USX Foundation, 3157
Ukiah Valley Association for Habilitation, 6671
The Ultimate Guide to Sex and Disability, 5179
Ultra-Lite XL Hand Control, 143
Ultratec, 497, 7577
Umpqua Valley Disabilities Network, 4413
Uncommon Fathers, 5242
Undercounter Lid Opener, 374
Understanding & Controlling Stuttering: A Comprehensive New Approach Based on the Valsa Hyp, 8763
Understanding ADHD, 7864
Understanding Asthma, 8584
Understanding Asthma: The Blueprint for Breathing, 8585
Understanding Attention Deficit Disorder, 7865
Understanding Autism, 7866, 8787
Understanding Cystic Fibrosis, 8586
Understanding Down Syndrome: An Introduction for Parents, 7817
Understanding Multiple Sclerosis, 8587
Understanding and Accommodating Physical Disabilities: Desk Reference, 5183
Understanding and Teaching Emotionally Disturbed Children & Adolescents, 2574
Underwood Books, 7722
Underwood-Miller, 7821
Uni-Turner, 375
Unicorn Keyboards, 1620
Union Pacific Foundation, 2998
Unisex Low Vision Watch, 640
United Access, 144
United Art and Education, 2010
United Brachial Plexus Network, Inc., 8303
United Cerebral Palsy, 2053, 7656, 4640
United Cerebral Palsy Association, 1849, 3381
United Cerebral Palsy Association New York, 1262, 8346
United Cerebral Palsy Associations of New Jersey, 6125
United Cerebral Palsy Associations of New Jersey, 3624
United Cerebral Palsy Of Delaware, 1030
United Cerebral Palsy of Texas, 3796
United Church of Christ, 1002
United Disability Services, 34
United Foundation for Disabled Archers, 8241
United Methodist Church, 1225, 7957
United Methodist Church: Eastern Pennsylvania, 1353
United Spinal Association, 1902, 4874, 8156
United States Access Board, 1885, 1886
United States Association of Blind Athletes, 8873
United States Association of Blind Athletes, 9085
United States Blind Golf Association, 9138
United States Blind Golfers Association, 8874
United States Braille Chess Association, 8875
United States Deaf Ski & Snowboard Associa tion, 7947
United States Department of the Interior National Park Service, 5495
United States Disabled Golf Association, 930
United States Trager Association, 931
United We Stand of New York, 3663
Unity, 244
Universal Attention Disorders, 1772
Universal Hand Cuff, 376
Universal Institute Rehabilitation & Fitne ss Center, 6380
Universal Pediatric Services, 932
Universal Switch Mounting System, 1540
University Afiliated Program/Rose F Kennedy Center, 3664
University Health Care Burn Camp Programs, 1403
University Healthcare-Rehabilitation Center, 6474
University Legal Services AT Program, 4644
University Medical Center, 6369, 6437
University Of Alabama at Birmingham, 6509
University Of Cincinnati Uap, 4884
University Of Iowa, 1113, 7709, 8705, 8715, 8899
University Of Tennessee, 1377
University Of Virginia School Of Engineering, 5549
University Press of Mississippi, 8586, 8587

University Press of New England, 8554
University of Alabama, 3313
University of Arkansas at Little Rock, 9076
University of California Memory and Aging Center, 7559
University of California Press, 7784
University of Chicago Press, 8060
University of Cincinnati Hospital, 6400
University of Colorado Health Sciences Center, 6272
University of Idaho, 4735
University of Illinois, 1080, 8163
University of Illinois Medical Center, 6876
University of Illinois Press, 8022
University of Illinois at Chicago, 4749
University of Illinois at Chicago: Lions of Illinois Eye Research Institute, 4749
University of Iowa, 4761
University of Kansas, 805, 3478
University of Maine at Augusta, 1582, 3502
University of Maryland Rehabilitation and Orthopaedic Institute, 2689
University of Miami, 6299
University of Miami: Bascom Palmer Eye Institute, 4715
University of Miami: Jackson Memorial Rehabilitation Center, 6299
University of Miami: Mailman Center for Child Development, 4716
University of Michigan, 2138
University of Michigan: Orthopaedic Research Laboratories, 4824
University of Minnesota, 4833
University of Minnesota at Crookston, 2720
University of Missouri, 4841
University of Missouri-Kansas City, 3567
University of Missouri: Columbia Arthritis Center, 4841
University of New Hampshire, 2148
University of New Mexico, 1874
University of North Carolina at Chapel Hill: Neuroscience Research Building, 4880
University of North Carolina at Chapel Hill, 7653, 8511
University of Oregon, 2721
University of Pennsylvania, 2708
University of Rochester Medical Center, 3665
University of South Carolina, 3174
University of South Florida, 4708
University of Texas, 3794
University of Texas Southwestern Medical Center/Allergy & Immunology, 4913
University of Texas at Austin, 1598
University of Texas at Austin Library, 4914
University of Virginia, 6477
University of Virginia Health System General Clinical Research Group, 4929
University of Virginia, Rehab Engineering Centers, 687
University of Washington PKU Clinic, 2478
University of Wisconsin, 2200
Unseen Minority: A Social History of Blindness in the United States, 9043
Unyeway, 5872
Up and Running, 1825
Upledger Institute, 933
Upper Coastal Plain Council of Governments Area Agency on Aging, 7560
Upper Peninsula Library for the Blind, 4825
Upper Pinellas Association for Retarded Citizens, 6783
Upper Valley Medical/Rehab Services, 6401
Uppertone, 546
Upstate Update, 9112
Upward Bound Camp for Persons With, 1334
Urologic Care of the Child with Spina Bifida, 8588
Usher Syndrome, 8589
Using the Dictionary of Occupational Titles in Career Decision Making, 2575
Utah Assistive Technology Program (UTAP) Utah State University, 4496
Utah Assistive Technology Projects, 3799
Utah Client Assistance Program, 3800

Utah Department of Aging, 3801
Utah Department of Human Services, 3802, 3803
Utah Department of Human Services: Division of Services for People with Disabilities, 3802
Utah Division Of Substance Abuse & Mental Health, 3803
Utah Division of Services for the Disabled, 3804
Utah Division of Veterans Affairs, 5766, 5766
Utah Employment Services, 6196
Utah Governor's Committee on Employment of the Handicapped, 6197
Utah Governor's Council for People with Disabilities, 3805
Utah Independent Living Center, 4497
Utah Independent Living Center: Minersville, 4498
Utah Independent Living Center: Tooele, 4499
Utah Labor Commission, 3806
Utah Protection & Advocacy Services for Persons with Disabilities, 3807
Utah State Library Division: Program for the Blind and Disabled, 4915
Utah State Office of Education, 2166
Utah State Office of Education: At-Risk and Special Education Service Unit, 2166
Utah State Office of Rehabilitation, 6199
Utah State University, 3799
Utah Veterans Centers, 6198
Utah Vocational Rehabilitation Agency, 6199

V

V A Montana Healthcare System, 5675
V Foundation for Cancer Research, 5447
V OR T Corporation, 1694, 1760
V XI Corporation Incorporated, 1638
V-Bar Enterprises, 5873
VA Ann Arbor Healthcare System, 5661
VA Boston Healthcare System: Brockton Division, 5653
VA Boston Healthcare System: Jamaica Plain Campus, 5654
VA Boston Healthcare System: West Roxbury Division, 5655
VA Central California Health Care System, 5584
VA Central Iowa Health Care System, 5631
VA Connecticut Healthcare System: Newington Division, 5594
VA Connecticut Healthcare System: West Haven, 5595
VA Greater Los Angeles Healthcare System, 5585
VA Hudson Valley Health Care System, 5708
VA Illiana Health Care System, 5622
VA Maryland Health Care System, 5649
VA Medical Center, Washington DC, 5601
VA Montana Healthcare System, 5676
VA Nebraska-Western Iowa Health Care System, 5681
VA North Indiana Health Care System: Fort Wayne Campus, 5625
VA North Texas Health Veterans Affairs Care System: Dallas VA Medical Center, 5763
VA Northern California Healthcare System, 5586
VA Northern Indiana Health Care System: Marion Campus, 5626
VA Pittsburgh Healthcare System, University Drive Division, 5742
VA Pittsburgh Healthcare System, Highland Drive Division, 5743
VA Puget Sound Health Care System, 5778
VA Salt Lake City Healthcare System, 5767
VA San Diego Healthcare System, 5587
VA Sierra Nevada Healthcare System, 5684
VA Southern Nevada Healthcare System, 5685
VA Western NY Healthcare System, Batavia, 5709
VA Western NY Healthcare System, Buffalo, 5710
VACC Camp, 1047, 8411
VAK Tasks Workbook: Visual, Auditory and Kinesthetic, 2011
VBS Special Education Teaching Guide, 2576
VCT/A Job Retention Skill Training Program, 5830
VESID, 3666
VIA Services West, 970

VIP Newsletter, 2269
VISIONS Center on Blindness, 1282, 8898
VISIONS Vacation Camp for the Blind, 1282, 8898
VOLAR Center for Independent Living, 4486
VSA - The International Organization on Arts and Disability, 68
VSA Arts of New York City, 3667
VSA Indiana, 6334
VSA arts, 69
VUE: Vision Use in Employment, 9144
Valir Health, 6407
Valley Associates for Independent Living (VAIL), 4523
Valley Associates for Independent Living: Lexington, 4524
Valley Association for Independent Living (VAIL), 4487
Valley Association for Independent Living: Harlingen, 4488
Valley Center for the Blind, 6672
Valley Forge Specialized Educational Services, 2690
Valley Garden Health Care and Rehabilitation Center, 7236
Valley Health Care and Rehabilitation Center, 7226
Valley Light Industries, 5874
Valley Memorial Health Center, 5904
Valley News Dispatch, 7818
Valley Regional Medical Center, 7400
Valley Regional Medical Center: RehabCare Unit, 6468
Valley View Regional Hospital-RehabCare Unit, 7124
Valpar International, 1818
ValueOptions, 5448
Van Ameringen Foundation, 3088
Van G Miller & Associates, 6892
VanMatre Rehabilitation Center, 6877
Vancouver Health & Rhabilitation Center, 7420
Vancouver Health and Rehabilitation Center, 7215
Vanderbilt Kennedy Center, 1373
Vanderbilt Rehabilitation Center, 7148
Vangater, Vangater II, Mini-Vangater, 435
Vanguard School, The, 2690
Vantage, 245
Vantage Mini-Vans, 145, 145
Variety Club Camp & Developmental, 1359
Vaughn-Blumberg Services, 6510
Vector Mobility, 738
Velcro Booties, 1458
Velcro Peel-Off Shoes, 146
Ventilator-Assisted Living, 8611
Ventura Enterprises, 668
Venture Publishing Inc., 4979
Ventures Travel, 5537
Verbal Behavior Approach: How to Teach Children with Autism & Related Disorders, 7819, 8764
Verbal View of the Web & Net, 7585
Verizon Foundation, 3089
Vermont Achievement Center, 6475
Vermont Assistive Technology Program, 4500
Vermont Assistive Technology Project: Department of Aging & Disabilities, 1605
Vermont Assistive Technology Projects, 3811
Vermont Assn for the Blind & Visually Impaired, 9114
Vermont Association for the Blind and Visually Impaired, 8876
Vermont Back Research Center, 8157
Vermont Center for Independent Living: Bennington, 4501
Vermont Center for Independent Living: Chittenden, 4502
Vermont Center for Independent Living: Montpelier, 4503
Vermont Client Assistance Program, 3812
Vermont Community Foundation, 3225
Vermont Department Of Health, 3816
Vermont Department of Aging, 3813
Vermont Department of Developmental and, 3814
Vermont Department of Disabilities, Aging and Independent Living, 3815

Vermont Department of Health: Children with Special Health Needs, 3816
Vermont Department of Libraries - Special Services Unit, 4916
Vermont Department of Libraries -Special Services Unit, 4917
Vermont Developmental Disabilities Council, 3817
Vermont Division for the Blind & Visually Impaired, 3818
Vermont Division of Disability & Aging Services, 3819
Vermont Employment Services and Job Training, 6202
Vermont Governor's Committee on Employment of People with Disabilities, 6203
Vermont Interdependent Services Team Approach (VISTA), 2577
Vermont VA Regional Office Center, 5768
Vermont Veterans Centers, 5769
Versatrainer, 436
Vertek, 1815
Vestibular Board, 437
Vestibular Disorders Association, 5184, 7948, 5184, 7993, 8088, 8111, 8112, 8113, 8519
Vet Center, 5666, 5677
Vet Center Readjustment Counseling Service, 5662
Vet Health Administration U S Department of VA, 5715
Veteran Benefits Administration Anchorage Regional Office, 5568
Veteran's Administration, 6038
Veterans Benefits Administration, 5700
Veterans Benefits Administration U S Deparment of, 5741
Veterans Benefits Administration U S Department V, 5768
Veterans Benefits Administration U S Department of, 5592, 5623, 5776
Veterans Benefits Administration U S Dept. of V A, 5580, 5589, 5596
Veterans Benefits Administration U S Deptartment o, 5683
Veterans Benefits Administration, U S Dept. of V A, 5575, 5578, 5583, 5607, 5609, 5615, 5617, 5628, 5634, 5638, 5642, 5644, 5650, 5660, 5665, 5668, 5672, 5679, 5686, 5692, 5704, 5716, 5718, 5721, 5724, 5729, 5739, 5745, 5747, 5751, 5755, 5764, 5772, 5779, 5787, 5791
Veterans Health Administration, 5591
Veterans Health Administration U S Department of V, 5582, 5620, 5722, 5749, 5784
Veterans Health Administration U S Department. of, 5594
Veterans Health Administration U S Deptartment of, 5585, 5651, 5697
Veterans Health Administration U.S. Dept. of VA, 5563
Veterans Health Administration, U S Department of, 5708, 5738
Veterans Health Administration, U S Dept. of V A, 5565, 5569, 5571, 5572, 5576, 5577, 5579, 5584, 5586, 5587, 5590, 5595, 5602, 5603, 5604, 5605, 5606, 5608, 5610, 5611, 5612, 5618, 5619, 5621, 5622, 5624, 5625, 5626, 5627, 5629, 5630, 5633, 5635, 5636, 5637, 5640, 5641, 5643, 5645, 5646, 5648, 5652, 5653, 5654, 5655, 5656, 5657, 5658, 5659, 5661, , 5663, 5664, 5667, 5669, 5670, 5671, 5673, 5676, 5678, 5680, 5681, 5684, 5685, 5687, 5691, 5695, 5698, 5699, 5701, 5702, 5703, 5705, 5706, 5709, 5710, 5711, 5713, 5714, 5717, 5719, 5720, 5723, 5726, 5726, 5730
Veterans Health Administration, U S Dept. of VA, 5750
Veterans Health Administration, U.S. Dept. of VA, 5564
Veterans Health Administration, US Dept. of VA, 5570, 5573, 5574, 5597, 5616, 5694, 5754, 5756
Vibes Bed Shaker, 196
Vibra Health Care, 6276
Vibrotactile Personal Alerting System, 246
Victor E Speas Foundation, 2993
Victoria Foundation, 3018
Victory Junction Gang Camp, 1295

Video Guide to Disability Awareness Aquarius Health Care Media, 5369
Video Intensive Parenting, 5370
Video Learning Library, 8100
Views from Our Shoes, 4969
Viking Books, 8942
Villa Esperanza Services, 6673
Village Square Nursing And Rehabilitation Center, 6674
Vinfen Corporation, 6988
Vinland Center Lake Independence, 4259
Vinsen Corporation, 6056
Vintage and Anchor Books, 8047
Vintage-Random House, 7794
Virginia Autism Resource Center, 4930
Virginia Beach Foundation, 3232
Virginia Beach Public Library Special Services Library, 4931
Virginia Chapter of the Arthtitis Foundation, 4932
Virginia Commonwealth University, 4924
Virginia Department Of Education, 2168
Virginia Department for the Blind and Vision Impaired, 3822
Virginia Department of Education: Division of Pre & Early Adolescent Education, 2168
Virginia Department of Mental Health, 3823
Virginia Department of Veterans Services, 5774
Virginia Developmental Disability Council, 3824
Virginia Office Protection and Advocacy for People with Disabilities, 3825
Virginia Office for Protection & Advocacy, 3826
Virginia Office for Protection and Advocacy, 3827
Virginia State Library for the Visually and Physically Handicapped, 4933
Virginia's Developmental Disabilities Plan ning Council, 3828
Visalia Workshop, 5875
Visi-Pitch III, 1773
Vision Enhancement, 9044
Vision Forward Association, 8877
Vision Foundation, 2954
Vision Loss Resources, 7015
Vision Magazine, 8099
Vision Northwest, 7130
Vision Rehabilitation Service, 6982
Vision World Wide, 8878
Visions & Values, 5185
Visions Center on Blindness (VCB), 8879
Visiting Nurse Association of America, 8670
Visiting Nurse Association of North Shore, 6989
Vista Center for the Blind & Visually Impaired, 6675
Vista Center for the Blind & Visually Impaired, 9105
Vista Wheelchair, 730
Visual Aids and Informational Material, 9113
Visual Alerting Guest Room Kit, 547
Visual Impairment: An Overview, 9045
Visual Impairments And Learning, 9046
Visually Impaired Center, 7009, 9079
Visually Impaired Persons of Southwest Florida, 6784
Visually Impaired Seniors as Senior Companions: A Reference Guide, 7522
Visually Impaired Veterans of America, 8880
Vital Signs: Crip Culture Talks Back Fanlight Productions/Icarus Films, 5371
Vocabulary Development, 1809
Vocational Rehabilitation Agency, 6059, 6133
Vocational Rehabilitation Service - Opelika, 5799
Vocational Rehabilitation Service - Dothan, 5800
Vocational Rehabilitation Service - Homewo od, 5801
Vocational Rehabilitation Service - Huntsv ille, 5802
Vocational Rehabilitation Service - Jackso n, 5803
Vocational Rehabilitation Service - Jasper, 5804
Vocational Rehabilitation Service - Mobile, 5805
Vocational Rehabilitation Service - Muscle Shoals, 5806
Vocational Rehabilitation Service - Selma, 5807
Vocational Rehabilitation Service - Tallad ega, 5808
Vocational Rehabilitation Service - Troy, 5809

Vocational Rehabilitation Service - Tuscal oosa, 5810
Vocational Rehabilitation Service- Gadsden, 5811
Vocational Rehabilitation Service: Scottsboro, 5812
Vocational Rehabilitation Services - Andal usia, 5813
Vocational Rehabilitation Services - Annis ton, 5814
Vocational Rehabilitation and Employment, 6387
Vocational Rehabilitation, Division of Department of Workforce Services, 6224
Vocational and Rehabilitation Agency, 5891, 5905, 5958, 5964, 5986, 6010, 6044, 6072, 6089, 6094, 6126, 6134, 6146, 6159, 6166, 6174, 6184, 6195
Vocational and Rehabilitation Agency Department of Education, 5945
Vocational and Rehabilitation Agency Division of Services for the Blind, 5831
Vocational and Rehabilitation Agency Massachusetts Commission for the Blind, 6060
Vocational and Rehabilitation Agency Rehabilitation Services Administrations, 5826
Vocational and Rehabilitation Agency for Persons Who Are Visually Impaired, 5832
Vocational and Rehabilitation Agency: Commission for the Blind, 6184
Vocational and Rehabilitation Agency: Department for the Blind/Visually Impaired, 6147, 6175, 6180, 6212
Vocational and Rehabilitation Agency: Division of Vocational Rehabilitation, 5946, 6200, 6218
Vocational and Rehabilitation Agency: Oregon Commission for the Blind, 6167
Vocational and Rehabilitation Agency: State Department of Social Services, 5906
Vocational and Rehabilitation Agency: State Rehabilitation Commission, 6195
Vocational and Rehabilitation Agency: Divi sion of Services to the Blind/Visually Impaired, 6188
Vocational and Rehabilitation Service - Decatur, 5815
Vocational and Rehabilitation Services - Montgomery, 5816
Vocational and Rehabilitation: State of Wisconsin, 6222
Voice, 8778, 9114
Voice Amplified Handsets, 247
Voice Choice, 147
Voice Scan, 148
Voice of Vision, 9115
Voice of the Diabetic, 8637
Voice-It, 1638
Voices for Independence, 4439
Voices of Vision Talking Book Center at DuPage Library System, 4750
Volta Review, 8072
Volta Voices, 8077
Volunteer Transcribing Services, 2012
Volunteers of America of Greater New Orlea ns, 4180
Volunteers of America: Western Washington, 1428

W

W GB H Educational Foundation, 6965
W Troy Cole Independent Living Specialist, 4181
WA Department of Services for the Blind, 3833
WAVE Work, Achievement, Value, & Education, 5918
WB Saunders Company, 8745
WCI/Weitbrecht Communications, 498
WCIB Heavy-Duty Folding Cane, 669
WG Hefner VA Medical Center Salisbury, 5715
WGBH Educational Foundation, 8693
WINGS for Learning, 1646, 1652, 1653, 1717, 1723, 1784
WM Keck Foundation, 2795
WP and HB White Foundation, 2899
WW Norton & Company, 5032, 8179
WX: Work Capacities, 6081
WY Department of Health: Mental Health and Substance Abuse Service Division, 3861

Waban Projects, Inc., 1134
Wabash Independent Living Center & Learning Center (WILL), 4108
Wabash/Employability Center, 6011
Waco Regional Office, 5764
Wage and Hour Division of the Employment Standards Administration, 3395
Wagon Road Camp, 1283
Wahiawa Family, 5959
Wakeman/Walworth, 3277
Walden Rehabilitation and Nursing Center, 7322
Walgreens Home Medical Center, 499
Walker Leg Support, 670
WalkerTalker, 248
Walking Alone and Marching Together, 9047
Wallace Memorial Library, 4875
Wallowa Lake Camp, 1335, 8412
Walter Winchell Foundation, 5403
Walton Options for Independent Living, 4036
Walton Options for Independent Living: Nor th Augusta, 4450
Walton Rehabilitation Health System, 6804, 7265
Walton Way Medical, 500
War Memorial Hospital, 7421
Wardrobe Wagon: The Special Needs Clothing Store, 5449
Warner Books, 7711
Warner Robins Rehabilitation and Nursing C enter, 7266
Warp Drive, 149
Warren Achievement Center, 6878
Warren Grant Magnuson Clinical Center, 4796
Warren Memorial Hospital, 7408
Wasatch Valley Rehabilitation, 7405
Wasatch Vision Clinic, 7185
Washable Shoes, 1459
Washington Client Assistance Program, 3834
Washington Connection, 9145
Washington County Disability, Aging and Veteran Services, 3716
Washington County Vocational Workshop, 5987
Washington DC VA Medical Center, 5602
Washington Department of Mental Health, 3835
Washington Developmental Disability, 3836
Washington Ear, 8881
Washington Governor's Committee on Disability Issues & Employment, 3837
Washington Hearing and Speech Society, 3396
Washington Memorial Library, 4726
Washington Office of Superintendent of Public Instruction, 3838
Washington Square Health Foundation, 2900
Washington State Developmental Disabilities Council, 3839
Washington Talking Book and Braille Library, 4936
Washtenaw County Library for the Blind & Physically Handicapped, 4826
Waterproof Bib, 1477
Waterproof Sheet-Topper Mattress and Chair Pad, 197
Waterville Public Library, 4786
Waupaca Elevator Company, 389
Waushers Industries, 7217
Wayne County Regional Educational Service Agency, 1635
Wayne County Regional Library for the Blind, 4827
Wayne State University, 838, 926
Wayne State University: CS Mott Center for Human Genetics and Development, 4828
We Are PHAMALY, 70
We CAN Hear and Speak, 8061
We Can Do it Together!, 9132
We Can Speak for Ourselves: Self Advocacy by Mentally Handicapped People, 5243
We Magazine, 5450
We Media, 5451
We're Not Stupid, 7867
WebABLE, 5452
Webster Enterprises Inc., 6148
Week the World Heard Gallaudet, The, 8062
Weekly Wisdom, 7846
Weiner's Herbal, 5186

Welcome Homes Retirement Community for the Visually Impaired, 7010
Weldon Center for Rehabilitation, 6990
Well Mind Association of Greater Washington, 3397
Wellsouth Health Systems, 7301
Wendell Johnson Speech & Hearing Clinic, 8715
Wendell Johnson Speech And Hearing Clinic, 1113, 7709, 8705, 8899
Wes Test Engineering Corporation, 1820
WesTest Engineering Corporation, 1515
Wesley Woods Camp and Retreat Center, 1114
West Central Illinois Center for Independent Living, 4093
West Central Illinois Center for Independe nt Living: Macomb, 4094
West Central Independent Living Solutions, 4289
West Essex Rehab Center, 6127
West Florida Hospital: The Rehabilitation Institute, 6785
West Florida Regional Library, 4717
West Gables Health Care Center, 6786
West Michigan Learning Disabilities Foundation, 2675
West Palm Beach VA Medical Center, 5608
West Suburban Hospital Medical Center, 6829
West Texas Lighthouse for the Blind, 7183
West Texas VA Healthcare System, 5765
West Virginia Advocates, 3844, 3845
West Virginia Autism Training Center, 4942
West Virginia Client Assistance Program, 3845
West Virginia Department of Aging, 3846
West Virginia Department of Children with Disabilities, 3847
West Virginia Department of Education: Office of Special Education, 2170
West Virginia Department of Health, 3848, 3854
West Virginia Developmental Disabilities Council, 3849
West Virginia Division of Rehabilitation Services, 3850, 6219
West Virginia Employment Services and Job Training Programs Liaison, 6220
West Virginia Library Commission, 4943
West Virginia Research and Training Center, 2625
West Virginia School for the Blind Library, 4944
West Virginia Vocational Rehabilitation, 6221
Westbank Sheltered Workshop, 6036
Westchester Disabled on the Move, 4374
Westchester Independent Living Center, 4375
Westchester Institute for Human Developmen t, 3668
Western Alliance Center for Independent Living, 4382
Western Alliance for Independent Living, 4383
Western Michigan University, 3528
Western NC Conference/United Methodist Church, 1292, 7967
Western New York Foundation, 3090
Western PA United Methodist Church, 1348
Western Psychological Services, 7863
Western Regional Vocational Rehabilitation Facility Clifford File, Jr., 6149
Western Resources for dis-ABLED Independence, 4459
Western Washington University, 2722
Westin Hotels and Resorts, 5512
Westpark Rehabilitation Center, 7293
Westside Center for Independent Living, 3965
Westside Opportunity Workshop, 5876
Westside Parents Work Activity Center, 5988
Westview Nursing and Rehabilitation Center, 7294
Weyerhaeuser Company Foundation, 3242
What About Me? Educational Productions, 5372
What About Me? Growing Up with a Developme ntally Disabled Sibling, 4970
What Do You Do When You See a Blind Person - and What Don't You Do?, 9048
What Everyone Needs to Know About Asthma, 8590
What It's Like to be Me, 4971
What Museum Guides Need to Know: Access for the Blind and Visually Impaired, 9049
What Psychotherapists Should Know about Disabilty, 5292

What School Counselors Need to Know, 2578
What Was That!, 1754
What is Auditory Processing?, 8063
Wheat Ridge Ministries, 2901
Wheel Life News, 687
Wheelchair Accessories, 688
Wheelchair Activity/Computer Table, 569
Wheelchair Aide, 689
Wheelchair Back Pack and Tote Bag, 690
Wheelchair Bowling, 8217
Wheelchair Carrier, 438
Wheelchair Getaways, 5538
Wheelchair Getaways Wheelchair/Scooter Accessible Van Rentals, 5550
Wheelchair Roller, 691
Wheelchair Sports, USA, 8242
Wheelchair Work Table, 692
A Wheelchair for Petronilia, 8211
Wheelchair with Shock Absorbers, 731
WheelchairNet, 5453
Wheelchairs of Kansas, 721
Wheelers Accessible Van Rentals, 150
Wheelers Handicapped Accessible Van Rental s, 5513, 5552
Wheelers Handicapped Accessible Van Rentals, 5496
Wheelers Marauatha Baptist Church, 5551
Wheelin Around, 5496
When Billy Broke His Head...and Other Fanlight Productions/Icarus Films, 5373
When I Grow Up, 5374
When Parents Can't Fix It Fanlight Productions/Icarus Films, 5375
When You Have a Visually Impaired Student in Your Classroom: A Guide for Teachers, 2579
When Your Student Has Arthritis, 8185
When the Brain Goes Wrong, 5187
When the Road Turns: Inspirational Stories About People with MS, 8591
Where to Stay USA, 5497
White Cane and Wheels Fanlight Productions/Icarus Films, 5376
Whittier Trust Company Foundations Office, 2773
Whittier Union High School District, 5839
Whole Person, The, 4290
Whole Person: Kansas City, 4291
Whole Person: Nortonville, 4160
Whole Person: Nortonville, The, 4161
Whole Person: Prairie Village, 4162
Whole Person: Prairie Village, The, 4163
Whole Person: Tonganoxie, 4164
Whoops, 1810
Why My Child, 5377
Why Won't My Child Pay Attention?, 7868
Wichita Public Library, 4771
Wichita Public Library/Talking Book Service, 4771
Wichita Public Library/Talking Book Servic e, 4772
Wilderness Inquiry, 5514, 5539
Wiley, 5277, 5301
Wiley & Sons, 32, 44
Wiley Publishers, 7732, 8722
Wiley Publishing, 4571, 7811, 8730
Wiley-Blackwell, 4976
Wilkes-Barre VA Medical Center, 5744
Will Grundy Center for Independent Living, 4095
Willam G Gilmore Foundation, 2796
Willamette Valley Rehabilitation Center, 7131
William B Dietrich Foundation, 3158
William H Honor Rehabilitation Center Henry Ford Wyanclotte Hospital, 7011
William Hein & Company, 4597, 4606, 4609, 4610, 4621
William J and Dorothy K O'Neill Foundation, 3129
William Jennings Bryan Dorn VA Medical Center, 5749
William Morrow & Company, 8738
William Morrow Paperbacks (HarperCollins), 5253, 5266
William N Pennington Foundation, 3002
William S Hein & Co Inc, 4601
William S Hein & Company, 4645, 4627

William S Middleton Memorial VA Hospital Center, 5786
William Stamps Farish Fund, 3221
William T Grant Foundation, 3091
William Talbott Hillman Foundation, 3159
William V and Catherine A McKinney Charitable Foundation, 3160
Willough at Naples, 6787
Wilmer Ophthalmology Institute, 4787
Wilmington VA Medical Center, 5597
Wilmington Vet Center, 5598
WinSCAN: The Single Switch Interface for PC's with Windows, 1541
Winchester Rehabilitation Center, 7409
Wind River Healthcare and Rehabilitation Center, 7437
Window-Ease, 548
Window-Eyes, 1639
Windsor Estates Health and Rehab Center, 7295
Windsor Mountain American Sign Language Camp Program, 1238
Windsor Mountain International, 1238
Windsor Rehabilitation and Healthcare Cent er, 7244
Winkler Court, 7259
Winston-Salem Industries for the Blind, 7087
Winston-Salem Regional Office, 5716
Winston-Salem Rehabilitation and Healthcar e Center, 7359
Winter Park Memorial Hospital, 6300, 7260
Winthrop Rockefeller Foundation, 2736
Winways at Orange County, 6676
Wiregrass Rehabilitation Center, Inc., 5817
Wisconsin Association of Homes and Service s for the Aging, 7492
Wisconsin Badger Camp, 1440
Wisconsin Board for People with Developmen tal Disabilities (WBPDD), 3855
Wisconsin Bureau of Aging, 3856
Wisconsin Coalition for Advocacy: Madison Office, 3857
Wisconsin Elks/Easter Seals Respite Camp, 1441
Wisconsin Governor's Committee for People with Disabilities, 3858
Wisconsin Lions Camp, 1442, 8413
Wisconsin Lions Foundation, 1442, 8413
Wisconsin Regional Library for the Blind & Physically Handicapped, 4948
Wisconsin VA Regional Office, 5787
Wisconson Badger Camp, 1443
Wise Enterprises, 186, 191, 192
Wishing Wells Collection, 1478, 1481
Without Reason: A Family Copes with two Ge nerations of Autism, 7820, 8765
Wivik 3, 1755
Wolfner Talking Book & Braille Library, 4842
A Woman's Guide to Living with HIV Infecti on, 8425
Women to Women, 934
Women with Attention Deficit Disorder: Embracing Disorganization at Home and Work, 7821
Women with Physical Disabilities: Achievin g & Maintaining Health & Well-Being, 5188
Women with Visible & Invisible Disabilitie es: Multiple Intersections, Issues, Therapies, 5293
Wonderland Camp Foundation, 1221
Woodbine House, 2108, 2377, 2550, 4961, 5242, 5249, 5252, 7742, 7771, 7816, 7998, 8457
Woodcock Reading Mastery Tests, 2657
Woodrow Wilson Rehabilitation Center, 7195
Woodrow Wilson Rehabilitation Center Training Program, 4525
Woodside Day Program, 6718
Woodstock Health and Rehabilitation Center, 7218
WordMaker, 1756
Wordly Wise 3000, 2013
Words+, 1529, 1539, 1542, 1619, 1621, 1622, 1636, 1685, 1715, 1765, 1824
Words+ IST (Infrared, Sound, Touch), 1542
Words+ Inc, 1522
Work Enhancement Center of Western Kentucky, 6031
Work Exploration Center, 5947
Work Inc., 6061

Work Sight, 9050
Work Training Center, 5877
Work and Disability: Contexts, Issues & St rategies for Enhancing Employment Outcomes, 5303
Work in the Context of Disability Culture, 5189
Work!, 2014
Work, Health and Income Among the Elderly, 7523
Work-Related Vocational Assessment Systems : Computer Based, 1818
Workers Compensation Board Alabama, 3320
Workers Compensation Board Illinois, 3461
Workers Compensation Board Iowa, 3477
Workers Compensation Board Louisiana, 3501
Workers Compensation Board Maryland, 3519
Workers Compensation Board Massachusetts, 3527
Workers Compensation Board Missouri, 3572
Workers Compensation Board Nevada, 3603
Workers Compensation Board New Hampshire, 3615
Workers Compensation Board New Mexico, 3636
Workers Compensation Board New York, 3669
Workers Compensation Board North Dakota, 3687
Workers Compensation Board Oklahoma, 3707
Workers Compensation Board Pennsylvania, 3728
Workers Compensation Board Rhode Island, 3740
Workers Compensation Board Vermont, 3820
Workers Compensation Board Washington, 3840
Workers Compensation Board Wisconsin, 3859
Workers Compensation Board Wyoming, 3862
Workers Compensation Board: District of Columbia, 3398
Workers Compensation Board: South Carolina, 3749
Workers Compensation Board: South Dakota, 3758
Workers Compensation Division, 3331
Workers Compensation Division Tennessee, 3768
Workforce and Technology Center, 6959
Working Bibliography on Behavioral and Emotional Disorders, 2580
Working Together & Taking Part, 2015
Working Together with Children and Families: Case Studies, 2581
Working with Visually Impaired Young Students: A Curriculum Guide for 3 to 5 Year Olds, 2582
Workplace Skills: Learning How to Function on the Job, 1819
Workshops, Inc., 5818
Worksight, 6076
World Association of Persons with Disabilities, 5454
A World Awaits You, 4992, 5486, 8201
World Chiropractic Alliance, 7886, 8158
World Experience Teenage Exchange Program, 2723
World Institute on Disability, 935, 2281, 2434, 2570, 5109, 5153, 5180, 5182
World Research Foundation, 4661
World Through Their Eyes, 9051
World of Options, 2724
Worldwide Mobility Products, 86
Worst Loss: How Families Heal from the Death of a Child, 5270

Worthmore Academy, 2691
Wright-Way, 144
Write: Out Loud, 1757
Write: OutLoud, 1826
Writer's Showcase Press, 5075
Wyman Center, 1218, 8380, 8392
Wyoming Client Assistance Program, 3863
Wyoming Department of Aging, 3864
Wyoming Department of Education, 2171, 4949
Wyoming Department of Employment Unemployment Insurance, 6225
Wyoming Department of Workforce Services, 6223
Wyoming Developmental Disability Council, 3865
Wyoming Governor's Committee on Employment of the Handicapped, 6226
Wyoming Protection & Advocacy for Persons with Disabilities, 3866
Wyoming Services for Independent Living, 4554
Wyoming Services for the Visually Impaired, 4949
Wyoming's New Options in Technology (WYNOT) - University of Wyoming, 4950
Wyoming/Colorado VA Regional Office, 5791

X

XL Steering, 151
Xavier Society for the Blind, 4876

Y

Y Camp, 1115, 8414
YAI: National Institute for People with Disabilities, 936
YMCA, 1000, 7692, 8712
YMCA Camp Burgess & Hayward, 1180
YMCA Camp Chandler, 945, 8374
YMCA Camp Chingachgook on Lake George, 1284, 8900
YMCA Camp Copneconic, 1197
YMCA Camp Duncan, 1082
YMCA Camp Erdman, 1060
YMCA Camp Fitch, 1360, 7980, 8165, 8415, 8716
YMCA Camp Glacier Hollow, 1439, 7707
YMCA Camp Horseshoe, 1433, 8416
YMCA Camp Ihduhapi, 1207, 8417
YMCA Camp Jewell, 1028
YMCA Camp Kitaki, 1231, 8418
YMCA Camp Orkila, 1431, 8419
YMCA Camp Shady Brook, 1020, 8420
YMCA Camp Weona, 1285, 8421
YMCA Camp jewell, 8422
YMCA Camp of Maine, 1145, 8423
YMCA Camping Services, 1188, 7667
YMCA Of Honolulu, 1060
YMCA Of Southern Arizona, 958
The YMCA Of Youngstown - Metro Office, 8415, 8716
YMCA Outdoor Center Campbell Gard, 1319, 8424
YMCA of Greater Buffalo, 1285, 8421
YMCA of Greater Des Moines, 1115, 8414
YMCA of Greater Hartford, 1028, 8422

YMCA of Greater Oklahoma City, 1320, 8328
YMCA of Greater Seattle, 1431, 8419
YMCA of Southern Arizona, 7708
YMCA of the Pikes Peak Region (PPYMCA), 1020, 8420
The YMCA's Camp Fitch On Lake Erie, 1360
The YMCA's Camp Fitch on Lake Erie, 7980
YWCA Camp Westwind, 1336, 7981
YWCA of Greater Portland, 1336, 7981
Yale New Haven Health System-Bridgeport Hospital, 6708
Yale University Press, 8556
Yale University: Vision Research Center, 4692
Yavapai Regional Medical Center-West, 5827
Yoga for Arthritis, 8218
Yoga for Fibromyalgia: Move, Breathe, and Relax to Improve Your Quality of Life, 8186
Yoga for MS and Related Conditions, 8219
You May Be Able to Adopt, 5244
You Mean I'm Not Lazy, Stupid or Crazy?!: A Self-Help Book for Adults with ADD, 7822
You Seem Like a Regular Kid to Me, 9052
You Tell Me: Learning Basic Information, 1758
You Will Dream New Dreams, 5245
You and Your ADD Child, 7823
You and Your Deaf Child: A Self-Help Guide for Parents of Deaf and Hard of Hearing Children, 8064
Young Adult Deaf Camp, 1162
Young Children with Special Needs: A Developmentally Appropriate Approach, 2658
Young Onset Parkinson Conference, 1876
Young Person's Guide to Spina Bifida, 8592
Younger Onset Dementia Association, 7657
Youngstown Foundation, 3130
Youngstown YMCA, 8165
Younker Rehabilitation Center of Iowa Methodist Medical Center, 6335
Your Child Has a Disability: A Complete So urcebook of Daily and Medical Care, 5246
Your Child and Asthma, 8593
Your Child in the Hospital: A Practical Guide for Parents (3rd Edition), 5254
Your Cleft Affected Child, 8594
Your Guide to Bowel Cancer, 8595
Youth Leadership Camp, 1163, 7982
Youth for Understanding International Exchange, 2725
Youville Hospital & Rehab Center, 6991
Yuma Center for the Visually Impaired, 6533
Yuma County Workshop, 5892

Z

ZoomText, 1628
Zygo-Usa Svc Corporation, 1623

Alabama

ADA Teen Adventure Camp, 937
ADA Triangle D Camp, 938
ADRS Lakeshore, 5792
Alabama Goodwill Industries, 5793
Alabama Institute for Deaf and Blind Library and Resource Center, 4646
Alabama Power Foundation, 2726
Alabama Radio Reading Service Network (ARRS), 4647
Alabama Regional Library for the Blind and Physically Handicapped, 4648
Alabama VA Benefits Regional Office - Montgomery, 5562
Alabama VA Medical Center - Birmingham, 5563
Andalusia Health Services, 2727
Arc Of Alabama, The, 2728
Arc of Jefferson County, 5794
Birdie Thornton Center, 3867
Camp Evoked Potential @ Camp ASCCA, 939
Camp Merrimack, 940
Camp Rap-A-Hope, 941
Camp Seale Harris, 942
Camp Shocco for the Deaf, 943
Camp Smile-A-Mile, 944
Camp WheezeAway, 945
Central Alabama Veterans Healthcare System, 5564
Coffee County Training Center, 5795
Dothan Houston County Library System, 4649
Easter Seals Camp ASCCA, 946
Easter Seals: Achievement Center, 5796
Easter Seals: Opportunity Center, 5797
Huntsville Subregional Library for the Blind & Physically Handicapped, 4650
Independent Living Center of Mobile, 3868
Independent Living Resources Of Greater Birmingham: Alabaster, 3869
Independent Living Resources of Greater Birmingham: Jasper, 3870
Independent Living Resources of Greater Birmingham, 3871
Montgomery Career Center: Alabama Employment Services Division, 5798
Montgomery Center for Independent Living, 3872
Public Library Of Anniston-Calhoun County, 4651
Technology Assistance for Special Consumers, 4652
Tuscaloosa VA Medical Center, 5565
Vocational Rehabilitation Service - Opelika, 5799
Vocational Rehabilitation Service - Dothan, 5800
Vocational Rehabilitation Service - Homewood, 5801
Vocational Rehabilitation Service - Huntsville, 5802
Vocational Rehabilitation Service - Jackson, 5803
Vocational Rehabilitation Service - Jasper, 5804
Vocational Rehabilitation Service - Mobile, 5805
Vocational Rehabilitation Service - Muscle Shoals, 5806
Vocational Rehabilitation Service - Selma, 5807
Vocational Rehabilitation Service - Tallad ega, 5808
Vocational Rehabilitation Service - Troy, 5809
Vocational Rehabilitation Service - Tuscaloosa, 5810
Vocational Rehabilitation Service- Gadsden, 5811
Vocational Rehabilitation Service: Scottsboro, 5812
Vocational Rehabilitation Services - Andalusia, 5813
Vocational Rehabilitation Services - Anniston, 5814
Vocational and Rehabilitation Service - Decatur, 5815
Vocational and Rehabilitation Services - Montgomery, 5816
Wiregrass Rehabilitation Center, Inc., 5817
Workshops, Inc., 5818

Alaska

ADA Camp Kushtaka, 947
Access Alaska: ADA Partners Project, 3873
Access Alaska: Fairbanks, 3874
Access Alaska: Mat-Su, 3875
Alaska Division of Vocational Rehabilitation, 5819
Alaska Fair Employment Practice Agency, 5820
Alaska Job Center Network, 5821
Alaska SILC, 3876
Alaska State Library Talking Book Center, 4653
Alaska VA Healthcare System - Anchorage, 5566
Arc of Alaska, 2729
Arctic Access, 3877
Camp Alpine, 948
Camp Birchwood, 949
DAV Department of Alaska, 5567
Hope Community Resources, 3878
Kenai Peninsula Independent Living Center, 3879
Kenai Peninsula Independent Living Center: Seward, 3880
Keni Peninsula Independent Living Center: Central Peninsula, 3881
Rasmuson Foundation, 2730
Southeast Alaska Independent Living, 3882
Southeast Alaska Independent Living: Ketch ikan, 3883
Southeast Alaska Independent Living: Sitka, 3884
Veteran Benefits Administration Anchorage Regional Office, 5568

Arizona

ASSIST! to Independence, 3885
American Foundation Corporation, 3105
Arizona Autism Resources, 2731
Arizona Braille and Talking Book Library Arizona State Library, 4654
Arizona Bridge to Independent Living, 3886
Arizona Bridge to Independent Living: Phoenix, 3887
Arizona Bridge to Independent Living: Mesa, 3888
Arizona Camp Sunrise, 950
Arizona Community Foundation, 2732
Arizona Instructional Resource Center for Students who are Blind or Visually Impaired, The, 2733
Bonnie Prudden Myotherapy, 807
Books for the Blind of Arizona, 4655
CARF Rehabilitation Accreditation Commission, 810
Camp Abilities Tucson, 951
Camp Candlelight, 952
Camp Civitan, 953
Camp Honor, 954
Camp Not-A-Wheeze, 955
Camp Rainbow, 956
Carl T Hayden VA Medical Center, 5569
Children's Center for Neurodevelopmental Studies, 4656
Community Outreach Program for the Deaf, 3889
DIRECT Center for Independence, 3890
Downtown Neighborhood Learning Center, 5822
Fair Employment Practice Agency: Arizona, 5823
Flagstaff City-Coconino County Public Library, 4657
Fountain Hills Lioness Braille Service, 4658
International Association of Yoga Therapists, 862
JOBS Administration Job Opportunities & Basic Skills, 5824
Lions Camp Tatiyee, 957
Margaret T Morris Foundation, 2734
Native American Protection and Advocacy, 906
New Horizons Independent Living Center: Prescott Valley, 3891
Northern Arizona VA Health Care System, 5570
Prescott Public Library, 4659
Services Maximizing Independent Living and Empowerment (SMILE), 3892
Southern Arizona VA Healthcare System, 5571
Special Needs Center/Phoenix Public Library, 4660
Sterling Ranch: Residence for Special Women, 3893
TETRA Services, 5825

Triangle Y Ranch YMCA, 958
Vocational and Rehabilitation Agency Rehabilitation Services Administrations, 5826
Wheelers Handicapped Accessible Van Rental s, 5552
Wheelers Marauatha Baptist Church, 5551
World Research Foundation, 4661
Yavapai Regional Medical Center-West, 5827

Arkansas

Arc of Arkansas, 2735
Arkansas Employment Service Agency and Job Training Program, 5828
Arkansas Independent Living Council, 3894
Arkansas Regional Library for the Blind and Physically Handicapped, 4662
Arkansas School for the Blind, 4663
Association of Disability Advocates, The, 800
Camp Aldersgate, 959
Camp Funshine, 960
Camp Kota, 961
Camp Quality Arkansas, 962
Case Management Society of America, 814
Delta Resource Center for Independent Living, 3895
Easter Seal Work Center, 5829
Educational Services for the Visually Impaired, 4664
Eugene J Towbin Healthcare Center, 5572
John L McClellan Memorial Hospital, 5574
Library for the Blind and Physically Handicapped SW Region of Arkansas, 4665
North Little Rock Regional Office, 5575
Northwest Ozarks Regional Library for the Blind and Handicapped, 4666
Sources for Community IL Services, 3898
Spa Area Independent Living Services, 3899
VCT/A Job Retention Skill Training Program, 5830
Vocational and Rehabilitation Agency Division of Services for the Blind, 5831
Vocational and Rehabilitation Agency for Persons Who Are Visually Impaired, 5832
Winthrop Rockefeller Foundation, 2736

California

AAO Annual Meeting, 1830
ABLE Industries, 5833
ARC-Adult Vocational Program, 5834
ASCCA, 963
Abilities Expo, 1842
Ability 1st, 3998
AbilityFirst, 5835
Access Center of San Diego, 3900
Access to Independence, 3901
Access to Independence of Imperial Valley, 3902
Access to Independence of North County, 3903
Achievement House & NCI Affiliates, 5836
Acupressure Institute, 763
Ahmanson Foundation, 2737
Alice Tweed Touhy Foundation, 2738
Anglo California Travel Service, 5519
Arc of California, 2740
Atkinson Foundation, 2741
Baker Commodities Corporate Giving Program, 2742
Bakersfield ARC, 5837
Balance Centers of America, 5993
Bank of America Foundation, 2743
Bearskin Meadow Camp, 964
Beaumont Senior Center: Community Access Center, 3904
Blind Babies Foundation, 2744
Blind Childrens Center Annual Meeting, 1851
Bothin Foundation, 2745
Braille Institute Library, 4667
Braille Institute Santa Barbara Center, 4668
Braille Institute Sight Center, 4669
Braille and Talking Book Library: California, 4670
Briggs Foundation, 2746
Burns-Dunphy Foundation, 2747

California Community Foundation, 2748
California Department of Fair Employment & Housing, 5838
California Endowment, 2749
California Foundation For Independent Living Centers, 3905
California Foundation for Independent Living Centers, 3906
California State Independent Living Counci l (SILC), 3907
California State Library Braille and Talking Book Library, 4671
Camp Beyond The Scars, 965
Camp Bloomfield, 966
Camp Christian Berets, 967
Camp Coelho, 968
Camp Conrad-Chinnock, 969
Camp Costanoan, 970
Camp Del Corazon, 971
Camp Firefly, 972
Camp Forrest, 973
Camp Grizzly, 974
Camp Krem, 976
Camp Okizu, 977
Camp Pacifica, Inc., 978
Camp Paivika, 979
Camp Quest, 980
Camp Ramah In California, 981
Camp ReCreation, 982
Camp Reach for the Sky, 983
Camp Ronald McDonald for Good Times, 984
Camp Ronald McDonald® at Eagle Lake, 985
Camp Rubber Soul, 986
Camp Sunburst, 987
Camp Sunshine Dreams, 988
Camp Taylor, Inc., 989
Camp Trinity, 990
Camp-A-Lot And Leisure Express (PALS Program), 991
Camping Unlimited, 992
Camping Unlimited-Camp Krem, 993
Canine Companions for Independence, 811
Career Connection Transition Program, 5839
Career Development Program (CDP), 5840
Carrie Estelle Doheny Foundation, 2750
Center for Independence of the Disabled, 3908
Center for Independence of the Disabled- Daly City, 3909
Center for Independent Living, 3910
Center for Independent Living: East Oakland, 3911
Center for Independent Living: Oakland, 3912
Center for Independent Living: Tri-County, 3913
Center for Independent Living:Fresno, 3914
Center for Independent Living; Oakland, 3915
Center of Independent Living: Visalia, 3916
Central Coast Center for IL: San Benito, 3917
Central Coast Center for Independent Living, 3918
Central Coast Center: Independent Living - Santa Cruz Office, 3919
Central Coast for Independent Living, 3920
Central Coast for Independent Living: Watsonville, 3921
Clearinghouse for Specialized Media and Translations, 4672
Coeta and Donald Barker Foundation, 2751
College Student's Guide to Merit and Other No-Need Funding, 3261
Colton-Redlands-Yucaipa Regional Occupational Programs, 5841
Communities Actively Living Independent and Free, 3922
Community Access Center, 3923
Community Access Center: Indio Branch, 3924
Community Access Center: Perris, 3925
Community Outpatient Rehabilitation Center, 5842
Community Rehabilitation Services, 3926
Community Resources for Independence: Mendocino/Lake Branch, 3927
Community Resources for Independence: Napa, 3928
Community Resources for Independent Living: Hayward, 3929
Community Resources for Independent Living, 3930

Conrad N Hilton Foundation, 2999
Crescent Porter Hale Foundation, 2752
Cunard Line, 5520
DRAIL (Disability Resource Agency for Independent Living), 3931
David and Lucile Packard Foundation, 2753
Dayle McIntosh Center: Laguna Niguel, 3932
Deaf Kid's Kamp, 994
Desert Haven Enterprises, 5843
Deutsch Foundation, 2754
Directory of Financial Aids for Women, 3263
Disability Resource Agency for Independent Living: Modesto, 3933
Disability Services & Legal Center, 3934
Disabled Businesspersons Association, 833
Disabled Resources Center, 3935
Dream Street Camp, 995
ESS Work Center, 5844
East Bay Community Foundation, 2755
Easter Seals Camp Harmon, 996
Employment Service: California, 5845
Enchanted Hills Camp for the Blind, 997
Environmental Traveling Companions, 5526
Esalen Institute, 841
Evelyn and Walter Hans Jr Haas Jr, 2756
FREED Center for Independent Living, 3936
FREED Center for Independent Living: Marys ville, 3937
Family Caregiver Alliance, 2757
Feather River Industries, 5846
Financial Aid for Asian Americans, 3267
Financial Aid for Hispanic Americans, 3268
Financial Aid for Native Americans, 3269
Financial Aid for Research and Creative Ac tivities Abroad, 3270
Financial Aid for Veterans, Military Personnel and their Dependents, 3271
Financial Aid for the Disabled and Their F amilies, 2758, 3272
Firefighters Kids Camp, 998
Firemans Fund Foundation, 2759
First Step Independent Living, 3938
Fit to Work, 5847
Fred Gellert Foundation, 2760
Fresno City College: Disabled Students Programs and Services, 5848
Fresno County Free Library Blind and Handicapped Services, 4674
Gallo Foundation, 2761
Glaucoma Research Foundation, 2762, 4675
Harden Foundation, 2763
Health Action, 855
Heartland Opportunity Center, 5849
Henry J Kaiser Family Foundation, 2764
Henry W Bull Foundation, 2765
Herrick Health Sciences Library, 4676
High School Senior's Guide to Merit and Ot her No-Need Funding, 3281
Hollister Workshop, 5850
Homeopathic Educational Services, 857
How to Pay for Your Degree in Business & Related Fields, 3282
How to Pay for Your Degree in Education & Related Fields, 3283
Independent Living Center of Kern County, 3939
Independent Living Center of Lancaster, 3940
Independent Living Resource Center: Santa Barbara, 3942
Independent Living Resource Center: San Fr ancisco, 3943
Independent Living Resource Center: Santa Maria Office, 3944
Independent Living Resource Center: Ventur a, 3945
Independent Living Resource of Contra Coast, 3946
Independent Living Resource of Fairfield, 3947
Independent Living Resource: Antioch, 3948
Independent Living Resource: Concord, 3949
Independent Living Resources (ILR), 3950
Independent Living Service Northern California: Redding Office, 3951
Independent Living Services of Northern California, 3952

Institute of Transpersonal Psychology, 860
Irvine Health Foundation, 2766
Jerry L Pettis Memorial VA Medical Center, 5576
Job Training Program Liaison: California, 5851
Joni and Friends, 868
Joseph Drown Foundation, 2767
Junior Blind of America, 2768
Kenneth T and Eileen L Norris Foundation, 2769
King's Rehabilitation Center, 5852
Koret Foundation, 2770
Kuzell Institute for Arthritis and Infectious Diseases, 4677
LA84 Foundation, 2771
LJ Skaggs and Mary C Skaggs Foundation, 2772
LK Whittier Foundation, 2773
Legler Benbough Foundation, 2774
Levi Strauss Foundation, 2775
Lions Wilderness Camp for Deaf Children, Inc., 999
Long Beach VA Medical Center, 5577
Los Angeles Regional Office, 5578
Louis R Lurie Foundation, 2776
Luke B Hancock Foundation, 2777
Marin Center for Independent Living, 3953
Marin Community Foundation, 2778
Martinez Outpatient Clinic, 5579
Mary A Crocker Trust, 2779
MedicAlert Foundation International, 5455
Morongo Basin Work Activity Center, 5853
Mother Lode Independent Living Center (DRAIL: Disability Resource Agency for Independent, 3954
Mother Lode Rehabilitation Enterprises, 5854
Napa Valley PSI Inc., 5855
National Center on Caregiving at Family Caregiver Alliance (FCA), 2780
National Foundation of Wheelchair Tennis, 2781
New Beginnings: The Blind Children's Center, 4678
New Directions For People With Disabilitie s, Inc., 5532
New Directions for People with Disabilities, 2714
New Horizons Summer Day Camp, 1000
Oakland VA Regional Office, 5580
Oakland Work Activity Area, 5856
Orange County ARC, 5858
Our Way: The Cottage Apt Homes, 3897
PRIDE Industries, 5859
PWI Profile, 6052
Pacific Institute of Aromatherapy, 913
Painted Turtle, The, 1001
Parents Helping Parents (PHP), 915
Parents and Friends, Inc, 5860
Parker Foundation, 2782
Pasadena Foundation, 2783
PathPoint, 5861
People Services, Inc, 5862
Pilgrim Pines Camp & Conference Center, 1002
Placer Independent Resource Services, 3955
Pomona Valley Workshop, 5863
Porterville Sheltered Workshop, 5864
Project Independence, 5865
Quan Yin Healing Arts Center, 920
Quest Camp, 1003
RC Baker Foundation, 2784
Ralph M Parsons Foundation, 2785
Regional Assessment and Training Center, 5889
Research & Training Center on Mental Health for Hard of Hearing Persons, 4679
Robert Ellis Simon Foundation, 2786
Rolling Start, 3957
Rolling Start: Victorville, 3958
Rosalind Russell Medical Research Center for Arthritis, 4680
Sacramento Medical Center, 5582
Sacramento Vocational Services, 5866
San Diego VA Regional Office, 5583
San Francisco Foundation, 2787
San Francisco Public Library for the Blind and Print Handicapped, 4681
San Francisco Vocational Services, 5867
San Jose State University Library, 4682
Santa Barbara Foundation, 2788
Services Center For Independent Living, 3959

Shasta County Opportunity Center, 5868
Sidney Stern Memorial Trust, 2789
Sierra Health Foundation, 2790
Silicon Valley Community Foundation, 2791
Silicon Valley Independent Living Center, 3960
Silicon Valley Independent Living Center: South
County Branch, 3961
Social Vocational Services, 5869
Sonora Area Foundation, 2792
South Bay Vocational Center, 5870
Southern California Rehabilitation Service s, 3962
Special Camp For Special Kids, 1004
Stella B Gross Charitable Trust C/O Bank of The
West Trust Department, 2793
Teichert Foundation, 2794
Through the Looking Glass, 3963
Tri-County Independent Living Center, 3964,
4495, 5871, 5871
Tuolumne Trails, 1005
US Healthworks, 6173
Unyeway, 5872
V-Bar Enterprises, 5873
VA Central California Health Care System, 5584
VA Greater Los Angeles Healthcare System, 5585
VA Northern California Healthcare System, 5586
VA San Diego Healthcare System, 5587
Valley Light Industries, 5874
Visalia Workshop, 5875
WM Keck Foundation, 2795
Westside Center for Independent Living, 3965
Westside Opportunity Workshop, 5876
Willam G Gilmore Foundation, 2796
Work Training Center, 5877
World Experience Teenage Exchange Program,
2723
World Institute on Disability, 935

Canada

Child and Parent Resource Institute, 820
Clay Tree Society, 823
Haldimand-Norfolk Resource Education and C
ounseling, 854
Lambton County Developmental Services, 870
LoSeCa Foundation, 874
MCC Supportive Care Services, 875
North Hastings Community Integration Assoc
iation, 909
People First of Canada, 916
St. Paul Abilities Network, 925

Colorado

AMC Cancer Research Center, 4683
AV Hunter Trust, 2797
Adam's Camp, 1006
Adolph Coors Foundation, 2798
American Society of Bariatric Physicians, 794
American Universities International Programs,
2694
Arc of Colorado, 2799
Aspen Camp of the Deaf & Hard of Hearing, 1007
Association for Applied Psychophysiology and
Biofeedback, 796
Atlantis Community, 3966
Blue Peaks Developmental Services, 5878
Bonfils-Stanton Foundation, 2800
Boulder Public Library, 4684
Boulder Vet Center, 5588
Breckenridge Outdoor Education Center, 1008
CNI Cochlear Kids Camp, 1009
Camp Paha Rise Above, 1010
Camp Rocky Mountain Village, 1011
Camp Wapiyapi, 1012
Center for Independence, 3967
Center for People with Disabilities, 3968
Center for People with Disabilities: Pueblo, 3969
Center for People with Disabilities: Bould er, 3970
Challenge Aspen, 1013
Champ Camp, 1014
Cheley/Children's Hospital Burn Camps Program,
1015
Cheyenne Village, 5879

Colorado Civil Rights Divsion, 5880
Colorado Employment Service, 5881
Colorado Lions Camp, 1016
Colorado Springs Independence Center, 3971
Colorado Talking Book Library, 4685
Colorado/Wyoming VA Medical Center, 5589
Comprecare Foundation, 2801
Connections for Independent Living, 3972
Denver CIL, 3973
Denver Foundation, 2802
Denver VA Medical Center, 5590
Disability Center for Independent Living, 3974
Disabled Resource Services, 3975
Disbled Resource Services, 3976
Dvorak Expeditions, 5525
El Pomar Foundation, 2803
First Descents, 1017
Grand Junction VA Medical Center, 5591
Gray Street Workcenter, 5884
Greeley Center for Independence, 3977
Helen K and Arthur E Johnson Foundation, 2804
Hope Center, 5885
Imagine: Innovative Resources for Cognitive &
Physical Challenges, 5886
Independent Life Center, 3978
Invisible Disabilities Association, 866
Las Animas County Rehabilitation Center, 5887
Mainstream, 876, 3896, 6047, 6047
NORESCO Workshop, 5888
National Association of Blind Merchants, 883
National Jewish Medical & Research Center, 4686
North America Riding for the Handicapped
Association, 908
PEAK Parent Center, 912
Rocky Mountain Village, 1018
Rolf Institute, 923
Roundup River Ranch, 1019
Southwest Center for Independence, 3980
Southwest Center for Independence: Cortez, 3981
Wyoming/Colorado VA Regional Office, 5791
YMCA Camp Shady Brook, 1020
Yuma County Workshop, 5892

Connecticut

Abilities Without Boundaries, 5893
Aetna Foundation, 2805
Allied Community Services, 5894
American Institute for Foreign Study, 2693
Arc of Connecticut, 2806
Area Cooperative Educational Services (ACES),
5895
Arthur C. Luf Children's Burn Camp, 1021
CW Resources, 5896
Camp Harkness, 1022
Camp Hemlocks, 1023
Camp Horizons, 1024
Camp Isola Bella, 1025
Center for Disability Rights, 3982
Center for Independent Living SC, 3983
Central Connecticut Association For Retarded
Citizens, 5897
Chapel Haven, 3984
Community Foundation of Southeastern
Connecticut, 2807
Connecticut Braille Association, 4687
Connecticut Governor's Committee on
Employment of People With Disabilities, 5899
Connecticut Library for the Blind and Phys ically
Handicapped, 4688
Connecticut Mutual Life Foundation, 2808
Connecticut State Library, 4689
Connecticut Tech Act Project: Connecticut
Department of Social Services, 4690
Cornelia de Lange Syndrome Foundation, 2809
Disabilities Network of Eastern Connecticu t, 3985
Disability Resource Center of Fairfield County,
3986
Favarh/Farmington Valley ARC, 844
Fidelco Guide Dog Foundation, 2810
Focus Alternative Learning Center, 850
Fotheringhay Farms, 5900
GE Foundation, 2811
George Hegyi Industrial Training Center, 5901

Hartford Foundation for Public Giving, 2812
Hartford Insurance Group, 2813
Hartford Regional Office, 5592
Hartford Vet Center, 5593
Henry Nias Foundation, 2814
Hole in the Wall Gang Camp, 1026
Independence Northwest Center for Independent
Living, 3987
Independence Unlimited, 3988
Jane Coffin Childs Memorial Fund for Medical
Research, 2815
Kennedy Center, 5902
Marvelwood Summer, 1027
New Horizons Village, 3989
Prevent Blindness Connecticut, 4691
Quaezar, 5903
Rich Foundation, 2856
Scheuer Associates Foundation, 2817
VA Connecticut Healthcare System: Newington
Division, 5594
VA Connecticut Healthcare System: West Haven,
5595
Valley Memorial Health Center, 5904
YMCA Camp Jewell, 1028
Yale University: Vision Research Center, 4692

Delaware

Arc of Delaware, 2819
Arc of Utah, 3222
Camp Fairlee Manor, 1029, 1147
Camp Manito/Camp Lenape, 1030
Childrens Beach House, 1031
Delaware Assistive Technology Initiative (DATI),
4693
Delaware Division of Vocational Rehabilita tion,
5907
Delaware Fair Employment Practice Agency, 5908
Delaware Job Training Program Liaison, 5909
Delaware Library for the Blind and Physically
Handicapped, 4694
Delaware VA Regional Office, 5596
Freedom Center for Independent Living, 3990
Independent Resource Georgetown, 3992
Independent Resources: Dover, 3993
Independent Resources: Wilmington, 3994
Longwood Foundation, 2820
Sandcastle Day Camp, 1032
Service Source, 5910
Wilmington VA Medical Center, 5597
Wilmington Vet Center, 5598

District of Columbia

AAIDD Annual Meeting, 1829
AG Bell Convention, 1836
Alexander and Margaret Stewart Trust, 2821
American Association of Oriental Medicine, 772
American Association of People with Disabilities,
773
American Public Health Association, 790
American Red Cross, 791
American The Beautiful; National Parks & Federal
Recreation Lands, 5518
Annual TASH Conference, The, 1846
Arc National Convention, The, 1847
Arc of the District of Columbia, 2822
Association for Persons with Severe Handicaps
(TASH), 798
Believable Hope Conference, 1849
Blinded Veterans Association National
Convention, 1852
Center for Mind/Body Studies, 817
Change, 819
Children's National Medical Center, 822
Chronicle Guide to Grants, 3260
Columbia Lighthouse for the Blind Summer Camp,
1033
DAV National Service Headquarters, 5553
Department of Medicine and Surgery Veterans
Administration, 5554
Department of Veterans Benefits, 5556

Disabled American Veterans, National Service & Legislative Headquarters, 5599
District of Columbia Center for Independen t Living, 3996
District of Columbia Department of Employment Services, 5911
District of Columbia Dept. of Employment Services: Office of Workforce Development, 5912
District of Columbia Fair Employment Practice Agencies, 5913
District of Columbia Public Library: Services for the Deaf Community, 4696
District of Columbia Regional Library for the Blind and Physically Handicapped, 4697
Eugene and Agnes E Meyer Foundation, 2823
Eye Bank Association of America Annual Meeting, 1857
Federal Benefits for Veterans and Dependents, 5558
Federal Student Aid Information Center, 2824
GEICO Philanthropic Foundation, 2825
George Washington University Health Resource Center, 851
Georgetown University Center for Child and Human Development, 4698
Goodwill of Greater Washington, 5914
Green Door, 5915
Guide Service of Washington, 5528
Jacob and Charlotte Lehrman Foundation, 2826
Joseph P Kennedy Jr Foundation, 2828
Kiplinger Foundation, 2829
Lab School of Washington, 1034
Montgomery County Arc, 3187
Morris and Gwendolyn Cafritz Foundation, 2830
NACDD Annual Conference, 1861
NADR Conference, 1863
NASPAC Annual Conference Association Annual Convention/Expo, 1864
National Association of Councils on Develo pmental Disabilities, 884
National Association of Developmental Disabilities Councils, 885
National Association of Disability Represe ntatives, 886
National Center for Education in Maternal and Child Health, 889
National Council on Disability, 891
National Council on Independent Living, 892, 3997
National Council on the Aging Conference, 1866
National Deaf Education Network and Clearinghouse/Info To Go, 893
National Disability Rights Network, 894
National Institute on Disability and Rehabilitation Research, 900, 4699
National Women's Health Network, 905
Operation Job Match, 5916
PVA Sports and Recreation Program, 5600
PVA Summit & Expo, 1867
Paul and Annetta Himmelfarb Foundation, 2831
President's Committee on Employment of Employment of the Disabled, 5981
Public Technology, 5548
Public Welfare Foundation, 2832
Rehabilitation Research and Development Center, 5581
Rehabilitation Services Administration, 5917
Sister Cities International, 2718
Small Business Development Center, 6067
Student Guide, 3286
Teacher Preparation and Special Education, 927
US Department of Veterans Affairs National Headquarters, 5560
US Veteran's Affairs, 5561
Utah Vocational Rehabilitation Agency, 6199
VA Medical Center, Washington DC, 5601
WAVE Work, Achievement, Value, & Education, 5918
Washington DC VA Medical Center, 5602

Florida

Abilities of Florida: An Affiliate of Service Source, 5919
Able Trust, 2833
Able Trust, The, 5920
Adult Day Training, 3999
Advocacy Center for Persons with Disabilit ites, 765
Alpha One: Bangar, 4182
American Disabled Golfers Association, 784
Arc of Florida, 2834
Bank of America Client Foundation, 2835
Barron Collier Jr Foundation, 2836
Bay Pines VA Medical Center, 5603
Birth Defect Research for Children, 806
Blazing Toward a Cure Annual Conference, 1850
Brevard County Talking Books Library, 4700
Broward County Talking Book Library, 4701
CIL of Central Florida, 4000
Camiccia-Arnautou Charitable Foundation, 2837
Camp Amigo Burn Camp, 1035
Camp Boggy Creek, 1036
Camp Thunderbird, 1038
Career Assessment & Planning Services, 5921
Caring and Sharing Center for Independent Living, 4001
Caring and Sharing Center: Pasco County, 4002
Center Academy at Pinellas Park, 1039
Center for Independent Living in Central Florida, 4003
Center for Independent Living of Broward, 4004
Center for Independent Living of Florida Keys, 4005
Center for Independent Living of N Florida, 4006
Center for Independent Living of NW Florid a, 4007
Center for Independent Living of North Central Florida, 4008
Center for Independent Living of North Cen tral Florida, 4009
Center for Independent Living of S Florida, 4010
Center for Independent Living of SW Florida, 4011
Chatlos Foundation, 2838
Chiles Foundation, 3134
Choices to Work Program, 5922
Coalition for Independent Living Options: Fort Pierce, 4013
Coalition for Independent Living Options, 4014
Coalition for Independent Living Options: Stuart, 4015
Coalition for Independent Living Options: Okeechobee, 4012
Consulting & Engineering for the Handicapp ed (CEH), 5543
Dade County Talking Book Library, 4702
Dialysis at Sea Cruises, 5523
Disabled Drummers Association, 835
Dream Oaks Camp, 1040
Edyth Bush Charitable Foundation, 2839
Enable America Inc., 840
FPL Group Foundation, 2840
Federal Grants & Contracts Weekly, 3266
Florida Diabetes Camp, 1041
Florida Division of Blind Services, 4703
Florida Division of Vocational Rehabilitation, 5923
Florida Fair Employment Practice Agency, 5924
Florida Instructional Materials Center for the Visually Impaired (FIMC-VI), 4704
Florida Lions Camp, 1042
Florida Sheriffs Caruth Camp, 1043
Foundation & Corporate Grants Alert, 3273
Gainesville Division, North Florida/South Georgia Veterans Healthcare System, 5604
Goodwill Industries-Suncoast Adult Day Training, 5925
Goodwill Industries-Suncoast Inc. Adult Day Training, 5926
Goodwill Industries-Suncoast Inc. Adult Day Training, 5927
Goodwill Industries-Suncoast Non-Residenti al Supports And Services Program, 5928
Goodwill Industries-Suncoast Supported Living, 5929

Goodwill Industries-Suncoast,Adult Day Training, 5930
Goodwill Temporary Staffing, 5931
Hands To Love, 1044
Hillsborough County Talking Book Library Tampa-Hillsborough County Public Library, 4705
Impact: Ocala Vocational Services, 5932
Jacksonville Public Library: Talking Books /Special Needs, 4706
James A Haley VA Medical Center, 5605
Jefferson Lee Ford III Memorial Foundation, 2841
Jessie Ball duPont Fund, 2842
JobWorks NISH Food Service, 5933
JobWorks NISH Postal Service, 5934
Kris' Camp, 1045
Lakeland Adult Day Training, 4017
Lee County Library System: Talking Books Library, 4707
Lighthouse Central Florida, 4018, 5935
Lost Tree Village Charitable Foundation, 2843
Louis de la Parte Florida Mental Health Institute Research Library, 4708
MAClown Vocational Rehabilitation Workshop, 5936
Miami Foundation, The, 2844
Miami VA Medical Center, 5606
Miami-Dade County Disability Services and Independent Living (DSAIL), 4019
Mount Sinai Medical Center, 3070
National Car Rental System, 5545
National Parkinson Foundation, 2845
Norwegian Cruise Line, 5533
Ocala Adult Day Training, 4020
One-Stop Service, 5937
Orange County Library System: Audio-Visual Department, 4709
Palm Beach Habilitation Center, 5938
Pearlman Biomedical Research Institute, 4710
Pinellas Park Adult Day Training, 4021
Pinellas Talking Book Library for the Blind and Physically Handicapped, 4711
Primrose Supported Employment Programs, 5939
Publix Super Markets Charities, 2846
Quest, 5940
Quest - Tampa Area, 5941
SCARC, Inc Evaluation, Training + Emplomen t Center, 5942
SCCIL at Titusville, 4022
Seagull Industries for the Disabled, 5943
Self Reliance, 4023
Sertoma Camp Endeavor, 1046
Space Coast Center for Independent Living, 4024
St. Petersburg Regional Office, 5607
Suncoast Center for Independent Living, Inc., 4025
Supported Employment Program, 5944
Talking Book Service: Mantatee County Central Library, 4712
Talking Books Library for the Blind and Physically Handicapped, 4713
Talking Books/Homebound Services, 4714
University of Miami: Bascom Palmer Eye Institute, 4715
University of Miami: Mailman Center for Child Development, 4716
Upledger Institute, 933
VACC Camp, 1047
Vocational and Rehabilitation Agency Department of Education, 5945
West Florida Regional Library, 4717
West Palm Beach VA Medical Center, 5608
Work Exploration Center, 5947
Young Onset Parkinson Conference, 1876
disAbility Solutions for Independent Living, 4026

Georgia

ASIA Annual Scientific Meeting, 1840
Aerie Experiences, 1048
Arc Of Georgia, 2847
Arms Wide Open, 4027
Athens Talking Book Center-Athens-Clarke County Regional Library, 4718
Atlanta Regional Office, 5609

Atlanta VA Medical Center, 5610
Augusta Talking Book Center, 4719
Augusta VA Medical Center, 5611
Bain, Inc. Center For Independent Living, 4028
Bainbridge Subregional Library for the Blind & Physically Handicapped, 4720
Camp Breathe Easy, 1049
Camp Caglewood, 1050
Camp Dream, 1051
Camp Esperanza, 1052
Camp Hawkins, 1053
Camp Juliana, 1054
Camp Kudzu, 1055
Camp Twin Lakes, 1057
Carl Vinson VA Medical Center, 5612
Center for Assistive Technology and Environmental Access, 815
Columbus Subregional Library For The Blind And Physically Handicapped, 4721
Community Foundation for Greater Atlanta, 2848
DisAbility LINK, 829
Disability Connections, 4029
Emory Autism Resource Center, 4722
Emory University Laboratory for Ophthalmic Research, 4723
Employment and Training Division, Region B, 5948
Fair Housing and Equal Employment, 5949
Florence C and Harry L English Memorial Fund, 2849
Georgia Library for the Blind and Physically Handicapped, 4724
Georgia Power, 2850
Griffin Area Resource Center Griffin Community Workshop Division, 5950
Hall County Library: East Hall Branch and Special Needs Library, 4725
Harriet McDaniel Marshall Trust in Memory of Sanders McDaniel, 2852
Human Ecology Action League (HEAL), 858
IBM National Support Center, 5951
John H and Wilhelmina D Harland Charitable Foundation, 2854
Kelley Diversified, 5952
Lettie Pate Whitehead Foundation, 2855
Living Independence for Everyone (LIFE), 4031
Macon Library for the Blind and Physically Handicapped, 4726
Multiple Choices Center for Independent Living, 4032
National Center on Birth Defects and Developmental Disabilities, 4727
New Ventures, 5953
North District Independent Living Program, 4033
North Georgia Talking Book Center, 4728
Oconee Regional Library, 4729
Rome Subregional Library for the Blind and Physically Handicapped, 4730
South Georgia Regional Library-Valdosta Talking Book Center, 4731
Southeastern Paralyzed Veterans of America (PVA), 5613
Southwest District Independent Living Program, 4034
Squirrel Hollow Summer Camp, 1058
Statewide Independent Living Council of Ge orgia, 4035
SunTrust Bank, Atlanta Foundation, 2857
Talking Book Center Brunswick-Glynn County Regional Library, 4732
Walton Options for Independent Living, 4036
disABILITY LINK: Rome, 4037

Hawaii

Arc of Hawaii, 2858
Assets School, 5954
Assistive Technology Resource Centers of Hawaii (ATRC), 4733
Atherton Family Foundation, 2859
Camp Anuenue, 1059
Center For Independent Living- Kauai, 4038
GN Wilcox Trust, 2860
Hawaii Center For Independent Living, 4039

Hawaii Center for Independent Living-Maui, 4040
Hawaii Centers for Independent Living, 4041
Hawaii Community Foundation, 2861
Hawaii Fair Employment Practice Agency, 5955
Hawaii State Library for the Blind and Physically Handicapped, 4734
Hawaii Vocational Rehabilitation Division, 5956
Hilo Vet Center, 5614
Honolulu VBA Regional Office, 5615
Kauai Center for Independent Living, 4042
Lanakila Rehabilitation Center, 5957
McInerny Foundation Bank Of Hawaii, Corporate Trustee, 2862
Over the Rainbow Disabled Travel Services & Wheelers Accessible Van Rentals, 5547
Pacific Islands Health Care System, 5616
Pacific Rim International Conference on Disability And Diversity, 1869
Sophie Russell Testamentary Trust Bank Of Hawaii, 2863
Wahiawa Family, 5959
YMCA Camp Erdman, 1060

Idaho

American Falls Office: Living Independently for Everyone (LIFE), 4043
Boise Regional Office, 5617
Boise VA Medical Center, 5618
Camp Hodia, 1061
Camp Rainbow Gold, 1062
Camp Sawtooth, 1063
Dawn Enterprises, 4044
Disability Action Center NW, 4045
Disability Action Center NW: Coeur D'Alene, 4046
Disability Action Center NW: Lewiston, 4047
Idaho Assistive Technology Project, 4735
Idaho Commission for Libraries: Talking Book Service, 4736
Idaho Employment Service and Job Training Program Liaison, 5960
Idaho Fair Employment Practice Agency, 5961
Idaho Falls Office: Living Independently for Everyone (LIFE), 4048
Idaho Governor's Committee on Employment of People with Disabilities, 5962
Idaho Vocational Rehabilitation Agency, 5963
Living Independence Network Corporation, 4050
Living Independence Network Corporation: Twin Falls, 4051
Living Independence Network Corporation: C aldwell, 4052
Living Independent for Everyone (LIFE): Pocatello Office, 4053
Living Independently for Everyone (LIFE): Blackfoot Office, 4054
Living Independently for Everyone: Burley, 4055
ROW Adventures, 5534
Southwestern Idaho Housing Authority, 4056

Illinois

ATIA Conference, 1841
Access Living of Metropolitan Chicago, 4057
Ada S McKinley Vocational Services, 5965
Alzheimer's Association, 2864
American Academy of Disability Evaluating Physicians, 768
American Academy of Pediatrics, 770
American Massage Therapy Association, 787
American Society of Clinical Hypnosis, 795
Amerock Corporation, 2866
Anixter Center, 5966
Arc of Illinois, 2867
Association of Assistive Technology Act Pr ograms, 799
Benjamin Benedict Green-Field Foundation, 2868
Blowitz-Ridgeway Foundation, 2869
C-4 Work Center, 5967
Camp Callahan, 1064
Camp Christmas Seal, 1065
Camp Easter Seals, 1067

Camp Hug The Bear, 1068
Camp I Am Me, 1069
Camp Little Giant, 1070
Camp Surefoot Center, 1346
Center on Deafness, 4058
Chaddick Institute for Metropolitan Development, 2870
Chicago Community Trust, 2871
Chicago Community Trust and Affiliates, 2872
Chicago Public Library Talking Book Center, 4737
Clearbrook, 5968
Community Foundation of Champaign County, 2873
Community Residential Alternative, 4059
Cornerstone Services, 5969
Department of Ophthalmology and Visual Science, 4738
Division of Rehabilitation Services, 4030, 4060
Dr Scholl Foundation, 2874
DuPage Center for Independent Living, 4061
Duchossois Foundation, 2875
Easter Seals, 837
Easter Seals Camp Sunnyside, 1073
Edward Hines Jr Hospital, 5619
Evenston Community Foundation, 2876
Family Resource Center on Disabilities, 842
Field Foundation of Illinois, 2877
Fite Center for Independent Living, 4062
Francis Beidler Charitable Trust, 2878
Fred J Brunner Foundation, 2879
Fulton County Rehab Center, 5970
George M Eisenberg Foundation for Charities, 2880
Glenkirk, 5971
Grover Hermann Foundation, 2881
Guild for the Blind, 4739
Health Resource Center for Women with Disabilities, 856
Horizons for the Blind, 4740
Illinois Department of Rehab Services, 4063
Illinois Early Childhood Intervention Clearinghouse, 4741
Illinois Employment Service, 5972
Illinois Machine Sub-Lending Agency, 4742
Illinois Regional Library for the Blind and Physically Handicapped, 4743
Illinois Valley Center for Independent Living, 4064
Illinois and Iowa Center for Independent L iving, 4065
Impact Center for Independent Living, 4066
JCYS Camp Red Leaf, 1074
Jacksonville Area CIL: Havana, 4067
Jacksonville Area Center for Independent Living, 4068
Jewish Vocational Services, 5973
JoDavies Workshop, 5974
John D and Catherine T MacArthur Foundation, 2882
Kennedy Job Training Center, 5975
Knox County Council for Developmental Disabilities, 5976
Kreider Services, 5977
LIFE Center for Independent Living, 4069
LINC-Monroe Randolph Center, 4070
Lake County Center for Independent Living, 4071
Lambs Farm, 5978
Land of Lincoln Goodwill Industries, 5979
Les Turne Amyotrophic Laterial Sclerosis Foundation, 2883
Life Center for Independent Living: Pontia c, 4072
Lions Clubs International, 2711
Little City Foundation, 2884
Living Independently Now Center (LINC), 4073
Living Independently Now Center: Sparta, 4074
Living Independently Now Center: Waterloo, 4075
MAGIC Foundation for Children's Growth, 2885
Marion VA Medical Center, 5620
McDonald's Corporation Contributions Program, 2886
Michael Reese Health Trust, 2887
Mid-Illinois Talking Book Center, 4744
Muscular Dystrophy Association - USA, 881
Muscular Dystrophy Association Free Camp, 1075
National Easter Seal Society, 897

National Eye Research Foundation, 2888
National Eye Research Foundation (NERF), 4745
National Foundation for Ectodermal Dysplasias, 2889
National Headache Foundation, 2890
National Lekotek Center, 4746
New Courier Travel, 5531
North Chicago VA Medical Center, 5621
Northwest Limousine Service, 5546
Northwestern University Multipurpose Arthritis & Musculoskeletal Center, 4747
OMRON Foundation OMRON Electronics, 2891
One Step At A Time Camp, 1076
Opportunities for Access: A Center for Independent Living, 4077
Options Center for Independent Living: Bourbonnais, 4078
Options Center for Independent Living: Watseka, 4079
Orchard Village, 5980
PACE Center for Independent Living, 4080
Patrick and Anna M Cudahy Fund, 3257
Peoria Area Community Foundation, 2893
Polk Brothers Foundation, 2894
Progress Center for Independent Living, 4081
Progress Center for Independent Living: Blue Island, 4082
Regional Access & Mobilization Project, 4083
Regional Access & Mobilization Project: Belvidere, 4084
Regional Access & Mobilization Project: De Kalb, 4085
Regional Access & Mobilization Project: Freeport, 4086
Retirement Research Foundation, 2895
Rimland Services for Autistic Citizens, 1077
Rotary Youth Exchange, 2716
Sears-Roebuck Foundation, 2896
Sertoma Centre, 5982
Shady Oaks Camp, 1078
Shore Training Center, 5983
Siragusa Foundation, 2897
Skokie Accessible Library Services, 4748
Soyland Access to Independent Living (SAIL), 4087
Soyland Access to Independent Living: Charleston, 4088
Soyland Access to Independent Living: Shelbyville, 4089
Soyland Access to Independent Living: Sullivan, 4090
Springfield Center for Independent Living, 4091
Square D Foundation, 2898
Stone-Hayes Center for Independent Living, 4092
Summer Camp for Children with Muscular Dystrophy, 1079
Summer Wheelchair Sport Camps, 1080
Thresholds AMISS, 5985
Thresholds Psychiatric Rehabilitation Centers, 929
Timber Pointe Outdoor Center, 1081
University of Illinois at Chicago: Lions of Illinois Eye Research Institute, 4749
VA Illiana Health Care System, 5622
Voices of Vision Talking Book Center at DuPage Library System, 4750
WP and HB White Foundation, 2899
Washington County Vocational Workshop, 5987
Washington Square Health Foundation, 2900
West Central Illinois Center for Independent Living, 4093
West Central Illinois Center for Independent Living: Macomb, 4094
Wheat Ridge Ministries, 2901
Will Grundy Center for Independent Living, 4095
YMCA Camp Duncan, 1082

Indiana

ADEC Resources for Independence, 5989
ARC of Allen County, 5990
Allen County Public Library, 4751
American Camping Association, 778
Anderson Woods, 1083
Arc Bridges, 5991

Arc of Indiana, 2902
Assistive Technology Training and Information Center (ATTIC), 4096
Autism Day Camp, 1084
BI-County Services, 5992
Ball Brothers Foundation, 2903
Bartholomew County Public Library, 4752
Bradford Woods: Camp Riley, 1085
Brave Heart's Camp, 1086
Bridge Pointe Services & Goodwill of Southern Indiana, Inc, 5994
CHAMP Camp, 1087
Camp About Face, 1088
Camp Alexander Mack, 1089
Camp Brave Eagle, 1090
Camp Crosley YMCA, 1092
Camp John Warvel, 1093
Camp Little Red Door, 1094
Camp Millhouse, 1095
Camp Red Cedar, 1096
Camp Riley, 1097
Career Connections, 6213
Carey Services, 5995
Community Foundation of Boone County, 2904
DAMAR Services, 4097
Elkhart Public Library for the Blind and Physiclly Handicapped, 4753
Englishton Park Academic Remediation, 1098
Evansville Association for the Blind, 5996
Everybody Counts Center for Independent Living, 4098
Feingold Association of the US, 848
Four Rivers Resource Services, 4099, 5997
Future Choices Independent Living Center, 4100
Gateway Services/JCARC, 5998
Goodwill Industries of Central Indiana, 5999
Happiness Bag, 1099
Hoosier Burn Camp, 1100
Independent Living Center of Eastern Indiana (ILCEIN), 4101
Indiana Children's Deaf Camp, 1101
Indiana Civil Rights Commission, 6000
Indiana Employment Services and Job Training Program Liaison, 6001
Indiana Resource Center for Autism, 4754
Indiana University: Multipurpose Arthritis Center, 4755
Indianapolis Regional Office, 5623
Indianapolis Resource Center for Independent Living, 4102
John W Anderson Foundation, 2905
Lake County Public Library Talking Books Service, 4756
League for the Blind and Disabled, 4103
Martin Luther Homes of Indiana, 4104
Michigan Resources, 6002
New Hope Services, 6003
New Horizons Rehabilitation, 6004
Noble Of Indiana, 6005
Office of State Coordinator of Vocational Education for Students with Disability, 6006
Putnam County Comprehensive Services, 6007
Residential Camp, 1102
Richard L Roudebush VA Medical Center, 5624
Ruben Center for Independent Living, 4105
SILC, Indiana Council on Independent Living (ICOIL), 4106
Southern Indiana Center for Independent Living, 4107
Southern Indiana Resource Solutions, 6008
Special Services Division: Indiana State Library, 4757
St. Joseph Hospital Rehabilitation Center, 4758
Sycamore Rehabilitation Services, 6009
Talking Books Service Evansville Vanderburgh County Public Library, 4759
Twin Lakes Camp, 1103
VA North Indiana Health Care System: Fort Wayne Campus, 5625
VA Northern Indiana Health Care System: Marion Campus, 5626
Wabash Independent Living Center & Learning Center (WILL), 4108

Iowa

ACT Assessment Test Preparation Reference Manual, 6012
Arc of Iowa, 2906
Black Hawk Center for Independent Living, 4109
Camp Albrecht Acres, 1104
Camp Courageous of Iowa, 1105
Camp Hertko Hollow, 1106
Camp L-Kee-Ta, 1107
Camp Quality Heartland, 1108
Camp Sunnyside, 1109
Camp Tanager, 1110
Camp Wyoming, 1111
Central Iowa Center for Independent Living, 4110
Des Moines VA Medical Center, 5627
Des Moines VA Regional Office, 5628
Diabetes Camp, 1112
Evert Conner Rights & Resources CIL, 4111
Franklin County Work Activity Center, 6013
Hall-Perrine Foundation, 2907
Hope Haven, 4112
Iowa City VA Medical Center, 5629
Iowa Civil Rights Commission, 6015
Iowa Department for the Blind Library, 4760
Iowa Employment Service, 6016
Iowa Job Training Program Liaison, 6017
Iowa Registry for Congenital and Inherited Disorders, 4761
Iowa Valley Community College, 6018
Iowa Vocational Rehabilitation Services, 6019
Knoxville VA Medical Center, 5630
League of Human Dignity, Center for Independent Living, 4113
Library Commission for the Blind, 4762
Mid-Iowa Health Foundation, 2908
New Focus, 6020
Principal Financial Group Foundation, 2909
Siouxland Community Foundation, 2910
South Central Iowa Center for Independent Living, 4115
Universal Pediatric Services, 932
VA Central Iowa Health Care System, 5631
Wendell Johnson Speech And Hearing Clinic, 1113
Wesley Woods Camp and Retreat Center, 1114
Y Camp, 1115

Kansas

Advocates for Better Living For Everyone (A.B.L.E.), 4117
American Academy of Environmental Medicine, 769
Arc of Kansas, 2911
Beach Center on Families and Disability, 805
Camp Discovery - Kansas, 1116
Camp Quality Kansas, 1117
Center for Independent Living SW Kansas: Liberal, 4118
Center for Independent Living Southwest Kansas, 4119
Center for Independent Living Southwest Kansas: Dodge City, 4120
Center for the Improvement of Human Functioning, 4763
Central Kansas Library Systems Headquarters (CSLS), 4764
Coalition for Independence, 4121
Colmery-O'Neil VA Medical Center, 5632
Cowley County Developmental Services, 4122
Dwight D Eisenhower VA Medical Center, 5633
Hospitalized Veterans Writing Project, 5559
Hutchinson Community Foundation, 2912
Independence, 4123
Independent Connection, 4124
Independent Connection: Abilene, 4125
Independent Connection: Beloit, 4126
Independent Connection: Concordia, 4127
Independent Living Resource Center, 3941, 4128
Kansas Fair Employment Practice Agency, 6023
Kansas Services for the Blind & Visually Impaired, 4129
Kansas State Library, 4765
Kansas Talking Books Regional Library, 4766

Kansas VA Regional Office, 5634
Kansas Vocational Rehabilitation Agency, 6024
LINK: Colby, 4130
Living Independently in Northwest Kansas: Hays, 4131
Manhattan Public Library, 4767
Northwest Kansas Library System Talking Books, 4768
Prairie IL Resource Center, 4132
Prairie Independent Living Resource Center, 4133
Resource Center for Independent Living: Emporia, 4136
Resource Center for Independent Living: Ar kansas City, 4137
Resource Center for Independent Living: Bu rlington, 4138
Resource Center for Independent Living: Co ffeyville, 4139
Resource Center for Independent Living: El Dorado, 4140
Resource Center for Independent Living: Ft Scott, 4141
Resource Center for Independent Living: Ot tawa, 4142
Resource Center for Independent Living: Ov erland Park, 4143
Resource Center for Independent Living: To peka, 4144
Richard W Higgins Charitable Foundation, 2913
Robert J Dole VA Medical Center, 5635
South Central Kansas Library System, 4769
Southeast Kansas Independent Living (SKIL), 4145
Southeast Kansas Independent Living: Independence, 4146
Southeast Kansas Independent Living: Chanu te, 4147
Southeast Kansas Independent Living: Colum bus, 4148
Southeast Kansas Independent Living: Fredo nia, 4149
Southeast Kansas Independent Living: Hays, 4150
Southeast Kansas Independent Living: Pitts burg, 4151
Southeast Kansas Independent Living: Sedan, 4152
Southeast Kansas Independent Living: Yates Center, 4153
Summer Camp for Physically & Mentally Chal lenged Children & Adults, 1118
Three Rivers Independent Living Center, 4154
Three Rivers Independent Living Center: Clay, 4155
Three Rivers Independent Living Center: Ma nhattan, 4156
Three Rivers Independent Living Center: Se neca, 4157
Three Rivers Independent Living Center: To peka, 4158
Topeka & Shawnee County Public Library Talking Books Service, 4770
Topeka Independent Living Resource Center, 4159
Whole Person: Nortonville, 4160
Whole Person: Nortonville, The, 4161
Whole Person: Prairie Village, 4162
Whole Person: Prairie Village, The, 4163
Whole Person: Tonganoxie, 4164
Wichita Public Library/Talking Book Service, 4771
Wichita Public Library/Talking Book Servic e, 4772

Kentucky

Arc of Kentucky, 2914
Bethel Mennonite Camp, 1119
Camp Quality Kentuckiana, 1120
Cedar Ridge Camp, 1121
Center For Courageous Kids, The, 1122
Center for Accessible Living, 4165
Center for Accessible Living: Murray, 4166
Center for Independent Living: Kentucky Department for the Blind, 4167
Children's Alliance, 821
Disability Coalition of Northern Kentucky, 4168

Disability Resource Initiative, 4169
EnTech: Enabling Technologies of Kentuckiana, 4773
Independence Place, 4170
Indian Summer Camp, 1123
Kentucky Committee on Employment of People with Disabilities, 6025
Kentucky Department for Employment Service and Job Training Program Liaison, 6026
Kentucky Department for the Blind, 6027
Kentucky Office for the Blind, 6028
Kentucky Talking Book Library Kentucky Dept. for Libraries and Archives, 4774
Kentucky Vocational Rehabilitation Agency, 6029
Lexington VA Medical Center, 5636
Lions Camp Crescendo, Inc., 1124
Louisville Free Public Library, 4775
Louisville VA Medical Center, 5637
Louisville VA Regional Office, 5638
Medical Camping, 1125
Pathfinders for Independent Living, 4171
Pioneer Vocational/Industrial Services, 6030
SILC Department of Vocational Rehabilitation, 4172
Work Enhancement Center of Western Kentucky, 6031

Louisiana

Alexandria VA Medical Center, 5639
Arc of Louisiana, 2915
Baton Rouge Area Foundation, 2916
Camp Bon Coeur, 1126
Camp Challenge, 1037, 1091, 1127, 1127
Camp Pelican, 1128
Camp Quality Louisiana, 1129
Central Louisiana State Hospital Medical and Professional Library, 4776
Community Foundation of Shreveport-Bossier, 2917
Community Opportunities of East Ascension, 6032
Dynamic Dimensions, 5883
Louisiana Employment Service and Job Training Program Liaison, 6033
Louisiana Lions Camp, 1131
Louisiana Lions Camp - Camp Pelican, 1132
Louisiana State Library, 4777
Louisiana State University Genetics Sectio n of Pediatrics, 4778
Louisiana Vocational Rehabilitation Agency, 6034
Med-Camps of Louisiana, 1133
New Horizons: Central Louisiana, 4173
New Horizons: Northeast Louisiana, 4174
New Horizons: Northwest Louisiana, 4175
New Orleans VA Medical Center, 5640
Resources for Independent Living: Baton Rouge, 4176
Resources for Independent Living: Metairie, 4177
Shreveport VA Medical Center, 5641
Southwest Louisiana Independence Center: L ake Charles, 4178
Southwest Louisians Independence Center: Lafayette, 4179
St. James Association for Retarded Citizens, 6035
State Library of Louisiana: Services for the Blind and Physically Handicapped, 4779
Volunteers of America of Greater New Orlea ns, 4180
W Troy Cole Independent Living Specialist, 4181
Westbank Sheltered Workshop, 6036

Maine

Addison Point Specialized Services, 6037
Alpha One: South Portland, 4183
BCR Foundation, 2918
Bangor Public Library, 4780
Bangor Veteran Center: Veterans Outreach Center, 6038
Camp Waban, 1134
Camp Bishopswood, 1135
Camp Capella, 1136
Camp Lawroweld, 1137

Camp No Limits, 1138
Camp Pinecone, 1139
Camp Sunshine, 1056, 1140
Camp Waziyatah, 1141
Cary Library, 4781
Creative Work Systems, 6039
High School Students Guide to Study, Travel, and Adventure Abroad, 2704
Indian Acres Camp for Boys, 1143
Lewiston Public Library, 4782
Maine Department Of Labor, 6040
Maine Governor's Committee on Employment of the Disabled, 6041
Maine Human Rights Commission, 6042
Maine State Library, 4783
Maine VA Regional Office, 5642
Motivational Services, 4184
Northeast Occupational Exchange, 6043
Pine Tree Camp, 1144
Portland Public Library, 4785
Shalom House, 4185
Togus VA Medical Center, 5643
UNUM Charitable Foundation, 2919
Waterville Public Library, 4786
Women to Women, 934
YMCA Camp of Maine, 1145

Maryland

AADB National Conference, 1828
APSE, 761
APSE Conference: Revitalizing Supported Employment, Climbing to the Future, 1838
ASHA Convention, 1839
ASL Camp, 1146
American Association on Health and Disabil ity, 774
American College of Nurse Midwives, 781
American Health Assistance Foundation, 2920
American Occupational Therapy Association, 788
American Occupational Therapy Foundation, 2921
Arc of Maryland, 2922
Ardmore Developmental Center, 6045
Association for International Practical Training, 2698
Association for Persons in Supported Employment, 797
Association of University Centers on Disabilities, 802
Baltimore Community Foundation, 2923
Baltimore Regional Office, 5644
Baltimore VA Medical Center, 5645
Broadmead, 4186
CASA Inc., 4329
CQL Accreditation, 1853
Camp Glyndon, 1148
Camp JCC, 1149
Camp Joy, 1150
Camp Milldale, 1151
Camp Quality George Washington University, 1152
Camp Roehr, 1153
Camp Sunrise, 1154
Camp Superkids, 1155
Candlelighters Childhood Cancer Foundation, 2924
Children's Fresh Air Society Fund, 2925
Clark-Winchcole Foundation, 2926
Columbia Foundation, 2927
Community Health Funding Report, 3262
Corporate Giving Program, 2928
Cystic Fibrosis Foundation, 2929
Deaf Camp, 1156
Department of Physical Medicine & Rehabilitation at Sinai Hospital, 828
Disability Funding News, 3264
Eastern Shore Center for Independent Living, 4187
Epilepsy Foundation of Southeast Texas, 3204
Federation of Families for Children's Mental Health, 847
Fort Howard VA Medical Center, 5646
Foundation Fighting Blindness, 2930
Freedom Center, 4188
George Wasserman Family Foundation, 2931
Giant Food Foundation, 2932

Goodwill Industries International, 852
HRSA Information Center, 853
Harry and Jeanette Weinberg Foundation, 2933
Hostelling North America, 5530
Housing Unlimited, 4189
IDF National Conference, 1858
Independence Now, 4190
Independence Now: Silver Spring, 4191
International Association of Machinists, 861
Job Opportunities for the Blind, 6046
Johns Hopkins University Dana Center for Preventive Ophthalmology, 4787
Johns Hopkins University: Asthma and Allergy Center, 4788
Kamp A-Komp-Plish, 1157
Kennedy Krieger Institute, 2934
League at Camp Greentop, 1158
Lions Camp Merrick, 1159
Making Choices for Independent Living, 4192
Maryland Employment Services and Job Training Program Liaison, 6048
Maryland Fair Employment Practice Agency, 6049
Maryland State Department of Education, 6050
Maryland State Library for the Blind and Physically Handicapped, 4789
Maryland Veterans Centers, 5647
Melwood, 6051
Mobile Care, 5544
Montgomery County Department of Public Libraries/Special Needs Library, 4790
National 4-H Council, 2713
National Epilepsy Library (NEL), 4791
National Federation of the Blind, 2936
National Federation of the Blind Jernigan Institute, 4792
National Rehabilitation Information Center (NARIC), 903, 4793
Optometric Extension Program Foundation, 2937
Perry Point VA Medical Center, 5648
Project LINK, 6053
Pueblo Goodwill Industries, 3979
Raven Rock Lutheran Camp, 1160
Red Notebook, 4794
Resources for Independence, 4193
Sjogren's Syndrome Foundation, 2938
Social Security Library, 4795
Southern Maryland Center for LIFE, 4194
TLC's Summer Programs, 1161
Treatment and Learning Centers (TLC), 6054
VA Maryland Health Care System, 5649
Warren Grant Magnuson Clinical Center, 4796
Young Adult Deaf Camp, 1162
Youth Leadership Camp, 1163
Youth for Understanding International Exchange, 2725

Massachusetts

Abbot and Dorothy H Stevens Foundation, 2939
Adlib, 4195
Agassiz Village Camp, 1164
Arc of Cape Cod, 4196
Arc of Massachusetts, The, 2940
Arc of Northern Bristol County, 2941
Becket Chimney Corners YMCA Camps and Outdoor Center, 1165
Boston Center for Independent Living, 4197
Boston Foundation, 2942
Boston Globe Foundation, 2943
Boston University Arthritis Center, 4797
Boston University Center for Human Genetics, 4798
Boston University Robert Dawson Evans Memorial Dept. of Clinical Research, 4799
Boston VA Regional Office, 5650
Braille and Talking Book Library, Perkins School for the Blind, 4800
Brigham and Women's Hospital: Asthma and Allergic Disease Research Center, 4801
Brigham and Women's Hospital: Robert B Brigham Multipurpose Arthritis Center, 4802
Bright Horizons Summer Camp, 1166
Bushrod H Campbell and Ada F Hall Charity Fund, 2944

CAPP National Parent Resource Center Federation for Children with Special Needs, 809
Camp Howe, 1167
Camp Jabberwocky, 1168
Camp Joslin, 1169
Camp New Connections, 1170
Camp Ramah in New England, 1171
Camp Starfish, 1172
Camp Wee-Kan-Tu, 1173
Cape Organization for Rights of the Disabled (CORD), 813
Cape Organization for Rights of the Disabl ed (CORD), 4198
Caption Center, 4803
Carroll School Summer Programs, 1174
Center for Interdisciplinary Research on Immunologic Diseases, 4804
Center for Living & Working: Fitchburg, 4199
Center for Living & Working: Framingham, 4200
Center for Living & Working: Worcester, 4201
Clara Barton Diabetes Camp, 1175
Clipper Ship Foundation, 2945
Community Enterprises, 824, 5898
Community Foundation of Western Massachusetts, 2946
Department Of Workforce Development, 6055
Developmental Evaluation and Adjustment Fa cilities, 4202
Eagle Hill School: Summer Program, 1176
Edith Nourse Rogers Memorial Veterans Hospital, 5651
Edward J Madden Open Hearts Camp, 1177
Federation for Children with Special Needs, 846
Feldenkrais Guild of North America (FGNA), 849
Frank R and Elizabeth Simoni Foundation, 2947
Frank Stanley Beveridge Foundation, 2948
Friendly Ice Cream Corp Contributions Prog ram, 2949
Gateway Arts Center: Studio, Craft Store & Gallery, 6056
Greater Worcester Community Foundation, 2950
Handi Kids, 1178
Harvard University Howe Laboratory of Ophthalmology, 4805
Hyams Foundation, 2951
Independence Associates, 4203
Independent Living Center of Stavros: Gree nfield, 4204
Independent Living Center of Stavros: Spri ngfield, 4205
Independent Living Center of the North Sho re & Cape Ann, 4206
Kamp for Kids: Camp Togowauk, 1179
Laboure College Library, 4806
Learning Disabilities Worldwide, 873
Massachusetts Fair Employment Practice Agency, 6057
Massachusetts Governor's Commission on Employment of Disabled Persons, 6058
Massachusetts Rehabilitation Commission, 4807
MetroWest Center for Independent Living, 4207
Multi-Cultural Independent Living Center of Boston, 4208
New England Regional Genetics Group, 4784
Northampton VA Medical Center, 5652
Northeast Independent Living Program, 4209
PKU Camp, 1180
Parent Professional Advocacy League, 914
Raytheon Company Contributions Program, 2952
Renaissance Clubhouse, 4210
Scandinavian Exchange, 2717
Schepens Eye Research Institute, 4808
Second Time Around, 6021
Skills Inc., 5984
Southeast Center for Independent Living, 4211
Student Independent Living Experience Massachusetts Hospital School, 4212
TJX Foundation, 2953
TSA CT Kid's Summer Event, 1181
Talking Book Library at Worcester Public Library, 4809
Tower Program at Regis College, 1182
VA Boston Healthcare System: Brockton Division, 5653

VA Boston Healthcare System: Jamaica Plain Campus, 5654
VA Boston Healthcare System: West Roxbury Division, 5655
Vocational and Rehabilitation Agency Massachusetts Commission for the Blind, 6060
Work Inc., 6061

Michigan

Aleda E Lutz VA Medical Center, 5656
Alternating Hemiplegia of Childhood Foundation, 2739
Ann Arbor Area Community Foundation, 2955
Ann Arbor Center for Independent Living, 4213
Arc Michigan, 4214
Arc of Michigan, 2956
Arc/Muskegon, 4215
Artificial Language Laboratory, 4810
Bad Axe: Blue Water Center for Independent Living, 4216
Battle Creek VA Medical Center, 5657
Bay Area Coalition for Independent Living, 4217
Berrien Community Foundation, 2957
Blind Children's Fund, 2958
Burger School for the Autistic, 4811
Camp Barakel, 1183
Camp Barefoot, 1184
Camp Catch-a-Rainbow, 1185
Camp Chris Williams, 1186
Camp Grace Bentley, 1187
Camp Nissokone, 1188
Camp Quality Illinois, 1072
Camp Quality Michigan, 1189
Camp Roger, 1190
Camp Tall Turf, 1191
Capital Area Center for Independent Living, 4218
Caro: Blue Water Center for Independent Li ving, 4219
Center for Independent Living of Mid-Michigan, 4220
Chi Medical Library, 4812
Community Connections of Southwest Michigan, 4221
Community Foundation of Monroe County, 2959
Cowan Slavin Foundation, 2960
Cristo Rey Handicappers Program, 4222
Daimler Chrysler, 2961
Department Of Human Services, 6062
Detroit Center for Independent Living, 4223
Disability Advocates of Kent County, 4224
Disability Connection, 4225
Disability Network Southwest Michigan, 4226
Disability Network of Mid-Michigan, 4227
Disability Network of Oakland & Macomb, 4228
Disability Network/Lakeshore, 4229
Echo Grove Camp, 1192
Educational Accessibility Services, 838
Frank & Mollie S VanDervoort Memorial Foun dation, 2962
Fremont Area Community Foundation, 2963
Glaucoma Laser Trial, 4813
Grand Rapids Foundation, 2964
Grand Traverse Area Community Living Management Corporation, 4230
Grand Traverse Area Library for the Blind and Physically Handicapped, 4814
Granger Foundation, 2965
Great Lakes/Macomb Rehabilitation Group, 4231
Harvey Randall Wickes Foundation, 2966
Havirmill Foundation, 2967
Indian Trails Camp, 1193
Iron Mountain VA Medical Center, 5658
JARC, 4232
John D Dingell VA Medical Center, 5659
Kelly Services Foundation, 2968
Kent County Arc, 3170
Kent District Library for the Blind and Physically Handicapped, 4815
Kresge Foundation, 2969
Lamplighter's Work Center, 6063
Lanting Foundation, 2970
Lapeer: Blue Water Center for Independent Living, 4233

Library of Michigan Service for the Blind, 4816
Livingston Center for Independent Living, 4234
Macomb Library for the Blind & Physically Handicapped, 4817
Michigan Commission for the Blind: Independent Living Rehabilitation Program, 4235
Michigan Commission for the Blind: Detroit, 4236
Michigan Department of Civil Rights, 6064
Michigan Employment Service, 6065
Michigan Rehabilitation Services: Dept of Labor & Regulatory Affairs, 6066
Michigan VA Regional Office, 5660
Michigan's Assistive Technology Resource, 4818
Mideastern Michigan Library Co-op, 4819
Monroe Center for Independent Living, 4237
Muskegon Area District Library for the Bli nd and Physically Handicapped, 4820
Northland Library Cooperative, 4821
Oakland County Library for the Visually & Physically Impaired, 4822
Port Huron: Blue Water Center for Independ ent Living, 4238
Rehabilitation Services, 922
Rollin M Gerstacker Foundation, 2971
Sandusky: Blue Water Center for Independen t Living, 4239
Sherman Lake YMCA Outdoor Center, 1194
Southeastern Michigan Commission for the Blind, 4240
St. Clair County Library Special Technologies Alternative Resources (S.T.A.R.), 4823
St. Francis Camp On The Lake, 1195
Steelcase Foundation, 2972
Student Disability Services, 926
Superior Alliance for Independent Living (SAIL), 4241
Trail's Edge Camp, 1196
University of Michigan: Orthopaedic Research Laboratories, 4824
Upper Peninsula Library for the Blind, 4825
VA Ann Arbor Healthcare System, 5661
Vet Center Readjustment Counseling Service, 5662
Washtenaw County Library for the Blind & Physically Handicapped, 4826
Wayne County Regional Library for the Blind, 4827
Wayne State University: CS Mott Center for Human Genetics and Development, 4828
YMCA Camp Copneconic, 1197
disAbility Connections, 4242

Minnesota

Accessible Space, Inc., 4243
Accessnorth CIL of Northeastern MN: Aitkin, 4244
Accessnorth CIL of Northeastern MN: Duluth, 4245
American Holistic Medical Association, 786
Arc of Minnesota, 2973
Burnett Foundation, 3194
Camp Benedict, 1198
Camp Buckskin, 1199
Camp Confidence, 1200
Camp Courage North, 1201
Camp Heartland, 1203
Camp Knutson, 1204
Camp Winnebago, 1142
Center for Independent Living of NE Minnesota, 4246
Century College, 4829
Closing the Gap's Annual Conference, 1854
Communication Center/Minnesota State Services for the Blind, 4830
Confidence Learning Center, 1205
Courage Center, 4247
Courage Center Camps, 1206
Deluxe Corporation Foundation, 2974
Duluth Public Library, 4831
Flying Wheels Travel, 5527
Freedom Resource Center for Independent Living: Fergus Falls, 4248
General Mills Foundation, 2975
Hugh J Andersen Foundation, 2976
Independent Life Styles, 4474

James R Thorpe Foundation, 2977
Jay and Rose Phillips Family Foundation, 2978
Jewish Vocational Service of Jewish Family and Children's Services, 6068
Metropolitan Center for Independent Living, 4249
Minneapolis Foundation, 2979
Minneapolis VA Medical Center, 5663
Minnesota Association of Centers for Independent Living, 4250
Minnesota Department of Employment and Economic Development - Vocational Rehab Services, 6069
Minnesota Employment Practice Agency, 6070
Minnesota Library for the Blind and Physically Handicapped, 4832
Miracle-Ear Children's Foundation, 2935
OPTIONS, 4251
Options Interstate Resource Center for Independent Living, 4252
Ordean Foundation, 2980
Otto Bremer Foundation, 2981
PACER Center (Parent Advocacy Coalition for Educational Rights), 911
PWI Forum, 6071
Perry River Home Care, 4253
Rochester Area Foundation, 2982
SMILES, 4254
SMILES: Mankato, 4255
Southeastern Minnesota Center for Independent Living: Red Wing, 4256
Southeastern Minnesota Center for Independent Living: Rochester, 4257
Special U, 4833
St. Cloud VA Medical Center, 5664
St. Paul Regional Office, 5665
University of Minnesota at Crookston, 2720
Ventures Travel, 5537
Vinland Center Lake Independence, 4259
Wilderness Inquiry, 5539
YMCA Camp Ihduhapi, 1207

Mississippi

Allied Enterprises of Tupelo, 6073
Alpha Home Royal Maid Association for the Blind, 4260
Arc of Mississippi, 2983
Biloxi/Gulfport VA Medical Center, 5667
Blind and Physically Handicapped Library Services, 4834
Gulf Coast Independent Living Center, 4261
Jackson Regional Office, 5668
LIFE of Mississippi, 4263
LIFE of Mississippi: Biloxi, 4264
LIFE of Mississippi: Greenwood, 4265
LIFE of Mississippi: Hattiesburg, 4266
LIFE of Mississippi: McComb, 4267
LIFE of Mississippi: Meridian, 4268
LIFE of Mississippi: Oxford, 4269
LIFE of Mississippi: Tupelo, 4270
Mississippi Department of Rehabilitation Services, 6074
Mississippi Employment Secutity Commission, 6075
Mississippi Library Commission, 4835
Mississippi Library Commission\Talking Book and Braille Services, 4836
Worksight, 6076

Missouri

Access II Independent Living Center, 4271
Allen P & Josephine B Green Foundation, 2984
Anheuser-Busch, 2985
Arc of the US Missouri Chapter, 2986
Assemblies of God Center for the Blind, 4837
Bootheel Area Independent Living Services, 4272
Camp Barnabas, 1209
Camp Encourage, 1210
Camp Hickory Hill, 1211
Camp MITIOG, 1212
Camp Quality Central Missouri, 1213
Camp Quality Greater Kansas City, 1214

Camp Quality Northwest Missouri, 1215
Camp Quality Ozarks, 1216
Church of the Nazarene, 4838
Coalition for Independence: Missouri Branc h Office, 4273
Concerned Care, Inc., 1217
Delta Center for Independent Living, 4274
Disability Resource Association, 4275
Disabled Athlete Sports Association, 832
Greater Kansas City Community Foundation & Affiliated Trusts, 2987
Greater St Louis Community Foundation, 2988
H&R Block Foundation, 2989
Harry S Truman Memorial Veterans' Hospital, 5669
Independent Living Center of Southeast Missouri, 4276
International Clinic of Biological Regeneration, 864
James S McDonnell Foundation, 2990
John J Pershing VA Medical Center, 5670
Judevine Center for Autism, 4839
Kansas City VA Medical Center, 5671
Kiwanis Camp Wyman, 1218
Life Skills Foundation, 4277
Lions Den Outdoor Learning Center, 1219
Lutheran Blind Mission, 4840
Lutheran Charities Foundation of St Louis, 2991
Midland Empire Resources for Independent Living (MERIL), 4278
Missouri Commission on Human Rights, 6077
Missouri Governor's Council on Disability, 6078
Missouri Job Training Program Liaison, 6079
Missouri Vocational Rehabilitation Agency, 6080
Northeast Independent Living Services, 4279
On My Own, 4280
Ozark Independent Living, 4281
Paraquad, 4282
People to People International, 2715
People-to-People Committee on Disability, 918
People-to-People International: Committee for the Handicapped, 919
Places for People, 4283
RA Bloch Cancer Foundation, 2992
RAIL, 4284
SEMO Alliance for Disability Independence, 4285
Southwest Center for Independent Living (S CIL), 4287
Southwestern Center for Independent Living, 4258
St. Louis Regional Office, 5672
St. Louis VA Medical Center, 5673
Sunnyhill Adventure Center, 1220
Tri-County Center for Independent Living, 4288
University of Missouri: Columbia Arthritis Center, 4841
Victor E Speas Foundation, 2993
WX: Work Capacities, 6081
West Central Independent Living Solutions, 4289
Whole Person, The, 4290
Whole Person: Kansas City, 4291
Wolfner Talking Book & Braille Library, 4842
Wonderland Camp Foundation, 1221

Montana

American College of Advancement in Medicine, 780
Big Sky Kids Cancer Camps, 1222
Camp Mak-A-Dream, 1223
Charles Campbell Childrens Camp, 1224
Living Independently for Today and Tomorro w, 4292
MonTECH, Montana's Statewide Assistive Tec hnology Program, 4843
Montana Fair Employment Practice Agency, 6082
Montana Governor's Committee on Employment of Disabled People, 6083
Montana Independent Living Project, Inc., 4293
Montana State Library-Talking Book Library, 4844
Montana VA Regional Office, 5674
North Central Independent Living Services, 4294
Summit Independent Living Center: Kalipsell, 4295

Summit Independent Living Center: Hamilton, 4296

Summit Independent Living Center: Missoula, 4297

Summit Independent Living Center: Ronan, 4298

V A Montana Healthcare System, 5675

VA Montana Healthcare System, 5676

Vet Center, 5666, 5677

Nebraska

Arc of Nebraska, 2994

Camp Comeca & Retreat Center, 1225

Camp Floyd Rogers, 1226

Camp Kindle, 975, 1227

Center for Independent Living of Central Nebraska, 4299

Cooper Foundation, 2995

Easter Seals Nebraska, 1228

Grand Island VA Medical System, 5678

Kamp Kaleo, 1229

League of Human Dignity: Lincoln, 4300

League of Human Dignity: Norfolk, 4301

League of Human Dignity: Omaha, 4302

Lincoln Regional Office, 5679

Lincoln VA Medical Center, 5680

Mosaic, 2996

Mosaic Of De, 3995

Mosaic of Axtell Bethpage Village, 4303

Mosaic of Beatrice, 4304

Mosaic: Pontiac, 4076

Mosiac: York, 4305

National Camps for Blind Children, 1230

Nebraska Assistive Technology Partnership Nebraska Department of Education, 4845

Nebraska Employment Services, 6084

Nebraska Fair Employment Practice Agency, 6085

Nebraska Library Commission: Talking Book and Braille Service, 4846

Nebraska Vocational Rehabilitation Agency, 6086

Slosburg Family Charitable Trust, 2997

Union Pacific Foundation, 2998

VA Nebraska-Western Iowa Health Care System, 5681

YMCA Camp Kitaki, 1231

Nevada

ABC Union, ACE, ANLV, Vegas Western Cab, 5540

Camp Buck, 1232

Camp Lotsafun, 1233

Camp SignShine, 1234

CampCare, 1235

Carson City Center for Independent Living, 4306

EL Wiegand Foundation, 3000

Las Vegas Veterans Center, 5682

Las Vegas-Clark County Library District, 4847

Nell J Redfield Foundation, 3001

Nevada Equal Rights Commission Department Of Employment,Training & Rehabilitation, 6087

Nevada Governor's Committee on Employment of Persons with Disabilities, 6088

Nevada State Library and Archives, 4848

Northern Nevada Center for Independent Liv ing: Fallon, 4307

Reno Regional Office, 5683

Rural Center for Independent Living, 4308

Southern Nevada Center for Independent Living: North Las Vegas, 4309

Southern Nevada Center for Independent Living: Las Vegas, 4310

VA Sierra Nevada Healthcare System, 5684

VA Southern Nevada Healthcare System, 5685

William N Pennington Foundation, 3002

New Hampshire

Agnes M Lindsay Trust, 3003

Camp Allen, 1236

Camp Sno Mo, 1237

Fit for Work at Exeter Hospital, 6090

Foundation for Seacoast Health, 3004

Granite State Independent Living Foundation, 4311

Manchester Regional Office, 5686

Manchester VA Medical Center, 5687

National Guild of Hypnotists, 898

New Hampshire Employment Security, 6091

New Hampshire Fair Employment Practice Agency, 6092

New Hampshire Job Training Program Liaison, 6093

New Hampshire State Library: Talking Book Services, 4849

New Hampshire Veterans Centers, 5688

Windsor Mountain American Sign Language Camp Program, 1238

New Jersey

ARC of Gloucester County, 6095

ARC of Hunterdon County, The, 6096

ARC of Mercer County, 6097

ARC of Monmouth, 6098

Abilities Center of New Jersey, 6099

Abilities of Northwest New Jersey, 6100

Alliance Center for Independance, 4312

Alliance for Disabled in Action New Jersey, 6101

Alternatives for Growth: New Jersey, 6102

American Organization for Bodywork Therapies of Asia, 789

American Self-Help Clearinghouse, 792

Arc of Bergen and Passaic Counties, 6103

Arc of New Jersey, 3005

Arnold A Schwartz Foundation, 3006

Avis Rent A Car, 5542

Camden City Independent Living Center, 4313

Camp Chatterbox, 1239

Camp Dream Street, 1208, 1240

Camp Jotoni, 1241

Camp Lou Henry Hoover, 1242

Camp Merry Heart, 1243

Camp Nejeda, 1244

Camp Oakhurst, 1245

Camp Quality New Jersey, 1246

Camp Sun'N Fun, 1247

Camp Vacamas, 1248

Campbell Soup Foundation, 3007

Career Opportunity Development of New Jersey, 6104

Center for Educational Advancement New Jersey, 6105

Center for Independent Living: Long Branch, 4314

Center for Independent Living: South Jersey, 4315

Cerebral Palsy Association of Middlesex County, 6106

Children's Hopes & Dreams Wish Fulfillment Foundation, 3008

Children's Specialized Hospital Medical Library - Parent Resource Center, 4850

Christopher & Dana Reeve Foundation Resour ce Center, 4851

Community Foundation of New Jersey, 3009

DAWN Center for Independent Living, 4316

Davis Center, The, 827

Dial: Disabled Information Awareness & Liv ing, 4317

Disability Matters, 1856

Disability Rights New Jersey, 4318

Disabled American Veterans: Ocean County, 5689

East Orange Campus of the VA New Jersey Healthcare System, 5690

Easter Seal Society of New Jersey Highlands Workshop, 6107

Easter Seal of Ocean County, 6108

Easter Seals New Jersey, 6109

Eden Acres Administrative Services, 6110

Edison Sheltered Workshop, 6111

Eye Institute of New Jersey, 4852

FM Kirby Foundation, 3010

Family Resource Associates, 4319

Fannie E Rippel Foundation, 3011

First Occupational Center of New Jersey, 6112

Fund for New Jersey, 3012

Goodwill Industries of Southern New Jersey, 6113

Happiness Is Camping, 1249

Hausmann Industries, 6114

Heightened Independence and Progress: Hack ensack, 4320

Heightened Independence and Progress: Jers ey City, 4321

Jersey Cape Diagnostic Training & Opportunity Center, 6115

Lyons Campus of the VA New Jersey Healthcare System, 5691

Martin Luther Homes of Iowa, 4114

Merck Company Foundation, 3013

Mycoclonus Research Foundation, 4853

Nabisco Foundation, 3014

National Dissemination Center for Children and Youth with Disabilities (NICHCY), 895

National Information Center for Children, 899

New Jersey Center for Outreach and Service s for the Autism Community (COSAC), 4854

New Jersey Commission for the Blind and Visually Impaired, 6116

New Jersey Employment Service and Job Training Program Services, 6117

New Jersey Library for the Blind and Handicapped, 4855

New Jersey YMHA/YWHA Camps Milford, 1251

Newark Regional Office, 5692

Occupational Center of Hudson County, 6118

Occupational Center of Union County, 6119

Occupational Training Center of Burlington County, 6120

Occupational Training Center of Camden County, New Jersey, 6121

Ostberg Foundation, 3015

Pathways to Independence, Inc., 6122

Progressive Center for Independent Living, 4322

Progressive Center for Independent Living: Flemington, 4323

Project Freedom, 4324

Project Freedom: Hamilton, 4325

Project Freedom: Lawrence, 4326

Prudential Foundation, 3016

Robert Wood Johnson Foundation, 3017

Rolling Hills Country Day Camp, 1252

Round Lake Camp, 1253

Somerset Training and Employment Program, 6123

St. John of God Community Services Vocational Rehabilitation, 6124

Summit Camp, 1254

Total Living Center, 4327

United Cerebral Palsy Associations of New Jersey, 6125

Verizon Foundation, 3089

Victoria Foundation, 3018

West Essex Rehab Center, 6127

New Mexico

Ability Center, 4328

Adelante Development Center, 6128

Arc of New Mexico, 3019

CHOICES Center for Independent Living, 4330

Camp for Kids With Diabetes, 1255

Dental Amalgam Syndrome (DAMS) Newsletter, 4673

Family Voices, 843

Frost Foundation, 3020

Goodwill Industries of New Mexico, 6129

McCune Charitable Foundation, 3021

Mind, Body, Health Sciences, 880

New Mexico Employment Services and Job Training Liaison, 6130

New Mexico State Library for the Blind and Physically Handicapped, 4856

New Mexico State Veterans' Home, 5693

New Mexico Technology Assistance Program, 4331

New Mexico VA Healthcare System, 5694

New Vistas, 4332

RCI, 6131

San Juan Center for Independence, 4333

Santa Fe Community Foundation, 3022

Southwest Conference On Disability, 1874

Tohatchi Area of Opportunity & Services, 6132

Vocational Rehabilitation Agency, 6059, 6133

New York

ADA Camp Sunshine, 1256
AFB Center on Vision Loss, 3188
AIM Independent Living Center: Corning, 4334
AIM Independent Living Center: Elmira, 4335
ARISE, 4336
ARISE: Oneida, 4337
ARISE: Oswego, 4338
ARISE: Pulaski, 4339
AT&T Foundation, 3023
Abilities!, 762
Access to Independence of Cortland County , Inc., 4340
Action Toward Independence: Middletown, 4341
Action Toward Independence: Monticello, 4342
Advocacy Center, 764
Advocates for Children of New York, 766
Albany VA Medical Center: Samuel S Stratton, 5695
Albany Vet Center, 5696
Altman Foundation, 3024
Ambrose Monell Foundation, 3025
American Chai Trust, 3026
American Foundation for the Blind, 3028
American-Scandinavian Foundation, 2695
Andrew Heiskell Braille and Talking Book Library, 4857
Annual Conference on Dyslexia and Related Learning Disabilities, 1845
Arthur Ross Foundation, 3029
Artists Fellowship, 3030
Basic Facts on Study Abroad, 2699
Bath VA Medical Center, 5697
Bodman Foundation, 3031
Bronx Independent Living Services, 4343
Bronx VA Medical Center, 5698
Brooklyn Campus of the VA NY Harbor Healthcare System, 5699
Brooklyn Center for Independence of the Disabled, 4344
Brooklyn Home for Aged Men, 3032
Buffalo Regional Office Department of Veterans Affairs, 5700
Buffalo State (SUNY), 2701
Camp Abilities Brockport, 1257
Camp Glengarra, 1258
Camp Good Days and Special Times, 1259
Camp Huntington, 1260
Camp Independence, 1261
Camp Jened, 1262
Camp Mark Seven, 1263
Camp Northwood, 1264
Camp Ramapo, 1265
Camp Sisol, 1266
Camp Tova, 1267
Camp Venture, Inc., 1268
Camp Whitman on Seneca Lake, 1269
Canandiagua VA Medical Center, 5701
Cancer Care, 3033
Canine Helpers for the Handicapped, 812
Capital District Center for Independence, 4345
Casowasco Camp, Conference and Retreat Center, 1270
Castle Point Campus of the VA Hudson Valley Healthcare System, 5702
Catskill Center for Independence, 4346
Center for Community Alternatives, 4347
Center for Independence of the Disabled of New York, 4348
Center for Independence of the Disabled of New York, 4349
Center on Human Policy: School of Educatio n, 4858
Children's Tumor Foundation, 3034
Clay Center Adult Training Center, 6022
Clover Patch Camp, 1271
Commonwealth Fund, 3035
Community Foundation for Greater Buffalo, 3036
Community Foundation of Herkimer & Oneida Counties, 3037
Community Foundation of the Capitol Region, 3038
Comsearch: Broad Topics, 3039

DD Center/St Lukes: Roosevelt Hospital Center, 4350
DE French Foundation, 3040
Dana Foundation, 3041
David J Green Foundation, 3042
Diabetic Cruise Desk, 5522
Directions Unlimited Acccessible Tours, 5524
Disability Rights Bar Association, 831
Disabled Children's Relief Fund, 834
Disabled and Alone/Life Services for the Handicapped, 836
Double H Ranch, 1272
Easter Seals New York, 3043
Edna McConnel Clark Foundation, 3044
Edward John Noble Foundation, 3045
Ehrman Medical Library, 4860
Epilepsy Foundation of Long Island, 3046
Episcopal Charities, 3047
Esther A & Joseph Klingenstein Fund, 3048
FC Search, 3265
Father Drumgoole Connelly Summer Camp, 1273
Fay J Lindner Foundation, 3049
Fedcap Rehabilitation Services, 845
Finger Lakes Developmental Disabilities Service Office, 4861
Finger Lakes Independence Center, 4351
Ford Foundation, 3050
Fortis Foundation, 3051
Foundation 1000, 3274
Foundation Center, 3052
Foundation Center Library Services, 3053
Foundation Directories, 3275
Foundation Grants to Individuals, 3276
Foundation for Advancement in Cancer Therapy, 3054
Friends Academy Summer Camps, 1274
Friendship Circle Summer Camp, 1275
Gebbie Foundation, 3055
Gladys Brooks Foundation, 3056
Glickenhaus Foundation, 3057
Gow School Summer Programs, 1276
Grant Guides, 3278
Guide Dog Foundation for the Blind, 3058
Guide to Funding for International and Foreign Programs, 3279
Guide to US Foundations their Trustees, Officers and Donors, 3280
Harlem Independent Living Center, 4352
Hearst Foundations, 3059
Helen Keller International, 4862
Helen Keller National Center for Deaf - Blind Youths And Adults, 4863
Hemophilia Camp, 1277
Henry and Lucy Moses Fund, 3060
Herman Goldman Foundation, 3061
IBM Corporation, 2853
Independent Living, 3991, 4353
Institute for Basic Research in Developmental Disabilities, 4864
Institute for Visual Sciences, 4865
International Christian Youth Exchange, 2705
International Women's Health Coalition, 865
JGB Cassette Library International, 4866
JOBS VI and SAGE, 6135
John Edward Fowler Memorial Foundation, 2827
John H and Ethel G Nobel Charitable Trust, 2816
Just One Break (JOBS), 6136
Juvenile Diabetes Research Foundation International, 869
Kamp Kiwanis, 1278
Kenneth & Evelyn Lipper Foundation, 3062
Learning Disabilities Association of New York State, 872
Long Island Alzheimer's Foundation, 3063
Long Island Center for Independent Living, 4354
Louis and Anne Abrons Foundation, 3064
Maplebrook School, 1279
March of Dimes Birth Defects Foundation, 877
Margaret L Wendt Foundation, 3065
Marist Brothers Mid-Hudson Valley Camp, 1280
Massena Independent Living Center, 4355
Merrill Lynch & Company Foundation, 3066
Metzger-Price Fund, 3067
Milbank Foundation for Rehabilitation, 3068

Morgan Stanley Foundation, 3069
NADD, 1862
NASW-NYS Chapter, 1865
NYS Independent Living Council, 4356
Nassau County Office for the Physically Challenged, 4357
Nassau Library System, 4867
National Braille Association, 4868
National Business & Disability Council, 888
National Directory of Corporate Giving, 3284
National Foundation for Facial Reconstruction, 3071
National Hemophilia Foundation, 3072
National Organization on Disability, 901
Neisloss Family Foundation, 3073
New York City Campus of the VA NY Harbor Healthcare System, 5703
New York Community Trust, 3074
New York Foundation, 3075
New York Regional Office, 5704
New York State Department of Labor, 6137
New York State Talking Book & Braille Library, 4869
New York Therapeutic Riding Center-Equestrian, 907
North Country Center for Independent Livin g, 4358
Northern New York Community Foundation, 3076
Northern Regional Center for Independent Living: Watertown, 4359
Northern Regional Center for Independent L iving: Lowville, 4360
Northport VA Medical Center, 5705
Nurse Healers: Professional Associates International, 910
Opportunities for the Handicapped, 5857
Options for Independence: Auburn, 4361
PWSA (USA) Conference, 1868
Parkinson's Disease Foundation, 2892, 3077
Postgraduate Center for Mental Health, 4870
Putnam Independent Living Services, 4362
Rational Effectiveness Training Systems, 6138
Reader's Digest Foundation, 3078
Regional Center for Independent Living, 4363
Rehabilitation International, 921, 1871
Rehabilitation Research Library, 4871
Research to Prevent Blindness, 3079
Resource Center for Accessible Living, 4364
Resource Center for Independent Living, 4134, 4365
Resource Center for Independent Living, In c. (RCIL), 4135
Rita J and Stanley H Kaplan Foundation, 3080
Robert Sterling Clark Foundation, 3081
Rockland Independent Living Center, 4366
Skadden Fellowship Foundation, 3082
Southern Adirondack Independent Living, 4367
Southern Adirondack Independent Living Cen ter, 4368
Southern Tier Independence Center, 4369
Southwestern Independent Living Center, 4370
Special Education and Vocational Rehabilitation Agency: New York, 6139
St George's Society of New York, 3083
Stanley W Metcalf Foundation, 3084
State University of New York, 2719
State University of New York Health Sciences Center, 4872
Staten Island Center for Independent Living, Inc., 4371
Stonewall Community Foundation, 3085
Suffolk Cooperative Library System: Long Island Talking Book Library, 4873
Suffolk Independent Living Organization (SILO), 4372
Sunshine Campus, 1281
Surdna Foundation, 3086
Syracuse VA Medical Center, 5706
TSA National Conference, 1875
Taconic Resources for Independence, 4373
Tisch Foundation, 3087
Torah Alliance of Families of Kids with Disabilities, 5707
United Spinal Association, 4874

VA Hudson Valley Health Care System, 5708
VA Western NY Healthcare System, Batavia, 5709
VA Western NY Healthcare System, Buffalo, 5710
VISIONS Vacation Camp for the Blind, 1282
Van Ameringen Foundation, 3088
Wabash/Employability Center, 6011
Wagon Road Camp, 1283
Wallace Memorial Library, 4875
Westchester Disabled on the Move, 4374
Westchester Independent Living Center, 4375
Western New York Foundation, 3090
William T Grant Foundation, 3091
Xavier Society for the Blind, 4876
YAI: National Institute for People with Disabilities, 936
YMCA Camp Chingachgook on Lake George, 1284
YMCA Camp Weona, 1285

North Carolina

AHEAD, 1837
AHEAD Association, 760
American Herbalists Guild, 785
Arc of North Carolina, 3092
Asheville VA Medical Center Charles George, 5711
Association on Higher Education and Disability (AHEAD), 803
Bob & Kay Timberlake Foundation, 3093
Camp Carefree, 1286
Camp Carolina Trails, 1287
Camp New Hope, 1071, 1288
Camp Royall, 1289
Camp Sertoma, 1290
Camp Sky Ranch, 1291
Camp Tekoa UMC, 1292
Center for Universal Design, 818
Charlotte Vet Center, 5712
Davidson College, Office of Study Abroad, 2703
Disability Awareness Network, 4376
Disability Rights & Resources, 4377
Division Of Workforce Development, 6140
Duke Endowment, 3094
Durham VA Medical Center, 5713
Fayetteville VA Medical Center, 5573, 5714
First Union Foundation, 3095
Foundation for the Carolinas, 3096
Genova Diagnostics, 4877
Grayson Foundation, 2851
Iredell Vocational Workshop, 6141
Joy: A Shabazz Center for Independent Living, 4378
Kate B Reynolds Charitable Trust, 3097
Live Independently Networking Center, 4379
Live Independently Networking Center: Hickory, 4380
Mary Reynolds Babcock Foundation, 3098
Metametrix Clinical Laboratory, 879
National Association for Holistic Aromatherapy, 882
National Early Childhood Technical Assistance Center, 896
North Carolina Division of Services for the Blind, 6142
North Carolina Library for the Blind and Physically Handicapped, 4878
Older Americans Report, 3285
Pathways for the Future Center for Independent Living, 4381
Pediatric Rheumatology Clinic, 4879
Rowan County Vocational Workshop, 6143
Rutherford Vocational Workshop, 6144
SOAR Summer Adventures, 1293
Talisman Summer Camp, 1294
Transylvania Vocational Services, 6145
Triangle Community Foundation, 3099
United States Disabled Golf Association, 930
University of North Carolina at Chapel Hill: Neuroscience Research Building, 4880
Victory Junction Gang Camp, 1295
WG Hefner VA Medical Center Salisbury, 5715
Webster Enterprises Inc., 6148

Western Alliance Center for Independent Living, 4382
Western Alliance for Independent Living, 4383
Western Regional Vocational Rehabilitation Facility Clifford File, Jr., 6149
Winston-Salem Regional Office, 5716

North Dakota

Alex Stern Family Foundation, 3100
Arc of North Dakota, 3101
Camp Sioux, 1296
Dakota Center for Independent Living: Dickinson, 4384
Dakota Center for Independent Living: Bism arck, 4385
Fargo VA Medical Center, 5717
Fraser, 4386
Freedom Resource Center for Independent Li ving: Fargo, 4387
North Dakota Community Foundation, 3102
North Dakota Department of Labor, Human Ri ghts Division, 6150
North Dakota Employment Service and Job Training Program Liaison, 6151
North Dakota State Library Talking Book Services, 4881
North Dakota VA Regional Office Fargo Regional Office, 5718
North Dakota Vocational Rehabilitation Agency, 6152
Resource Center for Independent Living: Minot, 4388

Ohio

Ability Center of Greater Toledo, 4389
Ability Center of Greater Toledo: Defiance, 4390
Ability Center of Greater Toledo: Port Cli nton, 4391
Access Center for Independent Living, 4392
Akron Community Foundation, 3103
Albert G and Olive H Schlink Foundation, 3104
American Board of Clinical Metal Toxicology, 775
American Society for the Alexander Technique, 793
Antioch College, 2696
Arc of Ohio, 3106
Bahmann Foundation, 3107
CYO Day Camp: Wickliffe, 1297
Camp Allyn, 1298
Camp Cheerful, 1299
Camp Courageous, 1300
Camp Emanuel, 1301
Camp Happiness, 1302
Camp Ho Mita Koda, 1303
Camp Ko-Man-She, 1304
Camp Libbey, 1305
Camp Nuhop, 1306
Camp Quality Ohio, 1307
Camp Stepping Stone, 1308
Case Western Reserve University, 4882
Case Western Reserve University Northeast Ohio Multipurpose Arthritis Center, 4883
Center for Independent Living Options, 4393
Chillicothe VA Medical Center, 5719
Cincinnati Children's Hospital Medical Center, 4884
Cincinnati VA Medical Center, 5720
Cleveland FES Center, 4885
Cleveland Foundation, 3108
Cleveland Public Library, 4886
Cleveland Regional Office, 5721
Columbus Foundation and Affiliated Organizations, 3109
Cornucopia, 6153
Dayton VA Medical Center, 5722
Disabled American Veterans, 5557
Echoing Hills, 1309
Eleanora CU Alms Trust, 3110
Eva L And Joseph M Bruening Foundation, 3111
Fairfield Center for Disabilities and Cerebral Palsy, 4394

Fred & Lillian Deeks Memorial Foundation, 3112
GAR Foundation, 3113
George Gund Foundation, 3114
Great Oaks Joint Vocational School, 6154
Greater Cincinnati Foundation, 3115
HCR Manor Care Foundation, 3116
Harry C Moores Foundation, 3117
Hearth Day Treatment and Vocational Services, 6155
Helen Steiner Rice Foundation, 3118
Herbert W Hoover Foundation, 3119
Highbrook Lodge, 1310
Highland Unlimited Business Enterprises of CRI, 6156
Innovative Industries, 6014
Lake Erie College, 2709
Leo Yassenoff JCC Specialty Day Camp, 1311
Linking Employment, Abilities and Potentia l, 4395
Louis Stokes VA Medical Center Wade Park Campus, 5723
Mid-Ohio Board for an Independent Living Environment (MOBILE), 4396
Nationwide Foundation, 3120
Nordson Corporate Giving Program, 3121
Ohio Civil Rights Commission, 6157
Ohio Commission On Minority Health, 6158
Ohio Regional Library for the Blind and Physically Handicapped, 4887
Ohio Statewide Independent Living Council, 4397
Parker-Hannifin Foundation, 3122
Recreation Unlimited: Day Camp, 1312
Recreation Unlimited: Residential Camp, 1313
Recreation Unlimited: Respite Weekend Camp, 1314
Recreation Unlimited: Specialty Camp, 1315
Rehabilitation Service of North Central Oh io, 4398
Reinberger Foundation, 3123
Robert Campeau Family Foundation, 3124
Rotary Camp, 1316
Samuel W Bell Home for Sightless, 4399
Services for Independent Living, 4286, 4400
Sisler McFawn Foundation, 3125
Society for Equal Access: Independent Living Center, 4401
St. Augustine Rainbow Camp, 1317
Stark Community Foundation, 3126
State Library of Ohio: Talking Book Program, 4888
Stocker Foundation, 3127
Toledo Community Foundation, 3128
Triangle D Camp, 1318
United States Trager Association, 931
William J and Dorothy K O'Neill Foundation, 3129
YMCA Outdoor Center Campbell Gard, 1319
Youngstown Foundation, 3130

Oklahoma

Ability Resources, 4402
Anne and Henry Zarrow Foundation, 3131
Camp Classen YMCA, 1320
Camp Perfect Wings, 1321
Easter Seals Oklahoma, 1322
Green County Independent Living Resource Center, 4403
Jack C. Montgomery VA Medical Center, 5724
Jack C. Montomery VA Medical Center, 5725
Oklahoma City VA Medical Center, 5726
Oklahoma Department of Rehabilitation Services, 6160
Oklahoma Employment Services and Job Training Program Liaison, 6161
Oklahoma Governor's Committee on Employment of People with Disabilities, 6162
Oklahoma Library for the Blind & Physically Handicapped, 4889
Oklahoma Medical Research Foundation, 4890
Oklahoma Veterans Centers Vet Center, 5727
Oklahomans for Independent Living, 4404
Progressive Independence, 4405
Sarkeys Foundation, 3132

Tulsa City-County Library System: Outreach Services, 4891

Oregon

A Guide to International Educational Excha nge, 2692
Abilitree, 4406
Adventures Without Limits, 1323
Arc of Oregon, 3133
Bend Work Activity Center, 6163
Building Bridges: Including People with Disabilities in International Programs, 2702
Camp Latgawa Special Needs, Inc., 1324
Camp Magruder, 1325
Camp Starlight, 1326
Camp Taloali, 1327
DB-Link, 826
Eastern Oregon Center for Independent Living, 4407
Gales Creek Diabetes Camp, 1328
HASL Independent Abilities Center, 4408
Hull Park, 1329
Independent Living Resources, 4409
International Partnership for Service-Learning and Leadership, 2706
Jackson Foundation, 3135
Lane Community College, 2710
Laurel Hill Center, 4410
Leslie G Ehmann Trust, 3136
Meadowood Springs Speech and Hearing Camp, 1330
Mt Hood Kiwanis Camp, 1331
National College of Naturopathic Medicine, 890
Oregon Fair Employment Practice Agency, 6164
Oregon Health Sciences University, 5728
Oregon Health Sciences University, Elks' Children's Eye Clinic, 4892
Oregon Talking Book & Braille Services, 4893
People First of Oregon, 917
Portland Regional Office, 5729
Portland VA Medical Center, 5730
Progressive Options, 4411
Roseburg VA Medical Center, 5731
SPOKES Unlimited, 4412
Southern Oregon Rehabilitation Center & Cl inics, 5732
State of Oregon Office of Vocational Rehabilitation Service, 6165
Strength for the Journey, 1332
Sundial Special Vacations, 5535
Suttle Lake Camp, 1333
Swindells Charitable Foundation Trust, 2818
Talking Book & Braille Services Oregon State Library, 4894
Trips Inc., 5536
Umpqua Valley Disabilities Network, 4413
University of Oregon, 2721
Upward Bound Camp for Persons With, 1334
Vocational and Rehabilitation Agency: Oregon Commission for the Blind, 6167
Wallowa Lake Camp, 1335
World of Options, 2724
YWCA Camp Westwind, 1336

Pennsylvania

ACLD/An Association for Children and Adult s with Learning Disabilities: Greater Pittsburgh, 6168
Abilities in Motion, 4414
AccessToThePlanet, 5516
Accessible Journeys, 5517
Achieva, 1337
Air Products Foundation, 3137
Anthracite Region Center for Independent Living, 4415
Arc of Pennsylvania, 3138
Arcadia Foundation, 3139
Associated Services For The Blind & Visually Impaired, 4895
Beaver College, 2700
Brachial Plexus Palsy Foundation, 3140

Brian's House, 4416
Butler VA Medical Center, 5733
Camp AIM, 1338
Camp Akeela, 1339
Camp Can Do, 1340
Camp Dunmore ia, 1341
Camp Kweebec, 1342
Camp Lee Mar, 1343
Camp Ramah in the Poconos Education, Inc., 1344
Camp Setebaid, 1345
Camp Victory, 1130, 1347
Camp Wesley Woods: Northeastern Pennsylvan, 1348
Camp Woodlands, 1349
Carnegie Library of Pittsburgh Library for the Blind & Physically Handicapped, 4896
Coatesville VA Medical Center, 5734
Columbia Gas of Pennsylvania Corporate Giv ing, 3141
Community Resources for Independence, 4417
Community Resources for Independence, Inc., Bradford, 4418
Community Resources for Independence: Lewistown, 4419
Community Resources for Independence: Alto ona, 4420
Community Resources for Independence: Clar ion, 4421
Community Resources for Independence: Clea rfield, 4422
Community Resources for Independence: Herm itage, 4423
Community Resources for Independence: Lewi sburg, 4424
Community Resources for Independence: Oil City, 4425
Community Resources for Independence: Warr en, 4426
Community Resources for Independence: Well sboro, 4427
Connelly Foundation, 3142
Dolfinger-McMahon Foundation, 3143
Dragonfly Forest Summer Camp, 1350
Elling Camps, 1351
Elwyn, 839
Elwyn Delaware, 4695
Erie VA Medical Center, 5735
Free Library of Philadelphia: Library for the Blind and Physically Handicapped, 4897
Freedom Valley Disability Center, 4428
Guided Tour for Persons 17 & Over with Developmental and Physical Challenges, 5529
Handi Camp, 1352
Heinz Endowments, 3144
Henry L Hillman Foundation, 3145
Innabah Camps, 1353
Institute on Disabilities At Temple Univ., 4429
International University Partnerships, 2708
James E Van Zandt VA Medical Center, 5736
Jewish Healthcare Foundation of Pittsburgh, 3146
Juliet L Hillman Simonds Foundation, 3147
Learning Disabilities Association of Ameri ca, 871
Lebanon VA Medical Center, 5737
Lehigh Valley Center for Independent Living, 4430
Liberty Resources, 4431
Life and Independence for Today, 4432
Lions Camp Kirby, 1354
Mainstay Life Services Summer Program, 1355
New Jersey Camp Jaycee, 1250
Northeastern Pennsylvania Center for Independent Living, 4433
Oberkotter Foundation, 3148
Office of Vocational Rehabilitation, 6169
Outside In School Of Experiential, 1356
PECO Energy Company Contributions Program, 3149
PNC Bank Foundation, 3150
Pennsylvania College of Optometry Eye Institute, 4898
Pennsylvania Employment Services and Job Training, 6170
Pennsylvania Governor's Committee on Employment of Disabled Persons, 6171

Pennsylvania Human Relations Commission Agency, 6172
Pennsylvania Veterans Centers, 5738
Phelps School Summer School, 1357
Philadelphia Foundation, 3151
Philadelphia Regional Office and Insurance Center, 5739
Philadelphia VA Medical Center, 5740
Pittsburgh Foundation, 3152
Pittsburgh Regional Office, 5741
Reading Rehabilitation Hospital, 4899
Sequanota Lutheran Conference Center and Camp, 1358
Shenango Valley Foundation, 3153
South Central Pennsylvania Center for Inde pendence Living, 4434
Staunton Farm Foundation, 3154
Stewart Huston Charitable Trust, 3155
Teleflex Foundation, 3156
Three Rivers Center for Independent Living: New Castle, 4435
Three Rivers Center for Independent Livi ng: Washington, 4436
Three Rivers Center for Independent Living, 4116, 4437
Tri-County Patriots for Independent Living, 4438
USX Foundation, 3157
VA Pittsburgh Healthcare System, University Drive Division, 5742
VA Pittsburgh Healthcare System, Highland Drive Division, 5743
Variety Club Camp & Developmental, 1359
Vocational and Rehabilitation Agency, 5891, 5905, 5958, 5958, 5964, 5986, 6010, 6044, 6072, 6089, 6094, 6126, 6134, 6146, 6159, 6166, 6174
Voices for Independence, 4439
Wilkes-Barre VA Medical Center, 5744
William B Dietrich Foundation, 3158
William Talbott Hillman Foundation, 3159
William V and Catherine A McKinney Charitable Foundation, 3160
YMCA Camp Fitch, 1360

Rhode Island

Arc South County Chapter, 3161
Arc of Blackstone, 4440
Arc of Blackstone Valley, 3162
Arc of Northern Rhode Island, 3163
Camp Mauchatea, 1361
Camp Ruggles, 1362
Canonicus Camp, 1363
Champlin Foundations, 3164
CranstonArc, 3165
Department of Veterans Affairs Regional Office - Vocational Rehab Division, 5555
Down Syndrome Society of Rhode Island, 3166
Frank Olean Center, 3167
Franklin Court Assisted Living, 4441
Goodwill Industries of RI, 6176
Groden Center, 6177
Hasbro Children's Hospital Asthma Camp, 1364
Horace A Kimball and S Ella Kimball Foundation, 3168
IN-SIGHT Independent Living, 4442
James L. Maher Center, 3169
Newport County Chapter of Retarded Citizens, 6178
Ocean State Center for Independent Living, 4443
Office Of Library & Information Services for the Blind and Physically Handicapped, 4900
Office of Rehabilitation Services, 4444, 6179
PARI Independent Living Center, 4445
Providence Regional Office, 5745
Providence VA Medical Center, 5746
Rhode Island Arc, 3171
Rhode Island Foundation, 3172
Talking Books Plus, 4901

South Carolina

Arc of South Carolina, 3173
Burnt Gin Camp, 1365

Camp Adam Fisher, 1366
Camp Debbie Lou, 1367
Camp Gravatt, 1368
Camp Spearhead, 1369
Center for Disability Resources, 816, 3174
Colonial Life and Accident Insurance Company
    Contributions Program, 3175
Columbia Disability Action Center, 4446
Columbia Regional Office, 5747
DREAMMS for Kids, 4859
Disability Action Center, 4447
Graham Street Community Resources, 4448
Medical University of South Carolina Arthritis
    Clinical/Research Center, 4902
Ralph H Johnson VA Medical Center, 5748
South Carolina Employment Security Commission
    South Carolina Center, 6181
South Carolina Governor's Committee on
    Employment of the Handicapped, 6182
South Carolina Independent Living Council, 4449
South Carolina State Library, 4903
South Carolina Vocational Rehabilitation
    Department, 6183
Vocational and Rehabilitation Agency:
    Commission for the Blind, 6184
Walton Options for Independent Living: Nor th
    Augusta, 4450
William Jennings Bryan Dorn VA Medical Center,
    5749

South Dakota

Adjustment Training Center, 4451
Black Hills Workshop & Training Center, 4452
Camp Friendship, 1202, 1370
Camp Gilbert, 1371
Dell Rapids Sportsmens Club, 5521
Native American Advocacy Program for Perso ns
    with Disabilities, 4454
NeSoDak, 1372
Prairie Freedom Center for Independent Living:
    Sioux Falls, 4455
Prairie Freedom Center for Independent Li ving:
    Madison, 4456
Prairie Freedom Center for Independent Liv ing:
    Yankton, 4457
Royal C Johnson Veterans Memorial Medical
    Center, 5750
Sioux Falls Regional Office, 5751
South Dakota Assistive Technology Project:
    DakotaLink, 4458
South Dakota Governor's Advisory Committee on
    Employment of the Disabled, 6185
South Dakota State Library, 4904
South Dakota State Vocational Rehabilitati on,
    6186
South Dakota Workforce Investment Act Training
    Programs, 6187
Vocational and Rehabilitation Agency: Divi sion of
    Services to the Blind/Visually Impaired, 6188
Western Resources for dis-ABLED Independence,
    4459

Tennessee

ABD Winter Conference, 1831
ACM Lifting Lives Music Camp, 1373
All Days Are Happy Days Summer Camp, 1374
Alliance for Technology Access, 767
Alvin C York VA Medical Center, 5752
American Board of Disability Analysts Annual
    Conference, 1844
American Board of Professional Disability
    Consultants, 776
Arc of Anderson County, 3176
Arc of Davidson County, 3177
Arc of Hamilton County, 3178
Arc of Tennessee, 3179
Arc of Washington County, 3180
Arc of Williamson County, 3181
Arc-Diversified, 3182
Benwood Foundation, 3183
Bill Rice Ranch, 1375

Camp Discovery, 1066, 1376
Camp Koinonia, 1377
Camp Okawehna, 1378
Camp Sugar Falls, 1379
Center for Independent Living of Middle
    Tennessee, 4460
Community Foundation of Greater Chattanooga,
    3184
DisAbility Resource Center: Knoxville, 4461
Division of Rehabilitative Services, 6189
Easter Seals Tennessee Camping Program, 1380
Education and Auditory Research Foundation,
    3185
Indian Creek Camp, 1381
International Paper Company Foundation, 3186
Jackson Center for Independent Living, 4462
Jackson Independent Living Center, 4262
Joint Conference with ABMPP Annual Conference,
    1859
LeBonheur Cardiac Kids Camp, 1382
Memphis Center for Independent Living, 4463
Memphis VA Medical Center, 5753
Mountain Home VA Medical Center James H
    Quillen VA Medical Center, 5754
Nasheville Regional Office, 5755
Nashville VA Medical Center, 5756
Paddy Rossbach Youth Camp, 1383
Tennessee Department of Labor: Job Training
    Program Liaison, 6190
Tennessee Fair Employment Practice Agency, 6191
Tennessee Library for the Blind and Physically
    Handicapped, 4905
Tennessee Technology Access Program (TTAP),
    4464
Tri-State Resource and Advocacy Corporation,
    4465
Vision Foundation, 2954

Texas

ABLE Center for Independent Living, 4466
Abell-Hangar Foundation, 3189
Albert & Bessie Mae Kronkosky Charitable
    Foundation, 3190
Amarillo VA Healthcare System, 5757
Amarillo Vet Center, 5758
American Botanical Council, 777
American Express Foundation, 3027
Arc of Texas, The, 3191
Army and Air Force Exchange Services, 2697
Attention Deficit Disorders Association, Southern
    Region: Annual Conference, 1848
Austin Resource Center for Independent Living,
    4467
Austin Resource Center: Round Rock, 4468
Austin Resource Center: San Marcos, 4469
BA and Elinor Steinhagen Benevolent Trust, 3192
Baylor College of Medicine Birth Defects Center,
    4906
Baylor College of Medicine: Cullen Eye Institute,
    4907
Brazoria County Center For Independent Living,
    4470
Brown Foundation, 3193
Brown-Heatly Library, 4908
C-CAD Center of United Cerebral Palsy of
    Metropolitan Dallas, 6192
CH Foundation, 3195
Camp Be An Angel, 1384
Camp CAMP, 1385
Camp Cpals, 1386
Camp John Marc, 1387
Camp Neuron, 1388
Camp Quality Texas, 1389
Camp Spike 'n' Wave, 1390
Camp Summit, 1391
Camp Sweeney, 1392
Camp for All, 1393
Center for Research on Women with Disabilities,
    4909
Centre, The, 4471
Children's Association for Maximum Potenti al
    Summer Camp, 1394
Christian Education for the Blind, 4910

Cockrell Foundation, 3196
Communication Service for the Deaf: Rapid City,
    4453
Communities Foundation of Texas, 3197
Community Foundation of North Texas, 3198
Crockett Resource Center for Independent Living,
    4472
Cullen Foundation, 3199
Curtis & Doris K Hankamer Foundation, 3200
Dallas Academy, 1395
Dallas Foundation, 3201
David D & Nona S Payne Foundation, 3202
El Paso Natural Gas Foundation, 3203
El Paso VA Healthcare Center, 5759
Epilepsy Foundation: Central and South Texas,
    3205
Growing Together Diabetes Camp, 1396
Handbook of Career Planning for Students with
    Special Needs, 6193
Harris and Eliza Kempner Fund, 3206
Hill School of Fort Worth, 1397
Hillcrest Foundation, 3207
Hoblitzelle Foundation, 3208
Houston Center for Independent Living, 4473
Houston Endowment, 3209
Houston Public Library: Access Center, 4911
Houston Regional Office, 5760
Independent Living Research Utilization Project,
    4475
John G & Marie Stella Kennedy Memorial
    Foundation, 3210
John S Dunn Research Foundation, 3211
Kamp Kaleidoscope, 1398
LIFE/ Run Centers for Independent Living, 4476
LIFE: Fort Hall, 4049
Lisle, 2712
Lola Wright Foundation, 3212
Lowe's Syndrome Conference, 1860
Meadows Foundation, 3213
Michael E. Debakey VA Medical Center, 5761
Moody Foundation, 3214
Office for Students with Disabilities, University of
    Texas at Arlington, 4477
Palestine Resource Center for Independent Living,
    4478
Panhandle Action Center for Independent Living
    Skills, 4479
Pearle Vision Foundation, 3215
REACH of Dallas Resource Center on Independent
    Living, 4480
REACH of Denton Resource Center on
    Independent Living, 4481
REACH of Fort Worth Resource Center on Ind
    ependent Living, 4482
RISE-Resource: Information, Support and
    Empowerment, 4483
SAILS, 4484
San Antonio Area Foundation, 3216
Shell Oil Company Foundation, 3217
South Texas Charitable Foundation, 3218
South Texas Veterans Healthcare System, 5762
Sterling-Turner Foundation, 3219
TLL Temple Foundation, 3220
Talking Book Program/Texas State Library, 4912
Texas Department of Assistive and Rehabili tative
    Services, 4485
Texas Employment Services and Job Training
    Program Liaison, 6194
Texas Lions Camp, 1399
University of Texas Southwestern Medical
    Center/Allergy & Immunology, 4913
University of Texas at Austin Library, 4914
VA North Texas Health Veterans Affairs Car e
    System: Dallas VA Medical Center, 5763
VOLAR Center for Independent Living, 4486
Valley Association for Independent Living (VAIL),
    4487
Valley Association for Independent Living:
    Harlingen, 4488
Vocational and Rehabilitation Agency: State
    Rehabilitation Commission, 5906, 6195
Waco Regional Office, 5764
West Texas VA Healthcare System, 5765
William Stamps Farish Fund, 3221

Utah

Active Re-Entry, 4489
Active Re-Entry: Vernal, 4490
Camp Giddy-Up, 1400
Camp Hobe, 1401
Camp Kostopulos, 1402
Camp Nah-Nah-Mah, 1403
Camp Vision, 1404
Camp X-Treme, 1405
Central Utah Independent Living Center, 4491
Discovery Camps, 1406
FCYD Camp, 1407
Marriner S Eccles Foundation, 3223
OPTIONS for Independence, 4492
OPTIONS for Independence: Brigham Satellit e, 4493
Overnight Camps, 1408
Questar Corporation Contributions Program, 3224
Red Rock Center for Independence, 4494
Utah Assistive Technology Program (UTAP) Utah State University, 4496
Utah Division of Veterans Affairs, 5766
Utah Employment Services, 6196
Utah Governor's Committee on Employment of the Handicapped, 6197
Utah Independent Living Center, 4497
Utah Independent Living Center: Minersville, 4498
Utah Independent Living Center: Tooele, 4499
Utah State Library Division: Program for the Blind and Disabled, 4915
Utah Veterans Centers, 6198
VA Salt Lake City Healthcare System, 5767

Vermont

Camp Betsey Cox, 1409
Camp Thorpe, 1410
Silver Towers Camp, 1411
State of Vermont Department of Disabilitie s, Aging and Independent Living, 6201
Vermont Assistive Technology Program, 4500
Vermont Center for Independent Living: Ben nington, 4501
Vermont Center for Independent Living: Chi ttenden, 4502
Vermont Center for Independent Living: Mon tpelier, 4503
Vermont Community Foundation, 3225
Vermont Department of Libraries - Special Services Unit, 4916
Vermont Department of Libraries -Special Services Unit, 4917
Vermont Employment Services and Job Training, 6202
Vermont Governor's Committee on Employment of People with Disabilities, 6203
Vermont VA Regional Office Center, 5768
Vermont Veterans Centers, 5769

Virginia

ACA Annual Conference, 1832
ACB Annual Convention, 1833
ACS Federal Healthcare, 759
ADA Annual Scientific Sessions, 1834
ADA Camp Grenada, 1412
AER Annual International Conference, 1835
Access Independence, 4504
Access Services, 4918
Adventure Camp, 1413
Adventure Day Camp, 1414
Alexandria Community Y Head Start, 6204
Alexandria Library Talking Book Service, 4919
American Chiropractic Association, 779
American Counseling Association, 782
American National Bank and Trust Company, 2865
Appalachian Independence Center, 4505
Arc of Virginia, 3226
Arlington County Department of Libraries, 4920
Blue Ridge Independent Living Center, 4506
Blue Ridge Independent Living Center: Christianburg, 4507

Blue Ridge Independent Living Center: Low Moor, 4508
Braille Circulating Library for the Blind, 4921
Brain Injury Association of America, 808
Camp Dickenson, 1415
Camp Easter Seals Virginia, 1416
Camp Foundation, 3227
Camp Holiday Trails, 1417
Camp Loud And Clear, 1418
Camp Virginia Jaycee, 1419
Camps for Children & Teens with Diabetes, 1420
Central Rappahannock Regional Library, 4922
Civitan Acres for the Disabled, 1421
Clinch Independent Living Services, 4509
Community Foundation of Richmond & Central Virginia, 3228
Council For Exceptional Children, 825
Council for Exceptional Children, 4923
Council for Exceptional Children Annual Convention and Expo, 1855
Department Of Rehabilitative Services, 6205
Developmental Training Services, 5882
Didlake, 6206
Disability Funders Network, 830
Disability Resource Center, 4016, 4510
ENDependence Center of Northern Virginia, 4511
Equal Access Center for Independence, 4512
From the State Capitals: Public Health, 3277
Hampton VA Medical Center, 5770
Hunter Holmes McGuire VA Medical Center, 5771
Independence Empowerment Center, 4513
Independence Resource Center, 4514
Independent Living Center Network: Department of the Visually Handicapped, 4515
International Chiropractors Association, 863
International Student Exchange Programs (I SEP), 2707
James Branch Cabell Library, 4924
John Randolph Foundation, 3229
Junction Center for Independent Living, 4516
Junction Center for Independent Living: Du ffield, 4517
Learning Services: Shenandoah, 6207
Loudoun County Special Recreation Programs, 1422
Lynchburg Area Center for Independent Living, 4518
Makemie Woods Camp, 1423
Mental Health America, 878
NISH, 6208
National Association of State Directors of Developmental Disabilities Services (NASDDDS), 887
National Rehabilitation Association (NRA), 902
National Vaccine Information Center, 904
Newport News Public Library System, 4925
Norfolk Foundation, 3230
Northern Virginia Resource Center for Deaf and Hard of Hearing Persons, 4926
Oakland School & Camp, 1424
Peidmont Independent Living Center, 4519
Peninsula Center for Independent Living, 4520
Piedmont Independent Living Center, 4521
RESNA Annual Conference, 1870
Rehabiliation Engineering Center for Personal Licensed Transportation, 5549
Resources for Independent Living, 3956, 4522
Richmond Research Training Center, 6209
Roanoke City Public Library System, 4927
Roanoke Regional Office, 5772
Robey W Estes Family Foundation, 3231
Salem VA Medical Center, 5773
ServiceSource, 6210
Sheltered Occupational Center of Virginia, 6211
Source-APTA Audio Conference, 1873
Staunton Public Library Talking Book Center, 4928
Technology and Media Division, 928
University of Virginia Health System General Clinical Research Group, 4929
Valley Associates for Independent Living (VAIL), 4523
Valley Associates for Independent Living: Lexington, 4524

Virginia Autism Resource Center, 4930
Virginia Beach Foundation, 3232
Virginia Beach Public Library Special Services Library, 4931
Virginia Chapter of the Arthtitis Foundation, 4932
Virginia Department of Veterans Services, 5774
Virginia State Library for the Visually and Physically Handicapped, 4933
Vocational and Rehabilitation Agency: Department for the Blind/Visually Impaired, 6147, 6175, 6180, 6180, 6212
Woodrow Wilson Rehabilitation Center Training Program, 4525

Washington

Alliance for People with Disabilities: Sea ttle, 4526
Alliance of People with Disabilities: Redmond, 4527
American Disability Association, 783
Arc of Washington State, 3233
Bastyr University Natural Health Clinic, 804
Ben B Cheney Foundation, 3234
Camp Fun in the Sun, 1425
Camp Killoqua, 1426
Camp Prime Time, 1427
Camp Volasuca, 1428
Coalition of Responsible Disabled, 4528
Community Foundation of North Central Washington, 3235
Community Services for the Blind and Parti ally Sighted Store: Sight Connection, 4529
Department of Services for the Blind National Business & Disability Council, 6214
DisAbility Resource Connection: Everett, 4530
Division of Developmental Disabilities: De partment of Social & Health Services, 6215
Easter Seals Camp Stand by Me, 1429
Glaser Progress Foundation, 3236
Greater Tacoma Community Foundation, 3237
Inland Northwest Community Foundation, 3238
Jonathan M Wainwright Memorial VA Medical Center, 5775
Kitsap Community Resources, 4531
Medina Foundation, 3239
Meridian Valley Clinical Laboratory, 4934
Norcliffe Foundation, 3240
Northwest Kiwanis Camp, 1430
Ophthalmic Research Laboratory Eye Institute/First Hill Campus, 4935
SL Start and Associates, 6216
School of Piano Technology for the Blind, 6217
Seattle Regional Office, 5776
Spokane VA Medical Center, 5777
Stewardship Foundation, 3241
Tacoma Area Coalition of Individuals with Disabilities, 4532
VA Puget Sound Health Care System, 5778
Vocational and Rehabilitation Agency: Division of Vocational Rehabilitation, 5946, 6200, 6218, 6218
Washington Talking Book and Braille Library, 4936
Western Washington University, 2722
Westside Parents Work Activity Center, 5988
Weyerhaeuser Company Foundation, 3242
Wheelchair Getaways, 5538
Wheelchair Getaways Wheelchair/Scooter Accessible Van Rentals, 5550
YMCA Camp Orkila, 1431

West Virginia

Appalachian Center for Independent Living, 4533
Appalachian Center for Independent Living: Spencer, 4534
Arc Of West Virginia, The, 3243
Bernard McDonough Foundation, 3244
Cabell County Public Library/Talking Book Department/Subregional Library for the Blind, 4937
Division of Rehabilitation Services: Staff Library, 4938

Huntington Regional Office, 5779
Huntington VA Medical Center, 5780
Institute for Scientific Research, 859
Job Accommodation Network, 867
Kanawha County Public Library, 4939
Louis A Johnson VA Medical Center, 5781
Martinsburg VA Medical Center, 5782
Mountain State Center for Independent Living, 4535
Mountain State Center for Independent Living, 4536
Mountaineer Spina Bifida Camp, 1432
Northern West Virginia Center for Independent Living, 4537
Ohio County Public Library Services for the Blind and Physically Handicapped, 4940
Rehabilitation Technology Association Conference, 1872
Ronald McDonald House, 924
Talking Book Department, Parkersburg and Wood County Public Library, 4941
US Department Veterans Affairs Beckley Vet Center, 5783
West Virginia Autism Training Center, 4942
West Virginia Division of Rehabilitation Services, 6219
West Virginia Employment Services and Job Training Programs Liaison, 6220
West Virginia Library Commission, 4943
West Virginia School for the Blind Library, 4944
West Virginia Vocational Rehabilitation, 6221
YMCA Camp Horseshoe, 1433

Wisconsin

AACRC Annual Meeting, 1827
Able Trek Tours, 5515
American Academy for Cerebral Palsy and Developmental Medicine Annual Conference, 1843
American Association of Children's Residential Centers, 771

Arc of Dunn County, 3245
Arc of Eau Claire, 3246
Arc of Fox Cities, 3247
Arc of Racine County, 3248
Arc of Wisconsin Disability Association, 3249
Arc-Dane County, 3250
Association of Educational Therapists, 801
Brown County Library, 4945
Camp Kee-B-Waw, 1434
Camp Needlepoint, 1435
Center for Independent Living of Western Wisconsin, 4538
Clement J Zablocki VA Medical Center, 5784
Easter Seal Camp Wawbeek, 1436
Eye Institute of the Medical College of Wisconsin and Froedtert Clinic, 4946
Faye McBeath Foundation, 3251
Helen Bader Foundation, 3252
Independence First, 4539
Independence First: West Bend, 4540
Inspiration Ministries, 4541
Johnson Controls Foundation, 3253
Lutherdale Bible Camp, 1437
Lynde and Harry Bradley Foundation, 3254
Mid-State Independent Living Consultants: Wausau, 4542
Mid-state Independent Living Consultants: Stevens Point, 4543
Milwaukee Foundation, 3255
North Country Independent Living, 4544
North Country Independent Living: Ashland, 4545
Northwestern Mutual Life Foundation, 3256
Options for Independent Living, 4546
Options for Independent Living: Fox Valley, 4547
Phantom Lake YMCA Camp, 1438
SB Waterman & E Blade Charitable Foundation, 3258
Society's Assets: Elkhorn, 4548
Society's Assets: Kenosha, 4549
Society's Assets: Racine, 4550
Timbertop Nature Adventure Camp, 1439
Tomah VA Medical Center, 5785
Trace Research and Development Center, 4947

Vocational and Rehabilitation: State of Wisconsin, 6222
William S Middleton Memorial VA Hospital Center, 5786
Wisconsin Badger Camp, 1440
Wisconsin Elks/Easter Seals Respite Camp, 1441
Wisconsin Lions Camp, 1442
Wisconsin Regional Library for the Blind & Physically Handicapped, 4948
Wisconsin VA Regional Office, 5787
Wisconson Badger Camp, 1443

Wyoming

Arc of Natrona County, 3259
Camp Hope, 1444
Casper Vet Center, 5788
Cheyenne VA Medical Center, 5789
Division of Vocational Rehabilitation of Wyoming, 6223
Eagle View Ranch, 1445
RENEW: Gillette, 4551
RENEW: Rehabilitation Enterprises of North Eastern Wyoming, 4552
Rehabilitation Enterprises of North Easter n Wyoming: Newcastle, 4553
Sheridan VA Medical Center, 5790
Vocational Rehabilitation, Division of Department of Workforce Services, 6224
Wyoming Department of Employment Unemployment Insurance, 6225
Wyoming Governor's Committee on Employment of the Handicapped, 6226
Wyoming Services for Independent Living, 4554
Wyoming Services for the Visually Impaired, 4949
Wyoming's New Options in Technology (WYNOT) - University of Wyoming, 4950

AIDS

AIDS Alert, 8614
AIDS Legal Council of Chicago, 4555
AIDS Sourcebook, 8427
AIDS United, 8245
AIDS and Other Manifestations of HIV Infection, 8428
AIDS in the Twenty-First Century: Disease and Globalization, 8429
AIDS: The Official Journal of the International AIDS Society, 8596
AIDSLAW of Louisiana, 4556
Camp Heartland, 1203
Camp Kindle, 1227
Caremark Healthcare Services, 6822
Children with Disabilities, 5199
FC Search, 3265
Glaser Progress Foundation, 3236
Guide to Living with HIV Infection: Developed at the Johns Hopkins AIDS Clinic, 8479
HEAL: Health Education AIDS Liaison, 2028
HIV Infection and Developmental Disabilities, 2409
Harborview Medical Center, Low Vision Aid Clinic, 7200
Legal Action Center, 4566
Legislative Network for Nurses, 4618
Levi Strauss Foundation, 2775
Living Well with Chronic Fatigue Syndrome and Fibromyalgia, 8507
Living Well with HIV and AIDS, 8508
Miami VA Medical Center, 5606
Michigan Association for Deaf, and Hard of Hearing, 3530
Michigan Protection & Advocacy Service, 3543
National AIDS Hotline, 8660
No Longer Immune: A Counselor's Guide to AIDS, 2473
POZ Magazine, 8608
Penitent, with Roses: An HIV+ Mother Reflects, 8554
Questions and Answers: The ADA and Persons with HIV/AIDS, 8561
Sight by Touch, 9130
Strength for the Journey, 1332, 8404
Vinfen Corporation, 6988
Visiting Nurse Association of North Shore, 6989

Accupressure

Acupressure Institute, 763

Aging

ADHD: What Can We Do?, 7850
ARC Of Southeast Los Angeles-Southeast Industries, 6546
Activities in Action, 7493
Administration on Aging, 3287
Aging & Vision News, 7527
Aging Brain, 2290
Aging News Alert, 7528, 7534
Aging Services of California, 7439
Aging Services of Michigan, 7440
Aging Services of South Carolina, 7441
Aging Services of Washington, 7442
Aging and Disability Services Division, 3593
Aging and Disability: Crossing Network Lines, 2291
Aging and Family Therapy: Practitioner Perspectives on Golden Pond, 7496
Aging and Rehabilitation II: The State of the Practice, 2292
Aging and Vision News, 7529
Aging and Vision: Declarations of Independence, 9118
Aging in America, 7443
Aging in Stride, 7497
Aging in the Designed Environment, 7498
Aging with a Disability, 7499
Alabama Department of Senior Services, 3312

Alabama VA Benefits Regional Office -Montgomery, 5562
Alaska Commission on Aging, 3322
Albany County Department for Aging and Albany Social Services, 3637
Albany VA Medical Center: Samuel S Stratton, 5695
Aleda E Lutz VA Medical Center, 5656
Alexandria VA Medical Center, 5639
Alvin C York VA Medical Center, 5752
Amarillo VA Healthcare System, 5757
American Association of Homes and Services for the Aging, 7447
American Wheelchair Bowling Association, 8223
Amyotrophic Lateral Sclerosis: A Guide for Patients and Families, 8437
Area Agency on Aging of Southwest Arkansas, 7548
Area Agency on Aging: Region One, 7549
Arizona Association of Homes and Housing for the Aging, 7451
Arizona Division of Aging and Adult Services, 3334
Arkansas Division of Aging & Adult Services, 3343
Asheville VA Medical Center Charles George, 5711
Association for International Practical Training, 2698
Association of Ohio Philanthropic Homes, Housing and Services for the Aging, 7453
Atlanta Regional Office, 5609
Atlanta VA Medical Center, 5610
Attention Getter, 1667
Attention Teens, 1668
Augusta VA Medical Center, 5611
Baltimore Regional Office, 5644
Baltimore VA Medical Center, 5645
Bath VA Medical Center, 5697
Battle Creek VA Medical Center, 5657
Bay Pines VA Medical Center, 5603
Biloxi/Gulfport VA Medical Center, 5667
Blindness, A Family Matter, 9119
Boise Regional Office, 5617
Boise VA Medical Center, 5618
Boston VA Regional Office, 5650
Bronx VA Medical Center, 5698
Brooklyn Campus of the VA NY Harbor Healthcare System, 5699
Buffalo Regional Office Department of Veterans Affairs, 5700
Building Blocks: Foundations for Learning for Young Blind and Visually Impaired Children, 9120
Butler VA Medical Center, 5733
CARF International (Commission on Accreditation of Rehabilitation Facilities), 2023
CARF Rehabilitation Accreditation Commission, 810
California Department of Aging, 3351
Can America Afford to Grow Old?, 4584
Canandiagua VA Medical Center, 5701
Caring for Those You Love: A Guide to Compassionate Care for the Aged, 7501
Carl T Hayden VA Medical Center, 5569
Carl Vinson VA Medical Center, 5612
Castle Point Campus of the VA Hudson Valley Healthcare System, 5702
Center for Disability and Elder Law, Inc., 4557
Change Your Brain, Change Your Life: The Breakthrough Program for Conquering Depression, 7740
Cheyenne VA Medical Center, 5789
Children of Aging Parents, 7455
Chillicothe VA Medical Center, 5719
Cincinnati VA Medical Center, 5720
Clement J Zablocki VA Medical Center, 5784
Cleveland Regional Office, 5721
Coatesville VA Medical Center, 5734
Colmery-O'Neil VA Medical Center, 5632
Colorado Association of Homes and Services for the Aging, 7456
Colorado Department of Aging & Adult Services, 3366
Colorado Springs Independence Center, 3971

Colorado/Wyoming VA Medical Center, 5589
Columbia Foundation, 2927
Columbia Regional Office, 5747
Communication Skills for Working with Elders, 2347
Complementary Alternative Medicine and Multiple Sclerosis, 8462
Connecticut Commission on Aging, 3375
Coping and Caring: Living with Alzheimer's Disease, 7503
Court-Related Needs of the Elderly and Persons with Disabilities, 4591
CurePSP Magazine, 8603
DSHS/Aging & Adult Disability Services Administration, 3829
Dayton VA Medical Center, 5722
Deaf-Blind Division of the National Federation of the Blind, 8827
Delaware Department of Health and Social Services, 3382
Delaware VA Regional Office, 5596
Denver VA Medical Center, 5590
Des Moines VA Medical Center, 5627
Des Moines VA Regional Office, 5628
District of Columbia Office on Aging, 3391
Duchenne Muscular Dystrophy, 8469
Durham VA Medical Center, 5713
Dwight D Eisenhower VA Medical Center, 5633
East Orange Campus of the VA New Jersey Healthcare System, 5690
Edith Nourse Rogers Memorial Veterans Hospital, 5651
Edward Hines Jr Hospital, 5619
Ehrman Medical Library, 4860
El Paso VA Healthcare Center, 5759
Elder Abuse and Mistreatment, 7504
ElderLawAnswers.com, 4602
Elgin Training Center, 6837
Employment for Individuals with Asperger Syndrome or Non-Verbal Learning Disability, 8736
Enabling News, 7530
Erie VA Medical Center, 5735
Eugene J Towbin Healthcare Center, 5572
Explore Your Options, 7505
Facilitating Self-Care Practices in the Elderly, 2397
Falling in Old Age, 7506
Family Intervention Guide to Mental Illness, 7507
Family-Guided Activity-Based Intervention for Toddlers & Infants, 5329
Fanlight Productions, 25
Fargo VA Medical Center, 5717
Fayetteville VA Medical Center, 5573, 5714
Federation for Children with Special Needs, 846
Films & Videos on Aging and Sensory Change, 5332
Florida Adult Services, 3405
Fort Howard VA Medical Center, 5646
Foundations of Orientation and Mobility, 8956
Gainesville Division, North Florida/South Georgia Veterans Healthcare System, 5604
Georgia Association of Homes and Services for the Aging, 7458
Georgia Department of Aging, 3421
Gerontology: Abstracts in Social Gerontology, 7524
Getting Better, 8111
Golf Xpress, 554
Goodwill Industries of Central Indiana, 5999
Grand Island VA Medical System, 5678
Grand Junction VA Medical Center, 5591
Gulf States Association of Homes and Services for the Aging, 7460
Hampton VA Medical Center, 5770
Handbook of Assistive Devices for the Handicapped Elderly, 7508
Handbook on Ethnicity, Aging and Mental Health, 7509
Harry S Truman Memorial Veterans' Hospital, 5669
Hartford Regional Office, 5592
Hawaii Executive Office on Aging, 3437
Health Care of the Aged: Needs, Policies, and Services, 7510

Health Promotion and Disease Prevention in Clinical Practice, 7511
Helping the Family Understand, 8112
Highlighter and Note Tape, 619
Honolulu VBA Regional Office, 5615
Houston Regional Office, 5760
Hunter Holmes McGuire VA Medical Center, 5771
Huntington Regional Office, 5779
Huntington VA Medical Center, 5780
Idaho Commission on Aging, 3442
Illinois Department on Aging, 3458
Increasing and Decreasing Behaviors of Persons with Severe Retardation and Autism, 2066, 7778
Independence Council for Economic Development, 4564
Independent Living Office, 5098
Independent Living Resources, 4409
Indiana Association of Homes and Services for the Aging, 7462
Indianapolis Regional Office, 5623
Innovations, 7541
Institute on Aging, 7551
Insurance Solutions: Plan Well, Live Better, 5102
Interstitial Cystitis Association, 5423
Iowa Association of Homes and Services for the Aging, 7463
Iowa City VA Medical Center, 5629
Iowa Department on Aging, 3474
Iron Mountain VA Medical Center, 5658
Jack C. Montgomery VA Medical Center, 5724
Jackson Regional Office, 5668
James A Haley VA Medical Center, 5605
James E Van Zandt VA Medical Center, 5736
Jerry L Pettis Memorial VA Medical Center, 5576
John D Dingell VA Medical Center, 5659
John J Pershing VA Medical Center, 5670
John L McClellan Memorial Hospital, 5574
Jonathan M Wainwright Memorial VA Medical Center, 5775
Kansas City VA Medical Center, 5671
Kansas Department on Aging, 3483
Kansas VA Regional Office, 5634
Kentucky Office of Aging Services, 3489
Knoxville VA Medical Center, 5630
Laurel Grove Hospital: Rehab Care Unit, 6251
Lebanon VA Medical Center, 5737
Lexington VA Medical Center, 5636
Life Planning for Adults with Developmental Disabilities, 7512
Life Services Network of Illinois, 7465
LifeSpan Network: Maryland, 7466
Lifestyles of Employed Legally Blind People, 8989
Lighthouse International, 8843
Lincoln Regional Office, 5679
Lincoln VA Medical Center, 5680
Long Beach VA Medical Center, 5577
Long-Term Care: How to Plan and Pay for It, 7513
Los Angeles Regional Office, 5578
Louis A Johnson VA Medical Center, 5781
Louis Stokes VA Medical CenterWade Park Campus, 5723
Louisiana Department of Aging, 3496
Louisville VA Medical Center, 5637
Louisville VA Regional Office, 5638
Lyons Campus of the VA New Jersey Healthcare System, 5691
Maine VA Regional Office, 5642
Making Wise Decisions for Long-Term Care, 5124
Managing Post Polio: A Guide to Living Well with Post Polio, 8518
Managing Your Symptoms, 8113
Manchester Regional Office, 5686
Manchester VA Medical Center, 5687
Marion VA Medical Center, 5620
Martinez Outpatient Clinic, 5579
Martinsburg VA Medical Center, 5782
Maryland Department of Aging, 3513
Massachusetts Aging Services Association, 7467
Math for Successful Living, 1650
MedEscort International, 5505
Memphis VA Medical Center, 5753
Mentally Impaired Elderly: Strategies and Interventions to Maintain Function, 7514
Mercy Medical Group, 6635

Michael E. Debakey VA Medical Center, 5761
Michigan Office of Services to the Aging, 3542
Michigan Psychological Association, 2035
Michigan VA Regional Office, 5660
Mid-Carolina Area Agency on Aging, 7554
Minneapolis VA Medical Center, 5663
Minnesota Board on Aging, 3549
Mirrored Lives: Aging Children and Elderly Parents, 7515
Mississippi Division of Aging and Adult Services, 3564
Missouri Association of Homes for the Aging, 7468
Monkeys Jumping on the Bed, 1714
Montana Department of Aging, 3578
Mountain Home VA Medical CenterJames H Quillen VA Medical Center, 5754
Muhlenberg County Opportunity Center, 6921
Multiple Sclerosis: 300 Tips for Making Life Easier, 8523
Multiple Sclerosis: The Guide to Treatment and Management, 8526
Muscular Dystrophies, 8527
Muscular Dystrophy in Children: A Guide for Families, 8528
Muscular Dystophy: The Facts, 8529
Nasheville Regional Office, 5755
Nashville VA Medical Center, 5756
National Association for Home Care & Hospice, 8282
National Association of Area Agencies on Aging, 7469
National Association of Counties, 7470
National Association of Nutrition and Aging Services Programs, 7472
National Association of State Units on Aging, 7473
National Council on Aging, 7475
National Council on the Aging Conference, 1866
National Hispanic Council on Aging, 7477
National Indian Council on Aging, 7478
National Senior Citizens Law Center, 7479
Nebraska Association of Homes and Services for the Aging, 7480
Nebraska Department of Health and Human Services, Division of Aging Services, 3588
Nevada Division for Aging: Las Vegas, 3599
New Hampshire Division of Elderly and Adult Services, 3611
New Jersey Association of Homes and Services for the Aging, 7481
New Jersey Department of Aging, 3619
New Mexico Aging and Long-Term Services Department, 3626
New Mexico VA Healthcare System, 5694
New Orleans VA Medical Center, 5640
New York Association of Homes and Services for the Aging, 7482
New York City Campus of the VA NY Harbor Healthcare System, 5703
New York Regional Office, 5704
Newark Regional Office, 5692
North Carolina Association of Non-Profit Homes for the Aging, 7483
North Carolina Division of Aging, 3677
North Chicago VA Medical Center, 5621
North Dakota Department of Human Resources, 3683
North Dakota VA Regional OfficeFargo Regional Office, 5718
North Little Rock Regional Office, 5575
Northampton VA Medical Center, 5652
Northern Arizona VA Health Care System, 5570
Northern New England Association of Homes and Services for the Aging, 7484
Northport VA Medical Center, 5705
Not Without Sight, 9125
Oakland VA Regional Office, 5580
Ohio Department of Aging, 3693
Oklahoma Association of Homes and Services for the Aging, 7485
Oklahoma City VA Medical Center, 5726
Oklahoma Department of Human Services Aging Services Division, 3703
Oxford Textbook of Geriatric Medicine, 2477

Pacific Islands Health Care System, 5616
Part B News, 7531
Passion for Justice, 5352
Pennsylvania Association of Nonprofit Senior Services, 7487
Pennsylvania Department of Aging, 3722
Perry Point VA Medical Center, 5648
Philadelphia Regional Office and Insurance Center, 5739
Philadelphia VA Medical Center, 5740
Physical & Mental Issues in Aging Sourcebook, 7516
Physical & Occupational Therapy in Geriatrics, 7525
Piedmont Triad Council of Governments Area Agency on Aging, 7555
Pittsburgh Regional Office, 5741
Portland Regional Office, 5729
Portland VA Medical Center, 5730
Practicing Rehabilitation with Geriatric Clients, 2490
Prescriptions for Independence: Working with Older People Who are Visually Impaired, 7517
Providence Regional Office, 5745
Providence VA Medical Center, 5746
Quality Healthcare Foundation of Wyoming, 7488
Ralph H Johnson VA Medical Center, 5748
Reading Rehabilitation Hospital, 4899
Recreation Activities for the Elderly, 2504
Rehabilitation Interventions for the Institutionalized Elderly, 2506
Rehabilitation Research and Development Center, 5581
Reno Regional Office, 5683
Resource Center for Independent Living(RCIL), 1594
Respiratory Disorders Sourcebook, 8564
Retirement Research Foundation, 2895
Rhode Island Association of Facilities and Services for the Aging, 7489
Rhode Island Department of Elderly Affairs, 3731
Richard L Roudebush VA Medical Center, 5624
Roanoke Regional Office, 5772
Robert J Dole VA Medical Center, 5635
Role Portrayal and Stereotyping on Television, 5166
Roseburg VA Medical Center, 5731
Royal C Johnson Veterans Memorial Medical Center, 5750
Sacramento Medical Center, 5582
Salem VA Medical Center, 5773
San Antonio Area Foundation, 3216
San Diego VA Regional Office, 5583
Seattle Regional Office, 5776
Sharing the Burden, 7518
Sheridan VA Medical Center, 5790
Shreveport VA Medical Center, 5641
Silent Call Communications, 228
Sioux Falls Regional Office, 5751
Sister Cities International, 2718
Social Security Bulletin, 7532
Social Security, Medicare, and Government Pensions, 7519
South Dakota Department of Aging, 3754
South Texas Veterans Healthcare System, 5762
Southern Arizona VA Healthcare System, 5571
Southern Oregon Rehabilitation Center & Clinics, 5732
Spokane VA Medical Center, 5777
St. Cloud VA Medical Center, 5664
St. Louis Regional Office, 5672
St. Louis VA Medical Center, 5673
St. Paul Regional Office, 5665
St. Petersburg Regional Office, 5607
Start-to-Finish Library, 1800
State of Vermont Department of Disabilities, Aging and Independent Living, 6201
Stickybear Typing, 1817
Storybook Maker Deluxe, 1736
Strategies for Teaching Students with Learning and Behavior Problems, 2533
Strides Magazine, 8193
Successful Models of Community Long Term Care Services for the Elderly, 7520

Syracuse VA Medical Center, 5706
Teaching Special Students in Mainstream, 2075
Tennessee Association of Homes and Services for the Aging, 7490
Tennessee Commission on Aging and Disability, 3763
Texas Association of Homes and Services for the Aging, 7491
Texas Department on Aging, 3788
Therapeutic Activities with Persons Disabled by Alzheimer's Disease, 7521
Togus VA Medical Center, 5643
Tomah VA Medical Center, 5785
Tomorrow's Promise: Language Arts, 1806
Tomorrow's Promise: Spelling, 1808
Tompkins County Office for the Aging, 7557
Tourette Syndrome: The Facts, 8580
US Department of Veterans Affairs National Headquarters, 5560
US Servas, 5511
University of California Memory and Aging Center, 7559
Utah Department of Aging, 3801
Utah Division of Veterans Affairs, 5766
V A Montana Healthcare System, 5675
VA Ann Arbor Healthcare System, 5661
VA Boston Healthcare System: Brockton Division, 5653
VA Boston Healthcare System: Jamaica Plain Campus, 5654
VA Boston Healthcare System: West Roxbury Division, 5655
VA Central California Health Care System, 5584
VA Connecticut Healthcare System: Newington Division, 5594
VA Connecticut Healthcare System: West Haven, 5595
VA Greater Los Angeles Healthcare System, 5585
VA Illiana Health Care System, 5622
VA Montana Healthcare System, 5676
VA Nebraska-Western Iowa Health Care System, 5681
VA North Indiana Health Care System: Fort Wayne Campus, 5625
VA Northern California Healthcare System, 5586
VA Northern Indiana Health Care System: Marion Campus, 5626
VA Pittsburgh Healthcare System, Highland Drive Division, 5743
VA Pittsburgh Healthcare System, University Drive Division, 5742
VA Puget Sound Health Care System, 5778
VA Salt Lake City Healthcare System, 5767
VA San Diego Healthcare System, 5587
VA Sierra Nevada Healthcare System, 5684
VA Southern Nevada Healthcare System, 5685
VA Western NY Healthcare System, Batavia, 5709
VA Western NY Healthcare System, Buffalo, 5710
Vermont Department of Aging, 3813
Vermont Department of Disabilities, Aging and Independent Living, 3815
Vermont Division of Disability & Aging Services, 3819
Vermont VA Regional Office Center, 5768
Veteran Benefits AdministrationAnchorage Regional Office, 5568
Visiting Nurse Association of America, 8670
Visually Impaired Seniors as Senior Companions: A Reference Guide, 7522
WG Hefner VA Medical CenterSalisbury, 5715
Waco Regional Office, 5764
Washington County Disability, Aging and Veteran Services, 3716
Washington DC VA Medical Center, 5602
We Can Do it Together!, 9132
West Palm Beach VA Medical Center, 5608
West Texas VA Healthcare System, 5765
West Virginia Department of Aging, 3846
Wilkes-Barre VA Medical Center, 5744
William Jennings Bryan Dorn VA Medical Center, 5749
William S Middleton Memorial VA Hospital Center, 5786
Wilmington VA Medical Center, 5597

Winston-Salem Regional Office, 5716
Wisconsin Association of Homes and Services for the Aging, 7492
Wisconsin Bureau of Aging, 3856
Wisconsin VA Regional Office, 5787
Work Exploration Center, 5947
Work, Health and Income Among the Elderly, 7523
Wyoming Department of Aging, 3864
Wyoming/Colorado VA Regional Office, 5791
Yoga for Fibromyalgia: Move, Breathe, and Relax to Improve Your Quality of Life, 8186
Young Person's Guide to Spina Bifida, 8592

Alternative Therapies

Academy for Guided Imagery, 2660
American Academy of Osteopathy, 8119
American Association of Oriental Medicine, 772
American Board of Clinical Metal Toxicology, 775
American College of Advancement in Medicine, 780
American College of Nurse Midwives, 781
American Council for Headache Education(ACHE), 2019
American Herb Association Newsletter, 5012
American Holistic Medical Association, 786
American Sexual Health Association, 8257
American Society for the Alexander Technique, 793
American Society of Clinical Hypnosis, 795
Aromatherapy Book: Applications and Inhalations, 5019
Aromatherapy for Common Ailments, 5020
Association for Applied Psychophysiology and Biofeedback, 796
Association on Higher Education and Disability, 2022
Ayurvedic Institute, 2665
Bach Flower Therapy: Theory and Practice, 5025
Bastyr University Natural Health Clinic, 804
Beliefs, Values, and Principles of Self Advocacy, 5027
Brain Allergies: The Psychonutrient and Magnetic Connections, 8446
Center for Mind/Body Studies, 817
Chinese Herbal Medicine, 5045
Chronic Fatigue Syndrome: Your Natural Gu ide to Healing with Diet, Herbs and Other Methods, 8458
Colon Health: Key to a Vibrant Life, 8461
Creating Wholeness: Self-Healing Workbook Using Dynamic Relaxation, Images and Thoughts, 5053
Curing MS: How Science is Solving the Mysteries of Multiple Sclerosis, 8465
Designing and Using Assistive Technology: The Human Perspective, 2360
Divided Legacy: A History of the Schism in Medical Thought, The Bacteriological Era, 2375
Environmental Health Center: Dallas, 8268
Esalen Institute, 841
Everybody's Guide to Homeopathic Medicines, 5072
Feldenkrais Guild of North America (FGNA), 849
Handbook of Chronic Fatigue Syndrome, 8480
Healing Herbs, 5086
Health Action, 855
Heart of the Mind, 8483
Herb Research Foundation, 5419
Homeopathic Educational Services, 857
Human Ecology Action League (HEAL), 858
Imagery in Healing Shamanism and Modern Medicine, 5094
Informed Touch; A Clinician's Guide To TheEvaluation Of Myofascial Disorders, 8489
Institute of Transpersonal Psychology, 860
International Association of Hygienic Physicians, 8274
International Association of Parents and Professionals for Safe Alternatives in Childbirth, 2029
International Association of Yoga Therapists, 862

International Childbirth Education Association, 2030
International Clinic of Biological Regeneration, 864
It's All in Your Head: The Link Between Mercury Amalgams and Illness, 8493
Living Beyond Multiple Sclerosis: A Woman's Guide, 8505
Living an Idea: Empowerment and the Evolution of an Alternative School, 1962
Long Beach Department of Health and Human Services, 3359
Los Angeles County Department of Health Services, 3360
Lupus: Alternative Therapies That Work, 8514
Mind, Body, Health Sciences, 880
National Association for Holistic Aromatherapy, 882
National Association to Advance Fat Acceptance, 8287
National Center for Homeopathy, 2042
National College of Naturopathic Medicine, 890
National Guild of Hypnotists, 898
National Headache Foundation, 2890
National Vaccine Information Center, 904
New York Therapeutic Riding Center-Equestria, 907
Nothing is Impossible: Reflections on a New Life, 5138
Nurse Healers: Professional Associates International, 910
Nutritional Desk Reference, 5139
Nutritional Influences on Illness:, 5140
Optometric Extension Program Foundation, 2937
Our Own RoadAquarius Health Care Media, 5350
PACER Center (Parent Advocacy Coalition for Educational Rights), 911
Pacific Institute of Aromatherapy, 913
Pain Erasure, 5221
Pain Erasure: the Bonnie Prudden Way, 9006
Pocket Guide to the ADA: Accessibility Guidelines for Buildings and Facilities, 4571
Quan Yin Healing Arts Center, 920
Rolf Institute, 923
Small Wonder, 1994
Solving the Puzzle of Chronic Fatigue, 8570
Tourette's Syndrome: Tics, Obsessions, Compulsions: Developmental Psychopathology, 8582
United States Trager Association, 931
Upledger Institute, 933
Weiner's Herbal, 5186

Amputation

American Amputee Foundation, Inc., 7872
Baylor Institute for Rehabilitation, 7160
Botsford Center For Rehabilitation & Health Improvement-Redford, 6992
Breaking New Ground Resource Center, 8647
Camp No Limits, 1138
Don't Feel Sorry for Paul, 7888
Functional Restoration of Adults and Children with Upper Extremity Amputation, 7889
Healthsouth Rehabilitation Hospital of Mechanicsburg, 6420
Healthsouth Rehabilitation Hospital of York, 6421
MossRehab ResourceNet, 5429
National Amputation Foundation, 7882
National Commission on Orthotic and Prosthetic Education, 7883
National Institute of Neurological Disorde Disorders & Stroke, 7884
Northeast Rehabilitation Clinic, 7332
Shands Rehab Hospital, 7257
Siskin Hospital For Physical Rehabilitation, 7156
Siskin Hospital for Physical Rehabilitation, 7398

Amythrophic Lateral Sclerosis

Amytrophic Lateral Sclerosis Association, 8126
Les Turne Amyotrophic Lateral Sclerosis Foundation, 2883

Art & Music Therapies

AbleArts, 1
American Art Therapy Association (AATA), 2
American Association of Cardiovascular and
　Pulmonary Rehabilitation, 8250
American Brain Tumor Association, 8251
American Thoracic Society, 8259
Art Therapy SourceBook, 7
Art and Disabilities, 8
Art and Healing: Using Expressive Art to Heal
　Your Body, Mind, and Soul, 9
Art for All the Children: Approaches to Art
　Therapy for Children with Disabilities, 10
Art-Centered Education and Therapy for Children
　with Disabilities, 2299
Arts Unbound, 11
The Arts of Life, 66
Awakenings Project, The, 13
Camping Unlimited, 992
Clinical Applications of Music Therapy in
　Developmental Disability, Pediatrics and
　Neurolog, 15
Contemporary Art Therapy with Adolescents, 16
Creative Arts Resources Catalog, 17
Creative Arts Therapy Catalogs, 1927
Creative Growth Art Center, 18
Creativity Explored, 19
Deaf West Theatre, 21
Dionysus Theatre, 22
Fountain House Gallery, 26
In-Definite Arts Society, 30
Infinity Dance Theater, 31
Interact Center for the Visual and Performing Arts,
　33
International Journal of Arts Medicine, 2438
Kaleidoscope: Exploring the Experience of
　Disability through Literature & the Fine Arts, 34
Keshet Dance Company, 35
Mad Hatters: Theatre That Makes a World of
　Difference, 2677
Manual of Sequential Art Activities for Classified
　Children and Adolescents, 37
Music Therapy and Leisure for Persons with
　Disabilities, 40
Music Therapy, Sensory Integration and the
　Autistic Child, 43
Music for the Hearing Impaired, 45
Music: Physician for Times to Come, 46
National Arts and Disability Center (NADC), 47
National Endowment for the Arts: Office for
　AccessAbility, 49
National Institute of Art and Disabilities, 50
National Library Service for the Blind And
　Physically Handicapped, 51
New Music Therapist's Handbook, 2nd Ed. Berklee
　School of Music, 54
No Limits, 55
Open Circle Theatre, 58
Pied Piper: Musical Activities to Develop Basic
　Skills, 59
A Practical Guide to Art Therapy Groups, 4991
Project Onward Gallery, 60
Pure Vision Arts, 61
Special Care in Dentistry, 8633
Survivors Art Foundation, 63
Teaching Basic Guitar Skills to Special Learners,
　65
VSA arts, 69
We Are PHAMALY, 70

Arthritis

American College of Rheumatology, Researchand
　Education Foundation, 5388
Arthritis Bible, 8167
Arthritis Foundation, 8127
Arthritis Foundation Great West Region, 8195
Arthritis Helpbook: A Tested Self Management
　Program for Coping with Arthritis, 8168
Arthritis Self-Management, 8616
Arthritis Sourcebook, 8169
Arthritis Sourcebook., 8438
Arthritis Today, 8187

Arthritis Update, 8196
Arthritis, What Exercises Work: Breakthrough
　Relief for the Rest of Your Life, 8170
Arthritis: A Take Care of Yourself Health Guide,
　8171
Back & Neck Sourcebook., 8441
Baptist Health Rehabilitation Institute, 3347
Big Lamp Switch, 504
Body Reflexology: Healing at Your Fingertips,
　5031
Boston University Arthritis Center, 4797
Boston University Robert Dawson Evans Memorial
　Dept. of Clinical Research, 4799
Brigham and Women's Hospital: Robert B
　Brigham Multipurpose Arthritis Center, 4802
Burke Rehabilitation Hospital, 6383
Camp Esperanza, 1052, 8160
Card Holder Deluxe, 5466
Carpal Tunnel Syndrome, 7887
Case Western Reserve University Northeast Ohio
　Multipurpose Arthritis Center, 4883
Challenge Golf, 9136
Checker Set: Deluxe, 5469
Daniel Freeman Rehabilitation Centers, 6585
Freedom from Arthritis Through Nutrition, 8174
Guide to Managing Your Arthritis, 8176
Health Resource Center for Women with
　Disabilities, 856
How to Deal with Back Pain and Rheumatoid Joint
　Pain: A Preventive and Self Treatment Manua,
　8177
Indiana University: Multipurpose Arthritis Center,
　4755
Information Hotline, 8243
Kids on the Block Programs, 8244
Kuzell Institute for Arthritis and Infectious
　Diseases, 4677
Loma Linda University Orthopedic and
　Rehabilitation Institute, 6623
Managing Your Activities, 5127
Managing Your Health Care, 5128
Medical University of South Carolina Arthritis
　Clinical/Research Center, 4902
New York Arthritis Reporter, 8209
Oklahoma Medical Research Foundation, 4890
Primer on the Rheumatic Diseases, 8182
RIC Northshore, 6858
RIC Windermere House, 6860
Raynaud's Phenomenon, 8562
Swedish Covenant Hospital Rehabilitation
　Services, 6870
Thumbs Up Cup, 373
University of Michigan: Orthopaedic Research
　Laboratories, 4824
University of Missouri: Columbia Arthritis Center,
　4841
Virginia Chapter of the Arthtitis Foundation, 4932
When Your Student Has Arthritis, 8185
Yoga for Arthritis, 8218
Yoga for MS and Related Conditions, 8219

Asthma

AAN's Toll-Free Hotline, 8646
ABC of Asthma, Allergies & Lupus, 8426
Allergies & Asthma: What Every Parent Needs To
　Know (2nd Edition), 8432
Allergies Sourcebook, 8433
Allergy & Asthma Today, 5255
American Academy of Allergy, Asthma &
　Immunology, 8246
Asthma & Allergy Education for Worksite
　Clinicians, 2662
Asthma & Allergy Essentials for Children's Care
　Provider, 2663
Asthma Action Cards: Child Care Asthma/Allergy
　Action Card, 1911
Asthma Action Cards: Student Asthma Action
　Card, 1912
Asthma Care Training for Kids (ACT), 2664
Asthma Management and Education, 2310
Asthma Sourcebook., 8439
Asthma and Allergy Answers: A Patient Education
　Library, 8440

Asthma and Allergy Foundation of America, 5396
Bakersfield Regional Rehabilitation Hospital, 6241
Becket Chimney Corners YMCA Camps and
　Outdoor Center, 1165, 8315
Being Close, 8442
Brigham and Women's Hospital: Asthma and
　Allergic Disease Research Center, 4801
Camp Breathe Easy, 1049, 8322
Camp Christmas Seal, 1065, 8327
Camp Glengarra, 1258, 8337
Camp L-Kee-Ta, 1107, 8352
Camp Not-A-Wheeze, 955, 8358
Camp Pelican, 1128, 8360
Camp Superkids, 1155
Camp Tall Turf, 1191, 8370
Camp Tekoa UMC, 1292, 7967
Camp Vacamas, 1248, 8372
Camp WheezeAway, 945, 8374
Canonicus Camp, 1363
Center for Interdisciplinary Research on
　Immunologic Diseases, 4804
Champ Camp, 1014, 8377
Hasbro Children's Hospital Asthma Camp, 1364
Johns Hopkins University: Asthma and Allergy
　Center, 4788
Let's Talk About Having Asthma, 8499
Living Well with Asthma, 8506
MA Report, 2252
Med-Camps of Louisiana, 1133, 8396
Meeting-in-a-Box, 1973
My House is Killing Me! The Home Guide for
　Families with Allergies and Asthma, 8530
Nocturnal Asthma, 8535
Parent's Guide to Allergies and Asthma, 8552
Power Breathing Program, 1983
Teens & Asthma, 8638
Toll-Free Information Line, 8669
Understanding Asthma, 8584
Understanding Asthma: The Blueprint for
　Breathing, 8585
What Everyone Needs to Know About Asthma,
　8590
YMCA Camp Ihduhapi, 1207, 8417
YMCA Camp of Maine, 1145, 8423
Your Child and Asthma, 8593

Attention Deficit Disorder

ADD, Stepping Out of the Dark, 7848
ADD: Helping Your Child, 7711
ADHD Report, 7829
ADHD in Adults, 7849
ADHD in the Classroom: Strategies for Teachers,
　2278
ADHD with Comorbid Disorders: Clinical
　Assessment and Management, 7714
ADHD: What Do We Know?, 7851
ALST: Adolescent Language Screening Test, 2589
Adapted Physical Education for Students with
　Autism, 2283
Adventure Learning Center at Eagle Village, 7658
All About Attention Deficit Disorders, Revised,
　5309, 7717
Around the Clock: Parenting the Delayed AD HD
　Child, 7852
Attention, 7828
Attention Deficit Disorder, 7719
Attention Deficit Disorder and Learning
　Disabilities, 7720
Attention Deficit Disorder in Adults Workbook,
　7721
Attention Deficit Disorder in Children, 2312
Attention Deficit Disorder: A Different Perception,
　7722
Attention Deficit Disorder: Adults, 7853
Attention Deficit Disorder: Children, 7854
Attention Deficit Disorders Association, Southern
　Region: Annual Conference, 1848
Attention Deficit Disorders: Assessment &
　Teaching, 7723
Attention-Deficit Hyperactivity Disorder:
　Symptoms and Suggestons for Treatment, 7724
Attention-Deficit/Hyperactivity Disorder, What
　Every Parent Wants to Know, 7725

Braille Book Bank, Music Catalog, 8924
Camp Betsey Cox, 1409, 7661
Camp Buckskin, 1199, 7662
Camp Northwood, 1264, 7668
Camp Ruggles, 1362, 7672
Camp World Light, 7674
Casowasco Camp, Conference and Retreat Center, 1270, 7677
Chadder, 7832
Clinical Connection, 2180
Clinical Management of Childhood Stuttering, 2nd Edition, 2340
Clinician's Practical Guide to Attention-Deficit/Hyperactivity Disorder, 5276
Cogrehab, 7847
Communication & Language Acquisition: Discoveries from Atypical Development, 2346
Community Signs, 1925
Comprehensive Assessment of Spoken Language (CASL), 1926
Comprehensive Guide to ADD in Adults: Research, Diagnosis & Treatment, 7745
Concentration Cockpit: Explaining Attention Deficits, 7746
Coping for Kids Who Stutter, 8734
Coping with ADD/ADHD, 7747
Counseling Persons with Communication Disorders and Their Families, 2352
Development of Language, 2364
Disorders of Motor Speech: Assessment, Treatment, and Clinical Characterization, 8735
Driven to Distraction, 7753
Eagle View Ranch, 1445
Educating Inattentive Children, 7859
Englishton Park Academic Remediation, 1098, 7683
Family Therapy for ADHD: Treating Children, Adolescents and Adults, 7759
Florida Sheriffs Caruth Camp, 1043, 7684
GO-MO Articulation Cards- Second Edition, 1941
Getting a Grip on ADD: A Kid's Guide to Understanding & Coping with ADD, 7763
Gillingham Manaual, 1942
Handbook for Speech Therapy, 2411
Helping Your Hyperactive: Attention Deficit Child, 7770
How to Own and Operate an Attention Deficit Disorder, 7773
Hyperactive Child, Adolescent, and Adult: ADD Through the Lifespan, 7774
Hyperactivity, Attention Deficits, and School Failure: Better Ways, 7775
Indian Acres Camp for Boys, 1143, 7687
It's Just Attention Disorder, 7863
Jumpin' Johnny Get Back to Work, A Child's Guide to ADHD/Hyperactivity, 7779
K-SEALS: Kaufman Survey of Early Academic and Language Skills, 2616
KLST-2: Kindergarten Language Screening Test Edition, 2nd Edition, 2617
Lollipop Lunch, 8743
Loudoun County Special Recreation Programs, 1422
Management of Children and Adolescents with AD-HD, 7788
Managing Attention Deficit Hyperactivity in Children: A Guide for Practitioners, 7789
Maplebrook School, 1279, 7690
Meeting the ADD Challenge: A Practical Guide for Teachers, 2464
Model Program Operation Manual: Business Enterprise Program Supervisors, 8998
New Jersey YMHA/YWHA Camps Milford, 1251, 7693
Out of the Corner of My Eye: Living with Macular Degeneration, 9005
Out of the Fog: Treatment Options and Coping Strategies for ADD, 7793
Outside In School Of Experiential, 1356
Outside In School Of Experiential Education, Inc., 7695
Parenting Attention Deficit Disordered Teens, 7797
Parents Helping Parents: A Directory of Support Groups for ADD, 7798

Readings on Research in Stuttering, 2503
Reference Manual for Communicative Sciences and Disorders, 2505
Rethinking Attention Deficit Disorder, 7805
Rolling Hills Country Day Camp, 1252, 7700
Rose-Colored Glasses, 9018
Sharing Solutions: A Newsletter for Support Groups, 9106
Slingerland Screening Tests, 2642
Solving Language Difficulties, 1995
Speech Bin, 1996, 2644
Speech-Language Pathology and Audiology: An Introduction, 2529
Stuttering, 8782
Stuttering & Your Child: Help For Parents, 8776
Stuttering Foundation of America, 8703
Stuttering Severity Instrument for Children and Adults, 2645
Summit Camp, 1254, 7704
Survey of Direct Labor Workers Who Are Blind & Employed by NIB, 9030
Taking Charge of ADHD Complete Authoritative Guide for Parents, 7812
Teenagers with ADD, 7816
Triangle Y Ranch YMCA, 958, 7708
Understanding ADHD, 7864
Understanding Attention Deficit Disorder, 7865
Why Won't My Child Pay Attention?, 7868
Women with Attention Deficit Disorder: Embracing Disorganization at Home and Work, 7821
You Seem Like a Regular Kid to Me, 9052
You and Your ADD Child, 7823

Autism

Aging and Developmental Disability: Current Research, Programming, and Practice, 7495
Anxiety-Free Kids: An Interactive Guide for Parents and Children, 2297
Arc of the United States, 5394
Arizona Autism Resources, 2731
Autism 24/7: A Family Guide to Learning at Home & in the Community, 7727, 8717
Autism Day Camp, 1084, 8159
Autism Handbook: Understanding & Treating Autism & Prevention Development, 7728, 8718
Autism Research Institute, 7612, 8676
Autism Research Review International, 7831, 8771
Autism Services Center, 7613, 8677
Autism Society of America, 7869, 8788
Autism Treatment Center of America, 7614, 8678
Autism and Learning, 7729, 8719
Autism in Adolescents and Adults, 7730, 8720
Autism...Nature, Diagnosis and Treatment, 7731, 8721
Autism: A World Apart, 7855, 8783
Autism: Explaining the Enigma, 7732, 8722
Autism: From Tragedy to Triumph, 7733, 8723
Autism: Identification, Education and Treatment, 7734, 8724
Autism: The Facts, 7735, 8725
Autism: the Unfolding Mystery, 7856, 8784
AutismAquarius Health Care Media, 5310
Autistic Adults at Bittersweet Farms, 7736, 8726
Breakthroughs: How to Reach Students with Autism, 7738, 8729
Burger School for the Autistic, 4811
CNS Camp New Connections, 7659, 8706
Camp Baker, 7660
Camp Eden Wood, 8334
Camp Encourage, 1210
Camp Friendship, 1202
Camp Horizons, 1024, 7665
Camp Hug The Bear, 1068
Camp Joy, 1150, 7961, 8349
Camp Merrimack, 940
Camp New Connections, 1170
Camp New Hope, 1071, 1288
Camp Royall, 1289, 7671, 8707
Camp Sisol, 1266, 7673, 8708
Camp Stepping Stone, 1308
Camp Tova, 1267

Camp-A-Lot And Leisure Express (PALS Program), 991, 7675
Child With Special Needs: Encouraging Intellectual and Emotional Growth, 5044
Children's Center for Neurodevelopmental Studies, 4656
Cognitive Behavioral Therapy for Adult Asperger Syndrome, 7743, 8731
Communication Unbound, 2348
Communication in Autism, 8681
Courage Center, 4247
Davis Center, The, 827, 7911, 8682
Developmental Disabilities: A Handbook for Occupational Therapists, 2366
Dogs for the Deaf, 7915
Easter Seals Camp ASCCA, 946
Emory Autism Resource Center, 4722
Encounters with Autistic States, 7756, 8737
Essential First Steps for Parents of Children with Autism, 5249
Exploring Autism: A Look at the Genetics of Autism, 5412
Families of Adults With Autism: Stories & Advice For the Next Generation, 7758
Fighting for Darla: Challenges for Family Care & Professional Responsibility, 7760
Filmakers Library: An Imprint Of AlexanderStreet Press, 5331
Focus Alternative Learning Center, 850, 7630
Focus Times Newsletter, 7842
Focus on Autism and Other Developmental Disabilities, 2192
Fragile Success, 7761
Fundamentals of Autism, 1940
Future Horizons, 28
Gateway Arts Center: Studio, Craft Store& Gallery, 6056
Getting Started with Facilitated Communication, 7860, 8785
Going to School with Facilitated Communication, 5082
Guide to Successful Employment for Individuals with Autism, 7766
Handbook of Autism and Pervasive Developmental Disorders, 7767
Heartspring, 6909
Helping People with Autism Manage Their Behavior, 7768
Hidden Child: The Linwood Method for Reaching the Autistic Child, 7771
Illinois Center for Autism, 6843
Imagery Procedures for People with Special Needs, 5339
Imagine: Innovative Resources for Cognitive & Physical Challenges, 5886
Indiana Resource Center for Autism, 4754
Judevine Center for Autism, 4839
Keys to Parenting the Child with Autism, 7782
Kris' Camp, 1045
Let Community Employment be the Goal for Individuals with Autism, 7785, 8742
Little City Foundation, 2884
Little Friends, Inc., 6846
Living with Spina Bifida: A Guide for Families and Professionals, 8511
Louis de la Parte Florida Mental Health Institute Research Library, 4708
Management of Autistic Behavior, 7787, 8516, 8744
Mount Sinai Medical Center, 3070
Music Therapy, 39
National Autism Association, 7643
National Autism Hotline, 7870
National Easter Seal Society, 897
National Institute on Deafness and Other Communication Disorder, 7647
Neurobiology of Autism, 7792, 8746
New England Center for Children, 6981
New Jersey Camp Jaycee, 1250
New Jersey Center for Outreach and Services for the Autism Community (COSAC), 4854
Northwest Kiwanis Camp, 1430, 8400
Oak Leyden Developmental Services, 7648
Parent Survival Manual, 7795, 8748

Please Don't Say Hello, 7799, 8750
Prufrock Press, 2102
Reaching the Autistic Child: A Parent Training Program, 8563
Reaching the Child with Autism Through Art, 62
Riddle of Autism: A Psychological Analysis, 7806, 8754
Rimland Services for Autistic Citizens, 1077, 7699
Schools And Services For Children With Autism Spectrum Disorders., 3656
Sex Education: Issues for the Person with Autism, 7808, 8756
Sometimes You Just Want to Feel Like a Human Being, 5172
Son Rise: The Miracle Continues, 8571
Son-Rise Program, 8666
Son-Rise: The Miracle Continues, 7809, 8757
Soon Will Come the Light, 7810
Special Needs Advocacy Resource Book, 2643
Special Needs Project, 2106
Sunnyhill Adventure Center, 1220, 7705
TEACCH, 7653
Teaching Asperger's Students Social Skills Through Acting, 64
Teaching Children With Autism in the General Classroom, 2542
Teaching Children with Autism: Strategies for Initiating Positive Interactions, 7813, 8760
Teaching Students with Moderate/Severe Disabilities, Including Autism, 2557
Teaching and Mainstreaming Autistic Children, 7814, 8761
Treating Disordered Speech Motor Control, 2572
Treatment and Learning Centers (TLC), 6054
Uncommon Fathers, 5242
Understanding Autism, 7866, 8787
Valley News Dispatch, 7818
Vanguard School, The, 2690
Virginia Autism Resource Center, 4930
Wendell Johnson Speech And Hearing Clinic, 1113, 7709, 8705, 8899
West Virginia Autism Training Center, 4942
Without Reason: A Family Copes with two Generations of Autism, 7820, 8765
YMCA Outdoor Center Campbell Gard, 1319, 8424

Behavioral Disorders

AACRC Annual Meeting, 1827
Alternative Teaching Strategies, 2295
American Academy of Child & Adolescent Psychiatry, 7607
American Group Psychotherapy Association, 8253
Behavior Analysis in Education: Focus on Measurably Superior Instruction, 2314
Behavior Modification, 2315
Behavioral Disorders, 2316
Center for Neuro Skills, 6571
Childhood Behavior Disorders: Applied Research & Educational Practice, 2331
Creating Positive Classroom Environments: Strategies for Behavior Management, 2354
Devereux Advanced Behavioral Health NewJersey, 7043
Groden Center, 6177
Journal of Emotional and Behavioral Disorders, 2204
Journal of Motor Behavior, 2206
Journal of Vocational Behavior, 2214
Lakeview NeuroRehabilitation Center, 6371
Progress Without Punishment: Approaches for Learners with Behavior Problems, 2497
Teaching Students with Learning and Behavior Problems, 2555
ValueOptions, 5448
Working Bibliography on Behavioral and Emotional Disorders, 2580

Birth Defects

BDRC Newsletter, 5398

Baylor College of Medicine Birth Defects Center, 4906
Birth Defect Research for Children, 806
Camp Bon Coeur, 1126, 8321
Camp Del Corazon, 971, 8331
Cornelia de Lange Syndrome Foundation, 2809
Dictionary of Congenital Malformations& Disorders, 5057
Division of Birth Defects and Developmental Disabilities, 3417
Edward J Madden Open Hearts Camp, 1177, 8382
Management of Genetic Syndromes, 8517
March of Dimes Birth Defects Foundation, 877
National Center on Birth Defects and Developmental Disabilities, 4727
National Fragile X Foundation, 8695
National Organization for Albinism and Hypopigmentation, 8294
National Organization on Fetal Alcohol Syndrome, 8295
University of Miami: Mailman Center for Child Development, 4716
Why My Child, 5377

Blind/Deaf

AADB National Conference, 1828
ASD Athletics, 7603
Alaska Center for the Blind and Visually Impaired, 6511
American Association of the Deaf-Blind, 7561
Arena Stage, 6, 7563
Canadian Deafblind Association (CDBA) National Office, 7565
Communicating with People Who Have Trouble Hearing & Seeing: A Primer, 7581
Deaf-Blind Perspective, 7590, 9077
Florida School for the Deaf and Blind, 7579
A Handbook for Writing Effective Psychoeducational Reports (2nd Edition), 7580
Hearing Loss Association of America, 7567, 7921
Helen Keller National Center for Deaf- Blind Youths And Adults, 7568
InFocus, 7591
National Consortium on Deaf-Blindness, 7572
National Family Association for Deaf-Blind, 7573
National Information Center for Children and Youth with Disabilities (NICHCY), 7575
National Information Clearinghouse on Children who are Deaf-Blind, 7576
Ultratec, 497, 7577

Brain Injuries

Bancroft, 7041
Before and After Zachariah, 5262
Brain Injury Association of New York State, 7619
Brain Injury Association of Texas, 7620
Camp Barefoot, 1184
Camp Hawkins, 1053
Center for Comprehensive Services, 6824
Center for Neuro-Rehabilitation, 6950
Devereux Advanced Behavioral HealthCalifornia, 6588
Easter Seals Superior California, 6594
The Education of Children with AcquiredBrain Injury, 2565
The Essential Brain Injury Guide (5th Edition), 5291
Hope Network Rehabilitation Services, 6999
Hospital For Special Care (HSC), 7241
Living with Brain Injury: A Guide for Families, 8510
Measure of Cognitive-Linguistic Abilities(MCLA), 2622
National Hydrocephalus Foundation, 7646
Neurobehavioral Medicine Center, 6765
North Broward Rehab Unit, 6766
Occupational Therapy Approaches to Traumatic Brain Injury, 2475
Preventable Brain Damage, 7800
Rasmussen's Syndrome and Hemispherectomy Support Network Newsletter, 8631

Rehabilitation Services, 922
Students with Acquired Brain Injury: The School's Response, 2534
Universal Institute Rehabilitation & Fitness Center, 6380
When Billy Broke His Head...and OtherFanlight Productions/Icarus Films, 5373

Cancer

AMC Cancer Research Center, 4683
Adult Leukemia: A Comprehensive Guide for Patients and Families, 8430
Advanced Breast Cancer: A Guide to Living with Metastic Disease, 8431
Adventure Day Camp, 1414, 8311
Alexander and Margaret Stewart Trust, 2821
American Society of Pediatric Hematology/Oncology, 8258
Aplastic Anemia and MDS International Foundation, 8260
Arbors at New Castle, 7245
Arizona Camp Sunrise, 950, 8313
Association for the Cure of Cancer of the Prostate (CaP CURE)-Prostate Cancer Foundation, 5395
Baxter Healthcare Corporation, 6817
Beliefs: Pathways to Health and Well Being, 5028
Big Sky Kids Cancer Camps, 1222
Breast Cancer Sourcebook, 8448
Camp Anuenue, 1059, 8318
Camp Barnabas, 1209
Camp Boggy Creek, 1036, 8320
Camp Can Do, 1340, 8323
Camp Catch-a-Rainbow, 1185, 8325
Camp Dream Street, 1208, 1240
Camp Firefly, 972
Camp Good Days and Special Times, 1259
Camp Hobe, 1401
Camp Little Red Door, 1094
Camp Magruder, 1325, 8356
Camp Mak-A-Dream, 1223
Camp Okizu, 977, 8359
Camp Quality Arkansas, 962
Camp Quality Central Missouri, 1213
Camp Quality George Washington University, 1152
Camp Quality Greater Kansas City, 1214
Camp Quality Heartland, 1108
Camp Quality Illinois, 1072
Camp Quality Kansas, 1117
Camp Quality Kentuckiana, 1120
Camp Quality Louisiana, 1129
Camp Quality Michigan, 1189
Camp Quality New Jersey, 1246
Camp Quality Northwest Missouri, 1215
Camp Quality Ohio, 1307
Camp Quality Ozarks, 1216
Camp Quality Texas, 1389
Camp Rainbow, 956, 8361
Camp Rap-A-Hope, 941, 8362
Camp Reach for the Sky, 983
Camp Ronald McDonald for Good Times, 984, 8363
Camp Smile-A-Mile, 944, 8367
Camp Sunrise, 1154, 8368
Camp Sunshine, 1056, 1140
Camp Sunshine Dreams, 988
Camp Wapiyapi, 1012
Canadian Cancer Society, 8261
Cancer Care, 3033
Cancer Clinical Trials: A CommonsenseGuide to Experimental Cancer Therapies and Trials, 5247
Cancer Immunology Research Foundation(CIRF) Cancer Research Institute National Headquar, 5399
Cancer Immunotherapy and Gene Therapy, 5400
Cancer Information Service, 8648
Cancer Research Institute, 5401
Cancer Sourcebook, 8450
Cancer Sourcebook for Women, 8451
Candlelighters Childhood Cancer Foundation, 2924
Childhood Cancer Canada Foundation, 8264
Childhood Cancer Survivors: A Practical Guide to Your Future, 8453

Childhood Cancer: A Parent's Guide to Solid Tumor Cancers, 8454
Childhood Leukemia Foundation, 8265
Colon & Rectal Cancer: A Comprehensive Guide for Patients & Families, 8460
Conquering the Darkness: One Story of Recovering from a Brain Injury, 8463
Coping with Cancer Magazine, 8602
Damon Runyon Cancer Research Foundation, 5403
Desert Regional Medical Center, 6587
Double H Ranch, 1272
Eastern Idaho Regional Medical Center, 7269
Fannie E Rippel Foundation, 3011
Foundation for Advancement in Cancer Therapy, 3054
Genetic Nutritioneering, 5081
Happiness Is Camping, 1249, 8389
Healthsouth Rehabilitation Hospital of Greater Pittsburgh, 6419
Hole in the Wall Gang Camp, 1026, 8391
Indian Summer Camp, 1123
Institute for Families, 8839
International Association for Cancer Victors & Friends, 8273
International Myeloma Foundation, 8276
Jane Coffin Childs Memorial Fund for Medical Research, 2815
Jane Phillips Medical Center, 6403
John Muir Medical Center Rehabilitation Services, Therapy Center, 6612
Leukemia & Lymphoma Society, 8277
Leukemia Sourcebook, 8500
Liver Disorders Sourcebook, 8504
Lung Cancer: Making Sense of Diagnosis, Treatment, and Options, 8512
Lymphoma Canada, 8279
Madonna Rehabilitation Hospital, 7328
Marist Brothers Mid-Hudson Valley Camp, 1280, 8395
Methodist Hospital Rehabilitation Institute, 6325
Multiple Sclerosis National Research Institute, 5430
National Association for Proton Therapy, 8284
National Cancer Institute, 8288
Northwest Hospital Center for Medical Rehabilitation, 6479
One Day at a Time: Children Living with Leukemia, 8549
Options, 8625
Options: Revolutionary Ideas in the War on Cancer, 8550
Painted Turtle, The, 1001
Parma Community General Hospital Acute Rehabilitation Center, 6395
Prostate and Urological Disorders Sourcebook, 8559
Psychology and Health, 5158
RA Bloch Cancer Foundation, 2992
Simonton Cancer Center, 8298
St. Anthony's Hospital, 7258
Sumner Regional Medical Center, 6439
V Foundation for Cancer Research, 5447
Victory Junction Gang Camp, 1295
YMCA Camp Horseshoe, 1433, 8416
YMCA Camp Jewell, 1028
YMCA Camp jewell, 8422
Your Guide to Bowel Cancer, 8595

Cerebral Palsy

American Academy for Cerebral Palsy and Developmental Medicine Annual Conference, 1843
Believable Hope Conference, 1849
Cerebral Palsy Associations of New York State, 7622
Cerebral Palsy: North County Center, 6574
Charles Campbell Childrens Camp, 1224
Children with Cerebral Palsy: A Parents' Guide, 8457
Coping with Cerebral Palsy, 8464
Echoing Hills, 1309, 8381
From Where I Sit: Making My Way with Cerebral Palsy, 8476

No Time for Jello: One Family's Experience, 8534
Ontario Cerebral Palsy Sports Association, 8238
Ontario Federation for Cerebral Palsy, 7649
Preventing Secondary Conditions Associated with Spina Bifida or Cerebral Palsy, 8558
Summer Camp for Physically & Mentally Challenged Children & Adults, 1118, 8406
Ten Things I Learned from Bill Porter, 8578
Treating Cerebral Palsy for Clinicians by Clinicians, 2571
United Cerebral Palsy, 2053, 7656
United Cerebral Palsy of Texas, 3796

Chiropractics

American Chiropractic Association, 779
International Chiropractors Association, 863

Chronic Disabilities

Access to Health Care: Number 3&4, 2281
Broken Dolls: Gathering the Pieces: Caringfor Chronically Ill Children, 5197
Burnt Gin Camp, 1365
Camp Holiday Trails, 1417
Caring for Children with Chronic Illness, 2324
Comprehensive Care Coordination for Chronically Ill Adults, 4976
Counseling Parents of Children with Chronic Illness or Disability, 5277
Developing Cross-Cultural Competence:Guideto Working with Young Children & Their Families, 2361
Family Interventions Throughout Disability, 5210
Living with a Brother or Sister with Special Needs: A Book for Sibs, 5214
National Association of Chronic Disease Directors, 8286
Screening in Chronic Disease, 5167
Treating Adults with Disabilities: Access and Communication, 2570
Usher Syndrome, 8589

Cleft Palate

Camp About Face, 1088
Cleft Palate-Craniofacial Journal, 8600
Nasometer, 1768
Your Cleft Affected Child, 8594

Cognitive Disorders

ADHD Book of Lists: A Practical Guide for Helping Children and Teens with ADDs, 7712
ADHD in the Schools: Assessment and Intervention Strategies, 2279, 7713
Adult ADD: The Complete Handbook: Everything You Need to Know About How to Cope with ADD, 7716
Arc Connection Newsletter, 5018, 7830
Arc Light, 7837
Assistive Technology for Individuals withCognitive Impairments Handbook, 7718
Augmenting Basic Communcation in Natural Contexts, 7726
Be Quiet, Marina!, 7737
Best Buddies, 7616
Biology Concepts Through Discovery, 7857
Camp Easter Seals Virginia, 1416
Camp Nissokone, 1188, 7667
Camp Nuhop, 1306, 7669
Camp Ramapo, 1265, 7670
Child and Adolescent Therapy: Cognitive-Behavioral Procedures, Third Edition, 7741
Concentration Video, 7858
Count Us In, 7748
Dallas Academy, 1395, 7680
Difficult Child, 7750
Disability Culture Perspective on Early Intervention, 7751
Dynamic Learning Center, 7628
Elling Camps, 1351

Embracing the Monster: Overcoming the Challenges of Hidden Disabilities, 7755
Equal Treatment for People With Mental Retardation: Having and Raising Children, 7757
Evaluation and Treatment of the Psychogeriatric Patient, 2394
Getting Our Heads Together, 7762
Helping Your Child with Attention-Deficit Hyperactivity Disorder, 7769
Hill School of Fort Worth, 1397, 7686
I Just Want My Little Boy Back, 7862, 8786
Imagine!, 7835
In Search of Wings: A Journey Back from Traumatic Brain Injury, 7776
In Their Own Way, 7777
Journal of Cognitive Rehabilitation, 7826
Keys to Parenting a Child with Attention Deficit Disorder, 7780
LD Child and the ADHD Child: Ways Parents & Professionals Can Help, 7783
Life Development Institute, 7632
Making the Writing Process Work, 7786
Marvelwood Summer, 1027, 7691
A Miracle to Believe In, 7710
NLP Comprehensive, 7635
National Association of Cognitive- Behavioral Therapists, 7639
New Horisons Summer Day Camp, 7692
New Horizons Summer Day Camp, 1000, 8712
Oakland School & Camp, 1424, 7694
Phelps School Summer School, 1357, 7696
Pure Facts, 7836
Quest Camp, 1003, 7697
Ramapo Training, 2681
Relationship Development Intervention with Young Children, 7803, 8753
SOAR Summer Adventures, 1293, 7701
Sherman Lake YMCA Outdoor Center, 1194, 7702
Squirrel Hollow Summer Camp, 1058, 7703
St. Francis Camp On The Lake, 1195
Successful Job Search Strategies for the Disabled: Understanding the ADA, 7811
Techniques for Aphasia Rehab: (TARGET) Generating Effective Treatment, 7815, 8762
Timbertop Nature Adventure Camp, 1439, 7707
Tower Program at Regis College, 1182
You Mean I'm Not Lazy, Stupid or Crazy?!: A Self-Help Book for Adults with ADD, 7822

Cystic Fibrosis

Bittersweet Chances: A Personal Journey o f Living and Learning in the Face of Illness, 8443
Camp Funshine, 960
Cystic Fibrosis Foundation, 2929
Cystic Fibrosis: Medical Care, 5279
Cystic Fibrosis: A Guide for Patient and Family, 8466
Official Patient's Sourcebook on Cystic Fibrosis, 8540
Understanding Cystic Fibrosis, 8586
YMCA Camp Kitaki, 1231, 8418

Dementia

Alzheimer Disease Sourcebook, 8435
Alzheimer Disease Sourcebook, 4th Edition, 8436
Alzheimer's Association, 2864
Bay View Nursing and Rehabilitation Center, 7228
Brain Disorders Sourcebook, 8447
Brewer Rehab and Living Center, 6350
Clinical Alzheimer Rehabilitation, 2339
Country Manor Rehabilitation and Nursing Center, 7316
Kennedy Park Medical Rehabilitation Center, 7427
Lafayette Nursing and Rehabilitation Center, 7262
Levindale Hebrew Geriatric Center, 6954
Mississippi Department of Mental Health, 3563
Music Therapy in Dementia Care, 42
Renaissance at South Shore, 7282
San Luis Medical and Rehabilitation Center, 7433

Dental Issues

International Academy of Biological Dentistry and Medicine, 8271
International Academy of Oral Medicine & Toxicology, 8272
International Medical and Dental Hypnotherapy Association, 8275
Special Care Dentistry Association, 8299

Depression

DAYS: Depression and Anxiety in Youth Scale, 2606
Florida CORF, 6744
Focal Group Psychotherapy, 2400
Menopause without Medicine, 8520
Motivator, 8208
Phenomenology of Depressive Illness, 2485
Social Security: Tampa Disability Determination, 3415
Stroke Connection Magazine, 7892, 8194
When the Brain Goes Wrong, 5187

Developmental Disabilities

AAIDD Annual Meeting, 1829
Abilities of Northwest New Jersey, 6100
Activities with Developmentally Disabled Elderly and Older Adults, 7494
Administration on Developmental Disabilities, 3289
Advocate Illinois Masonic Medical Center, 6812
Alliance for Disabled in Action New Jersey, 6101
Allied Enterprises of Tupelo, 6073
Arc National Convention, The, 1847
Arc South County Chapter, 3161
As I Am, 5021
Association of University Centers on Disabilities, 802
Bakersfield ARC, 5837
Berkshire Meadows, 6961
Breaking Ground, 8617
Brooklyn Bureau of Community Service, 7057
Builders of Skills, 6308
CYO Day Camp: Wickliffe, 1297
Camp Waban, 1134
Camp Abilities Tucson, 951
Camp Caglewood, 1050
Camp Callahan, 1064
Camp Cheerful, 1299, 8326
Camp Civitan, 953
Camp Courageous, 1300
Camp Dickenson, 1415
Camp Dream, 1051
Camp Happiness, 1302
Camp Killoqua, 1426
Camp Kota, 961
Camp Krem, 976
Camp Lee Mar, 1343
Camp ReCreation, 982
Camp Starfish, 1172
Camp Sun'N Fun, 1247
Camp Thunderbird, 1038
Camp Whitman on Seneca Lake, 1269
Camp Winnebago, 1142
Career Assessment & Planning Services, 5921
Catalog for Teaching Life Skills to Persons with Development Disability, 1921
Center for Disability Resources, 816, 3174
Cheyenne Village, 5879
Clausen House, 6578
Clay Tree Society, 823
Clearbrook, 5968
Colton-Redlands-Yucaipa Regional Occupational Programs, 5841
Communication Development and Disorders in African American Children, 8732
Community Opportunities of East Ascension, 6032
Comprehensive Rehabilitation Center of Naples Community Hospital, 6731
Concerned Care, Inc., 1217
Confidence Learning Center, 1205

DOCS: Developmental Observation Checklist System, 2607
Datahr Rehabilitation Institute, 6699
Developmental Disabilities in Infancy and Childhood, 5203
Developmental Disabilities: A Handbook for Interdisciplinary Practice, 2367
Developmental Services Center, 2609
Dictionary of Developmental Disabilities Terminology, 5058, 5204
Directory for Exceptional Children, 2062
Donaldsville Association for Retarded Citizens, 6929
Dynamic Dimensions, 5883
Easter Seals: Achievement Center, 5796
Family Support Project for the Developmentally Disabled, 8656
Family-Centered Service Coordination: A Manual for Parents, 5211
First Occupational Center of New Jersey, 6112
Foundation Industries, 6932
Fragile X Family, 8639
Gateway Center of Monterey County, 6600
Gateway Industries: Castroville, 6601
Glenkirk, 5971
Handbook of Developmental Education, 2414
Happiness Bag, 1099
Hartford Foundation for Public Giving, 2812
HealthSouth Sports Medicine & Rehabilitation Center, 6282
Hockanum Greenhouse, 6703
Information Services for People with Developmental Disabilities, 5100
Innabah Camps, 1353
JCYS Camp Red Leaf, 1074
Jersey Cape Diagnostic Training & Opportunity Center, 6115
Kennedy Job Training Center, 5975
Knox County Council for Developmental Disabilities, 5976
Lambs Farm, 5978
Lambton County Developmental Services, 870
Language, Learning & Living, 215
Life-Span Approach to Nursing Care for Individuals with Developmental Disabilities, 2458
Lifelong Leisure Skills and Lifestyles for Persons with Developmental Disabilities, 5114
LoSeCa Foundation, 874
Lutherdale Bible Camp, 1437
MAGIC Foundation for Children's Growth, 2885
MAGIC Touch, 8515
Medical Camping, 1125
Music Therapy for the Developmentally Disabled, 41
Napa Valley PSI Inc., 5855
National Association of Developmental Disabilities Councils, 885
National Association of State Directors of Developmental Disabilities Services (NASDDDS), 887
National Sports Center for the Disabled, 8235, 8643
National Theatre Workshop of the Handicapped (NTWH), 52
New Hampshire Bureau of Developmental Services, 3606
New Hampshire Developmental Disabilities Council, 3610
Nuvisions For Disabled Artists, Inc., 57
Orange County ARC, 5858
Parallels in Time, 5144
People First of Oregon, 917
Pilgrim Pines Camp & Conference Center, 1002
Porterville Sheltered Workshop, 5864
Professional Fit Clothing, 1470
Rational Effectiveness Training Systems, 6138
Rehabilitation Opportunities, 6956
Relaxation Techniques for People with Special Needs, 5358
Richmond Research Training Center, 6209
Sebasticook Farms-Great Bay Foundation, 6947
Sexuality and the Developmentally Handicapped, 5227

Sibpage, 2262
Spring Dell Center, 7944
Steps to Independence: Teaching Everyday Skills to Children with Special Needs, 8572
Sundial Special Vacations, 5535
Supported Employment Program, 5944
TERI, 5177
Thumb Industries, 7008
Torah Alliance of Families of Kids with Disabilities, 5707
Toyei Industries, 6532
Trips Inc., 5536
United Foundation for Disabled Archers, 8241
Vocational and Rehabilitation Agency: State Department of Social Services, 5906
Warren Achievement Center, 6878
Wesley Woods Camp and Retreat Center, 1114
YMCA Camp Erdman, 1060
Young Children with Special Needs: A Developmentally Appropriate Approach, 2658

Diabetes

ADA Annual Scientific Sessions, 1834
ADA Camp Grenada, 1412, 8304
ADA Camp Kushtaka, 947, 8305
ADA Camp Needlepoint, 8306
ADA Camp Sunshine, 1256
ADA Camp for Kids, 8307
ADA Teen Adventure Camp, 937, 8308
ADA Triangle D Camp, 938, 8309
American Diabetes Association, 8252
Bearskin Meadow Camp, 964, 8314
Camp Adam Fisher, 1366
Camp Aldersgate, 959
Camp Buck, 1232
Camp Carefree, 8324
Camp Carolina Trails, 1287
Camp Classen YMCA, 1320, 8328
Camp Comeca & Retreat Center, 1225, 7957
Camp Conrad-Chinnock, 969, 8329
Camp Crosley YMCA, 1092
Camp Discovery, 1376, 8332
Camp Discovery - Illinois, 8333
Camp Discovery - Kansas, 1116
Camp Floyd Rogers, 1226, 8335
Camp Fun in the Sun, 1425, 8336
Camp Gilbert, 1371
Camp Glyndon, 1148, 8338
Camp Hertko Hollow, 1106, 8340
Camp Hickory Hill, 1211, 8341
Camp Ho Mita Koda, 1303, 8342
Camp Hodia, 1061, 8343
Camp Hope, 1444
Camp John Warvel, 1093, 8347
Camp Joslin, 1169, 8348
Camp Ko-Man-She, 1304, 8350
Camp Kudzu, 1055
Camp Kweebec, 1342, 8351
Camp Libbey, 1305, 8354
Camp Needlepoint, 1435
Camp Nejeda, 1244, 8357
Camp Seale Harris, 942, 8365
Camp Setebaid, 1345, 8366
Camp Sioux, 1296
Camp Sugar Falls, 1379
Camp Sweeney, 1392, 8369
Camp Trinity, 990
Camp Victory, 1130
Camp Waziyatah, 1141, 8373
Camps for Children & Teens with Diabetes, 1420, 8375
Canadian Diabetes Association, 8262
Cedar Ridge Camp, 1121, 8376
Center for the Partially Sighted, 6572
Clara Barton Diabetes Camp, 1175, 8378
Coast to Coast Home Medical, 311
Comprehensive Rehabilitation Center at Lee Memorial Hospital, 6730
Diabetes Camp, 1112, 8379
Diabetes Network of East Hawaii, 3429
Diabetes Self-Management, 8619
Diabetes Sourcebook., 8467
Diabetic Cruise Desk, 5522

EDI Camp, 8380
FCYD Camp, 1407, 8383
Florida Diabetes Camp, 1041, 8385
Friends Academy Summer Camps, 1274, 8386
Gales Creek Diabetes Camp, 1328
Growing Together Diabetes Camp, 1396, 8388
Immune System Disorders Sourcebook., 8488
Joslin Guide to Diabetes: A Program for Managing
     Your Treatment, 8494
Juvenile Diabetes Research Foundation
     International, 869
Kiwanis Camp Wyman, 1218, 8392
Kluge Children's Rehabilitation Center, 6477
Lions Camp Merrick, 1159, 7973
Louisiana Lions Camp, 1131
Louisiana Lions Camp - Camp Pelican, 1132
Makemie Woods Camp, 1423, 8393
Makemie Woods Camp/Conference Retreat, 8394
Meeting the Needs of People with Vision Loss:
     Multidisciplinary Perspective, 8997
National Diabetes Action Network for the Blind,
     8862
NeSoDak, 1372, 8399
No More Allergies, 8533
Raleigh Rehabilitation and Healthcare Center, 7357
Resources for People with Disabilities and Chronic
     Conditions, 5165
Taking Control of Your Diabetes (TCOYD), 8302
Texas Lions Camp, 1399, 7979, 8409, 8897
Triangle D Camp, 1318
Tuolumne Trails, 1005
Voice of the Diabetic, 8637
Wisconsin Lions Camp, 1442, 8413
Y Camp, 1115, 8414
YMCA Camp Copneconic, 1197
YMCA Camp Fitch, 1360, 7980, 8165, 8415, 8716
YMCA Camp Orkila, 1431, 8419

Diet & Nutrition

Feingold Association of the US, 848
Metametrix Clinical Laboratory, 879
National Association of Anorexia Nervosa and
     Associated Disorders, 8285

Down Syndrome

Adam's Camp, 1006
Adolescents with Down Syndrome: Toward a More
     Fulfilling Life, 7715
Biomedical Concerns in Persons with Down's
     Syndrome, 2318
Bobby Dodd Institute (BDI), 6790
Bus Girl: Selected Poems, 7739
Camp Knutson, 1204
Camp Lotsafun, 1233
Clockworks, 5320
Communication Development in Children with
     Down Syndrome, 7744, 8733
Down Syndrome, 7752
Down Syndrome News, 7833
Down Syndrome Society of Rhode Island, 3166
Early Communication Skills for Children with
     Down Syndrome, 2377
Keys to Parenting a Child with Downs Syndrome,
     7781
National Association for Down Syndrome, 7637
National Down Syndrome Congress, 7644
National Down Syndrome Society, 7645
Parent's Guide to Down Syndrome: Toward a
     Brighter Future, 7796
Teaching Children with Down Syndrome about
     Their Bodies, Boundaries, and Sexuality, 5252
Teaching Reading to Children with Down
     Syndrome: A Guide for Parents and Teachers,
     2550
Understanding Down Syndrome: An Introduction
     for Parents, 7817

Dyslexia

Annals of Dyslexia, 7825

Annual Conference on Dyslexia and Related
     Learning Disabilities, 1845
Assets School, 5954
Dyslexia Training Program, 1933
Dyslexia over the Lifespan, 7754
Gow School Summer Programs, 1276, 7685
How To Reach and Teach Children and Teens with
     Dyslexia, 7772
Individualized Keyboarding, 1948
Instrumental Music for Dyslexics: A Teaching
     Handbook, 32
International Dyslexia Association, 2031
International Dyslexia Association of DC, 3394
International Dyslexia Association of NY: Buffalo
     Branch, 3638
International Dyslexia Association of New
     England, 3521
International Dyslexia Association: Arizona
     Branch, 3338
International Dyslexia Association: Austin Branch,
     3775
International Dyslexia Association: Central
     California Branch, 3358
International Dyslexia Association: Central Ohio
     Branch, 3689
International Dyslexia Association: Florida Branch,
     3411
International Dyslexia Association: Georgia
     Branch, 3425
International Dyslexia Association: Hawaii Branch,
     3439
International Dyslexia Association: Illinois Branch,
     3459
International Dyslexia Association: Indiana
     Branch, 3466
International Dyslexia Association: Iowa Branch,
     3468
International Dyslexia Association: Kansas/West
     Missouri Branch, 3479
International Dyslexia Association: Maryland
     Branch, 3511
International Dyslexia Association: Minnesota
     Branch, 3547
International Dyslexia Association: Mississippi
     Branch, 3559
International Dyslexia Association: Nebraska
     Branch, 3583
International Dyslexia Association: New Jersey
     Branch, 3617
International Dyslexia Association: North Carolina
     Branch, 3671
International Dyslexia Association: Oregon
     Branch, 3708
International Dyslexia Association: Pennsylvania
     Branch, 3717
International Dyslexia Association: Rocky
     Mountain Branch, 3372
International Dyslexia Association: Tennessee
     Branch, 3759
International Dyslexia Association: Virginia
     Branch, 3821
International Dyslexia Association: Washington
     State Branch, 3831
International Dyslexia Association: Wisconsin
     Branch, 3852
Language and the Developing Child, 8740
Learning Disabilities Sourcebook, 3rd Ed., 36
Let's Write Right: Teacher's Edition, 2456
Louisiana Center for Dyslexia and Related
     Learning Disorders, 3495
Many Faces of Dyslexia, 1968
Mozart Effect: Tapping the Power of Music to
     Heal the Body, Strengthen the Mind, 38
Multisensory Teaching of Basic Language Skills:
     Theory and Practice, 2471
Music and Dyslexia: A Positive Approach, 44
Overcoming Dyslexia, 7794
Overcoming Dyslexia in Children, Adolescents and
     Adults, 2476
Pre-Reading Screening Procedures, 2635
Reading, Writing and Speech Problems in
     Children, 7801, 8752
Reality of Dyslexia, 7802
Recording for the Blind & Dyslexic, 9015

Sandhills School, 2682
Southwest Branch of the International Dyslexia
     Association, 3635
Stern Center, 8702
TESTS, 2537
Teaching of Reading: A Continuum from
     Kindergarten through College, The, 2647
To Teach a Dyslexic, 2008
We're Not Stupid, 7867

Education & Counseling

ACS Federal Healthcare, 759
Adapting Early Childhood Curricula for Children
     with Special Needs (9th Edition), 2284
Advocacy Center, 764
Advocates for Children of New York, 766
Agassiz Village Camp, 1164
Alaska Department of Education:
     SpecialEducation, 2110
American Counseling Association, 782
American Occupational Therapy Association, 788
American Red Cross, 791
American Self-Help Clearinghouse, 792
Applied Rehabilitation Counseling (Springer Series
     on Rehabilitation), 2298
Association for Persons in Supported Employment,
     797
Association on Higher Education and Disability
     (AHEAD), 803
Breckenridge Outdoor Education Center, 1008
Brookline Books, 2082
Building the Healing Partnership: Parents,
     Professionals and Children with Chronic
     Illnesses, 2322
CAPP National Parent Resource Center Federation
     for Children with Special Needs, 809
Camp Independence, 1261, 8345
Camp Pinecone, 1139
Camp Sno Mo, 1237
Camp Thorpe, 1410
Cape Organization for Rights of the Disabled
     (CORD), 813, 4198
Case Management Society of America, 814
Center for Assistive Technology and
     Environmental Access, 815
Challenge Aspen, 1013
Childhood Disablity and Family
     Systems(Routledge Library Editions) (Volume
     5), 2332
Choices: A Guide to Sex Counseling with
     Physically Disabled Adults, 2335
Colorado Lions Camp, 1016
Community Enterprises, 824
Deciphering the System: A Guide for Families of
     Young Disabled Children, 2358
Department of Rehabilitation Services &Bureau of
     Education And Services for the Blind, 2115
Early Intervention: Implementing Child & Family
     Services for At-Risk Infants and Toddlers, 2378
Easter Seals, 8654
Easter Seals Nebraska, 1228
Educating Individuals with Disabilities:IDEIA
     2004 and Beyond (1st Edition), 2382
Favarh/Farmington Valley ARC, 844
George Washington University Health Resource
     Center, 851
Handi Camp, 1352
Images of the Disabled, Disabling Images, 2428
Inclusive Play People, 1947
Institute for Scientific Research, 859
The K&W Guide to Colleges for Studentswith
     Learning Disabilities (13th Edition), 2567
Library Manager's Guide to Hiring and Serving
     Disabled Persons, 2457
Mainstream, 876
National Council on Disability, 891, 3297
National Diabetes Information Clearinghouse, 8289
National Digestive Diseases Information
     Clearinghouse, 8290
National Kidney and Urologic Diseases
     Information Clearinghouse, 8293
National Organization on Disability, 901
National Rehabilitation Association (NRA), 902

National Rehabilitation Information Center(NARIC), 903
Native American Protection and Advocacy, 906
Nevada Department of Education: Special Eduction Branch, 2152
People-to-People International: Committee for the Handicapped, 919
Pine Tree Camp, 1144
Professional Development Programs, 2140
Rehabilitation Technology, 2509
South Dakota Division of Rehabilitation, 3757
Student Disability Services, 926
Teacher Preparation and Special Education, 927
Technology and Media Division, 928

Emergency Alert

Cornell Communications, 208
MedicAlert Foundation International, 5455
Sidney Stern Memorial Trust, 2789
Step-by-Step Communicator, 235
TalkTrac Wearable Communicator, 238

Environmental Disorders

Alternative Approach to Allergies, 8434
Protecting Against Latex Allergy, 8560

Epilepsy

Acting BlindFanlight Productions/Icarus Films, 5306
Boy Inside, TheFanlight Productions/Icarus Films, 5314
Camp Candlelight, 952, 7663
Camp Coelho, 968
Camp Evoked Potential @ Camp ASCCA, 939, 7664
Camp Quest, 980
Camp Roehr, 1153
Camp Wee-Kan-Tu, 1173
Easter Seals Camp Harmon, 996
Epilepsy Council of Greater Cincinnati, 3688
Epilepsy Foundation, 7629, 7878, 8135, 8655
Epilepsy Foundation of Long Island, 3046
Epilepsy Foundation of Southeast Texas, 3204
Epilepsy Foundation: Central and South Texas, 3205
Epilepsy, 199 Answers: A Doctor Responds to His Patients' Questions, 8473
Epilepsy: Patient and Family Guide, 8474
EpilepsyUSA, 8604
Father Drumgoole Connelly Summer Camp, 1273, 7970, 8384
Global Assistive Devices, Inc., 189
Growing Up with Epilepsy: A Pratical Guide for Parents, 8478
Ketogenic Diet: A Treatment for Children and Others with Epilepsy, 8496
Narcolepsy, 8641
National Association of Epilepsy Centers, 7641
Neuropsychiatry of Epilepsy, 8531
On The SpectrumFanlight Productions/Icarus Films, 5347
Outsider: The Life and Art of Judith ScottFanlight Productions/Icarus Films, 5351
Phantom Lake YMCA Camp, 1438, 8401
Pushin' ForwardFanlight Productions/Icarus Films, 5356
Seizures and Epilepsy in Childhood: A Guide, 8566
Twin Lakes Camp, 1103, 8164, 8410
White Cane and WheelsFanlight Productions/Icarus Films, 5376
YMCA Camp Weona, 1285, 8421

Head & Neck Injuries

American Academy of Otolaryngology - Head and Neck Surgery, 8247
American Head and Neck Society, 8254
Annals of Otology, Rhinology and Laryngology, 8598

Cervical Support Pillow, 186
Head Injury Hotline, 8657
Head Injury Rehabilitation: Children, 2416
Health and Rehabilitation Products, 473
IAL News, 8621
Injured Mind, Shattered Dreams: Brian's Survival from a Severe Head Injury, 8490
Jackson Cervipillo, 191
Journal of Head Trauma Rehabilitation, 8601
Life Line, 8502
NeckEase, 192

Hearing Impairments

ADA Hotel Built-In Alerting System, 198
AG Bell Convention, 1836
ASD Summer Camp, 7949
ASHA Leader, The, 8079
ASSISTECH Special Needs, 183
Academy of Rehabilitative Audiology, 7897
Access for All: Integrating Deaf, Hard of Hearing and Hearing Preschoolers, 7987
Access-USA, 501, 610
Addison Point Specialized Services, 6037
Advanced Sign Language Vocabulary: A Resource Text for Educators, 2288, 7988
Akron Resources, 201
Alexander Graham Bell Association for the Deaf and Hard of Hearing, 7898
Alternatives in Education for the Hearing Impaired (AEHI), 5384
American Academy of Audiology, 5385
American Academy of Environmental Medicine, 769
American Action Fund for Blind Children and Adults, 8798
American Annals of the Deaf, 8080
American Association of People with Disabilities, 773, 7899
American Hearing Impaired Hockey Association, 8114
American Journal of Audiology, 8065
American Sign Language Handshape Cards, 1910
American Sign Language Handshape Dictionary, 7989
American Sign Language Phrase Book, 7990
American Sign Language: A Look at Its History, Structure & Community, 7991
American Society for Deaf Children, 7562, 7901
American Speech-Language and Hearing Association, 5391
Americans with Disabilities Act: Selected Resources for Deaf, 4580
Amplified Handsets, 202
Amplified Phones, 203
Amplified Portable Phone, 204
Approaching Equality, 4581
Aspen Camp of the Deaf & Hard of Hearing, 1007, 7951
Assessment & Management of Mainstreamed Hearing-Impaired Children, 2301
Association of Late-Deafened Adults, 7564, 7905
At Home Among Strangers, 7992
Auditech: Personal FM Educational System, 1914
Auditech: Personal PA Value Pack System, 329
Auditory-Verbal Therapy for Parents and Professionals, 1915
Aural Habilitation, 2313
Aurora of Central New York, 7604
BPPV: What You Need to Know, 7993
A Basic Course in American Sign Language, 7983
Basic Course in American Sign Language, 8914
Basic Course in American Sign Language(B100) Harris Communications, Inc., 5311
A Basic Course in Manual Communication, 7984
A Basic Vocabulary: American Sign Languagefor Parents and Children, 7985
Bath and Shower Bench 3301B, 158
Battery Device Adapter, 331
Bed Rails, 310
Beginning ASL Video CourseHarris Communications, Inc., 5312
Belonging, 8916
Ben's Story: A Deaf Child's Right to Sign, 7994

Better Hearing Institute, 7906
Bold Tracks, 8224
Book of Name Signs: Naming in American Sign Language, 7995
CHAMP Camp, 1087, 7952
CNI Cochlear Kids Camp, 1009
Camp Abilities Brockport, 1257
Camp Alexander Mack, 1089, 7953
Camp Bishopswood, 1135, 7954
Camp Capella, 1136, 7955
Camp Chris Williams, 1186, 7956
Camp Emanuel, 1301, 7958
Camp Grizzly, 974, 7959
Camp Isola Bella, 1025
Camp Isola Bella On Twin Lakes,Salisbury, Ct., 7960
Camp Juliena, 1054, 7962
Camp Mark Seven, 1263, 7963
Camp Pacifica, Inc., 978, 7964
Camp Ramah in the Poconos Education, Inc., 1344
Camp Sertoma, 1290
Camp Shocco for the Deaf, 943, 7965
Camp SignShine, 1234
Camp Taloali, 1327, 7966
Center for Hearing and Communication, 7907
Challenge of Educating Together Deaf and Hearing Youth: Making Manistreaming Work, 2327
Chelsea: The Story of a Signal Dog, 7996
Children of a Lesser God, 7997
Choices in Deafness: A Parent's Guide to Communication Options, 7998
Christmas Stories, 8100
Clark-Winchcole Foundation, 2926
Classroom GOAL: Guide for Optimizing Auditory Learning Skills, 1922
Classroom Notetaker: How to Organize a Program Serving Students with Hearing Impairments, 1923
Cochlear Implants In Children: Ethics and Choices, 8093
Cochlear Implants for Kids, 7999
Cognition, Education and Deafness: Directions for Research and Instruction, 8000
College and University Programs for Deaf and Hard of Hearing Students, 8001
Come Sign with Us, 8002
Communication Service for the Deaf, 7908
Communique, 8094
Comprehensive Reference Manual for Signers and Interpreters, 8003
Comprehensive Signed English Dictionary, 8004
Conference of Educational Administrators of Schools and Programs for the Deaf, 7909
Connect, 8773
Connect - Commmunity News, 8082
Conversational Sign Language II: An Intermediate Advanced Manual, 8005
Council of American Instructors of the Deaf (CAID), 7910
Courage Center Camps, 1206
Crutches, 645
Custom Earmolds, 332
DB-Link, 826
Deaf Catholic, 8083
Deaf Children Signers, 5322
Deaf Culture Series, 5323
Deaf Empowerment: Emergence, Struggle and Rhetoric, 8006
Deaf History Unveiled: Interpretations from the New Scholarship, 8007
Deaf Kid's Kamp, 994, 7968
Deaf Like Me, 8008
Deaf Mosaic, 5324
Deaf Parents and Their Hearing Children, 8009
Deaf REACH, 7912
Deaf in America: Voices from a Culture, 8010
Deafness Research Foundation, 7914
Deafness and Communicative Disorders Branch of Rehab Services Administration Office, 8683
Dial-a-Hearing Screening Test, 8116
Digital Hearing Aids, 333
Do You Hear That?, 5325
Doorbell Signalers, 334
Double Gong Indoor/Outdoor Ringer, 335

Duracell & Rayovac Hearing Aid Batteries, 336
EASE Program: Emergency Access Self Evaluation, 8011
Ear Foundation, 7916
Education and Auditory Research Foundation, 3185
Education of the Handicapped: Laws, Legislative Histories and Administrative Document, 4601
Educational Audiology for the Limited Hearing Infant and Preschooler, 2385
Effectively Educating Handicapped Students, 2390
Enchanted Hills Camp for the Blind, 997, 8890
Encyclopedia of Deafness and Hearing Disorders, 8012
Evaluation and Educational Programming of Students with Deafblindness & Severe Disabilities, 2393
Expressive and Receptive Fingerspelling for Hearing Adults, 8013
Eye-Centered: A Study of Spirituality of Deaf People, 8014
Fantastic Series Videotape Set, 8101
Fantastic: Colonial Times, Chocolate, and Cars, 8102
Fantastic: Dogs at Work and Play, 8103
Fantastic: Exciting People, Places and Things!, 8104
Fantastic: From Post Offices to Dairy Goats, 8105
Fantastic: Imagination, Actors, and 'Deaf Way', 8106
Fantastic: Roller Coasters, Maps, and Ice Cream!, 8107
Fantastic: Skiing, Factories, and Race Hores, 8108
Fantastic: Wonderful Worlds of Sports and Travel, 8109
Fingerspelling: Expressive and Receptive Fluency, 8110
Flashing Lamp Telephone Ring Alerter, 210
Fold-Down 3-in-1 Commode, 317
For Hearing People Only, 8015
Free Hand: Enfranchising the Education of Deaf Children, 2401
Freedom Three Wheel Walker, 651
From Gesture to Language in Hearing and Deaf Children, 8016
From Mime to Sign Package, 8017
GA and SK Etiquette, 8018
Gallaudet Survival Guide to Signing, 8019
Gallaudet University Press, 2089, 5416
General Motors Mobility Program for Persons with Disabilities, 5503
Georgiana Institute, 7917
Goldilocks and the Three Bears: Told in Signed English, 8020
HAC Hearing Aid Centers of America: HARC Mercantile, 472
HEAR Center, 7918
Harc Mercantile Ltd, 211
Harris Communications, 337
Healing Dressing for Pressure Sores, 318
Hear You Are, 475
Hearing Aid Batteries, 338
Hearing Aid Battery Testers, 339
Hearing Aid Dehumidifier, 340
Hearing Education and Awareness for Rockers, 7919
Hearing Health Magazine, 8074
Hearing Impaired Children and Youth with Developmental Disabilities, 8021
Hearing Loss Magazine, 8075
Hearing, Speech & Deafness Center (HSDC), 8084
Hearing, Speech and Deafness Center (HSDC), 7922, 8685
Helen Beebe Speech and Hearing Center, 5418
Helen Keller National Center Newsletter, 8970
Hollywood Speaks: Deafness and the Film Entertainment Industry, 8022
House Ear Institute, 7923
How to Thrive, Not Just Survive, 8973
I Can't Hear You in the Dark: How to Lean and Teach Lipreading, 2424
I Have a Sister, My Sister is Deaf, 8023
I Heard That!, 2425
I Heard That!2, 2426

IBM National Support Center, 5951
In the Ear Hearing Aid Battery Extractor, 341
Independence Without Sight and Sound: Suggestions for Practitioners, 7583
Independence Without Sight or Sound, 8024
Innovative Practices for Teaching Sign Language Interpreters, 8025
Intermediate Conversational Sign Language, 8026
International Catholic Deaf Association, 7924
International Hearing Dog, 7925
International Hearing Society, 7570, 7926
International Organization for the Education of the Hearing Impaired, 2032
Interpretation: A Sociolinguistic Model, 8027
Interpreting: An Introduction, 8028
Invisible Children, 5342
JADARA, 8067
Jason & Nordic Publishers, Inc., 5107
Journal of the Academy of Rehabilitative Audiology, 8069
Journey, 7602
Joy of Signing, 8029
Joy of Signing Puzzle Book, 8030
Kid-Friendly Parenting with Deaf and Hard of Hearing Children, 8031
Knock Light, 525
LPB Communications, 214
Language Learning Practices with Deaf Children, 2448
Laurent Clerc: The Story of His Early Years, 8032
Learning American Sign Language, 1957
Learning to See: American Sign Language asa Second Language, 2455
Learning to Sign in My Neighborhood, 1959
Legal Right: The Guide for Deaf and Hard of Hearing People, 4616
Lexington School for the Deaf: Center for the Deaf, 7928
Liberty Lightweight Aluminum Stroll Walker, 652
Linguistics of American Sign Language: An Introduction, 8033
Lions Camp Crescendo, Inc., 1124, 7971
Lions Camp Kirby, 1354, 7972
Lions Wilderness Camp for Deaf Children, Inc., 999, 7974
Literacy & Your Deaf Child: What Every Parent Should Know, 8034
Literature Journal, The, 8070
A Loss for Words, 7986
MADAMIST 50/50 PSI Air Compressor, 320
Mainstreaming Deaf and Hard of Hearing Students: Questions and Answers, 2459
Mask of Benevolence: Disabling the Deaf Community, The, 8035
Meniere's Disease, 8519
Michigan Association for Deaf and Hard of Hearing, 3529, 7929
Michigan Commission for the Blind, 3534
Michigan Commission for the Blind - Gaylord, 3533
Michigan Commission for the Blind Training Center, 3535, 7003
Michigan Commission for the Blind: Escanaba, 3536
Michigan Commission for the Blind: Flint, 3537
Michigan Commission for the Blind: Grand Rapids, 3538
Micro Audiometrics Corporation, 342
Mini Teleloop, 221
Miracle-Ear Children's Foundation, 2935
Mother Father Deaf: Living Between Sound and Silence, 8036
Mushroom Inserts, 343
My First Book of Sign, 8037
My Signing Book of Numbers, 8038
NAD Broadcaster, 4629
National Association of Blind Educators, 8849
National Association of Blind Lawyers, 8850
National Association of Blind Secretaries and Transcribers, 8852
National Association of Hearing Officials, 7931
National Association of Special Education Teachers, 7933, 8691
National Association of the Deaf, 7934

National Black Association for Speech Language and Hearing, 7935
National Black Association for Speech-Language and Hearing, 8692
National Black Deaf Advocates, 7936
National Catholic Office of the Deaf, 7937
National Center for Accessible Media, 8693
National Deaf Education Network and Clearinghouse/Info To Go, 893
National Deaf Women's Bowling Association, 7939
National Division of the Blind and Visually Impaired, 3298
National Hearing Conservation Association, 7940
National Student Speech Language Hearing Association, 7941, 8697
News from Advocates for Deaf-Blind, 7592
Newsletter Bulletin, 8087
Nursery Rhymes from Mother Goose, 8039
On the Level, 8088
Outsiders in a Hearing World: A Sociology of Deafness, 8040
Oval Window Audio, 344
Parents and Teachers, 2481
Patient Transport Chair, 719
Patriot Extra Wide Folding Walkers, 655
Patriot Folding Walker Series, 656
Patriot Reciprocal Folding Walkers, 657
Paws for Silence, 8089
People with Disabilities Who Challenge the System, 5151
Perigee Visual Dictionary of Signing, 8041
Personal FM Systems, 223
Personal Infrared Listening System, 224
Phone of Our Own: The Deaf Insurrection Against Ma Bell, 8042
PhoneMax Amplified Telephone, 560
Place of Their Own: Creating the Deaf Community in America, 8043
Pocket Otoscope, 323
Potomac Technology, 490
PreReading Strategies, 8044
Products for People with Disabilities, 492
Push to Talk Amplified Handset, 226
Quad Canes, 660
Quad City Deaf & Hard of Hearing Youth Group: Tomorrow's Leaders for our Community, 8045
Ramah in the Poconos, 7976
Reading and Deafness, 2502
Registry of Interpreters for the Deaf, 7942
Religious Signing: A Comprehensive Guide for All Faiths, 8046
Say it with Sign, 9019
See What I'm Saying, 9127
Seeing Voices, 8047
Sertoma Camp Endeavor, 1046, 7978
Shape Up 'n Sign, 9129
Show Me How: A Manual for Parents of Preschool Blind Children, 9023
Sign Language Interpreting and Interpreter Education, 8048
Sign Language Studies, 8071
Sign of the Times, 9024
Signaling Wake-Up Devices, 539
Signed English Schoolbook, 2522
Signed English Starter, The, 8049
Signing Family: What Every Parent Should Know About Sign Communication, The, 8050
Signing Naturally Curriculum, 1993
Signing for Reading Success, 8051
Signing: How to Speak with Your Hands, 8052
Signs Across America, 8053
Signs for Me: Basic Sign Vocabulary for Children, Parents & Teachers, 8054
Signs for Sexuality: A Resource Manual, 8055
Signs of the Times, 8056
Silent Garden, The, 8057
Sing Praise Hymnal for the Deaf, 8058
Smoke Detector with Strobe, 540
Sonic Alert, 229
Sonic Alert Bed Shaker, 195
Sound & FuryAquarius Health Care Media, 5364
Sound Induction Receiver, 230
Soundings Newsletter, 8090

Speech and the Hearing-Impaired Child, 2528
Standard 3-in-1 Commode, 324
Standard Wheelchair, 727
Starkey Hearing Foundation, 7945
Stick Canes, 665
TDI National Directory & Resource Guide: Blue Book, 8059
TTY's: Telephone Device for the Deaf, 237
Talking Thermometers, 327
Telecaption Adapter, 242
Telecommunications for the Deaf and Hard of Hearing, 7946
Test of Early Reading Ability Deaf or Hard of Hearing, 2649
Texas School of the Deaf, 2165
Theoretical Issues in Sign Language Research, 8060
There's a Hearing Impaired Child in My Class, 2568
To Love this Life: Quotations by Helen Keller, 9039
Toward Effective Public School Program for Deaf Students, 2569
Transfer Bench, 328
USA Deaf Sports Federation, 8115
Vestibular Disorders Association, 7948
Vibes Bed Shaker, 196
Vibrotactile Personal Alerting System, 246
Vision Magazine, 8099
Visual Alerting Guest Room Kit, 547
Volta Review, 8072
Volta Voices, 8077
WCI/Weitbrecht Communications, 498
We CAN Hear and Speak, 8061
Week the World Heard Gallaudet, The, 8062
What is Auditory Processing?, 8063
Windsor Mountain American Sign Language Camp Program, 1238
YWCA Camp Westwind, 1336, 7981
You and Your Deaf Child: A Self-Help Guidefor Parents of Deaf and Hard of Hearing Children, 8064
Youth Leadership Camp, 1163, 7982

Hemophilia

Bright Horizons Summer Camp, 1166, 8316
Camp Brave Eagle, 1090
Camp Honor, 954, 8344
National Hemophilia Foundation, 3072, 8292

Herbal Medicine

American Botanical Council, 777
American Herbalists Guild, 785

Human Interaction Disabilities

Carroll School Summer Programs, 1174, 7676
Eagle Hill School: Summer Program, 1176, 7681
Taking Part: Introducing Social Skills to Young Children, 2646

Immune Deficiencies

Suttle Lake Camp, 1333, 8407
YMCA Camp Shady Brook, 1020, 8420

Incontinence

Adaptive Clothing: Adults, 442, 1461
Adult Absorbent Briefs, 1495
Care Electronics, 508
Duraline Medical Products Inc., 313
Informer, 8622
Kleinert's, 479
MOMS Catalog, 483
National Association for Continence, 8144
Quality Care Newsletter, 8630
Simon Foundation for Continence, 8154
Specialty Care Shoppe, 1474
Waterproof Sheet-Topper Mattress and Chair Pad, 197

Language Disorders

American Speech-Language-Hearing Association, 7902, 8672
Beyond Baby Talk: From Sounds to Sentences, a Parent's Guide to Language Development, 8727
Communication Help, Education, Research, Apraxia Base (CHERAB), 8680
International Fluency Association, 8687
Language Arts: Detecting Special Needs, 2447
Language Disabilities in Children and Adolescents, 8739
Language and Communication Disorders in Children, 2449
Lindamood-Bell Home Learning Process, 8688
OWLS: Oral and Written Language Scales LC/OE & WE, 2626
PAT-3: Photo Articulation Test, 2627
Peabody Early Experiences Kit (PEEK), 2628
Peabody Language Development Kits (PLDK), 2630
Perspectives: Whole Language Folio, 8749
Preventing Academic Failure - TeachersHandbook, 2493
RULES: Revised, 2638
Receptive-Expressive Emergent-REEL-2 Language Test, 2nd Edition, 2639
Teaching Language-Disabled Children: A Communication/Games Intervention, 2546
Teaching Reading to Disabled and Handicapped Learners, 2551
Test of Language Development: Primary, 2650
Test of Phonological Awareness, 2653
Woodcock Reading Mastery Tests, 2657

Learning Disabilities

ACLD/An Association for Children and Adults with Learning Disabilities: Greater Pittsburgh, 6168
AEPS Child Progress Record: For Children Ages Three to Six, 1903
AEPS Child Progress Report: For Children Ages Birth to Three, 2584
AEPS Curriculum for Birth to Three Years, 2280
AEPS Curriculum for Three to Six Years, 1904
AEPS Data Recording Forms: For Children Ages Birth to Three, 2585
AEPS Data Recording Forms: For Children Ages Three to Six, 1905
AEPS Family Interest Survey, 1906
AEPS Family Report: For Children Ages Birth to Three, 5000
AEPS Measurement for Birth to Three Years, 2586
AEPS Measurement for Three to Six Years, 2587
AHEAD Association, 760
AIR: Assessment of Interpersonal Relations, 2588
AVKO Educational Research Foundation, 2016
Activity-Based Approach to Early Intervention, 2nd Edition, 2282
Adaptive Education Strategies Building on Diversity, 2286
Adaptive Mainstreaming: A Primer for Teachers and Principals, 3rd Edition, 2590
Advanced Language Tool Kit, 1908
Ages & Stages Questionnaires, 2591
All Kinds of Minds, 1909
Alphabetic Phonics Curriculum, 2293
Alternative Educational Delivery Systems, 2294
American College Testing Program, 2592
American School Counselor Association, 2020
Arkansas Department of Special Education, 2111
Assessing Students with Special Needs, 2593
Assessment Log & Developmental Progress Charts for the CCPSN, 2302, 2594
Assessment of Learners with Special Needs, 2595
Assessment: The Special Educator's Role, 2308
Assistive Technology, 206
BOSC: Directory of Facilities for People with Learning Disabilities, 2055
Beacon Therapeutic Diagnostic and Treatment Center, 6818
Beginning Reasoning and Reading, 1919
Behind Special Education, 2317

Benchmark Measures, 2596
Buy!, 1920
CAI, Career Assessment Inventories for theLearning Disabled, 2323
CEC Catalog, 2175
CREVT: Comprehensive Receptive and Expressive Vocabulary Test, 2598
Carolina Curriculum for Infants and Toddlers with Special Needs (3rd Edition), 2325
Carolina Curriculum for Preschoolers with Special Needs, 2326
Catalyst, 2178
Center Academy At Pinellas Park, 7621
Center Academy at Pinellas Park, 1039, 7678
Children's Understanding of Disability, 4953
Christian Approach to Overcoming Disability: A Doctor's Story, 5046
Classroom Success for the LD and ADHD Child, 2338
Clovernook Printing House, The Clovernook Center for the Blind and Visually Impaired, 8822
Cognitive Approaches to Learning Disabilities, 2341
College Internship Program at the Berkshire Center, 6969
Colorado Department of Education: Special Education Service Unit, 2113
Communicating with Parents of Exceptional Children, 2345
Complete Directory for Pediatric Disorders, 2057
Complete Directory for People with Chronic Illness, 2058
Complete Handbook of Children's Reading Disorders: You Can Prevent or Correct LDs, 2349
Complete Learning Disabilities Directory, 2059
Computer Access/Computer Learning, 2350
Council for Exceptional Children, 2025
Critical Voices on Special Education: Problems & Progress Concerning the Mildly Handicapped, 2355
Department of Public Health Human Services, 2143
Developmental Disabilities of Learning, 2365
Developmental Variation and Learning Disorders, 2368
Early Childhood Reporter, 2239
Early Intervention, 2189
Educating all Students in the Mainstream, 2384
Educational Care, 2386
Educational Prescriptions, 2388
Educational Referral Service, 2027
Educators Resource Directory, 2063
Effective Instruction for Special Education, 2389
Explode the Code, 1937
Feeding Children with Special Needs, 2399
Florida Department of Education: Bureau of Exceptional Education And Student Services, 2121
Focus on Exceptional Children, 2193
Food!, 1938
Frames of Reference for the Assessment of Learning Disabilities, 2610
Global Perspectives on Disability: A Curriculum, 2406
Graduate Technological Education and the Human Experience of Disability, 2408
Guide to Teaching Phonics, 1943
Handbook for Implementing Workshops for Siblings of Special Children, 2410
Handbook for the Special Education Administrator, 2412
Hawaii Department of Education: Special Needs, 2122
Help Newsletter, 2247
Helping Learning- Disabled Gifted ChildrenLearn Through Compensatory Active Play, 2419
Helping Students Grow, 2420
How to Teach Spelling/How to Spell, 2422
Howard School, The, 2672
If It Is To Be, It Is Up To Me To Do It!, 1946
If It Is To Be, It Is Up To Us To Help!, 2427
Illinois State Board of Education: Department of Special Education, 2123

Including Students with Special Needs: A Practical Guide for Classroom Teachers, 2432
Indiana Department of Education: Special Education Division, 2124
Infant & Toddler Convection of Fairfield: Falls Church, 2613
Instructional Methods for Students, 2436
Intervention Research in Learning Disabilities, 2440
Intervention in School and Clinic, 2199
Introduction to Learning Disabilities, 2441
Introduction to Special Education: Teaching in an Age of Challenge, 4th Edition, 2443
Issues and Research in Special Education, 2445
Journal of Applied School Psychology, 2201
Journal of Learning Disabilities, 2205
Journal of Postsecondary Education & Disability, 2209
Journal of Reading, Writing and Learning Disabled International, 2211
Journal of Social Work in Disabilty & Rehabilitation, 5108
Journal of Special Education, 2213
K-BIT: Kaufman Brief Intelligence Test, 2614
K-FAST: Kaufman Functional Academic Skills Test, 2615
Kansas State Board of Education: Special Education Services, 2126
Kaufman Test of Educational Achievement(K-TEA), 2618
Keeping Ahead in School, 1951
Kendall Demonstration Elementary School Curriculum Guides, 2446
Kentucky Department of Education: Divisionof Exceptional Children's Services, 2127
KeyMath Teach and Practice, 1952
Keyboarding by Ability, 1705
LD OnLineWETA Public Television, 5424
Lab School of Washington, 1034, 7688
Lakeshore Learning Materials, 1953
Learning Disabilities Association of America, 871
Learning Disabilities Association of NewYork State, 872
Learning Disabilities Consultants Newsletter, 2251
Learning Disabilities, Literacy, and Adult Education, 2450
Learning Disabilities: Concepts and Characteristics, 2451
Learning Disability: Social Class and the Cons of Inequality In American Education, 2452
Learning and Individual Differences, 2453
Leo Yassenoff JCC Specialty Day Camp, 1311
Life Beyond the Classroom: Transition Strategies for Young People with Disabilities, 4958
Life Centered Career Education: A Contemporary Based Approach, 4th Edition, 2621
Literacy Program, 1960
Literature Based Reading, 1961
MTA Readers, 1964
Mainstreaming Exceptional Students: A Guide for Classroom Teachers, 2460
Making School Inclusion Work: A Guide to Everyday Practice, 1965
Making Self-Employment Work for People with Disabilities, 4987
Making the Writing Process Work: Strategies for Composition and Self-Regulation, 1966
Managing Diagnostic Tool of Visual Perception, 2462
Manual Alphabet Poster, 1967
Maryland State Department of Education: Division of Special Education, 2134
Match-Sort-Assemble Job Cards, 1969
Match-Sort-Assemble TOOLS, 1972
McGraw-Hill Company, 2097
Michigan Department of Education: Special Education Services, 2137
Mississippi Department of Education: Office of Special Services, 2142
Missouri Department of Elementary and Secondary Education: Special Education Programs, 2141
More Food!, 1974
More Work!, 1975
Multisensory Teaching Approach, 1976

National Clearinghouse on Family Support and Children's Mental Health, 2120
National Education Association of the United States, 2045
Nebraska Department of Education: Special Populations Office, 2147
New Hampshire Department of Education: Bureau for Special Education Services, 2149
New Mexico State Department of Education, 2151
New York State Education Department, 2153
North Dakota Department of Education: Special Education, 2146
Ohio Department of Education: Division of Special Education, 2154
Oklahoma State Department of Education, 2155
Oregon Department of Education: Office of Special Education, 2156
Our World, 2221
Peabody Articulation Decks, 1978
Peabody Individual Achievement Test-Revised Normative Update (PIAT-R-NU), 2629
Pennsylvania Department of Education: Bureau of Special Education, 2157
Phonemic Awareness in Young Children: A Classroom Curriculum, 1979
Phonics for Thought, 1980
Phonological Awareness Training for Reading, 1981
Play!, 1982
Pragmatic Approach, 2491
Preschoolers with Special Needs: Children At-Risk, Children with Disabilities, 2492
Preventing School Dropouts, 2494
Prevocational Assessment, 2495
Primary Phonics, 1984
Promoting Postsecondary Education for Students with Learning Disabilities, 2498
Reading for Content, 1985
Reading from Scratch, 1986
Recipe for Reading, 1987
Remedial and Special Education, 2226
Resource Room, The, 2511
Rewarding Speech, 1988
Rhode Island Department of Education: Office of Special Needs, 2158
SAYdee Posters, 1989
Sage Publications, 2105
Semiotics and Dis/ability: Interogating Categories of Difference, 2517
Sequential Spelling: 1-7 with 7 Student Response Books, 1992
Social Studies: Detecting and Correcting Special Needs, 2524
South Carolina Department of Education: Office of Exceptional Children, 2160
Special Education Report, 2264
Special Education Today, 2526
Special Education for Today, 2527
Special Siblings: Growing Up With Someone with A Disability, 5176
Spell of Words, 1998
Spellbound, 1999
Spelling Dictionary, 2000
Starting Over, 2001
Strategies for Teaching Learners with Special Needs, 2532
Students with Mild Disabilities in the Secondary School, 2535
Studio 49 Catalog, 2002
Syracuse Community-Referenced Curriculum Guide for Students with Disabilties, 2003
Teaching Adults with Learning Disabilities, 2541
Teaching Chemistry to Students with Disabilities: A Manual, 5302
Teaching Every Child Every Day: Integrated Learning in Diverse Classrooms, 2544
Teaching Exceptional Children, 2227
Teaching Infants and Preschoolers with Handicaps, 2545
Teaching Learners with Mild Disabilities: Integrating Research and Practice, 2547
Teaching Mathematics to Students with Learning Disabilities, 2548

Teaching Mildly and Moderately Handicapped Students, 2549
Teaching Reading to Handicapped Children, 2552
Teaching Students Ways to Remember, 2005
Teaching Students with Mild and Moderate Learning Problems, 2556
Teaching Students with Special Needs in Inclusive Settings, 2558
Teaching Test-Taking Skills: Helping Students Show What They Know, 2006
Teaching Young Children to Read, 2559
Teaching the Bilingual Special Education Student, 2560
Teaching the Learning Disabled Adolescent:Strategies and Methods, 2561
Tennessee Department of Education, 2162
Test Critiques: Volumes I-X, 2648
Test of Mathematical Abilities, 2nd Edition, 2651
Test of Nonverbal Intelligence, 3rd Edition, 2652
Test of Written Spelling, 3rd Edition, 2654
Texas Education Agency, 2163
Textbooks and the Student Who Can't Read Them: A Guide for Teaching Content, 2564
Tools for Transition, 2009
Topics in Early Childhood Special Education, 2267
Utah State Office of Education: At-Risk and Special Education Service Unit, 2166
VAK Tasks Workbook: Visual, Auditory and Kinesthetic, 2011
Virginia Department of Education: Divisionof Pre & Early Adolescent Education, 2168
West Virginia Department of Education: Office of Special Education, 2170
Wordly Wise 3000, 2013
Work!, 2014
Working Together & Taking Part, 2015
Worthmore Academy, 2691
Wyoming Department of Education, 2171

Lowe's Syndrome

Lowe's Syndrome Conference, 1860

Lung Disorders

American Lung Association, 8255
BIPAP S/T Ventilatory Support System, 309
Breathe Free, 8449
Canadian Lung Association, 8263
Emphysema Foundation for Our Right to Survive, 8267
Healthy Breathing, 8482
Lung Disorders Sourcebook, 8513
Lung Line Information Service, 8659

Massage Therapy

American Massage Therapy Association, 787
American Organization for Bodywork Therapies of Asia, 789
Bonnie Prudden Myotherapy, 807

Mental Disabilities

Addictive & Mental Disorders Division, 3573
Agnes M Lindsay Trust, 3003
Ahmanson Foundation, 2737
American Music Therapy Association (AMTA), 5
American Psychiatric Association, 7609
Anderson Woods, 1083
Arc of the Farmington Valley, 6697
Authoritative Guide to Self- Help Resourcein Mental Health, 5023
Bethy and the Mouse: A Father Remembers His Children with Disabilities, 5263
Camp Wesley Woods: Northeastern Pennsylvan, 1348
Cheaha Regional Mental Health Center, 6493
Children's Needs Psychological Perspective, 2334
Chilton-Shelby Mental Health Center, 6495
Colorado Division of Mental Health, 3368
Complete Mental Health Directory, 2060
Consulting Psychologists Press, 2351

Cornerstone Services, 5969, 8651
Counseling Psychologist, 2184
Criminal Law Handbook on Psychiatric &
    Psychological Evidence & Testimony, 4592
Culture and the Restructuring of Community
    Mental Health, 7749
Department Of Health& Social ServicesDivision
    Of Behaviorial Health, 3326
Department of Mental Health, Retardation and
    Hospitals of Rhode Island, 3729
Developmental Disability Services Section, 3670
Dimensions of State Mental Health Policy, 4594
Division of Mental Health and Substance Abuse,
    3680
Eating Disorders Sourcebook., 8471
Ecology of Troubled Children, 2379
Emotional Problems of Childhood and
    Adolescence, 2391
Florida Department of Mental Health and
    Rehabilitative Services, 3407
Georgia Division of Mental Health, Developmental
    Disabilities & Addictive Diseases, 3423
Giant Food Foundation, 2932
Green Door, 5915
Handbook on Supported Education for Peoplewith
    Mental Illness, 2415
Hawaii Department of Health, Adult Mental Health
    Division, 3433
Home Health Care Provider: A Guide to Essential
    Skills, 2421
Idaho Mental Health Center, 3447
Illinois Department of Mental Health and
    Developmental Disabilities, 3456
International Handbook on Mental Health Policy,
    4612
Journal of Counseling & Development, 2202
Judge David L Bazelon Center for Mental Health
    Law, 4565
Kentucky Department for Mental Health and
    Mental Retardation Services, 3486
Law Center Newsletter, 4614
Louisiana Division of Mental Health, 3498
Louisiana Employment Service and Job Training
    Program Liaison, 6033
Maine Department of Health and Human Services,
    3504
Maryland Division of Mental Health, 3516
Massachusetts Department of Mental Health, 3524
Mental & Physical Disability Law Digest, 2465
Mental Disabilities and the Americans with
    Disabilities Act, 4623
Mental Disability Law, Evidence and Testimony,
    4624
Mental Health America, 878, 7633
Mental Health Association in Pennysylvania, 3718
Mental Health Concepts and Techniques for the
    Occupational Therapy Assistant, 2466
Mental Health Law Reporter, 4625
Mental Health and Mental Illness, 2467
Mentally Ill Individuals, 2468
Minnesota Mental Health Division, 3554
NAMI Texas, 3776
National Alliance on Mental Illness(NAMI), 7636
National Association for the Dually Diagnosed,
    7638
National Association of School Psychologists,
    2098
Nebraska Department of Mental Health, 3589
Nevada Division of Mental Health and
    Developmental Services, 3600
New Hampshire Department of Mental Health,
    3609
New Jersey Division of Mental Health Services,
    3621
New State Office of Mental Health Agency, 3644
New York State Office of Mental Health, 3651
Occupational Center of Union County, 6119
Office of Rehabilitation Services, 6179
Ohio Department of Mental Health, 3694
Oklahoma Department of Mental Health &
    Substance Abuse Services, 3705
Orchard Village, 5980
Oregon Department of Mental Health, 3713
Palm Beach Habilitation Center, 5938

Parent Professional Advocacy League, 914
Parental Concerns in College Student Mental
    Health, 2480
Personality and Emotional Disturbance, 2484
Providing Services for People with Vision Loss:
    Multidisciplinary Perspective, 9065
Psychiatric Mental Health Nursing, 2499
Psychiatric Staffing Crisis in Community Mental
    Health, 2223
Psycho-Educational Assessment of Preschool
    Children, 2637
Psychological and Social Impact of Illness and
    Disability, 2501
Readings: A Journal of Reviews and Commentary
    in Mental Health, 2224
Rhode Island Department of Mental Health, 3732
SAMHSA News, 2260
Seagull Industries for the Disabled, 5943
Services for the Seriously Mentally Ill: A Survey of
    Mental Health Centers, 2519
Social and Emotional Development of Exceptional
    Students: Handicapped, 2525
South Carolina Department of Mental Healthand
    Mental Retardation, 3747
South Dakota Department of Human Services
    Division of Community Behavioral Health, 3755
St. James Association for Retarded Citizens, 6035
State Mental Health Representative for Children
    and Youth, 3661
Teaching Disturbed and Disturbing Students: An
    Integrative Approach, 2543
Tennessee Department of Mental Health, 3766
Texas Department of Mental Health & Mental
    Retardation, 3787
Texas Federation of Families for Children's Mental
    Health, 3789
Thresholds AMISS, 5985
Thresholds Psychiatric Rehabilitation Centers, 929
Treating Families of Brain Injury Survivors, 2573
Understanding and Teaching Emotionally
    Disturbed Children & Adolescents, 2574
Utah Division Of Substance Abuse &
    MentalHealth, 3803
VA Maryland Health Care System, 5649
Virginia Department of Mental Health, 3823
Vocational and Rehabilitation Agency: Department
    of Human Services, 6180
WY Department of Health: Mental Health and
    Substance Abuse Service Division, 3861
Washington Department of Mental Health, 3835
We Can Speak for Ourselves: Self Advocacy by
    Mentally Handicapped People, 5243
Well Mind Association of Greater Washington,
    3397

Mental Retardation

ARC, 7605
ARC Gateway, 3399
ARC's Government Report, 5001
American Journal on Mental Retardation, 7824
Arc of Alaska, 2729
Arc of Anderson County, 3176
Arc of Arkansas, 2735
Arc of Bergen and Passaic Counties, 6103
Arc of Blackstone Valley, 3162
Arc of California, 2740
Arc of Colorado, 2799
Arc of Connecticut, 2806
Arc of Davidson County, 3177
Arc of Delaware, 2819
Arc of Dunn County, 3245
Arc of Eau Claire, 3246
Arc of Florida, 2834
Arc of Fox Cities, 3247
Arc of Hamilton County, 3178
Arc of Hawaii, 2858
Arc of Illinois, 2867
Arc of Indiana, 2902
Arc of Iowa, 2906
Arc of Kansas, 2911
Arc of Kentucky, 2914
Arc of Louisiana, 2915
Arc of Maryland, 2922

Arc of Massachusetts, The, 2940
Arc of Michigan, 2956
Arc of Minnesota, 2973
Arc of Mississippi, 2983
Arc of Natrona County, 3259
Arc of Nebraska, 2994
Arc of New Jersey, 3005
Arc of New Mexico, 3019
Arc of North Carolina, 3092
Arc of North Dakota, 3101
Arc of Northern Bristol County, 2941
Arc of Northern Rhode Island, 3163
Arc of Ohio, 3106
Arc of Oregon, 3133
Arc of Pennsylvania, 3138
Arc of Racine County, 3248
Arc of South Carolina, 3173
Arc of Tennessee, 3179
Arc of Texas, The, 3191
Arc of Utah, 3222
Arc of Virginia, 3226
Arc of Washington County, 3180
Arc of Washington State, 3233
Arc of Williamson County, 3181
Arc of Wisconsin Disability Association, 3249
Arc of the District of Columbia, 2822
Arc-Dane County, 3250
Arc-Diversified, 3182
Ardmore Developmental Center, 6045
Assessing the Handicaps/Needs of Children, 2300
Assessment in Mental Handicap: A Guide to
    Assessment Practices & Tests, 2304
Beck Institute for Cognitive Therapy and Research,
    7615
Brain Injury Association of America, 808, 7618
Breaking the Speech Barrier: Language
    Develpment Through Augmented Means, 8728
Camp Huntington, 1260, 7666
Camp Virginia Jaycee, 1419
Camp Virginia Jaycee Newsletter, 2230
Children with Mental Retardation, 7742
Connecticut Office of Protection and Advocacy for
    Persons with Disabilities, 3378
Cornucopia, 6153
Council for Extended Care of Mentally Retarded
    Citizens, 7679
CranstonArc, 3165
Directory of Members, 5059
Farmington Valley ARC, 7834
Federal Laws of the Mentally Handicapped: Laws,
    Legislative Histories and Admin. Documents,
    4606
Frank Olean Center, 3167
Introduction to Mental Retardation, 2442
James L. Maher Center, 3169
Joseph P Kennedy Jr Foundation, 2828
Keep the Promise: Managed Care and People with
    Disabilities, 5110
Kennedy Center, 5902
Kent County Arc, 3170
Labeling the Mentally Retarded, 7784
Lions Den Outdoor Learning Center, 1219, 7689
Match-Sort-Assemble Pictures, 1970
Match-Sort-Assemble SCHEMATICS, 1971
Mental Retardation, 7790
Mental Retardation: A Life-Cycle Approach, 7791
Mississippi Bureau of Mental Retardation, 3561
Missouri Division Of Developmental Disabilities,
    3568
Montgomery County Arc, 3187
Multidisciplinary Assessment of Children With
    Learning Disabilities and Mental Retardation,
    2470
National Association of Cognitive-Behavioral
    Therapists, 7640
President's Committee for People with Intellectual
    Disabilities, 2047
President's Committee on People with Intellecutual
    Disabilities, 3302
Quaezar, 5903
Raven Rock Lutheran Camp, 1160, 7698
Retarded Isn't Stupid, Mom!, 7804
Rhode Island Arc, 3171
St. John Valley Associates, 7652

State Mental Retardation Program, 3662
TASH Connections, 4577
Teaching the Mentally Retarded Student:
   Curriculum, Methods, and Strategies, 2562
VBS Special Education Teaching Guide, 2576
Ventures Travel, 5537

Multiple Disabilities

Abilities Expo, 1842
Accessible Home of Your Own, 1889
Alternative Work Concepts, 2018
Annual TASH Conference, The, 1846
Bethel Mennonite Camp, 1119
Blood and Circulatory Disorders Sourcebook, 8444
Blowitz-Ridgeway Foundation, 2869
Bothin Foundation, 2745
Bradford Woods: Camp Riley, 1085
Buck and Buck Clothing, 1464
Burns-Dunphy Foundation, 2747
California Community Foundation, 2748
Camp AIM, 1338
Camp Allen, 1236
Camp Allyn, 1298
Camp Alpine, 948, 8317
Camp CAMP, 1385
Camp Costanoan, 970
Camp Courageous of Iowa, 1105
Camp Dunmoreia, 1341
Camp Easter Seals, 1067
Camp Forrest, 973
Camp Gravatt, 1368
Camp Hemlocks, 1023
Camp Howe, 1167
Camp JCC, 1149
Camp John Marc, 1387
Camp Kostopulos, 1402
Camp Little Giant, 1070
Camp Merry Heart, 1243
Camp Milldale, 1151
Camp Millhouse, 1095
Camp Paha Rise Above, 1010
Camp Paivika, 979
Camp Roger, 1190
Camp Ronald McDonald® at Eagle Lake, 985
Camp Sky Ranch, 1291
Camp Summit, 1391
Camp Surefoot Center, 1346
Camp Tanager, 1110
Camp Twin Lakes, 1057
Camp Venture, Inc., 1268
Camp Volasuca, 1428
Camp Wyoming, 1111
Camp for All, 1393
Camping Unlimited-Camp Krem, 993
Cardiovascular Diseases and Disorders
   Sourcebook, 3rd Edition, 8452
Center for Independence of the Disabled, 3908
Center for Independence of the Disabled- Daly
   City, 3909
Center for Independent Living: Oakland, 3912
Childhood Diseases and Disorders Sourcebook,
   2nd Edition, 8455
Children's Fresh Air Society Fund, 2925
Civitan Acres for the Disabled, 1421
Clover Patch Camp, 1271
Clovernook Center for the Blind and Visually
   Impaired, 8821
Community Resources for Independence:
   Mendocino/Lake Branch, 3927
Creative Designs, 1479
Cultural Diversity, Families and the Special
   Education System, 2356
Deutsch Foundation, 2754
Digestive Diseases & Disorders Sourcebook, 8468
Disability and Health: National Center for Birth
   Defects and Developmental Disabilities, 8653
Division for Physical, Health & Multiple
   Disabilities, 8266
Driving Systems Inc., 83
Ear, Nose, and Throat Disorders Sourcebook, 8470
Easter Seal Camp Wawbeek, 1436
Easter Seals Camp Sunnyside, 1073

Easter Seals Oklahoma, 1322, 7682, 7969, 8710,
   8889
Eastern Colorado Services for the Disabled, 3371
Educating Children with Multiple Disabilities: A
   Transdisciplinary Approach, 2381
Educating Students Who Have Visual Impairments
   with Other Disabilities, 2383
Enhancing Everyday Communication for Children
   with Disabilities, 5282
Equalizer 5000 Home Gym, 676
Ethnic Diseases Sourcebook, 8475
Eugene and Agnes E Meyer Foundation, 2823
Eunice Kennedy Shriver National Institute of Child
   Health and Human Development (NICHD), 8269
Financial Aid for the Disabled and Their Families,
   2758, 3272
Firemans Fund Foundation, 2759
Florida Lions Camp, 1042, 7578
Gallo Foundation, 2761
Goodwill Industries International, 852
Handi Kids, 1178
Hemophilia Camp, 1277, 8390
Henry W Bull Foundation, 2765
Hepatitis Sourcebook, 8484
Hypertension Sourcebook, 8487
Including All of Us: An Early Childhood
   Curriculum About Disability, 2430
Institute for Human Centered Design, 1879
Interdisciplinary Clinical Assessment of Young
   Children with Developmental Disabilities, 8491
International Center for the Disabled, 1578
John W Anderson Foundation, 2905
Joni and Friends, 868
Journal for Vocational Special Needs Education,
   2200
Kamp Kiwanis, 1278
Kamp for Kids: Camp Togowauk, 1179
Kenneth T and Eileen L Norris Foundation, 2769
League at Camp Greentop, 1158
Lions Camp Tatiyee, 957
Longwood Foundation, 2820
M&M Health Care Apparel Company, 1469
Mayor of the West Side, 4959
Mt Hood Kiwanis Camp, 1331
National Association for Parents of Children with
   Visual Impairments (NAPVI), 8847, 9143
North America Riding for the Handicapped
   Association, 908
Official Patient's Sourcebook on Bell's Palsy, 8539
Official Patient's Sourcebook on Osteoporosis,
   8542
Official Patient's Sourcebook on Sickle Cell
   Anemia, 8547
Official Patient's Sourcebook on Ulcerative Colitis,
   8548
Perkins Activity and Resource Guide: A Handbook
   for Teachers, 9009
Physical Management of Multiple Handicaps: A
   Professional's Guide, 2488
Protection & Advocacy System: Alaska, 3329
Recreation Unlimited: Day Camp, 1312
Recreation Unlimited: Residential Camp, 1313
Recreation Unlimited: Respite Weekend Camp,
   1314
Recreation Unlimited: Specialty Camp, 1315
Rotary Camp, 1316
Senior Program for Teens and Young Adults with
   Special Needs, 2683
Shady Oaks Camp, 1078, 8402
Social Security Administration, 3412
Social Security: Baltimore Disability
   Determination, 3518
Social Security: Maine Disability Determination,
   3509
St. Augustine Rainbow Camp, 1317
Starting Points, 9027
Steelcase Foundation, 2972
Sunshine Campus, 1281
Tennessee Division of Rehabilitation, 3767
Texas Speech-Language-Hearing Association,
   8704
Thyroid Disorders Sourcebook, 8579
Timber Pointe Outdoor Center, 1081
The Ultimate Guide to Sex and Disability, 5179

Upward Bound Camp for Persons With, 1334
Variety Club Camp & Developmental, 1359
Wage and Hour Division of the Employment
   Standards Administration, 3395
Wagon Road Camp, 1283
Weyerhaeuser Company Foundation, 3242
Wilderness Inquiry, 5514, 5539

Multiple Sclerosis

Blooming Where You're Planted: Stories From The
   Heart, 8445
Coffee in the Cereal: The First Year with Multiple
   Sclerosis, 8459
Consortium of Multiple Sclerosis Centers, 8132
Dressing Tips and Clothing Resources for Making
   Life Easier, 463
MSFOCUS Magazine, 8605
Momentum, 8624
Multiple Sclerosis Foundation, 8142
Multiple Sclerosis and Having a Baby, 8522
Multiple Sclerosis: A Guide for Families, 8524
Multiple Sclerosis: A Guide for the Newly
   Diagnosed, 8525
Understanding Multiple Sclerosis, 8587
When the Road Turns: Inspirational Stories About
   People with MS, 8591

Muscular Dystrophy

Camp Birchwood, 949, 8319
MDA Newsmagazine, 2218
Muscular Dystrophy Association - USA, 881
Muscular Dystrophy Association Free Camp, 1075,
   8398
Official Patient's Sourcebook on Muscular
   Dystrophy, 8541
Summer Camp for Children with Muscular
   Dystrophy, 1079, 8405

Neurological Impairments

Archives of Neurology, 8599
Association for Neurologically Impaired Brain
   Injured Children, 8128
Child Neurology Society, 7623
Digest of Neurology and Psychiatry, 2369
Pervasive Developmental Disorders: Findinga
   Diagnosis and Getting Help, 5251
Rehabilitation Nursing for the Neurological
   Patient, 2507

Obesity

American Society of Bariatric Physicians, 794
Obesity Sourcebook, 8537
Overeaters Anonymous World Service Office,
   8296

Orthopedical Disabilities

American Board for Certification in Orthotics &
   Prosthetics And Pedorthics, Inc., 7873
American Journal of Orthopsychiatry, 8597
Camp Manito/Camp Lenape, 1030
Doing Things Together, 5326
Orthotics and Prosthetics Almanac, 8606
Osteoporosis Sourcebook, 8551
Sun-Mate Seat Cushions, 296

Pain Management

AMI, 307
Foot Snugglers, 1455
TRU-Mold Shoes, 1457

Parkinson Disease

Allen P & Josephine B Green Foundation, 2984
Blazing Toward a Cure Annual Conference, 1850
Movement Disorders Sourcebook, 8521
National Parkinson Foundation, 2845

PDF News, 8607
PDF Newsletter, 8626
Parkinson's Disease Foundation, 2892, 3077
Parkinsons Report, 8627
Young Onset Parkinson Conference, 1876

Pediatric Issues

AEPS Family Report: Birth to Three Years, 5190
American Academy of Pediatrics, 770
American Association of Children's Residential
    Centers, 771
American SIDS Institute, 8256
Assessment of Children and Youth, 2305
Child and Parent Resource Institute, 820
Child with Disabling Illness, 2330
Childcare and the ADA, 4585
Children's Alliance, 821
Children's National Medical Center, 822
Choosing Options and Accommodations for
    Children, 2336
Commonly Asked Questions About Child Care
    Centers and the Americans with Disabilities Act,
    4587
Disabilities Sourcebook, 461
Family Voices, 843
Federation of Families for Children's Mental
    Health, 847
Formed Families: Adoption of Children with
    Handicaps, 4607
Handbook of Epilepsy, 8481
Human Exceptionality: School, Community, and
    Family (12th Edition), 2423, 4978
National Association for Children of Alcoholics,
    8281
National Center for Education in Maternal and
    Child Health, 889
National Dissemination Center for Children and
    Youth with Disabilities (NICHCY), 895
National Early Childhood Technical Assistance
    Center, 896
National Information Center for Children, 899
National Maternal and Child Health Bureau, 3517
Parents Helping Parents (PHP), 915
Pediatric Early Elementary (PEEX II) Examination,
    2631
Pediatric Exam of Educational-PEERAMID
    Readiness at Middle Childhood, 2632
Pediatric Examination of Educational Readiness,
    2633
Pediatric Extended Examination at-PEET Three,
    2634
Ronald McDonald House, 924
Universal Pediatric Services, 932

Phenylketonuria

PKU for Children: Learning to Measure, 2478
A Teacher's Guide to PKU, 2274

Physical Disabilities

ABC Union, ACE, ANLV, Vegas Western Cab,
    5540
ACPOC News, 8612
APSE, 761
ARJO Inc., 152
ASCCA, 963, 8310
Abilities!, 762
Ability Center, 71
Able Trek Tours, 5515
AbleApparelAffordable Adaptive Clothing and
    Accessories, 5380
Abledata, 5381
Accent on Living Magazine, 5003
Access America, 5498
Access Control Systems: NHX Nurse Call System,
    199
Access Design Services: CILs as Experts, 5004
Access Store Products for Barrier Free
    Environments, 439
Access To Independence Inc., 5005
Access Travel: Airports, 5487

Access Unlimited, 5382
Access Yosemite National Park, 5499
Access to Recreation, 440
Accessibility Lift, 377
Accessible Journeys, 5517
Accessible Vans Of America, 5541
Achievement Products, 441
Achieving Diversity and Independence, 5007
Achilles Track Club, 8221
Action Products, 270
Ad Lib Drop-In Center: Consumer Management,
    Ownership and Empowerment, 5009
Adapted Physical Activity, 5192
Adapted Physical Activity Programs, 2172
Adapted Physical Education and Sport, 8166
Adaptive Sports Center, 8222
Adaptive Tracks, 8615
Address Book, 611
Adjustable Bath Seat, 153
Adjustable Bed, 184
Adjustable Chair, 249
Adjustable Clear Acrylic Tray, 250
Adjustable Incline Board, 378
Adjustable Raised Toilet Seat & Guard, 154
Adjustable Rigid Chair, 251
Adjustable Tee Stool, 252
Adjustable Wedge, 271
Advantage Wheelchair & Walker Bags, 671
Advocacy Center for Persons with Disabilitites,
    765
Aerospace Compadre, 570
Air Lift Oxygen Carriers, 641
Alante, 571
Albany Vet Center, 5696
Alert, 2229
Alexian Brothers Medical Center, 6813
All View Mirror, 73
Alliance for Technology Access, 767
AlumiRamp, 379
Aluminum Crutches, 642
Aluminum Walking Canes, 643
American Academy of Physical Medicine and
    Rehabilitation, 8248
American Back Society, 8122
American Board of Professional Disability
    Consultants, 776
American Camping Association, 778
American Discount Medical, 447
American Hotel and Lodging Foundation, 5500
American Mobility: Personal Mobility Solutions,
    5390
Amigo Mobility International, 572
Amigo Mobility International Inc., 573
Amtrak, 5501
Anglo California Travel Service, 5519
Appliance 411, 5393
Applied Kinesiology: Muscle Response in
    Diagnosis, Therapy and Preventive Medicine,
    5017
Apria Healthcare, 448
Architectural Barriers Action League, 5488
Arcoa Travel Chair, 694
Arcola Mobility, 74
Area Access, 380
Armstrong Medical, 449
Assistive Technology Sourcebook, 451
Association of Mouth and Foot Painting Artists
    (AMPFA), 12
Automobile Lifts for Scooters, Wheelchairs and
    Powerchairs, 75
Avis Rent A Car, 5542
Back-Huggar Pillow, 272
BackSaver, 253
Backyards and Butterflies: Ways to Include
    Children with Disabilities in Outdoor Activities,
    5195
Bagel Holder, 345
Bailey, 452
Bariatric Wheelchairs Regency FL, 695
Barrier Free Travel: A Nuts and Bolts Guide for
    Wheelers and Slow Walkers (3rd Edition), 5026
Basement Motorhome Lift By Handicaps, Inc., 381
Bath Fixtures, 155
Bath Products, 156

BathEase, 159
Bathroom Transfer Systems, 160
Bathtub Safety Rail, 161
Battery Operated Cushion, 673
BeOK Key Lever, 503
Behavioral Vision Approaches for Persons with
    Physical Disabilities, 8915
Best 25 Catalog Resources for Making Life Easier,
    453
Better Back, 254
Beyond the Barriers, 8212
Big Red Switch, 207
Blinker Buddy II Electronic Turn Signal, 76
Bookholder: Roberts, 505
Boulder Vet Center, 5588
Bounder Plus Power Wheelchair, 742
Bounder Power Wheelchair, 743
Box Top Opener, 347
Braun Corporation, 77, 162
Braun Corporation, The, 382
Bravo! + Three-Wheel Scooter, 574
Breez 1025, 744
Breezy, 696
Bruno Independent Living Aids, 383
Bus and Taxi Sign, 507
Butlers Wheelchair Lifts, 384
Button Aid, 298
Bye-Bye Decubiti (BBD), 273
Bye-Bye Decubiti Air Mattress Overlay, 185
Camp Fairlee Manor, 1029, 1147
Camp Jotoni, 1241
Camp Ramah in New England, 1171
Camp Riley, 1097
Canine Companions for Independence, 811
Capscrew, 348
Carendo, 255
Carex Health Brands, 456
Center for Libraries and Educational Improvement,
    5041
Center for Universal Design, 818
Century 50/60XR Sit, 256
Champion 1000, 697
Champion 2000, 698
Champion 3000, 699
Charlotte Vet Center, 5712
Chevy Lowered Floor, 78
Child Convertible Balance Beam Set, 509
Child Variable Balance Beam, 510
Child's Mobility Crawler, 511
Childhood Leukemia: A Guide for Families,
    Friends & Caregivers, 8456
Choice Switch Latch and Timer, 512
Choosing a Wheelchair: A Guide for Optimal
    Independence, 700
Christopher & Dana Reeve Paralysis Resource
    Center, 8131
Clarke Healthcare Products, Inc., 164
Classic, 79
Classique, 385
Clip Board Notebook, 617
Columbus McKinnon Corporation, 386
Combination File/Reference Carousel, 549
Commode, 165
Communication Aids for Children and Adults, 458
Commuter & Kid's Commuter, 732
Compact Folding Travel Rollator, 644
Complete Armchair Fitness, 8214
Consulting & Engineering for the Handicapped
    (CEH), 5543
Consumer Buyer's Guide for Independent Living,
    5049
Convaid, 701, 733
Convert-Able Table, 257
Cool Handle, 349
Cordless Big Red Switch, 513
Cordless Receiver, 350
Crescent Porter Hale Foundation, 2752
Cruiser Bus Buggy 4MB, 575
Cunard Line, 5520
Cursive Writing Skills, 1928
Custom, 702
Custom Durable, 703
Custom Lift Residential Elevators, 389

DEUCE Environmental Control Unit, 514
DW Auto & Home Mobility, 80
Damaco D90, 745
Dancing from the Inside Out, 20
Danmar Products, 459
Dapper Folding Adustable Cane, 646
Dapper Walking Stick, 647
Dayspring Associates, 460
Deluxe Bath Bench with Adjustable Legs, 166
Deluxe Convertible Exercise Staircase, 390
Deluxe Nova Wheeled Walker & Avant Wheeled
    Walker, 648
Deluxe Roller Knife, 352
Deluxe Signature Guide, 618
Deluxe Sock and Stocking Aid, 299
Deluxe Standard Wood Cane, 649
Demand Response Transportation Through a Rural
    ILC, 5055
Developing Organized Coalitions and Strategic
    Plans, 5056
Dialysis at Sea Cruises, 5523
Digi-Flex, 516
Directions Unlimited Acccessible Tours, 5524
Directory of Travel Agencies for the Disabled,
    5489
Disability Bookshop Catalog, 462
Disability and Medical Resources Mall, 5407
Disability and Sport, 8172
DisabilityResources.org, 5408
Disabled Sports Program Center, 8226
Disabled Sports USA, 8227
Disabled Watersports Program, 8228
Dodge Lowered Floor, 81
Dorma Architectural Hardware, 517
Dressing Stick, 300
Drew Karol Industries, 312
Drive Master Company, 82
Dual Brake Control, 84
Dual Brush with Suction Base, 353
Dual Security Bed Rail, 187
Dual Switch Latch and Timer, 518
Dual-Mode Charger, 674
Duro-Med Industries, 314
Dvorak Expeditions, 5525
Dynamic Living, 5410
Dynamic Systems, 274
E-Z Access Van Ramp, 391
Eagle Sportschairs, LLC, 755
East Penn Manufacturing Company, 756
Easter Seals Camp Stand by Me, 1429, 8162
Easter Seals Project ACTION, 5502
Easy Pivot Transfer Machine, 392
Easy Pour Locking Lid Pot, 354
Easy Stand, 393
Easy Things to Make Things Simple: Do It
    Yourself Modifications for Disabled Persons,
    5068
Econo-Float Water Flotation Cushion, 275
Econo-Float Water Flotation Mattress, 276
Economical Liberty, 394
Edge, 704
Elastic Shoelaces, 301
Elderly Guide to Budget Travel/Europe, 5490
Electric Can Opener & Knife Sharpener, 355
Electric Leg Bag Emptier and Tub Slide Shower
    Chair, 167
Electric Mobility Corporation, 577
Enhancer Cushion, 277
Enrichments Catalog, 464
Environmental Traveling Companions, 5526
Equalizer 1000 Series, 675
Equipment Shop, 465
Escort II XL, 86
Essential Medical Supply, Inc., 466
Etac USA: F3 Wheelchair, 705
Evac + Chair Emergency Evacuation Chair, 258
Evacu-Trac, 706
Everest & Jennings, 467
Evio Plastics, 356
Explorer+ 4-Wheel Scooter, 578
Express Medical Supply, 468
Expressive Arts for the Very Disabled and
    Handicapped of All Ages, 24
Extensions for Independence, 551

Fairway Spirit Adaptive Golf Car: Model4852, 552
Family Resource Center on Disabilities, 842
Featherspring, 677
Featherweight Reachers, 302
Fedcap Rehabilitation Services, 845
Fitness Programming for Physical Disabilities,
    8173
FlagHouse Special Populations, 470
Florence C and Harry L English Memorial Fund,
    2849
Flying Wheels Travel, 5527
Foam Decubitus Bed Pads, 188
Folding Chair with a Rigid Feel, 707
Foot Inversion Tread, 520
Foot Pedal Extensions, 87
Foot Placement Ladder, 521
Foot Steering, 88
Foot Steering System, 89
Ford Lowered Floor, 90
Formula Series Active Mobility Wheelchairs, 708
Four-Ingredient Cookbook, 5078
Freedom Bath, 168
Freedom Ryder Handcycles, 553
Freedom Wheels, 398
Freestyle II, 709
Frequently Asked Questions About Multiple
    Chemical Sensitivity, 5079
Fresno City College: Disabled Students Programs
    and Services, 5848
Functional Forms, 278
GEICO Philanthropic Foundation, 2825
Gadabout Wheelchairs, 710
Galvin Health and Fitness Center, 8229
Gaymar Industries, 279
Gear Shift Adaptor By Handicaps, Inc., 91
Gem Wheelchair & Scooter Service: Mobility &
    Homecare, 678, 711, 746
Gendron, 712
Geo-Matt for High Risk Patients, 280
Geronimo, 747
Glendale Memorial Hospital and Health Center
    Rehabilitation Unit, 6604
Golden Technologies, 259
Good Grips Cutlery, 358
Great Big Safety Tub Mat, 169
Gresham Driving Aids, 92
Guide Service of Washington, 5528
A Guide for the Wheelchair Traveler, 5485
A Guide to International Educational Exchange,
    2692
Guide to Wheelchair Sports and Recreation, 8230
Guided Tour for Persons 17 & Over with
    Developmental and Physical Challenges, 5529
Guidelines on Disability, 5084
H.E.L.P. Knife, 359
HANDYBAR, The, 93
Hand Brake Control Only, 94
Hand Dimmer Switch, 95
Hand Dimmer Switch with Horn Button, 96
Hand Gas & Brake Control, 97
Hand Operated Parking Brake, 98
Hand Parking Brake, 99
Handi Home Lift, 399
Handi Lift, 400
Handi Prolift, 401
Handi-Ramp, 402
Handicapped Driving Aids, 100
Handicapped Scuba Association International,
    8231
Handicaps, Inc., 101
Hands-Free Controller, 5474
Handy-Helper Cutting Board, 360
Hard Manufacturing Company, 190
Hartford Vet Center, 5593
Headlight Dimmer Switch, 102
HealthCare Solutions, 474
HealthCraft SuperPole Traveller, 522
HealthSouth Rehab Hospital: South Carolina, 6428
HiRider, 713
Hig's Manufacturing, 476
High Profile Single Compartment Cushion, 281
High-Low Chair, 260
Hip Function & Ambulation, 8485
Home Bed Side Helper, 523

Home is in the Heart: Accommodating Peoplewith
    Disabilities in the Homestay Experience, 5335
Homemade Battery-Powered Toys, 1944
Homewaiter, 403
Horcher Lifting Systems, 404
Horizontal Steering, 103
Horn Control Switch, 104
Hospital Environmental Control System, 524
Hostelling North America, 5530
How Come You Walk Funny?, 8215
How We PlayFanlight Productions/Icarus Films,
    5337
Huntleigh Healthcare, 477
Hydrocephalus: A Guide for Patients, Families &
    Friends, 8486
I'm Not DisabledLandmark Media, Inc., 5338
Ideal-Phone, 212
Ideas for Kids on the Go, 5091
Imp Tricycle, 734
Inclinette, 405
Inclusive Games, 8178
Independent Living Centers and Managed Care:
    Results of an ILRU Study on Involvement, 5096
Independent Living Challenges the Blues, 5097
Independent Living for Persons with Disabilities
    and Elderly People, 4980
Indian Trails Camp, 1193
Inflatable Back Pillow, 282
Innerlip Plates, 361
Innovative Products, 714
Innovative Programs: An Example of How CILs
    Can Put Their Work in Context, 5101
Inside The Halo and Beyond: The Anatomy of a
    Recovery, 8179
International Association of Machinists, 861
Invacare Corporation, 319, 478
Invacare Fulfillment Center, 580
Invacare IVC Tracer EX2 Wheelchair with Legrest,
    748
Invacare Lynx L-3 Scooter, 581
Invacare Top End, 757
Invacare Top End Excelerator XLT Gold Handcyle,
    758
Issues in Independent Living, 5104
It isn't Fair!: Siblings of Children with Disabilities,
    4957
Jet 3 Ultra Power Wheelchair, 749
Job Accommodation Network, 867
Jobri, 283
Joey Interior Platform Lift, 407
John Edward Fowler Memorial Foundation, 2827
Joint Efforts, 8198
Journal of Musculoskeletal Pain, 2207
Journal of Prosthetics and Orthotics, 2210
Joystick Driving Control, 105
Julius and Betty Levinson Center, 6844
Just Like Everyone Else, 5109
Kenny Foundation, 5504
Kessler Institute for Rehabilitation, 106
Key Changes: A Portrait of Lisa Thorson, 8216
Key Holders, Ignition & Door Keys, 107
Kid's Custom, 735
Kid's Edge, 736
Kid's Liberty, 737
Kid-Friendly Chairs, 738
Kneelkar, 108
Koala Miniflex, 739
Koret Foundation, 2770
Ladybug Corner Chair, 261
Lakeshore Foundation, 8232
Land of Lincoln Goodwill Industries, 5979
Large Button Speaker Phone, 216
Large Print Telephone Dial, 217
Large Print Touch-Telephone Overlays, 218
Latchloc Automatic Wheelchair Tiedown, 109
Lectra-Lift, 408
Left Foot Accelerator, 110
Left Foot Gas Pedal, 111
Left Foot Gas Pedal by Handicaps, Inc., 112
Left Hand Shift Lever, 113
Leg Elevation Board, 526
Leisure Lift, 582
Letter Writing Guide, 620
Lettering Guide Value Pack, 621

Leveron, 527
Liberty, 715
Liberty LT, 409
Life on Wheels: For the Active Wheelchair User, 8180
Lifestand, 679
Lift-All, 410
Lifts for Swimming Pools and Spas, 411
Lightweight Breezy, 716
Little People of America, 8278
Living in the Community, 5117
Long Handled Bath Sponges, 170
Long Oven Mitts, 362
Longreach Reacher, 528
Loop Scissors, 529
Low Effort and No Effort Steering, 114
Low Tech Assistive Devices: A Handbook for the School Setting, 1963
Lumex Cushions and Mattresses, 284
Lumex Recliner, 262
MVP+ 3-Wheel Scooter, 583
Mac's Lift Gate, 412
Maddak Inc., 484
Majors Medical Equipment, 717
Making Informed Medical Decisions: Where to Look and How to Use What You Find, 5123
Mariner Shower and Commode Chair, 171
Maryland State Department of Education, 6050
Maxi Superior Cane, 653
MedDev Corporation, 321
Medi-Grip, 322
Medpro Static Air Chair Cushion, 285
Medpro Static Air Mattress Overlay, 286
Meeting the Needs of Employees with Disabilities, 5130
Mental and Physical Disability Law Reporter, 4626
Midland Treatment Furniture, 2469
Mini-Bus and Mini-Vans, 115
Mini-Max Cushion, 287
Mini-Rider, 116
Mirror Go Lightly, 303
Mobile Care, 5544
Mobility International USA, 8140
Modular QuadDesk, 263
Modular Wall Grab Bars, 172
Molded Sock and Stocking Aid, 304
Monarch Mark 1-A, 118
Monmouth Vans, Access and Mobility, 119
MonoMouse Electronic Magnifiers, 636
Motorhome Lift By Handicaps, Inc., 414
Mulholland Positioning Systems, 264
NEXUS Wheelchair Cushioning System, 288
Nantahala Outdoor Center, 5506
National Car Rental System, 5545
National Disability Sports Alliance, 8233
National Foundation of Wheelchair Tennis, 2781
National Hookup, 5134
National Library Services for the Blind& Physically Handicapped, 8866
National Mobility Equipment Dealers Association, 8148
National Skeet Shooting Association, 8234
National Wheelchair Poolplayers Association, 8236
Natural Access, 718
New Courier Travel, 5531
New Directions For People With Disabilities, Inc., 5532
New Hampshire Veterans Centers, 5688
New Mobility, 8189
New Quad Grip, 120
Nick Joins In, 8532
No BarriersAquarius Health Care Media, 5346
North American Riding for the Handicapped Association, 8237
Northwest Limousine Service, 5546
Norwegian Cruise Line, 5533
Nosey Cup, 365
O&P Almanac, 2254
Official Patient's Sourcebook on Scoliosis, 8546
One Thousand FS, 681, 750
Open for Business, 5348
Open to the PublicAquarius Health Care Media, 5349
Operation Job Match, 5916

Oregon Talking Book & Braille Services, 4893
Organ Transplants: Making the Most of Your Gift of Life, 5142
Out-N-About American Walker, 654
Outdoor Independence, 585
PAC Unit, 121
PALAESTRA: Forum of Sport, Physical Education and Recreation for Those with Disabilities, 8190
Pac-All Wheelchair Carrier, 682
Pace Saver Plus II, 586
Pain Centers: A Revolution in Health Care, 2479
Palmer Independence, 587
Palmer Twosome, 588
Parent Centers and Independent Living Centers: Collectively We're Stronger, 5222
Paring Boards, 366
Park Brake Extension By Handicaps, Inc., 122
Parker Bath, 418
Partial Seizure Disorders: A Guide for Patients and Families, 8553
Partnering with Public Health: Funding& Advocacy Opportunities for CILs and SILCs, 5146
Patient Lifting & Injury Prevention, 419
Pedal Ease, 123
Pediatric Seating System, 289
Peer Counseling: Roles, Functions, Boundaries, 5147
Peer Mentor Volunteers: Empowering People for Change, 5148
Pencil/Pen Weighted Holders, 558
People with Disabilities & Abuse: Implications for Center for Independent Living, 5150
People-to-People Committee on Disability, 918
Permaflex Home Care Mattress, 193
Permobil Max 90, 751
Permobil Super 90, 752
Personal Perspectives on Personal Assistance Services, 5153
Phantom Compact Size Scooter, 589
Physical Disabilities and Health Impairments: An Introduction, 2486
Physical Education and Sports for Exceptional Students, 2487
Physically Handicapped in Society, 2489
Plastic Card Holder, 532
Polaris Trail Blazer, 590
Portable Hand Controls, 124
Portable Hand Controls By Handicaps, Inc., 125
Portable Shampoo Bowl, 173
Portable Vehicle Controls, 126
Posture-Glide Lounger, 720
Power Door, 533
Power Seat Base (6-Way), 127
Power Wheelchairs, 753
Power for Off-Pavement, 754
PowerLink 2 Control Unit, 367
Prairie Cruiser, 721
Prelude, 174
Prime Engineering, 265
Prone Support Walker, 658
ProtectaCap, ProtectaCap+PLUS, ProtectaChin Guard and ProtectaHip, 534
Protection & Advocacy for People with Disabilities, 3741
Push-Button Quad Cane, 659
Quad Commander, 535
Quad Grip with Pin, 128
Quadtro Cushion, 290
Quickie 2, 591
ROW Adventures, 5534
Ragtime Industries, 6902
Raised Line Drawing Kit, 561
Ramplette Telescoping Ramp, 420
Rampvan, 129
Rand-Scot, 661
Rascal 3-Wheeler, 592
Rascal ConvertAble, 593
Redman Apache, 722
Redman Crow Line, 723
Reduced Effort Steering, 130
Regal Scooters, 594
Regent, 595

Rehabiliation Engineering Center for Personal Licensed Transportation, 5549
Rehabilitation Engineering and Assistive Technology Society of North America (RESNA), 493
Rehabilitation Gazette, 5163
Rehabilitation Institute of Chicago's Virginia Wadsworth Sports Program, 8644
Rehabilitation Institute of Southern California, 6654
Residential Camp, 1102
Resources for Independent Living, 4522
Ricon Corporation, 422
Right Hand Turn Signal Switch Lever, 131
Rocker Balance Square, 536
Roll Chair, 266
Rolls 2000 Series, 724
Room Valet Visual-Tactile Alerting System, 227
Safari Scooter, 597
Safari Tilt, 267
Safety Deck II, 683
Sammons Preston Enrichments Catalog, 494
Sammons Preston Rolyan, 368
Scoota Bug, 598
Scooter & Wheelchair Battery Fuel Gauges and Motor Speed Controllers, 684
Scott Sign Systems, 537
Seven Fifty-Five FS, 740
Sexual Adjustment, 5168
Sexuality and Disabilities: A Guide for Human Service Practitioners, 5169
Shilo Inns & Resorts, 5508
Shoe and Boot Valet: Decreased Mobility Aid, 306
Sierra 3000/4000, 599
Signature and Address Self-Inking Stamps, 564
Silicone Padding, 291
Skyway, 725
Slicing Aid, 369
Slim Line Brake Only, 132
Slim Line Control, 133
Slim Line Control: Brake and Throttle, 134
Small Appliance Receiver, 370
Smart Leg, 423
Smooth Mover, 424
Socialization Games for Persons with Disabilities, 5171, 5481
Society for Progressive Supranuclear Palsy, 8155
Soft-Touch Convertible Flotation Mattress, 292
Soft-Touch Gel Flotation Cushion, 293
Softfoot Ergomatta, 685
Solo Scooter, 600
SoloRider Industries, 601
Source-APTA Audio Conference, 1873
Spatial Tilt Custom Chair, 268
Spec-L Clothing Solutions, 1471
Special Children, 8667
Special Clothes for Children, 5446
Special Needs Trust Handbook, 5175
Special Olympics, 8239
Special Olympics International, 8240
SpectraLift, 425
Spectrum Products Catalog, 427
Spenco Medical Group, 294
Spirit Magazine, 8192
Sport Science Review: Adapted Physical Activity, 8183
Sportaid, 495
St. Clair County Library Special Technologies Alternative Resources (S.T.A.R.), 4823
StairClimber, 663
StairLIFT SC & SL, 428
Stairway Elevators, 429
Stand-Up Wheelchairs, 726
Standard Touch Turner Sip & Puff Switch, 234
Standing Aid Frame with Rear Entry, 664
Steady Write, 565
Steel Food Guard, 371
Steering Backup System, 135
Steering Device By Handicaps, Inc., 136
Still Me, 8184
Stop-Leak Gel Flotation Mattress, 295
Straight and Custom Curved Stairlifts, 430

Strengthening the Roles of Independent Living Centers Through Implementing Legal Service, 4575
Summer Wheelchair Sport Camps, 1080
Summer Wheelchair Sports Camp, 8163
Super Grade 4 Hand Controls By Handicaps, Inc., 137
Super Grade IV Hand Controls, 138
Super Light Folding Transport Chair with Carry Bag, 728
Superarm Lift for Vans By Handicaps, Inc., 431
SureHands Lift & Care Systems, 432
Suregrip Bathtub Rail, 176
Surf Chair, 729
Systems 2000, 603
TMX Tricycle, 741
TV & VCR Remote, 543
Talking Bathroom Scale, 177
Teaching Individuals with Physical and Multiple Disabilities, 2004
Technology and Handicapped People, 2563
Television Remote Controls with Large Numbers, 568
Terra-Jet: Utility Vehicle, 604
Terrier Tricycle, 605
Terry-Wash Mitt: Medium Size, 178
Texas Governor's Committee on People with Disabilities, 3790
Therapy Putty, 545
They Don't Come with Manuals, 5239
Thick-n-Easy, 372
Three Rivers News, 9038
Thyssen Krupp Access, 433
Tilt-N-Table, 686
Tim's Trim, 139
Toilet Guard Rail, 179
Torso Support, 666
Touch Turner-Page Turning Devices, 243
Touch/Ability Connects People with Disabilities & Alternative Health Care Pract., 5181
Tourette's Syndrome: Finding Answers and Getting Help, 8581
Transfer Bench with Back, 269
Transfer Tub Bench, 180
Transportation Equipment for People with Disabilities, 140
Travel Information Service/Moss Rehab Hospital, 5494
Travelers Aid International, 5509
Treating Epilepsy Naturally: A Guide to Alternative and Adjunct Therapies, 8583
Tri-Grip Bathtub Rail, 181
Tri-Lo's, 607
Tri-Post Steering Wheel Spinner, 141
Triumph 3000/4000, 608
Triumph Scooter, 609
Tub Slide Shower Chair, 182
Turn Signal Adapter By Handicaps, Inc., 142
Twin-Rest Seat Cushion & Glamour Pillow, 297
21st Century Scientific, Inc.Bounder Power Wheelchair, 693
U-Step Walking Stabilizer: Walker, 667
US Airways/America West Airlines, 5510
US Department Veterans Affairs Beckley Vet Center, 5783
US Paralympics, 8645
Ultra-Lite XL Hand Control, 143
Undercounter Lid Opener, 374
Understanding and Accommodating Physical Disabilities: Desk Reference, 5183
Uni-Turner, 375
United Access, 144
Universal Hand Cuff, 376
Uppertone, 546
Utah Veterans Centers, 6198
Vangater, Vangater II, Mini-Vangater, 435
Vantage Mini-Vans, 145
Velcro Peel-Off Shoes, 146
Ventura Enterprises, 668
Vermont Back Research Center, 8157
Versatrainer, 436
Vestibular Board, 437
Vista Wheelchair, 730
Voice Choice, 147

Voice Scan, 148
WA Department of Services for the Blind, 3833
WCIB Heavy-Duty Folding Cane, 669
Walgreens Home Medical Center, 499
Walker Leg Support, 670
Wardrobe Wagon: The Special Needs Clothing Store, 5449
Warp Drive, 149
Westin Hotels and Resorts, 5512
Westside Parents Work Activity Center, 5988
Wheel Life News, 687
Wheelchair Accessories, 688
Wheelchair Activity/Computer Table, 569
Wheelchair Aide, 689
Wheelchair Back Pack and Tote Bag, 690
Wheelchair Bowling, 8217
Wheelchair Carrier, 438
Wheelchair Getaways, 5538
Wheelchair Getaways Wheelchair/Scooter Accessible Van Rentals, 5550
Wheelchair Sports, USA, 8242
Wheelchair Work Table, 692
A Wheelchair for Petronilia, 8211
Wheelchair with Shock Absorbers, 731
WheelchairNet, 5453
Wheelers Handicapped Accessible Van Rentals, 5513, 5552
WheelersMarauatha Baptist Church, 5551
Where to Stay USA, 5497
Window-Ease, 548
Wonderland Camp Foundation, 1221
Work in the Context of Disability Culture, 5189
Workshops, Inc., 5818
World Chiropractic Alliance, 7886, 8158
World of Options, 2724
XL Steering, 151
Youville Hospital & Rehab Center, 6991

Polio

Official Patient's Sourcebook on Post-Polio Syndrome: A Revised and Updated Directory, 8543
Post-Polio Health, 8628
Post-Polio Health International, 8153
Post-Polio Support Group, 8664
Post-Polio Syndrome: A Guide for Polio Survivors and Their Families, 8556
Ventilator-Assisted Living, 8611

Prader-Willi Syndrome

PWSA (USA) Conference, 1868
Prader-Willi Alliance of New York Newsletter, 8629
Prader-Willi Syndrome Association USA, 8297
Prader-Willi Syndrome: Development and Manifestations, 8557

Rare Disabilities

Acid Maltase Deficiency Association, 8118
Alternating Hemiplegia of Childhood Foundation, 2739
Brachial Plexus Palsy Foundation, 3140
Children's Tumor Foundation, 3034
The Hemispherectomy Foundation, 7654
National Ataxia Foundation, 7642
Rettsyndrome.org, 7650
A Teacher's Guide to Isovaleric Acidemia, 2272
A Teacher's Guide to Methylmalonic Acidemia, 2273
United Brachial Plexus Network, Inc., 8303

Respiratory Disorders

Advances in Cardiac and Pulmonary Rehabilitation, 2289
American Association for Respiratory Care, 8249
National Association for Medical Direction of Respiratory Care, 8283
Official Patient's Sourcebook on Primary Pulmonary Hypertension, 8544

Official Patient's Sourcebook on Pulmonary Fibrosis, 8545
Sinus Survival: A Self-help Guide, 8568
VACC Camp, 1047, 8411

Severe Disabilites

Assessment of Individuals with Severe Disabilities, 2306
Association for Persons with Severe Handicaps (TASH), 798
Bodie, Dolina, Smith & Hobbs, P.C., 5030
Camp Jened, 1262, 8346
Collaborative Teams for Students with Severe Disabilities, 2344
Curriculum Decision Making for Students with Severe Handicaps, 2357
Department Of Rehabilitative Services, 6205
Including Students with Severe and Multiple Disabilites in Typical Classrooms, 2431
Instruction of Persons with Severe Handicaps, 1949
Life After Trauma: A Workbook for Healing, 8501

Sexual Abuse & Related Conditions

Herpes Resource Center, 8270
Prevent Child Abuse America, 8665
Shining Bright: Head Start Inclusion, 5361
Wilmington Vet Center, 5598

Sjogren's Syndrome

Moisture Seekers, 8623
Sjogren's Syndrome Foundation, 2938

Speech Disorders

ASHA Convention, 1839
Adaptive Technology Catalog, 443
American Journal of Speech-Language Pathology, 8766
Artificial Larynx, 205
Assessment and Remediation of Articulatoryand Phonological Disorders, 2303
Awareness Training, 8911
Camp Chatterbox, 1239
Childhood Speech, Language & Listening Problems, 8730
Childrens Beach House, 1031, 8709
Communication Outlook, 8769
Journal of Speech, Language and Hearing Research, 8068, 8767
Kitten Who Couldn't Purr, 8738
Language Parts Catalog, 1954
Language Tool Kit, 1955
Language, Speech and Hearing Services in School, 1956
Language, Speech, and Hearing Services in Schools, 8768
Late Talker: What to Do If Your Child Isn't Talking Yet, 8741
Liberator, 219
Luminaud, 482
Meadowood Springs Speech and Hearing Camp, 1330, 7975, 8711
Motor Speech Disorders, 8745
National Cued Speech Association, 7938, 8694
Nonverbal Learning Disabilities at Home: A Parent's Guide, 8747
Prentke Romich Company Product Catalog, 491
Promoting Communication in Infants and Young Children: 500 Ways to Succeed, 8751
Providence Speech and Hearing Center, 8700
Sandcastle Day Camp, 1032, 7977
Scottish Rite Center for Childhood Language Disorders, 8701
Sequanota Lutheran Conference Center and Camp, 1358, 8713
Sound Connections for the Adolescent, 8758
SpeakEasy Communication Aid, 231
Speech Discrimination Unit, 232
Speechmaker-Personal Speech Amplifier, 233

Take a Chance, 5482
Talisman Summer Camp, 1294, 7706, 8714
Talkable Tales, 8759
Talking Desktop Calculators, 566
Understanding & Controlling Stuttering: A
   Comprehensive New Approach Based on the
   Valsa Hyp, 8763
Unity, 244
Vantage, 245
Voice Amplified Handsets, 247
WalkerTalker, 248
Wendell Johnson Speech & Hearing Clinic, 8715

Spina Bifida

Agassiz Village, 8312
Camp Harkness, 1022, 8339
Camp MITIOG, 1212, 8355
Camp Oakhurst, 1245, 8161
Educational Issues Among Children with Spina
   Bifida, 8472
Genetics and Spina Bifida, 8477
In the Middle, 8640
Introduction to Spina Bifida, 8492
Latex Allergy in Spina Bifida Patients, 8497
Learning Among Children with Spina Bifida, 8498
Lipomas & Lipomyelomeningocele, 8503
Mountaineer Spina Bifida Camp, 1432, 8397
Obesity, 8536
Occulta, 8538
Plan Ahead: Do What You Can, 8555
SPINabilities: A Young Person's Guide to Spina
   Bifida, 8565
Sexuality and the Person with Spina Bifida, 8567
Sherman Lake YMCA Summer Camp, 8403
Social Development and the Person with Spina
   Bifida, 8569
Spina Bifida Association, 8300
Spina Bifida and Hydrocephalus Association of
   Canada, 8301
Symptomatic Chiari Malformation, 8576
Taking Charge, 8577
Urologic Care of the Child with Spina Bifida, 8588

Spinal Cord Injuries

ASIA Annual Scientific Meeting, 1840
Academy of Spinal Cord Injury Professionals, 8117
American Association of Spinal Cord Injury
   Psychologists & Social Workers, 8121
Cure SMA, 8133
Directions, 8620
Functional Electrical Stimulation for Ambulation
   by Paraplegics, 8175
Head Injury Rehabilitation And Referral Service,
   Inc. (HIRRS), 8137
Journey to Well: Learning to Live After Spinal
   Cord Injury, 8495
Living With Spinal Cord Injury Series, 8509
Multiple Sclerosis Association of America, 7634,
   8141
National Coalition for Assistive and Rehab
   Technology, 8145
National Council on Independent Living, 8146
National Fibromyalgia Association, 8147, 8291
NeuroControl Corporation, 5438
PVA Summit & Expo, 1867
Paralysis Resource Guide, 8181
Paralysis Society of America, 5507
Paralyzed Veterans of America, 8151
SCI Life, 8609
SCI Psychosocial Process, 8632
Spinal Cord Dysfunction, 2530
Spine, 8610
Sports n' Spokes Magazine, 5492
Tethering Cord, 8635
United Spinal Association, 8156
VA North Texas Health Veterans Affairs Care
   System: Dallas VA Medical Center, 5763

Stroke

American Stroke Association, 7875, 8125

Children's Hemiplegia & Stroke Association, 8130
National Stroke Association, 7885
Pedal-in-Place Exerciser, 530
Stroke Sourcebook, 2nd Edition, 8574

Theater & Dance Therapies

American Dance Therapy Association (ADTA), 4
Disability and Social Performance: Using Drama to
   Achieve Successful Acts, 23
National Association for Drama Therapy, 48
National Theatre of the Deaf, 53
Non-Traditional Casting Project, 56
Phoenix DanceFanlight Productions/Icarus Films,
   5353

Tinnitus

American Tinnitus Association, 7903
Tinnitus Today, 8076

Tourette Syndrome

TSA CT Kid's Summer Event, 1181, 8408
TSA National Conference, 1875
TSA Newsletter, 8634
Tourette Association of America, 7655
Tourette Syndrome Association Children's
   Newsletter, 8636
Twitch and Shout, 8642
YMCA Camp Duncan, 1082

Visual Impairments

AAO Annual Meeting, 1830
ACB Annual Convention, 1833
ACB Government Employees, 8793
ACB Radio Amateurs, 8794
ACB Social Service Providers, 8795
AER Annual International Conference, 1835
AFB Center on Vision Loss, 3188
AFB Directory of Services for Blind and Visually
   Impaired Persons in the US and Canada, 8902
AFB News, 9066
AFB Press, 2076
About Children's Eyes, 8903
About Children's Vision: A Guide for Parents,
   8904
Access to Art: A Museum Directory for Blind and
   Visually Impaired People, 8905
Achromatopsia Network, 8796
Adaptek Systems, 200
Adaptive Services Division, 9068
African Americans in the Profession of Blindness
   Services, 8906
Age-Related Macular Degeneration, 8907
Ai Squared, 5383
Aluminum Adjustable Support Canes for the Blind,
   622
American Academy of Ophthalmology, 8797
American Anals of the Deaf Reference, 8908
American Blind Bowling Association, 9133
American Council of Blind Lions, 8799
American Council of the Blind, 3, 8800
American Foundation for the Blind, 3028, 8801
American Optometric Association, 8802
American Printing House for the Blind, 8803
American The Beautiful; National Parks & Federal
   Recreation Lands, 5518
Americans with Disabilities Act Guide for Places
   of Lodging: Serving Guests Who Are Blind,
   8909
Amerock Corporation, 2866
Annual Report/Newsletter, 9070
Arizona Rehabilitation State Services for the Blind
   and Visually Impaired, 3335
Arkenstone: The Benetech Initiative, 1508
Art and Science of Teaching Orientation and
   Mobility to Persons with Visual Impairments,
   8910
Associated Blind, 8804
Associated Services for the Blind, 8805

Association for Education & Rehabilitationof the
   Blind & Visually Impaired, 8806
Association for Macular Diseases, 8807
Association for Macular Diseases Newsletter, 9071
Awareness, 9072
Babycare Assistive Technology, 8912
Babycare Assistive Technology for Parents with
   Physical Disabilties, 8913
Backgammon Set: Deluxe, 5460
Basketball: Beeping Foam, 9134
Beam, 7595
Berthold Lowenfeld on Blindness and Blind
   People, 8917
Beyond Sight, 624
Big Bold Timer Low Vision, 346
Big Number Pocket Sized Calculator, 625
Big Print Address Book, 612
Blind Babies Foundation, 2744
Blind Children's Fund, 2958
Blind Childrens Center, 8811
Blind Childrens Center Annual Meeting, 1851
Blind Educator, 9054
Blind Information Technology Specialists, 8812
Blind Outdoor Leisure Development, 9135
Blind and Vision-Impaired Individuals, 8918
Blinded Veterans Association, 8813
Blinded Veterans Association National
   Convention, 1852
Blindness and Early Childhood Development
   Second Edition, 8919
Blindness: What it is, What it Does and How to
   Live with it, 8920
BlindnessLandmark Media, Inc., 5313
Board Games: Solitaire, 5462
Bold Line Paper, 613
Books are Fun for Everyone, 8921
Books for Blind and Physically Handicapped
   Individuals, 8814, 8923
Braille Compass, 626
Braille Documents, 5315
Braille Forum, 9055
Braille Institute Orange County Center, 9139
Braille Institute of America, 8815
Braille Notebook, 614
Braille Plates for Elevator, 627
Braille Playing Cards: Plastic, 5463
Braille Touch-Time Watches, 628
Braille: An Extraordinary Volunteer Opportunity,
   8925
Braille: Bingo Cards, Boards and Call Numbers,
   5464
Braille: Desk Calendar, 615
Braille: Greeting Cards, 616
Braille: Rook Cards, 5465
Bureau Of Exceptional Education And Student
   Services, 3402
Burns Braille Transcription Dictionary, 8926
California Department of Education: Special
   Education Division, 2112
California State Library Braille and Talking Book
   Library, 8816
Camp Barakel, 1183, 8882
Camp Bloomfield, 966
Camp Challenge, 1091, 1127, 8883
Camp Courage North, 1201, 8330
Camp Lawroweld, 1137, 8884
Camp Lou Henry Hoover, 1242, 8885
Camp Merrick, 8886
Camp Winnekeag, 8887
Can't Your Child See? A Guide for Parents of
   Visually Impaired Children, 8927
Canine Helpers for the Handicapped, 812, 8817
Caption Center, 8818
Cards: Musical, 5467
Cards: UNO, 5468
Career Perspectives: Interviews with Blindand
   Visually Impaired Professionals, 8928
Careers in Blindness Rehabilitation Services, 8929
Carolyn's Catalog, 1465
Carolyn's Low Vision Products, 457
Cataracts, 8930
Characteristics, Services, & Outcomes of Rehab.
   Consumers who are Blind/Visually Impaired,
   8931

Chicago Lighthouse for People who are Blind and Visually Impaired, 8820
Childhood Glaucoma: A Reference Guide for Families, 8932
Children with Visual Impairments: A Guide For Parents, 8933
Choice Magazine Listening, 9121
A Christian Approach to Overcoming Disability: A Doctor's Story, 8901
Circline Illuminated Magnifier, 629
Classification of Impaired Vision, 8934
College of Optometrists in Vision Development, 8823
College of Syntonic Optometry, 8824
Columbia Lighthouse for the Blind, 8825
Columbia Lighthouse for the Blind Summer Camp, 1033, 8888
Committee for Purchase from People Who Are Blind or Severely Disabled, 3292
Communication Skills for Visually Impaired Learners, 8935
Community Services for the Blind and Partially Sighted Store: Sight Connection, 1924
Comprehensive Examination of Barriers to Employment Among Persons who are Blind or Impaire, 8936
Connecticut Board of Education and Servicefor the Blind, 3374
Consumer and Patient Information Hotline, 9140
Contrasting Characteristics of Blind and Visually Impaired Clients, 8937
Council of Families with Visual Impairments, 8826
DVH Quarterly, 9076
Dancing Cheek to Cheek, 8938
Dazor Manufacturing Corporation, 515
Defining Rehabilitation Agency Types, 2359
Delaware Division for the Visually Impaired, 3385
Delaware Industries for the Blind, 3386
Deluxe Long Ring Low Vision Timer, 351
Department Of Human Services, 6062
Department of Medicine and Surgery Veterans Administration, 5554
Department of Ophthalmology Information Line, 9141
Development of Social Skills by Blind and Visually Impaired Students, 8939
Diabetic Retinopathy, 8940
Dialogue Magazine, 9057
Dice: Jumbo Size, 5471
Diversity and Visual Impairment: The Influence of Race, Gender, Religion and Ethnicity, 8941
Division of Blind Services, 6739
Division of Vocational Rehabilitation of Wyoming, 6223
Do You Remember the Color Blue: The Questi Ons Children Ask About Blindness, 8942
Don't Lose Sight of Glaucoma, 8943
Early Focus: Working with Young Children Who Are Blind or Visually Impaired & Their Families, 8944
Encyclopedia of Blindness and Vision Impairment Second Edition, 8945
Equals in Partnership: Basic Rights for Families of Children with Blindness, 8946
Exceptional Teaching Inc, 1936
Extra Loud Alarm with Lighter Plug, 630
Eye Bank Association of America, 8829
Eye Bank Association of America Annual Meeting, 1857
Eye Research News, 8947
Eye and Your Vision, 8948
Eye-Q Test, 8949
Family Context and Disability Culture Reframing: Through the Looking Glass, 8950
Family Guide to Vision Care (FG1), 8951
Family Guide: Growth & Development of the Partially Seeing Child, 8952
Fathers: A Common Ground, 8953
Fidelco Guide Dog Foundation, 2810, 8830
Fight for Sight, 8831
Fighting Blindness News, 8954
First Steps, 8955
Focus, 8197, 9079
Food Markers/Rubberbands, 357

Foundation Fighting Blindness, 2930, 5414, 7566, 8832
Foundations of Rehabilitation Counseling with Persons Who Are Blind r Visually Impaired, 8957
Freedom Scientific, 5415
General Facts and Figures on Blindness, 8958
Get a Wiggle On, 8959
Gift of Sight, 8960
Glaucoma, 8961
Glaucoma Research Foundation, 2762, 5417
Glaucoma: The Sneak Thief of Sight, 8962
Gleams Newsletter, 9080
Guide Dog Foundation for the Blind, 3058
Guide Dog Users, 8833
Guide Dogs for the Blind, 8834
Guidelines and Games for Teaching Efficient Braille Reading, 8963
Guidelines for Comprehensive Low Vision Care, 8964
Guideway, 9082
Guiding Eyes for the Blind, 8835
Guiding Eyes for the Blind: Breeding and Placement Center, 8836
Guild Briefs, 9083
Handbook for Itinerant and Resource Teachers of Blind Students, 8965
Handbook of Information for Members of the Achromatopsia Network, 8966
Hawaii Department of Human Services, 3434
Health Care Professionals Who Are Blind or Visually Impaired, 8967
Heart to Heart, 8968
Heart to HeartBlind Childrens Center, Inc, 5333
Heartbreak of Being A Little Bit Blind, 8969
Helen and Teacher: The Story of Helen & Anne Sullivan Macy, 7582
Helping the Visually Impaired Child with Developmental Problems, 8971
Highbrook Lodge, 1310, 8891
History and Use of Braille, 8972
Hospitalized Veterans Writing Project, 5559
Hub, 8974
Huntsville Subregional Library for the Blind & Physically Handicapped, 4650
IAAIS Report, 9084
If Blindness Comes, 8975
Imagining the Possibilities: Creative Approaches to Orientation and Mobility Instructio, 8977
Increasing Literacy Levels: Final Report, 8978
Independent Visually Impaired Enterprisers, 8838
Indian Creek Camp, 1381, 8892
Information & Referral Center, 2435
Information Access Project, 8979
Information on Glaucoma, 8980
Insight, 9085
International Association of Audio Information Services (IAAIS), 8840
International Braille and Technology Center for the Blind, 8658
International Directory of Libraries for the Disabled, 5103
Intervention Practices in the Retention of Competitive Employment, 8981
Iowa Department for the Blind, 3472
JBI Voice, 9060
Jewish Braille Institute International, 8841
Jewish Braille Review, 9061
Jewish Guild for the Blind, 2033
Job Opportunities for the Blind, 6046
Journal of Visual Impairment and Blindness, 9053
Juggler, 9122
Junior Blind of America, 2768
Kamp A-Komp-Plish, 1157, 8893
Kamp Kaleo, 1229, 8894
Kentucky Office for the Blind, 6028
Know Your Eye, 8982
LS&S, 480
Large Print Loan Library, 8983
Large Print Loan Library Catalog, 8984
Large Print Recipies for a Healthy Life, 8985
Learning to Play, 8986
Let's Eat, 8987
Let's Eat Video, 9123

Library Services for the Blind, 8988
Library Users of America Newsletter, 9087
Light the Way, 9088
Lighthouse Central Florida, 5935
Lighthouse International Information and Resource Service, 9142
Lighthouse Low Vision Products, 481
Lion, 8990
Lions Clubs International, 2711, 8844
Living with Achromatopsia, 8991
Long Cane News, 9091
Look Out for Annie, 9124
Louis R Lurie Foundation, 2776
Low Vision Questions and Answers: Definitions, Devices, Services, 8992
Low Vision Telephones, 631
Low Vision: Reflections of the Past, Issues for the Future, 8993
Macular Degeneration Foundation, 8845
Magnetic Card Reader, 363
Magni-Cam & Primer, 632
Maine Division for the Blind and Visually Impaired, 3506
Mainstreaming and the American Dream, 8994
Mainstreaming the Visually Impaired Child, 8995
Making Life More Livable, 8996
Man's Low-Vision Quartz Watches, 634
Maxi Aids, 485
Maxi Marks, 557
Maxi-Aids Braille Timer, 364
Men's/Women's Low Vision Watches & Clocks, 635
Metropolitan Washington Ear, 220
Miami-Dade County Disability Services and Independent Living (DSAIL), 4019
Michigan Council of the Blind and Visually Impaired (MCBVI), 3539
Minnesota State Services for the Blind, 3557
Missouri Rehabilitation Services for the Blind, 3570
More Alike Than Different: Blind and Visually Impaired Children, 8999
Mothers with Visual Impairments who are Raising Young Children, 9000
Move With Me, 9001
Musical Mainstream, 9063
NISH, 6208
NLS News, 9095
NLS Newsletter, 9096
National Alliance of Blind Students NABS Liaison, 8846
National Association for Visually Handicapped (NAVH), 8848
National Association for Visually Handicapped Lighthouse International, 5432
National Association of Blind Merchants, 883, 8851
National Association of Blind Students, 8853
National Association of Blind Teachers, 8854
National Association of Guide Dog Users, 8856
National Association to Promote the Use of Braille, 8857
National Braille Association, 8859
National Braille Press, 8860
National Camp for Blind Children, 8895
National Camps for Blind Children, 1230, 8896
National Center for Vision and Child Development, 8861
National Eye Institute, 8863, 9002
National Eye Research Foundation, 2888
National Federation of the Blind, 2936, 7574, 8864
National Industries for the Blind, 8865
National Organization of Parents of Blind Children, 8867
Nebraska Commission for the Blind & Visually Impaired, 3586
Nevada Bureau of Vocational Rehabilitation, 3595
New Eyes for the Needy, 8868
New Jersey Commission for the Blind and Visually Impaired, 3618, 6116
New Mexico Commission for the Blind, 3628
New Vision Store, 486
New York State Commission for the Blind, 3647

North Carolina Division of Services for the Blind, 6142

North Dakota Vocational Rehabilitation Agency, 6152

North Georgia Talking Book Center, 4728

Oklahoma Department of Rehabilitation Services, 3706

Opportunity, 9064

Oregon Commission for the Blind, 3712

Oregon Health Sciences University, 5728

Orientation and Mobility Primer for Families and Young Children, 9003

Out of Left Field, 9126

Out of the Corner of My Eye: Living with Vision Loss in Later Life, 9004

PBA News, 9097

PXE International, 8662

Patient's Guide to Visual Aids and Illumination, 9007

Pearle Vision Foundation, 3215

Pediatric Visual Diagnosis Fact Sheets, 9008

Pennsylvania Bureau of Blindness & VisualServices, 3720

Perkins Brailler, 559

Personal Reader Update, 9010

Pet Partners, 531

Playback, 9099

Preschool Learning Activities for the Visually Impaired Child, 9011

Prevent Blindness America, 8869

Psychoeducational Assessment of Visually Impaired and Blind Students, 2500

Quantum Technologies, 5442

Quarterly Update, 9100

RP Messenger, 9101

Reaching, Crawling, Walking....Let's Get Moving, 9012

Reading Is for Everyone, 9013

Reading with Low Vision, 9014

Reference and Information Services From NLS, 9016

Rehabilitation Resource Manual: VISION, 2508

Reizen Braille Labeler, 562

Research to Prevent Blindness, 3079

Resource List for Persons with Low Vision, 9017

Rhode Island Services for the Blind and Visually Impaired, 3737

Rigid Aluminum Cane with Golf Grip, 637

Robert Ellis Simon Foundation, 2786

SCENE, 9102

Say What, 305

School of Piano Technology for the Blind, 6217

See A Bone, 9020

See What I Feel, 9021

See for Yourself, 9128

Seeing Eye Guide, 9104

Seeing Eye, The, 8870

Selecting a Program, 9022

Self-Therapy for the Stutterer, 8755

Services for the Blind and Visually Impaired, 3738

Services for the Visually Impaired, 8871

Shared Visions, 9105

Sharp Calculator with Illuminated Numbers, 563

Sightings Newsletter, 9107

Smith Kettlewell Rehabilitation Engineering Research Center, 9108

Society for the Blind, 8872

South Carolina Commission for the Blind, 3745

Special Technologies Alternative Resources, 9025

Standing on My Own Two Feet, 9026

State Library of Ohio: Talking Book Program, 4888

Step-By-Step Guide to Personal Management for Blind Persons, 9028

Stretch-View Wide-View Rectangular Illuminated Magnifier, 638

Student Teaching Guide for Blind and Visually Impaired College Students, 9029

TBC Focus, 9110

TLC: Treatment and Learning Centers, 6958

Tactile Thermostat, 544

Talk to Me, 9031

Talk to Me II, 9032

Talking Calculators, 239

Talking Clinical Thermometer, 326

Talking Clocks, 240

Talking Watches, 241

Taping for the Blind, 9131

Teaching Orientation and Mobility in the Schools: An Instructor's Companion, 9035

Teaching Visually Impaired Children, 9036

Technology Assistance for Special Consumers, 1603

Technology for the DisabledLandmark Media, Inc., 5366

Texas Commission for the Blind, 3783

Textbook Catalog, 9037

Tic Tac Toe, 5483

Timex Easy Reader, 639

Touch the Baby: Blind & Visually Impaired Children As Patients, 9040

Transition Activity Calendar for Students with Visual Impairments, 9041

Transition to College for Students with Visual Impairments: Report, 9042

Turnabout Game, 5484

US Association of Blind Athletes, 9137

Unisex Low Vision Watch, 640

United States Association of Blind Athletes, 8873

United States Blind Golf Association, 9138

Unseen Minority: A Social History of Blindness in the United States, 9043

Upstate Update, 9112

Utah Division of Services for the Disabled, 3804

Utah State Library Division: Program for the Blind and Disabled, 4915

VIP Newsletter, 2269

VISIONS Vacation Camp for the Blind, 1282, 8898

VUE: Vision Use in Employment, 9144

Vermont Association for the Blind and Visually Impaired, 8876

Vermont Division for the Blind & Visually Impaired, 3818

Virginia Department for the Blind and Vision Impaired, 3822

Vision Enhancement, 9044

Vision Foundation, 2954

Vision World Wide, 8878

Visions Center on Blindness (VCB), 8879

Visual Aids and Informational Material, 9113

Visual Impairment: An Overview, 9045

Visual Impairments And Learning, 9046

Visually Impaired Veterans of America, 8880

Vocational and Rehabilitation Agency, 5905, 5964, 6010, 6094, 6146

Vocational and Rehabilitation Agency Massachusetts Commission for the Blind, 6060

Vocational and Rehabilitation Agency: State Rehabilitation Commission, 6195

Vocational and Rehabilitation: State of Wisconsin, 6222

Voice of Vision, 9115

Volunteer Transcribing Services, 2012

WP and HB White Foundation, 2899

Walking Alone and Marching Together, 9047

Washington Connection, 9145

Washington Ear, 8881

West Virginia Vocational Rehabilitation, 6221

What Do You Do When You See a Blind Person- and What Don't You Do?, 9048

What Museum Guides Need to Know: Access for the Blind and Visually Impaired, 9049

When You Have a Visually Impaired Student in Your Classroom: A Guide for Teachers, 2579

Work Sight, 9050

Working with Visually Impaired Young Students: A Curriculum Guide for 3 to 5 Year Olds, 2582

World Through Their Eyes, 9051

YMCA Camp Chingachgook on Lake George, 1284, 8900

Women

International Women's Health Coalition, 865

National Women's Health Network, 905

A Woman's Guide to Living with HIV Infection, 8425

Women to Women, 934

Women with Visible & Invisible Disabilitiees: Multiple Intersections, Issues, Therapies, 5293